2000 Edition

Questionable Doctors

Sidney Wolfe, M.D.
Phyllis McCarthy
Alana Bame
Benita Marcus Adler

Disciplined by State and Federal Governments

Oklahoma, Texas

Public Citizen
Health Research Group

Public Citizen is a nonprofit membership organization in Washington, D.C., dedicated to advancing consumer rights through lobbying, litigation, research, publications and information services.

Since its founding by Ralph Nader in 1971, Public Citizen has fought for consumer rights in the marketplace, for safe and secure health care, for fair trade, for clean and safe energy sources, and for corporate and government accountability

First printing

Region 15: Texas, Oklahoma ISBN 1-58231-016-5

Acknowledgments

The authors would like to acknowledge the important efforts of many people and institutions which made this study possible.

First, we are grateful to the state licensing or disciplinary boards which cooperated with our requests for doctor-specific information by sending us lists which, in many cases, required them to reorganize data in a form which would be more useful to us. Similarly, the Inspector General's Office of the Department of Health and Human Services (HHS) has been extremely cooperative with our requests for information on those physicians who were sanctioned by the Peer Review Organizations and those who were the subject of other HHS sanctions. The Drug Enforcement Administration (DEA), initially, belatedly, incompletely and only in the face of a lawsuit from Public Citizen, gave us the data on doctors with uncontested restrictions or revocations of their narcotics licenses. Several consumer groups, including the New York Public Interest Research Group (NYPIRG) have also provided us with valuable information.

But the lion's share of time spent on this report was in the time-consuming process of data entry, checking, rechecking and *rechecking* for accuracy and editing of information. A group of Public Citizen employees and former Public Citizen employees assisted in this enormous task including Kimberly Ferlauto, Luisa Hegedus, Salwa Nassar, Demian Larry and Ragin Jennings.

Jason Stele, Public Citizen's Manager of Information Systems, spent many long hours desiging our programs and providing computer assistance. Sean R. Witte, our computer consultant offered valuable assistance.

David Vladeck, an attorney with and Director of the Public Citizen Litigation Group, spent many long hours going over our summaries of the legal actions taken by state boards to ensure that they correctly interpreted the lengthier statements we received from the states.

Previous authors of the first four editions were Nicole Simmons, Ingrid VanTuinen, Durrie McKnew, Mary Gabay and Katie Franklin. Other Public Citizen employees who worked on earlier editions include Toufic Rahman, Dana Hull, Lynn Soffer, Joan Stieber, Joanne Mott, Stephen Moore, Beverly Wellman, Kate Moore, Lauren Kanee, Kathy Cashel. Elizabeth Hanson, Edith T. Burpee, Christine E. Dehlendorf, Lauren Dame, and Elizabeth Schramm.

Table of Contents

Executive Summary

Information in the one federal repository of disciplinary actions by state medical boards and federal agencies--the National Practitioner Data Bank--is kept secret from both patients and from almost all physicians thanks to the American Medical Association's successful lobbying for secrecy when the legislation concerning the Data Bank was being considered. It is partially in protest to this congressionally-mandated secrecy that Public Citizen's Health Research Group has established our own publicly-available data bank of doctors who have been disciplined. What follows are just a few of the main findings from our study of the data as reported in the national version of *20,125 Questionable Doctors* and in the regional versions:

* 20,125 doctors disciplined by either state medical boards or federal agencies are listed in the national books. This represents an increase of 6,185 new physicians since the last version of this report.
* These 20,125 doctors had a total of 38,589 disciplinary actions taken against them, the most common of which were probation (7,431 times), license suspension (3,704 times), fine (3,708 times) and license revocation (3,045 times). (See other types of disciplinary actions in Table D, Findings, pg. 21.) Although these and other serious actions made up 70% of all actions, far too many physicians received slaps on the wrist in the form of fines or reprimands despite having committed serious offenses. (see Tables F through J, pages 24-28.)
* For those doctors with disciplinary actions for which the states or federal agencies supplied specific information on the offenses they had committed, the following numbers of doctors committed the five most serious offenses (see other types of offenses in Table E, Findings, pg. 23):
    1. Sexual abuse of or sexual misconduct with a patient: 547 doctors
    2. Substandard care, incompetence or negligence: 3,215 doctors
    3. Criminal Conviction (includes plea of guilty or no contest): 2,963 doctors
    4. Misprescribing or overprescribing of drugs: 1,318 doctors
    5. Substance abuse: 1,715 doctors

Of the 24,042 disciplinary actions for which offenses were listed (See Table E, pg. 23) for

7,132, the reason listed was "disciplinary action taken by another state or agency," leaving 16,910 offenses with specific details as to the nature of the offense. For 15,310 of these offenses or 90.6% of them, the offense was one of the five listed above or another serious offense such as providing false information, loss of hospital privileges or insurance fraud.

An analysis of the 2,366 doctors who were the subjects of DEA disciplinary actions revealed that hundreds were not the subject of any state disciplinary action even though their federal narcotics license had been revoked or restricted.

Similarly, of the 3,232 Medicare doctors who were the subjects of Medicare disciplinary actions, hundreds were not disciplined by their state boards even though most had involved exclusion from Medicare.

Thus, many states are not acting promptly, if at all, against physicians about whom a federal agency has already compiled sufficient information to discipline them for very serious offenses. Even for those states which do discipline these doctors, for most of the serious offenses involved in DEA or Medicare actions, some states frequently do little more than slap physicians on the wrist, leaving the majority free to practice with few if any restrictions.

Overall, the majority of physicians who were disciplined for the five most serious offenses--sexual abuse or sexual misconduct, substandard care, incompetence, or negligence, criminal conviction, misprescribing or overprescribing of drugs, or substance abuse were not required to stop practicing even temporarily. The most common disciplinary action for each of these five offenses was probation, the severity of which varies widely from state to state. Following are the percentages and numbers of physicians for each offense who did not have to stop practicing despite the offenses which they had committed:

* Sexual abuse of or sexual misconduct with a patient: 547 doctors.
  Only 52.3% of these physicians had to stop practicing, even temporarily. 47.7% or 261 doctors were not required to stop.
* Substandard care, incompetence or negligence: 3,215 doctors.
  Only 29.3% of these physicians had to stop practicing, even temporarily. 70.7% or 2,273 were not required to stop.
* Criminal conviction (includes plea of guilty or no contest): 2,963 doctors.
  Only 39.2% of these doctors had to stop practicing, even temporarily. 60.8% or 1,802 were not required to stop.
* Misprescribing or overprescribing of drugs: 1,318 doctors.
  Only 27.9% of these physicians had to stop practicing, even temporarily. 72.1% or 950

were not required to stop.

* Substance abuse: 1,715 doctors.

Only 32.4% of these doctors had to stop practicing, even temporarily. 67.6% or 1,159 were not required to stop.

(See Tables F through J pages 24-28.)

Thus, it is likely that most of the doctors in these above five categories of very serious offenses are currently practicing medicine, with few if any of their patients aware of these offenses.

Precisely because regulators provide so many protections for these health care practitioners, in 1988 the Congressional Office of Technology Assessment concluded that a formal disciplinary action against a doctor provides a good reason to question his or her care.

Our study of the nation's medical quality control system led us to conclude that:

* Too little discipline is still being done. The rate of serious disciplinary actions by state medical boards was only 3.50 serious actions per 1,000 doctors or 2,696 serious actions in 1999. Therefore only an extremely small fraction of the nation's doctors face any serious state sanctions each year despite the fact that at least 80,000 patients are killed and 234,000 injured as a result of negligence in hospitals, most cases involving doctors.
* Far too few state medical board disciplinary actions are for medical negligence or incompetence. Of the 16,910 disciplinary actions in which we knew the basis (the offense) for which the action was taken and for which the basis of the action was not an action by another state, only 3,184 of those cases (18.8%) were for substandard care, incompetence or negligence.

This country's system for ensuring medical quality needs to be made much stronger. We suggest several avenues towards improvement. Most states need to strengthen their medical practice statutes, restructure their medical boards, and dramatically increase both funding and staffing. Most states should also establish programs to audit and weed out bad doctors so that patient injuries can be prevented rather than simply reacted to.

The total number of serious state disciplinary actions against physicians decreased from 2,803 reported for 1995 to 2,696 in 1999 for a nationwide rate of 3.50 serious actions per 1,000 physicians. A difference greater than 10-fold exists between Alaska, the state with the highest rate (10.34 per 1,000), and Delaware, with the lowest rate, (0.96). (See Table A, pg. 14.)

It is clear that state-by-state performance is spotty. Only one of the nation's 15 largest states, Ohio, is represented among those 10 states with the highest disciplinary rates, as it also was in

1996, 1997 and 1998. Other large states such as, New York, Michigan and California (14th, 19th and 20th respectively in 1999) have shown improvement from 40th, 49th and 37th in 1991. But other large states such as Texas, Pennsylvania, Massachusetts and Illinois (34th, 36th, 39th and 43rd in 1999) have not done very much doctor discipline for many of the last 10 years. It is not unreasonable to estimate that a nationwide average rate of at least 10 serious disciplinary actions per 1,000 doctors can be attained (the number was 3.50 in 1999) since, in most years, one or more states (Alaska, in 1999) actually takes this many actions. This would amount to 7,703 serious disciplinary actions a year, far in excess of the 2,696 serious disciplinary actions in 1999. If this had occurred, there would have been 5,007 more serious disciplinary actions that year--almost three times the number of actions which actually were taken.

Recommendations

Congress should require cooperation and routine data-sharing between state medical boards, Medicare Peer Review Organizations, state Medicaid agencies, the Drug Enforcement Administration and hospitals in catching and sanctioning malfeasant physicians.

The National Practitioner Data Bank, which began collecting information on questionable doctors in September 1990, should be opened to the public. This change will require legislation. Although there have been Congressional hearings on this topic in 2000, there is not any evidence that Congress has enough guts to take on the A.M.A.

The Drug Enforcement Administration should routinely tell the public and pharmacists which doctors' controlled substances prescription licenses it has pulled or restricted.

State medical boards should be required to promptly make public all their disciplinary actions and the offenses for which their actions were taken, and to regularly distribute lists of actions to consumers, the press, and other health care consumer organizations. In addition, boards should publicly disclose information they have concerning final hospital disciplinary actions and malpractice payouts against doctors.

In the past two years, many medical boards have started putting varying degrees of disciplinary information on their web sites. (for a report on the status of these sites--with grades A to X for completeness--visit our web site at http://www.citizen.org/hrg/publications/1506.htm) Unfortunately, most states either have no web site with disciplinary information or an inadequate amount of information about this important topic. Combined with the fact that only slightly more than half of the people in this country have access to the internet, this means that probably 75% of the people in this country do not have internet access to an adequate amount of this information. It is inexcusable that all states do not have detailed information about actions and offenses about every doctor who has been disciplined, including a copy of the board's order spelling out the details as to why the action was taken.

How to Use This Report

Questionable Doctors was designed to assist consumers in making better informed health care choices. The individual doctor listings aid patients in understanding the quality of care they would potentially receive or have already received from a particular practitioner. The general discussion of disciplinary actions and offenses within a state and the nation help to interpret the information we received.

Please Note...

Names sound alike. Just because a doctor whose name resembles your doctor's is listed in this report doesn't mean your doctor has been sanctioned. Some states failed to give us much identifying information on each doctor, and of the half a million doctors in this country, at least two are bound to have the same name.

Many things change with time. While your doctor's license may be listed as having been revoked, suspended or restricted in this edition of the report, this doesn't necessarily mean those restrictions are still in effect. The information contained in this edition is information we received from the state medical boards by January 31, 2000. We also included information received through May 31, 2000 regarding previous actions which were either overturned or terminated, leaving the physician with an unrestricted license. However, the state may have fully reinstated a doctor's license or lifted their probation or other restrictions in materials received after our deadlines.

Boards don't always have the final say. Your doctor may have appealed his or her disciplinary action and had it overturned by a court. Although we strive to provide the most current information, we are unable to obtain information on many appeals.

If you are selecting a doctor...

* Call the medical board in the state where the doctor practices or used to practice. The board can frequently provide information on the physician's educational and specialty background, and whether the doctor has been disciplined or formally charged with misconduct. (Contact information for each state board is listed at the end of each state's introductory section

in this book.)

* Check to see if your local consumer group has published a guide to local doctors.

* Look your doctor up in the American Medical Association's American Medical Directory or the Directory of Medical Specialists, which can be found in all medical libraries and many large public libraries. These directories list the physician's educational background and whether or not he or she is board-certified in a specialty. You should not select a self-designated specialist who has not been trained in the specialty field.

* Ask the doctor for the names of hospitals where he or she has admitting privileges. Your local university teaching hospital will probably be the most selective about the physicians it admits to its staff. Also, should you need to be hospitalized, you will want a doctor who can admit you to the best hospital.

If your current doctor is on this list...

* Check which state(s) or federal agency has disciplined him or her.

* Request a copy of the doctor's disciplinary file from the state or federal agency. State agency addresses are listed in the "Addresses" section of each state section. Federal addresses are in Appendix 3, pg. 50.

* Read the file before making a decision about whether to switch doctors. Some of the information contained in our report is sketchy and may not include a full explanation of the reason for the disciplinary action because states may not have sent these details to us. Some of the actions taken involve offenses that were administrative in nature and do not necessarily reflect on the physician's ability to practice.

* Ask your doctor why he or she was disciplined. If your doctor can convince you that any problem that resulted in the disciplinary action has been resolved or is irrelevant to your future care, fine. Otherwise, you should consider switching.

If you have a complaint about a doctor...

Some examples of reportable actions are:

* if a doctor over-charged you or charged for treatment that was not delivered;
* if a physician failed to order or properly administer appropriate tests or treatment;
* if you suspect that a doctor may be abusing drugs or alcohol;
* if a physician inappropriately touched you in a sexual manner or conducted a sexual relationship with you while you were a patient;

* if you suspect a physician is unable to function mentally or physically.

* Find out what degree your doctor has, whether a medical doctor (M.D.), osteopathic physician (D.O.), chiropractor (D.C.), podiatrist (D.P.M.), or dentist (D.D.S. or D.M.D.). Different state agencies often regulate these different professionals.

* File your complaint with the state medical disciplinary agency. This agency is the only one that can remove dangerous or incompetent doctors from practice, impose limitations on a physician's license to practice, and truly protect other patients from being harmed. Your complaint could lead to the suspension or revocation of a doctor's license directly, or it could aid the medical board in detecting a pattern of poor medical care.

* File the complaint in the state where the doctor is licensed--i.e., where his or her office is located. Turn to that state's section under our "State by State Listings." Find the "Address" heading. Look for the address of the agency that regulates that type of doctor.

* If your care was within a hospital, you should also file a complaint with the hospital's peer review committee, which has the power to revoke or limit a doctor's privileges to practice there.

* You may also want to file a complaint with Medicare (Addresses, Appendix 3, pg. 50).

* Call the agency you have found to inquire about how to file a formal complaint. Some agencies have toll-free hotlines for complaints. Others require complaints to be filed on a specific form.

* Ask whether your complaint will remain confidential. State laws vary. If the agency intends to reveal your name to your doctor, you may want to consider switching to another physician before pursuing any action.

* File a written complaint containing as much information as possible. Make sure to include the doctor's full name, correctly spelled, office address, and the exact date when the conduct you are complaining of occurred. The state may also ask you to release your medical records for review.

* Ask the agency to notify you of the outcome of your complaint.

If you want to improve medical quality assurance in the state or the nation...

* Write your state representatives, your congressional representative, and your senators. Ask them to pass the legislation we recommend on pg. 32.

Introduction

For more than a quarter of a century, Public Citizen's Health Research Group has been providing consumers with information they can use to make educated choices about their doctors. It has not been an easy road. Doctors generally don't like comparative information on quality to be released.

In the nation's first consumer's directory of local physicians, which we published in 1974 for Prince Georges County, Maryland, we wrote, "Most people can find out more about a car they plan to buy than they can about a doctor who may hold their life in his or her hands."[1] Unfortunately, that statement is still largely true today. In the process of collecting information from doctors for that directory, the Maryland State Medical Association threatened doctors who cooperated with loss of their license, arguing that "information that would point out differences between doctors" is illegal.

Another example of the barriers to public access to information on specific doctors: the federal government began collecting information on state disciplinary actions, malpractice payments, and revocations and restrictions of hospital privileges for its National Practitioner Data Bank (NPDB) in September 1990. The problem is that consumers (and even doctors--except for information on themselves) are forbidden by law to have access to the data. This information is available only to hospitals, Health Maintenance Organizations, and state and federal government agencies that regulate the quality of medical care.[2,3,4]

In the wake of efforts to pass legislation to open up the NPDB, the American Medical Association, whose earlier efforts had succeeded in a prohibition against public disclosure when the law creating the NPDB was passed in 1986, passed a resolution at its 1993 annual convention stating: "Resolved, that the American Medical Association...call for the dissolution of the National Practitioner Data Bank." Now, as then, the AMA seems to want to protect the minority of American physicians about whom there is data in the NPDB from the scrutiny of their own patients and other physicians.

It should be noted that a number of states have been increasingly using their disciplinary power to address administrative issues. Illinois and Medicare are sanctioning many physicians for defaulting on student loans; the District of Columbia targets physicians who failed to renew their license before the expiration date; and Pennsylvania suspends doctors for not paying a liability insurance surcharge. Although we do not advocate physicians shirking financial responsibilities, we feel that the public would be better served if boards focused more of their resources on exposing and preventing more serious patient abuses. We include such actions in our book because the agencies supplying this information have labeled them "disciplinary;" consumers, however, can and should differentiate between physicians sanctioned for true quality of care issues and administrative violations. These administrative actions, however, make up only a small fraction of cases listed in *20,125 Questionable Doctors.*

There has been some progress in the area of informing the public about poorly practicing physicians. Much information on state and federal government discipline of physicians is now public, although often difficult to obtain, and we have used that data to compile this report. State medical boards, licensing bureaus, and medical societies have increased public access to physician sanctions and license status via toll-free numbers and Internet postings (See our report on State Medical Board Web Sites at www.citizen.org/hrg/1506.htm); New York and California have made concerted efforts to enhance the exchange of information with other medical boards.

The United States has approximately 770,320 licensed medical doctors, most of them competent and dedicated. *20,125 Questionable Doctors* includes only that 2.6% of physicians whose care or conduct was substandard enough to be cited by a state medical disciplinary board, Medicare, or the federal Drug Enforcement Administration, or whose eligibility to participate in Food and Drug Administration (FDA) experiments was rescinded.

In a 1988 study on medical care quality assessment, the Congressional Office of Technology Assessment concluded that "a sanction imposed on a physician by a state or a Medicare Peer Review Organization is good reason to question the quality of his or her care.[5] The rigorous due process followed by state medical boards lends credibility to the validity of their formal disciplinary actions against physicians," stated the report. "State boards are reluctant to censure physicians and accord accused physicians extensive opportunities for appeal."

But until the day that consumers can have access to as much information about their health care providers as they can about buying a car Public Citizen will continue to battle the shroud of secrecy in which the medical community envelops itself.

The U.S. "System" of Medical Quality Control

The United States has a patchwork system for protecting the public from poor quality health care that is still largely uncoordinated and ineffective.

The first lines of defense are the state medical boards, the state government agencies charged with licensing physicians who meet certain standards. These boards are also responsible for catching already-licensed doctors who fall below standards of conduct or competence in any of a number of areas. They are legally empowered to discipline these doctors: to reprimand them, require them to take course work, impose fines, place them on probation, and, in the worst cases, to suspend them from practice or revoke their licenses altogether.

These licensing and disciplinary systems vary from state to state. In some states the medical board is an independent state agency. In others, it is contained within the state department of licensing, of health, or of consumer affairs. In some states there is one board or agency for medical licensing and another for medical discipline. In a few states, one board or agency regulates all the health care professions--doctors, nurses, dentists, and so forth. In others, there are separate licensing and disciplinary boards for medical (allopathic) physicians, for osteopathic physicians, for dentists, and so on.[6]

In all states, the licensing boards are required to provide consumers with some disciplinary information about a specific doctor. The state agencies' addresses, including their website address if applicable, and phone numbers are listed in the "Addresses" section of each state's listing in this report.

The U.S. Department of Health and Human Services, through its Medicare and Medicaid programs, also disciplines health practitioners. It excludes doctors from participation in Medicare or Medicaid for specified periods of time, and may fine them for violations as well.

The Department's Inspector General must exclude a doctor for at least five years for a criminal conviction related to the Medicare or Medicaid programs and for patient abuse or neglect.[7] It may also impose sanctions based on other types of convictions, on license revocation or suspension by a state agency, or on a sanction by any state Medicaid program. The Inspector General may also sanction a doctor for fraud, for accepting kickbacks, for failing to cooperate with investigators, for failing to pay loans, and, based on a recommendation by the Medicare Peer Review Organizations for each state, for providing substandard or unnecessary care. The Inspector General's office accepts consumer complaints at the phone numbers and addresses listed in Appendix 3, pg. 50.

The Drug Enforcement Administration (DEA), which is part of the U.S. Department of

Justice, tracks down doctors who overprescribe or abuse the so-called "scheduled drugs"--drugs such as narcotics, tranquilizers, and amphetamines that may be addictive or otherwise abused. The DEA issues licenses to doctors and dentists that allow them to prescribe these "controlled dangerous substances." No doctor may legally prescribe drugs listed as controlled substances without a valid DEA license. Some states require a separate state controlled substance license as well.

The DEA may deny a license to prescribe these drugs, restrict a doctor's prescription privileges, or revoke his or her privileges to prescribe controlled substances. It publishes notices of such disciplinary actions in the *Federal Register* when the actions have been contested. The address to direct complaints to the DEA is listed in Appendix 3, pg. 50.

The Food and Drug Administration (FDA) sanctions physicians who violated FDA laws, regulations, or policies regarding clinical research on patients. In addition, the FDA permanently debars from ever working for an FDA-regulated company any one--including physicians--who was convicted of a felony related to FDA regulation of drugs.

State medical societies and specialty societies, both of which are unofficial trade associations for doctors, not government agencies, have peer review committees and have a role to play in medical discipline. However, they cannot prevent a doctor from continuing to practice, and their vested interest, in most cases, is in protecting their members, not the public.

Hospitals are required to have peer review committees to review the quality of medical care in their institutions. Consumers who have complaints about the quality of care in a hospital should file them with these committees. The committees may throw doctors off their staffs or restrict doctors' privileges to practice there. Unfortunately, most hospitals regard their peer review activities and disciplinary actions as confidential and will not inform patients about them. The National Practitioner Data Bank (NPDB), as of December 31, 1997, contained information on 6,793 clinical privilege actions against doctors[8] but, as mentioned above, these data are kept secret. There is also serious concern that hospitals are not reporting all of the hospital disciplinary actions against doctors as required by law. During the first three years and four months of operation of the NPDB, 75 percent of U.S. hospitals had not reported even one physician to the NPDB.[9] By 1996, according to NPDB staff, the situation had improved and "only" two-thirds of hospitals had not reported a single physician to the NPDB.By early 2000, almost 10 years after the NPDB had started its operations, 59% of U.S. hospitals, over 4000 hospitals, had still never reported any physicians to the data bank. One of the ways hospitals are said to be gaming the system and avoiding reporting doctors is related to the requirement that only those hospital disciplinary actions against doctors which are more than 30 days in duration need to be reported. Many hospitals are apparently taking a plethora of 27, 28 or 29-day actions so they will not have to report doctors whose cash flow of patient referrals they do not want to jeopardize.

Malpractice insurers can also play a role in quality control: they can cancel the policy of a physician who presents a bad risk, raise his or her rates, or offer coverage only if his or her practice is restricted.[10] Unfortunately, many states guarantee every doctor access to malpractice insurance, no matter how poor his or her record. Without an insurance policy, few doctors could afford to continue practicing and, in many states, would not be legally allowed to. Some state medical boards are informed when a doctor has had malpractice insurance canceled and will tell consumers.

The Magnitude of the Problem of Inadequate Doctor Discipline

Though it has improved during the past 15 years, the nation's system for protecting the public from medical incompetence and malfeasance is still far from adequate.

Gaps and breakdowns in communication still exist, although the National Practitioner Data Bank is helping to prevent doctors from being able to indiscriminately cross state lines to evade disciplinary boards. Those dangerous doctors who do fall through the cracks continue to kill, maim, defraud, and otherwise injure their unknowing patients.

Too many state medical boards, despite a clear duty to protect the public,[11] still believe their first responsibility is to rehabilitate "impaired physicians" and to protect them from the public's prying eyes. And the definition of "impaired" has expanded: it now covers doctors who may be drunk on the job, strung out on drugs, mentally ill, or habitual sex offenders.

Arizona, unlike any of the other state medical boards, states in its orders about doctors that it interprets the Americans with Disabilities Act as a reason for not "disciplining" physicians for substance abuse simply because they are already in or will be required to be in a rehabilitation program. Therefore, these actions are viewed as a "voluntary agreement" between the Board and the doctors, not as a disciplinary action.

While it is important for doctors who suffer from emotional problems or drug or alcohol addiction to receive appropriate treatment, this must be balanced with the state's responsibility to protect the public from doctors who are not able to deliver good medical care. Some states show a dangerous pattern of letting chemically dependent doctors return to practice after numerous failed attempts at rehabilitation. And while behavior that is sexually abusive may result from a mental illness, it is also a crime and is never acceptable in the context of patient care.

Although medical boards are now able to communicate with each other, at least indirectly, about doctors they have disciplined, the boards are often far too slow to act on what they have learned. And many state medical boards seldom communicate with the other agencies that guard against medical incompetence, fraud, and abuse--the federal Department of Health and Human Services, the Medicare Peer Review Organizations, the federal Drug Enforcement Administration, and the agencies that run state Medicaid programs.[12] Many of our recommendations to the states and federal government call for improved and regular communication between these groups.

Only a few of the country's medical boards, for example those in Utah, West Virginia, Georgia, Oregon, and a few others attempt to proactively sleuth out highly questionable physicians before receiving complaints, in order to prevent misconduct and poor care.

The College of Physicians and Surgeons in the Canadian province of Ontario, by contrast, visits physicians' offices and performs random audits of their care in order to "be assured that licensed physicians meet minimal requirements for safe practice."[13,14] Physicians who fail to meet those standards, as many as 12% of family doctors and 2% of specialists, must undergo intensive educational retraining and in rare cases face disciplinary action. To our knowledge, no American state has yet attempted such a far-reaching quality control program.

Most importantly, most state medical boards have not refined the art of speaking to their primary constituency: the public.

Because of a commendable increase in requirements to report malpractice information to them, states are now repositories of masses of information on the quality of individual doctors, but most states have not begun effective ways of disseminating all of it.

Many consumers when selecting a doctor still feel that they are floundering in the dark. They are unfamiliar with the role or the existence of medical boards. They are unaware that they can request disciplinary information, or that they can file complaints. Unwarned, too many of these people are treated by doctors guilty of previous acts of malpractice. And unwarned, too many of them are harmed.

Too little discipline is still being done. Fewer than one-half of 1% of the nation's doctors face any serious state sanctions each year. 2,696 total serious disciplinary actions a year, the number state medical boards took in 1999,[15] (see Table A, pg. 14) is a pittance compared to the volume of injury and death of patients caused by negligence of doctors. A recent study by the Institute of Medicine of the National Academy of Sciences estimated that as many as 98,000 patients may be killed each year in hospitals alone as a result of medical errors.[16] Earlier studies also found that this was a serious national problem.

* Harvard researchers found that 1% of a representative sample of patients treated in New York state hospitals in 1984 were injured, and one-quarter of those died, because of medical negligence.[17] Nationwide, that would have translated into 234,000 injuries and 80,000 deaths in 1988 from negligence in American hospitals. Most of this involves physicians. There is no clear evidence that there has been significant improvement since then.
* A similar study conducted in California in 1974 found that 0.8% of hospital patients had either been injured by negligence in the hospital or had been hospitalized because of negligent care.[18] Extrapolation of those findings would have yielded an estimate of 249,000 injuries and deaths from negligent medical practice in 1988.
* In 1976 the HEW Malpractice Commission estimated similarly that one-half of 1% of all patients entering hospitals are injured there due to negligence. That estimate would have indicated 156,000 injuries and deaths resulting from doctor negligence in 1988.[19]

Expanding these estimates to include general medical practice outside of a hospital, the potential abuse by physicians is even greater. An in-depth interview with 53 family physicians revealed that 47% of the doctors recalled a case in which the patient died due to physician error. Only four of the total reported errors led to malpractice suits, and none of these errors resulted in an action by a peer review organization.[20]

Medical students at SUNY-Buffalo were asked to recall incidents during their clinical training that raised ethical concerns. More than 200 students responded (40% of total sample); the majority of instances they reported (60%) did not in the researchers' opinions threaten the patient's life, health or welfare. This, however, implies that potentially 40% did.[21]

Systemic changes over time may also suggest a rise in physician malpractice. In a journal commentary, Dr. Alvan R. Feinstein reflects that in his 40 years of experience the manner in which medicine is now conducted may be sufficiently more complex as to contribute to an "epidemic of negligent medical errors."[22] A review of 43 malpractice insurance claims also indicates that systemic causes significantly contribute to pediatrician error; 91% of these claims, however, were also attributed to alleged errors of physician judgment involving diagnosis and treatment.[23] Even medical students and residents are now being held legally accountable for their mistakes,[24] thus broadening the pool of recognized physician error.

Given that many state medical boards now have the same information on claims and payments, they should be able to discipline at least as many doctors as malpractice carriers do. A 1989 Tufts University study found that physician-owned malpractice insurers sanctioned 13.6 of every 1,000 doctors they covered. The insurers terminated policies of 6.6 of every 1,000 policyholders in 1985 because of negligence-prone behavior, and they restricted the practice or imposed other sanctions on another 7 of every 1,000 doctors whose care was found to be substandard.[25] In an estimated population of 770,320 nonfederal doctors, this would translate to 10,476 doctors being disciplined a year.

The Impact of Substance Abuse

Specific physician attributes also contribute to this rate. Two studies surveyed residents to determine the incidence of substance use. Recent alcohol use was extremely high in both groups (87% within the last year for emergency medicine residents; 74% within the past 30 days for surgery residents).[26,27] Additional findings proved extremely disturbing; although the emergency medicine program directors accurately determined the incidence of alcohol use amongst residents, they dramatically underestimated the percent who were actually impaired by the substance as indicated by diagnostic tests (1% estimate impaired vs. 13% diagnosed.)[28]

This does not bode well for creating a medical system that prevents mishaps before they occur. And although the surgery residents reported negligible recent cocaine use, when employed, the drug was typically obtained from the hospital supply,[29] indicating a greater ease of access than for the general population.

Hughes reported that approximately 1-3% of physicians are disciplined or treated for substance abuse with an AMA estimated lifetime prevalence of 6-8% for alcoholism and 1-2% for drug dependency.[30] In 1985, Smith proposed that 17,000 doctors suffered from substance abuse.[31] Six percent of physicians indicated lifetime alcohol abuse and 1.6% reported either alcohol dependency or abuse within the last year alone.[32] If only 1% of physicians needed disciplining for chemical dependency, that alone would translate to 6,891 doctors.

Sexual Abuse or Misconduct

Sexual abuse of or sexual misconduct with a patient is also a serious issue. Six to ten percent of psychiatrists surveyed confessed to having engaged in sexual contact with a patient[33,34] and in a longitudinal study, Garfinkel at al. noted that of the original 70 psychiatrists they tracked, 2 (2.9%) had lost their medical licenses due to repeated violations of sexual boundaries with patients.[35] In reviewing their own rate of disciplinary actions for the years 1991-1995, the Oregon Board of Medical Examiners determined that of 100 open complaints investigated against 80 doctors during this time period, 5.9% were alleged to be sexual misconduct. More than one-third (39%) of these were classified as sexual impropriety, 31% were categorized as sexual transgression and 30% sexual violation. Disciplinary action was reported in 5%, 27%, and 54% of the instances, respectively. Twenty-five percent of the closed complaints also resulted in reportable disciplinary action.[36]

In light of these findings, it is not unreasonable to estimate that at least 1 percent of doctors in this country deserve some serious disciplinary action each year. This would amount to 7,703 physicians being disciplined each year, a number that, unfortunately far exceeds the actual number of physicians disciplined.

Findings

Public Citizen National Ranking of State Disciplinary Actions

Based on the Federation of State Medical Boards' (FSMB) data released annually on the number of disciplinary actions taken against doctors, Public Citizen calculated the rate of serious disciplinary actions per 1,000 doctors in each state and compiled a national report ranking state boards by the extent to which they are taking serious disciplinary actions against doctors in 1999 (See Table A, Findings, pg. 14).

Public Citizen has had and continues to have, two disputes with the FSMB over these data. First, we choose to look only at the most serious actions taken by state medical boards as a way of evaluating them, whereas the FSMB looks at "prejudicial" actions, a broader category which includes relative slaps on the wrist such as fines and reprimands as well as what we deem "serious" disciplinary actions. This category, in our view, should include only license revocations, suspensions or surrenders, plus probations, restrictions or other limitations on license (categories A & B in the FSMB data).

Second, the Federation states "it is virtually impossible to make sound comparisons of one medical board to another," and thereby avoids doing a ranking of state boards. We strongly disagree, and the Federation admits that the structure and funding of medical boards may have a direct impact on their effectiveness. Public Citizen believes that a valid uniform measure of board effectiveness is the rate of serious disciplinary actions per 1,000 doctors per year--a belief shared by Richard Kusserow, formerly Inspector General of the federal Department of Health and Human Services.

According to James R. Winn, M.D., the Federation's executive vice-president, "Boards that are independent or semi-autonomous, adopting their own budgets and allocating revenues to their operations, appear to perform their role of public protectors more effectively than those boards that are classified as subordinate or advisory." So, although the FSMB disagrees with the idea of our rankings based on their data, it admits to differences in structure and funding between boards which are amongst the probable causes of the differences in rates of serious disciplinary action.

Table A	Ranking of Serious Doctor Disciplinary Actions by State Medical Licensing Boards 1999			
1999 Rank	**State**	**Number Of Serious Actions 1999**	**Total Number of Nonfederal Doctors 1998**	**Serious Actions Per 1,000 Doctors**
1	Alaska	12	1160	10.34
2	North Dakota	14	1596	8.77
3	Wyoming	8	981	8.15
4	Idaho	16	2278	7.02
5	Oklahoma	37	6216	5.95
6	Kentucky	54	9115	5.92
7	Ohio	190	32220	5.90
8	Mississippi	30	5107	5.87
9	Vermont	11	2061	5.34
10	Colorado	59	11253	5.24
11	Iowa	33	6602	5.00
12	Arkansas	27	5486	4.92
13	Alabama	45	9559	4.71
14	New York	366	77781	4.71
15	Georgia	82	17961	4.57
16	Indiana	60	13267	4.52
17	West Virginia	19	4249	4.47
18	New Hampshire	14	3309	4.23
19	Michigan	101	24001	4.21
20	California	367	90940	4.04
21	Arizona	42	11025	3.81
22	Virginia	70	18441	3.80
23	Louisiana	43	11581	3.71
24	Maine	11	3195	3.44
25	Nevada	11	3373	3.26
26	North Carolina	62	19615	3.16
27	New Mexico	13	4138	3.14
28	New Jersey	89	28432	3.13
29	South Carolina	27	8923	3.03
30	Oregon	27	8984	3.01
31	Missouri	45	15211	2.96
32	Montana	6	2036	2.95
33	Utah	13	4770	2.73
34	Texas	124	45707	2.71
35	Rhode Island	10	3784	2.64
36	Pennsylvania	97	38080	2.55
37	Washington	38	15254	2.49
38	Florida	105	42169	2.49
39	Massachusetts	67	27622	2.43
40	Maryland	51	21116	2.42
41	District of Columbia	9	4121	2.18
42	Wisconsin	28	13567	2.06
43	Illinois	73	35581	2.05
44	South Dakota	3	1562	1.92
45	Kansas	12	6577	1.82
46	Connecticut	23	12910	1.78
47	Hawaii	6	3555	1.69
48	Minnesota	21	13275	1.58
49	Tennessee	18	14412	1.25
50	Nebraska	5	4070	1.23
51	Delaware	2	2092	0.96
	Total	**2696**	**770320**	**3.50**

Our calculation of rates of serious disciplinary actions per 1,000 doctors by state is created by taking the number of such actions (as defined above) and dividing it by the American Medical Association data on non-federal M.D.s, and then multiplying the result by 1,000 to get state disciplinary rates. Nationwide, there were 2,696 serious disciplinary actions in 1999 out of 770,320 nonfederal M.D.s, which is a rate of 3.50 serious disciplinary actions per 1,000 physicians. State rates ranged from 10.34 (Alaska) to 0.96 (Delaware).

Best States. The top 10 states, or those with the highest rate of serious disciplinary actions per 1,000 physicians are (in order): Alaska (10.34/1,000 physicians), North Dakota (8.77), Wyoming (8.15), Idaho (7.02), Oklahoma (5.95), Kentucky (5.92), Ohio (5.90), Mississippi (5.87), Vermont (5.34), and Colorado (5.24). Five of these 10 states (Alaska, Oklahoma, Mississippi, Wyoming, and Ohio) were also in the top 10 in 1997 and 1998 and two, (Mississippi and Alaska) have been in the top 10 for nine straight years. Oklahoma, 5th this year, has been in the top 10 states for eight of the last nine years. Wyoming, 3rd this year, has been in the top 10 for seven of the last nine years and Vermont, 9th this year and Ohio, 7th this year, have been in the top ten for five of the last nine years.

It is clear that state-by-state performance is spotty. Only one of the nation's 15 largest states, Ohio, is represented among those 10 states with the highest disciplinary rates, as it also was in 1996, 1997 and 1998. Other large states such as, New York, Michigan and California (14th, 19th and 20th respectively in 1999) have shown improvement from 40th, 49th and 37th in 1991. But other large states such as Texas, Pennsylvania, Massachusetts and Illinois (34th, 36th, 39th and 43rd in 1999) have not done very much doctor discipline for many of the last 10 years.

Worst States. The bottom 15 states, those with the lowest serious disciplinary rates in 1998, were, starting with the lowest: Delaware 0.96 per 1,000 physicians), Nebraska (1.23), Tennessee (1.25), Minnesota (1.58), Hawaii (1.69), Connecticut (1.78), Kansas (1.82), South Dakota (1.92), Illinois (2.05), Wisconsin (2.06), D.C. (2.18), Maryland (2.42), Massachusetts (2.43), Florida (2.49), and Washington (2.49). Massachusetts, Tennessee, Minnesota, Wisconsin, Kansas, Hawaii, and Delaware were also in the bottom 15 states in 1997 and 1998. In 1999, the bottom 20 states all had rates of serious disciplinary action that were one-half or less than the rate of all of the top five states.

Table B Ranking of States 1991-1999: Serious Disciplinary Actions

Rank 1999	Rank 1998	Rank 1997	Rank 1996	Rank 1995	Rank 1994	Rank 1993	Rank 1992	Rank 1992	State
1	1	2	6	8	2	8	7	6	Alaska
2	11	9	2	34	10	3	5	13	N. Dakota
3	7	3	31	3	1	21	4	9	Wyoming
4	25	30	21	36	30	37/38	23	34/35	Idaho
5	2	5	7	12	5	2	1	2	Oklahoma
6	14	7/8	14	14	4	4	16	5	Kentucky
7	10	7/8	8	9	24	22/23	19	23	Ohio
8	3	1	1	1	9	9	6	6	Mississippi
9	6	25/26	10	6	39	17	15	10	Vermont
10	18	6	4	5	12	6	8	17	Colorado
11	23	4	3	2	7	5	2	3	Iowa
12	4	13	15	23	28	26	18	29	Arkansas
13	17	23/24	38	30	43/44	29	30	31	Alabama
14	16	16	18	17	29	34	39	49	New York
15	12	23/24	19	4	8	10	9	4	Georgia
16	21	19/20	33	28	16	7	14	15	Indiana
17	5	12	11	7	6	1	3	8	W. Virginia
18	30	46	51	49	49	47	47	44	New Hampshire
19	13	15	28	21	34/35	35	40	40	Michigan
20	27	18	27	20	34/35	32	42	37	California
21	38	19/20	5	10	17	16	22	22	Arizona
22	40	34/35	50	41/42	32	30	37	32	Virginia
23	15	34/35	44	13	18	11	12	7	Louisiana
24	9	22	17	32	33	41	44	46	Maine
25	26	32	9	11	31	20	25	26	Nevada
26	43	33	48/49	35	36	40	34	42/43	N. Carolina
27	8	50	23	15	43/44	49	33	33	New Mexico
28	35	42	20	25	19	18	28	20	New Jersey
29	22	40	45	44	14	15	11	11	S. Carolina
30	31	28/29	29	16	20	22/23	24	14	Oregon
31	48	17	30	37	13	12	13	12	Missouri
32	34	11	13	18	3	14	10	19	Montana
33	20	25/26	16	38	46	39	43	18	Utah
34	28/29	37	35	19	23	28	29	21	Texas
35	24	10	25	26	26	42	41	50/51	Rhode Island
36	45	27	32	43	47	48	48	47	Pennsylvania
37	36/37	28/29	40	24	27	24	17	24	Washington
38	49	36	22	22	25	25	21	27	Florida
39	47	45	43	40	37	45	46	48	Massachusetts
40	36/37	38	41	29	21	19	27	42/43	Maryland
41	33	44	36	50	51	51	45	45	D. Columbia
42	46	39	34	47	41	27	26	34/35	Wisconsin
43	41	21	46	45	40	31	36	36	Illinois
44	19	14	42	33	11	13	32	50/51	S. Dakota
45	44	41	12	46	22	37/38	20	25	Kansas
46	32	31	37	27	42	36	35	30	Connecticut
47	39	49	39	51	50	46	50	41	Hawaii
48	42	51	47	39	45	33	31	28	Minnesota
49	51	48	48/49	31	38	44	49	38	Tennessee
50	28/29	43	24	41/42	15	50	38	39	Nebraska
51	50	47	26	48	48	43	51	16	Delaware

Table B, on pg. 16, shows the ranking of state boards for the last nine years. It can be seen that there are some states which have consistently been among the highest-ranking ones, others which have stayed consistently toward the bottom and yet others which have gone from better to worse or vice versa.

This analysis raises serious questions about the extent to which patients in many states with poorer records of serious doctor discipline are being protected from physicians who might well be barred from practice in states with boards that are doing a better job of disciplining physicians. It is likely, if not certain that patients are being injured or killed more often in states with poor doctor disciplinary records than in states with consistent top 10 performances. It is not unreasonable to estimate that at least 1 percent of doctors in this country deserve some serious disciplinary action each year, a number comparable to Alaska's rate of 10.32 actions per 1,000 doctors or 1.032 percent. In fact, each year one or more states achieves a rate of serious disciplinary actions of approximately 10 per 10,000 doctors. This would amount to 7,703 (1% of 770,320 non-federal doctors) serious actions a year, which cover only a small fraction of the 98,000 patient deaths thought to occur each year in American hospitals as a result of errors, almost all of it involving physicians. The current overall national rate of serious disciplinary actions, 3.50 per 1,000 or .350 percent is far short of the rate of 1.034 percent in Alaska. If the rate of serious disciplinary actions had been 10 per 1,000 (1 percent), the national total would have been 7,703 actions or 5,007 more actions in 1999 (2.8 times more) than the 2,696 that actually occurred in 1999.

Considering what is known about substandard doctoring, not even Alaska's disciplinary rate seems adequate. Most states have a long way to go before they even begin to offer serious protection for citizens from doctors who are incompetent, who sexually abuse patients or who otherwise have serious problems that interfere with delivery of high-quality medical care in a compassionate way. All states, even those with best records, need to strengthen the structure and functions of their licensing boards. The statement by the Federation that you cannot compare the disciplinary rates of boards with each other because they are set-up, structured and funded differently is preposterous.

Disciplinary Actions from Public Citizen's Database

As shown in Table C, pg. 19, of the 38,589 disciplinary actions reported by state boards or the federal government to Public Citizen (representing actions against 20,125 doctors), the majority (32,868 or 85.2%) of these were imposed by state medical boards. A description and statistical breakdown of the actions provided to Public Citizen by each state is provided in the "State by State Listings" section. These counts represent the two most serious disciplinary actions for each sanction reported. Some sanctions included more than two actions against the doctors. These less serious actions are not included in these counts. (For a more detailed discussion of how disciplinary actions are reported, refer to "How We Compiled This Report," Appendix 2, pg. 40.)

Please note that the period of years covered in the database varies from state to state. However, of the 50 states and the District of Columbia, for 44 of these jurisdictions, (86%), we have 10 years of data, from the beginning of 1990 through 1999. For the remaining 7 states, we have between 6 and 3/4 years of data (Arkansas) and 9 and 1/2 years of disciplinary data (Florida).

The federal agencies account for the remaining 5721 disciplinary actions imposed; 6.4% (2,462) were DEA sanctions in contested and uncontested cases, 8.3% (3,234) were fines and exclusions from the Medicare program, and 25 were restrictions placed on a physician's eligibility to participate as investigators in FDA experiments or to work for FDA-regulated companies.

An analysis of the 2,366 doctors who were the subject of DEA disciplinary actions revealed that hundreds were not the subject of any state disciplinary action even though their federal narcotics license had been revoked, surrendered, or restricted.

Similarly, of the 3,232 Medicare doctors who were the subjects of the 3,234 Medicare disciplinary actions, hundreds were not disciplined by their state boards even though most had involved exclusion from Medicare.

Table C Disciplinary Actions by State and Federal Agencies

State/Federal Agency	Number of Actions	State/Federal Agency	Number of Actions
Alabama	366	Mississippi	298
Alaska	161	Missouri	630
Arizona	942	Montana	97
Arkansas	168	Nebraska	114
California	2670	Nevada	151
Colorado	884	New Hampshire	117
Connecticut	440	New Jersey	1472
Delaware	44	New Mexico	145
District of Columbia	242	New York	2993
DEA	***2462***	North Carolina	523
Florida	2746	North Dakota	131
FDA	***25***	Ohio	1484
Georgia	855	Oklahoma	592
Hawaii	119	Oregon	344
Idaho	51	Pennsylvania	1230
Illinois	1390	Rhode Island	176
Indiana	556	South Carolina	389
Iowa	526	South Dakota	75
Kansas	250	Tennessee	409
Kentucky	595	Texas	2035
Louisiana	505	Utah	218
Maine	177	Vermont	132
Maryland	803	Virginia	567
Massachusetts	586	Washington	596
Medicare	***3234***	West Virginia	419
Michigan	1341	Wisconsin	501
Minnesota	493	Wyoming	68
		TOTAL	**38,589**

Thus, many states are not acting promptly, if at all, against physicians about whom a federal agency has already compiled sufficient information to discipline them for very serious offenses.

Types of Disciplinary Actions and Offenses

The following tables provide a statistical national look at the types of disciplinary actions and the offenses for which they were taken.

Table D, Types of Disciplinary Actions Reported to Public Citizen (pg. 21) shows that the most common type of state disciplinary action of those submitted to us was probation. States imposed probation 19.3% of the times (7,431 times) when practitioners were disciplined. They revoked licenses 7.9% of the time (3,045 times), suspended licenses 9.6% of the time (3,704 times), and accepted a doctor's surrender of his or her license 7.9% of the time (3,063 times). Cumulatively, only 9,812 or 25.4% of the actions against doctors listed in this report were ones which resulted in at least a temporary loss of ability to practice medicine (revocation, suspension and surrender). Most of the doctors who are listed in this book never had to stop practicing medicine and many more who had suspensions may once again be practicing. It is not likely that many of their patients are aware of these actions. **A total of 20,125 different physicians were the subject of the 38,589 disciplinary actions taken by state and federal agencies.**

Table D	Disciplinary Actions Reported to Public Citizen: A Breakdown of the Types of Disciplinary Actions Contained in This Report	
Disciplinary Action	**Number**	**Percent**
Probation	7431	19.3%
Suspension	3704	9.6%
Revocation	3045	7.9%
Fine	3708	9.6%
Surrender	3063	7.9%
Reprimand	3094	8.0%
Exclusion from the Medicare Program	3220	8.3%
Practice Restriction	2243	5.8%
Revocation, Surrender, Suspension of Controlled Substance License	2275	5.9%
Restriction of Controlled Substance License	1317	3.4%
Emergency Suspension	1231	3.2%
Education	1357	3.5%
Physician Monitoring	1251	3.2%
License Denial, Reinstatement or Nonrenewal	803	2.1%
Required to Enter an Impaired Physicians Program or Substance Abuse Treatment	266	0.7%
Other Actions	581	1.5%
Total Actions	**38589**	**100.0%**

Table E, Offenses for which Disciplinary Action was Taken (pg. 23). The reason an action was taken--the offense--was provided by state and federal authorities for 24,042 of the records in our database. For a number of offenses, more than one action was taken. In 7,132 cases, the stated reason for the listed actions was "disciplinary action taken by another state agency," leaving 16,910 offenses with specific details as to the nature of the offense. For 15,310 of these offenses or 90.6% of them, the offense was one of the five discussed previoiusly--substandard care, incompetence or negligence, criminal conviction, substance abuse, misprescribing or over prescribing of drugs or sex-related offenses--or another serious offense such as providing false information, loss of hospital privileges or fraud. Among those 16,910 actions for which specific reasons other than discipline by another state or agency were reported, the five most serious offenses were as follows.

Sexual abuse of or sexual misconduct with a patient accounted for 3.2% of the total known offenses for which doctors were disciplined. A total of 547 different doctors were disciplined for these offenses.

Substandard care, incompetence or negligence: The most common single reason for which states disciplined doctors was for offenses involving substandard care, incompetence or negligence. which accounted for 18.8% of all the 16,910 actions for which a specific offense was stated. A total of 3,215 different doctors were disciplined for this offense.

Criminal conviction, the second largest category, accounted for 17.2% of known offenses other than those listed as disciplinary action by another state. A total of 2,963 different doctors were disciplined for criminal conviction (plea of guilty or nolo contendere--no contest).

Disciplinary actions taken because of *misprescribing or overprescribing drugs* accounted for an additional 7.7% of known offenses. A total of 1,318 different doctors were disciplined for these offenses.

Substance abuse accounted for an additional 10.0% of known offenses for which doctors were disciplined. A total of 1,715 different doctors were disciplined for these offenses.

The five offenses listed above, all extremely serious, accounted for 56.9% or more than half of all of those disciplinary actions in which a specific offense other than discipline by another state or agency was listed.

Table E Offenses for which Disciplinary Action was Taken*		
Offense	**Number**	**Percent**
Criminal Conviction	2901	12.1%
Disciplinary Action Taken by Another State or Agency	7132	29.7%
Substandard Care, Incompetence, or Negligence	3184	13.2%
Misprescribing or Overprescribing Drugs	1302	5.4%
Substance Abuse	1683	7.0%
Professional Misconduct	2182	9.1%
Noncompliance with a Board Order	1274	5.3%
Noncompliance with a Professional Rule	2075	8.6%
Practicing without a License	420	1.7%
Practicing without a Controlled Substance License	70	0.3%
Providing False Information to Medical Board or Other Health Agency	417	1.7%
Sexual Abuse of or Sexual Misconduct with a Patient	536	2.2%
Physical or Mental Impairment	472	2.0%
Hospital Privilege Loss or Restriction	236	1.0%
Insurance or Medicare/Medicaid Fraud	72	0.3%
Falsifying/Altering Medical Records	38	0.2%
Overcharging	34	0.1%
Exceeding Professional Limitations	14	0.1%
Total Records With Offense Cited	**24042**	**100.0%**

* Frequencies and types of violations cited by states or federal government for disciplinary actions. Includes only those actions for which an offense was reported and for which we had a corresponding term in our database. This table does not include the 5,371 cases in which the stated reason was action by another state.

Table F, Disciplinary Actions Taken Against Doctors Cited for Sexual Abuse of or Sexual Misconduct with a Patient, below, shows that of the 547 different doctors who were disciplined for sexual abuse of or sexual misconduct with a patient, there were 302 actions (81 revocations, 46 surrenders, 130 suspensions plus 45 emergency suspensions) which required those doctors, at least temporarily, to stop practicing medicine. Switching from actions to doctors, there were 286 doctors (52.3%) who were, at least temporarily, removed from practice by license suspension, surrender or revocation. But this means that at least 47.7% of doctors (261 doctors) were allowed to continue practicing, their behavior probably unknown to most if not all of their patients. It is likely that other doctors, especially those whose licenses were only suspended temporarily, are once again practicing medicine.

Table F — Disciplinary Actions Taken Against Doctors Cited for Sexual Abuse of or Sexual Misconduct with a Patient

Action	Number	Percent
Revocation	81	10.3%
Surrender	46	5.9%
Suspension	130	16.6%
Emergency Suspension	45	5.7%
Probation	189	24.1%
Fine	77	9.8%
Other Actions	217	27.6%
Total Actions	**785**	**100.0%**

Table G, Disciplinary Actions Taken Against Doctors Cited for Substandard Care, Incompetence or Negligence, below, shows that of the 3,215 different doctors who were disciplined for substandard care, incompetence or negligence, there were 987 actions (315 revocations, 244 surrenders, 338 suspensions plus 90 emergency suspensions) which required those doctors, at least temporarily, to stop practicing medicine. Switching from actions to doctors, there were 942 doctors (29.3%) who were, at least temporarily, removed from practice by license suspension, surrender or revocation. But this means that at least 70.7% of doctors (2,273 doctors) were allowed to continue practicing, their behavior probably unknown to most if not all of their patients. It is likely that other doctors, especially those whose licenses were only suspended temporarily, are once again practicing medicine.

Table G Disciplinary Actions Taken Against Doctors Cited for Substandard Care, Incompetence or Negligence

Action	Number	Percent
Revocation	315	6.8%
Surrender	244	5.3%
Suspension	338	7.3%
Emergency Suspension	90	2.0%
Probation	1181	25.6%
Practice Restriction	359	7.8%
Fine	809	17.6%
Reprimand	491	10.7%
Other Actions	779	16.9%
Total Actions	**4606**	**100.0%**

Table H, Disciplinary Actions Taken Against Doctors Cited for Criminal Convictions, below, shows that of the 2,963 different doctors who were disciplined because of a criminal conviction, there were 1,363 actions (563 revocations, 159 surrenders, 491 suspensions plus 150 emergency suspensions) which required those doctors, at least temporarily, to stop practicing medicine. Switching from actions to doctors, there were 1,162 doctors (39.2%) who were, at least temporarily, removed from practice by license suspension, surrender or revocation. But this means that at least 60.8% of doctors (1,801 doctors) were allowed to continue practicing, their behavior probably unknown to most if not all of their patients. It is likely that other doctors, especially those whose licenses were only suspended temporarily, are once again practicing medicine.

Table H Disciplinary Actions Taken Against Doctors Cited for Criminal Convictions

Action	Number	Percent
Revocation	563	16.2%
Surrender	159	4.6%
Suspension	491	14.1%
Emergency Suspension	150	4.3%
Probation	587	16.9%
Fine	203	5.8%
Other Actions	1319	38.0%
Total Actions	**3472**	**100.0%**

Table I, Disciplinary Actions Taken Against Doctors Cited for Misprescribing or Overprescribing Drugs, below, shows that of the 1,318 different doctors who were disciplined because of misprescribing or overprescribing drugs, there were 378 actions (96 revocations, 85 surrenders, 155 suspensions plus 42 emergency suspensions) which required those doctors, at least temporarily, to stop practicing medicine. Switching from actions to doctors, there were 368 doctors (27.9%) who were, at least temporarily, removed from practice by license suspension, surrender or revocation. But this means that at least 72.1% of doctors (950 doctors) were allowed to continue practicing, their behavior probably unknown to most if not all of their patients. It is likely that other doctors, especially those whose licenses were only suspended temporarily, are once again practicing medicine.

Table I — Disciplinary Actions Taken Against Doctors Cited for Mispresribing or Overprescribing Drugs

Action	Number	Percent
Revocation	96	5.0%
Surrender	85	4.4%
Revocation, Surrender, or Suspension of Controlled Substance License	171	8.9%
Suspension	155	8.1%
Emergency Suspension	42	2.2%
Probation	486	25.2%
Restriction of Controlled Substance License	211	11.0%
Fine	200	10.4%
Education	141	7.3%
Other Actions	338	17.6%
Total Actions	**1925**	**100.0%**

Table J, Disciplinary Actions Taken Against Doctors Cited for Substance Abuse, below, shows that of the 1,715 different doctors who were disciplined because of substance abuse, there were 611 actions (71 revocations, 111 surrenders, 293 suspensions plus 136 emergency suspensions) which required those doctors, at least temporarily, to stop practicing medicine. Switching from actions to doctors, there were 556 doctors (32.4%) who were, at least temporarily, removed from practice by license suspension, surrender or revocation. But this means that at least 67.6% of doctors (1,159 doctors) were allowed to continue practicing, their behavior probably unknown to most if not all of their patients. It is likely that other doctors, especially those whose licenses were only suspended temporarily, are once again practicing medicine.

Table J Disciplinary Actions Taken Against Doctors Cited for Substance Abuse

Action	Number	Percent
Revocation	71	2.9%
Surrender	111	4.5%
Revocation, Surrender, or Suspension of Controlled Substance License	116	4.7%
Suspension	293	11.8%
Emergency Suspension	136	5.5%
Probation	741	29.9%
Restriction of Controlled Substance License	143	5.8%
Fine	43	1.7%
Required to Enter an Impaired Physician Program or Substance Abuse Treatment	161	6.5%
Other Actions	665	26.8%
Total Actions	**2480**	**100.0%**

Conclusions

1. The current rate of serious disciplinary actions is a dangerously small drop in the bucket of adequate, consumer-protective doctor discipline.
2. All states, especially those with the worst records, need to strengthen the structure and functions of their licensing boards.
3. The increase in the total number of disciplinary actions in a given state may not indicate that more doctors are being caught. Much of the disciplinary activity, in states such as New York, involves insuring that doctors, once caught by one state, are disciplined when they move to another. There has also been a noticeable increase in sanctioning doctors for administrative purposes.
4. Questionable doctors can still cross state borders, though with less impunity than before. The extent to which one board shares information with another still varies widely by state.

    * In many instances discipline is still too slow although the case backlogs in some states have been greatly reduced. Wisconsin sanctioned a number of doctors only after they had already retired from practice.

    * The vast majority of states continue to require reporting of hospital disciplinary actions and malpractice claims or payments to the medical board, but few check whether the required reports have actually been filed. And some still fail to act promptly, if at all, on the information they receive.

    * Medical boards are much too forgiving. Many still see their priority as "rehabilitation," and their disciplinary actions are too light. Probation is the most common sanction against doctors for all of the five most serious offenses: sexual abuse or misconduct; substandard care; conviction; prescription violations, or substance abuse. Arizona, for example, interprets the Americans with Disabilities Act to indicate that action for substance abuse is a "voluntary agreement" between the physician and the Board, not a disciplinary action.

    * Far too few board actions, only 18.8% of the 16,910 identified offenses (other than those listed as action by another state), were for medical negligence or incompetence. Instead boards focus on more easily documentable offenses such as

prescription violations and fraud convictions or disciplinary action in another state as potential indicators of substandard care. Other instances of incompetence may be overlooked because the investigations soak up resources like a sponge.

To date, legislation--mainly at the state level--on medical malpractice, the injury and death of patients caused by doctor negligence, has been to punish the victim instead of disciplining the perpetrator. Legislative attention must be given to requiring states to significantly improve the discipline of physicians in order to prevent future death and injury.

Recommendations for Action

Complain. As discussed in *How To Use This Report*, pg. 1, file your complaints about poor medical care or medical misconduct with your state medical board and with the federal Department of Health and Human Services. If the offense occurred in a hospital, also file a complaint with the hospital peer review committee. Your complaints are needed to protect others!

Organize. Form citizens' action or victims' rights groups to improve medical quality assurance in your area. The American Association of Retired Persons publishes a guide that can help you mobilize a group for reform.[37] Try to get a representative of your group appointed to the state medical board or the Medicare Peer Review Organization for your state.

Write to your Congresspersons, at both state and federal levels urging actions as listed below.

Recommendations for the Federal Government

Create grants and standards. Congress should create a small program of grants-in-aid to state medical boards. The grants should be tied to the boards' agreements to meet certain performance standards, which should be developed by the Public Health Service, as the Department of Health and Human Services Office of Inspector General recommended in 1990.[38]

In developing these standards, the Public Health Service should work with the Federation of State Medical Boards' Assessment Task Force. In September 1990 the FSMB received a federal contract for $200,000 to undertake the development of a self-assessment instrument for state medical boards. The goal of the task force was to produce a sound and objective means by which boards could assess their performance over time and in comparison with other boards.[39] In April 1992 the Federation released its "Self-Assessment Instrument for State Medical Boards" and the accompanying handbook. The Instrument is a survey that each board can fill out regarding its own activities, enabling boards to eventually share information with each other and compare resources and performance. The standards should include (but not be limited to) the following: processing complaints within a certain limited period of time; maintaining a certain level of staffing and having staff meet certain qualifications; disseminating disciplinary information to the public; having at least 30% of board members be consumer members; regularly publishing a newsletter that includes names of disciplined physicians and descriptions of the disciplinary actions taken against them; issuing an annual report that includes meaningful disciplinary statistics; and other standards.

The Medicare Peer Review Organizations (PRO), which have been practically moribund in disciplining physicians for substandard care, should become more aggressive. The PROs should hire investigators and advisers trained in law enforcement so that fewer of their sanctions will be overturned.

As a 1990 Institute of Medicine report noted, the PROs are not evaluated on their ability to detect and correct poor quality care.[40] The Department of Health and Human Services should change its evaluation procedures to place more emphasis on quality.

Open the National Practitioner Data Bank (NPDB). In 1986 Congress passed the Health Care Quality Improvement Act. This act mandated the establishment of a data bank containing information on adverse professional review actions taken against doctors, and on doctors who had been sued for malpractice and on whose behalf settlement or adjudicated payments had been made. Unfortunately, the law establishing the data bank also required that it be closed to the general public. Congress should pass legislation opening the data bank to consumers and loudly rebuke the American Medical Association's resolution to destroy the data bank. Although there have been Congressional hearings in 2000 on the topic of opening up the NPDB, as this report goes to press, there is no significant likelihood that such legislation is likely to become law.

The Drug Enforcement Administration should release a monthly list of all practitioners whose controlled substance prescription licenses have been revoked, surrendered, restricted, or denied. The list should be widely distributed to pharmacies, state pharmacy and medical boards, and the general public. Far too many doctors continue to prescribe controlled substances after their DEA licenses have expired or have been revoked. The DEA should consider requiring pharmacies to subscribe to an on-line service with which they could check the validity of these DEA license numbers.

Require doctor recertification. Congress should consider legislation proposed by Rep. Pete Stark, D-California, to require physicians who accept Medicare patients to be periodically recertified for competency.

Recommendations for States

Strengthen the statutes. States that have not already done so should adopt legislation at least as strong as that in the Model Medical Practice Act developed by the Federation of State Medical

Boards,[41] or, preferably, stronger laws.

Restructure the boards. States should sever any remaining formal, debilitating links between state licensing boards and state medical societies. Members of medical boards (and separate disciplinary boards, where present) should be appointed by the governor, and the governor's choice of appointees should not be limited to a medical society's nominees. At least 50% of the members of each state medical board and disciplinary board should be well-informed and well-trained public members who have no ties to health care providers and who, preferably, have a history of advocacy on behalf of patients. The governor should appoint members to the Medical Board whose top priority is protecting the public's health, not providing assistance to physicians who are trying to evade disciplinary actions.

Inform the public. Each state's Open Records Law and its Medical Practice Act should state that all formal disciplinary actions against licensed professionals are fully public records. Each legislature should require widespread dissemination of final disciplinary orders. Lists of those disciplined and full disciplinary orders should be promptly available by mail to all requesting them.

Notices of disciplinary actions should be sent to the local news media and to all hospitals, health maintenance organizations (HMOs), and other health care providers in the state, as well as to other state agencies, the federal Department of Health and Human Services, and the federal Drug Enforcement Administration. Federal law already requires that such information be reported to the National Practitioner Data Bank, which began operating on September 1, 1990.

As has already begun to happen in many states, all states should make disciplinary actions they take against physicians promptly available on their web sites and it should include all details such as the full text of the board order against the physician.

Strengthen board authority. Every medical board should have the authority to impose emergency suspensions pending formal hearing in cases where a doctor poses a potential danger to the public health. Boards should aggressively use this authority when they learn of a potentially dangerous doctor. The legal standard for disciplining physicians should be a preponderance of the evidence, not more difficult to accomplish standards.

Medical boards should have the authority to rapidly, after confirmation, accept the findings of other state boards and of the federal Department of Health and Human Services and the Drug Enforcement Administration. If a physician has been disciplined by another state, any subsequent state's medical board should be required to impose sanctions at least as stringent as those imposed by the first state. Each state should require physicians who have been licensed in other states and who seek licensure in a new state to submit affidavits that they are not under investigation elsewhere before being granted a new license. Physicians who are under investigation should not be permitted to practice until the board has heard the details of their case and can evaluate their competency. Each legislature should grant its state medical licensing board the authority to examine physicians for physical, mental and professional competence and to test them for alcohol and drug use upon reason to believe that a problem exists in one of these areas.

Encourage complaints. Each legislature should provide for the protection of confidentiality and immunity to those who report violations of the Medical Practice Act to a board. Such protections should also be extended to board members, their staff, and consultants.

Each legislature should require all licensed health care practitioners to report Medical Practice Act violations by other practitioners to the medical board, with large civil penalties for failure to do so. Boards should aggressively use their authority to enforce the requirement that all health care providers report such violations. Each legislature should also require hospitals to report all revocations, restrictions, or voluntary surrenders of privileges.

Courts should be required to report all indictments and convictions of physicians to the medical disciplinary board. In addition, each legislature should require liability insurers to report all claims, payments, and policy cancellations to state medical disciplinary boards. It should request reports from other state agencies, Medicare, the DEA and other federal agencies. It should also require impaired physicians' programs to report the names of doctors who fail to successfully complete their programs. Medical boards should conduct random audits of institutions to check compliance with these reporting requirements, and should fine those who fail to comply. After a doctor is disciplined, a board should fine any other practitioners who knew of that doctor's offense, but failed to report it.

Keep the courts in check. Each legislature should pass laws that make clear their intent that the judgements of the medical board be given extreme deference, and that, barring extraordinary circumstances, disciplinary actions should take immediate effect pending appeal.

Each legislature should adopt the 'preponderance of the evidence' standard of proof in medical disciplinary cases, replacing the tougher-to-meet 'clear and convincing evidence' standard now in effect in most states. According to the August 1990 report on state medical boards issued by the Office of the Inspector General, "The 'clear and convincing evidence' standard of proof is more rigorous than the 'preponderance of evidence' standard that is typically required to justify tort damages for negligence in civil cases. The more rigorous standard provides greater protection for physicians, but adds complexity to the investigative process and appears to make it less likely that a board will persevere on a case through a full evidentiary hearing."[42]

Furthermore, the Project Work Panel of the Federation of State Medical Boards, in its August 1989 report "Elements of a Modern State Medical Board: A Proposal," recommended that each state medical board "use preponderance of evidence as the standard of proof" and that they each have the power "to issue final decisions when acting as trier of fact in the performance of [their] adjudicatory duties."[43]

Beef up funding and staffing. Each legislature should permit the medical board to spend all the revenue from medical licensing fees, rather than being forced to give part to the state Treasury. The medical boards should raise their fees to $500 a year. All boards could benefit from hiring new investigators and legal staff. Boards should employ adequate staff to process and investigate all complaints within 30 days, to review all malpractice claims filed with the board, to monitor and regularly visit doctors who have been disciplined to ensure their compliance with the sanctions imposed, and to ensure compliance with reporting requirements. They should hire investigators to seek out errant doctors, through review of pharmacy records, consultation with medical examiners, and targeted office audits of those doctors practicing alone and suspected of poor care.

Require risk prevention. States should adopt a law, similar to one in Massachusetts, that requires all hospitals and other health care providers to have a meaningful, functioning risk prevention program designed to prevent injury to patients. Massachusetts also requires all adverse incidents occurring in hospitals or in doctors' offices to be reported to the medical board.

Require periodic recertification of doctors based on a written exam and audit of their patients' medical care records.

Appendix 1
Glossary

Controlled substances, controlled dangerous substances: drugs which are regulated under the federal Controlled Substances Act because of their potential for addiction or abuse.

D.O.: the academic degree awarded to osteopathic physicians.

DEA: the federal Drug Enforcement Administration, an agency of the U.S. Justice Department. Its mission is to enforce controlled substances laws.

DEA license, DEA registration, or DEA certificate: every person who handles or prescribes controlled substances, including physicians and dentists, must legally have a registration number issued by the Drug Enforcement Administration.

Disciplinary action: any of a number of ways a regulatory agency can limit or forbid a doctor's practice or formally indicate its displeasure. Includes license revocations, suspensions, and probations, consent agreements placing conditions on a doctor's continuing practice, monetary fines, and letters of reprimand.

Disciplinary action rate: total state disciplinary actions per 1,000 M.D.s practicing in a state.

Emergency suspension: a disciplinary action in which a medical board may remove a doctor from practice temporarily, without a formal disciplinary hearing, if it finds the doctor's continued practice could endanger the public health. Generally, boards are required to then hold a formal hearing on the case within a specified time period.

Impaired physicians program: a program to rehabilitate physicians suffering from an illness. Impaired physicians programs generally serve alcohol and drug abusers, but they have also been used to aid the mentally or physically ill, as well as habitual sex offenders.

Liability insurer: a company that insures doctors against malpractice lawsuits.

M.D.: the academic degree awarded to U.S. medical doctors, or allopathic physicians.

Medical Board: used generically, any state regulatory agency that licenses and/or disciplines M.D.s. Medical boards may also license other practitioners and health care paraprofessionals.

Osteopath: a physician who graduated from a school of osteopathic medicine. Osteopaths have training in skeletal manipulation in addition to their medical training.

Peer Review Committee: a hospital committee that reviews the quality of care in the institution. The committee may admit physicians to the hospital staff or revoke or limit their privileges.

Peer Review Organization: a state-based group under contract to the federal Medicare program to audit the necessity and quality of Medicare patients' care.

Probation: a disciplinary action or agreement wherein a doctor must abide by certain conditions for a definite or indefinite period of time, or face a more severe penalty. Probationary conditions are generally tailored to the individual.

Reinstatement: issuance of a new medical license to a doctor who previously surrendered his or her license or had it revoked.

Reprimand: a formal letter to a doctor criticizing a particular episode of misconduct or poor care. Sometimes called an admonition or letter of censure.

Restriction: a disciplinary action which limits the type of medicine a doctor may practice. For instance, a doctor's license may be restricted to prevent him or her from practicing surgery, or to limit practice to a certain clinic.

Revocation: the cancellation of a doctor's state or DEA license. State laws regarding revocations vary. In some states, revocations are permanent; in others, doctors may reapply for a new license immediately; in others, doctors must wait for a certain time period before reapplying.

Sanction: a formal disciplinary action.

Schedule I: controlled substances such as marijuana and heroin, which are usually held to have no approved medical purpose.

Schedule II: controlled substances with approved medical uses, but with high potential for addiction or abuse. This category includes raw opium, codeine, amphetamines, and some barbiturates.

Schedule III: controlled substances whose use may lead to low-moderate physical dependence or high psychological dependence and are therefore considered to have some potential for abuse. This category includes many barbiturates and other depressant drugs, and narcotics which include moderate amounts of codeine.

Schedule IV: controlled substances whose use may lead to limited physical and psychological dependence. This category includes Valium, Xanax, and other benzodiazepine tranquilizers, sleeping pills such as Halcion and anorectic stimulants, which are frequently used for weight loss.

Schedule V: controlled substances whose abuse potential is low. This category includes many non-prescription narcotic antidiarrheal drugs and cough suppressants.

Scheduled drugs: see Controlled Substances.

Serious disciplinary actions: Public Citizen's term for revocations, suspensions, surrenders, and probations, as they are reported by the Federation of State Medical Boards.

Serious disciplinary action rate: the number of revocations, suspensions, surrenders and probations per 1,000 M.D.s practicing in a state.

Summary suspension: see emergency suspension.

Surrender: a voluntary agreement by a doctor to give up his or her license to practice. Some surrender agreements permit a doctor to reapply for a new license; others are permanent.

State medical society: a local trade association of physicians. It serves no governmental function.

Stay: a stayed disciplinary action is like a suspended sentence: it does not take effect unless the doctor who has been disciplined disobeys the board or commits some further offense.

Suspension: the temporary removal of a doctor from practice. Some suspensions run for a definite period of time; others are indefinite, and a doctor must apply for the suspension to be lifted.

Triplicate prescription program: a program, now in effect in nine states, that requires copies of prescriptions for certain scheduled drugs to be sent to the state regulatory authority. Intended to prevent drug dealing and overprescribing of drugs that can easily be abused.

Appendix 2
How We Compiled This Report

Sources of Information

In the fall of 1989, using a list published by the Federation of State Medical Boards, Public Citizen contacted all the medical boards from the 50 states and the District of Columbia and requested the name of every physician the boards had disciplined since the beginning of 1985. We also asked at that time to be placed on the boards' mailing lists to receive notification of future disciplinary orders. Since that initial request, Public Citizen has periodically contacted these boards to obtain additional information on disciplinary actions. Most recently, we sent a letter to each state in March 2000 requesting updated information for this edition of *Questionable Doctors.*

This edition reflects disciplinary actions taken against doctors from all 50 states, the District of Columbia, the U.S. Department of Health and Human Services, the Drug Enforcement Administration, and the Food and Drug Administration. The extent of information each medical board provides regarding disciplinary actions varies by state; some boards enclose a detailed synopsis of the case history and findings, whereas others simply supply the physician's name and resulting action within a quarterly newsletter. A description of the information we received from each state is included in the "State by State Listing" section of this report

The time period reflected in this edition of *Questionable Doctors* spans from 1990 through 1999. Public Citizen made every effort to include information from every state for each of these years, but due to either periodic board inactivity or inoperation, data was not always available. The cutoff date for receipt of disciplinary materials in this report was January 31, 2000. Although the earliest editions of *Questionable Doctors* included disciplinary actions against dentists, chiropractors, and podiatrists if the state Board provided that information, because we did not consistently receive information on such health care providers from all medical boards, we decided to eliminate these entries on such professionals from our database.

Public Citizen obtained from the Inspector General's office of the U.S. Department of Health and Human Services a list of all health care providers excluded from the Medicare program for disciplinary purposes through December 1999. The list is called the

Medicare/Medicaid Sanction--Reinstatement Report. It includes the doctor's name, degree and/or specialty, address, date of the sanction notice, period of exclusion from the program, and section of the Social Security Act violated. We included all physicians (both M.D.s and D.O.s) listed in these reports in our database. Previously, from January 1990 through October 1990, the Inspector General's office also provided Public Citizen with copies of the notices of all sanctions, both fines and exclusions, imposed by the Department of Health and Human Services as a result of recommendations from Medicare Peer Review Organizations (PROs), which may sanction doctors for substandard or unnecessary care. The sanction notices included the physician's name, address, the PRO that recommended disciplinary action, the number of cases of substandard or unnecessary care for which the doctor was cited, sometimes the Department's findings about that care, the type of disciplinary action being taken, the length of an exclusion or the amount of a fine, and any information on appeals then available.

Public Citizen obtained from the *Federal Register* notices about doctors whose Drug Enforcement Administration registrations to prescribe controlled substances were revoked, restricted or denied following contested cases dated from 1990 through 1999. The *Federal Register* notices include the doctor's name, address, and DEA certificate number, a description of the conduct that led to the agency's action, the type of action taken, and the effective date. *20,125 Questionable Doctors* also includes most of the physicians who did not contest the DEA's decision and agreed to surrender or restrict their prescribing privilege. This information was obtained directly from the DEA.

From the Food and Drug Administration, Public Citizen obtained information on physicians who were sanctioned because they had violated FDA laws, regulations, or policies regarding clinical research on patients or were convicted of a crime regarding their contract. These physicians are ineligible to receive investigational products for research purposes. Our database includes actions taken through December 1999.

Generating the Database

From the information received from the states, the Drug Enforcement Administration, the Food and Drug Administration, and the Department of Health and Human Services, we created database entries on individual practitioners. Each entry included (when available) the doctor's full name, degree, license number, date of birth, and location (street address, city and state), the disciplinary state or agency, and the date of the disciplinary action. When it was unclear whether a physician was an M.D. or D.O., we listed the physician's degree as "DR".

We included up to two types of disciplinary actions taken on a given action date, and one violation or offense that served as the basis for that action (see below). Any additional actions were described in the "Notes" heading of items on individual doctors. Details and information on appeals, when available, are also included in this section. Information regarding appeals was not generally available, and hence it is possible that some doctors have had their sanctions stayed or overturned on appeal. Public Citizen made a special effort to obtain information on court actions/decisions that overrule or change previous disciplinary actions taken by state boards. In March 2000, we sent a letter to all boards requesting this information. Not all boards were able to fulfill this request, but of the information received, any actions that were overturned by the courts on appeal or for which litigation in the matter had ended in the physician's favor were deleted from the database.

Each disciplinary action was classified into one of 27 categories. For each disciplinary order, we chose what we viewed as the two most "severe" actions. These were included under the heading "Disciplinary Action:" on the individual doctor listings.

Following is a listing of our categories of disciplinary actions, in order of "severity."

* license revocation
* surrender of license
* nonrenewal of license
* revocation of license to prescribe controlled substances
* surrender of license to prescribe controlled substances
* nonrenewal of license to prescribe controlled substances
* denial of new license
* denial of license reinstatement (following surrender or revocation)
* license reinstatement (following surrender or revocation)
* license suspension
* suspension of authority to prescribe controlled substances
* emergency suspension (pending a formal disciplinary hearing)
* probation
* controlled substance license placed on probation
* fine
* restriction placed on license to practice
* restriction placed on license to prescribe controlled substances

* public reprimand
* required to take additional medical education
* required to enter an impaired physician program or substance abuse treatment
* required to enter an impaired physician program or treatment
* cease and desist order
* monitoring of physician performance
* community service

Medicare program sanctions and actions taken against physicians by the Food and Drug Administration were classified in the following three categories respectively:

* exclusion from the Medicare program
* investigator ineligible to receive investigational new drugs for experimental purposes
* debarment from the FDA's contract program

We placed any further details about disciplinary actions under the heading "Notes." Any disciplinary actions that do not fall into the above categories are detailed in the notes sections and classified as "Other Actions" in our charts and statistical summaries.

When a state provided information on the legal violation or offense that led them to discipline a doctor, we classified that violation into one of 18 categories. If several violations were listed by the Board, we chose the one that appeared to contribute the most to the disciplinary decision. If that choice was unclear, we selected the offense that ranked highest on our hierarchy of offenses as listed below. We included the violation under the heading "Offense" in the listings of individual doctors.

Following are the lists of our categories of offenses, and definitions as needed, in order of presumed importance:

* disciplinary action by another state or agency
* criminal conviction or plea of guilty, nolo contendere, or no contest to a crime
* practicing without a valid license
* practicing without a valid controlled substance license
* loss or restriction of hospital privileges
* failure to comply with a previous board order
* providing false information to the medical board or other health agency
* substandard care, incompetence or negligence
* sexual abuse of or sexual misconduct with a patient
* substance abuse

* overprescribing or misprescribing drugs
* physical or mental illness inhibiting the ability to practice with skill and safety
* insurance, Medicare or Medicaid fraud
* falsifying or altering patient records or medical reports
* overcharging
* exceeding professional limitations
* professional misconduct (see below)
* failure to comply with a professional rule (see below)

The category "professional misconduct" includes a variety of offenses that are more serious than the violation of a professional rule but do not fit into any of the other categories listed above. Some examples of offenses classified as professional misconduct are:

* "unprofessional conduct"
* a criminal offense of which the physician has not been actually convicted
* ordering or performing unnecessary or inappropriate procedures for a patient deliberately, rather than because of incompetence
* failing to supervise a physician's assistant, or other non-medical personnel
* permitting an unlicensed person to practice medicine
* tax violations
* intimidating a patient in an attempt to convince them not to seek a second opinion
* terminating a patient's medical care without transferring the patient to another's care
* abandonment of a patient
* making fraudulent representations in medical practice
* assuring a cure for an incurable disease
* offering to treat by a "secret method"
* accepting payments from laboratories for sending them patients' tests
* procuring a criminal abortion
* performing medical services that the board has declared to be of no value (frequently chelation therapy)
* soliciting patients in a deceitful manner
* disruption of residency program
* improperly transferring a patient from a treatment center to a hospital
* engaging in lewd conduct
* clearly excessive use of diagnostic procedures

* unlawful possession of a controlled substance outside the practice of medicine
* fraud in medical research
* operating an illegal drug lab
* unspecified perjury
* diversion of drugs (not specifically prescription drugs) or drug use
* presigning blank prescription pads so that an unlicensed person may practice medicine
* breaching physician-patient confidentiality
* charging for services as supervising physician even though not present during the course of treatment
* selling drugs and devices for financial gain
* sending out letters to request payment using an attorney's name without the attorney's knowledge or consent
* use of disposable syringes on multiple patients
* rendering a psychiatric evaluation without properly examining and treating the subject of said evaluation
* sexual abuse of a person other than a patient, or of an unspecified person
* not getting a consent form signed
* failing to provide information on license applications, renewals, etc., rather than actually giving false information
* unspecified malpractice settlement
* patient abuse

Examples of the types of violations included in the category "Failure to comply with a professional rule" are:

* violation of restrictions on advertising
* failure to respond to the board
* failure to maintain sanitary practice conditions
* violation of medical records laws (except for falsifying records) including failure to provide copies of records when requested or excessive charges for providing records
* requiring patients to purchase drugs or devices from physician
* failure to keep required documents on file
* employing an agent to solicit patients
* making excessive claims of expertise
* violating AMA ethics standards

* failure to report a disciplinary action in another state
* failure to report child abuse
* failure to pay fees
* failure to display a valid license
* endorsing a product
* keeping outdated or misbranded drugs
* failure to keep proper controlled substance records
* failure to report other medical personnel who are violating the Medical Practice Act to the medical board
* fee-splitting
* failure to report a suspicious death to the police
* failure to meet continuing medical education requirements
* allowing someone not in the doctor's employ and not under direct supervision to demonstrate a medical device to patients
* two-tiered billing
* failure to have liability insurance
* practicing under a name other than the one on his or her physician's license
* violating patient dumping regulations
* nonpayment of student loan

Counting Physicians and Actions

Counting physicians: It is impossible for us to know exactly how many physicians are in our database. There are two main reasons for this:

Many states are not consistent in how they list the names of physicians who have been disciplined, i.e. they may have reported only a first and last name in one newsletter, but included a middle initial and suffix (such as Jr. or Sr.) in another. We made numerous phone calls to try and resolve questions about multiple actions taken against what appeared to be a single physician by a single state and in some cases made calls regarding multiple actions taken against what appeared to be the same person by different states. We also used board web sites to try and verify middle initials, license numbers, etc. These attempts were not always successful.

Many states do not include license numbers or birth dates in their listings of disciplined doctors, which can quickly clarify situations in which names appear similar but are not exactly alike.

After entering the corrected information obtained through phone calls, we counted all the physicians in the database. This is done by using a computer program that compared physician identifying information. The program used six database fields to "match" entries: last name, first name, middle name, the suffix (Jr., Sr., etc.), license number, and birth date. It compared two entries with the same first and last name and "matched" them if one or more of the following was true:

* they had the same birth date;
* they were sanctioned by the same state and had the same license number;
* a middle name in one matched the middle name in the other;
* a middle name in one matched the middle initial in the other; or
* a suffix in one matched the suffix in the other.

Entries within the same state with the same first and last name were not matched if they had differing birth dates or license numbers. When one record included a middle name and the other did not, the records were not considered a match unless the birth dates or license numbers matched. The same is true if one record had a suffix (Jr., Sr., etc.) and another did not.

Counting actions: Although each sanction may consist of several disciplinary actions, we entered only the two most serious disciplinary actions in each case. Both of these disciplinary actions were included when generating counts of actions taken by the state boards or federal agencies. Because we calculated only the two most serious actions, the counts of the less serious actions (such as fines, restrictions, education, and monitoring) will not reveal the frequency with which these less serious actions were imposed. Rather, they will only demonstrate how often these actions were among the two most serious actions levied.

Generation of the State-by-State Lists

In the "Disciplinary Actions" sections of each state listing, we attempted to include all doctors who had any connection with the state. For example, the New York "Disciplinary Actions" section includes:

* All disciplinary actions taken by the New York State Board of Regents;
* All disciplinary actions by other states, the Drug Enforcement Administration, the Food and Drug Administration or Medicare/Medicaid against doctors for whom a New York state address is given;

* All other disciplinary actions against doctors with names like those included above, i.e., actions taken by another state or agency that the computer program described above "matched" to doctors disciplined by New York or located in New York.

Any time a doctor's license number is listed in an action, it is the license number of the state that is sanctioning the doctor.

Some state listings may include doctors with similar names who are not, in fact, the same doctor.

When we were informed by state medical boards or other sources that a physician listed in the book had died, we deleted all records for the deceased doctor from the database. Using the matching program we ensured that all records that matched to the physician's identifying information were also deleted.

Although we have made every effort to match physicians' names correctly, some materials we received did not include complete information on middle names, license numbers, or birth dates. Therefore, consumers should remember that non-disciplined physicians and physicians with different disciplinary actions may have similar names to those physicians listed in the state listing of disciplinary actions. Consumers should also remember that if they want the most current information on the status of a physician's license, they should contact the medical board of the state in which the physician practices or has practiced in the past.

Appeals, Reinstatements

While we attempted to acquire as much up-to-date information as possible on doctors whose disciplinary actions have been appealed to and/or overturned by the courts, we do not have information on all appellate actions. Therefore, we cannot guarantee that a doctor listed here as being disciplined has not had that action overturned or stayed by a court. We entered into our database all disciplinary actions we received by January 31, 2000 and all reinstatements to an unrestricted license and court appeals we received by May 31, 2000. Again, the medical board should be contacted for more detailed and up-to-date information.

Some states did not supply us with information on license reinstatements or the lifting of license restrictions. We cannot guarantee that a physician listed as being suspended or restricted has not had that suspension or restriction lifted, or that a physician whose license was revoked has not obtained a new license.

Charts, Tables, Statistics

This report uses data on disciplinary actions from two general sources: Public Citizen's analysis of information on disciplinary actions provided by each state; and, the 1999 statistical summaries of state serious disciplinary actions released by the Federation of State Medical Boards. This latter source is only used to generate Tables A and B (pgs. 14 and 16) in the national and regional reports.

These two data sources are not always comparable. States may not have published or sent Public Citizen all the disciplinary actions they counted in their statistical summaries or reported to the Federation of State Medical Boards. Furthermore, our categorization of disciplinary actions may differ from the Federation's.

In our rankings of the numbers of serious state disciplinary actions, we use the Federation statistics because they are the only statistics that are relatively uniform from state to state. However, the Federation is dependent on the states to supply it with disciplinary information, and the types of actions reported may be different from state to state. This may lead to inconsistencies in the rankings. In this report we have ranked states based on the total number of serious disciplinary actions reported to the Federation in 1999 (see Table A, pg. 14) and, in Table B, pg. 16, show the rankings of states for the past nine years as far as the rate of serious disciplinary actions per 1,000 physicians.

For the tables summarizing the disciplinary actions taken by a state over a period of several years, we used our own method of counting only those actions in our database. Therefore, the numbers in these tables may look different from the numbers the Federation has released.

Appendix 3
Addresses of Federal Agencies

Drug Enforcement Administration (DEA)

Drug Enforcement Administration
U.S. Department of Justice
1405 I Street, NW
Washington, D.C. 20005

For questions regarding Physician Registration of the Controlled Substances Act (CSA):

Drug Enforcement Administration

Office of Diversion Control
600 Army Navy Drive
Arlington, VA 22202

Information Services Section (CPI)
700 Army Navy Drive
Arlington, VA 22202

U.S. Department of Health and Human Services

Use these addresses and phone numbers for information on the Medicare/Medicaid sanctions program:

June Gibbs Brown
Inspector General
Department of Health and Human Services
330 Independence Ave. SW
Room 5246 Cohen Bldg.
Washington, DC 20201
(202) 619-3148

Judy Holtz
Public Affairs Office
Office of Inspector General
Department of Health and Human Services
330 Independence Ave. SW
Room 5246 Cohen Building
Washington DC 20201
(202) 619-1343

To get a current list of those sanctioned, contact:

William M. Libercci
Deputy Director
Health Care Administrative Sanctions
Office of Investigations
Office of Inspector General
Department of Health and Human Services
Room N2-01-26
7500 Security Boulevard
Baltimore MD 21244-1850
(410) 786-9603

Use these numbers and addresses to file complaints about health care providers with the Medicare sanctions program:

Nationwide, 24-hour complaints hotline
Toll free 1-800-447-8477

Region I - Boston
(Connecticut, Maine, Massachusetts, New Hampshire, Rhode Island, Vermont,)
Regional Inspector General
Room 2425, JFK Federal Bldg.
Boston, MA 02203
(617) 565-2689

Region II - New York
(New York, New Jersey, Puerto Rico, Virgin Islands)
Regional Inspector General
Room 3900B, Federal Bldg.
26 Federal Plaza
New York, NY 10278
(212) 264-1691

Region III - Philadelphia
(Pennsylvania, Delaware, Maryland, Virginia, West Virginia, District of Columbia)
Regional Inspector General
P.O. Box 13716
Mailstop #9
Philadelphia, PA 19101
(215) 861-4587

Region IV - Atlanta
(Alabama, Florida, Georgia, Kentucky, Mississippi, North Carolina, South Carolina, Tennessee)
Regional Inspector General
Atlanta Federal Center
61 Forsyth Street, SW
Suite 5T18
Atlanta, GA 30303-8909
(404) 562-7603

Region V - Chicago
(Illinois, Indiana, Michigan, Minnesota, Ohio, Wisconsin)
Regional Inspector General
233 North Michigan, Suite 1330
Chicago, IL 60601
(312) 353-2740

Region VI - Dallas
(Arkansas, Louisiana, Montana, New Mexico, Oklahoma, Texas)
Regional Inspector General
Room 6B-13, Federal Bldg.
1100 Commerce Street
Dallas, TX 75242
(214) 767-8406

Region VII - Kansas City
(Kansas, Nebraska, Missouri, Iowa)
Regional Inspector General
Room 284B Richard Bolling Federal Bldg.
601 E. 12th Street
Kansas City, MO 64106
(816) 426-5959

Region VIII - Denver
(Colorado, Montana, North Dakota, South Dakota, Utah, Wyoming)
Division of Health Standards and Quality
Federal Building 1961 Stout Street
Denver, CO 80294
(303) 844-2121

Region IX - San Francisco
(Arizona, California, Hawaii, Nevada, Guam, American Samoa)
Regional Inspector General
DHHS, OIG, OI
Room 174, Federal Office Bldg.
50 United Nations Plaza
San Francisco, CA 94102
(415) 437-7961

Region X - Seattle
Regional Inspector General
(Alaska, Washington, Oregon, Idaho)
2201 Sixth Avenue, MS/RX-40
Seattle, WA 98121-2500
(206) 615-2306

References

1. Public Citizen's Health Research Group. A Consumer's Directory of Prince George's County Doctors 1974.

2. Public Health Service, Department of Health and Human Services. National Practitioner Data Bank for Adverse Information on Physicians and Other Health Care Providers. 45 CFR Part 60, *Federal Register*, October 17, 1989.

3. The Health Care Quality Improvement Act of 1986. *New Jersey Medicine* June 1987;84 (6): 401-403.

4. Iglehart John K. Congress Moves to Bolster Peer Review: The Health Care Quality Improvement Act of 1986. *New England Journal of Medicine* 1987;316 (15):960-964.

5. Office of Technology Assessment. The Quality of Medical Care: Information for Consumers. OTA-H-386. Washington, DC: U.S. Government Printing Office June 1988.

6. Federation of State Medical Boards. Exchange. Section 3: Physician Licensing Boards and Physician Discipline 1989/1990 edition.

Federation of State Medical Boards. Exchange. Section 3: Physician Licensing Boards and Physician Discipline 1988 edition.

7. Title II of the Social Security Act in Compilation of Social Security Laws including Social Security Act as amended and related enactments through January 1, 1989, Vol. 1, U.S. Government Printing Office 1989.

8. Health Resources and Services Administration. National Practitioner Data Bank Statistical Summary, As of Month Ending December 31, 1997.

9. Office of the Inspector General, Department of Health and Human Services. Hospital Reporting to the National Practitioner Data Bank. OEI-01-94-00050 February 1995.

10. Quality-of-Care Data Bank for Patients Coming Soon. *Internal Medicine News* April 15-30, 1989; 22 (8):9.

11. *Dent v. West Virginia*, 127 U.S. 114 (1889); see also *Klafter v. State Board of Examiners of Architects*, 259 Ill. 15, 102 N.E. 193 (1913); *In re Polk License Revocation*, 90 N.J. 550, 449 A.2nd 7 (1982).

12. Office of Evaluation and Inspections, Office of the Inspector General, U.S. Department of Health and Human Services. State Medical Boards and Medical Discipline, draft report April 1990.

13. McAuley R.G. Letter to the Editor, *New England Journal of Medicine* August 8, 1985.

14. Kusserow Richard, Inspector General, U.S. Department of Health and Human Services. Testimony before the U.S. House of Representatives Committee on Small Business, Subcommittee on Regulation, Business Opportunities and Energy June 8, 1990.

15. Federation of State Medical Boards. 1999 Summary of Board Actions Reported by State Licensing and Disciplinary Boards April 2000.

16. To Err is Human: Institute of Medicine, Washington, D.C., 1999.

17. Harvard Medical Practice Study Group. Patients, Doctors and Lawyers: Medical Injury, Malpractice Litigation and Patient Compensation in New York 1990.

18. Mills, D.H. ed. California Medical Association and California Hospital Association Report on the Medical Insurance Feasibility Study. San Francisco: Sutter Publications 1977.

19. *Journal of Legal Medicine* February 1976.

20. Ely John W, Levinson Wendy, Elder Nancy C, Mainous Arch G III, Vinson Daniel C. Perceived Causes of Family Physicians' Errors. *The Journal of Family Practice* 1995;40(4):337-344.

21. Bissonette Raymond, O'Shea Robert M, Horwitz Mary, Route Cynde F. A Data-Generated Basis for Medical Ethics Education: Categorizing Issues Experienced by Students During Clinical Training. *Academic Medicine* 1995;70(11):1035-1037.

22. Feinstein Alvan R. System, Supervision, Standards, and the 'Epidemic' of Negligent Medical Errors. *Archives of Internal Medicine* 1997;157:1285-1289.

23. Pichert James W, Hickson Gerald B, Bledsoe Sandy, Trotter Tinsla, Quinn Doris. Understanding the Etiology of Serious Medical Events Involving Children: Implications for Pediatricians and Their Risk Managers. *Pediatric Annal* 1997;26(3):160-172.

24. Butters Janice M, Strope John L. Legal Standards of Conduct for Students and Residents: Implications for Health Profession Educators. *Academic Medicine* 1996;1(6):583-590.

25. Schwartz William B, Mendelson Daniel N. The Role of Physician-Owned Insurance Companies in the Detection and Deterrence of Negligence. *Journal of the American Medical Association* 1989;260(10):1342-1346.

26. McNamara Robert M, Margulies Jeffrey L. Chemical Dependency in Emergency Medicine Residency Programs: Perspective of the Program Directors. *Annals of Emergency Medicine* 1994;23(5):1072-1076.

27. Hyde Gordon L, Wolfe James. Alcohol and Drug Use by Surgery Residents. *Journal of the American College of Surgeons* 1995;181(1):1-5.

28. McNamara, op. cit.

29. Hyde, op. cit.

30. Hughes Patrick H, Brandenburg Nancy, Baldwin DeWitt C Jr, Storr Carla L, Williams Kristine M, Anthony James C, Sheehan David V. Prevalence of Substance Use Among US Physicians. *Journal of the American Medical Association* 1992;267(17):2333-2339.

31. Smith DE, Seymour R. A Clinical Approach to the Impaired Health Professional. *The International Journal of the Addictions* 1985;20(5):713-722, as cited in Centrella Michael. Physician Addiction and Impairment--Current Thinking: A Review. *Journal of Addictive Diseases* 1994;13:91-105.

32. Hughes, op. cit.

33. Gartrell N, Herman J, Olarte S, Feldsteing M, Localio R. Prevalence of Psychiatrist-Patient Sexual Contact. Sexual Exploitation in Professional Relationships. Washington, DC: American Psychiatric Press 1989:3-13, as cited in Garfinkel Paul E, Bagby RM, Waring EM, and Dorian Barbara. Boundary Violations and Personality Traits among Psychiatrists. *Canadian Journal of Psychiatry* 1997;42:758-763.

34. Kardener SH, Fuller M, Mensh IN. A Survey of Physician's Attitudes and Practices Regarding Erotic and Nonerotic Contact with Patients. *American Journal of Psychiatry* 1973;139:1077-81, as cited in Garfinkel, op. cit.

35. Garfinkel, op. cit.

36. Enbom John A, Thomas Claire D. Evaluation of Sexual Misconduct Complaints: The Oregon Board of Medical Examiners, 1991 to 1995. *American Journal of Obstetrics and Gynecology* 1997;176(6):1340-1348.

37. American Association of Retired Persons. Effective Physician Oversight: Prescription for Medical Licensing Board Reform 1987.

38. Lohr Kathleen N, Schroeder Steven A, Institute of Medicine. A Strategy for Quality Assurance in Medicare. *New England Journal of Medicine* 1990;322(10):707-712.

39. Federation Receives Federal Contract to Develop Self-Assessment Instrument for State Medical Boards. *FSMB Newsletter* September 1990;36.

40. Lohr, op. cit.

41. Federation of State Medical Boards. Elements of a Modern State Medical Board: A Proposal August 1989.

42. Office of Evaluation and Inspections, Office of the Inspector General, U.S. Department of Health and Human Services. State Medical Boards and Medical Discipline August 1990:9.

43. Federation of State Medical Boards August 1989, op. cit.

OKLAHOMA

1999 serious action rate: 5.95/1000

1999 ranking: 5th

The Oklahoma State Board of Medical Licensing and Supervision sent board orders from 1991 through 1999. These include the physician's name, degree, license number, date and type of action taken, the reason for the action, and the address (in some cases). They also include modifications and terminations of board actions, but not court decisions affecting board actions. Oklahoma informed us no such actions had taken place.

The Oklahoma Board of Osteopathic Examiners sent listings of board orders from 1990 through 1999. They include the physician's name, degree, license number, date and type of action taken and the reason for the action. They also include modifications and terminations of board actions but contain no information on court decisions affecting board actions.

The information provided covers disciplinary actions taken against allopathic physicians (MDs) and osteopathic physicians (DOs).

Besides disciplinary actions taken by the State Medical Boards, this listing also includes actions taken by the Medicare/Medicaid programs, the FDA, and the DEA against physicians located in this state. Disciplinary actions taken by other states against physicians located in Oklahoma or that match a physician disciplined by Oklahoma (see Appendix 2 for an explanation of the matching protocol) are also included.

Although we have made every effort to match physicians' names correctly, some materials we received did not include complete information on middle names, license numbers, birth dates or addresses. Therefore, consumers should remember that non-disciplined physicians and physicians with different disciplinary actions may have similar names to those disciplined physicians listed in this state. Consumers should also remember that if they want the most current information on the status on a physician's license, they should contact the medical board of the state in which the physician practices or had practiced. (See board address below.) Internet address: *http://www.osbmls.state.ok.us/*. This state has a web site which we have graded D on a scale of A (best) to X (worst). This is a measure of the completeness of the information on disciplined doctors. Internet address (Osteopathic Board): *http://www.docboard.org/ok/ok-htm.* We did not rate osteopathic boards in our survey. Those state licensing boards with web sites make independent choices about the type of information to be included on their site and how often it is updated.

According to the Federation of State Medical Boards, Oklahoma took 37 serious disciplinary actions against MDs in 1999. Compared to the 6,216 MDs licensed in the state, Oklahoma had a serious disciplinary action rate of 5.95 serious actions per 1,000 MDs and a ranking of 5th on that list (see Table A, Findings, pg. 14).

The tables below summarize the data Public Citizen received from Oklahoma.

Table 1. Disciplinary Actions Against MDs and DOs 1990 through 1999*

Action	Number	Percent**
Revocation	47	7.9%
Surrender	29	4.9%
Suspension	62	10.5%
Probation	185	31.3%
Practice Restriction	65	11.0%
Action Taken Against Controlled Substance License	40	6.8%
Other Actions	164	27.7%
Total Actions	**592**	**100.0%**

* This table lists only the two most serious disciplinary actions taken against a physician.
** Percentages may not total 100% due to rounding.

Table 2. Offenses for which MDs and DOs were Disciplined 1990 through 1999*

Offense	Number	Percent
Criminal Conviction	21	8.2%
Sexual Abuse of or Sexual Misconduct with a Patient	14	5.5%
Substandard Care, Incompetence or Negligence	5	2.0%
Misprescribing or Overprescribing Drugs	33	12.9%
Substance Abuse	56	22.0%
Disciplinary Action Taken Against License by Another State or Agency	41	16.1%
Other Offenses	85	33.3%
Total Records With Offense Listed	**255**	**100.0%**

* Includes only those actions for which an offense was listed and for which we had a corresponding term in our database.

Table 3. Disciplinary Actions Taken for Sexual Abuse of or Sexual Misconduct with a Patient

Action	Number	Percent
Revocation	5	23.8%
Suspension	5	23.8%
Probation	6	28.6%
Other Actions	5	23.8%
Total Actions	**21**	**100.0%**

Table 4. Disciplinary Actions Taken for Criminal Conviction

Action	Number	Percent
Revocation	7	22.6%
Suspension	9	29.0%
Probation	9	29.0%
Other Actions	6	19.4%
Total Actions	**31**	**100.0%**

Table 5. Disciplinary Actions Taken for Misprescribing or Overprescribing Drugs

Action	Number	Percent
Revocation	6	10.7%
Revocation, Surrender, or Suspension of Controlled Substance License	3	5.4%
Suspension	5	8.9%
Emergency Suspension	1	1.8%
Probation	20	35.7%
Restriction of Controlled Substance License	9	16.1%
Education	1	1.8%
Other Actions	11	19.6%
Total Actions	**56**	**100.0%**

Table 6. Disciplinary Actions Taken for Substance Abuse

Action	Number	Percent
Revocation	5	5.1%
Surrender	1	1.0%
Suspension	16	16.2%
Emergency Suspension	3	3.0%
Probation	34	34.3%
Restriction of Controlled Substance License	5	5.1%
Required to Enter an Impaired Physician Program or Substance Abuse Treatment	9	9.1%
Other Actions	26	26.3%
Total Actions	**99**	**100.0%**

If you feel that your doctor has not given you proper medical care or has mistreated you in any way--whether or not he or she is listed in this report--it is important that you let your state medical board know. Even if they do not immediately act on your complaint, it is important that the information be recorded in their files because it is possible that other people may have filed or will file complaints about the same doctor. Send a brief written description of what occurred to the addresses below or call the phone numbers listed for more information on how to file a complaint.

Addresses

Oklahoma State Board of Medical Licensure and Supervision
Carole A. Smith, Executive Director
PO Box 18256
Oklahoma City, OK 73154-0256
(405) 848-6841
Fax: (405) 848-8240

Oklahoma State Board of Osteopathic Examiners
Gary R Clark, Executive Director
4848 N. Lincoln Blvd., Suite 100
Oklahoma City, OK 73105-3321
(405) 528-8625

Listing of Doctors Sanctioned by Offense

Sexual Abuse of or Sexual Misconduct with a Patient

ANKLESARIA, MANEK E
BOTTLES, KURT D
CLEAVER, EDGAR M
DAVIS, MARTIN J
DUBE, PHILIPPE ABEL
ELLIOTT, CHARLES CALEB
FORSYTHE, JOHN T
HAMMOND, MICHAEL W
HARVEY, CHARLES F
HARWELL, PHILLIP R
KING, E KIM
LEE, EDWARD ALLEN
ROBINSON, MALCOLM G
YARBROUGH, ARDRY LANCE

Substandard Care, Incompetence, or Negligence

CONLEY, RICHARD A
CRITTENDON, WILLIAM F
GIBSON, ROBERT W
MASSAD, DALE GLEN
STOUT, HAROLD

Criminal Conviction or Plea of Guilty, Nolo Contendere, or No Contest to a Crime

AMIN, RAJENDRA
BUTT, MICHAEL J
COOKE, FRANCIS WARDELL
CRAMER, LEIGH E
CRASS, DAVID P
ERWIN, JEFFERSON DAVIS
FERGUSON, FREDERIC H
GOODLOE, ROBERT K
LAUGHLIN, SIDNEY C
LERA, THOMAS A
METCALF, JOE DAN
NEVREKAR, LILA V
REYNOLDS, JOE BILLS
SNIDER, GERALD A
SOMVONGSIRI, CHAROEN
TORRES, WILSON
TROMBKA, LAWRENCE HENRY
VEINTIMILLA, JAMES E
WIGGS, WILLIAM G
WILSON, J SCOT
WYLY, MICHAEL

Misprescribing or Overprescribing Drugs

COFFMAN, RICHARD D
COOKE, FRANCIS WARDELL
DICKERSON, CHARLES WAYNE
DUNCAN, KENNETH C
DUNFORD, WILLIAM W
ENGLISH, RONALD H
ENOS, JACK P
GILLIAM, MARY ANN
HANAN, STANLEY SCOTT
HENSON, EDWIN RAY
HERD, PATRICK S
LESLIE, PORTER B
LOERKE, JAMES R
MCDANIEL, JOSEPH C
MURPHY, TERRENCE E
NELSON, ARNOLD G
NGUYEN, THUONG VAN
PATZKOWSKY, PAUL DEAN
PENTECOST, RICHARD L
PICKETT, ROGER L
PORTER, WARREN H
RAMIREZ, MANUEL JOSEPH
REED, GUY D
ROSE, DAVID D
SCHOENDIENST, STEVEN PAUL
SERJEANT, MICHAEL EWART
SNIDER, GERALD A
SPEED, HENRY K
TRENT, DAVID LEE
WILLIAMS, JAMES R
WOOD, BRYAN SCOTT
WOODS, LUANN

Substance Abuse

AVERY, THOMAS A
BAGGETT, LYNN DEAN
BEASON, MICHAEL BRITTON
BREWER, MICHAEL A
CHANDLER, HAROLD MULLINS
CONWAY, JIMMY HAROLD
CORNELIUS, DOUGLAS HUGH
CRAWFORD, MICHAEL K

> Caution: This list is designed to be used only in conjunction with the rest of this book which includes additional information on each physician such as license number, date of action and more complete descriptions of the offenses.

Substance Abuse (cont'd)

DEASON, DEAN A
DIXON, THOMAS A
DORIA, ALBERTO
ERWIN, JEFFERSON DAVIS
FUCCI, JOHN C
GILBERT, JERALD MILTON
GLOMSET, JOHN
GOLDSTEIN, JOSEPH A
GRIGSBY, ORVILLE LEE
GRODE, TIMOTHY W
HASSMANN, GARY CHARLES
HENDERSON, JOSEPH S
HILL, WILLIAM ELLIOTT
HOLT, HUEY THOMAS
HUBBARD, FRANK LEROI
HUSEN, LUVERNE A
JOHNSON, PAUL DAVIS
KILBURY, MERLIN J
KNIGHT, PHILLIP JOSEPH
KOSTIUK, STEFAN A
LINDSEY, PHILLIP HARRIS
LOCKWOOD, RICHARD L
LYNN, MARK R
MAPPES, WILLIAM PATRICK
MILLER, DAVID DOW
MORTON, ROBERT O
MUELLER, LYNDA L
PEAKE, STEPHEN TRAVIS
POLLNOW, ROBERT EDWARD
PRICE, WILLIAM FRANKLIN
RICKETSON, ROBERT
ROBERTSON, LOWELL J
SCOTT, MICHAEL DEAN
STARR, DWIGHT BAILEY
SYNAR, PHIL H
VINSON, BILLY MICHAEL
WATSON, STEVEN E
WHEELER, PAUL E
WILLIAMS, JAMES MICHAEL
YARBOROUGH, WILLIAM H
YOUNG, JAMES A

Caution: This list is designed to be used only in conjunction with the rest of this book which includes additional information on each physician such as license number, date of action and more complete descriptions of the offenses.

AGARWAL, RAVINDRA MD, WAS DISCIPLINED BY OKLAHOMA ON MAY 3, 1990
DISCIPLINARY ACTION: 60-MONTH PROBATION; MONITORING OF PHYSICIAN PERFORMANCE

NOTES: VOLUNTARILY SUBMITS TO JURISDICTION OF THE BOARD AND CHOOSE NOT TO CONTEST THE ALLEGATIONS. PROBATION UNDER THE FOLLOWING TERMS AND CONDITIONS: SHALL NOT PRESCRIBE, ADMINISTER, OR DISPENSE ANY MEDICATIONS FOR HIS PERSONAL USE AND SHALL TAKE NONE UNLESS AUTHORIZED BY ANOTHER PHYSICIAN FOR LEGITIMATE MEDICAL NEED; SHALL ABSTAIN FROM CONSUMING ALCOHOL OR ANY SUBSTANCE, WHICH WOULD ADVERSELY AFFECT HIS ABILITY TO PRACTICE; SHALL SUBMIT BIOLOGICAL FLUID SPECIMENS; SHALL SUBMIT TO THE BOARD ADDRESS/CHANGE OF ADDRESS; SHALL APPEAR BEFORE THE BOARD UPON REQUEST AND SUBMIT ANY REQUIRED REPORTS; SHALL PAY COSTS; SHALL NOTIFY ANY HOSPITAL WHERE HE HOLDS STAFF PRIVILEGES, OR CLINIC, OR GROUPS WHERE HE PRACTICES, OF THE TERMS AND CONDITIONS OF THIS BOARD ORDER AND SUPPLY A COPY THEREOF; SHALL ACTIVELY PARTICIPATE IN SUPPORT PROGRAMS OPERATED THROUGH OR REFERRED BY THE PHYSICIAN RECOVERY COMMITTEE.

AHMAD, WAZIR S MD, LICENSE NUMBER 12461 OF 1216 N SHARTEL AVE #600, OKLAHOMA CITY, OK, WAS DISCIPLINED BY OKLAHOMA ON JUNE 5, 1997
DISCIPLINARY ACTION: REPRIMAND
OFFENSE: PROFESSIONAL MISCONDUCT

NOTES: ENGAGED IN INAPPROPRIATE PERSONAL AND SEXUAL RELATIONSHIPS WITH THREE MOTHERS OF HIS PEDIATRIC PATIENTS WHILE TREATING THEIR CHILDREN. A 9/9/93 RULING IN THE DISTRICT COURT OF OKLAHOMA COUNTY DECLARED HIM TO BE THE FATHER OF A CHILD BORN TO ONE OF THE MOTHERS ON 12/14/91. ON 6/13/96 THE BOARD SERVED HIM WITH A SUBPOENA FOR MEDICAL RECORDS AND HE FAILED TO COOPERATE WITH THE INVESTIGATION OR PROVIDE THE RECORDS.

AKBERZIE, MOHAMMAD EHSAN OF 6102 82ND STREET APT 6, TULSA, OK, WAS DISCIPLINED BY OKLAHOMA ON MARCH 31, 1994
DISCIPLINARY ACTION: DENIAL OF NEW LICENSE

NOTES: MEDICAL SCHOOL EDUCATION WAS 30 YEARS AGO AND FAILED TO PROVIDE EVIDENCE IT WAS EQUIVALENT TO THAT OFFERED AT THE UNIVERSITY OF OKLAHOMA; FORMAL TRAINING WAS 20 YEARS AGO IN PATHOLOGY; FAILED THE FLEX EXAM NINE TIMES BEFORE PASSING IN 6/80; ALL OF WHICH RAISE SERIOUS ISSUES AS TO CLINICAL COMPETENCY.

ALEXANDER, CATHERINE A MD OF 2103 W BRIGGS, NORMAN, OK, WAS DISCIPLINED BY DEA ON MARCH 18, 1999
DISCIPLINARY ACTION: SURRENDER OF CONTROLLED SUBSTANCE LICENSE

NOTES: IN LIEU OF PUBLIC INTEREST REVOCATION.

ALEXANDER, JOE BOB MD, LICENSE NUMBER E0780 OF ABILENE, TX, WAS DISCIPLINED BY TEXAS ON MAY 16, 1998
DISCIPLINARY ACTION: REPRIMAND
OFFENSE: PROFESSIONAL MISCONDUCT

NOTES: AT THE WEIGHT LOSS CLINIC HE OWNS, PROSPECTIVE PATIENTS ARE GIVEN A PAMPHLET PROVIDING INFORMATION ABOUT THE CLINIC AND OFFERING A $5.00 CREDIT ON THE NEXT VISIT UPON THE REFERRAL OF 3 ADDITIONAL PATIENTS, AND A PERMANENT $5.00 DECREASE IN OFFICE CHARGES UPON THE REFERRAL OF 10 NEW PATIENTS; BOARD FOUND THIS CONSTITUTES IMPERMISSIBLE DRUMMING OF PATIENTS; HE STOPPED THIS PRACTICE AFTER BEING INFORMED ABOUT THIS. SHALL COOPERATE WITH THE BOARD IN VERIFYING COMPLIANCE; SHALL GIVE A COPY OF THIS ORDER TO ANY HEALTH CARE ENTITY WHERE HE HAS PRIVILEGES.

ALEXANDER, JOE BOB MD, LICENSE NUMBER 10682 OF 1025 CYPRESS, ABILENE, TX, WAS DISCIPLINED BY OKLAHOMA ON JULY 28, 1999
DISCIPLINARY ACTION: REPRIMAND
OFFENSE: DISCIPLINARY ACTION BY ANOTHER STATE OR AGENCY

NOTES: ON 5/16/98 TEXAS BOARD REPRIMANDED LICENSE FINDING PATIENT SOLICITATION CONSTITUTING IMPERMISSIBLE DRUMMING OF PATIENTS FOR HIS WEIGHT LOSS CLINIC; MAINTAINS HE WAS NOT AWARE OF THE ACT PROHIBITING USE OF DISCOUNTS AND VOLUNTARILY AGREED TO DISCONTINUE THE PRACTICE OF OFFERING DISCOUNTS OF ANY KIND; ALTHOUGH THE LITERATURE IN HIS OFFICE STATES THAT HE WOULD SEE EVERY PATIENT AT EVERY VISIT, THAT PRACTICE DID NOT ALWAYS OCCUR; FAILED TO ADEQUATELY DOCUMENT PATIENT RECORDS. TERMS AND CONDITIONS: SHALL SUBMIT TO HOSPITALS, CLINICS OR OTHER INSTITUTIONS IN WHICH HE HOLDS OR ANTICIPATES HOLDING ANY FORM OF STAFF PRIVILEGE A COPY OF THIS ORDER.

ALLRED, ROBERT L MD, LICENSE NUMBER 0008460, WAS DISCIPLINED BY OKLAHOMA ON MARCH 25, 1995
OFFENSE: LOSS OR RESTRICTION OF HOSPITAL PRIVILEGES

NOTES: RESIGNED FROM THE STAFF OF PRESBYTERIAN HOSPITAL AFTER IT INITIATED A CREDENTIAL REVIEW; ON 1994-1995 RENEWAL APPLICATION SAID HE HAD NOT LOST PRIVILEGES AT ANY HOSPITAL; THE BOARD DETERMINED THAT THE REPORTING REQUIREMENTS FOR LICENSEES OF THE BOARD INCLUDES THE REPORTING OF VOLUNTARY SURRENDER OF PRIVILEGE WHILE A CREDENTIALS INVESTIGATION IS PENDING OR TO AVOID A FORMAL PEER REVIEW ACTION; ALLRED SHALL DO SO IN THE FUTURE; SHALL PAY COSTS.

AMIN, RAJENDRA MD, LICENSE NUMBER 11099, WAS DISCIPLINED BY OKLAHOMA ON JULY 29, 1999
DISCIPLINARY ACTION: LICENSE SUSPENSION
OFFENSE: CRIMINAL CONVICTION OR PLEA OF GUILTY, NOLO CONTENDERE, OR NO CONTEST TO A CRIME

NOTES: ON OR ABOUT 11/19/98 A SECURITY CAMERA AT THE HOSPITAL WHERE HE HAD MEDICAL STAFF PRIVILEGES VIDEO TAPED HIM AS HE STOLE PRESCRIPTION DRUGS FOR HIS PERSONAL USE; ON OR ABOUT 12/11/98 HE WAS CHARGED WITH ONE COUNT OF GRAND LARCENY; ON 5/21/99 PLED NO CONTEST AND ENTERED INTO A PLEA AGREEMENT. LICENSE SUSPENDED INDEFINITELY PENDING COMPLETION OF AN EVALUATION AT MENNINGER'S CLINIC.

AMIN, RAJENDRA MD, LICENSE NUMBER 11099, WAS DISCIPLINED BY OKLAHOMA ON SEPTEMBER 24, 1999
DISCIPLINARY ACTION: 60-MONTH PROBATION; MONITORING OF PHYSICIAN PERFORMANCE

NOTES: TERMS AND CONDITIONS: SHALL SUBMIT TO EVERY STATE IN WHICH HE HOLDS LICENSURE AND TO HOSPITALS, CLINICS OR OTHER INSTITUTIONS IN

WHICH HE HOLDS OR ANTICIPATES HOLDING ANY FORM OF STAFF PRIVILEGE A COPY OF THIS ORDER; SHALL NOT PRESCRIBE, ADMINISTER OR DISPENSE ANY MEDICATIONS FOR HIS PERSONAL USE OR FOR THAT OF ANY FAMILY MEMBER; SHALL OBTAIN TREATMENT FROM A BOARD-APPROVED PSYCHIATRIST FOR NO LESS THAN FIVE YEARS, WITH QUARTERLY REPORTS TO THE BOARD; SHALL KEEP THE BOARD INFORMED OF HIS ADDRESS AND PAY COSTS; SHALL APPEAR BEFORE THE BOARD UPON REQUEST.

ANDERSON, LANNY G MD, LICENSE NUMBER 0007810 OF 3435 NW 56 #210, OKLAHOMA CITY, OK, WAS DISCIPLINED BY OKLAHOMA ON JUNE 21, 1990
DISCIPLINARY ACTION: LICENSE SUSPENSION; REQUIRED TO ENTER AN IMPAIRED PHYSICIAN PROGRAM OR TREATMENT

NOTES: SUSPENSION UNTIL HE COMPLETES IN-PATIENT TREATMENT.

ANDERSON, LANNY G MD, LICENSE NUMBER 0007810 OF 3435 NW 56 #210, OKLAHOMA CITY, OK, WAS DISCIPLINED BY OKLAHOMA ON SEPTEMBER 13, 1990
DISCIPLINARY ACTION: 60-MONTH PROBATION; REQUIRED TO ENTER AN IMPAIRED PHYSICIAN PROGRAM OR SUBSTANCE ABUSE TREATMENT

NOTES: SUCCESSFULLY COMPLETED IN-PATIENT TREATMENT AT TALBOTT CENTER, GEORGIA. LICENSE REINSTATED FROM 06/08/90 SUSPENSION AND PUT ON PROBATION WITH FOLLOWING TERMS AND CONDITIONS: SHALL NOT PRESCRIBE, ADMINISTER OR DISPENSE ANY MEDICATIONS FOR HIS PERSONAL USE; SHALL TAKE NO MEDICATION EXCEPT THAT AUTHORIZED BY A PHYSICIAN TREATING HIM FOR A LEGITIMATE MEDICAL NEED; SHALL ABSTAIN FROM CONSUMING ALCOHOL OR ANY SUBSTANCE, WHICH WOULD ADVERSELY AFFECT HIS ABILITY TO PRACTICE. SHALL SUBMIT BIOLOGICAL FLUID SPECIMENS FOR ANALYSIS; SHALL NOTIFY ANY HOSPITAL WHERE HE HOLDS STAFF PRIVILEGES, OR CLINIC, OR GROUP OF THE TERMS AND CONDITIONS; SHALL CONTINUE ALL IN-PATIENT AND OUT-PATIENT TREATMENT BY AND THROUGH THE TALBOTT RECOVERY SYSTEM WITH REPORTS TO THE BOARD; SHALL FURNISH BOARD WITH CHANGE OF ADDRESS AND APPEAR BEFORE BOARD WHEN REQUESTED. ON 11/08/91, HE WAS RETAINED ON PROBATION WITH A REDUCTION OF THE LEVEL OF SUPERVISION FROM LEVEL I TO LEVEL II WITH THE SAME PROBATIONARY CONDITIONS AS LISTED ABOVE. ON 07/02/92, MOTION FOR TERMINATION OF PROBATION OVERRULED AND HE IS RETAINED ON PROBATION WITH SAME CONDITIONS AS ORIGINAL PROBATION IN PART BECAUSE OF PENDING CRIMINAL CHARGES. ON 2/17/94, MOTION FOR TERMINATION OF PROBATION DENIED. HE IS STILL UNDER TERMS AND CONDITIONS OF PROBATION.

ANDERSON, LANNY GORDON MD OF 3435 NW 56TH STREET, OKLAHOMA CITY, OK, WAS DISCIPLINED BY DEA ON NOVEMBER 19, 1990
DISCIPLINARY ACTION: SURRENDER OF CONTROLLED SUBSTANCE LICENSE
OFFENSE: OVERPRESCRIBING OR MISPRESCRIBING DRUGS

NOTES: CONTROLLED SUBSTANCE LICENSE SUSPENDED 08/30/90 IN OKLAHOMA CITY FOR 30 DAYS BEGINNING 11/01/90. AFTER THIS, HE MAY REGISTER FOR IN-HOSPITAL USE ONLY UNTIL 09/01/91. PROBATION ORDERED REDUCED FROM LEVEL I TO LEVEL II TO CONTINUE THROUGH 06/95 INCLUDING URINALYSIS AND OUTPATIENT TREATMENT FOR ADDICTION. PLED GUILTY TO FRAUDULENT PRESCRIPTION WRITING; SENTENCED 10/20/92 TO $10,000 FINE AND FOUR YEARS PROBATION.

ANKLESARIA, MANEK E MD, LICENSE NUMBER 0013574 OF 2325 S. HARVARD SUITE 104, TULSA, OK, WAS DISCIPLINED BY OKLAHOMA ON NOVEMBER 23, 1992
DISCIPLINARY ACTION: LICENSE SUSPENSION; REQUIRED TO ENTER AN IMPAIRED PHYSICIAN PROGRAM OR TREATMENT
OFFENSE: SEXUAL ABUSE OF OR SEXUAL MISCONDUCT WITH A PATIENT

NOTES: EXHIBITED INAPPROPRIATE SEXUAL BEHAVIOR WITH TWO OPHTHALMOLOGIC PATIENTS, ONE IN THE FALL OF 1990 AND THE OTHER MAY 6, 1991 INCLUDING SEXUAL COMMENTS, PLACING PATIENTS HAND ON HIS PENIS, AND FONDLING AND KISSING PATIENT. SUSPENSION IN EFFECT UNTIL PRESENTS EVIDENCE OF MEDICAL IN-PATIENT EVALUATION AND SUCCESSFUL COMPLETION OF TREATMENT. ON 5/20/93 SUSPENSION CONTINUED. HE WILL IMMEDIATELY UNDERGO FULL IN-PATIENT EVALUATION AND COMPLETE ANY NECESSARY TREATMENT; WILL NOT REAPPEAR BEFORE THE BOARD AND REQUEST TERMINATION OR MODIFICATION UNLESS HE CAN PROVIDE EVIDENCE OF SUCCESSFUL COMPLETION OF EVALUATION AND ANY NECESSARY TREATMENT AND ASSURANCE TO THE BOARD BY THE TREATMENT PROVIDER THAT HE MAY RETURN SAFELY TO PRACTICE MEDICINE.

ANKLESARIA, MANEK E MD, LICENSE NUMBER 0013574 OF 2325 S HARVARD AVE #104, TULSA, OK, WAS DISCIPLINED BY OKLAHOMA ON OCTOBER 11, 1993
DISCIPLINARY ACTION: 60-MONTH PROBATION; RESTRICTION PLACED ON LICENSE

NOTES: LICENSE REINSTATED FROM 11/21/92 SUSPENSION. CONDITIONS OF PROBATION BEGINNING 10/1/93: SHALL SUBMIT BIOLOGICAL FLUID SPECIMENS; SHALL FULFILL CONDITIONS RECOMMENDED BY SPECIFIED MD AND/OR THE STAFF OF SPECIFIED CENTER; SHALL ALLOW STAFF TO SPEAK WITH BOARD TO VERIFY COMPLIANCE; WHEN EXAMINING ANY FEMALE PATIENT SHALL HAVE A FEMALE MEDICAL PROFESSIONAL PRESENT; SHALL CONTINUE UNDER PSYCHIATRIC CARE WITH BOARD-APPROVED PHYSICIAN; SHALL NOTIFY ANY HEALTH CARE ENTITY WHERE HE HOLDS OR APPLIES FOR STAFF PRIVILEGES OF THE CONDITIONS OF THE ORDER; SHALL FURNISH BOARD WITH ADDRESS AND/OR CHANGE OF ADDRESS; SHALL APPEAR BEFORE THE BOARD UPON REQUEST AND SUBMIT REQUIRED REPORTS; SHALL PAY COSTS. ON 3/31/94 ORDER MODIFIED SUCH THAT BIOLOGICAL FLUID SPECIMENS WERE NO LONGER REQUIRED.

ANKLESARIA, MANEK E MD, LICENSE NUMBER 0141034 OF 2325 SOUTH HARVARD #206, TULSA, OK, WAS DISCIPLINED BY NEW YORK ON JANUARY 7, 1994
DISCIPLINARY ACTION: SURRENDER OF LICENSE
OFFENSE: DISCIPLINARY ACTION BY ANOTHER STATE OR AGENCY

NOTES: FOUND GUILTY OF IMPROPER PRACTICE BY THE OKLAHOMA BOARD.

ANKLESARIA, MANEK EDALJI MD, DATE OF BIRTH APRIL 15, 1949, LICENSE NUMBER 00F2155 OF 2325 SO HARVARD SUITE 104, TULSA, OK, WAS DISCIPLINED BY TEXAS ON APRIL 30, 1993
DISCIPLINARY ACTION: SURRENDER OF LICENSE

NOTES: LICENSE PERMANENTLY CANCELED.

ANKLESARIA, MANEK EDALJI MD, DATE OF BIRTH APRIL 15, 1949, LICENSE NUMBER 0020520 OF TULSA, OK, WAS DISCIPLINED BY NORTH CAROLINA ON DECEMBER 3, 1993
DISCIPLINARY ACTION: SURRENDER OF LICENSE

ANKLESARIA, MANEK EDALJI MD, DATE OF BIRTH APRIL 15, 1949, LICENSE NUMBER 0033882 OF 2325 S. HARVARD AVE., TULSA, OK, WAS DISCIPLINED BY NEW JERSEY ON DECEMBER 28, 1993
DISCIPLINARY ACTION: CEASE AND DESIST ORDER
OFFENSE: DISCIPLINARY ACTION BY ANOTHER STATE OR AGENCY

NOTES: DISCIPLINARY ACTION TAKEN IN OKLAHOMA. SHALL HAVE LEAVE TO SURRENDER HIS LICENSE TO PRACTICE MEDICINE AND SURGERY IN NEW JERSEY WITH PREJUDICE TO SEEKING REINSTATEMENT AT ANY FUTURE DATE.

ANTOINE, EWALD JONATHAN OF 1525 PINE GROVE AVENUE, RICE LAKE, WI, WAS DISCIPLINED BY OKLAHOMA ON OCTOBER 7, 1993
DISCIPLINARY ACTION: DENIAL OF NEW LICENSE
OFFENSE: PROVIDING FALSE INFORMATION TO THE BOARD OR OTHER HEALTH AGENCY

NOTES: FAILED TO ADVISE BOARD OF TWO FAILURES OF THE FLEX EXAM; TOLD THEM HE HAD FAILED ONCE WHEN IN FACT HE HAD FAILED THREE TIMES; FAILED TO PROVIDE BOARD WITH INFORMATION RELATED TO TWO RESIDENCY PROGRAMS HE HAD UNDERTAKEN. ON 12/9/93 BOARD AFFIRMED THIS DENIAL.

ANTONINI, AUDBERTO C MD, DATE OF BIRTH MAY 20, 1956, LICENSE NUMBER 1062716 OF 1611 MONROE, DEARBORN, MI, WAS DISCIPLINED BY MICHIGAN ON MAY 16, 1997
DISCIPLINARY ACTION: FINE; REPRIMAND
OFFENSE: SUBSTANDARD CARE, INCOMPETENCE OR NEGLIGENCE

NOTES: INCOMPETENCE. $250 FINE.

ANTONINI, AUDBERTO CESAR OF PO BOX 673, TALIHINA, OK, WAS DISCIPLINED BY OKLAHOMA ON FEBRUARY 17, 1994
DISCIPLINARY ACTION: DENIAL OF NEW LICENSE

NOTES: FAILED TO PASS THE FLEX EXAM ON THREE OCCASIONS WHICH RAISES SERIOUS ISSUES AS TO CLINICAL COMPETENCY AND FITNESS TO PRACTICE.

AVERY, BERT M MD, LICENSE NUMBER 11216 OF 3617 W. GORE BLVD. #C, LAWTON, OK, WAS DISCIPLINED BY OKLAHOMA ON MAY 15, 1997
DISCIPLINARY ACTION: 60-MONTH PROBATION; RESTRICTION PLACED ON LICENSE

NOTES: CONDITIONS OF PROBATION: SHALL NOT PRESCRIBE, ADMINISTER OR DISPENSE ANY MEDICATIONS FOR HIS PERSONAL USE AND SHALL TAKE NONE UNLESS AUTHORIZED BY ANOTHER PHYSICIAN FOR A LEGITIMATE MEDICAL NEED; SHALL ABSTAIN FROM CONSUMING ALCOHOL OR ANY SUBSTANCE WHICH WOULD ADVERSELY AFFECT HIS ABILITY TO PRACTICE MEDICINE; SHALL SUBMIT BIOLOGICAL FLUID SPECIMENS; SHALL SUBMIT TO HOSPITALS, CLINICS OR OTHER INSTITUTIONS IN WHICH HE HOLDS OR ANTICIPATES HOLDING ANY FORM OF STAFF PRIVILEGE A COPY OF THIS ORDER; SHALL NOT SUPERVISE A PHYSICIAN ASSISTANT; SHALL COMPLY WITH ALL TERMS AND CONDITIONS OF HIS CONTINUING CARE CONTRACT; SHALL KEEP THE BOARD INFORMED OF HIS ADDRESS AND PAY COSTS; SHALL APPEAR BEFORE THE BOARD AND SUBMIT REPORTS UPON REQUEST.

AVERY, BERT M MD, LICENSE NUMBER G44664 OF LAWTON, OK, WAS DISCIPLINED BY CALIFORNIA ON JULY 20, 1998
DISCIPLINARY ACTION: SURRENDER OF LICENSE

NOTES: WHILE CHARGES PENDING.

AVERY, THOMAS A MD, LICENSE NUMBER 0010046, WAS DISCIPLINED BY OKLAHOMA ON MAY 20, 1993
DISCIPLINARY ACTION: 60-MONTH PROBATION; MONITORING OF PHYSICIAN PERFORMANCE
OFFENSE: SUBSTANCE ABUSE

NOTES: PREVIOUS ALCOHOL DEPENDENCE AND RELATED PSYCHOLOGICAL PROBLEMS OF RECURRENT DEPRESSION IN SPITE OF COMPLETION OF INPATIENT TREATMENT. CONDITIONS OF PROBATION: SHALL NOT PRESCRIBE, ADMINISTER OR DISPENSE ANY MEDICATIONS FOR HIS PERSONAL USE; SHALL NOT TAKE ANY MEDICATION UNLESS AUTHORIZED BY TREATING PHYSICIAN; SHALL ABSTAIN FROM CONSUMING ALCOHOL OR ANY SUBSTANCE WHICH WOULD ADVERSELY AFFECT HIS ABILITY TO PRACTICE; SHALL SUBMIT BIOLOGICAL FLUID SPECIMENS; SHALL CONTINUE REGULAR ATTENDANCE AT PHYSICIAN RECOVERY COMMITTEE INCLUDING 90 AA MEETINGS IN 90 DAYS AND PARTICIPATE IN WEEKLY MEETINGS; SHALL FURNISH EVERY STATE WHERE HE HOLDS OR APPLIES FOR LICENSURE OR ANY HOSPITAL WHERE HE MAY HOLD STAFF PRIVILEGES A COPY OF THIS ORDER; SHALL FURNISH BOARD WITH ADDRESS/CHANGE OF ADDRESS; SHALL APPEAR BEFORE THE BOARD UPON REQUEST AND SUBMIT ANY REQUIRED REPORTS; SHALL NOT SUPERVISE A PHYSICIAN'S ASSISTANT; SHALL PAY COSTS.

AVERY, THOMAS A MD, LICENSE NUMBER 0010046, WAS DISCIPLINED BY OKLAHOMA ON OCTOBER 7, 1993
DISCIPLINARY ACTION: EMERGENCY SUSPENSION; REQUIRED TO ENTER AN IMPAIRED PHYSICIAN PROGRAM OR SUBSTANCE ABUSE TREATMENT
OFFENSE: SUBSTANCE ABUSE

NOTES: SUSPENSION IMPERATIVE ON AN EMERGENCY BASIS WHILE HE IS ATTENDING INPATIENT TREATMENT FOR SUBSTANCE ABUSE AND UNTIL A HEARING.

AVERY, THOMAS A MD OF 916 W FARRELL, SHAWNEE, OK, WAS DISCIPLINED BY DEA ON NOVEMBER 1, 1993
DISCIPLINARY ACTION: SURRENDER OF CONTROLLED SUBSTANCE LICENSE
OFFENSE: DISCIPLINARY ACTION BY ANOTHER STATE OR AGENCY

NOTES: MEDICAL BOARD ACTION/SUBSTANCE ABUSE.

AVERY, THOMAS A MD, LICENSE NUMBER 0010046, WAS DISCIPLINED BY OKLAHOMA ON FEBRUARY 17, 1994
DISCIPLINARY ACTION: 6-MONTH LICENSE SUSPENSION; PROBATION
OFFENSE: FAILURE TO COMPLY WITH PREVIOUS BOARD ORDER

NOTES: IN VIOLATION OF PREVIOUS ORDER HE INGESTED ALCOHOL AS SHOWN BY ANALYSIS OF URINE SAMPLE ON 8/25/93. CONDITIONS OF INDEFINITE PROBATION: SHALL NOT PRESCRIBE, ADMINISTER OR DISPENSE ANY MEDICATIONS FOR HIS PERSONAL USE AND WILL TAKE NONE UNLESS AUTHORIZED BY ANOTHER PHYSICIAN FOR LEGITIMATE MEDICAL NEED; SHALL ABSTAIN FROM CONSUMING ALCOHOL OR ANY SUBSTANCE WHICH WOULD ADVERSELY AFFECT HIS ABILITY TO PRACTICE; SHALL SUBMIT BIOLOGICAL FLUID SPECIMENS; SHALL CONTINUE REGULAR ATTENDANCE AT PHYSICIAN RECOVERY COMMITTEE AND SHALL SIGN A RECOVERY CONTRACT INCLUDING

90 AA MEETINGS IN 90 DAYS AND PARTICIPATION IN WEEKLY MEETINGS; SHALL FURNISH EVERY STATE WHERE HE HOLDS OR APPLIES FOR LICENSURE AND ANY HEALTH CARE ENTITY WHERE HE HAS PRIVILEGES A COPY OF THIS ORDER; SHALL FURNISH THE BOARD WITH ADDRESS/CHANGE OF ADDRESS; SHALL APPEAR BEFORE THE BOARD UPON REQUEST AND PROVIDE REQUIRED REPORTS; SHALL NOT SUPERVISE A PHYSICIAN'S ASSISTANT; SHALL PAY COSTS.

AZUBUIKE, KENNETH, WAS DISCIPLINED BY OKLAHOMA ON JULY 22, 1994
DISCIPLINARY ACTION: DENIAL OF NEW LICENSE

NOTES: EVIDENCE REFLECTS HE HAS NOT MADE SIGNIFICANT ATTEMPTS TO COMPLETE REQUIREMENTS FOR LICENSURE DESPITE BEING IN A FELLOWSHIP PROGRAM AND LICENSED AS A SUPERVISED MEDICAL DOCTOR FOR FOUR YEARS WHICH RAISE ISSUES AS TO HIS ABILITY TO PRACTICE WITH REASONABLE SKILL.

BABB, MICHAEL J MD, LICENSE NUMBER 14271, WAS DISCIPLINED BY OKLAHOMA ON MARCH 14, 1997
DISCIPLINARY ACTION: RESTRICTION PLACED ON LICENSE; RESTRICTION PLACED ON CONTROLLED SUBSTANCE LICENSE

NOTES: HE DENIES ALL MATERIAL ALLEGATIONS. FORMAL REPRIMAND; CONDITIONS ON LICENSE FOR THREE YEARS, UNLESS MODIFIED BY THE BOARD: SHALL PRACTICE WITH OVERSIGHT OF HIS MEDICAL PRACTICE; SHALL USE A FEMALE CHAPERONE WITHIN HIS MEDICAL PHYSICAL INTERACTIONS WITH FEMALE PATIENTS; SHALL HAVE REVIEW AND MONITORING OF HIS PRACTICE BY A PEER PHYSICIAN TO ENSURE COMPLIANCE; HE WILL IDENTIFY AND UTILIZE A BOARD APPROVED MENTOR; SHALL ENTER AND CONTINUE IN INDIVIDUAL PSYCHOTHERAPY WITH A BOARD APPROVED THERAPIST FOCUSING ON ETHICS WITHIN THE MEDICAL PROFESSION AND THE DISPARITY OF POWER AND POSITION IN THE PHYSICIAN PATIENT RELATIONSHIP WITH QUARTERLY REPORTS TO THE BOARD; SHALL ENGAGE IN CONTINUING MEDICAL EDUCATION INVOLVING BOUNDARY ISSUES, MEDICAL ETHICS, SIGNS AND SYMPTOMS OF DOMESTIC VIOLENCE AND SEXUAL ABUSE; SHALL NOTIFY HOSPITALS, CLINICS OR OTHER INSTITUTIONS IN WHICH HE HOLDS OR ANTICIPATES HOLDING ANY FORM OF STAFF PRIVILEGE OF THIS ORDER; SHALL KEEP THE BOARD INFORMED OF HIS ADDRESS AND PAY COSTS; SHALL APPEAR BEFORE THE BOARD AND SUBMIT REPORTS UPON REQUEST; SHALL KEEP DUPLICATE SERIALLY NUMBERED PRESCRIPTIONS OF ALL CONTROLLED SUBSTANCES; SHALL COOPERATE WITH THE BOARD IN VERIFYING COMPLIANCE INCLUDING ALLOWING THEM TO SPEAK TO STAFF AND COLLEAGUES.

BADZINSKI, GARY L DO, DATE OF BIRTH JANUARY 21, 1956, LICENSE NUMBER 0031226, WAS DISCIPLINED BY COLORADO ON APRIL 11, 1996
DISCIPLINARY ACTION: 3-MONTH LICENSE SUSPENSION; 60-MONTH PROBATION
OFFENSE: SEXUAL ABUSE OF OR SEXUAL MISCONDUCT WITH A PATIENT

NOTES: SEXUAL CONTACT WITH A PATIENT. 90 DAY PERIOD OF NO MEDICAL PRACTICE. TREATMENT MONITORING AND AN AGREEMENT TO HAVE A CHAPERONE PRESENT FOR ALL FEMALE PATIENTS.

BADZINSKI, GARY L DO, LICENSE NUMBER 0003416, WAS DISCIPLINED BY OKLAHOMA ON SEPTEMBER 19, 1996
DISCIPLINARY ACTION: 60-MONTH PROBATION; RESTRICTION PLACED ON LICENSE

NOTES: LICENSE GRANTED. SHALL SUBMIT TO THE OKLAHOMA BOARD DOCUMENTATION VERIFYING HIS SUCCESSFUL COMPLETION OF A PROGRAM ON BOUNDARY AND MEDICAL ETHICS ISSUES APPROVED BY THE COLORADO PHYSICIAN'S HEALTH PROGRAM (CPHP) AS REQUIRED BY THE COLORADO BOARD. SHALL RECEIVE SUCH MEDICAL TREATMENT, PARTICULARLY PERSONAL PSYCHOTHERAPY, AS IS DETERMINED TO BE APPROPRIATE BY CPHP; ALL TREATMENT RECOMMENDATIONS BY CPHP SHALL CONSTITUTE TERMS OF THIS ORDER; CPHP SHALL SUBMIT QUARTERLY WRITTEN REPORTS TO THE BOARD WHICH SHALL BRIEFLY DESCRIBE HIS TREATMENT AND STATE WHETHER HE IS COMPLIANCE WITH THIS ORDER; A CHAPERONE SHALL BE PRESENT DURING HIS PHYSICAL EXAMINATIONS OF ANY FEMALE PATIENT AND THE NAME SHALL BE RECORDED IN THE PATIENT'S RECORD; SHALL NOTIFY THE BOARD OF ANY CHANGE OF ADDRESS WITHIN 14 DAYS; SHALL APPEAR BEFORE THE BOARD UPON REQUEST AND SHALL RECEIVE UNANNOUNCED VISITS FROM THE BOARD AT ITS DISCRETION; MAY NOT APPLY FOR MODIFICATION OF THIS ORDER FOR THREE YEARS; SHALL COMPLETE A RELEASE PERMITTING CPHP TO DISCLOSE TO THE BOARD ALL PRIVILEGED INFORMATION CONCERNING HIM IN ITS POSSESSION, INCLUDING INFORMATION GENERATED BY OTHER SOURCES; THE EXPIRATION OF THE PROBATIONARY PERIOD WILL BE TOLLED AND THE PROBATIONARY PERIOD WILL BE EXTENDED FOR ANY PERIOD OF RESIDENCE OR PRACTICE OUTSIDE OF OKLAHOMA OR WHEN HE IS NOT PARTICIPATING WITH CPHP. ON 6/18/98 PROBATION TERMINATED.

BADZINSKI, GARY L DO, DATE OF BIRTH JANUARY 21, 1956, LICENSE NUMBER 1009464 OF 1060 ORCHARD AVENUE STE E, GRAND JUNCTION, CO, WAS DISCIPLINED BY MICHIGAN ON FEBRUARY 6, 1997
DISCIPLINARY ACTION: FINE; RESTRICTION PLACED ON LICENSE
OFFENSE: DISCIPLINARY ACTION BY ANOTHER STATE OR AGENCY

NOTES: FAILURE TO REPORT/COMPLY. $1000 FINE.

BAGGETT, LYNN D MD, DATE OF BIRTH JUNE 1, 1953 OF HC 79, BOX 84, HUGO, OK, WAS DISCIPLINED BY MEDICARE ON FEBRUARY 8, 1995
DISCIPLINARY ACTION: EXCLUSION FROM THE MEDICARE AND/OR MEDICAID PROGRAM
OFFENSE: DISCIPLINARY ACTION BY ANOTHER STATE OR AGENCY

NOTES: LICENSE REVOCATION OR SUSPENSION. REINSTATED ON 6/1/99.

BAGGETT, LYNN DEAN MD, LICENSE NUMBER 0014448, WAS DISCIPLINED BY OKLAHOMA ON SEPTEMBER 13, 1990
DISCIPLINARY ACTION: LICENSE SUSPENSION; REQUIRED TO ENTER AN IMPAIRED PHYSICIAN PROGRAM OR SUBSTANCE ABUSE TREATMENT
OFFENSE: FAILURE TO COMPLY WITH PREVIOUS BOARD ORDER

NOTES: ON 7/23/90 WILLFULLY, DELIBERATELY AND CONTEMPTUOUSLY REFUSED TO SUBMIT A BIOLOGICAL FLUID SPECIMEN UPON REQUEST OF A BOARD INVESTIGATOR, AS REQUIRED BY TERMS OF 10/27/89 PROBATION ORDER. SHALL BE SUSPENDED FOR A TERM UNTIL EVIDENCE PRESENTED OF SUCCESSFUL COMPLETION OF IN-PATIENT TREATMENT TO THE BOARD. MAY SEEK

REINSTATEMENT AT THIS TIME UNDER TERMS AND CONDITIONS OF PROBATION SET BY THE BOARD AT THAT TIME.

BAGGETT, LYNN DEAN MD, LICENSE NUMBER 0014448 OF RTE 2 BOX 109, HUGO, OK, WAS DISCIPLINED BY OKLAHOMA ON JANUARY 12, 1991
DISCIPLINARY ACTION: 60-MONTH PROBATION; RESTRICTION PLACED ON CONTROLLED SUBSTANCE LICENSE

NOTES: LICENSE REINSTATED ON PROBATION WITH FOLLOWING CONDITIONS: SHALL NOT PRESCRIBE, ADMINISTER OR DISPENSE ANY CONTROLLED DANGEROUS SUBSTANCES OR ANY MEDICATION FOR HIS PERSONAL USE OR TO OTHERS; REQUIRED TO ATTEND A MINIMUM OF THREE AA MEETINGS AND ONE PROFESSIONAL MEETING PER WEEK; SHALL ABSTAIN FROM CONSUMING ALCOHOL OR ANY SUBSTANCE, WHICH WOULD ADVERSELY AFFECT HIS ABILITY TO PRACTICE MEDICINE; SHALL TAKE NO MEDICATION EXCEPT THAT WHICH IS AUTHORIZED BY A PHYSICIAN TREATING HIM FOR A LEGITIMATE MEDICAL NEED; SHALL SUBMIT BIOLOGICAL FLUID SPECIMENS FOR ANALYSIS; SHALL NOTIFY ANY HOSPITAL WHERE HE HOLDS STAFF PRIVILEGES, OR CLINIC, OR GROUP WHERE HE PRACTICES OF TERMS AND CONDITIONS; SHALL FURNISH BOARD WITH ADDRESS AND/OR CHANGE OF ADDRESS AND APPEAR BEFORE BOARD WHEN REQUESTED. ON 11/8/91, ORDER STATING LICENSE RETAINED ON PROBATION WITH SAME CONDITIONS OF ORIGINAL ORDER.

BAGGETT, LYNN DEAN MD, LICENSE NUMBER 0014448 OF 5000 300 EAST SKELLY DR, TULSA, OK, WAS DISCIPLINED BY OKLAHOMA ON JUNE 28, 1992
DISCIPLINARY ACTION: 2-MONTH LICENSE SUSPENSION; 60-MONTH PROBATION
OFFENSE: FAILURE TO COMPLY WITH PREVIOUS BOARD ORDER

NOTES: ON 7/2/92 FOUND IN CONTEMPT OF BOARD ORDER ISSUED 1/12/91 IN THAT A URINE SAMPLE TESTED POSITIVE FOR PHENTERMINE, A CONTROLLED DANGEROUS SUBSTANCE FOR WHICH HE DIDN'T PRODUCE ANY PRESCRIPTION FROM A TREATING PHYSICIAN. PROBATION UNDER SAME TERMS AS 1/19/91 ORDER.

BAGGETT, LYNN DEAN MD, LICENSE NUMBER 0014448, WAS DISCIPLINED BY OKLAHOMA ON FEBRUARY 17, 1994
DISCIPLINARY ACTION: EMERGENCY SUSPENSION

NOTES: ALLEGATIONS AND PREVIOUS DISCIPLINARY ACTION CONSTITUTE GROUNDS THAT LICENSE SHOULD BE SUSPENDED PENDING HEARING. HEARING POSTPONED BY ORDER OF 3/31/94.

BAGGETT, LYNN DEAN MD, LICENSE NUMBER 0014448, WAS DISCIPLINED BY OKLAHOMA ON MAY 19, 1994
DISCIPLINARY ACTION: LICENSE REVOCATION
OFFENSE: PRACTICING WITHOUT A VALID CONTROLLED SUBSTANCE LICENSE

NOTES: FROM 3/23/93 THROUGH 5/28/93 DID POSSESS, ADMINISTER AND/OR DISPENSE VARIOUS CONTROLLED DANGEROUS SUBSTANCES IN HIS PRACTICE WITHOUT A STATE OR FEDERAL NARCOTICS PERMIT AND WHILE LICENSE WAS SUSPENDED.

BAGGETT, LYNN DEAN MD, LICENSE NUMBER 0014448 OF BOX 521, RYAN, OK, WAS DISCIPLINED BY OKLAHOMA ON OCTOBER 2, 1995
DISCIPLINARY ACTION: DENIAL OF LICENSE REINSTATEMENT

NOTES: FAILED TO PRODUCE EVIDENCE TO OVERCOME THE ISSUES AS TO HIS COMPETENCY AND FITNESS TO PRACTICE MEDICINE.

BAGGETT, LYNN DEAN MD, LICENSE NUMBER 0014448 OF BOX 521, RYAN, OK, WAS DISCIPLINED BY OKLAHOMA ON MARCH 28, 1996
DISCIPLINARY ACTION: LICENSE REINSTATEMENT; PROBATION

NOTES: REINSTATED AS A SPECIAL LICENSE WITH PROBATION OF INDEFINITE LENGTH BEGINNING 3/22/96: SHALL NOT PRESCRIBE, ADMINISTER, OR DISPENSE ANY CONTROLLED DANGEROUS SUBSTANCES; SHALL NOT PRESCRIBE, ADMINISTER, OR DISPENSE ANY MEDICATION FOR HIS PERSONAL USE; WILL ATTEND RECOVERY GROUP MEETINGS AND PROVIDE DOCUMENTATION OF ATTENDANCE MONTHLY; SHALL ABSTAIN FROM CONSUMING ALCOHOL OR ANY SUBSTANCE, WHICH WOULD ADVERSELY AFFECT HIS ABILITY TO PRACTICE; SHALL TAKE NO MEDICATION UNLESS AUTHORIZED BY ANOTHER PHYSICIAN FOR LEGITIMATE MEDICAL NEED; SHALL SUBMIT BIOLOGICAL FLUID SPECIMENS; SHALL SUBMIT TO THE BOARD ADDRESS/CHANGE OF ADDRESS; SHALL APPEAR BEFORE THE BOARD UPON REQUEST AND SUBMIT ANY REQUIRED REPORTS; SHALL PAY ANY BALANCE DUE TO THE BOARD; SHALL NOTIFY ANY HOSPITAL, CLINIC, OR PRACTICE WORK SITE WHERE HE HOLDS STAFF PRIVILEGES OR APPLIES FOR STAFF PRIVILEGES OF THE TERMS AND CONDITIONS OF THIS ORDER AND PROVIDE A COPY THEREOF; SHALL CONFINE HIS PRACTICE TO THE OKLAHOMA DEPARTMENT OF CORRECTIONS MAXIMUM SECURITY FACILITY AT MCALESTER, OKLAHOMA.

BAGGETT, LYNN DEAN MD, LICENSE NUMBER 14448 OF RT 3, BOX 130G, MCALESTER, OK, WAS DISCIPLINED BY OKLAHOMA ON JUNE 5, 1997
DISCIPLINARY ACTION: LICENSE REVOCATION
OFFENSE: FAILURE TO COMPLY WITH PREVIOUS BOARD ORDER

NOTES: ON 3/28/96, A SPECIAL LICENSE WAS GRANTED WITH TERMS OF PROBATION INCLUDING REQUIREMENTS THAT HE ABSTAIN FROM CONSUMING ALCOHOL OR ANY SUBSTANCE WHICH WOULD ADVERSELY AFFECT HIS ABILITY TO PRACTICE MEDICINE AND FROM TAKING ANY MEDICATION EXCEPT THAT WHICH IS PRESCRIBED TO HIM BY ANOTHER PHYSICIAN FOR A LEGITIMATE MEDICAL NEED. A URINE SAMPLE COLLECTED FROM HIM ON OR AROUND 11/21/96 TESTED POSITIVE FOR TRAMADOL (ULTRAM). HE DID NOT REPORT ANY MEDICATION HE WAS TAKING THAT WOULD TEST POSITIVE NOR DID HE PROVIDE EVIDENCE THAT SUCH MEDICATION WAS AUTHORIZED BY ANY TREATING PHYSICIAN FOR A LEGITIMATE MEDICAL NEED.

BAGGETT, LYNN DEAN MD, LICENSE NUMBER 14448, WAS DISCIPLINED BY OKLAHOMA ON OCTOBER 2, 1998
DISCIPLINARY ACTION: LICENSE REINSTATEMENT; PROBATION
OFFENSE: SUBSTANCE ABUSE

NOTES: ON 5/15/97, THE BOARD REVOKED A SPECIAL LICENSE ISSUED UNDER TERMS OF PROBATION 3/22/96 FOR HABITUAL INTEMPERANCE OR THE HABITUAL USE OF HABIT-FORMING DRUGS. ISSUED A SPECIAL LICENSE UNDER THE FOLLOWING CONDITIONS OF PROBATION: HE WILL NOT PRESCRIBE, ADMINISTER, DISPENSE, OR POSSESS ANY DRUGS IN SCHEDULES II-V; HE WILL NOT REAPPLY FOR STATE AND FEDERAL REGISTRATION FOR CONTROLLED DANGEROUS SUBSTANCES UNLESS AUTHORIZED TO DO SO BY THE BOARD; SHALL KEEP DUPLICATE, SERIALLY NUMBERED PRESCRIPTIONS OF ALL SUBSTANCES

AND WILL SUBMIT COPIES TO THE BOARD UPON REQUEST; SHALL NOT AUTHORIZE ANY PERSONNEL UNDER HIS SUPERVISION TO INITIATE AN ORDER FOR A PRESCRIPTION TO BE ISSUED; SHALL PRACTICE IN A CONTROLLED ENVIRONMENT APPROVED BY THE BOARD LIMITED TO THE OKLAHOMA STATE DEPARTMENT OF CORRECTIONS, MAXIMUM SECURITY FACILITY, MCALESTER, OKLAHOMA; SHALL SUBMIT BIOLOGICAL FLUID SPECIMENS AND SHALL NOT INGEST ANY SUBSTANCE WHICH WILL CAUSE A SPECIMEN TO TEST POSITIVE FOR PROHIBITED SUBSTANCES; SHALL REQUEST ALL HEALTH CARE FACILITIES IN WHICH HE ANTICIPATES PRACTICING TO FURNISH A STATEMENT REGARDING MONITORING OF HIS PRACTICE; SHALL SUBMIT TO EVERY STATE IN WHICH HE HOLDS LICENSURE AND TO HOSPITALS, CLINICS OR OTHER INSTITUTIONS IN WHICH HE HOLDS OR ANTICIPATES HOLDING ANY FORM OF STAFF PRIVILEGE A COPY OF THIS ORDER; SHALL NOT SUPERVISE ALLIED HEALTH PROFESSIONALS; SHALL DO OPEN OR INVASIVE SURGICAL PROCEDURES ONLY UNDER THE DIRECT SUPERVISION OF AND IN THE IMMEDIATE PRESENCE OF A LICENSED MEDICAL DOCTOR PRACTICING IN THE SAME SPECIALTY; SHALL NOT PRESCRIBE, ADMINISTER OR DISPENSE ANY MEDICATIONS FOR HIS PERSONAL USE AND SHALL TAKE NONE UNLESS AUTHORIZED BY ANOTHER PHYSICIAN FOR A LEGITIMATE MEDICAL NEED; SHALL ABIDE BY HIS POST-CARE CONTRACT; SHALL CONTINUE PSYCHIATRIC TREATMENT UNDER AN APPROVED PRACTITIONER FOR PSYCHOTHERAPY AND MEDICATION MANAGEMENT, FOLLOW THE TREATMENT REGIMEN SUGGESTED WITH QUARTERLY REPORTS TO THE BOARD AND WILL RELEASE ANY AND ALL RECORDS OF THAT TREATMENT TO THE BOARD; SHALL KEEP THE BOARD INFORMED OF HIS ADDRESS AND PAY COSTS; SHALL APPEAR BEFORE THE BOARD UPON REQUEST; SHALL EXECUTE THE RELEASE OF ANY MEDICAL, COUNSELING, AND PSYCHIATRIC RECORDS AS NECESSARY TO DISCUSS HIS CASE WITH TREATING PHYSICIANS AND/OR ANY PHYSICIANS HOLDING RECORDS; EACH WEEK HE WILL ATTEND THE WEEKLY MEETING OF THE PHYSICIANS' RECOVERY COMMITTEE AND AT LEAST THREE OTHER RECOVERY GROUP MEETINGS APPROVED BY THE BOARD. ON 11/19/98 THE BOARD DENIED HIS REQUEST FOR A MODIFICATION TO THIS ORDER TO ALLOW HIM TO PRACTICE AT SPECIFIED CLINIC DUE TO THE FAILURE OF THE OKLAHOMA DEPARTMENT OF CORRECTIONS TO OFFER HIM EMPLOYMENT AT THE AFOREMENTIONED FACILITY. ON 2/10/99 THE WESTERN STATE PSYCHIATRIC CENTER (WSPC) WAS ADDED AS AN APPROVED PRACTICE LOCATION; DURING PROBATION, WILL PRACTICE IN A BOARD- APPROVED CONTROLLED ENVIRONMENT, LIMITED TO THE WESTERN STATE PSYCHIATRIC CENTER UNDER THE FOLLOWING PRACTICE PARAMETERS: WILL CONDUCT PHYSICALS AND SICK CALL FOR WSPC SUBSTANCE ABUSE RESIDENTIAL PROGRAM AND WILL CONDUCT MEDICATION CLINICS AND REVIEWS FOR OUTPATIENT MENTAL HEALTH SATELLITES IN WOODWARD, GUYMON, BEAVER, AND SHATTUCK, OKLAHOMA; WILL NOT NEED A DEA NUMBER AND WILL WORK UNDER THE DIRECT SUPERVISION OF A BOARD-APPROVED PSYCHIATRIST; WILL VOLUNTARILY SUBMIT TO DRUG TESTING DURING HIS EMPLOYMENT IN ADDITION TO ANY RANDOM URINE SCREENS PERFORMED BY THE BOARD; DURING PROBATION: WILL TAKE NO MEDICATION EXCEPT THAT WHICH AUTHORIZED BY A BOARD APPROVED PHYSICIAN FOR A LEGITIMATE MEDICAL NEED; WILL OBTAIN AND UTILIZE A PERSONAL FAMILY PHYSICIAN LOCATED IN THE IMMEDIATE GEOGRAPHIC VICINITY; SHALL INFORM ANY AND EVERY DOCTOR TREATING HIM OF THE BOARD ORDER IMMEDIATELY UPON INITIATION OF TREATMENT. ON 9/24/99 REQUEST OF AN INTERDEPARTMENTAL TRANSFER TO CARL ALBERT HOSPITAL IN MCALESTER, OKLAHOMA GRANTED.

BAILEY, SHARON DO OF 1133 MADLYNNE, CEDAR HILL, TX, WAS DISCIPLINED BY OKLAHOMA ON DECEMBER 13, 1990
DISCIPLINARY ACTION: MONITORING OF PHYSICIAN PERFORMANCE

NOTES: LICENSE GRANTED WITH THE FOLLOWING STIPULATIONS: WEEKLY ATTENDANCE WITH DOCUMENTATION TO THE BOARD OF NARCOTICS ANONYMOUS, AA, AND THE OOA PHYSICIAN'S RECOVERY COMMITTEE MEETINGS; SHALL SUBMIT TO RANDOM DRUG SCREENS AT THE BOARD'S DISCRETION; SHALL CONTACT THE PHYSICIAN'S RECOVERY COMMITTEE OF THE OOA FOR INCORPORATION WITH THEM OF THE CONTRACT SIGNED REGARDING HER RECOVERY IN TEXAS.

BALDWIN, RICHARD E DO OF DAVIS, OK, WAS DISCIPLINED BY MISSOURI ON JULY 27, 1990
DISCIPLINARY ACTION: 2-MONTH LICENSE SUSPENSION; 22-MONTH PROBATION
OFFENSE: DISCIPLINARY ACTION BY ANOTHER STATE OR AGENCY

NOTES: TWO MONTH SUSPENSION RETROACTIVE TO 6/15/89, TWENTY-TWO MONTH PROBATION RETROACTIVE TO 8/16/89.

BALDWIN, RICHARD E DO, LICENSE NUMBER 00E3192 OF DAVIS, OK, WAS DISCIPLINED BY TEXAS ON AUGUST 18, 1990
OFFENSE: DISCIPLINARY ACTION BY ANOTHER STATE OR AGENCY

NOTES: STIPULATED ORDER. MUST COMPLY WITH OKLAHOMA BOARD ORDER, RECEIVE PERMISSION OF TEXAS BOARD BEFORE RETURNING TO PRACTICE MEDICINE IN TEXAS, AND BE SUBJECT TO ANY TERMS IMPOSED.

BALDWIN, RICHARD E DO, DATE OF BIRTH JULY 19, 1938, LICENSE NUMBER 0018743 OF DAVIS, OK, WAS DISCIPLINED BY COLORADO ON FEBRUARY 21, 1992
DISCIPLINARY ACTION: SURRENDER OF LICENSE
OFFENSE: CRIMINAL CONVICTION OR PLEA OF GUILTY, NOLO CONTENDERE, OR NO CONTEST TO A CRIME

NOTES: FELONY CONVICTION FOR MEDICAID FRAUD.

BANEZGUZMAN, CORAZON MD, LICENSE NUMBER 0008904, WAS DISCIPLINED BY OKLAHOMA ON FEBRUARY 18, 1991
DISCIPLINARY ACTION: 36-MONTH LICENSE SUSPENSION
OFFENSE: DISCIPLINARY ACTION BY ANOTHER STATE OR AGENCY

NOTES: ON 10/15/90 ENTERED A GUILTY PLEA TO FILING FALSE MEDICAID CLAIMS AND DEVISING A SCHEME TO DEFRAUD THE OKLAHOMA MEDICAL PROGRAM. ON 4/26/90 WAS EXCLUDED FROM MEDICAID PROGRAM. UNTIL SUSPENSION BEGINS, SHALL ONLY PRACTICE MEDICINE AND SURGERY TO TRANSFER CARE OF PEDIATRIC PATIENTS TO OTHER HEALTH CARE PROVIDERS. ON 03/05/92 REINSTATEMENT REQUEST DENIED.

BANEZGUZMAN, CORAZON MD, DATE OF BIRTH JUNE 1, 1929 OF 1010 EAST 20TH STREET, TULSA, OK, WAS DISCIPLINED BY MEDICARE ON JULY 23, 1991
DISCIPLINARY ACTION: 180-MONTH EXCLUSION FROM THE MEDICARE AND/OR MEDICAID PROGRAM
OFFENSE: CRIMINAL CONVICTION OR PLEA OF GUILTY, NOLO CONTENDERE, OR NO CONTEST TO A CRIME

NOTES: PROGRAM-RELATED CONVICTION.

BARBER, RONALD D MD, LICENSE NUMBER 0015264, WAS DISCIPLINED BY OKLAHOMA ON NOVEMBER 8, 1991
DISCIPLINARY ACTION: REPRIMAND
OFFENSE: PROFESSIONAL MISCONDUCT

NOTES: IN FEBRUARY OR MARCH 1991 GAVE BLANK, UNDATED, PRESIGNED PRESCRIPTION FORMS TO A DOCTOR IN ORDER TO ALLOW THE DOCTOR, WHO DID NOT POSSESS THE REQUIRED REGISTRATION FROM THE U.S. DRUG ENFORCEMENT ADMINISTRATION, TO PRESCRIBE CONTROLLED DANGEROUS SUBSTANCES; ALSO SIGNED HIS NAME AND NUMBER TO THIS DOCTOR'S PRESCRIPTIONS. NO MALICIOUS INTENT, INTENTIONAL CONSPIRACY, PATIENT HARM, PERSONAL DRUG USE, OR DELIBERATE DIVERSION FOUND.

BARKER, MARCUS S MD, LICENSE NUMBER 5894, WAS DISCIPLINED BY OKLAHOMA ON MAY 29, 1998
DISCIPLINARY ACTION: SURRENDER OF LICENSE

NOTES: VOLUNTARY SURRENDER IN LIEU OF PROSECUTION.

BAYLESS, JAMES M MD, DATE OF BIRTH JUNE 15, 1921, LICENSE NUMBER 0C27649 OF RIVERSIDE, CA, WAS DISCIPLINED BY CALIFORNIA ON MARCH 21, 1992
DISCIPLINARY ACTION: 3-MONTH LICENSE SUSPENSION; 57-MONTH PROBATION
OFFENSE: CRIMINAL CONVICTION OR PLEA OF GUILTY, NOLO CONTENDERE, OR NO CONTEST TO A CRIME

NOTES: MISDEMEANOR CONVICTION FOR UNLAWFULLY PRESCRIBING CONTROLLED SUBSTANCE NOT FOR A LEGITIMATE MEDICAL PURPOSE; EXCESSIVE, GROSSLY NEGLIGENT AND INCOMPETENT PRESCRIBING. REVOCATION, STAYED. PROBATION WITH TERMS AND CONDITIONS.

BAYLESS, JAMES M MD, LICENSE NUMBER 0005723 OF 10327 HOLE AVENUE, RIVERSIDE, CA, WAS DISCIPLINED BY OKLAHOMA ON JANUARY 15, 1993
DISCIPLINARY ACTION: LICENSE SUSPENSION; 60-MONTH PROBATION
OFFENSE: DISCIPLINARY ACTION BY ANOTHER STATE OR AGENCY

NOTES: ON 2/20/92 CALIFORNIA DISCIPLINED HIS LICENSE FOR EXCESSIVE PRESCRIBING OF CONTROLLED DANGEROUS SUBSTANCES WHICH AROSE OUT OF A CRIMINAL PROCEEDING WHERE HE PLED NOLO CONTENDERE TO ALLEGATIONS OF UNLAWFUL PRESCRIBING OF CONTROLLED DANGEROUS SUBSTANCES WITHOUT GOOD FAITH PRIOR EXAM AND MEDICAL INDICATION; SENTENCED TO THREE YEAR PROBATION, RESTITUTION AND SURRENDER OF DEA LICENSE. OKLAHOMA SUSPENSION UNTIL HE PASSES EXAM REQUIRED BY CALIFORNIA ORDER OR THE SPEX EXAM IN OKLAHOMA; PROBATION RETROACTIVE TO 3/21/92 AND IS COMMENSURATE WITH THE TERMS IMPOSED BY THE CALIFORNIA ORDER INCLUDING RESTRICTION ON DRUG PRESCRIBING, EDUCATION AND MEDICAL ETHICS COURSES, MONITORING BY ANOTHER PHYSICIAN, QUARTERLY REPORTS, PROBATION SURVEILLANCE AND INTERVIEWS WITH MEDICAL CONSULTANT.

BAYLESS, JAMES M MD, LICENSE NUMBER C27649 OF RIVERSIDE, CA, WAS DISCIPLINED BY CALIFORNIA ON JUNE 9, 1997
DISCIPLINARY ACTION: SURRENDER OF LICENSE

NOTES: WHILE CHARGES PENDING.

BAYLESS, JAMES M MD, DATE OF BIRTH JUNE 15, 1921 OF 3940 CHAPMAN PLACE, RIVERSIDE, CA, WAS DISCIPLINED BY MEDICARE ON FEBRUARY 19, 1998
DISCIPLINARY ACTION: EXCLUSION FROM THE MEDICARE AND/OR MEDICAID PROGRAM
OFFENSE: DISCIPLINARY ACTION BY ANOTHER STATE OR AGENCY

NOTES: LICENSE REVOKED, SUSPENDED, SURRENDERED OR OTHERWISE LOST FOR REASONS BEARING ON PROFESSIONAL PERFORMANCE, PROFESSIONAL COMPETENCE OR FINANCIAL INTEGRITY.

BEASON, MICHAEL B MD OF 921 14TH NW, ARDMORE, OK, WAS DISCIPLINED BY DEA ON APRIL 9, 1990
DISCIPLINARY ACTION: SURRENDER OF CONTROLLED SUBSTANCE LICENSE
OFFENSE: SUBSTANCE ABUSE

NOTES: PLACED ON TOTAL OF SIX YEARS PROBATION FOR HABITUALLY ABUSING CONTROLLED SUBSTANCES.

BEASON, MICHAEL BRITTON MD, LICENSE NUMBER 0014702 OF 921 14TH AVENUE, NW, ARDMORE, OK, WAS DISCIPLINED BY OKLAHOMA ON FEBRUARY 8, 1990
DISCIPLINARY ACTION: SURRENDER OF LICENSE; REQUIRED TO ENTER AN IMPAIRED PHYSICIAN PROGRAM OR SUBSTANCE ABUSE TREATMENT
OFFENSE: FAILURE TO COMPLY WITH PREVIOUS BOARD ORDER

NOTES: FAILED TO COMPLY WITH PROBATION OF 6/09/89 IN THAT ON 10/31/89 HIS LABORATORY URINE ANALYSIS TESTED POSITIVE FOR PROPOXYPHENE, A CONTROLLED DANGEROUS SUBSTANCE. ON 11/16/89 HE ADMITTED HE TOOK DARVON, OBTAINED FROM SAMPLE DRUGS, NOT PRESCRIPTION, FOR A BACK INJURY. HE VOLUNTARILY SURRENDERED HIS LICENSE ON 2/16/90 WHICH SHALL BE HELD BY THE BOARD UNTIL THE SUCCESSFUL COMPLETION OF IN-PATIENT TREATMENT.

BEASON, MICHAEL BRITTON MD, LICENSE NUMBER 0014702, WAS DISCIPLINED BY OKLAHOMA ON SEPTEMBER 13, 1990
DISCIPLINARY ACTION: LICENSE REINSTATEMENT; 60-MONTH PROBATION
OFFENSE: SUBSTANCE ABUSE

NOTES: REINSTATEMENT OF SURRENDERED LICENSE AFTER THE SUCCESSFUL COMPLETION OF IN-PATIENT TREATMENT. PROBATION BEGINNING 7/05/90 UNDER THE FOLLOWING TERMS AND CONDITIONS: SHALL NOT PRESCRIBE, ADMINISTER, OR DISPENSE ANY CONTROLLED DANGEROUS SUBSTANCES WITH THE EXCEPTION THAT HE MAY ADMINISTER/ORDER CONTROLLED DANGEROUS SUBSTANCES TO HOSPITAL IN-PATIENTS ONLY; SHALL TAKE NO MEDICATION UNLESS AUTHORIZED BY ANOTHER PHYSICIAN FOR LEGITIMATE MEDICAL NEED; SHALL NOT PRESCRIBE, ADMINISTER OR DISPENSE ANY MEDICATION FOR HIS PERSONAL USE; SHALL ABSTAIN FROM CONSUMING ALCOHOL OR ANY SUBSTANCE WHICH WOULD ADVERSELY AFFECT HIS ABILITY TO PRACTICE MEDICINE; SHALL SUBMIT BIOLOGICAL FLUID SPECIMENS; SHALL CONTINUE TO ACTIVELY PARTICIPATE IN SUPPORT PROGRAMS OPERATED THROUGH THE PHYSICIAN RECOVERY COMMITTEE AND ANY PSYCHOLOGICAL COUNSELING AS RECOMMENDED BY THE BOARD; SHALL SUBMIT TO THE BOARD ADDRESS/CHANGE OF ADDRESS; SHALL APPEAR BEFORE THE BOARD UPON REQUEST AND SUBMIT ANY REQUIRED REPORTS; SHALL PAY COSTS; SHALL GIVE BLANKET PERMISSION TO THE BOARD TO OBTAIN ALL OTHERWISE CONFIDENTAL INFORMATION PERTAINING TO HIS PHYSICAL, MENTAL, AND EMOTIONAL CONDITIONS; SHALL ADVISE THE BOARD OF ALL PHYSICIANS WHO HAVE TREATED HIM WITHIN

THE LAST FIVE YEARS; SHALL NOTIFY ANY HOSPITAL WHERE HE HOLDS STAFF PRIVILEGES OR CLINIC OR GROUP WHERE HE PRACTICES OF THE TERMS AND CONDITIONS AND SHALL SUPPLY A COPY THEREOF.

BEAVERS, JOHN E MD, DATE OF BIRTH APRIL 2, 1960 OF 4020 N W 26TH STREET, OKLAHOMA CITY, OK, WAS DISCIPLINED BY MEDICARE ON MAY 9, 1995
DISCIPLINARY ACTION: EXCLUSION FROM THE MEDICARE AND/OR MEDICAID PROGRAM
OFFENSE: NONCOMPLIANCE WITH A PROFESSIONAL RULE

NOTES: DEFAULTED ON PUBLIC HEALTH SERVICE EDUCATION LOAN. REINSTATED ON 5/16/95.

BOTTLES, KURT D MD, LICENSE NUMBER 0017375, WAS DISCIPLINED BY OKLAHOMA ON MAY 19, 1994
DISCIPLINARY ACTION: LICENSE REVOCATION
OFFENSE: SEXUAL ABUSE OF OR SEXUAL MISCONDUCT WITH A PATIENT

NOTES: DURING 1990 AND 1991 HE DID IMPROPERLY HANDLE A MINOR FEMALE PATIENT AND PURSUED A SEXUAL RELATIONSHIP WITH THIS PATIENT FOR SEVERAL MONTHS OUTSIDE OF A LAWFUL PHYSICIAN-PATIENT RELATIONSHIP; UNPROFESSIONAL ACTS INCLUDED THE FOLLOWING; SENDING SUGGESTIVE GREETING CARDS, FOLLOWING THE PATIENT WHEN SHE WENT OUT WITH FRIENDS, AND MAKING NUMEROUS PHONE CALLS TO PATIENT. IN 6/96 THIS ORDER WAS REVERSED BY THE SUPREME COURT, REMANDED TO THE BOARD FOR NEW ACTION AND LICENSE WAS ORDERED REINSTATED. ON 1/10/97, HE VOLUNTARILY SUBMITTED TO THE JURISDICTION OF THE BOARD, ADMITTED HE WAS IN VIOLATION OF THE OKLAHOMA MEDICAL PRACTICE ACT, AND AGREED TO THREE YEARS PROBATION. TERMS OF PROBATION INCLUDE: SHALL HAVE A FEMALE CHAPERONE PRESENT WHEN SEEING FEMALE PATIENTS; SHALL DEFINE BOUNDARIES WITH RESPECT TO PRACTICE, SEPARATING PERSONAL AND PROFESSIONAL RELATIONSHIPS; SHALL HAVE A BOARD APPROVED PEER PHYSICIAN REVIEW AND MONITOR HIS PRACTICE; SHALL CONTINUE PSYCHOTHERAPY WITH QUARTERLY REPORTS TO THE BOARD; SHALL ENGAGE IN MEDICAL EDUCATION INVOLVING APPROPRIATE PROFESSIONAL BOUNDARIES AND MEDICAL ETHICS; SHALL NOTIFY ANY HEALTH CARE ENTITY WHERE HE HAS PRIVILEGES OF THIS VOLUNTARY SUBMITTAL TO JURISDICTION; SHALL INFORM THE BOARD OF ANY CHANGE OF ADDRESS; SHALL APPEAR BEFORE THE BOARD UPON REQUEST. ON 2/12/99 REQUEST TO TERMINATE PROBATION GRANTED.

BOTTLES, KURT D MD, DATE OF BIRTH APRIL 17, 1961 OF 909 LINN LANE, YUKON, OK, WAS DISCIPLINED BY MEDICARE ON FEBRUARY 8, 1995
DISCIPLINARY ACTION: EXCLUSION FROM THE MEDICARE AND/OR MEDICAID PROGRAM
OFFENSE: DISCIPLINARY ACTION BY ANOTHER STATE OR AGENCY

NOTES: LICENSE REVOCATION OR SUSPENSION. REINSTATED ON 2/18/98.

BOWLAN, TIMOTHY MARK MD, WAS DISCIPLINED BY OKLAHOMA ON JULY 2, 1992
DISCIPLINARY ACTION: DENIAL OF NEW LICENSE
OFFENSE: FALSIFYING OR ALTERING PATIENT RECORDS

NOTES: TWO LETTERS WERE RECEIVED BY THE BOARD FROM TWO PHYSICIANS AT MASSACHUSETTS GENERAL HOSPITAL WHICH INDICATED THAT HE FALSIFIED PATIENT ADMISSIONS BY PUTTING AN EVALUATION AND MEDICATION ORDERS IN THE CHART FOR TWO PATIENTS WHO DID NOT GET ADMITTED TO THE HOSPITAL; SIGNED OUT ONE DAY A WEEK FOR OVER A YEAR FROM INPATIENT SERVICE AND USED THIS TIME FOR HIS PRIVATE PRACTICE BY CLAIMING TO BE WORKING IN RESEARCH. ON 07/02/92, BOARD ORDER ISSUED DENYING MOTION FOR RECONSIDERATION.

BOWLAN, TIMOTHY MARK MD, DATE OF BIRTH AUGUST 14, 1957 OF 3124 QUAIL CREEK ROAD, OKLAHOMA CITY, OK, WAS DISCIPLINED BY MEDICARE ON FEBRUARY 22, 1995
DISCIPLINARY ACTION: 36-MONTH EXCLUSION FROM THE MEDICARE AND/OR MEDICAID PROGRAM
OFFENSE: CRIMINAL CONVICTION OR PLEA OF GUILTY, NOLO CONTENDERE, OR NO CONTEST TO A CRIME

NOTES: CONVICTED OF A CRIME RELATED TO THE DELIVERY OF HEALTH CARE OR FINANCIAL MISCONDUCT INVOLVING A GOVERNMENT-OPERATED PROGRAM.

BOWLAN, TIMOTHY MARK MD, LICENSE NUMBER 0056848 OF 1905 MISSION HILLS CIRCLE, EDMOND, OK, WAS DISCIPLINED BY MASSACHUSETTS ON SEPTEMBER 27, 1995
DISCIPLINARY ACTION: NONRENEWAL OF LICENSE
OFFENSE: DISCIPLINARY ACTION BY ANOTHER STATE OR AGENCY

NOTES: DISCIPLINARY ACTION IN OKLAHOMA. REVOCATION OF INCHOATE RIGHT TO RENEW.

BREWER, MICHAEL A DO, LICENSE NUMBER 0002307, WAS DISCIPLINED BY OKLAHOMA ON MARCH 29, 1990
DISCIPLINARY ACTION: 60-MONTH PROBATION; RESTRICTION PLACED ON CONTROLLED SUBSTANCE LICENSE
OFFENSE: SUBSTANCE ABUSE

NOTES: SUFFERED A RELAPSE IN HIS RECOVERY FROM DRUG ADDICTION IN THE LATE MONTHS OF 1988. SHALL ATTEND FOUR AA OR NARCOTICS ANONYMOUS MEETINGS PER WEEK AND DOCUMENT SUCH ATTENDANCE FOR THE BOARD; SHALL SUBMIT URINE SPECIMENS FOR DRUG SCREENING AT SUCH TIMES AND PLACES AS DESIGNATED BY THE BOARD; SHALL APPEAR BEFORE THE BOARD AT SIX MONTH INTERVALS TO REPORT ON THE PROGRESS OF HIS RECOVERY; SHALL NOT PRESCRIBE, DISPENSE OR ADMINISTER SCHEDULED CONTROLLED DANGEROUS SUBSTANCE DRUGS; SHALL NOT PERSONALLY USE OR CONSUME ALCOHOLIC BEVERAGES OR ANY CONTROLLED DANGEROUS SUBSTANCES EXCEPT AS PRESCRIBED BY A PHYSICIAN IN THE PHYSICIAN RECOVERY NETWORK. ON 3/18/93 HIS REQUEST FOR TERMINATION OF PROBATION DENIED. TO BE RECONSIDERED AFTER ONE ADDITIONAL YEAR OF PROBATION; IT WAS RECOMMENDED TO THE DEA AND THE OKLAHOMA BUREAU OF DRUG CONTROL THAT HIS NARCOTICS PERMITS FOR SCHEDULE III, IV, AND V DRUGS BE APPROVED. ON 9/15/94 THE CONDITIONS ON HIS LICENSE WERE TERMINATED.

BREWER, MICHAEL ANDREW DO OF 1015 WASHBURN, PO BOX 350, JAY, OK, WAS DISCIPLINED BY DEA ON APRIL 4, 1990
DISCIPLINARY ACTION: SURRENDER OF CONTROLLED SUBSTANCE LICENSE
OFFENSE: SUBSTANCE ABUSE

NOTES: MEDICAL LICENSE PLACED ON PROBATION FOR TWO YEARS DUE TO DEMEROL ADDICTION. REGISTRATION SURRENDERED DUE TO RELAPSE IN RECOVERY FROM DRUG ADDICTION. TESTED POSITIVE FOR OPIATES ON 01/06/89.

BREWER, MICHAEL ANDREW DO OF 1015 WASHBOURNE P.O BOX 350, JAY, OK, WAS DISCIPLINED BY DEA ON MARCH 30, 1994
DISCIPLINARY ACTION: RESTRICTION PLACED ON CONTROLLED SUBSTANCE LICENSE
OFFENSE: SUBSTANCE ABUSE

BROADIE, LARRY MD, DATE OF BIRTH FEBRUARY 25, 1940, LICENSE NUMBER 041520 OF 11520 SURREY LANE, MIDWEST CITY, OK, WAS DISCIPLINED BY GEORGIA ON APRIL 1, 1998
DISCIPLINARY ACTION: LICENSE REVOCATION

NOTES: VOLUNTARY SURRENDER; SAME AS REVOCATION.

BROADIE, LARRY L MD, LICENSE NUMBER 12218, WAS DISCIPLINED BY OKLAHOMA ON JULY 3, 1997
DISCIPLINARY ACTION: LICENSE REVOCATION
OFFENSE: LOSS OR RESTRICTION OF HOSPITAL PRIVILEGES

NOTES: HIS PRIVILEGES TO PRACTICE MEDICINE AT A MILITARY BASE WERE REVOKED ON 12/20/95 DUE TO MULTIPLE EPISODES OF FAILURE TO TAKE AN ADEQUATE HISTORY AND FAILURE TO PERFORM AN ADEQUATE PHYSICAL EXAM. ON 6/21/96, HE SIGNED AN APPLICATION FOR RENEWAL OF OKLAHOMA MEDICAL LICENSE ON WHICH HE INDICATED THAT HE HAD NOT BEEN REPORTED TO THE NATIONAL PRACTITIONER DATA BANK AND THAT HE HAD NOT BEEN DENIED PRIVILEGES, LOST PRIVILEGES, OR RECEIVED DISCIPLINE BY ANY HOSPITAL OR OTHER PROFESSIONAL MEDICAL ORGANIZATION.

BROWN, WILLIAM DO OF 101 S PECAN, TUSHKA, OK, WAS DISCIPLINED BY DEA ON AUGUST 2, 1999
DISCIPLINARY ACTION: SURRENDER OF CONTROLLED SUBSTANCE LICENSE
OFFENSE: DISCIPLINARY ACTION BY ANOTHER STATE OR AGENCY

NOTES: STATE BOARD.

BROWN, WILLIAM E DO OF OKLAHOMA CITY, OK, WAS DISCIPLINED BY DEA ON DECEMBER 3, 1993
DISCIPLINARY ACTION: RESTRICTION PLACED ON CONTROLLED SUBSTANCE LICENSE
OFFENSE: SUBSTANCE ABUSE

NOTES: FROM 1977 THROUGH 1981 HE WAS LISTED BY THE DEA AS AN "EXCESSIVE PURCHASER" OF CONTROLLED SUBSTANCES AND IN FEBRUARY 1983 HE ISSUED PRESCRIPTIONS FOR CONTROLLED SUBSTANCES WHILE UNREGISTERED. IN 10/84 HE WAS CONVICTED OF FIFTEEN FELONY COUNTS INVOLVING THE RECEIPT OF CONTROLLED SUBSTANCES BY FRAUD. HIS OKLAHOMA OSTEOPATHIC LICENSE WAS REVOKED AS A RESULT OF THIS CONVICTION AND HIS CONTROLLED SUBSTANCES PRIVILEGES SUSPENDED. IN 9/86 HIS PROBATION WAS REVOKED BASED UPON A VIOLATION OF BEING INTOXICATED IN THE WORKPLACE. IN 6/87 HIS OSTEOPATHIC LICENSE WAS REINSTATED AND HE WAS AUTHORIZED UNDER STATE LAW TO HANDLE SCHEDULE III THROUGH V CONTROLLED SUBSTANCES, WITH CERTAIN LIMITATIONS, INCLUDING THAT HE UTILIZE TRIPLICATE SERIALLY NUMBERED PRESCRIPTIONS; ACCEPT NO SAMPLES; NOT DISPENSE ANY SCHEDULED DRUGS FROM HIS OFFICE; AND SUBMIT COPIES OF SAID PRESCRIPTIONS MONTHLY TO THE BOARD AND DOCUMENTATION OF HIS ATTENDANCE AT AA. RESTRICTIONS ON DEA LICENSE CONSISTENT WITH THOSE IMPOSED BY OKLAHOMA BOARD.

BROWN, WILLIAM E DO, LICENSE NUMBER 1490, WAS DISCIPLINED BY OKLAHOMA ON MARCH 19, 1998
DISCIPLINARY ACTION: LICENSE SUSPENSION

BROWN, WILLIAM E DO, DATE OF BIRTH DECEMBER 8, 1938 OF PO BOX 237, ATOKA, OK, WAS DISCIPLINED BY MEDICARE ON NOVEMBER 19, 1998
DISCIPLINARY ACTION: EXCLUSION FROM THE MEDICARE AND/OR MEDICAID PROGRAM
OFFENSE: DISCIPLINARY ACTION BY ANOTHER STATE OR AGENCY

NOTES: LICENSE REVOKED, SUSPENDED, SURRENDERED OR OTHERWISE LOST FOR REASONS BEARING ON PROFESSIONAL PERFORMANCE, PROFESSIONAL COMPETENCE OR FINANCIAL INTEGRITY.

BRUMMELL, DARLA MD OF 2815 S. SHERIDAN, TULSA, OK, WAS DISCIPLINED BY DEA ON JUNE 29, 1999
DISCIPLINARY ACTION: SURRENDER OF CONTROLLED SUBSTANCE LICENSE

NOTES: IN LIEU OF PUBLIC INTEREST REVOCATION.

BULLOCK, WILLIAM R MD, LICENSE NUMBER 0008754, WAS DISCIPLINED BY OKLAHOMA ON FEBRUARY 17, 1994
DISCIPLINARY ACTION: 24-MONTH PROBATION; RESTRICTION PLACED ON LICENSE
OFFENSE: PROFESSIONAL MISCONDUCT

NOTES: FROM 1/6/93 THROUGH 10/4/93 SIGNED 20 PRESCRIPTIONS TO VARIOUS PATIENTS AND DIRECTED OTHER OFFICE PERSONNEL INCLUDING AN INSURANCE CLERK AND BOOKKEEPER, A FIRST YEAR PA STUDENT, A LAB TECHNICIAN AND A LICENSED PRACTICAL NURSE TO SIGN HIS NAME TO AT LEAST 11 ADDITIONAL PRESCRIPTIONS; NONE OF THESE PEOPLE WERE AUTHORIZED TO WRITE PRESCRIPTIONS. CONDITIONS OF PROBATION TO BEGIN 2/11/94: SHALL PRESCRIBE CONTROLLED DANGEROUS SUBSTANCES ONLY ON SERIALLY-NUMBERED, DUPLICATE PRESCRIPTION PADS WITH COPIES AVAILABLE FOR INSPECTION; SHALL COMPLETE 50 HOURS OF BOARD APPROVED CONTINUING MEDICAL EDUCATION ON CONTROLLED DANGEROUS SUBSTANCES AND PRESCRIBING PRACTICES; SHALL FURNISH THE BOARD WITH ADDRESS AND/OR CHANGE OF ADDRESS; SHALL APPEAR BEFORE THE BOARD UPON REQUEST AND SUBMIT REQUIRED REPORTS; SHALL NOT SUPERVISE A PHYSICIAN'S ASSISTANT; SHALL FURNISH EACH STATE WHERE HE HOLDS OR APPLIES FOR LICENSURE AND ANY HEALTH CARE ENTITY WHERE HE HOLDS PRIVILEGES A COPY OF THIS ORDER; SHALL PAY COSTS.

BUTT, MICHAEL J MD, LICENSE NUMBER 17948, WAS DISCIPLINED BY OKLAHOMA ON MARCH 5, 1999
DISCIPLINARY ACTION: LICENSE REVOCATION
OFFENSE: CRIMINAL CONVICTION OR PLEA OF GUILTY, NOLO CONTENDERE, OR NO CONTEST TO A CRIME

NOTES: ON OR ABOUT 7/15/98 PLED NOLO CONTENDRE TO SEXUAL BATTERY.

CARPENTER, BYRON L MD, LICENSE NUMBER 6041 OF PO BOX 771, TULSA, OK, WAS DISCIPLINED BY OKLAHOMA ON JUNE 19, 1998
DISCIPLINARY ACTION: RESTRICTION PLACED ON LICENSE

NOTES: QUESTIONS RAISED IN APPLICATION CONCERNING HIS FITNESS OR ABILITY TO PRACTICE. GRANTED A SPECIAL TRAINING LICENSE WITH FOLLOWING TERMS AND CONDITIONS: SHALL SUBMIT TO BOARD THE NAME OF A PSYCHIATRIST, AND UPON APPROVAL, SHALL SUBMIT HIMSELF FOR EVALUATION AND

TREATMENT WITH QUARTERLY REPORTS TO BOARD; SHALL SUBMIT TO EVERY STATE IN WHICH HE HOLDS LICENSURE AND TO HOSPITALS, CLINICS OR OTHER INSTITUTIONS IN WHICH HE HOLDS OR ANTICIPATES HOLDING ANY FORM OF STAFF PRIVILEGE A COPY OF THIS ORDER; SHALL REQUEST ALL HEALTH CARE FACILITIES IN WHICH HE ANTICIPATES PRACTICING TO FURNISH A STATEMENT REGARDING MONITORING OF HIS PRACTICE; SHALL SUBMIT BIOLOGICAL FLUID SPECIMENS; SHALL NOT PRESCRIBE, ADMINISTER OR DISPENSE ANY MEDICATIONS FOR HIS PERSONAL USE AND SHALL TAKE NONE UNLESS AUTHORIZED BY ANOTHER PHYSICIAN FOR A LEGITIMATE MEDICAL NEED; SHALL NOT INGEST ANY SUBSTANCE WHICH WILL CAUSE A SPECIMEN TO TEST POSITIVE FOR PROHIBITED SUBSTANCES; WILL COMPLY WITH THE RECOMMENDATIONS OF AND ABIDE BY THE TERMS CONTAINED IN THE POST-CARE CONTRACT FROM THE WILLIAM J. FARLEY CENTER, AND WILL UNDERTAKE ALL NECESSARY OR RECOMMENDED SUBSEQUENT TREATMENT; WILL AFFILIATE WITH AA AND THE OKLAHOMA MEDICAL ASSOCIATION PHYSICIAN RECOVERY PROGRAM WITH REPORTS TO THE BOARD UPON REQUEST, AND SUBMIT MONTHLY SELF-REPORTS ON HIS PROGRESS AND ATTENDANCE; SHALL EXECUTE ALL RELEASES OF MEDICAL AND PSYCHIATRIC RECORDS AS NECESSARY TO DISCUSS HIS CASE WITH HIS TREATING PHYSICIANS AND/OR ANY PHYSICIANS HOLDING RECORDS; SHALL KEEP THE BOARD INFORMED OF HIS ADDRESS.

CAVENDER, LUNDY E JR MD, LICENSE NUMBER 00H7711 OF FORT WORTH, TX, WAS DISCIPLINED BY TEXAS ON MAY 11, 1995
DISCIPLINARY ACTION: 60-MONTH PROBATION; RESTRICTION PLACED ON LICENSE
OFFENSE: LOSS OR RESTRICTION OF HOSPITAL PRIVILEGES

NOTES: BETWEEN APPROXIMATELY THE FALL OF 1990 AND 11/93, ENGAGED IN INAPPROPRIATE PHYSICAL CONTACT WITH THE MOTHERS OF VARIOUS PEDIATRIC PATIENTS WHICH INCLUDED IN SOME INSTANCES KISSING, HUGGING AND OTHER INAPPROPRIATE TOUCHING; IN 5/94, HOSPITAL PRIVILEGES WERE SUSPENDED AND HE WAS ADMITTED TO TREATMENT PROGRAM TO ADDRESS ISSUES OF SEXUAL COMPULSIVITY; SUSPENSION OF HOSPITAL PRIVILEGES WAS LIFTED UPON COMPLETION OF TREATMENT AND HE WAS PLACED ON A TWO YEAR PROBATION PERIOD WITH RESTRICTIONS INCLUDING A CHAPERONE REQUIREMENT; HAS ENTERED INTO A PROFESSIONAL RE-ENTRY PLAN WITH A TREATING PSYCHIATRIST INCLUDING PRACTICE REVIEW AND A 12-STEP RECOVERY PROGRAM FOR SEXUAL ADDICTION. SUSPENSION STAYED. PROBATION WITH TERMS: SHALL SUBMIT HIMSELF FOR EVALUATION AND TREATMENT BY A BOARD-APPROVED PSYCHIATRIST AT LEAST ONCE A MONTH WHO SHALL SUBMIT REPORTS TO THE BOARD; SHALL HAVE A CHAPERONE PRESENT ANYTIME HE PERFORMS A PHYSICAL EXAMINATION ON ANY PATIENT; SHALL COMPLY WITH ALL TERMS OF THE PROFESSIONAL RE-ENTRY PLAN AND THE AGREEMENT FOR HOSPITAL PRIVILEGES; SHALL MAINTAIN ADEQUATE MEDICAL RECORDS WHICH SHALL BE AVAILABLE FOR REVIEW; SHALL APPEAR BEFORE BOARD AT LEAST ONCE EACH YEAR OR AT BOARD REQUEST; SHALL FULLY COOPERATE WITH BOARD IN VERIFYING COMPLIANCE INCLUDING PROVIDING ANY MEDICAL RELEASES AND PEER REVIEW RECORDS UPON REQUEST; SHALL GIVE A COPY OF THIS ORDER TO ANY HEALTH CARE ENTITY WHERE HE HAS PRIVILEGES; TIME PERIOD OUT OF TEXAS DOES NOT COUNT TOWARD PROBATION; SHALL INFORM BOARD OF CHANGE OF ADDRESS WITHIN 10 DAYS OR IF HE LEAVES THE STATE. SHALL NOT SEEK MODIFICATION FOR ONE YEAR. ON 8/22/98 ORDER TERMINATED.

CAVENDER, LUNDY E JR MD OF FORT WORTH, TX, WAS DISCIPLINED BY LOUISIANA ON DECEMBER 7, 1995
DISCIPLINARY ACTION: 60-MONTH PROBATION; RESTRICTION PLACED ON LICENSE
OFFENSE: DISCIPLINARY ACTION BY ANOTHER STATE OR AGENCY

NOTES: ACTION IN TEXAS. PROHIBITED FROM PRACTICING IN LOUISIANA DURING PROBATION; SHALL COMPLY WITH THE TEXAS PROBATIONARY ORDER; SHALL APPEAR BEFORE THE BOARD PRIOR TO PRACTICING IN LOUISIANA.

CAVENDER, LUNDY E JR MD, LICENSE NUMBER 0013744 OF 11803 S FREEWAY #204, FORT WORTH, TX, WAS DISCIPLINED BY OKLAHOMA ON DECEMBER 21, 1995
DISCIPLINARY ACTION: EMERGENCY SUSPENSION
OFFENSE: DISCIPLINARY ACTION BY ANOTHER STATE OR AGENCY

NOTES: ON 5/11/95 TEXAS BOARD PLACED LICENSE ON PROBATION BASED ON HIS ENGAGING IN INAPPROPRIATE PHYSICAL CONDUCT WITH MOTHERS OF PEDIATRIC PATIENTS; TWO HOSPITALS TEMPORARILY SUSPENDED PRIVILEGES AS A RESULT OF THIS CONDUCT.

CAVENDER, LUNDY E JR MD, LICENSE NUMBER 0013744 OF 11803 S. FREEWAY, SUITE 204, OKLAHOMA CITY, OK, WAS DISCIPLINED BY OKLAHOMA ON JANUARY 25, 1996
DISCIPLINARY ACTION: LICENSE REVOCATION
OFFENSE: DISCIPLINARY ACTION BY ANOTHER STATE OR AGENCY

NOTES: ACTION IN TEXAS ON 5/11/95 PLACING HIM ON FIVE YEAR PROBATION. THIS ORDER STATED THAT HE ENGAGED IN INAPPROPRIATE PHYSICAL CONTACT WITH MOTHERS OF VARIOUS PEDIATRIC PATIENTS. AS A RESULT OF HIS CONDUCT, HUGULEY HOSPITAL AND HARRIS SOUTHWEST HOSPITAL TEMPORARILY SUSPENDED HIS LICENSE.

CHANDLER, HAROLD MULLINS MD, LICENSE NUMBER 0007636 OF 11101 MAPLE GROVE, OKLAHOMA CITY, OK, WAS DISCIPLINED BY OKLAHOMA ON MAY 20, 1993
DISCIPLINARY ACTION: 12-MONTH LICENSE SUSPENSION
OFFENSE: SUBSTANCE ABUSE

NOTES: IN 1992 WAS USING ALCOHOL IN EXCESSIVE AMOUNTS AND IN 9/92 ADMITTED HIMSELF FOR ASSESSMENT AND TREATMENT; CONTINUED OUTPATIENT TREATMENT INCLUDING AA PARTICIPATION, PSYCHIATRIC TREATMENT AND ADDITIONAL HOSPITALIZATION; ALSO WAS DIAGNOSED WITH A BRAIN TUMOR AND UNDERWENT SURGERY FOR REMOVAL. WHEN HE APPLIES FOR REINSTATEMENT MUST PROVIDE COPIES OF ALL EVALUATIONS, REPORTS AND PROGNOSIS FROM RECOVERY CENTER AND EVALUATIONS OF RECOVERY FROM BRAIN SURGERY.

CHANDLER, HAROLD MULLINS MD, LICENSE NUMBER 0007636, WAS DISCIPLINED BY OKLAHOMA ON FEBRUARY 17, 1994
DISCIPLINARY ACTION: 60-MONTH PROBATION; RESTRICTION PLACED ON LICENSE

NOTES: IN COMPLIANCE WITH 5/14/93 SUSPENSION ORDER HAS COMPLETED IN-PATIENT EVALUATION AND TREATMENT AND PROVIDED DISCHARGE SUMMARY AND LETTERS OF SUPPORT AND AN MRI DATED 2/2/94. LICENSE REINSTATED FROM SUSPENSION. PROBATION TO BEGIN 2/11/94. CONDITIONS OF

PROBATION: SHALL MEET REGULARLY WITH PHYSICIAN RECOVERY COMMITTEE; SHALL NOT PRESCRIBE, ADMINISTER OR DISPENSE ANY MEDICATIONS FOR HIS PERSONAL USE AND TAKE NO MEDICATION UNLESS IT IS AUTHORIZED BY ANOTHER PHYSICIAN FOR A LEGITIMATE MEDICAL NEED; SHALL ABSTAIN FROM THE CONSUMPTION OF ALCOHOL OR ANY SUBSTANCE WHICH WOULD ADVERSELY AFFECT HIS ABILITY TO PRACTICE MEDICINE; SHALL NOT INGEST ANY SUBSTANCE THAT WOULD TEST POSITIVE FOR ALCOHOL OR ANY CONTROLLED SUBSTANCE; SHALL SUBMIT BIOLOGICAL FLUID SPECIMENS; SHALL HAVE HIS PHYSICIAN MONITOR LITHIUM LEVELS AND PROVIDE QUARTERLY REPORTS; SHALL PRACTICE UNDER A BOARD-APPROVED MONITOR; SHALL HAVE HIS PATIENTS SIGN A PATIENT'S RIGHTS STATEMENT; SHALL FURNISH BOARD WITH ADDRESS AND/OR CHANGE OF ADDRESS; SHALL APPEAR BEFORE THE BOARD UPON REQUEST AND PROVIDE REQUIRED REPORTS; SHALL PAY COSTS; SHALL SUPPLY A COPY OF THIS ORDER TO ANY HEALTH CARE ENTITY WHERE HE HAS PRIVILEGES; SHALL NOT SUPERVISE A PHYSICIAN'S ASSISTANT.

CHANDLER, HAROLD MULLINS MD, LICENSE NUMBER 00H5382 OF BEAUMONT, TX, WAS DISCIPLINED BY TEXAS ON APRIL 15, 1994
DISCIPLINARY ACTION: 60-MONTH PROBATION; REQUIRED TO TAKE ADDITIONAL MEDICAL EDUCATION
OFFENSE: DISCIPLINARY ACTION BY ANOTHER STATE OR AGENCY

NOTES: ON 5/20/93 OKLAHOMA SUSPENDED HIS LICENSE FOR ONE YEAR BASED ON INTEMPERATE USE OF ALCOHOL; ADMITS HE IS AN ALCOHOLIC AND HAS SOUGHT IN-PATIENT TREATMENT ON HIS OWN INITIATIVE IN THE PAST; HAS BEEN SOBER SINCE 9/8/92; HE IS CURRENTLY PRACTICING PSYCHIATRY IN TEXAS AND BEING TREATED BY HIS PHYSICIAN IN OKLAHOMA; OKLAHOMA REINSTATED HIS LICENSE ON PROBATION ON 2/11/94. SUSPENSION STAYED. CONDITIONS OF PROBATION: SHALL ABSTAIN FROM THE CONSUMPTION OF ALCOHOL/CHEMICAL SUBSTANCES IN ANY FORM UNLESS PRESCRIBED BY ANOTHER PHYSICIAN FOR A LEGITIMATE AND THERAPEUTIC PURPOSE; SHALL NOT TREAT OR OTHERWISE SERVE AS PHYSICIAN, PRESCRIBE, DISPENSE OR ADMINISTER DRUGS THAT MAY BE SUBJECT TO ABUSE TO HIMSELF OR ANY MEMBER OF HIS FAMILY; SHALL SUBMIT HIMSELF FOR APPROPRIATE EXAMS INCLUDING DRUG AND ALCOHOL SCREENS; SHALL PARTICIPATE IN AA'S PROGRAM NOT LESS THAN TWO TIMES A WEEK WITH QUARTERLY REPORTS TO THE BOARD; SHALL CONTINUE TREATMENT WITH HIS PRESENT PHYSICIAN AND MONITORING WITH HIS PRESENT SUPERVISOR WITH QUARTERLY REPORTS; SHALL ATTEND AT LEAST 50 HOURS PER YEAR OF CONTINUING MEDICAL EDUCATION INCLUDING COURSES ADDRESSING ADDICTIONOLOGY, DRUG ABUSE, AND CO-DEPENDENCY; SHALL PERFORM TWO HOURS PER WEEK OF COMMUNITY SERVICE FOR FIVE YEARS; SHALL FOLLOW ALL TERMS OF OKLAHOMA ORDER AND PROVIDE TEXAS BOARD ALL DOCUMENTS SUBMITTED TO OKLAHOMA BOARD; SHALL APPEAR BEFORE THE BOARD TWICE A YEAR; SHALL GIVE A COPY OF THIS ORDER TO ANY HEALTH CARE ENTITY WHERE HE HAS PRIVILEGES; SHALL COOPERATE WITH THE BOARD IN VERIFYING COMPLIANCE; SHALL INFORM BOARD OF CHANGE OF ADDRESS WITHIN 10 DAYS OR IF HE LEAVES THE STATE; TIME SPENT OUT OF TEXAS DOES NOT COUNT TOWARD PROBATION. SHALL NOT SEEK MODIFICATION FOR ONE YEAR. ON 5/11/95 REQUEST FOR TERMINATION DENIED AND ORDER MODIFIED AS FOLLOWS: NO LONGER HAS TO CONTINUE TO RECEIVE TREATMENT FROM BOARD APPROVED PHYSICIAN; NO LONGER HAS TO PERFORM TWO HOURS PER WEEK OF COMMUNITY SERVICE; SHALL APPEAR BEFORE THE BOARD AT LEAST ONE TIME PER YEAR; ALL OTHER CONDITIONS REMAIN IN EFFECT.

CHANG, JONATHAN H MD, LICENSE NUMBER 0016997 OF 6602 59TH ST. COURT WEST, TACOMA, WA, WAS DISCIPLINED BY OKLAHOMA ON OCTOBER 22, 1995
DISCIPLINARY ACTION: LICENSE REVOCATION
OFFENSE: DISCIPLINARY ACTION BY ANOTHER STATE OR AGENCY

NOTES: ON 11/23/93 THE UNITED STATES ARMY REVOKED HIS CLINICAL PRIVILEGES FOR HIS UNSATISFACTORY PERFORMANCE OF HIS DUTIES AS AN ANESTHESIOLOGIST.

CHOUTEAU, ROBERT MICHAEL DO, LICENSE NUMBER 00E9578 OF DALLAS, TX, WAS DISCIPLINED BY TEXAS ON JANUARY 6, 1995
DISCIPLINARY ACTION: REPRIMAND
OFFENSE: NONCOMPLIANCE WITH A PROFESSIONAL RULE

NOTES: INADEQUATELY DOCUMENTED THE CARE AND TREATMENT OF A PATIENT. SHALL GIVE A COPY OF THIS ORDER TO ANY HEALTH CARE ENTITY WHERE HE HAS PRIVILEGES.

CHOUTEAU, ROBERT MICHAEL DO, LICENSE NUMBER 0001998, WAS DISCIPLINED BY OKLAHOMA ON APRIL 2, 1996
DISCIPLINARY ACTION: REPRIMAND
OFFENSE: DISCIPLINARY ACTION BY ANOTHER STATE OR AGENCY

NOTES: ON 1/06/95 THE TEXAS BOARD ORDERED A PUBLIC REPRIMAND FOR FAILING TO ADEQUATELY DOCUMENT CARE AND TREATMENT RENDERED. SHALL GIVE A COPY OF THIS ORDER TO ANY HEALTH CARE ENTITY WHERE HE HAS PRIVILEGES; SHALL APPEAR BEFORE THE BOARD BEFORE PRACTICING IN OKLAHOMA; $925 ADMINISTRATIVE COSTS.

CLARAVALL, LEONARDO H MD, LICENSE NUMBER 10412 OF 100 W RIDGEWOOD DRIVE, MIDWEST CITY, OK, WAS DISCIPLINED BY OKLAHOMA ON JANUARY 23, 1998
DISCIPLINARY ACTION: 2-MONTH LICENSE SUSPENSION; 60-MONTH PROBATION
OFFENSE: PROFESSIONAL MISCONDUCT

NOTES: FROM 1994-96 HE OPERATED AND MAINTAINED A CLINIC LOCATED IN DEL CITY, OKLAHOMA, PRIMARILY TREATING PATIENTS FOR WEIGHT LOSS WHICH REGULARLY DISPENSED CONTROLLED DRUGS, INCLUDING PHENTERMINE, PONDIMIN, AND PHENDIMETRAZINE, AMONG OTHERS, TO PATIENTS; ON OCCASION, HE ALLOWED HIS SISTERS TO HOLD THEMSELVES OUT TO PATIENTS AS BEING LICENSED MEDICAL DOCTORS, SEE AND EXAMINE PATIENTS, AND DISPENSE MEDICATION TO PATIENTS. THIS WAS DONE PRIMARILY WHEN HE WAS NOT ON THE PREMISES. THEY CHARGED PATIENTS FOR MEDICAL SERVICES RENDERED AND FOR CONTROLLED AND NON-CONTROLLED DRUGS THAT WERE DISPENSED WITHIN THE CLINIC BY THEMSELVES. AT TIMES, HE ALLOWED HIS BROTHER-IN-LAW TO EXAMINE PATIENTS AND DISPENSE MEDICATION, REPRESENTING HIMSELF TO BE A DOCTOR, WHEN IN FACT HE WAS NOT. HE EASED THIS MANNER OF PRACTICE IN 8/96, AND, SINCE THAT TIME, HAS OPERATED HIS CLINIC IN A LEGAL AND ACCEPTABLE MANNER. CONDITIONS OF PROBATION: SHALL SUBMIT TO AND MAKE HIMSELF AVAILABLE FOR ALL TYPES OF MONITORING DEEMED APPROPRIATE BY THE BOARD; MUST BE PHYSICALLY PRESENT DURING THE

EXAMINATION OF PATIENTS, CONDUCT THE EXAMINATION AND EVALUATION AND PRESCRIBE AND DEVISE ALL TREATMENT PLANS; SHALL ENSURE THAT ONLY HEALTH CARE PROFESSIONALS WHO ARE LICENSED IN OKLAHOMA WILL ASSIST IN THE EXAM, CARE, AND TREATMENT OF PATIENTS; NO MODIFICATIONS IN MEDICATIONS PRESCRIBED BY HIM SHALL EVER BE MADE WITHOUT HIS PERSONALLY SEEING AND EXAMINING THE PATIENT, AND PERSONALLY MODIFYING THE TREATMENT PLANS AND/OR PRESCRIPTIONS; SHALL IMMEDIATELY DIVEST HIMSELF OF ALL QUANTITIES OF WEIGHT-CONTROL MEDICATIONS NOW IN HIS POSSESSION AND/OR CONTROL BY DELIVERING ALL SUCH QUANTITIES TO THE FEDERAL DRUG ENFORCEMENT AGENCY OR THE OKLAHOMA BUREAU OF NARCOTICS AND DANGEROUS DRUGS; SHALL NOT ADMINISTER AND/OR DISPENSE ANY CONTROLLED SUBSTANCES FOR WEIGHT CONTROL PROBLEMS TO ANY PATIENTS; RATHER, THE ONLY METHOD BY WHICH HE WILL MAKE CONTROLLED SUBSTANCES FOR WEIGHT PROBLEMS AVAILABLE TO HIS PATIENTS IS BY MEANS OF WRITTEN OR TELEPHONE CALL-IN PRESCRIPTIONS, PERSONALLY MADE BY HIM; THESE PRESCRIPTIONS WILL BE KEPT ON DUPLICATE NUMERICALLY SEQUENTIAL PRESCRIPTION ORDERS AND WILL BE AVAILABLE FOR REVIEW BY THE BOARD UPON REQUEST; SHALL KEEP THE BOARD INFORMED OF HIS ADDRESS AND PAY COSTS; SHALL MAKE ALL PATIENT RECORDS AVAILABLE TO THE BOARD UPON REQUEST; SHALL APPEAR BEFORE THE BOARD UPON REQUEST.

CLARK, FRANK WILSON MD, LICENSE NUMBER 0006326, WAS DISCIPLINED BY OKLAHOMA ON MARCH 16, 1991
DISCIPLINARY ACTION: SURRENDER OF CONTROLLED SUBSTANCE LICENSE; 36-MONTH PROBATION

NOTES: PROBATION UNDER FOLLOWING TERMS AND CONDITIONS: HE MAY NOT PRESCRIBE, ADMINISTER, OR DISPENSE ANY SCHEDULED DRUGS OR CONTROLLED DANGEROUS SUBSTANCES; MAY PRESCRIBE OTHER NON-SCHEDULED DRUGS ONLY ON DUPLICATE PRESCRIPTION PADS; SHALL IMMEDIATELY SURRENDER HIS REGISTRATION FOR CONTROLLED DANGEROUS SUBSTANCES UNTIL PROBATIONARY TERM HAS EXPIRED; SHALL LIMIT AND SCHEDULE HIS PROFESSIONAL ACTIVITIES TO ALLOW ADEQUATE TIME FOR PATIENT RECORD-KEEPING; SHALL BE REEVALUATED BY BOARD IN ONE YEAR; SHALL FURNISH BOARD WITH ADDRESS AND/OR CHANGE OF ADDRESS; SHALL APPEAR BEFORE BOARD UPON REQUEST.

CLEAVER, EDGAR MD OF 1795 EAST 71ST STREET, TULSA, OK, WAS DISCIPLINED BY DEA ON MAY 31, 1995
DISCIPLINARY ACTION: SURRENDER OF CONTROLLED SUBSTANCE LICENSE
OFFENSE: DISCIPLINARY ACTION BY ANOTHER STATE OR AGENCY

NOTES: STATE BOARD.

CLEAVER, EDGAR M MD, LICENSE NUMBER 0012107 OF 3442 E 8TH PLACE, TULSA, OK, WAS DISCIPLINED BY OKLAHOMA ON MAY 19, 1995
DISCIPLINARY ACTION: SURRENDER OF CONTROLLED SUBSTANCE LICENSE; 60-MONTH PROBATION
OFFENSE: SEXUAL ABUSE OF OR SEXUAL MISCONDUCT WITH A PATIENT

NOTES: FROM ABOUT 1992 UNTIL MAY 1995 HE PRESCRIBED, ADMINISTERED, DISTRIBUTED, OR ORDERED CONTROLLED DANGEROUS SUBSTANCES OR DRUGS RECOGNIZED AS ADDICTIVE OR DANGEROUS FOR REASONS OTHER THAN MEDICALLY ACCEPTED THERAPEUTIC PURPOSES TO PERSONS WHO ARE ADDICTED, HABITUATED, OR CHEMICALLY DEPENDENT; DURING 1994 HE MAINTAINED A ROMANTIC RELATIONSHIP WITH A DRUG DEPENDENT PATIENT TO WHOM HE PRESCRIBED CONTROLLED DANGEROUS SUBSTANCES. PROBATION UNDER THE FOLLOWING TERMS AND CONDITIONS: WILL IMMEDIATELY SURRENDER TO THE PROPER AUTHORITIES ANY PERMIT POSSESSED BY HIM TO ALLOW HIS PRESCRIPTION, SALE, ADMINISTRATION, DISTRIBUTION, OR ORDER OF CONTROLLED DANGEROUS DRUGS, SPECIFICALLY TO INCLUDE, BUT NOT LIMITED TO HIS OKLAHOMA BUREAU OF NARCOTICS AND DANGEROUS DRUGS PERMIT AND HIS UNITED STATES DRUG ENFORCEMENT ADMINISTRATION PERMIT; SHALL NOT PRESCRIBE, ADMINISTER, OR DISPENSE ANY CONTROLLED DANGEROUS SUBSTANCES; SHALL APPEAR BEFORE THE BOARD UPON REQUEST AND SUBMIT ANY REQUIRED REPORTS; SHALL PAY COSTS; SHALL NOTIFY ANY HOSPITAL WHERE HE HOLDS STAFF PRIVILEGES, OR CLINIC, OR GROUP WHERE HE PRACTICES OF THE TERMS AND CONDITIONS OF THIS ORDER AND PROVIDE A COPY THEREOF; SHALL NOT SUPERVISE A PHYSICIAN ASSISTANT; SHALL MEET NO LESS THAN QUARTERLY WITH THE BOARD AND DURING SUCH MEETINGS SHALL PROVIDE ANY AND ALL CHARTS AND PATIENT RECORDS UPON REQUEST; SHALL IMMEDIATELY TERMINATE HIS PERSONAL RELATIONSHIP WITH THE PATIENT REFERRED TO ABOVE AND REFRAIN PERMANENTLY FROM RE-ENGAGING IN SUCH RELATIONSHIP; REPRIMAND. ON 5/10/96 ORDER MODIFIED SUCH THAT HE MAY APPLY FOR PERMITS FROM OKLAHOMA BUREAU OF NARCOTICS AND DANGEROUS DRUGS AND THE DRUG ENFORCEMENT ADMINISTRATION; SHALL NOT PRESCRIBE, ADMINISTER OR DISPENSE CONTROLLED DANGEROUS SUBSTANCES WITHOUT PROPER PERMITS; MAY WRITE PRESCRIPTIONS FOR SPECIFIED DRUGS ON SERIALLY NUMBERED DUPLICATE PRESCRIPTION PADS TO BE SUBMITTED MONTHLY; ALL OTHER CONDITIONS OF THIS ORDER REMAIN IN EFFECT.

CLEAVER, EDGAR M MD, WAS DISCIPLINED BY NEBRASKA ON MAY 12, 1998
DISCIPLINARY ACTION: RESTRICTION PLACED ON LICENSE; REPRIMAND
OFFENSE: DISCIPLINARY ACTION BY ANOTHER STATE OR AGENCY

NOTES: OTHER STATE ACTION.

CLEAVER, EDGAR M MD, LICENSE NUMBER 16375 OF TULSA, OK, WAS DISCIPLINED BY IOWA ON AUGUST 26, 1999
DISCIPLINARY ACTION: PROBATION; RESTRICTION PLACED ON LICENSE
OFFENSE: DISCIPLINARY ACTION BY ANOTHER STATE OR AGENCY

NOTES: ON OR ABOUT 5/13/95, OKLAHOMA PLACED HIS LICENSE ON PROBATION FOR FIVE YEARS UNDER CERTAIN TERMS AND CONDITIONS FOR INAPPROPRIATELY PRESCRIBING CONTROLLED SUBSTANCES AND ENGAGING IN A ROMANTIC RELATIONSHIP WITH A PATIENT; HE FAILED TO NOTIFY IOWA OF SAID ACTION. HIS IOWA MEDICAL LICENSE SHALL BE ON PROBATION FOR A PERIOD OF TIME CONCURRENT WITH THE OKLAHOMA BOARD, UNDER THE FOLLOWING TERMS AND CONDITIONS: WHILE ENGAGED IN THE PRACTICE OF MEDICINE IN OKLAHOMA HE SHALL COMPLY WITH ALL TERMS AND CONDITIONS OF THE 5/13/95 ORDER; SHALL NOTIFY

THE BOARD IN WRITING AND PROVIDE DOCUMENTATION FROM THE OKLAHOMA BOARD UPON SUCCESSFUL COMPLETION OF THE TERMS OF THE OKLAHOMA ORDER; SHOULD HE ELECT TO ENGAGE IN THE PRACTICE OF MEDICINE IN IOWA DURING THE TIME OF PROBATION HE SHALL, NOT LESS THAN 30 DAYS PRIOR TO BEGINNING PRACTICE, NOTIFY THE BOARD IN WRITING OF HIS INTENDED PRACTICE LOCATION. UPON BEGINNING PRACTICE IN IOWA: SHALL BE PROHIBITED FROM PRESCRIBING, ADMINISTERING OR DISPENSING ANY CONTROLLED SUBSTANCES; SHALL REFRAIN FROM ENGAGING IN A ROMANTIC OR SEXUAL RELATIONSHIP WITH ANY PATIENT; SHALL INFORM ANY FUTURE EMPLOYER, HOSPITAL, CLINIC OR GROUP WITH WHICH HE PRACTICES OF THIS ORDER; SHALL NOT SUPERVISE A PHYSICIAN ASSISTANT; SHALL FILE SWORN QUARTERLY REPORTS TO THE BOARD ATTESTING TO HIS COMPLIANCE WITH ALL THE TERMS AND CONDITIONS OF THIS ORDER; SHALL MAKE APPEARANCES BEFORE THE BOARD ANNUALLY OR UPON REQUEST.

COFFMAN, RICHARD D DO, LICENSE NUMBER 0002778, WAS DISCIPLINED BY OKLAHOMA ON JUNE 20, 1996
DISCIPLINARY ACTION: 12-MONTH PROBATION; REPRIMAND
OFFENSE: OVERPRESCRIBING OR MISPRESCRIBING DRUGS

NOTES: BETWEEN 10/28/95 AND 3/23/96 FAILED TO ESTABLISH A LEGITIMATE PHYSICIAN/PATIENT RELATIONSHIP WITH TWO PATIENTS FOR WHOM HE IS THE LEGAL GUARDIAN WHEN HE ISSUED PRESCRIPTIONS FOR SOMA, VALIUM, AND DHC PLUS; FAILED TO UNDERTAKE A SUFFICIENT EXAMINATION FOR TWO PATIENTS BEFORE PRESCRIBING DRUGS; FAILED TO KEEP COMPLETE AND/OR ACCURATE MEDICAL RECORDS OF THE DISPOSAL OF THESE PRESCRIPTION DRUGS TO TWO PATIENTS. SHALL ATTEND AND SUCCESSFULLY COMPLETE A COURSE ENTITLED "THE PROPER PRESCRIBING OF CONTROLLED DANGEROUS SUBSTANCES" AND SHALL REPORT SUCCESSFUL COMPLETION OF THAT COURSE TO THE BOARD; $725 ADMINISTRATIVE COSTS; MAY NOT PETITION THE BOARD FOR MODIFICATION OF THIS ORDER; SHALL APPEAR BEFORE THE BOARD UPON REQUEST.

COFFMAN, RICHARD D DO OF 5350 SOUTH WESTERN #555, OKLAHOMA CITY, OK, WAS DISCIPLINED BY DEA ON APRIL 9, 1998
DISCIPLINARY ACTION: SURRENDER OF CONTROLLED SUBSTANCE LICENSE

NOTES: IN LIEU OF PUBLIC INTEREST REVOCATION.

COFFMAN, RICHARD D DO, LICENSE NUMBER 2778, WAS DISCIPLINED BY OKLAHOMA ON SEPTEMBER 17, 1998
DISCIPLINARY ACTION: 60-MONTH PROBATION

COLE, GEORGE MARTIN DO, LICENSE NUMBER 00F5175 OF AMARILLO, TX, WAS DISCIPLINED BY TEXAS ON NOVEMBER 13, 1992
DISCIPLINARY ACTION: 36-MONTH RESTRICTION PLACED ON LICENSE

NOTES: PROFESSIONAL FAILURE TO PRACTICE MEDICINE IN AN ACCEPTABLE MANNER CONSISTENT WITH PUBLIC HEALTH AND WELFARE. ON 6/28/95 HIS PETITION FOR TERMINATION WAS DENIED.

COLE, GEORGE MARTIN DO, LICENSE NUMBER 0002071, WAS DISCIPLINED BY OKLAHOMA ON JANUARY 11, 1994
DISCIPLINARY ACTION: RESTRICTION PLACED ON LICENSE; MONITORING OF PHYSICIAN PERFORMANCE
OFFENSE: DISCIPLINARY ACTION BY ANOTHER STATE OR AGENCY

NOTES: ON 11/13/92 HIS TEXAS LICENSE TO PRACTICE OSTEOPATHIC MEDICINE WAS RESTRICTED FOR THREE YEARS UNDER TERMS AND CONDITIONS. OKLAHOMA LICENSE PLACED ON INDEFINITE RESTRICTION UNDER THE FOLLOWING TERMS AND CONDITIONS: SHALL NOT PETITION THE BOARD FOR A MODIFICATION FOR AT LEAST ONE YEAR; SHALL NOT PERFORM CERVICAL SPINE SURGERY IN OKLAHOMA; SHALL NOTIFY AND PROVIDE A COPY OF THIS ORDER TO ALL HEALTH CARE ENTITIES WHERE HE HAS PRIVILEGES; SHALL NOTIFY THE BOARD IN WRITING OF ANY CHANGES IN ADDRESS, EMPLOYMENT, EMPLOYMENT TERMINATION OR HOSPITAL OR HEALTH CARE ENTITIES PRIVILEGE RESTRICTION OR ANY ADMINISTRATIVE PROCEEDING INITIATED AGAINST HIM BY ANY OTHER STATE OR FEDERAL REGULATORY BODY WITHIN 14 DAYS OF SUCH ACTION; SHALL COOPERATE WITH THE BOARD AND PROVIDE ANY REQUIRED REPORTS; MUST APPEAR BEFORE THE BOARD PRIOR TO PRACTICING IN OKLAHOMA WITH HIS PLANS AND HIS COMPLIANCE WITH THE TERMS AND CONDITIONS OF THE TEXAS ORDER; SHALL PAY THE COST OF ADMINISTRATIVE PROCEEDING OF $1,525.50.

COLE, GEORGE MARTIN DO, LICENSE NUMBER F5175 OF AMARILLO, TX, WAS DISCIPLINED BY TEXAS ON AUGUST 9, 1997
DISCIPLINARY ACTION: RESTRICTION PLACED ON LICENSE
OFFENSE: SUBSTANDARD CARE, INCOMPETENCE OR NEGLIGENCE

NOTES: FROM APPROXIMATELY 1991 THROUGH APPROXIMATELY 1995, HE PERFORMED VARIOUS BACK, KNEE AND ANKLE SURGERIES WHICH RESULTED IN ADVERSE MEDICAL OUTCOMES, INCLUDING REQUIRING SEVERAL PATIENTS TO UNDERGO ADDITIONAL SURGERIES BY OTHER PHYSICIANS TO CORRECT HIS ALLEGED SURGICAL DEFICIENCIES; HE REPORTS THAT HE VOLUNTARILY CEASED PERFORMING SURGERIES IN 6/95, DUE TO THE CHANGE IN HIS PRACTICE PHILOSOPHY AND HIS EMPHASIS ON PREVENTATIVE MEDICINE; HE DENIES THE CHARGES. HE SHALL NOT PERFORM ANY INVASIVE SURGICAL PROCEDURE AS DEFINED IN THE ORDER; SHALL COOPERATE WITH THE BOARD IN VERIFYING COMPLIANCE INCLUDING PROVIDING COPIES OF MEDICAL RELEASES UPON REQUEST; SHALL GIVE A COPY OF THIS ORDER TO ANY HEALTH CARE ENTITY WHERE HE HAS PRIVILEGES; SHALL PROVIDE A COPY OF THIS ORDER TO ANYONE REQUESTING IT WITHIN 10 DAYS; SHALL INFORM THE BOARD OF CHANGE OF ADDRESS WITHIN 10 DAYS; SHALL NOT SEEK MODIFICATION FOR ONE YEAR; SHALL APPEAR BEFORE THE BOARD UPON REQUEST.

COLLAZO, LUIS, WAS DISCIPLINED BY OKLAHOMA ON JANUARY 27, 1995
DISCIPLINARY ACTION: DENIAL OF NEW LICENSE

NOTES: FAILED THE FLEX EXAM REPEATEDLY AND HAD LOW GRADES IN MEDICAL SCHOOL COURSES FACTORS WHICH RAISE SERIOUS ISSUES AS TO HIS ABILITY TO PRACTICE WITH REASONABLE SKILL AND SAFETY.

COLLETT, MICHAEL G DO, LICENSE NUMBER 3107, WAS DISCIPLINED BY OKLAHOMA ON OCTOBER 23, 1996
DISCIPLINARY ACTION: SURRENDER OF LICENSE

CONLEY, RICHARD MD OF 405 NORTH HARMON STREET #400, WATONGA, OK, WAS DISCIPLINED BY DEA ON JULY 6, 1999
DISCIPLINARY ACTION: SURRENDER OF CONTROLLED SUBSTANCE

LICENSE
OFFENSE: DISCIPLINARY ACTION BY ANOTHER STATE OR AGENCY

NOTES: STATE BOARD.

CONLEY, RICHARD A MD, LICENSE NUMBER 7424, WAS DISCIPLINED BY OKLAHOMA ON MARCH 4, 1999
DISCIPLINARY ACTION: LICENSE REVOCATION
OFFENSE: SUBSTANDARD CARE, INCOMPETENCE OR NEGLIGENCE

NOTES: UNPROFESSIONAL CONDUCT IN SIX PATIENT CASES BETWEEN 3/95 AND 12/97 INCLUDING FAILED TO PROPERLY DIAGNOSE, TREAT AND CARE FOR: A PATIENT WHO SUBSEQUENTLY DIED FROM POST-SURGICAL COMPLICATIONS, A FEMALE WHO UNDERWENT A HYSTERECTOMY WHEREIN HER URETERS WERE OBSTRUCTED DUE TO SUTURE PLACEMENT PREVENTING HER FROM URINATING, A PATIENT WHO SUFFERED A MYOCARDIAL INFARCTION WHICH WENT UNTREATED AND LED TO HIS DEATH SHORTLY THEREAFTER, A PATIENT WHO UNDERWENT A HERNIA OPERATION WHEREIN HIS BLADDER WAS INADVERTENTLY PERFORATED SEVERAL TIMES, A CEREBRAL PALSY PATIENT WHO SUFFERED A WRIST FRACTURE WITH TWO UNSUCCESSFUL REDUCTIONS ATTEMPTED; AND ANOTHER PATIENT WHO WAS TREATED FOR NICOTINE DEPENDENCE DESPITE THE FACT HE HAD NOT SMOKED IN OVER 10 YEARS. SHALL PAY COSTS.

CONLEY, ROBERT L MD OF 2808 S. SHERIDAN ROAD, TULSA, OK, WAS DISCIPLINED BY DEA ON SEPTEMBER 21, 1994
DISCIPLINARY ACTION: RESTRICTION PLACED ON CONTROLLED SUBSTANCE LICENSE
OFFENSE: SUBSTANCE ABUSE

CONLEY, ROBERT LEE MD OF 3101 TWIN CIRCLE, MOORE, OK, WAS DISCIPLINED BY OKLAHOMA ON DECEMBER 2, 1993
DISCIPLINARY ACTION: DENIAL OF LICENSE REINSTATEMENT

NOTES: HAD PREVIOUSLY OBTAINED A SUPERVISED MEDICAL DOCTOR CERTIFICATE; HAS NOT YET COMPLETED ONE YEAR OF SUCCESSFUL WORK UNDER THIS CERTIFICATE AND THERE IS NO SUBSTANTIAL CHANGE IN HIS STATUS. ANY CONSIDERATION OF AN APPLICATION FOR REINSTATEMENT IS PREMATURE AT THIS TIME. HIS SUPERVISED MEDICAL DOCTOR CERTIFICATE REMAINS IN GOOD STANDING AND IN FULL FORCE AND EFFECT.

CONLEY, ROBERT LEE MD, LICENSE NUMBER 0012219 OF 3101 TWIN CIRCLE, OK, WAS DISCIPLINED BY OKLAHOMA ON MAY 19, 1994
DISCIPLINARY ACTION: LICENSE REINSTATEMENT; PROBATION

NOTES: FOLLOWING A HIATUS FROM PRACTICE DID OBTAIN AND DOES HOLD IN GOOD STANDING A SUPERVISED MEDICAL DOCTOR CERTIFICATE; IS NEARING COMPLETION OF PG1 TRAINING AND PURSUING TRAINING IN ADDICTIONOLOGY AND IS WORKING WITH THE PHYSICIAN RECOVERY COMMITTEE. CONDITIONS OF INDEFINITE PROBATION: SHALL NOT PRESCRIBE, ADMINISTER OR DISPENSE ANY MEDICATION FOR HIS PERSONAL USE AND SHALL TAKE NO MEDICATIONS OR ANY SUBSTANCES WHICH WILL TEST POSITIVE FOR ALCOHOL OR ANY CONTROLLED DANGEROUS SUBSTANCE UNLESS AUTHORIZED BY ANOTHER PHYSICIAN FOR A LEGITIMATE MEDICAL NEED; SHALL ABSTAIN FROM CONSUMING ALCOHOL OR ANY SUBSTANCES WHICH WOULD ADVERSELY AFFECT HIS ABILITY TO PRACTICE; SHALL SUBMIT BIOLOGICAL FLUID SPECIMENS; SHALL MAINTAIN A PROGRAM OF ABSTINENCE THROUGH PARTICIPATION WITH BOARD APPROVED GROUPS; SHALL ATTEND WEEKLY MEETINGS WITH PHYSICIAN'S RECOVERY COMMITTEE, ONE NARCOTICS MEETING PER WEEK, AND ONE AA MEETING PER WEEK; SHALL SIGN A RELEASE TO ALLOW BOARD TO OBTAIN REPORTS FROM THESE PROGRAMS; SHALL NOT RECEIVE, ACCEPT OR SIGN FOR IN ANY MANNER ANY SAMPLES OF CONTROLLED DANGEROUS SUBSTANCES; SHALL NOT ADMINISTER OR DISPENSE SCHEDULES II THROUGH V DRUGS; MAY PRESCRIBE SCHEDULES IV AND V ONLY ON SERIALLY-NUMBERED DUPLICATE PRESCRIPTION PADS WITH COPIES AVAILABLE UPON REQUEST; SHALL PRACTICE IN A CONTROLLED, BOARD-APPROVED ENVIRONMENT; SHALL NOT AUTHORIZE ANY PERSONNEL UNDER HIS SUPERVISION TO INITIATE AN ORDER FOR A PRESCRIPTION; SHALL FURNISH BOARD WITH ADDRESS AND/OR CHANGE OF ADDRESS; SHALL APPEAR BEFORE THE BOARD UPON REQUEST AND SUBMIT ANY REQUIRED REPORTS; SHALL PAY COSTS; SHALL NOTIFY ANY HEALTH CARE ENTITY WHERE HE HOLDS PRIVILEGES OF THIS ORDER; ; SHALL NOT SUPERVISE A PHYSICIAN'S ASSISTANT; SHALL COMPLETE 20 HOURS OF CONTINUING MEDICAL EDUCATION IN PHARMACOLOGY AND RELATED ISSUES WITHIN ONE YEAR. ON 9/9/94 ORDER MODIFIED SUCH THAT MEETINGS OF PHYSICIAN RECOVERY NETWORK MAY BE ANYWHERE OF HIS CHOOSING. PROBATION MODIFIED ON 10/2/95 BY ALLOWING HIM TO PRESCRIBE SCHEDULES II AND III SUBSTANCES AS WELL AS SCHEDULES IV AND V ALL ONLY ON SERIALLY-NUMBERED, DUPLICATE PRESCRIPTION PADS WITH COPIES AVAILABLE TO INVESTIGATORS.

CONWAY, JIMMY HAROLD MD, LICENSE NUMBER 0016834 OF 3301 NW 50TH, OKLAHOMA CITY, OK, WAS DISCIPLINED BY OKLAHOMA ON MARCH 8, 1996
DISCIPLINARY ACTION: EMERGENCY SUSPENSION

NOTES: 5/16/96 CONTINUANCE OF SUMMARY SUSPENSION UNTIL HEARING ON 7/25-27/96. 8/15/96 CONTINUANCE OF SUMMARY SUSPENSION UNTIL HEARING ON 9/26-28/96.

CONWAY, JIMMY HAROLD JR MD OF 3301 N.W. 50TH, OKLAHOMA CITY, OK, WAS DISCIPLINED BY DEA ON MARCH 29, 1996
DISCIPLINARY ACTION: SURRENDER OF CONTROLLED SUBSTANCE LICENSE

NOTES: IN LIEU OF ORDER TO SHOW CAUSE.

CONWAY, JIMMY HAROLD MD, LICENSE NUMBER 0016834 OF 3301 N.W. 50TH, OKLAHOMA CITY, OK, WAS DISCIPLINED BY OKLAHOMA ON SEPTEMBER 22, 1996
DISCIPLINARY ACTION: 60-MONTH PROBATION; RESTRICTION PLACED ON LICENSE
OFFENSE: SUBSTANCE ABUSE

NOTES: ON 3/04/96 PRACTICED MEDICINE AND SURGERY WHILE UNDER THE INFLUENCE OF DRUGS; HABITUAL OR EXCESSIVE USE OF ANY DRUG WHICH IMPAIRS THE ABILITY TO PRACTICE MEDICINE WITH REASONABLE SKILL AND SAFETY TO THE PATIENT; PURCHASED A REGULATED SUBSTANCE SCHEDULE I THROUGH V FOR PERSONAL USE; ON 3/08/96 ENTERED RUSH BEHAVIORAL CENTER FOR TREATMENT OF DRUG ADDICTION; AND SINCE COMPLETING TREATMENT HAS ADHERED TO THE AFTER-CARE TREATMENT CONTRACT. PROBATION BEGINNING 3/08/96: SHALL KEEP DUPLICATE, SERIALLY NUMBERED PRESCRIPTIONS OF ALL CONTROLLED DANGEROUS SUBSTANCES READILY RETRIEVABLE, IN NUMERICAL ORDER AND WILL FURNISH COPIES TO THE BOARD UPON REQUEST;

SHALL NOT AUTHORIZE ANY PERSONNEL UNDER HIS SUPERVISION TO INITIATE AN ORDER FOR A PRESCRIPTION; SHALL NOT PRESCRIBE, ADMINISTER, OR DISPENSE ANY AMPHETAMINE OR AMPHETAMINE-LIKE SUBSTANCES, ANOREXIC DRUGS, AND ANABOLIC STEROIDS; APPROVED TO PRACTICE WITH OKLAHOMA SPORTS SCIENCE AND ORTHOPEDIC; SHALL REQUEST ALL HOSPITALS IN WHICH HE ANTICIPATES TO PRACTICE TO FURNISH THE BOARD WITH A WRITTEN STATEMENT REGARDING MONITORING OF HIS PRACTICE WHILE PERFORMING SERVICES IN THAT HOSPITAL; SHALL FURNISH EACH STATE IN WHICH HE HOLDS OR APPLIES FOR LICENSURE AND ALL HEALTH CARE ENTITIES IN WHICH HE HOLDS STAFF PRIVILEGES A COPY OF THE ORDER; SHALL NOT EMPLOY A PHYSICIAN'S ASSISTANT; SHALL SUBMIT BIOLOGICAL FLUID SPECIMENS; SHALL NOT PRESCRIBE, ADMINISTER, OR DISPENSE ANY MEDICATIONS FOR PERSONAL USE; SHALL TAKE NO MEDICATION UNLESS AUTHORIZED BY A TREATING PHYSICIAN FOR LEGITIMATE MEDICAL NEED; SHALL CONTINUE HIS CONTRACT WITH RUSH BEHAVIORAL HEALTH CENTER INCLUDING ATTENDANCE AT 12-STEP MEETINGS WEEKLY, OBTAIN AND WORK WITH A 12-STEP SPONSOR; RANDOM, OBSERVED, URINE MONITORING FOR A PERIOD OF NOT LESS THAN TWO YEARS OF THE PROBATION, WEEKLY ATTENDANCE AT CADUCEUS GROUP; COMPLIANCE WITH THE OKLAHOMA PHYSICIAN RECOVERY PROGRAM, RETURN TO RUSH BEHAVIORAL HEALTH IN 3-6 MONTHS FOR FOLLOW UP VISIT; SHALL KEEP THE BOARD INFORMED OF HIS CURRENT ADDRESS; AND SHALL KEEP CURRENT PAYMENT OF ALL PROSECUTION, INVESTIGATION, AND MONITORING COSTS OF HIS CASE.

CONWAY, JIMMY HAROLD JR MD OF OKLAHOMA CITY, OK, WAS DISCIPLINED BY DEA ON JULY 16, 1999
DISCIPLINARY ACTION: MONITORING OF PHYSICIAN PERFORMANCE
OFFENSE: CRIMINAL CONVICTION OR PLEA OF GUILTY, NOLO CONTENDERE, OR NO CONTEST TO A CRIME

NOTES: IN AN INVESTIGATION STARTING IN 2/96 IT WAS DISCOVERED THAT A PHARMACY COMPUTER PRINTOUT BETWEEN 6/1/95 AND 2/26/96 REVEALED 13 PRESCRIPTIONS FILLED WITH THE NAME "JIM CONWAY;" A SURVEY OF OTHER PHARMACIES REVEALED PRESCRIPTIONS ISSUED TO HIM BY VARIOUS PHYSICIANS FOR 5,973 DOSAGE UNITS OF CONTROLLED SUBSTANCES; TWO PHYSICIANS WHOSE NAMES WERE LISTED SAID THEY DID NOT WRITE THE PRESCRIPTIONS; ON 3/4/96 HE ADMITTED TO INVESTIGATOR FORGING THE PRESCRIPTIONS AND THAT HE WAS ADDICTED TO ALCOHOL AND CONTROLLED SUBSTANCES; STARTED IN 1992 AND 1993 CONSUMING SAMPLES OF LORTAB AND SOMA; THEN BEGAN FORGING PRESCRIPTIONS; SURRENDERED DEA REGISTRATION ON 3/29/96 OKLAHOMA BOARD SUMMARILY SUSPENDED HIS LICENSE; ENTERED TREATMENT AT THAT TIME AND HAS A CONTRACT WITH PHYSICIANS RECOVERY PROGRAM; OKLAHOMA BOARD IN 9/96 OKLAHOMA LICENSE PLACED O N PROBATION WITH CONDITIONS ON HANDLING CONTROLLED SUBSTANCES AND OTHER MONITORING CONDITIONS; ON 10/31/96 PLED GUILTY TO TWO COUNTS OF OBTAINING CONTROLLED SUBSTANCES BY FORGED OR ALTERED PRESCRIPTIONS; URINE SCREENS HAVE BEEN CLEAR SINCE 3/4/96; DEA FOUND HE HAS ACCEPTED RESPONSIBILITY FOR HIS CONDUCT. DEA REGISTRATION GRANTED ON CONDITIONS: MUST MAINTAIN CONTRACTUAL RELATIONSHIP WITH THE OKLAHOMA PHYSICIANS RECOVERY PROGRAM; SHALL CONTINUE TO UNDERGO RANDOM URINALYSIS AT LEAST MONTHLY; SHALL MAKE COPIES OF HIS PRESCRIPTIONS AVAILABLE FOR REVIEW; SHALL NOTIFY DEA OF ANY CHANGE IN EMPLOYMENT; SHALL CONSENT TO PERIODIC INSPECTIONS BY DEA.

COOKE, FRANCIS W MD, DATE OF BIRTH MARCH 25, 1922 OF PO BOX 280, GUTHRIE, OK, WAS DISCIPLINED BY MEDICARE ON DECEMBER 5, 1994
DISCIPLINARY ACTION: EXCLUSION FROM THE MEDICARE AND/OR MEDICAID PROGRAM
OFFENSE: DISCIPLINARY ACTION BY ANOTHER STATE OR AGENCY

NOTES: LICENSE REVOKED FOR REASONS BEARING ON PROFESSIONAL PERFORMANCE.

COOKE, FRANCIS WARDELL MD, LICENSE NUMBER 0008964 OF PO BOX 280, GUTHRIE, OK, WAS DISCIPLINED BY OKLAHOMA ON NOVEMBER 1, 1990
DISCIPLINARY ACTION: 60-MONTH PROBATION; REPRIMAND
OFFENSE: CRIMINAL CONVICTION OR PLEA OF GUILTY, NOLO CONTENDERE, OR NO CONTEST TO A CRIME

NOTES: ON 7/23/90 PLED GUILTY TO FOUR FELONY CHARGES WHICH CONSISTED OF THE COUNT OF CONSPIRACY TO PRESENT A FALSE CLAIM AND THREE COUNTS OF OBTAINING MONEY UNDER FALSE PRETENSES. SENTENCED TO FIVE YEARS ON EACH COUNT, TO RUN CONCURRENTLY. PROBATION BEGINNING 10/26/90 UNDER THE FOLLOWING TERMS AND CONDITIONS: SHALL APPEAR BEFORE THE BOARD UPON REQUEST AND SUBMIT ANY REQUIRED REPORTS; SHALL SUBMIT TO THE BOARD ADDRESS/CHANGE OF ADDRESS; SHALL PAY COSTS; SHALL NOTIFY ANY HOSPITAL WHERE HE HOLDS STAFF PRIVILEGES, OR CLINIC, OR GROUP WHERE HE PRACTICES, OF THE TERMS AND CONDITIONS OF THIS BOARD ORDER AND SUPPLY A COPY THEREOF.

COOKE, FRANCIS WARDELL MD, LICENSE NUMBER 0008964 OF PO BOX 280, GUTHRIE, OK, WAS DISCIPLINED BY OKLAHOMA ON FEBRUARY 18, 1994
DISCIPLINARY ACTION: LICENSE REVOCATION
OFFENSE: OVERPRESCRIBING OR MISPRESCRIBING DRUGS

NOTES: ADMITTED THAT BETWEEN 8/92 AND 2/93 IN THE CASE OF SEVEN PATIENTS HE PRESCRIBED CONTROLLED SUBSTANCES NOT NEEDED IN THE AMOUNT PRESCRIBED AND THAT THESE PRESCRIPTIONS WERE NOT DOCUMENTED IN ANY MEDICAL CHARTS AND THAT PATIENTS WERE "SCAMMING" HIM.

COOPER, WILLIAM I MD, DATE OF BIRTH MARCH 20, 1942 OF 300 N 14TH STREET, EASTON, PA, WAS DISCIPLINED BY MEDICARE ON NOVEMBER 8, 1994
DISCIPLINARY ACTION: EXCLUSION FROM THE MEDICARE AND/OR MEDICAID PROGRAM
OFFENSE: DISCIPLINARY ACTION BY ANOTHER STATE OR AGENCY

NOTES: LICENSE SUSPENDED FOR REASONS BEARING ON PROFESSIONAL PERFORMANCE.

COOPER, WILLIAM ISAAC MD OF EASTON, PA, WAS DISCIPLINED BY PENNSYLVANIA ON MARCH 22, 1994
DISCIPLINARY ACTION: CEASE AND DESIST ORDER
OFFENSE: PROFESSIONAL MISCONDUCT

NOTES: ALLEGATIONS OF UNPROFESSIONAL CONDUCT. AGREEMENT TO PERMANENTLY CEASE AND DESIST FROM PRACTICING IN PENNSYLVANIA ON OR BEFORE 6/20/94.

COOPER, WILLIAM ISAAC MD, LICENSE NUMBER 15621 OF 2448

EAST 81 #1600, TULSA, OK, WAS DISCIPLINED BY OKLAHOMA ON FEBRUARY 19, 1998
DISCIPLINARY ACTION: LICENSE REVOCATION
OFFENSE: DISCIPLINARY ACTION BY ANOTHER STATE OR AGENCY

NOTES: IN 4/96 HE PERFORMED IN-OFFICE SURGICAL PROCEDURES ON A PATIENT, INCLUDING LAPAROSCOPY AND LAPAROTOMY, IN ORDER TO REVERSE A PREVIOUS TUBAL LIGATION. THE RETENTION OF THE PATIENT, THE TREATMENT OF THE PATIENT, THE PROCEDURES UTILIZED AND THE CONDUCT OF THE DOCTOR, INCLUDING FAILURE TO PROVIDE PROPER SETTING AND ASSISTANT PERSONNEL, CONSTITUTED UNPROFESSIONAL CONDUCT. IN 1994 THE PENNSYLVANIA BOARD HAD TAKEN ACTION AGAINST HIM INVOLVING SURRENDER OF HIS LICENSE ON GROUNDS PERTAINING TO HIS INABILITY TO PRACTICE MEDICINE WITH REASONABLE SKILL AND SAFETY AND FRAUD AND CONDUCT LIKELY TO DECEIVE, DEFRAUD, OR HARM THE PUBLIC; WAS SUSPENDED FROM A RESIDENCY PROGRAM IN GEORGIA IN 1980; HE FAILED TO DISCLOSE COMPLETE AND ACCURATE INFORMATION REGARDING THE PENNSYLVANIA AND GEORGIA ACTIONS ON APPLICATIONS FOR MEMBERSHIP AND/OR RENEWAL TO MEDICAL SOCIETY AND MEDICAL CENTER. HE HAS BEEN SUBJECT TO 11 DIFFERENT ADVERSE JUDGMENTS, AWARDS, OR SETTLEMENTS ARISING FROM MEDICAL LIABILITY CLAIMS RELATED TO PROHIBITED ACTS; HE UTILIZED FALSE AND MISLEADING INFORMATION CONCERNING HIS QUALIFICATIONS AND CERTIFICATIONS FOR THE PURPOSE OF SOLICITING PATIENTS; SHALL PAY COSTS.

CORDOVA, EDMUND S MD, WAS DISCIPLINED BY NEW MEXICO ON FEBRUARY 16, 1995
DISCIPLINARY ACTION: LICENSE REVOCATION
OFFENSE: PROFESSIONAL MISCONDUCT

NOTES: SEXUAL MISCONDUCT; UNPROFESSIONAL CONDUCT.

CORDOVA, EDMUND S MD, LICENSE NUMBER 0D25096 OF 4231 POSTAL COURT, STE 102, PASADENA, MD, WAS DISCIPLINED BY MARYLAND ON MARCH 22, 1995
DISCIPLINARY ACTION: EMERGENCY SUSPENSION
OFFENSE: DISCIPLINARY ACTION BY ANOTHER STATE OR AGENCY

NOTES: BASED ON REVOCATION OF LICENSE IN NEW MEXICO FOR SEXUAL MISCONDUCT WITH PATIENTS IN THAT STATE AND A 1984 REPRIMAND BY THE U.S. ARMY FOR "UNPROFESSIONAL AND INDECENT CONDUCT DURING HIS MEDICAL EXAMINATION OF SEVERAL WOMEN PATIENTS;" AND A 1986 REPRIMAND FROM THE ARMY FOR UNPROFESSIONAL CONDUCT IN THE PRACTICE OF MEDICINE.

CORDOVA, EDMUND S MD OF 4231 POSTAL COURT, PASADENA, MD, WAS DISCIPLINED BY DEA ON APRIL 24, 1995
DISCIPLINARY ACTION: SURRENDER OF CONTROLLED SUBSTANCE LICENSE
OFFENSE: DISCIPLINARY ACTION BY ANOTHER STATE OR AGENCY

NOTES: STATE BOARD.

CORDOVA, EDMUND S MD, LICENSE NUMBER 0D25096 OF 7669 RONA COURT, APT. J, GLEN BURNIE, MD, WAS DISCIPLINED BY MARYLAND ON AUGUST 1, 1995
DISCIPLINARY ACTION: SURRENDER OF LICENSE
OFFENSE: DISCIPLINARY ACTION BY ANOTHER STATE OR AGENCY

NOTES: INVESTIGATION CONDUCTED BASED ON ACTIONS THE UNITED STATES ARMY TOOK AGAINST HIM FOR UNPROFESSIONAL AND INDECENT CONDUCT DURING MEDICAL EXAMINATIONS OF WOMEN PATIENTS AT ARMY HOSPITALS IN ALASKA AND OKLAHOMA; ALSO HAD LICENSE REVOKED IN NEW MEXICO FOR SEXUAL ABUSE OF TWO WOMEN PATIENTS.

CORDOVA, EDMUND S MD, LICENSE NUMBER 0016849 OF PO BOX 1296, PASADENA, MD, WAS DISCIPLINED BY OKLAHOMA ON OCTOBER 2, 1995
DISCIPLINARY ACTION: LICENSE REVOCATION
OFFENSE: DISCIPLINARY ACTION BY ANOTHER STATE OR AGENCY

NOTES: ACTION IN NEW MEXICO ON 2/23/95 WHICH REVOKED HIS LICENSE FOR INAPPROPRIATE CONDUCT WITH TWO FEMALE PATIENTS. IN 1990 WHILE IN THE MILITARY FORCES OF THE UNITED STATES, THE MILITARY RECEIVED COMPLAINTS THAT HE HAD FONDLED WOMEN IN ALASKA AND OKLAHOMA AND THAT THE COMPLAINTS HAD ADDRESSED HIS USE OF A STETHOSCOPE WHEN EXAMINING FEMALE PATIENTS' HEARTS. THE MILITARY REQUIRED HIM TO HAVE CHAPERONES PRESENT FOR EXAMINATIONS UNLESS DURING EXTREME EMERGENCY. STAFF PRIVILEGES WERE SUSPENDED IN A HOSPITAL IN 10/93 BASED ON THIS TYPE OF COMPLAINT.

CORDOVA, EDMUND S MD, DATE OF BIRTH JANUARY 5, 1947 OF C/O 4231 POSTAL COURT, PASADENA, MD, WAS DISCIPLINED BY MEDICARE ON DECEMBER 20, 1995
DISCIPLINARY ACTION: EXCLUSION FROM THE MEDICARE AND/OR MEDICAID PROGRAM
OFFENSE: DISCIPLINARY ACTION BY ANOTHER STATE OR AGENCY

NOTES: LICENSE SUSPENDED FOR REASONS BEARING ON PROFESSIONAL PERFORMANCE.

CORNELIUS, DOUGLAS HUGH MD, WAS DISCIPLINED BY OKLAHOMA ON SEPTEMBER 13, 1990
DISCIPLINARY ACTION: 60-MONTH PROBATION; MONITORING OF PHYSICIAN PERFORMANCE
OFFENSE: SUBSTANCE ABUSE

NOTES: PREVIOUS ALCOHOL ABUSE. PROBATION BEGINNING 9/01/90 UNDER THE FOLLOWING TERMS AND CONDITIONS: SHALL TAKE NO MEDICATION UNLESS AUTHORIZED BY ANOTHER PHYSICIAN FOR LEGITIMATE MEDICAL NEED; SHALL ABSTAIN FROM CONSUMING ALCOHOL OR ANY SUBSTANCES WHICH WOULD ADVERSELY AFFECT HIS ABILITY TO PRACTICE; SHALL SUBMIT BIOLOGICAL FLUID SPECIMENS; SHALL CONTINUE REGULAR ATTENDANCE AND PARTICIPATION IN EITHER AA MEETINGS OR THE PHYSICIAN RECOVERY COMMITTEE OR SIMILAR ORGANIZATION AND SHALL REPORT PERIODICALLY UPON BOARD REQUEST ON HIS PROOF OF ATTENDANCE AND SHALL CONTINUE ALL SUPPORTIVE PROGRAMS RECOMMENDED; SHALL APPEAR BEFORE THE BOARD UPON REQUEST AND SUBMIT ALL REQUIRED REPORTS; SHALL FURNISH TO THE BOARD ADDRESS/CHANGE OF ADDRESS; SHALL PAY COSTS; SHALL NOTIFY ANY HOSPITAL WHERE HE HOLDS STAFF PRIVILEGES, OR CLINIC, OR GROUP WHERE HE PRACTICES, OF THE TERMS AND CONDITIONS OF THIS ORDER.

CORNELIUS, DOUGLAS HUGH MD, DATE OF BIRTH OCTOBER 14, 1948, LICENSE NUMBER 0028256 OF 801 FIFTH STREET, SIOUX CITY, IA, WAS DISCIPLINED BY IOWA ON JULY 16, 1991

NOTES: LICENSE ISSUED PURSUANT TO TERMS OF A CONSENT AGREEMENT. CONSENT AGREEMENT TERMINATED ON 5/1/93; LICENSE FREE AND CLEAR OF RESTRICTIONS.

CORNELIUS, GEORGE ROBERT MD OF 4215 CLASSEN, OKLAHOMA CITY, OK, WAS DISCIPLINED BY DEA ON APRIL 3, 1990
DISCIPLINARY ACTION: SURRENDER OF CONTROLLED SUBSTANCE LICENSE
OFFENSE: DISCIPLINARY ACTION BY ANOTHER STATE OR AGENCY

NOTES: ON 1/31/90 OKLAHOMA BOARD SUSPENDED HIS STATE CONTROLLED SUBSTANCES REGISTRATION FOR SIX MONTHS; HE THEN SURRENDERED HIS DEA REGISTRATION ON 4/3/90.

CORNELIUS, SAM G DO, LICENSE NUMBER 0001768, WAS DISCIPLINED BY OKLAHOMA ON APRIL 11, 1995
DISCIPLINARY ACTION: REQUIRED TO TAKE ADDITIONAL MEDICAL EDUCATION; 12-MONTH MONITORING OF PHYSICIAN PERFORMANCE

NOTES: ALLEGED VIOLATIONS OF THE OSTEOPATHIC ACT. THE BOARD DEFERRED PROSECUTION OF THE SECOND AMENDED COMPLAINT FOR A ONE YEAR PERIOD DURING WHICH TIME HIS PRACTICE WILL BE MONITORED; WITHIN THIS YEAR SHALL ATTEND A SPECIFIED COURSE SPONSORED BY THE DIRECTOR OF THE CONTROLLED DANGEROUS SUBSTANCES PROGRAM AT THE UNIVERSITY OF MEDICINE AND DENTISTRY, AND WILL REPORT THE SUCCESSFUL COMPLETION OF THIS COURSE TO THE BOARD; SHALL ATTEND A BOARD APPROVED ETHICS COURSE AND REPORT HIS SUCCESSFUL COMPLETION TO THE BOARD; SHALL COOPERATE WITH RANDOM REVIEW BY THE BOARD; SHALL PROVIDE THE BOARD WITH A COPY OF ALL PRESCRIPTIONS AND/OR CONTROLLED DANGEROUS SUBSTANCES DISPENSED, PRESCRIBED, ADMINISTERED, OR OTHERWISE DISTRIBUTED. ON 6/96 ORDER TERMINATED.

CRAMER, LEIGH E DO, LICENSE NUMBER 0001302, WAS DISCIPLINED BY OKLAHOMA ON DECEMBER 30, 1992
DISCIPLINARY ACTION: LICENSE REVOCATION
OFFENSE: CRIMINAL CONVICTION OR PLEA OF GUILTY, NOLO CONTENDERE, OR NO CONTEST TO A CRIME

NOTES: CONVICTED OF ATTEMPTED POSSESSION OF MARIJUANA WITH INTENT TO DISTRIBUTE AND UNLAWFUL POSSESSION OF A CONTROLLED DRUG. SHALL PAY INVESTIGATION AND PROSECUTION COSTS.

CRASS, DAVID P MD, LICENSE NUMBER 0011365 OF 1725 EAST 19TH ST #604, TULSA, OK, WAS DISCIPLINED BY OKLAHOMA ON FEBRUARY 4, 1991
DISCIPLINARY ACTION: LICENSE SUSPENSION; 24-MONTH PROBATION
OFFENSE: CRIMINAL CONVICTION OR PLEA OF GUILTY, NOLO CONTENDERE, OR NO CONTEST TO A CRIME

NOTES: ON 11/1/90, HE VOLUNTARILY ENTERED A PLEA OF GUILTY IN THE U.S. DISTRICT COURT FOR THE WESTERN DISTRICT OF OKLAHOMA TO FIVE COUNTS OF SUBMITTING AND RECEIVING PAYMENT ON FALSE CLAIMS AGAINST MEDICAID. COURT IMPOSED A TWO-YEAR SUSPENDED SENTENCE AND PROBATION, RESTITUTION OF $2,850 AND A $10,000 FINE. BOARD SUSPENSION FOR A TEN DAY PERIOD. PUT ON PROBATION WITH FOLLOWING CONDITIONS: SHALL NOTIFY ANY HOSPITAL WHERE HE HOLDS STAFF PRIVILEGES, OR CLINIC, OR GROUP WHERE HE PRACTICES OF HIS TERMS AND CONDITIONS; SHALL COMPLETE 100 HOURS OF COMMUNITY SERVICE ACCEPTABLE TO THE BOARD; SHALL FURNISH BOARD WITH ADDRESS AND/OR CHANGE OF ADDRESS; SHALL APPEAR BEFORE BOARD UPON REQUEST. PROBATION TERMINATED ON 1/15/93.

CRASS, DAVID P MD, LICENSE NUMBER 0C40488 OF TULSA, OK, WAS DISCIPLINED BY CALIFORNIA ON APRIL 11, 1993
DISCIPLINARY ACTION: LICENSE REVOCATION

CRASS, DAVID PAUL MD, DATE OF BIRTH MAY 4, 1948 OF 1145 SOUTH UTICA #416, TULSA, OK, WAS DISCIPLINED BY MEDICARE ON JULY 23, 1991
DISCIPLINARY ACTION: 60-MONTH EXCLUSION FROM THE MEDICARE AND/OR MEDICAID PROGRAM
OFFENSE: CRIMINAL CONVICTION OR PLEA OF GUILTY, NOLO CONTENDERE, OR NO CONTEST TO A CRIME

NOTES: PROGRAM-RELATED CONVICTION. REINSTATED ON 2/12/97.

CRAWFORD, MICHAEL K MD, LICENSE NUMBER 14749 OF 4108 NW 144TH TERRACE, OKLAHOMA CITY, OK, WAS DISCIPLINED BY OKLAHOMA ON MAY 7, 1999
DISCIPLINARY ACTION: 2-MONTH LICENSE SUSPENSION; 60-MONTH PROBATION
OFFENSE: SUBSTANCE ABUSE

NOTES: DURING 1997 AND 1998 SEVERAL PROBLEMS FOUND WITH HIS PRESCRIBING PRACTICES: ON OR ABOUT 3/19/98 USED A BLANK PHARMACY PRESCRIPTION PAD TO WRITE HIMSELF A PRESCRIPTION FOR DIDREX USING ANOTHER DOCTORS NAME AND LICENSE NUMBER WHO DENIED AUTHORIZING THE PRESCRIPTION; PHARMACY RECORDS SHOW THAT HE WROTE HIMSELF ANOTHER PRESCRIPTION ON 12/31/97; IN 11/97 HAD ONE OF HIS OFFICE ASSISTANTS CALL IN AN UNAUTHORIZED PRESCRIPTION USING THE NAME OF THE SAME DOCTOR; ON 12/10/97 AND 1/7/98 HE FILLED PRESCRIPTIONS ALLEGEDLY AUTHORIZED BY THE DOCTOR WHO DENIES HAVING AUTHORIZED THE PRESCRIPTIONS ALTHOUGH HIS RECORDS SHOW PRESCRIPTIONS FOR THE SAME DRUGS ON DIFFERENT DATES; ON OR AROUND 4/98 ONE OF HIS TREATING PHYSICIANS CEASED PRESCRIBING HIM DIDREX WHEN HE LEARNED THAT HE WAS GETTING PRESCRIPTIONS FOR THE SAME SUBSTANCE DURING THAT SAME TIME FROM ANOTHER DOCTOR; THE TREATING PHYSICIANS CONFRONTED HIM AND CONTACTED THE OKLAHOMA PHYSICIAN'S RECOVERY GROUP; ADMITTED ABUSING DIDREX AND HAS BEEN ASSESSED FOR POSSIBLE TREATMENT OF WHICH HE DECLINED, ELECTING TO SEEK TREATMENT ON HIS OWN; ADMITTED GIVING PRESCRIPTIONS FOR CONTROLLED SUBSTANCES TO TWO FRIENDS OF A PATIENT; ADMITTED THAT HE WROTE PRESCRIPTIONS TO HIS WIFE AND MOTHER-IN LAW; TREATED HIS PERSONAL FRIEND FOR NARCOLEPSY DESPITE HIS BELIEF THAT SHE HAD A DRUG PROBLEM; WROTE PRESCRIPTIONS FOR A PATIENT'S GRANDMOTHER, AT THE PATIENT'S REQUEST, EVEN THOUGH HE HAD NOT SEEN THE GRANDMOTHER AND HEARD THAT SHE DIED; FAILED TO MAINTAIN OFFICE RECORDS FOR EACH PATIENT WHICH ACCURATELY REFLECTS THE EVALUATION, TREATMENT, AND MEDICAL NECESSITY OF TREATMENT. LICENSE LIMITED AS FOLLOWS: SHALL KEEP DUPLICATE, SERIALLY NUMBERED PRESCRIPTIONS OF ALL CONTROLLED DANGEROUS SUBSTANCES AND WILL SUBMIT COPIES TO THE BOARD UPON REQUEST; SHALL NOT PRESCRIBE, ADMINISTER, OR DISPENSE ANY AMPHETAMINES OR ANY OTHER ANOREXICS; SHALL REQUEST ALL HEALTH CARE FACILITIES IN WHICH HE ANTICIPATES PRACTICING TO FURNISH A STATEMENT REGARDING MONITORING OF HIS PRACTICE; SHALL SUBMIT TO EVERY STATE IN WHICH HE HOLDS LICENSURE AND TO HOSPITALS, CLINICS OR OTHER INSTITUTIONS IN

WHICH HE HOLDS OR ANTICIPATES HOLDING ANY FORM OF STAFF PRIVILEGE A COPY OF THIS ORDER; SHALL NOT SUPERVISE ALLIED HEALTH PROFESSIONALS; SHALL SUBMIT BIOLOGICAL FLUID SPECIMENS; SHALL NOT PRESCRIBE, ADMINISTER OR DISPENSE ANY MEDICATIONS FOR HIS PERSONAL USE OR FOR THAT OF ANY FAMILY MEMBER, AND SHALL TAKE NONE UNLESS AUTHORIZED BY ANOTHER PHYSICIAN FOR A LEGITIMATE MEDICAL NEED; SHALL NOT INGEST ANY SUBSTANCE WHICH WILL CAUSE A SPECIMEN TO TEST POSITIVE FOR PROHIBITED SUBSTANCES; SHALL EXECUTE ALL RELEASES OF MEDICAL AND PSYCHIATRIC RECORDS AS NECESSARY TO DISCUSS HIS CASE WITH HIS TREATING PHYSICIANS AND/OR ANY PHYSICIANS HOLDING RECORDS; SHALL ABIDE BY THE TERMS AND CONDITIONS OF HIS POSTCARE CONTRACT; SHALL KEEP THE BOARD INFORMED OF HIS ADDRESS AND PAY COSTS; SHALL APPEAR BEFORE THE BOARD UPON REQUEST.

CRITTENDON, WILLIAM F MD, LICENSE NUMBER 0006708, WAS DISCIPLINED BY OKLAHOMA ON JULY 7, 1991
DISCIPLINARY ACTION: LICENSE REVOCATION
OFFENSE: SUBSTANDARD CARE, INCOMPETENCE OR NEGLIGENCE

NOTES: ON 7/30/90, DR. CRITTENDON AND U.S. ARMY REACHED AGREEMENT TO VOLUNTARILY SETTLE HIS APPEAL OF THE U.S. ARMY'S DECISION TO REMOVE HIM FROM THE POSITION OF MEDICAL OFFICER FOR FAILURE TO MAINTAIN CLINICAL PRIVILEGES AND FAILURE TO PROVIDE COMPETENT CARE. AGREES NEVER AGAIN TO APPLY OR PRACTICE MEDICINE IN THE U.S. FOUND TO BE UNABLE TO PRACTICE MEDICINE WITH REASONABLE SKILL AND SAFETY TO PATIENTS BY REASON OF AGE, ILLNESS, DRUNKENNESS, EXCESSIVE USE OF DRUGS, NARCOTICS, CHEMICALS, OR ANY OTHER TYPE OF MATERIAL OR AS A RESULT OF ANY MENTAL OR PHYSICAL CONDITION. ON 9/19/90, OKLAHOMA BOARD RECEIVED DR. CRITTENDON'S VOLUNTARY RETIREMENT AND REQUEST FOR REVOCATION OF LICENSE TO PRACTICE MEDICINE.

CUNNINGHAM, DARRIN D DO OF OKLAHOMA CITY, OK, WAS DISCIPLINED BY ILLINOIS ON SEPTEMBER 1, 1994
DISCIPLINARY ACTION: 6-MONTH PROBATION
OFFENSE: DISCIPLINARY ACTION BY ANOTHER STATE OR AGENCY

NOTES: DISCIPLINED IN OKLAHOMA. LIMITED TEMPORARY LICENSE ISSUED.

CUNNINGHAM, DARRIN DOUGLAS DO, LICENSE NUMBER 0003069, WAS DISCIPLINED BY OKLAHOMA ON JULY 6, 1992
DISCIPLINARY ACTION: 60-MONTH PROBATION; MONITORING OF PHYSICIAN PERFORMANCE

NOTES: LICENSE GRANTED. CONDITIONS OF PROBATION: SHALL PARTICIPATE IN ALCOHOLICS ANONYMOUS AND HAVE THE BOARD RECEIVE REGULAR REPORTS REGARDING HIS ATTENDANCE; SHALL PARTICIPATE IN THE OKLAHOMA PHYSICIAN'S RECOVERY PROGRAM; SHALL APPEAR BEFORE THE BOARD UPON REQUEST BUT, AT LEAST ONCE EACH YEAR; AGREES TO RECEIVE UNANNOUNCED BOARD VISITS AT SUCH TIMES AND PLACES AT BOARD DISCRETION; SHALL SUBMIT TO THE BOARD BIOLOGICAL FLUID SPECIMENS AT ANY TIME, UPON REQUEST, FOR LABORATORY ANALYSIS; IN CONNECTION WITH AT LEAST ONE BOARD APPEARANCE PER YEAR HIS DRIVING RECORD SHALL BE REVIEWED AND HE WILL COOPERATE TO THE EXTENT THAT ANY RELEASE FOR RECORDS THAT MAY BECOME NECESSARY; SHALL NOTIFY THE BOARD IN WRITING OF ANY CHANGE OF ADDRESS WITHIN 14 DAYS; TERMS OF RESIDENCE OR PRACTICE OUTSIDE OF OKLAHOMA WILL RESULT IN THE TOLLING OF THIS ORDER AND WILL NOT APPLY TO THE REDUCTION OF THIS PROBATIONARY PERIOD. ON 9/21/95 THE PROBATIONARY CONDITIONS WERE REMOVED.

DAVIDSON, CHORDE W DO, LICENSE NUMBER 1336, WAS DISCIPLINED BY OKLAHOMA ON JUNE 20, 1996
DISCIPLINARY ACTION: SURRENDER OF LICENSE

DAVIDSON, CHORDE W DO, DATE OF BIRTH OCTOBER 26, 1933 OF 108 SOUTH B STREET, OILTON, OK, WAS DISCIPLINED BY MEDICARE ON AUGUST 13, 1996
DISCIPLINARY ACTION: 60-MONTH EXCLUSION FROM THE MEDICARE AND/OR MEDICAID PROGRAM
OFFENSE: CRIMINAL CONVICTION OR PLEA OF GUILTY, NOLO CONTENDERE, OR NO CONTEST TO A CRIME

NOTES: CONVICTED OF A CRIME INVOLVING THE MEDICARE, MEDICAID, MATERNAL AND CHILD HEALTH SERVICES BLOCK GRANT OR BLOCK GRANTS TO STATES FOR SOCIAL SERVICES PROGRAMS.

DAVIS, MARTIN J DO, LICENSE NUMBER 0002516, WAS DISCIPLINED BY OKLAHOMA ON OCTOBER 23, 1996
DISCIPLINARY ACTION: 60-MONTH PROBATION; RESTRICTION PLACED ON LICENSE
OFFENSE: SEXUAL ABUSE OF OR SEXUAL MISCONDUCT WITH A PATIENT

NOTES: IN 1989 ENGAGED IN SEXUAL ACTIVITY WITHIN A PHYSICIAN-PATIENT RELATIONSHIP; AUTHORIZED THE ISSUANCE OF PRESCRIPTION DRUGS TO SOME PATIENTS, SCHEDULES II-V, WITHOUT SUFFICIENTLY EXAMINING THESE PATIENTS ON A REGULAR BASIS OR IN A TIMELY MANNER. FOR 90 DAYS IS PRECLUDED FROM ALL ACTIVITY AUTHORIZED PURSUANT TO THE ISSUANCE OF A LICENSE; PROBATION UNDER THE FOLLOWING TERMS AND CONDITIONS: DURING THE FIRST YEAR OF PROBATION, SHALL SUCCESSFULLY COMPLETE A COURSE ENTITLED "THE PROPER PRESCRIBING OF CONTROLLED DANGEROUS SUBSTANCES"; SHALL ATTEND A BOARD APPROVED COURSE IN MEDICAL ETHICS; SHALL ESTABLISH WRITTEN POLICIES AND PROCEDURES TO USE WHEN PRESCRIBING, DISPENSING, OR ADMINISTERING PRESCRIPTION DRUGS TO HIS PATIENTS TO BE SUBMITTED TO THE BOARD FOR APPROVAL; SHALL SUBMIT REPORTS TO THE BOARD DETAILING HOW HIS OFFICE HELP IS OPERATING AND COMPLIANCE WITH THIS ORDER ON A QUARTERLY BASIS; SHALL HAVE A FEMALE STAFF MEMBER PRESENT WHEN EXAMINING AND/OR TREATING A FEMALE PATIENT WHO MUST DISROBE; MAY NOT PETITION THE BOARD FOR MODIFICATION OF THIS ORDER FOR AT LEAST TWO YEARS; THE BOARD MAY MAKE UNANNOUNCED VISITS TO HIS OFFICE TO RANDOMLY MONITOR HIS PRESCRIBING OPERATIONS AND COMPLIANCE; SHALL APPEAR BEFORE THE BOARD UPON REQUEST; $2,475.00 ADMINISTRATIVE COSTS.

DAVIS, MICHAEL ROY DO, LICENSE NUMBER 0003011, WAS DISCIPLINED BY OKLAHOMA ON APRIL 6, 1992
DISCIPLINARY ACTION: 60-MONTH PROBATION; MONITORING OF PHYSICIAN PERFORMANCE

NOTES: LICENSE GRANTED. PROBATION EFFECTIVE 3/19/92 UNDER THE FOLLOWING TERMS AND CONDITIONS: SHALL NOTIFY THE BOARD IN WRITING OF ANY

CHANGE IN ADDRESS WITHIN 14 DAYS; SHALL APPEAR BEFORE THE BOARD UPON REQUEST; AGREES TO HAVE UNANNOUNCED VISITS FROM THE BOARD AT BOARD DISCRETION; TIME SPENT OUT OF OKLAHOMA WILL RESULT IN THE TOLLING OF THIS AGREEMENT AND WILL NOT REDUCE PROBATION; SHALL PARTICIPATE IN THE PHYSICIAN'S RECOVERY PROGRAM AND AGREES TO COMPLY WITH ALL TERMS OF HIS CONTRACT WITH THEM; SHALL PROVIDE BIOLOGICAL FLUID SPECIMENS FOR LABORATORY ANALYSIS.

DAVIS, MICHAEL ROY DO, DATE OF BIRTH APRIL 29, 1956, LICENSE NUMBER 0040871 OF 1700 NORTH DUPONT HIGHWAY, F304, DOVER, DE, WAS DISCIPLINED BY NEW JERSEY ON AUGUST 18, 1994
OFFENSE: DISCIPLINARY ACTION BY ANOTHER STATE OR AGENCY
NOTES: SANCTIONED BY THE OKLAHOMA BOARD OF OSTEOPATHIC EXAMINERS; MUST PRODUCE A LETTER FROM THE BOARD INDICATING THAT HE HAS COMPLIED WITH ALL REQUIREMENTS OF THE BOARD PRIOR TO THE SCHEDULING OF A STATUS CONFERENCE. MAY NOT ENGAGE IN THE PRACTICE OF MEDICINE AND SURGERY IN NEW JERSEY UNTIL HE APPEARS FOR A STATUS CONFERENCE BEFORE A COMMITTEE OF THE BOARD.

DEASON, DEAN A MD, LICENSE NUMBER 19457 OF 6001 N BROOKLINE #502, OKLAHOMA CITY, OK, WAS DISCIPLINED BY OKLAHOMA ON JANUARY 10, 1997
DISCIPLINARY ACTION: 12-MONTH LICENSE SUSPENSION; MONITORING OF PHYSICIAN PERFORMANCE
OFFENSE: SUBSTANCE ABUSE
NOTES: ON OR ABOUT 5/96 AND 6/96, AND THEREAFTER, HE PRACTICED MEDICINE WHEN HE WAS UNDER THE INFLUENCE OF ALCOHOL AND/OR DRUGS; HE ALSO WAS PRESCRIBING, SELLING, ADMINISTERING, DISTRIBUTING, ORDERING OR GIVING ANY DRUG LEGALLY CLASSIFIED AS A CONTROLLED SUBSTANCE OR RECOGNIZED AS AN ADDICTIVE DANGEROUS DRUG TO A FAMILY MEMBER OR TO HIMSELF. CONDITIONS OF SUSPENSION AS FOLLOWS: SHALL NOT ENGAGE IN THE PRACTICE OF MEDICINE UNTIL REINSTATEMENT BY THE BOARD; HE SHALL DEMONSTRATE COMPLIANCE WITH LOCAL OUTPATIENT PROGRAMS, HIS TWELVE STEP PROGRAM, COUNSELING AND MONITORING THROUGH AND AS DIRECTED BY THE OKLAHOMA PHYSICIANS' RECOVERY PROGRAM; AGREES TO UNDERGO REASSESSMENT AS NECESSARY AT OR BEFORE THE END OF HIS PERIOD OF SUSPENSION AND PRESENT SUCH EVIDENCE OF SUCCESSFUL COMPLETION OF ALL TERMS AND CONDITIONS TO THE BOARD; SHALL NOT PRESCRIBE, ADMINISTER OR DISPENSE ANY MEDICATIONS FOR HIS PERSONAL USE AND SHALL TAKE NONE UNLESS AUTHORIZED BY ANOTHER PHYSICIAN FOR A LEGITIMATE MEDICAL NEED; SHALL ABSTAIN FROM CONSUMING ALCOHOL OR ANY SUBSTANCE WHICH WOULD ADVERSELY AFFECT HIS ABILITY TO PRACTICE MEDICINE; SHALL SUBMIT BIOLOGICAL FLUID SPECIMENS; SHALL CONTINUE REGULAR PARTICIPATION IN THE OKLAHOMA STATE MEDICAL ASSOCIATION'S PHYSICIAN RECOVERY MEETINGS AND RECOVERY PROGRAM AND WILL PARTICIPATE IN REGULAR PSYCHIATRIC COUNSELING AS RECOMMENDED WITH REPORTS TO THE BOARD ON A REGULAR BASIS; SHALL COMPLY WITH ALL TERMS AND CONDITIONS OF HIS POST-TREATMENT CONTRACT; SHALL KEEP THE BOARD INFORMED OF HIS ADDRESS AND PAY COSTS; SHALL APPEAR BEFORE THE BOARD AND SUBMIT REPORTS UPON REQUEST.

DEASON, DEAN A MD, LICENSE NUMBER 19457 OF 2813 NW 59TH #119, OKLAHOMA CITY, OK, WAS DISCIPLINED BY OKLAHOMA ON MARCH 26, 1998
DISCIPLINARY ACTION: SURRENDER OF LICENSE
NOTES: VOLUNTARILY SURRENDERED HIS OKLAHOMA LICENSE FOLLOWING THE COMPLETION OF A ONE-YEAR SUSPENSION FROM PRACTICE BY ORDER OF THE BOARD. REINSTATEMENT, IF ANY, TO BE CONTINGENT UPON PROOF TO THE BOARD THAT HE HAS SUCCESSFULLY ADDRESSED ALL ISSUES RAISED IN THE COMPLAINT AND CITATION FILED IN THIS CAUSE AND HAS SATISFIED ALL OTHER ELIGIBILITY REQUIREMENTS FOR REINSTATEMENT.

DICKERSON, CHARLES WAYNE MD, LICENSE NUMBER 0014590, WAS DISCIPLINED BY OKLAHOMA ON JUNE 27, 1992
DISCIPLINARY ACTION: 60-MONTH PROBATION; RESTRICTION PLACED ON CONTROLLED SUBSTANCE LICENSE
OFFENSE: OVERPRESCRIBING OR MISPRESCRIBING DRUGS
NOTES: IN AT LEAST FOUR CASES FROM NOVEMBER 1990 THROUGH APRIL 1991 PATIENTS WERE BEING PRESCRIBED CONTROLLED DANGEROUS SUBSTANCES IN EXCESS OF THE AMOUNT CONSIDERED FOR MEDICAL NEED. LICENSE PLACED ON PROBATION UNDER FOLLOWING TERMS AND CONDITIONS: SHALL NOT PRESCRIBE, ADMINISTER OR DISPENSE ANY SCHEDULE II OR III DRUGS OR CONTROLLED DANGEROUS SUBSTANCES; MAY PRESCRIBE, ADMINISTER OR DISPENSE SCHEDULE IV OR V CONTROLLED DANGEROUS SUBSTANCES ONLY ON SERIALLY-NUMBERED, DUPLICATE PRESCRIPTION PADS WITH COPIES AVAILABLE TO BOARD. SHALL NOTIFY ANY HOSPITAL WHERE HE HOLDS STAFF PRIVILEGES, OR CLINIC, OR GROUP OF THE TERMS AND CONDITIONS; SHALL KEEP SUBSTANTIAL AND ADEQUATE MEDICAL RECORDS IN ORDER TO SUPPORT ALL DIAGNOSIS, TREATMENT, AND PRESCRIPTION, ADMINISTRATION AND DISPENSING OF CONTROLLED DANGEROUS SUBSTANCES AND NARCOTIC DRUGS; SHALL NOT SUPERVISE A PHYSICIAN'S ASSISTANT. SHALL FURNISH BOARD WITH ADDRESS AND/OR CHANGE OF ADDRESS; SHALL APPEAR BEFORE THE BOARD UPON REQUEST. PREVIOUS ORDER OF CONTINUANCE FROM 3/5/92 REQUIRED HIM TO USE DUPLICATE, SERIALLY-NUMBERED PRESCRIPTION PADS FOR ALL PRESCRIPTIONS OF CONTROLLED DANGEROUS SUBSTANCES, AND TO CONDUCT INTERNAL INVESTIGATION OF HIS OFFICE PRACTICE WITH RESPECT TO DOCUMENTING MEDICATIONS PRESCRIBED. AS OF 7/1/93 MODIFICATION OF TERMS AND CONDITIONS OF PROBATION GRANTED TO ALLOW HIM TO PRESCRIBE, ADMINISTER AND DISPENSE SCHEDULE II AND III CONTROLLED DANGEROUS SUBSTANCES ON SERIALLY-NUMBERED, DUPLICATE PRESCRIPTION PADS AND SHALL MAKE COPIES AVAILABLE TO THE OKLAHOMA BOARD TO INCLUDE ALL DISPENSING RECORDS ON CONTROLLED DANGEROUS SUBSTANCES AND TO INCLUDE SAMPLE MEDICATIONS. OTHER CONDITIONS OF PROBATION REMAIN THE SAME. ON 10/2/95 HIS MOTION TO AMEND, MODIFY, OR TERMINATE THIS PROBATION WAS DENIED.

DIXON, THOMAS A MD, LICENSE NUMBER 0011395 OF PO BOX 125, WEATHERFORD, OK, WAS DISCIPLINED BY OKLAHOMA ON MAY 19, 1994
DISCIPLINARY ACTION: LICENSE REVOCATION
OFFENSE: SUBSTANCE ABUSE

NOTES: FROM 1992 TO DATE HE DID HABITUALLY USE CONTROLLED DANGEROUS SUBSTANCES INCLUDING VALIUM, VICODIN, LORTAB, XANAX, ESGIC, DIAZEPAM, ALPRAZOLAM, BUTALBITOL, APAP WITH CAFFEINE, PHENTERIMINE, LORCET PLUS AND HYDROCODONE TO THE EXTENT THAT HE WAS IMPAIRED IN THE DISCHARGE OF HIS DUTIES AND WAS UNABLE TO PRACTICE; DURING THIS PERIOD UNDERTOOK VARIOUS SCHEMES AND PRACTICES TO UNLAWFULLY OBTAIN CONTROLLED SUBSTANCES FOR HIS OWN USE BY WRITING FALSE PRESCRIPTIONS TO FAMILY MEMBERS AND EMPLOYEES WITHOUT MEDICAL NEED.

DIXON, THOMAS A MD, LICENSE NUMBER 0011395, WAS DISCIPLINED BY OKLAHOMA ON DECEMBER 7, 1995
DISCIPLINARY ACTION: LICENSE REINSTATEMENT; 60-MONTH PROBATION
OFFENSE: SUBSTANCE ABUSE

NOTES: REINSTATEMENT OF HIS LICENSE REVOKED ON 5/14/94 FOR HIS PERSONAL USE OF NUMEROUS CONTROLLED DANGEROUS SUBSTANCES WHICH IMPAIRED HIS DUTIES AS PHYSICIAN AND SURGEON. HAS SINCE THEN PROVIDED EVIDENCE OF SUCCESSFUL TREATMENT OF INPATIENT TREATMENT AND CONTINUED AFFILIATION WITH THE PHYSICIANS RECOVERY PROGRAM. PROBATION BEGINNING 11/17/95 UNDER THE FOLLOWING TERMS AND CONDITIONS: SHALL NOT PRESCRIBE, ADMINISTER, OR DISPENSE ANY MEDICATIONS FOR HIS PERSONAL USE AND SHALL TAKE NONE UNLESS AUTHORIZED BY ANOTHER PHYSICIAN FOR LEGITIMATE MEDICAL NEED; SHALL ABSTAIN FROM CONSUMING ALCOHOL OR ANY SUBSTANCE WHICH WOULD ADVERSELY AFFECT HIS ABILITY TO PRACTICE; SHALL SUBMIT BIOLOGICAL FLUID SPECIMENS; SHALL CONTINUE HIS ACTIVE AFFILIATION WITH THE PHYSICIAN RECOVERY COMMITTEE AND SHALL COMPLY WITH ALL RECOMMENDATIONS AND DIRECTIONS; MAY PRESCRIBE CONTROLLED DANGEROUS SUBSTANCES ONLY ON SERIALLY-NUMBERED, DUPLICATE PRESCRIPTION PADS AND SHALL MAKE THE COPIES AVAILABLE TO THE BOARD UPON REQUEST; SHALL NOT ENGAGE IN ANY ACTIVITIES OR INGEST ANY MEDICATION OR SUBSTANCE OF ANY NATURE THAT WILL TEST POSITIVE FOR ALCOHOL OR ANY CONTROLLED DANGEROUS SUBSTANCE; SHALL NOT ALLOW THE INITIATION OF ANY THERAPEUTIC REGIMEN BY ANY OTHER PERSONNEL UNDER HIS SUPERVISION UNLESS HE IS IN THE IMMEDIATE VICINITY; SHALL NOTIFY ANY HOSPITAL WHERE HE HOLDS STAFF PRIVILEGES, OR CLINIC, OR GROUP WHERE HE PRACTICES, OF THE TERMS AND CONDITIONS OF THIS ORDER AND SUPPLY A COPY THEREOF; SHALL NOT SUPERVISE A PHYSICIAN ASSISTANT; SHALL SUBMIT TO THE BOARD ADDRESS/CHANGE OF ADDRESS; SHALL APPEAR BEFORE THE BOARD UPON REQUEST AND SUBMIT ANY REQUIRED REPORTS.

DIXON, THOMAS ANDREW MD OF P.O. BOX 625 MAIN & WASHINGTON, WEATHERFORD, OK, WAS DISCIPLINED BY DEA ON APRIL 29, 1994
DISCIPLINARY ACTION: SURRENDER OF CONTROLLED SUBSTANCE LICENSE

NOTES: IN LIEU OF PUBLIC INTEREST REVOCATION.

DOMBEK, STANLEY MD OF MIDWEST CITY, OK, WAS DISCIPLINED BY MISSOURI ON AUGUST 7, 1992
DISCIPLINARY ACTION: 24-MONTH PROBATION
OFFENSE: DISCIPLINARY ACTION BY ANOTHER STATE OR AGENCY

DORIA, ALBERTO MD OF HUGO, OK, WAS DISCIPLINED BY MISSOURI ON FEBRUARY 16, 1990
OFFENSE: DISCIPLINARY ACTION BY ANOTHER STATE OR AGENCY

NOTES: MUST APPEAR BEFORE BOARD BEFORE RETURNING TO PRACTICE IN MISSOURI.

DORIA, ALBERTO MD, LICENSE NUMBER 0016297, WAS DISCIPLINED BY OKLAHOMA ON JUNE 27, 1992
DISCIPLINARY ACTION: 60-MONTH PROBATION; RESTRICTION PLACED ON LICENSE
OFFENSE: SUBSTANCE ABUSE

NOTES: SINCE 6/90 HABITUALLY AND REGULARLY USED ALCOHOL AND IS PRESENTLY IN A STATE OF SOBRIETY; NEEDS ADEQUATE SUPERVISION FOR AN EXTENDED PERIOD OF TIME IN ORDER TO INSURE SOBRIETY AND TO PROTECT PUBLIC HEALTH, SAFETY AND WELFARE. PROBATION WITH FOLLOWING CONDITIONS: MUST ABSTAIN FROM CONSUMING ALCOHOL OR ANY SUBSTANCE WHICH WOULD ADVERSELY AFFECT HIS ABILITY TO PRACTICE; MUST SUBMIT BIOLOGICAL FLUID SPECIMENS FOR ANALYSIS; WILL MAINTAIN FORMAL RELATIONSHIP AND REGULAR PARTICIPATION IN ALCOHOLICS ANONYMOUS AND NARCOTICS ANONYMOUS; SHALL NOTIFY ANY HOSPITAL WHERE HE HOLDS STAFF PRIVILEGES, OR CLINIC, OR GROUP WHERE HE PRACTICES OF THE TERMS AND CONDITIONS; SHALL NOT SUPERVISE A PHYSICIAN'S ASSISTANT; SHALL FURNISH BOARD WITH ADDRESS AND/OR CHANGE OF ADDRESS; SHALL APPEAR BEFORE BOARD UPON REQUEST. TWO PREVIOUS ORDERS OF CONTINUANCE ON 11/8/91 AND 3/5/92 REQUIRED HIM TO SUBMIT TO PHYSICAL, PSYCHOLOGICAL AND/OR PSYCHIATRIC EXAMS, TO PROVIDE RANDOM FLUID TESTING, TO USE DUPLICATE SERIALLY NUMBERED PRESCRIPTION PADS FOR ALL CONTROLLED DANGEROUS SUBSTANCES, AND TO CONTINUE PARTICIPATION IN ALL RECOMMENDED FOLLOW-UP AND SUPPORT PROGRAMS. ON 7/22/94 AND 9/10/94 HIS MOTION TO MODIFY THE TERM OF HIS PROBATION DENIED.

DOUGLAS, HOWARD T MD, LICENSE NUMBER 12539 OF 4255 S BUCKLEY ROAD #130, AURORA, CO, WAS DISCIPLINED BY OKLAHOMA ON JUNE 26, 1998
DISCIPLINARY ACTION: DENIAL OF NEW LICENSE
OFFENSE: DISCIPLINARY ACTION BY ANOTHER STATE OR AGENCY

NOTES: LICENSE IN TEXAS WAS SUSPENDED ON 5/12/97 FOR UNPROFESSIONAL CONDUCT, INCLUDING HIS PRESCRIBING WITHOUT EXAMINATION OR EVALUATION AND HIS FAILURE TO CONFORM TO MINIMAL STANDARDS OF ACCEPTABLE MEDICAL PRACTICE. THE LICENSE REMAINS UNDER SUSPENSION AS OF THE DATE OF THIS ORDER. REINSTATEMENT DENIED.

DOWLING, WILLIAM J MD, LICENSE NUMBER 0005554, WAS DISCIPLINED BY OKLAHOMA ON JULY 22, 1994
DISCIPLINARY ACTION: 60-MONTH PROBATION; REPRIMAND
OFFENSE: PROFESSIONAL MISCONDUCT

NOTES: ALLEGATIONS THAT DURING 1993 AND 1994 HE AIDED AND ABETTED THE PRACTICE OF MEDICINE BY UNLICENSED PERSONS IN THAT HE DID NOT SPEND FULL TIME AT WORK AT HIS CLINIC AND THAT IN HIS ABSENCE UNLICENSED STAFF MEMBERS ROUTINELY SAW HIS PATIENTS, ADMINISTERED A REGIMEN OF DRUGS AND CONTROLLED SUBSTANCES TO PATIENTS FOR THE PURPOSE OF WEIGHT CONTROL AND THAT HE DID NOT MAINTAIN PROPER RECORDS

OF THE PURCHASE AND DISPOSAL OF CONTROLLED DRUGS OR NARCOTIC DRUGS; HE SUBMITS TO JURISDICTION OF BOARD WITHOUT ADMITTING OR DENYING THESE ALLEGATIONS. PROBATION TO BEGIN 7/23/94. CONDITIONS OF PROBATION: SHALL PERSONALLY SEE ALL NEW PATIENTS, PRESCRIBE THEIR MEDICATIONS PERSONALLY AND INITIAL THEIR CHARTS EVEN IF INFORMATION IS PROVIDED BY ANOTHER PERSON; FOR CURRENT PATIENTS CLINICAL STAFF MAY, PURSUANT TO HIS PRESCRIBED REGIMEN, SEE THESE PATIENTS, CONTINUE THEIR MEDICATIONS AND DOCUMENT THIS IN CHART AND SHALL INFORM HIM IF ANY CHANGE APPEARS IN THESE PATIENTS; IN PATIENTS WHO ARE ENDING THEIR TREATMENT HE SHALL PERSONALLY SEE SUCH PATIENT, DIAGNOSE THEIR CURRENT CONDITION, INITIAL THE CHART REGARDLESS IF THE INFORMATION WAS PROVIDED BY ANOTHER PERSON, PERSONALLY OVERSEE TERMINATION AND ANY CONTINUATION OR CESSATION OF ANY MEDICATIONS; SHALL PROVIDE BOARD WITH ANY REQUESTED REPORTS; SHALL PAY COSTS.

DUBE, PHILIPPE ABEL MD, LICENSE NUMBER 19237 OF 215 COLLEGE STREET SE, EDISON, GA, WAS DISCIPLINED BY OKLAHOMA ON APRIL 24, 1997
DISCIPLINARY ACTION: LICENSE REVOCATION
OFFENSE: SEXUAL ABUSE OF OR SEXUAL MISCONDUCT WITH A PATIENT

NOTES: FROM 2/95 THROUGH 6/95, HE INAPPROPRIATELY AND FREQUENTLY COMMENTED UPON OR INQUIRED ABOUT SEX, BREASTS, AND OTHER BODY PARTS TO PATIENTS AND STAFF AT A MEDICAL CLINIC; ROUTINELY PERFORMED PELVIC EXAMS ON ATTRACTIVE FEMALE PATIENTS WHO SOUGHT MEDICAL ATTENTION FOR UNRELATED COMPLAINTS AND ALSO CONDUCTED UNASSISTED BREAST EXAMS UPON A GROUP OF MINOR CHEERLEADERS, AGED 14 TO 18 YEARS OF AGE. HIS LICENSE EXPIRED IN NOVEMBER 1996 AND WAS AUTOMATICALLY SUSPENDED FOR FAILURE TO RENEW; BOARD CONTINUED HEARING FROM ORIGINAL DATE OF 1/9/97 TO 3/13/97 DUE TO HIS FAILURE TO EITHER RESPOND OR APPEAR TO DISCUSS THE COMPLAINT; FAILED TO SUBMIT TO THE BOARD HIS CURRENT ADDRESS UPON RELOCATION; FAILED TO FILE HIS WRITTEN RESPONSE AS REQUIRED BY BOARD RULES OR TO MAKE ANY OTHER RESPONSE OR APPEARANCE.

DUNCAN, KENNETH C MD, LICENSE NUMBER 0006838 OF 5555 E 71 #6105 BLDG 6, TULSA, OK, WAS DISCIPLINED BY OKLAHOMA ON NOVEMBER 23, 1992
DISCIPLINARY ACTION: EMERGENCY SUSPENSION; MONITORING OF PHYSICIAN PERFORMANCE
OFFENSE: OVERPRESCRIBING OR MISPRESCRIBING DRUGS

NOTES: FROM 1/91 THROUGH 3/92 WAS PRESCRIBING, DISPENSING OR ADMINISTERING CONTROLLED SUBSTANCES OR NARCOTIC DRUGS IN EXCESS OF THE AMOUNT CONSIDERED GOOD MEDICAL PRACTICE, OR WITHOUT MEDICAL NEED IN ACCORDANCE WITH PUBLISHED STANDARDS TO AT LEAST FOUR PATIENTS. SUSPENSION TO CONTINUE UNTIL BOARD MEETING 1/8-9/93. BY THAT DATE HE SHALL FURNISH BOARD WITH PROOF OF MENTAL AND PHYSICAL CAPACITY TO PRACTICE, INCLUDING REPORTS FROM EXAMINING PHYSICIAN AND PSYCHIATRIST.

DUNCAN, KENNETH C MD, LICENSE NUMBER 0006838 OF 5555 E 71 #6105 BLDG 6, TULSA, OK, WAS DISCIPLINED BY OKLAHOMA ON JANUARY 15, 1993
DISCIPLINARY ACTION: 60-MONTH PROBATION; RESTRICTION PLACED ON LICENSE

NOTES: IN COMPLIANCE WITH 11/23/92 SUSPENSION ORDER HE HAS PROVIDED PROOF OF MENTAL AND PHYSICAL CAPACITY TO PRACTICE INCLUDING LETTERS FROM A PHYSICIAN AND FROM A PSYCHIATRIST. SUSPENSION LIFTED. PROBATION TO BEGIN 1/8/93. CONDITIONS OF PROBATION: SHALL NOT PRESCRIBE, ADMINISTER OR DISPENSE ANY SCHEDULE II CONTROLLED DANGEROUS SUBSTANCES EXCEPT TO HOSPITAL IN-PATIENTS; MAY PRESCRIBE SCHEDULE III, IV AND V DRUGS ONLY ON SERIALLY-NUMBERED DUPLICATE PRESCRIPTION PADS COPIES OF WHICH SHALL BE AVAILABLE FOR INSPECTION; SHALL FURNISH BOARD ADDRESS/CHANGE OF ADDRESS; SHALL APPEAR BEFORE BOARD UPON REQUEST AND SUBMIT REQUIRED REPORTS; SHALL PAY COSTS; SHALL FURNISH EVERY STATE IN WHICH HE HOLDS OR APPLIES FOR LICENSURE AND ANY HEALTH CARE ENTITY WHERE HE HAS STAFF PRIVILEGES A COPY OF THIS ORDER; SHALL NOT SUPERVISE A PHYSICIAN'S ASSISTANT.

DUNFORD, WILLIAM W DO, LICENSE NUMBER 0001458, WAS DISCIPLINED BY OKLAHOMA ON FEBRUARY 9, 1993
DISCIPLINARY ACTION: LICENSE SUSPENSION; REQUIRED TO TAKE ADDITIONAL MEDICAL EDUCATION
OFFENSE: OVERPRESCRIBING OR MISPRESCRIBING DRUGS

NOTES: FAILED TO KEEP COMPLETE AND ACCURATE RECORDS OF PURCHASE AND DISPOSAL OF CONTROLLED DRUGS OR NARCOTICS; PRESCRIBED OR ADMINISTERED DRUGS OR TREATMENT WITHOUT SUFFICIENT EXAMINATION AND THE ESTABLISHMENT OF A VALID PHYSICIAN-PATIENT RELATIONSHIP IN THAT HIS OFFICE HAD AT LEAST 100-150 PATIENTS PER DAY, SAW THE PATIENT ON THE FIRST VISIT AND WOULD DEVELOP A DIET PLAN; RARELY SAW PATIENTS ON SUBSEQUENT VISITS WHEN FURTHER MEDICATIONS INCLUDING PHENDIMETRAZINE AND THYROID PILLS WERE DISPENSED; BETWEEN 1/90 AND 7/90 AT LEAST 384 PATIENTS RECEIVED CONTROLLED DANGEROUS SUBSTANCES; ALLOWED PATIENTS TO RECEIVE DRUGS UNTIL THEY WANTED TO STOP. INDEFINITE SUSPENSION WITH TERMS FOR REINSTATEMENT INCLUDING COMPLETING A COURSE IN "THE PROPER PRESCRIBING OF CONTROLLED DANGEROUS SUBSTANCES, AND A ONE YEAR POST-GRADUATE COURSE IN GENERAL PRACTICE RESIDENCY. $9,317.00 ADMINISTRATIVE COSTS.

EITEL, JOHN BEN DO, LICENSE NUMBER 00B8453 OF PORT NECHES, TX, WAS DISCIPLINED BY TEXAS ON APRIL 15, 1994
DISCIPLINARY ACTION: SURRENDER OF CONTROLLED SUBSTANCE LICENSE
OFFENSE: NONCOMPLIANCE WITH A PROFESSIONAL RULE

NOTES: FAILED TO MAINTAIN ADEQUATE RECORDS RELATING TO CONTROLLED SUBSTANCES; PLED GUILTY TO A PORTION OF THE CHARGES AGAINST HIM, LEADING TO THE IMPOSITION OF A FINE AND SURRENDER OF DEA AND TEXAS CONTROLLED SUBSTANCES CERTIFICATES. SHALL NOT HOLD THESE CERTIFICATES AND SHALL NOT REAPPLY WITHOUT BOARD APPROVAL; SHALL GIVE A COPY OF THIS ORDER TO ANY HEALTH CARE ENTITY WHERE HE HAS PRIVILEGES; SHALL COOPERATE WITH THE BOARD IN VERIFYING COMPLIANCE; SHALL INFORM BOARD OF CHANGE OF ADDRESS WITHIN 10 DAYS. SHALL NOT SEEK MODIFICATION FOR ONE YEAR.

EITEL, JOHN BEN DO, LICENSE NUMBER 0000577, WAS

DISCIPLINED BY OKLAHOMA ON MARCH 24, 1995
DISCIPLINARY ACTION: SURRENDER OF LICENSE
OFFENSE: DISCIPLINARY ACTION BY ANOTHER STATE OR AGENCY

NOTES: ALLEGATIONS OF ACTION IN TEXAS. HAD SURRENDERED HIS OKLAHOMA LICENSE AND CURRENT RENEWAL CERTIFICATE TO THE BOARD; LICENSE CANCELED.

ELLIOTT, CHARLES CALEB MD, LICENSE NUMBER 0007914, WAS DISCIPLINED BY OKLAHOMA ON JUNE 21, 1991
DISCIPLINARY ACTION: 24-MONTH LICENSE SUSPENSION
OFFENSE: SEXUAL ABUSE OF OR SEXUAL MISCONDUCT WITH A PATIENT

NOTES: PREVIOUS ACTIONS: SUSPENDED FROM 1/18/85-5/24/85 AND ON PROBATION FOR FIVE YEARS THEREAFTER FOR IMPROPERLY RENDERING MEDICAL SERVICES. ON 3/11/89, PRESENTED TO EMERGENCY ROOM AND DIAGNOSED WITH ACUTE SYNCOPE, UNKNOWN CAUSE, AND SECONDARILY AN ILLNESS REQUIRING LITHIUM THERAPY. INABILITY TO PRACTICE MEDICINE WITH REASONABLE SKILL AND SAFETY TO PATIENTS. DURING 1987-89, SEXUALLY HARASSED AND IMPROPERLY HANDLED FEMALE PATIENTS AND HOSPITAL STAFF MEMBERS. COMPLAINT AND CITATION WERE DISMISSED WITHOUT PREJUDICE 6/9/90, AND BOARD AGREED TO ACCEPT HIS LICENSE RESIGNATION WITHIN SIX MONTHS. HE SUBSEQUENTLY DEMANDED CASE BE HEARD, AND COMPLAINT WAS REFILED. SUSPENSION TO CONTINUE UNTIL HE CAN PRESENT PSYCHIATRIC TESTIMONY THAT HIS PHYSICAL AND MENTAL CONDITION DOES NOT REPRESENT A THREAT TO THE PUBLIC.

ELLIOTT, CHARLES CALEB MD, LICENSE NUMBER 0007914, WAS DISCIPLINED BY OKLAHOMA ON NOVEMBER 1, 1991
DISCIPLINARY ACTION: 60-MONTH PROBATION; RESTRICTION PLACED ON LICENSE

NOTES: WRITTEN REPORTS PROVIDED BY TWO PSYCHIATRISTS. SUSPENSION TERMINATED, PLACED ON PROBATION UNDER TERMS AND CONDITIONS: CONTINUED MONITORING AND TREATMENT BY PSYCHIATRIST WITH QUARTERLY REPORTS TO BOARD; MAY PRACTICE RADIOLOGY IN A HOSPITAL SETTING SUPERVISED BY CHIEF OF STAFF; NO DIRECT PERSONAL CONTACT WITH PATIENTS OF A SEXUAL NATURE; SHALL NOT PRESCRIBE, ADMINISTER OR DISPENSE ANY MEDICATIONS FOR PERSONAL USE, TO SPECIFICALLY INCLUDE CONTROLLED DANGEROUS SUBSTANCES; SHALL TAKE NO MEDICATION UNLESS AUTHORIZED BY TREATING PSYCHIATRIST; SHALL ABSTAIN FROM ALCOHOL; SHALL SUBMIT BIOLOGICAL FLUID SPECIMENS FOR ANALYSIS; SHALL NOT SUPERVISE A PHYSICIAN ASSISTANT; SHALL NOTIFY ANY HOSPITAL WHERE HE HOLDS STAFF PRIVILEGES, OR CLINIC, OR GROUP WHERE HE PRACTICES OF THE TERMS AND CONDITIONS; SHALL FURNISH BOARD WITH ADDRESS AND/OR CHANGE OF ADDRESS; SHALL APPEAR BEFORE BOARD UPON REQUEST. ON 11/1/96 PROBATION EXPIRED; LICENSE IS UNMODIFIED AND IN GOOD STANDING.

ENGLISH, RONALD H MD, LICENSE NUMBER 0017248 OF 543 EAST APACHE #201, TULSA, OK, WAS DISCIPLINED BY OKLAHOMA ON OCTOBER 2, 1995
DISCIPLINARY ACTION: 60-MONTH PROBATION; RESTRICTION PLACED ON CONTROLLED SUBSTANCE LICENSE
OFFENSE: OVERPRESCRIBING OR MISPRESCRIBING DRUGS

NOTES: A PRESCRIPTION SURVEY REVEALED THAT SCHEDULE DRUGS WERE BEING PRESCRIBED REGULARLY IN EXCESS OF THE AMOUNT CONSIDERED FOR THE MEDICAL NEED PRESENTED AND HIS PATIENT RECORDS MAINTAINED WERE INADEQUATE IN THE CASE OF AT LEAST FOUR PATIENTS BETWEEN 1/1/94 AND 11/16/94. PROBATION BEGINNING 9/16/95 UNDER THE FOLLOWING TERMS AND CONDITIONS: SHALL KEEP SERIALLY-NUMBERED, DUPLICATE PRESCRIPTIONS FOR ALL CONTROLLED DANGEROUS SUBSTANCES PRESCRIBED AND SHALL MAKE SUCH RECORDS AVAILABLE TO THE BOARD UPON REQUEST; SHALL SUBMIT TO THE BOARD ADDRESS/ CHANGE IN ADDRESS; SHALL APPEAR BEFORE THE BOARD UPON REQUEST AND SUBMIT ANY REQUIRED REPORTS; SHALL SUBSTANTIALLY REDUCE THE NUMBER OF CONTROLLED DANGEROUS SUBSTANCES PRESCRIPTIONS BEING WRITTEN; SHALL PAY COSTS; SHALL NOTIFY ANY HOSPITAL WHERE HE HOLDS STAFF PRIVILEGES, OR CLINIC, OR GROUP WHERE HE PRACTICES OF THE TERMS AND CONDITIONS OF THIS ORDER AND PROVIDE A COPY THEREOF; SHALL MEET WITH THE BOARD NO LESS THAN QUARTERLY AND SHALL BRING WITH HIM 10 MEDICAL RECORDS RANDOMLY SELECTED BY THE COMPLIANCE COORDINATOR.

ENOS, JACK P MD, LICENSE NUMBER 0006106, WAS DISCIPLINED BY OKLAHOMA ON OCTOBER 11, 1993
DISCIPLINARY ACTION: 1-MONTH LICENSE SUSPENSION; 60-MONTH PROBATION
OFFENSE: OVERPRESCRIBING OR MISPRESCRIBING DRUGS

NOTES: A PRESCRIPTION SURVEY REVEALED THAT DURING 1992 IN THE CASE OF FIVE PATIENTS HE PRESCRIBED CONTROLLED DANGEROUS SUBSTANCES IN EXCESSIVE AMOUNTS; NATURE AND EXTENT OF OMISSIONS IN PATIENT CHARTS RAISE ISSUES AS TO HIS COMPETENCY TO CONTINUE TO PRACTICE. 30 DAY SUSPENSION RETROACTIVE TO 10/9/93. CONDITIONS OF PROBATION: SHALL NOT PRESCRIBE, ADMINISTER OR DISPENSE ANY SCHEDULE II, III OR IV CONTROLLED DANGEROUS SUBSTANCES; MAY PRESCRIBE SCHEDULE V DRUGS ONLY ON SERIALLY-NUMBERED DUPLICATE PRESCRIPTION PADS WITH COPIES AVAILABLE TO THE BOARD; SHALL FURNISH BOARD WITH ADDRESS AND/OR CHANGE OF ADDRESS; SHALL APPEAR BEFORE THE BOARD UPON REQUEST AND PROVIDE ANY REPORTS REQUESTED; SHALL NOT SUPERVISE A PHYSICIAN'S ASSISTANT; SHALL PAY COSTS; SHALL FURNISH EVERY STATE WHERE HE IS LICENSED OR APPLIES FOR LICENSURE AND ALL HEALTH CARE ENTITIES WHERE HE ANTICIPATES HOLDING PRIVILEGES A COPY OF THIS ORDER.

ENOS, JACK P MD OF 331 MAIN ST, YUKON, OK, WAS DISCIPLINED BY DEA ON NOVEMBER 8, 1993
DISCIPLINARY ACTION: RESTRICTION PLACED ON CONTROLLED SUBSTANCE LICENSE
OFFENSE: DISCIPLINARY ACTION BY ANOTHER STATE OR AGENCY

NOTES: OKLAHOMA STATE MEDICAL LICENSE SUSPENDED ON 10/09/93 FOR OVERPRESCRIBING.

ERWIN, JEFFERSON D MD, LICENSE NUMBER A040468 OF LAWTON, OK, WAS DISCIPLINED BY CALIFORNIA ON JANUARY 30, 1992
DISCIPLINARY ACTION: LICENSE REVOCATION
OFFENSE: DISCIPLINARY ACTION BY ANOTHER STATE OR AGENCY

NOTES: DISCIPLINED BY OKLAHOMA BOARD FOR CHEMICAL DEPENDENCY. DEFAULT DECISION.

ERWIN, JEFFERSON DAVIS MD, LICENSE NUMBER 0015856 OF 7020 EAST RENO #203, MIDWEST CITY, OK, WAS DISCIPLINED BY OKLAHOMA ON DECEMBER 2, 1993
DISCIPLINARY ACTION: LICENSE SUSPENSION
OFFENSE: SUBSTANCE ABUSE

NOTES: ON 6/9/89 BOARD SUSPENDED HIS LICENSE IN ORDER TO ALLOW HIM TO FULFILL REQUIREMENTS OF PHYSICIAN RECOVERY COMMITTEE; ENTERED TREATMENT FOR CHEMICAL DEPENDENCY ON 6/20/89 FOLLOWED BY AN OUTPATIENT PROGRAM; ON 9/18/89 LEFT TREATMENT AGAINST MEDICAL ADVICE; HAS NOT COMPLETED THIS TREATMENT. LICENSE SHALL REMAIN SUSPENDED UNTIL HE PRESENTS EVIDENCE OF SUCCESSFUL COMPLETION OF TREATMENT.

ERWIN, JEFFERSON DAVIS MD, LICENSE NUMBER 0015856 OF 1000 NE 10, OKLAHOMA CITY, OK, WAS DISCIPLINED BY OKLAHOMA ON APRIL 1, 1994
DISCIPLINARY ACTION: PROBATION; RESTRICTION PLACED ON LICENSE
OFFENSE: SUBSTANCE ABUSE

NOTES: IN COMPLIANCE WITH 11/20/93 SUSPENSION HE PRESENTED EVIDENCE OF SUCCESSFUL COMPLETION OF EVALUATION AND IN-PATIENT TREATMENT; WITH REGARD TO GUARDIANSHIP, COURT FOUND HE WAS NO LONGER AN INCAPACITATED PERSON AND GUARDIAN WAS DISCHARGED. SUPERVISED MEDICAL DOCTOR CERTIFICATE GRANTED UNDER PROBATION. INDEFINITE PROBATION BEGINNING 2/12/94. CONDITIONS OF PROBATION: SHALL NOT PRESCRIBE, ADMINISTER OR DISPENSE ANY MEDICATIONS FOR HIS PERSONAL USE AND SHALL TAKE NONE UNLESS AUTHORIZED BY ANOTHER PHYSICIAN FOR A LEGITIMATE MEDICAL NEED; SHALL ABSTAIN FROM THE CONSUMPTION OF ALCOHOL OR ANY SUBSTANCE WHICH WOULD ADVERSELY AFFECT HIS ABILITY TO PRACTICE; SHALL NOT INGEST ANYTHING THAT WILL TEST POSITIVE FOR ALCOHOL OR ANY CONTROLLED SUBSTANCE; SHALL SUBMIT BIOLOGICAL FLUID SPECIMENS; TREATING PHYSICIANS SHALL SUBMIT QUARTERLY REPORTS; SHALL NOT PRESCRIBE, ADMINISTER OR DISPENSE ANY CONTROLLED DANGEROUS SUBSTANCES TO ANY PERSONS OR AUTHORIZE ANY PERSONNEL UNDER HIS SUPERVISION TO DO SO; SHALL PRACTICE IN A CONTROLLED, BOARD-APPROVED ENVIRONMENT; SHALL NOT ALLOW THE INDEPENDENT PRACTICE OF MEDICINE BY ANY PERSONNEL UNDER HIS SUPERVISION, EMPLOYMENT OR CONTROL NOR ALLOW THE INITIATION OF ANY THERAPEUTIC REGIMEN BY THEM IF HE IS NOT IN THE IMMEDIATE VICINITY; SHALL HAVE ANY HEALTH CARE ENTITY WHERE HE ANTICIPATES PRACTICE TO SUBMIT A WRITTEN STATEMENT REGARDING MONITORING HIS PRACTICE; SHALL FURNISH TO EVERY STATE WHERE HE HOLDS OR APPLIES FOR LICENSURE AND ANY HEALTH CARE ENTITY WHERE HE HAS PRIVILEGES A COPY OF THIS ORDER; SHALL NOT PERFORM ANY OPEN OR INVASIVE SURGICAL PROCEDURES UNTIL AUTHORIZED BY THE BOARD; SHALL PLACE HIMSELF IN A BOARD APPROVED REHABILITATION PROGRAM FOR AFTER-CARE TREATMENT; SHALL ENTER AND CONTINUE PSYCHIATRIC TREATMENT AND AUTHORIZE RELEASE OF THESE RECORDS TO THE BOARD; SHALL NOT SUPERVISE A PHYSICIAN'S ASSISTANT; SHALL FURNISH BOARD WITH CURRENT AND/OR CHANGE OF ADDRESS; SHALL APPEAR BEFORE THE BOARD UPON REQUEST AND SUBMIT ANY REQUIRED REPORTS; SHALL PAY COSTS. ON 9/9/94 REQUEST TO MODIFY THIS ORDER WAS DENIED. ON 3/27/97 APPLICATION FOR A SPECIAL LICENSE FOR SPECIFIED EMPLOYMENT IS GRANTED.

ERWIN, JEFFERSON DAVIS MD, LICENSE NUMBER 0015856, WAS DISCIPLINED BY OKLAHOMA ON OCTOBER 2, 1995
DISCIPLINARY ACTION: REPRIMAND
OFFENSE: CRIMINAL CONVICTION OR PLEA OF GUILTY, NOLO CONTENDERE, OR NO CONTEST TO A CRIME

NOTES: ON 8/23/94 PLED GUILTY TO THE CRIMES OF ASSAULT AND ASSAULT AND BATTERY; FAILED TO INFORM THE BOARD OF THE CRIMINAL ASSAULT AND BATTERY THAT OCCURRED ON 5/29/94, WHICH RESULTED IN HIS ARREST, CRIMINAL CHARGES, AND COURT DISPOSITION.

FERGUSON, FREDERIC H DO, LICENSE NUMBER 0001520, WAS DISCIPLINED BY OKLAHOMA ON MARCH 22, 1993
DISCIPLINARY ACTION: 6-MONTH LICENSE SUSPENSION; REQUIRED TO TAKE ADDITIONAL MEDICAL EDUCATION
OFFENSE: CRIMINAL CONVICTION OR PLEA OF GUILTY, NOLO CONTENDERE, OR NO CONTEST TO A CRIME

NOTES: CONVICTED OF UNLAWFUL DISPENSING OF A CONTROLLED SUBSTANCE. SHALL ATTEND AND SUCCESSFULLY COMPLETE A COURSE IN THE PROPER METHOD OF PRESCRIBING CONTROLLED DANGEROUS SUBSTANCES AND SHALL PROVIDE THE BOARD WITH DOCUMENTS INDICATING SUCCESSFUL COMPLETION OF SAID COURSE; SHALL ATTEND 100 HOURS OF CONTINUING MEDICAL EDUCATION; AFTER THE SIX MONTH SUSPENSION SHALL APPEAR BEFORE THE BOARD TO DEMONSTRATE HIS COMPLIANCE WITH THE TERMS AND CONDITIONS; $2,157.35 ADMINISTRATIVE COSTS.

FERGUSON, FREDERIC H DO, LICENSE NUMBER 0001520, WAS DISCIPLINED BY OKLAHOMA ON DECEMBER 29, 1993
DISCIPLINARY ACTION: 24-MONTH PROBATION; RESTRICTION PLACED ON CONTROLLED SUBSTANCE LICENSE

NOTES: LICENSE REISSUED UNDER THE FOLLOWING TERMS AND CONDITIONS: SHALL NOT DISPENSE ANY CONTROLLED DANGEROUS SUBSTANCES AND WILL PRESCRIBE ONLY THOSE FOR WHICH HE HAS AUTHORITY FROM THE BUREAU OF NARCOTICS AND DANGEROUS DRUGS; SHALL PROVIDE DUPLICATE COPIES OF ALL THESE PRESCRIPTIONS WRITTEN BY HIM, TO THE BOARD, ON A MONTHLY BASIS; SHALL PARTICIPATE IN 50 HOURS OF CONTINUING MEDICAL EDUCATION IN GENERAL AND FAMILY MEDICINE; PROOF OF THE ACHIEVEMENT OF THESE 50 HOURS MUST ACCOMPANY THE APPLICATION FOR ANNUAL LICENSE RENEWAL; SHALL NOTIFY THE BOARD, IN WRITING, OF ANY CHANGE OF ADDRESS WITHIN 14 DAYS; SHALL APPEAR BEFORE THE BOARD UPON REQUEST; AGREES TO RECEIVE UNANNOUNCED VISITS FROM THE BOARD AT ITS DISCRETION; TERMS OF RESIDENCE OR PRACTICE OUTSIDE OF OKLAHOMA WILL RESULT IN THE TOLLING OF THE AGREEMENT AND WILL NOT APPLY TO THE REDUCTION OF THE PROBATIONARY PERIOD. ON 12/19/95 PROBATION TERMINATED AND LICENSE REINSTATED IN GOOD STANDING.

FERMO, JOE C JR MD, DATE OF BIRTH AUGUST 31, 1930 OF 1145 SOUTH UTICA, SUITE 460, TULSA, OK, WAS DISCIPLINED BY MEDICARE ON JUNE 20, 1990
DISCIPLINARY ACTION: 180-MONTH EXCLUSION FROM THE MEDICARE AND/OR MEDICAID PROGRAM
OFFENSE: CRIMINAL CONVICTION OR PLEA OF GUILTY, NOLO CONTENDERE, OR NO CONTEST TO A CRIME

NOTES: PROGRAM-RELATED CONVICTION.

FERMO, JOSE CRUZ JR MD, LICENSE NUMBER 0011069, WAS DISCIPLINED BY OKLAHOMA ON JUNE 8, 1990
DISCIPLINARY ACTION: 57-MONTH PROBATION
OFFENSE: DISCIPLINARY ACTION BY ANOTHER STATE OR AGENCY

NOTES: FROM 5/6/87 THROUGH 5/15/89 PRESENTED CLAIMS FOR PAYMENT TO MEDICAID FOR SERVICES NOT RENDERED IN THE AMOUNT CLAIMED; ON 2/23/90 PLED GUILTY TO 10 COUNTS OF FILING A FALSE CLAIM. CONDITIONAL COURT ORDER WILL BE DISMISSED UPON COMPLETION OF SPECIFIED TERMS; MUST PAY A $100,000 FINE AND MAKE RESTITUTION OF $350,000; LOST PROVIDER AGREEMENT WITH MEDICARE/MEDICAID. PROBATIONARY TERMS AND CONDITIONS: SHALL COMPLY WITH ALL TERMS AND CONDITIONS OF DEFERRED SENTENCE ENTERED ON 2/23/90 IN OKLAHOMA COUNTY DISTRICT COURT; SHALL CREATE AND KEEP IN PLACE AN IN-HOUSE BILLING SYSTEM THAT WILL PREVENT INAPPROPRIATE CHARGES TO PATIENTS OR THIRD PARTY PAYERS; SHALL NOTIFY BOARD OF ANY APPLICATION FOR REINSTATEMENT OF PROVIDER STATUS.

FERMO, MERLI G MD, LICENSE NUMBER 0010751, WAS DISCIPLINED BY OKLAHOMA ON JUNE 8, 1990
DISCIPLINARY ACTION: 57-MONTH PROBATION; FINE
OFFENSE: DISCIPLINARY ACTION BY ANOTHER STATE OR AGENCY

NOTES: FROM 5/6/87 THROUGH 5/15/89 PRESENTED CLAIMS FOR PAYMENT TO MEDICAID FOR SERVICES NOT RENDERED IN THE AMOUNT CLAIMED; ON 2/23/90 PLED GUILTY TO FIVE COUNTS OF FILING A FALSE CLAIM. CONDITIONAL COURT ORDER WILL BE DISMISSED UPON COMPLETION OF SPECIFIED TERMS; MUST PAY A $50,000 FINE AND MAKE RESTITUTION OF $150,000; LOST PROVIDER AGREEMENT WITH MEDICARE/MEDICAID. PROBATIONARY TERMS AND CONDITIONS: SHALL COMPLY WITH ALL TERMS AND CONDITIONS OF DEFERRED SENTENCE ENTERED ON 2/23/90 IN OKLAHOMA COUNTY DISTRICT COURT; SHALL CREATE AND KEEP IN PLACE AN IN-HOUSE BILLING SYSTEM THAT WILL PREVENT INAPPROPRIATE CHARGES TO PATIENTS OR THIRD PARTY PAYERS; SHALL NOTIFY BOARD OF ANY APPLICATION FOR REINSTATEMENT OF HER PROVIDER STATUS WITH MEDICARE; SHALL NOTIFY ANY HOSPITAL WHERE SHE HOLDS STAFF PRIVILEGES, OR CLINIC OR GROUP OF THE TERMS AND CONDITIONS; SHALL FURNISH BOARD WITH ADDRESS AND/OR CHANGE OF ADDRESS; SHALL APPEAR BEFORE BOARD UPON REQUEST. SHE AND HER SPOUSE CONTRACTED WITH WESTERN STATE HOSPITAL TO PRACTICE THERE AND AFTER HER HUSBAND MOVED TO WESTERN STATE, THE PRACTICE WAS SHUT DOWN AND THEY ARE NOW IN CONSULTATION WITH LEGAL COUNSEL CONCERNING THEIR CONTRACT RIGHTS AGAINST THE OKLAHOMA DEPARTMENT OF MENTAL HEALTH.

FERMO, MERLI G MD, DATE OF BIRTH JULY 11, 1929 OF 1145 SOUTH UTICA, SUITE 460, TULSA, OK, WAS DISCIPLINED BY MEDICARE ON JUNE 20, 1990
DISCIPLINARY ACTION: 120-MONTH EXCLUSION FROM THE MEDICARE AND/OR MEDICAID PROGRAM
OFFENSE: CRIMINAL CONVICTION OR PLEA OF GUILTY, NOLO CONTENDERE, OR NO CONTEST TO A CRIME

NOTES: PROGRAM-RELATED CONVICTION.

FINCHER, MARK LYNN MD, LICENSE NUMBER 0014822 OF 1512 BARWICK, NORMAN, OK, WAS DISCIPLINED BY OKLAHOMA ON JUNE 22, 1991
DISCIPLINARY ACTION: 24-MONTH LICENSE SUSPENSION
OFFENSE: PROVIDING FALSE INFORMATION TO THE BOARD OR OTHER HEALTH AGENCY

NOTES: ON 5/31/90, ARRESTED IN STEPHENS COUNTY, OKLAHOMA, AND CHARGED WITH TWO COUNTS OF LARCENY OF DOMESTIC ANIMALS. FORMALLY CHARGED ON 6/1/90. ON 10/2/90, SUBMITTED AN APPLICATION FOR REINSTATEMENT OF LICENSE, AND FALSELY ANSWERED TWO QUESTIONS; SPECIFICALLY, ANSWERED "NO" TO "HAVE YOU EVER BEEN CHARGED WITH OR CONVICTED OF A FELONY OR MISDEMEANOR?" BEFORE NEXT BOARD APPEARANCE, SHALL PRESENT EVIDENCE FROM PSYCHIATRIST THAT HE IS FREE OF ANY MENTAL CONDITION THAT WOULD PREVENT HIM FROM PRACTICING WITH REASONABLE SKILL AND SAFETY.

FINCHER, MARK LYNN MD, LICENSE NUMBER 00H7413 OF NORMAN, OK, WAS DISCIPLINED BY TEXAS ON JUNE 17, 1992
DISCIPLINARY ACTION: SURRENDER OF LICENSE
OFFENSE: DISCIPLINARY ACTION BY ANOTHER STATE OR AGENCY

FINCHER, MARK LYNN MD OF 1512 BARWICK, NORMAN, OK, WAS DISCIPLINED BY DEA ON JUNE 22, 1992
DISCIPLINARY ACTION: REVOCATION OF CONTROLLED SUBSTANCE LICENSE
OFFENSE: DISCIPLINARY ACTION BY ANOTHER STATE OR AGENCY

NOTES: EFFECTIVE 06/22/91 OKLAHOMA SUSPENDED HIS MEDICAL LICENSE FOR TWO YEARS BASED ON HIS FRAUDULENT MISREPRESENTATION OF HIS PREVIOUS CRIMINAL RECORD IN AN APPLICATION THAT HE SUBMITTED FOR REINSTATEMENT OF HIS MEDICAL LICENSE. ALSO, AS OF 01/28/92 HE CONTINUED TO BE UNREGISTERED WITH THE CONTROLLED SUBSTANCES LICENSING AUTHORITY IN OKLAHOMA.

FINKLE, ROBERT H DR OF BOX 436, CAMERON, MO, WAS DISCIPLINED BY OKLAHOMA ON JANUARY 12, 1991
DISCIPLINARY ACTION: 36-MONTH PROBATION; MONITORING OF PHYSICIAN PERFORMANCE

NOTES: DISCUSSED WITH BOARD A RECENT HIATUS IN HIS PROFESSIONAL PRACTICE AND SEVERAL LOCATIONS OF PRACTICE WITHIN THE LAST FOUR YEARS. LICENSE GRANTED UNDER PROBATIONARY TERMS AND CONDITIONS: MONTHLY REPORTS ON HIS OVERALL PERFORMANCE TO BE SUBMITTED BY THE CHIEF OF STAFF OF SURGERY AT THE OKLAHOMA HOSPITAL WHERE HE PRACTICES; SHALL NOTIFY ANY HOSPITAL WHERE HE HOLDS STAFF PRIVILEGES, OR CLINIC, OR GROUP WHERE HE PRACTICES OF THE TERMS AND CONDITIONS; SHALL FURNISH BOARD WITH ADDRESS AND/OR CHANGE OF ADDRESS; SHALL APPEAR BEFORE BOARD UPON REQUEST.

FLOREZ, JUAN B G MD, WAS DISCIPLINED BY ARIZONA ON OCTOBER 8, 1991
DISCIPLINARY ACTION: REQUIRED TO TAKE ADDITIONAL MEDICAL EDUCATION
OFFENSE: FAILURE TO COMPLY WITH PREVIOUS BOARD ORDER

NOTES: FAILED THE BOARD-ORDERED SPEX EXAMINATION FOR THE SECOND TIME. BOARD SHALL CONTINUE ITS INVESTIGATION IN THIS MATTER AND HE SHALL COMPLETE A MINI-RESIDENCY COURSE IN PHARMACOLOGY, WITH EMPHASIS ON PSYCHOTROPIC DRUGS WITHIN SIX MONTHS; SHALL TAKE AND PASS THE SPEX EXAM ON 12/5/91. HE SHALL APPEAR FOR FURTHER INTERVIEW BEFORE THE BOARD AT A FUTURE MEETING WHEN THE ABOVE HAS

BEEN COMPLETED. HE VOLUNTARILY AGREED NOT TO PRACTICE IN THE STATE UNTIL HE COMPLETED THE ABOVE.

FLOREZ, JUAN BAUTISTA MD, LICENSE NUMBER 0015040, WAS DISCIPLINED BY ARIZONA ON JULY 19, 1993
DISCIPLINARY ACTION: LICENSE SUSPENSION; RESTRICTION PLACED ON LICENSE
OFFENSE: PROFESSIONAL MISCONDUCT
NOTES: INADEQUATE DOCUMENTATION AND INAPPROPRIATE PSYCHO-PHARMACOLOGICAL PRACTICES IN TREATING TWO PSYCHIATRIC PATIENTS; PRESCRIBED AND/OR DISPENSED XANAX TO HIS WIFE; BOARD ORDERED HIM TO TAKE THE SPEX EXAM WHICH HE FAILED 4 TIMES. TEMPORARILY SUSPENDED EXCEPT, HE MAY BE RETAINED OR EMPLOYED TO ENGAGE IN ADMINISTRATIVE MEDICINE WHICH DOES NOT INVOLVE DIRECT PATIENT CARE. SHALL TAKE AND PASS THE SPEX WITH A SCORE OF 75 OR MORE IN ONE ATTEMPT WITHIN ONE YEAR AFTER THE EFFECTIVE DATE OF THIS ORDER. IF HE FAILS TO COMPLY WITH THIS, BOARD MAY REVOKE HIS LICENSE TO PRACTICE MEDICINE IN ARIZONA.

FLOREZ, JUAN BAUTISTA MD, LICENSE NUMBER 0014204 OF 333 EAST MEDLOCK DRIVE, PHOENIX, AZ, WAS DISCIPLINED BY OKLAHOMA ON JULY 31, 1995
DISCIPLINARY ACTION: LICENSE REVOCATION
OFFENSE: DISCIPLINARY ACTION BY ANOTHER STATE OR AGENCY
NOTES: ON 7/20/93 ARIZONA SUSPENDED HIS LICENSE UNTIL HE PASSED THE SPEX EXAMINATION WITH A SCORE OF 75 BASED ON HIS ALLEGEDLY PRESCRIBING AND/OR DISPENSING XANAX TO HIS WIFE, INAPPROPRIATE TREATMENT OF TWO PSYCHIATRIC PATIENTS, FOCUSING ON INADEQUATE DOCUMENTATION AND INAPPROPRIATE PSYCO-PHARMACOLOGICAL PRACTICES.

FLOREZ, JUAN BAUTISTA MD, LICENSE NUMBER 0015040, WAS DISCIPLINED BY ARIZONA ON APRIL 19, 1996
DISCIPLINARY ACTION: LICENSE REVOCATION
OFFENSE: FAILURE TO COMPLY WITH PREVIOUS BOARD ORDER
NOTES: VIOLATION OF 7/93 BOARD ORDER IN THAT HE FAILED THE SPECIAL PURPOSE EXAMINATION WITH A SCORE OF 72. ON 4/19/96 MOTION FOR REHEARING/REVIEW DENIED.

FLYNN, JAMES PATRICK MD, DATE OF BIRTH NOVEMBER 30, 1936, LICENSE NUMBER 0028544 OF 8181 S LEWIS AVE DEPT OF RAD/ONC, TULSA, OK, WAS DISCIPLINED BY GEORGIA ON MARCH 5, 1992
DISCIPLINARY ACTION: FINE; REPRIMAND
OFFENSE: DISCIPLINARY ACTION BY ANOTHER STATE OR AGENCY
NOTES: DISCIPLINARY ACTION IN NEW JERSEY. $1000 FINE.

FORSYTHE, JOHN T MD OF TULSA, OK, WAS DISCIPLINED BY KANSAS ON JANUARY 5, 1990
DISCIPLINARY ACTION: DENIAL OF NEW LICENSE
OFFENSE: DISCIPLINARY ACTION BY ANOTHER STATE OR AGENCY
NOTES: SUSPENSION IN ANOTHER STATE.

FORSYTHE, JOHN T MD, LICENSE NUMBER 7562, WAS DISCIPLINED BY OKLAHOMA ON AUGUST 31, 1998
DISCIPLINARY ACTION: EMERGENCY SUSPENSION

FORSYTHE, JOHN T MD, LICENSE NUMBER 7562 OF 2733 S. HARVARD, TULSA, OK, WAS DISCIPLINED BY OKLAHOMA ON SEPTEMBER 30, 1998
DISCIPLINARY ACTION: LICENSE REVOCATION
OFFENSE: SEXUAL ABUSE OF OR SEXUAL MISCONDUCT WITH A PATIENT
NOTES: UNTIL 8/12/98 HE WAS REGISTERED TO DISPENSE CONTROLLED SUBSTANCES AT 3606 N. CINCINNATI, TULSA, OKLAHOMA, UNDER HIS DEA NUMBER AND HIS OBN NUMBER. IN DECEMBER 1996 HE MOVED HIS PRACTICE TO PRESENT ADDRESS BUT DID NOT CHANGE HIS REGISTERED LOCATION FOR CONTROLLED DRUGS WITH THE DEA AND OBN AS REQUIRED BY OKLAHOMA STATUTE AND IGNORED REPEATED ADVICE FROM THE BOARD INVESTIGATOR TO CHANGE HIS REGISTRATION SO THAT HE COULD LAWFULLY ADMINISTER, DISPENSE, OR STORE CONTROLLED DRUGS AT HIS CURRENT PRACTICE LOCATION. HE PERFORMED MANY VIOLATIONS OF PRESCRIBING AND DISPENSING REGULATIONS INCLUDING PROVIDING PRESCRIPTIONS OR CONTROLLED SUBSTANCES IN THE FOLLOWING CASES: HE FURNISHED TO AN OBN AGENT ON 5/7/97 TWO VIALS OF DEMEROL, 50 MG/ML (SCHEDULE C-II) WHICH HAD BEEN STORED IN AN UNLOCKED DRAWER IN A PATIENT EXAMINATION AREA OF HIS CLINIC; ON 10/7/97 AN INSPECTION OF THIS CLINIC REVEALED THAT HE ILLEGALLY WAS IN POSSESSION OF DRUG SAMPLES FOR LORTAB (C-III) AND LORTAB ELIXIR (C-III). HE RECEIVED SAMPLES OF CONTROLLED SUBSTANCES IN APRIL, MAY, AND JUNE 1997 AT ONE OF HIS CLINICS EVEN THOUGH HE DID NOT SEE ANY PATIENTS THERE BUT ONLY READ RADIOGRAPHS FOR A FEW HOURS PER WEEK. HE DID NOT MAINTAIN ANY DISPENSING OR INVENTORY RECORDS FOR THE SAMPLES. HE ILLEGALLY SUPPLIED ADDICTED PATIENTS WITH CONTROLLED SUBSTANCES BY WRITING PRESCRIPTIONS IN ANOTHER NAME AND CREATED A FALSE PATIENT CHART AS A COVER FOR THE DIVERSION OF DRUGS TO ANOTHER INDIVIDUAL ON AT LEAST ONE OCCASION; ON 5/7/97 AND 10/7/97 HE WAS SERVED WITH SUBPOENAS FOR PATIENT RECORDS AND FOR DISPENSING RECORDS, ADMINISTRATION RECORDS AND INVOICES OR OTHER RECORDS PERTAINING TO THE PURCHASE OR DISPOSITION OF CONTROLLED DANGEROUS SUBSTANCES AND WAS UNABLE TO PROVIDE MANY OF THE RECORDS ASKED FOR. HE ALSO MAINTAINED THE ADDICTION OF ANOTHER SPECIFIED PATIENT TO LORTAB AND PROVIDED HIM WITH OTHER SCHEDULE C-III DRUGS WITHOUT CONDUCTING PHYSICAL EXAMINATIONS AND AT A $75.00 COST PER VISIT; IN 1996 HE BEGAN PARTICIPATING IN A SCHEME TO SELL CONTROLLED SUBSTANCES FOR CASH OR IN SOME CASES TRADED DRUGS FOR SEX; BETWEEN 1/97 AND 5/97 SUBMITTED INSURANCE CLAIMS FOR OFFICE VISITS THAT NEVER OCCURRED. IN 1997 AND 1998 ON NUMEROUS OCCASIONS MADE INAPPROPRIATE SEXUAL REMARKS AND ADVANCES TOWARDS FEMALE PATIENTS, INCLUDING GROPING OF PATIENTS' BREASTS AND BUTTOCKS, AND PHOTOGRAPHING PATIENTS IN SUGGESTIVE POSES OR PARTIALLY UNDRESSED. HE ALSO EXPOSED HIS GENITALS TO ONE PATIENT ON AT LEAST TWO OCCASIONS AND FOLLOWED THIS PATIENT AROUND, MAKING UNANNOUNCED APPEARANCES AT HER HOME AND OFFICE AND OFFERING PRESCRIPTION DRUGS IN EXCHANGE FOR SEX; FAILED TO PROVIDE A PROPER SETTING FOR EXAMINATION OR TREATMENT OF HIS PATIENTS.

FORSYTHE, JOHN T MD OF 3606 N CINCINNATI, TULSA, OK, WAS DISCIPLINED BY DEA ON NOVEMBER 2, 1998
DISCIPLINARY ACTION: SURRENDER OF CONTROLLED SUBSTANCE

LICENSE

FORSYTHE, JOHN T MD, LICENSE NUMBER R1853 OF TULSA, OK, WAS DISCIPLINED BY ARKANSAS ON FEBRUARY 5, 1999
DISCIPLINARY ACTION: LICENSE REVOCATION

FOSTER, KENNETH W MD, LICENSE NUMBER G042475 OF RED BLUFF, CA, WAS DISCIPLINED BY CALIFORNIA ON SEPTEMBER 11, 1991
DISCIPLINARY ACTION: 2-MONTH LICENSE SUSPENSION; 58-MONTH PROBATION
OFFENSE: OVERPRESCRIBING OR MISPRESCRIBING DRUGS

NOTES: PRESCRIBED CONTROLLED SUBSTANCES TO ADDICTS OR HABITUAL USERS; EXCESSIVE PRESCRIBING; REPEATED NEGLIGENT ACTS IN PRESCRIBING TWO ANTIDEPRESSANTS CONCURRENTLY. REVOCATION STAYED.

FOSTER, KENNETH W MD, LICENSE NUMBER 0015885, WAS DISCIPLINED BY OKLAHOMA ON MAY 20, 1993
DISCIPLINARY ACTION: 60-MONTH PROBATION; 60-MONTH RESTRICTION PLACED ON LICENSE
OFFENSE: DISCIPLINARY ACTION BY ANOTHER STATE OR AGENCY

NOTES: ON 9/11/91 THE CALIFORNIA BOARD ADOPTED AN ORDER IN WHICH HE ADMITTED TO PRESCRIBING VICODIN, HYDROCODONE, BENZODIAZEPINES, PROZAC AND AMITRIPTYLINE TO ADDICTS OR HABITUAL USERS OR TO OTHER PATIENTS IN AMOUNTS THAT CONSTITUTE EXCESSIVE PRESCRIBING; CALIFORNIA LICENSE SUSPENDED FOR 60 DAYS AND PLACED ON PROBATION FOR FIVE YEARS. CONDITIONS OF PROBATION: PRACTICE LIMITED TO THE INSTITUTIONS OF THE OKLAHOMA DEPARTMENT OF CORRECTIONS; SHALL NOT PRESCRIBE, ADMINISTER OR DISPENSE ANY SCHEDULE II OR III CONTROLLED DANGEROUS SUBSTANCES; SHALL FURNISH EACH STATE WHERE HE HOLDS OR APPLIES FOR LICENSURE AND ALL HEALTH CARE ENTITIES WHERE HE HAS PRIVILEGES A COPY OF THIS ORDER; SHALL FURNISH BOARD WITH ADDRESS AND/OR CHANGE OF ADDRESS; SHALL APPEAR BEFORE THE BOARD UPON REQUEST AND SUBMIT ANY REPORTS AND FORMS REQUESTED; SHALL NOT SUPERVISE A PHYSICIAN'S ASSISTANT; SHALL PAY COSTS.

FOSTER, KENNETH W MD OF 600 EAST HICKORY STREET, HOLDENVILLE, OK, WAS DISCIPLINED BY DEA ON SEPTEMBER 7, 1993
DISCIPLINARY ACTION: RESTRICTION PLACED ON CONTROLLED SUBSTANCE LICENSE
OFFENSE: DISCIPLINARY ACTION BY ANOTHER STATE OR AGENCY

NOTES: CALIFORNIA MEDICAL LICENSE REVOKED ON 01/02/92 DUE TO FAILURE TO DISCLOSE INVOLVEMENT AS SUBJECT OF ACCUSATION REGARDING PREVIOUS DISCIPLINARY ACCUSATIONS ON 05/02/89. IN VIOLATION OF OKLAHOMA MEDICAL PRACTICE ACT 05/15/93. PLACED ON PROBATION. LIMITED TO SCHEDULE IV AND V CONTROLLED SUBSTANCES. ALIAS KENNETH MARIE.

FOSTER, KENNETH W MD, LICENSE NUMBER 0G42475 OF HOLDENVILLE, OK, WAS DISCIPLINED BY CALIFORNIA ON NOVEMBER 26, 1993
DISCIPLINARY ACTION: LICENSE REVOCATION
OFFENSE: DISCIPLINARY ACTION BY ANOTHER STATE OR AGENCY

NOTES: DISCIPLINED BY LOUISIANA BOARD FOR FALSE APPLICATION. VIOLATED PROBATION OF PRIOR DISCIPLINE. FALSE STATEMENTS IN APPLICATIONS. DEFAULT DECISION.

FOSTER, KENNETH W MD, LICENSE NUMBER 0015885, WAS DISCIPLINED BY OKLAHOMA ON MARCH 24, 1994
DISCIPLINARY ACTION: LICENSE REVOCATION
OFFENSE: DISCIPLINARY ACTION BY ANOTHER STATE OR AGENCY

NOTES: ON 3/26/91 FALSELY RESPONDED TO THREE QUESTIONS ON OKLAHOMA RENEWAL APPLICATION IN THAT HE SAID NO TO EVER HAVING BEEN CONVICTED OF A FELONY OR MISDEMEANOR, DENIED PRIVILEGES OR THE SUBJECT OF A DISCIPLINARY ACTION BY A HOSPITAL; ON 1/2/92 LOUISIANA REVOKED HIS LICENSE; ON 11/26/93 CALIFORNIA REVOKED HIS LICENSE; PLED GUILTY OR CONVICTED OF DRIVING UNDER THE INFLUENCE ON 1/27/84 IN OKLAHOMA, IN 1990 IN CALIFORNIA AND 12/15/93 IN OKLAHOMA; WAS ISSUED A WARNING AND TERMINATED FROM THE LAS VEGAS, NEW MEXICO, MEDICAL CENTER ALL RELATED TO HABITUAL, EXCESSIVE USE OF ALCOHOL. ON 6/22/94 THIS ORDER WAS MODIFIED TO ALLOW HIM TO PROVIDE PSYCHIATRIC SERVICES TO THE OKLAHOMA DEPARTMENT OF CORRECTIONS AT SPECIFIED LOCATIONS.

FOSTER, KENNETH W MD OF 600 EAST HICKORY ST P.O. BOX 347, HOLDENVILLE, OK, WAS DISCIPLINED BY DEA ON JUNE 16, 1994
DISCIPLINARY ACTION: SURRENDER OF CONTROLLED SUBSTANCE LICENSE
OFFENSE: DISCIPLINARY ACTION BY ANOTHER STATE OR AGENCY

NOTES: STATE BOARD.

FOSTER, KENNETH W MD, WAS DISCIPLINED BY ALASKA ON AUGUST 28, 1998
DISCIPLINARY ACTION: DENIAL OF NEW LICENSE
OFFENSE: DISCIPLINARY ACTION BY ANOTHER STATE OR AGENCY

NOTES: LICENSES REVOKED IN CALIFORNIA AND LOUISIANA.

FOSTER, KENNETH WASHIE MD OF RED BLUFF, CA, WAS DISCIPLINED BY LOUISIANA ON JANUARY 2, 1991
DISCIPLINARY ACTION: LICENSE REVOCATION
OFFENSE: DISCIPLINARY ACTION BY ANOTHER STATE OR AGENCY

NOTES: FRAUD, DECEIT OR PERJURY IN OBTAINING A LICENSE; ACTION TAKEN AGAINST LICENSE BY CALIFORNIA.

FREIDENBERGER, JOHN B MD, LICENSE NUMBER 0003008 OF 500 LOU S. ALLARD DRIVE, DRUMRIGHT, OK, WAS DISCIPLINED BY OKLAHOMA ON JULY 1, 1993
DISCIPLINARY ACTION: 60-MONTH PROBATION; RESTRICTION PLACED ON LICENSE

NOTES: ON 10/16/92 BOARD VOTED TO EXTEND HIS SUPERVISED MEDICAL DOCTOR CERTIFICATE FOR ONE YEAR AND PLACED HIM ON PROBATION FOR FIVE YEARS; HAS COMPLIED WITH THE TERMS OF THIS PROBATION AND COMPLETED FOUR YEARS OF SOBRIETY IN 9/93. LICENSE GRANTED ON PROBATION RETROACTIVE TO 10/16/92. CONDITIONS OF PROBATION: SHALL NOT PRESCRIBE, ADMINISTER OR DISPENSE ANY MEDICATIONS FOR HIS PERSONAL USE; SHALL TAKE NO MEDICATION UNLESS IT IS AUTHORIZED BY A TREATING PHYSICIAN FOR A LEGITIMATE MEDICAL NEED; SHALL ABSTAIN FROM THE CONSUMPTION OF ALCOHOL OR ANY SUBSTANCE WHICH WOULD ADVERSELY AFFECT HIS ABILITY TO PRACTICE; SHALL SUBMIT BIOLOGICAL FLUID SPECIMENS; SHALL MAINTAIN A PROGRAM OF ABSTINENCE BY PARTICIPATING IN BOARD-APPROVED

ORGANIZATIONS APPROPRIATE FOR ASSESSMENT, TREATMENT, OR SUPPORT; SHALL SECURE WEEKLY OR BI-MONTHLY BOARD-APPROVED OUTPATIENT COUNSELING WITH A CHEMICAL DEPENDENCY THERAPIST; SHALL FURNISH BOARD WITH ADDRESS AND/OR CHANGE OF ADDRESS; SHALL APPEAR BEFORE THE BOARD UPON REQUEST AND SUBMIT REQUIRED REPORTS; SHALL PAY COSTS; SHALL NOTIFY ANY HEALTH CARE ENTITY WHERE HE HAS PRIVILEGES OF THE TERMS OF THIS ORDER; SHALL NOT SUPERVISE A PHYSICIAN'S ASSISTANT. ON 9/9/94 PROBATION MODIFIED TO ALLOW SUPPORT MEETINGS TO BE ATTENDED ON AN "AS NEEDED" BASIS AND LEVEL OF PROBATION REDUCED FROM LEVEL I TO LEVEL II.

FUCCI, JOHN C MD, LICENSE NUMBER 19139, WAS DISCIPLINED BY OKLAHOMA ON FEBRUARY 5, 1998
DISCIPLINARY ACTION: 60-MONTH PROBATION; RESTRICTION PLACED ON LICENSE
OFFENSE: SUBSTANCE ABUSE

NOTES: FROM APPROXIMATELY 9/96 THROUGH 9/97 HE WROTE FALSE AND FICTITIOUS PRESCRIPTIONS FOR CONTROLLED DANGEROUS SUBSTANCES IN THE NAMES OF FORMER PATIENTS FOR HIS OWN PERSONAL USE AND CONSUMPTION; HE SUFFERED A SUBSTANCE ABUSE PROBLEM WHICH IMPAIRED HIS ABILITY TO PRACTICE MEDICINE AND SURGERY WITH REASONABLE SKILL AND SAFETY TO HIS PATIENTS. HE WAS ADMITTED TO A PROGRAM ON 9/29/97 FOR IN-PATIENT TREATMENT OF CHEMICAL DEPENDENCY AND WAS RELEASED ON 1/10/98. CONDITIONS OF PROBATION: SHALL NOT PRESCRIBE, ADMINISTER, POSSESS, OR DISPENSE ANY DRUGS IN SCHEDULES II OR III EXCEPT TO IN-HOSPITAL PATIENTS, OUT-PATIENTS, OR EMERGENCY ROOM PATIENTS. HE MAY DIRECT THE ADMINISTRATION BUT NOT PERSONALLY ADMINISTER THESE DRUGS TO SUCH PATIENTS; SHALL KEEP DUPLICATE, SERIALLY NUMBERED PRESCRIPTIONS OF ALL SCHEDULE IV AND V CONTROLLED DANGEROUS SUBSTANCES WHICH SHALL BE AVAILABLE TO THE BOARD UPON REQUEST; SHALL SUBMIT TO EVERY STATE IN WHICH HE HOLDS LICENSURE AND TO HOSPITALS, CLINICS OR OTHER INSTITUTIONS IN WHICH HE HOLDS OR ANTICIPATES HOLDING ANY FORM OF STAFF PRIVILEGE A COPY OF THIS ORDER; SHALL SUBMIT BIOLOGICAL FLUID SPECIMENS AND SHALL NOT INGEST ANY SUBSTANCE WHICH WILL CAUSE A SPECIMEN TO TEST POSITIVE FOR PROHIBITED SUBSTANCES; SHALL NOT PRESCRIBE, ADMINISTER OR DISPENSE ANY MEDICATIONS FOR HIS PERSONAL USE AND SHALL TAKE NONE UNLESS AUTHORIZED BY ANOTHER PHYSICIAN FOR A LEGITIMATE MEDICAL NEED; SHALL ABIDE BY HIS POST-CARE CONTRACT FROM TREATMENT PROGRAM AND THE OKLAHOMA PHYSICIAN RECOVERY PROGRAM; SHALL KEEP THE BOARD INFORMED OF HIS ADDRESS AND PAY COSTS; SHALL REQUEST ALL HOSPITALS IN WHICH HE ANTICIPATES PRACTICING TO FURNISH A STATEMENT REGARDING MONITORING OF HIS PRACTICE; SHALL NOT SUPERVISE ALLIED HEALTH PROFESSIONALS; SHALL APPEAR BEFORE THE BOARD AND SUBMIT REPORTS UPON REQUEST; SHALL EXECUTE ALL RELEASES OF MEDICAL AND PSYCHIATRIC RECORDS AS NECESSARY TO DISCUSS HIS CASE WITH HIS TREATING PHYSICIANS AND/OR ANY PHYSICIANS HOLDING RECORDS.

FUCCI, JOHN C MD, LICENSE NUMBER 146608 OF SOUTH 84TH E AVENUE, TULSA, OK, WAS DISCIPLINED BY NEW YORK ON JULY 10, 1998
DISCIPLINARY ACTION: SURRENDER OF LICENSE
OFFENSE: DISCIPLINARY ACTION BY ANOTHER STATE OR AGENCY

NOTES: DISCIPLINED BY THE OKLAHOMA BOARD FOR PRACTICING THE PROFESSION WHILE HIS ABILITY WAS IMPAIRED DUE TO SUBSTANCE ABUSE.

GALUSICK, JOSEPH ANTHONY MD, LICENSE NUMBER 6107, WAS DISCIPLINED BY OKLAHOMA ON MAY 14, 1999
DISCIPLINARY ACTION: SURRENDER OF LICENSE
OFFENSE: PHYSICAL OR MENTAL ILLNESS INHIBITING THE ABILITY TO PRACTICE WITH SKILL AND SAFETY

NOTES: IN APPROXIMATELY 1993, WHILE IN MEDICAL SCHOOL, DIAGNOSED WITH MAJOR DEPRESSIVE DISORDER; ON 10/8/98 PLACED ON PROBATION FOR SIX WEEKS DURING A ROTATION AT THE UNIVERSITY OF OKLAHOMA; FAILED HIS FIRST TWO ROTATIONS AND WAS THEN REMOVED FROM THE SURGERY ROTATION; ON 11/30/98 DISMISSED FROM THE RESIDENCY PROGRAM ON ACADEMIC GROUNDS. SURRENDERED HIS SPECIAL LICENSE FOR TRAINING.

GANACIAS, ADELA RAMIREZ OF 1619 KINGSPOINT DRIVE, CARROLLTON, TX, WAS DISCIPLINED BY OKLAHOMA ON JULY 1, 1993
DISCIPLINARY ACTION: DENIAL OF NEW LICENSE

NOTES: HAS FAILED THE FLEX EXAM 10 TIMES, WHICH RAISES SERIOUS ISSUES AS TO CLINICAL COMPETENCY AND FITNESS TO PRACTICE. DENIAL REAFFIRMED ON 12/2/93.

GARBER, GEORGE MD, LICENSE NUMBER 0018794 OF MCALESTER, OK, WAS DISCIPLINED BY COLORADO ON JULY 17, 1990
DISCIPLINARY ACTION: RESTRICTION PLACED ON LICENSE; MONITORING OF PHYSICIAN PERFORMANCE
OFFENSE: SUBSTANDARD CARE, INCOMPETENCE OR NEGLIGENCE

NOTES: INABILITY TO PRACTICE WITH REASONABLE SKILL AND SAFETY TO PATIENTS. CONSENT ORDER MANDATING FAVORABLE PHYSICAL/MENTAL EXAMINATIONS, PRACTICE MONITORING, AND A GENERAL SURGERY PROHIBITION.

GASTINEAU, G KIRK DO, LICENSE NUMBER 0002275, WAS DISCIPLINED BY OKLAHOMA ON APRIL 3, 1995
DISCIPLINARY ACTION: EMERGENCY SUSPENSION
OFFENSE: LOSS OR RESTRICTION OF HOSPITAL PRIVILEGES

NOTES: FROM 9/94 TO 2/95 HE WAS LATE ON MANY OCCASIONS FOR EMERGENCY ROOM CALLS CREATING SIGNIFICANT PROBLEMS FOR THE HOSPITAL HE WAS WORKING AT; FAILED TO RESPOND TO CALLS FOR MEDICAL ASSISTANCE FROM A RETIREMENT AND HEALTH CARE CENTER FROM WHICH HE WAS SUSPENDED AND EVENTUALLY TERMINATED; DID NOT FULFILL MANY APPOINTMENTS HE HAD SCHEDULED AT HIS OWN OFFICE AND PERMITTED NURSES TO GIVE ALLERGY AND/OR HORMONAL SHOTS TO PATIENTS ALTHOUGH HE WAS NOT PRESENT AND HAD NOT EXAMINED THE PATIENTS; FROM 4/15/94 THROUGH 2/2/95 HE PURCHASED 5,781 DOSAGE UNITS OF DIDREX AND 203 VIALS OF NALBUPHINE AND NUBAIN WITHOUT PROVIDING ANY PATIENT NAMES TO VARIOUS PHARMACIES OR PROVIDING APPROPRIATE PATIENT INFORMATION; INITIALLY FAILED TO PROVIDE PATIENT WITH A COPY OF HER RECORDS; COPY WAS EVENTUALLY PROVIDED. ON 9/21/95 SUSPENSION REMAINED IN EFFECT.

GASTINEAU, G KIRK DO, LICENSE NUMBER 2275, WAS DISCIPLINED

BY OKLAHOMA ON MARCH 11, 1998
DISCIPLINARY ACTION: 60-MONTH PROBATION

GASTINEAU, GLENN K DO OF 814 FRISCO, CLINTON, OK, WAS DISCIPLINED BY DEA ON JUNE 7, 1995
DISCIPLINARY ACTION: SURRENDER OF CONTROLLED SUBSTANCE LICENSE

NOTES: IN LIEU OF ORDER TO SHOW CAUSE.

GAVANKAR, SHALINI S MD OF 2711 WINFIELD STREET, JOPLIN, MO, WAS DISCIPLINED BY MISSOURI ON JUNE 28, 1993
DISCIPLINARY ACTION: DENIAL OF NEW LICENSE
OFFENSE: DISCIPLINARY ACTION BY ANOTHER STATE OR AGENCY

NOTES: DENIAL TAKEN IN ANOTHER STATE.

GAVANKAR, SHALINI SHARAD OF 2711 WINFIELD SOUTH, JOPLIN, MO, WAS DISCIPLINED BY OKLAHOMA ON DECEMBER 2, 1993
DISCIPLINARY ACTION: DENIAL OF NEW LICENSE

NOTES: FAILED TO PASS THE FLEX EXAM 14 TIMES BEFORE PASSING WHICH RAISES SERIOUS ISSUES AS TO HER EDUCATION, CLINICAL COMPETENCY AND FITNESS TO PRACTICE. DENIAL FOR CERTIFICATE AS SUPERVISED MEDICAL DOCTOR.

GIBSON, ROBERT W MD, LICENSE NUMBER 5958, WAS DISCIPLINED BY OKLAHOMA ON NOVEMBER 23, 1999
DISCIPLINARY ACTION: LICENSE REVOCATION
OFFENSE: SUBSTANDARD CARE, INCOMPETENCE OR NEGLIGENCE

NOTES: DURING 1997 AND 1998 ILLEGALLY PROCURED AND ADMINISTERED LAETRILE TO NUMEROUS PATIENTS AND RECEIVED COMPENSATION; HAS BEEN USING LAETRILE TO TREAT PATIENTS FOR 20 YEARS; LAETRILE IS CLASSIFIED AS AN UNAPPROVED NEW DRUG AND MANUFACTURED OUTSIDE THE U.S. AND MAY NOT LEGALLY BE SHIPPED IN INTERSTATE COMMERCE WITHOUT AN APPROVED NEW DRUG APPLICATION FROM THE FDA; HE DISTRIBUTED AND/OR SOLD LAETRILE TO NUMEROUS THIRD PARTIES WITHIN THE U.S., ALL WITHIN INTERSTATE COMMERCE; CONSISTENTLY AND REPEATEDLY, IN A DECEPTIVE AND DECEITFUL MANNER, ADVISED PATIENTS, ORALLY AND IN WRITING, THAT HE WOULD ADMINISTER LAETRILE TO THE PATIENTS KNOWING THAT THE PATIENTS WERE COMING TO HIM FOR THE TREATMENT OF CANCER; HE ACCEPTED REMUNERATION IN THE AMOUNT OF $3,000 PER PATIENT REGARDING THE ADMINISTRATION OF LAETRILE FOR CANCER PATIENTS, WHILE AT THE SAME TIME ADVISING THE PATIENTS IN WRITING THAT HE WOULD NOT TREAT THEM FOR CANCER OR ANY OTHER SPECIFIC DISEASES; CONSISTENTLY PRESCRIBED CONTROLLED DRUGS WITHOUT ESTABLISHING A MEDICAL NEED FOR SUCH DRUGS; FROM 1/96-3/99 MEDICAL CHARTS REVEAL THAT HE KNOWINGLY PRESCRIBED CONTROLLED DRUGS TO ADDICTS, REFERRING TO VARIOUS PATIENTS AS "MY LITTLE DEMEROL ADDICT", "HOOKED ON HYDROCODONE", "IS ADDICTED TO TYLENOL #4"; PATIENT RECORDS FROM 1991-1999 REFLECT LITTLE OR NO PHYSICAL EXAMINATION FINDINGS, FEW RECORDS OF VITAL SIGNS AND LITTLE OR NO HISTORY, FOLLOWED MOSTLY BY NOTATIONS OF PRESCRIPTIONS WRITTEN OR AUTHORIZED WITH LITTLE FOLLOW-UP AND ALMOST NO DOCUMENTATION OF MEDICAL NEED; SPECIFIC AND ACCURATE QUANTITIES OF CONTROLLED DRUG MEDICATIONS AND NON-CONTROLLED DRUG MEDICATIONS ARE NOT RECORDED, AND MEDICATIONS THAT ARE RECORDED DO NOT CORRELATE WITH PUBLISHED STANDARDS OF MEDICAL CARE.

GILBERT, JERALD M MD OF 7530 N.W. 23 STREET, BETHANY, OK, WAS DISCIPLINED BY DEA ON DECEMBER 5, 1995
DISCIPLINARY ACTION: SURRENDER OF CONTROLLED SUBSTANCE LICENSE
OFFENSE: DISCIPLINARY ACTION BY ANOTHER STATE OR AGENCY

NOTES: STATE BOARD.

GILBERT, JERALD MILTON MD, LICENSE NUMBER 0010960, WAS DISCIPLINED BY OKLAHOMA ON JULY 31, 1995
DISCIPLINARY ACTION: LICENSE SUSPENSION; REQUIRED TO ENTER AN IMPAIRED PHYSICIAN PROGRAM OR SUBSTANCE ABUSE TREATMENT
OFFENSE: SUBSTANCE ABUSE

NOTES: GUILTY OF THE HABITUAL OR EXCESSIVE USE OF ANY DRUG WHICH IMPAIRS THE ABILITY TO PRACTICE MEDICINE WITH REASONABLE SKILL AND SAFETY TO THE PATIENT AND IMPROPER MANAGEMENT OF MEDICAL RECORDS. SINCE MAY 1994 HE UNLAWFULLY USED CERTAIN HABIT-FORMING DRUGS AND CERTAIN ADDICTIVE DRUGS FOR MIGRAINE HEADACHES WHILE IN THE PRACTICE OF MEDICINE AND SURGERY. IN 6/95 VOLUNTARILY ADMITTED HIMSELF TO THE TALBOTT-MARSH TREATMENT CENTER IN ATLANTA, GEORGIA FOR IN-PATIENT TREATMENT FOR SUBSTANCE ABUSE. HE AGREES TO COMPLETE AN IN-PATIENT PROGRAM, TO BE FOLLOWED BY NORMAL AFTER-CARE AND FOLLOW-UP CARE AS PRESCRIBED BY THE PROFESSIONAL STAFF OF THE TREATMENT PROGRAM AND FURTHER AGREES TO FULLY PARTICIPATE IN ANY AND ALL AFTER-CARE PROGRAMS ORDERED BY THE BOARD. MAY PETITION FOR REINSTATEMENT IN SIX MONTHS.

GILBERT, JERALD MILTON MD, LICENSE NUMBER 0010960 OF 7530 NW 23 GILBERT MEDICAL, BETHANY, OK, WAS DISCIPLINED BY OKLAHOMA ON SEPTEMBER 5, 1996
DISCIPLINARY ACTION: 60-MONTH PROBATION; 60-MONTH RESTRICTION PLACED ON LICENSE
OFFENSE: SUBSTANCE ABUSE

NOTES: CONDITIONS OF PROBATION: SHALL LIMIT HIS WORK WEEK TO 40 HOURS PER WEEK, NOT TO INCLUDE ANY HOSPITAL WORK OR NIGHT CALLS; SHALL NOT PRESCRIBE, ADMINISTER, DISPENSE, OR POSSESS ANY DRUGS IN SCHEDULES II THROUGH V; SHALL NOT AUTHORIZE ANY PERSONNEL UNDER HIS SUPERVISION TO INITIATE AN ORDER FOR A PRESCRIPTION TO BE ISSUED; SHALL NOT ALLOW THE INDEPENDENT PRACTICE OF MEDICINE BY ANY PERSONNEL UNDER HIS SUPERVISION OR EMPLOY; SHALL NOT ALLOW THE INITIATION OF ANY THERAPEUTIC REGIME BY ANY PERSONNEL UNDER HIS SUPERVISION UNLESS HE IS IN THE IMMEDIATE GEOGRAPHIC VICINITY; SHALL FURNISH EACH STATE IN WHICH HE HOLDS OR APPLIES FOR LICENSURE AND ANY HEALTH CARE ENTITIES IN WHICH HE HOLDS PRIVILEGES A COPY OF THIS ORDER; SHALL NOT SUPERVISE A PHYSICIAN ASSISTANT; SHALL SUBMIT BIOLOGICAL FLUID SPECIMENS UPON BOARD REQUEST; SHALL NOT PRESCRIBE, ADMINISTER, OR DISPENSE, ANY MEDICATIONS FOR PERSONAL USE; SHALL NOT TAKE ANY MEDICATIONS UNLESS PRESCRIBED BY AN AUTHORIZED TREATING PHYSICIAN FOR LEGITIMATE MEDICAL NEED; SHALL CONTINUE MONTHLY VISITS WITH HIS PSYCHIATRIST WHO SHALL SUBMIT MONTHLY REPORTS TO THE BOARD; THE COMPLIANCE COORDINATOR FOR THE BOARD SHALL SUBMIT PROGRESS REPORTS EVERY

SIX MONTHS TO THE BOARD; SHALL KEEP THE BOARD INFORMED OF HIS CURRENT ADDRESS; SHALL KEEP CURRENT ALL PROSECUTION, INVESTIGATION, AND MONITORING COSTS. ON 9/26/97 REQUEST TO MODIFY ORDER GRANTED ALLOWING HIS 40 HOURS OF PRACTICE TO INCLUDE HOSPITAL WORK AND NIGHT CALL. ON 10/2/98 REQUEST TO MODIFY ORDER GRANTED ALLOWING HIM TO PRESCRIBE CONTROLLED SUBSTANCES IN SCHEDULES II, III, IV AND V AS LONG AS HE USES DUPLICATE, SERIALLY-NUMBERED PRESCRIPTION PADS TO BE MADE AVAILABLE TO THE BOARD UPON REQUEST.

GILLIAM, DAVID THOMAS MD, LICENSE NUMBER 38060 OF PADUCAH, KY, WAS DISCIPLINED BY OHIO ON AUGUST 18, 1998
DISCIPLINARY ACTION: 1-MONTH LICENSE SUSPENSION
OFFENSE: PROVIDING FALSE INFORMATION TO THE BOARD OR OTHER HEALTH AGENCY

NOTES: CERTIFIED ON HIS LICENSE RENEWAL APPLICATION THAT HE HAD COMPLETED THE REQUIRED CONTINUING MEDICAL EDUCATION HOURS WHEN, IN FACT, HE HAD NOT COMPLETED THOSE HOURS AT THE TIME OF CERTIFICATION. REQUIRED HOURS WERE COMPLETED SUBSEQUENTLY. SUBSEQUENT TO REINSTATEMENT, REQUIRED TO DOCUMENT COMPLIANCE WITH CONTINUING MEDICAL EDUCATION REQUIREMENTS FOR THREE REGISTRATION PERIODS. PROBATIONARY TERMS IMPOSED FOR SIX YEARS.

GILLIAM, DAVID THOMAS MD, WAS DISCIPLINED BY OKLAHOMA ON SEPTEMBER 30, 1998
DISCIPLINARY ACTION: DENIAL OF NEW LICENSE
OFFENSE: PROVIDING FALSE INFORMATION TO THE BOARD OR OTHER HEALTH AGENCY

NOTES: ON HIS APPLICATION FOR LICENSURE HE ANSWERED "NO" TO THE FOLLOWING: "HAS YOUR LICENSE EVER BEEN REVOKED?"; "HAVE YOU EVER BEEN SUBJECT TO DISCIPLINARY ACTION?"; "HAVE YOU EVER BEEN REQUESTED TO APPEAR BEFORE A LICENSING OR DISCIPLINARY AGENCY?". AT THE TIME OF THIS APPLICATION HE WAS THE SUBJECT OF DISCIPLINARY ACTION IN OHIO FOR FAILURE TO COMPLY WITH CONTINUING MEDICAL EDUCATION REQUIREMENTS, RESULTING IN THE SUSPENSION OF HIS OHIO LICENSE (REINSTATED 9/17/98). HE ADMITTED HE HAD MADE A FALSE STATEMENT ON HIS APPLICATION AT THE TIME HE FILED IT AND HIS APPLICATION CONTAINED ADDITIONAL MISSTATEMENTS RELATING TO LICENSURE EXAMINATIONS.

GILLIAM, DAVID THOMAS MD, LICENSE NUMBER 38060 OF PADUCAH, KY, WAS DISCIPLINED BY OHIO ON NOVEMBER 19, 1999
DISCIPLINARY ACTION: LICENSE SUSPENSION; PROBATION
OFFENSE: DISCIPLINARY ACTION BY ANOTHER STATE OR AGENCY

NOTES: DENIAL OF HIS LICENSURE APPLICATION BY OKLAHOMA'S BOARD DUE TO HIS FAILURE TO REVEAL ON LICENSURE APPLICATION THAT HE HAD BEEN THE SUBJECT OF DISCIPLINARY ACTION IN OHIO FOR FAILING TO COMPLY WITH CONTINUING MEDICAL EDUCATION REQUIREMENTS. PERMANENT REVOCATION STAYED; SUSPENSION FOR AT LEAST 18 MONTHS; CONDITIONS FOR REINSTATEMENT AND SUBSEQUENT PROBATIONARY TERMS, CONDITIONS AND LIMITATIONS ESTABLISHED FOR AT LEAST FIVE YEARS. NOTICE OF APPEAL TO FRANKLIN COUNTY COURT OF COMMON PLEAS OF BOARD'S SUSPENSION ORDER FILED BY HIM ON OR ABOUT 12/2/99.

GILLIAM, MARY ANN MD, LICENSE NUMBER 0009089 OF 1627 N KLEIN AVE, OKLAHOMA CITY, OK, WAS DISCIPLINED BY OKLAHOMA ON OCTOBER 26, 1990
DISCIPLINARY ACTION: SURRENDER OF CONTROLLED SUBSTANCE LICENSE; 60-MONTH PROBATION
OFFENSE: OVERPRESCRIBING OR MISPRESCRIBING DRUGS

NOTES: FROM 6/23/87 TO 3/1/90 PRESCRIBED SCHEDULED DRUGS TO AT LEAST FIVE PATIENTS IN EXCESS OF THE AMOUNT CONSIDERED FOR THE MEDICAL NEED PRESENTED. PROBATION UNDER TERMS AND CONDITIONS: SHALL NOT PRESCRIBE, ADMINISTER OR DISPENSE ANY SCHEDULED DRUGS OR CONTROLLED DANGEROUS SUBSTANCES; SHALL IMMEDIATELY SURRENDER REGISTRATION FOR STATE AND FEDERAL CONTROLLED DANGEROUS SUBSTANCES AND WILL NOT REAPPLY UNTIL PROBATION EXPIRES; SHALL SUCCESSFULLY COMPLETE 20 HOURS OF CONTINUING MEDICAL EDUCATION ON PROPER PRESCRIPTION WRITING OR AN EQUIVALENT AMOUNT OF COUNSELING BY BOARD STAFF WITHIN TWO YEARS; SHALL NOTIFY ANY HOSPITAL WHERE SHE HOLDS STAFF PRIVILEGES, OR CLINIC OR GROUP OF THE TERMS AND CONDITIONS; SHALL FURNISH BOARD WITH ADDRESS AND/OR CHANGE OF ADDRESS; SHALL APPEAR BEFORE BOARD UPON REQUEST. ON 11/8/91 SUPERVISION REDUCED FROM LEVEL I TO LEVEL II. ON 10/11/93 PROBATION TERMINATED.

GILLIAM, MARY ANN MD OF 1629 N KLEIN, OKLAHOMA CITY, OK, WAS DISCIPLINED BY DEA ON NOVEMBER 20, 1990
DISCIPLINARY ACTION: SURRENDER OF CONTROLLED SUBSTANCE LICENSE
OFFENSE: DISCIPLINARY ACTION BY ANOTHER STATE OR AGENCY

NOTES: PLACED ON PROBATION BY OKLAHOMA MEDICAL BOARD ON 10/26/90 AS A RESULT OF EXCESSIVE AND INDISCRIMINATE PRESCRIBING OF CONTROLLED SUBSTANCES. ONE OF THE TERMS OF THE PROBATION WAS THAT SHE COULD NOT PRESCRIBE, ADMINISTER, OR DISPENSE CONTROLLED SUBSTANCES.

GILLIAM, MARY ANN MD, LICENSE NUMBER 0009089 OF PO BOX 2239, ADA, OK, WAS DISCIPLINED BY OKLAHOMA ON OCTOBER 2, 1995
DISCIPLINARY ACTION: EMERGENCY SUSPENSION

NOTES: LICENSE IS TEMPORARILY SUSPENDED UNTIL THE NEXT MEETING OF THE BOARD. SHALL NOT PRACTICE MEDICINE AND SURGERY IN OKLAHOMA UNTIL FURTHER NOTICE. SUSPENSION EXTENDED ON 1/25/96 AND 3/29/96. 5/16/96 CONTINUANCE OF SUSPENSION UNTIL HEARING ON 7/25-27/96.

GILLIAM, MARY ANN MD, DATE OF BIRTH NOVEMBER 10, 1943 OF PO BOX 2239, ADA, OK, WAS DISCIPLINED BY MEDICARE ON APRIL 23, 1996
DISCIPLINARY ACTION: 60-MONTH EXCLUSION FROM THE MEDICARE AND/OR MEDICAID PROGRAM
OFFENSE: CRIMINAL CONVICTION OR PLEA OF GUILTY, NOLO CONTENDERE, OR NO CONTEST TO A CRIME

NOTES: CONVICTED OF A CRIME INVOLVING THE MEDICARE, MEDICAID, MATERNAL AND CHILD HEALTH SERVICES BLOCK GRANT OR BLOCK GRANTS TO STATES FOR SOCIAL SERVICES PROGRAMS.

GILSON, MAYO D MD, LICENSE NUMBER 0008854 OF 8277 SOUTH WALKER, OKLAHOMA CITY, OK, WAS DISCIPLINED BY OKLAHOMA ON MAY 16, 1996
DISCIPLINARY ACTION: RESTRICTION PLACED ON LICENSE; MONITORING OF PHYSICIAN PERFORMANCE

NOTES: FOLLOWING TERMS AND CONDITIONS: HIS ORDERS FOR THE ADMINISTRATION OF ENEMAS TO PATIENTS SHALL BE FOR SELF-ADMINISTRATION BY THE PATIENT OR ADMINISTRATION BY AN INDIVIDUAL, OTHER THAN A PHYSICIAN, COMPETENT IN ADMINISTRATION OF ENEMAS; FOR A PERIOD OF SIX MONTHS, SHALL PAY $100 PER MONTH FOR A BOARD COMPLIANCE CONSULTANT WHO SHALL MAKE UNANNOUNCED VISITS TO ANY OF HIS MEDICAL PRACTICE SITES TO DETERMINE HIS FULFILLMENT OF THESE TERMS AND CONDITIONS.

GLOMSET, JOHN MD, LICENSE NUMBER 8092 OF 4221 S WESTERN #5010, OKLAHOMA CITY, OK, WAS DISCIPLINED BY OKLAHOMA ON JULY 25, 1997
DISCIPLINARY ACTION: 60-MONTH PROBATION; RESTRICTION PLACED ON LICENSE
OFFENSE: SUBSTANCE ABUSE

NOTES: HABITUAL INTEMPERANCE OR THE HABITUAL USE OF HABIT-FORMING DRUGS AND THE INABILITY TO PRACTICE MEDICINE WITH REASONABLE SKILL AND SAFETY TO PATIENTS BY REASON OF AGE, ILLNESS, DRUNKENNESS, EXCESSIVE USE OF DRUGS, NARCOTICS, CHEMICALS, OR ANY OTHER TYPE OF MATERIAL OR AS A RESULT OF ANY MENTAL OR PHYSICAL CONDITION. CONDITIONS OF PROBATION: SHALL SUBMIT TO EVERY STATE IN WHICH HE HOLDS LICENSURE AND TO HOSPITALS, CLINICS OR OTHER INSTITUTIONS IN WHICH HE HOLDS OR ANTICIPATES HOLDING ANY FORM OF STAFF PRIVILEGE A COPY OF THIS ORDER; SHALL SUBMIT BIOLOGICAL FLUID SPECIMENS; SHALL NOT PRESCRIBE, ADMINISTER OR DISPENSE ANY MEDICATIONS FOR HIS PERSONAL USE AND SHALL TAKE NONE UNLESS AUTHORIZED BY ANOTHER PHYSICIAN FOR A LEGITIMATE MEDICAL NEED; SHALL ABIDE BY HIS POST CARE CONTRACT FROM RECOVERY PROGRAM; SHALL KEEP THE BOARD INFORMED OF HIS ADDRESS AND PAY COSTS; SHALL REQUEST ALL HOSPITALS IN WHICH HE ANTICIPATES PRACTICING TO FURNISH A STATEMENT REGARDING MONITORING OF HIS PRACTICE; SHALL PLACE HIMSELF IN A BOARD APPROVED REHABILITATION PROGRAM FOR INPATIENT EVALUATION AND SUBSEQUENT TREATMENT; WILL AUTHORIZE THE RELEASE OF ANY AND ALL INFORMATION REGARDING TREATMENT TO THE BOARD. SHALL ABSTAIN FROM CONSUMING ALCOHOL OR ANY SUBSTANCE WHICH WOULD ADVERSELY AFFECT HIS ABILITY TO PRACTICE MEDICINE; SHALL NOT SUPERVISE A PHYSICIAN ASSISTANT; SHALL APPEAR BEFORE THE BOARD UPON REQUEST.

GLOMSET, JOHN MD, LICENSE NUMBER 8092 OF 4221 S WESTERN #5010, OKLAHOMA CITY, OK, WAS DISCIPLINED BY OKLAHOMA ON DECEMBER 11, 1997
DISCIPLINARY ACTION: MONITORING OF PHYSICIAN PERFORMANCE
OFFENSE: FAILURE TO COMPLY WITH PREVIOUS BOARD ORDER

NOTES: ON OR AROUND 10/23/97, HE DRANK BETWEEN A HALF-PINT AND ONE PINT OF VODKA AND THEN WAS STOPPED BY POLICE AND CHARGED WITH DRIVING UNDER THE INFLUENCE FOR A BLOOD ALCOHOL LEVEL OF .22 OR .23. HE WAS PLACED IN JAIL IN NORMAN, OKLAHOMA AND ADMITTED TO A DRUG TREATMENT PROGRAM ON 11/3/97. UNDERWENT EVALUATION, AND WAS DISCHARGED ON11/5/97. RETAINED ON PROBATION FOR FIVE YEARS UNDER ALL CONDITIONS OF 7/25/97 ORDER WITH THE FOLLOWING ADDITIONAL CONDITIONS: HE WILL EXECUTE ALL RELEASES OF MEDICAL AND PSYCHIATRIC RECORDS NECESSARY TO DISCUSS THE CASE WITH HIS TREATING PHYSICIANS AND/OR ANY PHYSICIANS HOLDING HIS RECORDS; HE WILL ATTEND REGULAR THERAPY BY BOARD APPROVED THERAPIST WITH PERIODIC REPORTS TO THE BOARD; SHALL SIGN ANY CONSENT NECESSARY TO ALLOW THE PHYSICIAN OR COUNSELOR TO DISCUSS HIS CASE WITH THE BOARD.

GOLDSTEIN, JOSEPH A DO, LICENSE NUMBER 0002615, WAS DISCIPLINED BY OKLAHOMA ON APRIL 17, 1996
DISCIPLINARY ACTION: 48-MONTH PROBATION; MONITORING OF PHYSICIAN PERFORMANCE
OFFENSE: SUBSTANCE ABUSE

NOTES: IN AUGUST AND SEPTEMBER 1990 WAS TREATED FOR SUBSTANCE ABUSE AND ADDICTION AT TIMBERLAWN PSYCHIATRIC HOSPITAL AND PARTICIPATED IN A RECOVERY PROGRAM THAT WAS MONITORED BY THE TEXAS OSTEOPATHIC MEDICAL ASSOCIATION. THESE PROGRAMS WERE SUCCESSFULLY COMPLETED ON 9/26/92 WHICH HE ADMITTED ON HIS OKLAHOMA 1991 RENEWAL APPLICATION. IN 1995 HE VOLUNTARILY ADMITTED HIMSELF IN RUSH BEHAVIORAL CENTER IN CHIGAGO, ILLINOIS, FOR HABITUAL DRUNKENNESS OR HABITUAL ADDICTION TO THE USE OF HABIT-FORMING DRUGS. CONDITIONS OF OKLAHOMA PROBATION; SHALL PARTICIPATE IN THE OKLAHOMA PHYSICIAN'S RECOVERY PROGRAM WHO SHALL SUBMIT REPORTS TO THE BOARD ON A QUARTERLY BASIS DESCRIBING HIS COMPLIANCE WITH THE PROGRAM; SHALL SUBMIT TO RANDOM URINALYSIS ADMINISTERED BY THE BOARD; $565.00 ADMINISTRATIVE COSTS; MAY NOT PETITION FOR MODIFICATION OF THIS ORDER FOR TWO YEARS; SHALL APPEAR BEFORE THE BOARD UPON REQUEST. ON 6/19/97 PROBATION RESCINDED.

GOLDSTEIN, JOSEPH A DO, LICENSE NUMBER 2615, WAS DISCIPLINED BY OKLAHOMA ON NOVEMBER 20, 1998
DISCIPLINARY ACTION: SURRENDER OF LICENSE

GOLDSTEIN, JOSEPH A DO, LICENSE NUMBER 2615, WAS DISCIPLINED BY OKLAHOMA ON JUNE 17, 1999
DISCIPLINARY ACTION: LICENSE REINSTATEMENT; 60-MONTH PROBATION

GOODLOE, ROBERT K DO, LICENSE NUMBER 0001338, WAS DISCIPLINED BY OKLAHOMA ON SEPTEMBER 19, 1991
DISCIPLINARY ACTION: 12-MONTH PROBATION; REQUIRED TO TAKE ADDITIONAL MEDICAL EDUCATION
OFFENSE: CRIMINAL CONVICTION OR PLEA OF GUILTY, NOLO CONTENDERE, OR NO CONTEST TO A CRIME

NOTES: CONVICTED OF HAVING IMPROPERLY PRESCRIBED CONTROLLED SUBSTANCES TO HIS FORMER WIFE; SENTENCED TO 18 MONTHS PROBATION. THE OKLAHOMA BUREAU OF NARCOTICS AND DANGEROUS DRUGS CONTROL SUSPENDED HIS REGISTRATION FOR THREE DAYS BEGINNING 10/11/91. CONDITIONS OF PROBATION: SHALL WITHIN SIX MONTHS ENROLL IN AND ATTEND A COURSE ENTITLED "THE PROPER PRESCRIBING OF CONTROLLED DANGEROUS SUBSTANCES"; AND HIS LICENSE IS DEVOID OF ANY RESTRICTIONS. PROBATION TERMINATED ON 9/17/92, THE BOARD APPROVED A LETTER TO THE DRUG ENFORCEMENT ADMINISTRATION RECOMMENDING THAT HIS SCHEDULE II NARCOTIC AUTHORITY BE REINSTATED.

GOODLOE, ROBERT K DO, DATE OF BIRTH OCTOBER 4, 1937, LICENSE NUMBER 0028511 OF MUSTANG, OK, WAS DISCIPLINED BY COLORADO ON JUNE 19, 1992
DISCIPLINARY ACTION: SURRENDER OF LICENSE

OFFENSE: CRIMINAL CONVICTION OR PLEA OF GUILTY, NOLO CONTENDERE, OR NO CONTEST TO A CRIME

NOTES: CONVICTION OF A FELONY WITH RESPECT TO FURNISHING OF FALSE INFORMATION ON A DOCUMENT PERTAINING TO DEMEROL DISTRIBUTION.

GOODLOE, ROBERT K DO OF MUSTANG, OK, WAS DISCIPLINED BY MISSOURI ON APRIL 27, 1993
DISCIPLINARY ACTION: LICENSE REVOCATION
OFFENSE: CRIMINAL CONVICTION OR PLEA OF GUILTY, NOLO CONTENDERE, OR NO CONTEST TO A CRIME

NOTES: FELONY CONVICTION. NO REINSTATEMENT OF LICENSE FOR SEVEN YEARS.

GOODMON, ROBERT L DO, LICENSE NUMBER 1553, WAS DISCIPLINED BY OKLAHOMA ON JUNE 19, 1997
DISCIPLINARY ACTION: 60-MONTH PROBATION

GREEN, FRANK D JR MD OF 10705 FARRAGUT HILLS BOULEVARD, KNOXVILLE, TN, WAS DISCIPLINED BY DEA ON DECEMBER 11, 1995
DISCIPLINARY ACTION: SURRENDER OF CONTROLLED SUBSTANCE LICENSE

NOTES: IN LIEU OF ORDER SHOW TO CAUSE.

GREEN, FRANK D JR MD, DATE OF BIRTH OCTOBER 14, 1927, LICENSE NUMBER 1054086 OF 10705 FARRGOUT HILLS BLVD, KNOXVILLE, TN, WAS DISCIPLINED BY MICHIGAN ON DECEMBER 15, 1995
DISCIPLINARY ACTION: 6-MONTH LICENSE SUSPENSION
OFFENSE: DISCIPLINARY ACTION BY ANOTHER STATE OR AGENCY

NOTES: FAILURE TO REPORT/COMPLY.

GREEN, FRANK D JR MD, DATE OF BIRTH OCTOBER 14, 1927 OF 10705 FARRAGUT HILLS BLVD., KNOXVILLE, TN, WAS DISCIPLINED BY MEDICARE ON JANUARY 30, 1997
DISCIPLINARY ACTION: EXCLUSION FROM THE MEDICARE AND/OR MEDICAID PROGRAM
OFFENSE: DISCIPLINARY ACTION BY ANOTHER STATE OR AGENCY

NOTES: LICENSE SUSPENDED FOR REASONS BEARING ON PROFESSIONAL PERFORMANCE.

GREEN, FRANK DELAPLAINE JR MD, DATE OF BIRTH OCTOBER 11, 1927 OF 10705 FARRAGUT HILLS BLVD, KNOXVILLE, TN, WAS DISCIPLINED BY OKLAHOMA ON JULY 1, 1993
DISCIPLINARY ACTION: DENIAL OF NEW LICENSE
OFFENSE: PROFESSIONAL MISCONDUCT

NOTES: EVIDENCE INDICATED NO VALIDATION OF MEDICAL PRACTICE SKILLS SINCE 1987, FAILED TO PROVIDE EVIDENCE OF SUCCESSFUL COMPLETION OF THE FLEX OR NATIONAL BOARD EXAM, AND HAS A SIGNIFICANT MALPRACTICE HISTORY WHICH RAISES SERIOUS ISSUES AS TO CLINICAL COMPETENCY.

GREEN, FRANK DELAPLAINE JR MD, DATE OF BIRTH OCTOBER 14, 1927 OF 10705 FARRAGUT HILLS BLVD, KNOXVILLE, TN, WAS DISCIPLINED BY NORTH DAKOTA ON NOVEMBER 18, 1994
DISCIPLINARY ACTION: LICENSE REVOCATION
OFFENSE: PROVIDING FALSE INFORMATION TO THE BOARD OR OTHER HEALTH AGENCY

NOTES: MADE A FALSE STATEMENT ON HIS NORTH DAKOTA LICENSE RENEWAL APPLICATION.

GREEN, FRANK DELAPLAINE JR MD, DATE OF BIRTH OCTOBER 14, 1927, LICENSE NUMBER 1039962 OF 10705 FARRAGUT HILLS BLVD, KNOXVILLE, TN, WAS DISCIPLINED BY INDIANA ON OCTOBER 26, 1995
DISCIPLINARY ACTION: SURRENDER OF LICENSE
OFFENSE: DISCIPLINARY ACTION BY ANOTHER STATE OR AGENCY

NOTES: ON 7/1/93, OKLAHOMA DENIED HIM MEDICAL LICENSURE BASED ON FAILURE TO UPDATE MEDICAL SKILLS SINCE 1987, FAILURE TO SUCCESSFULLY COMPLETE NATIONAL BOARD EXAMINATION, AND SERIOUS ISSUES REGARDING HIS CLINICAL COMPETENCY; IN 1994, HE SUBMITTED A MEDICAL LICENSE RENEWAL APPLICATION TO NORTH DAKOTA AND FAILED TO REPORT THAT HE HAD BEEN DENIED A LICENSE IN OKLAHOMA; ON 11/18/94, NORTH DAKOTA REVOKED HIS MEDICAL LICENSE; HIS LICENSE TO PRACTICE MEDICINE IN INDIANA EXPIRED ON 6/30/95 AND HE DID NOT FILE A RENEWAL APPLICATION OR INFORM THE INDIANA BOARD THAT HE WAS PREVIOUSLY DISCIPLINED IN TWO OTHER STATES. IMMEDIATE AND PERMANENT SURRENDER OF HIS LICENSE, AND CONTROLLED SUBSTANCES PERMIT. ASSESSED COSTS OF $195.

GREEN, LAWRENCE C MD, LICENSE NUMBER 9260 OF 102 WEST ASH, #1219, CARNEGIE, OK, WAS DISCIPLINED BY OKLAHOMA ON JANUARY 21, 1997
DISCIPLINARY ACTION: 60-MONTH PROBATION; RESTRICTION PLACED ON LICENSE
OFFENSE: PROFESSIONAL MISCONDUCT

NOTES: IN OR ABOUT 3/95 HE OPENED A CLINIC IN CARNEGIE OKLAHOMA, AND IN 11/95 OPENED A SECOND CLINIC IN WEATHERFORD, OKLAHOMA. IN THE FIRST CLINIC HE DID BUT IN THE SECOND DID NOT OBTAIN DEA REGISTRATION TO DISPENSE CONTROLLED SUBSTANCES. DURING THIS TIME, HE OFFICED PRIMARILY IN CARNEGIE, WHILE HIS SPOUSE PRIMARILY STAFFED THE WEATHERFORD OFFICE WITH A RECEPTIONIST WHO HAD NO MEDICAL TRAINING UNTIL SOMETIME IN 5/96. CONTROLLED SUBSTANCES WERE ROUTINELY DISPENSED TO PATIENTS AT THE WEATHERFORD CLINIC BY HIS SPOUSE WITHOUT THEIR EVER BEING EXAMINED BY THE DOCTOR HIMSELF. IN ADDITION TO THE UNAUTHORIZED DISPENSING OF CONTROLLED SUBSTANCES AT AN UNREGISTERED LOCATION, HE HAS IMPROPERLY TRANSPORTED THESE SUBSTANCES AND FAILED TO MAINTAIN ADEQUATE RECORDS. CONDITIONS OF PROBATION: SHALL SUBMIT TO AND MAKE HIMSELF AVAILABLE FOR ALL TYPES OF MONITORING DEEMED APPROPRIATE BY THE BOARD; MUST BE PHYSICALLY PRESENT DURING THE EXAMINATION OF PATIENTS BEING SEEN FOR WEIGHT CONTROL PROBLEMS, CONDUCT THE EXAMINATION AND EVALUATION OF SUCH PATIENTS AND PRESCRIBE AND DEVISE ALL TREATMENT PLANS PERTAINING TO SUCH PATIENTS; NO MODIFICATIONS IN MEDICATIONS PRESCRIBED BY HIM SHALL EVER BE MADE WITHOUT HIM PERSONALLY SEEING AND EXAMINING THE PATIENT AND PERSONALLY MODIFYING THE TREATMENT PLANS AND/OR PRESCRIPTIONS; MUST DIVEST HIMSELF OF ALL QUANTITIES OF PONDIMIN AND PHENTERMINE NOW IN HIS POSSESSION AND/OR CONTROL BY DELIVERING SUCH QUANTITIES TO THE FEDERAL DRUG ENFORCEMENT AGENCY (DEA) OR THE OKLAHOMA BUREAU OF NARCOTICS AND DANGEROUS DRUGS (OBNDD); SHALL NOT ADMINISTER OR DISPENSE ANY CONTROLLED SUBSTANCES FOR WEIGHT CONTROL PROBLEMS TO ANY PATIENTS; RATHER, THE ONLY METHOD BY WHICH HE WILL MAKE CONTROLLED SUBSTANCES FOR WEIGHT CONTROL PROBLEMS AVAILABLE TO HIS PATIENTS IS BY MEANS OF WRITTEN PRESCRIPTIONS OR TELEPHONE CALL-IN PRESCRIPTIONS, PERSONALLY MADE BY HIM, ALL OF

WHICH SHALL BE RECORDED ON DUPLICATE, NUMERICALLY SEQUENTIAL PRESCRIPTION ORDERS WHICH WILL BE AVAILABLE FOR THE BOARD TO REVIEW; SHALL MAKE AVAILABLE FOR REVIEW BY THE BOARD ANY AND ALL PATIENT RECORDS AND ALL OTHER DOCUMENTATION RELATING TO HIS PATIENTS AS MAY BE DEEMED NECESSARY; SHALL KEEP THE BOARD INFORMED OF HIS ADDRESS AND PAY COSTS; WILL BE ALLOWED TO MAINTAIN ONLY HIS CLINICS LOCATED IN CARNEGIE AND WEATHERFORD, OKLAHOMA, DURING PROBATION, EXCEPT THAT HE CAN MAINTAIN HIS CLINIC IN GUYMON, OKLAHOMA, THROUGH 6/30/97, THE DATE OF TERMINATION OF HIS CURRENT LEASE, PROVIDED THAT HE BE PERSONALLY PRESENT AT ALL TIMES DURING WHICH THE GUYMON CLINIC IS OPEN; SHALL APPEAR BEFORE THE BOARD UPON REQUEST.

GRIGSBY, ORVILLE LEE MD, LICENSE NUMBER 0005392, WAS DISCIPLINED BY OKLAHOMA ON DECEMBER 3, 1992
DISCIPLINARY ACTION: REPRIMAND
OFFENSE: SUBSTANCE ABUSE

NOTES: FROM 1/1/92 TO 9/30/92, PRESCRIBED CONTROLLED DANGEROUS SUBSTANCES TO HIS BUSINESS MANAGER, ATTORNEY'S WIFE, DAUGHTER AND SON, AMONG OTHERS. INITIALLY DENIED HAVING RECORDS ON THESE PATIENTS; RECORDS LATER FOUND IN GARAGE BUT HAD NO ENTRIES SINCE 1989. AT LEAST SOME OF THESE PATIENTS WERE RETURNING THE MEDICATIONS TO DR. GRIGSBY FOR HIS PERSONAL USE. IN LIEU OF ADDITIONAL SANCTION, BOARD AGREES TO ACCEPT HIS REQUEST FOR PHYSICIAN EMERITUS STATUS; MUST FILE WITHIN TEN DAYS OF ORDER DATE.

GRIGSBY, ORVILLE LEE MD, LICENSE NUMBER 0005392, WAS DISCIPLINED BY OKLAHOMA ON MARCH 11, 1993
DISCIPLINARY ACTION: LICENSE SUSPENSION
OFFENSE: PHYSICAL OR MENTAL ILLNESS INHIBITING THE ABILITY TO PRACTICE WITH SKILL AND SAFETY

NOTES: ON 11/21/92 HE AGREED TO ACCEPT PHYSICIAN EMERITUS STATUS IN LIEU OF FURTHER PROCEEDINGS. ON 12/17/92 HE WITHDREW HIS APPLICATION FOR PHYSICIAN EMERITUS STATUS SAYING IT WAS OBTAINED UNDER DURESS AND THREATENED TO SUE THE BOARD; THIS CONSTITUTES GROUNDS FOR THE CASE TO BE REOPENED; HE HAS A PAST HISTORY OF PRACTICING MEDICINE OUT OF HIS HOME AND OF SELF-MEDICATING HIMSELF FOR AN UNDOCUMENTED MEDICAL CONDITION; ON 2/8/93 HE WAS DECLARED A WARD UNDER A GUARDIANSHIP. HE IS PRESENTLY UNABLE TO PRACTICE WITH REASONABLE SKILL AND SAFETY TO THE PUBLIC BUT HIS FAMILY SEES PROGRESS AND HOPES FOR A EVENTUAL COMPLETE RECOVERY. SUSPENSION SHALL RUN UNTIL THIS GUARDIANSHIP IS TERMINATED AND HE PROVIDES EVIDENCE OF MENTAL AND PHYSICAL ABILITY.

GRODE, TIMOTHY W MD, LICENSE NUMBER 0012230, WAS DISCIPLINED BY OKLAHOMA ON DECEMBER 2, 1994
DISCIPLINARY ACTION: LICENSE SUSPENSION; 60-MONTH PROBATION
OFFENSE: SUBSTANCE ABUSE

NOTES: FROM 2/01/94 TO 6/28/94 HE PRESCRIBED, ADMINISTERED, TOOK OR USED HIMSELF WITHOUT MEDICAL NECESSITY CONTROLLED DANGEROUS SUBSTANCES WHICH MADE HIM UNABLE TO PRACTICE MEDICINE WITH REASONABLE SKILL AND SAFETY. HIS LICENSE IS SUSPENDED DURING HIS IN-PATIENT TREATMENT. PROBATION BEGINNING 12/2/94 UNDER THE FOLLOWING TERMS AND CONDITIONS: SHALL NOT PRESCRIBE, ADMINISTER, OR DISPENSE ANY MEDICATIONS FOR HIS PERSONAL USE AND SHALL TAKE NONE UNLESS AUTHORIZED BY ANOTHER PHYSICIAN FOR LEGITIMATE MEDICAL NEED; SHALL ABSTAIN FROM CONSUMING ANY SUBSTANCE WHICH ADVERSELY AFFECTS HIS ABILITY TO PRACTICE; SHALL SUBMIT BIOLOGICAL FLUID SPECIMENS; SHALL NOT ENGAGE IN ANY ACTIVITY OR INGEST ANY MEDICATION OR SUBSTANCE THAT WILL TEST POSITIVE FOR ANY CONTROLLED DANGEROUS SUBSTANCE EXCEPT FOR MEDICATION PROPERLY PRESCRIBED BY A PHYSICIAN FOR A LEGITIMATE MEDICAL NEED DOCUMENTED TO THE BOARD; SHALL MAINTAIN A PROGRAM OF ABSTINENCE THROUGH PARTICIPATION IN AND/OR ASSOCIATION WITH ANY OR ALL ORGANIZATIONS, GROUPS, OR INDIVIDUALS SELECTED BY THE BOARD; SHALL ATTEND WEEKLY MEETINGS OF THE PHYSICIAN'S RECOVERY COMMITTEE; SHALL FULFILL ALL OF THE TERMS AND CONDITIONS OF HIS AFTER-CARE PROGRAMS OF HIS IN-PATIENT TREATMENT; SHALL PRESCRIBE CONTROLLED DANGEROUS SUBSTANCES ONLY UPON DUPLICATE, SEQUENTIALLY NUMBERED PRESCRIPTION FORMS; SHALL NOT CALL IN ANY PRESCRIPTIONS NOR ADMINISTER OR DISPENSE CONTROLLED DANGEROUS SUBSTANCES; SHALL NOT ACCEPT, RECEIVE, OR SIGN FOR IN ANY MANNER ANY SAMPLES OF ANY DRUGS, EXCEPT THOSE WHICH ARE BOARD APPROVED; SHALL APPEAR BEFORE THE BOARD UPON REQUEST AND SUBMIT ANY REQUIRED REPORTS; SHALL PAY COSTS; SHALL NOTIFY ANY HOSPITAL WHERE HE HOLDS STAFF PRIVILEGES, OR CLINIC, OR GROUPS WHERE HE PRACTICES OF THE TERMS AND CONDITIONS OF THIS ORDER AND PROVIDE A COPY THEREOF; SHALL NOT SUPERVISE A PHYSICIAN ASSISTANT; SHALL MEET NOT LESS THAN QUARTERLY WITH THE BOARD AND SHALL PROVIDE UPON REQUEST ANY AND ALL CHARTS AND PATIENT RECORDS.

GUIJARRO, JOSE J MD OF SOUTHSIDE MEDICAL CLINIC, MARLOW, OK, WAS DISCIPLINED BY DEA ON OCTOBER 29, 1990
DISCIPLINARY ACTION: RESTRICTION PLACED ON CONTROLLED SUBSTANCE LICENSE

NOTES: SURRENDER OF SCHEDULE II AND IIN. PLACED ON THREE YEAR MEDICAL BOARD PROBATION FROM 01/11/88 TO 01/11/91; CANNOT BE AUTOMATICALLY RENEWED; RENEWED CONTROLLED SUBSTANCES LICENSE 09/27/90.

GUJRAL, INDER SINGH OF 48615 LAKE VIEW CIRCLE, EAST LIVERPOOL, OH, WAS DISCIPLINED BY OKLAHOMA ON JANUARY 26, 1994
DISCIPLINARY ACTION: DENIAL OF NEW LICENSE

NOTES: HAS FAILED THE FLEX EXAM ON SEVEN OCCASIONS RAISING ISSUES AS TO HIS CLINICAL COMPETENCY AND FITNESS TO PRACTICE. LICENSURE ALSO DENIED ON 3/31/94.

GUZMAN, VIRGILIO T DR OF GLEN CARBON, IL, WAS DISCIPLINED BY ILLINOIS ON MAY 1, 1992
DISCIPLINARY ACTION: 36-MONTH PROBATION
OFFENSE: SUBSTANDARD CARE, INCOMPETENCE OR NEGLIGENCE

NOTES: ALLEGEDLY FAILED TO PROPERLY MONITOR POSTOPERATIVE RECOVERY OF PATIENT.

GUZMAN, VIRGILIO T MD, LICENSE NUMBER 0010982, WAS DISCIPLINED BY OKLAHOMA ON OCTOBER 7, 1993

DISCIPLINARY ACTION: SURRENDER OF LICENSE

GUZMAN, VIRGILIO T MD OF GRANITE CITY, IL, WAS DISCIPLINED BY MISSOURI ON DECEMBER 28, 1993
DISCIPLINARY ACTION: 36-MONTH PROBATION
OFFENSE: DISCIPLINARY ACTION BY ANOTHER STATE OR AGENCY

HAGGLUND, HOWARD MD, LICENSE NUMBER 9798 OF 1818 W LINDSEY SUITE C100, NORMAN, OK, WAS DISCIPLINED BY OKLAHOMA ON MAY 29, 1998
DISCIPLINARY ACTION: REPRIMAND
OFFENSE: PROFESSIONAL MISCONDUCT

NOTES: WAS THE SUPERVISING PHYSICIAN FOR A PHYSICIAN'S ASSISTANT FROM 3/13/97 TO 6/16/97. HE NOTIFIED THE BOARD OF HIS TERMINATION AS SUPERVISING PHYSICIAN ON 3/23/98 AFTER THE QUESTION AROSE WHETHER THE BOARD HAD BEEN NOTIFIED THAT HE HAD TERMINATED HIS RESPONSIBILITIES. THE PHYSICIAN'S ASSISTANT HAD BEGUN WORKING IN HIS CLINIC IN 2/97 PRIOR TO RECEIVING APPROVAL FROM THE BOARD. HE SIGNED AND LEFT BLANK PRESCRIPTIONS FOR USE BY THE PHYSICIAN'S ASSISTANT TO PRESCRIBE CONTROLLED DRUGS TO PATIENTS WHEN HE WAS OUT OF TOWN. SHALL NOT SUPERVISE ALLIED HEALTH PROFESSIONALS WITHOUT FIRST OBTAINING A COPY OF THE APPLICABLE PRACTICE ACT AND REGULATIONS AND DILIGENTLY ADHERING TO THE OBLIGATIONS AND RESPONSIBILITIES OF SUPERVISING PHYSICIANS; SHALL PAY COSTS.

HAGGLUND, HOWARD MD, DATE OF BIRTH MARCH 17, 1999, LICENSE NUMBER 185620 OF 1818 WEST LINDSEY SUITE C100, NORMAN, OK, WAS DISCIPLINED BY NEW YORK ON MARCH 17, 1999
DISCIPLINARY ACTION: REPRIMAND
OFFENSE: DISCIPLINARY ACTION BY ANOTHER STATE OR AGENCY

NOTES: DISCIPLINED BY THE OKLAHOMA BOARD FOR SIGNING BLANK PRESCRIPTION FORMS AND LEAVING THE FORMS FOR HIS PHYSICIAN ASSISTANT'S USE WHEN HE WAS OUT OF TOWN.

HALL, BRIAN K MD, LICENSE NUMBER 13764 OF 7134 S YALE AVENUE #300, TULSA, OK, WAS DISCIPLINED BY OKLAHOMA ON JANUARY 16, 1997
DISCIPLINARY ACTION: 36-MONTH PROBATION; RESTRICTION PLACED ON LICENSE
OFFENSE: NONCOMPLIANCE WITH A PROFESSIONAL RULE

NOTES: WROTE PRESCRIPTIONS FOR CONTROLLED DANGEROUS SUBSTANCES TO A FAMILY MEMBER AND FAILED TO MAINTAIN A MEDICAL CHART SUPPORTING MEDICAL NEED FOR THE PRESCRIPTIONS. FORMAL REPRIMAND AND CONDITIONS OF PROBATION: SHALL KEEP DUPLICATE, SERIALLY NUMBERED PRESCRIPTIONS OF ALL CONTROLLED DANGEROUS SUBSTANCES AND WILL SUBMIT COPIES TO THE BOARD UPON REQUEST; SHALL SUBMIT BIOLOGICAL FLUID SPECIMENS ALTHOUGH THERE IS NO EVIDENCE OF HIS PERSONAL USE OF CONTROLLED DANGEROUS SUBSTANCES; WILL NOT ALLOW THE INITIATION OF ANY THERAPEUTIC REGIMEN BY ANY PERSONNEL UNDER HIS SUPERVISION UNLESS HE IS IN THE IMMEDIATE VICINITY; SHALL SUBMIT TO EVERY STATE IN WHICH HE HOLDS LICENSURE AND TO HOSPITALS, CLINICS OR OTHER INSTITUTIONS IN WHICH HE HOLDS OR ANTICIPATES HOLDING ANY FORM OF STAFF PRIVILEGE A COPY OF THIS ORDER; SHALL NOT SUPERVISE A PHYSICIAN ASSISTANT; SHALL KEEP THE BOARD INFORMED OF HIS ADDRESS AND PAY COSTS. ON 6/4/98 THIS ORDER IS MODIFIED TO DELETE THE PROBATIONARY TERM OF TESTING OF BIOLOGICAL FLUID SPECIMENS; REQUEST TO TERMINATE THE REMAINDER OF PROBATIONARY PERIOD AS A WHOLE DENIED.

HALL, JAMES N III DO, LICENSE NUMBER 0002951, WAS DISCIPLINED BY OKLAHOMA ON APRIL 14, 1995
DISCIPLINARY ACTION: REPRIMAND
OFFENSE: PROVIDING FALSE INFORMATION TO THE BOARD OR OTHER HEALTH AGENCY

NOTES: ON 1/19/94 WAS SUSPENDED FROM RESIDENT DUTIES AT THE UNIVERSITY OF OKLAHOMA HEALTH SCIENCES CENTER, COLLEGE OF MEDICINE, TULSA CAMPUS. ON 1/26/94 WAS DISMISSED FROM HIS RESIDENT TRAINING PROGRAM AT UNIVERSITY OF OKLAHOMA HEALTH SCIENCES CENTER. ON 5/25/94 ON HIS LICENSURE RENEWAL APPLICATION HE ANSWERED THAT NO DISCIPLINARY ACTION HAD BEEN TAKEN AGAINST HIM BY ANY SOCIETY, HOSPITAL STAFF, OR OTHER PEER REVIEW COMMITTEE. HE CONTENDS THIS WAS A MISTAKE, NOT AN EFFORT TO MISLEAD THE BOARD.

HALL, JAMES N III DO, LICENSE NUMBER 0002951, WAS DISCIPLINED BY OKLAHOMA ON APRIL 11, 1996
DISCIPLINARY ACTION: EMERGENCY SUSPENSION
OFFENSE: LOSS OR RESTRICTION OF HOSPITAL PRIVILEGES

NOTES: ON 12/20/90 PLACED ON PROBATION BY THE HILLCREST HEALTH CENTER FOR THE REMAINDER OF HIS INTERNSHIP AND ON 3/21/91 THEY TERMINATED HIS INTERN CONTRACT. ON 1/19/94 SUSPENDED FROM HIS RESIDENCY DUTIES AT THE UNIVERSITY OF OKLAHOMA HEALTH SERVICES CENTER AND ON 1/26/94 WAS OFFICIALLY DISMISSED FROM THE TRAINING PROGRAM. ON 6/06/95 HE WAS NOTIFIED THAT HIS EMPLOYMENT WITH THE MCCURTAIN MEMORIAL HOSPITAL WAS BEING TERMINATED 7/06/95 AND RELIEVED OF ALL PATIENT RESPONSIBILITIES, INCLUDING THE CLINIC AT WRIGHT CITY. HAD ORDERED CONTROLLED SUBSTANCES DURING 5/94 BEFORE HIS EMPLOYMENT STARTED AT MCCURTAIN HOSPITAL CLINIC AT WRIGHT CITY AND IN 7/95 AFTER HE WAS RELIEVED OF ALL PATIENT RESPONSIBILITIES AT HIS EMPLOYMENT AT MCCURTAIN HOSPITAL; ALSO DURING THE TIME HE WAS EMPLOYED BY THE CLINIC FROM 2/95 THROUGH 6/95 ORDERED CONTROLLED SUBSTANCES WHICH HE KEPT FOR HIMSELF; ON 9/12/95 MCCURTAIN HOSPITAL NOTIFIED HIM TO COMPLETE AND RETURN CERTAIN PATIENT MEDICAL RECORDS THAT HE HAD REMOVED FROM THE HOSPITAL WHEN HIS ADMISSION PRIVILEGES HAD BEEN SUSPENDED FOR FAILURE TO TIMELY COMPLETE MEDICAL RECORDS. ON 9/22/95 A DRUG TEST WAS POSITIVE FOR BUTALBITAL AND PHENTERMINE, EPHEDRINE/PSEUDOEPHEDRINE, ACETAMINOPHEN, AND PHENOTHIAZINE METABOLITES. ON 9/15/95 SUBMITTED AN APPLICATION FOR APPOINTMENT TO THE MEDICAL STAFF OF EASTERN OKLAHOMA MEDICAL CENTER AND STATED THAT HE HAD NOT HAD ACTION TAKEN AGAINST HIS LICENSE. A 3/96 EVALUATION BY RUSH BEHAVIORAL HEALTH CENTER-DUPAGE RECOMMENDED THAT HE ENTER A RESIDENTIAL, PARTIAL OR DAY HOSPITAL PROGRAM FOR THE TREATMENT AND ASSESSMENT OF IMPAIRED CHEMICALLY DEPENDENT PROFESSIONALS.

HALL, JAMES N III DO, LICENSE NUMBER 2951, WAS DISCIPLINED BY OKLAHOMA ON MARCH 19, 1998
DISCIPLINARY ACTION: 60-MONTH PROBATION; RESTRICTION

PLACED ON LICENSE

NOTES: RESTRICTED TO FAMILY MEDICINE RESIDENCY AT SPECIFIED FACILITY.

HALL, JAMES N III DO, LICENSE NUMBER 2951, WAS DISCIPLINED BY OKLAHOMA ON DECEMBER 20, 1999
DISCIPLINARY ACTION: SURRENDER OF LICENSE

HAMMOND, MICHAEL W MD, LICENSE NUMBER 15215, WAS DISCIPLINED BY OKLAHOMA ON JULY 23, 1998
DISCIPLINARY ACTION: 5-MONTH LICENSE SUSPENSION; 60-MONTH PROBATION
OFFENSE: SEXUAL ABUSE OF OR SEXUAL MISCONDUCT WITH A PATIENT

NOTES: ENGAGED IN INAPPROPRIATE AND UNPROFESSIONAL SEXUAL RELATIONS WITH ONE PATIENT. ALLOWED, AIDED, AND ABETTED THE PRACTICE OF MEDICINE BY AN UNAUTHORIZED INDIVIDUAL IN HIS OFFICE AND IMPROPERLY DELEGATED AUTHORITY FOR THE SIGNING OF PRESCRIPTIONS FOR REDUX, PONDIMIN, PREMARIN, AND AMBIEN ON BEHALF OF THE DOCTOR. HE UNDERWENT PSYCHIATRIC AND PSYCHOLOGICAL EVALUATION IN 2/98, AND UNDERWENT TREATMENT ON 5/25/98, 6/24/98, AND 7/9/98. SUSPENSION RETROACTIVE TO 2/21/98. CONDITIONS OF PROBATION: SHALL KEEP THE BOARD INFORMED OF HIS ADDRESS AND PAY COSTS; SHALL APPEAR BEFORE THE BOARD AND SUBMIT REPORTS UPON REQUEST; SHALL CONTINUE TO UNDERGO PSYCHIATRIC THERAPY FOR ONE YEAR; SHALL AUTHORIZE THE RELEASE OF REPORTS AND/OR THE CONDUCTION OF CONFERENCES BETWEEN THE TREATING PSYCHIATRIST AND THE BOARD FOR PURPOSES OF MONITORING; SHALL SUBMIT TO EVERY STATE IN WHICH HE HOLDS LICENSURE AND TO HOSPITALS, CLINICS OR OTHER INSTITUTIONS IN WHICH HE HOLDS OR ANTICIPATES HOLDING ANY FORM OF STAFF PRIVILEGE A COPY OF THIS ORDER; SHALL HAVE A LICENSED HEALTHCARE PROFESSIONAL PHYSICALLY PRESENT AT ALL TIMES THAT A FEMALE PATIENT IS EXAMINED OR TREATED; SHALL KEEP DUPLICATE, SERIALLY-NUMBERED PRESCRIPTIONS OF ALL PRESCRIPTIVE SUBSTANCES AND WILL SUBMIT COPIES TO THE BOARD UPON REQUEST; SHALL NOT PRESCRIBE, ADMINISTER OR DISPENSE ANY MEDICATIONS FOR HIS PERSONAL USE AND SHALL TAKE NONE UNLESS AUTHORIZED BY ANOTHER PHYSICIAN FOR A LEGITIMATE MEDICAL NEED; SHALL SUBMIT BIOLOGICAL FLUID SPECIMENS AND SHALL NOT INGEST ANY SUBSTANCE WHICH WILL CAUSE A SPECIMEN TO TEST POSITIVE FOR PROHIBITED SUBSTANCES; SHALL NOT AUTHORIZE ANY PERSONNEL UNDER HIS SUPERVISION (OTHER THAN AN APPROPRIATELY LICENSED PHYSICIAN) TO INITIATE AN ORDER FOR A PRESCRIPTION TO BE ISSUED; SHALL NOT ALLOW THE INDEPENDENT PRACTICE OF MEDICINE BY ANY PERSONNEL UNDER HIS SUPERVISION OR EMPLOY, EXCEPT AN APPROPRIATELY LICENSED PHYSICIAN; WILL NOT ALLOW THE INITIATION OF ANY THERAPEUTIC REGIMEN BY ANY PERSONNEL UNDER HIS SUPERVISION UNLESS HE IS IN THE IMMEDIATE VICINITY.

HANAN, STANLEY SCOTT MD, LICENSE NUMBER 11542 OF 4019 SHADOWALK DRIVE, VAN BUREN, AR, WAS DISCIPLINED BY OKLAHOMA ON JANUARY 10, 1997
DISCIPLINARY ACTION: REPRIMAND
OFFENSE: OVERPRESCRIBING OR MISPRESCRIBING DRUGS

NOTES: PRESCRIBED SIGNIFICANT AMOUNTS OF CONTROLLED SUBSTANCES TO EIGHT PATIENTS; HAS FAILED TO COMPLY WITH REQUESTS FROM THE BOARD TO PROVIDE PATIENT RECORDS AND LOGS FOR ACQUIRING AND DISPENSING CONTROLLED AND DANGEROUS DRUGS; HE EXPLAINS THIS WAS THE RESULT OF A FINANCIAL INSTITUTION WHICH TOOK POSSESSION OF HIS OFFICE. HE HAS DECIDED NOT TO RENEW HIS OKLAHOMA LICENSE; IF HE EVER ATTEMPTS TO RENEW IT, HE WILL BE SUBJECT TO IMMEDIATE PROBATION AND MONITORING. IN ADDITION, HE WILL NOT CONTRACT WITH ANY NURSING HOME OR OTHER HEALTH CARE FACILITY IN OKLAHOMA AND WILL NOT PRACTICE MEDICINE IN THE STATE WITHOUT FIRST RENEWING HIS LICENSE AND COMPLYING WITH THE ABOVE PROVISIONS.

HANAN, STANLEY SCOTT MD, LICENSE NUMBER 11542 OF 411 N 11TH STREET, PERRY, OK, WAS DISCIPLINED BY OKLAHOMA ON JULY 23, 1998
DISCIPLINARY ACTION: 60-MONTH PROBATION; RESTRICTION PLACED ON LICENSE

NOTES: FAILED TO RENEW LICENSE FOLLOWING AN OFFICIAL REPRIMAND IN 1/97 FOR UNPROFESSIONAL CONDUCT. REINSTATEMENT OF LICENSE UNDER THE FOLLOWING CONDITIONS OF PROBATION: SHALL WILL KEEP DUPLICATE, SERIALLY NUMBERED PRESCRIPTIONS OF ALL CONTROLLED DANGEROUS SUBSTANCES AND WILL SUBMIT COPIES TO THE BOARD UPON REQUEST; SHALL PRACTICE IN A CONTROLLED ENVIRONMENT APPROVED BY THE BOARD; SHALL REQUEST ALL HEALTH CARE FACILITIES IN WHICH HE ANTICIPATES PRACTICING TO FURNISH A STATEMENT REGARDING MONITORING OF HIS PRACTICE; SHALL SUBMIT TO EVERY STATE IN WHICH HE HOLDS LICENSURE AND TO HOSPITALS, CLINICS OR OTHER INSTITUTIONS IN WHICH HE HOLDS OR ANTICIPATES HOLDING ANY FORM OF STAFF PRIVILEGE A COPY OF THE 1997 ORDER AND THIS ORDER; SHALL NOT SUPERVISE ALLIED HEALTH PROFESSIONALS; SHALL KEEP THE BOARD INFORMED OF HIS ADDRESS AND PAY COSTS; SHALL APPEAR BEFORE THE BOARD UPON REQUEST; SHALL NOT PRESCRIBE, ADMINISTER, OR DISPENSE ANY MEDICATION FOR PERSONAL USE OR FOR USE BY HIS FAMILY MEMBERS; SHALL GENERATE AND MAINTAIN COMPLETE, ACCURATE MEDICAL RECORDS WHICH SHALL BE AVAILABLE TO THE BOARD UPON REQUEST.

HARDER, JACK A MD, LICENSE NUMBER 0001017 OF PO BOX 250, TEMPLE, OK, WAS DISCIPLINED BY OKLAHOMA ON JANUARY 18, 1990
DISCIPLINARY ACTION: 60-MONTH PROBATION; RESTRICTION PLACED ON CONTROLLED SUBSTANCE LICENSE

NOTES: FULL MEDICAL LICENSE REINSTATED ON PROBATION RETROACTIVE TO 3/22/89 UNDER THE FOLLOWING TERMS AND CONDITIONS: SHALL IMMEDIATELY BRING CURRENT THE PRESENT ARREARAGE OF COSTS IN THE AMOUNT OF $1,573.87; SHALL NOT PRESCRIBE, ADMINISTER, OR DISPENSE ANY MEDICATIONS FOR HIS PERSONAL USE AND SHALL TAKE NONE UNLESS AUTHORIZED BY ANOTHER PHYSICIAN FOR LEGITIMATE MEDICAL NEED; SHALL ABSTAIN FROM CONSUMING ALCOHOL OR ANY SUBSTANCES WHICH WOULD ADVERSELY AFFECT HIS ABILITY TO PRACTICE; SHALL ADVISE THE BOARD OF ALL PHYSICIANS WHO HAVE TREATED HIM WITHIN THE LAST FIVE YEARS AND SHALL SIGN A RELEASE ALLOWING THE BOARD TO OBTAIN AND REVIEW THOSE RECORDS; SHALL SUBMIT BIOLOGICAL FLUID SPECIMENS; SHALL REGULARLY ATTEND MEETINGS OF THE PHYSICIAN RECOVERY COMMITTEE AND/OR

OTHER ALCOHOL AND DRUG SUPPORT GROUPS; SHALL NOT PRESCRIBE, ADMINISTER OR DISPENSE ANY SCHEDULE DRUGS OR CONTROLLED SUBSTANCES; SHALL NOT APPLY FOR STATE AND FEDERAL CONTROLLED DANGEROUS SUBSTANCES REGISTRATION; SHALL SUBMIT TO THE BOARD ADDRESS/CHANGE OF ADDRESS; SHALL APPEAR BEFORE THE BOARD UPON REQUEST AND SUBMIT ANY REQUIRED REPORTS; SHALL PAY COSTS. ON 5/31/90 PROBATION MODIFIED AUTHORIZING HIM TO PRESCRIBE, ADMINISTER OR DISPENSE ANY SCHEDULE DRUGS OR CONTROLLED DANGEROUS SUBSTANCES ONLY ON SERIALLY-NUMBERED, DUPLICATE PRESCRIPTION PADS AND SHALL MAKE THE COPIES AVAILABLE TO THE BOARD UPON REQUEST.

HARRISON, WILLIAM JOSEPH DO, LICENSE NUMBER 0019919 OF DURANT, OK, WAS DISCIPLINED BY KANSAS ON FEBRUARY 12, 1991

NOTES: STIPULATION AND ENFORCEMENT ORDER. MODIFIED ON 3/10/92 TO INCLUDE THE FOLLOWING: SHALL ENTER INTO A PSYCHOLOGICAL/PSYCHIATRIC COUNSELING MONITORING PROGRAM WITH A BOARD APPROVED HEALTH CARE PRACTITIONER FOR A PERIOD ENDING NO SOONER THAN 2/12/94 WITH QUARTERLY REPORTS TO THE BOARD. PROGRAM SHALL INCLUDE INDIVIDUAL AND GROUP PSYCHOTHERAPY SESSIONS AS WELL AS ACTIVE PARTICIPATION IN A 12-STEP TYPE PROGRAM OR PEER SUPPORT GROUP. ON 11/2/92 COUNSELING REQUIREMENTS WERE REDUCED. ON 2/2/95 ORDER AND MODIFICATIONS TERMINATED AND LICENSE PLACED IN AN INACTIVE STATUS.

HARRISON, WILLIAM JOSEPH DO, LICENSE NUMBER 0002926, WAS DISCIPLINED BY OKLAHOMA ON JUNE 18, 1992
DISCIPLINARY ACTION: 48-MONTH PROBATION; RESTRICTION PLACED ON LICENSE
OFFENSE: DISCIPLINARY ACTION BY ANOTHER STATE OR AGENCY

NOTES: ON 2/12/91 THE KANSAS BOARD RESTRICTED HIS LICENSE FOR THREE YEARS AND PLACED ADDITIONAL TERMS OF PROBATION. CONDITIONS OF OKLAHOMA PROBATION: AFTER COMPLETION OF HIS AFTERCARE TREATMENT HE MAY PETITION THE BOARD FOR MODIFICATION OF THE LENGTH OF HIS PROBATION; SHALL STRICTLY COMPLY WITH THE AFTERCARE PROGRAM ESTABLISHED BY GOLDEN VALLEY HEALTH CENTER AND SHALL ATTEND AND SUCCESSFULLY COMPLETE ANY TREATMENT, COUNSELING, AND THERAPY ESTABLISHED AS A RESULT OF HIS EVALUATION AND ASSESSMENT; SHALL ACTIVELY PURSUE FORMAL PARTICIPATION IN THE OKLAHOMA PHYSICIAN'S RECOVERY PROGRAM AND AGREES TO COMPLY WITH ALL TERMS THEY SET FORTH; SHALL HAVE A FEMALE NURSE/EMPLOYEE PRESENT WHEN EXAMINING OR CONSULTING WITH ANY FEMALE PATIENT IN HIS OFFICE OR EXAMINING ROOM; SHALL SUBMIT QUARTERLY REPORTS TO THE BOARD VERIFYING HIS COMPLIANCE WITH THE AFTERCARE PROGRAM; AND SHALL NOTIFY THE BOARD IN WRITING OF ANY CHANGE IN ADDRESS, EMPLOYMENT, EMPLOYMENT TERMINATION, OR HOSPITAL PRIVILEGE RESTRICTION AND ANY ADMINISTRATIVE PROCEEDING INITIATED AGAINST HIM BY ANY OTHER STATE OR FEDERAL REGULATORY BODY WITHIN 14 DAYS; SHALL APPEAR BEFORE THE BOARD UPON REQUEST; AGREES TO RANDOM, UNANNOUNCED VISITS FROM THE BOARD AT HIS PLACE OF BUSINESS FOR OBSERVATION AND ACCESS TO ANY APPROPRIATE RECORDS IN HIS POSSESSION, PROVIDED THAT THESE VISITS WILL NOT INTERRUPT HIS MEDICAL SERVICES; PERIOD OF PROBATION SHALL NOT INCLUDE ANY PERIODS OF RESIDENCE OR PRACTICE OUTSIDE OF OKLAHOMA; ADMINISTRATIVE COSTS OF $2,405.76. ON 12/30/92 ADDENDUM TO THIS ORDER TO INCLUDE: MONTHLY PARTICIPATION IN THE OKLAHOMA PHYSICIAN RECOVERY PROGRAM; ONE HOUR OF INDIVIDUAL PSYCHOTHERAPY PER WEEK; ONE GROUP PSYCHOTHERAPY SESSION PER WEEK; ACTIVE PARTICIPATION IN SEX ADDICTS ANONYMOUS' 12 STEP PROGRAM; SHALL ARRANGE FOR REPORTS OF HIS PARTICIPATION IN THIS COUNSELING PROGRAM TO BE SUBMITTED WITH HIS CONTINUING MEDICAL EDUCATION AND NURSE ATTENDANT VERIFICATION REPORTS ON OR BEFORE 12/30/92 AND QUARTERLY THEREAFTER. ON 9/15/94 PROBATION TERMINATED.

HARVEY, CHARLES F DO, LICENSE NUMBER 0002953, WAS DISCIPLINED BY OKLAHOMA ON JUNE 16, 1995
DISCIPLINARY ACTION: 24-MONTH PROBATION; REQUIRED TO TAKE ADDITIONAL MEDICAL EDUCATION
OFFENSE: SEXUAL ABUSE OF OR SEXUAL MISCONDUCT WITH A PATIENT

NOTES: ON 1/31/94 ISSUED A PRESCRIPTION IN THE NAME OF A PATIENT AND EMPLOYEE FOR TEMAZEPAM, A SCHEDULE IV CONTROLLED DANGEROUS SUBSTANCE. SHE THEN DELIVERED THIS DRUG BACK TO HIM AND HE GAVE THIS DRUG TO HIS WIFE; ISSUED A PRESCRIPTION IN THIS PATIENT'S NAME TWICE; ALSO HAD SEXUAL ACTIVITY WITH THIS PATIENT; ADMITTED TO PROVIDING NALBUPHINE TO HIS WIFE; HE DID NOT HAVE A PHYSICIAN-PATIENT RELATIONSHIP WITH HIS WIFE. CONDITIONS OF PROBATION: SHALL ATTEND AND SUCCESSFULLY COMPLETE A COURSE "THE PROPER PRESCRIBING OF CONTROLLED DANGEROUS SUBSTANCES" AND SHALL COMPLETE AN ETHICS COURSE; AND SHALL REPORT TO THE BOARD SUCCESSFUL COMPLETION OF THOSE COURSES; SHALL GIVE A COPY OF THIS ORDER TO ANY HEALTH CARE ENTITY WHERE HE HAS PRIVILEGES; SHALL NOTIFY THE BOARD IN WRITING OF ANY CHANGE IN ADDRESS, EMPLOYMENT, EMPLOYMENT TERMINATION OR HOSPITAL OR HEALTH CARE ENTITIES PRIVILEGE RESTRICTION OR ANY ADMINISTRATIVE PROCEEDING INITIATED AGAINST HIM BY ANY OTHER STATE OR FEDERAL REGULATORY BODY WITHIN 14 DAYS; $1,450.00 ADMINISTRATIVE COSTS.

HARVEY, CHARLES F DO, LICENSE NUMBER 2953, WAS DISCIPLINED BY OKLAHOMA ON JULY 6, 1996
DISCIPLINARY ACTION: SURRENDER OF LICENSE

HARVEY, CHARLES F DO, LICENSE NUMBER 2953, WAS DISCIPLINED BY OKLAHOMA ON MARCH 24, 1997
DISCIPLINARY ACTION: LICENSE REINSTATEMENT; 60-MONTH PROBATION

HARWELL, PHILLIP R MD, LICENSE NUMBER 0009695, WAS DISCIPLINED BY OKLAHOMA ON OCTOBER 30, 1995
DISCIPLINARY ACTION: LICENSE REVOCATION
OFFENSE: SEXUAL ABUSE OF OR SEXUAL MISCONDUCT WITH A PATIENT

NOTES: ON 1/20/93 WHEN CONDUCTING A FOLLOW-UP EXAM HE LOWERED HIS PANTS AND SHOWED A PATIENT HIS TATTOO OF A DRAGON LOCATED ON HIS HIP. THIS OCCURRED WHILE THE PATIENT WAS MERELY CLOTHED WITH A DRAPE GOWN AND NO NURSE OR ASSISTANT WAS PRESENT; AT ANOTHER FOLLOW UP EXAMINATION HE TALKED TO THE SAME PATIENT

ABOUT A WOMAN IN A PORNOGRAPHIC VIDEO TAPE WHO HAD A TATTOO OF A SERPENT. LATER THAT SAME DAY HE DROVE TO THE PATIENT'S RESIDENCE AND DELIVERED A PORNOGRAPHIC VIDEO TAPE TO THE PATIENT.

HASSMAN, GARY C MD, DATE OF BIRTH APRIL 6, 1941, LICENSE NUMBER 0028004 OF 3207 RIVERSIDE DRIVE #112, TULSA, OK, WAS DISCIPLINED BY NEW JERSEY ON MARCH 18, 1991
DISCIPLINARY ACTION: LICENSE REVOCATION
OFFENSE: DISCIPLINARY ACTION BY ANOTHER STATE OR AGENCY

NOTES: ACTION BASED UPON REVOCATION OF LICENSE IN TEXAS BASED UPON A CRIMINAL CONVICTION FOR ILLEGAL DISTRIBUTION OF COCAINE.

HASSMANN, GARY C MD OF TULSA, OK, WAS DISCIPLINED BY DEA ON SEPTEMBER 24, 1998
DISCIPLINARY ACTION: DENIAL OF LICENSE REINSTATEMENT
OFFENSE: PROVIDING FALSE INFORMATION TO THE BOARD OR OTHER HEALTH AGENCY

NOTES: BETWEEN 2/87 AND 8/87 MET WITH DEA AGENTS ON AT LEAST FIVE OCCASIONS FOR THE PURPOSE OF INVESTING IN A COCAINE SMUGGLING OPERATION WHEN HE SUPPLIED THEM WITH $99,200 TO FINANCE THE PURCHASE OF 14 KILOGRAMS FOR DISTRIBUTION; ON 2/19/88 HE PLED GUILTY IN U.S. DISTRICT COURT IN TEXAS OF ONE FELONY COUNT OF TRAVELING IN INTERSTATE AND FOREIGN COMMERCE FOR THE PURPOSE OF DISTRIBUTING THE PROCEEDS OF AN UNLAWFUL ACTIVITY AND SURRENDERED HIS DEA REGISTRATION AT THIS TIME; ON 9/24/88 THE TEXAS BOARD REVOKED HIS LICENSE, ON 2/21/91 THE OKLAHOMA BOARD PLACED HIS LICENSE ON PROBATION AND ON 3/18/91 THE NEW JERSEY BOARD REVOKED HIS LICENSE; IN 1994 HE PLED GUILTY TO RESIDENTIAL BURGLARY AND DRIVING UNDER THE INFLUENCE OF ALCOHOL; ON 12/23/95 APPLICATION FOR DEA REGISTRATION ANSWERED NO TO WHETHER ANY DISCIPLINARY ACTION HAD BEEN TAKEN AGAINST HIS LICENSE; APPLIED FOR REGISTRATION IN SCHEDULES II THROUGH V EVEN THOUGH HIS OKLAHOMA LICENSE COULD NOT HANDLE SCHEDULE II SUBSTANCES.

HASSMANN, GARY CHARLES MD, LICENSE NUMBER 0017579 OF 3207 RIVERSIDE DR, TULSA, OK, WAS DISCIPLINED BY OKLAHOMA ON FEBRUARY 1, 1991
DISCIPLINARY ACTION: 60-MONTH PROBATION; RESTRICTION PLACED ON LICENSE

NOTES: LICENSED UNDER PROBATIONARY TERMS AND CONDITIONS: MUST NOT PRESCRIBE, ADMINISTER OR DISPENSE ANY MEDICATIONS, INCLUDING CONTROLLED DANGEROUS SUBSTANCES, FOR HIS PERSONAL USE; MUST NOT PRESCRIBE, ADMINISTER OR DISPENSE ANY SCHEDULE DRUGS, OR ANY LEGEND DRUGS PRIOR TO OBTAINING PERMISSION FROM BOARD; MUST ABSTAIN FROM ALCOHOL OR ANY SUBSTANCE WHICH WOULD ADVERSELY AFFECT HIS ABILITY TO PRACTICE OR ANY MEDICATION NOT PRESCRIBED BY HIS DOCTOR; MUST SUBMIT BIOLOGICAL FLUID SPECIMENS FOR ANALYSIS; MUST TAKE SPEX; SHALL COMPLETE 50 HOURS OF CONTINUING MEDICAL EDUCATION EACH YEAR OF PROBATION; SHALL NOT PERFORM ANY SURGERY OR SURGICAL PROCEDURES UNTIL FURTHER ORDER; SHALL NOTIFY ANY HOSPITAL WHERE HE HOLDS STAFF PRIVILEGES, OR CLINIC OR GROUP OF THE TERMS AND CONDITIONS; SHALL FURNISH BOARD WITH ADDRESS AND/OR CHANGE OF ADDRESS; SHALL APPEAR BEFORE BOARD UPON REQUEST. ON 3/11/93 MOTION TO TERMINATE PROBATION DENIED. ON 2/18/94 ORDER MODIFIED ALLOWING HIM TO PRESCRIBE, ADMINISTER OR DISPENSE LEGEND DRUGS BUT ONLY ON SERIALLY NUMBERED DUPLICATE PRESCRIPTION PADS WITH COPIES AVAILABLE TO THE BOARD; PROVISIONS REQUIRING HIM TO SUBMIT BIOLOGICAL FLUID SPECIMENS FOR ANALYSIS WERE DROPPED.

HASSMANN, GARY CHARLES MD, LICENSE NUMBER 0017579, WAS DISCIPLINED BY OKLAHOMA ON NOVEMBER 18, 1994
DISCIPLINARY ACTION: MONITORING OF PHYSICIAN PERFORMANCE
OFFENSE: SUBSTANCE ABUSE

NOTES: ON 2/11/94 BOARD HAD MODIFIED TERMS OF PREVIOUS PROBATION DELETING REQUIREMENTS THAT HE ABSTAIN FROM THE CONSUMPTION OF ALCOHOL AND TO SUBMIT BIOLOGICAL FLUID SPECIMENS; WAS ARRESTED FOR DRIVING UNDER THE INFLUENCE OF ALCOHOL ON 3/25/94. THESE TWO REQUIREMENTS WERE REINSTATED AND ALL OTHER TERMS OF PROBATION STILL IN EFFECT.

HAWKINS, CHARLES G DO, DATE OF BIRTH DECEMBER 5, 1948, LICENSE NUMBER D0R0138 OF 2900 WEBER ROAD, CLAREMORE, OK, WAS DISCIPLINED BY IOWA ON OCTOBER 8, 1992
DISCIPLINARY ACTION: 48-MONTH PROBATION
OFFENSE: SUBSTANCE ABUSE

NOTES: PREVIOUS ALCOHOL PROBLEM. RESIDENT MEDICAL LICENSE GRANTED UNDER CONSENT AGREEMENT.

HAWKINS, CHARLES G DO, LICENSE NUMBER 0002458, WAS DISCIPLINED BY OKLAHOMA ON DECEMBER 11, 1992
DISCIPLINARY ACTION: 48-MONTH PROBATION; MONITORING OF PHYSICIAN PERFORMANCE
OFFENSE: DISCIPLINARY ACTION BY ANOTHER STATE OR AGENCY

NOTES: ON 8/27/91 PLED GUILTY TO DRIVING UNDER THE INFLUENCE OF ALCOHOL AND RECEIVED A THREE YEAR DEFERRED SENTENCE. ON 8/31/92 HIS HOSPITAL EMPLOYMENT AND PRIVILEGES AT EASTERN STATE HOSPITAL IN VINITA, OKLAHOMA WERE ADMINISTRATIVELY SUSPENDED. ON 10/08/92 WAS LICENSED FOUR YEARS UNDER CERTAIN TERMS AND CONDITIONS BY THE IOWA BOARD. CONDITIONS OF OKLAHOMA PROBATION: SHALL COMPLETELY ABSTAIN FROM THE PERSONAL USE OF ALL CONTROLLED OR PRESCRIPTION DRUGS UNLESS PRESCRIBED FOR HIM BY ANOTHER DULY, LICENSED, TREATING PHYSICIAN AND SHALL ADVISE THE PHYSICIAN OF HIS PREVIOUS HISTORY OF CHEMICAL ABUSE; SHALL ABSTAIN FROM THE CONSUMPTION OF ALCOHOL; THE RESULT OF BLOOD OR URINE SAMPLES TAKEN FOR SCREENING PURPOSES BY THE IOWA BOARD SHALL BE PROVIDED TO THE OKLAHOMA BOARD; SHALL PROVIDE THE BOARD WITH DOCUMENTS INDICATING HIS ATTENDANCE OF NOT LESS THAN ONE MEETING OF AA OR A SIMILAR ORGANIZATION EACH WEEK AS REQUIRED BY THE IOWA BOARD; SHALL FURNISH THE BOARD WITH A COPY OF THE QUARTERLY PHYSICIAN OR COUNSELOR'S REPORT FROM TREATMENT OR COUNSELING REQUIRED BY THE IOWA BOARD; SHALL CONTINUE TREATMENT OR COUNSELING UNTIL DISCHARGED BY THE IOWA BOARD APPROVED PHYSICIAN OR COUNSELOR AND UNTIL THE DISCHARGE HAS BEEN APPROVED BY THE IOWA BOARD; SHALL FURNISH THE BOARD WITH A COPY OF THE QUARTERLY REPORTS REGARDING COMPLIANCE WITH ALL THE TERMS OF THE CONSENT ORDER AS REQUIRED BY THE IOWA BOARD; $1,268.54 ADMINISTRATIVE COSTS; SHALL NOTIFY THE BOARD

IN WRITING OF HIS CURRENT ADDRESS AND OF ANY CHANGE OF ADDRESS, EMPLOYMENT, EMPLOYMENT TERMINATION OR HOSPITAL PRIVILEGE RESTRICTION AND ANY ADMINISTRATIVE PROCEEDING INITIATED AGAINST HIM BY ANY OTHER STATE OR FEDERAL REGULATORY BODY WITHIN 14 DAYS; SHALL NOT PETITION THE BOARD FOR MODIFICATION FOR AT LEAST ONE YEAR; SHALL APPEAR BEFORE THE BOARD PRIOR TO PRACTICING OSTEOPATHIC MEDICINE IN OKLAHOMA.

HAWKINS, CHARLES G DO, DATE OF BIRTH DECEMBER 5, 1948, LICENSE NUMBER DOR0138 OF 729 WEST CEDAR, APT. 302, CHEROKEE, IA, WAS DISCIPLINED BY IOWA ON DECEMBER 28, 1993
DISCIPLINARY ACTION: SURRENDER OF LICENSE
OFFENSE: FAILURE TO COMPLY WITH PREVIOUS BOARD ORDER

NOTES: SETTLEMENT TO CHARGES OF VIOLATING THE TERMS OF HIS CONSENT AGREEMENT BY CONSUMING ALCOHOL.

HAWKINS, CHARLES G DO OF 1200 W CEDAR, CHEROKEE, IA, WAS DISCIPLINED BY DEA ON FEBRUARY 7, 1994
DISCIPLINARY ACTION: SURRENDER OF CONTROLLED SUBSTANCE LICENSE
OFFENSE: DISCIPLINARY ACTION BY ANOTHER STATE OR AGENCY

NOTES: ACTION TAKEN BY IOWA BOARD OF MEDICAL EXAMINERS.

HAWKINS, CHARLES G DO, LICENSE NUMBER 2458, WAS DISCIPLINED BY OKLAHOMA ON MARCH 20, 1997
DISCIPLINARY ACTION: LICENSE SUSPENSION
OFFENSE: DISCIPLINARY ACTION BY ANOTHER STATE OR AGENCY

NOTES: MIRRORED FROM IOWA.

HENDERSON, JOSEPH S MD, LICENSE NUMBER 0009231, WAS DISCIPLINED BY OKLAHOMA ON OCTOBER 29, 1992
DISCIPLINARY ACTION: LICENSE SUSPENSION
OFFENSE: SUBSTANCE ABUSE

NOTES: MET WITH BOARD INVESTIGATORS ON 5/19/92 30-45 MINUTES AFTER FINISHING A SURGICAL CASE, AT WHICH TIME HE EXHIBITED THICK-TONGUED AND SLURRED SPEECH, DRY MOUTH, DISORIENTATION, AND DIFFICULTY IN THINKING OR REMEMBERING. ALSO HAD WHAT APPEARED TO BE NEEDLE MARKS ON INSIDE ELBOW. SUSPENDED UNTIL HE PRESENTS EVIDENCE OF MEDICAL EVALUATION AND COMPLETION OF ANY RECOMMENDED TREATMENT.

HENDERSON, JOSEPH S MD, LICENSE NUMBER 0009231, WAS DISCIPLINED BY OKLAHOMA ON NOVEMBER 21, 1992
DISCIPLINARY ACTION: 60-MONTH PROBATION; RESTRICTION PLACED ON LICENSE

NOTES: A PREVIOUS PARTIAL ASSESSMENT AND AN IN-PATIENT EVALUATION RELEASED ON 11/10/92 INDICATED CERTAIN AREAS IN HIS PERSONALITY AND PROFESSIONAL WORK HABITS THAT RAISE ISSUES THAT MUST BE ADDRESSED. LICENSE REINSTATED FROM 10/29/92 SUSPENSION, PLACED ON PROBATION UNDER TERMS AND CONDITIONS: SHALL LIMIT PRACTICE TO AN AVERAGE OF 44 HOURS PER WEEK, WITH CEILING OF 60 HOURS IN ANY ONE WEEK; SHALL NOT PRESCRIBE, ADMINISTER OR DISPENSE ANY MEDICATIONS, INCLUDING CONTROLLED DANGEROUS SUBSTANCES, FOR HIS PERSONAL USE; SHALL TAKE NO MEDICATION UNLESS AUTHORIZED BY TREATING PHYSICIAN; SHALL ABSTAIN FROM ALCOHOL OR ANY SUBSTANCE WHICH WOULD ADVERSELY AFFECT HIS ABILITY TO PRACTICE; SHALL SUBMIT BIOLOGICAL FLUID SPECIMENS FOR ANALYSIS; SHALL MAINTAIN REGULAR PSYCHOTHERAPY; SHALL NOT SUPERVISE A PHYSICIAN ASSISTANT OR ALLOW THE INITIATION OF ANY THERAPEUTIC REGIMEN BY ANY PERSONNEL UNDER HIS SUPERVISION UNLESS HE'S IN THE IMMEDIATE VICINITY; SHALL NOTIFY ANY HOSPITAL WHERE HE HOLDS STAFF PRIVILEGES, OR CLINIC, OR GROUP WHERE HE PRACTICES OR OTHER STATES WHERE HE'S LICENSED OF THE TERMS AND CONDITIONS; SHALL FURNISH BOARD WITH ADDRESS AND/OR CHANGE OF ADDRESS; SHALL APPEAR BEFORE BOARD UPON REQUEST.

HENSON, EDWIN R III MD OF 3201 W GORE BLVD SUITE 100, LAWTON, OK, WAS DISCIPLINED BY DEA ON MAY 17, 1994
DISCIPLINARY ACTION: SURRENDER OF CONTROLLED SUBSTANCE LICENSE

NOTES: IN LIEU OF PUBLIC INTEREST REVOCATION.

HENSON, EDWIN RAY MD, LICENSE NUMBER 0016952, WAS DISCIPLINED BY OKLAHOMA ON SEPTEMBER 9, 1994
DISCIPLINARY ACTION: 1-MONTH LICENSE SUSPENSION; 60-MONTH PROBATION
OFFENSE: OVERPRESCRIBING OR MISPRESCRIBING DRUGS

NOTES: ALLEGATIONS THAT FROM 5/93 THROUGH 4/94 HE WROTE AND CALLED IN FALSE AND FICTITIOUS PRESCRIPTIONS IN THE NAMES OF THREE PEOPLE WHO WERE NOT PATIENTS WHICH WERE PROVIDED TO HIS WIFE; AMOUNT OBTAINED FOR HIS WIFE WAS IN EXCESS OF THE AMOUNT CONSIDERED GOOD MEDICAL PRACTICE; FAILED TO KEEP COMPLETE AND ACCURATE RECORDS OF THESE DRUGS; HE SUBMITS TO JURISDICTION OF BOARD WITHOUT ADMITTING OR DENYING ALLEGATIONS. BOTH SUSPENSION AND PROBATION TO BEGIN 9/12/94. CONDITIONS OF PROBATION: SHALL NOT PRESCRIBE, DISPENSE OR ADMINISTER ANY SCHEDULE II OR III CONTROLLED SUBSTANCES EXCEPT IN EMERGENCY SITUATION WHERE HE WILL OBTAIN COSIGNATURE WITHIN 24 HOURS; SHALL CONTINUE TO ABIDE BY ALL TERMS OF TREATMENT SET BY THE BEHAVIORAL HEALTH CENTER; SHALL PROVIDE BOARD WITH ANY REQUESTED REPORTS; SHALL PAY COSTS.

HERD, PATRICK S MD, LICENSE NUMBER 18233 OF RR1 BOX 67D, MCALESTER, OK, WAS DISCIPLINED BY OKLAHOMA ON MAY 7, 1998
DISCIPLINARY ACTION: 60-MONTH PROBATION; RESTRICTION PLACED ON LICENSE
OFFENSE: OVERPRESCRIBING OR MISPRESCRIBING DRUGS

NOTES: FROM APPROXIMATELY 7/95 TO 11/97 HE PRESCRIBED, ADMINISTERED, OR DISPENSED CONTROLLED DANGEROUS SUBSTANCES AND OTHER DRUGS TO PATIENTS AND MAINTAINED PATIENTS ON THOSE DRUGS FOR LONG PERIODS OF TIME IN EXCESS OF THE AMOUNT CONSIDERED GOOD MEDICAL PRACTICE AND WITHOUT MEDICAL NEED. THE CONTROLLED DANGEROUS SUBSTANCES PRESCRIBED, ADMINISTERED, OR DISPENSED INCLUDED SCHEDULE II, III, AND IV DRUGS, FOR 13 PATIENTS. HE DID NOT MAINTAIN COMPLETE MEDICAL RECORDS AND CHARTS THAT CONTAINED ALL PERTINENT MEDICAL INFORMATION ON HIS PATIENTS AND THEY FAILED TO DEMONSTRATE THAT HE PRESCRIBED, ADMINISTERED, OR DISPENSED CONTROLLED DANGEROUS SUBSTANCES WITH SUFFICIENT EXAMINATION AND THE ESTABLISHMENT OF A VALID PHYSICIAN-PATIENT RELATIONSHIP. REPRIMAND. CONDITIONS OF PROBATION: SHALL NOT PRACTICE ANY WEIGHT CONTROL OR PAIN MANAGEMENT; SHALL KEEP AND MAINTAIN ADEQUATE MEDICAL

RECORDS TO SUPPORT ANY PRESCRIPTION OF CONTROLLED AND NON-CONTROLLED ADDICTIVE SUBSTANCES TO ANY PATIENT AND SHALL MAKE THOSE RECORDS AVAILABLE TO HE BOARD UPON REQUEST TO INCLUDE QUARTERLY REVIEW; SHALL LIMIT HIS PRACTICE TO PSYCHIATRY FOR PATIENTS OF A SPECIFIED MENTAL HEALTH CENTER IN MCALESTER, OKLAHOMA, AND THE BOARD STAFF WILL OBTAIN REPORTS FROM THE CHIEF OF PSYCHIATRY THERE REGARDING HIS CLINICAL PERFORMANCE; SHALL KEEP DUPLICATE, SERIALLY NUMBERED PRESCRIPTIONS OF ALL ADDICTIVE SUBSTANCES AND WILL SUBMIT COPIES TO THE BOARD UPON REQUEST; SHALL SUBMIT TO EVERY STATE IN WHICH HE HOLDS LICENSURE AND TO HOSPITALS, CLINICS OR OTHER INSTITUTIONS IN WHICH HE HOLDS OR ANTICIPATES HOLDING ANY FORM OF STAFF PRIVILEGE A COPY OF THIS ORDER; SHALL NOT SUPERVISE ALLIED HEALTH PROFESSIONALS; SHALL KEEP THE BOARD INFORMED OF HIS ADDRESS AND PAY COSTS. ON 10/2/98 HIS REQUEST TO CHANGE HIS PRACTICE LOCATION WAS GRANTED.

HERNDON, NOEL ELWOOD MD, LICENSE NUMBER 0006808 OF 2907 LAKESIDE CIRCLE, OKLAHOMA CITY, OK, WAS DISCIPLINED BY OKLAHOMA ON NOVEMBER 1, 1990
DISCIPLINARY ACTION: 36-MONTH PROBATION; RESTRICTION PLACED ON CONTROLLED SUBSTANCE LICENSE

NOTES: PROBATION BEGINNING 10/26/90 UNDER THE FOLLOWING TERMS AND CONDITIONS: MUST UTILIZE SERIALLY-NUMBERED, DUPLICATE PRESCRIPTION BLANKS FOR ALL CONTROLLED DANGEROUS SUBSTANCES SCHEDULES II THROUGH IV AND MUST SUBMIT ONE COPY OF EACH PRESCRIPTION TO THE BOARD MONTHLY; SHALL NOT ALLOW HIS STAFF TO INDEPENDENTLY PRESCRIBE OR AUTHORIZE REFILLS OF CONTROLLED DANGEROUS SUBSTANCES AND MUST MAINTAIN VALID PATIENT RECORDS SHOWING CONTROL OF PRESCRIBING CONTROLLED DANGEROUS SUBSTANCES; MUST PROVIDE PROOF WITHIN SIX MONTHS OF OBTAINING 20 HOURS OF CONTINUING EDUCATION ON PRESCRIBING CONTROLLED SUBSTANCES; SHALL APPEAR BEFORE THE BOARD UPON REQUEST AND SUBMIT REQUIRED REPORTS; SHALL SUBMIT TO THE BOARD ADDRESS/CHANGE IN ADDRESS; SHALL PAY COSTS; SHALL NOTIFY ANY HOSPITAL WHERE HE HOLDS STAFF PRIVILEGES, OR CLINIC, OR GROUP WHERE HE PRACTICES, OF THE TERMS AND CONDITIONS OF THIS ORDER AND SUPPLY A COPY THEREOF.

HERNDON, NOEL ELWOOD MD, LICENSE NUMBER 0006808 OF 2907 LAKESIDE CIRCLE, OKLAHOMA CITY, OK, WAS DISCIPLINED BY OKLAHOMA ON JUNE 26, 1992
DISCIPLINARY ACTION: 60-MONTH PROBATION; RESTRICTION PLACED ON CONTROLLED SUBSTANCE LICENSE

NOTES: PROBATIONARY TERMS AND CONDITIONS: SHALL NOT PRESCRIBE, ADMINISTER OR DISPENSE ANY SCHEDULED DRUGS, SUBSTANCE OR PHARMACEUTICAL AGENT, EXCEPT TO PRESCRIBE SCHEDULE II, IIN, III, IIIN TO IN-PATIENTS AT A NURSING HOME AND SCHEDULE IV, V FOR OFFICE PATIENTS, FOR WHICH HE SHALL USE SERIALLY-NUMBERED DUPLICATE PRESCRIPTION BLANKS; ALSO MAY PRESCRIBE, ADMINISTER OR DISPENSE DEPO-TESTADIOL WITH PROPER DIAGNOSIS AND APPROPRIATE DOCUMENTATION OF MEDICAL NEED; SHALL NOT ALLOW STAFF TO INDEPENDENTLY PRESCRIBE OR AUTHORIZE REFILLS OF CONTROLLED SUBSTANCES; SHALL NOTIFY ANY HOSPITAL WHERE HE HOLDS STAFF PRIVILEGES, OR CLINIC OR GROUP OF THE TERMS AND CONDITIONS; SHALL FURNISH BOARD WITH ADDRESS AND/OR CHANGE OF ADDRESS; SHALL APPEAR BEFORE BOARD UPON REQUEST. HAD PREVIOUSLY BEEN PLACED ON PROBATION FOR 3 YEARS ON 10/26/90.

HILL, WILLIAM ELLIOTT MD OF 320 S W 5TH STREET, ROOM 156, OKLAHOMA CITY, OK, WAS DISCIPLINED BY DEA ON JUNE 22, 1990
DISCIPLINARY ACTION: SURRENDER OF CONTROLLED SUBSTANCE LICENSE
OFFENSE: CRIMINAL CONVICTION OR PLEA OF GUILTY, NOLO CONTENDERE, OR NO CONTEST TO A CRIME

NOTES: OKLAHOMA MEDICAL LICENSE SUSPENDED 11/01/90. ARRESTED AND PLED GUILTY 08/16/91 TO KNOWINGLY AND INTENTIONALLY FURNISHING FALSE OR FRAUDULENT MATERIAL INFORMATION IN OR THE OMISSION OF MATERIAL INFORMATION FROM CONTROLLED SUBSTANCE RECORDS REQUIRED TO BE KEPT OR MADE UNDER THE DRUG ABUSE PREVENTION AND CONTROL ACT. CHARGED WITH DISTRIBUTION OF DEMEROL 08/16/91; CONVICTED; SENTENCED ON 10/25/91 TO SIX MONTHS PRISON AND 208 HOURS OF COMMUNITY SERVICE.

HILL, WILLIAM ELLIOTT MD, LICENSE NUMBER 0013169, WAS DISCIPLINED BY OKLAHOMA ON NOVEMBER 1, 1990
DISCIPLINARY ACTION: LICENSE SUSPENSION; REQUIRED TO ENTER AN IMPAIRED PHYSICIAN PROGRAM OR SUBSTANCE ABUSE TREATMENT
OFFENSE: SUBSTANCE ABUSE

NOTES: BEGAN IN-PATIENT TREATMENT FOR SUBSTANCE ABUSE AT AN INSTITUTION ACCEPTABLE TO THE BOARD. LICENSE SUSPENSION UNTIL HE PRODUCES EVIDENCE TO THE BOARD OF SUCCESSFUL COMPLETION OF IN-PATIENT TREATMENT AND RELATED RESIDENTIAL OUTPATIENT TREATMENT.

HILST, WILBUR MD, LICENSE NUMBER 412627 OF 1821 N CALHOUN AVENUE, LIBERAL, KS, WAS DISCIPLINED BY KANSAS ON JULY 16, 1997
DISCIPLINARY ACTION: LICENSE REVOCATION
OFFENSE: FAILURE TO COMPLY WITH PREVIOUS BOARD ORDER

NOTES: VIOLATED THE TERMS OF 10/22/96 ORDER AND HIS CONTRACT WITH THE KANSAS IMPAIRED PHYSICIANS PROGRAM.

HILST, WILBUR D MD, LICENSE NUMBER 0412627 OF TOPEKA, KS, WAS DISCIPLINED BY KANSAS ON FEBRUARY 10, 1990
DISCIPLINARY ACTION: LICENSE REVOCATION

HILST, WILBUR D MD, LICENSE NUMBER 0412627 OF 3724 SOUTHWEST 29TH, TOPEKA, KS, WAS DISCIPLINED BY KANSAS ON MARCH 14, 1994
DISCIPLINARY ACTION: LICENSE REINSTATEMENT; RESTRICTION PLACED ON LICENSE

NOTES: ALCOHOLISM PROBLEMS WHICH RESULTED IN A PATTERN OF BEHAVIOR CLEARLY DEMONSTRATING AN INCOMPETENCE TO PRACTICE MEDICINE. LED TO 2/10/90 ORDER OF REVOCATION. LICENSE REINSTATED UNDER THE FOLLOWING CONDITIONS: AGREES TO COMPLETELY ABSTAIN FROM THE CONSUMPTION OR USE OF ANY ALCOHOL OR CEREAL MALT BEVERAGE; SHALL NOT ADMINISTER TO HIMSELF OR ALLOW TO BE DISPENSED OR PRESCRIBED TO HIM ANY CONTROLLED SUBSTANCES OR ANY OTHER MOOD ALTERING SUBSTANCE OR POTENTIALLY ADDICTING SUBSTANCE WITHOUT

FIRST OBTAINING A WRITTEN PRESCRIPTION BY A DULY-LICENSED PHYSICIAN; AGREES TO COMPLY WITH ALL TERMS AND CONDITIONS OF HIS REVISED CONTRACT WITH THE KANSAS MEDICAL SOCIETY IMPAIRED PHYSICIANS PROGRAM AND TO FOLLOW ALL RECOMMENDATIONS MADE BY SUCH PROGRAM FOR SUBSEQUENT TREATMENT, MONITORING AND SUPPORT; AGREES TO SUBMIT TO RANDOM URINALYSIS; AGREES TO ATTEND ALCOHOLICS ANONYMOUS MEETINGS AT A MINIMUM OF FOUR TIMES PER WEEK; AGREES HIS PRACTICE OF MEDICINE IS LIMITED TO PERFORMING SERVICES WITHIN THE SCOPE OF HIS EMPLOYMENT AT SOUTHWEST MEDICAL CENTER IN LIBERAL AND AT A.H. THIEMANN MEMORIAL CLINIC IN SUBLETTE; HIS PRACTICE IS LIMITED TO EMERGENCY MEDICINE AND FAMILY PRACTICE, AND SHALL NOT PERFORM GENERAL SURGERY, EXCEPT TO THE EXTENT REQUIRED IN THE COURSE OF PERFORMANCE OF EMERGENCY ROOM SERVICES; MAY PERFORM MINOR CUTANEOUS INCISIONS AND THOSE PROCEDURES PERFORMED UNDER LOCAL ANESTHESIA; SHALL NOT ENGAGE IN THE PRACTICE OF OBSTETRICS, PRENATAL, POSTPARTUM OR NEWBORN MEDICAL CARE; AGREES TO SHOW PROOF OF COMPLETION OF A WEEK-LONG REVIEW SESSION IN FAMILY MEDICINE AT LEAST ONCE A YEAR, THE FIRST SESSION TO BE COMPLETED BY 09/01/94; AGREES TO FOCUS CONTINUING MEDICAL EDUCATION IN THE FOLLOWING AREAS: PEDIATRICS, OFFICE GYNECOLOGY, MODERN IMAGING TECHNIQUES, ACUTE ASTHMA, HYPERTENSION, ANTIMICROBIAL THERAPY, DIABETES, PHYSICIAN-PATIENT COMMUNICATIONS AND MEDICAL DOCUMENTATION; MUST HAVE HIS PATIENT CHARTS REVIEWED; IF FAVORABLE REPORTS WITH RESPECT TO CHART REVIEW ARE DEEMED SATISFACTORY, SUCH REVIEW WILL BE REDUCED TO 10 CHARTS PER MONTH AFTER SIX MONTHS; IF FAVORABLE REPORTS ARE DEEMED SATISFACTORY AFTER THE NEXT SIX MONTHS, SUCH CHART REVIEW MAY BE DISCONTINUED; STIPULATION TO BE IN EFFECT FOR AT LEAST FIVE YEARS; HE MAY PETITION FOR MODIFICATION AFTER ONE YEAR. ON 3/14/94 AN ADDITIONAL HOSPITAL WAS ADDED TO WHERE HE COULD PRACTICE WITH THE SAME CONDITIONS OF CHART MONITORING.

HILST, WILBUR D MD, DATE OF BIRTH DECEMBER 7, 1931, LICENSE NUMBER 0014776 OF TOPEKA, KS, WAS DISCIPLINED BY COLORADO ON NOVEMBER 3, 1994
DISCIPLINARY ACTION: SURRENDER OF LICENSE
OFFENSE: SUBSTANCE ABUSE

NOTES: HABITUAL INTEMPERANCE OR EXCESSIVE USE OF ANY HABIT-FORMING DRUG OR CONTROLLED SUBSTANCE.

HILST, WILBUR D MD, LICENSE NUMBER 0412627 OF 1821 N. CALHOUN AVENUE, LIBERAL, KS, WAS DISCIPLINED BY KANSAS ON JULY 13, 1995
DISCIPLINARY ACTION: EMERGENCY SUSPENSION
OFFENSE: FAILURE TO COMPLY WITH PREVIOUS BOARD ORDER

NOTES: ON 6/24/95 THROUGH 6/27/95 CONSUMED AND WAS UNDER THE INFLUENCE OF ALCOHOL ON SEVERAL OCCASIONS WHERE HE TREATED PATIENTS IN VIOLATION OF HIS PREVIOUS STIPULATION AGREEMENT OF 3/14/94; FAILED TO SUBMIT TO A URINALYSIS ON TWO OCCASIONS. ON 8/29/96 THE EMERGENCY SUSPENSION WAS TERMINATED; HE REMAINS SUBJECT TO THE TERMS OF THE 3/14/94 ORDER.

HILST, WILBUR D MD, LICENSE NUMBER 0412627, WAS DISCIPLINED BY KANSAS ON OCTOBER 22, 1996
DISCIPLINARY ACTION: 14-MONTH LICENSE SUSPENSION; RESTRICTION PLACED ON LICENSE
OFFENSE: FAILURE TO COMPLY WITH PREVIOUS BOARD ORDER

NOTES: VIOLATED A PREVIOUS ORDER BY CONSUMING ALCOHOL ON 6/24 AND 6/25/95; FAILING TO SUBMIT TO REQUESTED URINALYSIS ON THREE OCCASIONS BETWEEN 6/30 AND 7/4/95, TESTING POSITIVE FOR BARBITURATES AND BENZODIAZEPINES ON 7/7/95, AND FAILING TO REPORT HIS POSITIVE TESTING. SUSPENSIONS RETROACTIVE TO 7/07/95 UNTIL 9/01/96. FINAL ORDER: SHALL ABSTAIN FROM THE CONSUMPTION OR USE OF ANY ALCOHOL OR CEREAL MALT BEVERAGE; SHALL NOT ADMINISTER TO HIMSELF OR ALLOW TO BE DISPENSED OR PRESCRIBED TO HIM ANY SUBSTANCES IN ANY SCHEDULE OF THE UNIFORM CONTROLLED SUBSTANCES ACT OR ANY OTHER MOOD OR MIND ALTERING SUBSTANCE OR POTENTIALLY ADDICTING SUBSTANCE WITHOUT FIRST OBTAINING A WRITTEN PRESCRIPTION BY A DULY LICENSED PHYSICIAN FOR MEDICAL NEED; SHALL LIMIT HIS PRACTICE TO EMERGENCY MEDICINE AND FAMILY PRACTICE; SHALL NOT HOLD HIMSELF OUT TO THE PUBLIC AS A GENERAL SURGEON, BUT MAY APPLY FOR PRIVILEGES AS A GENERAL SURGEON; SHALL NOT PERFORM GENERAL SURGERY, EXCEPT TO THE EXTENT REQUIRED IN THE COURSE OF PERFORMANCE OF EMERGENCY ROOM SERVICES; MAY PERFORM MINOR CUTANEOUS INCISIONS, THOSE PERFORMED UNDER LOCAL ANESTHESIA, AND MAY ASSIST AT A SURGERY ONLY IN THE PRESENCE OF A GENERAL OR OTHER SURGEON WITH SURGICAL PRIVILEGES; SHALL NOT ENGAGE IN THE PRACTICE OF OBSTETRICS, PRENATAL, POSTPARTUM, OR NEWBORN MEDICAL CARE; SHALL COMPLY WITH THE RECOMMENDATIONS FROM THE COLORADO PERSONALIZED EDUCATION FOR PHYSICIANS, EXCEPT TO THE EXTENT INCONSISTENT WITH THIS ORDER; SHALL COMPLY WITH ANY REASONABLE PEER REVIEW REPORTS AT ANY HEALTH CARE FACILITY WITH WHICH HE IS AFFILIATED; MAY SEEK EMPLOYMENT AND/OR STAFF PRIVILEGES AS HE DEEMS APPROPRIATE AND NOTIFY THE BOARD OF ANY CHANGE; MUST COMPLETE A CURRENT PSYCHIATRIC EVALUATION AND REPORT RESULTS TO THE BOARD; AND SHALL SEEK ON-GOING PSYCHOTHERAPY, AS A TERM AND CONDITION OF HIS KMS-MAP MONITORING CONTRACT. MUST SEEK ONGOING PSYCHOTHERAPY.

HILST, WILBUR D MD, LICENSE NUMBER 6037 OF 1821 NORTH CALHOUN, LIBERAL, KS, WAS DISCIPLINED BY OKLAHOMA ON JULY 7, 1998
DISCIPLINARY ACTION: 60-MONTH PROBATION; RESTRICTION PLACED ON LICENSE
OFFENSE: DISCIPLINARY ACTION BY ANOTHER STATE OR AGENCY

NOTES: HISTORY OF ALCOHOL ABUSE AND PRIOR DISCIPLINARY ACTION IN COLORADO AND KANSAS. HE PLANS TO LIMIT HIS OKLAHOMA PRACTICE TO EMERGENCY MEDICINE AT A HOSPITAL IN GUYMON, OKLAHOMA. GRANTED LICENSURE WITH CONDITIONS OF PROBATION: SHALL PRACTICE IN A CONTROLLED ENVIRONMENT APPROVED BY THE BOARD LIMITED TO EMERGENCY MEDICINE AT THE SPECIFIED HOSPITAL IN GUYMON, OKLAHOMA AND WILL NOT PRACTICE MORE THAN 60 HOURS IN ANY GIVEN WEEK; MUST OBTAIN APPROVAL FROM THE BOARD PRIOR TO MAKING ANY CHANGE IN HIS PRACTICE OR LOCATION; SHALL REQUEST THE SPECIFIED HOSPITAL AND PRACTICE GROUP, AND ANY AND ALL HOSPITALS

SUBSEQUENTLY APPROVED BY THE BOARD TO FURNISH TO THE BOARD A WRITTEN QUARTERLY STATEMENT MONITORING HIS PRACTICE; SHALL SUBMIT TO EVERY STATE IN WHICH HE HOLDS LICENSURE AND TO HOSPITALS, CLINICS OR OTHER INSTITUTIONS IN WHICH HE HOLDS OR ANTICIPATES HOLDING ANY FORM OF STAFF PRIVILEGE A COPY OF THIS ORDER; SHALL NOT SUPERVISE ALLIED HEALTH PROFESSIONALS; SHALL SUBMIT BIOLOGICAL FLUID SPECIMENS AND SHALL NOT INGEST ANY SUBSTANCE WHICH WILL CAUSE A SPECIMEN TO TEST POSITIVE FOR PROHIBITED SUBSTANCES; SHALL SUBMIT HIS WRITTEN WORK SCHEDULE TO THE BOARD AS OFTEN AS NECESSARY TO KEEP THE BOARD INFORMED, AT ALL TIMES, OF THE DATES AND TIMES THAT HE WILL BE PROVIDING MEDICAL SERVICES TO OKLAHOMA; SHALL NOT PRESCRIBE, ADMINISTER OR DISPENSE ANY MEDICATIONS FOR HIS PERSONAL USE AND SHALL TAKE NONE UNLESS AUTHORIZED BY ANOTHER PHYSICIAN FOR A LEGITIMATE MEDICAL NEED; SHALL AFFILIATE WITH THE OKLAHOMA PHYSICIANS' RECOVERY PROGRAM AND AA AND WILL ASK THOSE SUPPORT GROUPS TO SUBMIT QUARTERLY REPORTS ON HIS PROGRESS TO THE BOARD; SHALL MEET PERIODICALLY WITH A BOARD APPROVED PSYCHIATRIST AND SHALL AUTHORIZE THEM TO SUBMIT WRITTEN REPORTS TO THE BOARD FOLLOWING SUCH CONSULTATIONS AND SHALL COMPLY WITH ALL TREATMENT RECOMMENDATIONS; SHALL KEEP THE BOARD INFORMED OF HIS ADDRESS AND PAY COSTS; SHALL APPEAR BEFORE THE BOARD UPON REQUEST; SHALL EXECUTE THE RELEASE OF ANY MEDICAL, COUNSELING, AND PSYCHIATRIC RECORDS AS NECESSARY TO DISCUSS HIS CASE WITH TREATING PHYSICIANS AND/OR ANY PHYSICIANS HOLDING RECORDS; SHALL NOTIFY THE BOARD OF ANY ENTRY, OR RE-ENTRY, INTO AN INPATIENT REHABILITATION, ASSESSMENT, OR EVALUATION PROGRAM AND SHALL PROVIDE AUTHORIZATION FOR ANY AND ALL RECORDS ASSOCIATED WITH TREATMENT. ON 10/2/98 HIS REQUEST TO ADD A SECOND PRACTICE LOCATION WHICH WOULD ALLOW HIM TO PRACTICE IN THE ER OF SPECIFIED MUNICIPAL HOSPITAL, STILL AS AN EMPLOYEE OF THE SAME PRACTICE GROUP WAS GRANTED SUBJECT TO ALL OTHER TERMS OF THIS ORDER.

HILST, WILBUR DEAN MD, DATE OF BIRTH DECEMBER 7, 1931 OF 1821 NORTH CALHOUN AVENUE, LIBERAL, KS, WAS DISCIPLINED BY MEDICARE ON JULY 20, 1998
DISCIPLINARY ACTION: EXCLUSION FROM THE MEDICARE AND/OR MEDICAID PROGRAM
OFFENSE: DISCIPLINARY ACTION BY ANOTHER STATE OR AGENCY

NOTES: LICENSE REVOKED, SUSPENDED, SURRENDERED OR OTHERWISE LOST FOR REASONS BEARING ON PROFESSIONAL PERFORMANCE, PROFESSIONAL COMPETENCE OR FINANCIAL INTEGRITY.

HINMAN, ROBERT CHARLES MD, LICENSE NUMBER 18322 OF 4300 THOMAS, LAWTON, OK, WAS DISCIPLINED BY OKLAHOMA ON NOVEMBER 19, 1998
DISCIPLINARY ACTION: 3-MONTH LICENSE SUSPENSION; COMMUNITY SERVICE
OFFENSE: PROVIDING FALSE INFORMATION TO THE BOARD OR OTHER HEALTH AGENCY

NOTES: ON 5/24/93 AND 5/17/94, HE SUBMITTED APPLICATIONS FOR RENEWAL OF HIS MEDICAL LICENSE TO THE BOARD AND ANSWERED "NO" TO QUESTIONS ASKING IF HE HAD BEEN TREATED FOR MENTAL OR EMOTIONAL DISORDERS AND IF HE HAD BEEN DENIED PRIVILEGES, LOST PRIVILEGES, OR BEEN DISCIPLINED BY ANY HOSPITAL OR OTHER PROFESSIONAL MEDICAL ORGANIZATION. IN 1/93 THE U.S. ARMY REVIEWED HIS CHARTS. OF 55 REVIEWED, 20 WERE DEEMED UNACCEPTABLE. HIS CLINICAL PRIVILEGES WERE SUSPENDED AND HE WAS ORDERED TO UNDERGO A NEUROPSYCHIATRIC EVALUATION. IN 3/93 A CREDENTIALS HEARING WAS HELD AND THE RECOMMENDATION FOLLOWING THE HEARING WAS TO SUSTAIN REVOCATION OF HIS CLINICAL PRIVILEGES. THE US ARMY MEDICAL COMMAND REPORTED HIM TO THE NATIONAL PRACTITIONER DATA BANK ON 12/9/97 AS HAVING LOST HIS CLINICAL PRIVILEGES AS OF 1/7/93 FOR SUBSTANDARD CARE AND MENTAL IMPAIRMENT. ON 6/11/93 HIS PRIVILEGES WERE REINSTATED ON A PROVISIONAL BASIS. HE WAS PLACED UNDER THE IMPAIRED PROVIDER PROGRAM; SHALL COMPLETE 250 HOURS OF COMMUNITY SERVICE APPROVED BY THE BOARD DURING THE NEXT YEAR; SHALL PAY COSTS.

HOLT, HUEY THOMAS JR DR OF 4749 TOWERING OAKS DR #2, MEMPHIS, TN, WAS DISCIPLINED BY OKLAHOMA ON JULY 1, 1992
DISCIPLINARY ACTION: 36-MONTH PROBATION; MONITORING OF PHYSICIAN PERFORMANCE
OFFENSE: SUBSTANCE ABUSE

NOTES: PREVIOUS HISTORY OF SUBSTANCE ABUSE, FOLLOWED BY LENGTHY PERIOD OF SOBRIETY. LICENSE GRANTED UNDER TERMS AND CONDITIONS: SHALL ABSTAIN FROM ALCOHOL OR ANY SUBSTANCE WHICH WOULD ADVERSELY AFFECT HIS ABILITY TO PRACTICE; SHALL SUBMIT BIOLOGICAL FLUID SPECIMENS FOR ANALYSIS; SHALL MAINTAIN A FORMAL RELATIONSHIP WITH PHYSICIAN RECOVERY COMMITTEE AND PARTICIPATE IN THEIR MEETINGS AND ACTIVITIES.

HONEYWELL, ROY W DO, LICENSE NUMBER 0001417, WAS DISCIPLINED BY OKLAHOMA ON MARCH 22, 1993
DISCIPLINARY ACTION: SURRENDER OF LICENSE

NOTES: VOLUNTARY RESIGNATION IN LIEU OF A HEARING. SHOULD NOT BE CONSTRUED AS AN ADMISSION OF ANY OF THE COMPLAINTS FILED AGAINST HIM.

HORANZY, ROBERT R MD, LICENSE NUMBER 054672 OF FAIRVIEW, OK, WAS DISCIPLINED BY VIRGINIA ON JULY 21, 1997
DISCIPLINARY ACTION: REPRIMAND
OFFENSE: EXCEEDING PROFESSIONAL LIMITATIONS

NOTES: MATTER CONTINUED ON TERMS AND CONDITIONS FOR TREATING AN INDIVIDUAL OUTSIDE OF A BONA FIDE PHYSICIAN/PATIENT RELATIONSHIP, AND PRESCRIBING OUTSIDE THE SCOPE OF PRACTICE OF AN INTERN/RESIDENT.

HORN, STEVEN CRAIG DO, DATE OF BIRTH AUGUST 12, 1964 OF 1836 11TH STREET NW, OKLAHOMA CITY, OK, WAS DISCIPLINED BY MEDICARE ON NOVEMBER 19, 1998
DISCIPLINARY ACTION: EXCLUSION FROM THE MEDICARE AND/OR MEDICAID PROGRAM
OFFENSE: NONCOMPLIANCE WITH A PROFESSIONAL RULE

NOTES: DEFAULTED ON PUBLIC HEALTH SERVICE EDUCATION LOAN.

HOUGHTON, MICHAEL A MD, LICENSE NUMBER 0014523 OF TRICITIES MED & SURG POB 1221, WEWOKA, OK, WAS DISCIPLINED BY OKLAHOMA ON FEBRUARY 2, 1991
DISCIPLINARY ACTION: 60-MONTH PROBATION; RESTRICTION PLACED ON LICENSE

NOTES: PROBATIONARY CONDITIONS AS FOLLOWS: SHALL MAKE ALL HOSPITAL ROUNDS IN PERSON OR MAKE ARRANGEMENTS FOR ANOTHER PHYSICIAN TO MAKE ROUNDS IN HIS ABSENCE; SHALL NOT PRACTICE ANY OBSTETRICS OR TRAUMA SURGERY AT ANY HOSPITAL, CLINIC OR INSTITUTION; BASED UPON THE ALLEGATION THAT HE EXHIBITS SYMPTOMS CONSISTENT WITH A HEALTH CONDITION WHICH HE DENIES, SHALL UNDERGO A COMPLETE PHYSICAL AND PSYCHIATRIC EXAMINATION BY A PHYSICIAN CHOSEN BY THE OKLAHOMA BOARD; BASED UPON THE ALLEGATION THAT HE WAS INGESTING A NON-SCHEDULED MEDICATION WHICH HE ALSO DENIES, SAID DENIAL SUPPORTED BY VOLUNTARY FLUID TESTS, SHALL TAKE NO MEDICATION EXCEPT THAT WHICH IS AUTHORIZED BY A PHYSICIAN TREATING HIM FOR A LEGITIMATE MEDICAL NEED; SHALL CONTINUE HIS CURRENT VOLUNTARY PRACTICE AND PRESCRIBE CONTROLLED DANGEROUS SUBSTANCES ONLY ON SERIALLY-NUMBERED DUPLICATE PRESCRIPTION PADS AND SHALL MAKE COPIES AVAILABLE TO BOARD; SHALL CONTINUE TO MAINTAIN RECORDS ON AND REDUCE TOTAL NUMBERS OF CONTROLLED DANGEROUS SUBSTANCES PRESCRIBED, ADMINISTERED AND DISPENSED; BASED UPON ALLEGED HEALTH CONDITION, WHICH HE DENIES, SHALL SUBMIT BIOLOGICAL FLUID SPECIMENS FOR ANALYSIS; SHALL FURNISH BOARD WITH ADDRESS AND/OR CHANGE OF ADDRESS; SHALL APPEAR BEFORE BOARD UPON REQUEST; SHALL NOTIFY ANY HOSPITAL WHERE HE HOLDS STAFF PRIVILEGES, OR CLINIC OR GROUP OF THE TERMS AND CONDITIONS. ON 3/5/92, THE PROVISIONS REQUIRING HIM TO SUBMIT BIOLOGICAL FLUID SPECIMENS AND NOT TO TAKE MEDICATION NOT PRESCRIBED BY HIS DOCTOR WERE REMOVED. BODILY FLUID SPECIMENS HAD TESTED NEGATIVE FOR ALCOHOL AND CONTROLLED DANGEROUS SUBSTANCES. ON 7/2/92 HIS REQUEST TO TERMINATE PROBATION WAS DENIED. ON 10/7/93 AND ON 9/9/94 HIS REQUESTS TO TERMINATE OR MODIFY PROBATION WERE DENIED AND THE TERMS AND CONDITIONS OF HIS PROBATION REMAIN IN EFFECT. ON 8/30/95 PROBATION TERMINATED.

HOUGHTON, MICHAEL A MD, DATE OF BIRTH MARCH 17, 1945, LICENSE NUMBER 0023729 OF PO BOX 1221, WEWOKA, OK, WAS DISCIPLINED BY IOWA ON JULY 23, 1992
DISCIPLINARY ACTION: PROBATION
OFFENSE: DISCIPLINARY ACTION BY ANOTHER STATE OR AGENCY

NOTES: INDEFINITE PROBATION.

HUBBARD, FRANK LEROI DO, LICENSE NUMBER 0002700, WAS DISCIPLINED BY OKLAHOMA ON SEPTEMBER 16, 1993
DISCIPLINARY ACTION: 60-MONTH PROBATION; REQUIRED TO ENTER AN IMPAIRED PHYSICIAN PROGRAM OR SUBSTANCE ABUSE TREATMENT
OFFENSE: SUBSTANCE ABUSE

NOTES: IN 4/93 CHARGED WITH UNLAWFUL POSSESSION OF CONTROLLED DANGEROUS SUBSTANCES; VOLUNTARILY ENTERED INTO TALBOT RECOVERY CENTER IN ATLANTA GEORGIA FOR THE TREATMENT OF CHEMICAL DEPENDENCE. CONDITIONS OF PROBATION: SHALL NOT PETITION THE BOARD FOR A MODIFICATION OF THIS ORDER FOR AT LEAST ONE YEAR; SHALL CONTINUE TO BE ACTIVELY INVOLVED IN THE OKLAHOMA PHYSICIAN'S RECOVERY PROGRAM (PRP) AND AGREES TO COMPLY WITH ALL THE TERMS AND CONDITIONS OF ANY CONTRACT HE ENTERS INTO WITH PRP; SHALL STRICTLY COMPLY WITH ANY AFTERCARE PROGRAM OR PROGRAMS ESTABLISHED BY TALBOT RECOVERY CENTER AND/OR OKLAHOMA PRP AND MUST ATTEND AND SUCCESSFULLY COMPLETE ANY TREATMENT, COUNSELING THERAPY ESTABLISHED BY THEM; SHALL SUBMIT QUARTERLY REPORTS TO THE BOARD VERIFYING COMPLIANCE WITH THIS PROGRAM; $565 ADMINISTRATIVE COSTS; SHALL SUBMIT TO RANDOM DRUG SCREENING AS REQUESTED BY THE BOARD AND/OR PRC; SHALL NOTIFY THE BOARD IN WRITING OF ANY CHANGE IN ADDRESS, EMPLOYMENT, EMPLOYMENT TERMINATION OR HOSPITAL PRIVILEGE RESTRICTION AND ANY ADMINISTRATIVE PROCEEDING INITIATED AGAINST HIM BY ANY OTHER STATE OR FEDERAL REGULATORY BODY WITHIN 14 DAYS; SHALL APPEAR BEFORE THE BOARD UPON REQUEST; AGREES TO RANDOM, UNANNOUNCED BOARD VISITS AT HIS PLACE OF BUSINESS FOR OBSERVATION AND ACCESS TO ANY APPROPRIATE RECORDS, PROVIDED HOWEVER THAT THESE VISITS WILL NOT INTERRUPT HIS MEDICAL SERVICES; THE TIME PERIOD DURING WHICH THE PROBATION RESTRICTIONS, LIMITATIONS, OR CONDITIONS ARE ASSESSED SHALL NOT INCLUDE ANY PERIODS OF RESIDENCE OR PRACTICE OUTSIDE OKLAHOMA. ON 6/20/96 PROBATION AND ALL OTHER RESTRICTIONS TERMINATED.

HUDSON, RICHARD C DO, DATE OF BIRTH OCTOBER 22, 1946, LICENSE NUMBER 00E9485 OF BRIDGEPORT, TX, WAS DISCIPLINED BY TEXAS ON AUGUST 24, 1991
DISCIPLINARY ACTION: 60-MONTH PROBATION; RESTRICTION PLACED ON LICENSE
OFFENSE: DISCIPLINARY ACTION BY ANOTHER STATE OR AGENCY

NOTES: DISCIPLINARY ACTION TAKEN BY THE U.S. AIR FORCE. CONDITIONS OF PROBATION: SHALL APPEAR BEFORE THE BOARD ONCE A YEAR; SUBMIT FOR EVALUATION AND TREATMENT OF A PSYCHIATRIST APPROVED BY THE BOARD; MUST NOT CONDUCT ANY EXAMINATION UPON ANY FEMALE PATIENT UNLESS A THIRD PARTY IS PRESENT DURING EXAMINATION.

HUDSON, RICHARD C DO, DATE OF BIRTH OCTOBER 22, 1946, LICENSE NUMBER 0001802, WAS DISCIPLINED BY OKLAHOMA ON MARCH 18, 1993
DISCIPLINARY ACTION: 48-MONTH RESTRICTION PLACED ON LICENSE; MONITORING OF PHYSICIAN PERFORMANCE
OFFENSE: DISCIPLINARY ACTION BY ANOTHER STATE OR AGENCY

NOTES: ON 8/24/91 TEXAS LICENSE PLACED ON FIVE YEAR PROBATION UNDER TERMS AND CONDITIONS. SHALL NOT PETITION FOR MODIFICATION FOR AT LEAST ONE YEAR; SHALL COMPLY WITH PSYCHIATRIC EVALUATION, TREATMENT, AND RECOMMENDATIONS AS REQUIRED BY THE TEXAS BOARD AND SHALL SUBMIT A COPY OF SAID PSYCHIATRIST REPORTS TO THE OKLAHOMA BOARD; SHALL NOT CONDUCT ANY EXAMINATION UPON ANY FEMALE PATIENT UNLESS A FEMALE NURSE OR EMPLOYEE IS PRESENT DURING THE EXAMINATION; AND THIS SHALL BE ENTERED IN THE MEDICAL RECORDS; SHALL FURNISH WRITTEN REPORTS TO THE BOARD REGARDING HIS MEDICAL CONDITION AND COMPLIANCE WITH THIS ORDER UPON REQUEST; SHALL NOTIFY THE BOARD IN WRITING, OF ANY CHANGE IN ADDRESS, EMPLOYMENT, EMPLOYMENT TERMINATION OR HOSPITAL PRIVILEGE RESTRICTION AND ANY ADMINISTRATIVE PROCEEDING INITIATED AGAINST HIM BY ANY OTHER STATE OR FEDERAL REGULATORY BODY WITHIN 14 DAYS; SHALL APPEAR BEFORE THE BOARD UPON REQUEST; AGREES TO RANDOM, UNANNOUNCED VISITS FROM THE BOARD AT HIS PLACE OF BUSINESS FOR OBSERVATION AND ACCESS TO ANY APPROPRIATE RECORDS, PROVIDED

HOWEVER THAT THESE VISITS WILL NOT INTERRUPT HIS MEDICAL SERVICES; THE TIME PERIOD OF MONITORING THE RESTRICTIONS, LIMITATIONS, OR CONDITIONS ASSESSED SHALL NOT INCLUDE ANY PERIODS OF RESIDENCE OR PRACTICE OUTSIDE OF OKLAHOMA; $2,460.75 ADMINISTRATIVE COSTS. ON 3/17/94 PROVISION REQUESTING THAT HE NOT PETITION FOR MODIFICATION FOR ONE YEAR DROPPED; ON 6/20/96 ALL RESTRICTIONS ON LICENSE TERMINATED.

HUDSON, RICHARD C DO, DATE OF BIRTH OCTOBER 22, 1946, LICENSE NUMBER 00E9485 OF 4001 NW OZMUN, LAWTON, OK, WAS DISCIPLINED BY TEXAS ON JUNE 15, 1993
DISCIPLINARY ACTION: SURRENDER OF LICENSE
OFFENSE: NONCOMPLIANCE WITH A PROFESSIONAL RULE

NOTES: BOARD HAS RECEIVED ALLEGATIONS CONCERNING POSSIBLE VIOLATIONS OF THE MEDICAL PRACTICE ACT; WHILE NOT ADMITTING THESE HE VOLUNTARILY SURRENDERS HIS LICENSE IN LIEU OF FURTHER INVESTIGATION OR A HEARING. SHALL NOT PETITION THE BOARD FOR REINSTATEMENT.

HUDSON, RICHARD C DO, LICENSE NUMBER 1802, WAS DISCIPLINED BY OKLAHOMA ON JUNE 19, 1997
DISCIPLINARY ACTION: SURRENDER OF LICENSE

HUNT, ROBERT RANDALL DO, WAS DISCIPLINED BY OKLAHOMA ON DECEMBER 9, 1993
DISCIPLINARY ACTION: 60-MONTH PROBATION; REQUIRED TO ENTER AN IMPAIRED PHYSICIAN PROGRAM OR TREATMENT

NOTES: LICENSE GRANTED ON CONDITIONS OF PROBATION: MAY NOT PETITION FOR MODIFICATION FOR ONE YEAR; SHALL CONTINUE TO BE ACTIVELY INVOLVED IN THE OKLAHOMA PHYSICIAN'S RECOVERY PROGRAM (PRP) AND AGREES TO COMPLY WITH ALL THE TERMS AND CONDITIONS OF ANY CONTRACT HE ENTERS INTO WITH PRP; SHALL COMPLY WITH AFTERCARE TREATMENT PROGRAMS ESTABLISHED BY THEM; SHALL SUBMIT QUARTERLY REPORTS TO THE BOARD VERIFYING HIS COMPLIANCE WITH THIS; SHALL SUBMIT TO RANDOM DRUG SCREENING AS REQUESTED BY THE BOARD AND/OR THE PRP; SHALL NOTIFY THE BOARD IN WRITING OF ANY CHANGE OF ADDRESS, EMPLOYMENT, EMPLOYMENT TERMINATION OR HOSPITAL PRIVILEGE RESTRICTION AND ANY ADMINISTRATIVE PROCEEDING INITIATED AGAINST HIM BY ANY OTHER STATE OR FEDERAL REGULATORY BODY WITHIN 14 DAYS; SHALL APPEAR BEFORE THE BOARD UPON REQUEST; AGREES TO RANDOM, UNANNOUNCED VISITS FROM THE BOARD AT HIS PLACE OF BUSINESS FOR OBSERVATION AND ACCESS TO ANY APPROPRIATE RECORDS, PROVIDED, HOWEVER THAT THESE VISITS DO NOT INTERRUPT HIS MEDICAL SERVICES; THE TIME PERIOD DURING WHICH THE PROBATION RESTRICTIONS, LIMITATIONS, OR CONDITIONS ARE ASSESSED SHALL NOT INCLUDE ANY PERIODS OF TIME DURING WHICH HE RESIDES OR PRACTICES MEDICINE OUTSIDE OKLAHOMA.

HUSEN, LUVERNE A MD, LICENSE NUMBER 8191 OF BOX 386, MEAD, OK, WAS DISCIPLINED BY OKLAHOMA ON JULY 25, 1997
DISCIPLINARY ACTION: 60-MONTH PROBATION; RESTRICTION PLACED ON LICENSE
OFFENSE: SUBSTANCE ABUSE

NOTES: HABITUAL INTEMPERANCE OR THE HABITUAL USE OF HABIT-FORMING DRUGS AND THE INABILITY TO PRACTICE MEDICINE WITH REASONABLE SKILL AND SAFETY TO PATIENTS BY REASON OF AGE, ILLNESS, DRUNKENNESS, EXCESSIVE USE OF DRUGS, NARCOTICS, CHEMICALS, OR ANY OTHER TYPE OF MATERIAL OR AS A RESULT OF ANY MENTAL OR PHYSICAL CONDITION. WAS ADMITTED FOR INPATIENT TREATMENT FOR SUBSTANCE ABUSE ON 3/27/97 AND RELEASED ON 7/19/97. CONDITIONS OF PROBATION: SHALL SUBMIT TO EVERY STATE IN WHICH HE HOLDS LICENSURE AND TO HOSPITALS, CLINICS OR OTHER INSTITUTIONS IN WHICH HE HOLDS OR ANTICIPATES HOLDING ANY FORM OF STAFF PRIVILEGE A COPY OF THIS ORDER; SHALL SUBMIT BIOLOGICAL FLUID SPECIMENS; SHALL NOT PRESCRIBE, ADMINISTER OR DISPENSE ANY MEDICATIONS FOR HIS PERSONAL USE AND SHALL TAKE NONE UNLESS AUTHORIZED BY ANOTHER PHYSICIAN FOR A LEGITIMATE MEDICAL NEED; SHALL ABIDE BY HIS POST CARE CONTRACT FROM RECOVERY PROGRAM; SHALL KEEP THE BOARD INFORMED OF HIS ADDRESS AND PAY COSTS; SHALL REQUEST ALL HOSPITALS IN WHICH HE ANTICIPATES PRACTICING TO FURNISH A STATEMENT REGARDING MONITORING OF HIS PRACTICE; SHALL PLACE HIMSELF IN A BOARD APPROVED REHABILITATION PROGRAM FOR INPATIENT EVALUATION AND SUBSEQUENT TREATMENT; WILL AUTHORIZE THE RELEASE OF ANY AND ALL INFORMATION REGARDING TREATMENT TO THE BOARD; SHALL ABSTAIN FROM CONSUMING ALCOHOL OR ANY SUBSTANCE WHICH WOULD ADVERSELY AFFECT HIS ABILITY TO PRACTICE MEDICINE; SHALL NOT SUPERVISE A PHYSICIAN ASSISTANT; SHALL APPEAR BEFORE THE BOARD UPON REQUEST.

JARVIS, JAMES N MD, LICENSE NUMBER 20522 OF 940 NE 13TH, OKLAHOMA CITY, OK, WAS DISCIPLINED BY OKLAHOMA ON JANUARY 23, 1998
DISCIPLINARY ACTION: 60-MONTH PROBATION; RESTRICTION PLACED ON CONTROLLED SUBSTANCE LICENSE
OFFENSE: PROFESSIONAL MISCONDUCT

NOTES: IN APPROXIMATELY 9/97 HE DID VOLUNTARILY SUBMIT TO AN EVALUATION BY THE MENNINGER CLINIC DUE TO PROFESSIONAL SEXUAL MISCONDUCT. AS A RESULT OF THAT EVALUATION, HE ENTERED INTO A FORMAL CONTRACT AND AGREEMENT BETWEEN HIMSELF AND THE OKLAHOMA STATE MEDICAL ASSOCIATION RECOVERY COMMITTEE ON OR AROUND 12/8/97, SETTING FORTH TERMS AND CONDITIONS THAT WOULD GOVERN ANY PRACTICE OF MEDICINE IN OKLAHOMA. LICENSURE GRANTED SUBJECT TO THE FOLLOWING PROBATIONARY CONDITIONS: SHALL REMAIN ABSTINENT FROM ALL PSYCHO-ACTIVE SUBSTANCES, LEGAL OR ILLEGAL, INCLUDING ALCOHOL; TO VALIDATE THAT ABSTINENCE, RANDOM URINE DRUG SCREENS WILL BE OBTAINED; SHALL ATTEND THE OKLAHOMA CITY MEDICAL PROFESSIONAL SUPPORT GROUP AS WELL AS OTHER COMMUNITY 12-STEP MEETINGS ON A WEEKLY BASIS; SHALL SUBMIT TO EVERY STATE IN WHICH HE HOLDS LICENSURE AND TO HOSPITALS, CLINICS OR OTHER INSTITUTIONS IN WHICH HE HOLDS OR ANTICIPATES HOLDING ANY FORM OF STAFF PRIVILEGE A COPY OF THIS ORDER; SHALL NOT PRESCRIBE, ADMINISTER, OR DISPENSE ANY MEDICATION FOR PERSONAL USE; SHALL ABIDE BY HIS POST CARE CONTRACT FROM RECOVERY PROGRAM; SHALL KEEP THE BOARD INFORMED OF HIS ADDRESS AND PAY COSTS; SHALL EXECUTE THE RELEASE OF ANY MEDICAL AND PSYCHIATRIC RECORDS AS NECESSARY TO DISCUSS HIS CASE WITH TREATING PHYSICIANS AND/OR ANY PHYSICIANS HOLDING RECORDS.

JARVIS, JAMES N MD, DATE OF BIRTH OCTOBER 28, 1952, LICENSE

NUMBER 1055417 OF 13900 PLYMOUTH CROSSING, OKLAHOMA CITY, OK, WAS DISCIPLINED BY MICHIGAN ON JULY 15, 1998
DISCIPLINARY ACTION: 6-MONTH LICENSE SUSPENSION; 60-MONTH PROBATION
OFFENSE: SUBSTANDARD CARE, INCOMPETENCE OR NEGLIGENCE

NOTES: NEGLIGENCE.

JENNINGS, JEFF S DO, LICENSE NUMBER 2827, WAS DISCIPLINED BY OKLAHOMA ON APRIL 14, 1997
DISCIPLINARY ACTION: SURRENDER OF LICENSE

JENNINGS, JEFF S DO, LICENSE NUMBER 2827, WAS DISCIPLINED BY OKLAHOMA ON SEPTEMBER 17, 1998
DISCIPLINARY ACTION: LICENSE REINSTATEMENT; 60-MONTH PROBATION

NOTES: RESTRICTED TO RADIOLOGY RESIDENCY.

JOHNSON, HAROLD Z MD, LICENSE NUMBER 00D0926 OF ADA, OK, WAS DISCIPLINED BY TEXAS ON JUNE 10, 1991
OFFENSE: DISCIPLINARY ACTION BY ANOTHER STATE OR AGENCY

NOTES: SHOULD HE DESIRE TO PRACTICE MEDICINE IN TEXAS, MUST DEMONSTRATE TO BOARD HIS CAPACITY TO PRACTICE WITH REASONABLE SKILL AND SAFETY AND PROVIDE STATUS REPORT OF WASHINGTON LICENSE; IF TEXAS GRANTS HIM PERMISSION TO PRACTICE, TEXAS BOARD MAY IMPOSE ADDITIONAL PROBATIONARY TERMS.

JOHNSON, HAROLD ZAY MD, LICENSE NUMBER 0G18683 OF LONG BEACH, CA, WAS DISCIPLINED BY CALIFORNIA ON MAY 1, 1994
DISCIPLINARY ACTION: LICENSE REVOCATION
OFFENSE: DISCIPLINARY ACTION BY ANOTHER STATE OR AGENCY

NOTES: DISCIPLINED BY WASHINGTON STATE BOARD BASED ON ALLEGED IMPAIRMENT DUE TO ALCOHOLISM. TEXAS DISCIPLINE BASED ON ABOVE ACTION. DEFAULT DECISION.

JOHNSON, PAUL DAVIS MD, LICENSE NUMBER 0014767, WAS DISCIPLINED BY OKLAHOMA ON SEPTEMBER 7, 1994
DISCIPLINARY ACTION: SURRENDER OF LICENSE
OFFENSE: SUBSTANCE ABUSE

NOTES: AGREES THAT SURRENDER SHALL CONTINUE UNTIL HE PROVIDES SATISFACTORY EVIDENCE THAT HE HAS SUCCESSFULLY COMPLETED A BOARD-APPROVED PROGRAM FOR TREATMENT OF ALCOHOL DEPENDENCY AND ENTERED AN AFTERCARE PROGRAM.

JOHNSON, PAUL DAVIS MD, LICENSE NUMBER 0014767, WAS DISCIPLINED BY OKLAHOMA ON JANUARY 5, 1995
DISCIPLINARY ACTION: LICENSE REINSTATEMENT; 60-MONTH PROBATION

NOTES: ON 9/09/94 HE VOLUNTARILY SURRENDERED HIS LICENSE. REINSTATEMENT WITH PROBATION BEGINNING UNDER THE FOLLOWING TERMS AND CONDITIONS: SHALL ABSTAIN FROM CONSUMING ALCOHOL; SHALL SUBMIT BIOLOGICAL FLUID SPECIMENS; SHALL MAINTAIN A PROGRAM OF ABSTINENCE THROUGH PARTICIPATION IN AND/OR ASSOCIATION WITH ANY OR ALL ORGANIZATIONS, GROUPS, OR INDIVIDUALS SELECTED BY THE BOARD; SHALL ATTEND WEEKLY MEETINGS OF THE PHYSICIAN'S RECOVERY COMMITTEE AND SHALL SUBMIT TO THE BOARD PROOF OF ATTENDANCE; SHALL ATTEND 90 MEETINGS OF ALCOHOLICS ANONYMOUS IN THE FIRST 90 DAYS FOLLOWING THE ADOPTION OF THIS ORDER; SHALL FULFILL ALL TERMS AND CONDITIONS OF HIS AFTER-CARE PROGRAMS AND HIS IN-PATIENT TREATMENT; SHALL APPEAR BEFORE THE BOARD UPON REQUEST AND SUBMIT ANY REQUIRED REPORTS; SHALL PAY COSTS; SHALL NOTIFY ANY HOSPITAL WHERE HE HOLDS STAFF PRIVILEGES, OR CLINIC, OR GROUPS WHERE HE PRACTICES OF THE TERMS AND CONDITIONS OF THIS ORDER AND PROVIDE A COPY THEREOF. TIME SPENT NOT PRACTICING IN OKLAHOMA DOESN'T COUNT TOWARD PROBATION. ON 11/14/98 REQUEST FOR EARLY TERMINATION OF ORDER GRANTED; SHALL HAVE A FULL UNRESTRICTED LICENSE BEGINNING 11/30/98.

JONES, TIMOTHY BRIAN MD, LICENSE NUMBER 0015714 OF 2233 HICKORY DRIVE, ARDMORE, OK, WAS DISCIPLINED BY OKLAHOMA ON OCTOBER 7, 1993
DISCIPLINARY ACTION: FINE
OFFENSE: NONCOMPLIANCE WITH A PROFESSIONAL RULE

NOTES: BOARD WAS ADVISED ON 3/22/93 THAT HIS MAILING ADDRESS WAS NOT CURRENT AND HE HAD FAILED TO REPORT THIS TO THE BOARD; HE REQUESTED A HEARING AFTER BEING FINED ON 5/19/93. $75.00 FINE AND SHALL PAY COSTS.

KANG, BOBBY C DO, DATE OF BIRTH AUGUST 16, 1950, LICENSE NUMBER 0026022 OF COLORADO SPRINGS, CO, WAS DISCIPLINED BY COLORADO ON JANUARY 17, 1992
DISCIPLINARY ACTION: LICENSE REVOCATION

NOTES: FAILURE TO MEET GENERALLY ACCEPTED STANDARDS OF MEDICAL PRACTICE. REVOCATION VACATED BY COURT OF APPEALS ON 8/13/92; CASE REMANDED WITH DIRECTIONS. SECOND FINAL BOARD ORDER ISSUED 12/11/92 REVOKING HIS MEDICAL LICENSE.

KANG, BOBBY CHU DO, LICENSE NUMBER 0002373, WAS DISCIPLINED BY OKLAHOMA ON APRIL 6, 1992
DISCIPLINARY ACTION: LICENSE REINSTATEMENT; 60-MONTH PROBATION

NOTES: PROBATION UNDER THE FOLLOWING TERMS AND CONDITIONS: THE FIRST TWO YEARS OF THIS PERIOD MUST BE SPENT AS A FAMILY PRACTICE RESIDENT UNDER SUPERVISION; HIS LICENSE WILL BE CANCELED IF HE LEAVES THE RESIDENCY PROGRAM PRIOR TO COMPLETION; MUST CONFINE HIS PRACTICE ACTIVITY TO PARTICIPATION IN THE RESIDENCY PROGRAM. SHALL NOTIFY THE BOARD IN WRITING OF ANY CHANGE OF ADDRESS WITHIN 14 DAYS; SHALL APPEAR BEFORE THE BOARD UPON REQUEST; AGREES TO UNANNOUNCED VISITS FROM THE BOARD AT SUCH TIMES AND PLACES AS WILL BE DETERMINED AT BOARD DISCRETION; TERMS OF RESIDENCE OR PRACTICE OUTSIDE OKLAHOMA WILL RESULT IN THE TOLLING OF THE AGREEMENT AND WILL NOT APPLY TO THE REDUCTION OF PROBATION; SHALL NOT SEEK ANY AUTHORITY FROM THE STATE BUREAU OF NARCOTICS AND DANGEROUS DRUGS OR THE DRUG ENFORCEMENT ADMINISTRATION TO PRESCRIBE, DISPENSE, OR ADMINISTER CONTROLLED DANGEROUS SUBSTANCES, NOR SHALL HE ENGAGE IN THE PRESCRIPTION, DISPENSING, OR ADMINISTRATION OF SUCH CONTROLLED DANGEROUS SUBSTANCES; WITHIN 180 DAYS HE MUST FURNISH EVIDENCE THAT HE HAS COMPLETED A COURSE IN MEDICAL ETHICS; SHALL PROVIDE THE BOARD WITH QUARTERLY REPORTS OF HIS PROGRESS THROUGH THE RESIDENCY PROGRAM. ON 3/17/94 PROBATION AND RESTRICTIONS TERMINATED.

KANTZLER, MARK G DO, LICENSE NUMBER 0002565 OF 1400 GULF BOULEVARD #702, CLEARWATER, FL, WAS DISCIPLINED BY OKLAHOMA ON JULY 20, 1992
DISCIPLINARY ACTION: RESTRICTION PLACED ON CONTROLLED SUBSTANCE LICENSE; REQUIRED TO ENTER AN IMPAIRED PHYSICIAN PROGRAM OR SUBSTANCE ABUSE TREATMENT
OFFENSE: DISCIPLINARY ACTION BY ANOTHER STATE OR AGENCY

NOTES: ACTION IN FLORIDA ON 8/26/91. SHALL APPEAR BEFORE THE BOARD UPON REQUEST; AGREES TO UNANNOUNCED VISITS FROM THE BOARD AT SUCH TIMES AT BOARD DISCRETION; SHALL REMAIN IN COMPLIANCE WITH THE FLORIDA BOARD ORDER WHICH INCLUDES PROVISIONS THAT HE SHALL NOT USE PRESCRIPTION DRUGS UNLESS AUTHORIZED BY A PRACTITIONER FOR A LEGITIMATE MEDICAL PURPOSE; SHALL PARTICIPATE WITH THE FLORIDA PHYSICIANS RECOVERY NETWORK, SHALL UTILIZE SEQUENTIALLY NUMBERED TRIPLICATE PRESCRIPTION FORMS FOR PRESCRIBED DRUGS; SHALL NOTIFY THE OKLAHOMA BOARD OF CHANGE OF ADDRESS WITHIN 14 DAYS; SHALL EXECUTE A RELEASE FOR THE FLORIDA PHYSICIAN'S RECOVERY NETWORK (PRN) TO AUTHORIZE THEM TO RELEASE INFORMATION RELATING TO THE TREATMENT AND AFTERCARE TREATMENT FOR DRUG DEPENDENCE TO THE OKLAHOMA BOARD AS NEEDED TO MONITOR THE PROGRESS WITH THE PRN.

KILBURY, MERLIN J MD OF 2219 E 21ST, TULSA, OK, WAS DISCIPLINED BY DEA ON FEBRUARY 12, 1990
DISCIPLINARY ACTION: SURRENDER OF CONTROLLED SUBSTANCE LICENSE
OFFENSE: CRIMINAL CONVICTION OR PLEA OF GUILTY, NOLO CONTENDERE, OR NO CONTEST TO A CRIME

NOTES: LICENSE SUSPENDED 11/03/89. PLED GUILTY TO OBTAINING CONTROLLED SUBSTANCES BY FRAUD IN TULSA, OKLAHOMA.

KILBURY, MERLIN J MD, LICENSE NUMBER 0009907 OF 1529 LAKEVIEW DRIVE, CUSHING, OK, WAS DISCIPLINED BY OKLAHOMA ON JANUARY 25, 1996
DISCIPLINARY ACTION: LICENSE REVOCATION
OFFENSE: SUBSTANCE ABUSE

NOTES: GUILTY OF GIVING PRESCRIPTIONS FOR CONTROLLED DANGEROUS SUBSTANCES TO PATIENTS AND HAVING THE PATIENTS FILL THE PRESCRIPTIONS AND RETURN MEDICATION TO HIM FOR PERSONAL USE; MADE TELEPHONE ORDERS FOR CONTROLLED DANGEROUS SUBSTANCES USING THE NAME OF HIS OFFICE MATE WHEN IN FACT THAT PHYSICIAN DID NOT INITIATE THE PRESCRIPTION; TELEPHONED IN PRESCRIPTIONS TO THE PHARMACY FOR ONE OF HIS PATIENTS, BUT THEN HE PICKED UP THE DRUGS HIMSELF FOR PERSONAL USE; PRACTICED MEDICINE IN THE EMERGENCY ROOM OF THE CUSHING REGIONAL HOSPITAL IN AN IMPAIRED STATE AND THEN REFUSED TO PROVIDE A URINE SAMPLE ON DEMAND OF THE HOSPITAL ADMINISTRATOR AS PER HIS HOSPITAL CONTRACT; FAILED TO KEEP ACCURATE PATIENT RECORDS ON CONTROLLED DANGEROUS SUBSTANCES OBTAINED BY FRAUD; WROTE FALSE PRESCRIPTIONS FOR CONTROLLED DANGEROUS SUBSTANCES TO HIS HOUSE-KEEPER, THE SECRETARY OF A PHYSICIAN FRIEND, VARIOUS PATIENTS, AND HIS WIFE, FOR THE PURPOSE OF OBTAINING CONTROLLED DANGEROUS SUBSTANCES FOR HIS PERSONAL USE AND ADDICTION; WROTE PRESCRIPTIONS FOR CONTROLLED DANGEROUS SUBSTANCES FOR PATIENTS WITHOUT SUFFICIENT EXAMINATION AND THE ESTABLISHMENT OF A VALID PHYSICIAN/PATIENT RELATIONSHIP; ACTED AS THE PRINCIPAL IN A SCHEME TO DEFRAUD THE PUBLIC, USE OF HABIT-FORMING DRUGS, AND PRACTICE MEDICINE AND SURGERY WITHOUT REASONABLE SKILL AND SAFETY; PRESCRIBED CONTROLLED DANGEROUS SUBSTANCES IN EXCESS AMOUNTS FOR HIMSELF AND OTHERS WITHOUT MEDICAL NEED AND CLEARLY IN EXCESS OF THE AMOUNT CONSIDERED GOOD MEDICAL PRACTICE AND IN ACCORD WITH PUBLISHED STANDARDS IN THAT THERE WAS NO MEDICAL NEED AND THUS ANY AMOUNT OF CONTROLLED DANGEROUS SUBSTANCES PRESCRIBED WAS EXCESSIVE.

KILBURY, MERLIN J MD OF 1102 G 2ND STREET, CUSHING, OK, WAS DISCIPLINED BY DEA ON FEBRUARY 29, 1996
DISCIPLINARY ACTION: SURRENDER OF CONTROLLED SUBSTANCE LICENSE
OFFENSE: DISCIPLINARY ACTION BY ANOTHER STATE OR AGENCY

NOTES: STATE BOARD.

KILBURY, MERLIN J MD, LICENSE NUMBER 9907 OF 4308 SOUTH PEORIA BOX 72, TULSA, OK, WAS DISCIPLINED BY OKLAHOMA ON JANUARY 30, 1997
DISCIPLINARY ACTION: LICENSE REINSTATEMENT; PROBATION
OFFENSE: SUBSTANCE ABUSE

NOTES: HIS OKLAHOMA LICENSE WAS REVOKED FOR EVIDENCE OF ADDICTION TO CONTROLLED SUBSTANCES. HE APPLIED FOR REINSTATEMENT AND PRESENTED EVIDENCE OF REHABILITATION. LICENSE IS REINSTATED UNDER THE FOLLOWING CONDITIONS OF PROBATION: CONDITIONS OF TERMS: SHALL NOT PRESCRIBE, ADMINISTER, DISPENSE, OR POSSESS ANY CONTROLLED DANGEROUS SUBSTANCES; SHALL NOT AUTHORIZE ANY PERSONNEL UNDER HIS SUPERVISION TO INITIATE AN ORDER FOR A PRESCRIPTION TO BE ISSUED; SHALL NOT ALLOW THE INDEPENDENT PRACTICE OF MEDICINE BY ANY PERSONNEL UNDER HIS SUPERVISION OR EMPLOY; SHALL REQUEST ALL HOSPITALS IN WHICH HE ANTICIPATES PRACTICING TO FURNISH A STATEMENT REGARDING MONITORING OF HIS PRACTICE; SHALL SUBMIT TO EVERY STATE IN WHICH HE HOLDS LICENSURE AND TO HOSPITALS, CLINICS OR OTHER INSTITUTIONS IN WHICH HE HOLDS OR ANTICIPATES HOLDING ANY FORM OF STAFF PRIVILEGE A COPY OF THIS ORDER; SHALL SUBMIT BIOLOGICAL FLUID SPECIMENS; SHALL NOT PRESCRIBE, ADMINISTER OR DISPENSE ANY MEDICATIONS FOR HIS PERSONAL USE AND SHALL TAKE NONE UNLESS AUTHORIZED BY ANOTHER PHYSICIAN FOR A LEGITIMATE MEDICAL NEED; SHALL AFFILIATE WITH A BOARD APPROVED PROGRAM FOR CONTINUING REHABILITATION AND WILL AUTHORIZE THE RELEASE OF ANY AND ALL INFORMATION INCLUDING BUT NOT LIMITED TO MEDICAL AND/OR PSYCHIATRIC RECORDS, REGARDING TREATMENT OR REHABILITATION TO THE BOARD; SHALL KEEP THE BOARD INFORMED OF HIS ADDRESS AND PAY COSTS; SHALL PRACTICE MEDICINE ONLY WITHIN THE DEPARTMENT OF CORRECTIONS FACILITIES. ON 10/2/98, THE PROBATION ORDER WAS MODIFIED TO ALLOW HIM TO PRACTICE AT THE VETERANS HOSPITAL IN MUSKOGEE, OKLAHOMA, IN ADDITION TO THE DEPARTMENT OF CORRECTIONS. ON 2/12/99 PROBATION MODIFIED TO ALLOW HIM TO PRESCRIBE CONTROLLED SUBSTANCES IN AN INSTITUTIONAL SETTING FOR HIS SURGICAL PATIENTS REQUIRING HIM TO KEEP DUPLICATE, SERIALLY NUMBERED PRESCRIPTIONS WHICH SHALL BE AVAILABLE FOR REVIEW.

KINCAID, JEAN W MD, DATE OF BIRTH AUGUST 15, 1937 OF P.O. BOX 714, ADA, OK, WAS DISCIPLINED BY IOWA ON DECEMBER 20, 1993
DISCIPLINARY ACTION: DENIAL OF NEW LICENSE
OFFENSE: PROVIDING FALSE INFORMATION TO THE BOARD OR OTHER HEALTH AGENCY

NOTES: FRAUD IN PROCURING A MEDICAL LICENSE. DENIAL AFFIRMED BY A HEARING 11/23/94.

KING, E KIM DO, LICENSE NUMBER 0002534, WAS DISCIPLINED BY OKLAHOMA ON SEPTEMBER 19, 1996
DISCIPLINARY ACTION: 60-MONTH PROBATION; REQUIRED TO TAKE ADDITIONAL MEDICAL EDUCATION
OFFENSE: SEXUAL ABUSE OF OR SEXUAL MISCONDUCT WITH A PATIENT

NOTES: AT LEAST FROM 12/94 TO 6/95 HE ESTABLISHED A PHYSICIAN/PATIENT RELATIONSHIP WITH A FEMALE WITH WHOM HE HAD A PRIOR PERSONAL RELATIONSHIP STARTING IN 1970 TO 1981 AND FOR WHOM HE WROTE PRESCRIPTIONS WITHOUT ESTABLISHING A PATIENT RECORD TO REFLECT ANY EXAMINATION, DIAGNOSIS AND/OR PRESCRIPTIONS ISSUED. AT LEAST DURING THIS PERIOD OF TIME HE ENGAGED IN SEXUAL ACTIVITY WITH THIS PATIENT. WROTE PRESCRIPTIONS TO A PATIENT IN ABSENCE OF MEDICAL EXAMINATION, MEDICAL RECORDS, AND CHARTS. BACKDATED RECORDS ON A PATIENT'S MEDICAL RECORD AND FAILED TO NOTE THIS. FOR 90 DAYS IS PRECLUDED FROM ALL ACTIVITY AUTHORIZED PURSUANT TO THE ISSUANCE OF A LICENSE. CONDITIONS OF PROBATION: SHALL ATTEND, AND SUCCESSFULLY COMPLETE A COURSE ENTITLED "THE PROPER PRESCRIBING OF CONTROLLED DANGEROUS SUBSTANCES" AND SHALL REPORT TO THE BOARD THE SUCCESSFUL COMPLETION OF THE COURSE; SHALL ATTEND A BOARD APPROVED COURSE IN MEDICAL ETHICS. THE BOARD MAY MAKE UNANNOUNCED VISITS TO HIS OFFICE; SHALL APPEAR BEFORE THE BOARD UPON REQUEST; MAY NOT PETITION THE BOARD FOR MODIFICATION FOR AT LEAST TWO YEARS; $8,400 ADMINISTRATIVE COSTS.

KINNEY, ROGER LEE MD OF SAPULPA, OK, WAS DISCIPLINED BY DEA ON SEPTEMBER 7, 1999
DISCIPLINARY ACTION: 36-MONTH MONITORING OF PHYSICIAN PERFORMANCE
OFFENSE: CRIMINAL CONVICTION OR PLEA OF GUILTY, NOLO CONTENDERE, OR NO CONTEST TO A CRIME

NOTES: DURING THE EARLY 1980S HE PURCHASED AND INGESTED COCAINE; ACCORDING TO HIM THE LAST TIME WAS 8/8/85; ADMITTED ON HIS 1990 APPLICATION THAT HE HAD BEEN CONVICTED OF ILLEGAL DISTRIBUTION OF CONTROLLED SUBSTANCES WHICH STEMMED FROM A PROBLEM OF SUBSTANCE ABUSE; ON 2/24/86 OKLAHOMA SUSPENDED HIS LICENSE WHILE HE WAS IN PRISON; UPON HIS RELEASE HE UNDERWENT TREATMENT AND MONITORING FOR SUBSTANCE ABUSE; ON 5/19/87 THE OKLAHOMA BOARD PLACED HIS LICENSE ON PROBATION WITH THE PROVISION THAT HE COULD NOT HANDLE CONTROLLED SUBSTANCES WITHOUT APPROVAL FROM THE BOARD; ON 10/26/89 ALL CONDITIONS WERE TERMINATED; DEA FOUND THAT IT IS CLEAR HE RECOGNIZES THE UNLAWFULNESS OF HIS PRIOR CONDUCT AND APPRECIATES THE CONSEQUENCE OF SUCH ACTIVITIES. DEA ISSUED REGISTRATION WITH THE FOLLOWING CONDITIONS FOR THREE YEARS: SHALL PROVIDE THE DEA WITH A LOG OF HIS HANDLING OF CONTROLLED SUBSTANCES QUARTERLY; SHALL INFORM DEA OF ANY STATE ACTION TAKEN AGAINST HIS LICENSE OR ANY CHANGE IN EMPLOYMENT WITHIN 30 DAYS.

KNIGHT, PHILLIP J MD, DATE OF BIRTH JULY 3, 1950, LICENSE NUMBER 0022197 OF PONCA CITY, OK, WAS DISCIPLINED BY COLORADO ON JULY 12, 1991
DISCIPLINARY ACTION: 60-MONTH PROBATION; REQUIRED TO ENTER AN IMPAIRED PHYSICIAN PROGRAM OR SUBSTANCE ABUSE TREATMENT
OFFENSE: SUBSTANCE ABUSE

NOTES: HABITUAL INTEMPERANCE OR EXCESSIVE USE OF CONTROLLED SUBSTANCES. ALCOHOL AND SUBSTANCE ABUSE TREATMENT, AND PRACTICE AND TREATMENT MONITORS. IN ABEYANCE. ORDER BECOMES EFFECTIVE UPON HIS RETURN TO COLORADO.

KNIGHT, PHILLIP JOSEPH MD, LICENSE NUMBER 0012150, WAS DISCIPLINED BY OKLAHOMA ON SEPTEMBER 27, 1990
DISCIPLINARY ACTION: LICENSE SUSPENSION; REQUIRED TO ENTER AN IMPAIRED PHYSICIAN PROGRAM OR SUBSTANCE ABUSE TREATMENT
OFFENSE: SUBSTANCE ABUSE

NOTES: ON 2/26/90 LEFT INPATIENT TREATMENT FOR SUBSTANCE ABUSE BEFORE TREATMENT WAS COMPLETED AGAINST MEDICAL ADVICE. SUSPENSION UNTIL HE CAN PROVIDE TO THE BOARD EVIDENCE OF SUCCESSFUL COMPLETION OF IN-PATIENT TREATMENT AND RELATED RESIDENTIAL OUT-PATIENT TREATMENT FROM THE PHYSICIAN RECOVERY CENTER IN JACKSON, MISSISSIPPI, OR AN EQUIVALENT BOARD APPROVED PROGRAM. ON 11/1/90 SUSPENSION WAS RETAINED.

KNIGHT, PHILLIP JOSEPH MD, LICENSE NUMBER 0012150, WAS DISCIPLINED BY OKLAHOMA ON MARCH 6, 1991
DISCIPLINARY ACTION: 60-MONTH PROBATION; RESTRICTION PLACED ON CONTROLLED SUBSTANCE LICENSE
OFFENSE: SUBSTANCE ABUSE

NOTES: IN 1990 WAS PLACED ON SUSPENSION WHILE SUCCESSFULLY COMPLETING IN-PATIENT TREATMENT FOR SUBSTANCE ABUSE. CONDITIONS OF PROBATION: SHALL NOT PRESCRIBE, ADMINISTER OR DISPENSE ANY MEDICATIONS FOR HIS PERSONAL USE AND SHALL TAKE NONE UNLESS AUTHORIZED BY ANOTHER PHYSICIAN FOR LEGITIMATE MEDICAL NEED; SHALL NOT PRESCRIBE, ADMINISTER OR DISPENSE ANY CONTROLLED DANGEROUS SUBSTANCES OR NARCOTIC DRUGS TO ANY PATIENT FOR ANY CONDITION; SHALL ABSTAIN FROM CONSUMING ALCOHOL OR ANY SUBSTANCE WHICH WOULD ADVERSELY AFFECT HIS ABILITY TO PRACTICE; SHALL SUBMIT BIOLOGICAL FLUID SPECIMENS; SHALL CONTINUE REGULAR PARTICIPATION IN PHYSICIAN RECOVERY COMMITTEE AND AA OR NARCOTICS ANONYMOUS; SHALL FURNISH TO BOARD ADDRESS AND/OR CHANGE OF ADDRESS; SHALL APPEAR BEFORE BOARD UPON REQUEST; SHALL NOTIFY ANY HOSPITAL WHERE HE HOLDS STAFF PRIVILEGES OR CLINIC OR GROUP, OF THE TERMS AND CONDITIONS.

KNIGHT, PHILLIP JOSEPH MD, LICENSE NUMBER 0012150 OF 400 FAIRVIEW AVE, PONCA CITY, OK, WAS DISCIPLINED BY OKLAHOMA ON NOVEMBER 8, 1991
DISCIPLINARY ACTION: 6-MONTH PROBATION; REPRIMAND
OFFENSE: FAILURE TO COMPLY WITH PREVIOUS BOARD ORDER

NOTES: FAILED TO APPEAR BEFORE BOARD; FAILED TO PAY

COSTS WITHIN 30 DAYS. REPRIMAND FOR NON-PAYMENT OF COSTS; PROBATION OF 3/6/91 EXTENDED AN ADDITIONAL SIX MONTHS. ON 10/22/92 ORDER MODIFIED TO ALLOW HIM TO PRESCRIBE, ADMINISTER OR DISPENSE SCHEDULE III, IV OR V DRUGS TO HOSPITAL IN-PATIENTS, HOSPITAL EMERGENCY ROOM PATIENTS, AND NURSING HOME PATIENTS, AND TO REDUCE HIS LEVEL OF PROBATION FROM LEVEL I TO LEVEL II AND TO APPLY FOR STATE AND FEDERAL REGISTRATION FOR CONTROLLED DANGEROUS SUBSTANCES. ON 7/23/94, THE PROBATION IF FURTHER MODIFIED TO ALLOW HIM TO PRESCRIBE SCHEDULE III, IV AND V CONTROLLED DANGEROUS SUBSTANCES ON AN OUTPATIENT BASIS USING SEQUENTIALLY NUMBERED, DUPLICATE PRESCRIPTION FORMS, COPIES OF WHICH SHALL BE SUBMITTED MONTHLY TO THE BOARD. OTHER TERMS AND CONDITIONS REMAIN IN EFFECT. ON 12/7/95 PROBATION MODIFIED ALLOWING HIM TO PRESCRIBE, ADMINISTER OR DISPENSE SCHEDULE II SUBSTANCES TO INPATIENTS IN AN INSTITUTIONAL SETTING BY WAY OF A SPECIFIC WRITTEN ORDER UNTIL 9/6/96 UNDER THE REMAINING CONDITIONS.

KOSTIUK, STEFAN A MD, LICENSE NUMBER 0013231, WAS DISCIPLINED BY OKLAHOMA ON JUNE 21, 1990
DISCIPLINARY ACTION: LICENSE SUSPENSION; REQUIRED TO ENTER AN IMPAIRED PHYSICIAN PROGRAM OR TREATMENT

NOTES: SUSPENDED UNTIL SUCCESSFUL COMPLETION OF IN-PATIENT TREATMENT AS DEMONSTRATED TO THE BOARD.

KOSTIUK, STEFAN A MD OF 3229 RAINTREE RD, OKLAHOMA CITY, OK, WAS DISCIPLINED BY DEA ON AUGUST 29, 1990
DISCIPLINARY ACTION: SURRENDER OF CONTROLLED SUBSTANCE LICENSE
OFFENSE: SUBSTANCE ABUSE

NOTES: MEDICAL LICENSE SUSPENDED 06/08/90 FOR PERSONAL DRUG ABUSE.

KOSTIUK, STEFAN A MD, LICENSE NUMBER 0013231 OF PO BOX 20364, OKLAHOMA CITY, OK, WAS DISCIPLINED BY OKLAHOMA ON OCTOBER 26, 1990
DISCIPLINARY ACTION: 60-MONTH PROBATION; RESTRICTION PLACED ON CONTROLLED SUBSTANCE LICENSE

NOTES: ON 06/08/90 LICENSE WAS SUSPENDED UNTIL HE PRODUCED EVIDENCE OF SUCCESSFUL COMPLETION OF INPATIENT TREATMENT, WHICH HE DID. PROBATION UNDER TERMS AND CONDITIONS: SHALL NOT PRESCRIBE, ADMINISTER OR DISPENSE CONTROLLED DANGEROUS SUBSTANCES; SHALL NOT PRESCRIBE, ADMINISTER OR DISPENSE ANY MEDICATION FOR HIS PERSONAL USE; SHALL TAKE NO MEDICATION UNLESS AUTHORIZED BY TREATING PHYSICIAN; SHALL ABSTAIN FROM ALCOHOL OR ANY SUBSTANCE WHICH WOULD ADVERSELY AFFECT HIS ABILITY TO PRACTICE; SHALL SUBMIT BIOLOGICAL FLUID SPECIMENS FOR ANALYSIS; AGREES TO PARTICIPATE IN SUCH RECOVERY PROGRAMS AS MAY BE RECOMMENDED BY THE DIRECTOR OF THE PHYSICIAN RECOVERY PROGRAM; SHALL NOTIFY ANY HOSPITAL WHERE HE HOLDS STAFF PRIVILEGES OR CLINIC OR GROUP WHERE HE PRACTICES OF TERMS AND CONDITIONS. SHALL FURNISH BOARD WITH ADDRESS AND/OR CHANGE OF ADDRESS; SHALL APPEAR BEFORE BOARD UPON REQUEST. ON 03/12/92 SUPERVISION REDUCED FROM LEVEL I TO LEVEL II AND IS ALLOWED TO PRESCRIBE CONTROLLED DANGEROUS SUBSTANCES IN THE HOSPITAL EMERGENCY ROOM ON DUPLICATE, SERIALLY-NUMBERED PRESCRIPTION PADS WITH COPIES AVAILABLE TO THE BOARD. ON 3/11/93 HE IS RETAINED ON PROBATION WITH THE SAME CONDITIONS AND TERMS EXCEPT AS MODIFIED: HE IS ABLE TO PRESCRIBE CONTROLLED DANGEROUS SUBSTANCES TO PATIENTS HE SEES IN THE CLINIC UNDER THE SAME CONDITIONS AS ABOVE, AND ON 7/7/93 ORDER FURTHER MODIFIED TO ALLOW HIM TO PRESCRIBE, ADMINISTER OR DISPENSE CONTROLLED DANGEROUS SUBSTANCES TO HOSPITAL IN-PATIENTS UNDER THE SAME CONDITIONS.

KOSTIUK, STEFAN A MD, LICENSE NUMBER 13231 OF 3229 RAINTREE ROAD, OKLAHOMA CITY, OK, WAS DISCIPLINED BY OKLAHOMA ON APRIL 23, 1998
DISCIPLINARY ACTION: 1-MONTH LICENSE SUSPENSION; PROBATION
OFFENSE: SUBSTANCE ABUSE

NOTES: SINCE APPROXIMATELY 10/96 AND UNTIL 8/97, HE RE-STARTED THE PERSONAL USE AND ABUSE OF CONTROLLED DANGEROUS SUBSTANCES WITH NO DOCUMENTED MEDICAL NEED, AND HE USED A SERIES OF PRESCRIPTIONS WRITTEN TO DIFFERENT FRIENDS AND ACQUAINTANCES TO ASSIST HIM IN OBTAINING THESE DRUGS FOR HIS PERSONAL USE. THE CONTROLLED DANGEROUS SUBSTANCES HE OBTAINED FOR HIS PERSONAL USE INCLUDED, BUT WAS NOT LIMITED TO, VICODIN, LORTAB, HYDROCODONE, AND CARISOPRODOL FROM 23 SPECIFIED PHARMACIES. HE HAS A HISTORY OF SUBSTANCE ABUSE PROBLEMS AND HAS BEEN THE SUBJECT OF PRIOR BOARD ACTION. SUSPENSION RETROACTIVE TO 11/21/97. CONDITIONS OF PROBATION: SHALL NOT PRESCRIBE, ADMINISTER, POSSESS, OR DISPENSE ANY DRUGS IN SCHEDULES II, III, IV, AND V; WILL SURRENDER HIS REGISTRATION FOR STATE AND FEDERAL CONTROLLED DANGEROUS SUBSTANCES TO THE PROPER AUTHORITIES AND WILL NOT APPLY FOR STATE AND FEDERAL REGISTRATION UNTIL THE TERM OF HIS PROBATION HAS EXPIRED UNLESS AUTHORIZED TO DO SO BY THE BOARD; SHALL NOT AUTHORIZE ANY PERSONNEL UNDER HIS SUPERVISION TO INITIATE AN ORDER FOR A PRESCRIPTION; SHALL PRACTICE IN A CONTROLLED ENVIRONMENT APPROVED BY THE BOARD; SHALL REQUEST ALL HOSPITALS IN WHICH HE ANTICIPATES PRACTICING TO FURNISH A STATEMENT REGARDING MONITORING OF HIS PRACTICE; SHALL NOT PRESCRIBE, ADMINISTER OR DISPENSE ANY MEDICATIONS FOR HIS PERSONAL USE AND SHALL TAKE NONE UNLESS AUTHORIZED BY ANOTHER PHYSICIAN FOR A LEGITIMATE MEDICAL NEED; SHALL NOT SUPERVISE ALLIED HEALTH PROFESSIONALS; SHALL SUBMIT BIOLOGICAL FLUID SPECIMENS AND NOT INGEST ANY SUBSTANCE WHICH WILL CAUSE A SPECIMEN TO TEST POSITIVE FOR PROHIBITED SUBSTANCES; SHALL SUBMIT TO EVERY STATE IN WHICH HE HOLDS LICENSURE AND TO HOSPITALS, CLINICS OR OTHER INSTITUTIONS IN WHICH HE HOLDS OR ANTICIPATES HOLDING ANY FORM OF STAFF PRIVILEGE A COPY OF THIS ORDER; SHALL PLACE HIMSELF IN A BOARD APPROVED REHABILITATION PROGRAM FOR INPATIENT EVALUATION AND SUBSEQUENT TREATMENT; WILL AUTHORIZE THE RELEASE OF ANY AND ALL INFORMATION REGARDING TREATMENT TO THE BOARD; SHALL ABIDE BY HIS POST CARE CONTRACT; SHALL KEEP THE BOARD INFORMED OF HIS ADDRESS AND PAY COSTS; SHALL EXECUTE ALL RELEASES OF MEDICAL AND PSYCHIATRIC RECORDS AS NECESSARY FOR USE TO DISCUSS HIS CASE WITH HIS TREATING PHYSICIANS AND/OR ANY PHYSICIANS HOLDING HIS RECORDS; SHALL PARTICIPATE FULLY IN THE OSMA PHYSICIAN

RECOVERY PROGRAM AND TO AUTHORIZE THE RELEASE OF ANY AND ALL INFORMATION TO THE BOARD. ON 2/11/99 PROBATION MODIFIED TO ALLOW HIM TO PRESCRIBE CONTROLLED SUBSTANCES IN SCHEDULES II, III, IV AND V SOLELY TO INPATIENTS IN AN INSTITUTIONAL SETTING SUCH AS A NURSING HOME OR HOSPITAL; SHALL KEEP DUPLICATE, SERIALLY NUMBERED PRESCRIPTIONS WHICH SHALL BE AVAILABLE FOR REVIEW..

KREBSBACH, ROBERT LEO MD, LICENSE NUMBER 0010091, WAS DISCIPLINED BY OKLAHOMA ON NOVEMBER 1, 1990
DISCIPLINARY ACTION: EMERGENCY SUSPENSION

NOTES: VOLUNTARY SUSPENSION DURING HEARING CONTINUANCE.

KREBSBACH, ROBERT LEO MD OF 5507 E 32ND PLACE, TULSA, OK, WAS DISCIPLINED BY DEA ON JUNE 14, 1991
DISCIPLINARY ACTION: DENIAL OF NEW LICENSE
OFFENSE: DISCIPLINARY ACTION BY ANOTHER STATE OR AGENCY

NOTES: ON 11/1/90 THE OKLAHOMA BOARD SUSPENDED HIS LICENSE. SINCE 8/1/90 HE HAS NOT BEEN AUTHORIZED TO PRACTICE MEDICINE IN KANSAS.

KREBSBACH, ROBERT LEO MD, LICENSE NUMBER 0010091 OF 7416 E 19TH ST, TULSA, OK, WAS DISCIPLINED BY OKLAHOMA ON OCTOBER 10, 1991
OFFENSE: PHYSICAL OR MENTAL ILLNESS INHIBITING THE ABILITY TO PRACTICE WITH SKILL AND SAFETY

NOTES: PSYCHIATRIC AND MEDICAL RECORDS FROM 3/90 TO 6/91 REVEALED CLEAR EVIDENCE THAT HIS ABILITY TO PRACTICE WAS IMPAIRED. AS OF THE LATER RECORDS, THERE WAS NO EVIDENCE DOCUMENTING ANY RECOVERY. CANNOT PRESENTLY PRACTICE WITH REASONABLE SKILL AND SAFETY TO PATIENTS. IN THE EVENT OF RECOVERY AND CHANGE OF CIRCUMSTANCES, MAY RENEW APPLICATION. HAD VOLUNTARILY AGREED TO SUSPEND LICENSE BEFORE HEARING.

KRUK, KATHLEEN ADELE DR, LICENSE NUMBER 0017571 OF 10 HAPPY HILL, WICHITA FALLS, TX, WAS DISCIPLINED BY OKLAHOMA ON JANUARY 12, 1991
DISCIPLINARY ACTION: 60-MONTH PROBATION; MONITORING OF PHYSICIAN PERFORMANCE
OFFENSE: PHYSICAL OR MENTAL ILLNESS INHIBITING THE ABILITY TO PRACTICE WITH SKILL AND SAFETY

NOTES: HISTORY OF TREATMENT FOR DEPRESSION STARTING IN 1989. CURRENTLY UNDERGOING OUT-PATIENT TREATMENT. ISSUES RAISED AS TO HER PHYSICAL AND MENTAL FITNESS TO PRACTICE. LICENSE GRANTED UNDER PROBATIONARY TERMS AND CONDITIONS: SHALL CONTINUE PSYCHIATRIC/PSYCHOLOGICAL CARE AND MAKE RECORDS AVAILABLE TO BOARD; SHALL SUBMIT BIOLOGICAL FLUID SPECIMENS FOR ANALYSIS; SHALL NOTIFY ANY HOSPITAL WHERE SHE HOLDS STAFF PRIVILEGES, OR CLINIC OR GROUP OF THE TERMS AND CONDITIONS; SHALL FURNISH BOARD WITH ADDRESS AND/OR CHANGE OF ADDRESS; SHALL APPEAR BEFORE BOARD UPON REQUEST.

LAMB, KERBY W DO, LICENSE NUMBER 0003075, WAS DISCIPLINED BY OKLAHOMA ON OCTOBER 21, 1992
DISCIPLINARY ACTION: MONITORING OF PHYSICIAN PERFORMANCE

NOTES: GRANTING OF LICENSE UNDER TERMS AND CONDITIONS: SHALL NOTIFY THE BOARD IN WRITING OF ANY CHANGE OF ADDRESS WITHIN 14 DAYS; SHALL APPEAR BEFORE THE BOARD UPON REQUEST; AGREES TO UNANNOUNCED VISITS AT BOARD DISCRETION; SHALL PARTICIPATE IN THE PHYSICIAN'S RECOVERY PROGRAM (PRP) AND AGREES TO COMPLY WITH ALL TERMS OF HIS CONTRACT; SHALL PROVIDE BIOLOGICAL FLUID SPECIMENS FOR LABORATORY ANALYSIS UPON REQUEST.

LANE, KEVIN B DO OF 422 S. MAIN P.O. BOX 1303, NEWCASTLE, OK, WAS DISCIPLINED BY DEA ON MARCH 14, 1994
DISCIPLINARY ACTION: RESTRICTION PLACED ON CONTROLLED SUBSTANCE LICENSE

NOTES: SELF ABUSE PROBLEM.

LAUGHLIN, SIDNEY C DO, DATE OF BIRTH OCTOBER 12, 1951 OF PO BOX 11500, EL RENO, OK, WAS DISCIPLINED BY MEDICARE ON AUGUST 3, 1993
DISCIPLINARY ACTION: 120-MONTH EXCLUSION FROM THE MEDICARE AND/OR MEDICAID PROGRAM
OFFENSE: CRIMINAL CONVICTION OR PLEA OF GUILTY, NOLO CONTENDERE, OR NO CONTEST TO A CRIME

NOTES: CONVICTED OF SUBMITTING FALSE CLAIMS TO THE MEDICAID PROGRAM FOR SURGERY SERVICES.

LAUGHLIN, SIDNEY C DO, LICENSE NUMBER 0002215, WAS DISCIPLINED BY OKLAHOMA ON SEPTEMBER 21, 1995
DISCIPLINARY ACTION: REQUIRED TO TAKE ADDITIONAL MEDICAL EDUCATION
OFFENSE: CRIMINAL CONVICTION OR PLEA OF GUILTY, NOLO CONTENDERE, OR NO CONTEST TO A CRIME

NOTES: IN 1992 CONVICTED OF FOUR COUNTS OF MAIL FRAUD. ALLOWED HIS OSTEOPATHIC MEDICAL LICENSE TO LAPSE BY NOT REAPPLYING. REINSTATED UNDER THE FOLLOWING CONDITIONS: COMPLETION OF APPLICATION AND PAYMENT TO THE BOARD OF FEES DUE; SHALL NOT PRACTICE UNTIL HE PROVIDES SATISFACTORY EVIDENCE OF SUCCESSFUL COMPLETION OF A RESIDENCY PROGRAM ACCREDITED BY THE AMERICAN OSTEOPATHIC ASSOCIATION; $5,650.00 ADMINISTRATIVE COSTS; SHALL APPEAR BEFORE THE BOARD UPON REQUEST. ON 4/08/96 REQUEST FOR AMENDMENT OF THIS ORDER DENIED.

LAUGHLIN, SIDNEY C DO, DATE OF BIRTH OCTOBER 12, 1951, LICENSE NUMBER 004889L OF FAIRFIELD INN ROOM 188, KING OF PRUSSIA, PA, WAS DISCIPLINED BY PENNSYLVANIA ON JANUARY 16, 1997
DISCIPLINARY ACTION: PROBATION; RESTRICTION PLACED ON LICENSE
OFFENSE: DISCIPLINARY ACTION BY ANOTHER STATE OR AGENCY

NOTES: ON 10/29/92 CONVICTED OF FOUR COUNTS OF MAIL FRAUD FOR BILLING THE OKLAHOMA STATE MEDICAID PROGRAM FOR MEDICAL PROCEDURES AND SERVICES NOT PERFORMED BETWEEN APRIL AND OCTOBER 1990. FIVE YEAR SUSPENSION RETROACTIVE TO 3/5/93, STAYED IN FAVOR OF PROBATION. TERMS OF PROBATION AS FOLLOWS: HE MAY PRACTICE OSTEOPATHIC MEDICINE AND SURGERY ONLY UNDER THE SUPERVISION OF A LICENSED PHYSICIAN. IF HE PERFORMS AN INVASIVE PROCEDURE, HIS SUPERVISOR MUST BE ON THE PREMISES. HE SHALL PROVIDE A COPY OF THIS ORDER TO HIS SUPERVISOR AND EMPLOYER. HE SHALL HAVE HIS SUPERVISOR SUBMIT MONTHLY REPORTS ON HIS ACTIVITIES TO THE BOARD, BEGINNING 2/15/97. HE SHALL COMPLETE 100 HOURS OF CONTINUING MEDICAL EDUCATION WITHIN ONE YEAR. HE SHALL PROVIDE ANY FURTHER

INFORMATION REQUESTED BY THE BOARD AND SHALL MEET WITH THE BOARD ON 7/9/97 TO REPORT ON HIS ACTIVITIES.

LAUGHLIN, SIDNEY C DO, DATE OF BIRTH OCTOBER 12, 1951, LICENSE NUMBER 1009405 OF 2700 MARTIN LUTHER KING JR BLVD, DETROIT, MI, WAS DISCIPLINED BY MICHIGAN ON APRIL 19, 1999
DISCIPLINARY ACTION: RESTRICTION PLACED ON LICENSE

NOTES: EDUCATIONAL LIMITED LICENSE FOR THE SOLE PURPOSE OF PARTICIPATING IN A RESIDENCY PROGRAM.

LEBAUD, PIERRE MD, LICENSE NUMBER 17183, WAS DISCIPLINED BY OKLAHOMA ON AUGUST 13, 1997
DISCIPLINARY ACTION: REPRIMAND
OFFENSE: LOSS OR RESTRICTION OF HOSPITAL PRIVILEGES

NOTES: ON OR AROUND 1/17/95 HOSPITAL PRIVILEGES WERE REVOKED BASED ON AN INTERNAL PEER REVIEW WHICH ESTABLISHED A CLEAR PATTERN OF HIS FAILING TO EXERCISE APPROPRIATE JUDGMENT IN SELECTING THOSE PROCEDURES WHICH HE WAS COMPETENT TO PERFORM AND FAILING TO RECOGNIZE HIS LACK OF COMPETENCE WHILE CONTINUING SUCH PROCEDURES; IN MAKING APPLICATION FOR LICENSURE IN OKLAHOMA HE FAILED AND REFUSED TO DISCLOSE TO THE OKLAHOMA BOARD THAT HE WAS PREVIOUSLY THE SUBJECT OF DISCIPLINARY ACTION BY JURISDICTIONAL AGENCY OR HOSPITAL OR NAMED AS A DEFENDANT IN A CIVIL SUIT; SINCE HIS ORIGINAL OKLAHOMA LICENSURE HE WAS NAMED IN A SERIES OF MALPRACTICE ACTIONS AND CLAIMS THAT RAISE ADDITIONAL QUESTIONS OF HIS CLINICAL COMPETENCE. HE IS ENCOURAGED TO CONTINUE UNDER MONITORING BY PEER REVIEW AND TO SUCCESSFULLY COMPLETE CONTINUING MEDICAL EDUCATION IN HIS FIELD.

LEE, EDWARD MD OF 1401 NORTH 4TH, PURCELL, OK, WAS DISCIPLINED BY DEA ON JULY 27, 1999
DISCIPLINARY ACTION: SURRENDER OF CONTROLLED SUBSTANCE LICENSE
OFFENSE: DISCIPLINARY ACTION BY ANOTHER STATE OR AGENCY

NOTES: STATE BOARD.

LEE, EDWARD ALLEN MD, LICENSE NUMBER 11807, WAS DISCIPLINED BY OKLAHOMA ON MAY 6, 1999
DISCIPLINARY ACTION: LICENSE REVOCATION
OFFENSE: SEXUAL ABUSE OF OR SEXUAL MISCONDUCT WITH A PATIENT

NOTES: SEXUAL MISBEHAVIOR WITH FOUR PATIENTS. SHALL PAY COSTS.

LERA, THOMAS A JR MD, LICENSE NUMBER 14097, WAS DISCIPLINED BY OKLAHOMA ON JULY 22, 1999
DISCIPLINARY ACTION: LICENSE REVOCATION
OFFENSE: CRIMINAL CONVICTION OR PLEA OF GUILTY, NOLO CONTENDERE, OR NO CONTEST TO A CRIME

NOTES: ON 3/1/99 PLED GUILTY TO: SEXUAL ABUSE OF A CHILD; PROCURING OR CAUSING PARTICIPATION OF A CHILD IN LEWD PHOTOGRAPHS; INDECENT OR LEWD ACTS WITH A CHILD; PROCURING OR CAUSING PARTICIPATION OF A CHILD IN LEWD PHOTOGRAPHS. SHALL PAY COSTS.

LESLIE, PORTER B MD, LICENSE NUMBER 0010616, WAS DISCIPLINED BY OKLAHOMA ON NOVEMBER 23, 1992
DISCIPLINARY ACTION: 2-MONTH LICENSE SUSPENSION; PROBATION
OFFENSE: OVERPRESCRIBING OR MISPRESCRIBING DRUGS

NOTES: FROM 1/1/91 THROUGH 3/5/92, PRESCRIBED, DISPENSED OR ADMINISTERED CONTROLLED SUBSTANCES OR NARCOTIC DRUGS IN EXCESS OF THE AMOUNT CONSIDERED GOOD MEDICAL PRACTICE, OR WITHOUT MEDICAL NEED IN ACCORDANCE WITH PUBLISHED STANDARDS IN AT LEAST 5 CASES. ALSO WROTE PRESCRIPTIONS UNDER DEA LICENSE NUMBER WHICH HAD BEEN REVOKED 11/88, AND WROTE NONE UNDER DEA LICENSE NUMBER ISSUED 2/28/90. PROBATION INDEFINITE, UNDER TERMS AND CONDITIONS: MAY NOT PRESCRIBE, ADMINISTER, DISPENSE OR POSSESS ANY CONTROLLED DANGEROUS SUBSTANCES OR SCHEDULE DRUGS, EXCEPT MAY PRESCRIBE THEM FOR HOSPITAL IN-PATIENTS FOR USE WHILE IN HOSPITAL; SHALL NOT SUPERVISE A PHYSICIAN ASSISTANT; SHALL NOT ALLOW INITIATION OF ANY THERAPEUTIC REGIMEN BY ANY PERSONNEL UNDER HIS SUPERVISION UNLESS HE IS IN THE IMMEDIATE GEOGRAPHIC VICINITY; SHALL FURNISH BOARD WITH ADDRESS AND/OR CHANGE OF ADDRESS; SHALL APPEAR BEFORE BOARD UPON REQUEST; SHALL NOTIFY ANY HOSPITAL WHERE HE HOLDS STAFF PRIVILEGES, OR CLINIC OR GROUP, AND EVERY STATE WHERE HE IS LICENSED OF THE TERMS AND CONDITIONS.

LEVALLEY, STEVE A MD, LICENSE NUMBER 0008158 OF 185 S ELM STREET, DENVER, CO, WAS DISCIPLINED BY OKLAHOMA ON FEBRUARY 8, 1990
DISCIPLINARY ACTION: 7-MONTH PROBATION; MONITORING OF PHYSICIAN PERFORMANCE
OFFENSE: DISCIPLINARY ACTION BY ANOTHER STATE OR AGENCY

NOTES: CURRENTLY PRACTICING MEDICINE AND SURGERY IN COLORADO. THE COLORADO BOARD FOUND THAT FROM 3/84 TO 2/01/88 HE DID NOT PRACTICE MEDICINE AND SURGERY. WAS DETERMINED TO HAVE A DISABILITY WHICH RENDERED HIM UNABLE TO PERFORM MEDICAL SERVICES WITH REASONABLE SKILL AND SAFETY TO THE PATIENTS. ON 8/12/88 THE COLORADO BOARD FOUND THAT HE HAD NO DIAGNOSIS OR PSYCHOPATHOLOGY THAT PREVENTED HIM FROM PRACTICING WITH REASONABLE SKILL AND SAFETY TO PATIENTS, BUT FOUND A CASE OF UNPROFESSIONAL CONDUCT AND PLACED HIM ON TWO YEAR PROBATION. OKLAHOMA PLACES HIM ON PROBATION BEGINNING 2/2/90 UNDER THE FOLLOWING TERMS AND CONDITIONS: HIS MEDICAL PRACTICE IN COLORADO SHALL BE MONITORED BY A BOARD APPROVED LICENSED COLORADO PHYSICIAN WHO SHALL BE RESPONSIBLE FOR OVERSIGHT OF THE HIS ENTIRE MEDICAL PRACTICE WHICH INCLUDES, BUT IS NOT LIMITED TO ANY HOSPITAL WHERE HE PRACTICES; SHALL REVIEW A RANDOM SAMPLING OF ANY RECORDS MAINTAINED, TO DETERMINE WHETHER HE HAS PRACTICED IN ACCORDANCE WITH THE GENERALLY ACCEPTED STANDARD OF MEDICAL CARE; THE MONITOR SHALL REPORT QUARTERLY TO THE BOARD; SHALL OBTAIN PSYCHIATRIC TREATMENT ON A REGULAR, CONTINUING BASIS, NO LESS THAN ONCE EVERY 30 DAYS, BY A BOARD APPROVED PHYSICIAN WHO SHALL SUBMIT TO THE BOARD IN WRITING, ON A REGULAR BASIS, A REPORT CONCERNING HIS MENTAL STABILITY; SHALL UNDERGO AN EVALUATION FOR SUBSTANCE ABUSE AT ANY TIME THAT THE PRACTICE MONITOR OR TREATMENT MONITOR BELIEVES IT TO BE APPROPRIATE; SHALL NOTIFY THE BOARD OF HIS CHANGE IN ADDRESS SHOULD HE

RELOCATE TO ANOTHER STATE; IF HE RETURNS TO THE ACTIVE PRACTICE OF MEDICINE AND SURGERY IN OKLAHOMA, HE SHALL REAPPEAR BEFORE THE BOARD AND SHALL PROVIDE THE BOARD WITH A COPY OF THE FINAL REPORT FROM HIS PSYCHIATRIST THAT WAS SUBMITTED TO THE COLORADO BOARD IN 8/90.

LEWIS, JIM E DO, LICENSE NUMBER 3423, WAS DISCIPLINED BY OKLAHOMA ON DECEMBER 12, 1996
DISCIPLINARY ACTION: 24-MONTH PROBATION

LEWIS, JIM E DO, LICENSE NUMBER 3423, WAS DISCIPLINED BY OKLAHOMA ON MARCH 19, 1998
DISCIPLINARY ACTION: SURRENDER OF LICENSE

LEWIS, JIM EARL DO, DATE OF BIRTH JUNE 12, 1954, LICENSE NUMBER 0006123 OF 711 MAIN STREET SW, RONAN, MT, WAS DISCIPLINED BY MONTANA ON MAY 20, 1991

NOTES: UNSPECIFIED AGREEMENT AND ORDER.

LEWIS, JIM EARL DO, DATE OF BIRTH JUNE 12, 1954, LICENSE NUMBER 0AA1903 OF PO BOX 82931, FAIRBANKS, AK, WAS DISCIPLINED BY ALASKA ON JUNE 6, 1991
DISCIPLINARY ACTION: 60-MONTH PROBATION; MONITORING OF PHYSICIAN PERFORMANCE

NOTES: PRIOR PSYCHIATRIC TREATMENT AND CHEMICAL DEPENDENCY EVALUATION. CONDITIONS OF PROBATION: MUST CONSUME NO CONTROLLED DRUGS OR ALCOHOL; MUST PARTICIPATE IN BOARD APPROVED MONITORING PROGRAM; MUST RECEIVE PSYCHIATRIC CARE; MUST NOTIFY EMPLOYER/HOSPITALS OF ORDER; REPORTS TO BOARD; MUST NOTIFY BOARD OF CHANGE IN PERSONAL PHYSICIAN AND ABSENCES FROM STATE. ON 9/23/94 ORDER AMENDED TO DE-EMPHASIZE SUBSTANCE ABUSE AS IT RELATES TO HIS UNDERLYING MENTAL CONDITION.

LEWIS, JIM EARL DO, DATE OF BIRTH JUNE 12, 1954 OF PO BOX 1390, NOME, AK, WAS DISCIPLINED BY MEDICARE ON DECEMBER 20, 1998
DISCIPLINARY ACTION: EXCLUSION FROM THE MEDICARE AND/OR MEDICAID PROGRAM
OFFENSE: DISCIPLINARY ACTION BY ANOTHER STATE OR AGENCY

NOTES: LICENSE REVOKED, SUSPENDED, SURRENDERED OR OTHERWISE LOST FOR REASONS BEARING ON PROFESSIONAL PERFORMANCE, PROFESSIONAL COMPETENCE OR FINANCIAL INTEGRITY.

LIGHTFOOT, STANLEY AUGUSTUS MD, LICENSE NUMBER 00D0946 OF TYLER, TX, WAS DISCIPLINED BY TEXAS ON DECEMBER 1, 1990
DISCIPLINARY ACTION: LICENSE SUSPENSION
OFFENSE: CRIMINAL CONVICTION OR PLEA OF GUILTY, NOLO CONTENDERE, OR NO CONTEST TO A CRIME

NOTES: LICENSE SUSPENDED WHILE PHYSICIAN SERVES PRISON TERM IN PENITENTIARY.

LIGHTFOOT, STANLEY AUGUSTUS MD, LICENSE NUMBER 00D0946, WAS DISCIPLINED BY TEXAS ON SEPTEMBER 16, 1991
DISCIPLINARY ACTION: 60-MONTH PROBATION; RESTRICTION PLACED ON LICENSE

NOTES: SUSPENSION OF LICENSE TERMINATED. CONDITIONS OF PROBATION: SHALL APPEAR BEFORE THE BOARD TWICE A YEAR; SHALL NOT PETITION FOR MODIFICATION FOR AT LEAST ONE YEAR; PRACTICE LIMITED TO PATHOLOGY; SHALL COMPLY WITH TERMS OF PROBATION UNDER THE U.S. DISTRICT COURT OR FEDERAL CORRECTIONAL SYSTEM; SHALL GIVE A COPY OF ORDER TO ALL INSTITUTIONS WHERE HE HAS PRIVILEGES; SHALL COOPERATE WITH BOARD IN VERIFYING COMPLIANCE; SHALL ADVISE THE BOARD OF CHANGE OF ADDRESS WITHIN 10 DAYS; TIME SPENT OUT OF TEXAS DOES NOT COUNT TOWARDS PROBATION.

LIGHTFOOT, STANLEY AUGUSTUS MD OF 119 EAST HOUSTON, TYLER, TX, WAS DISCIPLINED BY OKLAHOMA ON MAY 9, 1992
DISCIPLINARY ACTION: 60-MONTH PROBATION; RESTRICTION PLACED ON LICENSE
OFFENSE: DISCIPLINARY ACTION BY ANOTHER STATE OR AGENCY

NOTES: ON 2/25/78, LICENSE REVOKED BY TEXAS, REVOCATION STAYED, PLACED ON FIVE YEARS PROBATION; FULLY REINSTATED 3/83. ON 5/15/90, PLED GUILTY TO FOUR COUNTS OF MAKING FALSE STATEMENTS TO BANKS FOR LOANS, SENTENCED TO TWO YEARS IN PRISON AND FIVE YEARS PROBATION; TEXAS LICENSE SUSPENDED 8/18/90. ON 8/23/91, TEXAS LICENSE REINSTATED UNDER FIVE YEARS PROBATION. OKLAHOMA LICENSE GRANTED WITH TEXAS TERMS AND CONDITIONS IMPOSED. SHALL APPEAR BEFORE BOARD TWICE A YEAR; SHALL NOT PETITION FOR MODIFICATION FOR ONE YEAR; PRACTICE LIMITED TO PATHOLOGY; SHALL NOT SUPERVISE A PHYSICIAN ASSISTANT; SHALL FURNISH BOARD WITH ADDRESS AND/OR CHANGE OF ADDRESS; SHALL APPEAR BEFORE BOARD UPON REQUEST; SHALL NOTIFY ANY HOSPITAL WHERE HE HOLDS STAFF PRIVILEGES, OR CLINIC OR GROUP OF THE TERMS AND CONDITIONS. ON 3/29/96 PROBATION TERMINATED.

LINDSEY, PHILLIP H MD OF 1001 SW 44TH, OKLAHOMA CITY, OK, WAS DISCIPLINED BY DEA ON DECEMBER 28, 1993
DISCIPLINARY ACTION: SURRENDER OF CONTROLLED SUBSTANCE LICENSE
OFFENSE: DISCIPLINARY ACTION BY ANOTHER STATE OR AGENCY

NOTES: STATE ACTION REVOKING MEDICAL LICENSE.

LINDSEY, PHILLIP HARRIS MD, LICENSE NUMBER 0013244, WAS DISCIPLINED BY OKLAHOMA ON OCTOBER 7, 1993
DISCIPLINARY ACTION: EMERGENCY SUSPENSION

NOTES: SUSPENDED IN THE INTEREST OF PROTECTION OF PUBLIC HEALTH, SAFETY AND WELFARE UNTIL THIS MATTER COMES ON FOR HEARING ON THE MERITS AT THE BOARD'S NEXT MEETING.

LINDSEY, PHILLIP HARRIS MD, LICENSE NUMBER 0013244, WAS DISCIPLINED BY OKLAHOMA ON DECEMBER 2, 1993
DISCIPLINARY ACTION: LICENSE REVOCATION
OFFENSE: SUBSTANCE ABUSE

NOTES: BETWEEN 8/90 AND 7/93 WROTE OR CALLED IN PRESCRIPTIONS FOR CONTROLLED DANGEROUS SUBSTANCES WITHOUT SUFFICIENT EXAMINATION AND THE ESTABLISHMENT OF A VALID PHYSICIAN-PATIENT RELATIONSHIP IN TWO CASES AND FOR A NONEXISTENT PATIENT IN ONE CASE; FROM 1/93 TO 4/93 HE HAD A HABITUAL PATTERN AND PRACTICE OF PERSONALLY TAKING CONTROLLED DANGEROUS SUBSTANCES PRESCRIBED TO OR TELEPHONED IN ON BEHALF OF THREE PATIENTS.

LINDSEY, PHILLIP HARRIS MD, LICENSE NUMBER 0013244, WAS DISCIPLINED BY OKLAHOMA ON JANUARY 27, 1995

DISCIPLINARY ACTION: LICENSE REINSTATEMENT; PROBATION

NOTES: REINSTATED WITH INDEFINITE PROBATION UNDER THE FOLLOWING TERMS AND CONDITIONS: GRANTED A SPECIAL LICENSE TO PRACTICE MEDICINE SOLELY AND EXCLUSIVELY AT THE OKLAHOMA DEPARTMENT OF HEALTH FOR HIS EMPLOYMENT AS AN ASSISTANT TUBERCULOSIS CONTROL OFFICES; SHALL NOT PRESCRIBE, DISPENSE, OR ADMINISTER ANY MEDICATION FOR HIS PERSONAL USE AND SHALL TAKE NONE UNLESS AUTHORIZED BY ANOTHER PHYSICIAN FOR LEGITIMATE MEDICAL NEED; SHALL NOT CONSUME OR USE IN ANY WAY ANY SUBSTANCE WHICH WOULD ADVERSELY AFFECT HIS ABILITY TO PRACTICE; SHALL SUBMIT BIOLOGICAL FLUID SPECIMENS; SHALL SUBMIT TO AND COOPERATE WITH PERIODIC INTERVIEWS AND/OR EVALUATIONS CONDUCTED BY THE BOARD; SHALL APPEAR BEFORE THE BOARD UPON REQUEST AND SUBMIT REQUIRED REPORTS; SHALL NOT SUPERVISE A PHYSICIAN'S ASSISTANT; SHALL PAY COSTS; SHALL INFORM ANY PLACE WHERE HE HAS PRIVILEGES OR PRACTICES OF TERMS AND CONDITIONS AND SUPPLY A COPY THEREOF. SHALL MAINTAIN A CONTINUED PROGRAM OF PHYSICIAN RECOVERY AS PRESCRIBED BY THE BOARD; SUPERVISOR SHALL SUBMIT QUARTERLY REPORTS TO THE BOARD; SHALL NOT ALLOW THE INITIATION OF ANY THERAPEUTIC REGIMEN BY ANY PERSONNEL UNDER HIS SUPERVISION UNLESS HE IS IN THE IMMEDIATE VICINITY; SHALL NOT BE CONSIDERED BY THE BOARD FOR ANY EXPANSION OF THIS SPECIAL LICENSE. ON 6/5/97 PETITION TO MODIFY ORDER DENIED. ON 6/4/98 REQUEST FOR MODIFICATION OF SPECIAL LICENSE GRANTED ALLOWING HIM TO PERFORM BACK UP SERVICES AS A TUBERCULOSIS ASSISTANT CONTROL OFFICER FOR SPECIFIED HEALTH DEPARTMENT.

LIU, KUO TAI MD, LICENSE NUMBER 00E3047 OF MARLIN, TX, WAS DISCIPLINED BY TEXAS ON DECEMBER 4, 1991
DISCIPLINARY ACTION: 60-MONTH PROBATION; RESTRICTION PLACED ON LICENSE
OFFENSE: SUBSTANDARD CARE, INCOMPETENCE OR NEGLIGENCE

NOTES: FAILED TO DEMONSTRATE ADEQUATE KNOWLEDGE AND SKILLS IN TREATING FOUR PATIENTS AND PREPARING THEIR MEDICAL RECORDS. SUSPENSION STAYED; CONDITIONS OF PROBATION: SHALL LIMIT PRACTICE TO TREATING PATIENTS AT GOLDEN YEARS AND ELMWOOD NURSING HOMES ONLY; SHALL OBTAIN A BOARD APPROVED MONITORING PHYSICIAN WHO SHALL REPORT TO THE BOARD EVERY SIX MONTHS; A COPY OF THIS ORDER SHALL BE PROVIDED TO THE MONITOR AND ALL INSTITUTIONS WHERE HE HAS PRIVILEGES; SHALL REFRAIN FROM PRESCRIBING ANY DRUG UNLESS MEDICALLY INDICATED AND IN THERAPEUTIC DOSES, AND WITH AN APPROPRIATE MEDICAL HISTORY AND EXAM; SHALL CONDUCT FOLLOW-UP EXAMS TO DETERMINE IF DRUG REGIMEN IS WORKING AND IF IT SHOULD BE ALTERED; WITHIN THREE MONTHS SHALL COMPLETE A TWO WEEK MINIRESIDENCY COURSE; WITHIN NINE MONTHS MUST PASS THE SPEX EXAM; WITHIN SIX MONTHS SHALL COMPLETE A REMEDIAL PHARMACOLOGY COURSE; SHALL COOPERATE WITH BOARD IN VERIFYING COMPLIANCE; SHALL ADVISE THE BOARD OF A CHANGE OF ADDRESS WITHIN 10 DAYS; TIME SPENT OUT OF TEXAS DOES NOT COUNT TOWARDS PROBATION; SHALL APPEAR BEFORE THE BOARD TWICE A YEAR; SHALL NOT APPLY FOR MODIFICATION OF ORDER FOR ONE YEAR.

LIU, KUO TAI MD, LICENSE NUMBER 0010449, WAS DISCIPLINED BY OKLAHOMA ON JANUARY 15, 1993

NOTES: IN LIEU OF ANY FURTHER FORMAL PROCEEDINGS BOARD AGREED TO ACCEPT APPLICATION FOR PHYSICIAN EMERITUS STATUS (RETIRED STATUS, NOT ACTIVE TO PRACTICE) WITH THE PROVISION THAT HE FILES WITHIN 10 DAYS.

LOCKWOOD, RICHARD L MD, LICENSE NUMBER 0017165 OF 1404 MISSOURI, HOUSTON, TX, WAS DISCIPLINED BY OKLAHOMA ON JUNE 21, 1990
DISCIPLINARY ACTION: LICENSE REVOCATION
OFFENSE: SUBSTANCE ABUSE

NOTES: GUILTY OF HABITUAL INTEMPERANCE OR THE HABITUAL USE OF HABIT-FORMING DRUGS WHICH IMPAIRS THE ABILITY TO PRACTICE MEDICINE WITH REASONABLE SKILL AND SAFETY TO THE PATIENT. ON 2/8/90 HOSPITAL WHERE HE WORKED AS AN ANESTHESIOLOGIST REQUESTED HIM TO STOP DELIVERING ANESTHETICS TO PATIENTS AND TO UNDERGO A MEDICAL EVALUATION; EVALUATOR AT HIS REQUEST WOULD NOT REVEAL RESULTS BUT SAID AT THAT TIME SHOULD NOT BE GIVING ANESTHESIA; AT ANOTHER HOSPITAL IN TEXAS HE EXPERIENCED SIMILAR PROBLEMS. HE RESIGNED WHEN ASKED TO UNDERGO A PHYSICAL EXAM INCLUDING TESTING FOR SUBSTANCE ABUSE.

LOCKWOOD, RICHARD L MD, LICENSE NUMBER 00G7083 OF HOUSTON, TX, WAS DISCIPLINED BY TEXAS ON AUGUST 18, 1990
DISCIPLINARY ACTION: LICENSE SUSPENSION; REQUIRED TO TAKE ADDITIONAL MEDICAL EDUCATION
OFFENSE: SUBSTANCE ABUSE

NOTES: STIPULATED ORDER. LICENSE INDEFINITELY SUSPENDED COMMENCING UPON BOARD VERBAL APPROVAL OF ORDER (8/17/90). MUST SUBMIT FOR PSYCHIATRIC EVALUATIONS AND RECOMMENDED TREATMENTS, PARTICIPATE IN HARRIS COUNTY MEDICAL SOCIETY COMMITTEE ON PHYSICIAN HEALTH AND REHABILITATION AND AA, SUBMIT FOR APPROPRIATE EXAMINATIONS TO DETERMINE FREEDOM FROM DRUGS AND ALCOHOL, AND OBTAIN CONTINUING MEDICAL EDUCATION.

LOCKWOOD, RICHARD L MD OF 1404 MISSOURI ST, HOUSTON, TX, WAS DISCIPLINED BY DEA ON OCTOBER 2, 1990
DISCIPLINARY ACTION: SURRENDER OF CONTROLLED SUBSTANCE LICENSE
OFFENSE: SUBSTANCE ABUSE

NOTES: OKLAHOMA MEDICAL LICENSE REVOKED 06/08/90; TESTED POSITIVE ON URINE DRUG SCREEN FOR BENZODIAZEPINE METABOLITES 11/10/89 AND 04/04/90; TREATED FOR ABUSE OF FENTANYL AND SODIUM PENTOTHAL 12/87.

LOCKWOOD, RICHARD L MD, LICENSE NUMBER 00G7083 OF IRVING, TX, WAS DISCIPLINED BY TEXAS ON APRIL 29, 1991
DISCIPLINARY ACTION: PROBATION; REQUIRED TO TAKE ADDITIONAL MEDICAL EDUCATION

NOTES: REINSTATED FROM SUSPENSION; PROBATION CONDITIONS INCLUDE: PARTICIPATION IN IMPAIRED PHYSICIANS PROGRAM; MUST PARTICIPATE IN AA; MUST SUBMIT TO ALCOHOL OR DRUG SCREENS; SHALL ATTEND AT LEAST 50 HOURS OF CONTINUING MEDICAL EDUCATION IN FAMILY PRACTICE.

LOCKWOOD, RICHARD L MD, LICENSE NUMBER G7083 OF HOUSTON, TX, WAS DISCIPLINED BY TEXAS ON AUGUST 9, 1997
DISCIPLINARY ACTION: LICENSE SUSPENSION

OFFENSE: FAILURE TO COMPLY WITH PREVIOUS BOARD ORDER

NOTES: HE VIOLATED 8/18/90 AND 4/29/91 BOARD ORDERS IN THAT HE FAILED TO PARTICIPATE IN ACTIVITIES OF A PHYSICIANS HEALTH AND REHABILITATION COMMITTEE OR IN AA; FAILED TO PROVIDE REQUIRED QUARTERLY REPORTS; FAILED TO ATTEND OR SHOW PROOF OF ATTENDANCE AT REQUIRED CONTINUING MEDICAL EDUCATION COURSES. SUSPENSION UNTIL HE REQUESTS TO HAVE THE SUSPENSION STAYED OR APPEARS BEFORE THE BOARD WITH SUFFICIENT EVIDENCE THAT HE IS PHYSICALLY, MENTALLY AND OTHERWISE COMPETENT TO SAFELY PRACTICE MEDICINE INCLUDING AT A MINIMUM: COMPLETE COPIES OF MEDICAL RECORDS AND REPORTS OF PSYCHOLOGICAL AND NEUROPSYCHIATRIC EVALUATIONS, INCLUDING A 96-HOUR INPATIENT EVALUATION CONDUCTED BY A BOARD-APPROVED CERTIFIED PSYCHIATRIST; SHALL INFORM THE BOARD OF CHANGE OF ADDRESS WITHIN 10 DAYS OR IF HE LEAVES THE STATE; SHALL NOT SEEK MODIFICATION FOR ONE YEAR.

LOCKWOOD, RICHARD L MD, LICENSE NUMBER G7083, WAS DISCIPLINED BY TEXAS ON AUGUST 22, 1998
DISCIPLINARY ACTION: 120-MONTH PROBATION; RESTRICTION PLACED ON LICENSE
OFFENSE: SUBSTANCE ABUSE

NOTES: SUCCESSFULLY COMPLETED A 96 HOUR INPATIENT EVALUATION AS REQUIRED BY 8/9/97 ORDER WHICH INDICATED THAT HIS OPIATE DEPENDENCE IS IN COMPLETE REMISSION; HE ATTENDS AA FOUR TIMES A WEEK AND HAS A SPONSOR; HE REPORTS A SOBRIETY DATE OF 3/3/93. SUSPENSION STAYED FOR PROBATION WITH FOLLOWING TERMS AND CONDITIONS AS SOON AS HE PASSES THE SPEX AND JURISPRUDENCE EXAM WITH A SCORE OF 75 OR ABOVE, WITHIN 3 ATTEMPTS. SHALL BE RESTRICTED TO A BOARD-APPROVED OUTPATIENT PRACTICE AND/OR CLINICAL SETTING; SHALL NOT PRACTICE IN A HOSPITAL SETTING; SHALL ABSTAIN FROM THE CONSUMPTION OF ALCOHOL/DRUGS IN ANY FORM UNLESS PRESCRIBED BY ANOTHER PHYSICIAN FOR A LEGITIMATE AND THERAPEUTIC PURPOSE; SHALL SUBMIT HIMSELF FOR APPROPRIATE EXAMS INCLUDING DRUG OR ALCOHOL SCREENS; SHALL PARTICIPATE IN THE ACTIVITIES OF A PHYSICIAN HEALTH AND REHABILITATION COMMITTEE AND ATTEND WEEKLY MEETINGS WITH QUARTERLY REPORTS; SHALL PARTICIPATE IN AA'S PROGRAM NOT LESS THAN THREE TIMES A WEEK; SHALL REPORT ON HIS ATTENDANCE; SHALL NOT TREAT OR OTHERWISE SERVE AS PHYSICIAN, PRESCRIBE, DISPENSE OR ADMINISTER DRUGS THAT MAY BE SUBJECT TO ABUSE TO HIMSELF OR TO ANY MEMBER OF HIS FAMILY; SHALL SURRENDER DEA AND TEXAS DEPARTMENT OF PUBLIC SAFETY CONTROLLED SUBSTANCE CERTIFICATES AND ANY DRUGS REMAINING IN HIS POSSESSION INCLUDING SAMPLES; SEPARATE FROM PATIENT RECORDS, SHALL MAINTAIN A LOGBOOK OF EVERY PRESCRIPTION WRITTEN BY HIM FOR DANGEROUS DRUGS WITH ADDICTIVE POTENTIAL WHICH SHALL BE MADE AVAILABLE FOR REVIEW; HIS MEDICAL PRACTICE SHALL BE MONITORED BY A BOARD APPROVED TEXAS PHYSICIAN WHO SHALL PROVIDE QUARTERLY REPORTS TO THE BOARD; SHALL MAINTAIN ADEQUATE MEDICAL RECORDS WHICH SHALL BE AVAILABLE FOR REVIEW; SHALL OBTAIN 50 HOURS PER YEAR OF CONTINUING MEDICAL EDUCATION WITH 1 COURSE IN GENERAL MEDICINE AND 1 COURSE IN PRIMARY CARE; SHALL APPEAR BEFORE THE BOARD UPON REQUEST; SHALL COOPERATE WITH THE BOARD IN VERIFYING COMPLIANCE INCLUDING PROVIDING COPIES OF MEDICAL RELEASES UPON REQUEST; SHALL GIVE A COPY OF THIS ORDER TO ANY HEALTH CARE ENTITY WHERE HE HAS PRIVILEGES; SHALL PROVIDE A COPY OF THIS ORDER TO ANYONE REQUESTING IT WITHIN 10 DAYS; TIME SPENT OUT OF TEXAS DOES NOT COUNT TOWARD PROBATION; SHALL INFORM THE BOARD OF CHANGE OF ADDRESS WITHIN 10 DAYS OR IF HE LEAVES THE STATE; SHALL NOT SEEK MODIFICATION FOR ONE YEAR.

LOERKE, JAMES R DO, LICENSE NUMBER 0002289, WAS DISCIPLINED BY OKLAHOMA ON NOVEMBER 6, 1995
DISCIPLINARY ACTION: SURRENDER OF CONTROLLED SUBSTANCE LICENSE; 36-MONTH PROBATION
OFFENSE: OVERPRESCRIBING OR MISPRESCRIBING DRUGS

NOTES: PRIOR TO 9/21/95 GAVE PRESCRIPTIONS TO A SERIES OF PATIENTS WHO MAY HAVE USED THEM TO SECURE CONTROLLED DANGEROUS SUBSTANCES OR EXCHANGED PRESCRIPTIONS FOR THINGS OF VALUE OR BENEFIT TO THE DOCTOR AND NOT IN CONNECTION WITH ANY PHYSICIAN/PATIENT RELATIONSHIP; PRESCRIPTIONS GIVEN WITHOUT EXAMINATION AND A GOOD FAITH BELIEF THEY WOULD BE USED BY THE PATIENT TO RELIEVE PAIN AND SUFFERING, OR TO TREAT AN AILMENT, PHYSICAL INFIRMITY, OR DISEASE. SHALL NOT PETITION THE BOARD FOR MODIFICATION OF THIS ORDER FOR ONE YEAR; VOLUNTARILY OFFERED TO SURRENDER HIS LICENSE TO DISPENSE CONTROLLED DANGEROUS SUBSTANCES TO THE DRUG ENFORCEMENT AGENCY AND MAY NOT APPLY FOR REINSTATEMENT FOR ONE YEAR; DURING THE FIRST SIX MONTHS OF PROBATION SHALL ATTEND A COURSE ENTITLED "THE PROPER PRESCRIBING OF CONTROLLED DANGEROUS SUBSTANCES" AND ATTEND ONE BOARD APPROVED COURSE IN ETHICS AND SHALL REPORT TO THE BOARD SUCCESSFUL COMPLETION OF THESE COURSES; SHALL GIVE A COPY OF THIS ORDER TO ANY HEALTH CARE ENTITY WHERE HE HAS PRIVILEGES; SHALL NOTIFY THE BOARD IN WRITING OF ANY CHANGE IN ADDRESS, EMPLOYMENT, EMPLOYMENT TERMINATION OR HOSPITAL OR HEALTH CARE PROVIDERS PRIVILEGE RESTRICTION OR ANY ADMINISTRATIVE PROCEEDING INITIATED AGAINST HIM BY ANY OTHER STATE OR FEDERAL REGULATORY BODY WITHIN 14 DAYS; ADMINISTRATIVE COSTS OF $1,650. ON 12/10/98 PROBATION TERMINATED.

LOERKE, JAMES R DO OF 18 N NORWOOD SHERIDAN VILLAGE W, TULSA, OK, WAS DISCIPLINED BY DEA ON MAY 8, 1996
DISCIPLINARY ACTION: SURRENDER OF CONTROLLED SUBSTANCE LICENSE
OFFENSE: PROFESSIONAL MISCONDUCT

NOTES: ILLEGAL DISPENSING. VOLUNTARY SURRENDER.

LYNN, MARK MD OF 316 NW 18, OKLAHOMA CITY, OK, WAS DISCIPLINED BY OKLAHOMA ON AUGUST 8, 1996
DISCIPLINARY ACTION: 60-MONTH PROBATION; RESTRICTION PLACED ON LICENSE

NOTES: ISSUED FULL LICENSURE IN OKLAHOMA. CONDITIONS OF PROBATION: SHALL NOT PRESCRIBE, ADMINISTER, OR DISPENSE ANY MEDICATIONS FOR HIS PERSONAL USE, TO SPECIFICALLY INCLUDE CONTROLLED DANGEROUS SUBSTANCES; SHALL TAKE NO MEDICATION UNLESS PRESCRIBED BY AN AUTHORIZED TREATING PHYSICIAN FOR LEGITIMATE MEDICAL NEED; SHALL ABSTAIN FROM CONSUMING

ALCOHOL OR ANY SUBSTANCE, SPECIFICALLY INCLUDING, BUT NOT LIMITED TO CONTROLLED DANGEROUS SUBSTANCES, WHICH WOULD ADVERSELY AFFECT HIS ABILITY TO PRACTICE MEDICINE OR SURGERY; SHALL SUBMIT BIOLOGICAL FLUID SPECIMENS UPON BOARD REQUEST; SHALL NOT ENGAGE IN ANY ACTIVITY OR INGEST ANY MEDICATION OR SUBSTANCE OF ANY NATURE THAT WILL TEST POSITIVE FOR ALCOHOL OR ANY CONTROLLED DANGEROUS SUBSTANCE; SHALL MAINTAIN A PROGRAM OF ABSTINENCE THROUGH PARTICIPATION IN AND/OR ASSOCIATION WITH ANY AND ALL ORGANIZATIONS, GROUPS, OR INDIVIDUALS SELECTED BY THE BOARD AND DEEMED APPROPRIATE FOR ASSESSMENT, TREATMENT, AND SUPPORT; SHALL NOT ORDER, DISPENSE, OR ADMINISTER ANY CONTROLLED DANGEROUS SUBSTANCES OR LEGEND DRUGS, EXCEPT HE MAY ORDER, DISPENSE, OR ADMINISTER LIFE-SAVING DRUGS TO A PATIENT IN AN EMERGENCY, LIFE-THREATENING SITUATION AND SHALL NOTIFY THE BOARD OF SUCH CASES; SHALL SUBMIT TO THE BOARD ADDRESS/CHANGE OF ADDRESS; SHALL APPEAR BEFORE THE BOARD UPON REQUEST AND SUBMIT REQUIRED REPORTS; SHALL NOT ALLOW THE INITIATION OF ANY THERAPEUTIC REGIMEN BY ANY PERSONNEL UNDER HIS SUPERVISION UNLESS HE IS IN THE IMMEDIATE GEOGRAPHIC VICINITY; SHALL FURNISH ALL STATES IN WHICH HE HOLDS OR APPLIES FOR LICENSURE AND ALL HEALTH CARE ENTITIES IN WHICH HE HOLDS PRIVILEGES A COPY OF THIS ORDER; AND SHALL NOT SUPERVISE A PHYSICIAN ASSISTANT. ON 1/30/98 REQUEST TO MODIFY TERMS OF PROBATION GRANTED IN THAT HE WILL KEEP DUPLICATE, SERIALLY NUMBERED PRESCRIPTIONS WHICH SHALL BE AVAILABLE FOR REVIEW. ON 3/12/99 REQUEST TO MODIFY TERMS OF PROBATION GRANTED SUCH THAT HE SHALL LIMIT HIS PRACTICE TO FAMILY PRACTICE.

LYNN, MARK R MD, LICENSE NUMBER 0014916 OF 1000 SW 44 #200, OKLAHOMA CITY, OK, WAS DISCIPLINED BY OKLAHOMA ON MAY 20, 1993
DISCIPLINARY ACTION: LICENSE REVOCATION
OFFENSE: SUBSTANCE ABUSE

NOTES: BEGINNING IN 1/93 HE MAINTAINED A REGULAR PATTERN OF LEAVING PRE-SIGNED BLANK PRESCRIPTION FORMS FOR THE USE OF ANOTHER DOCTOR WHICH WERE USED FOR PRESCRIPTIONS FOR PATIENTS WITH WHOM HE HAD NOT ESTABLISHED A PHYSICIAN/PATIENT RELATIONSHIP; IN 1992 HE ADMITTED HIMSELF FOR TREATMENT OF ALCOHOL AND DRUG ADDICTION, SPECIFICALLY FENTANYL AND SUFENTA; IS ATTENDING AA MEETINGS AND WEEKLY MEETINGS OF THE PHYSICIANS RECOVERY COMMITTEE.

LYNN, MARK R MD, LICENSE NUMBER 0014916, WAS DISCIPLINED BY OKLAHOMA ON JANUARY 27, 1995
DISCIPLINARY ACTION: LICENSE REINSTATEMENT; 3-MONTH PROBATION

NOTES: GRANTED A SPECIAL LICENSE FOR THREE MONTHS DURING WHICH HE SHALL PRACTICE SOLELY AND EXCLUSIVELY IN A "MINI-INTERNSHIP" UNDER THE FOLLOWING TERMS AND CONDITIONS: SHALL REAPPEAR BEFORE THE BOARD WITHIN THREE MONTHS TO PRESENT FUTURE PRACTICE PLANS AT WHICH TIME HIS APPLICATION FOR REINSTATEMENT SHALL BE CONSIDERED; SHALL NOT ENTER ANY INTERNSHIP WHICH INVOLVES EMERGENCY ROOM PRACTICE OR ANESTHESIOLOGY; SHALL CONTINUE IN THE RECOMMENDED RECOVERY STEPS OF THE PHYSICIAN'S RECOVERY GROUP WHICH INCLUDE SHALL NOT RETURN TO THE PRACTICE OF ANESTHESIOLOGY, SHALL OBTAIN 30 HOURS OF CONTINUING MEDICAL EDUCATION, SHALL WORK UNPAID UNDER A PRECEPTOR FOR THREE MONTHS, SHALL WORK HALF TIME IN THE INITIAL SIX MONTHS OF PRIMARY CARE PRACTICE, SHALL SUBMIT TO WEEKLY URINE MONITORING, SHALL CONTINUE PSYCHIATRIC MONITORING AND WEEKLY GROUP THERAPY, SHALL ATTEND A MINIMUM OF THREE AA MEETINGS PER WEEK, SHALL CONTINUE ATTENDANCE OF THE CADUCEUS GROUP; SHALL NOT PRESCRIBE, DISPENSE OR ADMINISTER ANY NARCOTICS; SHALL SUBMIT TO THE BOARD THE SPECIFIC DETAILS OF HIS INTERNSHIP AND PROVIDE ADDITIONAL INFORMATION UPON REQUEST.

MALONEY, GREGORY P DO, LICENSE NUMBER 3609, WAS DISCIPLINED BY OKLAHOMA ON JUNE 18, 1998
DISCIPLINARY ACTION: PROBATION

MAPPES, WILLIAM PATRICK MD, LICENSE NUMBER 0010934, WAS DISCIPLINED BY OKLAHOMA ON JANUARY 16, 1990
DISCIPLINARY ACTION: 6-MONTH LICENSE SUSPENSION; REQUIRED TO ENTER AN IMPAIRED PHYSICIAN PROGRAM OR SUBSTANCE ABUSE TREATMENT
OFFENSE: SUBSTANCE ABUSE

NOTES: ON 9/11/87 PLACED ON TWO DAY SUSPENSION AND ON 9/13/87 PLACED ON FIVE YEAR PROBATION; SINCE 2/23/88 HE HAS CONTINUED A REGULAR PATTERN AND PRACTICE OF HABITUALLY USING VARIOUS CONTROLLED DANGEROUS SUBSTANCES, WHEN PRESCRIBED BY DIFFERENT PHYSICIANS AS DETERMINED BY TESTS OF BODILY FLUIDS. SUSPENSION BEGINNING ON 10/20/89. SHALL MEET WITH THE PHYSICIAN RECOVERY COMMITTEE AND WORK OUT DETAILS FOR A SUCCESSFUL COMPLETION OF IN-PATIENT, SUBSTANCE ABUSE TREATMENT IN A PHYSICIAN-ORIENTED REHABILITATION PROGRAM; UPON SUCCESSFUL COMPLETION OF A REHABILITATION PROGRAM THE BOARD WILL CONSIDER TERMINATION OF THE ORDER AND ALLOW HIM PRACTICE MEDICINE AND SURGERY WITH PROBATION UNDER CERTAIN TERMS AND CONDITIONS.

MAPPES, WILLIAM PATRICK MD, LICENSE NUMBER 0010934 OF 300 UNITED FOUNDERS BLVD, OKLAHOMA CITY, OK, WAS DISCIPLINED BY OKLAHOMA ON SEPTEMBER 27, 1990
DISCIPLINARY ACTION: 60-MONTH PROBATION; RESTRICTION PLACED ON CONTROLLED SUBSTANCE LICENSE
OFFENSE: SUBSTANCE ABUSE

NOTES: REINSTATEMENT FROM SUSPENSION AFTER SUCCESSFUL COMPLETION OF IN-PATIENT, SUBSTANCE ABUSE TREATMENT IN A PHYSICIAN-ORIENTED REHABILITATION PROGRAM. PROBATION BEGINNING 9/01/90 UNDER THE FOLLOWING TERMS AND CONDITIONS: SHALL NOT PRESCRIBE, ADMINISTER, OR DISPENSE ANY MEDICATIONS FOR HIS PERSONAL USE AND SHALL TAKE NONE UNLESS AUTHORIZED BY ANOTHER PHYSICIAN FOR LEGITIMATE MEDICAL NEED; SHALL ABSTAIN FROM CONSUMING ALCOHOL OR ANY SUBSTANCE WHICH WOULD ADVERSELY AFFECT HIS ABILITY TO PRACTICE; MAY PRESCRIBE CONTROLLED DANGEROUS SUBSTANCES ONLY ON SERIALLY NUMBERED, DUPLICATE PRESCRIPTION PADS AND SHALL MAKE THE COPIES AVAILABLE TO THE BOARD UPON REQUEST; SHALL NOT ADMINISTER OR DISPENSE ANY CONTROLLED DANGEROUS

SUBSTANCE; SHALL SUBMIT BIOLOGICAL FLUID SPECIMENS; SHALL CONTINUE UNDER REGULAR, PSYCHIATRIC CARE; SHALL WAIVE THE NORMAL PHYSICIAN/PATIENT CONFIDENTIAL RELATIONSHIP INSOFAR AS AUTHORIZING THE PSYCHIATRIST TO COMMUNICATE RECORDS OF TREATMENT TO THE BOARD; SHALL SUBMIT TO THE BOARD ADDRESS/ CHANGE OF ADDRESS; SHALL APPEAR BEFORE THE BOARD UPON REQUEST AND SUBMIT ANY REQUIRED REPORTS; SHALL PAY COSTS; SHALL NOTIFY ANY HOSPITAL WHERE HE HOLDS STAFF PRIVILEGES, OR CLINIC, OR GROUP WHERE HE PRACTICES OF THE TERMS AND CONDITIONS OF THIS BOARD ORDER AND SUPPLY A COPY THEREOF.

MAPPES, WILLIAM PATRICK MD, LICENSE NUMBER 0010934 OF 3000 UNITED FOUNDERS BLV STE 228, OKLAHOMA CITY, OK, WAS DISCIPLINED BY OKLAHOMA ON OCTOBER 10, 1991
DISCIPLINARY ACTION: LICENSE REVOCATION
OFFENSE: FAILURE TO COMPLY WITH PREVIOUS BOARD ORDER

NOTES: SINCE 9/27/85, HAS CONTINUALLY BEEN UNDER SOME FORM OF PROBATION OR SUSPENSION, AND HAS BEEN IN CONTEMPT OF NUMEROUS BOARD ORDERS AND HAD ADDITIONAL TERMS IMPOSED. SINCE 9/85, HAS CONTINUED PERIODIC USE OF OPIATES, COCAINE AND OTHER CONTROLLED DANGEROUS SUBSTANCES, CONFIRMED BY LAB TESTS, DESPITE BOARD ORDERS PROHIBITING THEIR USAGE. PROBLEM PERSISTS DESPITE ATTEMPTS AT DIFFERENT TREATMENT REGIMENS. LICENSE SUSPENDED 6/21/91 FOR SIX MONTHS FOLLOWED BY FIVE YEARS PROBATION. AT THE HEARING, NOTED THAT HE HAD SUFFERED RELAPSE OF SUBSTANCE ABUSE AND WAS IN TREATMENT. SINCE THAT DATE, HE HAS ADMITTED THAT HE IS NOT "COMFORTABLE WITH HIS LEVEL OF SOBRIETY" AND IS NOT READY TO RE-ENTER PRACTICE. SINCE 10/87, HAS INCURRED $4,234.99 IN FEES OWED BOARD, WHICH HE HAS NOT PAID.

MARTIN, JIMMY C MD OF 4100 EAST 51ST STREET SUITE 110, TULSA, OK, WAS DISCIPLINED BY DEA ON JANUARY 24, 1995
DISCIPLINARY ACTION: RESTRICTION PLACED ON CONTROLLED SUBSTANCE LICENSE
OFFENSE: PROFESSIONAL MISCONDUCT

NOTES: PAST ALLEGED CONTROLLED SUBSTANCE VIOLATIONS.

MASSAD, DALE G MD, LICENSE NUMBER 0030749 OF CORAL GABLES, FL, WAS DISCIPLINED BY FLORIDA ON DECEMBER 10, 1992
DISCIPLINARY ACTION: SURRENDER OF LICENSE
OFFENSE: SUBSTANDARD CARE, INCOMPETENCE OR NEGLIGENCE

NOTES: CHARGED WITH FAILING TO PRACTICE MEDICINE WITH AN ACCEPTABLE LEVEL OF CARE AND SKILL; FAILING TO KEEP MEDICAL RECORDS JUSTIFYING THE COURSE OF TREATMENT OF A PATIENT; PERFORMING ANY PROCEDURE OR PRESCRIBING ANY THERAPY WHICH, BY THE PREVAILING STANDARDS OF MEDICAL PRACTICE IN THE COMMUNITY, WOULD CONSTITUTE EXPERIMENTATION ON A HUMAN SUBJECT, WITHOUT FIRST OBTAINING FULL, INFORMED AND WRITTEN CONSENT; DELEGATING PROFESSIONAL RESPONSIBILITIES TO A PERSON WHOM HE KNEW OR HAD REASON TO KNOW IS NOT QUALIFIED BY TRAINING, EXPERIENCE, OR LICENSURE TO PERFORM THEM. IN LIEU OF FURTHER PROSECUTION, ACCEPTED A VOLUNTARY RELINQUISHMENT OF LICENSE AND AGREED NEVER AGAIN TO APPLY FOR LICENSURE IN FLORIDA.

MASSAD, DALE GLEN MD, WAS DISCIPLINED BY OKLAHOMA ON MAY 20, 1993
DISCIPLINARY ACTION: DENIAL OF NEW LICENSE
OFFENSE: SUBSTANDARD CARE, INCOMPETENCE OR NEGLIGENCE

NOTES: FLORIDA BOARD FILED A COMPLAINT AGAINST HIM ARISING OUT OF THE DEATH OF A THREE YEAR OLD PATIENT FOLLOWING SURGICAL PROCEDURE IN LIDOCAINE DENTAL BLOCK ADMINISTERED BY A DENTIST; INCIDENT INDICATES HE FAILED TO DEMONSTRATE ADEQUATE MEDICAL KNOWLEDGE AND JUDGMENT.

MCCALL, VICTOR EUGENE MD, LICENSE NUMBER 00D3509 OF DUNCANVILLE, TX, WAS DISCIPLINED BY TEXAS ON FEBRUARY 22, 1991
DISCIPLINARY ACTION: 120-MONTH PROBATION; REQUIRED TO TAKE ADDITIONAL MEDICAL EDUCATION

NOTES: MUST COMPLETE COURSE IN GENERAL PHARMACOLOGY; COMPLETE COURSE IN ADVANCED CARDIAC LIFE SUPPORT; RESEARCH AND WRITE A PAPER SUITABLE FOR PUBLICATION REGARDING RADIOLOGICAL TECHNICIANS AND THE PROCEDURES OR TREATMENTS THAT CAN BE DELEGATED FROM A PHYSICIAN TO A TECHNICIAN; MAINTAIN ADEQUATE MEDICAL RECORDS FOR A RADIOLOGIST ON ALL PATIENT OFFICE VISITS; ADEQUATELY SUPERVISE ALL "EMPLOYEES OR DELEGATES"; APPEAR FOR SEMIANNUAL REPORTS TO BOARD. ON 11/3/94 PROBATION TERMINATED.

MCCALL, VICTOR EUGENE MD, LICENSE NUMBER 0015667 OF 6236 INDIAN CREEK DRIVE, FORT WORTH, TX, WAS DISCIPLINED BY OKLAHOMA ON SEPTEMBER 9, 1994
DISCIPLINARY ACTION: 60-MONTH PROBATION; MONITORING OF PHYSICIAN PERFORMANCE
OFFENSE: DISCIPLINARY ACTION BY ANOTHER STATE OR AGENCY

NOTES: ON 2/22/91 THE TEXAS BOARD ISSUED AN ORDER PLACING LICENSE ON PROBATION FOR 10 YEARS WITH CONDITIONS FOR DELEGATING TO A RADIOLOGIC TECHNICIAN THE RESPONSIBILITY FOR CALCULATING A DOSAGE FOR CHLORAL HYDRATE WHICH WAS INCORRECTLY CALCULATED AND LED TO THE DEATH OF THE PATIENT. EXPECTS TEXAS TO VACATE ITS ORDER; AGREES TO SUBMIT TO PROBATION IN OKLAHOMA. CONDITIONS OF PROBATION: SHALL PROVIDE THE BOARD WITH ANY DOCUMENTATION REQUESTED RELATED TO HIS PRACTICE AND SHALL PAY COSTS.

MCCANN, BERYL DR OF DURANT, OK, WAS DISCIPLINED BY ILLINOIS ON JULY 1, 1994
DISCIPLINARY ACTION: LICENSE SUSPENSION
OFFENSE: DISCIPLINARY ACTION BY ANOTHER STATE OR AGENCY

NOTES: DISCIPLINED IN OKLAHOMA. INDEFINITE SUSPENSION.

MCCORMICK, MICHAEL B MD OF 920 STANTON L. YOUNG RM 920BMS, OKLAHOMA CITY, OK, WAS DISCIPLINED BY DEA ON APRIL 7, 1995
DISCIPLINARY ACTION: RESTRICTION PLACED ON CONTROLLED SUBSTANCE LICENSE
OFFENSE: CRIMINAL CONVICTION OR PLEA OF GUILTY, NOLO CONTENDERE, OR NO CONTEST TO A CRIME

NOTES: CONTROLLED SUBSTANCE CONVICTION.

MCCORMICK, MICHAEL W B MD, DATE OF BIRTH MARCH 17, 1952, LICENSE NUMBER 0026445 OF 2825 GETTYSBURG, EDMOND, OK, WAS DISCIPLINED BY IOWA ON APRIL 6, 1990
DISCIPLINARY ACTION: 39-MONTH PROBATION

NOTES: ON 11/15/91, AMENDMENT TO CURRENT PROBATION; ALLOWED TO POSSESS TWO SYRINGES OF DIAZEPAM, AS PART OF A BANYAN STAT KIT. EFFECTIVE 11/29/93 PROBATION TERMINATED AND MEDICAL LICENSE RESTORED TO FULL PRIVILEGES.

MCCORMICK, MICHAEL W BYRON MD, LICENSE NUMBER 0011875 OF 1108 11TH AVE, DEWITT, IA, WAS DISCIPLINED BY OKLAHOMA ON OCTOBER 5, 1991
DISCIPLINARY ACTION: 24-MONTH PROBATION; MONITORING OF PHYSICIAN PERFORMANCE

NOTES: FOLLOWING FEDERAL INCARCERATION HIS LICENSE WAS SUSPENDED ON 1/18/85 FOR THE PERIOD OF HIS INCARCERATION; WHEN HE WAS RELEASED, LICENSE REINSTATED TO FIVE YEAR PROBATION; PROBATION ENDED ON 1/22/88; LICENSE LAPSED BECAUSE OF NONRENEWAL; NOW WANTS TO SEEK TRAINING IN PATHOLOGY. PROBATION WITH FOLLOWING CONDITIONS: SHALL NOT PRESCRIBE, ADMINISTER OR DISPENSE ANY SCHEDULED DRUGS OR CONTROLLED DANGEROUS SUBSTANCES FOR HIS PERSONAL USE OR FOR OTHERS; SHALL NOTIFY ANY HOSPITAL WHERE HE HOLDS STAFF PRIVILEGES OR CLINIC OR GROUP OF THESE TERMS AND CONDITIONS; SHALL BE MONITORED ON PROFESSIONAL ACTIVITIES ON LEVEL III PROBATION; SHALL FURNISH BOARD WITH ADDRESS AND/OR CHANGE OF ADDRESS; SHALL APPEAR BEFORE BOARD UPON REQUEST.

MCCORMICK, MICHAEL W B MD, DATE OF BIRTH MARCH 17, 1952, LICENSE NUMBER 0004383 OF 1108 11TH STREET, DEWITT, IA, WAS DISCIPLINED BY MONTANA ON DECEMBER 31, 1991
DISCIPLINARY ACTION: FINE
OFFENSE: NONCOMPLIANCE WITH A PROFESSIONAL RULE

NOTES: FAILED TO DISCLOSE IOWA DISCIPLINARY ACTION ON 1991 MONTANA RENEWAL APPLICATION. LETTER OF CENSURE. AGREED HE WILL NOT SEEK RENEWAL OF MONTANA LICENSE IN 1992 OR THEREAFTER, NOR REAPPLY OR SEEK REINSTATEMENT OF LICENSE. $500 FINE.

MCCORMICK, MICHAEL W B MD OF 920 STANTON L. YOUNG RM. 920 BMS, OKLAHOMA CITY, OK, WAS DISCIPLINED BY DEA ON FEBRUARY 1, 1994
DISCIPLINARY ACTION: RESTRICTION PLACED ON CONTROLLED SUBSTANCE LICENSE
OFFENSE: CRIMINAL CONVICTION OR PLEA OF GUILTY, NOLO CONTENDERE, OR NO CONTEST TO A CRIME

NOTES: CONVICTED 11/19/84 FOR KNOWINGLY AND INTENTIONALLY OMITTING MATERIAL INFORMATION FROM WRITTEN PRESCRIPTION FOR DILAUDID. RESTRICTION PLACED ON REGISTRATION. REGISTRATION PLACED ON PROBATION 04/06/90. FINED. IN 11/09/93 HEARING IN OKLAHOMA REGARDING FELONY COCAINE CONVICTION IN 1984, WAS PLACED ON PROBATION ENDING 11/9/94.

MCDANIEL, JOSEPH C MD, LICENSE NUMBER 0014623 OF 2327 NW NOTTINGHAM ROAD, LAWTON, OK, WAS DISCIPLINED BY OKLAHOMA ON MARCH 28, 1996
OFFENSE: OVERPRESCRIBING OR MISPRESCRIBING DRUGS

NOTES: THE BOARD ISSUED A LETTER OF CONCERN LISTING THE FOLLOWING CONCERNS: RECORD KEEPING INCLUDING THE NOTATION OF APPROPRIATE PHYSICAL EXAMINATION AND LABORATORY DATA OBTAINED ON THE PATIENT; THE EXTENT OF NARCOTICS ADMINISTRATION BOTH IN THE OFFICE AND THROUGH PRESCRIPTION WRITING; PATIENT COUNSELING ABOUT MEDICAL SIDE-EFFECTS OF THE MEDICATIONS PRESCRIBED; BETTER COMMUNICATION WITH CONSULTANTS.

MCINNIS, ALICE E MD, LICENSE NUMBER 11880, WAS DISCIPLINED BY OKLAHOMA ON JULY 10, 1997
DISCIPLINARY ACTION: 60-MONTH PROBATION; RESTRICTION PLACED ON LICENSE
OFFENSE: PHYSICAL OR MENTAL ILLNESS INHIBITING THE ABILITY TO PRACTICE WITH SKILL AND SAFETY

NOTES: FROM ABOUT 11/95 THROUGH 5/96 SHE SUFFERED FROM AND WAS DIAGNOSED WITH MANIC/DEPRESSIVE, BIPOLAR MENTAL ILLNESS WHICH MANIFESTED ITSELF IN BEHAVIOR INDICATIVE OF IMPAIRMENT AT HER FAMILY PRACTICE RESIDENCY PROGRAM AND AT SPECIFIED MEDICAL CENTERS AND CLINICS. CONDITIONS OF PROBATION: SHALL NOT PRACTICE MORE THAN 40 HOURS PER WEEK NOR PRACTICE AT NIGHT; SHALL WORK WITH A MENTOR; SHALL REGULARLY RECEIVE PSYCHIATRIC TREATMENT WITH MONTHLY REPORTS TO THE BOARD FOR THE FIRST SIX MONTHS OF THIS PROBATIONARY TERM. AND AFTER THAT AT THE DISCRETION OF THE BOARD; THE MENTOR WILL PROVIDE REPORTS TO THE BOARD ON A SIMILAR SCHEDULE; SHALL SUBMIT TO MONTHLY MEDICATION LEVEL TESTING; WILL NOTIFY THE BOARD OF ANY CHANGE IN TREATING PHYSICIANS, MENTORS, OR PLACE OF EMPLOYMENT; BOARD SHALL BE ALLOWED TO CONFER WITH THE MENTOR AT ITS DISCRETION; SHALL KEEP THE BOARD INFORMED OF HER ADDRESS AND PAY COSTS; SHALL APPEAR BEFORE THE BOARD AND SUBMIT REPORTS UPON REQUEST. ON 3/12/99 PROBATION TERMINATED.

MCKENZIE, STEVE LEWIS DO, WAS DISCIPLINED BY OKLAHOMA ON DECEMBER 8, 1994
DISCIPLINARY ACTION: DENIAL OF NEW LICENSE
OFFENSE: PHYSICAL OR MENTAL ILLNESS INHIBITING THE ABILITY TO PRACTICE WITH SKILL AND SAFETY

NOTES: ENGAGED IN UNPROFESSIONAL CONDUCT IN THE FORM OF PERSONAL OFFENSIVE BEHAVIOR, INCLUDING OBSCENITY, AND HE IS INCAPABLE, FOR MEDICAL OR PSYCHIATRIC CAUSES, OF DISCHARGING THE FUNCTIONS OF AN OSTEOPATHIC PHYSICIAN IN A MANNER CONSISTENT WITH THE PUBLIC'S HEALTH, SAFETY, AND WELFARE.

MCKNIGHT, MARTHA ANNE MD OF CHARLOTTE, NC, WAS DISCIPLINED BY NORTH CAROLINA ON JANUARY 27, 1990
DISCIPLINARY ACTION: LICENSE REINSTATEMENT; SURRENDER OF LICENSE

NOTES: ON 2/12/90 CONSENT ORDER, UNSPECIFIED. LICENSE SURRENDERED, TEMPORARY LICENSE ISSUED.

MCKNIGHT, MARTHA ANNE MD OF DOROTHEA DIX HOSPITAL, RALEIGH, NC, WAS DISCIPLINED BY DEA ON MARCH 8, 1990
DISCIPLINARY ACTION: SURRENDER OF CONTROLLED SUBSTANCE LICENSE
OFFENSE: SUBSTANCE ABUSE

NOTES: SURRENDER OF REGISTRATION DUE TO ABUSE OF XANAX, 01/27/90, AND ISSUED ONE YEAR TEMPORARY LICENSE LIMITED TO EMPLOYER. RESTRICTED PER MEMORANDUM OF AGREEMENT IN LIEU OF PUBLIC INTEREST SHOW CAUSE PROCEEDINGS.

MCKNIGHT, MARTHA ANNE MD, LICENSE NUMBER 0017877 OF OKLAHOMA CITY, OK, WAS DISCIPLINED BY OKLAHOMA ON

OCTOBER 10, 1991
DISCIPLINARY ACTION: RESTRICTION PLACED ON LICENSE; MONITORING OF PHYSICIAN PERFORMANCE

NOTES: APPLICATION FOR LICENSURE GRANTED. TO CONTINUE ON FIVE YEAR PROBATION BEGUN 7/12/91 UNDER TERMS AND CONDITIONS: SHALL NOT PRESCRIBE, ADMINISTER OR DISPENSE ANY MEDICATIONS FOR HER PERSONAL USE; SHALL TAKE NO MEDICATION UNLESS AUTHORIZED BY TREATING PHYSICIAN; SHALL ABSTAIN FROM ALCOHOL OR ANY SUBSTANCE WHICH WOULD ADVERSELY AFFECT HER ABILITY TO PRACTICE; SHALL SUBMIT BIOLOGICAL FLUID SPECIMENS FOR ANALYSIS; SHALL PARTICIPATE ACTIVELY WITH PHYSICIAN RECOVERY COMMITTEE; SHALL FURNISH BOARD WITH ADDRESS AND/OR CHANGE OF ADDRESS; SHALL APPEAR BEFORE BOARD UPON REQUEST; SHALL NOTIFY ANY HOSPITAL WHERE SHE HOLDS STAFF PRIVILEGES OR CLINIC OR GROUP OF THE TERMS AND CONDITIONS; MAY NOT FUNCTION AS A SUPERVISING PHYSICIAN FOR ANY PHYSICIAN'S ASSISTANT.

MCKNIGHT, MARTHA ANNE MD, LICENSE NUMBER 0017877, WAS DISCIPLINED BY OKLAHOMA ON MARCH 5, 1992
DISCIPLINARY ACTION: EMERGENCY SUSPENSION
OFFENSE: LOSS OR RESTRICTION OF HOSPITAL PRIVILEGES

NOTES: AGREED TO FIVE YEAR PROBATION ON 07/12/91. ON 01/10/92 RELIEVED OF DUTIES AT UNIVERSITY OF OKLAHOMA COLLEGE OF MEDICINE. VOLUNTARILY ADMITTED HERSELF TO THE CARE OF BOARD-CERTIFIED PSYCHIATRIST AND ADDICTIONOLOGIST WHO DOES NOT "FEEL COMFORTABLE IN RETURNING HER TO WORK."

MCKNIGHT, MARTHA ANNE MD, DATE OF BIRTH SEPTEMBER 29, 1955, LICENSE NUMBER 0026571 OF CHARLOTTE, NC, WAS DISCIPLINED BY NORTH CAROLINA ON APRIL 19, 1997
DISCIPLINARY ACTION: SURRENDER OF LICENSE

NOTES: VOLUNTARY SURRENDER OF LICENSE. ON 5/21/99, FULL AND UNRESTRICTED LICENSE REINSTATED.

MCKNIGHT, MARTHA ANNE MD OF 3621 RANDOLPH ROAD, CHARLOTTE, NC, WAS DISCIPLINED BY DEA ON AUGUST 22, 1997
DISCIPLINARY ACTION: SURRENDER OF CONTROLLED SUBSTANCE LICENSE

NOTES: IN LIEU OF PUBLIC INTEREST REVOCATION.

MEDCALF, WINFRED L MD, LICENSE NUMBER 0007115, WAS DISCIPLINED BY OKLAHOMA ON NOVEMBER 15, 1990
DISCIPLINARY ACTION: 36-MONTH PROBATION; RESTRICTION PLACED ON CONTROLLED SUBSTANCE LICENSE

NOTES: PROBATION BEGINNING 10/27/90 UNDER THE FOLLOWING TERMS AND CONDITIONS: SHALL PRESCRIBE CONTROLLED DANGEROUS SUBSTANCES ONLY ON SERIALLY-NUMBERED, DUPLICATE PRESCRIPTION PADS AND SHALL MAKE THE COPIES AVAILABLE TO THE BOARD UPON REQUEST; SHALL DOCUMENT IN PATIENT RECORDS HIS EFFORTS TO RE-ESTABLISH A DIAGNOSIS IN WRITING ON AN ANNUAL BASIS, BUT NOT NECESSARILY INCLUDE LABORATORY WORK ON AN ANNUAL BASIS; SHALL DOCUMENT IN PATIENT CHARTS HIS EFFORTS TO CHANGE THE PATIENT'S MEDICATION FROM CONTROLLED DANGEROUS SUBSTANCES TO NON-CONTROLLED DANGEROUS SUBSTANCES; ANYTIME HE PRESCRIBES CONTROLLED DANGEROUS SUBSTANCES IN EXCESS OF FOUR DOSES WITHIN 24 HOURS IT MUST BE STRICTLY BASED ON THE PATIENT'S DOCUMENTED NEED FOR THE MEDICATION AND HE SHOULD DOCUMENT HIS ADVICE TO THE PATIENT CONCERNING RISKS OF MEDICATION AND POSSIBLE NON-CONTROLLED PHARMACEUTICAL AGENTS AS ALTERNATIVES; SHALL SUBMIT TO THE BOARD ADDRESS/CHANGE OF ADDRESS; SHALL APPEAR BEFORE THE BOARD UPON REQUEST AND SUBMIT REQUIRED REPORTS; SHALL PAY COSTS; WILL RECEIVE EDUCATION FROM THE BOARD ON STANDARDS FOR PRESCRIPTION WRITING.

METCALF, JOE DAN MD, LICENSE NUMBER 0008629 OF 2610 NW EXPRESSWAY #B, OKLAHOMA CITY, OK, WAS DISCIPLINED BY OKLAHOMA ON DECEMBER 11, 1996
DISCIPLINARY ACTION: 12-MONTH LICENSE SUSPENSION; 60-MONTH PROBATION
OFFENSE: CRIMINAL CONVICTION OR PLEA OF GUILTY, NOLO CONTENDERE, OR NO CONTEST TO A CRIME

NOTES: ON 11/13/95 PLED GUILTY TO INTERSTATE COMMERCE VIOLATION, A FELONY; ON 3/05/96 FINED $5,000.00 PAYABLE TO THE U.S. GOVERNMENT AND SENTENCED TO SIX MONTHS IN FEDERAL PRISON BEGINNING 4/05/96. ONE YEAR SUSPENSION AFTER HIS RELEASE FROM INCARCERATION. DURING HIS PROBATION, A RANDOM SELECTION OF HIS PATIENT RECORDS SHALL BE REVIEWED BY THE BOARD ON A QUARTERLY BASIS; SHALL PROVIDE THE BOARD WITH ANY REQUESTED REPORTS; SHALL KEEP THE BOARD INFORMED OF HIS CURRENT ADDRESS; SHALL KEEP CURRENT PAYMENT OF PROSECUTION, INVESTIGATION, AND MONITORING OF HIS CASE; AND SHALL FURNISH EACH STATE IN WHICH HE HOLDS OR APPLIES FOR LICENSURE AND ANY HEALTH CARE ENTITY WHERE HE HAS PRIVILEGES WITH A COPY OF THIS ORDER.

MEYER, PHILIP J DO, DATE OF BIRTH MARCH 25, 1952, LICENSE NUMBER 0001756 OF 1200 N 7TH STREET, CHARITON, IA, WAS DISCIPLINED BY IOWA ON DECEMBER 21, 1992
DISCIPLINARY ACTION: 48-MONTH PROBATION
OFFENSE: PROFESSIONAL MISCONDUCT

NOTES: ALLEGED UNLAWFUL POSSESSION AND USE OF MARIJUANA.

MEYER, PHILIP J DO, WAS DISCIPLINED BY OKLAHOMA ON JULY 2, 1993
DISCIPLINARY ACTION: 48-MONTH PROBATION; MONITORING OF PHYSICIAN PERFORMANCE
OFFENSE: DISCIPLINARY ACTION BY ANOTHER STATE OR AGENCY

NOTES: PROBATIONARY ACTION IN IOWA. LICENSE ISSUED IN OKLAHOMA ON PROBATION UNDER CONDITIONS: MAY PETITION THE BOARD FOR TERMINATION PRIOR TO THE EXPIRATION DATE; SHALL PARTICIPATE IN THE PHYSICIAN'S RECOVERY PROGRAM AND ATTEND AT LEAST ONE MEETING PER WEEK; SHALL ATTEND THREE AA AND/OR NARCOTICS ANONYMOUS MEETINGS EACH WEEK; SHALL ABSTAIN FROM THE USE OF ALCOHOL; SHALL NOT POSSESS OR USE ANY CONTROLLED OR PRESCRIPTION DRUG IN ANY FORM UNLESS PRESCRIBED FOR HIM BY A TREATING PHYSICIAN, OR OTHER QUALIFIED MEDICAL PRACTITIONER; NOTHING IN THIS ORDER SHALL BE CONSTRUED TO PROHIBIT HIM FROM ADMINISTERING MEDICATION TO HIS DAUGHTER THAT HAS BEEN PRESCRIBED FOR HER BY ANOTHER TREATING PHYSICIAN; SHALL SUBMIT TO WITNESSED BLOOD OR URINE SAMPLES; SHALL SUBMIT QUARTERLY REPORTS UNDER PENALTY OF PERJURY STATING THAT THERE HAS BEEN COMPLIANCE WITH THE CONDITIONS OF THIS ORDER; SHALL MAKE ANNUAL APPEARANCES AND/OR UPON REQUEST BEFORE THE

BOARD. PROBATIONARY PERIOD TERMINATED ON 12/08/94.

MEYER, PHILIP J DO, DATE OF BIRTH MARCH 25, 1952, LICENSE NUMBER 0036774 OF 1200 EAST PECAN, ALTUS, OK, WAS DISCIPLINED BY NEW JERSEY ON APRIL 19, 1994
DISCIPLINARY ACTION: 48-MONTH PROBATION
OFFENSE: SUBSTANCE ABUSE

NOTES: SHALL NOT COMMENCE THE ACTIVE PRACTICE OF MEDICINE UNTIL HE HAS COMPLIED WITH ALL REQUIREMENTS EMBODIED IN THE ORDER FILED BY THE IOWA BOARD OF MEDICAL EXAMINERS AND UNTIL HE APPEARS FOR A STATUS CONFERENCE BEFORE A COMMITTEE OF THIS BOARD. PROBATION RETROACTIVE TO 12/21/92.

MILES, PATRICK KELLY DO, LICENSE NUMBER 00D8037 OF ABELINE, TX, WAS DISCIPLINED BY TEXAS ON OCTOBER 27, 1993
DISCIPLINARY ACTION: EMERGENCY SUSPENSION
OFFENSE: PHYSICAL OR MENTAL ILLNESS INHIBITING THE ABILITY TO PRACTICE WITH SKILL AND SAFETY

NOTES: HISTORICALLY SUFFERS FROM CONFIRMED BIPOLAR DISORDER AND PROBABLE CYCLOTHYMIC DISORDER WHICH IS NOT ADEQUATELY CONTROLLED AS REPRESENTED BY BEHAVIORS AND ACTIVITIES INCLUDING THE FOLLOWING: ON 9/16/93 ATTEMPTED TO HAVE A PATIENT RELEASED WHO HAD BEEN INVOLUNTARILY COMMITTED TO A STATE HOSPITAL BECAUSE OF A CASE INVOLVING THE CHARGE OF MURDER AGAINST THE PATIENT; FROM INVOLUNTARY COMMITMENT BECAUSE OF A CASE INVOLVING MURDER; FALSE REPRESENTATIONS TO MEMBERS OF THE MEDICAL COMMUNITY AND OTHERS REGARDING HIS PROFESSIONAL EXPERIENCE AND ASSOCIATIONS; REPRESENTATIONS TO MEMBERS OF THE MEDICAL COMMUNITY WHICH DEMONSTRATE FAILURE TO MAINTAIN ADEQUATE BOUNDARIES IN PHYSICIAN-PATIENT RELATIONSHIPS; EXTREME AND INAPPROPRIATE REACTION TO NORMAL EVENTS AND CIRCUMSTANCES.

MILES, PATRICK KELLY DO, LICENSE NUMBER 00D8037 OF ABILENE, TX, WAS DISCIPLINED BY TEXAS ON MARCH 5, 1994
DISCIPLINARY ACTION: 60-MONTH PROBATION; RESTRICTION PLACED ON LICENSE
OFFENSE: PHYSICAL OR MENTAL ILLNESS INHIBITING THE ABILITY TO PRACTICE WITH SKILL AND SAFETY

NOTES: AFTER 10/27/93 EMERGENCY SUSPENSION, HE WAS EVALUATED BY A BOARD APPROVED PSYCHIATRIST ON 1/26/94 WHO MADE A DIAGNOSIS OF AN ATYPICAL CYCLOTHYMIA AND SIGNIFICANT ANXIETY BUT FELT THAT DR. MILES' CONDITION DID NOT PREVENT HIM FROM PRACTICING ALTHOUGH WITH RESTRICTIONS. FIVE YEAR SUSPENSION STAYED. CONDITIONS OF PROBATION: PRACTICE RESTRICTED TO THAT ASSOCIATED WITH A BOARD-APPROVED INSTITUTIONAL OR RESEARCH SETTING; SUPERVISOR WILL MAKE QUARTERLY REPORTS TO THE BOARD; SHALL CONTINUE TO RECEIVE TREATMENT FROM A PSYCHIATRIST WITH QUARTERLY REPORTS; SHALL APPEAR BEFORE THE BOARD ONCE A YEAR; SHALL GIVE A COPY OF THIS ORDER TO ANY HEALTH CARE ENTITY WHERE HE HAS PRIVILEGES; SHALL COOPERATE WITH THE BOARD IN VERIFYING COMPLIANCE; SHALL INFORM BOARD OF CHANGE OF ADDRESS WITHIN 10 DAYS OR IF HE LEAVES THE STATE; TIME SPENT OUT OF TEXAS DOES NOT COUNT TOWARD PROBATION. SHALL NOT SEEK MODIFICATION FOR ONE YEAR. ON 2/7/98 PETITION TO TERMINATE ORDER DENIED.

MILES, PATRICK KELLY DO, LICENSE NUMBER 0001579, WAS DISCIPLINED BY OKLAHOMA ON MARCH 17, 1994
DISCIPLINARY ACTION: 60-MONTH PROBATION; RESTRICTION PLACED ON LICENSE
OFFENSE: DISCIPLINARY ACTION BY ANOTHER STATE OR AGENCY

NOTES: ON 3/05/94 TEXAS LICENSE SANCTIONED WITH FIVE YEAR SUSPENSION STAYED AS PROBATION. IN OKLAHOMA FIVE YEAR SUSPENSION, STAYED AS PROBATION: SHALL NOT PETITION THE BOARD FOR MODIFICATION FOR AT LEAST ONE YEAR; SHALL SUBMIT TO PSYCHIATRIC EVALUATION AND TREATMENT, SHALL COMPLY WITH SAID PSYCHIATRIST'S RECOMMENDATIONS, IF ANY, REGARDING CONTINUING CARE AND TREATMENT, AND SHALL FURNISH THE BOARD WITH A COPY OF THESE RECOMMENDATIONS AND AUTHORIZE THE PSYCHIATRIST TO MAKE REPORTS TO THE BOARD; HIS PRACTICE SHALL BE RESTRICTED TO A BOARD APPROVED INSTITUTION OR RESEARCH SETTING UNDER THE SUPERVISION OF THE A MEDICAL DIRECTOR WHO SHALL MAKE QUARTERLY REPORTS; SHALL FURNISH THE BOARD WITH WRITTEN REPORTS REGARDING HIS MEDICAL CONDITION AND COMPLIANCE WITH THIS ORDER; SHALL NOTIFY THE BOARD IN WRITING OF ANY CHANGE OF ADDRESS, EMPLOYMENT, EMPLOYMENT TERMINATION OR HOSPITAL PRIVILEGE RESTRICTION AND ANY ADMINISTRATIVE PROCEEDING INITIATED AGAINST HIM BY ANY OTHER STATE OR FEDERAL REGULATORY BODY WITHIN 14 DAYS; SHALL APPEAR BEFORE THE BOARD UPON REQUEST; AGREES TO RANDOM, UNANNOUNCED VISITS FROM THE BOARD FOR OBSERVATION AND ACCESS TO ANY APPROPRIATE RECORDS, HOWEVER, THESE VISITS WILL NOT INTERRUPT HIS MEDICAL SERVICES; THE TIME PERIOD OF PROBATION SHALL NOT INCLUDE ANY PERIODS OF RESIDENCE OR PRACTICE OUTSIDE OF OKLAHOMA; SHALL INFORM THE BOARD IF HE LEAVES OKLAHOMA. ADMINISTRATIVE COSTS $435.

MILLER, DAVID DOW MD, LICENSE NUMBER 0012785, WAS DISCIPLINED BY OKLAHOMA ON DECEMBER 4, 1992
DISCIPLINARY ACTION: EMERGENCY SUSPENSION
OFFENSE: SUBSTANCE ABUSE

NOTES: ON 9/1/92, DELIVERED 1/8 OUNCE OF MARIJUANA TO UNDERCOVER AGENT OF OKLAHOMA BUREAU OF NARCOTICS AND DANGEROUS DRUGS. ON 10/1/92, SURRENDERED 2-3 OUNCES OF MARIJUANA TO AGENT. ADMITTED PREVIOUS POSSESSION OF MARIJUANA, USE OF THE DRUG SINCE COLLEGE, AND THAT HE HAD A PROBLEM WITH IT. IN 10/92, VOLUNTARILY CEASED RENDERING MEDICAL SERVICES TO ANY PATIENTS AND ADMITTED HIMSELF TO IN-PATIENT EVALUATION AND TREATMENT WHERE HE IS TO-DATE. NO EVIDENCE AS TO ANY DIRECT PATIENT HARM CAUSED BY HIS DRUG USE. ON 1/15/93 SUSPENSION EXTENDED UNTIL NEXT BOARD MEETING OF 2/27/93.

MILLER, DAVID DOW MD, LICENSE NUMBER 0012785, WAS DISCIPLINED BY OKLAHOMA ON MAY 20, 1993
DISCIPLINARY ACTION: 60-MONTH PROBATION; RESTRICTION PLACED ON LICENSE

NOTES: IN COMPLIANCE WITH 11/21/92 ORDER PRESENTED EVIDENCE OF COMPLETION OF INPATIENT TREATMENT AND PARTICIPATION IN THE PHYSICIAN RECOVERY COMMITTEE. LICENSE REINSTATED FROM SUSPENSION. CONDITIONS OF PROBATION: SHALL NOT PRESCRIBE, ADMINISTER OR DISPENSE ANY MEDICATIONS FOR HIS PERSONAL USE NOR TAKE ANY

EXCEPT THAT WHICH IS AUTHORIZED BY A TREATING PHYSICIAN FOR LEGITIMATE MEDICAL NEED; SHALL ABSTAIN FROM CONSUMING ALCOHOL OR ANY SUBSTANCE WHICH WOULD ADVERSELY AFFECT HIS ABILITY TO PRACTICE; SHALL SUBMIT BIOLOGICAL FLUID SPECIMENS UPON REQUEST; SHALL PROVIDE PROOF OF PARTICIPATION IN PHYSICIAN RECOVERY COMMITTEE AND NARCOTICS ANONYMOUS AND/OR AA; SHALL COOPERATE WITH THE BOARD WITH INTERVIEWS AND EVALUATIONS AND APPEAR BEFORE THEM WHEN REQUESTED; SHALL FURNISH BOARD WITH ADDRESS AND/OR CHANGE OF ADDRESS AND ANY REQUESTED REPORTS AND FORMS; SHALL NOT SUPERVISE PHYSICIANS' ASSISTANTS; SHALL SUPPLY A COPY OF THIS ORDER TO ANY HEALTH CARE ENTITY WHERE HE HAS PRIVILEGES.

MILLER, DAVID DOW MD OF BARTLESVILLE, OK, WAS DISCIPLINED BY DEA ON NOVEMBER 24, 1995
DISCIPLINARY ACTION: 36-MONTH RESTRICTION PLACED ON CONTROLLED SUBSTANCE LICENSE; MONITORING OF PHYSICIAN PERFORMANCE
OFFENSE: CRIMINAL CONVICTION OR PLEA OF GUILTY, NOLO CONTENDERE, OR NO CONTEST TO A CRIME

NOTES: ON 10/14/92 HE ENTERED A PLEA OF NOLO CONTENDERE TO A FELONY CHARGE OF UNLAWFUL DISTRIBUTION OF A CONTROLLED DANGEROUS SUBSTANCE-MARIJUANA, PLACING HIM ON FIVE YEAR PROBATION; ON 12/3/92 THE OKLAHOMA BOARD SUSPENDED HIS LICENSE TO PRACTICE MEDICINE, AND ON 2/8/93 PLACED HIM ON FIVE YEAR PROBATION; SURRENDERED PREVIOUS DEA CERTIFICATE ON 1/93. ACKNOWLEDGED HIS LONG-TERM SUBSTANCE ABUSE PROBLEM IN 1992; HAS SOUGHT IN-PATIENT TREATMENT AND LONG-TERM FOLLOW-ON OUTPATIENT TREATMENT OF HIS PROBLEM; SINCE 4/93 NO ADVERSE REPORTS HAVE BEEN SUBMITTED CONCERNING HIS QUALITY OF CARE. DEA REGISTRATION WITH THE FOLLOWING LIMITATIONS: HIS CONTROLLED SUBSTANCE HANDLING AUTHORITY SHALL BE LIMITED TO THE WRITING OF PRESCRIPTIONS ONLY; SHALL NOT DISPENSE, POSSESS, OR STORE ANY CONTROLLED SUBSTANCES, EXCEPT HE MAY ADMINISTER CONTROLLED SUBSTANCES IN A HOSPITAL AND MAY POSSESS CONTROLLED SUBSTANCES WHICH ARE MEDICALLY NECESSARY FOR HIS OWN USE AND WHICH HE HAS OBTAINED FROM ANOTHER LICENSED PRACTITIONER; SHALL NOT PRESCRIBE ANY CONTROLLED SUBSTANCES FOR HIS OWN USE; SHALL MAINTAIN A LOG RECORDING PRESCRIPTIONS WRITTEN WHICH SHALL BE MADE AVAILABLE FOR INSPECTION; SHALL COMPLY WITH CONDITIONS IMPOSED BY OKLAHOMA UNTIL REMOVED; UNTIL THE OKLAHOMA BOARD TERMINATES HIS PROBATIONARY PERIOD ON HIS MEDICAL LICENSE, HE SHALL SUBMIT, UPON DEA REQUEST, COPIES OF THE RESULTS OF HIS RANDOM URINE OR BLOOD SCREENING TESTS.

MILLER, SUSAN M DO, DATE OF BIRTH FEBRUARY 3, 1949 OF 1435 41ST STREET, TULSA, OK, WAS DISCIPLINED BY MEDICARE ON APRIL 16, 1994
DISCIPLINARY ACTION: EXCLUSION FROM THE MEDICARE AND/OR MEDICAID PROGRAM
OFFENSE: NONCOMPLIANCE WITH A PROFESSIONAL RULE

NOTES: DEFAULTED ON PUBLIC HEALTH SERVICE EDUCATION LOAN.

MITCHELL, WILLIAM B MD, LICENSE NUMBER 0009317 OF CLAREMORE, OK, WAS DISCIPLINED BY WASHINGTON ON JUNE 19, 1992
DISCIPLINARY ACTION: PROBATION

NOTES: ALLEGATIONS OF ACTION TAKEN IN ANOTHER STATE. ON 5/11/95 HIS REQUEST TO TERMINATE THIS PROBATION GRANTED.

MOLINE, LESTER L MD, LICENSE NUMBER 0006738, WAS DISCIPLINED BY OKLAHOMA ON JANUARY 13, 1990
DISCIPLINARY ACTION: SURRENDER OF CONTROLLED SUBSTANCE LICENSE; LICENSE SUSPENSION

NOTES: HE ACKNOWLEDGED ALLEGATIONS RAISED ISSUES AS TO HIS FITNESS TO PRACTICE, BUT VOLUNTARILY WAIVED EVIDENTIARY HEARING AND AGREED TO ENTER INTO STIPULATIONS. FOURTEEN DAY SUSPENSION BEGINNING 1/15/90. PROBATION UNDER THE FOLLOWING TERMS AND CONDITIONS: SHALL NOT PRESCRIBE, ADMINISTER, OR DISPENSE ANY CONTROLLED DANGEROUS SUBSTANCES OR SCHEDULE DRUGS, BUT MAY APPLY FOR MODIFICATION AFTER SUCCESSFUL COMPLETION OF ONE YEAR PROBATION; WILL NOT ALLOW ANY UNLICENSED PERSON TO PRACTICE MEDICINE OR REPRESENT THEMSELF AS A PHYSICIAN IN HIS OFFICE OR ANY OFFICE WHERE HE HAS A PROPRIETARY INTEREST; SHALL BRING COSTS CURRENT WITHIN 60 DAYS; SHALL NOTIFY ANY HOSPITAL WHERE HE HOLDS STAFF PRIVILEGES, OR CLINIC, OR GROUP WHERE HE PRACTICES, OF THE TERMS AND CONDITIONS OF THIS BOARD ORDER AND SUPPLY A COPY THEREOF; WILL IMMEDIATELY SURRENDER HIS REGISTRATION FOR STATE AND FEDERAL CONTROLLED DANGEROUS SUBSTANCES TO THE PROPER AUTHORITIES AND WILL NOT APPLY UNTIL THE TERMS OF HIS PROBATION HAS EXPIRED OR SPECIFICALLY AUTHORIZED BY THE BOARD; SHALL SUBMIT TO THE BOARD ADDRESS/CHANGE OF ADDRESS; SHALL APPEAR BEFORE THE BOARD UPON REQUEST AND SUBMIT ANY REQUIRED REPORTS; SHALL PAY COSTS.

MOLINE, LESTER L MD, LICENSE NUMBER 0006738, WAS DISCIPLINED BY OKLAHOMA ON FEBRUARY 4, 1991
DISCIPLINARY ACTION: 24-MONTH LICENSE SUSPENSION
OFFENSE: FAILURE TO COMPLY WITH PREVIOUS BOARD ORDER

NOTES: DELIBERATELY AND WILLFULLY FAILED AND NEGLECTED TO PROMPTLY PAY UPON RECEIPT OF INVOICE FROM THE INVESTIGATION DIVISION THE COSTS IN THE AMOUNT OF $3,309.71 FOR INVESTIGATION, PROSECUTION AND PROBATION OF A CASE DECIDED 5/13/88. AMOUNT OF COSTS WAS A CONDITION OF A THREE-YEAR PROBATION.

MOLINE, LESTER L MD, LICENSE NUMBER 0006738, WAS DISCIPLINED BY OKLAHOMA ON MARCH 16, 1991
DISCIPLINARY ACTION: 36-MONTH PROBATION; RESTRICTION PLACED ON CONTROLLED SUBSTANCE LICENSE

NOTES: SINCE 2/4/91 SUSPENSION PEOPLE HAVE CONTRIBUTED MONEY TO PAY OFF COSTS OF THIS CASE THAT WERE DUE AND OWING. SUSPENSION TERMINATED; PLACED ON PROBATION UNDER TERMS AND CONDITIONS: MAY PRESCRIBE CONTROLLED DANGEROUS SUBSTANCES ONLY ON SERIALLY-NUMBERED, DUPLICATE PRESCRIPTION PADS WITH COPIES AVAILABLE TO BOARD; SHALL SUBSTANTIALLY REDUCE THE NUMBER OF CONTROLLED DANGEROUS SUBSTANCE PRESCRIPTIONS WRITTEN AND SIGNIFICANTLY REDUCE THE DURATION OF TIME THAT PATIENTS ARE RETAINED ON THEM; SHALL FURNISH BOARD WITH ADDRESS AND/OR CHANGE OF ADDRESS; SHALL APPEAR BEFORE BOARD UPON

REQUEST.

MOLINE, LESTER LEE MD OF 807 E BROADWAY, HOLLIS, OK, WAS DISCIPLINED BY DEA ON JANUARY 24, 1990
DISCIPLINARY ACTION: SURRENDER OF CONTROLLED SUBSTANCE LICENSE
OFFENSE: DISCIPLINARY ACTION BY ANOTHER STATE OR AGENCY
NOTES: SUSPENDED LICENSE ON 01/13/89 FOR 14 DAYS AND FIVE YEARS PROBATION. PLED GUILTY ON 03/90 AND SENTENCED TO ONE YEAR WHICH WAS DEFERRED.

MORRISON, JOHN WILDEY MD OF 12620 TRIAL OAKS DRIVE, OKLAHOMA CITY, OK, WAS DISCIPLINED BY DEA ON SEPTEMBER 11, 1995
DISCIPLINARY ACTION: SURRENDER OF CONTROLLED SUBSTANCE LICENSE
NOTES: IN LIEU OF PUBLIC INTEREST REVOCATION.

MORTON, ROBERT O MD, LICENSE NUMBER 0010500 OF PO BOX 58, WAURIKA, OK, WAS DISCIPLINED BY OKLAHOMA ON MAY 20, 1993
DISCIPLINARY ACTION: LICENSE REVOCATION
OFFENSE: FAILURE TO COMPLY WITH PREVIOUS BOARD ORDER
NOTES: IN VIOLATION OF PREVIOUS BOARD ORDER, ON 3/2/93 HE PERSONALLY USED A CONTROLLED DANGEROUS SUBSTANCE (NUBAIN) OR A FORM OF MEPROBAMATE AND WAS IMPAIRED THEREBY AT LEAST TO THE EXTENT OF DRIVING HIS CAR INTO A DITCH AND TWICE WAS NOT AVAILABLE TO BOARD COMPLIANCE ORDER FOR OBTAINING FLUID SAMPLES.

MORTON, ROBERT O MD, LICENSE NUMBER 0010500 OF 1334 NORMANDY ROAD, DUNCAN, OK, WAS DISCIPLINED BY OKLAHOMA ON MAY 19, 1994
DISCIPLINARY ACTION: LICENSE REINSTATEMENT; PROBATION
NOTES: PROVIDED EVIDENCE SUPPORTING REINSTATEMENT OF LICENSE ON PROBATION. CONDITIONS OF INDEFINITE PROBATION: SHALL NOT PRESCRIBE, ADMINISTER OR DISPENSE ANY MEDICATIONS FOR HIS OWN PERSONAL USE AND SHALL TAKE NO MEDICATION UNLESS AUTHORIZED BY ANOTHER PHYSICIAN FOR A LEGITIMATE MEDICAL NEED; SHALL ABSTAIN FROM CONSUMING ALCOHOL AND ANY SUBSTANCE WHICH WOULD ADVERSELY AFFECT HIS ABILITY TO PRACTICE; SHALL SUBMIT BIOLOGICAL FLUID SPECIMENS; SHALL NOT INGEST ANY SUBSTANCE THAT WILL TEST POSITIVE FOR ALCOHOL OR ANY CONTROLLED SUBSTANCE; SHALL MAINTAIN A PROGRAM OF ABSTINENCE THROUGH PARTICIPATION IN BOARD-APPROVED ORGANIZATIONS INCLUDING WEEKLY MEETINGS OF THE PHYSICIAN'S RECOVERY COMMITTEE, ONE NARCOTICS ANONYMOUS MEETING PER WEEK AND TWO AA MEETINGS PER WEEK; SHALL MAINTAIN WEEKLY OUTPATIENT COUNSELING; SHALL SIGN A RELEASE TO ALLOW BOARD TO OBTAIN DOCUMENTS REGARDING TREATMENT; SHALL NOT ACCEPT SAMPLES OF ANY DRUGS; SHALL NOT ORDER, DISPENSE OR ADMINISTER ANY CONTROLLED DANGEROUS SUBSTANCES EXCEPT IN AN EMERGENCY LIFE-THREATENING SITUATION; MAY ONLY PRESCRIBE LEGEND DRUGS THE BOARD HAS APPROVED AND THESE ON SERIALLY-NUMBERED, DUPLICATE PRESCRIPTION PADS WITH COPIES AVAILABLE FOR INSPECTION ON A MONTHLY BASIS; SHALL FURNISH THE BOARD WITH ADDRESS AND/OR CHANGE OF ADDRESS; SHALL APPEAR BEFORE THE BOARD UPON REQUEST AND PROVIDE REQUIRED REPORTS; SHALL PAY COSTS; SHALL NOTIFY ANY HEALTH CARE ENTITY WHERE HE HAS PRIVILEGES OF THE TERMS OF THIS ORDER; SHALL NOT SUPERVISE A PHYSICIAN'S ASSISTANT.

MORTON, ROBERT O MD, LICENSE NUMBER 0010500 OF P.O. BOX 1305, DUNCAN, OK, WAS DISCIPLINED BY OKLAHOMA ON OCTOBER 3, 1996
DISCIPLINARY ACTION: LICENSE REVOCATION
OFFENSE: FAILURE TO COMPLY WITH PREVIOUS BOARD ORDER
NOTES: ON 5/19/94 PLACED ON PROBATION AND AGREED NOT TO CONSUME ANY MEDICATION OR SUBSTANCE THAT WOULD TEST POSITIVE FOR ALCOHOL OR ANY CONTROLLED DANGEROUS SUBSTANCE. ON 7/02/96 HE TESTED POSITIVE FOR NUBAIN.

MORTON, ROBERT O MD, LICENSE NUMBER 10500 OF 1007 1/2 ASH, DUNCAN, OK, WAS DISCIPLINED BY OKLAHOMA ON NOVEMBER 20, 1998
DISCIPLINARY ACTION: LICENSE REINSTATEMENT; PROBATION
OFFENSE: SUBSTANCE ABUSE
NOTES: APPLIED FOR REINSTATEMENT OF HIS OKLAHOMA MEDICAL LICENSE TO ENTER A SECOND-YEAR PSYCHIATRY RESIDENCY TRAINING POSITION AT THE UNIVERSITY OF OKLAHOMA COLLEGE OF MEDICINE-TULSA WHICH HAD BEEN REVOKED ON 9/26/96 FOR HABITUAL INTEMPERANCE OR THE HABITUAL USE OF HABIT-FORMING DRUGS. REINSTATED WITH A SPECIAL TRAINING LICENSE UNDER THE TERMS SET FORTH BELOW, FOR THE PURPOSE OF HIS RESIDENCY TRAINING PROGRAM. THE PROBATIONARY TERMS ARE TO EXTEND FOR THE DURATION OF HIS SPECIAL TRAINING LICENSE: SHALL NOT PRESCRIBE, ADMINISTER OR DISPENSE ANY MEDICATIONS FOR HIS PERSONAL USE AND SHALL TAKE NONE UNLESS AUTHORIZED BY ANOTHER PHYSICIAN FOR A LEGITIMATE MEDICAL NEED; SHALL. ABSTAIN FROM CONSUMING ALCOHOL OR ANY SUBSTANCE WHICH WOULD ADVERSELY AFFECT HIS ABILITY TO PRACTICE MEDICINE; SHALL SUBMIT BIOLOGICAL FLUID SPECIMENS AND SHALL NOT INGEST ANY SUBSTANCE WHICH WILL CAUSE A SPECIMEN TO TEST POSITIVE FOR ANY PROHIBITED SUBSTANCES; SHALL MAINTAIN A PROGRAM OF ABSTINENCE THROUGH PARTICIPATION IN AND/OR ASSOCIATION WITH ANY AND ALL ORGANIZATIONS, GROUPS, OR INDIVIDUALS SELECTED BY THE BOARD AND DEEMED APPROPRIATE FOR ASSESSMENT, TREATMENT, OR SUPPORT; SHALL ATTEND WEEKLY MEETING OF THE PHYSICIANS RECOVERY COMMITTEE, ONE NARCOTICS ANONYMOUS MEETING PER WEEK, AND TWO AA MEETINGS PER WEEK; SHALL NOT RECEIVE, ACCEPT OR SIGN FOR, IN ANY MANNER, ANY SAMPLES OF ANY DRUG, EXCEPT THOSE DRUGS APPROVED BY THE BOARD; SHALL NOT ORDER, DISPENSE, OR ADMINISTER ANY CONTROLLED DANGEROUS SUBSTANCES, EXCEPT IN AN EMERGENCY, LIFE-THREATENING SITUATION; SHALL NOT ADMINISTER OR DISPENSE LEGEND DRUGS, EXCEPT DRUGS THAT ARE ESSENTIAL TO HIS PRACTICE OF MEDICINE WHICH HAVE BEEN APPROVED FOR THIS PURPOSE BY THE BOARD AND THEN ONLY ON DUPLICATE, SERIALLY NUMBERED PRESCRIPTION PADS WHICH SHALL BE SUBMITTED TO THE BOARD MONTHLY; SHALL PRACTICE IN A CONTROLLED ENVIRONMENT APPROVED BY THE BOARD LIMITED TO DUTIES THAT ARE A PART OF THE PSYCHIATRY RESIDENCY TRAINING POSITION; SHALL SUBMIT TO EVERY STATE IN WHICH HE HOLDS LICENSURE AND TO HOSPITALS, CLINICS OR OTHER INSTITUTIONS IN WHICH HE HOLDS OR ANTICIPATES HOLDING ANY FORM OF STAFF PRIVILEGE A COPY OF THIS ORDER; SHALL NOT SUPERVISE ALLIED HEALTH

PROFESSIONALS; SHALL ABIDE BY HIS POST-CARE CONTRACT FROM THE OKLAHOMA PHYSICIAN RECOVERY PROGRAM AND WILL COMPLY WITH THE CONDITIONS FOR RESIDENCY; SHALL AUTHORIZE THE BOARD TO DISCUSS HIS PARTICIPATION AND PERFORMANCE WITH APPROPRIATE REPRESENTATIVES FROM BOTH PROGRAMS AND WILL AUTHORIZE THE BOARD TO OBTAIN RECORDS FROM BOTH PROGRAMS; SHALL CONTINUE TREATMENT WITH A BOARD APPROVED PSYCHOTHERAPIST AND WILL FOLLOW ALL TREATMENT RECOMMENDATIONS WITH QUARTERLY REPORTS TO THE BOARD; SHALL KEEP THE BOARD INFORMED OF HIS ADDRESS AND PAY COSTS; SHALL APPEAR BEFORE THE BOARD UPON REQUEST; SHALL EXECUTE THE RELEASE OF ANY MEDICAL, COUNSELING AND PSYCHIATRIC RECORDS AS NECESSARY TO DISCUSS HIS CASE WITH TREATING PHYSICIANS AND/OR ANY PHYSICIANS HOLDING THE RECORDS.

MORTON, ROBERT OLIVER MD, DATE OF BIRTH MARCH 21, 1947 OF PO BOX 1305, DUNCAN, OK, WAS DISCIPLINED BY MEDICARE ON SEPTEMBER 20, 1998
DISCIPLINARY ACTION: EXCLUSION FROM THE MEDICARE AND/OR MEDICAID PROGRAM
OFFENSE: DISCIPLINARY ACTION BY ANOTHER STATE OR AGENCY

NOTES: LICENSE REVOKED, SUSPENDED, SURRENDERED OR OTHERWISE LOST FOR REASONS BEARING ON PROFESSIONAL PERFORMANCE, PROFESSIONAL COMPETENCE OR FINANCIAL INTEGRITY.

MOULTRIE, ROBERT LEE OF HC 73 BOX 272, PARK HILL, OK, WAS DISCIPLINED BY OKLAHOMA ON DECEMBER 2, 1993
DISCIPLINARY ACTION: DENIAL OF NEW LICENSE
OFFENSE: LOSS OR RESTRICTION OF HOSPITAL PRIVILEGES

NOTES: ONE HOSPITAL HAD DENIED HIM ICU CARE PRIVILEGES, HAD PREVIOUSLY SUSPENDED HIM FROM THE HOSPITAL FOR NOT RESPONDING TO HIS PAGER, AND DENIED HIM PRIVILEGES BASED ON INADEQUATE ADMINISTRATIVE DUTIES. HE FAILED TO PROVIDE SUFFICIENT RESPONSES TO BOARD ON THESE PROCEEDINGS; FAILED TO UTILIZE HIS SMD CERTIFICATE IN A PROPER MANNER IN PRACTICE.

MUELLER, LYNDA L MD, LICENSE NUMBER 0019565 OF 4611 WINDCASTLE DRIVE #1028, ARLINGTON, TX, WAS DISCIPLINED BY OKLAHOMA ON DECEMBER 12, 1996
DISCIPLINARY ACTION: 60-MONTH PROBATION; RESTRICTION PLACED ON CONTROLLED SUBSTANCE LICENSE
OFFENSE: SUBSTANCE ABUSE

NOTES: ESTABLISHED A PATTERN OF ABUSE OF ALCOHOL AND DRIVING UNDER THE INFLUENCE ARRESTS; ON 9/15/95 ENTERED INTO A WRITTEN AGREEMENT WITH THE BOARD; ON 1/04/96 ENTERED FULL-TIME IN-PATIENT TREATMENT AT COPAC; AND DISCHARGED FROM COPAC ON 4/12/96 UNDER A CONTINUING CARE ADVOCACY CONTRACT. TIMING OF PROBATION SHALL START WHEN SHE REPORTS TO THE BOARD REGARDING HER PRACTICE OF MEDICINE AND SURGERY IN OKLAHOMA; SHALL NOT PRESCRIBE, ADMINISTER, OR DISPENSE ANY MEDICATIONS FOR HER PERSONAL USE, TO SPECIFICALLY INCLUDE CONTROLLED DANGEROUS SUBSTANCES; SHALL TAKE NO MEDICATION UNLESS AUTHORIZED BY A PHYSICIAN FOR A LEGITIMATE MEDICAL NEED; SHALL SUBMIT BIOLOGICAL FLUID SPECIMENS; SHALL PRESENT HERSELF TO A PHYSICAL AND/OR PSYCHIATRIC EXAMINATION BY A BOARD APPROVED DOCTOR WITH A REPORT SUBMITTED TO THE BOARD; SHALL COMPLY WITH ALL TERMS AND CONDITIONS OF HER CONTINUING CARE ADVOCACY CONTRACT; SHALL NOT PRESCRIBE, ADMINISTER, OR DISPENSE ANY SCHEDULE DRUGS OR CONTROLLED DANGEROUS SUBSTANCES UNTIL AUTHORIZED BY THE BOARD; SHALL FURNISH THE BOARD WITH ADDRESS/CHANGE OF ADDRESS; SHALL APPEAR BEFORE THE BOARD UPON REQUEST AND SUBMIT ANY REQUIRED REPORTS; SHALL PAY COSTS; AND SHALL FURNISH EACH STATE IN WHICH SHE HOLDS OR APPLIES FOR LICENSURE AND ALL HEALTH CARE ENTITIES WHERE SHE HAS PRIVILEGES A COPY OF THIS ORDER. ON 4/10/98 REQUEST TO WAIVE THE TERMS AND CONDITIONS OF PROBATION AND RESTORE TO HER A FULL AND UNRESTRICTED LICENSE IS DENIED. ON 5/6/99 REQUEST TO MODIFY TERMS OF HER PROBATION IS GRANTED ALLOWING HER TO PRESCRIBE CONTROLLED SUBSTANCES IN SCHEDULES II-V, USING DUPLICATE, SERIALLY NUMBERED PRESCRIPTION PADS TO BE MADE AVAILABLE TO THE BOARD UPON REQUEST; SHALL COMPLY WITH ALL TERMS AND CONDITIONS OF HER CONTRACT WITH THE PHYSICIANS RECOVERY NETWORK.

MUNCRIEF, KIM I DO, LICENSE NUMBER 2425, WAS DISCIPLINED BY OKLAHOMA ON SEPTEMBER 17, 1998
DISCIPLINARY ACTION: 60-MONTH PROBATION

MUNCRIEF, KIM IVAN DO, LICENSE NUMBER 00G7284 OF COLBERT, OK, WAS DISCIPLINED BY TEXAS ON JANUARY 27, 1990
DISCIPLINARY ACTION: PROBATION
OFFENSE: DISCIPLINARY ACTION BY ANOTHER STATE OR AGENCY

NOTES: STIPULATED ORDER. REVOCATION STAYED, INDEFINITE PROBATION. SHALL COMPLY WITH CONDITIONS OF OKLAHOMA BOARD ORDER, SUBMIT REPORTS TO TEXAS BOARD AS SUBMITTED TO OKLAHOMA BOARD, AND MUST SECURE BOARD APPROVAL BEFORE PRACTICING. PROBATION TERMINATED EFFECTIVE 1/9/92; LICENSE FREE OF ANY RESTRICTION OR LIMITATION.

MUNCRUIEF, KIM IVAN DO, DATE OF BIRTH FEBRUARY 3, 1957 OF 1010 ELMWOOD STREET, NORMAN, OK, WAS DISCIPLINED BY MEDICARE ON DECEMBER 20, 1998
DISCIPLINARY ACTION: 60-MONTH EXCLUSION FROM THE MEDICARE AND/OR MEDICAID PROGRAM
OFFENSE: CRIMINAL CONVICTION OR PLEA OF GUILTY, NOLO CONTENDERE, OR NO CONTEST TO A CRIME

NOTES: CONVICTED OF A CRIME INVOLVING THE MEDICARE, MEDICAID, MATERNAL AND CHILD HEALTH SERVICES BLOCK GRANT OR BLOCK GRANTS TO STATES FOR SOCIAL SERVICES PROGRAMS.

MURPHY, TERRENCE E MD, LICENSE NUMBER 0051286 OF STILLWATER, OK, WAS DISCIPLINED BY FLORIDA ON FEBRUARY 18, 1991
DISCIPLINARY ACTION: PROBATION; FINE
OFFENSE: DISCIPLINARY ACTION BY ANOTHER STATE OR AGENCY

NOTES: $500 FINE. UPON REACTIVATION OF FLORIDA MEDICAL LICENSE, LICENSE SHALL BE PLACED ON PROBATION WITH TERMS AND CONDITIONS TO BE SET BY THE BOARD.

MURPHY, TERRENCE E MD, LICENSE NUMBER 0014919, WAS DISCIPLINED BY OKLAHOMA ON JANUARY 22, 1996
DISCIPLINARY ACTION: EMERGENCY SUSPENSION
OFFENSE: PHYSICAL OR MENTAL ILLNESS INHIBITING THE ABILITY TO PRACTICE WITH SKILL AND SAFETY

NOTES: SUFFERS FROM A MENTAL DISABILITY MAKING HIM INCOMPETENT TO PRACTICE MEDICINE.

MURPHY, TERRENCE E MD OF TULSA, OK, WAS DISCIPLINED BY DEA ON FEBRUARY 28, 1996
DISCIPLINARY ACTION: REVOCATION OF CONTROLLED SUBSTANCE LICENSE
OFFENSE: DISCIPLINARY ACTION BY ANOTHER STATE OR AGENCY

NOTES: ON 10/26/88 THE ALABAMA BOARD SUSPENDED HIS MEDICAL LICENSE FOR ONE YEAR, AND THEREAFTER PLACED HIS MEDICAL LICENSE ON INDEFINITE PROBATION FOR PRESCRIBING, DISPENSING, FURNISHING, OR SUPPLYING CONTROLLED SUBSTANCES TO PERSONS FOR OTHER THAN A LEGITIMATE MEDICAL PURPOSE; LICENSE STILL RESTRICTED TO SCHEDULES IV AND V; ON 2/12/91 FLORIDA CONSENT ORDER FINED HIM AND REQUIRED THAT IF HE EVER WAS TO SEEK REACTIVATION OF HIS FLORIDA LICENSE IT WOULD BE PLACED ON PROBATION WITH CONDITIONS. ON 6/11/90 HE MATERIALLY FALSIFIED AN APPLICATION FOR A CONTROLLED SUBSTANCE LICENSE IN OKLAHOMA BOARD BY INDICATING THAT HE HAD NEVER HAD A PREVIOUS REGISTRATION SUSPENSION; ON 12/27/90 HE MATERIALLY FALSIFIED AN APPLICATION FOR A DEA CERTIFICATE OF REGISTRATION BY INDICATING THAT HE HAD NEVER HAD A STATE PROFESSIONAL LICENSE OR CONTROLLED SUBSTANCE REGISTRATION SUSPENDED; FAILED TO TAKE RESPONSIBILITY FOR REVIEWING HIS APPLICATION. ON 1/11/91 THE DEA RENEWED HIS DEA REGISTRATION FOR THREE YEARS.

MURPHY, TERRENCE E MD, LICENSE NUMBER 0014919 OF 401 SOUTH RIDGE ROAD, STILLWATER, OK, WAS DISCIPLINED BY OKLAHOMA ON AUGUST 29, 1996
DISCIPLINARY ACTION: LICENSE REVOCATION
OFFENSE: OVERPRESCRIBING OR MISPRESCRIBING DRUGS

NOTES: GUILTY OF UNPROFESSIONAL CONDUCT IN THAT IN 6/95 AIDED AND ABETTED THE PRACTICE OF MEDICINE WITHOUT A LICENSE, BY ALLOWING A CHIROPRACTOR, NOT LICENSED AS A MEDICAL DOCTOR, IN HIS OFFICE TO TREAT PATIENTS AS A MEDICAL DOCTOR; FROM 12/01/93 THROUGH 08/16/94 PRESCRIBED MEDICATIONS WITHOUT A MEDICAL NEED, OVER PRESCRIBING MEDICATIONS, AND/OR ENGAGING IN THE INDISCRIMINATE AND/OR EXCESSIVE PRESCRIBING OF MEDICATIONS.

MURPHY, TERRENCE E MD, LICENSE NUMBER 14919 OF 401 SOUTH RIDGE ROAD, STILLWATER, OK, WAS DISCIPLINED BY OKLAHOMA ON OCTOBER 2, 1998
DISCIPLINARY ACTION: LICENSE REVOCATION
OFFENSE: OVERPRESCRIBING OR MISPRESCRIBING DRUGS

NOTES: FROM 12/1/93 THROUGH 8/16/94 HE ENGAGED IN UNPROFESSIONAL CONDUCT BY OVERPRESCRIBING MEDICATIONS, AND/OR ENGAGING IN THE INDISCRIMINATE AND/OR EXCESSIVE PRESCRIBING OF MEDICATIONS.

MUSCARI, PIETRO J DO, DATE OF BIRTH DECEMBER 14, 1930 OF 514 N FOREST RIDGE BLVD, BROKEN ARROW, OK, WAS DISCIPLINED BY MEDICARE ON APRIL 12, 1995
DISCIPLINARY ACTION: 120-MONTH EXCLUSION FROM THE MEDICARE AND/OR MEDICAID PROGRAM
OFFENSE: CRIMINAL CONVICTION OR PLEA OF GUILTY, NOLO CONTENDERE, OR NO CONTEST TO A CRIME

NOTES: CONVICTED OF A CRIME INVOLVING THE MEDICARE, MEDICAID, MATERNAL AND CHILD HEALTH SERVICES BLOCK GRANT OR BLOCK GRANTS TO STATES FOR SOCIAL SERVICES PROGRAMS.

MUSCARI, PIETRO J DO, LICENSE NUMBER 0003757 OF BROKEN ARROW, OK, WAS DISCIPLINED BY OHIO ON JULY 18, 1995
DISCIPLINARY ACTION: LICENSE REVOCATION
OFFENSE: CRIMINAL CONVICTION OR PLEA OF GUILTY, NOLO CONTENDERE, OR NO CONTEST TO A CRIME

NOTES: PLED GUILTY TO ONE FELONY COUNT OF MAIL FRAUD. PERMANENT REVOCATION.

MUSCARI, PIETRO J JR DO OF BROKEN ARROW, OK, WAS DISCIPLINED BY MISSOURI ON MAY 16, 1997
DISCIPLINARY ACTION: LICENSE REVOCATION
OFFENSE: DISCIPLINARY ACTION BY ANOTHER STATE OR AGENCY

NOTES: PLED GUILTY TO ONE COUNT OF FELONY MAIL FRAUD IN THE US DISTRICT COURT, SOUTHERN DISTRICT OF OHIO. FINAL AND UNCONDITIONAL REVOCATION OF HIS OHIO LICENSE. NO APPLICATION FOR REINSTATEMENT FOR TWO YEARS AND ONE DAY.

NELSON, ARNOLD G MD, LICENSE NUMBER 0006416 OF 2820 PARKLAWN DR, MIDWEST CITY, OK, WAS DISCIPLINED BY OKLAHOMA ON MARCH 16, 1991
DISCIPLINARY ACTION: 60-MONTH PROBATION; RESTRICTION PLACED ON CONTROLLED SUBSTANCE LICENSE
OFFENSE: OVERPRESCRIBING OR MISPRESCRIBING DRUGS

NOTES: FROM 7/1/90 THROUGH 11/15/90, PRESCRIBED CONTROLLED DANGEROUS SUBSTANCES TO AT LEAST 5 PATIENTS IN EXCESS OF THE AMOUNT CONSIDERED GOOD MEDICAL PRACTICE FOR THE MEDICAL NEED PRESENTED. PROBATION UNDER TERMS AND CONDITIONS: MAY PRESCRIBE CONTROLLED DANGEROUS SUBSTANCES ONLY ON SERIALLY-NUMBERED, DUPLICATE PRESCRIPTION PADS WITH COPIES AVAILABLE TO BOARD; SHALL REDUCE THE NUMBER OF CONTROLLED DANGEROUS SUBSTANCES PRESCRIPTIONS BEING WRITTEN, AND WILL REDUCE THE LENGTH OF TIME PATIENTS ARE RETAINED ON THESE DRUGS; SHALL FURNISH BOARD WITH ADDRESS AND/OR CHANGE OF ADDRESS; SHALL APPEAR BEFORE BOARD UPON REQUEST; SHALL NOTIFY ANY HOSPITAL WHERE HE HOLDS STAFF PRIVILEGES, OR CLINIC OR GROUP OF THE TERMS AND CONDITIONS.

NEVREKAR, LILA V MD, LICENSE NUMBER 0010357, WAS DISCIPLINED BY OKLAHOMA ON MAY 20, 1993
DISCIPLINARY ACTION: LICENSE SUSPENSION
OFFENSE: CRIMINAL CONVICTION OR PLEA OF GUILTY, NOLO CONTENDERE, OR NO CONTEST TO A CRIME

NOTES: ON 1/21/93 VOLUNTARILY ENTERED A PLEA OF GUILTY TO THE FELONY CHARGE OF MEDICAID FRAUD; FORMAL SENTENCING DEFERRED UNTIL 3/4/96 AND SHE WAS ORDERED TO PAY A FINE OF $17,000. LICENSE SUSPENDED FOR 3 DAYS AS OF 5/14/93 AND SHALL PAY COSTS.

NEVREKAR, LILA V MD, DATE OF BIRTH JANUARY 5, 1941 OF 6 CASTLE CREEK PLACE, SHAWNEE, OK, WAS DISCIPLINED BY MEDICARE ON OCTOBER 11, 1993
DISCIPLINARY ACTION: 60-MONTH EXCLUSION FROM THE MEDICARE AND/OR MEDICAID PROGRAM
OFFENSE: CRIMINAL CONVICTION OR PLEA OF GUILTY, NOLO CONTENDERE, OR NO CONTEST TO A CRIME

NOTES: CONVICTED OF SUBMITTING FALSE CLAIMS TO MEDICAID FOR HIGHER CODED SERVICES THAN THOSE PROVIDED. REINSTATED ON 11/20/98.

NEVREKAR, LILA V MD, LICENSE NUMBER 0117145 OF 1902 GORDON COOPER DRIVE, SHAUNEE, OK, WAS DISCIPLINED BY NEW YORK ON SEPTEMBER 30, 1994
DISCIPLINARY ACTION: LICENSE REVOCATION
OFFENSE: DISCIPLINARY ACTION BY ANOTHER STATE OR AGENCY

NOTES: GUILTY OF MISCONDUCT BY OKLAHOMA BOARD AND CONVICTED OF MEDICAID FRAUD.

NGUYEN, THUONG MD OF 1908 N.W. 23RD, OKLAHOMA CITY, OK, WAS DISCIPLINED BY DEA ON DECEMBER 16, 1994
DISCIPLINARY ACTION: SURRENDER OF CONTROLLED SUBSTANCE LICENSE

NOTES: IN LIEU OF PUBLIC INTEREST REVOCATION.

NGUYEN, THUONG VAN MD, LICENSE NUMBER 14885 OF 1908 N.W. 23RD STREET, OKLAHOMA CITY, OK, WAS DISCIPLINED BY OKLAHOMA ON SEPTEMBER 24, 1999
DISCIPLINARY ACTION: 36-MONTH PROBATION; RESTRICTION PLACED ON CONTROLLED SUBSTANCE LICENSE
OFFENSE: OVERPRESCRIBING OR MISPRESCRIBING DRUGS

NOTES: ON OR ABOUT 12/16/94 SURRENDERED HIS DEA CERTIFICATE OF REGISTRATION IN LIEU OF PROSECUTION BY THE DEA FOR ILLEGALLY DISTRIBUTING CONTROLLED SUBSTANCES; FROM 7/95-5/22/98 DID NOT REGISTER TO DISPENSE DANGEROUS DRUGS ON HIS APPLICATIONS FOR RENEWAL OF LICENSE; DESPITE NOT REGISTERING DURING THIS PERIOD HE CONTINUED TO DISPENSE DANGEROUS DRUGS WITH EXAMPLES AS FOLLOWS: AROUND 2/97 PRESCRIBED AND DISPENSED MEDICATION TO THREE MINOR PATIENTS; THE MEDICATION WAS DISPENSED BY HIM IN BOTTLES CONTAINING NO PRESCRIPTION LABEL, NO NAME OF THE MEDICATION, NO NAME OF THE PATIENT, AND NO INSTRUCTIONS FOR TAKING THE MEDICATION EXCEPT A MARK ON THE LID TELLING THE PATIENT HOW OFTEN TO TAKE THE MEDICATION, ALL IN VIOLATION OF THE OKLAHOMA PHARMACY ACT; IN OR AROUND 9/97-EARLY 1998 PRESCRIBED AND DISPENSED TO OTHER MINORS WITH SAME LABELING PROBLEMS; IN 5/98 INVESTIGATORS FOUND SIMILAR PROBLEMS WITH TWO PATIENTS LEAVING HIS OFFICE; ON 9/15/98 ISSUED A PRESCRIPTION FOR IDA NOT KNOWING WHAT IT WAS BUT BECAUSE THE PATIENT WANTED IT; DURING OR JUST PRIOR TO 5/99 SEVERAL PRESCRIPTION MEDICATIONS WERE CONFISCATED BY THE SCHOOL NURSE AT A MIDDLE SCHOOL: A TUBE OF BETAMETHASONE CREAM, COMPLETELY UNLABELED, AND A BOTTLE OF "PROMETH 26" AND A BOTTLE OF "MOTRIN 600", BOTH OF WHICH CONTAINED HIS NAME, ADDRESS AND TELEPHONE NUMBER; AND A DROPPER BOTTLE CONTAINING AN UNKNOWN MEDICATION (NAME WAS ILLEGIBLE) WITH HIS NAME, ADDRESS AND TELEPHONE NUMBER. REPRIMAND; LICENSE LIMITED AS FOLLOWS: SHALL IMMEDIATELY CEASE DISPENSING MEDICATIONS FROM HIS OFFICE; SHALL SUBMIT TO EVERY STATE IN WHICH HE HOLDS LICENSURE AND TO HOSPITALS, CLINICS OR OTHER INSTITUTIONS IN WHICH HE HOLDS OR ANTICIPATES HOLDING ANY FORM OF STAFF PRIVILEGE A COPY OF THIS ORDER; SHALL ALLOW THE BOARD ACCESS TO ALL PATIENT CHARTS FOR RANDOM PERIODIC REVIEWS; SHALL KEEP THE BOARD INFORMED OF HIS ADDRESS; SHALL APPEAR BEFORE THE BOARD UPON REQUEST.

NOVOSAD, CHARLES L JR MD, DATE OF BIRTH DECEMBER 19, 1930 OF PO BOX 3498, POJOAQUE, NM, WAS DISCIPLINED BY MEDICARE ON SEPTEMBER 15, 1996
DISCIPLINARY ACTION: EXCLUSION FROM THE MEDICARE AND/OR MEDICAID PROGRAM
OFFENSE: DISCIPLINARY ACTION BY ANOTHER STATE OR AGENCY

NOTES: LICENSE REVOKED FOR REASONS BEARING ON PROFESSIONAL PERFORMANCE.

NOVOSAD, CHARLES LOUIS JR MD OF 210 NORTH HIGHWAY 285, POJOAQUE, NM, WAS DISCIPLINED BY NEW MEXICO ON MAY 20, 1994
DISCIPLINARY ACTION: LICENSE REVOCATION
OFFENSE: OVERPRESCRIBING OR MISPRESCRIBING DRUGS

NOTES: UNPROFESSIONAL CONDUCT; INJUDICIOUS PRESCRIBING.

NOVOSAD, CHARLES LOUIS JR MD, LICENSE NUMBER 0008996, WAS DISCIPLINED BY OKLAHOMA ON SEPTEMBER 9, 1994
DISCIPLINARY ACTION: LICENSE REVOCATION
OFFENSE: DISCIPLINARY ACTION BY ANOTHER STATE OR AGENCY

NOTES: ON 5/20/94 NEW MEXICO BOARD REVOKED HIS LICENSE BASED ON OVER-PRESCRIPTION AND IMPROPER PRESCRIPTION OF CONTROLLED DANGEROUS SUBSTANCES.

NOVOSAD, CHARLES LOUIS JR MD, LICENSE NUMBER 00C4483 OF POJOAQUE, NM, WAS DISCIPLINED BY TEXAS ON JANUARY 6, 1995
OFFENSE: DISCIPLINARY ACTION BY ANOTHER STATE OR AGENCY

NOTES: ON 5/20/94 NEW MEXICO BOARD REVOKED HIS LICENSE ON THE GROUNDS OF INJUDICIOUS PRESCRIBING TO SEVERAL PATIENTS; PRESENTLY SEEKING JUDICIAL REVIEW OF THIS ORDER. SHALL NOT PRACTICE IN TEXAS UNTIL HE REQUESTS PERMISSION IN WRITING FROM THE TEXAS BOARD TO RESUME PRACTICE, PERSONALLY APPEARS BEFORE THE BOARD AND PROVIDES SUFFICIENT EVIDENCE THAT HE IS PHYSICALLY, MENTALLY AND OTHERWISE COMPETENT TO PRACTICE INCLUDING AT A MINIMUM CERTIFICATION OF REVERSAL OF THE NEW MEXICO REVOCATION; SHALL COOPERATE WITH THE BOARD IN VERIFYING COMPLIANCE; SHALL INFORM BOARD OF CHANGE OF ADDRESS WITHIN 10 DAYS.

NOVOSAD, CHARLES LOUIS JR MD OF POJOAQUE, NM, WAS DISCIPLINED BY DEA ON OCTOBER 11, 1995
DISCIPLINARY ACTION: REVOCATION OF CONTROLLED SUBSTANCE LICENSE
OFFENSE: DISCIPLINARY ACTION BY ANOTHER STATE OR AGENCY

NOTES: ON 5/20/94 NEW MEXICO BOARD ORDERED THE REVOCATION OF HIS LICENSE; ON 9/15/94 THE NEW MEXICO PHARMACY BOARD REVOKED HIS STATE REGISTRATION TO HANDLE CONTROLLED SUBSTANCES.

OLIVEROS, DANILO E MD, LICENSE NUMBER 0028176 OF MEDFORD, WI, WAS DISCIPLINED BY FLORIDA ON AUGUST 16, 1990
DISCIPLINARY ACTION: REQUIRED TO TAKE ADDITIONAL MEDICAL EDUCATION
OFFENSE: DISCIPLINARY ACTION BY ANOTHER STATE OR AGENCY

NOTES: BEFORE PRACTICING MEDICINE IN FLORIDA, MUST APPEAR BEFORE THE BOARD AND DEMONSTRATE ABILITY TO PRACTICE WITH SKILL AND SAFETY INCLUDING, BUT NOT LIMITED TO, DOCUMENTATION THAT WISCONSIN LICENSE IS UNENCUMBERED; MUST COMPLETE ONE YEAR OF AN APPROVED FAMILY PRACTICE RESIDENCY PROGRAM; OR AS AN ALTERNATIVE, COMPLETE 70 HOURS CONTINUING MEDICAL EDUCATION, 30 HOURS OF WHICH SHALL PERTAIN TO THE USE OF ANTICOAGULANTS, 30 HOURS SHALL PERTAIN TO THE USE OF DIURETICS

AND HYPERTENSION, AND 10 HOURS IN RISK MANAGEMENT AND MEDICAL RECORDKEEPING.

OLIVEROS, DANILO E MD, DATE OF BIRTH NOVEMBER 10, 1941, LICENSE NUMBER 0021408 OF 129 SOUTH BERKSHIRE WAY, LAWTON, OK, WAS DISCIPLINED BY WISCONSIN ON OCTOBER 26, 1995
DISCIPLINARY ACTION: REPRIMAND
OFFENSE: SUBSTANDARD CARE, INCOMPETENCE OR NEGLIGENCE

NOTES: REPORT OF AN INCIDENT ON 12/26/89 CONCERNING HIS DELIVERY OF OBSTETRICAL CARE; IN 4/90 HE WITHDREW OBSTETRIC PRIVILEGES AT THAT HOSPITAL; THIS INCIDENT CONSTITUTED NEGLIGENCE. $570 PARTIAL COSTS.

OLSON, DONALD C JR DO OF TAHLEQUAH, OK, WAS DISCIPLINED BY MISSOURI ON APRIL 10, 1990
DISCIPLINARY ACTION: LICENSE REVOCATION

ORTEGA, JUAN B MD, LICENSE NUMBER 0010918, WAS DISCIPLINED BY OKLAHOMA ON JUNE 21, 1990
DISCIPLINARY ACTION: REPRIMAND
OFFENSE: PROFESSIONAL MISCONDUCT

NOTES: ALLEGATIONS THAT HE ENGAGED IN UNWISE AND INAPPROPRIATE PERSONAL CONDUCT WITH A NURSE EMPLOYED AT THE CLINTON HOSPITAL. NO CRIMINAL CHARGES WERE PROSECUTED AFTER HE AGREED TO RELOCATE HIS MEDICAL PRACTICE OUTSIDE OKLAHOMA. HIS ACTIONS DID NOT AT ANY TIME ENDANGER OR THREATEN THE MEDICAL CARE OR WELFARE OF ANY PATIENT, NOR CONSTITUTE OR INDICATE ANY LACK OF DIAGNOSTIC, CLINICAL, OR TREATMENT SKILLS; THIS ORDER IS NOT TO BE CONSTRUED AS ADMISSION BY HIM OF ANY ALLEGATIONS WHICH HE EXPRESSLY DENIES. SHALL PAY COSTS.

OSTER, ELLIS MD OF 400 FAIRVIEW SUITE 9, PONCA CITY, OK, WAS DISCIPLINED BY DEA ON DECEMBER 21, 1999
DISCIPLINARY ACTION: SURRENDER OF CONTROLLED SUBSTANCE LICENSE
OFFENSE: DISCIPLINARY ACTION BY ANOTHER STATE OR AGENCY

NOTES: STATE BOARD.

PACE, SCOTT MD, LICENSE NUMBER 0018169 OF 3369 WEST BROADWAY, MUSKOGEE, OK, WAS DISCIPLINED BY OKLAHOMA ON MAY 16, 1996
DISCIPLINARY ACTION: 60-MONTH PROBATION; RESTRICTION PLACED ON LICENSE

NOTES: PROBATION BEGINNING 5/09/96 UNDER THE FOLLOWING TERMS AND CONDITIONS: SHALL KEEP DUPLICATE SERIALLY NUMBERED PRESCRIPTIONS OF ALL CONTROLLED DANGEROUS SUBSTANCES AND WILL SUBMIT COPIES TO THE BOARD UPON REQUEST; SHALL SUBMIT BIOLOGICAL FLUID SPECIMENS; SHALL NOT PRESCRIBE, ADMINISTER, OR DISPENSE ANY MEDICATIONS FOR HIS PERSONAL USE AND SHALL TAKE NONE UNLESS AUTHORIZED BY ANOTHER PHYSICIAN FOR A LEGITIMATE MEDICAL NEED; SHALL PARTICIPATE IN THE OKLAHOMA STATE MEDICAL ASSOCIATION PHYSICIAN RECOVERY COMMITTEE MEETINGS AND RECOVERY PROGRAM AS DESIGNATED BY ITS LEADERSHIP; WILL STRICTLY ADHERE TO HIS AFTER-CARE CONTRACT; WILL NOT ALLOW THE INITIATION OF ANY THERAPEUTIC REGIMEN BY ANY PERSONNEL UNDER HIS SUPERVISION UNLESS HE IS IN THE IMMEDIATE GEOGRAPHIC VICINITY; SHALL SUBMIT TO EVERY STATE IN WHICH HE HOLDS LICENSURE OR APPLIES FOR LICENSURE AND HOSPITALS, CLINICS, OR OTHER INSTITUTIONS IN WHICH HE HOLDS OR ANTICIPATES HOLDING ANY FORM OF STAFF PRIVILEGE, A COPY OF THE BOARD ORDER; SHALL NOT SUPERVISE A PHYSICIAN ASSISTANT; SHALL KEEP THE BOARD INFORMED OF HIS ADDRESS AND PAY COSTS.

PARKISON, GARY A MD, LICENSE NUMBER 0015420, WAS DISCIPLINED BY OKLAHOMA ON JUNE 26, 1992
DISCIPLINARY ACTION: 36-MONTH PROBATION; RESTRICTION PLACED ON CONTROLLED SUBSTANCE LICENSE

NOTES: PROBATION UNDER TERMS AND CONDITIONS: MAY NOT PRESCRIBE CLASS II CONTROLLED DANGEROUS SUBSTANCES EXCEPT FOR HOSPITALIZED PATIENTS, AND MAY PRESCRIBE CONTROLLED DANGEROUS SUBSTANCES ONLY ON SERIALLY-NUMBERED, DUPLICATE PRESCRIPTION PADS, WITH COPIES AVAILABLE TO BOARD; SHALL NOT SUPERVISE ANY PHYSICIAN ASSISTANT; SHALL FURNISH BOARD WITH ADDRESS AND/OR CHANGE OF ADDRESS; SHALL APPEAR BEFORE BOARD UPON REQUEST; SHALL NOTIFY ANY HOSPITAL WHERE HE HOLDS STAFF PRIVILEGES, OR CLINIC OR GROUP OF THE TERMS AND CONDITIONS.

PARKISON, GARY ALAN MD, LICENSE NUMBER 0A49604 OF CONCORD, CA, WAS DISCIPLINED BY CALIFORNIA ON APRIL 23, 1994
DISCIPLINARY ACTION: 36-MONTH PROBATION; RESTRICTION PLACED ON CONTROLLED SUBSTANCE LICENSE
OFFENSE: DISCIPLINARY ACTION BY ANOTHER STATE OR AGENCY

NOTES: DISCIPLINED BY OKLAHOMA MEDICAL BOARD FOR EXCESSIVE PRESCRIBING AND PRESCRIBING OF CONTROLLED SUBSTANCES OR NARCOTIC DRUGS WITHOUT MEDICAL NEED. REVOCATION STAYED IN CALIFORNIA AND CONDITIONS OF PROBATION INCLUDE SHALL NOT PRESCRIBE CONTROLLED SUBSTANCES EXCEPT FOR INPATIENTS IN A HOSPITAL OR HOSPICE.

PARKISON, GARY ALAN MD, LICENSE NUMBER 0A49604 OF ANTIOCH, CA, WAS DISCIPLINED BY CALIFORNIA ON OCTOBER 26, 1994
DISCIPLINARY ACTION: 36-MONTH PROBATION
OFFENSE: DISCIPLINARY ACTION BY ANOTHER STATE OR AGENCY

NOTES: DISCIPLINED BY OKLAHOMA BOARD RELATED TO CHARGES OF EXCESSIVE PRESCRIBING AND PRESCRIBING WITHOUT MEDICAL NEED. REVOCATION STAYED.

PATEL, NARESHKUMAR G MD, LICENSE NUMBER 0014640, WAS DISCIPLINED BY OKLAHOMA ON JULY 12, 1990
DISCIPLINARY ACTION: REPRIMAND; MONITORING OF PHYSICIAN PERFORMANCE
OFFENSE: PROFESSIONAL MISCONDUCT

NOTES: FAILED TO MAINTAIN DISPENSING RECORDS FOR DANGEROUS DRUGS AND FAILED TO KEEP COMPLETE AND ACCURATE RECORDS OF THE PURCHASE AND DISPENSING OF CONTROLLED DRUGS OR NARCOTIC DRUGS. ON 6/10/89 PERFORMED A SURGICAL PROCEDURE ON A PATIENT IN AN UNPROFESSIONAL MANNER AND IN AN UNPROFESSIONAL SETTING. SHALL MEET WITH THE BOARD AND IMPLEMENT A PROPER RECORD-KEEPING SYSTEM FOR CONTROLLED AND NARCOTIC DRUGS AND APPEAR BEFORE THE BOARD WITHIN ONE YEAR FROM 6/09/90 TO DEMONSTRATE THE SYSTEM; SHALL IMPLEMENT A FORMAL, WRITTEN, PROCEDURE TO INCLUDE

QUALIFICATIONS OF HIS PROFESSIONAL AND NON-PROFESSIONAL EMPLOYEES AND JOB DESCRIPTIONS THEREFORE, AND TO PROVIDE A COPY TO THE BOARD WITHIN 60 DAYS OF 6/09/90. HE MAY CONSULT WITH THE BOARD FOR ASSISTANCE IN PREPARING THE FORMAL PROCEDURES MANUAL.

PATEL, NARESHKUMAR G MD, LICENSE NUMBER 0051343 OF SHAWNEE, OK, WAS DISCIPLINED BY OHIO ON MARCH 24, 1992
DISCIPLINARY ACTION: REPRIMAND
OFFENSE: DISCIPLINARY ACTION BY ANOTHER STATE OR AGENCY

NOTES: FORMAL REPRIMAND AND IMPOSITION OF CONDITIONS ON OKLAHOMA LICENSE BY OKLAHOMA'S MEDICAL BOARD; REQUIRED TO PROVIDE WRITTEN DOCUMENTATION OF COMPLIANCE WITH CONDITIONS PLACED ON OKLAHOMA LICENSE.

PATZKOWSKY, PAUL DEAN MD, LICENSE NUMBER 0007588 OF 2915 PINE RIDGE ROAD, OKLAHOMA CITY, OK, WAS DISCIPLINED BY OKLAHOMA ON NOVEMBER 1, 1990
DISCIPLINARY ACTION: 36-MONTH PROBATION; RESTRICTION PLACED ON CONTROLLED SUBSTANCE LICENSE
OFFENSE: OVERPRESCRIBING OR MISPRESCRIBING DRUGS

NOTES: GUILTY OF INDISCRIMINATE OR EXCESSIVE PRESCRIBING, DISPENSING, OR ADMINISTERING OF A CONTROLLED OR NARCOTIC DRUG IN EXCESS OF THE AMOUNT CONSIDERED GOOD MEDICAL PRACTICE OR WITHOUT MEDICAL NEED IN FIVE PATIENTS HE SAW BETWEEN 2/84 AND 4/90; PRESCRIBED OR ADMINISTERED A DRUG WITHOUT SUFFICIENT EXAMINATION AND ESTABLISHMENT OF A VALID PHYSICIAN-PATIENT RELATIONSHIP IN THREE CASES FROM 3/88 THROUGH 4/90 WHERE PATIENTS RECEIVED NUMEROUS PRESCRIPTIONS WITHOUT SEEING THE DOCTOR OR GETTING A PHYSICAL EXAM. PROBATION BEGINNING 10/26/90 UNDER THE FOLLOWING TERMS AND CONDITIONS: MAY PRESCRIBE CONTROLLED DANGEROUS SUBSTANCES ONLY ON SERIALLY-NUMBERED, DUPLICATE PRESCRIPTION PADS AND SHALL MAKE THE COPIES AVAILABLE UPON BOARD REQUEST; SHALL ABSTAIN FROM CONSUMING ALCOHOL OR ANY SUBSTANCE WHICH WOULD ADVERSELY AFFECT HIS ABILITY TO PRACTICE; SHALL SUBMIT BIOLOGICAL FLUID SPECIMENS; NO PERSON IN HIS OFFICE SHALL BE ALLOWED TO AUTHORIZE PRESCRIPTION REFILLS EXCEPT HIMSELF IN PERSON; SHALL PRESENT EVIDENCE OF SUCCESSFUL COMPLETION OF 20 HOURS OF CONTINUING MEDICAL EDUCATION ON PROPER PRESCRIPTION WRITING OR AN EQUIVALENT AMOUNT OF COUNSELING BY BOARD STAFF WITHIN TWO YEARS; SHALL APPEAR BEFORE THE BOARD UPON REQUEST AND SUBMIT ANY REQUIRED REPORTS; SHALL SUBMIT ADDRESS/CHANGE OF ADDRESS; SHALL APPEAR BEFORE THE BOARD UPON REQUEST; SHALL PAY COSTS; SHALL NOTIFY ANY HOSPITAL WHERE HE HOLDS STAFF PRIVILEGES, OR CLINIC, OR GROUP WHERE HE PRACTICES, OF THE TERMS AND CONDITIONS OF THIS BOARD ORDER AND SUPPLY A COPY THEREOF.

PEAKE, STEPHEN TRAVIS MD, LICENSE NUMBER 0017254, WAS DISCIPLINED BY OKLAHOMA ON MARCH 28, 1996
DISCIPLINARY ACTION: 60-MONTH PROBATION; 12-MONTH RESTRICTION PLACED ON LICENSE
OFFENSE: SUBSTANCE ABUSE

NOTES: DURING 1995 HE PERSONALLY USED, WITHOUT A THIRD-PARTY PRESCRIPTION, A TOTAL OF THREE ONE OUNCE SAMPLES OF HISTUSSIN, A SCHEDULE III CONTROLLED DANGEROUS SUBSTANCE, OVER A FIVE DAY PERIOD FOR AN ALLEGED PROPER MEDICAL PRACTICE. HIS HISTORY OF PERSONAL CHEMICAL DEPENDENCY, FOR WHICH HE WAS RECOVERING DURING 1995, CONSTITUTES A DIRECT THREAT OF SAFETY AND WELFARE TO THE CITIZENS OF OKLAHOMA. PROBATION UNDER THE FOLLOWING TERMS AND CONDITIONS: SHALL NOT PRESCRIBE, ADMINISTER, OR DISPENSE ANY CONTROLLED DANGEROUS SUBSTANCES, PRESCRIPTIVE OR OTHER HABIT FORMING MEDICATIONS FOR PERSONAL USE AND SHALL TAKE NONE UNLESS AUTHORIZED BY ANOTHER PHYSICIAN FOR LEGITIMATE MEDICAL NEED; SHALL ABSTAIN FROM ALCOHOL AND ANY SUBSTANCE WHICH WOULD ADVERSELY AFFECT HIS ABILITY TO PRACTICE MEDICINE; SHALL SUBMIT BIOLOGICAL FLUID SPECIMENS; SHALL NOT SUPERVISE A PHYSICIAN'S ASSISTANT; SHALL INFORM THE BOARD OF ADDRESS/CHANGE OF ADDRESS; SHALL APPEAR BEFORE THE BOARD UPON REQUEST AND SUBMIT ALL REQUIRED REPORTS; SHALL NOT ISSUE PRESCRIPTIONS FOR CONTROLLED DANGEROUS SUBSTANCES TO PATIENTS WHO ARE NOT IN A HOSPITAL OR IN-PATIENT TYPE SETTING AT THE TIME THE PRESCRIPTION IS ISSUED; HOWEVER, HE SHALL BE PERMITTED TO PRESCRIBE CONTROLLED INVESTIGATIONAL DRUGS AND ANABOLIC STEROIDS TO PATIENTS FREE AND CLEAR OF THIS LIMITATION; SHALL KEEP CURRENT THE PAYMENT OF ALL ASSESSMENT BY THE BOARD; SHALL FURNISH EACH STATE IN WHICH HE HOLDS LICENSE OR APPLIES FOR LICENSURE, AND ALL HOSPITALS, CLINICS, OR ANY WORKPLACE AT WHICH HE RECEIVES ANY FORM OF STAFF PRIVILEGES, A COPY OF THIS BOARD ORDER; TO THESE CONDITIONS RUSH BEHAVIORAL HEALTH CENTER ADDS THE FOLLOWING: SHALL REFRAIN FROM THE PRACTICE OF ANESTHESIOLOGY FOR AT LEAST ONE YEAR FROM 7/94; SHALL RETURN TO MONITORED MEDICAL PRACTICE IN AREAS OTHER THAN ANESTHESIOLOGY; SHALL ATTEND NO LESS THAN THREE 12-STEP MEETINGS PER WEEK; SHALL PARTICIPATE IN WEEKLY CADUCEUS GROUP MEETINGS; SHALL SUBMIT TO RANDOM, OBSERVED URINE MONITORING; SHALL HAVE NO PERSONAL HANDLING OF MOOD-ALTERING CHEMICALS IN THE WORK PLACE; SHALL OBTAIN A PRIMARY CARE PHYSICIAN; SHALL ADHERE TO A STRICT POLICY OF NOT SELF-PRESCRIBING MEDICATION; SHALL RETURN TO RUSH BEHAVIORAL HEALTH CENTER FOR REASSESSMENT IN THREE TO SIX MONTHS FROM 7/94; SHALL COMPLY WITH ALL STIPULATIONS OF THE OKLAHOMA PHYSICIAN RECOVERY PROGRAM. ON 3/27/97 REQUEST TO MODIFY ORDER GRANTED ALLOWING HIM TO ISSUE PRESCRIPTIONS FOR CONTROLLED SUBSTANCES TO OUTPATIENTS ON DUPLICATE SERIALLY NUMBERED PRESCRIPTIONS WHICH SHALL BE AVAILABLE FOR REVIEW.

PEARMAN, DARRELL W MD, DATE OF BIRTH AUGUST 13, 1958 OF 8905 DANLEY DRIVE, OKLAHOMA CITY, OK, WAS DISCIPLINED BY MEDICARE ON MAY 9, 1995
DISCIPLINARY ACTION: EXCLUSION FROM THE MEDICARE AND/OR MEDICAID PROGRAM
OFFENSE: NONCOMPLIANCE WITH A PROFESSIONAL RULE

NOTES: DEFAULTED ON PUBLIC HEALTH SERVICE EDUCATION LOAN. REINSTATED ON 6/22/95.

PENNINGTON, KAREN MD, DATE OF BIRTH SEPTEMBER 21, 1940 OF 703 N W 64TH STREET, OKLAHOMA CITY, OK, WAS DISCIPLINED BY MEDICARE ON APRIL 9, 1996
DISCIPLINARY ACTION: EXCLUSION FROM THE MEDICARE AND/OR MEDICAID PROGRAM

OFFENSE: DISCIPLINARY ACTION BY ANOTHER STATE OR AGENCY

NOTES: LICENSE SUSPENDED FOR REASONS BEARING ON PROFESSIONAL PERFORMANCE.

PENTECOST, RICHARD L MD, LICENSE NUMBER 0008068, WAS DISCIPLINED BY OKLAHOMA ON JANUARY 15, 1993
DISCIPLINARY ACTION: REPRIMAND
OFFENSE: OVERPRESCRIBING OR MISPRESCRIBING DRUGS

NOTES: A PRESCRIPTION SURVEY CONDUCTED IN REFERENCE TO CERTAIN SCHEDULED DRUGS FROM 6/5/90 THROUGH 9/28/92 INDICATES THAT IN THE CASE OF SEVERAL PATIENTS SCHEDULED DRUGS WERE BEING PRESCRIBED IN EXCESS OF THE AMOUNT CONSIDERED FOR THE MEDICAL NEED PRESENTED; ALSO LACK OF ADEQUATE IN-OFFICE CONTROL OF THE ISSUANCE OF PRESCRIPTIONS BOTH BY TELEPHONE AND IN PERSON. IT IS SUGGESTED BUT NOT ORDERED THAT HE NOT RELY ON TELEPHONE PRESCRIPTIONS, THAT HE REVIEW THE STREET VALUE OF CERTAIN CONTROLLED DANGEROUS SUBSTANCES REGULARLY PRESCRIBED BY HIM, AND THAT HE REMOVE HIS PRE-PRINTED DEA NUMBER FROM PRESCRIPTION PADS.

PENTECOST, RICHARD L MD, LICENSE NUMBER 0C19974 OF MUSKOGEE, OK, WAS DISCIPLINED BY CALIFORNIA ON APRIL 15, 1995
DISCIPLINARY ACTION: 60-MONTH PROBATION
OFFENSE: DISCIPLINARY ACTION BY ANOTHER STATE OR AGENCY

NOTES: DISCIPLINED BY OKLAHOMA BOARD FOR INDISCRIMINATE PRESCRIBING. REVOCATION STAYED.

PERSHICA, BILLY MD OF 105 S KEMP, TISHOMINGO, OK, WAS DISCIPLINED BY DEA ON JUNE 7, 1999
DISCIPLINARY ACTION: SURRENDER OF CONTROLLED SUBSTANCE LICENSE
OFFENSE: DISCIPLINARY ACTION BY ANOTHER STATE OR AGENCY

NOTES: STATE BOARD.

PHILPOTT, WILLIAM H MD, LICENSE NUMBER 0010713 OF 17171 SE 29, CHOCTAW, OK, WAS DISCIPLINED BY OKLAHOMA ON JUNE 21, 1990
DISCIPLINARY ACTION: SURRENDER OF LICENSE
OFFENSE: DISCIPLINARY ACTION BY ANOTHER STATE OR AGENCY

NOTES: ALLEGATIONS OF UNPROFESSIONAL CONDUCT ON MINOR PATIENTS; VOLUNTARILY ENTERED INTO A STIPULATION WITH THE FLORIDA BOARD; HE PROVIDED WRITTEN RESIGNATION FROM THE PRACTICE OF MEDICINE ON 5/21/90. MAY NOT RE-APPLY FOR LICENSURE AS A PHYSICIAN AND SURGEON IN OKLAHOMA.

PHILPOTT, WILLIAM H MD, LICENSE NUMBER 0031212 OF 17171 SE 29TH STREET, CHOCTAW, OK, WAS DISCIPLINED BY MASSACHUSETTS ON DECEMBER 29, 1993
DISCIPLINARY ACTION: SURRENDER OF LICENSE

NOTES: RESIGNATION.

PICKETT, ROGER L MD, LICENSE NUMBER 0008166, WAS DISCIPLINED BY OKLAHOMA ON JUNE 26, 1992
DISCIPLINARY ACTION: 60-MONTH PROBATION; RESTRICTION PLACED ON LICENSE
OFFENSE: OVERPRESCRIBING OR MISPRESCRIBING DRUGS

NOTES: FROM 6/23/91 THROUGH 12/23/91, WROTE PRESCRIPTIONS FOR CONTROLLED DANGEROUS SUBSTANCES FOR AT LEAST SIX PATIENTS IN EXCESS OF THE AMOUNT CONSIDERED GOOD MEDICAL PRACTICE FOR THE MEDICAL NEED PRESENTED. PROBATION UNDER TERMS AND CONDITIONS: MAY PRESCRIBE, ADMINISTER OR DISPENSE CONTROLLED DANGEROUS SUBSTANCES ONLY ON SERIALLY-NUMBERED, DUPLICATE PRESCRIPTION PADS, WITH COPIES AVAILABLE TO BOARD; SHALL CEASE USING ANY UNDATED OR UNSIGNED PRESCRIPTIONS FOR CONTROLLED DANGEROUS SUBSTANCES; SHALL SUCCESSFULLY COMPLETE AT LEAST 60 HOURS OF CONTINUING MEDICAL EDUCATION ON THE ISSUE OF PAIN MANAGEMENT; SHALL NOT SUPERVISE A PHYSICIAN ASSISTANT; SHALL FURNISH BOARD WITH ADDRESS AND/OR CHANGE OF ADDRESS; SHALL APPEAR BEFORE BOARD UPON REQUEST; SHALL NOTIFY ANY HOSPITAL WHERE HE HOLDS STAFF PRIVILEGES OR CLINICS OR GROUP OF THE TERMS AND CONDITIONS.

POLLNOW, ROBERT E MD, DATE OF BIRTH JANUARY 30, 1946, LICENSE NUMBER 0027751 OF 4205 SQUIRE DRIVE, BETTENDORF, IA, WAS DISCIPLINED BY IOWA ON FEBRUARY 4, 1992
DISCIPLINARY ACTION: 60-MONTH PROBATION
OFFENSE: SUBSTANCE ABUSE

NOTES: ALLEGATIONS OF EXCESSIVE USE OF ALCOHOL.

POLLNOW, ROBERT EDWARD MD, DATE OF BIRTH JANUARY 30, 1946, LICENSE NUMBER 0018141, WAS DISCIPLINED BY OKLAHOMA ON JUNE 26, 1992
DISCIPLINARY ACTION: 60-MONTH PROBATION; RESTRICTION PLACED ON LICENSE
OFFENSE: SUBSTANCE ABUSE

NOTES: EVIDENCE INDICATED THAT HE PREVIOUSLY MISUSED ALCOHOL; HAS COMPLETED APPROPRIATE SUBSTANCE ABUSE TREATMENT; PRESENTLY IN RECOVERY. LICENSE GRANTED UNDER PROBATIONARY TERMS AND CONDITIONS: SHALL NOT PRESCRIBE, ADMINISTER OR DISPENSE ANY MEDICATIONS FOR HIS PERSONAL USE; SHALL TAKE NO MEDICATION UNLESS PRESCRIBED BY TREATING PHYSICIAN; SHALL ABSTAIN FROM ALCOHOL OR ANY SUBSTANCE WHICH WOULD ADVERSELY AFFECT HIS ABILITY TO PRACTICE; SHALL SUBMIT BIOLOGICAL FLUID SPECIMENS FOR ANALYSIS; SHALL MAINTAIN FORMAL RELATIONSHIP WITH PHYSICIAN RECOVERY COMMITTEE AND PARTICIPATE IN THEIR MEETINGS AND ACTIVITIES; SHALL NOT SUPERVISE A PHYSICIAN ASSISTANT; SHALL FURNISH BOARD WITH ADDRESS AND/OR CHANGE OF ADDRESS; SHALL APPEAR BEFORE BOARD UPON REQUEST; SHALL NOTIFY ANY HOSPITAL WHERE HE HOLDS STAFF PRIVILEGES OR CLINIC OR GROUP OF THE TERMS AND CONDITIONS. ON 8/9/96 HIS REQUEST FOR EARLY TERMINATION OF PROBATION DENIED.

POLLNOW, ROBERT EDWARD MD, DATE OF BIRTH JANUARY 30, 1946, LICENSE NUMBER 00E2321 OF 4205 SQUIRE DRIVE, BETTENDORF, IA, WAS DISCIPLINED BY TEXAS ON APRIL 30, 1993
DISCIPLINARY ACTION: 60-MONTH PROBATION; MONITORING OF PHYSICIAN PERFORMANCE
OFFENSE: DISCIPLINARY ACTION BY ANOTHER STATE OR AGENCY

NOTES: ON 1/23/92 PLACED ON PROBATION WITH CONDITIONS BY IOWA BOARD DUE TO ALCOHOL ABUSE; ON 7/2/92 HE WAS GRANTED LICENSURE BY OKLAHOMA ON PROBATION WITH CONDITIONS. FIVE YEAR SUSPENSION STAYED. CONDITIONS OF PROBATION: PRIOR TO PRACTICING IN TEXAS SHALL APPEAR BEFORE THE BOARD; SHALL PROVIDE THE TEXAS BOARD COPIES OF REPORTS SUBMITTED TO IOWA AND OKLAHOMA UPON REQUEST; SHALL PARTICIPATE

IN ACTIVITIES OF A PHYSICIAN HEALTH AND REHABILITATION COMMITTEE AND ATTEND WEEKLY MEETINGS WITH QUARTERLY REPORTS; SHALL PARTICIPATE IN AA OR ANY SUBSTANTIALLY SIMILAR PROGRAM NOT LESS THAN TWICE A WEEK WITH QUARTERLY REPORTS TO THE BOARD; SHALL SUBMIT HIMSELF FOR APPROPRIATE EXAMS INCLUDING DRUG OR ALCOHOL SCREENS; SHALL SUBMIT HIMSELF FOR EVALUATION AND TREATMENT TO A BOARD-APPROVED PSYCHIATRIST; SHALL ABSTAIN FROM THE CONSUMPTION OF ALCOHOL/CHEMICAL SUBSTANCES IN ANY FORM; SHALL NOT TREAT OR OTHERWISE SERVE AS THE PHYSICIAN, PRESCRIBE, DISPENSE OR ADMINISTER DRUGS THAT MAY BE SUBJECT TO ABUSE FOR HIMSELF OR ANY MEMBER OF HIS FAMILY; SHALL FURNISH WRITTEN REPORTS TO THE BOARD REGARDING HIS MEDICAL CONDITION UPON REQUEST; SHALL GIVE A COPY OF THIS ORDER TO ANY HEALTH CARE ENTITY WHERE HE HAS PRIVILEGES; SHALL COOPERATE WITH THE BOARD IN VERIFYING COMPLIANCE; SHALL INFORM BOARD OF CHANGE OF ADDRESS WITHIN 10 DAYS OR IF HE LEAVES THE STATE; TIME SPENT OUT OF TEXAS DOES NOT COUNT TOWARD PROBATION. SHALL NOT SEEK MODIFICATION FOR ONE YEAR.

POLLNOW, ROBERT EDWARD MD, DATE OF BIRTH JANUARY 30, 1946, LICENSE NUMBER 0018141, WAS DISCIPLINED BY OKLAHOMA ON NOVEMBER 19, 1994
OFFENSE: FAILURE TO COMPLY WITH PREVIOUS BOARD ORDER

NOTES: CURRENTLY ON LEVEL II PROBATION WHICH REQUIRES HIM TO SUBMIT MONTHLY COMPLIANCE REPORTS ON A TIMELY BASIS; HAS FAILED TO SUBMIT REPORTS ON A TIMELY BASIS. LICENSE PLACED ON LEVEL I PROBATION AND SHALL BE REVIEWED IN SIX MONTHS.

PORTER, JOHN F DO OF 1200 WEST 4TH, TAHLEQUAH, OK, WAS DISCIPLINED BY DEA ON NOVEMBER 10, 1994
DISCIPLINARY ACTION: SURRENDER OF CONTROLLED SUBSTANCE LICENSE
OFFENSE: PROFESSIONAL MISCONDUCT

NOTES: ALLEGED VIOLATION OF CONTROLLED SUBSTANCE ACT.

PORTER, STEVEN B DO, LICENSE NUMBER 3411, WAS DISCIPLINED BY OKLAHOMA ON SEPTEMBER 14, 1999
DISCIPLINARY ACTION: SURRENDER OF LICENSE

PORTER, STEVEN B DO, LICENSE NUMBER 3411, WAS DISCIPLINED BY OKLAHOMA ON DECEMBER 11, 1999
DISCIPLINARY ACTION: LICENSE REINSTATEMENT

NOTES: TERMS AND CONDITIONS FOR THREE YEARS.

PORTER, WARREN H MD, LICENSE NUMBER 0006287 OF PO BOX 15568, DEL CITY, OK, WAS DISCIPLINED BY OKLAHOMA ON FEBRUARY 1, 1991
DISCIPLINARY ACTION: 60-MONTH PROBATION; RESTRICTION PLACED ON CONTROLLED SUBSTANCE LICENSE
OFFENSE: OVERPRESCRIBING OR MISPRESCRIBING DRUGS

NOTES: FROM 7/1/90 THROUGH 11/15/90, WROTE PRESCRIPTIONS FOR CONTROLLED DANGEROUS SUBSTANCES FOR AT LEAST FIVE PATIENTS IN EXCESS OF THE AMOUNT CONSIDERED MEDICALLY NECESSARY FOR THE MEDICAL NEED PRESENTED. PROBATION UNDER TERMS AND CONDITIONS: MAY PRESCRIBE CONTROLLED DANGEROUS SUBSTANCES ONLY ON SERIALLY-NUMBERED, DUPLICATE PRESCRIPTION PADS, WITH COPIES AVAILABLE FOR BOARD; SHALL FURNISH BOARD WITH ADDRESS AND/OR CHANGE OF ADDRESS; SHALL APPEAR BEFORE BOARD UPON REQUEST; SHALL NOTIFY ANY HOSPITAL WHERE HE HOLDS STAFF PRIVILEGES OR CLINIC OR GROUP OF THE TERMS AND CONDITIONS.

PRICE, WILLIAM FRANKLIN MD, LICENSE NUMBER 18087 OF HC 71, BOX 160 P, KINGSTON, OK, WAS DISCIPLINED BY OKLAHOMA ON JULY 29, 1999
DISCIPLINARY ACTION: 2-MONTH LICENSE SUSPENSION; PROBATION
OFFENSE: SUBSTANCE ABUSE

NOTES: FROM 12/2/98-4/19/99 ADMITTED THAT HE WROTE PRESCRIPTIONS FOR TUSSIONEX SUSPENSION, AS WELL AS OTHER CONTROLLED DANGEROUS DRUGS, FOR HIS AUNT; FURTHER ADMITS THAT HE PICKED UP THESE MEDICATIONS FOR HIS OWN PERSONAL USE; FROM 4/14/98-5/12/99 ADMITTED THAT HE WROTE PRESCRIPTIONS FOR CONTROLLED DANGEROUS DRUGS FOR VARIOUS RELATIVES, HIS WIFE, HIS STEP-SON-IN-LAW AND HIS STEP-GRANDSON, SOME OF WHICH WERE FOR HIS OWN PERSONAL USE; FROM 4/17/98-4/6/99 ADMITTED THAT HE WROTE OR CALLED IN PRESCRIPTIONS FOR CONTROLLED DANGEROUS DRUGS ALLEGEDLY AUTHORIZED BY ANOTHER DOCTOR (WHO DENIED AUTHORIZING THE PRESCRIPTIONS) FOR HIS WIFE AND SON AND ADMITS THAT THE DRUGS WERE FOR HIS OWN PERSONAL USE; FROM 5/24/99-7/10/99 HE WAS TREATED FOR OPIOID DEPENDENCE WITH RELAPSE. SUSPENSION RETROACTIVE TO 5/24/99; TERMS AND CONDITIONS OF PROBATION: SHALL REQUEST ALL HEALTH CARE FACILITIES IN WHICH HE ANTICIPATES PRACTICING TO FURNISH A STATEMENT REGARDING MONITORING OF HIS PRACTICE; SHALL SUBMIT TO EVERY STATE IN WHICH HE HOLDS LICENSURE AND TO HOSPITALS, CLINICS OR OTHER INSTITUTIONS IN WHICH HE HOLDS OR ANTICIPATES HOLDING ANY FORM OF STAFF PRIVILEGE A COPY OF THIS ORDER; SHALL NOT SUPERVISE ALLIED HEALTH PROFESSIONALS; SHALL NOT PRESCRIBE, ADMINISTER, OR DISPENSE OR POSSESS ANY DRUGS IN SCHEDULES I-V, EXCEPT THAT HE MAY WRITE ORDERS FOR THE ADMINISTRATION OF PAIN MEDICATION FOR EMERGENCY ROOM PATIENTS OR FOR HOSPITAL INPATIENTS; SHALL SUBMIT BIOLOGICAL FLUID SPECIMENS; SHALL NOT PRESCRIBE, ADMINISTER, OR DISPENSE ANY MEDICATIONS FOR PERSONAL USE, OR FOR THAT OF ANY FAMILY MEMBER, AND SHALL TAKE NONE UNLESS AUTHORIZED BY ANOTHER PHYSICIAN FOR A LEGITIMATE MEDICAL NEED; SHALL NOT INGEST ANY SUBSTANCE WHICH WILL CAUSE A SPECIMEN TO TEST POSITIVE FOR PROHIBITED SUBSTANCES; SHALL EXECUTE ALL RELEASES OF MEDICAL AND PSYCHIATRIC RECORDS AS NECESSARY TO DISCUSS HIS CASE WITH HIS TREATING PHYSICIANS AND/OR ANY PHYSICIANS HOLDING RECORDS; SHALL ABIDE BY HIS POSTCARE CONTRACT; SHALL ATTEND THREE MEETINGS PER WEEK OF A LOCAL 12-STEP PROGRAM; SHALL KEEP THE BOARD INFORMED OF HIS ADDRESS AND PAY COSTS; SHALL APPEAR BEFORE THE BOARD AND SUBMIT REPORTS UPON REQUEST. ON 9/24/99 ORDER MODIFIED ALLOWING HIM TO WRITE ORDERS FOR SCHEDULES II THROUGH V DRUGS FOR HOSPITAL INPATIENTS AND EMERGENCY ROOM PATIENTS.

PUGH, ROBERT LEWIS JR OF 902 KENTUCKY TOWERS, LOUISVILLE, KY, WAS DISCIPLINED BY OKLAHOMA ON DECEMBER 2, 1993
DISCIPLINARY ACTION: DENIAL OF NEW LICENSE

NOTES: PAST ACADEMIC AND PERSONAL RECORD RAISE SERIOUS ISSUES AS TO CLINICAL COMPETENCY AND FITNESS TO PRACTICE.

PULUM, RICHARD W DO, LICENSE NUMBER 0002506 OF 918 ASH STREET, OSAGE, IA, WAS DISCIPLINED BY OKLAHOMA ON DECEMBER 12, 1991
DISCIPLINARY ACTION: SURRENDER OF LICENSE
OFFENSE: DISCIPLINARY ACTION BY AÑOTHER STATE OR AGENCY

NOTES: IN 1989 SANCTIONED BY THE U.S. ARMY. VOLUNTARY SURRENDER.

RAJPUT, MOHAMMAD SHABBIR AHMED OF 2601 GABRIEL AVENUE, PARSONS, KS, WAS DISCIPLINED BY OKLAHOMA ON DECEMBER 2, 1993
DISCIPLINARY ACTION: DENIAL OF NEW LICENSE

NOTES: FAILED TO PASS FLEX EXAM ON TEN SEPARATE OCCASIONS BEFORE FINALLY OBTAINING A MINIMUM PASSING SCORE, WHICH RAISES SERIOUS ISSUES AS TO HIS EDUCATION AND CLINICAL COMPETENCY TO PRACTICE.

RAMIREZ, MANUEL J MD, LICENSE NUMBER 0136841 OF PO BOX 2120, GUYMON, OK, WAS DISCIPLINED BY NEW YORK ON SEPTEMBER 30, 1993
DISCIPLINARY ACTION: SURRENDER OF LICENSE
OFFENSE: NONCOMPLIANCE WITH A PROFESSIONAL RULE

NOTES: DID NOT CONTEST CHARGES THAT HE WILLFULLY FAILED TO COMPLY WITH PROVISIONS OF FEDERAL, STATE OR LOCAL LAWS, RULES OR REGULATIONS GOVERNING THE PRACTICE OF MEDICINE.

RAMIREZ, MANUEL JOSEPH MD, LICENSE NUMBER 0014479, WAS DISCIPLINED BY OKLAHOMA ON MARCH 22, 1990
DISCIPLINARY ACTION: 36-MONTH PROBATION; RESTRICTION PLACED ON CONTROLLED SUBSTANCE LICENSE
OFFENSE: OVERPRESCRIBING OR MISPRESCRIBING DRUGS

NOTES: GUILTY OF PRESCRIBING OR ADMINISTERING A DRUG OR TREATMENT WITHOUT SUFFICIENT EXAMINATION AND THE ESTABLISHMENT OF A VALID PHYSICIAN-PATIENT RELATIONSHIP OR WITHOUT MEDICAL NEED TO THREE NARCOTICS AGENTS POSING AS PATIENTS IN JULY AND AUGUST 1989. THREE YEAR PROBATION RETROACTIVE TO 11/14/88 UNDER THE FOLLOWING MODIFIED TERMS AND CONDITIONS: SHALL NOT PRESCRIBE, ADMINISTER, OR DISPENSE ANY CONTROLLED DANGEROUS SUBSTANCES, SCHEDULES II, III, IV, AND V, EXCEPT TO HOSPITAL IN-PATIENTS AND TO EMERGENCY ROOM PATIENTS AND THEN ONLY AT THE TIME THE TREATMENT IS RECEIVED; ANY SUBSTANCES PRESCRIBED, ADMINISTERED, OR DISPENSED IN THESE LIMITED SETTINGS MUST BE ON SERIALLY-NUMBERED, DUPLICATE PRESCRIPTION PADS AND HE SHALL MAKE COPIES AVAILABLE TO THE BOARD UPON REQUEST; SHALL SUBSTANTIALLY REDUCE THE NUMBER OF CONTROLLED DANGEROUS SUBSTANCE PRESCRIPTIONS BEING WRITTEN, THE DURATION OF TIME THAT PATIENTS ARE RETAINED ON CONTROLLED DANGEROUS SUBSTANCES PRESCRIBED AND THE NUMBER OF PATIENTS HE SEES ON A DAILY BASIS; SHALL SUBMIT TO THE BOARD ADDRESS/ CHANGE OF ADDRESS; SHALL APPEAR BEFORE THE BOARD UPON REQUEST AND SUBMIT ANY REQUIRED REPORTS TO INCLUDE, BUT NOT LIMITED TO MONTHLY SELF-REPORT FORMS, COPIES OF DUPLICATE, SERIALLY-NUMBERED PRESCRIPTIONS OF ALL CONTROLLED DANGEROUS SUBSTANCES PRESCRIBED, ADMINISTERED, OR DISPENSED, POST-OPERATION SUMMARY REPORTS AND ANY OTHER BOARD REQUIRED REPORTS; THE REFERRED TO REPORTS SHALL BE SUBMITTED MONTHLY TO THE BOARD AND REVIEWED EVERY SIX MONTHS; SHALL PAY COSTS; SHALL FURNISH ANY HOSPITAL WHERE HE HOLDS STAFF PRIVILEGES OR CLINIC OR GROUP WHERE HE PRACTICES WITH A COPY OF THE ORDER. ON 6/21/90 RECONSIDERATION DENIED.

RAY, ARLES GAREL MD, LICENSE NUMBER 0011310, WAS DISCIPLINED BY OKLAHOMA ON JUNE 22, 1991
DISCIPLINARY ACTION: 2-MONTH LICENSE SUSPENSION; 60-MONTH PROBATION
OFFENSE: PROVIDING FALSE INFORMATION TO THE BOARD OR OTHER HEALTH AGENCY

NOTES: ON 12/2/89, PROVIDED 8 PRESCRIPTIONS FOR NON-CONTROLLED SUBSTANCES FOR ONE PATIENT, 6 OF WHICH WERE UNDATED. ON 10/31/90, LICENSURE APPLICATION DENIED IN FLORIDA DUE TO HISTORY OF CHEMICAL ADDICTION; DENIAL OF PREVIOUS SUBSTANCE ABUSE PROBLEMS; SUBSTANCE-INDUCED BLACKOUTS AS RECENTLY AS 1988; MARIJUANA USE AS RECENTLY AS 1989; CONTINUED CONSUMPTION OF ALCOHOL, THOUGH CLAIMING NOT TO HAVE BEEN INTOXICATED SINCE 1988; HISTORY OF DEPRESSIVE EPISODES INCLUDING AN ATTEMPTED SUICIDE; ADMITS TO SELF-MEDICATING; UNCOOPERATIVE WITH PHYSICIANS RECOVERY NETWORK IN EFFORTS TO SECURE PSYCHIATRIC EVALUATION. ON 3/20/91, SUBMITTED APPLICATION FOR OKLAHOMA LICENSE RENEWAL AND LIED AS TO HISTORY OF DRUG OR ALCOHOL ADDICTION, HISTORY OF TREATMENT IN DRUG OR ALCOHOL REHABILITATION PROGRAM OR HISTORY OF TREATMENT FOR EMOTIONAL OR MENTAL DISORDERS. PROBATION UNDER TERMS AND CONDITIONS: MAY PRESCRIBE CONTROLLED DANGEROUS SUBSTANCES ONLY ON SERIALLY-NUMBERED, DUPLICATE PRESCRIPTION PADS, WITH COPIES AVAILABLE TO BOARD; SHALL NOT AUTHORIZE ANY STAFF TO PRESCRIBE, ADMINISTER OR DISPENSE ANY CONTROLLED DANGEROUS SUBSTANCES IN HIS PLACE; SHALL SUBMIT BIOLOGICAL FLUID SPECIMENS FOR ANALYSIS; SHALL NOT PRESCRIBE, ADMINISTER OR DISPENSE ANY MEDICATIONS FOR HIS PERSONAL USE; SHALL TAKE NO MEDICATION UNLESS PRESCRIBED BY TREATING PHYSICIAN; SHALL ABSTAIN FROM ALCOHOL OR ANY SUBSTANCE WHICH WOULD ADVERSELY AFFECT HIS ABILITY TO PRACTICE; SHALL NOTIFY ANY HOSPITAL WHERE HE HOLDS STAFF PRIVILEGES OR CLINIC OR GROUP OF THE TERMS AND CONDITIONS; SHALL REQUEST HOSPITALS WHERE HE HAS STAFF PRIVILEGES TO SUPPLY WRITTEN REPORTS TO THE BOARD; SHALL FURNISH BOARD WITH ADDRESS AND/OR CHANGE OF ADDRESS; SHALL APPEAR BEFORE BOARD UPON REQUEST; SHALL PARTICIPATE IN ACTIVITIES OF PHYSICIAN RECOVERY COMMITTEE. MOTION FOR MODIFICATION OF PROBATION DENIED ON 7/2/92, BUT PROBATIONARY LEVEL OF SUPERVISION REDUCED FROM LEVEL I TO LEVEL II. TERMS AND CONDITIONS REMAIN THE SAME.

REED, GUY D DO OF 6109 EAST ADMIRAL PLACE, TULSA, OK, WAS DISCIPLINED BY DEA ON JUNE 16, 1994
DISCIPLINARY ACTION: SURRENDER OF CONTROLLED SUBSTANCE LICENSE

NOTES: IN LIEU OF PUBLIC INTEREST REVOCATION.

REED, GUY D DO, LICENSE NUMBER 0001021, WAS DISCIPLINED BY OKLAHOMA ON JUNE 30, 1994

DISCIPLINARY ACTION: LICENSE REVOCATION
OFFENSE: OVERPRESCRIBING OR MISPRESCRIBING DRUGS

NOTES: BETWEEN 2/93 AND 1/94 FAILED TO KEEP COMPLETE AND ACCURATE RECORDS OF PURCHASE AND DISPOSAL OF CONTROLLED DRUGS; IN ONE CASE EXCESSIVELY AND INAPPROPRIATELY DISPENSED CONTROLLED DRUGS; BETWEEN 1/93 AND 1/94 PRESCRIBED MEDICATION WITHOUT A VALID PHYSICIAN/PATIENT RELATIONSHIP IN ONE CASE AND MEDICAL EXAMINATION IN NINE CASES. ALSO DISPENSED EXCESSIVE AND INAPPROPRIATE AMOUNT OF CONTROLLED DRUGS IN EIGHT OF THESE CASES.

REED, GUY D DO OF TULSA, OK, WAS DISCIPLINED BY MISSOURI ON JANUARY 24, 1995
DISCIPLINARY ACTION: LICENSE REVOCATION
OFFENSE: DISCIPLINARY ACTION BY ANOTHER STATE OR AGENCY

NOTES: OKLAHOMA FINALLY AND UNCONDITIONALLY REVOKED LICENSE FOR EXCESSIVELY AND INAPPROPRIATELY PRESCRIBING CONTROLLED SUBSTANCES WITHOUT MEDICAL NEED. NO REAPPLICATION FOR SEVEN YEARS.

REED, GUY D DO, DATE OF BIRTH NOVEMBER 4, 1922 OF 6775 S ATLANTA PL, TULSA, OK, WAS DISCIPLINED BY MEDICARE ON FEBRUARY 8, 1995
DISCIPLINARY ACTION: EXCLUSION FROM THE MEDICARE AND/OR MEDICAID PROGRAM
OFFENSE: DISCIPLINARY ACTION BY ANOTHER STATE OR AGENCY

NOTES: LICENSE REVOCATION OR SUSPENSION.

REED, GUY D DO, LICENSE NUMBER 20A3938 OF TULSA, OK, WAS DISCIPLINED BY CALIFORNIA ON AUGUST 14, 1995
DISCIPLINARY ACTION: LICENSE REVOCATION
OFFENSE: DISCIPLINARY ACTION BY ANOTHER STATE OR AGENCY

NOTES: ACTION IN OKLAHOMA FOR INABILITY TO ACCOUNT FOR CONTROLLED SUBSTANCES.

REED, GUY DEAN DO, LICENSE NUMBER 0000426 OF TULSA, OK, WAS DISCIPLINED BY OHIO ON NOVEMBER 8, 1995
DISCIPLINARY ACTION: LICENSE REVOCATION
OFFENSE: DISCIPLINARY ACTION BY ANOTHER STATE OR AGENCY

NOTES: OKLAHOMA LICENSE REVOKED FOR REASONS INCLUDING, BUT NOT LIMITED TO, FAILURE TO KEEP ACCURATE CONTROLLED SUBSTANCE RECORDS, FAILURE TO ACCOUNT FOR ADMINISTRATION AND/OR DISPENSING OF CONTROLLED SUBSTANCES, AND EXCESSIVE AND/OR INAPPROPRIATE PRESCRIBING; MISSOURI LICENSE REVOKED ON THE BASIS OF THE OKLAHOMA ACTION. PERMANENT REVOCATION.

REYNOLDS, JOE BILLS MD, LICENSE NUMBER 0007938 OF 4720 S WESTERN, OKLAHOMA CITY, OK, WAS DISCIPLINED BY OKLAHOMA ON MARCH 22, 1990
DISCIPLINARY ACTION: EMERGENCY SUSPENSION
OFFENSE: PROFESSIONAL MISCONDUCT

NOTES: SURGICAL PROCEDURES ON THREE PATIENTS, ONE OF WHOM WAS FOR LIPOSUCTION AND DIED AS A RESULT OF THE SURGERY BEING DONE OUTSIDE OF A HOSPITAL SETTING, WERE DONE IN AN UNPROFESSIONAL MANNER AND IN AN UNPROFESSIONAL SETTING WHICH CONSTITUTE CLEAR AND IMMEDIATE DANGER TO PUBLIC HEALTH, SAFETY, AND WELFARE.

REYNOLDS, JOE BILLS MD, LICENSE NUMBER 0007938, WAS DISCIPLINED BY OKLAHOMA ON NOVEMBER 8, 1991
DISCIPLINARY ACTION: LICENSE REVOCATION
OFFENSE: CRIMINAL CONVICTION OR PLEA OF GUILTY, NOLO CONTENDERE, OR NO CONTEST TO A CRIME

NOTES: ON 6/18/91, CONVICTED OF SECOND DEGREE MANSLAUGHTER IN THE DISTRICT COURT OF OKLAHOMA COUNTY. LICENSE HAD BEEN SUSPENDED SINCE 3/17/90. VOLUNTARILY SURRENDERED ON 6/19/91.

RICKETSON, ROBERT MD, LICENSE NUMBER 16569 OF PO BOX 7086, EDMOND, OK, WAS DISCIPLINED BY OKLAHOMA ON JANUARY 21, 1999
DISCIPLINARY ACTION: 2-MONTH LICENSE SUSPENSION; 60-MONTH PROBATION
OFFENSE: SUBSTANCE ABUSE

NOTES: WROTE MULTIPLE PRESCRIPTIONS FOR LORTAB IN THE NAME OF THE EDMOND SPINE CENTER RATHER THAN A PARTICULAR PATIENT; PRESCRIPTIONS WERE FILLED AND RETURNED TO HIS OFFICE WHERE HE TOOK CUSTODY OF THEM, AND INGESTED SOME OF THEM FROM THE IMPROPERLY WRITTEN PRESCRIPTIONS; ADMITTED WRITING HYDROCODONE PRESCRIPTIONS FOR HIS WIFE AND PERSONALLY INGESTING SOME OF HER HYDROCODONE; ADMITTED INGESTING HYDROCODONE SAMPLES; FROM APPROXIMATELY 1/97-6/98 REGULARLY TOOK HYDROCODONE WHILE SELF-TREATING HIS CHRONIC BACK PAIN; FROM 11/2/98-12/11/98 RECEIVED INPATIENT TREATMENT AND UPON LEAVING, ENTERED INTO AN AFTER-CARE CONTRACT AND HAS BEEN AN ACTIVE PARTICIPANT IN THE OKLAHOMA PHYSICIANS RECOVERY GROUP. LICENSE SHALL BE AUTOMATICALLY REINSTATED ON PROBATION EFFECTIVE 2/1/99 WITH FOLLOWING TERMS AND CONDITIONS: SHALL NOT RECEIVE, POSSESS, DISPENSE OR ADMINISTER ANY CONTROLLED DRUGS IN SCHEDULES II-V OR ANY ADDICTIVE DRUGS, INCLUDING ANY SAMPLES, IN AN OFFICE OR OUT-PATIENT SETTING BUT MAY POSSESS SUCH DRUGS IN A HOSPITAL OR OTHER INSTITUTIONAL SETTING; MAY PRESCRIBE THESE DRUGS ONLY IF HE KEEPS DUPLICATE, SERIALLY NUMBERED PRESCRIPTIONS OF AND SUBMITS COPIES TO THE BOARD UPON REQUEST; SHALL REQUEST ALL HEALTH CARE FACILITIES IN WHICH HE ANTICIPATES PRACTICING TO FURNISH A STATEMENT REGARDING MONITORING OF HIS PRACTICE; SHALL SUBMIT BIOLOGICAL FLUID SPECIMENS; SHALL NOT PRESCRIBE, ADMINISTER OR DISPENSE ANY MEDICATIONS FOR HIS PERSONAL USE, OR FOR USE BY HIS FAMILY OR FRIENDS, AND SHALL TAKE NONE UNLESS AUTHORIZED BY ANOTHER PHYSICIAN FOR A LEGITIMATE MEDICAL NEED; SHALL NOT INGEST ANY SUBSTANCE WHICH WILL CAUSE A SPECIMEN TO TEST POSITIVE FOR PROHIBITED SUBSTANCES; SHALL ABIDE BY HIS POST CARE CONTRACT AND ATTEND AT LEAST THREE WEEKLY 12-STEP MEETINGS; SHALL OBTAIN A PRACTICE MONITOR; SHALL BEGIN COUNSELING; SHALL EXECUTE ALL RELEASES OF MEDICAL AND PSYCHIATRIC RECORDS AS NECESSARY TO DISCUSS HIS CASE WITH HIS TREATING PHYSICIANS AND/OR ANY PHYSICIANS HOLDING RECORDS; SHALL SUBMIT TO EVERY STATE IN WHICH HE HOLDS LICENSURE AND TO HOSPITALS, CLINICS OR OTHER INSTITUTIONS IN WHICH HE HOLDS OR ANTICIPATES HOLDING ANY FORM OF STAFF PRIVILEGE A COPY OF THIS ORDER; SHALL NOT SUPERVISE ALLIED HEALTH PROFESSIONALS; SHALL KEEP THE BOARD INFORMED OF HIS ADDRESS AND PAY COSTS; SHALL APPEAR BEFORE THE BOARD UPON REQUEST.

RIPKA, JAY WALTER MD, LICENSE NUMBER 0011413, WAS DISCIPLINED BY OKLAHOMA ON JULY 22, 1994
DISCIPLINARY ACTION: LICENSE SUSPENSION; REPRIMAND
OFFENSE: NONCOMPLIANCE WITH A PROFESSIONAL RULE

NOTES: DURING ANNUAL RENEWAL PROCESS FOR 1994/1995 LICENSE HE FAILED TO PROVIDE THE BOARD WITH NOTICE THAT HE HAD LOST PRIVILEGES FROM A HOSPITAL ON 3/9/94. SUSPENSION FOR THREE WEEKS.

RIPKA, JAY WALTER MD, DATE OF BIRTH JANUARY 12, 1933, LICENSE NUMBER 0028796 OF PELL CITY, AL, WAS DISCIPLINED BY NORTH CAROLINA ON MARCH 13, 1995

NOTES: PUBLIC ADMONISHMENT.

RIPKA, JAY WALTER MD, DATE OF BIRTH JANUARY 12, 1933, LICENSE NUMBER 0027111 OF 2811 HOSPITAL DR, PELL CITY, AL, WAS DISCIPLINED BY GEORGIA ON JULY 7, 1995
DISCIPLINARY ACTION: REPRIMAND
OFFENSE: DISCIPLINARY ACTION BY ANOTHER STATE OR AGENCY

NOTES: DISCIPLINARY ACTION IN OKLAHOMA.

RITTENHOUSE, LEE C MD, LICENSE NUMBER 12365 OF 1114 FENWICK PLACE, OKLAHOMA CITY, OK, WAS DISCIPLINED BY OKLAHOMA ON MAY 29, 1998
DISCIPLINARY ACTION: REPRIMAND
OFFENSE: PROFESSIONAL MISCONDUCT

NOTES: HE WAS THE SUPERVISING PHYSICIAN FOR A PHYSICIAN'S ASSISTANT FROM 1/5/95 TO 1/31/97. HE SIGNED AND LEFT BLANK PRESCRIPTIONS FOR USE BY THE PHYSICIAN'S ASSISTANT TO PRESCRIBE CONTROLLED DRUGS TO PATIENTS. AFTER THE PHYSICIAN'S ASSISTANT LEFT HIS PRACTICE, HE REVIEWED SEVERAL CHARTS OF PATIENTS AND DISCOVERED THAT SHE HAD AUTHORIZED LARGE NUMBERS OF CONTROLLED DRUG PRESCRIPTIONS FOR MANY PATIENTS. ALTHOUGH HE ADDRESSED THIS SITUATION WITH THE AFFECTED PATIENTS, HE NEVER ADVISED THE BOARD UNTIL INTERVIEWED BY BOARD STAFF. HE SHALL NOT SUPERVISE ALLIED HEALTH PROFESSIONALS WITHOUT FIRST OBTAINING A COPY OF THE APPLICABLE PRACTICE ACT AND REGULATIONS AND DILIGENTLY ADHERING TO THE OBLIGATIONS AND RESPONSIBILITIES OF SUPERVISING PHYSICIANS; SHALL PAY COSTS.

ROBBERSON, JAMES MD OF 116 E ROBERT S KERR, WYNNEWOOD, OK, WAS DISCIPLINED BY DEA ON OCTOBER 7, 1999
DISCIPLINARY ACTION: SURRENDER OF CONTROLLED SUBSTANCE LICENSE
OFFENSE: DISCIPLINARY ACTION BY ANOTHER STATE OR AGENCY

NOTES: STATE BOARD.

ROBERTSON, LOWELL J MD, LICENSE NUMBER 17290 OF 2944 SOUTH BOSTON PLACE, TULSA, OK, WAS DISCIPLINED BY OKLAHOMA ON JANUARY 16, 1997
DISCIPLINARY ACTION: 60-MONTH PROBATION; RESTRICTION PLACED ON LICENSE
OFFENSE: SUBSTANCE ABUSE

NOTES: HE ADMITS THAT DUE TO THE USE OF ALCOHOL HE WAS ADMITTED FOR RELAPSE TREATMENT FROM 9/9/96 TO 9/29/96. HE ALSO NOTES THAT HE HAS BEEN OUT OF PRACTICE FOR SEVEN MONTHS. CONDITIONS OF PROBATION: SHALL PROVIDE TO THE BOARD COPIES OF ALL AFTERCARE CONTRACTS AND ANY SUBSEQUENT CHANGES TO THEM AND SHALL COMPLY WITH THEIR TERMS AND CONDITIONS; SHALL KEEP DUPLICATE, SERIALLY NUMBERED PRESCRIPTIONS OF ALL CONTROLLED DANGEROUS SUBSTANCES AND WILL SUBMIT COPIES TO THE BOARD UPON REQUEST; WILL NOT ALLOW THE INITIATION OF ANY THERAPEUTIC REGIMEN BY ANY PERSONNEL UNDER HIS SUPERVISION UNLESS HE IS IN THE IMMEDIATE VICINITY; SHALL SUBMIT TO EVERY STATE IN WHICH HE HOLDS LICENSURE AND TO HOSPITALS, CLINICS OR OTHER INSTITUTIONS IN WHICH HE HOLDS OR ANTICIPATES HOLDING ANY FORM OF STAFF PRIVILEGE A COPY OF THIS ORDER; SHALL NOT SUPERVISE A PHYSICIAN ASSISTANT; SHALL SUBMIT BIOLOGICAL FLUID SPECIMENS; SHALL NOT PRESCRIBE, ADMINISTER OR DISPENSE ANY MEDICATIONS FOR HIS PERSONAL USE AND SHALL TAKE NONE UNLESS AUTHORIZED BY ANOTHER PHYSICIAN FOR A LEGITIMATE MEDICAL NEED; SHALL PROVIDE EVIDENCE OF PARTICIPATION IN AN AFTERCARE PROGRAM APPROVED BY THE BOARD, UPON REQUEST; SHALL KEEP THE BOARD INFORMED OF HIS ADDRESS AND PAY COSTS; SHALL APPEAR BEFORE THE BOARD UPON REQUEST.

ROBERTSON, LOWELL J MD, LICENSE NUMBER 17290 OF 2940 SOUTH BOSTON PLACE, TULSA, OK, WAS DISCIPLINED BY OKLAHOMA ON OCTOBER 5, 1998
DISCIPLINARY ACTION: SURRENDER OF LICENSE
OFFENSE: FAILURE TO COMPLY WITH PREVIOUS BOARD ORDER

NOTES: ALLEGATIONS THAT HE VIOLATED THE 1/17/97 ORDER OF PROBATION BY TESTING POSITIVE FOR SUBSTANCE ABUSE. SURRENDER IN LIEU OF PROSECUTION OF THE CHARGES. HE WILL NOT RE-APPLY FOR LICENSURE IN OKLAHOMA FOR AT LEAST ONE YEAR; SHALL PAY COSTS.

ROBINETT, JAMES KEVIN DO OF PO BOX 579, MCALESTER, OK, WAS DISCIPLINED BY DEA ON OCTOBER 10, 1990
DISCIPLINARY ACTION: RESTRICTION PLACED ON CONTROLLED SUBSTANCE LICENSE
OFFENSE: SUBSTANCE ABUSE

NOTES: ANSWERED YES TO A QUESTION ON DEA REGISTRATION APPLICATION THAT HE OBTAINED DRUGS ILLEGALLY FOR HIS OWN PERSONAL USE. SINCE HE HAS BEEN SUCCESSFUL IN HIS LONG-TERM NARCOTIC TREATMENT REHABILITATION PROGRAM AND CURRENTLY HOLDS THE REQUIRED STATE LICENSE, THE OKLAHOMA CITY RESIDENT OFFICE REQUESTS THAT DEA APPROVE HIS APPLICATION FOR SCHEDULES III THROUGH V.

ROBINSON, MALCOLM G MD, LICENSE NUMBER 0009063 OF 711 STANTON YOUNG BLVD SUITE 501, OKLAHOMA CITY, OK, WAS DISCIPLINED BY OKLAHOMA ON OCTOBER 9, 1996
DISCIPLINARY ACTION: 2-MONTH LICENSE SUSPENSION; 60-MONTH PROBATION
OFFENSE: SEXUAL ABUSE OF OR SEXUAL MISCONDUCT WITH A PATIENT

NOTES: FAILING TO KEEP COMPLETE AND ACCURATE RECORDS OF PURCHASE AND DISPOSAL OF CONTROLLED OR NARCOTIC DRUGS DURING 1993; ENGAGED IN NONCONSENSUAL PHYSICAL OR VERBAL CONDUCT WHICH IS SEXUAL IN NATURE FROM 1991 THROUGH 1995; PERFORMED MULTIPLE PELVIC, VAGINAL FIBEROPTIC EXAMS AND BREAST EXAMS ON FEMALE PATIENTS WITHOUT MEDICAL NEED AND IN SOME CASES WITHOUT PATIENT CONSENT. SUSPENSION RETROACTIVE TO 8/24/96; SHALL SUBMIT HIMSELF FOR EXAMINATION AND TREATMENT IF ANY RECOMMENDED BEFORE EXPIRATION OF SUSPENSION; SHALL IMMEDIATELY CEASE FROM CONDUCTING BREAST AND/OR VAGINAL EXAMS WITHOUT A CHAPERONE AND AMEND HIS CONSENT

FORMS; SHALL FURNISH A COPY OF THIS ORDER TO ANY STATE WHERE HE IS LICENSED. THE STAFF APPLICATION TO SETTLE TERMS OF THE FINAL ORDER IS SUSTAINED; HIS APPLICATION TO STAY THE SUSPENSION IS DENIED; THE 8/23/96 ORDER SHALL BE MODIFIED IN THAT THE TERM OF SUSPENSION SHALL REMAIN IN FULL FORCE AND EFFECT UNTIL HE SUBMITS HIMSELF TO EVALUATION AND TREATMENT BY A PERSON OF HIS CHOICE FROM THREE RECOMMENDATIONS; AND THE EXAMINATION AND TREATMENT SHALL NOT BE CONDUCTED BY DR. RICHARD IRONS. ON 9/11/97 PROBATION TERMINATED AND SUSPENSION LIFTED.

ROGERS, DAVID LINCOLN MD OF 14209 MIDDLEBERRY, EDMOND, OK, WAS DISCIPLINED BY OKLAHOMA ON NOVEMBER 14, 1996
DISCIPLINARY ACTION: 60-MONTH PROBATION; RESTRICTION PLACED ON LICENSE
NOTES: CONDITIONS OF PROBATION: SHALL FULFILL THE TERMS AND CONDITIONS OF ALL RECOMMENDATIONS BY THE ARKANSAS MEDICAL SOCIETY'S PHYSICIAN'S HEALTH COMMITTEE; SHALL ADHERE TO THE BOUNDARIES SUGGESTED IN HIS EVALUATION AND TREATMENT PROGRAM, INCLUDING A FEMALE CHAPERONE PRESENT FOR ALL ENCOUNTERS WITH FEMALE PATIENTS; SHALL ALLOW HIS STAFF TO SPEAK WITH THE BOARD TO HELP MONITOR HIS COMPLIANCE; WHEN EXAMINING ANY FEMALE PATIENT IN ANY PRACTICE SETTING, IN OR OUTSIDE THE OFFICE, SHALL HAVE A FEMALE ASSISTANT PRESENT WHO SHALL REMAIN PERSONALLY PRESENT DURING THE ENTIRETY OF THE EXAMINATION AND SHALL PLACE HERSELF IN A POSITION TO OBSERVE ALL PHYSICIAN-PATIENT CONTACT; SHALL CONTINUE CARE PROVIDED BY BOARD APPROVED THERAPIST AND SHALL REQUIRE THAT THERAPIST TO PROVIDE REGULAR WRITTEN REPORTS TO THE BOARD ON A QUARTERLY BASIS; SHALL NOTIFY ALL HEALTH CARE ENTITIES WHERE HE HOLDS STAFF PRIVILEGES OF THIS ORDER; SHALL AUTHORIZE ALL HOSPITAL OFFICIALS TO MEET WITH THE BOARD TO MONITOR HIS PROFESSIONAL ACTIVITIES; SHALL FURNISH THE BOARD WITH ADDRESS/ OR CHANGE OF ADDRESS; SHALL APPEAR BEFORE THE BOARD UPON REQUEST AND SUBMIT ALL REQUIRED REPORTS. SHALL PAY COSTS.

ROLDAN, ERNESTO OF 326 PIERMONT AVENUE, HILLSDALE, NJ, WAS DISCIPLINED BY OKLAHOMA ON JULY 1, 1993
DISCIPLINARY ACTION: DENIAL OF NEW LICENSE
NOTES: HAD MULTIPLE FAILURES OF FLEX EXAM WHICH RAISED ISSUES OF CLINICAL COMPETENCY.

ROSE, DAVID D MD, LICENSE NUMBER 0007472, WAS DISCIPLINED BY OKLAHOMA ON FEBRUARY 14, 1991
DISCIPLINARY ACTION: 12-MONTH RESTRICTION PLACED ON CONTROLLED SUBSTANCE LICENSE; REPRIMAND
OFFENSE: OVERPRESCRIBING OR MISPRESCRIBING DRUGS
NOTES: FROM 6/1/90 THROUGH 10/31/90, WROTE PRESCRIPTIONS FOR CONTROLLED DANGEROUS SUBSTANCES FOR AT LEAST FOUR PATIENTS IN EXCESS OF THE AMOUNT CONSIDERED MEDICALLY NECESSARY FOR THE MEDICAL NEED PRESENTED. MAY PRESCRIBE CONTROLLED DANGEROUS SUBSTANCES ONLY ON SERIALLY-NUMBERED, DUPLICATE PRESCRIPTION PADS, WITH COPIES AVAILABLE TO BOARD; SHALL FURNISH BOARD WITH ADDRESS AND/OR CHANGE OF ADDRESS; SHALL APPEAR BEFORE BOARD UPON REQUEST; SHALL NOTIFY ANY HOSPITAL WHERE HE HOLDS STAFF PRIVILEGES OR CLINIC OR GROUP OF THE TERMS AND CONDITIONS.

RUGGLES, RANDALL DO OF 527 W. 3RD, KONAWA, OK, WAS DISCIPLINED BY DEA ON AUGUST 4, 1999
DISCIPLINARY ACTION: SURRENDER OF CONTROLLED SUBSTANCE LICENSE

RUGGLES, RANDALL KING DO, LICENSE NUMBER 3532, WAS DISCIPLINED BY OKLAHOMA ON DECEMBER 11, 1997
DISCIPLINARY ACTION: 36-MONTH PROBATION

RUGGLES, RANDALL KING DO, LICENSE NUMBER 3532, WAS DISCIPLINED BY OKLAHOMA ON MARCH 19, 1998
DISCIPLINARY ACTION: SURRENDER OF LICENSE

RUGGLES, RANDALL KING DO, LICENSE NUMBER 3532, WAS DISCIPLINED BY OKLAHOMA ON JUNE 18, 1998
DISCIPLINARY ACTION: LICENSE REINSTATEMENT; 36-MONTH PROBATION

RUGGLES, RANDALL KING DO, LICENSE NUMBER 3532, WAS DISCIPLINED BY OKLAHOMA ON JULY 21, 1999
DISCIPLINARY ACTION: SURRENDER OF LICENSE

SABORIO, JORGE A MD OF 1705 NORTH WASHINGTON, DURANT, OK, WAS DISCIPLINED BY DEA ON MARCH 25, 1996
DISCIPLINARY ACTION: SURRENDER OF CONTROLLED SUBSTANCE LICENSE
OFFENSE: DISCIPLINARY ACTION BY ANOTHER STATE OR AGENCY
NOTES: STATE BOARD.

SABORIO, JORGE A MD, LICENSE NUMBER 0127089 OF P.O. BOX 6070, MANAGUA, NICARAGUA, WAS DISCIPLINED BY NEW YORK ON AUGUST 8, 1996
DISCIPLINARY ACTION: LICENSE REVOCATION
OFFENSE: DISCIPLINARY ACTION BY ANOTHER STATE OR AGENCY
NOTES: ACTION IN OKLAHOMA FOR HABITUAL USE OF DRUGS WHICH IMPAIR THE ABILITY TO PRACTICE MEDICINE; PRACTICED MEDICINE WHILE IMPAIRED; NEGLIGENCE AND INCOMPETENCE ON MORE THAN ONE OCCASION; SEXUAL MISCONDUCT OR EXPLOITATION OF A PATIENT; AND FAILURE TO TRANSFER MEDICAL RECORDS UPON REQUEST.

SABORIO, JORGE ANTONI0 MD, LICENSE NUMBER 0018393 OF 1705 NORTH WASHINGTON, DURANT, OK, WAS DISCIPLINED BY OKLAHOMA ON JANUARY 25, 1996
DISCIPLINARY ACTION: LICENSE REVOCATION
OFFENSE: LOSS OR RESTRICTION OF HOSPITAL PRIVILEGES
NOTES: REVOKED FOR REASONS LISTED IN 12/21/95 EMERGENCY SUSPENSION ORDER.

SABORIO, JORGE ANTONIO MD, LICENSE NUMBER 0018393 OF 1705 NORTH WASHINGTON, DURANT, OK, WAS DISCIPLINED BY OKLAHOMA ON DECEMBER 21, 1995
DISCIPLINARY ACTION: EMERGENCY SUSPENSION
OFFENSE: LOSS OR RESTRICTION OF HOSPITAL PRIVILEGES
NOTES: ON 11/18/94 REPRIMANDED BY HOSPITAL FOR ABANDONING A PATIENT WITHOUT ARRANGING FOR COVERAGE; ON 12/20/94 SUSPENDED FROM THE HOSPITAL STAFF FOR INCOMPLETE DELINQUENT MEDICAL RECORDS; IN 9/95 AGAIN SUSPENDED BASED ON PATIENT CONTACT INCLUDING PERFORMANCE OF SURGICAL PROCEDURES WHILE IN

AN IMPAIRED CONDITION; HOSPITAL STATED HE WAS CONSTANTLY LATE FOR SURGERY, SMELLED OF ALCOHOL AND KEPT CHANGING DIRECTION TO THE STAFF; HISTORY OF PERSONAL CHEMICAL DEPENDENCY AND THREAT TO THE PUBLIC HEALTH.

SANDHU, GURSEWAK SINGH OF 48 GRANDVIEW AVENUE BOX 1797, RUXBURY, MA, WAS DISCIPLINED BY OKLAHOMA ON MARCH 11, 1993
DISCIPLINARY ACTION: DENIAL OF NEW LICENSE
OFFENSE: PROVIDING FALSE INFORMATION TO THE BOARD OR OTHER HEALTH AGENCY

NOTES: PROVIDED FALSE INFORMATION TO THE BOARD; FAILED THE FLEX EXAM FOUR TIMES BEFORE PASSING; DID NOT PROVIDE TRANSCRIPT OF MEDICAL SCHOOL GRADES; A RESPONSE FROM HIS MEDICAL SCHOOL WAS NOT RECEIVED AND HE WAS NOT CERTIFIED IN ORTHOPEDICS.

SANDS, ABEL J MD, DATE OF BIRTH MARCH 10, 1920 OF 13213 CEDAR SPRINGS RD, OKLAHOMA CITY, OK, WAS DISCIPLINED BY MEDICARE ON FEBRUARY 8, 1995
DISCIPLINARY ACTION: EXCLUSION FROM THE MEDICARE AND/OR MEDICAID PROGRAM
OFFENSE: DISCIPLINARY ACTION BY ANOTHER STATE OR AGENCY

NOTES: LICENSE REVOCATION OR SUSPENSION.

SANDS, ABEL JAY MD OF 316 S MIDWEST BLVD, MIDWEST CITY, OK, WAS DISCIPLINED BY DEA ON JANUARY 29, 1990
DISCIPLINARY ACTION: SURRENDER OF CONTROLLED SUBSTANCE LICENSE
OFFENSE: DISCIPLINARY ACTION BY ANOTHER STATE OR AGENCY

NOTES: OKLAHOMA LICENSE SUSPENDED FOR FIVE YEARS 10/26/90.

SANDS, ABEL JAY MD, LICENSE NUMBER 0005560, WAS DISCIPLINED BY OKLAHOMA ON MARCH 29, 1990
DISCIPLINARY ACTION: RESTRICTION PLACED ON CONTROLLED SUBSTANCE LICENSE

NOTES: DURING THE PERIOD UNTIL THE HEARING OF THIS CASE: HE SHALL PARTICIPATE IN A FULL AND COMPLETE EMOTIONAL, INTELLECTUAL, AND PHYSICAL EXAMINATION AND EVALUATION BY APPROPRIATE MEDICAL EXPERTS THAT MAY INCLUDE, BUT SHALL NOT BE LIMITED TO, EXAMINATION AND EVALUATION BY A FORENSIC CLINICAL PSYCHOLOGIST AND A GENERAL INTERNIST; SHALL NOT PRESCRIBE, ADMINISTER, OR DISPENSE ANY CONTROLLED DANGEROUS SUBSTANCES.

SANDS, ABEL JAY MD, LICENSE NUMBER 0005560, WAS DISCIPLINED BY OKLAHOMA ON NOVEMBER 1, 1990
DISCIPLINARY ACTION: 60-MONTH PROBATION; RESTRICTION PLACED ON CONTROLLED SUBSTANCE LICENSE

NOTES: DOES NOT ADMIT NOR DENY THE ALLEGATIONS. PROBATION BEGINNING 10/26/90 UNDER THE FOLLOWING TERMS AND CONDITIONS: WILL NOT PRESCRIBE, ADMINISTER, OR DISPENSE ANY SCHEDULE II OR SCHEDULE III DRUGS OR CONTROLLED DANGEROUS SUBSTANCES; MAY PRESCRIBE, ADMINISTER, OR DISPENSE SCHEDULE IV AND SCHEDULE V CONTROLLED DANGEROUS SUBSTANCES, ONLY ON SERIALLY-NUMBERED, DUPLICATE PRESCRIPTION PADS AND SHALL MAKE THE COPIES AND PATIENT RECORDS AVAILABLE TO THE BOARD UPON REQUEST; SHALL PRESENT EVIDENCE OF SUCCESSFUL COMPLETION OF 20 HOURS CONTINUING MEDICAL EDUCATION ON PROPER PRESCRIPTION WRITING OR AN EQUIVALENT AMOUNT OF COUNSELING BY BOARD STAFF WITHIN TWO YEARS; SHALL SUBMIT TO THE BOARD ADDRESS/CHANGE OF ADDRESS; SHALL APPEAR BEFORE THE BOARD UPON REQUEST AND SUBMIT ANY REQUIRED REPORTS; SHALL PAY COSTS; SHALL NOTIFY ANY HOSPITAL WHERE HE HOLDS STAFF PRIVILEGES, OR CLINIC, OR GROUP WHERE HE PRACTICES OF THE TERMS AND CONDITIONS OF THIS BOARD ORDER AND SUPPLY A COPY THEREOF.

SANDS, ABEL JAY MD, LICENSE NUMBER 0005560 OF 316 S MIDWEST BLVD, MIDWEST CITY, OK, WAS DISCIPLINED BY OKLAHOMA ON NOVEMBER 8, 1991
DISCIPLINARY ACTION: 6-MONTH PROBATION; REPRIMAND
OFFENSE: FAILURE TO COMPLY WITH PREVIOUS BOARD ORDER

NOTES: CONTEMPT OF 10/26/90 BOARD ORDER IN THAT HE PAID COSTS LATE AND FAILED TO PROVIDE EVIDENCE OF SOME BASIS FOR NONPAYMENT THAT WAS NOT CONTEMPTUOUS. WAS PLACED ON PROBATION FOR FIVE YEARS BEGINNING 10/26/90, NOW EXTENDED SIX MONTHS, UNDER THE FOLLOWING TERMS AND CONDITIONS: SHALL NOT PRESCRIBE, ADMINISTER OR DISPENSE ANY SCHEDULE II OR SCHEDULE III DRUGS OR CONTROLLED DANGEROUS SUBSTANCES; MAY PRESCRIBE, ADMINISTER OR DISPENSE SCHEDULE IV AND SCHEDULE V CONTROLLED DANGEROUS SUBSTANCES ONLY ON SERIALLY-NUMBERED, DUPLICATE PRESCRIPTION PADS WITH COPIES AVAILABLE FOR BOARD; SHALL MAINTAIN PATIENT RECORDS TO DOCUMENT DIAGNOSIS AND MEDICAL NEED FOR ANY PRESCRIPTIONS OF SCHEDULE IV OR V CONTROLLED DANGEROUS SUBSTANCES; SHALL PRESENT EVIDENCE OF SUCCESSFUL COMPLETION OF 20 HOURS OF CONTINUING MEDICAL EDUCATION ON PROPER PRESCRIPTION WRITING OR AN EQUIVALENT AMOUNT OF COUNSELING BY BOARD STAFF; SHALL NOTIFY ANY HOSPITAL WHERE HE HOLDS STAFF PRIVILEGES, OR CLINIC, OR GROUP WHERE HE PRACTICES OF TERMS AND CONDITIONS; SHALL FURNISH BOARD WITH ADDRESS AND/OR CHANGE OF ADDRESS; SHALL APPEAR BEFORE BOARD UPON REQUEST. ON 5/20/93 HIS REQUEST FOR TERMINATION OF PROBATION IS DENIED BUT REQUEST FOR REDUCTION IN LEVEL OF PROBATION FROM LEVEL I TO LEVEL III IS GRANTED. ALL OTHER TERMS AND CONDITIONS OF PROBATION REMAIN IN EFFECT.

SANDS, ABEL JAY MD OF 316 SOUTH MIDWEST BOULEVARD, MIDWEST CITY, OK, WAS DISCIPLINED BY DEA ON JANUARY 6, 1994
DISCIPLINARY ACTION: DENIAL OF LICENSE REINSTATEMENT
OFFENSE: PROFESSIONAL MISCONDUCT

NOTES: ON SEVEN OCCASIONS STARTING 12/14/88 WROTE PRESCRIPTIONS FOR XANAX TO UNDERCOVER AGENTS IN THE ABSENCE OF A LEGITIMATE MEDICAL PURPOSE; TAPED TRANSCRIPTS REVEALED HE WAS AWARE OF THE ILLEGITIMACY OF THESE PRESCRIPTIONS; MEDICAL BOARD INVESTIGATION REVEALED THAT HE HAD FAILED TO KEEP ACCURATE RECORDS OF HIS PURCHASE AND DISPENSING OF CONTROLLED SUBSTANCES; ON 1/29/90 DEA CERTIFICATE WAS SURRENDERED AND IN 6/90 HE WAS STILL FOUND TO BE IN POSSESSION OF CONTROLLED SUBSTANCES; OKLAHOMA BOARD PUT HIM ON PROBATION FOR FIVE YEARS DURING WHICH HE WAS PROHIBITED FROM PRESCRIBING, ADMINISTERING OR DISPENSING ANY SCHEDULE II OR III CONTROLLED SUBSTANCES.

SANDS, ABEL JAY MD, LICENSE NUMBER 0005560, WAS

DISCIPLINED BY OKLAHOMA ON MARCH 18, 1994
DISCIPLINARY ACTION: SURRENDER OF LICENSE
OFFENSE: PROVIDING FALSE INFORMATION TO THE BOARD OR OTHER HEALTH AGENCY

NOTES: ON 1/4/94 COMPLAINT ISSUED THAT HE MISREPRESENTED SUCCESSFUL COMPLETION OF CONTINUING MEDICAL EDUCATION AS ORDERED BY THE BOARD; ON 2/1/94 HE OFFERED TO SURRENDER HIS MEDICAL LICENSE.

SARFO, JOSEPH K MD OF ROUTE 2 BOX 1660, TALIHINA, OK, WAS DISCIPLINED BY MARYLAND ON NOVEMBER 10, 1998
DISCIPLINARY ACTION: DENIAL OF LICENSE REINSTATEMENT
OFFENSE: DISCIPLINARY ACTION BY ANOTHER STATE OR AGENCY

NOTES: THE ACTION IS BASED ON ACTION IN NEW YORK: (1) BY THE MEDICAID PROGRAM TO EXCLUDE HIS PARTICIPATION FOR FIVE YEARS (2) BY A NEW YORK HOSPITAL TO TERMINATE TEMPORARY PRIVILEGES AND TO DENY HIS APPLICATION FOR PRIVILEGES FOR FURNISHING THE HOSPITAL FALSE INFORMATION ABOUT THE MEDICAID EXCLUSION; AND (3) BY THE NEW YORK MEDICAL BOARD TO PUT HIM ON PROBATION WHEN HE RETURNS TO THAT STATE.

SARTOR, WILLIAM DO OF 1414 NORTH KENNEDY #105, SHAWNEE, OK, WAS DISCIPLINED BY DEA ON NOVEMBER 16, 1999
DISCIPLINARY ACTION: SURRENDER OF CONTROLLED SUBSTANCE LICENSE
OFFENSE: DISCIPLINARY ACTION BY ANOTHER STATE OR AGENCY

NOTES: STATE BOARD.

SARTOR, WILLIAM A DO, LICENSE NUMBER 2674, WAS DISCIPLINED BY OKLAHOMA ON MARCH 18, 1999

NOTES: STOPPED PRACTICE UNDER BOARD ORDER; MUST PASS COMVEX EXAM AND RETURN TO BOARD FOR HEARING.

SCHACHT, FREDERICK W JR MD, DATE OF BIRTH APRIL 30, 1934, LICENSE NUMBER 15735, WAS DISCIPLINED BY COLORADO ON JULY 17, 1997
DISCIPLINARY ACTION: 60-MONTH PROBATION; REQUIRED TO TAKE ADDITIONAL MEDICAL EDUCATION
OFFENSE: SUBSTANDARD CARE, INCOMPETENCE OR NEGLIGENCE

NOTES: SUBSTANDARD CARE (PRIMA FACIE TYPE ADMISSION ONLY). TERMS OF PROBATION INCLUDE REEDUCATION ACTIVITIES AND PRACTICE MONITORING.

SCHACHT, FREDERICK W JR MD, DATE OF BIRTH APRIL 30, 1934, LICENSE NUMBER 15735, WAS DISCIPLINED BY COLORADO ON SEPTEMBER 18, 1997
DISCIPLINARY ACTION: EMERGENCY SUSPENSION
OFFENSE: FAILURE TO COMPLY WITH PREVIOUS BOARD ORDER

NOTES: FAILURE TO COMPLY WITH A LAWFUL ORDER OF THE BOARD. ON 9/23/97 SUSPENSION LIFTED.

SCHACHT, FREDERICK W JR MD, DATE OF BIRTH APRIL 30, 1934, LICENSE NUMBER 15735, WAS DISCIPLINED BY COLORADO ON MARCH 19, 1998
DISCIPLINARY ACTION: RESTRICTION PLACED ON LICENSE; CEASE AND DESIST ORDER
OFFENSE: SUBSTANDARD CARE, INCOMPETENCE OR NEGLIGENCE

NOTES: SUBSTANDARD CARE (PRIMA FACIE TYPE ADMISSION ONLY). MAY NOT PERFORM OBSTETRICS OR SURGERY EXCEPT FOR SPECIFICALLY IDENTIFIED CURRENT OBSTETRICAL PATIENTS. HE AGREES TO CEASE THE PRACTICE OF MEDICINE BY 2/28/99.

SCHACHT, FREDERICK WILLIAM JR MD, LICENSE NUMBER 8473 OF 1907 N. BOISE AVENUE, LOVELAND, CO, WAS DISCIPLINED BY OKLAHOMA ON SEPTEMBER 24, 1998
DISCIPLINARY ACTION: 60-MONTH PROBATION; RESTRICTION PLACED ON LICENSE
OFFENSE: DISCIPLINARY ACTION BY ANOTHER STATE OR AGENCY

NOTES: ON 7/17/97 THE COLORADO BOARD PLACED HIS LICENSE ON PROBATION FOR FIVE YEARS AFTER REVIEWING A MALPRACTICE SETTLEMENT HE ENTERED INTO. HE WAS ALSO ORDERED TO HAVE HIS PRACTICE, AND PARTICULARLY HIS GYNECOLOGICAL CARE AND SURGERY PRACTICE, EVALUATED. HE HAD FAILED TO MEET THE GENERALLY ACCEPTED STANDARDS OF MEDICAL PRACTICE IN THE TREATMENT OF ONE PATIENT BY FAILING TO OBTAIN AN APPROPRIATE CONSULTATION AND MEDICAL CLEARANCE PRIOR TO PERFORMING SURGERY ON A PATIENT WHO HAD SEVERE ALCOHOLIC LIVER DISEASE, WHICH REMAINED UNDIAGNOSED AT THE TIME OF SURGERY, AND FAILED TO DOCUMENT THE PATIENT'S HEAVY ALCOHOL USE IN EITHER HIS OFFICE CHART OR PREOPERATIVE HISTORY AND PHYSICAL. ON 3/19/98 THE COLORADO BOARD TOOK FURTHER ACTION AGAINST HIM AFTER LEARNING THAT HIS PRIVILEGES HAD BEEN LIMITED BY A MEDICAL CENTER IN LOVELAND, COLORADO. THE 3/19/98 ORDER PROHIBITS HIM FROM PERFORMING SURGERY OR OBSTETRICS IN THE FUTURE. EFFECTIVE 2/28/99, THE COLORADO BOARD ENTIRELY BARS HIM FROM PRACTICING. CONDITIONS OF OKLAHOMA PROBATION: HE WILL COMPLY WITH ALL TERMS, INCLUDING THOSE WITHOUT LIMITATION, THOSE OF EDUCATION AND MONITORING, DESCRIBED IN COLORADO ORDERS UP TO HIS RETIREMENT ON 2/28/99, HE MAY CONTINUE THE PRACTICE OF MEDICINE EXCEPT THAT HE MAY NOT PERFORM SURGERY OR OBSTETRICS UNLESS AS PART OF CONTINUING CARE FOR CURRENT PATIENTS. AFTER 2/28/99, HE SHALL PERFORM NO ACT REQUIRING A LICENSE ISSUED BY THE BOARD. UPON SUCCESSFUL COMPLETION OF THE CPEP LEARNING PLAN, HE MAY PETITION THE COLORADO BOARD TO RETURN TO PRACTICE IN A LIMITED CAPACITY SUCH AS AT A CLINIC OR OFFICE SETTING. SHALL SUBMIT TO EVERY STATE IN WHICH HE HOLDS LICENSURE AND TO HOSPITALS, CLINICS OR OTHER INSTITUTIONS IN WHICH HE HOLDS OR ANTICIPATES HOLDING ANY FORM OF STAFF PRIVILEGE A COPY OF THIS ORDER; SHALL NOT SUPERVISE ALLIED HEALTH PROFESSIONALS; SHALL KEEP THE BOARD INFORMED OF HIS ADDRESS AND PAY COSTS; SHALL APPEAR BEFORE THE BOARD UPON REQUEST. THE PROBATION IS TOLLED UNTIL HE BEGINS PRACTICING IN OKLAHOMA OR IN ANY FEDERAL OR NATIVE AMERICAN FACILITY LOCATED WITHIN ITS BOUNDARIES. SHOULD HE DESIRE TO ESTABLISH ACTIVE PRACTICE OR CONSULTATION PRIVILEGES IN OKLAHOMA, HE SHALL FIRST NOTIFY THE BOARD IN WRITING OF HIS INTENTIONS AND PERSONALLY APPEAR FOR A REVIEW OF THESE MATTERS AND HIS PRESENT STATE OF MEDICAL TRAINING AND COMPETENCE.

SCHEER, BRYAN E MD OF 1701 CRAIG BLVD., EDMOND, OK, WAS DISCIPLINED BY OKLAHOMA ON JUNE 19, 1998
DISCIPLINARY ACTION: MONITORING OF PHYSICIAN PERFORMANCE

NOTES: QUESTIONS RAISED IN HIS APPLICATION CONCERNING HIS FITNESS OR ABILITY TO PRACTICE. GRANTED SPECIAL TRAINING LICENSE WITH

FOLLOWING TERMS AND CONDITIONS: SHALL SUBMIT BIOLOGICAL FLUID SPECIMENS; SHALL NOT INGEST ANY SUBSTANCE WHICH WILL CAUSE A SPECIMEN TO TEST POSITIVE FOR PROHIBITED SUBSTANCES; SHALL NOT TAKE ANY MEDICATION UNLESS AUTHORIZED BY ANOTHER PHYSICIAN FOR A LEGITIMATE MEDICAL NEED; SHALL EXECUTE ALL RELEASES OF MEDICAL AND PSYCHIATRIC RECORDS AS NECESSARY TO DISCUSS HIS CASE WITH HIS TREATING PHYSICIANS AND/OR ANY PHYSICIANS HOLDING RECORDS; SHALL SUBMIT TO EVERY HOSPITAL, CLINIC OR OTHER INSTITUTION IN WHICH HE HOLDS OR ANTICIPATES HOLDING ANY FORM OF STAFF PRIVILEGE A COPY OF THIS ORDER.

SCHIMANDLE, JEFFREY H MD, LICENSE NUMBER 00P1517, WAS DISCIPLINED BY MARYLAND ON SEPTEMBER 24, 1990
DISCIPLINARY ACTION: PROBATION; MONITORING OF PHYSICIAN PERFORMANCE
OFFENSE: FAILURE TO COMPLY WITH PREVIOUS BOARD ORDER

NOTES: VIOLATED PREVIOUS BOARD ORDER 2/27/89 BY NOT SUBMITTING REQUIRED URINE SCREENS. REVOCATION STAYED. CONDITIONS OF PROBATION: HE MUST HAVE URINE TESTS THREE TIMES A WEEK FOR 18 MONTHS; PAY THE COST OF THESE TESTS; AND CANNOT POSSESS, DISPENSE, USE OR PROVIDE ANY PERSON ANY CONTROLLED DANGEROUS SUBSTANCE; SUPERVISOR SHALL PROVIDE QUARTERLY REPORTS TO THE BOARD; NOTIFY ANY EMPLOYER DURING THE PERIOD THIS CONSENT ORDER IS IN EFFECT, OF THE TERMS OF THIS CONSENT ORDER; ONLY ADMINISTER SCHEDULE II NARCOTICS INTRAVENOUSLY IF IT IS WITNESSED BY ANOTHER HEALTH CARE PROFESSIONAL, AND SUCH TREATMENTS MUST BE ADEQUATELY DOCUMENTED IN THE PATIENT'S CHARTS; MUST ATTEMPT TO INITIATE DRUG INTERVENTION PROGRAM FOR ANY PATIENT HE FEELS IS ADDICTED TO NARCOTICS. ON 12/15/92 PROBATION TERMINATED AND REGISTRATION REINSTATED WITHOUT ANY CONDITIONS OR RESTRICTIONS WHATSOEVER BUT SINCE HE IS NO LONGER IN A POST GRADUATE TEACHING PROGRAM IN MARYLAND HIS REGISTRATION HAS EXPIRED.

SCHIMANDLE, JEFFREY H MD, LICENSE NUMBER 00P1517, WAS DISCIPLINED BY MARYLAND ON OCTOBER 6, 1992
DISCIPLINARY ACTION: REPRIMAND
OFFENSE: PROVIDING FALSE INFORMATION TO THE BOARD OR OTHER HEALTH AGENCY

NOTES: PROVIDED MISLEADING, INCOMPLETE AND INACCURATE ANSWERS TO QUESTIONS ON HIS 10/25/90 PENNSYLVANIA RENEWAL APPLICATION WITH REGARD TO PREVIOUS DISCIPLINARY ACTIONS TAKEN IN MARYLAND. HE IS A REGISTERED, UNLICENSED MEDICAL PRACTITIONER WHO RECENTLY COMPLETED A POST-GRADUATE TRAINING PROGRAM IN MARYLAND.

SCHIMANDLE, JEFFREY H MD, LICENSE NUMBER D44215 OF 5810 N. PENN AVENUE, #206B, OKLAHOMA CITY, OK, WAS DISCIPLINED BY MARYLAND ON NOVEMBER 17, 1999
OFFENSE: SUBSTANCE ABUSE

NOTES: PROHIBITION AGAINST PRACTICE IN MARYLAND PENDING RESOLUTION OF OKLAHOMA CHARGES IN REGARD TO PERSONAL SUBSTANCE ABUSE.

SCHIMANDLE, JEFFREY H MD, LICENSE NUMBER 19233, WAS DISCIPLINED BY OKLAHOMA ON NOVEMBER 18, 1999
DISCIPLINARY ACTION: LICENSE REVOCATION
OFFENSE: DISCIPLINARY ACTION BY ANOTHER STATE OR AGENCY

NOTES: ON 6/21/88 MARYLAND LICENSE SUSPENDED DUE TO INAPPROPRIATE HANDLING OF DEMEROL; ON 8/22/88 ENTERED INTO A THREE MONTH CONSENT ORDER DURING WHICH TIME HE TESTED POSITIVE FOR DEMEROL; ON 11/16/88 MARYLAND LICENSE AGAIN SUSPENDED DUE TO DRUG SCREEN; ON 2/27/89 ENTERED INTO A THREE YEAR CONSENT ORDER, AGREEING TO RANDOM DRUG SCREENS; IN 1992, MOVED TO GEORGIA AND ON 11/5/92 ENTERED INTO A CONSENT ORDER WITH A ONE YEAR LICENSE WITH THE GEORGIA BOARD; ON 12/15/92 MARYLAND LICENSE WAS REINSTATED WITHOUT RESTRICTIONS; IN OR AROUND 11/93 THE GEORGIA BOARD ELECTED NOT TO RENEW HIS LICENSE DUE TO VIOLATIONS OF HIS CONSENT ORDER; SUBSEQUENTLY OBTAINED AN UNRESTRICTED LICENSE IN OKLAHOMA; ON 8/25/98 AND 11/9/98 A REGISTERED NURSE OBSERVED HIM FILLING SYRINGES WITH DEMEROL AND PUTTING THEM IN HIS POCKET (WITH ANOTHER SYRINGE) UNDER PRETENSE OF ADMINISTERING TO PATIENTS; ON 11/13/98 A TOXICOLOGY LAB REPORTED THAT THE SYRINGE GIVEN BY HIM TO THE NURSE TO BE ADMINISTERED TO THE PATIENT CONTAINED NO DEMEROL; ON 11/16/98 SUSPENDED BY A HEALTH CENTER FOR INAPPROPRIATE AND UNPROFESSIONAL HANDLING AND ADMINISTRATION OF CONTROLLED DANGEROUS SUBSTANCES; ON 11/20/98 SUSPENDED FROM A HOSPITAL FOR REPEATED MEDICALLY QUESTIONABLE HANDLING AND ADMINISTRATION OF DEMEROL; ON 11/20/98 TESTED POSITIVE FOR DEMEROL AND DILANTIN; SHALL PAY COSTS.

SCHIMANDLE, JEFFREY HOWARD MD, DATE OF BIRTH FEBRUARY 14, 1957, LICENSE NUMBER 0036329 OF 3131 N DRUID HILLS RD APT 3109, DECATUR, GA, WAS DISCIPLINED BY GEORGIA ON NOVEMBER 5, 1992
DISCIPLINARY ACTION: 12-MONTH PROBATION; REPRIMAND
OFFENSE: SUBSTANCE ABUSE

NOTES: CHEMICAL IMPAIRMENT. LICENSED SUBJECT TO TERMS AND CONDITIONS. LICENSED FOR ONE YEAR; MUST APPLY FOR CONTINUATION THEREAFTER.

SCHOENDIENST, STEVEN PAUL MD OF 22999 US HIGHWAY 59, KINGWOOD, TX, WAS DISCIPLINED BY DEA ON SEPTEMBER 4, 1997
DISCIPLINARY ACTION: SURRENDER OF CONTROLLED SUBSTANCE LICENSE

SCHOENDIENST, STEVEN PAUL MD, LICENSE NUMBER 17808 OF PO BOX 14544, OKLAHOMA CITY, OK, WAS DISCIPLINED BY OKLAHOMA ON FEBRUARY 11, 1998
DISCIPLINARY ACTION: 60-MONTH PROBATION; SURRENDER OF CONTROLLED SUBSTANCE LICENSE
OFFENSE: OVERPRESCRIBING OR MISPRESCRIBING DRUGS

NOTES: ON OR ABOUT 10/25/94 THROUGH 2/25/96 HE WRONGFULLY WROTE PRESCRIPTIONS FOR CONTROLLED DANGEROUS SUBSTANCES, WITHOUT MEDICAL NEED, TO PATIENTS WHO WERE NOT HIS PATIENTS, UPON WHOM HE PERFORMED NO PHYSICAL EXAMS AND FOR PURPOSES OTHER THAN THE RENDITION OF PROPER MEDICAL CARE. ADMITTED BOTH ORALLY AND IN WRITING THE VIOLATIONS OF STATE AND FEDERAL LAW AND OKLAHOMA BOARD RULES FOR THE IMPROPER WRITING OF PRESCRIPTIONS FOR CONTROLLED DANGEROUS SUBSTANCES TO PEOPLE OUTSIDE THE SCOPE OF THE DOCTOR/PATIENT RELATIONSHIP AND WITHOUT ESTABLISHED MEDICAL PROTOCOL OR NEED. CONDITIONS OF PROBATION AS FOLLOWS: SHALL NOT PRESCRIBE, ADMINISTER, OR DISPENSE ANY CONTROLLED AND DANGEROUS SUBSTANCES

OR NARCOTICS IN SCHEDULES II THROUGH V; SHALL, ON 9/12/97, SURRENDER HIS REGISTRATION FOR STATE AND FEDERAL CONTROLLED DANGEROUS SUBSTANCES TO PROPER AUTHORITIES AND WILL NOT APPLY FOR REINSTATEMENT UNTIL THE TERM OF HIS PROBATION HAS EXPIRED UNLESS AUTHORIZED TO DO SO BY THE OKLAHOMA BOARD; SHALL PRACTICE IN A CONTROLLED ENVIRONMENT APPROVED BY THE BOARD LIMITED TO THE OKLAHOMA CITY VETERANS ADMINISTRATION HOSPITAL AND ASSOCIATED CLINICS; SHALL NOT ALLOW THE INDEPENDENT PRACTICE OF MEDICINE BY ANY PERSONNEL UNDER HIS SUPERVISION OR EMPLOY; SHALL REQUEST ALL HOSPITALS IN WHICH HE ANTICIPATES PRACTICING TO FURNISH A STATEMENT REGARDING MONITORING OF HIS PRACTICE; SHALL SUBMIT TO EVERY STATE IN WHICH HE HOLDS LICENSURE AND TO HOSPITALS, CLINICS OR OTHER INSTITUTIONS IN WHICH HE HOLDS OR ANTICIPATES HOLDING ANY FORM OF STAFF PRIVILEGE A COPY OF THIS ORDER; SHALL NOT SUPERVISE ALLIED HEALTH PROFESSIONALS; SHALL NOT PRESCRIBE, ADMINISTER OR DISPENSE ANY MEDICATIONS FOR HIS PERSONAL USE AND SHALL TAKE NONE UNLESS AUTHORIZED BY ANOTHER PHYSICIAN FOR A LEGITIMATE MEDICAL NEED; SHALL KEEP THE BOARD INFORMED OF HIS ADDRESS AND PAY COSTS.

SCOTT, MICHAEL D MD, DATE OF BIRTH JUNE 30, 1954 OF 106 BRIAR LAKE DRIVE, ATMORE, AL, WAS DISCIPLINED BY MEDICARE ON JULY 8, 1996
DISCIPLINARY ACTION: EXCLUSION FROM THE MEDICARE AND/OR MEDICAID PROGRAM
OFFENSE: NONCOMPLIANCE WITH A PROFESSIONAL RULE
NOTES: DEFAULTED ON PUBLIC HEALTH SERVICE EDUCATION LOAN. REINSTATED ON 10/15/96.

SCOTT, MICHAEL DEAN DO, LICENSE NUMBER 0002112, WAS DISCIPLINED BY OKLAHOMA ON AUGUST 1, 1990
DISCIPLINARY ACTION: SURRENDER OF LICENSE
NOTES: ENTERED INTO A DEFERRED PROSECUTION AGREEMENT WITH THE DISTRICT ATTORNEY; ONE CONDITION WAS SURRENDER OF LICENSE.

SCOTT, MICHAEL DEAN DO, LICENSE NUMBER 0002112, WAS DISCIPLINED BY OKLAHOMA ON AUGUST 16, 1990
DISCIPLINARY ACTION: LICENSE REINSTATEMENT; 24-MONTH PROBATION
OFFENSE: SUBSTANCE ABUSE
NOTES: PARTICIPATED IN AN EXTENSIVE REHABILITATION PROGRAM IN JACKSON, MISSISSIPPI, PARTICIPATES IN AL-ANON MEETINGS, AND COUNSELS ADOLESCENTS WITH CHEMICAL DEPENDENCY. REINSTATEMENT SUBJECT TO PROBATION EFFECTIVE 7/01/90: SHALL LIMIT HIS MEDICAL PRACTICE TO FOUR DAYS AND 35 HOURS A WEEK TO BE PERFORMED UNDER SUPERVISION; SHALL CONTINUE HIS CURRENT COUNSELING ACTIVITIES; SHALL CONTINUE HIS PARTICIPATION IN DEPENDENCY MEETINGS; SHALL VOLUNTARILY SUBMIT TO RANDOM OR PERIODIC DRUG SCREENING TESTS; SHALL NOT USE OR CONSUME ANY ALCOHOLIC BEVERAGE OR CONTROLLED DANGEROUS SUBSTANCES EXCEPT UPON THE PRESCRIPTION BY A PHYSICIAN WHO IS A MEMBER OF THE PHYSICIAN RECOVERY NETWORK; SHALL NOT ALTER THE NATURE OF HIS MEDICAL PRACTICE IN ANY MANNER WITHOUT FIRST DESCRIBING SUCH CHANGE TO THE BOARD AND OBTAINING WRITTEN PERMISSION; SHALL COMPLETE 32 CONTINUING MEDICAL EDUCATION HOURS WITHIN A YEAR; SHALL OBTAIN AND SUBMIT TO THE BOARD QUARTERLY SUPERVISION REPORTS CONCERNING HIS CONDUCT AND PERFORMANCE; SHALL APPEAR BEFORE THE BOARD UPON REQUEST; SHALL NOT PRESCRIBE, ADMINISTER, OR DISPENSE ANY CONTROLLED DANGEROUS SUBSTANCE NOR SHALL SUCH BE STORED AT THE MEDFORD CLINIC WHERE HE PRACTICES UNLESS THEY BE STRICTLY SECURED; SHALL NOT REQUEST NOR ACCEPT CONTROLLED DANGEROUS SUBSTANCE MEDICATION SAMPLES FROM REPRESENTATIVES OF DRUG MANUFACTURERS, EXCEPT ANTIBIOTIC SAMPLES; $828.69 ADMINISTRATIVE COSTS.

SCOTT, MICHAEL DEAN DO, LICENSE NUMBER 0002112, WAS DISCIPLINED BY OKLAHOMA ON DECEMBER 1, 1990
DISCIPLINARY ACTION: SURRENDER OF LICENSE

SCOTT, MICHAEL DEAN DO, LICENSE NUMBER 0002112, WAS DISCIPLINED BY OKLAHOMA ON SEPTEMBER 15, 1994
DISCIPLINARY ACTION: LICENSE REINSTATEMENT; PROBATION
NOTES: REINSTATEMENT SUBJECT TO PROBATION: SHALL PARTICIPATE IN FAMILY PRACTICE RESIDENCY PROGRAM AND CONFINE HIS PRACTICE TO THIS RESIDENCY UNTIL THE BOARD GRANTS PERMISSION TO PRACTICE IN ANOTHER SETTING; DURING THIS RESIDENCY SHALL ATTEND AND SATISFACTORILY COMPLETE BASIC AND ADVANCED COURSES AT THE INSTITUTE OF BASIC LIFE PRINCIPLES AND NOTIFY THE BOARD UPON COMPLETION; SHALL CAUSE THE DIRECTOR OF HIS RESIDENCY PROGRAM TO SUBMIT QUARTERLY PROGRESS REPORTS CONCERNING PARTICIPATION IN PROGRAM ACTIVITIES; SHALL CONTINUE HIS PARTICIPATION IN THE OKLAHOMA PHYSICIAN RECOVERY PROGRAM (OPERA) AND CONTINUE HIS ATTENDANCE AT AA, NARCOTICS ANONYMOUS AND CADUCEUS CLUB PROGRAMS AND OTHER SUCH PROGRAMS AS REQUIRED BY OPERA WITH MONTHLY REPORTS OF THIS ACTIVITY; SHALL NOT USE OR CONSUME ANY ALCOHOLIC BEVERAGE OR CONTROLLED DANGEROUS SUBSTANCE EXCEPT UPON THE WRITTEN PRESCRIPTION OF ANOTHER PHYSICIAN; SHALL PROVIDE RANDOM BIOLOGICAL FLUID SPECIMENS FOR LABORATORY ANALYSIS; SHALL NOT APPLY FOR OR OBTAIN A LICENSE TO PRESCRIBE CONTROLLED DANGEROUS SUBSTANCES FROM THE DRUG ENFORCEMENT AGENCY, THE OKLAHOMA BUREAU OF NARCOTICS AND DANGEROUS DRUGS OR ANY OTHER LICENSING OR LAW ENFORCEMENT AGENCY; MUST NOTIFY THE BOARD IN WRITING OF ANY CHANGE OF ADDRESS WITHIN 14 DAYS; SHALL APPEAR BEFORE THE BOARD UPON REQUEST; SHALL RECEIVE UNANNOUNCED VISITS FROM THE BOARD; TERMS OF RESIDENCE OR PRACTICE OUTSIDE OF OKLAHOMA WILL RESULT IN THE TOLLING OF THIS ORDER AND NOT APPLY TO THE REDUCTION OF THIS PROBATIONARY PERIOD; THE BOARD WILL NOT CONSIDER THE TERMINATION OF THESE CONDITIONS FOR FIVE YEARS.

SCOTT, MICHAEL DEAN DO, LICENSE NUMBER 0002112, WAS DISCIPLINED BY OKLAHOMA ON JUNE 16, 1995
DISCIPLINARY ACTION: LICENSE REVOCATION
OFFENSE: FAILURE TO COMPLY WITH PREVIOUS BOARD ORDER
NOTES: IN 12/94 POSING AND USING ANOTHER DOCTORS NAME AND DEA NUMBER CALLED IN A FRAUDULENT PRESCRIPTION FOR CLASS II NARCOTICS DRUGS, TUSSIONEX, AND TETRACYCLINE WITH INTENT TO USE THIS MEDICATION FOR HIMSELF. ON 1/17/95 USED THE SAME DOCTOR'S NAME AND DEA NUMBER FOR A

REFILL; THE PHARMACIST CALLED TO VERIFY THIS REQUEST; ON 1/20/95 WAS SUSPENDED WITH PAY FROM THE RESIDENCY PROGRAM AT OKLAHOMA STATE UNIVERSITY COLLEGE OF OSTEOPATHIC MEDICINE DUE TO THESE ACTIONS; IN THE SPRING OF 1995 HE WAS CHARGED WITH OBTAINING CONTROLLED DANGEROUS SUBSTANCES BY FRAUD.

SEARS, RICHARD MARK MD, LICENSE NUMBER 0014357, WAS DISCIPLINED BY OKLAHOMA ON OCTOBER 1, 1993
DISCIPLINARY ACTION: 60-MONTH PROBATION; RESTRICTION PLACED ON LICENSE

NOTES: CONDITIONS OF PROBATION; SHALL NOT PRESCRIBE, ADMINISTER OR DISPENSE ANY MEDICATIONS FOR HIS PERSONAL USE AND SHALL TAKE NO MEDICATION NOT AUTHORIZED BY A TREATING PHYSICIAN; SHALL ABSTAIN FROM CONSUMING ALCOHOL OR ANY SUBSTANCE WHICH WOULD ADVERSELY AFFECT HIS ABILITY TO PRACTICE; SHALL SUBMIT BIOLOGICAL FLUID SPECIMENS; SHALL DOCUMENT PROOF OF PARTICIPATION IN AND COMPLIANCE WITH PHYSICIAN RECOVERY COMMITTEE AND NARCOTICS ANONYMOUS OR AA; SHALL SUBMIT TO INTERVIEWS/EVALUATIONS RECOMMENDED BY BOARD; SHALL FURNISH TO BOARD ADDRESS AND/OR CHANGE OF ADDRESS; SHALL APPEAR BEFORE BOARD UPON REQUEST AND SUBMIT REQUESTED REPORTS; SHALL NOT SUPERVISE A PHYSICIAN'S ASSISTANT; SHALL PAY COSTS; SHALL NOTIFY ANY STATE WHERE HE IS LICENSED OR HEALTH CARE ENTITY WHERE HE HAS PRIVILEGES OF THIS ORDER.

SEARS, RICHARD MARK MD, LICENSE NUMBER 0014357, WAS DISCIPLINED BY OKLAHOMA ON MARCH 22, 1996
DISCIPLINARY ACTION: PROBATION; RESTRICTION PLACED ON LICENSE
OFFENSE: FAILURE TO COMPLY WITH PREVIOUS BOARD ORDER

NOTES: VIOLATED PREVIOUS PROBATION. SHALL CONTINUE TO ABIDE BY THE TERMS OF PROBATION SET FORTH IN THE 10/18/93 FINAL ORDER; SHALL SUBMIT HIMSELF FOR VOLUNTARY SUBSTANCE ABUSE EVALUATION; SHALL SUBMIT TO FOUR ADDITIONAL RANDOM URINALYSIS DRUG SCREENS PER MONTH; SHALL HAVE A NURSE PRESENT WITH HIM AT ALL TIMES WHILE TREATING A PATIENT.

SEELIG, DARRELL A MD, LICENSE NUMBER 6539 OF 416 S OAK AVENUE, CHANDLER, OK, WAS DISCIPLINED BY OKLAHOMA ON MAY 29, 1998
DISCIPLINARY ACTION: 60-MONTH RESTRICTION PLACED ON LICENSE; REPRIMAND
OFFENSE: PROFESSIONAL MISCONDUCT

NOTES: WAS THE SUPERVISING PHYSICIAN FOR A PHYSICIAN'S ASSISTANT FROM 10/30/97 TO 3/19/98. BOTH WERE EMPLOYEES OF A HEALTH CLINIC IN GUTHRIE, OKLAHOMA. HE REVIEWED THE PHYSICIAN'S ASSISTANT'S CHARTS ONE MORNING PER WEEK. AT THE PHYSICIAN'S ASSISTANT'S REQUEST, HE SIGNED AND LEFT BLANK PRESCRIPTIONS FOR USE BY THE PHYSICIAN'S ASSISTANT TO PRESCRIBE CONTROLLED DRUGS TO PATIENTS WITHOUT CONSULTING HIM. HE DID NOT PREPARE A POLICY OR PROTOCOL FOR THE PHYSICIAN'S ASSISTANT TO OPERATE UNDER OR PROVIDE PROPER SUPERVISION. HE SIGNED, AGAIN AT THE PHYSICIAN'S ASSISTANT'S REQUEST, AN OPEN LETTER AUTHORIZING HER TO TREAT HER FAMILY IN A PROFESSIONAL MANNER ALTHOUGH THE DOCTOR HAD NEVER SEEN THE PHYSICIAN'S ASSISTANT OR ANY OF HER FAMILY MEMBERS AS PATIENTS. SHALL NOT SUPERVISE ALLIED HEALTH PROFESSIONALS FOR FIVE YEARS, AFTER WHICH TIME HE SHALL NOT DO SO WITHOUT FIRST OBTAINING A COPY OF THE APPLICABLE PRACTICE ACT AND REGULATIONS AND DILIGENTLY ADHERING TO THE OBLIGATIONS AND RESPONSIBILITIES OF SUPERVISING PHYSICIANS; SHALL PAY COSTS.

SEIKEL, STACY E MD, LICENSE NUMBER 0015792 OF 1111 LUCERNE TERRACE, ORLANDO, FL, WAS DISCIPLINED BY OKLAHOMA ON MARCH 5, 1992
DISCIPLINARY ACTION: 4-MONTH LICENSE SUSPENSION
OFFENSE: DISCIPLINARY ACTION BY ANOTHER STATE OR AGENCY

NOTES: ON 2/12/90 FLORIDA GRANTED LICENSURE CONTINGENT UPON PARTICIPATION IN PHYSICIAN'S RECOVERY NETWORK FOR AT LEAST FIVE YEARS DUE TO HER HAVING A HISTORY OF PREVIOUS CHEMICAL DEPENDENCE AND THE DIRECTOR OF THE PHYSICIAN'S RECOVERY NETWORK HAS RECOMMENDED THAT THERE BE CONTINUED PARTICIPATION IN THE PROGRAM TO ENSURE CONTINUED RECOVERY AND ABILITY TO PRACTICE MEDICINE WITH REASONABLE SKILL AND SAFETY. OKLAHOMA BOARD ATTEMPTED TO REACH HER THROUGHOUT JANUARY 1992 WITH NOTICE OF THIS HEARING. SUSPENDED UNTIL 7/1/92.

SELF, JANE MD, LICENSE NUMBER 0007763, WAS DISCIPLINED BY OKLAHOMA ON JUNE 21, 1990
DISCIPLINARY ACTION: 60-MONTH PROBATION; RESTRICTION PLACED ON CONTROLLED SUBSTANCE LICENSE

NOTES: PROBATION BEGINNING 6/09/90 UNDER THE FOLLOWING TERMS AND CONDITIONS: SHALL NOT PRESCRIBE, ADMINISTER, OR DISPENSE ANY MEDICATIONS FOR HER PERSONAL USE AND SHALL TAKE NONE UNLESS AUTHORIZED BY ANOTHER PHYSICIAN FOR LEGITIMATE MEDICAL NEED; SHALL SUBMIT BIOLOGICAL FLUID SPECIMENS; SHALL PRESENT HERSELF FOR A PHYSICAL AND/OR PSYCHIATRIC EVALUATION BY A BOARD SELECTED DOCTOR OR DOCTORS AT HER EXPENSE. THE HISTORY GIVEN SUCH DOCTOR OR DOCTORS SHALL BE PRIVILEGED AND CONFIDENTIAL BUT A REPORT CONTAINING THE DIAGNOSIS, RECOMMENDED TREATMENT AND PROGNOSIS WILL BE SUBMITTED TO THE BOARD. SUCH REPORT SHALL BE CONFIDENTIAL EXCEPT TO HER, THE BOARD AND ITS STAFF; SHALL CARRY OUT RECOMMENDED TREATMENT; SHALL NOT PRESCRIBE, ADMINISTER OR DISPENSE ANY SCHEDULE DRUGS UNTIL AUTHORIZED BY BOARD; HER STATE AND FEDERAL REGISTRATION FOR THE PRESCRIBING OF CONTROLLED DANGEROUS SUBSTANCES WILL EXPIRE IN JUNE OF 1990. SHE AGREES THAT SHE WILL NOT REAPPLY UNTIL THE TERMS OF HER PROBATION HAVE EXPIRED OR BEEN MODIFIED BY THE BOARD; SHALL SUBMIT TO THE BOARD ADDRESS/CHANGE OF ADDRESS; SHALL APPEAR BEFORE THE BOARD UPON REQUEST AND SUBMIT ANY REQUESTED REPORTS; SHALL PAY COSTS.

SELF, JANE MD OF 11434 SOUTH YALE, TULSA, OK, WAS DISCIPLINED BY DEA ON AUGUST 3, 1990
DISCIPLINARY ACTION: SURRENDER OF CONTROLLED SUBSTANCE LICENSE
OFFENSE: DISCIPLINARY ACTION BY ANOTHER STATE OR AGENCY

NOTES: MEDICAL LICENSE PLACED ON FIVE YEAR PROBATION 06/09/90.

SELF, JANE MD, LICENSE NUMBER 0007763, WAS DISCIPLINED BY OKLAHOMA ON NOVEMBER 15, 1990
DISCIPLINARY ACTION: 60-MONTH PROBATION; MONITORING OF PHYSICIAN PERFORMANCE
OFFENSE: PHYSICAL OR MENTAL ILLNESS INHIBITING THE ABILITY TO PRACTICE WITH SKILL AND SAFETY

NOTES: RETAINED ON TERMS OF 6/9/90 PROBATION WITH THE ADDITION THAT SHE SHALL NOT PRACTICE MEDICINE DURING PROBATION UNTIL SHE APPEARS BEFORE THE BOARD AND PROVIDES EVIDENCE OF PHYSICAL AND MENTAL ABILITY TO PRACTICE. BASED ON EVALUATION REQUIRED BY 6/90 ORDER WHICH SUGGESTED POSSIBLE ORGANIC MENTAL DISORDER AND DEPRESSION.

SERJEANT, MICHAEL E MD OF 1501 SOUTHEAST 4TH SUITE C, MOORE, OK, WAS DISCIPLINED BY DEA ON APRIL 2, 1990
DISCIPLINARY ACTION: SURRENDER OF CONTROLLED SUBSTANCE LICENSE
OFFENSE: FAILURE TO COMPLY WITH PREVIOUS BOARD ORDER

NOTES: FOUND GUILTY OF VIOLATING CONSENT ORDER AND ORDERED TO SURRENDER CONTROLLED SUBSTANCE PRIVILEGES EFFECTIVE 02/02/90.

SERJEANT, MICHAEL EWART MD, LICENSE NUMBER 0010691, WAS DISCIPLINED BY OKLAHOMA ON MARCH 22, 1990
DISCIPLINARY ACTION: 60-MONTH PROBATION; RESTRICTION PLACED ON CONTROLLED SUBSTANCE LICENSE
OFFENSE: FAILURE TO COMPLY WITH PREVIOUS BOARD ORDER

NOTES: NONCOMPLIANCE WITH A PREVIOUS CONSENT ORDER OF 1/23/88 IN THAT IN THE CASE OF EIGHT PATIENTS BETWEEN 3/89 AND 7/89 PRESCRIBED ALPRAZOLAM IN A DOSAGE THAT EXCEEDED 4 MILLIGRAMS PER DAY FOR A PERIOD EXCEEDING 120 DAYS WITHOUT A REVIEW AND CONCURRING DIAGNOSIS BY A BOARD CERTIFIED PSYCHIATRIST AND HE FAILED TO PROVIDE COPIES OF ANY REVIEW AS ORDERED. CONTINUED FIVE YEAR PROBATION RETROACTIVE TO 9/05/86 UNDER THE FOLLOWING MODIFIED TERMS AND CONDITIONS: DURING THE ONE YEAR PERIOD FROM 2/02/90 TO 2/02/91, SHALL NOT PRESCRIBE, ADMINISTER OR DISPENSE ANY SCHEDULE DRUGS OR CONTROLLED DANGEROUS SUBSTANCES; BEGINNING ON 2/02/91 HE MAY PRESCRIBE, ADMINISTER, AND DISPENSE CONTROLLED DANGEROUS SUBSTANCES ONLY ON SERIALLY-NUMBERED, DUPLICATE PRESCRIPTION PADS AND SHALL MAKE THE COPIES AVAILABLE TO THE BOARD UPON REQUEST; AFTER 2/02/91 SHALL NOT PRESCRIBE ALPRAZOLAM TO ANY PATIENT IN A DOSAGE THAT EXCEEDS ON AVERAGE OF 4 MG. PER DAY FOR A PERIOD EXCEEDING 120 DAYS WITHOUT REVIEW AND CONCURRING DIAGNOSIS BY A BOARD-CERTIFIED PSYCHIATRIST WITH COPIES OF THE REPORT TO THE BOARD; IF HE RECEIVES APPROVAL FROM THE UNITED STATES FOOD AND DRUG ADMINISTRATION TO PRESCRIBE ALPRAZOLAM IN EXCESS OF THEIR CURRENT GUIDELINES THE RESTRICTION SHALL BE RECONSIDERED BY THE BOARD; ON 2/02/91 AND FOR THE REMAINDER OF THE PROBATION, SHALL NOT PRESCRIBE ANY OTHER CONTROLLED DANGEROUS SUBSTANCES IN EXCESS OF THE GUIDELINES SET FORTH BY THE UNITED STATES FOOD AND DRUG ADMINISTRATION; SHALL SUBMIT TO THE BOARD ADDRESS/CHANGE IN ADDRESS; SHALL APPEAR BEFORE THE BOARD UPON REQUEST; SHALL KEEP THE BOARD APPRISED OF HIS STATUS AND THE BOARD RETAINS CONTINUING JURISDICTION TO REVIEW PRESCRIPTIONS OF CONTROLLED DANGEROUS SUBSTANCES PRESCRIBED, ADMINISTERED, OR DISPENSED BY THE DEFENDANT AFTER 2/02/91; SHALL SUBMIT ANY REQUIRED REPORTS; SHALL PAY COSTS.

SERJEANT, MICHAEL EWART MD, LICENSE NUMBER 0010691, WAS DISCIPLINED BY OKLAHOMA ON NOVEMBER 15, 1996
DISCIPLINARY ACTION: LICENSE REVOCATION
OFFENSE: OVERPRESCRIBING OR MISPRESCRIBING DRUGS

NOTES: PRESCRIBED KETALAR, AN ANESTHETIC, NOT APPROVED FOR THE TREATMENT OF MIGRAINE HEADACHES, FOR THIS TREATMENT IN ONE PATIENT; PRESCRIBED KETALAR FOR HOME HEALTH CARE ADMINISTRATION TO PATIENT WITHOUT THE AVAILABILITY OF PROPER RESUSCITATION EQUIPMENT AND FOR ADMINISTRATION BY A PERSON NOT LICENSED TO ADMINISTER KETALAR; PRESCRIBED KETALAR FOR USE IN CONJUNCTION WITH XANAX, CARISPRODOL AND NUBAIN WITHOUT PROPER REGARD FOR THE CONDITION OF HIS PATIENT; AND UNTIL EMERGENCY SUSPENSION ON 8/15/94 CONTINUED TO PRESCRIBED KETALAR TO OTHER PATIENTS FOR MIGRAINES AND PAIN CONTROL CONTRARY TO THE APPROVED AND ACCEPTED USE OF KETALAR WITH RECKLESS DISREGARD FOR THE WELFARE OF HIS PATIENTS.

SHELDON, WILMER G MD, LICENSE NUMBER 0006869, WAS DISCIPLINED BY OKLAHOMA ON JUNE 27, 1991
OFFENSE: PHYSICAL OR MENTAL ILLNESS INHIBITING THE ABILITY TO PRACTICE WITH SKILL AND SAFETY

NOTES: IN 2/89 THE VETERANS ADMINISTRATION IN FAYETTEVILLE, ARKANSAS BEGAN INVESTIGATING HIS CARE OF A PATIENT WHO PRESENTED SYMPTOMS OF SEVERE NECK PAIN; IT WAS RECOMMENDED DISCIPLINARY ACTION BE TAKEN AGAINST HIM. ON 4/17/89 A PHYSICIAN WHO EXAMINED DR. SHELDON DECIDED THAT HE WOULD CONSIDER HIM TOTALLY INCAPACITATED FROM PERFORMING THE NORMAL DUTIES OF HIS JOB IF EXAMPLES HE CITED WHERE HIS LACK OF RECENT MEMORY HAVE ADVERSELY AFFECTED PATIENT CARE WERE TYPICAL. FURTHERMORE, HE SAID THAT IF ALLOWED TO CONTINUE TO PRACTICE MEDICINE, HE THOUGHT DR. SHELDON'S PATIENTS MIGHT SUFFER INJURY OR HARM. APPLIED FOR AND RECEIVED MEDICAL DISABILITY RETIREMENT FROM THE FEDERAL SERVICE. OKLAHOMA BOARD DECIDED THAT RENEWAL OF LICENSE SHALL BE GRANTED AFTER THEY RECEIVE COMMUNICATION FROM THE VETERANS ADMINISTRATION THAT HIS MEDICAL DISABILITY IS NO LONGER IN EFFECT.

SHERRILL, HARRIETT C DO, WAS DISCIPLINED BY OKLAHOMA ON AUGUST 25, 1993
DISCIPLINARY ACTION: SURRENDER OF LICENSE

NOTES: RETIRED. IN LIEU OF HEARING.

SIEGEL, PHILIP, WAS DISCIPLINED BY OKLAHOMA ON JULY 22, 1994
DISCIPLINARY ACTION: DENIAL OF NEW LICENSE
OFFENSE: LOSS OR RESTRICTION OF HOSPITAL PRIVILEGES

NOTES: EVIDENCE REFLECTS HE HAS A PROTRACTED HISTORY OF DISCIPLINARY ACTIONS AGAINST HIM GENERALLY IN THE FORM OF DENIAL OR LOSS OF HOSPITAL PRIVILEGES; LOSS OF HOSPITAL PRIVILEGES RELATED FREQUENTLY TO HIS ABILITY TO WORK WITHIN A HOSPITAL AND CONDUCT HIMSELF APPROPRIATELY WITH OTHER STAFF; FAILED TO PROVIDE BOARD WITH ADEQUATE EXPLANATION FOR HISTORY OF DISCIPLINARY ACTION

SIMMONS, JOSEPH B MD, LICENSE NUMBER 0016721 OF POB 1290 805 W 23 ST N, CLAREMORE, OK, WAS DISCIPLINED BY OKLAHOMA ON JULY 9, 1992
DISCIPLINARY ACTION: LICENSE REVOCATION
OFFENSE: LOSS OR RESTRICTION OF HOSPITAL PRIVILEGES

NOTES: ON 8/15/91 NOBLE ARMY COMMUNITY HOSPITAL IN ALABAMA FOUND THAT HE MEDICALLY MANAGED THREE PATIENTS INAPPROPRIATELY: DID NOT FULLY DOCUMENT THE MEDICAL RECORDS OF ALL THREE PATIENTS, DID NOT PERFORM PHYSICAL EXAMINATIONS THAT ALL THREE PATIENTS REQUIRED AND FAILED TO DIAGNOSE IN ALL THREE CASES. HOSPITAL THEN LIMITED HIS PRIVILEGES. ON 11/13/91 AN AUDIT BY THE HOSPITAL FOUND NO IMPROVEMENT AND THEY SUSPENDED HIS PRIVILEGES.

SIMPSON, DAVID W DO, WAS DISCIPLINED BY OKLAHOMA ON FEBRUARY 22, 1996
DISCIPLINARY ACTION: SURRENDER OF LICENSE

NOTES: VOLUNTARY SURRENDER.

SIMPSON, DAVID W D0, LICENSE NUMBER 0001307, WAS DISCIPLINED BY OKLAHOMA ON JUNE 20, 1996
DISCIPLINARY ACTION: LICENSE REINSTATEMENT; 48-MONTH PROBATION

NOTES: REINSTATEMENT WITH PROBATION ON CONDITIONS: BOARD SHALL NOT CONSIDER MODIFICATION FOR 20 MONTHS; SHALL SUBMIT BODILY FLUIDS FOR TESTING UPON BOARD REQUEST; SHALL COMPLY WITH ALL THE TERMS OF HIS CADUCEUS AFTERCARE AGREEMENT WITH RUSH HEALTH CENTER AND SHALL AUTHORIZE THEM TO SUBMIT TO THE BOARD QUARTERLY REPORTS ON HIS PERFORMANCE; SHALL NOTIFY THE BOARD IN WRITING OF ANY CHANGE OF ADDRESS WITHIN 14 DAYS; SHALL RECEIVE UNANNOUNCED VISITS FROM THE BOARD FOR THE PURPOSE OF REVIEWING HIS PRACTICE AND OF OBTAINING THE SAMPLES OF BODILY FLUIDS; TERMS OF RESIDENCE OR PRACTICE OUTSIDE OF THE STATE OF OKLAHOMA WILL RESULT IN THE TOLLING OF THE PROBATIONARY TIME PERIODS AND WILL NOT APPLY TO THE COMPLETION OF PROBATION. ON 6/18/98 PROBATION TERMINATED.

SIMPSON, DAVID W DO, LICENSE NUMBER 5302 OF OKLAHOMA CITY, OK, WAS DISCIPLINED BY FLORIDA ON OCTOBER 6, 1997
DISCIPLINARY ACTION: 60-MONTH LICENSE SUSPENSION
OFFENSE: DISCIPLINARY ACTION BY ANOTHER STATE OR AGENCY

NOTES: ACTION TAKEN BY ANOTHER BOARD.

SIMS-FORD, CHERYL D MD, DATE OF BIRTH SEPTEMBER 25, 1951 OF ROUTE 1, BOX 80, ELMORE CITY, OK, WAS DISCIPLINED BY MEDICARE ON OCTOBER 20, 1999
DISCIPLINARY ACTION: EXCLUSION FROM THE MEDICARE AND/OR MEDICAID PROGRAM
OFFENSE: NONCOMPLIANCE WITH A PROFESSIONAL RULE

NOTES: DEFAULTED ON PUBLIC HEALTH SERVICE EDUCATION LOAN.

SMITH, CARL ROY MD OF 320 NW 10TH STREET, OKLAHOMA CITY, OK, WAS DISCIPLINED BY DEA ON FEBRUARY 26, 1990
DISCIPLINARY ACTION: SURRENDER OF CONTROLLED SUBSTANCE LICENSE
OFFENSE: DISCIPLINARY ACTION BY ANOTHER STATE OR AGENCY

NOTES: SURRENDERED MEDICAL LICENSE 12/05/87 IN MISSOURI. PLACED ON TWO YEAR PROBATION ON 02/02/90 IN OKLAHOMA AND ORDERED TO SURRENDER STATE AND FEDERAL CONTROLLED SUBSTANCE REGISTRATION. DENIAL OF LOUISIANA LICENSE.

SMITH, CARL ROY MD, LICENSE NUMBER 0007402, WAS DISCIPLINED BY OKLAHOMA ON MARCH 1, 1990
DISCIPLINARY ACTION: SURRENDER OF CONTROLLED SUBSTANCE LICENSE; 24-MONTH PROBATION

NOTES: PROBATION BEGINNING ON 2/02/90 UNDER THE FOLLOWING TERMS AND CONDITIONS: SHALL CONTINUE TO SEE TWO SPECIFIED PHYSICIANS AND COMPLY WITH ALL TREATMENT, RECOMMENDATIONS, AND PRESCRIPTIONS MADE BY THEM; SHALL AUTHORIZE DOCTORS TO FORWARD PERIODIC REPORTS ON HIS CONDITION, PROGRESS, AND PROGNOSIS TO THE BOARD; SHALL NOT PRESCRIBE, ADMINISTER, OR DISPENSE ANY DRUGS; SHALL VOLUNTARILY SURRENDER REGISTRATION WITH THE OKLAHOMA BUREAU OF NARCOTICS AND DANGEROUS DRUGS AND THE UNITED STATES DRUG ENFORCEMENT AUTHORITY; SHALL NOT PRACTICE MEDICINE OR SURGERY IN OKLAHOMA EXCEPT AS SPECIFICALLY AUTHORIZED BY THE BOARD; SHALL NOT PRESCRIBE, ADMINISTER OR DISPENSE ANY MEDICATIONS FOR HIS PERSONAL USE AND SHALL TAKE NONE UNLESS AUTHORIZED BY ANOTHER PHYSICIAN FOR LEGITIMATE MEDICAL NEED; SHALL ABSTAIN FROM CONSUMING ALCOHOL OR ANY SUBSTANCE WHICH WOULD ADVERSELY AFFECT HIS ABILITY TO PRACTICE; SHALL SUBMIT BIOLOGICAL FLUID SPECIMENS; SHALL SUBMIT TO THE BOARD ADDRESS/CHANGE OF ADDRESS; SHALL APPEAR BEFORE THE BOARD UPON REQUEST AND SUBMIT ANY REQUIRED REPORTS; SHALL PAY COSTS; SHALL NOTIFY ANY HOSPITAL WHERE HE HOLDS STAFF PRIVILEGES, OR CLINIC, OR GROUP WHERE HE PRACTICES, OF THE TERMS AND CONDITIONS OF THIS BOARD ORDER AND SUPPLY A COPY THEREOF. AT THE END OF TWO YEAR PROBATION MUST PERSONALLY APPEAR BEFORE THE BOARD BEFORE RESUMING ACTIVE PRACTICE OF MEDICINE AND SURGERY IN OKLAHOMA.

SMITH, RENE Z DO, DATE OF BIRTH JANUARY 25, 1945, LICENSE NUMBER 0007854 OF 3313 NORTH COUNTRY CLUB RD, NEWCASTLE, OK, WAS DISCIPLINED BY MICHIGAN ON OCTOBER 13, 1992
DISCIPLINARY ACTION: EMERGENCY SUSPENSION
OFFENSE: SUBSTANDARD CARE, INCOMPETENCE OR NEGLIGENCE

NOTES: NEGLIGENCE AND INCOMPETENCE.

SMITH, RENE Z DR OF NEWCASTLE, OK, WAS DISCIPLINED BY ILLINOIS ON OCTOBER 1, 1993
DISCIPLINARY ACTION: LICENSE SUSPENSION
OFFENSE: DISCIPLINARY ACTION BY ANOTHER STATE OR AGENCY

NOTES: DISCIPLINED IN MISSOURI. INDEFINITE SUSPENSION FOR A MINIMUM OF 5 YEARS.

SMITH, RENE Z DO, DATE OF BIRTH JANUARY 25, 1945, LICENSE NUMBER 0007854 OF C/O BECHTEL PO BOX 9729, AHMADI 61008 KUWAIT, WAS DISCIPLINED BY MICHIGAN ON NOVEMBER 24, 1993
DISCIPLINARY ACTION: LICENSE REVOCATION
OFFENSE: SUBSTANDARD CARE, INCOMPETENCE OR NEGLIGENCE

NOTES: NEGLIGENCE/INCOMPETENCE; LACK OF GOOD MORAL CHARACTER.

SMITH, RENE Z DO, DATE OF BIRTH JANUARY 25, 1945 OF 248 EAST KEY BOULEVARD, MIDWEST CITY, OK, WAS DISCIPLINED BY MONTANA ON SEPTEMBER 26, 1996

DISCIPLINARY ACTION: DENIAL OF NEW LICENSE
OFFENSE: DISCIPLINARY ACTION BY ANOTHER STATE OR AGENCY

NOTES: DISCIPLINE IN OTHER STATE; UNPROFESSIONAL CONDUCT.

SNEED, NORMA L MD, DATE OF BIRTH FEBRUARY 11, 1928 OF ROUTE 2 BOX 1750, CHECOTAH, OK, WAS DISCIPLINED BY MEDICARE ON OCTOBER 6, 1994
DISCIPLINARY ACTION: 60-MONTH EXCLUSION FROM THE MEDICARE AND/OR MEDICAID PROGRAM
OFFENSE: CRIMINAL CONVICTION OR PLEA OF GUILTY, NOLO CONTENDERE, OR NO CONTEST TO A CRIME

NOTES: CONVICTED OF A CRIME INVOLVING THE MEDICARE, MEDICAID, MATERNAL AND CHILD HEALTH SERVICES BLOCK GRANT OR BLOCK GRANTS TO STATES FOR SOCIAL SERVICES PROGRAMS.

SNEED, NORMA LEE MD, LICENSE NUMBER 0007698, WAS DISCIPLINED BY OKLAHOMA ON JULY 22, 1994
DISCIPLINARY ACTION: 1-MONTH LICENSE SUSPENSION; PROBATION
OFFENSE: PROFESSIONAL MISCONDUCT

NOTES: ALLEGATIONS THAT DURING 1992 AND 1993 SHE AIDED AND ABETTED UNLICENSED PERSONS IN THE PRACTICE OF MEDICINE IN THAT SHE LEFT WRITTEN INSTRUCTIONS FOR HER STAFF AND A SUPPLY OF PRE-SIGNED, BLANK PRESCRIPTION PADS FOR USE OF HER UNLICENSED STAFF; THEY DID RENDER MEDICAL SERVICES IN HER ABSENCE; ON 2/17/94 PLED GUILTY TO MEDICAID FRAUD; SHE SUBMITS TO THE JURISDICTION OF THE BOARD WITHOUT ADMITTING OR DENYING THESE ALLEGATIONS. FOR FOUR MONTHS AFTER ONE MONTH ACTIVE SUSPENSION SHE SHALL PERFORM 20 HOURS PER WEEK OF PRO BONO PUBLIC SERVICE; MAY CONTINUE TO SEE MEDICAID, MEDICARE AND CHAMPUS PATIENTS ONLY; PLACED ON PERMANENT PROBATION; SHALL MAINTAIN NO MORE THAN ONE OFFICE AND IMMEDIATELY NOTIFY BOARD OF A CHANGE OF OFFICE LOCATION; NO MEDICAL SERVICE SHALL BE PERFORMED AT HER OFFICE UNLESS SHE OR ANOTHER LICENSED PRACTITIONER IS PRESENT; SHALL PROVIDE BOARD WITH REQUESTED REPORTS; SHALL PAY COSTS. A MOTION TO MODIFY THE TERMS OF THIS ORDER WERE DENIED ON 11/19/94.

SNEED, NORMA LEE MD, LICENSE NUMBER 0001141, WAS DISCIPLINED BY HAWAII ON OCTOBER 30, 1996
DISCIPLINARY ACTION: LICENSE REVOCATION; FINE
OFFENSE: DISCIPLINARY ACTION BY ANOTHER STATE OR AGENCY

NOTES: ON 7/22/94 TEMPORARILY SUSPENDED FROM THE PRACTICE OF MEDICINE IN OKLAHOMA. PLED GUILTY TO A PENAL OFFENSE SUBSTANTIALLY RELATED TO THE FUNCTIONS OF A PHYSICIAN; FAILED TO REPORT BOTH OF THESE ACTIONS TO THE BOARD. MAY NOT APPLY FOR REINSTATEMENT FOR AT LEAST FIVE YEARS; AND SHALL TURN IN ALL INDICIA OF LICENSURE TO THE BOARD WITHIN 30 DAYS. $10,000 FINE.

SNIDER, GERALD A MD, LICENSE NUMBER 0009483, WAS DISCIPLINED BY OKLAHOMA ON AUGUST 26, 1993
DISCIPLINARY ACTION: REPRIMAND; MONITORING OF PHYSICIAN PERFORMANCE
OFFENSE: OVERPRESCRIBING OR MISPRESCRIBING DRUGS

NOTES: RESULTS OF A PATIENT SURVEY SHOWED THAT BETWEEN 1/1/92 THROUGH 9/30/92 IN THE CASE OF THREE PATIENTS PRESCRIBED, DISPENSED OR ADMINISTERED CONTROLLED SUBSTANCES OR NARCOTIC DRUGS IN EXCESS OF THE AMOUNT CONSIDERED GOOD MEDICAL PRACTICE OR WITHOUT MEDICAL NEED. HE IS URGED BUT NOT ORDERED TO OBTAIN INDEPENDENT CONSULTATION WITH A QUALIFIED ADDICTIONOLOGIST FOR ANY PATIENT REQUIRING CONTROLLED DANGEROUS SUBSTANCES OVER A LONG PERIOD; BOARD WILL CONDUCT A FOLLOW-UP PRESCRIPTION SURVEY. ON 6/6/97 SUSPENSION ORDERED TO EXPIRE ON 5/26/97 ON THE CONDITION THAT ALL COURT COSTS ASSESSED HAVE BEEN PAID AND TO BEGIN A FIVE YEAR PROBATION UNDER THE FOLLOWING TERMS AND CONDITIONS: SHALL SERVE TEN HOURS A WEEK COMMUNITY SERVICE WITH REPORTS TO THE BOARD; SHALL NOT ACT AS A CONSULTANT ON ANY PATIENT HE HAS TREATED DURING THE PAST FIVE YEARS; SHALL PROVIDE THE BOARD WITH ANY REQUESTED REPORTS OR FILES IMMEDIATELY UPON REQUEST; SHALL KEEP BOARD INFORMED OF HIS CURRENT ADDRESS; SHALL KEEP CURRENT PAYMENT OF ALL ASSESSMENT BY THE BOARD FOR PROSECUTION, INVESTIGATION AND MONITORING OF HIS CASE; UNTIL SUCH TIME AS ALL INDEBTEDNESS TO THE BOARD HAS BEEN SATISFIED, HE SHALL REAFFIRM SAID INDEBTEDNESS IN ANY AND ALL BANKRUPTCY PROCEEDINGS; SHALL CONDUCT HIS PRACTICE IN COMPLIANCE WITH THE OKLAHOMA ALLOPATHIC MEDICAL AND SURGICAL LICENSURE AND SUPERVISION ACT; SHALL FURNISH TO EACH AND EVERY STATE IN WHICH HE HOLDS LICENSURE OR APPLIES FOR LICENSURE AND ANY HEALTHCARE ENTITY WHERE HE HAS PRIVILEGES, A COPY OF THIS ORDER.

SNIDER, GERALD A MD, DATE OF BIRTH SEPTEMBER 22, 1943 OF PO BOX 1500, EL RENO, OK, WAS DISCIPLINED BY MEDICARE ON DECEMBER 30, 1996
DISCIPLINARY ACTION: 120-MONTH EXCLUSION FROM THE MEDICARE AND/OR MEDICAID PROGRAM
OFFENSE: CRIMINAL CONVICTION OR PLEA OF GUILTY, NOLO CONTENDERE, OR NO CONTEST TO A CRIME

NOTES: CONVICTED OF A CRIME INVOLVING THE MEDICARE, MEDICAID, MATERNAL AND CHILD HEALTH SERVICES BLOCK GRANT OR BLOCK GRANTS TO STATES FOR SOCIAL SERVICES PROGRAMS.

SNIDER, GERALD A MD, LICENSE NUMBER 9483 OF 1500 N MAIN, MUSKOGEE, OK, WAS DISCIPLINED BY OKLAHOMA ON JANUARY 16, 1997
DISCIPLINARY ACTION: 2-MONTH LICENSE SUSPENSION; 60-MONTH PROBATION
OFFENSE: CRIMINAL CONVICTION OR PLEA OF GUILTY, NOLO CONTENDERE, OR NO CONTEST TO A CRIME

NOTES: ON 12/1/95 HE WAS FOUND GUILTY OF CONSPIRING TO RECEIVE FEES FOR REFERRAL OF MEDICARE PATIENTS AND ON 5/14/96 HE WAS SENTENCED TO A 12-MONTH AND ONE DAY PRISON TERM TO BE FOLLOWED BY THREE YEARS' SUPERVISED RELEASE. UPON RELEASE FROM PRISON, SUSPENSION WILL COMMENCE. SHALL SERVE 10 HOURS A WEEK OF COMMUNITY SERVICE DURING THE SUSPENSION PERIOD AND WILL MAKE A PERSONAL APPEARANCE BEFORE THE BOARD PRIOR TO THE END OF THE SUSPENSION AND SUBMIT A REPORT REGARDING THE COMMUNITY SERVICE. DURING PROBATION, THE FOLLOWING CONDITIONS APPLY: MAY NOT ACT AS A CONSULTANT ON ANY PATIENT HE HAS TREATED DURING THE PAST FIVE YEARS; SHALL KEEP THE BOARD INFORMED OF HIS ADDRESS AND PAY COSTS; SHALL SUBMIT REPORTS TO THE BOARD UPON REQUEST; SHALL SUBMIT TO EVERY STATE IN WHICH

HE HOLDS LICENSURE AND TO HOSPITALS, CLINICS OR OTHER INSTITUTIONS IN WHICH HE HOLDS OR ANTICIPATES HOLDING ANY FORM OF STAFF PRIVILEGE A COPY OF THIS ORDER; SHALL SUBMIT REPORTS TO THE BOARD UPON REQUEST; ON 6/6/97 SUSPENSION LIFTED AND LICENSE PLACED ON PROBATION EVEN THOUGH HE HAD BEEN UNABLE TO SERVE THE REQUIRED COMMUNITY SERVICE. INSTEAD A CONDITION WAS ADDED REQUIRING 10 HOURS A WEEK COMMUNITY SERVICE; THE OTHER CONDITIONS OF THIS ORDER REMAIN IN EFFECT.

SNIDER, GERALD ALBERT MD OF 1500 NORTH MAIN, MUSKOGEE, OK, WAS DISCIPLINED BY DEA ON JANUARY 21, 1997
DISCIPLINARY ACTION: SURRENDER OF CONTROLLED SUBSTANCE LICENSE

SNYDER, DAVID D MD, LICENSE NUMBER 0007094, WAS DISCIPLINED BY OKLAHOMA ON NOVEMBER 1, 1991
DISCIPLINARY ACTION: 24-MONTH PROBATION; MONITORING OF PHYSICIAN PERFORMANCE

NOTES: PROBATION UNDER TERMS AND CONDITIONS: SHALL NOT PRESCRIBE, ADMINISTER OR DISPENSE ANY MEDICATIONS FOR HIS PERSONAL USE, TO SPOUSE OR ANY IMMEDIATE FAMILY MEMBER; SHALL TAKE NO MEDICATION EXCEPT THAT WHICH IS AUTHORIZED BY A PHYSICIAN TREATING HIM FOR A LEGITIMATE MEDICAL NEED; SHALL FURNISH BOARD WITH ADDRESS AND/OR CHANGE OF ADDRESS; SHALL APPEAR BEFORE BOARD UPON REQUEST.

SOMVONGSIRI, CHAROEN MD, LICENSE NUMBER 0014682, WAS DISCIPLINED BY OKLAHOMA ON FEBRUARY 29, 1992
DISCIPLINARY ACTION: 3-MONTH LICENSE SUSPENSION; 54-MONTH PROBATION
OFFENSE: CRIMINAL CONVICTION OR PLEA OF GUILTY, NOLO CONTENDERE, OR NO CONTEST TO A CRIME

NOTES: ON 11/15/91 FOUND GUILTY OF THE FELONY CRIME OF MAKING A FALSE CLAIM UNDER THE OKLAHOMA MEDICAID PROGRAM IN OKLAHOMA COUNTY AND RECEIVED A TWO YEAR SUSPENDED SENTENCE, $5,000 FINE, $10,000 PAYMENT TO THE VICTIM'S COMPENSATION FUND AND $35,000 RESTITUTION. LICENSE SHALL BE REINSTATED FOLLOWING SUSPENSION ONLY TO ALLOW DR. SOMVONGSIRI TO PERFORM COMMUNITY SERVICE AS A PHYSICIAN AND SURGEON WITHOUT RECEIVING REMUNERATION. PERIOD OF PRACTICE WITHOUT REMUNERATION SHALL RUN FROM 6/1/92 TO 09/01/92. LICENSE THEN PUT ON PROBATION UNDER FOLLOWING CONDITIONS: MUST PROVIDE PROOF OF PERFORMANCE OF AT LEAST 100 HOURS OF UNPAID COMMUNITY SERVICE EVERY THREE MONTHS; SHALL NOTIFY ANY HOSPITAL WHERE HE HOLDS STAFF PRIVILEGES, OR CLINIC, OR GROUP WHERE HE PRACTICES OF THE TERMS AND CONDITIONS; SHALL FURNISH BOARD WITH ADDRESS AND/OR CHANGE OF ADDRESS; SHALL APPEAR BEFORE BOARD UPON REQUEST.

SPEED, HENRY K III MD, LICENSE NUMBER 0007960, WAS DISCIPLINED BY OKLAHOMA ON FEBRUARY 12, 1991
DISCIPLINARY ACTION: LICENSE REVOCATION
OFFENSE: OVERPRESCRIBING OR MISPRESCRIBING DRUGS

NOTES: FROM 3/30/78 TO 4/25/90 WROTE PRESCRIPTIONS FOR CONTROLLED SUBSTANCES TO AT LEAST 11 PATIENTS IN EXCESS OF THE AMOUNT CONSIDERED GOOD MEDICAL PRACTICE OR WITHOUT MEDICAL NEED IN ACCORDANCE WITH PUBLISHED STANDARDS. ON 3/21/91 BOARD DENIED A MOTION TO STAY THE REVOCATION.

SPEED, HENRY K III MD, LICENSE NUMBER 0007960 OF 5555 E 71ST ST #6112, TULSA, OK, WAS DISCIPLINED BY OKLAHOMA ON OCTOBER 5, 1991
DISCIPLINARY ACTION: LICENSE REINSTATEMENT; 60-MONTH PROBATION

NOTES: ON 2/27/91 VOLUNTARILY ENTERED TREATMENT AND ON 6/15/91 COMPLETED TREATMENT AT THE TALBOTT RECOVERY SYSTEM AND HAS PRODUCED EVIDENCE OF SUCCESSFUL COMPLETION IN THE FORM OF A LETTER SIGNED BY THE CONTINUING CARE COORDINATOR OF THE FACILITY. LICENSE REINSTATED UNDER TERMS AND CONDITIONS OF PROBATION: SHALL NOT PRESCRIBE, ADMINISTER OR DISPENSE ANY CONTROLLED DANGEROUS SUBSTANCES FOR OTHERS OR FOR HIMSELF; SHALL TAKE NO MEDICATION EXCEPT THAT WHICH IS AUTHORIZED BY A PHYSICIAN TREATING HIM FOR A LEGITIMATE MEDICAL NEED; SHALL ABSTAIN FROM CONSUMING ALCOHOL OR ANY SUBSTANCE, WHICH WOULD ADVERSELY AFFECT HIS ABILITY TO PRACTICE; SHALL SUBMIT BIOLOGICAL FLUID SPECIMENS FOR ANALYSIS; SHALL NOTIFY ANY HOSPITAL WHERE HE HOLDS STAFF PRIVILEGES, OR CLINIC, OR GROUP WHERE HE PRACTICES OF THE TERMS AND CONDITIONS; AGREES TO PARTICIPATE IN SUCH RECOVERY PROGRAM AS RECOMMENDED BY PHYSICIANS RECOVERY PROGRAM; SHALL FURNISH BOARD WITH ADDRESS AND/OR CHANGE OF ADDRESS; SHALL APPEAR BEFORE BOARD UPON REQUEST. AS OF 1/15/93 HIS REQUEST TO MODIFY TERMS OF PROBATION TO ALLOW HIM TO PRESCRIBE CONTROLLED DANGEROUS SUBSTANCES IS DENIED. HE MUST SUCCESSFULLY COMPLETE BOARD APPROVED CONTINUING MEDICAL EDUCATION ON THE PRESCRIBING OF CONTROLLED DANGEROUS SUBSTANCES BEFORE CONSIDERATION IS GIVEN TO REQUESTS TO MODIFY HIS PROBATION. HIS LEVEL OF SUPERVISION WHILE UNDER PROBATION IS REDUCED FROM LEVEL I TO LEVEL II. ON 7/1/93 BOARD GRANTED HIS REQUEST TO MODIFY PROBATION TO ALLOW HIM TO PRESCRIBE, ADMINISTER OR DISPENSE CONTROLLED DANGEROUS SUBSTANCES SCHEDULES II THROUGH V ONLY ON SERIALLY-NUMBERED, DUPLICATE PRESCRIPTION PADS WITH COPIES AVAILABLE TO THE BOARD. OTHER TERMS AND CONDITIONS OF PROBATION REMAIN IN EFFECT.

ST VILLE, JOSEPH M MD OF TULSA, OK, WAS DISCIPLINED BY MISSOURI ON FEBRUARY 16, 1994
DISCIPLINARY ACTION: NONRENEWAL OF LICENSE
OFFENSE: NONCOMPLIANCE WITH A PROFESSIONAL RULE

NOTES: DURING 1992 HE FAILED TO OBTAIN THE REQUIRED 25 HOURS OF CONTINUING MEDICAL EDUCATION CREDITS AND FAILED TO REPORT OBTAINING SUCH HOURS BY 05/20/93 AS REQUIRED BY BOARD RULE.

STARR, DWIGHT BAILEY MD OF 2915 PINE RIDGE ROAD, OKLAHOMA CITY, OK, WAS DISCIPLINED BY DEA ON OCTOBER 15, 1990
DISCIPLINARY ACTION: SURRENDER OF CONTROLLED SUBSTANCE LICENSE
OFFENSE: PROFESSIONAL MISCONDUCT

NOTES: ARRESTED 9/28/90 IN OKLAHOMA CITY FOR ILLEGAL DISTRIBUTION OF CONTROLLED SUBSTANCES AND OBTAINING CONTROLLED SUBSTANCES BY FRAUD. PLED GUILTY 11/08/91 TO THESE CHARGES.

STARR, DWIGHT BAILEY MD, LICENSE NUMBER 0013239, WAS DISCIPLINED BY OKLAHOMA ON NOVEMBER 1, 1990
DISCIPLINARY ACTION: LICENSE SUSPENSION; REQUIRED TO ENTER AN IMPAIRED PHYSICIAN PROGRAM OR SUBSTANCE ABUSE TREATMENT
OFFENSE: SUBSTANCE ABUSE

NOTES: BEGAN INPATIENT TREATMENT FOR SUBSTANCE ABUSE. SUSPENSION SHALL RUN UNTIL HE PRODUCES EVIDENCE OF SUCCESSFUL COMPLETION OF IN-PATIENT TREATMENT AND RELATED RESIDENTIAL OUT-PATIENT TREATMENT FROM A PHYSICIAN TREATMENT PROGRAM APPROVED BY THE BOARD.

STARR, DWIGHT BAILEY MD, LICENSE NUMBER 0013239 OF 1004 NW 39, OKLAHOMA CITY, OK, WAS DISCIPLINED BY OKLAHOMA ON FEBRUARY 28, 1991
DISCIPLINARY ACTION: 60-MONTH PROBATION; RESTRICTION PLACED ON CONTROLLED SUBSTANCE LICENSE

NOTES: PROVIDED EVIDENCE OF SUCCESSFUL COMPLETION OF IN-PATIENT TREATMENT. SUSPENSION OF 10/26/90 LIFTED. PROBATIONARY TERM UNDER FOLLOWING CONDITIONS: SHALL NOT PRESCRIBE, ADMINISTER, OR DISPENSE ANY MEDICATION FOR HIS PERSONAL USE OR ANY CONTROLLED DANGEROUS SUBSTANCES OR NARCOTICS TO HIS PATIENTS FOR ANY CONDITION; SHALL TAKE NO MEDICATION EXCEPT THAT WHICH IS AUTHORIZED BY A PHYSICIAN TREATING HIM FOR A LEGITIMATE MEDICAL NEED; SHALL ABSTAIN FROM CONSUMING ALCOHOL OR ANY SUBSTANCE, WHICH WOULD ADVERSELY AFFECT HIS ABILITY TO PRACTICE; SHALL SUBMIT BIOLOGICAL FLUID SPECIMENS FOR ANALYSIS; SHALL CONTINUE REGULAR PARTICIPATION IN THE OKLAHOMA STATE MEDICAL ASSOCIATION PHYSICIAN RECOVERY COMMITTEE AND ALCOHOLICS ANONYMOUS OR NARCOTICS ANONYMOUS; SHALL NOTIFY ANY HOSPITAL WHERE HE HOLDS STAFF PRIVILEGES, OR CLINIC OR GROUP OF THE TERMS AND CONDITIONS; SHALL FURNISH BOARD WITH ADDRESS AND/OR CHANGE OF ADDRESS; SHALL APPEAR BEFORE BOARD UPON REQUEST. ON 1/15/93 BOARD GRANTED HIS REQUEST TO MODIFY PROBATION TO ALLOW HIM TO PRESCRIBE SCHEDULE III, IV AND V CONTROLLED DANGEROUS SUBSTANCES FOR EMERGENCY ROOM PATIENTS AND HOSPITAL IN-PATIENTS WRITTEN ON DUPLICATE, SERIALLY-NUMBERED FORMS WITH COPIES AVAILABLE TO THE BOARD AND ALLOWS HIM TO ORDER SCHEDULE II CONTROLLED DANGEROUS SUBSTANCES FOR ADMINISTRATION BY HOSPITAL PERSONNEL ON SITE. ALL OTHER TERMS AND CONDITIONS OF PROBATION REMAIN IN EFFECT.

STARR, DWIGHT BAILEY MD, LICENSE NUMBER 0013239 OF 1004 NW 39TH, OKLAHOMA CITY, OK, WAS DISCIPLINED BY OKLAHOMA ON MAY 20, 1993
DISCIPLINARY ACTION: LICENSE SUSPENSION
OFFENSE: PRACTICING WITHOUT A VALID CONTROLLED SUBSTANCE LICENSE

NOTES: ON 1/27/93 WROTE A PRESCRIPTION FOR LORTAB USING A PRESCRIPTION SLIP THAT WAS PRESIGNED BY ANOTHER PHYSICIAN; HAD NO VALID DEA REGISTRATION WHEN HE WROTE THIS PRESCRIPTION; PERSONALLY DROVE THE PATIENT TO PHARMACY WHERE AN UNSUCCESSFUL ATTEMPT TO FILL THE PRESCRIPTION WAS MADE; DID NOT MAINTAIN MEDICAL RECORDS ON THIS PATIENT OR ESTABLISH A VALID PHYSICIAN/PATIENT RELATIONSHIP; PRESCRIBED IN A SIMILAR MANNER FOR FOUR OTHER PATIENTS IN 1/93 AND ONE IN 7/93.

STARR, DWIGHT BAILEY MD, LICENSE NUMBER 0013239 OF 1004 NW 39TH STREET, OKLAHOMA CITY, OK, WAS DISCIPLINED BY OKLAHOMA ON JULY 1, 1993
DISCIPLINARY ACTION: 60-MONTH PROBATION; RESTRICTION PLACED ON LICENSE

NOTES: LICENSE SUSPENDED ON 5/14/93 REINSTATED TO SUPERVISED MEDICAL DOCTOR LICENSE; SINCE THE DATE OF SUSPENSION UNDERWENT REEVALUATION IN HOSPITAL AND APPLIED FOR A PSYCHIATRIC RESIDENCY; THE DOCTOR WHO EXAMINED HIM REPORTED NO NEW PSYCHO-PATHOLOGY AND NO PROOF OF RELAPSE BUT EXAM DID RAISE SOME ISSUES OF IMMATURITY AND FACTORS COMMON TO DEPENDENCY. PROBATION TO BEGIN WITH THE ISSUANCE DATE OF HIS SUPERVISED MEDICAL DOCTOR CERTIFICATE. CONDITIONS OF PROBATION: SHALL NOT PRESCRIBE, ADMINISTER OR DISPENSE CONTROLLED DANGEROUS SUBSTANCES; SHALL NOT PRESCRIBE, ADMINISTER OR DISPENSE ANY MEDICATIONS FOR HIS PERSONAL USE AND SHALL TAKE NONE UNLESS AUTHORIZED BY ANOTHER PHYSICIAN FOR A LEGITIMATE MEDICAL NEED; SHALL ABSTAIN FROM CONSUMING ALCOHOL AND ANY SUBSTANCE WHICH WOULD ADVERSELY AFFECT HIS ABILITY TO PRACTICE; SHALL SUBMIT BIOLOGICAL FLUID SPECIMENS; SHALL CONTINUE PARTICIPATION IN PHYSICIAN RECOVERY COMMITTEE AND AA OR NARCOTICS ANONYMOUS AND ATTEND 90 MEETINGS WITHIN 90 DAYS; SHALL PARTICIPATE IN REGULAR PSYCHIATRIC COUNSELING WITH REPORTS; SHALL COMPLY WITH ALL TERMS OF HIS HOSPITAL POST-TREATMENT CONTRACT; SHALL FURNISH BOARD WITH ADDRESS/CHANGE OF ADDRESS; SHALL APPEAR BEFORE THE BOARD UPON REQUEST AND SUBMIT REQUIRED REPORTS; SHALL PAY COSTS; SHALL FURNISH EVERY STATE IN WHICH HE HOLDS OR APPLIES FOR LICENSURE AND ANY HEALTH CARE ENTITY WHERE HE HAS PRIVILEGES WITH A COPY OF THE ORDER; SHALL NOT SUPERVISE A PHYSICIAN'S ASSISTANT. ON 3/31/94 HIS LICENSE WAS REINSTATED AS A SUPERVISED MEDICAL DOCTOR.

STARR, DWIGHT BAILEY MD, LICENSE NUMBER 0013239, WAS DISCIPLINED BY OKLAHOMA ON FEBRUARY 14, 1996
DISCIPLINARY ACTION: EMERGENCY SUSPENSION
OFFENSE: FAILURE TO COMPLY WITH PREVIOUS BOARD ORDER

NOTES: 0N 2/6/96 FAILED TO PROVIDE URINE SAMPLE UPON REQUEST IN VIOLATION OF PREVIOUS ORDER.

STARR, DWIGHT BAILEY MD, LICENSE NUMBER 0013239, WAS DISCIPLINED BY OKLAHOMA ON MARCH 28, 1996
DISCIPLINARY ACTION: LICENSE REVOCATION
OFFENSE: FAILURE TO COMPLY WITH PREVIOUS BOARD ORDER

NOTES: HIS LICENSE WAS TEMPORARILY SUSPENDED UNTIL AN EMERGENCY HEARING ON 2/14/96. HE FAILED TO PROVIDE A URINE SPECIMEN UPON BOARD REQUEST ON 2/6/96 RESULTING IN VIOLATION OF TERMS OF PROBATION.

STOCKARD, REX E JR MD OF 4417 WEST GORE BLVD, LAWTON, OK, WAS DISCIPLINED BY DEA ON NOVEMBER 21, 1991
DISCIPLINARY ACTION: DENIAL OF NEW LICENSE
OFFENSE: DISCIPLINARY ACTION BY ANOTHER STATE OR AGENCY

NOTES: ON 4/18/89 SURRENDERED HIS DEA CERTIFICATE FOLLOWING HIS ADMISSION OF A SUBSTANCE ABUSE PROBLEM WITH DIDREX, A SCHEDULE III CONTROLLED SUBSTANCE, AND THE SUSPENSION OF HIS OKLAHOMA CONTROLLED SUBSTANCE REGISTRATION BY THE OKLAHOMA BUREAU OF NARCOTICS AND

DANGEROUS DRUGS CONTROL. THE BUREAU ALSO FOUND THAT HE FAILED TO MAINTAIN ADEQUATE CONTROLS AGAINST THE DIVERSION OF CONTROLLED SUBSTANCES TO UNAUTHORIZED ENTITIES. ADMINISTRATIVE LAW JUDGE FOUND HE AUTHORIZED AT LEAST 57 PRESCRIPTIONS FOR CONTROLLED SUBSTANCES AFTER THE SURRENDER OF HIS DEA LICENSE. HAS FULFILLED THE REQUIREMENTS OF A SUBSTANCE ABUSE PROGRAM IN CUSHING, OKLAHOMA AND HIS OKLAHOMA PRESCRIBING PRIVILEGES WERE REINSTATED FOR SCHEDULE II THROUGH V ON THE CONDITION THAT HE USE DUPLICATE, SERIALLY-NUMBERED PRESCRIPTION PADS. THE ADMINISTRATOR DENIED THE APPLICATION BUT WILL GIVE FAVORABLE CONSIDERATION TO A NEW APPLICATION IF NOT FILED WITHIN A YEAR AND IF ACCOMPANIED BY EVIDENCE THAT HE HAS COMPLETED CONTINUING EDUCATION COURSES TOTALING AT LEAST 30 HOURS OF INSTRUCTION.

STOCKTON, ROBERT LOUIS MD, LICENSE NUMBER 00C8855 OF WACO, TX, WAS DISCIPLINED BY TEXAS ON JANUARY 26, 1990
DISCIPLINARY ACTION: 60-MONTH PROBATION; RESTRICTION PLACED ON LICENSE

NOTES: STIPULATED ORDER. MUST OBTAIN CONCURRING NEUROLOGICAL CONSULTATION PRIOR TO SURGERY ON ANY CASE WHICH HAS OR MAY HAVE NEUROSURGICAL IMPLICATIONS.

STOCKTON, ROBERT LOUIS MD, LICENSE NUMBER 0007457, WAS DISCIPLINED BY OKLAHOMA ON NOVEMBER 8, 1991
DISCIPLINARY ACTION: 60-MONTH PROBATION; MONITORING OF PHYSICIAN PERFORMANCE

NOTES: PROBATION RETROACTIVE TO 1/26/90 WITH FOLLOWING TERMS AND CONDITIONS: PRIOR TO PERFORMING SURGERY ON ANY CASE WHICH HAS OR MAY HAVE NEUROSURGICAL IMPLICATIONS, SHALL FIRST OBTAIN A WRITTEN CONCURRING NEUROLOGICAL CONSULTATION FROM AN ABMS BOARD-CERTIFIED NEUROSURGEON OR NEUROLOGIST; SHALL NOTIFY ANY HOSPITAL WHERE HE HOLDS STAFF PRIVILEGES OR CLINIC OR GROUP WHERE HE PRACTICES OF TERMS AND CONDITIONS; SHALL FURNISH BOARD WITH ADDRESS AND/OR CHANGE OF ADDRESS; SHALL APPEAR BEFORE BOARD UPON REQUEST. THIS PROBATION SHALL RUN CONCURRENTLY WITH THE EXISTING PROBATION TO THE TEXAS STATE BOARD OF MEDICAL EXAMINERS WITH REPORTS TO OKLAHOMA BOARD; SHALL APPEAR BEFORE OKLAHOMA BOARD BEFORE RESUMING PRACTICE IN THE STATE. ON 6/5/97 PROBATION TERMINATED AS HE RETIRED AND APPLIED FOR PHYSICIAN EMERITUS STATUS. IF REACTIVATE/REINSTATE LICENSE IN OKLAHOMA, TERMS OF PROBATION WOULD BE REINSTATED.

STOCKTON, ROBERT LOUIS MD, LICENSE NUMBER 00C8855 OF WACO, TX, WAS DISCIPLINED BY TEXAS ON JANUARY 14, 1994
DISCIPLINARY ACTION: SURRENDER OF LICENSE

NOTES: DOES NOT ADMIT ALLEGATIONS BUT SURRENDERS LICENSE IN LIEU OF FURTHER INVESTIGATION. SHALL NOT PETITION THE BOARD FOR REINSTATEMENT.

STOCKTON, ROBERT LOUIS MD OF 824 N 18TH STREET, WACO, TX, WAS DISCIPLINED BY DEA ON FEBRUARY 14, 1994
DISCIPLINARY ACTION: SURRENDER OF CONTROLLED SUBSTANCE LICENSE
OFFENSE: DISCIPLINARY ACTION BY ANOTHER STATE OR AGENCY

STOOPS, DONALD E DO, LICENSE NUMBER 0001315, WAS DISCIPLINED BY OKLAHOMA ON MARCH 17, 1994
DISCIPLINARY ACTION: LICENSE SUSPENSION
OFFENSE: DISCIPLINARY ACTION BY ANOTHER STATE OR AGENCY

NOTES: ON 5/06/93 ON HIS APPLICATION FOR LICENSURE RENEWAL INDICATED THAT HE HAD NOT BEEN DISCIPLINED IN THE PAST YEAR. NEW MEXICO SUSPENDED HIS LICENSE FOR ONE YEAR EFFECTIVE 1993 AND HE IS EXCLUDED FROM PARTICIPATION IN MEDICARE FOR 10 YEARS. INDEFINITE SUSPENSION. $485.00 ADMINISTRATIVE COSTS.

STOOPS, DONALD E DO, LICENSE NUMBER 0051969, WAS DISCIPLINED BY NEW MEXICO ON NOVEMBER 19, 1994
DISCIPLINARY ACTION: LICENSE REVOCATION
OFFENSE: PROFESSIONAL MISCONDUCT

NOTES: UNPROFESSIONAL CONDUCT.

STOOPS, DONALD E DO OF TRUTH OR CONSEQUENCES, NM, WAS DISCIPLINED BY DEA ON SEPTEMBER 9, 1996
DISCIPLINARY ACTION: REVOCATION OF CONTROLLED SUBSTANCE LICENSE
OFFENSE: DISCIPLINARY ACTION BY ANOTHER STATE OR AGENCY

NOTES: ON 11/19/94 THE NEW MEXICO BOARD REVOKED HIS STATE LICENSE TO PRACTICE OSTEOPATHIC MEDICINE.

STOTTS, STEPHEN MD, LICENSE NUMBER 10878 OF 908 OVERBROOK AVENUE, PONCA CITY, OK, WAS DISCIPLINED BY OKLAHOMA ON JULY 23, 1999
DISCIPLINARY ACTION: REPRIMAND
OFFENSE: PROVIDING FALSE INFORMATION TO THE BOARD OR OTHER HEALTH AGENCY

NOTES: SINCE 7/92 EACH RENEWAL APPLICATION SHOWS HIM AS "RETIRED" OR "NOT CURRENTLY PRACTICING"; DURING THIS SAME TIME PERIOD, PHARMACY RECORDS SHOW HE ISSUED MANY CONTROLLED DRUG PRESCRIPTIONS FOR PERSONAL FRIENDS AND AT LEAST ONE FAMILY MEMBER; FAILED TO KEEP RECORDS OF THESE PRESCRIPTIONS OR PATIENT RECORDS OR CHARTS; FAILED TO CONDUCT A HISTORY, PHYSICAL OR EXAMINATION OF ANY OF THESE FRIENDS PRIOR TO PRESCRIBING THEM CONTROLLED DRUGS BUT PRESCRIBED THE DRUGS THAT THE PATIENTS TOLD HIM WORKED BEST FOR THEIR SELF-DESCRIBED MEDICAL PROBLEMS. PLACED ON PERMANENT PHYSICIAN EMERITUS STATUS; SHALL NOT APPLY FOR ADDITIONAL LICENSURE STATUS; SHALL PAY COSTS.

STOTTS, STEPHEN MD OF 908 E OVERBROOK, PONCA CITY, OK, WAS DISCIPLINED BY DEA ON SEPTEMBER 9, 1999
DISCIPLINARY ACTION: SURRENDER OF CONTROLLED SUBSTANCE LICENSE
OFFENSE: DISCIPLINARY ACTION BY ANOTHER STATE OR AGENCY

NOTES: STATE BOARD.

STOUT, HAROLD MD, LICENSE NUMBER 7602 OF PO BOX 207, WAURIKA, OK, WAS DISCIPLINED BY OKLAHOMA ON MARCH 27, 1998
DISCIPLINARY ACTION: 4-MONTH PROBATION; REPRIMAND
OFFENSE: SUBSTANDARD CARE, INCOMPETENCE OR NEGLIGENCE

NOTES: ON OR AROUND 3/27/97 HE SAW A TWO-YEAR-OLD FEMALE CHILD IN THE EMERGENCY ROOM AT A HOSPITAL IN WAURIKA, OKLAHOMA. SUBSEQUENT EXAMINATION AT A SUBSEQUENT HOSPITAL BY

OTHER PHYSICIANS SHOWED THAT SHE WAS SEVERELY BRUISED, HAD A FRACTURE OF THE ARM, AND DISLOCATED SHOULDER. HE DID NOT THOROUGHLY EXAMINE THE CHILD, DID NOT ORDER NECESSARY X-RAYS, DID NOT DETECT FRACTURE OR DISLOCATION, DID NOT TREAT THE CHILD, BUT RELEASED THE CHILD BACK TO THE PARENTS AND FAILED TO RECOGNIZE AND REPORT SUSPECTED CHILD ABUSE. ON OR AROUND 6/9/92, HE SAW A SEVEN-MONTH-OLD FEMALE CHILD IN HIS OFFICE AT WAURIKA, OKLAHOMA. SUBSEQUENT EXAMINATION AT A SUBSEQUENT HOSPITAL SHOWED THAT THE CHILD WAS BLIND AND SUFFERED PERMANENT BRAIN DAMAGE. HE DID NOT THOROUGHLY EXAMINE THE CHILD, DID NOT ORDER NECESSARY X-RAYS, DID NOT DETECT ANY SERIOUS INJURY, DID NOT RENDER TREATMENT, BUT RELEASED THE CHILD BACK TO THE PARENTS AND FAILED TO RECOGNIZE AND REPORT SUSPECTED CHILD ABUSE. THE PARENTS OF THIS SECOND PATIENT WERE LATER CONVICTED OF THE CRIME OF CHILD ABUSE AND SENTENCED TO TEN YEARS IN PRISON. CONDITIONS OF PROBATION: SHALL REQUEST ALL HOSPITALS IN WHICH HE ANTICIPATES PRACTICING TO FURNISH A STATEMENT REGARDING MONITORING OF HIS PRACTICE; SHALL SUBMIT TO EVERY STATE IN WHICH HE HOLDS LICENSURE AND TO HOSPITALS, CLINICS OR OTHER INSTITUTIONS IN WHICH HE HOLDS OR ANTICIPATES HOLDING ANY FORM OF STAFF PRIVILEGE A COPY OF THIS ORDER; SHALL KEEP THE BOARD INFORMED OF HIS ADDRESS AND PAY COSTS; SHALL ATTEND A TWO-DAY PROGRAM ON CHILD ABUSE MEDICAL EXAMINER TRAINING AND ATTEND CHILD PROTECTION COMMITTEE MEETINGS FOUR TIMES WITHIN THREE MONTHS; THE CHILD PROTECTION PROGRAM DIRECTOR WILL PROVIDE A WRITTEN PROGRESS REPORT TO THE BOARD.

STUBBLEFIELD, WAYNE MD, LICENSE NUMBER 00F2955 OF OKLAHOMA CITY, OK, WAS DISCIPLINED BY TEXAS ON AUGUST 18, 1990
OFFENSE: DISCIPLINARY ACTION BY ANOTHER STATE OR AGENCY

NOTES: STIPULATED ORDER. MUST COMPLY WITH TENNESSEE BOARD AGREED ORDER AND OKLAHOMA BOARD FINAL ORDER. IF DESIRING TO PRACTICE MEDICINE IN TEXAS, MUST DEMONSTRATE TO BOARD CAPACITY TO PRACTICE MEDICINE WITH REASONABLE SKILL AND SAFETY. IF AUTHORIZED TO PRACTICE IN TEXAS, MUST FOLLOW ANY ADDITIONAL TERMS OF PROBATION AS MAY BE IMPOSED.

STUBBLEFIELD, WAYNE MD, LICENSE NUMBER 0005893 OF OKLAHOMA CITY, OK, WAS DISCIPLINED BY TENNESSEE ON FEBRUARY 8, 1994
DISCIPLINARY ACTION: LICENSE REVOCATION; FINE
OFFENSE: FAILURE TO COMPLY WITH PREVIOUS BOARD ORDER

NOTES: VIOLATION OF TERMS OF PROBATION; MAKING FALSE STATEMENTS IN OBTAINING ADMISSION TO PRACTICE IN ANOTHER STATE; FAILURE TO RENEW TENNESSEE LICENSE. ASSESSED $1400 IN CIVIL PENALTIES.

STUBBLEFIELD, WAYNE MD, LICENSE NUMBER 0016809 OF 1001 SW 44, OKLAHOMA CITY, OK, WAS DISCIPLINED BY OKLAHOMA ON FEBRUARY 17, 1994
DISCIPLINARY ACTION: 24-MONTH PROBATION; MONITORING OF PHYSICIAN PERFORMANCE
OFFENSE: FAILURE TO COMPLY WITH PREVIOUS BOARD ORDER

NOTES: IN VIOLATION OF 1/12/89 PROBATION ORDER HE FAILED TO PRODUCE DUPLICATE PRESCRIPTIONS TO THE BOARD AND ON ONE OCCASION RECEIVED NECESSARY SCHEDULED DRUGS FROM A DENTIST BUT DID NOT INFORM THE DENTIST OF HIS HISTORY OF ADDICTION. PROBATION EXTENDED FOR TWO YEARS. CONDITIONS OF EXTENDED PROBATION: SHALL NOT PRESCRIBE, ADMINISTER OR DISPENSE ANY MEDICATIONS FOR HIS PERSONAL USE; SHALL NOT TAKE ANY MEDICATION UNLESS AUTHORIZED BY ANOTHER PHYSICIAN FOR A LEGITIMATE MEDICAL NEED; SHALL ABSTAIN FROM THE CONSUMPTION OF ALCOHOL OR ANY SUBSTANCE WHICH WOULD ADVERSELY AFFECT HIS ABILITY TO PRACTICE; SHALL SUBMIT BIOLOGICAL FLUID SPECIMENS; SHALL ONLY PRESCRIBE, ADMINISTER OR DISPENSE CONTROLLED SUBSTANCES ON DUPLICATE, SERIALLY-NUMBERED PRESCRIPTION PADS WITH COPIES AVAILABLE FOR INSPECTION; SHALL CONTINUE SUPPORTIVE PROGRAMS INCLUDING PHYSICIANS RECOVERY COMMITTEE AND PSYCHIATRIC CARE IF ORDERED; SHALL FURNISH BOARD WITH ADDRESS AND/OR CHANGE OF ADDRESS; SHALL APPEAR BEFORE THE BOARD UPON REQUEST AND PROVIDE REQUIRED REPORTS; SHALL PAY COSTS. LEVEL OF SUPERVISION REDUCED FROM LEVEL I TO LEVEL II.

STULL, DANA DUBER MD OF 118 LAKE ALUMA DRIVE, OKLAHOMA CITY, OK, WAS DISCIPLINED BY OKLAHOMA ON AUGUST 1, 1996
DISCIPLINARY ACTION: 60-MONTH PROBATION; RESTRICTION PLACED ON LICENSE

NOTES: IN 1/95 COMPLETED A THREE YEAR MONITORING AGREEMENT WITH THE PHYSICIANS' HEALTH PROGRAM IN PENNSYLVANIA AS WELL AS AN INPATIENT TREATMENT PROGRAM AT RUSH BEHAVIORAL TREATMENT CENTER FROM 3/11/96 TO 5/15/96. PROBATION BEGINNING 7/27/96 WITH CONDITIONS: SHALL NOT PRESCRIBE, ADMINISTER, DISPENSE, OR POSSESS ANY DRUGS IN SCHEDULES II THROUGH V; SHALL NOT ALLOW THE INITIATION OF ANY THERAPEUTIC REGIMEN BY ANY PERSONNEL UNDER HER SUPERVISION UNLESS SHE IS IN THE IMMEDIATE GEOGRAPHIC VICINITY; SHALL FURNISH EACH STATE IN WHICH SHE HOLDS OR APPLIES TO HOLD LICENSURE AND ANY HEALTH CARE ENTITIES IN WHICH SHE HOLDS PRIVILEGES A COPY OF THIS ORDER; SHALL NOT SUPERVISE A PHYSICIAN ASSISTANT; SHALL SUBMIT BIOLOGICAL FLUID SPECIMENS UPON BOARD REQUEST; SHALL NOT PRESCRIBE, ADMINISTER, OR DISPENSE, ANY MEDICATIONS FOR PERSONAL USE; SHALL TAKE NO MEDICATION UNLESS PRESCRIBED BY AN AUTHORIZED TREATING PHYSICIAN FOR LEGITIMATE MEDICAL NEED; SHALL PARTICIPATE IN THE OKLAHOMA STATE MEDICAL ASSOCIATION PHYSICIAN RECOVERY COMMITTEE MEETINGS AND RECOVERY PROGRAM AND FULFILL THE TERMS OF THE RUSH BEHAVIORAL HEALTH CENTER DISCHARGE AGREEMENT; SHALL KEEP THE BOARD INFORMED OF HER CURRENT ADDRESS; SHALL KEEP CURRENT PAYMENT OF ALL PROSECUTION, INVESTIGATION, AND MONITORING COSTS. ON 6/12/98 REQUEST TO MODIFY TERMS OF PROBATION GRANTED ALLOWING HER TO PRESCRIBE CONTROLLED SUBSTANCES IN SCHEDULES II-V, USING DUPLICATE, SERIALLY NUMBERED PRESCRIPTION PADS TO BE MADE AVAILABLE TO BOARD UPON REQUEST. ON 5/7/99 PROBATION TERMINATED.

SWYDEN, JOHN L DO, LICENSE NUMBER 2304, WAS DISCIPLINED BY OKLAHOMA ON JUNE 19, 1997
DISCIPLINARY ACTION: LICENSE SUSPENSION

SYNAR, PHIL H MD, LICENSE NUMBER 11405 OF 2809 NORTH

EDMOND ST., MUSKOGEE, OK, WAS DISCIPLINED BY OKLAHOMA ON FEBRUARY 5, 1998
DISCIPLINARY ACTION: 60-MONTH PROBATION; RESTRICTION PLACED ON LICENSE
OFFENSE: SUBSTANCE ABUSE

NOTES: ON OR ABOUT THE LAST WEEK OF 10/96 HE WAS UNDER THE INFLUENCE OR INTOXICATED WHILE ON DUTY AS A PHYSICIAN ON STAFF AT A HOSPITAL IN WAGONER, OKLAHOMA. DURING THIS SAME TIME PERIOD HE WAS SUFFERING A RELAPSE OF HIS SUBSTANCE ABUSE PROBLEM WHICH IMPAIRED HIS ABILITY TO PRACTICE MEDICINE AND SURGERY WITH REASONABLE SKILL AND SAFETY TO HIS PATIENTS. HE WAS ADMITTED TO A TREATMENT CENTER ON OR AROUND 9/3/97 FOR INPATIENT TREATMENT FOR SUBSTANCE ABUSE AND WAS RELEASED APPROXIMATELY 1/3/98. CONDITIONS OF PROBATION: SHALL SUBMIT TO EVERY STATE HE HOLDS LICENSURE AND HOSPITALS, CLINICS OR OTHER INSTITUTIONS IN WHICH HE HOLDS OR ANTICIPATES HOLDING ANY FORM OF STAFF PRIVILEGE A COPY OF THIS ORDER; SHALL SUBMIT BIOLOGICAL FLUID SPECIMENS AND SHALL NOT INGEST ANY SUBSTANCE WHICH WILL CAUSE A SPECIMEN TO TEST POSITIVE FOR PROHIBITED SUBSTANCES; SHALL NOT PRESCRIBE, ADMINISTER OR DISPENSE ANY MEDICATIONS FOR HIS PERSONAL USE AND SHALL TAKE NONE UNLESS AUTHORIZED BY ANOTHER PHYSICIAN FOR A LEGITIMATE MEDICAL NEED; SHALL ABIDE BY HIS POST-CARE CONTRACT FROM TREATMENT PROGRAM; SHALL KEEP THE BOARD INFORMED OF HIS ADDRESS AND PAY COSTS; SHALL REQUEST ALL HOSPITALS IN WHICH HE ANTICIPATES PRACTICING TO FURNISH A STATEMENT REGARDING MONITORING OF HIS PRACTICE; SHALL APPEAR BEFORE THE BOARD AND SUBMIT REPORTS UPON REQUEST; SHALL ENTER AND CONTINUE PSYCHIATRIC TREATMENT UNDER A BOARD APPROVED DOCTOR AND WILL AUTHORIZE THE RELEASE OF ALL RECORDS OF THAT TREATMENT TO THE BOARD; SHALL NOT SUPERVISE ALLIED HEALTH PROFESSIONALS; SHALL EXECUTE ALL RELEASES OF MEDICAL AND PSYCHIATRIC RECORDS AS NECESSARY TO DISCUSS HIS CASE WITH HIS TREATING PHYSICIANS AND/OR ANY PHYSICIANS HOLDING RECORDS.

TALBOTT, NEAL BEVAN MD, LICENSE NUMBER 0017448, WAS DISCIPLINED BY OKLAHOMA ON NOVEMBER 8, 1991
DISCIPLINARY ACTION: REPRIMAND
OFFENSE: PRACTICING WITHOUT A VALID CONTROLLED SUBSTANCE LICENSE

NOTES: FROM 12/90 THROUGH 2/91, ISSUED AND SIGNED AT LEAST 17 PRESCRIPTIONS FOR PATIENTS HE SAW IN THE EMERGENCY ROOM FOR VARIOUS CONTROLLED DANGEROUS SUBSTANCES AT A TIME WHEN HE DID NOT POSSESS THE REQUIRED REGISTRATION FROM THE U.S. DRUG ENFORCEMENT ADMINISTRATION; HE HAD APPLIED FOR DEA REGISTRATION; NO MALICIOUS INTENT WAS EVIDENT AND THERE WERE NO PRIOR COMPLAINTS AGAINST HIM; NO EVIDENCE OF PATIENT HARM, PERSONAL USE, OR DELIBERATE DIVERSION.

THOMAS-MCCAULEY, TINA MARIE MD, LICENSE NUMBER 0063897 OF CLEVELAND, OH, WAS DISCIPLINED BY OHIO ON DECEMBER 5, 1996
DISCIPLINARY ACTION: LICENSE SUSPENSION; PROBATION
OFFENSE: CRIMINAL CONVICTION OR PLEA OF GUILTY, NOLO CONTENDERE, OR NO CONTEST TO A CRIME

NOTES: IMPAIRMENT OF ABILITY TO PRACTICE ACCORDING TO ACCEPTABLE AND PREVAILING STANDARDS OF CARE BECAUSE OF HABITUAL OR EXCESSIVE USE OR ABUSE OF DRUGS; AND CONVICTION OF ONE MISDEMEANOR COUNT OF POSSESSION OF COCAINE. PERMANENT REVOCATION, STAYED SUBJECT TO INDEFINITE SUSPENSION FOR AT LEAST TWO YEARS. CONDITIONS DURING SUSPENSION AND SUBSEQUENT PROBATIONARY TERMS ESTABLISHED FOR AT LEAST FIVE YEARS; AND INELIGIBLE TO HOLD OR APPLY FOR DEA REGISTRATION WITHOUT BOARD APPROVAL.

THOMAS-MCCAULEY, TINA MARIE MD, LICENSE NUMBER 63897 OF OKLAHOMA CITY, OK, WAS DISCIPLINED BY OHIO ON MARCH 13, 1998
DISCIPLINARY ACTION: LICENSE REVOCATION
OFFENSE: FAILURE TO COMPLY WITH PREVIOUS BOARD ORDER

NOTES: VIOLATION OF CONDITIONS OF LIMITATION IMPOSED ON LICENSE BY 12/5/96 CONSENT AGREEMENT DUE TO A CHEMICAL DEPENDENCY RELAPSE. PERMANENT REVOCATION. NOTICE OF APPEAL OF BOARD'S 3/11/98 PERMANENT REVOCATION ORDER FILED WITH FRANKLIN COUNTY COURT OF COMMON PLEAS ON 3/17/98. ON 9/2/98 THE COURT AFFIRMED THE BOARD'S ORDER.

THOMAS-MCCAULEY, TINA MARIE MD, DATE OF BIRTH DECEMBER 26, 1962 OF 2101 N E 20TH, OKLAHOMA CITY, OK, WAS DISCIPLINED BY MEDICARE ON JULY 20, 1999
DISCIPLINARY ACTION: EXCLUSION FROM THE MEDICARE AND/OR MEDICAID PROGRAM
OFFENSE: DISCIPLINARY ACTION BY ANOTHER STATE OR AGENCY

NOTES: LICENSE REVOKED, SUSPENDED, SURRENDERED OR OTHERWISE LOST FOR REASONS BEARING ON PROFESSIONAL PERFORMANCE, PROFESSIONAL COMPETENCE OR FINANCIAL INTEGRITY.

THOMPSON, BOB DO OF 403 N TIMMONS, SEMINOLE, OK, WAS DISCIPLINED BY DEA ON JULY 13, 1999
DISCIPLINARY ACTION: SURRENDER OF CONTROLLED SUBSTANCE LICENSE
OFFENSE: DISCIPLINARY ACTION BY ANOTHER STATE OR AGENCY

NOTES: STATE BOARD.

THOMPSON, BOB J DO, LICENSE NUMBER 2030, WAS DISCIPLINED BY OKLAHOMA ON DECEMBER 12, 1996
DISCIPLINARY ACTION: 36-MONTH PROBATION

THOMPSON, BOB J DO, LICENSE NUMBER 2030, WAS DISCIPLINED BY OKLAHOMA ON JUNE 18, 1998
DISCIPLINARY ACTION: SURRENDER OF LICENSE

THOMPSON, BOB J DO, LICENSE NUMBER 2030, WAS DISCIPLINED BY OKLAHOMA ON SEPTEMBER 23, 1999
DISCIPLINARY ACTION: LICENSE REINSTATEMENT; 60-MONTH PROBATION

THOMPSON, SHANNON PAUL MD, LICENSE NUMBER 0019506 OF 24902 BUENA VISTA CIRCLE, BROKEN ARROW, OK, WAS DISCIPLINED BY OKLAHOMA ON DECEMBER 26, 1996
DISCIPLINARY ACTION: EMERGENCY SUSPENSION
OFFENSE: LOSS OR RESTRICTION OF HOSPITAL PRIVILEGES

NOTES: ON 11/13/96 WAS SUMMARILY TERMINATED AS A RESIDENT IN TRAINING WITH THE OKLAHOMA COLLEGE OF MEDICINE FOR ABANDONMENT OF POSITION WITH SUSPECTED SUBSTANCE ABUSE.

THOMPSON, SHANNON PAUL MD, LICENSE NUMBER 19506 OF

24902 BUENA VISTA CIRCLE, BROKEN ARROW, OK, WAS DISCIPLINED BY OKLAHOMA ON JANUARY 17, 1997
DISCIPLINARY ACTION: LICENSE REVOCATION

NOTES: HE WAS DECLARED PHYSICALLY OR MENTALLY UNABLE TO PRACTICE MEDICINE AND SURGERY WITH REASONABLE SKILL AND SAFETY; GUILTY OF PRACTICE OR OTHER BEHAVIOR THAT DEMONSTRATES AN INCAPACITY OR INCOMPETENCE TO PRACTICE MEDICINE AND SURGERY; AND THE INABILITY TO PRACTICE MEDICINE AND SURGERY WITH REASONABLE SKILL AND SAFETY TO PATIENTS BY REASON OF AGE, ILLNESS, DRUNKENNESS, EXCESSIVE USE OF DRUGS, NARCOTICS, CHEMICALS, OR ANY OTHER TYPE OF MATERIAL OR AS A RESULT OF ANY MENTAL OR PHYSICAL CONDITION.

TILLER, GEORGE RICHARD OF 5101 EAST KELLOGG, WICHITA, KS, WAS DISCIPLINED BY OKLAHOMA ON MAY 24, 1990
DISCIPLINARY ACTION: 60-MONTH PROBATION; RESTRICTION PLACED ON CONTROLLED SUBSTANCE LICENSE
OFFENSE: DISCIPLINARY ACTION BY ANOTHER STATE OR AGENCY

NOTES: LICENSE GRANTED. HE WAS PLACED ON PROBATION IN KANSAS FROM 2/84 UNTIL 4/86 FOR DRUG ABUSE AND ALCOHOLISM. COLORADO PLACED HIM ON PROBATION IN 5/89, BASED ON THE KANSAS ACTION. HE COMPLETED LONG TERM REHABILITATION IN GEORGIA, FROM 1/84 UNTIL 7/84, PLUS 20 MONTHS AFTERCARE TREATMENT. HE HAS BEEN RELEASED FROM THE KANSAS PROBATION AND HAS AN UNRESTRICTED KANSAS LICENSE. PROBATION BEGINNING 3/26/90 UNDER THE FOLLOWING TERMS AND CONDITIONS: SHALL NOT PRESCRIBE, ADMINISTER, OR DISPENSE ANY MEDICATIONS FOR HIS PERSONAL USE AND SHALL TAKE NONE UNLESS AUTHORIZED BY ANOTHER PHYSICIAN FOR LEGITIMATE MEDICAL NEED; SHALL ABSTAIN FROM CONSUMING ALCOHOL, OR ANY SUBSTANCE WHICH WOULD ADVERSELY AFFECT HIS ABILITY TO PRACTICE; SHALL SUBMIT BIOLOGICAL FLUID SPECIMENS; MAY PRESCRIBE CONTROLLED DANGEROUS SUBSTANCES ONLY ON SERIALLY-NUMBERED, DUPLICATE PRESCRIPTION PADS AND SHALL MAKE THE COPIES AVAILABLE TO THE BOARD UPON REQUEST; SHALL SUBMIT TO THE BOARD ADDRESS/CHANGE OF ADDRESS; SHALL APPEAR BEFORE THE BOARD UPON REQUEST AND SUBMIT ANY REQUIRED REPORTS; SHALL PAY COSTS; SHALL NOTIFY ANY HOSPITAL WHERE HE HOLDS STAFF PRIVILEGES, OR CLINIC, OR GROUP WHERE HE PRACTICES, OF THE TERMS AND CONDITIONS OF THIS VOLUNTARY SUBMITTAL TO JURISDICTION AND SUPPLY A COPY THEREOF.

TORRES, WILSON MD, LICENSE NUMBER 0016775, WAS DISCIPLINED BY OKLAHOMA ON JANUARY 27, 1995
DISCIPLINARY ACTION: LICENSE REVOCATION
OFFENSE: CRIMINAL CONVICTION OR PLEA OF GUILTY, NOLO CONTENDERE, OR NO CONTEST TO A CRIME

NOTES: ON 3/16/94 WAS CONVICTED BY MILITARY COURT MARTIAL OF NUMEROUS CHARGES OF INDECENT ACTS RELATED TO HIS PRACTICE OF MEDICINE IN THE MILITARY. HE SHALL PAY COSTS.

TRAMMELL, STEPHEN BRUCE DO, LICENSE NUMBER 0003321, WAS DISCIPLINED BY OKLAHOMA ON SEPTEMBER 21, 1995
DISCIPLINARY ACTION: 36-MONTH PROBATION; MONITORING OF PHYSICIAN PERFORMANCE

NOTES: CONDITIONS OF PROBATION: SHALL REGULARLY PARTICIPATE IN AND ATTEND NARCOTICS/ALCOHOLICS ANONYMOUS SESSIONS AND CAUSE WRITTEN DOCUMENTATION EVIDENCING HIS PARTICIPATION AND ATTENDANCE TO THE BOARD EVERY SIX MONTHS; SHALL REGULARLY PARTICIPATE IN AND ATTEND SESSIONS OF THE OKLAHOMA PHYSICIANS RECOVERY PROGRAM AND CAUSE WRITTEN DOCUMENTATION EVIDENCING HIS PARTICIPATION AND ATTENDANCE TO THE BOARD EVERY SIX MONTHS; SHALL RECEIVE UNANNOUNCED VISITS FROM THE BOARD; SHALL FURNISH BIOLOGICAL FLUID SPECIMENS UPON BOARD REQUEST; SHALL NOTIFY THE BOARD IN WRITING OF ANY CHANGE IN ADDRESS WITHIN 14 DAYS; TERMS OF RESIDENCE OR PRACTICE OUTSIDE OF OKLAHOMA WILL TOLL THE EXPIRATION OF THE PROBATIONARY PERIOD, EXTENDING THE PERIOD BEYOND THREE YEARS FROM THIS DATE.

TRENT, DAVID LEE MD, LICENSE NUMBER 0010794, WAS DISCIPLINED BY OKLAHOMA ON JANUARY 15, 1993
DISCIPLINARY ACTION: 60-MONTH PROBATION; RESTRICTION PLACED ON LICENSE
OFFENSE: OVERPRESCRIBING OR MISPRESCRIBING DRUGS

NOTES: ALLEGED THAT IN 1/92 HE ISSUED TWO PRESCRIPTIONS FOR CONTROLLED DANGEROUS SUBSTANCES TO A DEA UNDERCOVER AGENT WITHOUT KEEPING REQUIRED RECORDS AND WITHOUT SUFFICIENT EXAMINATION AND ESTABLISHMENT OF A VALID PHYSICIAN/PATIENT RELATIONSHIP; DURING 1991 AND 1992 HE PRESCRIBED, ADMINISTERED AND DISPENSED CONTROLLED DANGEROUS SUBSTANCES TO ADDITIONAL PATIENTS WITHOUT SUFFICIENT EXAMS AND ESTABLISHMENT OF A VALID PHYSICIAN/PATIENT RELATIONSHIP AND WITHOUT MEDICAL NEED. PROBATION TO BEGIN 1/8/93. CONDITIONS OF PROBATION: MAY PRESCRIBE CONTROLLED DANGEROUS SUBSTANCES ONLY ON SERIALLY-NUMBERED, DUPLICATE PRESCRIPTION PADS COPIES OF WHICH SHALL BE AVAILABLE FOR INSPECTION; SHALL NOT PRESCRIBE, ADMINISTER OR DISPENSE ANY MEDICATION FOR HIMSELF OR ANY FAMILY MEMBER; SHALL MEET QUARTERLY WITH BOARD TO REVIEW MEDICAL CHARTS; SHALL INITIATE AND CONTINUE REGULAR COUNSELING WITH BOARD APPROVED PHYSICIAN; SHALL COMPLETE 50 HOURS OF CONTINUING MEDICAL EDUCATION ON PHARMACOLOGY AND RELATED ISSUES 2O OF WHICH SHALL BE COMPLETED WITHIN ONE YEAR; SHALL NOT ALLOW INITIATION OF ANY THERAPEUTIC REGIMEN BY ANY PERSONNEL UNDER HIS SUPERVISION UNLESS HE IS IN THE IMMEDIATE GEOGRAPHIC VICINITY; SHALL NOT SUPERVISE A PHYSICIAN'S ASSISTANT; SHALL FURNISH THE BOARD WITH ADDRESS/CHANGE OF ADDRESS; SHALL APPEAR BEFORE BOARD UPON REQUEST AND SUBMIT REQUIRED REPORTS; SHALL PAY COSTS; SHALL PROVIDE EVERY STATE WHERE HE HOLDS LICENSURE OR APPLIES FOR LICENSURE AND ANY HEALTH CARE ENTITY WHERE HE HOLDS STAFF PRIVILEGES A COPY OF THIS ORDER.

TRENT, DAVID LEE MD, LICENSE NUMBER 0010794, WAS DISCIPLINED BY OKLAHOMA ON JANUARY 25, 1996
DISCIPLINARY ACTION: REPRIMAND
OFFENSE: PRACTICING WITHOUT A VALID CONTROLLED SUBSTANCE LICENSE

NOTES: ON 9/13/93 THE OKLAHOMA BUREAU OF NARCOTICS AND DANGEROUS DRUGS REVOKED HIS REGISTRATION TO PRESCRIBE, ADMINISTER, OR DISPENSE CONTROLLED DANGEROUS SUBSTANCES. A SUBSEQUENT PHARMACY SURVEY DISCLOSED THAT HE DID WRITE OR TELEPHONE IN SEVEN

PRESCRIPTIONS FOR VARIOUS CONTROLLED DANGEROUS SUBSTANCES DURING THE PERIOD OF TIME HE HAD NO LAWFUL REGISTRATION. FIVE YEAR PROBATION BEGINNING 1/8/93 REMAINS IN EFFECT UNDER TERMS AND CONDITIONS ISSUED.

TRINH, HOANG-LAN THI, WAS DISCIPLINED BY OKLAHOMA ON JULY 22, 1994
DISCIPLINARY ACTION: DENIAL OF NEW LICENSE
OFFENSE: LOSS OR RESTRICTION OF HOSPITAL PRIVILEGES

NOTES: SHE WAS "NOT CONTINUED" IN A FAMILY PRACTICE RESIDENCY BECAUSE OF ACADEMIC REASONS AND WAS REQUIRED TO REPEAT THE PROGRAM; AFTER 18 MONTHS SHE WAS APPROVED AS HAVING COMPLETED FIRST YEAR TRAINING BUT CONTRACT WAS NOT RENEWED; RAISES SERIOUS ISSUES AS TO ABILITY TO PRACTICE.

TROMBKA, LAWRENCE H MD, DATE OF BIRTH JANUARY 24, 1958 OF 10109 SOUTH 72ND EAST AVE, TULSA, OK, WAS DISCIPLINED BY MEDICARE ON FEBRUARY 10, 1992
DISCIPLINARY ACTION: 120-MONTH EXCLUSION FROM THE MEDICARE AND/OR MEDICAID PROGRAM
OFFENSE: CRIMINAL CONVICTION OR PLEA OF GUILTY, NOLO CONTENDERE, OR NO CONTEST TO A CRIME

NOTES: PROGRAM-RELATED CONVICTION.

TROMBKA, LAWRENCE H MD, DATE OF BIRTH JANUARY 24, 1958, LICENSE NUMBER 0025750 OF 10109 S 72ND AVENUE, TULSA, OK, WAS DISCIPLINED BY IOWA ON NOVEMBER 19, 1992
DISCIPLINARY ACTION: PROBATION
OFFENSE: DISCIPLINARY ACTION BY ANOTHER STATE OR AGENCY

NOTES: ACTION TAKEN IN OKLAHOMA. PROBATIONS TO RUN CONCURRENTLY. ON 8/26/97 REQUEST TO REMOVE PROBATION AND RESTRICTIONS PLACED UPON HIS LICENSE GRANTED.

TROMBKA, LAWRENCE HENRY MD, LICENSE NUMBER 0016300 OF 10109 S 72ND E AVE, TULSA, OK, WAS DISCIPLINED BY OKLAHOMA ON NOVEMBER 4, 1991
DISCIPLINARY ACTION: 6-MONTH LICENSE SUSPENSION; 60-MONTH PROBATION
OFFENSE: CRIMINAL CONVICTION OR PLEA OF GUILTY, NOLO CONTENDERE, OR NO CONTEST TO A CRIME

NOTES: ON 8/2/91 FOUND GUILTY OF THE FELONY CRIME OF MEDICAID FRAUD; RECEIVED THREE YEAR SUSPENDED SENTENCE, $15,000 FINE, $10,000 REIMBURSEMENT TO VICTIM'S COMPENSATION FUND, $75,000 RESTITUTION. SUSPENSION MODIFIED 3/5/92 TO ALLOW HIM TO PRACTICE MEDICINE WITHOUT REMUNERATION AT THE BEHAVIOR HEALTH UNIT, MUSKOGEE REGIONAL MEDICAL CENTER. IN ALL OTHER RESPECTS, SUSPENSION REMAINS IN FULL FORCE AND EFFECT. PROBATION WITH FOLLOWING CONDITIONS: PROVIDE PROOF OF PERFORMANCE OF AT LEAST 100 HOURS OF UNPAID COMMUNITY SERVICE EVERY THREE MONTHS; SHALL NOTIFY ANY HOSPITAL WHERE HE HOLDS STAFF PRIVILEGES OR CLINIC OR GROUP WHERE HE PRACTICES OF THE TERMS AND CONDITIONS; SHALL FURNISH BOARD WITH ADDRESS AND/OR CHANGE OF ADDRESS; SHALL APPEAR BEFORE BOARD UPON REQUEST.

TULEY, BARBARA K MD, DATE OF BIRTH JANUARY 25, 1959 OF 307 NORTH MONTE VISTA STREET, ADA, OK, WAS DISCIPLINED BY MEDICARE ON JULY 20, 1998
DISCIPLINARY ACTION: EXCLUSION FROM THE MEDICARE AND/OR MEDICAID PROGRAM
OFFENSE: NONCOMPLIANCE WITH A PROFESSIONAL RULE

NOTES: DEFAULTED ON PUBLIC HEALTH SERVICE EDUCATION LOAN. REINSTATED ON 8/6/98.

TURLEY, LOREN M DO, LICENSE NUMBER 0002638, WAS DISCIPLINED BY ARIZONA ON SEPTEMBER 14, 1992
DISCIPLINARY ACTION: LICENSE SUSPENSION; MONITORING OF PHYSICIAN PERFORMANCE
OFFENSE: PROFESSIONAL MISCONDUCT

NOTES: ON 9/10/92 ADMITTED TO THE BOARD THAT HE HAD SELF-MEDICATED WITH CONTROLLED AND/OR PRESCRIPTION ONLY MEDICATIONS (FLEXERIL) ON ONE OR MORE OCCASIONS PRIOR TO THAT DATE WHILE NOT UNDER THE CARE AND TREATMENT OF A PHYSICIAN AND NOT PRESCRIBED AS PART OF A RECOGNIZED COURSE OF TREATMENT. SHALL UNDERGO AN IN-PATIENT EVALUATION PROGRAM FOR SUSPECTED ALCOHOL AND SUBSTANCE ABUSE AND CHEMICAL DEPENDENCE FOR NOT LESS THAN FIVE DAYS; SHALL AUTHORIZE TREATING PERSONNEL AT THE IN-PATIENT EVALUATION PROGRAM TO RELEASE TO THE BOARD FINDINGS OF HIS EVALUATION AND ANY NECESSARY RECOMMENDATIONS FOR TREATMENT; SHALL MEET WITH THE BOARD FOLLOWING THE COMPLETION OF THE EVALUATION PROGRAM TO DETERMINE WHETHER OR NOT ANY ADDITIONAL ACTIONS ARE REQUIRED; SHALL USE NO CONTROLLED SUBSTANCES OR PRESCRIPTION-ONLY MEDICATIONS UNLESS PRESCRIBED BY HIS ATTENDING PHYSICIAN; SHALL REFRAIN FROM THE USE OF ALCOHOL.

TURLEY, LOREN M DO, LICENSE NUMBER 0002638, WAS DISCIPLINED BY ARIZONA ON SEPTEMBER 19, 1992
DISCIPLINARY ACTION: PROBATION; RESTRICTION PLACED ON LICENSE
OFFENSE: PROFESSIONAL MISCONDUCT

NOTES: SUBMITTED DOCUMENTATION OF COMPLIANCE WITH TERMS OF 9/14/92 ORDER. REINSTATED WITH MINIMUM THREE YEAR PROBATION UNDER TERMS AND CONDITIONS: SHALL COMPLETE AN INTENSIVE OUTPATIENT CHEMICAL DEPENDENCE PROGRAM; SHALL SECURE AND MAINTAIN A SPONSOR FOR 12 STEP RECOVERY PROGRAM; SHALL ATTEND AT LEAST FOUR 12 STEP MEETINGS PER WEEK FOR THE FIRST 12 MONTHS; SHALL MEET REGULARLY WITH HIS ATTENDING PHYSICIAN; SHALL ATTEND NO LESS THAN THREE GROUP THERAPY MEETINGS PER MONTH WITH A BOARD APPROVED COUNSELOR; SHALL SUBMIT TO RANDOM BODY FLUID TESTING UPON BOARD REQUEST; SHALL MEET WITH THE BOARD REGULARLY UPON REQUEST; SHALL USE NO CONTROLLED SUBSTANCE OR PRESCRIPTION-ONLY MEDICATION UNLESS PRESCRIBED BY HIS ATTENDING PHYSICIAN; SHALL REFRAIN FROM THE USE OF ALCOHOL; SHALL WORK NO MORE THAN 14 EMERGENCY DEPARTMENT SHIFTS PER MONTH UNLESS AUTHORIZED BY THE BOARD; SHALL AUTHORIZE ALL TREATING PERSONNEL INVOLVED IN HIS CARE TO RELEASE INFORMATION ON HIS PROGRESS AND PROGNOSIS TO THE BOARD UPON REQUEST. ORDER AMENDED ON 1/14/94 ALLOWING HIM TO WORK 17 RATHER THAN 14 EMERGENCY DEPARTMENT SHIFTS PER MONTH. OTHER PROVISIONS REMAIN IN FULL FORCE AND EFFECT.

TURLEY, LOREN M DO, LICENSE NUMBER 0002331 OF 19155 NORTH 94TH PLACE, SCOTTSDALE, AZ, WAS DISCIPLINED BY OKLAHOMA ON MARCH 12, 1993
DISCIPLINARY ACTION: 60-MONTH PROBATION

OFFENSE: DISCIPLINARY ACTION BY ANOTHER STATE OR AGENCY

NOTES: LICENSE SUSPENSION IN ARIZONA ON 9/14/92 WHICH WAS REINSTATED SUBJECT TO TERMS AND CONDITIONS. CONDITIONS OF PROBATION: SHALL REMAIN IN STRICT COMPLIANCE WITH THE ARIZONA ORDER; SHALL APPEAR BEFORE THE BOARD UPON REQUEST AND BEFORE HE REENTERS PRACTICE IN OKLAHOMA.

TURLEY, LOREN M MD, DATE OF BIRTH MARCH 7, 1945, LICENSE NUMBER 0028104 OF SCOTTSDALE, AZ, WAS DISCIPLINED BY COLORADO ON NOVEMBER 19, 1993
DISCIPLINARY ACTION: 60-MONTH PROBATION; MONITORING OF PHYSICIAN PERFORMANCE
OFFENSE: SUBSTANCE ABUSE

NOTES: EXCESSIVE USE OF A CONTROLLED SUBSTANCE AND HABITUAL INTEMPERANCE. PROBATIONARY PERIOD INCLUDES TREATMENT AND PRACTICE MONITORING.

TYSON, JOHN T OF 701 SOLANO SE, ALBUQUERQUE, NM, WAS DISCIPLINED BY OKLAHOMA ON JULY 1, 1993
DISCIPLINARY ACTION: DENIAL OF NEW LICENSE

NOTES: EVIDENCE INDICATES THAT HE HAD BEEN PRESCRIBED VARIOUS ANTIDEPRESSANTS FOR THE PAST 10 YEARS AND ALSO HAD A MALPRACTICE LITIGATION HISTORY; THOSE ELEMENTS RAISED ISSUES AS TO HIS CLINICAL COMPETENCY. EVIDENCE DID NOT SHOW HE HAS THE MENTAL AND PSYCHIATRIC ABILITY TO PRACTICE.

VANCE, RICARDO B MD OF 9209 S DARLINGTON, TULSA, OK, WAS DISCIPLINED BY OKLAHOMA ON JULY 24, 1998
DISCIPLINARY ACTION: DENIAL OF NEW LICENSE
OFFENSE: DISCIPLINARY ACTION BY ANOTHER STATE OR AGENCY

NOTES: LICENSE IN NEW YORK SUSPENDED FOR UNPROFESSIONAL CONDUCT.

VANCE, RICARDO BRUCE MD, LICENSE NUMBER 0156327 OF 1000 GRAND CONCOURSE, BRONX, NY, WAS DISCIPLINED BY NEW YORK ON JANUARY 7, 1994
DISCIPLINARY ACTION: LICENSE SUSPENSION; 24-MONTH PROBATION
OFFENSE: SUBSTANDARD CARE, INCOMPETENCE OR NEGLIGENCE

NOTES: PRACTICED WITH NEGLIGENCE ON MORE THAN ONE OCCASION; ORDERED EXCESSIVE TESTS; FAILED TO MAINTAIN ADEQUATE RECORDS. SUSPENSION PENDING EVALUATION OF MEDICAL SKILLS AND ANY RETRAINING NECESSARY; MAY PRACTICE TO THE EXTENT NECESSARY TO COMPLETE THESE REQUIREMENTS.

VARK, LAWRENCE E DO OF SEMINOLE, OK, WAS DISCIPLINED BY MISSOURI ON JANUARY 28, 1991
DISCIPLINARY ACTION: 60-MONTH PROBATION
OFFENSE: DISCIPLINARY ACTION BY ANOTHER STATE OR AGENCY

NOTES: OTHER STATE LIMITATION OF CONTROLLED SUBSTANCE AUTHORITY; HAS PRESCRIBED, DISPENSED OR ADMINISTERED DRUGS TO PERSONS WITH WHOM HE DID NOT HAVE A PHYSICIAN/PATIENT RELATIONSHIP AND HAS FAILED TO MAINTAIN PROPER INVENTORIES AND RECORDS OF CONTROLLED SUBSTANCES THAT HE HAS PRESCRIBED, DISPENSED, OR ADMINISTERED.

VARK, LAWRENCE EDWARD DO, LICENSE NUMBER 0002932 OF 1807 NEVA, SEMINOLE, OK, WAS DISCIPLINED BY OKLAHOMA ON DECEMBER 13, 1990
DISCIPLINARY ACTION: 60-MONTH PROBATION; RESTRICTION PLACED ON CONTROLLED SUBSTANCE LICENSE

NOTES: THE MISSOURI BUREAU OF NARCOTICS AND DANGEROUS DRUGS' ORDER OF 7/19/90 IS INCORPORATED INTO THIS ORDER. SHALL PRESCRIBE NO ANORECTIC DRUGS; SHALL APPEAR BEFORE THE BOARD UPON REQUEST; SHALL RECEIVE UNANNOUNCED VISITS FROM THE BOARD AT ANY TIME; SHALL PROVIDE BIOLOGICAL FLUID SPECIMENS FOR LABORATORY ANALYSIS UPON REQUEST; SHALL TREAT STADOL AND NUBAIN AS IF THEY WERE CONTROLLED SUBSTANCES; IF GRANTED AUTHORITY BY OKLAHOMA BUREAU OF NARCOTICS AND DANGEROUS DRUGS TO PRESCRIBE CONTROLLED DANGEROUS SUBSTANCES SHALL MAINTAIN A LOG OF SUCH SUBSTANCES; TERMS OF RESIDENCE OR PRACTICE OUTSIDE OF OKLAHOMA WILL RESULT IN THE TOLLING OF THIS ORDER AND NOT APPLY TO THE REDUCTION OF THIS PROBATIONARY PERIOD. ON 4/02/96 ALL RESTRICTIONS ON LICENSE REMOVED.

VEINTIMILLA, JAMES E MD, DATE OF BIRTH FEBRUARY 8, 1927, LICENSE NUMBER 0024804 OF 122 SOUTH THIRD STREET, MUSKOGEE, OK, WAS DISCIPLINED BY NEW JERSEY ON MAY 4, 1990
DISCIPLINARY ACTION: SURRENDER OF LICENSE
OFFENSE: SUBSTANDARD CARE, INCOMPETENCE OR NEGLIGENCE

NOTES: PROFESSIONAL MISCONDUCT, GROSS NEGLIGENCE/MALPRACTICE/INCOMPETENCE, AND INABILITY TO DISCHARGE FUNCTIONS OF A LICENSEE IN A MANNER CONSISTENT WITH THE PUBLIC'S HEALTH, SAFETY, AND WELFARE. PRECLUDED FROM APPLYING FOR LICENSE REINSTATEMENT.

VEINTIMILLA, JAMES E MD, LICENSE NUMBER 0015576 OF 403 SOUTH BROADWAY, COALGATE, OK, WAS DISCIPLINED BY OKLAHOMA ON JUNE 21, 1990
DISCIPLINARY ACTION: LICENSE REVOCATION
OFFENSE: CRIMINAL CONVICTION OR PLEA OF GUILTY, NOLO CONTENDERE, OR NO CONTEST TO A CRIME

NOTES: ON 2/17/90 PLED GUILTY TO VIOLATION OF FEDERAL ANTI-NARCOTICS LAWS TO INCLUDE: WILLFULLY CONSPIRING TO UNLAWFULLY POSSESS WITH INTENT TO DISTRIBUTE WITHOUT LEGITIMATE MEDICAL PURPOSE CERTAIN CONTROLLED DANGEROUS SUBSTANCES INCLUDING PRELUDIN, MEPERGAN, FORTIS AND DILAUDID; WILLFULLY AND UNLAWFULLY DISTRIBUTING PRELUDIN AND DILAUDID TO AN OKLAHOMA BUREAU OF NARCOTICS AND DANGEROUS DRUGS OFFICER BY DELIVERING A PRESCRIPTION TO HER NOT IN THE USUAL COURSE OF PROFESSIONAL PRACTICE AND WAS NOT FOR A LEGITIMATE MEDICAL NEED. SENTENCED TO 16 MONTHS FEDERAL PRISON TO BE FOLLOWED WITH A FIVE YEAR SUPERVISED PROBATION.

VENTIMILLA, JAMES EFRAIN DR OF 403 S BROADWAY, COALGATE, OK, WAS DISCIPLINED BY DEA
DISCIPLINARY ACTION: SURRENDER OF CONTROLLED SUBSTANCE LICENSE
OFFENSE: CRIMINAL CONVICTION OR PLEA OF GUILTY, NOLO CONTENDERE, OR NO CONTEST TO A CRIME

NOTES: PLED GUILTY 02/27/90 TO CONSPIRACY TO POSSESS WITH INTENT TO DISTRIBUTE AND DISTRIBUTION OF CONTROLLED SUBSTANCES WITHOUT LEGITIMATE MEDICAL PURPOSE AND NOT IN THE USUAL COURSE OF PROFESSIONAL MEDICAL PRACTICE, DELIVERY OF PRELUDIN AND DELIVERY OF DILAUDID. SENTENCED TO ONE YEAR 4 MONTHS PRISON, FIVE YEARS SUPERVISED RELEASE AND FINE OF $150.

VINSON, BILLY MICHAEL MD, LICENSE NUMBER 0012367 OF 1322 A AVE, PRAGUE, OK, WAS DISCIPLINED BY OKLAHOMA ON MARCH 5, 1992
DISCIPLINARY ACTION: EMERGENCY SUSPENSION
OFFENSE: SUBSTANCE ABUSE

NOTES: ON 2/13/92 ADMITTED TAKING DESYREL SINCE 1980 OR 1981 AND ALSO, A FEW YEARS LATER, BEGAN TAKING LITHIUM AND WAS IN FACT TAKING BOTH MEDICATIONS PRESENTLY ON A PROGRAM OF SELF-ADMINISTRATION, WITHOUT A TREATING PHYSICIAN; APPEARED IMPAIRED OR LETHARGIC ON A COUPLE OF OCCASIONS; PRESCRIBED CERTAIN SCHEDULED DRUGS WITH NO RECORDS. SUSPENSION REMAINS IN FULL FORCE AND EFFECT UNTIL HE PRESENTS EVIDENCE OF PSYCHIATRIC EVALUATION AND TREATMENT BY A PSYCHIATRIST MUTUALLY ACCEPTABLE TO THE BOARD AND HIMSELF. ORDER OF 07/09/92, ACKNOWLEDGES HIS SURRENDER OF LICENSURE BY REMOVING HIS WALLET IDENTIFICATION CARD AND THROWING IT ON THE FLOOR IN FRONT OF THE BOARD MEMBERS.

VINSON, BILLY MICHAEL MD, LICENSE NUMBER 0012367 OF GENERAL DELIVERY, TISHOMINGO, OK, WAS DISCIPLINED BY OKLAHOMA ON SEPTEMBER 12, 1992
DISCIPLINARY ACTION: 60-MONTH PROBATION; RESTRICTION PLACED ON LICENSE

NOTES: MET CONDITIONS OF PREVIOUS SUSPENSION BY UNDERGOING A COMPREHENSIVE ADDICTIVE DISEASE AND PSYCHIATRIC ASSESSMENT. PROBATION WITH FOLLOWING CONDITIONS: MAY PRESCRIBE CONTROLLED DANGEROUS SUBSTANCES ONLY ON SERIALLY-NUMBERED, DUPLICATE PRESCRIPTION PADS AND SHALL MAKE COPIES AVAILABLE TO THE BOARD; SHALL ABSTAIN FROM CONSUMING ALCOHOL OR ANY SUBSTANCE WHICH WOULD ADVERSELY AFFECT HIS ABILITY TO PRACTICE; SHALL SUBMIT BIOLOGICAL FLUID SPECIMENS FOR ANALYSIS; SHALL NOT PRESCRIBE, ADMINISTER OR DISPENSE ANY MEDICATIONS FOR HIS PERSONAL USE AND WILL TAKE NO MEDICATION EXCEPT THAT WHICH IS AUTHORIZED BY A PHYSICIAN TREATING HIM FOR A LEGITIMATE MEDICAL NEED; SHALL NOTIFY ANY HOSPITAL WHERE HE HOLDS STAFF PRIVILEGES OR CLINIC OR GROUP OF TERMS AND CONDITIONS; SHALL CONTINUE UNDER PSYCHIATRIC CARE WITH REPORTS TO THE BOARD; SHALL NOT SUPERVISE A PHYSICIAN ASSISTANT; SHALL FURNISH BOARD WITH ADDRESS AND/OR CHANGE OF ADDRESS; SHALL APPEAR BEFORE BOARD UPON REQUEST. ON 7/22/94 HIS REQUEST TO VACATE THIS ORDER DENIED. ON 7/31/95 HIS RECORDS MODIFIED TO SHOW HIS NAME AS BILLY MICHAEL PERSHICA; ALL OTHER TERMS AND CONDITIONS REMAIN IN EFFECT WITH THE EXCEPTION THAT THE SUBMITTING OF BIOLOGICAL FLUID SPECIMENS IS ELIMINATED.

VINSON, BILLY MICHAEL MD, LICENSE NUMBER 12367, WAS DISCIPLINED BY OKLAHOMA ON MAY 14, 1999
DISCIPLINARY ACTION: LICENSE SUSPENSION
OFFENSE: PRACTICING WITHOUT A VALID CONTROLLED SUBSTANCE LICENSE

NOTES: ALSO KNOWN AS BILLY MICHAEL PERSHICA; ON 5/29/97 FAILED TO FURNISH INFORMATION REQUESTED BY THE BOARD; FAILED TO COOPERATE WITH A LAWFUL INVESTIGATION CONDUCTED BY THE BOARD; VIOLATED PROVISIONS OF 9/12/92 BOARD ORDER; FAILED TO PAY ALL OUTSTANDING COSTS ASSESSED AGAINST HIM AS ORDERED BY THE BOARD: AS OF 11/98 OWED THE BOARD $6,833.49; ON OR ABOUT 3/21/98 FORCED HIS WAY INTO HIS ESTRANGED WIFE'S HOME, ARMED WITH A SHOTGUN AND A SEMIAUTOMATIC PISTOL; WHEN CONFRONTED BY A SHERIFF'S DEPUTY, HE RAN OUT OF THE HOUSE STILL ARMED WITH BOTH GUNS AND THREATENED TO SHOOT THE DEPUTY'S CAR; AFTER HE POINTED THE SHOTGUN AT THE DEPUTY, THE DEPUTY SHOT AND WOUNDED HIM; CONTINUED TO PRESCRIBE CONTROLLED DANGEROUS SUBSTANCES TO OVER 200 DIFFERENT PATIENTS EVEN THOUGH IN 11/96 HIS OKLAHOMA STATE BUREAU OF NARCOTICS AND DANGEROUS DRUGS REGISTRATION HAD LAPSED. LICENSE INDEFINITELY SUSPENDED PENDING COMPLETION OF THE FOLLOWING: PAYMENT OF ALL FEES TO THE BOARD; A FULL PSYCHIATRIC EXAMINATION AND TREATMENT COORDINATED THROUGH AND APPROVED BY THE BOARD. ANY REINSTATEMENT WILL BE CONTINGENT UPON HIS OBTAINING A JOB OFFER IN A STRUCTURED, CONTROLLED, SUPERVISED, NON-SOLO ENVIRONMENT; SHALL PAY COSTS.

VINSON, BILLY MICHAEL MD, LICENSE NUMBER 12367, WAS DISCIPLINED BY OKLAHOMA ON JULY 29, 1999
DISCIPLINARY ACTION: PROBATION; RESTRICTION PLACED ON LICENSE

NOTES: ALSO KNOWN AS BILLY MICHAEL PERSHICA. LICENSE REINSTATED ON CONDITIONS: SHALL NOT PRESCRIBE, ADMINISTER, DISPENSE OR POSSESS ANY DRUGS IN SCHEDULES I-V; SHALL NOT APPLY FOR STATE AND FEDERAL REGISTRATION OF CONTROLLED DANGEROUS SUBSTANCES UNTIL THE TERM OF HIS PROBATION HAS EXPIRED UNLESS AUTHORIZED TO DO SO BY THE BOARD; SHALL NOT PRESCRIBE, ADMINISTER OR DISPENSE ANY MEDICATIONS FOR HIS PERSONAL USE AND SHALL TAKE NONE UNLESS AUTHORIZED BY ANOTHER PHYSICIAN FOR A LEGITIMATE MEDICAL NEED; SHALL REQUEST ALL HEALTH CARE FACILITIES IN WHICH HE ANTICIPATES PRACTICING TO FURNISH A STATEMENT REGARDING MONITORING OF HIS PRACTICE; SHALL CONTINUE PSYCHIATRIC TREATMENT WITH QUARTERLY REPORTS TO THE BOARD; SHALL PRACTICE IN A STRUCTURED, CONTROLLED, SUPERVISED, NON-SOLO ENVIRONMENT APPROVED IN ADVANCE BY THE BOARD; SHALL EXECUTE ALL RELEASES OF MEDICAL AND PSYCHIATRIC RECORDS AS NECESSARY TO DISCUSS HIS CASE WITH HIS TREATING PHYSICIANS AND/OR ANY PHYSICIANS HOLDING RECORDS; SHALL SUBMIT TO EVERY STATE IN WHICH HE HOLDS LICENSURE AND TO HOSPITALS, CLINICS OR OTHER INSTITUTIONS IN WHICH HE HOLDS OR ANTICIPATES HOLDING ANY FORM OF STAFF PRIVILEGE A COPY OF THIS ORDER; SHALL NOT SUPERVISE ALLIED HEALTH PROFESSIONALS; SHALL KEEP THE BOARD INFORMED OF HIS ADDRESS AND WILL SUBMIT ANY REQUIRED REPORTS AND FORMS ON A TIMELY AND PROMPT BASIS; SHALL APPEAR BEFORE THE BOARD UPON REQUEST AND PAY COSTS

WAJSBORT, RICHARD RANI MD, LICENSE NUMBER 0019240 OF 3716 NW EXPRESSWAY #315, OKLAHOMA CITY, OK, WAS DISCIPLINED BY OKLAHOMA ON APRIL 18, 1996
DISCIPLINARY ACTION: LICENSE REVOCATION
OFFENSE: FAILURE TO COMPLY WITH PREVIOUS BOARD ORDER

NOTES: FAILURE TO SEEK OUT A PERSONAL PHYSICIAN, REFUSAL TO PROVIDE A URINE SPECIMEN UPON REPEATED REQUESTS AND SUBSEQUENT POSITIVE TEST FOR COCAINE IN JANUARY 1996 CONSTITUTES VIOLATION OF THE TERMS OF 12/5/94 PROBATION.

WALKER, DENNIS LYNN MD, LICENSE NUMBER 0012236 OF 427 EAST CHEROKEE AVENUE, ENID, OK, WAS DISCIPLINED BY OKLAHOMA ON JULY 31, 1995
DISCIPLINARY ACTION: RESTRICTION PLACED ON LICENSE

NOTES: AN EMERGENCY HEARING ON 5/19/95 ORDERED HIM TO: CEASE PERFORMING ANY SURGICAL PROCEDURE; ALLOWED HIM TO ORDER INJECTIONS SO LONG AS ANOTHER QUALIFIED AND TRAINED PERSON PERFORMED THE INJECTION; SHALL SUBMIT HIMSELF TO COMPLETE MEDICAL EXAMINATION AND EVALUATION TO A BOARD APPROVED NEUROLOGIST TO DETERMINE HIS ABILITY TO PRACTICE MEDICINE AND SURGERY WITH REASONABLE SKILL AND SAFETY. HE VOLUNTARILY AGREED THAT EFFECTIVE 9/30/95 HE WOULD PERMANENTLY RETIRE FROM THE PRACTICE OF MEDICINE AND SURGERY IN ANY CAPACITY IN OKLAHOMA, AND EFFECTIVE 10/01/95 HE WOULD ACCEPT THE STATUS OF PHYSICIAN EMERITUS.

WALKER, JAMES C MD, LICENSE NUMBER 0008186 OF 3601 E 70TH, TULSA, OK, WAS DISCIPLINED BY OKLAHOMA ON FEBRUARY 8, 1990
DISCIPLINARY ACTION: 60-MONTH LICENSE SUSPENSION; REQUIRED TO ENTER AN IMPAIRED PHYSICIAN PROGRAM OR SUBSTANCE ABUSE TREATMENT
OFFENSE: FAILURE TO COMPLY WITH PREVIOUS BOARD ORDER

NOTES: ON 1/23/88 HE WAS PLACED ON FIVE YEAR PROBATION OF WHICH HE VIOLATED SEVERAL OF THE TERMS AND CONDITIONS. ON 10/27/89 A ROUTINE FLUID SAMPLE TESTED POSITIVE FOR BARBITURATES. HE STATED THAT IT WAS NOT PRESCRIBED BUT TAKEN FROM SAMPLES STORED AT HIS HOME. ON 12/06/89 HE ADMITTED TO TAKING PARAFON FORTE EVERY SIX HOURS FOR ABOUT FOUR DAYS WITHOUT ANY PRESCRIPTION. ON 12/06/89 HE REFUSED A ROUTINE REQUEST BY A BOARD AGENT FOR FLUID SAMPLES. ABOUT 12/22/89 HE ENTERED AN INPATIENT TREATMENT PROGRAM AT TALBOT RECOVERY CENTER IN ATLANTA, GEORGIA. SUSPENSION BEGINNING 2/02/90. IN THE EVENT OF SUCCESSFUL COMPLETION OF IN-PATIENT TREATMENT FOR SUBSTANCE ABUSE BEFORE THE FIVE YEAR SUSPENSION HAS ELAPSED, HE MAY APPEAR BEFORE THE BOARD AND SEEK REINSTATEMENT OF HIS LICENSE.

WALKER, JAMES C MD, DATE OF BIRTH JUNE 22, 1932 OF 3233 EAST 31ST STREET, TULSA, OK, WAS DISCIPLINED BY MINNESOTA ON SEPTEMBER 15, 1990
DISCIPLINARY ACTION: LICENSE SUSPENSION
OFFENSE: DISCIPLINARY ACTION BY ANOTHER STATE OR AGENCY

NOTES: SUSPENSION TO PRACTICE IN MINNESOTA UNTIL DR. WALKER PETITIONS BOARD TO REMOVE THE SUSPENSION FOLLOWING THE UNCONDITIONAL REINSTATEMENT OF LICENSE TO PRACTICE MEDICINE IN OKLAHOMA.

WALLOCH, BETSY O MD, LICENSE NUMBER 0008791, WAS DISCIPLINED BY OKLAHOMA ON NOVEMBER 15, 1990
DISCIPLINARY ACTION: 48-MONTH LICENSE SUSPENSION
OFFENSE: FAILURE TO COMPLY WITH PREVIOUS BOARD ORDER

NOTES: NONCOMPLIANCE WITH HER PROBATION STARTED 2/05/89 BY FAILING TO MAKE PAYMENTS FOR THE COST OF INVESTIGATION, PROSECUTION AND PROBATION IN THE AMOUNT OF $21,519.69. RETROACTIVE TO 10/26/90.

WATSON, STEVEN E DO, LICENSE NUMBER 0001983, WAS DISCIPLINED BY OKLAHOMA ON SEPTEMBER 16, 1993
DISCIPLINARY ACTION: 60-MONTH PROBATION; RESTRICTION PLACED ON CONTROLLED SUBSTANCE LICENSE
OFFENSE: SUBSTANCE ABUSE

NOTES: GUILTY OF HABITUAL DRUNKENNESS, OR HABITUAL ADDICTION TO THE USE OF MORPHINE, COCAINE, OR OTHER HABIT-FORMING DRUGS. ABOUT 3/93 VOLUNTARILY ENTERED INTO TALBOT RECOVERY CENTER IN ATLANTA, GEORGIA FOR A CHEMICAL DEPENDENCY PROBLEM. CONDITIONS OF PROBATION: MAY NOT PETITION THE BOARD FOR MODIFICATION FOR ONE YEAR; SHALL CONTINUE TO BE ACTIVELY INVOLVED IN THE OKLAHOMA PHYSICIAN'S RECOVERY PROGRAM (PRP) AND AGREES TO COMPLY WITH ALL THE TERMS AND CONDITIONS OF ANY CONTRACT HE ENTERS INTO WITH THE PRP; SHALL COMPLY STRICTLY WITH ANY AFTERCARE PROGRAM OR PROGRAMS ESTABLISHED BY TALBOT RECOVERY CENTER OR PRP AND MUST ATTEND AND SUCCESSFULLY COMPLETE ANY TREATMENT, COUNSELING, AND THERAPY ESTABLISHED BY THEM; THEY SHALL SUBMIT QUARTERLY REPORTS TO THE BOARD; SHALL SUBMIT TO RANDOM DRUG SCREENING UPON BOARD REQUEST; SHALL USE DUPLICATE, SERIALLY NUMBERED PRESCRIPTIONS FOR CONTROLLED DANGEROUS SUBSTANCES IN SCHEDULES II-V AND WILL SUBMIT, ON A MONTHLY BASIS, A COPY OF EVERY SUCH PRESCRIPTION; SHALL NOTIFY THE BOARD IN WRITING OF ANY CHANGE OF ADDRESS, EMPLOYMENT, EMPLOYMENT TERMINATION OR HOSPITAL PRIVILEGE RESTRICTION AND ANY ADMINISTRATIVE PROCEEDING INITIATED AGAINST HIM BY ANY OTHER STATE OR FEDERAL REGULATORY BODY WITHIN 14 DAYS; SHALL APPEAR BEFORE THE BOARD UPON REQUEST; AGREES TO RANDOM, UNANNOUNCED VISITS FROM THE BOARD AT HIS PLACE OF BUSINESS FOR OBSERVATION AND ACCESS TO ANY APPROPRIATE RECORDS, PROVIDED THAT THESE VISITS DO NOT INTERRUPT HIS MEDICAL SERVICES; PROBATIONARY TIME SHALL NOT INCLUDE ANY PERIODS OF RESIDENCE OR PRACTICE OUTSIDE OF OKLAHOMA; SHALL INFORM THE BOARD IF HE LEAVES OKLAHOMA. $565.00 ADMINISTRATIVE COSTS.

WATSON, STEVEN E DO, LICENSE NUMBER 0001983, WAS DISCIPLINED BY OKLAHOMA ON MARCH 31, 1995
DISCIPLINARY ACTION: REPRIMAND
OFFENSE: FAILURE TO COMPLY WITH PREVIOUS BOARD ORDER

NOTES: NONCOMPLIANCE WITH THE ORDER OF 9/93 BY FAILING TO PROVIDE THE BOARD WITH QUARTERLY REPORTS VERIFYING COMPLIANCE.

WEBB, FLOYD E MD, LICENSE NUMBER 0007217 OF PO BOX 368, TISHOMINGO, OK, WAS DISCIPLINED BY OKLAHOMA ON FEBRUARY 4, 1991
DISCIPLINARY ACTION: 1-MONTH LICENSE SUSPENSION; 60-MONTH PROBATION

NOTES: PROBATION WITH CONDITIONS: SHALL NOT PRESCRIBE, ADMINISTER OR DISPENSE ANY MEDICATIONS FOR PERSONAL USE; SHALL NOT PRESCRIBE, ADMINISTER OR DISPENSE ANY SCHEDULE II DRUGS OR CONTROLLED DANGEROUS SUBSTANCES, EXCEPT FOR HOSPITAL IN-PATIENTS; MAY PRESCRIBE SCHEDULES III, IV OR V CONTROLLED DANGEROUS SUBSTANCES ONLY ON SERIALLY-NUMBERED, DUPLICATE PRESCRIPTION PADS AND SHALL MAKE COPIES AVAILABLE TO THE BOARD; SHALL CONTINUE TO MAINTAIN RECORDS ON CONTROLLED DANGEROUS SUBSTANCES PRESCRIBED, ADMINISTERED AND DISPENSED AND

SHALL REDUCE THESE TOTAL NUMBERS; SHALL NOTIFY ANY HOSPITAL WHERE HE HOLDS STAFF PRIVILEGES OR CLINIC OR GROUP OF TERMS AND CONDITIONS; SHALL FURNISH BOARD WITH ADDRESS AND/OR CHANGE OF ADDRESS; SHALL APPEAR BEFORE BOARD UPON REQUEST.

WELDEN, SHIRLEY J MD, DATE OF BIRTH OCTOBER 28, 1957 OF 2140 SOUTH HARVARD #105, TULSA, OK, WAS DISCIPLINED BY MEDICARE ON AUGUST 26, 1997
DISCIPLINARY ACTION: EXCLUSION FROM THE MEDICARE AND/OR MEDICAID PROGRAM
OFFENSE: NONCOMPLIANCE WITH A PROFESSIONAL RULE

NOTES: DEFAULTED ON PUBLIC HEALTH SERVICE EDUCATION LOAN. REINSTATED ON 10/29/97.

WESTCOTT, ROBERT MICHAEL MD, LICENSE NUMBER 0018951 OF 9100 RED OAK LANE, EDMOND, OK, WAS DISCIPLINED BY OKLAHOMA ON DECEMBER 21, 1995
DISCIPLINARY ACTION: EMERGENCY SUSPENSION
OFFENSE: PROVIDING FALSE INFORMATION TO THE BOARD OR OTHER HEALTH AGENCY

NOTES: IN 5/95 HE SUFFERED FROM ADVANCED CHEMICAL DEPENDENCY AND DEPRESSION AND REQUESTED AND RECEIVED A LEAVE OF ABSENCE FROM THE UNIVERSITY OF OKLAHOMA, HEALTH SCIENCE CENTER, FAMILY PRACTICE RESIDENCY. FROM MAY TO SEPTEMBER 1995 WAS AN IN-PATIENT AT RUSH BEHAVIORAL HEALTH CENTER, DOWNERS GROVE, ILLINOIS. HIS 1995 CHEMICAL DEPENDENCY AND DEPRESSION CONSTITUTE A PATTERN OF PERSONAL SUBSTANCE ABUSE THAT BEGAN IN 1982; ON 5/9/95 HE LIED ABOUT PRESENT CHEMICAL ABUSE ON HIS RENEWAL FORM. ON 1/25/96 EMERGENCY SUSPENSION CONTINUED UNTIL FURTHER NOTICE OF THE BOARD.

WESTCOTT, ROBERT MICHAEL MD, LICENSE NUMBER 18951 OF 212 N CREST ROAD #B, CHATTANOOGA, TN, WAS DISCIPLINED BY OKLAHOMA ON JUNE 19, 1998
DISCIPLINARY ACTION: 60-MONTH PROBATION; RESTRICTION PLACED ON LICENSE
OFFENSE: PROVIDING FALSE INFORMATION TO THE BOARD OR OTHER HEALTH AGENCY

NOTES: ON 12/21/95 LICENSE TO PRACTICE WAS SUSPENDED BY EMERGENCY ORDER OF THE BOARD FOR UNPROFESSIONAL CONDUCT INVOLVING PERSONAL SUBSTANCE ABUSE. HE NOW SEEKS REINSTATEMENT OF HIS LICENSE IN ANTICIPATION OF STARTING A RESIDENCY PROGRAM IN TENNESSEE. HE HAS A HISTORY OF PERSONAL SUBSTANCE ABUSE WHICH BEGAN IN APPROXIMATELY 1982. HE SUFFERED FROM ADVANCED CHEMICAL DEPENDENCY AND DEPRESSION AROUND 5/1/95 WHEN HE REQUESTED AND RECEIVED A LEAVE OF ABSENCE FROM A FAMILY PRACTICE RESIDENCY. HE RECEIVED INPATIENT TREATMENT FROM APPROXIMATELY 5/95 TO 9/95 AND CONTINUED INPATIENT TREATMENT. IN 6/96, HE BEGAN TREATMENT AT ANOTHER FACILITY. ON 5/9/95, HE ANSWERED THE FOLLOWING QUESTION IN THE NEGATIVE ON HIS LICENSE RENEWAL FORM: "ARE YOU USING ANY DRUG OR CHEMICAL SUBSTANCE INCLUDING ALCOHOL WHICH HAS AN ADVERSE IMPACT ON YOUR ABILITY TO PRACTICE MEDICINE AND SURGERY?". THE NEXT DAY, HE WAS ADMITTED AS AN INPATIENT. LICENSE REINSTATED WITH CONDITIONS OF PROBATION; SHALL COMPLY WITH THE RECOMMENDATIONS OF AND WILL ABIDE BY THE POST-CARE CONTRACT FROM TREATMENT CENTER AND WILL UNDERTAKE ALL NECESSARY OR RECOMMENDED SUBSEQUENT TREATMENT; SHALL AFFILIATE WITH A PHYSICIANS RECOVERY OR CADUCEUS SUPPORT GROUP IN EVERY STATE IN WHICH HE PRACTICES AND WILL ASK THOSE SUPPORT GROUPS TO SUBMIT QUARTERLY REPORTS ON HIS PROGRESS TO THE BOARD; SHALL NOTIFY THE BOARD OF ANY ENTRY OR RE-ENTRY INTO AN INPATIENT REHABILITATION, ASSESSMENT, OR EVALUATION PROGRAM AND SHALL PROVIDE AUTHORIZATION FOR ANY AND ALL RECORDS ASSOCIATED WITH TREATMENT; SHALL NOT PRESCRIBE, ADMINISTER, DISPENSE, OR POSSESS ANY DRUGS IN SCHEDULES III, IV, OR V OR ANY ADDICTIVE DRUGS, EXCEPT TO HOSPITAL, INPATIENTS, OR ER PATIENTS; NO CONTROLLED DANGEROUS SUBSTANCES OR ADDICTIVE DRUGS WILL BE PRESCRIBED, ADMINISTERED, OR DISPENSED TO OUTPATIENTS; SHALL PRACTICE IN A CONTROLLED ENVIRONMENT APPROVED BY THE BOARD; SHALL REQUEST ALL HOSPITALS IN WHICH HE ANTICIPATES TO PRACTICE TO FURNISH A STATEMENT REGARDING MONITORING OF HIS PRACTICE; SHALL SUBMIT TO EVERY STATE IN WHICH HE HOLDS LICENSURE AND TO HOSPITALS, CLINICS OR OTHER INSTITUTIONS IN WHICH HE HOLDS OR ANTICIPATES HOLDING ANY FORM OF STAFF PRIVILEGE A COPY OF THIS ORDER; SHALL NOT SUPERVISE ALLIED HEALTH PROFESSIONALS; SHALL SUBMIT BIOLOGICAL FLUID SPECIMENS AND SHALL NOT INGEST ANY SUBSTANCE WHICH WILL CAUSE A SPECIMEN TO TEST POSITIVE FOR PROHIBITED SUBSTANCES; SHALL NOT PRESCRIBE, ADMINISTER OR DISPENSE ANY MEDICATIONS FOR HIS PERSONAL USE AND SHALL TAKE NONE UNLESS AUTHORIZED BY ANOTHER PHYSICIAN FOR A LEGITIMATE MEDICAL NEED; SHALL KEEP THE BOARD INFORMED OF HIS ADDRESS AND PAY COSTS; SHALL EXECUTE THE RELEASE OF ANY MEDICAL, COUNSELING AND PSYCHIATRIC RECORDS AS NECESSARY TO DISCUSS HIS CASE WITH TREATING PHYSICIANS AND/OR ANY PHYSICIANS HOLDING RECORDS; SHALL NOTIFY THE BOARD OF ENTRY OR RE-ENTRY INTO AN INPATIENT REHABILITATION, ASSESSMENT OR EVALUATION PROGRAM AND PROVIDE TO THE BOARD AUTHORIZATION FOR ALL RECORDS ASSOCIATED WITH TREATMENT. THE PROBATIONARY PERIOD IS TOLLED UNTIL HE RETURNS TO PRACTICE IN OKLAHOMA, OR IN ANY FEDERAL OR NATIVE AMERICAN FACILITY LOCATED WITHIN ITS BORDERS. SHOULD HE DESIRE TO ESTABLISH ACTIVE MEDICAL PRACTICE OR CONSULTATION PRIVILEGES WITHIN OKLAHOMA SHALL FIRST NOTIFY THE BOARD OF HIS INTENTIONS AND PERSONALLY APPEAR BEFORE THE BOARD FOR A REVIEW OF THESE MATTERS AND HIS PRESENT STATE OF MEDICAL TRAINING AND COMPETENCE.

WHEELER, PAUL E MD, LICENSE NUMBER 0017806 OF 8820 FAIRFIELD GREENS DRIVE, MIDWEST CITY, OK, WAS DISCIPLINED BY OKLAHOMA ON MAY 19, 1994
DISCIPLINARY ACTION: 60-MONTH PROBATION; RESTRICTION PLACED ON LICENSE
OFFENSE: SUBSTANCE ABUSE

NOTES: FROM 7/20/92 TO DATE HE HAS HABITUALLY USED ALCOHOL AND/OR HABIT-FORMING DRUGS TO THE EXTENT THAT HE VOLUNTARILY SEPARATED FROM THE U.S. ARMY AND WAS UNABLE TO PRACTICE WITH REASONABLE SAFETY AND SKILL. PROBATION TO BEGIN 5/14/94. CONDITIONS OF PROBATION: SHALL NOT PRESCRIBE, ADMINISTER OR DISPENSE ANY MEDICATIONS FOR HIS PERSONAL USE; SHALL TAKE NO MEDICATION UNLESS AUTHORIZED BY ANOTHER PHYSICIAN FOR A LEGITIMATE MEDICAL NEED; SHALL

ABSTAIN FROM CONSUMING ALCOHOL OR ANY SUBSTANCE WHICH WOULD ADVERSELY AFFECT HIS ABILITY TO PRACTICE; SHALL NOT INGEST ANY SUBSTANCE THAT WILL TEST POSITIVE FOR ALCOHOL OR ANY CONTROLLED SUBSTANCE; SHALL SUBMIT BIOLOGICAL FLUID SPECIMENS; SHALL SUBMIT MONTHLY DOCUMENTATION OF ATTENDANCE AT AA AND PHYSICIAN'S RECOVERY COMMITTEE MEETINGS; SHALL FURNISH BOARD WITH ADDRESS AND/OR CHANGE OF ADDRESS; SHALL APPEAR BEFORE THE BOARD UPON REQUEST AND PROVIDE REQUIRED REPORTS; SHALL PAY COSTS; SHALL PROVIDE ANY HEALTH CARE ENTITY WHERE HE HAS PRIVILEGES WITH A COPY OF THIS ORDER; SHALL NOT SUPERVISE A PHYSICIAN'S ASSISTANT.

WHEELER, PAUL EDWARD MD, LICENSE NUMBER 17806 OF PO BOX 188, BOISE CITY, OK, WAS DISCIPLINED BY OKLAHOMA ON JULY 31, 1998
DISCIPLINARY ACTION: PROBATION; RESTRICTION PLACED ON LICENSE
OFFENSE: FAILURE TO COMPLY WITH PREVIOUS BOARD ORDER

NOTES: ON 9/26/96 HIS LICENSE TO PRACTICE MEDICINE AND SURGERY IN OKLAHOMA WAS SUSPENDED FOR UNPROFESSIONAL CONDUCT INVOLVING PERSONAL SUBSTANCE ABUSE AND THE VIOLATION OF A PREVIOUS BOARD ORDER FOR PROBATION ENTERED 5/14/94. HE RECEIVED AN ADDITIONAL FIVE YEARS' PROBATION FOLLOWING THE SUSPENSION. HIS PROBATION COMMENCED 3/26/97. AFTER SERVING NEARLY SIX MONTHS OF THE TERM, HE CEASED PRACTICING MEDICINE IN OKLAHOMA AND MOVED TO ALASKA. AT HIS REQUEST, THE PROBATIONARY TERM WAS TOLLED ON 9/18/97. SINCE HE HAS RETURNED TO OKLAHOMA TO PRACTICE MEDICINE, HE MUST COMPLETE THE REMAINDER OF HIS PROBATIONARY TERM. CONDITIONS OF PROBATION: SHALL ATTEND NO LESS THAN THREE 12-STEP MEETINGS WEEKLY AND WILL OBTAIN, MAINTAIN, AND WORK WITH A 12-STEP SPONSOR. HE WILL ATTEND WEEKLY CADUCEUS OR SIMILAR MEETINGS FOR RECOVERING PROFESSIONALS; SHALL MAINTAIN REASONABLE WORK HOURS CONDUCIVE TO THE LIFESTYLE OF A RECOVERING PHYSICIAN AND ACKNOWLEDGES THE BOARD'S RECOMMENDATION OF A 36-40 HOUR WORK WEEK; SHALL COMPLY WITH ALL RECOMMENDATIONS FOR DRUG THERAPY AND OTHER TREATMENT MADE BY HIS TREATING PHYSICIANS AND WILL CONTINUE UNDER THE CARE OF A PRIMARY CARE PHYSICIAN FOR ROUTINE HEALTH MAINTENANCE NEEDS AND INTERMITTENT EVALUATION; SHALL CONTINUE PROFESSIONAL COUNSELING WITH AN APPROVED PRACTITIONER AND WILL COMPLY WITH ALL TREATMENT RECOMMENDATIONS; SHALL COMPLY WITH ALL REQUIREMENTS OF THE OKLAHOMA PHYSICIANS' RECOVERY PROGRAM; SHALL NOT SUPERVISE ALLIED HEALTH PROFESSIONALS; SHALL REQUEST ALL HEALTH CARE FACILITIES IN WHICH HE ANTICIPATES PRACTICING TO FURNISH A STATEMENT REGARDING MONITORING OF PRACTICE; SHALL SUBMIT BIOLOGICAL FLUID SPECIMENS AND SHALL NOT INGEST ANY SUBSTANCE WHICH WILL CAUSE A SPECIMEN TO TEST POSITIVE FOR PROHIBITED SUBSTANCES; SHALL NOT PRESCRIBE, ADMINISTER OR DISPENSE ANY MEDICATIONS FOR HIS PERSONAL USE AND SHALL TAKE NONE UNLESS AUTHORIZED BY ANOTHER PHYSICIAN FOR A LEGITIMATE MEDICAL NEED; SHALL ABSTAIN FROM CONSUMING ALCOHOL OR ANY SUBSTANCE WHICH WOULD ADVERSELY EFFECT HIS ABILITY TO PRACTICE MEDICINE; SHALL FURNISH THE BOARD WITH MONTHLY DOCUMENTATION OF HIS REGULAR ATTENDANCE AT AA MEETINGS AND THE PHYSICIAN'S RECOVERY COMMITTEE PROGRAM MEETINGS; SHALL AUTHORIZE THE BOARD TO MAKE RANDOM, UNANNOUNCED VISITS TO HIS PLACE OF EMPLOYMENT AND WILL KEEP THE BOARD FULLY INFORMED OF HIS WORK SCHEDULE AT ALL TIMES; SHALL KEEP THE BOARD INFORMED OF HIS ADDRESS AND PAY COSTS; SHALL APPEAR BEFORE THE BOARD AND SUBMIT REPORTS UPON REQUEST; SHALL EXECUTE ALL RELEASES OF MEDICAL, COUNSELING AND PSYCHIATRIC RECORDS AS NECESSARY TO DISCUSS HIS CASE WITH TREATING PHYSICIANS AND/OR ANY PHYSICIANS HOLDING RECORDS; SHALL NOTIFY THE BOARD OF ANY ENTRY OR RE-ENTRY INTO AN INPATIENT REHABILITATION, ASSESSMENT, OR EVALUATION PROGRAM AND SHALL PROVIDE AUTHORIZATION FOR ANY AND ALL RECORDS ASSOCIATED WITH TREATMENT.

WHINERY, MICHAEL A DO, LICENSE NUMBER 2122, WAS DISCIPLINED BY OKLAHOMA ON OCTOBER 14, 1998
DISCIPLINARY ACTION: 48-MONTH PROBATION

NOTES: VOLUNTARILY STOPPED PRACTICE 9/17/98.

WICKER, WALTER JR MD, DATE OF BIRTH JUNE 27, 1919 OF PO BOX 759, APACHE, OK, WAS DISCIPLINED BY MEDICARE ON OCTOBER 29, 1992
DISCIPLINARY ACTION: EXCLUSION FROM THE MEDICARE AND/OR MEDICAID PROGRAM
OFFENSE: CRIMINAL CONVICTION OR PLEA OF GUILTY, NOLO CONTENDERE, OR NO CONTEST TO A CRIME

NOTES: PROGRAM-RELATED CONVICTION.

WIGGS, WILLIAM G MD, LICENSE NUMBER 14806 OF 1124 NORTH PORTER AVENUE, NORMAN, OK, WAS DISCIPLINED BY OKLAHOMA ON NOVEMBER 12, 1998
DISCIPLINARY ACTION: LICENSE SUSPENSION; 60-MONTH PROBATION
OFFENSE: CRIMINAL CONVICTION OR PLEA OF GUILTY, NOLO CONTENDERE, OR NO CONTEST TO A CRIME

NOTES: ON 1/9/97 HE WAS ARRESTED IN THE OKLAHOMA DISTRICT COURT ON TWO FELONY COUNTS. HE PLED NO CONTEST TO THE CHARGES OF UNLAWFUL DELIVERY OF A CONTROLLED DANGEROUS SUBSTANCE (HYDROCODONE, SCHEDULE C-III) ON TWO SEPARATE OCCASIONS TO A POLICE INFORMANT IN ADA, OKLAHOMA WHO OBTAINED A PRESCRIPTION FOR LORTAB PILLS FROM THE DOCTOR IN EXCHANGE FOR $100 CASH. ON 1/16/98 HE RECEIVED A DEFERRED SENTENCE OF 18 MONTHS FROM THE COURT UNDER THE FOLLOWING SPECIAL CONDITIONS: HE SHALL NOT APPLY OR REAPPLY FOR NOR POSSESS A NARCOTICS LICENSE FOR 18 MONTHS. HE SHALL PROVIDE THE BOARD WITH A COPY OF ANY AND ALL PRESCRIPTIONS HE WRITES FOR 18 MONTHS. HE VOLUNTARILY SURRENDERED HIS STATE NARCOTICS LICENSE TO THE OKLAHOMA BUREAU OF NARCOTICS AND DANGEROUS DRUGS IN 1/97 AND SURRENDERED HIS FEDERAL NARCOTICS LICENSE TO THE DRUG ENFORCEMENT AGENCY IN 2/98 PURSUANT TO COURT ORDER. DID NOT PROVIDE THE BOARD WITH DUPLICATE PRESCRIPTIONS AS REQUIRED IN THE ORDER UNTIL AFTER THE BOARD'S COMPLAINT AND CITATION WERE SERVED. A REVIEW OF 13 PATIENT CHARTS REVEALED A PATTERN OF IMPROPERLY PRESCRIBING LARGE NUMBERS OF CONTROLLED DRUGS FOR A NUMBER OF YEARS; CHARTS REFLECT LITTLE FOLLOWUP AND ALMOST NO DOCUMENTATION OF MEDICAL NEED. SUSPENSION TO LAST A MINIMUM OF 90 DAYS OR UNTIL HE COMPLETES A COURSE APPROVED BY THE BOARD

ON PAIN MANAGEMENT AND RECORD KEEPING. SUBSEQUENT CONDITIONS OF PROBATION: SHALL NOT PRESCRIBE, ADMINISTER, POSSESS, OR DISPENSE ANY DRUGS IN SCHEDULES II-V OR ANY ADDICTIVE DRUGS; SHALL SUBMIT TO EVERY STATE IN WHICH HE HOLDS LICENSURE AND TO HOSPITALS, CLINICS OR OTHER INSTITUTIONS IN WHICH HE HOLDS OR ANTICIPATES HOLDING ANY FORM OF STAFF PRIVILEGE A COPY OF THIS ORDER; SHALL NOT SUPERVISE ALLIED HEALTH PROFESSIONALS; SHALL KEEP THE BOARD INFORMED OF HIS ADDRESS AND PAY COSTS; SHALL APPEAR BEFORE THE BOARD UPON REQUEST.

WILLIAMS, GAIL ROGER MD, DATE OF BIRTH JANUARY 10, 1938, LICENSE NUMBER 0017467 OF 3196 W ROCK CREEK RD #1402, NORMAN, OK, WAS DISCIPLINED BY OKLAHOMA ON SEPTEMBER 1, 1990
DISCIPLINARY ACTION: 60-MONTH PROBATION; RESTRICTION PLACED ON LICENSE
OFFENSE: DISCIPLINARY ACTION BY ANOTHER STATE OR AGENCY

NOTES: STIPULATED TO A REVOCATION OF MICHIGAN LICENSE ARISING OUT OF A SEXUAL RELATIONSHIP WITH A FEMALE PATIENT; HAS PRODUCED EVIDENCE TO DEMONSTRATE THAT ANY PAST MISJUDGMENTS WILL NOT BE REPEATED. LICENSURE GRANTED WITH PROBATION UNDER TERMS AND CONDITIONS: WILL PRACTICE ONLY IN A SUPERVISED SETTING OF A PUBLIC AGENCY AND SHALL NOT ENGAGE IN UNSUPERVISED PRIVATE PRACTICE; ANY TIME HE EXAMINES A FEMALE PATIENT, SHALL HAVE ANOTHER FEMALE PRESENT TO ASSIST AND WITNESS THE PROCEDURE; SHALL NOTIFY ANY HOSPITAL WHERE HE HOLDS STAFF PRIVILEGES, OR CLINIC OR GROUP OF THE TERMS AND CONDITIONS; SHALL FURNISH BOARD WITH ADDRESS AND/OR CHANGE OF ADDRESS; SHALL APPEAR BEFORE BOARD UPON REQUEST. ON 3/5/92 SUPERVISION REDUCED FROM LEVEL I TO LEVEL II. ON 5/20/93 IT WAS FOUND THAT HIS INDEPENDENT CONTRACT RELATIONSHIP AND CONDUCTING OF PRE-ADMISSION SCREENING AND ANNUAL RESIDENT REVIEW EXAMS (PASSAR) IS SPECIFICALLY EXEMPTED FROM THE PROHIBITION OF UNSUPERVISED PRACTICE AND THIS EXEMPTION IS SPECIFICALLY LIMITED TO PASARR DUTIES AS AN INDEPENDENT CONTRACTOR AND SHALL NOT EXTEND TO OR ALLOW HIM TO PRACTICE MEDICINE OR SUPERVISION IN ANY OTHER SETTING OUTSIDE THE OKLAHOMA DEPARTMENT OF CORRECTIONS.

WILLIAMS, GAIL ROGER MD, DATE OF BIRTH JANUARY 10, 1938, LICENSE NUMBER 0017467, WAS DISCIPLINED BY OKLAHOMA ON DECEMBER 2, 1993
DISCIPLINARY ACTION: LICENSE REVOCATION
OFFENSE: PROFESSIONAL MISCONDUCT

NOTES: DURING 1992 AND 1993 IN THE COURSE OF HIS PRACTICE DID SEXUALLY BATTER AND HARASS FEMALE PROFESSIONAL STAFF AND SUPPORT STAFF MEMBERS AT A CORRECTIONAL CENTER.

WILLIAMS, GAIL ROGER MD, DATE OF BIRTH JANUARY 10, 1938 OF BOX 548, LEXINGTON, OK, WAS DISCIPLINED BY DEA ON JANUARY 26, 1994
DISCIPLINARY ACTION: SURRENDER OF CONTROLLED SUBSTANCE LICENSE
OFFENSE: DISCIPLINARY ACTION BY ANOTHER STATE OR AGENCY

NOTES: MEDICAL LICENSE REVOKED IN OKLAHOMA ON 12/02/93 FOR HARASSMENT OF FEMALE PROFESSIONAL STAFF AND SUPPORT STAFF MEMBERS.

WILLIAMS, GAIL ROGER MD, DATE OF BIRTH JANUARY 10, 1938 OF 2215 MORGAN DRIVE, NORMAN, OK, WAS DISCIPLINED BY KANSAS ON JUNE 20, 1994
DISCIPLINARY ACTION: DENIAL OF NEW LICENSE
OFFENSE: DISCIPLINARY ACTION BY ANOTHER STATE OR AGENCY

NOTES: ON 06/19/85 MICHIGAN STATE BOARD OF MEDICINE REVOKED HIS MEDICAL LICENSE BASED UPON HIS SEXUAL RELATIONSHIP WITH A FEMALE PATIENT FROM LATE 1981 TO MID-1983 AND HIS SEXUAL ACTIVITY WITH THE PATIENT DURING BIWEEKLY COUNSELING THERAPY SESSIONS; FURTHER FOUND TO HAVE ENGAGED IN UNETHICAL BUSINESS PRACTICE BY OBTAINING THIRD PARTY INSURANCE REIMBURSEMENT BY FRAUD OR DECEIT. MICHIGAN DENIED REINSTATEMENT IN 1987, 1989 AND 1990. THE OKLAHOMA BOARD REVOKED HIS LICENSE ON 12/3/93 BECAUSE HE SEXUALLY BATTERED AND HARASSED FEMALE PROFESSIONAL STAFF AND SUPPORT STAFF MEMBERS AT HIS WORKPLACE.

WILLIAMS, GAIL ROGER MD, LICENSE NUMBER 0018659 OF MT. MEIGS, AL, WAS DISCIPLINED BY ALABAMA ON DECEMBER 7, 1994
DISCIPLINARY ACTION: RESTRICTION PLACED ON LICENSE

NOTES: ENTERED AGAINST HIS CERTIFICATE OF QUALIFICATION. RESTRICTED TO THE PRACTICE OF PSYCHIATRY AT STATE PENAL INSTITUTIONS UNDER THE SUPERVISION AND ADMINISTRATION OF THE STATE DEPARTMENT OF CORRECTIONS.

WILLIAMS, GAIL ROGER MD, DATE OF BIRTH JANUARY 10, 1938 OF 305 ARROWHEAD DRIVE, MONTGOMERY, AL, WAS DISCIPLINED BY MISSISSIPPI ON SEPTEMBER 21, 1995
DISCIPLINARY ACTION: RESTRICTION PLACED ON LICENSE

NOTES: LICENSE ISSUED SUBJECT TO THE FOLLOWING RESTRICTIONS: LICENSE LIMITED SOLELY TO THE MISSISSIPPI PRISON SYSTEM; CANNOT ATTEND OR TREAT FEMALE PATIENTS WITHOUT PRESENCE OF A FEMALE ESCORT; APPLICATION MUST BE COMPLETED AND ALL OTHER LICENSURE REQUIREMENTS FULFILLED.

WILLIAMS, JAMES MICHAEL MD OF 6754 NW WILLOW WOOD, LAWTON, OK, WAS DISCIPLINED BY OKLAHOMA ON JULY 1, 1992
DISCIPLINARY ACTION: 60-MONTH PROBATION; RESTRICTION PLACED ON LICENSE
OFFENSE: SUBSTANCE ABUSE

NOTES: IS A RECOVERING ALCOHOLIC AND HAS BEEN INVOLVED IN AA SINCE 1/84 AND IS PRESENTLY ACTIVELY ASSOCIATED WITH THE NEW JERSEY MEDICAL SOCIETY'S PHYSICIAN HEALTH PROGRAM. LICENSE IN OKLAHOMA GRANTED UNDER FOLLOWING CONDITIONS: SHALL NOT PRESCRIBE, ADMINISTER OR DISPENSE ANY MEDICATIONS FOR HIS PERSONAL USE; SHALL TAKE NO MEDICATION EXCEPT THAT WHICH IS AUTHORIZED BY A PHYSICIAN TREATING HIM FOR A LEGITIMATE MEDICAL NEED; SHALL ABSTAIN FROM CONSUMING ALCOHOL OR ANY SUBSTANCE WHICH WOULD ADVERSELY AFFECT ABILITY TO PRACTICE; SHALL SUBMIT BIOLOGICAL FLUID SPECIMENS FOR ANALYSIS; SHALL MAINTAIN FORMAL RELATIONSHIP WITH THE PHYSICIAN RECOVERY COMMITTEE OF OSMA AND PARTICIPATE IN THEIR MEETINGS AND ACTIVITIES; SHALL NOTIFY ANY HOSPITAL WHERE HE HOLDS STAFF PRIVILEGES OR CLINIC OR GROUP WHERE HE PRACTICES OF TERMS AND CONDITIONS; SHALL NOT SUPERVISE A PHYSICIAN'S ASSISTANT; SHALL FURNISH BOARD WITH ADDRESS AND/OR CHANGE OF ADDRESS; SHALL APPEAR BEFORE BOARD UPON REQUEST. AS OF

10/11/93 PROBATION TERMINATED.

WILLIAMS, JAMES R MD, LICENSE NUMBER 0010260 OF 309 W GENTRY STREET PO BOX 500, CHECOTAH, OK, WAS DISCIPLINED BY OKLAHOMA ON MAY 19, 1995
DISCIPLINARY ACTION: 36-MONTH PROBATION; RESTRICTION PLACED ON LICENSE
OFFENSE: OVERPRESCRIBING OR MISPRESCRIBING DRUGS

NOTES: FROM JUNE THROUGH OCTOBER 1994, HE PRESCRIBED, ADMINISTERED, DISTRIBUTED, OR ORDERED CONTROLLED DANGEROUS SUBSTANCES TO HIS WIFE. FROM APRIL 1994 TO APRIL 1995 HE PRESCRIBED, ADMINISTERED, DISTRIBUTED, OR ORDERED CONTROLLED DANGEROUS SUBSTANCES WITHOUT SUFFICIENT EXAMINATION AND ESTABLISHMENT OF VALID PHYSICIAN/PATIENT RELATIONSHIP AND IN EXCESS OF AMOUNT CONSIDERED GOOD MEDICAL PRACTICE. PROBATION BEGINNING 4/13/95 UNDER THE FOLLOWING TERMS AND CONDITIONS: SHALL IMMEDIATELY AND PERMANENTLY CEASE PRESCRIBING ANY DRUG OR MEDICATION TO HIS WIFE FOR ANY REASON WHATSOEVER; SHALL NOT PRESCRIBE, ADMINISTER, OR DISPENSE ANY CONTROLLED DANGEROUS SUBSTANCES EXCEPT UPON SEQUENTIALLY NUMBERED, DUPLICATE PRESCRIPTION FORMS, A COPY OF WHICH SHALL BE PRESENTED UPON BOARD REQUEST; SHALL ESTABLISH WRITTEN OFFICE PROTOCOLS PURSUANT TO WHICH ONLY HE SHALL ISSUE PRESCRIPTIONS A COPY OF WHICH SHALL BE DELIVERED TO THE BOARD; NO PERSONNEL SHALL ISSUE OR AUTHORIZE THE ISSUANCE OF ANY PRESCRIPTION WHATSOEVER; SHALL APPEAR BEFORE THE BOARD UPON REQUEST AND SUBMIT ANY REQUIRED REPORTS; SHALL PAY COSTS; SHALL NOTIFY ANY HOSPITAL WHERE HE HOLDS STAFF PRIVILEGES, OR CLINIC, OR GROUP, WHERE HE PRACTICES OF THE TERMS AND CONDITIONS OF THIS ORDER AND PROVIDE A COPY THEREOF; SHALL NOT SUPERVISE A PHYSICIAN ASSISTANT; SHALL MEET NO LESS THAN QUARTERLY WITH THE BOARD AND SHALL PROVIDE ANY AND ALL REQUESTED CHARTS AND PATIENTS RECORDS; SHALL NOT ALLOW THE INITIATION OF ANY THERAPEUTIC REGIMEN BY ANY PERSONNEL UNDER HIS SUPERVISION UNLESS HE IS IN THE IMMEDIATE VICINITY; REPRIMAND. ON 1/30/97 REQUEST TO MODIFY ORDER GRANTED PERMITTING HIM LESS FREQUENT APPEARANCES BEFORE THE BOARD.

WILLIAMSON, LINDA D MD, LICENSE NUMBER 00J3678 OF LAWTON, OK, WAS DISCIPLINED BY TEXAS ON JUNE 28, 1995
DISCIPLINARY ACTION: REPRIMAND
OFFENSE: DISCIPLINARY ACTION BY ANOTHER STATE OR AGENCY

NOTES: DISCIPLINED BY THE AIR FORCE WITH A FINE OF $750 FOR NOT TELLING THE TRUTH TO A SENIOR OFFICER ABOUT TAKING AND PASSING A PORTION OF THE NATIONAL MEDICAL BOARD EXAMINATION; SUBSEQUENT AIR FORCE REPORTS INDICATE THAT SHE RENDERED A HIGH QUALITY OF MEDICAL CARE AS A MILITARY PHYSICIAN; SHE WAS HONORABLY DISCHARGED FROM MILITARY SERVICE ON 6/30/94. SHALL GIVE A COPY OF THIS ORDER TO ANY HEALTH CARE ENTITY WHERE SHE HAS PRIVILEGES; SHALL INFORM BOARD OF CHANGE OF ADDRESS WITHIN 10 DAYS.

WILSON, J SCOT MD OF 1607 S MUSKOGEE, TAHLEQUAH, OK, WAS DISCIPLINED BY DEA ON NOVEMBER 10, 1997
DISCIPLINARY ACTION: SURRENDER OF CONTROLLED SUBSTANCE LICENSE

NOTES: IN LIEU OF PUBLIC INTEREST REVOCATION.

WILSON, J SCOT MD, LICENSE NUMBER 17703 OF 1607 SOUTH MUSKOGEE, TAHLEQUAH, OK, WAS DISCIPLINED BY OKLAHOMA ON NOVEMBER 12, 1998
DISCIPLINARY ACTION: LICENSE REVOCATION
OFFENSE: CRIMINAL CONVICTION OR PLEA OF GUILTY, NOLO CONTENDERE, OR NO CONTEST TO A CRIME

NOTES: HE PLED NO CONTEST TO FOUR FELONY CHARGES THAT HE ENGAGED IN THE ACT OF SODOMY AFTER ADMINISTERING A NARCOTIC SUBSTANCE TO RENDER HIS VICTIMS INCAPABLE OF CONSENTING OR REFUSING TO CONSENT AND WAS FOUND GUILTY ON 7/20/98. HE RECEIVED 10 YEARS IMPRISONMENT ON EACH OF THREE COUNTS TO BE SERVED CONCURRENTLY AND 20 YEAR SUSPENDED SENTENCE ON ONE COUNT TO BE SERVED CONSECUTIVELY FOLLOWING COMPLETION OF THE FIRST THREE SENTENCES; SHALL PAY COSTS.

WILSON, JAMES S MD OF 6710 OLD ZARING BOARD, CRESTWOOD, KY, WAS DISCIPLINED BY INDIANA ON NOVEMBER 24, 1999

NOTES: UNSPECIFIED ORDER.

WILSON, JAMES STEPHEN WALTER OF PO BOX 382 MAIN CROSS STREET, BROWNSVILLE, KY, WAS DISCIPLINED BY OKLAHOMA ON APRIL 1, 1993
DISCIPLINARY ACTION: DENIAL OF LICENSE REINSTATEMENT
OFFENSE: PHYSICAL OR MENTAL ILLNESS INHIBITING THE ABILITY TO PRACTICE WITH SKILL AND SAFETY

NOTES: HAS NOT BEEN INVOLVED IN ACTIVE PRACTICE SINCE 1984 AND HAD PREVIOUS TREATMENT FOR EMOTIONAL ILLNESS AND THERE WAS A BASIS FOR ISSUE AS TO WHETHER HE COULD PRACTICE WITH REASONABLE SKILL AND SAFETY.

WIMBLY, TIMOTHY TYRONE, WAS DISCIPLINED BY OKLAHOMA ON JULY 22, 1994
DISCIPLINARY ACTION: DENIAL OF NEW LICENSE

NOTES: TOOK FLEX EXAM AT LEAST EIGHT TIMES BETWEEN 6/89 AND 12/92 BEFORE PASSING; FAILURE IN SO MANY ATTEMPTS RAISES SERIOUS ISSUES AS TO HIS ABILITY TO PRACTICE WITH REASONABLE SKILL AND SAFETY.

WOLF, GARY DUKE DO, LICENSE NUMBER 00E9029 OF MANSFIELD, TX, WAS DISCIPLINED BY TEXAS ON JANUARY 6, 1995
DISCIPLINARY ACTION: REQUIRED TO TAKE ADDITIONAL MEDICAL EDUCATION; MONITORING OF PHYSICIAN PERFORMANCE
OFFENSE: OVERPRESCRIBING OR MISPRESCRIBING DRUGS

NOTES: FROM 1985 TO 1993 PRESCRIBED CONTROLLED SUBSTANCES TO VARIOUS PATIENTS WITHOUT ADEQUATE INDICATIONS AND SUFFICIENT MONITORING OR FOLLOW-UP; CARE AND TREATMENT APPEARS TO BE WELL DOCUMENTED AND HE REPORTS THAT PATIENTS HAVE BEEN WEANED OFF THE DRUGS PRESCRIBED; AGREEMENT IN LIEU OF FURTHER INVESTIGATION OR A HEARING. CONDITIONS OF THREE YEAR RESTRICTION: SHALL OBTAIN AT LEAST 50 HOURS PER YEAR OF CONTINUING MEDICAL EDUCATION INCLUDING 25 HOURS IN PHARMACOLOGY, SUBSTANCE ABUSE OR PAIN MANAGEMENT IN THE FIRST YEAR; SEPARATE FROM PATIENT RECORDS, SHALL MAINTAIN A FILE OF EVERY PRESCRIPTION WRITTEN FOR CONTROLLED SUBSTANCES OR DANGEROUS DRUGS WHICH SHALL BE AVAILABLE FOR INSPECTION; SHALL MAINTAIN A LOGBOOK FOR ALL PRESCRIPTIONS OR REFILLS OF

SUCH DRUGS TELEPHONED IN, WHICH SHALL BE AVAILABLE FOR INSPECTION; SHALL APPEAR BEFORE THE BOARD ONCE A YEAR OR UPON REQUEST; SHALL COOPERATE WITH THE BOARD IN VERIFYING COMPLIANCE; SHALL EXECUTE RELEASES NECESSARY TO OBTAIN PEER REVIEW RECORDS; SHALL GIVE A COPY OF THIS ORDER TO ANY HEALTH CARE ENTITY WHERE HE HAS OR HAS APPLIED FOR PRIVILEGES OR ANYONE ELSE WHO REQUESTS IT; SHALL ENSURE INQUIRIES REGARDING HIS TEXAS LICENSURE STATUS ARE ANSWERED BY REFERENCING THIS ORDER; SHALL INFORM BOARD OF CHANGE OF ADDRESS WITHIN 10 DAYS OR IF HE LEAVES THE STATE; TIME SPENT OUT OF TEXAS DOES NOT COUNT TOWARD RESTRICTION. SHALL NOT SEEK MODIFICATION FOR ONE YEAR. ON 1/27/96 ORDER TERMINATED.

WOLF, GARY DUKE DO, LICENSE NUMBER 0002560, WAS DISCIPLINED BY OKLAHOMA ON JULY 14, 1995
DISCIPLINARY ACTION: 36-MONTH PROBATION; REQUIRED TO TAKE ADDITIONAL MEDICAL EDUCATION
OFFENSE: DISCIPLINARY ACTION BY ANOTHER STATE OR AGENCY

NOTES: THREE YEAR RESTRICTION PLACED ON LICENSE IN TEXAS UNDER TERMS AND CONDITIONS ON 1/06/95. OKLAHOMA LIMITED LICENSE: SHALL OBTAIN AT LEAST 50 HOURS PER YEAR OF CONTINUING MEDICAL EDUCATION DURING THE FIRST YEAR OF LIMITATION, AT LEAST 25 HOURS OF WHICH SHOULD BE IN PHARMACOLOGY, SUBSTANCE ABUSE OR PAIN MANAGEMENT; SHALL EACH YEAR SUBMIT PROOF TO THE BOARD OF THE PRIOR YEAR'S ATTENDANCE; SHALL REFRAIN FROM THE PRESCRIPTION OR ADMINISTRATION OF ANY DRUG UNLESS THE DRUG IS ISSUED TO HIS PATIENTS AND ONLY FOR THE EXPRESSED PURPOSE OF SERVING THE BEST INTERESTS AND PROMOTING THE WELFARE OF HIS PATIENTS; SHALL GIVE A COPY OF THIS ORDER TO ANY HEALTH CARE ENTITY WHERE HE HAS PRIVILEGES; SHALL NOTIFY THE BOARD IN WRITING OF ANY CHANGE IN ADDRESS, EMPLOYMENT, EMPLOYMENT TERMINATION OR HOSPITAL OR HEALTH CARE ENTITIES PRIVILEGE RESTRICTION OR ANY ADMINISTRATIVE PROCEEDING INITIATED AGAINST HIM BY ANY OTHER STATE OR FEDERAL REGULATORY BODY WITHIN 14 DAYS; SHALL APPEAR BEFORE THE BOARD BEFORE PRACTICING OSTEOPATHIC MEDICINE IN OKLAHOMA; $275.00 ADMINISTRATIVE COSTS. ON 12/10/98 PROBATION TERMINATED.

WOLF, GARY DUKE DO OF MANSFIELD, TX, WAS DISCIPLINED BY LOUISIANA ON AUGUST 24, 1995
DISCIPLINARY ACTION: 36-MONTH PROBATION
OFFENSE: DISCIPLINARY ACTION BY ANOTHER STATE OR AGENCY

NOTES: DISCIPLINARY ACTION BY TEXAS; PRESCRIBING, DISPENSING OR ADMINISTERING CONTROLLED SUBSTANCES IN OTHER THAN A LEGAL OR LEGITIMATE MANNER. CONDITIONS OF PROBATION: MUST COMPLY WITH TERMS OF PRIOR PROBATIONARY ORDER IMPOSED BY TEXAS; MUST COMPLETE TEXAS PROBATION AND APPEAR BEFORE BOARD PRIOR TO PRACTICING IN LOUISIANA.

WOOD, BRYAN S MD, LICENSE NUMBER TP214 OF PULASKI COUNTY, KY, WAS DISCIPLINED BY KENTUCKY ON FEBRUARY 1, 1999
DISCIPLINARY ACTION: 60-MONTH PROBATION; RESTRICTION PLACED ON CONTROLLED SUBSTANCE LICENSE

NOTES: TERMS AND CONDITIONS OF PROBATION INCLUDE: MAINTAINING CONTRACTUAL RELATIONSHIP WITH IMPAIRED PHYSICIANS PROGRAM; SUCCESSFUL COMPLETION OF CONTINUING MEDICAL EDUCATION; MAY NOT REAPPLY FOR DEA PERMIT UNTIL SPECIFIC CONDITIONS MET.

WOOD, BRYAN SCOTT MD, LICENSE NUMBER 18662, WAS DISCIPLINED BY OKLAHOMA ON SEPTEMBER 24, 1998
DISCIPLINARY ACTION: 1-MONTH LICENSE SUSPENSION; 60-MONTH PROBATION
OFFENSE: OVERPRESCRIBING OR MISPRESCRIBING DRUGS

NOTES: DURING 1997 USING A VARIETY OF METHODS HE OBTAINED FOR HIS WIFE, OR ASSISTED HIS WIFE IN OBTAINING, PRESCRIPTIONS FOR HYDROCODONE, A SCHEDULE III CONTROLLED SUBSTANCE (C-III) AND OXYCONTIN, A CONTROLLED SUBSTANCE (C-II). HIS ACTIONS WERE TAKEN WITH KNOWLEDGE OF HIS WIFE'S HYDROCODONE ADDICTION AND OCCURRED IN PART WHILE HIS WIFE WAS PREGNANT. HE HAS WRITTEN PRESCRIPTIONS FOR HYDROCODONE IN THE NAME OF HIS WIFE'S SISTER TO BE FILLED AND USED BY HIS WIFE. HE HAS FORGED THE SIGNATURE AND DEA NUMBER OF A COLLEAGUE; ASKED FIVE OTHER PHYSICIANS TO WRITE HIM PRESCRIPTIONS; HE ALSO SUPPLIED HYDROCODONE TO HIS WIFE BY ASKING PHYSICIANS UNDER HIS SUPERVISION TO PRESCRIBE IT FOR HER WITHOUT FIRST ESTABLISHING A VALID PHYSICIAN-PATIENT RELATIONSHIP. IN THE FALL OF 1997, HE UNSUCCESSFULLY ATTEMPTED TO DETOXIFY HIS WIFE AT HOME USING OXYCONTIN CONTROLLED RELEASED TABLETS, A SCHEDULE II CONTROLLED DANGEROUS SUBSTANCE AND INVOLVED OTHER PHYSICIANS IN THIS UNLAWFUL DETOXIFICATION TREATMENT. HE HAS BEEN RECOMMENDED FOR EVALUATION FOR POSSIBLE PERSONAL IMPAIRMENT OR DRUG ADDICTION AND FOR CO-DEPENDENCE GIVEN THE NATURE OF HIS UNPROFESSIONAL CONDUCT INVOLVING CONTROLLED SUBSTANCES. ON 7/21/98 THE BOARD GRANTED A CONTINUANCE IN THIS CASE. PRIOR TO AND DURING A CONTINUANCE, HE DELIVERED HIS NARCOTICS PERMITS TO THE BOARD FOR SURRENDER AND COMPLETED AN INPATIENT EVALUATION FOR POSSIBLE ADDICTION AND CODEPENDENCY. CONDITIONS OF PROBATION: SHALL NOT RE-APPLY FOR STATE AND FEDERAL REGISTRATION FOR CONTROLLED DANGEROUS SUBSTANCES FOR AT LEAST ONE YEAR . HE MAY NOT PETITION THE BOARD FOR REMOVAL OF THIS RESTRICTION PRIOR TO MAY 1999. ASSUMING HE VALIDLY OBTAINS HIS STATE OR FEDERAL REGISTRATION FOR CONTROLLED DANGEROUS SUBSTANCES DURING THE PERIOD OF PROBATION, HE WILL NOT PRESCRIBE, SELL, ADMINISTER, DISPENSE, ORDER, GIVE, OR DISTRIBUTE ANY DRUG LEGALLY CLASSIFIED AS A CONTROLLED SUBSTANCE OR RECOGNIZED AS AN ADDICTIVE DRUG TO A FAMILY MEMBER OR TO HIMSELF. HE WILL NOT AUTHORIZE OR REQUEST ANY PERSONNEL UNDER HIS SUPERVISION TO INITIATE OR ORDER A PRESCRIPTION TO BE ISSUED TO HIS FAMILY MEMBERS AND WILL NOT REQUEST COLLEAGUES TO DO THE SAME. HE WILL LIMIT HIS PRACTICE TO EMERGENCY MEDICINE AT HOSPITALS IN ADA AND BETHANY, OKLAHOMA; SHALL SUBMIT TO EVERY STATE IN WHICH HE HOLDS LICENSURE AND TO HOSPITALS, CLINICS OR OTHER INSTITUTIONS IN WHICH HE HOLDS OR ANTICIPATES HOLDING ANY FORM OF STAFF PRIVILEGE A COPY OF THIS ORDER; SHALL NOT SUPERVISE ALLIED HEALTH PROFESSIONALS; SHALL AUTHORIZE IN WRITING THE RELEASE OF ANY AND ALL INFORMATION REGARDING HIS MEDICAL, EMOTIONAL, OR PSYCHIATRIC

TREATMENT TO THE BOARD; SHALL ABIDE BY THE RECOMMENDATIONS OF TREATMENT CENTER, INCLUDING PSYCHIATRIC TREATMENT OR COUNSELING WITH A BOARD APPROVED DOCTOR OR THERAPIST; SHALL PARTICIPATE IN AN OUTPATIENT PSYCHIATRIC PROGRAM WITH A BOARD CERTIFIED PRACTITIONER WHICH ADDRESSES INDIVIDUAL AND FAMILY ISSUES IDENTIFIED BY THE TREATMENT CENTER AND HE WILL ABIDE BY ALL RECOMMENDATIONS MADE IN SUCH TREATMENT; SHALL ATTEND MONTHLY MEETINGS OF THE PHYSICIANS RECOVERY PROGRAM OR ANOTHER BOARD APPROVED SUPPORT GROUP; SHALL ATTEND AL-ANON MEETINGS; SHALL KEEP THE BOARD INFORMED OF HIS ADDRESS AND PAY COSTS; SHALL APPEAR BEFORE THE BOARD UPON REQUEST.

WOODRIDGE, CHARLES A DR OF CHICAGO, IL, WAS DISCIPLINED BY ILLINOIS ON MAY 1, 1996
DISCIPLINARY ACTION: NONRENEWAL OF LICENSE
OFFENSE: NONCOMPLIANCE WITH A PROFESSIONAL RULE

NOTES: DEFAULTED ON ILLINOIS STUDENT ASSISTANCE LOANS. PLACED IN A REFUSE TO RENEW STATUS.

WOODRIDGE, CHARLES A DR OF SOUTH HOLLAND, IL, WAS DISCIPLINED BY ILLINOIS ON AUGUST 1, 1996
DISCIPLINARY ACTION: PROBATION
OFFENSE: NONCOMPLIANCE WITH A PROFESSIONAL RULE

NOTES: DEFAULTED ON ILLINOIS STUDENT ASSISTANCE LOANS. ACTION DATE 8/96.

WOODRIDGE, CHARLES ANTHONY OF 10230 SOUTH WALLACE, CHICAGO, IL, WAS DISCIPLINED BY OKLAHOMA ON JULY 1, 1993
DISCIPLINARY ACTION: DENIAL OF NEW LICENSE

NOTES: HAD MULTIPLE FAILURES OF FLEX EXAM AND THAT AND OTHER EVIDENCE RAISED ISSUES AS TO HIS ABILITY TO PRACTICE WITH REASONABLE SKILL.

WOODRIDGE, CHARLES ANTHONY MD, DATE OF BIRTH FEBRUARY 20, 1950 OF 15635 DANTE DRIVE, S HOLLAND, IL, WAS DISCIPLINED BY MEDICARE ON NOVEMBER 7, 1996
DISCIPLINARY ACTION: EXCLUSION FROM THE MEDICARE AND/OR MEDICAID PROGRAM
OFFENSE: NONCOMPLIANCE WITH A PROFESSIONAL RULE

NOTES: DEFAULTED ON PUBLIC HEALTH SERVICE EDUCATION LOAN. REINSTATED ON 9/4/97.

WOODS, LUANN DO, LICENSE NUMBER 0002822, WAS DISCIPLINED BY OKLAHOMA ON DECEMBER 9, 1993
DISCIPLINARY ACTION: 24-MONTH PROBATION; RESTRICTION PLACED ON CONTROLLED SUBSTANCE LICENSE
OFFENSE: OVERPRESCRIBING OR MISPRESCRIBING DRUGS

NOTES: INDISCRIMINATELY AND EXCESSIVELY PRESCRIBED CONTROLLED DANGEROUS SUBSTANCES WITHOUT LEGITIMATE MEDICAL NEED TO 10 PATIENTS BETWEEN 10/92 AND 10/93. CONDITIONS OF PROBATION: SHALL NOT PETITION THE BOARD FOR MODIFICATION FOR AT LEAST ONE YEAR; SHALL ATTEND AND SUCCESSFULLY COMPLETE A COURSE ENTITLED "THE PROPER PRESCRIBING OF CONTROLLED DANGEROUS SUBSTANCES" AND SHALL REPORT THE SUCCESSFUL COMPLETION TO THE BOARD; SHALL MAKE DUPLICATE PRESCRIPTIONS FOR ANY CONTROLLED DANGEROUS SUBSTANCES SHE PRESCRIBES, ADMINISTERS, OR DISPENSES WITH ONE SET SENT TO THE BOARD ON A MONTHLY BASIS; SHALL NOTIFY AND PROVIDE A COPY OF THIS ORDER TO ALL HEALTH CARE ENTITIES WHERE SHE HAS PRIVILEGES; SHALL NOTIFY THE BOARD IN WRITING OF ANY CHANGE IN ADDRESS, EMPLOYMENT, EMPLOYMENT TERMINATION OR HOSPITAL OR HEALTH CARE ENTITIES OR PRIVILEGE RESTRICTION AGAINST HER BY ANY OTHER STATE OR FEDERAL REGULATORY BODY WITHIN 14 DAYS; SHALL OBTAIN AN ADDITIONAL 50 HOURS OF CONTINUED MEDICAL EDUCATION FOR EACH YEAR OF PROBATION AND SHALL REPORT EVIDENCE OF COMPLETION. $1,350 ADMINISTRATIVE COSTS. ON 12/19/95 PROBATION ENDED AND LICENSE REINSTATED IN GOOD STANDING.

WYLY, MICHAEL DO, LICENSE NUMBER 0001828 OF REYNOLDS FAM PRACT CLINIC #2, FORT SILL, OK, WAS DISCIPLINED BY OKLAHOMA ON SEPTEMBER 16, 1992
DISCIPLINARY ACTION: SURRENDER OF LICENSE

NOTES: IN LIEU OF A COMPLAINT AND EVIDENTIARY HEARING.

WYLY, MICHAEL DO, LICENSE NUMBER 0001828 OF REYNOLDS FAM PRACT CLINIC #2, FORT SILL, OK, WAS DISCIPLINED BY OKLAHOMA ON SEPTEMBER 17, 1993
DISCIPLINARY ACTION: LICENSE REINSTATEMENT; 60-MONTH PROBATION
OFFENSE: CRIMINAL CONVICTION OR PLEA OF GUILTY, NOLO CONTENDERE, OR NO CONTEST TO A CRIME

NOTES: SURRENDERED HIS LICENSE ON 9/16/92. ON 9/30/92 PLED GUILTY TO FIVE COUNTS OF OBTAINING PERCOCET, A SCHEDULE II CONTROLLED SUBSTANCE, BY MISREPRESENTATION, FRAUD, OR SUBTERFUGE. ON 11/17/92 SENTENCED TO FOUR YEAR PROBATION WHICH EXPIRED ON 11/16/96. CONDITIONS OF BOARD PROBATION: MAY NOT PETITION THE BOARD FOR MODIFICATION FOR ONE YEAR; SHALL CONTINUE TO BE ACTIVELY INVOLVED IN THE OKLAHOMA PHYSICIAN'S RECOVERY PROGRAM (PRP) AND AGREES TO COMPLY WITH ANY AFTERCARE PROGRAM ESTABLISHED BY THE OAKS REHABILITATIVE SERVICES CENTER AND THE PRP; SHALL SUBMIT QUARTERLY REPORTS TO THE BOARD VERIFYING HIS COMPLIANCE WITH ANY PROGRAM ESTABLISHED BY THE PRP; SHALL SUBMIT TO RANDOM DRUG SCREENINGS UPON REQUEST; SHALL NOTIFY THE BOARD IN WRITING OF ANY CHANGE IN ADDRESS, EMPLOYMENT, EMPLOYMENT, TERMINATION, OR HOSPITAL PRIVILEGE RESTRICTION AND ANY ADMINISTRATIVE PROCEEDING INITIATED AGAINST HIM BY ANY OTHER STATE OR FEDERAL REGULATORY BODY WITHIN 14 DAYS; SHALL APPEAR BEFORE THE BOARD UPON REQUEST; AGREES TO RANDOM, UNANNOUNCED BOARD VISITS AT HIS PLACE OF BUSINESS FOR OBSERVATION AND ACCESS TO ANY APPROPRIATE RECORDS, PROVIDED THESE VISITS DO NOT INTERRUPT HIS MEDICAL SERVICES; PROBATIONARY TIME SHALL NOT INCLUDE ANY PERIODS OF TIME OF RESIDENCE OR PRACTICE OUTSIDE OF OKLAHOMA; SHALL INFORM THE BOARD IF HE LEAVES OKLAHOMA; SHALL COMPLETE 50 HOURS OF CONTINUING MEDICAL EDUCATION; $565.00 ADMINISTRATIVE COSTS.

YAHNKE, DAVID MD OF TULSA, OK, WAS DISCIPLINED BY MISSOURI ON DECEMBER 20, 1991
DISCIPLINARY ACTION: 36-MONTH PROBATION
OFFENSE: DISCIPLINARY ACTION BY ANOTHER STATE OR AGENCY

NOTES: PERSONAL IMPAIRMENT.

YAHNKE, DAVID GROSS MD, LICENSE NUMBER 0017257, WAS DISCIPLINED BY OKLAHOMA ON JUNE 21, 1990
DISCIPLINARY ACTION: 60-MONTH PROBATION; RESTRICTION

PLACED ON LICENSE
OFFENSE: DISCIPLINARY ACTION BY ANOTHER STATE OR AGENCY

NOTES: ACTION IN INDIANA. ON 10/26/89 HE ADMITTED TO IMPROPER SEXUAL CONTACT WITH VARIOUS FEMALE PATIENTS AND THAT HE HAD RESIGNED HIS PRIVILEGES AT BARTHOLOMEW COUNTY HOSPITAL AND ENTERED TREATMENT AT GOLDEN VALLY HEALTH CENTER IN JANUARY 1989. PROBATION BEGINNING 6/08/90 UNDER THE FOLLOWING TERMS AND CONDITIONS: MAY NOT EXAMINE OR TREAT FEMALE PATIENTS WITHOUT A FEMALE R.N., L.P.N., OR TECHNICIAN IN THE ROOM, EXCEPT IN EMERGENCY SITUATIONS; MAY NOT ENGAGE IN SOLO PRACTICE OF MEDICINE AND SURGERY; SHALL CONTINUE HIS REGULAR THERAPY SESSIONS WITH A BOARD APPROVED PROFESSIONAL PHYSICIAN OR THERAPIST UNTIL FURTHER DECISION FROM THE BOARD; SHALL AUTHORIZE HIS THERAPIST TO SUBMIT RECORDS; SHALL AUTHORIZE HIS PRIOR THERAPIST TO PROVIDE COPIES OF HIS ADMISSION AND DISCHARGE SUMMARY, PROGRESS NOTES, AND PROGNOSIS TO THE BOARD; SHALL CONTINUE TO ATTEND SEX ADDICTS ANONYMOUS MEETINGS AT LEAST ONE TIME PER WEEK, WITH MONTHLY REPORTS SUBMITTED TO THE BOARD; SHALL SUBMIT TO THE BOARD ADDRESS/CHANGE OF ADDRESS; SHALL APPEAR BEFORE THE BOARD UPON REQUEST AND SUBMIT REQUIRED REPORTS; SHALL PAY COSTS; SHALL NOTIFY ANY HOSPITAL WHERE HE HOLDS STAFF PRIVILEGES, OR CLINIC, OR GROUP WHERE HE PRACTICES, OF THE TERMS AND CONDITIONS OF THIS ORDER AND SUPPLY A COPY THEREOF.

YARBOROUGH, WILLIAM H MD, LICENSE NUMBER 0011837 OF 7310 E 75TH ST, TULSA, OK, WAS DISCIPLINED BY OKLAHOMA ON JANUARY 16, 1990
DISCIPLINARY ACTION: 12-MONTH LICENSE SUSPENSION; REQUIRED TO ENTER AN IMPAIRED PHYSICIAN PROGRAM OR SUBSTANCE ABUSE TREATMENT
OFFENSE: SUBSTANCE ABUSE

NOTES: IN EARLY 1987 ABUSED ALCOHOL AND CERTAIN CHEMICAL SUBSTANCES AND WAS HOSPITALIZED FOR INPATIENT TREATMENT; SINCE MAY AND JUNE 1987 HE HAS FROM TIME TO TIME CONTINUED HIS USE OF ALCOHOL AND CONTROLLED DANGEROUS SUBSTANCE; FROM 11/88 TO 4/89 HE WROTE NUMEROUS FALSE AND FICTITIOUS PRESCRIPTIONS FOR CONTROLLED DANGEROUS SUBSTANCES IN THE NAMES OF PERSONS WHO DID NOT RECEIVE THE MEDICATION; ON 9/15/88 PLACED ON TWO YEAR PROBATION WITH CONDITIONS ALL OF WHICH ARE STILL IN EFFECT; PHYSICIAN'S RECOVERY COMMITTEE DETERMINED HE WAS STILL IN NEED OF SOME FORM OF INPATIENT THERAPY. PRESCRIBED CONTROLLED OR NARCOTIC DRUGS IN EXCESS OF THE AMOUNT CONSIDERED GOOD MEDICAL PRACTICE. SUSPENSION BEGINNING 10/20/89. DURING SUSPENSION HE SHALL COMPLY WITH THE FOLLOWING TERMS AND CONDITIONS: SHALL TAKE NO MEDICATION UNLESS AUTHORIZED BY ANOTHER PHYSICIAN FOR LEGITIMATE MEDICAL NEED; SHALL ABSTAIN FROM CONSUMING ALCOHOL OR ANY SUBSTANCE WHICH WOULD ADVERSELY AFFECT HIS ABILITY TO PRACTICE; SHALL SUBMIT BIOLOGICAL FLUID SPECIMENS; SHALL PAY COSTS. MAY PETITION FOR EARLY RELEASE FROM SUSPENSION UPON SUCCESSFUL COMPLETION OF INPATIENT TREATMENT.

YARBOROUGH, WILLIAM H MD, LICENSE NUMBER 0011837 OF 2853 S 96TH E PLACE, TULSA, OK, WAS DISCIPLINED BY OKLAHOMA ON SEPTEMBER 1, 1990
DISCIPLINARY ACTION: 60-MONTH PROBATION; MONITORING OF PHYSICIAN PERFORMANCE

NOTES: ON 10/20/89 LICENSE SUSPENDED FOR ONE YEAR WITH CONDITION THAT IF HE COMPLETED INPATIENT OR OUTPATIENT TREATMENT SATISFACTORY TO PHYSICIAN'S RECOVERY COMMITTEE HE COULD ASK FOR REMAINDER OF SUSPENSION TO BE SET ASIDE; HE HAS NOW DONE SO. REINSTATED WITH PROBATION UNDER TERMS AND CONDITIONS: SHALL TAKE NO MEDICATION UNLESS PRESCRIBED BY TREATING PHYSICIAN; SHALL ABSTAIN FROM ALCOHOL OR ANY SUBSTANCE WHICH WOULD ADVERSELY AFFECT HIS ABILITY TO PRACTICE; SHALL SUBMIT BIOLOGICAL FLUID SPECIMENS FOR ANALYSIS; SHALL CONTINUE REGULAR ATTENDANCE AND PARTICIPATION IN MEETINGS OF THE PHYSICIAN RECOVERY COMMITTEE OR SIMILAR ORGANIZATIONS WITH REPORTS TO BOARD; SHALL FURNISH BOARD WITH ADDRESS AND/OR CHANGE OF ADDRESS; SHALL APPEAR BEFORE BOARD UPON REQUEST; SHALL NOTIFY ANY HOSPITAL WHERE HE HOLDS STAFF PRIVILEGES, OR CLINIC OR GROUP, OF THE TERMS AND CONDITIONS. ON 11/6/91 SUPERVISION REDUCED FROM LEVEL I TO LEVEL II.

YARBROUGH, ARDRY LANCE MD, LICENSE NUMBER 5623 OF 5932 S. ROCKFORD, TULSA, OK, WAS DISCIPLINED BY OKLAHOMA ON JANUARY 21, 1999
DISCIPLINARY ACTION: LICENSE SUSPENSION
OFFENSE: SEXUAL ABUSE OF OR SEXUAL MISCONDUCT WITH A PATIENT

NOTES: IN 2/97 ENGAGED IN SEXUAL MISCONDUCT WITH A PATIENT AFTER SHE WAS DISCHARGED FROM A PSYCHIATRIC HOSPITAL WHERE HE WAS TREATING HER; HAS NEVER BEEN REGISTERED TO PRESCRIBE CONTROLLED SUBSTANCES; IN 8/98 WROTE THE SAME WOMAN A PRESCRIPTION FOR XANAX BY FORGING THE SIGNATURE OF ANOTHER DOCTOR; ON OR ABOUT 7/98 HE SAW AND TREATED ANOTHER FEMALE WHO, AT THE TIME, HAD OBTAINED A XANAX PRESCRIPTION FROM ANOTHER DOCTOR OF WHICH HE SUBSEQUENTLY FORGED THE DOCTOR'S SIGNATURE FOR AN ADDITIONAL 60 XANAX; ABOUT THREE WEEKS LATER, HE MET THE SAME PATIENT AT A RESTAURANT AND AGAIN FORGED PRESCRIPTIONS FOR HER FOR XANAX, AND VALIUM WITH ANOTHER DOCTOR'S NAME; AT THAT TIME, HE ADVISED HER THAT SHE NEEDED TO FIND A PHYSICIAN TO HELP HER WITH HER ADDICTION AND THAT HE WOULD NOT WRITE ADDITIONAL PRESCRIPTIONS FOR HER. SUSPENDED UNTIL 7/1/99 OR LONGER UNTIL HE SUBMITS EVIDENCE OF THE FOLLOWING: A FULL ASSESSMENT FOR POSSIBLE SEXUAL AND/OR CHEMICAL ADDICTION AT A BOARD-APPROVED EVALUATION FACILITY; ABIDES BY ALL THE RECOMMENDATIONS; SHALL ENTER AND COMPLETE COUNSELING AND/OR EDUCATIONAL COURSES ON STRESS MANAGEMENT AND PATIENT BOUNDARIES AND WILL RELEASE ALL MEDICAL RECORDS.

YARBROUGH, ARDRY LANCE MD, LICENSE NUMBER 5623 OF 5932 SOUTH ROCKFORD AVENUE, TULSA, OK, WAS DISCIPLINED BY OKLAHOMA ON JULY 29, 1999
DISCIPLINARY ACTION: PROBATION; RESTRICTION PLACED ON LICENSE

NOTES: LICENSE REINSTATED AND LIMITED AS FOLLOWS: SHALL NOT APPLY FOR REGISTRATION WITH THE OKLAHOMA BUREAU OF NARCOTICS AND DANGEROUS DRUGS CONTROL (OBN) OR THE DEA TO PRESCRIBE, DISPENSE, ADMINISTER OR POSSESS

ANY CONTROLLED DANGEROUS DRUGS FOR ONE YEAR; IF OBTAINS REGISTRATION WITH OBN AND DEA, SHALL KEEP DUPLICATE, SERIALLY NUMBERED PRESCRIPTIONS OF ALL CONTROLLED DANGEROUS SUBSTANCES AND WILL SUBMIT COPIES TO THE BOARD UPON REQUEST; SHALL REQUEST ALL HEALTH CARE FACILITIES IN WHICH HE ANTICIPATES PRACTICING TO FURNISH A STATEMENT REGARDING MONITORING OF HIS PRACTICE; SHALL EXECUTE ALL RELEASES OF MEDICAL AND PSYCHIATRIC RECORDS AS NECESSARY TO DISCUSS HIS CASE WITH HIS TREATING PHYSICIANS AND/OR ANY PHYSICIANS HOLDING RECORDS; SHALL CONTINUE TREATMENT WITH PSYCHOTHERAPIST WITH QUARTERLY REPORTS TO THE BOARD; SHALL SUBMIT QUARTERLY REPORTS FROM THE DIRECTOR OF HIS RESIDENCY PROGRAM; SHALL ABIDE BY ALL RECOMMENDATIONS OF ASSESSMENT TEAM AT MENNINGER'S; SHALL SUBMIT TO EVERY STATE IN WHICH HE HOLDS LICENSURE AND TO HOSPITALS, CLINICS OR OTHER INSTITUTIONS IN WHICH HE HOLDS OR ANTICIPATES HOLDING ANY FORM OF STAFF PRIVILEGE A COPY OF THIS ORDER; SHALL NOT SUPERVISE ALLIED HEALTH PROFESSIONALS; SHALL KEEP THE BOARD INFORMED OF HIS ADDRESS AND PAY COSTS; SHALL APPEAR BEFORE THE BOARD UPON REQUEST; SHALL LIMIT HIS DUTIES TO THE DUTIES REQUIRED OF RESIDENTS IN THE FAMILY MEDICINE RESIDENCY PROGRAM AT THE UNIVERSITY OF OKLAHOMA HEALTH SCIENCES CENTER; SHALL FORFEIT ANY CREDIT EARNED AS A RESIDENT DURING THE 1998-99 RESIDENCY YEAR AND REPEAT HIS ENTIRE PGY-2 RESIDENCY YEAR FOLLOWING REINSTATEMENT.

YATES, LOUISE T DO, LICENSE NUMBER 3065, WAS DISCIPLINED BY OKLAHOMA ON SEPTEMBER 17, 1998
DISCIPLINARY ACTION: REPRIMAND

YATES, LOUISE T DO, LICENSE NUMBER 3065, WAS DISCIPLINED BY OKLAHOMA ON MARCH 18, 1999
DISCIPLINARY ACTION: LICENSE SUSPENSION; 12-MONTH PROBATION

YOUNG, JAMES A DO, LICENSE NUMBER 0001073, WAS DISCIPLINED BY OKLAHOMA ON SEPTEMBER 20, 1990
DISCIPLINARY ACTION: 18-MONTH LICENSE SUSPENSION; REQUIRED TO ENTER AN IMPAIRED PHYSICIAN PROGRAM OR SUBSTANCE ABUSE TREATMENT
OFFENSE: SUBSTANCE ABUSE

NOTES: FROM 2/88 THROUGH 4/90 WROTE PRESCRIPTIONS TO HIS WIFE FOR INJECTABLE NUBAIN THAT IN FACT WAS FOR HIS OWN PERSONAL USE; INJECTED OR ADMINISTERED NUBAIN FOR HIS OWN PERSONAL USE. REFERRED TO THE IMPAIRED PHYSICIANS COMMITTEE OF THE OKLAHOMA OSTEOPATHIC ASSOCIATION AND THE OKLAHOMA STATE MEDICAL ASSOCIATION; BEFORE HE CAN ASK FOR REMOVAL OF THE SUSPENSION MUST COMPLETE A DRUG ABUSE PROGRAM AND BE IN RECOVERY SUCCESSFULLY WITH THE IMPAIRED PHYSICIANS COMMITTEE.

ZIELINSKI, RICHARD MD, LICENSE NUMBER 0018795 OF 519 EAST STATE ROAD, FAIRVIEW, OK, WAS DISCIPLINED BY OKLAHOMA ON FEBRUARY 18, 1994
DISCIPLINARY ACTION: 60-MONTH PROBATION; RESTRICTION PLACED ON LICENSE

NOTES: PREVIOUSLY HAD A SUPERVISED MEDICAL DOCTOR LICENSE ON PROBATION. IS NOW GRANTED A PHYSICIAN AND SURGEON LICENSE WHICH WILL REMAIN ON PROBATION. CONDITIONS OF PROBATION: SHALL NOT PRESCRIBE, ADMINISTER OR DISPENSE ANY MEDICATIONS FOR HIS PERSONAL USE; SHALL TAKE NO MEDICATION UNLESS AUTHORIZED BY ANOTHER PHYSICIAN FOR A LEGITIMATE MEDICAL NEED; SHALL ABSTAIN FROM THE CONSUMPTION OF ALCOHOL OR ANY SUBSTANCE WHICH WOULD ADVERSELY AFFECT HIS ABILITY TO PRACTICE; SHALL SUBMIT BIOLOGICAL FLUID SPECIMENS; SHALL PROVIDE DOCUMENTATION OF REGULAR PARTICIPATION WITH THE PHYSICIAN'S RECOVERY COMMITTEE AND THREE TIMES PER WEEK ATTENDANCE AT AA AND/OR NARCOTICS ANONYMOUS MEETINGS; SHALL FURNISH BOARD WITH ADDRESS AND/OR CHANGE OF ADDRESS; SHALL APPEAR BEFORE THE BOARD UPON REQUEST AND SUBMIT REQUIRED REPORTS; SHALL PAY COSTS; SHALL SUPPLY A COPY OF THIS ORDER TO ANY HEALTH CARE ENTITY WHERE HE HAS PRIVILEGES; SHALL NOT SUPERVISE A PHYSICIAN'S ASSISTANT.

ZIELINSKI, RICHARD MD, LICENSE NUMBER 18795 OF 900 17TH STREET, WOODWARD, OK, WAS DISCIPLINED BY OKLAHOMA ON JULY 28, 1999
DISCIPLINARY ACTION: PROBATION; RESTRICTION PLACED ON LICENSE
OFFENSE: LOSS OR RESTRICTION OF HOSPITAL PRIVILEGES

NOTES: IN OR AROUND 1/99, AFTER AN INCIDENT THAT OCCURRED IN THE EMERGENCY ROOM WHERE HE WAS WORKING, ADMITTED TO HIS EMPLOYER THAT HE HAD UTILIZED DRUGS WHILE ON DUTY; ADDITIONALLY, HAD A POSITIVE DRUG SCREEN AND ATTEMPTED TO COVER UP HIS MISCONDUCT; HIS EMPLOYMENT WAS SUBSEQUENTLY TERMINATED 2/12/99; FROM 1/26/99-1/29/99 UNDERWENT A MULTIDISCIPLINARY ASSESSMENT WHERE IT WAS RECOMMENDED THAT HE COMPLETE A RELAPSE "AUTOPSY"; FROM 2/8/99-3/5/99 TREATED FOR OPIOID DEPENDENCE WITH RELAPSE. LICENSE LIMITED AS FOLLOWS: SHALL SUBMIT TO EVERY STATE IN WHICH HE HOLDS LICENSURE AND TO HOSPITALS, CLINICS OR OTHER INSTITUTIONS IN WHICH HE HOLDS OR ANTICIPATES HOLDING ANY FORM OF STAFF PRIVILEGE A COPY OF THIS ORDER; SHALL NOT SUPERVISE ALLIED HEALTH PROFESSIONALS; SHALL NOT PRESCRIBE, ADMINISTER, DISPENSE OR POSSESS ANY DRUGS IN SCHEDULE II; SHALL KEEP DUPLICATE, SERIALLY NUMBERED PRESCRIPTIONS OF ALL CONTROLLED DANGEROUS SUBSTANCES AND WILL SUBMIT COPIES TO THE BOARD UPON REQUEST; SHALL SUBMIT BIOLOGICAL FLUID SPECIMENS; SHALL NOT PRESCRIBE, ADMINISTER OR DISPENSE ANY MEDICATIONS FOR HIS PERSONAL USE, OR FOR THAT OF ANY FAMILY MEMBER, AND SHALL TAKE NONE UNLESS AUTHORIZED BY ANOTHER PHYSICIAN FOR A LEGITIMATE MEDICAL NEED; SHALL NOT INGEST ANY SUBSTANCE WHICH WILL CAUSE A SPECIMEN TO TEST POSITIVE FOR PROHIBITED SUBSTANCES; SHALL ABIDE BY TERMS AND RECOMMENDATIONS OF POSTCARE CONTRACTS; SHALL EXECUTE ALL RELEASES OF MEDICAL AND PSYCHIATRIC RECORDS AS NECESSARY TO DISCUSS HIS CASE WITH HIS TREATING PHYSICIANS AND/OR ANY PHYSICIANS HOLDING RECORDS; SHALL ATTEND PERIODIC MEETING OF A LOCAL 12-STEP PROGRAM AND ATTEND 1 MEETING PER WEEK OF THE CADUCEUS GROUP; SHALL ENTER AND CONTINUE COUNSELING, THERAPY OR PSYCHIATRIC TREATMENT AND AUTHORIZE THE RELEASE OF ANY AND ALL RECORDS; SHALL PRACTICE IN A CONTROLLED ENVIRONMENT AND LIMIT HIS PRACTICE TO A MULTI-DOCTOR, GENERAL MEDICINE CLINIC; SHALL NOT PRACTICE IN AN EMERGENCY SETTING OF ANY KIND; SHALL NOT ALLOW THE INDEPENDENT PRACTICE OF MEDICINE BY

ANY PERSONNEL UNDER HIS SUPERVISION; SHALL KEEP THE BOARD INFORMED OF HIS ADDRESS AND PAY COSTS; SHALL APPEAR BEFORE THE BOARD AND SUBMIT REPORTS UPON REQUEST.

TEXAS

1999 serious action rate: 2.71/1000
1999 ranking: 34th

The Texas State Board of Medical Examiners sent newsletters dated from 1990 to the winter of 1992. The disciplinary actions were not individually dated, but they cover roughly through October 1992. The listed action date for these records is the date of the newsletter. The newsletters listed the physician's name, degree, license number, city and state of residence, the date and type of action taken, and usually the reason for the action. In 1992, the board started sending copies of disciplinary orders and they are included through 1999. These orders contain the physician's name, degree, license number, date and type of action taken, and the reason for the action. The orders contain information on modifications and terminations of board actions but not on court decisions affecting board actions. Texas gave us additional information on these actions.

The information provided covers disciplinary actions taken against both allopathic physicians (MDs) and osteopathic physicians (DOs).

Besides disciplinary actions taken by the State Medical Board, this listing also includes actions taken by the Medicare/Medicaid programs, the FDA, and the DEA against physicians located in this state. Disciplinary actions taken by other states against physicians located in Texas or that match a physician disciplined by Texas (see Appendix 2 for an explanation of the matching protocol) are also included.

Although we have made every effort to match physicians' names correctly, some materials we received did not include complete information on middle names, license numbers, birth dates or addresses. Therefore, consumers should remember that non-disciplined physicians and physicians with different disciplinary actions may have similar names to those disciplined physicians listed in this state. Consumers should also remember that if they want the most current information on the status on a physician's license, they should contact the medical board of the state in which the physician practices or had practiced. (See board address below.) Internet address: *http://www.tsbme.state.tx.us/*. This state has a web site which we have graded C on a scale of A (best) to X (worst). This is a measure of the completeness of the information on disciplined doctors. Those state licensing boards with web sites make independent choices about the type of information to be included on their site and how often it is updated.

According to the Federation of State Medical Boards, Texas took 124 serious disciplinary actions against MDs and DOs in 1999. Compared to the 45,707 MDs in the state, Texas had a serious disciplinary action rate of 2.71 serious actions per 1,000 MDs and a ranking of 34th on that list (see Table A, Findings, pg. 14).

The tables below summarize the data Public Citizen received from Texas.

Table 1. Disciplinary Actions Against MDs and DOs 1990 through 1999*

Action	Number	Percent**
Revocation	72	3.5%
Surrender	130	6.4%
Suspension	161	7.9%
Probation	463	22.8%
Practice Restriction	217	10.7%
Action Taken Against Controlled Substance License	160	7.9%
Other Actions	832	40.9%
Total Actions	**2035**	**100.0%**

* This table lists only the two most serious disciplinary actions taken against a physician.
** Percentages may not total 100% due to rounding.

Table 2. Offenses for which MDs and DOs were Disciplined 1990 through 1999*

Offense	Number	Percent
Criminal Conviction	68	5.7%
Sexual Abuse of or Sexual Misconduct with a Patient	46	3.8%
Substandard Care, Incompetence or Negligence	125	10.4%
Misprescribing or Overprescribing Drugs	99	8.2%
Substance Abuse	196	16.3%
Disciplinary Action Taken Against License by Another State or Agency	159	13.2%
Other Offenses	508	42.3%
Total Records With Offense Listed	**1201**	**100.0%**

*Includes only those actions for which an offense was listed and for which we had a corresponding term in our database.

Table 3. Disciplinary Actions Taken for Sexual Abuse of or Sexual Misconduct with a Patient		
Action	**Number**	**Percent**
Revocation	1	1.3%
Surrender	5	6.7%
Suspension	3	4.0%
Emergency Suspension	2	2.7%
Probation	12	16.0%
Fine	6	8.0%
Other Actions	46	61.3%
Total Actions	**75**	**100.0%**

Table 4. Disciplinary Actions Taken for Substandard Care, Incompetence or Negligence		
Action	**Number**	**Percent**
Revocation	3	1.5%
Suspension	4	2.0%
Emergency Suspension	3	1.5%
Probation	45	22.0%
Practice Restriction	39	19.0%
Fine	19	9.3%
Reprimand	30	14.6%
Other Actions	62	30.2%
Total Actions	**205**	**100.0%**

Table 5. Disciplinary Actions Taken for Criminal Conviction

Action	Number	Percent
Revocation	18	20.9%
Surrender	6	7.0%
Suspension	19	22.1%
Emergency Suspension	2	2.3%
Probation	11	12.8%
Fine	6	7.0%
Other Actions	24	27.9%
Total Actions	**86**	**100.0%**

Table 6. Disciplinary Actions Taken for Misprescribing or Overprescribing Drugs

Action	Number	Percent
Revocation	3	1.9%
Surrender	8	5.0%
Revocation, Surrender, or Suspension of Controlled Substance License	6	3.7%
Suspension	6	3.7%
Emergency Suspension	1	0.6%
Probation	34	21.1%
Restriction of Controlled Substance License	22	13.7%
Fine	7	4.3%
Education	27	16.8%
Other Actions	47	29.2%
Total Actions	**161**	**100.0%**

Table 7. Disciplinary Actions Taken for Substance Abuse

Action	Number	Percent
Revocation	5	1.6%
Surrender	2	0.6%
Revocation, Surrender, or Suspension of Controlled Substance License	21	6.5%
Suspension	40	12.5%
Emergency Suspension	18	5.6%
Probation	111	34.6%
Restriction of Controlled Substance License	34	10.6%
Required to Enter an Impaired Physician Program or Substance Abuse Treatment	10	3.1%
Other Actions	80	24.9%
Total Actions	**321**	**100.0%**

If you feel that your doctor has not given you proper medical care or has mistreated you in any way--whether or not he or she is listed in this report--it is important that you let your state medical board know. Even if they do not immediately act on your complaint, it is important that the information be recorded in their files because it is possible that other people may have filed or will file complaints about the same doctor. Send a brief written description of what occurred to the addresses below or call the phone numbers listed for more information on how to file a complaint.

Address

Texas State Board of Medical Examiners
Bruce A. Levy, MD, JD, Executive Secretary
PO Box 2018
Austin, TX 78768-2018
(512) 305-7010
(888) 201-9353

Listing of Doctors Sanctioned by Offense

Sexual Abuse of or Sexual Misconduct with a Patient

ABRANTES, ANTHONY CLARK
AGUIRRE-MORAN, RAFAEL AUGUSTO
ATHARI, MOHAMMAD
BASS, ROBERT K
BROWN, BARRY M
CASEY, JAMES GORDON
FILARDI, HECTOR HIRAM
FINK, JOHN MARK
GOLDMAN, EUGENE JEROME
HICKS, RAYMOND D
HIDALGO, CARLOS H
HULL, JAIME J
JOHNSTON, JAMES CHRISTOPHER
KATZEN, KENNETH LEE
KELLUM, DANIEL H
KORMAN, DAVID JOEL
LEATH, MICHAEL CARTER
LEE, CHUN SHON
LOGAN, WILLIAM M
LOPEZ, LOUIS ALFRED
MARKUS, GEORGE M
MCCLELLAN, DAVID MARK
MIRON, MORTON ARTHUR
MONTOYA, JUAN S
MORRIS, BROCK A
OVERTON, MARVIN C
PAYNE, STEVEN M
PENCE, RONALD M
PRUETT, CHESTER E
RAMIREZ, JOHN P
RAYMOND, DENNIS MICHAEL
RINGER, B R
ROBERTS, GARY F
ROMEU, DELIO G
SINGH, JASBIR BHATIA
SMITH, ART GLENN
TOWNSEND-PARCHMAN, WALLACE
TREVINO, RODOLFO
VILLARREAL, CESAR Q
WARE, STEPHEN HARRISON
WARREN, BRUCE HUNTINGTON
WEBSTER, CHARLES L
WHEELER, JAMES M

Substandard Care, Incompetence, or Negligence

ALLAS, JOSE O
ALMOND, THOMAS HENRY
ANGLE, JOHN FRANKLIN
ASHBY, CHARLES HENRY
AZIM, MOHAMMAD
BAGWELL, JERRY GLYN
BANJO, CHAIM
BELUE, JOE BILL
BEREZOSKI, ROBERT N
BITTLE, CHARLES CARROLL
BLAIR, DONALD LEVESTER
BOGER, JAMES ROBERT
BORDELON, JERRY PHILLIP
BOUDREAU, DANIEL ALEXANDER
BRENNER, JOHN FREDERICK
BROXTON, KYREL DARICE
CHANEY, MARTIN HESTER
CHERIAN, FRANCIS
CHONG, JUAN A
CLAYTON, EUGENE N
CLYNCH, MICHAEL RICHARD
COLE, GEORGE MARTIN
CORMIA, FRANK EDWARD
COSTA, FELIX AUGUSTO
DE LOS SANTOS, RAMIRO
DELGADILLO, FRANCISCO PEDRO
DESHEFY, ALAN N
DIXON, JOSEPH ANDREW
DRISCOLL, STEPHEN EDWARD
FAM, FATHI
FERNANDEZ, CARLOS H
FINCH, ALBERT B
FISCHER, ROY LEE
FISHER, ROY RAY
FONG, ROBERT Y
FRY, LEE PAUL
GAGLIANO, ANGELO VINCENT
GALLOWAY, ROBERT E
GARCIA, EDUARDO I
GOAL, JAY C
GOH, EWE GHEE
GOLDEN, MITCHELL KEITH
GOSWAMI, ANILKUMAR P
GROSSMAN, MAURICE SIDNEY
GUILLERMO, ROMEO DUNGCA
GUIMBARDA, LUIS A
HAMAMCY, THARWAT M
HAMPTON, RAYMOND MADISON
HARRISON, JACK WINFRED
HEAD, WILLIAM JUSTUS
HOBBS, BOBBY R
HOLMES, MICHAEL WESLEY
HOLT, CECIL ZENO
HOUSE, CHARLES HAROLD
HOWELL, SHELLEY M
HUFF, JOHN D

Caution: This list is designed to be used only in conjunction with the rest of this book which includes additional information on each physician such as license number, date of action and more complete descriptions of the offenses.

Substandard Care, Incompetence, or Negligence (cont'd)

ILAHI, MOHAMMAD ARIF
JACKSON, JOSEPH JORDAN
JAMES, JOCELYN LEAH
JAVIER, RICARDO R
JOHNSON, GERALD WAYNE
JOHNSON, HOOPER D
JOHNSON, NEAL D
KASNETZ, HERBERT ROY
KENNADY, DONALD SCOTT
KEY, LUTHER S
KIM, MYUNG JIN
KIRKPATRICK, JAMES L
KOROMPAI, FERENC L
LANGLEY, LAURA LYNN
LARA, FERNAN
LEE, HOWARD MONROE
LESHNOWER, ALAN C
LEVY, JAIME
LIU, KUO TAI
LONG, WALTER KEIRN
LOPEZ, VICTOR M
MABRAY, CHARLES R
MALABANAN, BEN C
MARASIGAN, FREDDIE P
MARTINEZ, MANUEL A
MEHARRY, ROGER ALVIN
MIMS, ROBERT LEWIS
MOAYAD, HAMID
MURRAY, ROBERT VINCENT
NAJERA, MIGUEL E
NIMCHAN, RALPH
NIX, DARRYL D
PARIKH, KIRAN RAJEN
PHILLIPS, TREVOR
POAGE, MARY MARGARET
POEHLMANN, KURT S
PRATUMRAT, PAIROJ
RAMPOLDI, JAMES MOSES
READING, WILLIAM H
RENSHAW, RALPH R
REYES, LUCIO ARTURO
ROBINSON, DANIEL D
SANDERS, MARK S
SCHACHAR, LESLIE
SCHEFFEY, ERIC HESTON
SILVA, MARCELINO S
SOTOODEH, BAGHER
SPEAK, KENNETH EDWIN
SPINKS, DAVID WAYNE
SWATE, TOMMY ERNEST
TALMADGE, JOHN MILLS
TEEL, THEODORE T
THOMAS, FITZGERALD M
THOMPSON, WALTER FRED
TRAN, PAUL CHI
TUCKER, THOMAS ANDREW
TYSON, SAMUEL TILDEN
VAUSE, DAVID DWIGHT
VEGGEBERG, KERMIT ROGER
VERDUZCO, RAFAEL
WASSERMAN, ALAN S
WHITE, DEZRA
WIGG, CINDY LOU
WINSLOW, DAVID EVERETT
WOMACK, JAMES CHANSLOR

Criminal Conviction or Plea of Guilty, Nolo Contendere, or No Contest to a Crime

ABUD-SANCHEZ, DANILO
AGUIRRE-MORAN, RAFAEL AUGUSTO
BACHYNSKY, NICHOLAS
BARTH, THOMAS LESLIE
BONHAM, HENRY EDWARD
BONILLA, JAIME
BOWLER, DONALD L
BRANCH, THOMAS COE
BROWN, JONEL LEONARD
BROWN, WILLIAM C
BURGOS, HERNAN ENRIQUE
CHRIST, JOHN ERNEST
DAVIS, ANTHONY A
EARGLE, CANTRAL L
EMERSON, TIMOTHY JOE
FLEMING, JAMES MICHAEL
GARZA, JUAN JOEL
GIFFORD, LORING A
GINTHER, CLARK E
GOLD, JACOB CHARLES
GONZALEZ, ALPHONSO
GRIFFIN, STEVEN WAYNE
GUERRERO, JORGE
GUO, GEORGE S
HALEY, RICHARD K
HERLIHY, DANIEL JAMES
HIDALGO, CARLOS H
HSU, YU-TO
HUSSEIN, RUQAIYA
INGRAM, CHESTER WILLIAM
JUST, ROBERT JOSEPH
KAUFMAN, IRA S
KEATTS, JAMES G
KIEPFER, RICHARD FRANCIS
LAMURE, DAVID S
LEGGETT, JOSEPH EDWARD
LEVIN, IRA MARK
LIBERMAN, ALBERTO J
LIGHTFOOT, STANLEY AUGUSTUS
LINSTRUM, TOM ELTON

Caution: This list is designed to be used only in conjunction with the rest of this book which includes additional information on each physician such as license number, date of action and more complete descriptions of the offenses.

Criminal Conviction or Plea of Guilty, Nolo Contendere, or No Contest to a Crime (cont'd)

LOFTIS, M DEAN
MARES, ALBERTO
MCLAUGHLIN, RICHARD A
MESSER, DALE L
PATTEN, EDWARD LEE
PAYNE, STEVEN M
RAMAHI, MICHAEL RANDY
REECE, DOUGLAS L
REYES, LUCIO ARTURO
SANDS, LARRY REX
SANTIBANEZ, ALFREDO LUIS
SCHULTZE, JORGE
SHAUGHNESSY, DENNIS M
SHIN, UN KYO
SILBERMAN, MICHAEL K
STENGER, EARL MARTIN
THOMPSON, LLOYD GILBERT
THOMSON, MARY E
TRAN, PAUL CHI
WHITE, JAMES HARRISON
WILLIAMS, ALFRED VAUGHN
WINTEROWD, KEITH GENE
YENTIS, RICHARD DAVID

Misprescribing or Overprescribing Drugs

ADELMAN, JACK ARNOLD
ALFORD, JACK ALLEN
ANDERSON, BERNICE
ANDREWS, RAWLE
AXELROD, WILLIAM
BASPED, BEAUFORD
BENZAQUEN, MATHEWS
BERNATH, ALEXANDER SANDOR
BERRY, SHELLIE J
BILSING, WILLIAM ALBERT
BOONE, GEORGE DANIEL
BORCHERDING, HARLAN JAMES
BRICE, NELSON
BROOKS, JESSE MILES
BROOKS, MARSHALL JAMES
BUCKLEY, THOMAS P
BURLESON, JAMES D
BYRNE, MICHAEL EDWARD
BYRNES, ROBERT J
CANNON, RICHARD A
CARPENTER, CHARLES
CASTANEDA, MANUEL FRANCO
CHAPPELL, TIMOTHY RAE
CHEN, RAY HUANG
CLARK, GEORGE B
COGBURN, CLARENCE G
COX, JOHNSTON STEWART
CRENWELGE, WILBUR E
DOTSON, RODNEY NORMAN
DOUGLAS, HOWARD THOMAS
DUBIN, JOSEPH
DUNN, FRANK LANIER
DWYER, PATRICK DAVID
EASTER, THOMAS GLENN
EDWARDSON, DELBERT L
FABIAN, HAROLD FRANK
FONTANIER, CHARLES EUGENE
FROELICH, JAMES EUGENE
GARDNER, ROBERT L
GIPSON, EDDIE MACK
GIRTANNER, ROBERT EDWARD
GUSTAFSON, WESLEY C
HEALING, ROBERT DYSON
HERNAL, PETER L
HUDDLESTON, WILLIAM E
HUNT, JOHN D
JOHNSON, WILLIAM R
JONES, JAMES HOLLIS
JUNG, ANTHONY CHARLES
KANTOR, JOHN R
KATERNDAHL, DAVID A
KILIAN, ROBERT JACK
LADLEY, DAVID MARK
LONG, JOSEPH MERL
MARES, ALBERTO
MASSAD, EUGENE MASSAD
MAZIQUE, EMORY E
MCCORKLE, RICKY ALLEN
MCELROY, DELMER GUINN
MCLEAN, JAMES R
MELCH, HERBERT R
MOORE, JOSEPH W
MOWATT, IBRAHIM GARCIA
NORRID, HENRY
PARKER, WAYLON MORRIS
PRANGLE, ROBERT E
REES, SEARLE BEAUFORT
REISCHMANN, EDDY
RHOADES, JOE WALKER
RICHTER, JAMES K
RUBINSTEIN, BARNEY
RUDY, ROBERT PATRICK
SAMUELS, MICHAEL G
SARGENT, MICHAEL G
SAYERS, STEPHEN C
SCHULZE, JOHN P
SCHWARTZ, HAROLD ROBERT
SIMON, JEAN-CHARLES
SPAIN, MICHAEL D
SPRINGER, TERRY W
STAYER, DAVID SHELLENBERGE

Caution: This list is designed to be used only in conjunction with the rest of this book which includes additional information on each physician such as license number, date of action and more complete descriptions of the offenses.

Misprescribing or Overprescribing Drugs (cont'd)

STAYER, DAVID SHELLENBERGER
STEGMAN, RONALD REGIS
STERN, STEVEN EMERY
STRINGER, DRENNON DURWOOD
TALMAGE, EDWARD ARTHUR
THOMPSON, FRANK WILLIAM
TITUS, PATRICK A
TUCKER, DONALD TOMMY
UY, SING DY
VANBUSKIRK, RONALD
WALKER, LOUIS E
WILSON, W BRAD
WITHERSPOON, ROBERT GLYNN
WOLF, GARY DUKE
ZEPEDA, RUSSELL WAYNE
ZINGERY, LEWIS W

Substance Abuse

ANDERSON, BERNICE
ANDERSON, VICKI SPARKS
ARCHER, JIM PAUL
BAILEY, SHARON ANNE
BAKER, JACK L
BAKER, JOHN SCOTT
BALLARD, CHARLES DONALD
BALLI, EDWARD A
BARBA, PEDRO
BARTLEY, MICHAEL ALAN
BECK, KEITH DEXTER
BEDNER, TOM DAVID
BENTLEY, GEORGE N
BERRY, G L
BERRY, RICHARD WILLIAM
BIRDWELL, LARRY RAY
BOLIN, DANIEL HUFFMAN
BOONE, MICHAEL KEVIN
BOWLES, THEODORE A
BREITENSTEIN, LARRY JACK
BRINER, BARBARA HADEN
BRITTAIN, ROBERT D
BROUGH, ROYCE DONALD
BROWNE, DUNCAN JAMES
BRUNKEN, ROBERT B
BUTLER, WELDON FRED
CAMMACK, JAMES THOMAS
CARTWRIGHT, GREGORY B
CAYLOR, ARTHUR BERNARD
CHAMBERLAIN, CHARLES D
CHESTER, JEREMY DAVID
CONRAD, EDGAR DONALD
CROPPER, KENNETH R
CURVIN, THOMAS J
CZEKAJ, PHILIP STEPHEN
DARBY, CASTILLA ADOLPHUS
DOTSON, BEVERLY ANN
DOWD, DONNA CATHERINE
DUNCAN, JOHN DAVID
DUNEGAN, MARK ALAN
DYKE, MARSHALL JAMES
EARL, GENE MARKLEY
EIBAND, JOHN M
ELLIS, NEELY JOE
EPPS, DEBRA KENNAMER
ERICKSON, CARL F
FALBEY, ROBERT JOSEPH
FAUST, HARRY LOUIS
FINLEY, OLIVIA I
FOWLER, STEPHEN RICE
GALLMAN, DOYLE F
GARNER, JAMES FRANCIS
GEMOETS, THOMAS HENRY
GILLILAND, MARK B
GLIDDEN, WELDON EDWARD
GORMAN, MARY GWEN
GREEN, DEMETRIS ALLEN
GREEN, KENNETH WAYNE
HARGETT, JOHN M
HEAD, WILLIAM JUSTUS
HINKLEY, BRUCE STANTON
HOUSE, FLOYD LEON
HOWARD, JAMES MARSHALL
HOWELL, WYATT ALLEN
HUBBARD, GREGORY GERARD
HUMMER, MICHAEL GORMAN
HUNTER, RICHARD BROOKSHIRE
JACKSON, NICHOLAS M
JOHNSON, SHEILA MOLLY
JONES, ROLAND WARD
KAUFFMAN, ROBERT P
KENNEDY, JERETTA IRENE
KETTERER, CYNTHIA LEE
KIMMONS, JOHN HENRY
KING, CLARENCE GORDON
KING, DENNIS MAURICE
KRAUS, VERNON J
KUHL, PETER VAN DOREN
KUO, LIMEI
KURTZ, IRWIN
LECONEY, THOMAS RATCLIFF
LEDLIE, WILLIAM BOYER
LEHMILLER, JOHN ERICH
LETT, CHARLES REGINALD
LEVIN, IRA MARK
LEWIS, EDWARD A
LEWIS, ELBERT HAMPTON
LOCKWOOD, RICHARD L
LOVELACE, CHARLES RAY
MAGEE, DOUGLAS LEE

Caution: This list is designed to be used only in conjunction with the rest of this book which includes additional information on each physician such as license number, date of action and more complete descriptions of the offenses.

Substance Abuse (cont'd)

MANION, ROBERT A
MARKSTROM, CARL ERIC
MARTINEZ, ALBERTO NOE
MASSEY, CHARLES R
MCCALLUM, MICHAEL H
MCCORKLE, ALLAN JAMES
MCCORKLE, BRANDT HALBERT
MCDANIEL, BRIAN D
MCFARLAND, BRUCE ROBIN
MCGINNESS, JOHN E
MCLEAN, PAUL EUGENE
MICHAELIS, MICHAEL LYNN
MOORE, M J
MORGAN, MICKEY D
MORRISON, RICHARD FRANK
MURPHY, FRANK STUART
NEWMAN, NICK JAY
O'BRYAN, ROBERT KEENE
OFFUTT, DONALD NIXON
PENNINGTON, KAREN
PHILLIPS, GREGGORY K
PRATER, WILLIAM WARREN
PUGH, MARION C
PULLIAM, KATHY A
QUENNEVILLE, KENNETH BRUCE
RANELLE, JOHN BARRY
RANKIN, DOUGLAS HALL
RATLIFF, HUBERT WESLEY
REYNOLDS, JARRELL PAUL
RHODES, THOMAS P
RICE, KARL WOODS
RIEDWEG, EDWARD ALBERT
ROBINETT, KELLY EUGENE
ROBINSON, LUKE E
RUSH, AVRIL BRICKLEY
RYAN, ANDREW JACK
SABATES, FELIX NABOR
SAUCEDA, FRANCISCO BASIL
SEGGER, FRANZJOSEF
SERRANO, ANTONIO P
SHARP, DOUGLAS ROBERT
SHARY, JOHN H
SHAUGHNESSY, DENNIS M
SHERP, GARY ALLAN
SHIELDS, FREDERICK S
SLUSHER, KEVIN D
SMITH, GEORGE ROBERT
SMITH, MONTE KEITH
SORIANO, SALVADOR L
STANTON, JAMES MICHAEL
STEELE, JOHN GILBERT
STILL, ROBERT LYLE
TAMEZ, RICHARD JOSEPH
THOMAS, STEPHEN C
TICAS, ROBERTO A
TODD, WILLIAM DAVID
ULDRICH, DENNIS ALAN
VICKERS, FRANK ALLEN
VILLEGAS, LEOPOLD
WALLACE, C B
WEST, PATRICIA BEATY
WESTBROOK, MARK DENTON
WHITMAN, PAUL F
WILLIAMSON, MARK A
WILSON, ROBERT STOREY
WIMBERLY, DAVID M
WIMPEE, MARC W

Caution: This list is designed to be used only in conjunction with the rest of this book which includes additional information on each physician such as license number, date of action and more complete descriptions of the offenses.

ABADIER, ABDALLA MD, LICENSE NUMBER 00G8662 OF E GREENWICK, RI, WAS DISCIPLINED BY TEXAS ON JANUARY 6, 1995
DISCIPLINARY ACTION: LICENSE REVOCATION
OFFENSE: PROFESSIONAL MISCONDUCT

NOTES: VOLUNTARILY SURRENDERED RHODE ISLAND LICENSE IN 5/93 FOR UNPROFESSIONAL OR DISHONORABLE CONDUCT AND PROFESSIONAL FAILURE TO PRACTICE MEDICINE IN AN ACCEPTABLE MANNER CONSISTENT WITH PUBLIC HEALTH AND WELFARE; VIOLATED TERMS OF AGREEMENTS WITH TWO HOSPITALS RESTRICTING HIS ADMITTING AND SURGICAL PRIVILEGES. ORDER WILL BECOME FINAL WHEN ADMINISTRATIVE APPEALS HAVE BEEN EXHAUSTED; HAS 20 DAYS TO FILE A MOTION FOR REHEARING.

ABDAL-ALIM, KHALID B DO, DATE OF BIRTH FEBRUARY 28, 1953 OF 4807 FITCH STREET, HOUSTON, TX, WAS DISCIPLINED BY MEDICARE ON AUGUST 10, 1995
DISCIPLINARY ACTION: EXCLUSION FROM THE MEDICARE AND/OR MEDICAID PROGRAM
OFFENSE: NONCOMPLIANCE WITH A PROFESSIONAL RULE

NOTES: DEFAULTED ON PUBLIC HEALTH SERVICE EDUCATION LOAN.

ABLE, ANTOINNE MD, DATE OF BIRTH FEBRUARY 28, 1958 OF 4041 MEDICAL DRIVE, SAN ANTONIO, TX, WAS DISCIPLINED BY MEDICARE ON MAY 23, 1993
DISCIPLINARY ACTION: EXCLUSION FROM THE MEDICARE AND/OR MEDICAID PROGRAM
OFFENSE: NONCOMPLIANCE WITH A PROFESSIONAL RULE

NOTES: DEFAULTED ON HEALTH EDUCATION ASSISTANCE LOAN. REINSTATED ON 7/5/95.

ABRAHAM, MALOUF JR MD, DATE OF BIRTH MARCH 29, 1939, LICENSE NUMBER 00D1528 OF 720 ASH, CANADIAN, TX, WAS DISCIPLINED BY TEXAS ON APRIL 30, 1993
DISCIPLINARY ACTION: REPRIMAND
OFFENSE: NONCOMPLIANCE WITH A PROFESSIONAL RULE

NOTES: FAILED TO DOCUMENT THE HISTORY AND PHYSICAL OF SEVERAL PATIENTS INCLUDING REASON FOR ADMINISTERING MEDICATIONS.

ABRANTES, ANTHONY CLARK MD, LICENSE NUMBER F6375 OF SHERMAN, TX, WAS DISCIPLINED BY TEXAS ON AUGUST 9, 1997
DISCIPLINARY ACTION: 60-MONTH PROBATION; RESTRICTION PLACED ON LICENSE
OFFENSE: SEXUAL ABUSE OF OR SEXUAL MISCONDUCT WITH A PATIENT

NOTES: IN 7/93 HE PRESCRIBED FASTIN TO A PATIENT WITHOUT ANY OR ADEQUATE INDICATION; IN 1993 HE ENGAGED IN SEXUAL RELATIONS WITH THIS PATIENT WHO HE HAD BEEN TREATING SINCE 1991. SUSPENSION STAYED FOR PROBATION WITH FOLLOWING TERMS AND CONDITIONS: SHALL NOT TREAT ANY PATIENT FOR WEIGHT CONTROL OR OBESITY; SHALL NOMINATE THREE CERTIFIED PSYCHIATRISTS FOR BOARD SELECTION OF A THERAPIST AND SHALL EXPEDITIOUSLY SUBMIT HIMSELF TO EVALUATION AND TREATMENT BY THE APPROVED PRACTITIONER; SHALL HAVE A FEMALE CHAPERONE ANYTIME HE EXAMINES A FEMALE PATIENT; SHALL NOT TREAT OR OTHERWISE SERVE AS PHYSICIAN, PRESCRIBE, DISPENSE OR ADMINISTER DRUGS THAT MAY BE SUBJECT TO ABUSE TO HIMSELF OR TO ANY MEMBER OF HIS FAMILY; SHALL NOT POSSESS, ADMINISTER, DISPENSE OR SUPPLY PHARMACEUTICAL SAMPLES WITH POTENTIAL FOR ABUSE TO ANY PATIENT; SEPARATE FROM PATIENT RECORDS, SHALL MAINTAIN A FILE OF EVERY PRESCRIPTION WRITTEN BY HIM FOR DANGEROUS DRUGS WITH ADDICTIVE POTENTIAL WHICH SHALL BE MADE AVAILABLE FOR REVIEW; $5,000 FINE; SHALL OBTAIN AT LEAST 50 HOURS PER YEAR OF CONTINUING MEDICAL EDUCATION; SHALL OBTAIN SIX HOURS OF ETHICS THROUGH COURSES OR PROGRAMS AND SHALL SUCCESSFULLY COMPLETE A COURSE IN THE AREA OF PHARMACOLOGY WITHIN ONE YEAR; SHALL APPEAR BEFORE THE BOARD AT LEAST ONCE A YEAR; SHALL COOPERATE WITH THE BOARD IN VERIFYING COMPLIANCE; TIME SPENT OUT OF TEXAS DOES NOT COUNT TOWARD PROBATION; SHALL INFORM THE BOARD OF CHANGE OF ADDRESS WITHIN 10 DAYS OR IF HE LEAVES THE STATE; SHALL NOT SEEK MODIFICATION FOR ONE YEAR; REPRIMAND. ON 8/22/98 BOARD ORDER TERMINATED.

ABUD-SANCHEZ, DANILO MD, LICENSE NUMBER 00H1545 OF EL PASO, TX, WAS DISCIPLINED BY TEXAS ON OCTOBER 9, 1992
DISCIPLINARY ACTION: 60-MONTH PROBATION
OFFENSE: CRIMINAL CONVICTION OR PLEA OF GUILTY, NOLO CONTENDERE, OR NO CONTEST TO A CRIME

NOTES: CONVICTION OF FELONY FOR FILING FALSE, FICTITIOUS OR FRAUDULENT CLAIMS. SUSPENSION, STAYED. PROBATION UNDER TERMS AND CONDITIONS

ABUD-SANCHEZ, DANILO MD, LICENSE NUMBER 00H1545 OF EL PASO, TX, WAS DISCIPLINED BY TEXAS ON JANUARY 6, 1995
DISCIPLINARY ACTION: SURRENDER OF LICENSE

NOTES: ALLEGATIONS OF POSSIBLE VIOLATIONS OF MEDICAL PRACTICE ACT; HE DOES NOT ADMIT VIOLATIONS; SURRENDER IN LIEU OF FURTHER INVESTIGATION AND TO EFFECTUATE HIS RETIREMENT. SHALL NOT PETITION FOR REINSTATEMENT.

ACREMAN, ANNE ELIZABETH MD, LICENSE NUMBER G3100 OF ODESSA, TX, WAS DISCIPLINED BY TEXAS ON AUGUST 22, 1998
DISCIPLINARY ACTION: FINE
OFFENSE: NONCOMPLIANCE WITH A PROFESSIONAL RULE

NOTES: ON 11/25/97 SHE WAS NOTIFIED BY BOARD LETTER OF A PENDING INVESTIGATION, WHICH INVOLVED ALLEGATIONS OF A PRACTICE INCONSISTENT WITH THE PUBLIC HEALTH AND WELFARE; ON 1/27/98 SHE EXPLAINED TO THE BOARD THAT SHE WAS ENCOUNTERING DIFFICULTIES IN OBTAINING CERTAIN BILLING DOCUMENTATION IN ORDER TO PROVIDE THE BOARD WITH A COMPLETE RECORD; A SUBPOENA WAS ISSUED AND WAS RECEIVED BY HER OFFICE ON 3/15/98; SHE FAILED TO RESPOND TO THE SUBPOENA OR TO THE PREVIOUS REQUESTS UNTIL 4/20/98. $1,000 FINE; SHALL INFORM THE BOARD OF CHANGE OF ADDRESS WITHIN 10 DAYS.

ADAMS, BARTON J DO, LICENSE NUMBER 00G7150 OF KAHULUI, HI, WAS DISCIPLINED BY TEXAS ON OCTOBER 9, 1992
DISCIPLINARY ACTION: SURRENDER OF LICENSE
OFFENSE: DISCIPLINARY ACTION BY ANOTHER STATE OR AGENCY

NOTES: UNPROFESSIONAL OR DISHONORABLE CONDUCT LIKELY TO DECEIVE, DEFRAUD OR INJURE THE PUBLIC; CONVICTION OF A FELONY OR A CRIME OF A LESSER DEGREE THAT INVOLVES MORAL TURPITUDE; SUSPENSION, REVOCATION OR RESTRICTION BY ANOTHER STATE. LICENSE PERMANENTLY RETIRED.

ADAMS, BARTON J DO OF SAN JOSE, CA, WAS DISCIPLINED BY VERMONT ON DECEMBER 3, 1996

DISCIPLINARY ACTION: EMERGENCY SUSPENSION
OFFENSE: DISCIPLINARY ACTION BY ANOTHER STATE OR AGENCY

NOTES: IN 1992 LICENSES REVOKED IN HAWAII AND TEXAS BECAUSE HE ENGAGED IN SEXUAL CONTACT WITH PATIENTS.

ADAMS, BARTON JOSEPH DO, DATE OF BIRTH NOVEMBER 17, 1951, LICENSE NUMBER 0000516, WAS DISCIPLINED BY HAWAII ON FEBRUARY 24, 1992
DISCIPLINARY ACTION: EMERGENCY SUSPENSION
OFFENSE: SEXUAL ABUSE OF OR SEXUAL MISCONDUCT WITH A PATIENT

NOTES: IN 3/90 SEXUALLY ASSAULTED A FEMALE EMPLOYEE WHILE EXAMINING HER; IN 6/91 PERFORMED A BREAST EXAMINATION ON ONE PATIENT WHO REQUESTED TREATMENT FOR FACIAL ACNE; IN 1991, DURING THE EXAMINATION OF ANOTHER PATIENT FOR AN EAR INFECTION, RESTED HIS HAND ON HER BREAST. SUMMARY SUSPENSION EXTENDED 3/13/92.

ADAMS, BARTON JOSEPH DO, DATE OF BIRTH NOVEMBER 17, 1951, LICENSE NUMBER 0000516 OF 261 LALO STREET, KAHULUI, HI, WAS DISCIPLINED BY HAWAII ON JULY 10, 1992
DISCIPLINARY ACTION: 24-MONTH LICENSE REVOCATION
OFFENSE: SEXUAL ABUSE OF OR SEXUAL MISCONDUCT WITH A PATIENT

NOTES: IN 3/90 SEXUALLY ASSAULTED A FEMALE EMPLOYEE WHILE EXAMINING HER; IN 6/91 PERFORMED A BREAST EXAMINATION ON ONE PATIENT WHO REQUESTED TREATMENT FOR FACIAL ACNE; IN 1991 DURING THE EXAMINATION OF ANOTHER PATIENT FOR AN EAR INFECTION, RESTED HIS HAND ON HER BREAST. REVOCATION RETROACTIVE TO 5/15/92.

ADAMS, BARTON JOSEPH DO, DATE OF BIRTH NOVEMBER 17, 1951, LICENSE NUMBER 0000923, WAS DISCIPLINED BY WEST VIRGINIA ON JANUARY 14, 1993
DISCIPLINARY ACTION: LICENSE REVOCATION

ADAMS, BARTON JOSEPH DO, DATE OF BIRTH NOVEMBER 17, 1951, LICENSE NUMBER 0027020 OF 99902 MOANAHIA HIGHWAY, AIEA, HI, WAS DISCIPLINED BY GEORGIA ON NOVEMBER 9, 1993
DISCIPLINARY ACTION: LICENSE REVOCATION
OFFENSE: DISCIPLINARY ACTION BY ANOTHER STATE OR AGENCY

NOTES: BASED ON ACTION BY HAWAII BOARD, SEXUAL ASSAULT OF FEMALE PATIENTS. CONVICTED OF THREE COUNTS OF SEXUAL ASSAULT IN HAWAII. ON 9/9/94 THE INTERMEDIATE COURT OF APPEALS OF HAWAII VACATED THE JUDGMENT OF CONVICTION WHICH SERVED AS ONE OF THE BASES FOR THE HAWAII BOARD ACTION AND REMANDED THE MATTER TO THE LOWER COURT FOR FURTHER PROCEEDINGS CONSISTENT WITH THIS OPINION. ON 10/16/95 THE CIRCUIT COURT OF THE SECOND CIRCUIT GRANTED HIS MOTION TO DISMISS BASED ON VIOLATION OF SPEEDY TRIAL. HE WILL NEVER BE RETRIED FOR THESE CHARGES. BASED ON THIS DECISION, THE HAWAII BOARD REDACTED ITS ORDER AND EXPUNGED THE CONVICTIONS AS ONE OF THE BASES OF THE REVOCATION.

ADAMS, BARTON JOSEPH DO, DATE OF BIRTH NOVEMBER 17, 1951 OF 261 LALO STREET, KAHULUI, HI, WAS DISCIPLINED BY DEA ON JANUARY 28, 1994
DISCIPLINARY ACTION: REVOCATION OF CONTROLLED SUBSTANCE LICENSE
OFFENSE: DISCIPLINARY ACTION BY ANOTHER STATE OR AGENCY

NOTES: ON 3/29/90 HE SEXUALLY ASSAULTED A PATIENT AND ON 1/30/92 WAS CONVICTED OF THREE COUNTS OF SEXUAL ASSAULT IN THE SECOND DEGREE. AS A RESULT OF THE CONVICTION AND OTHER ALLEGATIONS OF SEXUAL ASSAULT, HAWAII REVOKED HIS LICENSE ON 7/10/92. ON 6/30/92 HIS STATE CONTROLLED SUBSTANCE REGISTRATION EXPIRED. DEA CERTIFICATE OF REGISTRATION REVOKED DUE TO HIS LACK OF AUTHORIZATION TO HANDLE CONTROLLED SUBSTANCES IN HAWAII. ON 9/9/94 THE INTERMEDIATE COURT OF APPEALS OF HAWAII VACATED THE JUDGMENT OF CONVICTION WHICH SERVED AS ONE OF THE BASES FOR THE HAWAII BOARD ACTION AND REMANDED THE MATTER TO THE LOWER COURT FOR FURTHER PROCEEDINGS CONSISTENT WITH THIS OPINION. ON 10/16/95 THE CIRCUIT COURT OF THE SECOND CIRCUIT GRANTED HIS MOTION TO DISMISS BASED ON VIOLATION OF SPEEDY TRIAL. HE WILL NEVER BE RETRIED FOR THESE CHARGES. BASED ON THIS DECISION, THE HAWAII BOARD REDACTED ITS ORDER AND EXPUNGED THE CONVICTIONS AS ONE OF THE BASES OF THE REVOCATION.

ADAMS, BARTON JOSEPH DO, DATE OF BIRTH NOVEMBER 17, 1951, LICENSE NUMBER 0026287 OF COLORADO SPRINGS, CO, WAS DISCIPLINED BY COLORADO ON AUGUST 19, 1994
DISCIPLINARY ACTION: LICENSE REVOCATION
OFFENSE: SEXUAL ABUSE OF OR SEXUAL MISCONDUCT WITH A PATIENT

NOTES: FELONY CONVICTION IN HAWAII. SEXUAL ACT WITH A PATIENT. ON 12/9/96 COLORADO BOARD RECEIVED REQUEST FOR RECONSIDERATION AS APPELLATE COURT HAD OVERTURNED THE CONVICTION AND REMANDED IT FOR A NEW TRIAL; CHARGES WERE THEN DISMISSED DUE TO A VIOLATION OF A RIGHT TO A SPEEDY TRIAL. HE WILL NOT BE RETRIED ON THOSE CHARGES. HOWEVER, COLORADO BOARD DETERMINED THAT BASED ON HAVING ENGAGED IN A SEXUAL ACT WITH A PATIENT IN THE COURSE OF PATIENT CARE, HE HAD ENGAGED IN UNPROFESSIONAL CONDUCT AND ISSUED A FINAL BOARD ORDER AFTER RECONSIDERATION ON 2/14/97 AFFIRMING THE REVOCATION. REVOCATION STANDS AS OF 2/14/97.

ADAMS, GEORGE L MD, LICENSE NUMBER 00E4982 OF CENTRE HARBOR, NH, WAS DISCIPLINED BY TEXAS ON APRIL 10, 1992

NOTES: FINAL ACTION DEFERRED FOR ONE YEAR PENDING RESOLUTION OF CRIMINAL CASE. AGREED NOT TO PRACTICE MEDICINE IN TEXAS IN THE INTERIM. ON 1/29/99 ORDER TERMINATED.

ADEGBITE, SAMSON G MD, LICENSE NUMBER 175350 OF 28 STONELEDGE COURT, WILLIAMSVILLE, NY, WAS DISCIPLINED BY NEW YORK ON JULY 8, 1998
DISCIPLINARY ACTION: 36-MONTH PROBATION; FINE
OFFENSE: PROFESSIONAL MISCONDUCT

NOTES: CONDUCT DURING THE PRACTICE OF MEDICINE WHICH EVIDENCES MORAL UNFITNESS. $14,000 FINE; REPRIMAND.

ADEGBITE, SAMSON G MD, LICENSE NUMBER J6843 OF BUFFALO, NY, WAS DISCIPLINED BY TEXAS ON MAY 14, 1999
DISCIPLINARY ACTION: LICENSE SUSPENSION
OFFENSE: DISCIPLINARY ACTION BY ANOTHER STATE OR AGENCY

NOTES: HE IS UNDER A CONSENT AGREEMENT EFFECTIVE 7/8/98 WITH THE NEW YORK BOARD FOR UNPROFESSIONAL CONDUCT ARISING OUT OF ALLEGED SEXUAL HARASSMENT OF TWO NURSES; HE

CONTESTED ALLEGATIONS THAT HE ENGAGED IN INAPPROPRIATE PHYSICAL CONDUCT WITH THE TWO NURSES BUT DID NOT CONTEST THAT HE MADE LEWD AND SEXUALLY SUGGESTIVE REMARKS, GESTURES, AND COMMENTS DIRECTED TO THESE TWO NURSES. SUSPENSION UNTIL HE REQUESTS TO HAVE THE SUSPENSION STAYED OR APPEARS BEFORE THE BOARD WITH SUFFICIENT EVIDENCE THAT HE IS PHYSICALLY, MENTALLY OR OTHERWISE COMPETENT TO PRACTICE SAFELY INCLUDING AT A MINIMUM: A NEURO-PSYCHIATRIC EVALUATION; AND THAT TERMS OF PROBATION HAVE EXPIRED AND HE HAS AN UNRESTRICTED LICENSE IN GOOD STANDING IN NEW YORK, OR THAT HE IS IN FULL COMPLIANCE WITH ALL TERMS OF PROBATION; SHALL COOPERATE WITH THE BOARD IN VERIFYING COMPLIANCE; SHALL INFORM THE BOARD OF CHANGE OF ADDRESS WITHIN 10 DAYS; SHALL NOT SEEK MODIFICATION FOR ONE YEAR.

ADEGBITE, SAMSON G MD, LICENSE NUMBER 175350 OF 28 STONELEDGE COURT, WILLIAMSVILLE, NY, WAS DISCIPLINED BY NEW YORK ON SEPTEMBER 9, 1999
DISCIPLINARY ACTION: 48-MONTH PROBATION; FINE
OFFENSE: PROFESSIONAL MISCONDUCT

NOTES: CONDUCT DURING THE PRACTICE OF MEDICINE WHICH EVIDENCES MORAL UNFITNESS INVOLVING FEMALE STAFF MEMBERS. TWO YEAR SUSPENSION STAYED; $2,500 FINE; THREE MONTHS OF INTENSIVE THERAPY AND TREATMENT.

ADELMAN, JACK ARNOLD MD, LICENSE NUMBER 00B6953, WAS DISCIPLINED BY TEXAS ON AUGUST 20, 1993
DISCIPLINARY ACTION: 36-MONTH PROBATION; REQUIRED TO TAKE ADDITIONAL MEDICAL EDUCATION
OFFENSE: OVERPRESCRIBING OR MISPRESCRIBING DRUGS

NOTES: ON VARIOUS OCCASIONS OVER SEVERAL YEARS, PRESCRIBED THE CONTROLLED SUBSTANCES TEMAZEPAM AND MORPHINE TO ONE PATIENT WITHOUT PROPERLY DOCUMENTING INTRACTABLE PAIN SO AS TO PROVIDE SUFFICIENT MEDICAL JUSTIFICATION; DID NOT DOCUMENT ADEQUATE FOLLOW-UP EXAMS AND MONITORING. SUSPENSION STAYED. CONDITIONS OF PROBATION: SHALL ATTEND AT LEAST 50 HOURS PER YEAR OF CONTINUING MEDICAL EDUCATION; IN ADDITION SHALL, WITHIN ONE YEAR, ENROLL IN AND SUBSEQUENTLY COMPLETE A PHARMACOLOGY COURSE FOR 10 HOURS OF CREDITS; SEPARATE FROM PATIENT RECORDS SHALL MAINTAIN A FILE OF EVERY PRESCRIPTION WRITTEN FOR CONTROLLED SUBSTANCES OR DANGEROUS DRUGS WHICH SHALL BE AVAILABLE FOR INSPECTION; SHALL NOT TELEPHONE ANY PRESCRIPTIONS FOR THESE DRUGS; SHALL APPEAR BEFORE THE BOARD ONCE A YEAR; SHALL COOPERATE WITH THE BOARD IN VERIFYING COMPLIANCE; SHALL INFORM BOARD OF CHANGE OF ADDRESS WITHIN 10 DAYS OR IF HE LEAVES THE STATE; TIME SPENT OUT OF TEXAS DOES NOT COUNT TOWARD PROBATION NOR WILL ANY PERIODS OF TIME AFTER WHICH HE RETIRES FROM THE PRACTICE OF MEDICINE. SHALL NOT SEEK MODIFICATION FOR ONE YEAR.

ADELMAN, NEIL H MD, DATE OF BIRTH SEPTEMBER 18, 1950, LICENSE NUMBER 0036574 OF 116 WALNUT DRIVE, PAMPA, TX, WAS DISCIPLINED BY NEW JERSEY ON SEPTEMBER 26, 1996

NOTES: RECEIPT OF PATIENT COMPLAINTS CONCERNING TREATMENT FOR LYME DISEASE. AGREES TO REFRAIN FROM THE PRACTICE OF MEDICINE AND SURGERY IN NEW JERSEY UNTIL MATTERS PENDING BEFORE THE BOARD HAVE BEEN SATISFACTORILY RESOLVED. SHALL IMMEDIATELY NOTIFY THE BOARD OF HIS RETURN TO NEW JERSEY AND HIS PRACTICE PLANS.

ADEN, GARY CARL MD, DATE OF BIRTH NOVEMBER 18, 1935 OF 2403 CORONA CT, LA JOLLA, CA, WAS DISCIPLINED BY MEDICARE ON MAY 23, 1990
DISCIPLINARY ACTION: EXCLUSION FROM THE MEDICARE AND/OR MEDICAID PROGRAM
OFFENSE: DISCIPLINARY ACTION BY ANOTHER STATE OR AGENCY

NOTES: LICENSE REVOCATION OR SUSPENSION.

ADEN, GARY CARL MD, DATE OF BIRTH NOVEMBER 18, 1935, LICENSE NUMBER 0014167 OF LA JOLLA, CA, WAS DISCIPLINED BY COLORADO ON JUNE 7, 1991
DISCIPLINARY ACTION: SURRENDER OF LICENSE
OFFENSE: DISCIPLINARY ACTION BY ANOTHER STATE OR AGENCY

NOTES: GROSSLY NEGLIGENT MEDICAL PRACTICE, ENGAGING IN A SEXUAL ACT WITH A PATIENT DURING THE COURSE OF PATIENT CARE, AND STIPULATED TO REVOCATION OF HIS CALIFORNIA LICENSE EFFECTIVE 10/9/89 ALTHOUGH HE SPECIFICALLY DENIED ALL CHARGES. AGREEMENT WITH COLORADO NEVER TO REQUEST REINSTATEMENT OR APPLY FOR A NEW LICENSE.

ADEN, GARY CARL MD, DATE OF BIRTH NOVEMBER 18, 1935, LICENSE NUMBER 00D2974 OF 2403 CORONA COURT, LA JOLLA, CA, WAS DISCIPLINED BY TEXAS ON OCTOBER 5, 1991
DISCIPLINARY ACTION: LICENSE REVOCATION
OFFENSE: DISCIPLINARY ACTION BY ANOTHER STATE OR AGENCY

NOTES: CALIFORNIA LICENSE WAS REVOKED BECAUSE OF SEXUALLY ABUSIVE AND VIOLENT TREATMENT OF SEVEN PATIENTS UNDER HIS PSYCHIATRIC CARE; ALSO FAILED TO COMPLY WITH CALIFORNIA BOARD ORDER OF 10/9/89 TO UNDERGO A PSYCHIATRIC EVALUATION.

ADKINS, MARGO M MD, DATE OF BIRTH JANUARY 13, 1960 OF 2500 E 22ND STREET #213, AUSTIN, TX, WAS DISCIPLINED BY MEDICARE ON APRIL 16, 1994
DISCIPLINARY ACTION: EXCLUSION FROM THE MEDICARE AND/OR MEDICAID PROGRAM
OFFENSE: NONCOMPLIANCE WITH A PROFESSIONAL RULE

NOTES: DEFAULTED ON PUBLIC HEALTH SERVICE EDUCATION LOAN.

AGBEBIYI, JONATHAN A MD, LICENSE NUMBER 0013271, WAS DISCIPLINED BY ARIZONA ON JANUARY 24, 1991
OFFENSE: SUBSTANDARD CARE, INCOMPETENCE OR NEGLIGENCE

NOTES: CHARGED WITH UNPROFESSIONAL CONDUCT: GROSS MALPRACTICE, REPEATED MALPRACTICE, OR ANY MALPRACTICE RESULTING IN THE DEATH OF A PATIENT; KNOWINGLY MAKING ANY FALSE OR FRAUDULENT STATEMENT IN CONNECTION WITH THE PRACTICE OF MEDICINE; AND FAILING TO FURNISH INFORMATION IN A TIMELY MANNER FOR THE BOARD. ISSUED A DECREE OF CENSURE AND MUST REPORT BACK TO THE BOARD WITHIN 30 DAYS THAT HE HAS CORRECTED MATTERS; SHALL NOT UTILIZE VITAMIN B12 INJECTIONS, EXCEPT FOR MEDICALLY INDICATED REASONS.

AGBEBIYI, JONATHAN A MD, LICENSE NUMBER 0013271, WAS DISCIPLINED BY ARIZONA ON JUNE 19, 1991

DISCIPLINARY ACTION: 60-MONTH PROBATION; FINE
OFFENSE: OVERCHARGING

NOTES: BOARD INVESTIGATED POSSIBLE OVERCHARGING OF THREE PATIENTS. ORDERED TO PAY RESTITUTION TO TWO PATIENTS DESCRIBED. DURING PROBATION THE BOARD WILL CONDUCT A REEVALUATION OF HIS BILLING PROCEDURES. $2,500 FINE. ORDER MODIFIED ON 10/11/91: ORDER OF PROBATION AND FINE CANCELED; ONLY ONE CASE OF OVERCHARGING WAS CONSIDERED. SHALL PAY RESTITUTION; SURVEY WILL BE CONDUCTED OF PRACTICE WITHIN ONE YEAR.

AGBEBIYI, JONATHAN A MD, LICENSE NUMBER 0013271 OF PHOENIX, AZ, WAS DISCIPLINED BY ARIZONA ON JANUARY 26, 1994
DISCIPLINARY ACTION: LICENSE REVOCATION
OFFENSE: SUBSTANDARD CARE, INCOMPETENCE OR NEGLIGENCE

NOTES: IN 3/91 PERFORMED A HYSTERECTOMY DURING WHICH HE SHOULD HAVE BEEN MORE AGGRESSIVE IN STOPPING BLOOD LOSS WHICH WAS A HEALTH-THREATENING SITUATION. IN 7/91 MEDICAL MANAGEMENT AND CLINICAL JUDGMENT IN HANDLING A PATIENT WERE INADEQUATE AND PATIENT WAS PLACED IN SERIOUS JEOPARDY DUE TO THE UNEXPLAINED DELAY BETWEEN DIAGNOSIS AND SURGERY. IN BOTH CASES OPERATIVE REPORTS AND DISCHARGE SUMMARIES WERE NOT FILLED OUT IN A TIMELY MANNER. HOSPITAL PRIVILEGES WERE SUSPENDED ON 12/20/91 PARTIALLY BECAUSE OF UNWILLINGNESS TO ACCEPT RESPONSIBILITY FOR ACTIONS OR MAINTAIN MALPRACTICE INSURANCE; ENTERED INTO AGREEMENT WITH HOSPITAL ON 2/19/92. DID NOT PROPERLY HANDLE HIS OFFICE CLOSURE WITH REGARD TO ONE PATIENT WHO HAD PAID HIM IN ADVANCE FOR A DELIVERY AND WHOM HE DID NOT INFORM HE WAS CLOSING HIS PRACTICE NOR HAD HE REFERRED HER TO ANOTHER PHYSICIAN; ONLY ABOUT 1/2 OF PATIENT RECORDS WERE RETRIEVED AFTER HIS OFFICE CLOSED. AS OF DATE OF ORDER WAS WORKING IN CORPUS CHRISTI, TEXAS. ORDER OF REVOCATION AFFIRMED BY COURT ON 4/28/95; TIME TO APPEAL HAS RUN.

AGBEBIYI, JONATHAN A MD, LICENSE NUMBER 0G46725 OF CORPUS CHRISTI, TX, WAS DISCIPLINED BY CALIFORNIA ON JUNE 30, 1995
DISCIPLINARY ACTION: 60-MONTH PROBATION
OFFENSE: DISCIPLINARY ACTION BY ANOTHER STATE OR AGENCY

NOTES: DISCIPLINE BY ARIZONA BOARD FOR OB-GYN PRACTICE THAT WAS HARMFUL OR DANGEROUS TO PATIENTS. REVOCATION STAYED.

AGBEBIYI, JONATHAN ADESHINA MD, DATE OF BIRTH SEPTEMBER 7, 1949, LICENSE NUMBER 1041053 OF PO BOX 181135, CORPUS CHRISTI, TX, WAS DISCIPLINED BY MICHIGAN ON AUGUST 7, 1995
DISCIPLINARY ACTION: EMERGENCY SUSPENSION
OFFENSE: SUBSTANDARD CARE, INCOMPETENCE OR NEGLIGENCE

NOTES: NEGLIGENCE; INCOMPETENCE.

AGBEBIYI, JONATHAN ADESHINA MD, DATE OF BIRTH SEPTEMBER 7, 1949, LICENSE NUMBER 1041053 OF PO BOX 181135, CORPUS CHRISTI, TX, WAS DISCIPLINED BY MICHIGAN ON JANUARY 12, 1996
DISCIPLINARY ACTION: LICENSE REVOCATION; FINE
OFFENSE: SUBSTANDARD CARE, INCOMPETENCE OR NEGLIGENCE

NOTES: NEGLIGENCE; INCOMPETENCE. $1,000 FINE.

AGBEBIYI, JONATHAN ADESHINA MD, DATE OF BIRTH SEPTEMBER 7, 1949 OF PO BOX 181298, CORPUS CHRISTI, TX, WAS DISCIPLINED BY MEDICARE ON APRIL 23, 1996
DISCIPLINARY ACTION: EXCLUSION FROM THE MEDICARE AND/OR MEDICAID PROGRAM
OFFENSE: DISCIPLINARY ACTION BY ANOTHER STATE OR AGENCY

NOTES: LICENSE REVOKED FOR REASONS BEARING ON PROFESSIONAL PERFORMANCE.

AGUIRRE-MORAN, RAFAEL AUGUSTO MD, DATE OF BIRTH SEPTEMBER 26, 1937, LICENSE NUMBER 00D6922 OF HWY 124 AND OAK STREET, WINNIE, TX. WAS DISCIPLINED BY TEXAS ON SEPTEMBER 20, 1994
DISCIPLINARY ACTION: EMERGENCY SUSPENSION
OFFENSE: CRIMINAL CONVICTION OR PLEA OF GUILTY, NOLO CONTENDERE, OR NO CONTEST TO A CRIME

NOTES: THE FOLLOWING ALLEGATIONS WERE MADE: ON 6/17/94 A COMPLAINT WAS FILED WITH SHERIFF'S DEPARTMENT BY A PATIENT WHO ALLEGED INAPPROPRIATE AND UNSOLICITED TOUCHING BY HIM DURING AN EXAM; ON 6/22/94 AN ASSAULT CLASS C MISDEMEANOR WAS FILED AGAINST HIM TO WHICH HE PLED GUILTY; ON 8/30/94 HE WAS ARRESTED AND CHARGED WITH ONE COUNT OF INDECENCY WITH A MINOR WHOM HE MOLESTED DURING AN EXAM; FROM 1992 TO 1994 HE PRESCRIBED LARGE QUANTITIES OF CONTROLLED SUBSTANCES TO FOUR PATIENTS WITHOUT ADEQUATE DOCUMENTED EVALUATION AND NO APPARENT MEDICAL INDICATION OR ADEQUATE LEGITIMATE MEDICAL BASIS; HAD SOME FORM OF SEXUAL ENCOUNTER WITH THREE PATIENTS IN EXCHANGE FOR CONTROLLED SUBSTANCES AND PRESCRIPTION PADS.

AGUIRRE-MORAN, RAFAEL AUGUSTO MD, DATE OF BIRTH SEPTEMBER 26, 1937, LICENSE NUMBER 00D6922 OF HWY 124 AND OAK STREET, WINNIE, TX, WAS DISCIPLINED BY TEXAS ON MARCH 3, 1995
DISCIPLINARY ACTION: LICENSE SUSPENSION
OFFENSE: SEXUAL ABUSE OF OR SEXUAL MISCONDUCT WITH A PATIENT

NOTES: UNPROFESSIONAL CONDUCT IN THAT HE VIOLATED BOUNDARIES IN A SOCIAL/SEXUAL RELATIONSHIP WITH A PATIENT WITHOUT PROPER TERMINATION OF THE DOCTOR/PATIENT RELATIONSHIP AND KISSING A SECOND PATIENT; PRESCRIBED VARIOUS CONTROLLED SUBSTANCES TO MULTIPLE PATIENTS OVER A PROLONGED PERIOD WITHOUT ADEQUATE MEDICAL INDICATION AND WITHOUT SUFFICIENT DOCUMENTATION; EMPLOYED A NON-REGISTERED, NON-CERTIFIED INDIVIDUAL TO PERFORM RADIOLOGICAL TESTING IN HIS OFFICE. SUSPENSION UNTIL HE REQUESTS TO HAVE SUSPENSION STAYED OR LIFTED AND PERSONALLY APPEARS BEFORE BOARD WITH SUFFICIENT EVIDENCE INDICATING THAT HE IS PHYSICALLY, MENTALLY AND OTHERWISE COMPETENT TO SAFELY PRACTICE MEDICINE INCLUDING BUT NOT LIMITED TO COPIES OF MEDICAL RECORDS AND REPORTS OF PSYCHOLOGICAL AND NEUROPSYCHIATRIC EVALUATIONS CONDUCTED BY A BOARD CERTIFIED PSYCHIATRIST. UPON AN ADEQUATE SHOWING BEFORE THE BOARD THAT HE IS ABLE TO SAFELY PRACTICE MEDICINE, THE SUSPENSION SHALL BE STAYED AND HE SHALL BE PLACED ON SEVEN YEARS PROBATION.

AGUIRRE-MORAN, RAFAEL AUGUSTO MD, DATE OF BIRTH SEPTEMBER 26, 1937 OF PO BOX 695, WINNIE, TX, WAS DISCIPLINED BY MEDICARE ON APRIL 23, 1996
DISCIPLINARY ACTION: EXCLUSION FROM THE MEDICARE AND/OR MEDICAID PROGRAM
OFFENSE: DISCIPLINARY ACTION BY ANOTHER STATE OR AGENCY

NOTES: LICENSE SUSPENDED FOR REASONS BEARING ON

PROFESSIONAL PERFORMANCE.

AL MARASHI, ABDUL-HUSEIN S H MD, LICENSE NUMBER E5664 OF DALLAS, TX, WAS DISCIPLINED BY TEXAS ON AUGUST 22, 1998
DISCIPLINARY ACTION: SURRENDER OF LICENSE

NOTES: ALLEGATIONS OF VIOLATIONS OF THE MEDICAL PRACTICE ACT. VOLUNTARY AND PERMANENT SURRENDER.

ALDERMAN, JOHN A DO, LICENSE NUMBER E3639 OF ODESSA, TX, WAS DISCIPLINED BY TEXAS ON OCTOBER 24, 1998
DISCIPLINARY ACTION: SURRENDER OF LICENSE

NOTES: VOLUNTARY AND PERMANENT SURRENDER IN LIEU OF FURTHER INVESTIGATION.

ALDERMAN, JOHN ALLEN DO, DATE OF BIRTH SEPTEMBER 11, 1940 OF PO BOX 5000, FLORENCE, CO, WAS DISCIPLINED BY MEDICARE ON JUNE 17, 1999
DISCIPLINARY ACTION: EXCLUSION FROM THE MEDICARE AND/OR MEDICAID PROGRAM
OFFENSE: CRIMINAL CONVICTION OR PLEA OF GUILTY, NOLO CONTENDERE, OR NO CONTEST TO A CRIME

NOTES: CONVICTED OF A CRIME INVOLVING THE MEDICARE, MEDICAID, MATERNAL AND CHILD HEALTH SERVICES BLOCK GRANT OR BLOCK GRANTS TO STATES FOR SOCIAL SERVICES PROGRAMS.

ALEXANDER, JAMES ALAN MD, LICENSE NUMBER 00C9263 OF HOUSTON, TX, WAS DISCIPLINED BY TEXAS ON OCTOBER 27, 1993
DISCIPLINARY ACTION: 60-MONTH PROBATION; REQUIRED TO TAKE ADDITIONAL MEDICAL EDUCATION
OFFENSE: PROFESSIONAL MISCONDUCT

NOTES: IN SEVERAL CASES DURING LATE 1989 AND EARLY 1990 PERSISTENTLY AND FLAGRANTLY OVERCHARGED AND OVERTREATED PATIENTS INCLUDING PERFORMING UNNECESSARY PROCEDURES; IN SOME OF THESE CASES THERE WAS INADEQUATE DOCUMENTATION. SUSPENSION STAYED. CONDITIONS OF PROBATION: SHALL PERFORM 10 HOURS PER MONTH OF COMMUNITY SERVICE FOR FIVE YEARS; SHALL ATTEND AT LEAST 50 HOURS PER YEAR OF CONTINUING MEDICAL EDUCATION AND DURING THE FIRST YEAR OF PROBATION SHALL COMPLETE A BOARD-APPROVED ETHICS COURSE OR PROGRAM; SHALL UTILIZE A SYSTEM OF PATIENT RECORDKEEPING THAT ACCURATELY REFLECTS INFORMATION AND SHALL BE MONITORED BY A PHYSICIAN WHO SHALL CONDUCT RANDOM REVIEWS OF THESE RECORDS AND PROVIDE REPORTS EVERY FOUR MONTHS; SHALL GIVE A COPY OF THIS ORDER TO ANY HEALTH CARE ENTITY WHERE HE HAS PRIVILEGES; SHALL COOPERATE WITH THE BOARD IN VERIFYING COMPLIANCE; SHALL INFORM BOARD OF CHANGE OF ADDRESS WITHIN 10 DAYS OR IF HE LEAVES THE STATE; TIME SPENT OUT OF TEXAS DOES NOT COUNT TOWARD PROBATION. HAS 20 DAYS TO FILE A MOTION FOR REHEARING. ORDER WILL BECOME FINAL WHEN ALL APPEALS HAVE BEEN EXHAUSTED.

ALEXANDER, JAMES ALAN MD, LICENSE NUMBER 00C9263 OF HOUSTON, TX, WAS DISCIPLINED BY TEXAS ON JUNE 27, 1995
DISCIPLINARY ACTION: LICENSE REVOCATION
OFFENSE: FAILURE TO COMPLY WITH PREVIOUS BOARD ORDER

NOTES: COMPLIED WITH TERMS OF 10/27/93 BOARD ORDER EXCEPT THAT HE FAILED TO OBTAIN A MONITORING PHYSICIAN FOR HIS OFFICE PRACTICE; REQUESTED FOUR HOSPITALS AND A MEDICAL SOCIETY TO LOCATE HIM A MONITOR, BUT DID NOT APPROACH ANY OF THE PHYSICIANS AT THESE INSTITUTIONS INDIVIDUALLY AND AFTER 5/94 ONLY CONTACTED THE BOARD REGARDING THE APPOINTMENT OF A MONITOR; BETWEEN 6/94 AND 11/94, WROTE APPROXIMATELY 26 LETTERS TO THE BOARD PROPOSING THAT A MEMBER OF THE BOARD SERVE AS HIS MONITOR OR THAT THE BOARD DIRECTOR APPOINT HIM A MONITOR.

ALEXANDER, JOE BOB MD, LICENSE NUMBER E0780 OF ABILENE, TX, WAS DISCIPLINED BY TEXAS ON MAY 16, 1998
DISCIPLINARY ACTION: REPRIMAND
OFFENSE: PROFESSIONAL MISCONDUCT

NOTES: AT THE WEIGHT LOSS CLINIC HE OWNS, PROSPECTIVE PATIENTS ARE GIVEN A PAMPHLET PROVIDING INFORMATION ABOUT THE CLINIC AND OFFERING A $5.00 CREDIT ON THE NEXT VISIT UPON THE REFERRAL OF 3 ADDITIONAL PATIENTS, AND A PERMANENT $5.00 DECREASE IN OFFICE CHARGES UPON THE REFERRAL OF 10 NEW PATIENTS; BOARD FOUND THIS CONSTITUTES IMPERMISSIBLE DRUMMING OF PATIENTS; HE STOPPED THIS PRACTICE AFTER BEING INFORMED ABOUT THIS. SHALL COOPERATE WITH THE BOARD IN VERIFYING COMPLIANCE; SHALL GIVE A COPY OF THIS ORDER TO ANY HEALTH CARE ENTITY WHERE HE HAS PRIVILEGES.

ALEXANDER, JOE BOB MD, LICENSE NUMBER 10682 OF 1025 CYPRESS, ABILENE, TX, WAS DISCIPLINED BY OKLAHOMA ON JULY 28, 1999
DISCIPLINARY ACTION: REPRIMAND
OFFENSE: DISCIPLINARY ACTION BY ANOTHER STATE OR AGENCY

NOTES: ON 5/16/98 TEXAS BOARD REPRIMANDED LICENSE FINDING PATIENT SOLICITATION CONSTITUTING IMPERMISSIBLE DRUMMING OF PATIENTS FOR HIS WEIGHT LOSS CLINIC; MAINTAINS HE WAS NOT AWARE OF THE ACT PROHIBITING USE OF DISCOUNTS AND VOLUNTARILY AGREED TO DISCONTINUE THE PRACTICE OF OFFERING DISCOUNTS OF ANY KIND; ALTHOUGH THE LITERATURE IN HIS OFFICE STATES THAT HE WOULD SEE EVERY PATIENT AT EVERY VISIT, THAT PRACTICE DID NOT ALWAYS OCCUR; FAILED TO ADEQUATELY DOCUMENT PATIENT RECORDS. TERMS AND CONDITIONS: SHALL SUBMIT TO HOSPITALS, CLINICS OR OTHER INSTITUTIONS IN WHICH HE HOLDS OR ANTICIPATES HOLDING ANY FORM OF STAFF PRIVILEGE A COPY OF THIS ORDER.

ALFORD, JACK A MD OF 7602 BELLFORT AVENUE, HOUSTON, TX, WAS DISCIPLINED BY DEA ON SEPTEMBER 30, 1994
DISCIPLINARY ACTION: RESTRICTION PLACED ON CONTROLLED SUBSTANCE LICENSE
OFFENSE: DISCIPLINARY ACTION BY ANOTHER STATE OR AGENCY

NOTES: STATE BOARD.

ALFORD, JACK ALLEN MD, DATE OF BIRTH APRIL 2, 1930, LICENSE NUMBER 00C4971 OF 6550 MAPLERIDGE, SUITE 101C, HOUSTON, TX, WAS DISCIPLINED BY TEXAS ON JUNE 17, 1992
DISCIPLINARY ACTION: 60-MONTH PROBATION
OFFENSE: OVERPRESCRIBING OR MISPRESCRIBING DRUGS

NOTES: NONTHERAPEUTIC PRESCRIBING. SUSPENSION, STAYED. PROBATION UNDER TERMS AND CONDITIONS. ON 8/20/93 ORDER TERMINATED; LICENSE FREE AND CLEAR OF ANY PREVIOUS RESTRICTIONS.

ALLAS, JOSE O MD, LICENSE NUMBER 00H9589, WAS DISCIPLINED BY TEXAS ON AUGUST 17, 1996
DISCIPLINARY ACTION: REPRIMAND
OFFENSE: SUBSTANDARD CARE, INCOMPETENCE OR NEGLIGENCE

NOTES: IN MARCH 1995 FAILED TO INSTITUTE LIDOCAINE TREATMENT TO A PATIENT AFTER AN EPISODE OF VENTRICULAR FIBRILLATION AND FAILED TO DISCLOSE TO THE CARDIOLOGIST REQUESTED BY THE PATIENT'S FAMILY THAT THE PATIENT WAS IN FACT PRESENT AT THE HOSPITAL. SHALL GIVE A COPY OF THIS ORDER TO ANY HEALTH CARE ENTITY WHERE HE HAS PRIVILEGES; SHALL PROVIDE A COPY OF THIS ORDER TO ANYONE REQUESTING IT WITHIN 10 DAYS.

ALLEN, BRADY L MD, DATE OF BIRTH JANUARY 7, 1944 OF DALLAS, TX, WAS DISCIPLINED BY FDA ON DECEMBER 11, 1990
DISCIPLINARY ACTION: INELIGIBLE TO RECEIVE INVESTIGATIONAL NEW DRUGS FOR EXPERIMENTAL PURPOSES

ALLEN, GWENDOLYN JOYCE MD, LICENSE NUMBER 00G4784 OF SAN SABA, TX, WAS DISCIPLINED BY TEXAS ON JUNE 10, 1991
DISCIPLINARY ACTION: 36-MONTH PROBATION; RESTRICTION PLACED ON LICENSE
OFFENSE: PROFESSIONAL MISCONDUCT

NOTES: AIDING OR ABETTING, DIRECTLY OR INDIRECTLY, THE PRACTICE OF MEDICINE BY ANY PERSON, PARTNERSHIP, ASSOCIATION, OR CORPORATION NOT DULY LICENSED TO PRACTICE MEDICINE BY THE BOARD. CONDITIONS OF PROBATION INCLUDE: SHALL NOT ACCEPT EMPLOYMENT OR ENTER INTO CONTRACTUAL RELATIONSHIPS WHEREIN LICENSEE WOULD BE COMPENSATED TO DIAGNOSE AND/OR TREAT PATIENTS BY A LAYPERSON, CORPORATION, OR OTHER ENTITY NOT COMPRISED EXCLUSIVELY OF TEXAS LICENSED PHYSICIANS; SHALL NOT ALLOW SIGNATURE TO BE DUPLICATED AND USED AS A RUBBER STAMP OR ANY DOCUMENT UTILIZED IN HER PRACTICE OF MEDICINE FOR EITHER TREATMENT OF PATIENTS OR BILLING PURPOSES.

ALLEN, RUTH P MD, WAS DISCIPLINED BY TEXAS ON AUGUST 16, 1996

NOTES: SHALL SUBMIT TO A COMPLETE PSYCHIATRIC EVALUATION WITHIN 30 DAYS.

ALLGOOD, HOMER JR MD, DATE OF BIRTH DECEMBER 5, 1924, LICENSE NUMBER 00D7517 OF 708 S FIRST STREET, MULESHOE, TX, WAS DISCIPLINED BY TEXAS ON JUNE 12, 1990
DISCIPLINARY ACTION: 60-MONTH PROBATION; RESTRICTION PLACED ON CONTROLLED SUBSTANCE LICENSE

NOTES: STIPULATED ORDER. MUST COMPLETE PRECEPTORSHIP ON PREVENTION AND TREATMENT OF DRUG ABUSE, SURRENDER ALL UNUSED TRIPLICATE PRESCRIPTION FORMS, NOT TREAT ANY PATIENT FOR WEIGHT CONTROL OR OBESITY WITH ANY CONTROLLED SUBSTANCE OR OVER THE COUNTER DRUGS BUT MAY TREAT WITH COUNSELING, DIET, AND EXERCISE REGIMEN, NOT PRESCRIBE, ADMINISTER OR POSSESS SCHEDULE II CONTROLLED DRUG EXCEPT FOR ORDERING FOR HOSPITALIZED PATIENTS, ATTEND CONTINUING MEDICAL EDUCATION COURSES, MAINTAIN SEPARATE FILE OF COPY OF EVERY PRESCRIPTION WRITTEN FOR CONTROLLED SUBSTANCES, AND APPEAR BEFORE BOARD SEMI-ANNUALLY. ON 1/29/93, HIS REQUEST FOR TERMINATION OF PROBATION IS DENIED, HOWEVER, HE IS GRANTED PERMISSION TO REAPPLY TO THE DRUG ENFORCEMENT ADMINISTRATION AND THE TEXAS DEPARTMENT OF PUBLIC SAFETY FOR SCHEDULE II CONTROLLED SUBSTANCE REGISTRATION AND FOR TRIPLICATE PRESCRIPTION FORMS. RESTRICTIONS ON PRESCRIBING, ADMINISTERING OR POSSESSING ANY DRUGS CLASSIFIED AS SCHEDULE II CONTROLLED SUBSTANCES EXCEPT FOR ORDERING SUCH DRUGS FOR HOSPITALIZED PATIENTS ARE LIFTED. ON 8/20/93, ORDER MODIFIED SO HE SHALL ATTEND 50 HOURS PER YEAR OF CONTINUING MEDICAL EDUCATION. ALL OTHER TERMS AND CONDITIONS REMAIN IN EFFECT. ON 6/22/94 BOARD DENIED HIS REQUEST FOR TERMINATION OF THIS ORDER.

ALLISON, DALE CRAWFORD MD, LICENSE NUMBER E2435 OF WACO, TX, WAS DISCIPLINED BY TEXAS ON DECEMBER 11, 1999
DISCIPLINARY ACTION: FINE
OFFENSE: FAILURE TO COMPLY WITH PREVIOUS BOARD ORDER

NOTES: A PHYSICIAN ASSISTANT SHE WAS SUPERVISING WAS SELF-PRESCRIBING CONTROLLED SUBSTANCES FOR NON-THERAPEUTIC PURPOSES AND IN NON-THERAPEUTIC QUANTITIES; THE PHYSICIAN ASSISTANT DEVELOPED A DEPENDENCY ON STADOL; MEDICAL RECORDS WRITTEN BY PHYSICIAN ASSISTANT DID NOT PROPERLY DOCUMENT MEDICATIONS ADMINISTERED TO PATIENTS; $5,000 FINE; SHALL COOPERATE WITH THE BOARD IN VERIFYING COMPLIANCE INCLUDING PROVIDING COPIES OF PEER REVIEW RECORDS UPON REQUEST; SHALL GIVE A COPY OF THIS ORDER TO ANY HEALTH CARE ENTITY WHERE HE HAS PRIVILEGES; SHALL PROVIDE A COPY OF THIS ORDER TO ANYONE REQUESTING IT WITHIN 10 DAYS; TIME SPENT OUT OF TEXAS DOES NOT COUNT TOWARD RESTRICTION; SHALL INFORM THE BOARD OF CHANGE OF ADDRESS WITHIN 10 DAYS OR IF SHE LEAVES THE STATE; SHALL NOT SEEK MODIFICATION FOR ONE YEAR.

ALMARASHI, ABDUL-HUSEIN S H MD, LICENSE NUMBER 00E5664 OF GLADEWATER, TX, WAS DISCIPLINED BY TEXAS ON MARCH 31, 199(
OFFENSE: OVERCHARGING

NOTES: MUST ADJUST CHARGES AND CEASE CHARGING FOR CERTAIN EXTRANEOUS MATTERS. ON 6/22/94 ORDER TERMINATED DUE TO SUCCESSFUL COMPLETION AND COMPLIANCE WITH TERMS.

ALMOND, THOMAS HENRY MD, LICENSE NUMBER 00D4908 OF WIMBERLEY, TX, WAS DISCIPLINED BY TEXAS ON DECEMBER 4, 1991
DISCIPLINARY ACTION: RESTRICTION PLACED ON CONTROLLED SUBSTANCE LICENSE
OFFENSE: SUBSTANDARD CARE, INCOMPETENCE OR NEGLIGENCE

NOTES: WAS RESPONSIBLE FOR AVAILABILITY OF EQUIPMENT NECESSARY TO ADMINISTER ANESTHESIA AND FOR DEVELOPMENT OF SAFETY REGULATIONS AT BRAZOSPORT MEMORIAL HOSPITAL IN 3/88; ADEQUATE RULES AND PROCEDURES TO ENSURE SAFETY OF ANESTHESIA WERE NOT ESTABLISHED; ON 3/31/88 A PATIENT AND HER FETUS DIED APPARENTLY AS A RESULT OF IMPROPER INTUBATION BY A CRNA. INDEFINITELY EXCLUDED FROM ADMINISTERING ANY ANESTHETIC DRUGS; SHALL COOPERATE WITH BOARD IN VERIFYING COMPLIANCE; SHALL ADVISE THE BOARD OF CHANGE OF ADDRESS WITHIN 10 DAYS.

ALTER, DON E MD, DATE OF BIRTH NOVEMBER 7, 1957 OF 5018 92ND STREET, LUBBOCK, TX, WAS DISCIPLINED BY MEDICARE ON NOVEMBER 20, 1997
DISCIPLINARY ACTION: EXCLUSION FROM THE MEDICARE AND/OR

MEDICAID PROGRAM
OFFENSE: NONCOMPLIANCE WITH A PROFESSIONAL RULE

NOTES: DEFAULTED ON PUBLIC HEALTH SERVICE EDUCATION LOAN. REINSTATED ON 12/23/97.

ALVORD, REX JR MD OF 407A IRONDALE DRIVE, EL PASO, TX, WAS DISCIPLINED BY NEW MEXICO ON OCTOBER 6, 1994
OFFENSE: SUBSTANCE ABUSE

NOTES: LICENSE PLACED UNDER UNSPECIFIED CONDITIONS. IN 5/98 ALL STIPULATIONS REMOVED; UNRESTRICTED LICENSE.

AMARO, MICHAEL ANTHONY MD, DATE OF BIRTH JULY 6, 1956, LICENSE NUMBER 00G6431 OF 3807 FM 1092 SUITE 310, MISSOURI CITY, TX, WAS DISCIPLINED BY TEXAS ON JUNE 15, 1993
DISCIPLINARY ACTION: 60-MONTH PROBATION; RESTRICTION PLACED ON CONTROLLED SUBSTANCE LICENSE
OFFENSE: LOSS OR RESTRICTION OF HOSPITAL PRIVILEGES

NOTES: IN 10/91 WHILE HOLDING TEMPORARY PRIVILEGES AT A HOSPITAL HE WAS REQUIRED TO PARTICIPATE IN A MONITORING PROGRAM REQUIRING RANDOM DRUG SCREENS; SCREEN ON 9/14/92 WAS POSITIVE FOR COCAINE METABOLITES AND HIS HOSPITAL PRIVILEGES WERE SUSPENDED AT TWO HOSPITALS; COMPLETED INPATIENT TREATMENT AND CONTINUES TO PARTICIPATE IN OUTPATIENT TREATMENT AND AA, AND SEE A PSYCHIATRIST; HOSPITAL PRIVILEGES HAVE BEEN REINSTATED UNDER CONDITIONS. SUSPENSION STAYED. CONDITIONS OF PROBATION: SHALL ATTEND AT LEAST 50 HOURS PER YEAR OF CONTINUING MEDICAL EDUCATION; SHALL CONTINUE TO RECEIVE PSYCHIATRIC TREATMENT WITH QUARTERLY REPORTS TO THE BOARD; SHALL ABSTAIN FROM THE CONSUMPTION OF ALCOHOL/DRUGS IN ANY FORM UNLESS PRESCRIBED BY ANOTHER PHYSICIAN FOR A LEGITIMATE AND THERAPEUTIC PURPOSE; SHALL SURRENDER ALL UNUSED TRIPLICATE PRESCRIPTION FORMS AND SHALL NOT ATTEMPT TO ORDER MORE; SHALL NOT PRESCRIBE, ADMINISTER OR DISPENSE SCHEDULE II CONTROLLED SUBSTANCES EXCEPT TO HOSPITAL PATIENTS AND SHALL KEEP A LOG OF THESE PRESCRIPTIONS SUBJECT TO REVIEW; SHALL KEEP A SEPARATE LOG OF ALL PRESCRIPTIONS FOR OTHER CONTROLLED SUBSTANCES SUBJECT TO REVIEW; SHALL PARTICIPATE IN ACTIVITIES OF AN IMPAIRED PHYSICIAN'S GROUP AND ATTEND WEEKLY MEETINGS WITH QUARTERLY REPORTS; SHALL SUBMIT HIMSELF FOR APPROPRIATE EXAMS INCLUDING DRUG OR ALCOHOL SCREENS; SHALL PARTICIPATE IN AA'S PROGRAM NOT LESS THAN ONCE A WEEK WITH QUARTERLY REPORTS TO THE BOARD; SHALL COMPLY WITH CONDITIONS REQUIRED FOR HOSPITAL PRIVILEGES REINSTATEMENT; SHALL APPEAR BEFORE THE BOARD ONCE A YEAR; SHALL GIVE A COPY OF THIS ORDER TO ANY HEALTH CARE ENTITY WHERE HE HAS PRIVILEGES; SHALL COOPERATE WITH THE BOARD IN VERIFYING COMPLIANCE; SHALL INFORM BOARD OF CHANGE OF ADDRESS WITHIN 10 DAYS OR IF HE LEAVES THE STATE; TIME SPENT OUT OF TEXAS DOES NOT COUNT TOWARD PROBATION. SHALL NOT SEEK MODIFICATION FOR ONE YEAR. REQUEST FOR TERMINATION WAS DENIED ON 8/19/94. ON 8/17/96 PROBATION TERMINATED.

AMARO, MICHAEL ANTHONY MD, DATE OF BIRTH JULY 6, 1956, LICENSE NUMBER 0029835 OF 15700 LEXINGTON SUITE 1108, SUGAR LAND, TX, WAS DISCIPLINED BY GEORGIA ON DECEMBER 1, 1993
DISCIPLINARY ACTION: PROBATION
OFFENSE: DISCIPLINARY ACTION BY ANOTHER STATE OR AGENCY

NOTES: ACTION BASED ON ACTION TAKEN BY TEXAS BOARD. IMPAIRMENT.

AMAYO, EMMANUEL P K MD, DATE OF BIRTH JULY 13, 1943, LICENSE NUMBER 0039094 OF 30840 NORTHWESTERN HWY, FARMINGTON HILLS, MI, WAS DISCIPLINED BY MICHIGAN ON NOVEMBER 20, 1991
DISCIPLINARY ACTION: 24-MONTH LICENSE SUSPENSION; FINE
OFFENSE: SUBSTANDARD CARE, INCOMPETENCE OR NEGLIGENCE

NOTES: $20,945 FINE.

AMAYO, EMMANUEL P K MD, LICENSE NUMBER 00F4737 OF FARMINGTON HILLS, MI, WAS DISCIPLINED BY TEXAS ON JUNE 17, 1992
DISCIPLINARY ACTION: 24-MONTH LICENSE SUSPENSION
OFFENSE: DISCIPLINARY ACTION BY ANOTHER STATE OR AGENCY

NOTES: ACTION TAKEN BY ANOTHER STATE BOARD FOR UNPROFESSIONAL OR DISHONORABLE CONDUCT LIKELY TO DECEIVE, DEFRAUD OR INJURE THE PUBLIC; AND PROFESSIONAL FAILURE TO PRACTICE MEDICINE IN AN ACCEPTABLE MANNER CONSISTENT WITH PUBLIC HEALTH AND WELFARE. SUBJECT TO TERMS AND CONDITIONS OF MICHIGAN BOARD ORDER

AMAYO, EMMANUEL P MD, LICENSE NUMBER 0004462 OF PONTIAC, MI, WAS DISCIPLINED BY VIRGINIA ON FEBRUARY 1, 1993
DISCIPLINARY ACTION: REPRIMAND
OFFENSE: PROVIDING FALSE INFORMATION TO THE BOARD OR OTHER HEALTH AGENCY

NOTES: MISREPRESENTATION ON APPLICATION FOR INTERN/RESIDENT'S LICENSE; LICENSE EXPIRED 06/30/92.

AMICK, ROGER MD, LICENSE NUMBER 00F4739 OF LITTLE ROCK, AR, WAS DISCIPLINED BY TEXAS ON AUGUST 24, 1991
DISCIPLINARY ACTION: LICENSE REVOCATION; SURRENDER OF CONTROLLED SUBSTANCE LICENSE
OFFENSE: FAILURE TO COMPLY WITH PREVIOUS BOARD ORDER

NOTES: VIOLATION OF TERMS AND CONDITIONS OF PREVIOUS BOARD ORDER. SHALL NOT ATTEMPT TO REREGISTER OR OTHERWISE OBTAIN CONTROLLED SUBSTANCES REGISTRATION WITHOUT APPROVAL FROM THE BOARD; SHALL SURRENDER ALL UNUSED TRIPLICATE PRESCRIPTION FORMS AND NOT ATTEMPT TO ORDER MORE WITHOUT BOARD APPROVAL.

AMMETER, LESLIE FRANK MD OF 2718 PLEASANTON ROAD, SAN ANTONIO, TX, WAS DISCIPLINED BY DEA ON MAY 4, 1998
DISCIPLINARY ACTION: SURRENDER OF CONTROLLED SUBSTANCE LICENSE

NOTES: IN LIEU OF PUBLIC INTEREST REVOCATION.

ANASCO, REYNALDO MD, LICENSE NUMBER 1026058 OF 920 SOUTH HEBRON, EVANSVILLE, IN, WAS DISCIPLINED BY INDIANA ON OCTOBER 17, 1996
DISCIPLINARY ACTION: 3-MONTH EMERGENCY SUSPENSION
OFFENSE: SUBSTANCE ABUSE

NOTES: IN 8/96 SUBMITTED TO A RANDOM URINE DRUG SCREEN BY THE COMMISSION ON PHYSICIAN ASSISTANCE WHICH TESTED POSITIVE FOR TRAMADOL; RUSH BEHAVIORAL HEALTH CENTER IN CHICAGO CONCLUDED THAT HE MAY BE IN RELAPSE AND THAT HIS RECOVERY PROGRAM IS INADEQUATE AND RECOMMENDED THAT HE ATTEND COUNSELING, INCREASE HIS 12-STEP MEETING ATTENDANCE, AND

INCREASE THE FREQUENCY OF URINE MONITORING; ANOTHER SCREEN IN 10/96 TESTED POSITIVE FOR HYDROCODONE; DENIED HIS RELAPSE ALTHOUGH HE IS CURRENTLY HOSPITALIZED FOR DETOXIFICATION; HIS RELAPSE INTO THE USE OF MOOD ALTERING CHEMICALS IN VIOLATION OF HIS INDIANA STATE MEDICAL ASSOCIATION CONTRACT; AND CONTINUED TO PRACTICE ALTHOUGH HE HAS BECOME UNFIT TO PRACTICE DUE TO HIS CHEMICAL DEPENDENCY. SHALL SURRENDER HIS LICENSE, CONTROLLED SUBSTANCE REGISTRATION, ALL CONTROLLED SUBSTANCES, AND ALL PRESCRIPTION PADS IN HIS POSSESSION TO THE BOARD.

ANASCO, REYNALDO MD, LICENSE NUMBER 1026058 OF 10419 HORN BLVD, SAN ANTONIO, TX, WAS DISCIPLINED BY INDIANA ON JUNE 4, 1997
DISCIPLINARY ACTION: 1-MONTH LICENSE SUSPENSION; PROBATION
OFFENSE: SUBSTANCE ABUSE

NOTES: HAD PREVIOUSLY BEEN DISCIPLINED BY THE BOARD DUE TO SUBSTANCE ABUSE DURING 1983 AND 1984; ON 2/97 LICENSE WAS REINSTATED FROM 10/96 EMERGENCY SUSPENSION BY AN INTERIM ORDER. THE BOARD WITHDREW THE PROBATION ON HIS LICENSE ON 1/24/91. A MEMBER OF THE PHYSICIANS ASSISTANCE COMMISSION TELEPHONED HIM AT HIS OFFICE ON 10/15/96 ABOUT HIS POSITIVE DRUG SCREEN FOR HYDROCONE AND ULTRAM; HE SPOKE WITH SLURRED SPEECH, WAS INCOHERENT AND RAMBLED DURING THE CONVERSATION. HE ENTERED INPATIENT TREATMENT ON 10/24/96. COMPLIANCE WITH HIS INDIANA STATE MEDICAL ASSOCIATION CONTRACT WAS DESCRIBED AS "MARGINAL, AT BEST". HE TESTIFIED THAT HE HAS A HISTORY OF SUBSTANCE ABUSE PROBLEMS. REMAINDER OF INDEFINITE SUSPENSION STAYED. TERMS AND CONDITIONS OF PROBATION ARE AS FOLLOWS: SHALL KEEP THE BOARD ADVISED OF HIS ADDRESS, PHONE AND EMPLOYER; SHALL PRACTICE ONLY UNDER DIRECT SUPERVISION AND SHALL HAVE HIS SUPERVISOR SUBMIT MONTHLY REPORTS; SHALL MAINTAIN A MONITORING CONTRACT WITH THE PHYSICIAN'S ASSISTANCE COMMISSION WITH MONTHLY REPORTS; SHALL WORK NO MORE THAN 40 HOURS PER WEEK; SHALL APPEAR BEFORE THE BOARD MONTHLY; SHALL NOT HAVE ACCESS TO SAMPLE MEDICATIONS; SHALL SURRENDER HIS DRUG ENFORCEMENT ADMINISTRATION AND STATE CONTROLLED SUBSTANCES PERMITS; ASSESSED COSTS OF $75.

ANASCO, REYNALDO MD, LICENSE NUMBER 1026058 OF 10419 HORN BOULEVARD, SAN ANTONIO, TX, WAS DISCIPLINED BY INDIANA ON JANUARY 12, 1998
DISCIPLINARY ACTION: LICENSE REVOCATION
OFFENSE: FAILURE TO COMPLY WITH PREVIOUS BOARD ORDER

NOTES: HISTORY OF SUBSTANCE ABUSE PROBLEMS; DISCIPLINED ON 10/19/83, 11/23/83, 2/29/84, 5/17/84, 8/16/84 & 10/22/84 BY THE BOARD BECAUSE OF HIS SUBSTANCE ABUSE; ON 10/19/87 REINSTATED, AND ON 1/24/91 PROBATION WAS WITHDRAWN FROM HIS LICENSE; ON 10/17/96 LICENSE SUMMARILY SUSPENDED DUE TO RELAPSE; ON 5/22/97 BOARD FOUND THAT HE CONTINUED TO PRACTICE ALTHOUGH UNFIT DUE TO ADDICTION TO, ABUSE, OR SEVERE DEPENDENCY UPON ALCOHOL OR OTHER DRUGS; ON 6/22/97 LICENSE REINSTATED WITH INDEFINITE PROBATION; ON 12/4/97 VIOLATED 6/22/97 ORDER BY FAILING TO COMPLY WITH HIS CONTRACT WITH THE INDIANA PHYSICIANS HEALTH PROGRAM; FAILED TO KEEP THE BOARD INFORMED OF HIS WHEREABOUTS AND PRACTICE LOCATION; AND FAILED TO PERSONALLY APPEAR BEFORE THE BOARD FOR HIS REGULAR SCHEDULED APPEARANCES. SHALL PAY $658 IN COSTS.

ANDERS, STEPHEN O DO, DATE OF BIRTH SEPTEMBER 24, 1952, LICENSE NUMBER 1007801 OF 4101 AIRPORT FWY #101, BEDFORD, TX, WAS DISCIPLINED BY MICHIGAN ON AUGUST 1, 1996
DISCIPLINARY ACTION: 6-MONTH LICENSE SUSPENSION
OFFENSE: DISCIPLINARY ACTION BY ANOTHER STATE OR AGENCY

NOTES: ACTION IN OTHER STATE.

ANDERS, STEPHEN ODELL DO, DATE OF BIRTH SEPTEMBER 24, 1952, LICENSE NUMBER 00F5452 OF 4101 AIRPORT FREEWAY #101, BEDFORD, TX, WAS DISCIPLINED BY TEXAS ON JUNE 15, 1993
DISCIPLINARY ACTION: RESTRICTION PLACED ON LICENSE
OFFENSE: PHYSICAL OR MENTAL ILLNESS INHIBITING THE ABILITY TO PRACTICE WITH SKILL AND SAFETY

NOTES: CURRENTLY SUFFERS FROM AN ILLNESS AND HAS NOT PRACTICED SINCE 10/91 DUE TO THAT ILLNESS; AGREES TO REFRAIN FROM PRACTICE UNTIL BOARD DETERMINES HIS HEALTH ALLOWS HIM TO PRACTICE WITH REASONABLE SAFETY AND SKILL. SHALL PROVIDE ADEQUATE DOCUMENTATION TO THE BOARD ESTABLISHING THIS; SHALL GIVE A COPY OF THIS ORDER TO ANY HEALTH CARE ENTITY WHERE HE HAS PRIVILEGES.

ANDERS, STEPHEN ODELL DO, DATE OF BIRTH SEPTEMBER 24, 1952, LICENSE NUMBER 00F5452 OF BEDFORD, TX, WAS DISCIPLINED BY TEXAS ON JANUARY 6, 1995
DISCIPLINARY ACTION: SURRENDER OF LICENSE
OFFENSE: PHYSICAL OR MENTAL ILLNESS INHIBITING THE ABILITY TO PRACTICE WITH SKILL AND SAFETY

NOTES: HAS UNDERGONE THERAPY SINCE ENTRY OF 6/15/93 ORDER; CONTINUES TO SUFFER FROM A DISABLING ILLNESS WHICH PREVENTS HIM FROM RETURNING TO THE PRACTICE OF MEDICINE. MAY SEEK REINSTATEMENT.

ANDERSON, BERNICE DO, DATE OF BIRTH MAY 23, 1955, LICENSE NUMBER 00H9489, WAS DISCIPLINED BY TEXAS ON OCTOBER 16, 1991
DISCIPLINARY ACTION: EMERGENCY SUSPENSION
OFFENSE: SUBSTANCE ABUSE

NOTES: ALLEGED INTEMPERATE USE OF DRUGS AND DIVERSION OF CONTROLLED SUBSTANCES THROUGH FALSE PRESCRIPTIONS AND OTHER MISREPRESENTATIONS. MUST HAVE A PSYCHIATRIC EXAMINATION, INCLUDING NEUROPSYCHOLOGIC EVALUATION WITH COGNITIVE EVALUATIONS, FROM A BOARD-APPROVED PSYCHIATRIST.

ANDERSON, BERNICE DO, DATE OF BIRTH MAY 23, 1955, LICENSE NUMBER 00H9489 OF PO BOX 1050, PALACIOS, TX, WAS DISCIPLINED BY TEXAS ON JANUARY 24, 1992
DISCIPLINARY ACTION: LICENSE SUSPENSION; 60-MONTH PROBATION
OFFENSE: OVERPRESCRIBING OR MISPRESCRIBING DRUGS

NOTES: WROTE FALSE OR FICTITIOUS PRESCRIPTIONS FOR DANGEROUS DRUGS; AND UNPROFESSIONAL OR DISHONORABLE CONDUCT LIKELY TO DECEIVE, DEFRAUD OR INJURE THE PUBLIC. SUSPENDED UNTIL SUCH TIME AS SHE IS EVALUATED BY A PSYCHIATRIST SPECIALIZING IN ADDICTIONOLOGY SATISFACTORY TO THE EXECUTIVE DIRECTOR OF THE BOARD AND FURNISHES REPORTS TO THE BOARD FROM THE

PSYCHIATRIST INDICATING THAT SHE IS BOTH MENTALLY AND PHYSICALLY ABLE TO SAFELY PRACTICE MEDICINE. UPON RECEIPT AND VERIFICATION OF SUCH REPORTS, THE SUSPENSION SHALL BE STAYED AND PLACED ON PROBATION UNDER TERMS AND CONDITIONS. PROBATION MODIFIED 12/10/92: DUE TO WORK LOCATION AND PLACE OF RESIDENCE HAD DIFFICULTY COMPLYING WITH REQUIREMENT TO PARTICIPATE IN COUNTY MEDICAL SOCIETY COMMITTEE ON PHYSICIAN HEALTH AND REHABILITATION; THEREFORE, PERMISSION GRANTED TO MEET THE REQUIREMENT BY PARTICIPATION IN EITHER COUNTY MEDICAL SOCIETY OR A REHABILITATION GROUP OF THE TEXAS OSTEOPATHIC MEDICAL ASSOCIATION UNDER THE SAME TERMS AND CONDITIONS.

ANDERSON, BERNICE DO, DATE OF BIRTH MAY 23, 1955, LICENSE NUMBER 00H9489 OF PO BOX 1050, PALACIOS, TX, WAS DISCIPLINED BY TEXAS ON MAY 10, 1993
DISCIPLINARY ACTION: LICENSE SUSPENSION
OFFENSE: FAILURE TO COMPLY WITH PREVIOUS BOARD ORDER

NOTES: ON 1/24/92 SHE ENTERED INTO AN AGREEMENT WITH THE BOARD TO ADDRESS HER DIVERSION OF CONTROLLED SUBSTANCES; ONE OF THE CONDITIONS OF PROBATION WAS THAT SHE ABSTAIN FROM THE CONSUMPTION OF CONTROLLED SUBSTANCES IN ANY FORM AND THAT SHE SHALL NOT POSSESS, ADMINISTER DISPENSE OR PRESCRIBE THEM; DURING THE FIRST QUARTER OF 1993 SHE INGESTED CONTROLLED SUBSTANCES; THERE IS NO INDICATION THAT SHE HARMED ANY PATIENTS DUE TO THIS FAILURE TO COMPLY.

ANDERSON, BERNICE DO, DATE OF BIRTH MAY 23, 1955, LICENSE NUMBER 00H9489 OF SAN ANTONIO, TX, WAS DISCIPLINED BY TEXAS ON APRIL 22, 1994
DISCIPLINARY ACTION: SURRENDER OF CONTROLLED SUBSTANCE LICENSE; 120-MONTH PROBATION

NOTES: AS REQUIRED BY THE PREVIOUS ORDER HAS APPEARED BEFORE BOARD AND PROVIDED SUFFICIENT EVIDENCE TO SHOW SHE IS PHYSICALLY, MENTALLY AND OTHERWISE COMPETENT TO PRACTICE. CONDITIONS OF PROBATION: SHALL NOT PRACTICE AS A SOLO PRACTITIONER OR IN ANY SETTING NOT PREAPPROVED BY THE BOARD; SHALL BE SUPERVISED BY BOARD-APPROVED PHYSICIAN WITH REPORTS THREE TIMES A YEAR; SHALL ABSTAIN FROM THE CONSUMPTION OF ALCOHOL/CHEMICAL SUBSTANCES IN ANY FORM UNLESS PRESCRIBED BY ANOTHER PHYSICIAN FOR A LEGITIMATE AND THERAPEUTIC PURPOSE; SHALL SUBMIT HERSELF FOR APPROPRIATE EXAMS INCLUDING DRUG OR ALCOHOL SCREENS; SHALL NOT TREAT OR OTHERWISE SERVE AS PHYSICIAN, PRESCRIBE, DISPENSE OR ADMINISTER DRUGS THAT MAY BE SUBJECT TO ABUSE TO HERSELF OR ANY MEMBER OF HER FAMILY; SHALL SURRENDER DEA AND TEXAS CONTROLLED SUBSTANCES CERTIFICATES, ALL UNUSED TRIPLICATE PRESCRIPTION FORMS AND ALL UNUSED CONTROLLED SUBSTANCES INCLUDING SAMPLES IN HER POSSESSION; SHALL NOT REREGISTER FOR THESE CERTIFICATES WITHOUT PERMISSION; SEPARATE FROM PATIENT RECORDS SHALL MAINTAIN A FILE OF EVERY PRESCRIPTION WRITTEN FOR DANGEROUS DRUGS WITH POTENTIAL FOR ABUSE WHICH SHALL BE AVAILABLE FOR INSPECTION; SHALL PARTICIPATE IN ACTIVITIES OF A PHYSICIAN HEALTH AND REHABILITATION COMMITTEE AND ATTEND WEEKLY MEETINGS WITH QUARTERLY REPORTS; SHALL PARTICIPATE IN AA'S PROGRAM NOT LESS THAN THREE TIMES A WEEK WITH QUARTERLY REPORTS TO THE BOARD; SHALL SUBMIT HERSELF FOR EXAMINATION AND TREATMENT TO A BOARD-APPROVED PSYCHIATRIST; SHALL ATTEND AT LEAST 50 HOURS PER YEAR OF CONTINUING MEDICAL EDUCATION; SHALL APPEAR BEFORE THE BOARD TWICE A YEAR; SHALL GIVE A COPY OF THIS ORDER TO ANY HEALTH CARE ENTITY WHERE SHE HAS PRIVILEGES; SHALL COOPERATE WITH THE BOARD IN VERIFYING COMPLIANCE; SHALL INFORM BOARD OF CHANGE OF ADDRESS WITHIN 10 DAYS OR IF SHE LEAVES THE STATE; TIME SPENT OUT OF TEXAS DOES NOT COUNT TOWARD PROBATION. SHALL NOT SEEK MODIFICATION FOR ONE YEAR. ON 6/28/95 ORDER MODIFIED AS FOLLOWS: MAY REAPPLY TO THE DEA AND TO THE TEXAS DEPARTMENT OF PUBLIC SAFETY TO OBTAIN AUTHORIZATION TO PRESCRIBE SCHEDULES III, III-N, IV AND V; SEPARATE FROM PATIENT RECORDS, SHALL MAINTAIN FILE OF EVERY PRESCRIPTION WRITTEN FOR CONTROLLED SUBSTANCES WITH ADDICTIVE POTENTIAL WHICH SHALL BE AVAILABLE FOR REVIEW; SHALL NOT TELEPHONE TO A PHARMACY A PRESCRIPTION OR REFILL FOR CONTROLLED SUBSTANCES OR PERMIT ANY ONE UNDER HIS SUPERVISION TO DO SO; SHALL NOT PRESCRIBE, DISPENSE, ADMINISTER OR POSSESS HALCION OR ANY AMPHETAMINE-LIKE ACTION DRUGS UNDER ANY CIRCUMSTANCE. ON 5/10/97 PETITION TO TERMINATE ORDER DENIED; ORDER MODIFIED ALLOWING HER TO REAPPLY FOR FULL PRESCRIBING AUTHORITY AND, REQUIRING THAT SHE MAINTAIN A LOGBOOK OF ALL PRESCRIPTIONS WRITTEN FOR CONTROLLED SUBSTANCES AND DANGEROUS DRUGS WITH ADDICTIVE POTENTIAL. ON 11/22/97 PETITION TO TERMINATE ORDER DENIED; ORDER MODIFIED DELETING RESTRICTION TO PRACTICE ONLY IN A GROUP OR INSTITUTIONAL SETTING, TO HAVE PRACTICE MONITORED, AND TO PARTICIPATE IN A COUNTY MEDICAL SOCIETY COMMITTEE; REDUCTION OF AA PARTICIPATION FROM THREE TIMES TO TWICE A WEEK; TREATING PSYCHIATRIST SHALL OBTAIN RANDOM ALCOHOL OR DRUG SCREEN NO LESS THAN ONCE EVERY TWO MONTHS; AND SHALL APPEAR BEFORE THE BOARD UPON REQUEST INSTEAD OF TWICE A YEAR. ON 1/29/99 ORDER TERMINATED.

ANDERSON, BERNICE L DO OF 410 COMMERCE STREET, PALACIOS, TX, WAS DISCIPLINED BY DEA ON JULY 21, 1993
DISCIPLINARY ACTION: SURRENDER OF CONTROLLED SUBSTANCE LICENSE
OFFENSE: DISCIPLINARY ACTION BY ANOTHER STATE OR AGENCY

NOTES: TEXAS LICENSE SUSPENDED PENDING PSYCHIATRIC EXAM AND REHEARING AND PUBLIC INTEREST REVOCATION PROCEEDINGS TO BE INITIATED UNLESS BOARD SURRENDERED.

ANDERSON, BERNICE L DO OF 2601 HOSPITAL BLVD, SUITE 117, CORPUS CHRISTI, TX, WAS DISCIPLINED BY DEA ON SEPTEMBER 22, 1995
DISCIPLINARY ACTION: RESTRICTION PLACED ON CONTROLLED SUBSTANCE LICENSE
OFFENSE: DISCIPLINARY ACTION BY ANOTHER STATE OR AGENCY

NOTES: STATE BOARD.

ANDERSON, CHARLES P MD, LICENSE NUMBER 00E1801 OF SAN MARCOS, TX, WAS DISCIPLINED BY TEXAS ON MARCH 2, 1996
DISCIPLINARY ACTION: FINE
OFFENSE: PROFESSIONAL MISCONDUCT

NOTES: IN 9/94 SUBMITTED A BILL FOR A HISTORY AND

PHYSICAL ON A HOSPITALIZED PATIENT FOR WHICH HE WAS NOT THE ATTENDING PHYSICIAN. SHALL PAY AN $1,000 ADMINISTRATIVE PENALTY; SHALL COOPERATE WITH THE BOARD IN VERIFYING COMPLIANCE.

ANDERSON, FRANKLIN LEE MD, LICENSE NUMBER G7978, WAS DISCIPLINED BY TEXAS ON APRIL 4, 1997
DISCIPLINARY ACTION: 120-MONTH PROBATION; RESTRICTION PLACED ON LICENSE
OFFENSE: FAILURE TO COMPLY WITH PREVIOUS BOARD ORDER

NOTES: ENGAGED IN THE INTEMPERATE USE OF HYDROCODONE, TYLENOL 3, AND FENTANYL, FOR APPROXIMATELY SIX TO NINE MONTHS DURING 1994 AND 1995. HE SOUGHT TREATMENT FOR SUBSTANCE ABUSE IN 2/95 AND 6/95, AND UNDERWENT INPATIENT TREATMENT IN BOTH INSTANCES. HE SELF-REPORTED HIS ABUSE AND RECOVERY HISTORY TO REPRESENTATIVES OF THE BOARD IN 10/95. ON 3/2/96 HE ENTERED INTO AN "AGREED REHABILITATION ORDER" WITH THE BOARD, REPORTING AT THAT TIME A SOBRIETY DATE OF 6/24/95. HE REPORTS THAT IN 11/95 HE INGESTED NYQUIL, AN OVER-THE-COUNTER MEDICATION, TO HELP HIM SLEEP. IN 1996, HE FAILED TO PROVIDE SEVERAL RANDOM URINE DRUG SCREENS WHEN REQUESTED; FROM 4/1/96 TO 6/20/96 HE RECEIVED ADDITIONAL INPATIENT TREATMENT FOR CHEMICAL DEPENDENCY. REVOCATION STAYED FOR PROBATION UNDER THE FOLLOWING TERMS: SHALL NOT PRACTICE ANESTHESIOLOGY UNTIL SUCH TIME AS HE PERSONALLY APPEARS BEFORE THE BOARD AND SUBMITS SUFFICIENT EVIDENCE THAT HE IS PHYSICALLY, MENTALLY, AND OTHERWISE COMPETENT TO PRACTICE; SHALL ABSTAIN FROM THE CONSUMPTION OF ALCOHOL/DRUGS IN ANY FORM UNLESS PRESCRIBED BY ANOTHER PHYSICIAN FOR A LEGITIMATE AND THERAPEUTIC PURPOSE; SHALL SUBMIT HIMSELF FOR APPROPRIATE EXAMS INCLUDING DRUG OR ALCOHOL SCREENS; SHALL NOMINATE THREE CERTIFIED PSYCHIATRISTS FOR BOARD SELECTION OF A THERAPIST AND SHALL EXPEDITIOUSLY SUBMIT HIMSELF TO EVALUATION AND TREATMENT BY THE APPROVED PRACTITIONER; SHALL COOPERATE WITH THE BOARD IN VERIFYING COMPLIANCE; SHALL PARTICIPATE IN THE ACTIVITIES OF A PHYSICIAN HEALTH AND REHABILITATION COMMITTEE AND ATTEND WEEKLY MEETINGS WITH QUARTERLY REPORTS; SHALL PARTICIPATE IN AA'S PROGRAM NOT LESS THAN FIVE TIMES A WEEK; SHALL REPORT ON HIS ATTENDANCE; SHALL COMPLY WITH HIS CONTINUING CARE CONTRACT; SHALL APPEAR BEFORE THE BOARD AT LEAST TWICE YEARLY; SHALL NOT POSSESS ALCOHOL, CONTROLLED SUBSTANCES, OR DRUGS WITH ADDICTIVE POTENTIAL OR POTENTIAL FOR ABUSE; HE SHALL SURRENDER ANY SUCH DRUGS IN HIS POSSESSION; SHALL NOT TREAT OR OTHERWISE SERVE AS PHYSICIAN, PRESCRIBE, DISPENSE OR ADMINISTER DRUGS THAT MAY BE SUBJECT TO ABUSE TO HIMSELF OR TO ANY MEMBER OF HIS FAMILY; SHALL NOT TELEPHONE TO A PHARMACY A PRESCRIPTION OR REFILL FOR CONTROLLED SUBSTANCES OR DANGEROUS DRUGS AND SHALL NOT PERMIT ANY INDIVIDUAL UNDER HIS SUPERVISION TO TELEPHONE SUCH A PRESCRIPTION OR REFILL; SEPARATE FROM PATIENT RECORDS, SHALL MAINTAIN A FILE OF EVERY PRESCRIPTION WRITTEN BY HIM FOR DANGEROUS DRUGS WITH ADDICTIVE POTENTIAL WHICH SHALL BE MADE AVAILABLE FOR REVIEW; HIS MEDICAL PRACTICE SHALL BE MONITORED BY A BOARD APPROVED TEXAS PHYSICIAN WHO SHALL PROVIDE QUARTERLY REPORTS TO THE BOARD; SHALL MAINTAIN ADEQUATE MEDICAL RECORDS WHICH SHALL BE AVAILABLE FOR REVIEW; SHALL OBTAIN AT LEAST 50 HOURS PER YEAR OF CONTINUING MEDICAL EDUCATION; SHALL COOPERATE WITH THE BOARD IN VERIFYING COMPLIANCE INCLUDING PROVIDING COPIES OF MEDICAL RELEASES UPON REQUEST; SHOULD HE ENTER A RESIDENCY PROGRAM, HE SHALL IMMEDIATELY SUBMIT THE NAME OF THE PROGRAM FOR APPROVAL; SHALL GIVE A COPY OF THIS ORDER TO ANY HEALTH CARE ENTITY WHERE HE HAS PRIVILEGES; SHALL PROVIDE A COPY OF THIS ORDER TO ANYONE REQUESTING IT WITHIN 10 DAYS; TIME SPENT OUT OF TEXAS DOES NOT COUNT TOWARD PROBATION; SHALL INFORM THE BOARD OF CHANGE OF ADDRESS WITHIN 10 DAYS OR IF HE LEAVES THE STATE; SHALL NOT SEEK MODIFICATION FOR ONE YEAR. ON 5/10/97 PERMISSION GRANTED FOR MODIFICATION OF ORDER; THE REQUIREMENT THAT HE NOT PRACTICE ANESTHESIOLOGY UNTIL HE RECEIVED AUTHORITY FROM THE BOARD IS DELETED; THE FOLLOWING SHALL BE INCLUDED INTO THE ORDER: SHALL NOT POSSESS, PRESCRIBE, DISPENSE, OR ADMINISTER CONTROLLED SUBSTANCES EXCEPT AS PROVIDED FOR IN THIS ORDER; SHALL MAINTAIN A LOGBOOK OF ALL MEDICATIONS ADMINISTERED OR ORDERED; ANY DISPOSAL OR EXCESS MEDICATIONS OR DRUG WASTAGE SHALL BE PERFORMED BY HIM IN THE PRESENCE OF A NURSE, CERTIFIED NURSE ANESTHETIST, OR LICENSED TEXAS PHYSICIAN AND RECORDED IN THE LOGBOOK; THE DISPOSAL OF ANY WASTAGE SHALL BE INITIALED AND DATED IN THE LOGBOOK; SHALL MAINTAIN A SEPARATE NOTEBOOK CONTAINING COPIES OF ALL PATIENT ANESTHESIA RECORDS; SHALL MAKE THE REQUIRED NOTEBOOK AND LOGBOOK AVAILABLE FOR INSPECTION BY THE BOARD; ALL OTHER PROVISIONS OF THE ORDER REMAIN IN FULL FORCE AND EFFECT UNTIL SUPERSEDED BY A SUBSEQUENT BOARD ORDER. ON 5/14/99 THE ORDER WAS MODIFIED AS FOLLOWS: REQUIREMENT OF FIVE TIMES A WEEK AA PARTICIPATION LESSENED TO THREE TIMES A WEEK; REQUIREMENT OF 2 APPEARANCES PER YEAR BEFORE THE BOARD MODIFIED TO REQUIRED APPEARANCES UPON REQUEST OF THE BOARD; ALL OTHER PROVISIONS OF THE ORDER REMAIN IN FULL FORCE AND EFFECT UNTIL SUPERSEDED BY A SUBSEQUENT BOARD ORDER.

ANDERSON, KENNETH CARL MD, LICENSE NUMBER 00F0855 OF HUMBLE, TX, WAS DISCIPLINED BY TEXAS ON MARCH 5, 1994
DISCIPLINARY ACTION: REPRIMAND
OFFENSE: PROFESSIONAL MISCONDUCT

NOTES: IN 7/92 AFTER ESTABLISHING A PHYSICIAN-PATIENT RELATIONSHIP WITH ONE PATIENT WITH AN ECTOPIC PREGNANCY FAILED TO TREAT HER OR PROPERLY REFER HER TO ANOTHER PHYSICIAN. HAD HIS OFFICE STAFF DISMISS THIS PATIENT, RESULTING IN ABANDONMENT OF THE PATIENT. SHALL GIVE A COPY OF THIS ORDER TO ANY HEALTH CARE ENTITY WHERE HE HAS PRIVILEGES; SHALL COOPERATE WITH THE BOARD IN VERIFYING COMPLIANCE; SHALL INFORM BOARD OF CHANGE OF ADDRESS WITHIN 10 DAYS. SHALL NOT SEEK MODIFICATION FOR ONE YEAR.

ANDERSON, VICKI SPARKS MD, LICENSE NUMBER 00E6215 OF PFLUGERVILLE, TX, WAS DISCIPLINED BY TEXAS ON MARCH 5, 1994
DISCIPLINARY ACTION: LICENSE SUSPENSION
OFFENSE: SUBSTANCE ABUSE

NOTES: SHE HAS ADMITTED TO A DECLINE IN HER COGNITIVE ABILITIES AND DEXTERITY DUE TO A CONTUSION OF

THE RIGHT FRONTAL LOBE OF THE BRAIN WHICH SHE SUFFERED AS A RESULT OF AN AUTO ACCIDENT IN 1983; HOSPITALIZED DURING 1/93 PURSUANT TO AN INVOLUNTARY COMMITMENT DUE TO SUICIDAL IDEATION AND DISCHARGED IN 2/93 WITH A DIAGNOSIS OF BIPOLAR DISORDER; HAS ADMITTED A LONG HISTORY OF ALCOHOL ABUSE; CLAIMS A SOBRIETY DATE OF 3/90 BUT ADMITS A RELAPSE FROM SPRING TO JULY OF 1993. SUSPENSION UNTIL SHE CAN APPEAR BEFORE THE BOARD AND DEMONSTRATE SHE IS ABLE TO PRACTICE WITH REASONABLE SKILL AND SAFETY. IF SHE IS ALLOWED TO PRACTICE IT WILL BE UNDER SPECIFIED CONDITIONS; SHALL COOPERATE WITH THE BOARD IN VERIFYING COMPLIANCE; SHALL INFORM BOARD OF CHANGE OF ADDRESS WITHIN 10 DAYS AND IF SHE LEAVES THE STATE; TIME SPENT OUT OF TEXAS DOES NOT COUNT TOWARD SUSPENSION. SHALL NOT SEEK MODIFICATION FOR ONE YEAR.

ANDERSON, VICKI SPARKS MD OF 206 WEST HOOPES, PFLUGERVILLE, TX, WAS DISCIPLINED BY DEA ON MAY 24, 1994
DISCIPLINARY ACTION: SURRENDER OF CONTROLLED SUBSTANCE LICENSE
OFFENSE: DISCIPLINARY ACTION BY ANOTHER STATE OR AGENCY
NOTES: STATE BOARD.

ANDERSON, VICKI SPARKS MD, LICENSE NUMBER 00E6215 OF AUSTIN, TX, WAS DISCIPLINED BY TEXAS ON AUGUST 19, 1994
DISCIPLINARY ACTION: 120-MONTH PROBATION; RESTRICTION PLACED ON CONTROLLED SUBSTANCE LICENSE
NOTES: HAS SATISFIED THE MINIMUM REQUIREMENTS OF AGREED ORDER OF 3/5/94 AND SUSPENSION IS NOW STAYED. CONDITIONS OF PROBATION: SHALL TREAT NO PATIENTS UNTIL SHE PASSES THE EXAMS NECESSARY FOR OBTAINING ACLS AND ATLS CERTIFICATION; SHALL ATTEND AT LEAST 50 HOURS PER YEAR OF CONTINUING MEDICAL EDUCATION IN EMERGENCY OR FAMILY MEDICINE; SHALL SUBMIT HERSELF FOR EVALUATION AND TREATMENT BY A BOARD-APPROVED PSYCHIATRIST WITH REPORTS TO THE BOARD; SHALL ABSTAIN FROM THE CONSUMPTION OF ALCOHOL/CHEMICAL SUBSTANCES IN ANY FORM UNLESS PRESCRIBED BY ANOTHER PHYSICIAN FOR A LEGITIMATE AND THERAPEUTIC PURPOSE; SHALL SUBMIT HERSELF FOR APPROPRIATE EXAMS INCLUDING ALCOHOL OR DRUG SCREENS; SHALL NOT TREAT OR OTHERWISE SERVE AS PHYSICIAN, PRESCRIBE, DISPENSE OR ADMINISTER DRUGS THAT MAY BE SUBJECT TO ABUSE TO HERSELF OR ANY MEMBER OF HER FAMILY; SEPARATE FROM PATIENT RECORDS, SHALL MAINTAIN A FILE OF EVERY PRESCRIPTION WRITTEN FOR CONTROLLED SUBSTANCES OR DANGEROUS DRUGS WHICH SHALL BE AVAILABLE FOR INSPECTION; SHALL NOT TELEPHONE PRESCRIPTIONS TO A PHARMACY FOR CONTROLLED SUBSTANCES OR DANGEROUS DRUGS OR PERMIT ANYONE NOT LICENSED BY THIS BOARD TO DO SO ON HER BEHALF; SHALL PARTICIPATE IN AA'S PROGRAM NOT LESS THAN THREE TIMES A WEEK WITH QUARTERLY REPORTS TO BOARD; SHALL PARTICIPATE IN THE ACTIVITIES OF A PHYSICIAN HEALTH AND REHABILITATION COMMITTEE AND ATTEND WEEKLY MEETINGS WITH QUARTERLY REPORTS; SHALL PASS THE SPEX EXAM WITHIN ONE YEAR; SHALL APPEAR BEFORE THE BOARD TWICE A YEAR; SHALL COOPERATE WITH THE BOARD IN VERIFYING COMPLIANCE; SHALL INFORM BOARD OF CHANGE OF ADDRESS WITHIN 10 DAYS OR IF SHE LEAVES THE STATE; TIME SPENT OUT OF TEXAS DOES NOT COUNT TOWARD PROBATION. SHALL NOT SEEK MODIFICATION FOR ONE YEAR. ON 10/5/96 ORDER MODIFIED SUCH THAT SHE MAY MAINTAIN A LOGBOOK OF PRESCRIPTIONS FOR DANGEROUS DRUGS RATHER THAN A COPY OF EVERY PRESCRIPTION. ON 8/22/98 PETITION TO TERMINATE ORDER DENIED; ORDER MODIFIED DELETING CONTINUING MEDICAL EDUCATION REQUIREMENT, PRESCRIPTION LOGBOOK REQUIREMENT, RESTRICTION FROM CALLING IN PRESCRIPTIONS, PARTICIPATION WITH THE COUNTY MEDICAL SOCIETY COMMITTEE, AND REQUIREMENT TO PASS THE SPEX WITHIN ONE YEAR; REDUCTION IN APPEARANCES BEFORE THE BOARD FROM BIANNUAL TO ANNUAL. ON 10/15/99 PETITION TO TERMINATE ORDER DENIED.

ANDRABI, TAYAB R MD, LICENSE NUMBER J3961 OF HOUSTON, TX, WAS DISCIPLINED BY TEXAS ON DECEMBER 11, 1999
DISCIPLINARY ACTION: 60-MONTH RESTRICTION PLACED ON LICENSE; RESTRICTION PLACED ON CONTROLLED SUBSTANCE LICENSE
OFFENSE: FAILURE TO COMPLY WITH PREVIOUS BOARD ORDER
NOTES: ON 4/10/99 BOARD ENTERED A NONDISCIPLINARY, NON PUBLIC ORDER WHICH RESTRICTED HIS LICENSE FOR FIVE YEARS BASED ON HIS ADMITTED SUBSTANCE ABUSE PROBLEM INCLUDING INTRAVENOUS USE OF SUFENTANYL, A NARCOTIC , FROM 9/97 TO 4/98; RECEIVED TREATMENT AND SIGNED A CONTRACT WITH THE PHYSICIAN'S HEALTH PROGRAM; VIOLATED 4/4/99 ORDER BY TESTING POSITIVE FOR FENTANYL ON 8/25/99; ON OR ABOUT 9/4/99 HIS EMPLOYMENT WAS TERMINATED BASED ON ABOVE DRUG TEST; HE REPORTS THAT HE RELAPSED INTO THE USE OF FENTANYL APPROXIMATELY 2 MONTHS PRIOR TO THE DRUG SCREEN; REPORTS THAT HE HAS AGAIN ATTAINED SOBRIETY AND HAS BEGUN THE RE-ESTABLISHMENT OF HIS RECOVERY PROGRAM BY: EXTENSIVE ATTENDANCE AT AA MEETINGS; SPECIAL MEETINGS WITH HIS AA SPONSOR; WEEKLY MEETINGS WITH HIS TREATING PSYCHIATRIST; ENROLLMENT IN AN INTENSIVE REHABILITATION PROGRAM; AND ACCEPTANCE INTO THE STANFORD UNIVERSITY PAIN MANAGEMENT FELLOWSHIP PROGRAM. LICENSE LIMITED AS FOLLOWS: SHALL ABSTAIN FROM THE CONSUMPTION OF ALCOHOL/DRUGS IN ANY FORM UNLESS PRESCRIBED BY ANOTHER PHYSICIAN FOR A LEGITIMATE AND THERAPEUTIC PURPOSE; SHALL SUBMIT HIMSELF FOR APPROPRIATE EXAMS INCLUDING DRUG OR ALCOHOL SCREENS; SHALL NOMINATE THREE CERTIFIED PSYCHIATRISTS FOR BOARD SELECTION OF A THERAPIST AND SHALL EXPEDITIOUSLY SUBMIT HIMSELF TO EVALUATION AND TREATMENT BY THE APPROVED PRACTITIONER; SHALL PARTICIPATE IN THE ACTIVITIES OF A PHYSICIAN HEALTH AND REHABILITATION COMMITTEE AND ATTEND WEEKLY MEETINGS WITH QUARTERLY REPORTS; SHALL PARTICIPATE IN AA'S PROGRAM NOT LESS THAN FIVE TIMES A WEEK; SHALL REPORT ON HIS ATTENDANCE; SHALL NOT POSSESS ALCOHOL, CONTROLLED SUBSTANCES, OR DANGEROUS DRUGS WITH ADDICTIVE POTENTIAL OR POTENTIAL FOR ABUSE AND SHALL SURRENDER ALL SAMPLES IN HIS POSSESSION; SHALL NOT TREAT OR OTHERWISE SERVE AS PHYSICIAN, PRESCRIBE, DISPENSE OR ADMINISTER DRUGS THAT MAY BE SUBJECT TO ABUSE TO HIMSELF OR TO ANY MEMBER OF HIS FAMILY; SHALL IMMEDIATELY SURRENDER DEA AND TEXAS DEPARTMENT OF PUBLIC SAFETY CONTROLLED SUBSTANCES REGISTRATION CERTIFICATES, AND ANY UNUSED TRIPLICATE PRESCRIPTION FORMS; SHALL LIMIT PRACTICE TO A GROUP OR INSTITUTIONAL SETTING; ANY

RESTRICTIONS WILL NOT HAMPER HIS PARTICIPATION IN THE STANFORD PAIN MANAGEMENT FELLOWSHIP; SHALL APPEAR BEFORE THE BOARD UPON REQUEST; SHALL COOPERATE WITH THE BOARD IN VERIFYING COMPLIANCE INCLUDING PROVIDING COPIES OF MEDICAL RELEASES AND PEER REVIEW RECORDS UPON REQUEST; SHALL GIVE A COPY OF THIS ORDER TO ANY HEALTH CARE ENTITY WHERE HE HAS PRIVILEGES; SHALL PROVIDE A COPY OF THIS ORDER TO ANYONE REQUESTING IT WITHIN 10 DAYS; TIME SPENT OUT OF TEXAS DOES NOT COUNT TOWARD RESTRICTION; SHALL INFORM THE BOARD OF CHANGE OF ADDRESS WITHIN 10 DAYS OR IF HE LEAVES THE STATE; SHALL NOT SEEK MODIFICATION FOR SIX MONTHS.

ANDREWS, RAWLE MD, LICENSE NUMBER 00D1963 OF HOUSTON, TX, WAS DISCIPLINED BY TEXAS ON APRIL 15, 1994
DISCIPLINARY ACTION: REQUIRED TO TAKE ADDITIONAL MEDICAL EDUCATION; MONITORING OF PHYSICIAN PERFORMANCE
OFFENSE: OVERPRESCRIBING OR MISPRESCRIBING DRUGS

NOTES: PRESCRIBED CONTROLLED SUBSTANCES AND SUBSTANCES WITH ADDICTIVE POTENTIAL TO TWO PATIENTS FOR EXTENDED PERIODS OF TIME WITHOUT ADEQUATE INDICATION. LICENSE RESTRICTED FOR FIVE YEARS WITH THE FOLLOWING CONDITIONS: WITHIN ONE YEAR WILL ENROLL IN, AND SUBSEQUENTLY COMPLETE, A TWO WEEK PRECEPTORSHIP ON THE PREVENTION AND TREATMENT OF DRUG ABUSE AND ONE ON PAIN MANAGEMENT; SHALL MAINTAIN ADEQUATE, LEGIBLE MEDICAL RECORDS ON ALL PATIENT OFFICE VISITS AND MAKE THESE AVAILABLE FOR INSPECTION; SHALL REFRAIN FROM THE PRESCRIPTION OR ADMINISTRATION OF ANY DRUG THAT IS NOT MEDICALLY INDICATED; SEPARATE FROM PATIENT RECORDS SHALL MAINTAIN A FILE OF EVERY PRESCRIPTION WRITTEN FOR ANY DANGEROUS DRUG WHICH MAY BE HABIT-FORMING WHICH SHALL BE AVAILABLE FOR INSPECTION; SHALL APPEAR BEFORE THE BOARD ONCE A YEAR; SHALL GIVE A COPY OF THIS ORDER TO ANY HEALTH CARE ENTITY WHERE HE HAS PRIVILEGES; SHALL COOPERATE WITH THE BOARD IN VERIFYING COMPLIANCE; SHALL INFORM BOARD OF CHANGE OF ADDRESS WITHIN 10 DAYS OR IF HE LEAVES THE STATE; TIME SPENT OUT OF TEXAS DOES NOT COUNT TOWARD PROBATION. SHALL NOT SEEK MODIFICATION FOR ONE YEAR. ON 5/10/97 PETITION TO MODIFY ORDER GRANTED DELETING ANNUAL APPEARANCES BEFORE THE BOARD. ON 1/29/99 ORDER TERMINATED.

ANDREWS, RAWLE MD, LICENSE NUMBER 0D00272 OF 7901 W MONTGOMERY RD, HOUSTON, TX, WAS DISCIPLINED BY MARYLAND ON FEBRUARY 22, 1995
DISCIPLINARY ACTION: PROBATION
OFFENSE: DISCIPLINARY ACTION BY ANOTHER STATE OR AGENCY

NOTES: AGREED ORDER WITH THE TEXAS BOARD AS A RESULT OF PRESCRIBING CONTROLLED SUBSTANCES WITH ADDICTIVE POTENTIAL FOR TWO PATIENTS FOR EXTENDED PERIODS WITHOUT ADEQUATE INDICATION. PROBATION TO RUN CONCURRENT WITH THE PROBATION SET FORTH IN THE CONSENT AGREEMENT OF 4/15/94 WITH TEXAS.

ANDREWS, RAWLE MD, LICENSE NUMBER 0C26336 OF HOUSTON, TX, WAS DISCIPLINED BY CALIFORNIA ON DECEMBER 13, 1995
DISCIPLINARY ACTION: LICENSE REVOCATION
OFFENSE: DISCIPLINARY ACTION BY ANOTHER STATE OR AGENCY

NOTES: ACTION IN TEXAS FOR PRESCRIBING CONTROLLED SUBSTANCES AND SUBSTANCES WITH ADDICTIVE POTENTIAL TO TWO PATIENTS FOR EXTENDED PERIODS OF TIME WITHOUT ADEQUATE INDICATION. DEFAULT ACTION.

ANGLE, JOHN FRANKLIN MD, LICENSE NUMBER 00D3132, WAS DISCIPLINED BY TEXAS ON AUGUST 17, 1996
DISCIPLINARY ACTION: 48-MONTH RESTRICTION PLACED ON LICENSE; REQUIRED TO TAKE ADDITIONAL MEDICAL EDUCATION
OFFENSE: SUBSTANDARD CARE, INCOMPETENCE OR NEGLIGENCE

NOTES: ON 3/03/95 DURING AN OPERATIVE HYSTEROSCOPY, STERILE WATER WAS USED AS A DISTENDING MEDIUM UNDER PRESSURE, INPUT AND OUTPUT OF THE FLUID DISTENDING MEDIUM WAS NOT ADEQUATELY MONITORED, INDICATIONS OF HYPONATREMIA WERE NOT SUFFICIENTLY MONITORED AND THE HYSTEROSCOPY WAS NOT COMPLETED OR OTHERWISE TERMINATED IN A TIMELY MANNER, AND AS A RESULT OF SOME OF THESE FACTORS THE PATIENT DIED; HE NEITHER ADMITS NOR DENIES THE ALLEGATIONS. FOUR YEAR RESTRICTION UNDER TERMS AND CONDITIONS: SHALL NOT PERFORM ANY OPERATIVE HYSTEROSCOPIC PROCEDURES WITHOUT AN ASSISTING SURGEON WHO HAS SPECIFIC TRAINING AND EXPERIENCE IN HYSTEROSCOPY; PRIOR TO UTILIZING ANY HYPOTONIC SOLUTION AS A DISTENDING MEDIUM IN HYSTEROSCOPIC PROCEDURES, SHALL CONSULT WITH AND OBTAIN THE AGREEMENT OF A MONITORING PHYSICIAN; WITHIN 90 DAYS SHALL SUBMIT IN WRITING TO THE BOARD A CORRECTIVE ACTION PLAN DETAILING HIS GENERAL PLAN FOR CONDUCTING FUTURE OPERATIVE HYSTEROCOPIC PROCEDURES; HIS MEDICAL PRACTICE, INCLUDING ANY OFFICE, HOSPITAL, AND SURGICAL PRACTICE, SHALL BE MONITORED BY A BOARD APPROVED TEXAS PHYSICIAN WHO SHALL SUBMIT QUARTERLY REPORTS TO THE BOARD; SHALL MAINTAIN ADEQUATE MEDICAL RECORDS WHICH SHALL BE AVAILABLE FOR REVIEW; SHALL ADEQUATELY SUPERVISE THE ACTIVITIES OF ALL HIS EMPLOYEES AND OTHER INDIVIDUALS UNDER HIS SUPERVISION TO ENSURE THAT SUCH INDIVIDUALS ARE COMPLYING WITH THE LAWS RELATING TO HIS PRACTICE OF MEDICINE; SHALL ATTEND AT LEAST 50 HOURS PER YEAR OF CONTINUING MEDICAL EDUCATION AT LEAST 10 OF WHICH SHALL BE IN RISK MANAGEMENT; EACH YEAR SHALL PERFORM 100 HOURS OF HUMANITARIAN SERVICE FOR A BOARD APPROVED NON-PROFIT CHARITABLE ORGANIZATION AND SUBMIT PROOF TO THE BOARD; SHALL APPEAR BEFORE THE BOARD ONCE PER YEAR OR UPON REQUEST; SHALL COOPERATE WITH THE BOARD IN VERIFYING COMPLIANCE INCLUDING PROVIDING COPIES OF PEER REVIEW RECORDS UPON REQUEST; SHALL GIVE A COPY OF THIS ORDER TO ANY HEALTH CARE ENTITY WHERE HE HAS PRIVILEGES; SHALL PROVIDE A COPY OF THIS ORDER TO ANYONE REQUESTING IT WITHIN 10 DAYS; TIME PERIOD OUT OF TEXAS DOES NOT COUNT TOWARD RESTRICTION; SHALL INFORM THE BOARD OF CHANGE OF ADDRESS WITHIN 10 DAYS OF IF HE LEAVES THE STATE; SHALL NOT SEEK MODIFICATION FOR ONE YEAR. ON 9/20/97 THE BOARD GRANTED HIS PETITION FOR TERMINATION OF THIS ORDER BASED ON COMPLIANCE WITH CONDITIONS.

ANID, ANTUN GEORGE MD, LICENSE NUMBER E7362 OF BAYTOWN, TX, WAS DISCIPLINED BY TEXAS ON OCTOBER 15, 1999
DISCIPLINARY ACTION: FINE; REPRIMAND
OFFENSE: OVERCHARGING

NOTES:

DURING 1992 - 1993 HE FLAGRANTLY OVERCHARGED 9 PATIENTS FOR GYNECOLOGICAL SERVICES. $1000 FINE; SHALL INFORM THE BOARD OF CHANGE OF ADDRESS WITHIN 10 DAYS; SHALL COOPERATE WITH THE BOARD IN VERIFYING COMPLIANCE; SHALL GIVE A COPY OF THIS ORDER TO ANY HEALTH CARE ENTITY WHERE HE HAS PRIVILEGES; SHALL PROVIDE A COPY OF THIS ORDER TO ANYONE REQUESTING IT WITHIN 10 DAYS.

ANKLESARIA, MANEK E MD, LICENSE NUMBER 0013574 OF 2325 S. HARVARD SUITE 104, TULSA, OK, WAS DISCIPLINED BY OKLAHOMA ON NOVEMBER 23, 1992
DISCIPLINARY ACTION: LICENSE SUSPENSION; REQUIRED TO ENTER AN IMPAIRED PHYSICIAN PROGRAM OR TREATMENT
OFFENSE: SEXUAL ABUSE OF OR SEXUAL MISCONDUCT WITH A PATIENT

NOTES: EXHIBITED INAPPROPRIATE SEXUAL BEHAVIOR WITH TWO OPHTHALMOLOGIC PATIENTS, ONE IN THE FALL OF 1990 AND THE OTHER MAY 6, 1991 INCLUDING SEXUAL COMMENTS, PLACING PATIENTS HAND ON HIS PENIS, AND FONDLING AND KISSING PATIENT. SUSPENSION IN EFFECT UNTIL PRESENTS EVIDENCE OF MEDICAL IN-PATIENT EVALUATION AND SUCCESSFUL COMPLETION OF TREATMENT. ON 5/20/93 SUSPENSION CONTINUED. HE WILL IMMEDIATELY UNDERGO FULL IN-PATIENT EVALUATION AND COMPLETE ANY NECESSARY TREATMENT; WILL NOT REAPPEAR BEFORE THE BOARD AND REQUEST TERMINATION OR MODIFICATION UNLESS HE CAN PROVIDE EVIDENCE OF SUCCESSFUL COMPLETION OF EVALUATION AND ANY NECESSARY TREATMENT AND ASSURANCE TO THE BOARD BY THE TREATMENT PROVIDER THAT HE MAY RETURN SAFELY TO PRACTICE MEDICINE.

ANKLESARIA, MANEK E MD, LICENSE NUMBER 0013574 OF 2325 S HARVARD AVE #104, TULSA, OK, WAS DISCIPLINED BY OKLAHOMA ON OCTOBER 11, 1993
DISCIPLINARY ACTION: 60-MONTH PROBATION; RESTRICTION PLACED ON LICENSE

NOTES: LICENSE REINSTATED FROM 11/21/92 SUSPENSION. CONDITIONS OF PROBATION BEGINNING 10/1/93: SHALL SUBMIT BIOLOGICAL FLUID SPECIMENS; SHALL FULFILL CONDITIONS RECOMMENDED BY SPECIFIED MD AND/OR THE STAFF OF SPECIFIED CENTER; SHALL ALLOW STAFF TO SPEAK WITH BOARD TO VERIFY COMPLIANCE; WHEN EXAMINING ANY FEMALE PATIENT SHALL HAVE A FEMALE MEDICAL PROFESSIONAL PRESENT; SHALL CONTINUE UNDER PSYCHIATRIC CARE WITH BOARD-APPROVED PHYSICIAN; SHALL NOTIFY ANY HEALTH CARE ENTITY WHERE HE HOLDS OR APPLIES FOR STAFF PRIVILEGES OF THE CONDITIONS OF THE ORDER; SHALL FURNISH BOARD WITH ADDRESS AND/OR CHANGE OF ADDRESS; SHALL APPEAR BEFORE THE BOARD UPON REQUEST AND SUBMIT REQUIRED REPORTS; SHALL PAY COSTS. ON 3/31/94 ORDER MODIFIED SUCH THAT BIOLOGICAL FLUID SPECIMENS WERE NO LONGER REQUIRED.

ANKLESARIA, MANEK E MD, LICENSE NUMBER 0141034 OF 2325 SOUTH HARVARD #206, TULSA, OK, WAS DISCIPLINED BY NEW YORK ON JANUARY 7, 1994
DISCIPLINARY ACTION: SURRENDER OF LICENSE
OFFENSE: DISCIPLINARY ACTION BY ANOTHER STATE OR AGENCY

NOTES: FOUND GUILTY OF IMPROPER PRACTICE BY THE OKLAHOMA BOARD.

ANKLESARIA, MANEK EDALJI MD, DATE OF BIRTH APRIL 15, 1949, LICENSE NUMBER 00F2155 OF 2325 SO HARVARD SUITE 104, TULSA, OK, WAS DISCIPLINED BY TEXAS ON APRIL 30, 1993
DISCIPLINARY ACTION: SURRENDER OF LICENSE

NOTES: LICENSE PERMANENTLY CANCELED.

ANKLESARIA, MANEK EDALJI MD, DATE OF BIRTH APRIL 15, 1949, LICENSE NUMBER 0020520 OF TULSA, OK, WAS DISCIPLINED BY NORTH CAROLINA ON DECEMBER 3, 1993
DISCIPLINARY ACTION: SURRENDER OF LICENSE

ANKLESARIA, MANEK EDALJI MD, DATE OF BIRTH APRIL 15, 1949, LICENSE NUMBER 0033882 OF 2325 S. HARVARD AVE., TULSA, OK, WAS DISCIPLINED BY NEW JERSEY ON DECEMBER 28, 1993
DISCIPLINARY ACTION: CEASE AND DESIST ORDER
OFFENSE: DISCIPLINARY ACTION BY ANOTHER STATE OR AGENCY

NOTES: DISCIPLINARY ACTION TAKEN IN OKLAHOMA. SHALL HAVE LEAVE TO SURRENDER HIS LICENSE TO PRACTICE MEDICINE AND SURGERY IN NEW JERSEY WITH PREJUDICE TO SEEKING REINSTATEMENT AT ANY FUTURE DATE.

ARCHER, JIM PAUL DO OF 4242 MEDICAL DR #7150, SAN ANTONIO, TX, WAS DISCIPLINED BY DEA ON OCTOBER 26, 1990
DISCIPLINARY ACTION: SURRENDER OF CONTROLLED SUBSTANCE LICENSE
OFFENSE: PROFESSIONAL MISCONDUCT

NOTES: VIOLATIONS OF OBTAINING CONTROLLED SUBSTANCES BY FRAUD.

ARCHER, JIM PAUL DO, LICENSE NUMBER 00D2978 OF 8434 FREDERICKSBURG RD., SAN ANTONIO, TX, WAS DISCIPLINED BY TEXAS ON DECEMBER 4, 1991
DISCIPLINARY ACTION: PROBATION; RESTRICTION PLACED ON CONTROLLED SUBSTANCE LICENSE
OFFENSE: SUBSTANCE ABUSE

NOTES: ADDICTION TO DEMEROL, MORPHINE, DILAUDID, VICODIN, AND TALWIN, WHICH RENDERS HIM UNABLE TO PRACTICE MEDICINE WITH REASONABLE SKILL AND SAFETY TO PATIENTS; ISSUED FALSE OR FICTITIOUS TRIPLICATE PRESCRIPTIONS; FAILED TO KEEP ADEQUATE INVENTORY OR DISPENSATION RECORDS; FAILED TO KEEP ADEQUATE PATIENT RECORDS REGARDING PRESCRIBING PRACTICES. REVOCATION STAYED; PLACED ON INDEFINITE PROBATION UNDER THE FOLLOWING TERMS AND CONDITIONS: SHALL ABSTAIN FROM THE CONSUMPTION OF ALCOHOL/CHEMICAL SUBSTANCES IN ANY FORM, EXCEPT AS PRESCRIBED BY ANOTHER PHYSICIAN; SHALL PARTICIPATE IN THE ACTIVITIES OF AN IMPAIRED PHYSICIANS PROGRAM, INCLUDING WEEKLY MEETINGS, WITH QUARTERLY REPORTS TO THE BOARD; SHALL PARTICIPATE IN AA NOT LESS THAN THREE TIMES A WEEK FOR THE FIRST YEAR OF PROBATION, AND TWO TIMES THEREAFTER, WITH QUARTERLY REPORTS TO THE BOARD; SHALL SUBMIT TO RANDOM TESTS OF BODILY FLUIDS; SHALL ABIDE BY RECOMMENDATIONS OF A BOARD APPROVED PSYCHIATRIST; SHALL REFRAIN FROM THE USE OF AND SHALL NOT POSSESS, ADMINISTER, OR PRESCRIBE ANY CONTROLLED SUBSTANCE OR ANY OTHER DRUG REQUIRING A PRESCRIPTION; SHALL APPEAR BEFORE THE BOARD TWICE A YEAR; SHALL NOT ATTEMPT TO REREGISTER CONTROLLED SUBSTANCES LICENSES WITHOUT BOARD PERMISSION; SHALL GIVE A COPY OF THIS ORDER TO ANY HOSPITAL WHERE HE HAS PRIVILEGES; SHALL COOPERATE WITH THE BOARD IN VERIFYING COMPLIANCE; SHALL ADVISE THE BOARD OF A

CHANGE IN ADDRESS WITHIN 10 DAYS; TIME SPENT OUT OF TEXAS DOES NOT COUNT TOWARDS PROBATION. ON 8/19/94 HIS REQUEST FOR TERMINATION OF THIS ORDER DENIED.

ARCHER, JIM PAUL DO, LICENSE NUMBER 00D2978 OF SAN ANTONIO, TX, WAS DISCIPLINED BY TEXAS ON AUGUST 18, 1995
DISCIPLINARY ACTION: LICENSE SUSPENSION
OFFENSE: FAILURE TO COMPLY WITH PREVIOUS BOARD ORDER

NOTES: IN VIOLATION OF 12/4/91 ORDER DURING 1995, SUBMITTED INTENTIONALLY INACCURATE OR FRAUDULENT REPORTS OF HIS PARTICIPATION IN THE COUNTY MEDICAL SOCIETY'S WEEKLY CADUCEUS MEETINGS; DURING 1994 AND 1995 SUBMITTED INTENTIONALLY INACCURATE OR FRAUDULENT REPORTS OF HIS PARTICIPATION IN AA; IN 6/95 HE INGESTED ALCOHOL. SUSPENSION UNTIL HE APPEARS BEFORE BOARD WITH SUFFICIENT EVIDENCE THAT HE IS PHYSICALLY, MENTALLY AND OTHERWISE COMPETENT TO SAFELY PRACTICE MEDICINE INCLUDING AT A MINIMUM COPIES OF MEDICAL RECORDS OR REPORTS OF PSYCHOLOGICAL AND NEUROPSYCHIATRIC EVALUATIONS INCLUDING A 96-HOUR INPATIENT EVALUATION BY A BOARD-APPROVED PSYCHIATRIST.

ARNDT-HAGAN, MARY L MD, DATE OF BIRTH AUGUST 26, 1956 OF 13510 TOM FIELD ROAD, DALLAS, TX, WAS DISCIPLINED BY MEDICARE ON AUGUST 13, 1993
DISCIPLINARY ACTION: EXCLUSION FROM THE MEDICARE AND/OR MEDICAID PROGRAM
OFFENSE: NONCOMPLIANCE WITH A PROFESSIONAL RULE

NOTES: DEFAULTED ON HEALTH EDUCATION ASSISTANCE LOAN. REINSTATED ON 9/28/93.

ARORA, MUKAND LAL MD, LICENSE NUMBER 130350 OF 83 HOMESTEAD RD. #3, HOUSTON, TX, WAS DISCIPLINED BY NEW YORK ON OCTOBER 3, 1997
DISCIPLINARY ACTION: SURRENDER OF LICENSE
OFFENSE: DISCIPLINARY ACTION BY ANOTHER STATE OR AGENCY

NOTES: DISCIPLINED BY THE TEXAS BOARD FOR PRESCRIBING CONTROLLED SUBSTANCES WITHOUT MEDICAL JUSTIFICATION AND MAKING FALSE ENTRIES INTO A PATIENT RECORD.

ASENDIO, DONNA MD, LICENSE NUMBER 00H7380 OF DALLAS, TX, WAS DISCIPLINED BY TEXAS ON MAY 15, 1996
DISCIPLINARY ACTION: FINE
OFFENSE: OVERCHARGING

NOTES: PERSISTENTLY OR FLAGRANTLY OVERCHARGING OR OVERTREATING PATIENTS IN THAT DURING 1994, SHE BILLED FOR CARE AND TREATMENT IN A MANNER THAT REFLECTED THAT THE SERVICES WERE MORE COMPLEX OR TIME CONSUMING THAN THE CARE ACTUALLY RENDERED; ERRORS WERE APPARENTLY MADE IN SOME OF THE BILLINGS BY HER EMPLOYEE; SHE MAINTAINS THAT SERVICES PROVIDED WERE NECESSARY AND THAT ANY EXCESSIVE BILLINGS WERE A RESULT OF CODING ERRORS OR DUE TO MISINFORMATION RECEIVED FROM A CODING SEMINAR; REPORTS THAT SHE HAS IMPLEMENTED REMEDIAL MEASURES TO ELIMINATE FUTURE CODING ERRORS. SHALL PAY $5,000 FINE; SHALL COOPERATE WITH THE BOARD IN VERIFYING COMPLIANCE.

ASHBY, CHARLES HENRY MD, LICENSE NUMBER 00B6292, WAS DISCIPLINED BY TEXAS ON AUGUST 17, 1996
DISCIPLINARY ACTION: REQUIRED TO TAKE ADDITIONAL MEDICAL EDUCATION; MONITORING OF PHYSICIAN PERFORMANCE
OFFENSE: SUBSTANDARD CARE, INCOMPETENCE OR NEGLIGENCE

NOTES: FAILED TO ADEQUATELY MANAGE THE CARE OF THREE PATIENTS; MAY BE A RESULT OF A DECLINE IN HIS HEALTH. DOES NOT ADMIT VIOLATION. ON OR BEFORE 11/30/96 SHALL CEASE THE PRACTICE OF MEDICINE UNTIL HE REQUESTS PERMISSION IN WRITING TO RESUME PRACTICE AND PERSONALLY APPEAR BEFORE THE BOARD AND PROVIDES SUFFICIENT EVIDENCE TO INDICATE HE IS PHYSICALLY, MENTALLY, AND OTHERWISE COMPETENT TO SAFELY PRACTICE MEDICINE INCLUDING AT A MINIMUM A FAVORABLE WRITTEN ASSESSMENT BASED ON A NEURO-PSYCHIATRIC EXAMINATION BY A CERTIFIED PSYCHIATRIST; DOCUMENTATION OF CONTINUING MEDICAL EDUCATION WHICH AT LEAST MEETS THE MINIMUM REQUIREMENTS FOR LICENSURE RENEWAL; SHALL PASS THE SPEX WITHIN THREE MONTHS PRIOR TO HIS REQUEST TO RESUME PRACTICE; SHALL SUBMIT A TYPE-WRITTEN NARRATIVE DESCRIBING PATIENT CARE RENDERED AND A DETAILED CORRECTIVE ACTION PLAN TO AVOID SIMILAR DIFFICULTIES AND POSSIBLE ADVERSE OUTCOMES; SHALL COOPERATE WITH THE BOARD IN VERIFYING COMPLIANCE INCLUDING PROVIDING COPIES OF MEDICAL RELEASES AND PEER REVIEW RECORDS UPON REQUEST; SHALL GIVE A COPY OF THIS ORDER TO ANY HEALTH CARE ENTITY WHERE HE HAS PRIVILEGES; SHALL PROVIDE A COPY OF THIS ORDER TO ANYONE REQUESTING IT WITHIN 10 DAYS; TIME PERIOD OUT OF TEXAS DOES NOT COUNT TOWARD RESTRICTION; SHALL INFORM THE BOARD OF CHANGE OF ADDRESS WITHIN 10 DAYS OF IF HE LEAVES THE STATE; SHALL NOT SEEK MODIFICATION FOR ONE YEAR.

ATHARI, MOHAMMAD MD, LICENSE NUMBER E6718 OF BAYTOWN, TX, WAS DISCIPLINED BY TEXAS ON SEPTEMBER 20, 1997
DISCIPLINARY ACTION: REPRIMAND; REQUIRED TO TAKE ADDITIONAL MEDICAL EDUCATION
OFFENSE: SEXUAL ABUSE OF OR SEXUAL MISCONDUCT WITH A PATIENT

NOTES: IN 1993 ENGAGED IN SEXUAL RELATIONS WITH A PATIENT; FAILED TO PROPERLY TERMINATE THE RELATIONSHIP OR TO AWAIT A SUFFICIENT PERIOD OF TIME BEFORE ENGAGING IN A SEXUAL RELATIONSHIP WITH THE PATIENT; HE MAINTAINS THAT THE PHYSICIAN-PATIENT RELATIONSHIP WAS A PRETEXT ON THE PART OF THE ALLEGED PATIENT AND IT APPEARS THE PATIENT WAS MANIPULATIVE. TERMS AND CONDITIONS ON LICENSE FOR ONE YEAR: SHALL OBTAIN 24 HOURS OF AN ETHICS COURSE WITHIN 12 MONTHS; SHALL PERSONALLY APPEAR BEFORE THE BOARD AT LEAST ONCE DURING THE YEAR; SHALL COOPERATE WITH THE BOARD IN VERIFYING COMPLIANCE; SHALL GIVE A COPY OF THIS ORDER TO ANY HEALTH CARE ENTITY WHERE HE HAS PRIVILEGES; TIME SPENT OUT OF TEXAS DOES NOT COUNT TOWARD RESTRICTION; SHALL INFORM THE BOARD OF CHANGE OF ADDRESS WITHIN 10 DAYS OR IF HE LEAVES THE STATE; SHALL NOT SEEK MODIFICATION FOR ONE YEAR.

ATKINSON, WILLIAM HUDSON MD, LICENSE NUMBER 00E2448 OF WAXAHACHIE, TX, WAS DISCIPLINED BY TEXAS ON APRIL 10, 1992
DISCIPLINARY ACTION: 60-MONTH PROBATION

NOTES: PROFESSIONAL FAILURE TO PRACTICE MEDICINE IN AN ACCEPTABLE MANNER CONSISTENT WITH PUBLIC HEALTH AND WELFARE. LICENSE SUSPENDED, SUSPENSION STAYED; PROBATION UNDER TERMS

AND CONDITIONS. ON 5/15/96 HIS PETITION FOR TERMINATION DENIED AND ORDER MODIFIED AS FOLLOWS: PETITIONS FOR TERMINATION OR MODIFICATION MAY BE FILED ONCE EVERY SIX MONTHS; TERMINATION MAY BE GRANTED BASED UPON DOCUMENTATION THAT HE HAS ASSISTED IN INVASIVE SURGICAL PROCEDURES; ALL OTHER PROVISION OF THIS ORDER REMAIN IN EFFECT.

ATLAS, RUTH M MD, LICENSE NUMBER 00G7616 OF HOUSTON, TX, WAS DISCIPLINED BY TEXAS ON AUGUST 24, 1991
DISCIPLINARY ACTION: REPRIMAND
OFFENSE: PROFESSIONAL MISCONDUCT

NOTES: UNPROFESSIONAL OR DISHONORABLE CONDUCT LIKELY TO DECEIVE, DEFRAUD, OR INJURE THE PUBLIC.

AVERYT, ELMORE M JR MD OF 7930 FLOYD CURL, SAN ANTONIO, TX, WAS DISCIPLINED BY DEA ON JULY 23, 1996
DISCIPLINARY ACTION: SURRENDER OF CONTROLLED SUBSTANCE LICENSE

AVILES, WILFREDO A MD, LICENSE NUMBER 00E6719 OF WESLACO, TX, WAS DISCIPLINED BY TEXAS ON AUGUST 18, 1995
DISCIPLINARY ACTION: FINE; REPRIMAND
OFFENSE: PROFESSIONAL MISCONDUCT

NOTES: FAILED TO ADEQUATELY SUPERVISE THE ACTIVITIES OF HIS PHYSICIAN ASSISTANT, WHO ALLEGEDLY HELD HIMSELF OUT AS A LICENSED TEXAS PHYSICIAN ON OFFICE PAMPHLETS, A BUSINESS CARD AND AN OFFICE SIGN; HE CONTENDS THAT HE DID NOT FAIL TO ADEQUATELY SUPERVISE HIS ASSISTANT AND DID NOT AUTHORIZE HIM TO HOLD HIMSELF OUT AS A PHYSICIAN. SHALL PAY $5,000 FINE.

AXELROD, WILLIAM MD, DATE OF BIRTH JANUARY 9, 1918, LICENSE NUMBER 00B6608 OF 1109 MEDICAL TOWERS 1700 DRYDEN, HOUSTON, TX, WAS DISCIPLINED BY TEXAS ON APRIL 30, 1993
DISCIPLINARY ACTION: 60-MONTH PROBATION; RESTRICTION PLACED ON CONTROLLED SUBSTANCE LICENSE
OFFENSE: OVERPRESCRIBING OR MISPRESCRIBING DRUGS

NOTES: FROM 2/3/89 THROUGH 7/20/92 HE COMMITTED SEVERAL PRESCRIPTION VIOLATIONS INCLUDING FAILING TO JUSTIFY IN HIS MEDICAL RECORDS THE USE OF INJECTABLE DEMEROL FOR TWO PATIENTS FOR WHOM HE WAS NOT THEIR TREATING PHYSICIAN; PRESCRIBED DEMEROL FOR ONE OF THESE PATIENTS WHICH WAS ADMINISTERED TO THE OTHER; FAILED TO KEEP COMPLETE AND ACCURATE RECORDS OF PURCHASES AND DISPOSALS OF DANGEROUS DRUGS AND/OR CONTROLLED SUBSTANCES; FAILED TO MAINTAIN ACQUISITION AND DISPENSING RECORDS FOR TALWIN; ON 8/17/92 HE SURRENDERED DEA AND DPS REGISTRATIONS WHICH WERE THEN REVOKED. FIVE YEAR SUSPENSION STAYED. CONDITIONS OF PROBATION: MAY APPLY FOR REINSTATEMENT OF CONTROLLED SUBSTANCE REGISTRATIONS FOR SCHEDULES III, IV AND V BUT NOT SCHEDULE II; SHALL APPEAR BEFORE THE BOARD ONCE A YEAR; SHALL GIVE A COPY OF THIS ORDER TO ANY HEALTH CARE ENTITY WHERE HE HAS PRIVILEGES; SHALL COOPERATE WITH THE BOARD IN VERIFYING COMPLIANCE; SHALL INFORM THE BOARD OF CHANGE OF ADDRESS WITHIN 10 DAYS OR IF HE LEAVES THE STATE; TIME SPENT OUT OF TEXAS DOES NOT COUNT TOWARD PROBATION. SHALL NOT SEEK MODIFICATION FOR ONE YEAR.

AXELROD, WILLIAM MD, DATE OF BIRTH JANUARY 9, 1918 OF 1109 MEDICAL TOWERS, HOUSTON, TX, WAS DISCIPLINED BY DEA ON SEPTEMBER 20, 1993
DISCIPLINARY ACTION: RESTRICTION PLACED ON CONTROLLED SUBSTANCE LICENSE
OFFENSE: NONCOMPLIANCE WITH A PROFESSIONAL RULE

NOTES: EXCESSIVE PURCHASE REPORT. ORDERED EXCESSIVE AMOUNTS OF DEMEROL WITHOUT MAINTAINING RECORDS. VOLUNTARY SURRENDER OF REGISTRATION ON 08/17/92. SEIZED 9 MLS DEMEROL AND 10 MLS TALWIN. SUBMITTED APPLICATION FOR REGISTRATION ON 07/01/93. APPROVAL OF APPLICATION.

AYAD, FOUAD M MD, LICENSE NUMBER E5472 OF TYLER, TX, WAS DISCIPLINED BY TEXAS ON AUGUST 22, 1998
DISCIPLINARY ACTION: SURRENDER OF LICENSE

NOTES: IN CONTEMPLATION OF RETIREMENT, HE HAS CHOSEN TO VOLUNTARILY AND PERMANENTLY SURRENDER HIS LICENSE.

AYER, MAX E DO OF ATHENS, TX, WAS DISCIPLINED BY MISSOURI ON NOVEMBER 12, 1997
DISCIPLINARY ACTION: 60-MONTH PROBATION
OFFENSE: DISCIPLINARY ACTION BY ANOTHER STATE OR AGENCY

NOTES: ACTION BASED ON DISCIPLINE TAKEN BY THE TEXAS BOARD FOR FAILURE TO MAINTAIN ADEQUATE RECORDS RELATING TO A NUMBER OF PATIENTS TREATED FOR WEIGHT LOSS WITH PRESCRIPTION MEDICATIONS. PROBATION RETROACTIVE TO 6/22/96.

AYOUB, SAMY YOUSSEF MD, LICENSE NUMBER E5473 OF BEEVILLE, TX, WAS DISCIPLINED BY TEXAS ON APRIL 4, 1998
DISCIPLINARY ACTION: FINE
OFFENSE: LOSS OR RESTRICTION OF HOSPITAL PRIVILEGES

NOTES: IN 5/97 AN INSPECTION FOUND VIOLATIONS REGARDING HIS DUTIES AS A RADIATION SAFETY OFFICER AND SUPERVISING PHYSICIAN WHICH WERE REPEATS OF 4/96 VIOLATIONS AND INVOLVED: HIS RESPONSIBILITY TO REVIEW THE TECHNOLOGIST'S QUALITY CONTROL TESTS AT LEAST EVERY 3 MONTHS; RESPONSIBILITY TO PERFORM A QUARTERLY AUDIT AT EACH FACILITY FOR WHICH HE HAS BEEN DESIGNATED RADIATION SAFETY OFFICER; HE DID NOT OBTAIN 16 ADDITIONAL HOURS OF TRANING IN QUALITY ASSURANCE BY THE 5/97 INSPECTION AS WAS REQUIRED BY ENFORCEMENT CONFERENCES; HE CONTENDS THAT NO DEADLINE WAS PROVIDED FOR COMPLETING THE TRAINING AND THAT HE COMPLETED SAID TRAINING BY 9/97, THAT HE PERFORMS A MONTHLY REVIEW OF THE TECHNOLOGISTS' QUALITY CONTROL TEST, AND HE DID NOT FAIL TO PERFORM ANY QUARTERLY AUDIT, BUT RATHER FAILED TO PERFORM THE AUDIT WHICH PRECEDED THE REINSPECTION; HE WAS REMOVED BY THE HOSPITAL AS RADIATION SAFETY OFFICER AND THE HOSPITAL WAS REQUIRED TO NOTIFY MORE THAN 2,000 PATIENTS OF THE POSSIBILITY THAT THEIR MAMMOGRAMS WERE NOT OF SUFFICIENT QUALITY DUE TO THE VIOLATIONS; THERE WAS NO EVIDENCE THAT ANY OF THE PERFORMED MAMMOGRAMS LED TO PATIENT HARM. $3,500 FINE.

AYUB, PABLO MD OF 5301 ALAMEDA AVENUE, EL PASO, TX, WAS DISCIPLINED BY DEA ON JANUARY 19, 1999
DISCIPLINARY ACTION: SURRENDER OF CONTROLLED SUBSTANCE LICENSE

NOTES: IN LIEU OF PUBLIC INTEREST REVOCATION.

AYUB, PABLO MD, LICENSE NUMBER C1579 OF EL PASO, TX, WAS DISCIPLINED BY TEXAS ON DECEMBER 11, 1999
DISCIPLINARY ACTION: REPRIMAND
OFFENSE: PROFESSIONAL MISCONDUCT

NOTES: ON 1/14/99 A DRUG AUDIT OF HIS OFFICE FOUND THAT HE FAILED TO MAINTAIN ADEQUATE RECORDS FOR THE CONTROLLED SUBSTANCES FOUND ON THE PREMISES; UNABLE TO EXPLAIN HOW OR FROM WHOM HIS OFFICE ORDERS CONTROLLED SUBSTANCES; IMPROPERLY DELEGATED AND FAILED TO SUPERVISE THE RESPONSIBILITY FOR THE SAFEKEEPING AND RECORDKEEPING OF PURCHASES AND DISPOSALS OF CONTROLLED SUBSTANCES AND DANGEROUS DRUGS TO HIS WIFE WHO HOLDS NO MEDICAL LICENSE; AND ADMITTED THAT HE FAILED TO COMPLY WITH THE LAWS REGARDING CONTROL OVER CERTAIN DRUGS; SURRENDERED HIS CONTROLLED SUBSTANCES CERTIFICATES.

AZEVEDO, FERNANDO W MD, LICENSE NUMBER 00D8138 OF MISSOURI CITY, TX, WAS DISCIPLINED BY TEXAS ON JANUARY 24, 1992
DISCIPLINARY ACTION: SURRENDER OF LICENSE

NOTES: LICENSE PLACED ON RETIREMENT STATUS IN LIEU OF FURTHER INVESTIGATION AND DISCIPLINARY ACTION.

AZIM, MOHAMMAD MD, LICENSE NUMBER 00J3398, WAS DISCIPLINED BY TEXAS ON NOVEMBER 16, 1996
DISCIPLINARY ACTION: REPRIMAND
OFFENSE: SUBSTANDARD CARE, INCOMPETENCE OR NEGLIGENCE

NOTES: IN 9/95 HE FAILED TO ADEQUATELY DIAGNOSE AND TREAT AN 11 YEAR OLD PATIENT; HE FAILED TO OBTAIN A REPEAT SERUM GLUCOSE IN A PATIENT WITH CONTINUING WEIGHT LOSS, VOMITING AND KNOWN GLUCOSURIA; PATIENT WAS LATER DIAGNOSED WITH DIABETIC KETOACIDOSIS; FAILED TO ADEQUATELY COMMUNICATE WITH A PREVIOUS TREATING PHYSICIAN OR THE PATIENT'S PARENTS IN REGARD TO THE ABOVE MATTER. SHALL GIVE A COPY OF THIS ORDER TO ANY HEALTH CARE ENTITY WHERE HE HAS PRIVILEGES.

BACHYNSKY, NICHOLAS MD, LICENSE NUMBER 00E1495 OF HOUSTON, TX, WAS DISCIPLINED BY TEXAS ON JANUARY 26, 1990
DISCIPLINARY ACTION: LICENSE REVOCATION
OFFENSE: CRIMINAL CONVICTION OR PLEA OF GUILTY, NOLO CONTENDERE, OR NO CONTEST TO A CRIME

NOTES: PLEADED GUILTY 7/13/89 TO FRAUD IN U.S. DISTRICT COURT FOR THE SOUTHERN DISTRICT OF TEXAS

BACHYNSKY, NICHOLAS MD, LICENSE NUMBER 0168030 OF HOUSTON, TX, WAS DISCIPLINED BY NEW YORK ON MAY 13, 1991
DISCIPLINARY ACTION: LICENSE REVOCATION

BACHYNSKY, NICHOLAS MD, LICENSE NUMBER 0047143 OF FT WORTH, TX, WAS DISCIPLINED BY FLORIDA ON DECEMBER 30, 1991
DISCIPLINARY ACTION: LICENSE REVOCATION; FINE
OFFENSE: DISCIPLINARY ACTION BY ANOTHER STATE OR AGENCY

NOTES: LICENSE REVOKED IN ANOTHER STATE; CONVICTED OR FOUND GUILTY OF, OR ENTERED PLEA OF NOLO CONTENDERE TO, REGARDLESS OF ADJUDICATION, A CRIME IN ANY JURISDICTION WHICH DIRECTLY RELATES TO THE PRACTICE OF MEDICINE OR THE ABILITY TO PRACTICE MEDICINE. $10,000 FINE.

BAERTL, JUAN M MD, DATE OF BIRTH MARCH 14, 1926, LICENSE NUMBER 038088L OF MORRIS ROAD RD#1, BOX 220, FAWN GROVE, PA, WAS DISCIPLINED BY PENNSYLVANIA ON JULY 25, 1995
DISCIPLINARY ACTION: SURRENDER OF LICENSE

NOTES: IN LIEU OF PROSECUTION. VOLUNTARY SURRENDER. MAY NEVER RENEW, REACTIVATE OR REINSTATE HIS LICENSE.

BAERTL, JUAN M MD, LICENSE NUMBER 0D20881 OF 438 PINE SHADOWS DR, SOUR LAKE, TX, WAS DISCIPLINED BY MARYLAND ON NOVEMBER 28, 1995
DISCIPLINARY ACTION: SURRENDER OF LICENSE
OFFENSE: DISCIPLINARY ACTION BY ANOTHER STATE OR AGENCY

NOTES: SURRENDER OF LICENSE IN PENNSYLVANIA.

BAGWELL, JERRY GLYN MD, LICENSE NUMBER 00D1130 OF GATESVILLE, TX, WAS DISCIPLINED BY TEXAS ON NOVEMBER 3, 1994
DISCIPLINARY ACTION: 120-MONTH PROBATION; REQUIRED TO TAKE ADDITIONAL MEDICAL EDUCATION
OFFENSE: SUBSTANDARD CARE, INCOMPETENCE OR NEGLIGENCE

NOTES: TREATED A 28 YEAR OLD FEMALE ON MARCH 15 AND 16, 1993; HER MEDICAL RECORDS SHOW A HISTORY OF SEIZURES, PEPTIC ULCER DISEASE, CERVICAL DYSPLASIA AND LOWER EXTREMITY DEEP VEIN THROMBOSIS; ALSO NOTED IN HER RECORDS WAS ONGOING COUMADIN THERAPY; ON 3/16/93 HE NOTED BLEEDING INTO HER SKIN AND ORDERED LAB TESTING; HER PROTHROMBIN TIME WAS GREATER THAN 50; HE FAILED TO ALTER THE DOSAGE OF, OR TO DISCONTINUE, HER COUMADIN; WAS PLACED ON PROBATION BECAUSE OF THIS BY THE TEXAS DEPARTMENT OF CRIMINAL JUSTICE PEER REVIEW COMMITTEE FOR TWO MONTHS WHICH ENDED 12/26/93. SUSPENSION STAYED. CONDITIONS OF PROBATION: SHALL MAINTAIN ADEQUATE MEDICAL RECORDS ON ALL PATIENT VISITS WHICH SHALL BE AVAILABLE FOR INSPECTION; SHALL NOT SIGN ANY PATIENT RECORD UNLESS HE HAS PERSONALLY EXAMINED THE PATIENT OR CLEARLY NOTES IN THE RECORD THAT HE DID NOT; SHALL ATTEND AT LEAST 50 HOURS PER YEAR OF CONTINUING MEDICAL EDUCATION, 10 HOURS OF WHICH SHALL BE IN RISK MANAGEMENT AND 40 HOURS OF WHICH SHALL BE IN FAMILY PRACTICE; WITHIN SIX MONTHS SHALL PASS THE SPEX EXAM AND THE MEDICAL JURISPRUDENCE EXAM; SHALL APPEAR BEFORE THE BOARD TWICE A YEAR; SHALL GIVE A COPY OF THIS ORDER TO ANY HEALTH CARE ENTITY WHERE HE HAS PRIVILEGES; SHALL COOPERATE WITH THE BOARD IN VERIFYING COMPLIANCE; SHALL INFORM BOARD OF CHANGE OF ADDRESS WITHIN 10 DAYS OR IF HE LEAVES THE STATE; TIME SPENT OUT OF TEXAS DOES NOT COUNT TOWARD PROBATION. SHALL NOT SEEK MODIFICATION FOR ONE YEAR.

BAILEY, SHARON DO OF 1133 MADLYNNE, CEDAR HILL, TX, WAS DISCIPLINED BY OKLAHOMA ON DECEMBER 13, 1990
DISCIPLINARY ACTION: MONITORING OF PHYSICIAN PERFORMANCE

NOTES: LICENSE GRANTED WITH THE FOLLOWING STIPULATIONS: WEEKLY ATTENDANCE WITH DOCUMENTATION TO THE BOARD OF NARCOTICS ANONYMOUS, AA, AND THE OOA PHYSICIAN'S RECOVERY COMMITTEE MEETINGS; SHALL SUBMIT TO RANDOM DRUG SCREENS AT THE BOARD'S DISCRETION; SHALL CONTACT THE PHYSICIAN'S RECOVERY COMMITTEE OF THE OOA FOR INCORPORATION WITH THEM OF THE CONTRACT SIGNED REGARDING HER RECOVERY IN TEXAS.

BAILEY, SHARON ANNE DO, LICENSE NUMBER 00G0654 OF DALLAS,

TX, WAS DISCIPLINED BY TEXAS ON APRIL 20, 1991
DISCIPLINARY ACTION: 120-MONTH PROBATION; REQUIRED TO ENTER AN IMPAIRED PHYSICIAN PROGRAM OR SUBSTANCE ABUSE TREATMENT
OFFENSE: SUBSTANCE ABUSE

NOTES: SHALL COMPLY WITH TERMS OF IMPAIRED HEALTH PROFESSIONAL'S TREATMENT CONTRACT OF THE TEXAS OSTEOPATHIC MEDICAL ASSOCIATION; AFTER EXPIRATION OF THIS CONTRACT, SHALL PARTICIPATE IN AA ON A REGULAR BASIS; SHALL SUBMIT TO ALCOHOL OR DRUG SCREENS; SHALL CONTINUE TREATMENT WITH A BOARD-APPROVED PHYSICIAN, WITH TWICE YEARLY REPORTS TO THE BOARD; SHALL OBTAIN AND CONTINUE TO HAVE A RECOVERING ABUSE SPONSOR WHO IS A HEALTH CARE PROFESSIONAL. PROBATION TERMINATED ON 5/15/96.

BAIRD, DAVID BIRCH JR MD, DATE OF BIRTH MAY 11, 1937, LICENSE NUMBER 0024835 OF 76773 CHRYSANTHEMUM WAY, PALM DESERT, CA, WAS DISCIPLINED BY NEW JERSEY ON JULY 9, 1992
DISCIPLINARY ACTION: LICENSE REVOCATION
OFFENSE: INSURANCE, MEDICARE OR MEDICAID FRAUD

NOTES: SEXUAL MISCONDUCT AND SUBMISSION OF FRAUDULENT INSURANCE CLAIMS FOR OFFICE VISITS, WHEN THE PURPOSE OF THOSE OFFICE VISITS WAS OTHER THAN MEDICAL.

BAIRD, DAVID BIRCH JR MD, LICENSE NUMBER 0063410 OF TOWANDA, PA, WAS DISCIPLINED BY OHIO ON NOVEMBER 21, 1992
DISCIPLINARY ACTION: LICENSE REVOCATION

NOTES: PERMANENTLY REVOKED.

BAIRD, DAVID BIRCH JR MD, DATE OF BIRTH MAY 11, 1937 OF 1212 A CROSS HILL COURT, LANSDALE, PA, WAS DISCIPLINED BY MEDICARE ON APRIL 10, 1995
DISCIPLINARY ACTION: 60-MONTH EXCLUSION FROM THE MEDICARE AND/OR MEDICAID PROGRAM
OFFENSE: CRIMINAL CONVICTION OR PLEA OF GUILTY, NOLO CONTENDERE, OR NO CONTEST TO A CRIME

NOTES: CONVICTED OF A CRIME INVOLVING THE MEDICARE, MEDICAID, MATERNAL AND CHILD HEALTH SERVICES BLOCK GRANT OR BLOCK GRANTS TO STATES FOR SOCIAL SERVICES PROGRAMS.

BAIRD, DAVID BIRCH JR MD, DATE OF BIRTH MAY 11, 1937, LICENSE NUMBER 007458E OF 76773 CHRYSANTHEMUM WAY, PALM DESERT, CA, WAS DISCIPLINED BY PENNSYLVANIA ON FEBRUARY 20, 1996
DISCIPLINARY ACTION: LICENSE REVOCATION
OFFENSE: DISCIPLINARY ACTION BY ANOTHER STATE OR AGENCY

NOTES: DISCIPLINARY ACTION TAKEN BY NEW JERSEY; SUBMITTING A FALSIFIED LICENSURE CERTIFICATE TO EMPLOYERS; PRACTICING ON AN EXPIRED LICENSE/NOTIFICATION OF CHANGE OF ADDRESS AND PLED GUILTY TO A FELONY.

BAIRD, DAVID BIRCH JR MD, DATE OF BIRTH MAY 11, 1937, LICENSE NUMBER 24835 OF 2426 COMMUNICATIONS PKWY.#914, PLANO, TX, WAS DISCIPLINED BY NEW JERSEY ON APRIL 20, 1999
DISCIPLINARY ACTION: DENIAL OF LICENSE REINSTATEMENT
OFFENSE: SEXUAL ABUSE OF OR SEXUAL MISCONDUCT WITH A PATIENT

NOTES: 1/90 COMPLAINT ALLEGED NUMEROUS INAPPROPRIATE SEXUAL ACTS, INCLUDING ENGAGING IN SEXUAL HARASSMENT, INAPPROPRIATELY TOUCHING CO-WORKERS AND ENTERING INTO A SEXUAL RELATIONSHIP WITH A PATIENT; SUBMITTING FRAUDULENT BILLS TO INSURANCE COMPANIES; MAKING TERRORIST THREATS AGAINST ANOTHER PHYSICIAN; AND IMPROPERLY REQUESTING THAT A PATIENT WRITE EXCULPATORY LETTERS FOR HIM; HE INITIALLY CONTESTED THE ALLEGATIONS, BUT LEFT THE STATE AND NEITHER HE NOR HIS ATTORNEY APPEARED FOR THE BOARD HEARING, AT WHICH TIME HIS LICENSE WAS REVOKED WITH FINDINGS THAT THE ALLEGATIONS WERE TRUE; IN 12/96 PETITIONED FOR RESTORATION OF HIS LICENSE; THE BOARD SUBSEQUENTLY RECEIVED INFORMATION ALLEGING THAT HE DID NOT NOTIFY THE PENNSYLVANIA EMPLOYEE'S RETIREMENT SYSTEM WHEN HIS MOTHER DIED; HIS MOTHER'S CHECKS WERE DIRECTLY DEPOSITED INTO AN ACCOUNT HELD JOINTLY BY HIM AND HER; HE CASHED SEVERAL SOCIAL SECURITY CHECKS MADE OUT TO HIS MOTHER AFTER HER DEATH.

BAKER, JACK L MD, LICENSE NUMBER J2489 OF FRIENDSWOOD, TX, WAS DISCIPLINED BY TEXAS ON AUGUST 9, 1997
DISCIPLINARY ACTION: 84-MONTH PROBATION; RESTRICTION PLACED ON CONTROLLED SUBSTANCE LICENSE
OFFENSE: SUBSTANCE ABUSE

NOTES: ENGAGED IN INTEMPERATE USE OF ALCOHOL AND DRUGS; VOLUNTARILY SOUGHT TREATMENT; REPORTS SOBRIETY DATE OF 1/2/97. SUSPENSION STAYED WITH FOLLOWING TERMS AND CONDITIONS: SHALL ABSTAIN FROM THE CONSUMPTION OF ALCOHOL/DRUGS IN ANY FORM UNLESS PRESCRIBED BY ANOTHER PHYSICIAN FOR A LEGITIMATE AND THERAPEUTIC PURPOSE; SHALL SUBMIT HIMSELF FOR APPROPRIATE EXAMS INCLUDING DRUG OR ALCOHOL SCREENS; SHALL NOMINATE THREE CERTIFIED PSYCHIATRISTS FOR BOARD SELECTION OF A THERAPIST AND SHALL EXPEDITIOUSLY SUBMIT HIMSELF TO EVALUATION AND TREATMENT BY THE APPROVED PRACTITIONER; SHALL PARTICIPATE IN THE ACTIVITIES OF A PHYSICIAN HEALTH AND REHABILITATION COMMITTEE AND ATTEND WEEKLY MEETINGS WITH QUARTERLY REPORTS; SHALL PARTICIPATE IN AA'S PROGRAM NOT LESS THAN THREE TIMES A WEEK; SHALL REPORT ON HIS ATTENDANCE; SHALL NOT TREAT OR OTHERWISE SERVE AS PHYSICIAN, PRESCRIBE, DISPENSE OR ADMINISTER DRUGS THAT MAY BE SUBJECT TO ABUSE TO HIMSELF OR TO ANY MEMBER OF HIS FAMILY; SHALL IMMEDIATELY SURRENDER DEA CERTIFICATE AND TEXAS CONTROLLED SUBSTANCES REGISTRATION CERTIFICATE; SEPARATE FROM PATIENT RECORDS, SHALL MAINTAIN A LOGBOOK OF EVERY PRESCRIPTION WRITTEN BY HIM FOR DANGEROUS DRUGS WITH ADDICTIVE POTENTIAL WHICH SHALL BE MADE AVAILABLE FOR REVIEW; SHALL COOPERATE WITH THE BOARD IN VERIFYING COMPLIANCE INCLUDING PROVIDING COPIES OF MEDICAL RELEASES UPON REQUEST; SHALL GIVE A COPY OF THIS ORDER TO ANY HEALTH CARE ENTITY WHERE HE HAS PRIVILEGES; TIME SPENT OUT OF TEXAS DOES NOT COUNT TOWARD PROBATION; SHALL INFORM THE BOARD OF CHANGE OF ADDRESS WITHIN 10 DAYS OR IF HE LEAVES THE STATE; SHALL NOT SEEK MODIFICATION FOR ONE YEAR; SHALL OBTAIN AT LEAST 50 HOURS PER YEAR OF CONTINUING MEDICAL EDUCATION; SHALL COMPLY WITH ANY RECOMMENDATIONS MADE BY THE TALBOTT-MARSH RECOVERY SYSTEM. ON 8/22/98 THE ORDER WAS MODIFIED AS FOLLOWS: HE IS HEREBY AUTHORIZED TO REAPPLY TO THE DEA AND THE TEXAS DEPARTMENT OF PUBLIC SAFETY TO OBTAIN CONTROLLED SUBSTANCE REGISTRATIONS; SHALL APPLY FOR, BECOME PART OF, AND FOLLOW THE TEXAS MEDICAL ASSOCIATION'S PHYSICIAN HEALTH AND REHABILITATION COMMITTEE'S RANDOM URINE

DRUG SCREENING PROGRAM AND BE TESTED NO LESS THAN 8 TIMES PER MONTH WITH QUARTERLY REPORTS.

BAKER, JACK L MD OF 12853 GULF FREEWAY, HOUSTON, TX, WAS DISCIPLINED BY DEA ON SEPTEMBER 19, 1997
DISCIPLINARY ACTION: SURRENDER OF CONTROLLED SUBSTANCE LICENSE
NOTES: IN LIEU OF PUBLIC INTEREST REVOCATION.

BAKER, JACK L MD OF FRIENDSWOOD, TX, WAS DISCIPLINED BY MISSOURI ON AUGUST 17, 1998
DISCIPLINARY ACTION: 84-MONTH PROBATION
OFFENSE: DISCIPLINARY ACTION BY ANOTHER STATE OR AGENCY
NOTES: BASED UPON ACTION TAKEN BY THE TEXAS BOARD DUE TO HIS INTEMPERATE USE OF ALCOHOL AND DRUGS. PROBATION RETROACTIVE TO 8/7/97.

BAKER, JOHN A MD OF ARGYLE, TX, WAS DISCIPLINED BY MISSOURI ON FEBRUARY 16, 1994
DISCIPLINARY ACTION: NONRENEWAL OF LICENSE
OFFENSE: NONCOMPLIANCE WITH A PROFESSIONAL RULE
NOTES: DURING 1992 HE FAILED TO OBTAIN THE REQUIRED 25 HOURS OF CONTINUING MEDICAL EDUCATION CREDITS AND FAILED TO REPORT OBTAINING SUCH HOURS BY 05/20/93 AS REQUIRED BY BOARD RULE.

BAKER, JOHN SCOTT MD, LICENSE NUMBER 00J1853 OF WINSTON-SALEM, NC, WAS DISCIPLINED BY TEXAS ON NOVEMBER 19, 1993
DISCIPLINARY ACTION: MONITORING OF PHYSICIAN PERFORMANCE
OFFENSE: SUBSTANCE ABUSE
NOTES: IN 11/92 WAS GRANTED LICENSURE; BOARD LATER RECEIVED INFORMATION THAT HE HAD PROVIDED FALSE INFORMATION ABOUT HIS ABUSE OF ALCOHOL; IN 1/93 REPORTED HIMSELF TO THE BOARD AND SUPERVISING PHYSICIANS IN NORTH CAROLINA; COMPLETED INPATIENT TREATMENT AND ENTERED THREE MONTHS OF EXTENDED CARE; HAS SIGNED A CONTRACT WITH NORTH CAROLINA IMPAIRED PHYSICIANS PROGRAM; FULL LICENSURE STATUS WITH NORTH CAROLINA IS PENDING AS OF THE DATE OF THE ORDER. PRIOR TO PRACTICING IN TEXAS SHALL APPEAR BEFORE THE BOARD TO RECEIVE APPROVAL; SHALL PROVIDE TO TEXAS BOARD ANY REQUESTED COPIES OF REPORTS SUBMITTED TO NORTH CAROLINA; SHALL FOLLOW THE TERMS OF THE NORTH CAROLINA CONTRACT AND ALL CONDITIONS IMPOSED BY THE NORTH CAROLINA BOARD; SHALL GIVE A COPY OF THIS ORDER TO ANY HEALTH CARE ENTITY WHERE HE HAS PRIVILEGES; SHALL COOPERATE WITH THE BOARD IN VERIFYING COMPLIANCE; SHALL INFORM THE BOARD OF CHANGE OF ADDRESS WITHIN 10 DAYS. SHALL NOT SEEK MODIFICATION FOR ONE YEAR.

BALDWIN, RICHARD E DO OF DAVIS, OK, WAS DISCIPLINED BY MISSOURI ON JULY 27, 1990
DISCIPLINARY ACTION: 2-MONTH LICENSE SUSPENSION; 22-MONTH PROBATION
OFFENSE: DISCIPLINARY ACTION BY ANOTHER STATE OR AGENCY
NOTES: TWO MONTH SUSPENSION RETROACTIVE TO 6/15/89, TWENTY-TWO MONTH PROBATION RETROACTIVE TO 8/16/89.

BALDWIN, RICHARD E DO, LICENSE NUMBER 00E3192 OF DAVIS, OK, WAS DISCIPLINED BY TEXAS ON AUGUST 18, 1990
OFFENSE: DISCIPLINARY ACTION BY ANOTHER STATE OR AGENCY
NOTES: STIPULATED ORDER. MUST COMPLY WITH OKLAHOMA BOARD ORDER, RECEIVE PERMISSION OF TEXAS BOARD BEFORE RETURNING TO PRACTICE MEDICINE IN TEXAS, AND BE SUBJECT TO ANY TERMS IMPOSED.

BALDWIN, RICHARD E DO, DATE OF BIRTH JULY 19, 1938, LICENSE NUMBER 0018743 OF DAVIS, OK, WAS DISCIPLINED BY COLORADO ON FEBRUARY 21, 1992
DISCIPLINARY ACTION: SURRENDER OF LICENSE
OFFENSE: CRIMINAL CONVICTION OR PLEA OF GUILTY, NOLO CONTENDERE, OR NO CONTEST TO A CRIME
NOTES: FELONY CONVICTION FOR MEDICAID FRAUD.

BALLARD, CHARLES DONALD MD, DATE OF BIRTH JULY 19, 1952, LICENSE NUMBER 00F9165 OF 15187 HILLVIEW ROAD, TYLER, TX, WAS DISCIPLINED BY TEXAS ON JUNE 17, 1992
DISCIPLINARY ACTION: 60-MONTH PROBATION
OFFENSE: SUBSTANCE ABUSE
NOTES: INTEMPERATE USE OF DRUGS. SUSPENSION, STAYED. PROBATION UNDER TERMS AND CONDITIONS. ON 6/15/93 BOARD MODIFIED THIS ORDER AS FOLLOWS: HE MAY SEEK TO OBTAIN HIS DRUG ENFORCEMENT ADMINISTRATION AND TEXAS DEPARTMENT OF PUBLIC SAFETY CONTROLLED SUBSTANCES REGISTRATION CERTIFICATE; UPON OBTAINING THESE CERTIFICATES, HE MAY POSSESS, ADMINISTER, AND PRESCRIBE DRUGS ONLY IN HOSPITALS FOR INPATIENTS OR IN HOSPITAL EMERGENCY ROOMS FOR EMERGENCY ROOM PATIENTS. IN THE CASE OF ER PATIENTS, CAN ONLY PRESCRIBE IN QUANTITIES LIMITED TO ADDRESS THE IMMEDIATE NEEDS OF THE PATIENTS TO PROVIDE THERAPEUTIC CARE OF EMERGENCY CONDITIONS UNTIL SUCH TIME AS THE PATIENT CAN BE SEEN BY A TREATING OR ATTENDING PHYSICIAN FOR CONTINUED CARE. ON 8/17/96 THE BOARD DENIED HIS PETITION FOR TERMINATION OF THIS ORDER.

BALLI, EDWARD A MD, LICENSE NUMBER 00H5691 OF SAN ANTONIO, TX, WAS DISCIPLINED BY TEXAS ON SEPTEMBER 9, 1991
DISCIPLINARY ACTION: 60-MONTH PROBATION; REQUIRED TO ENTER AN IMPAIRED PHYSICIAN PROGRAM OR SUBSTANCE ABUSE TREATMENT
OFFENSE: SUBSTANCE ABUSE
NOTES: FROM LATE 1989 TO 5/24/90 HE ABUSED RITALIN AND VICODIN FOR NON-MEDICAL PURPOSES WHILE ACTIVELY ENGAGED IN THE PRACTICE OF MEDICINE; ENTERED A TREATMENT PROGRAM 5/24/90 FOR TREATMENT OF CHEMICAL DEPENDENCY AND WAS DISCHARGED 7/4/90; EXECUTED A 2 YEAR AFTERCARE CONTRACT. SUSPENSION STAYED; CONDITIONS OF PROBATION INCLUDE: REFRAINING FROM USE OF ALCOHOL OR DRUGS EXCEPT MEDICATION PRESCRIBED BY HIS PRIMARY CARE PHYSICIAN; SHALL SUBMIT FOR ALCOHOL OR DRUG SCREENS; SHALL PARTICIPATE IN BEXAR COUNTY MEDICAL SOCIETY COMMITTEE ON PHYSICIAN HEALTH AND REHABILITATION, WITH WEEKLY REPORTS TO THE BOARD; SHALL PARTICIPATE IN AA NOT LESS THAN TWICE A WEEK; SHALL COMPLY WITH THE TERMS AND CONDITIONS OF THE AFTERCARE CONTRACT EXECUTED WITH LAUREL RIDGE PSYCHIATRIC HOSPITAL; SHALL APPEAR BEFORE THE BOARD TWICE YEARLY; SHALL ADVISE THE BOARD OF A CHANGE IN ADDRESS; TIME SPENT OUT OF TEXAS DOES NOT COUNT TOWARD PROBATION. SHALL NOT PETITION THE BOARD FOR MODIFICATION OF ORDER FOR AT LEAST ONE YEAR.

BALLI, EDWARD A MD, LICENSE NUMBER 00H5691 OF SEGUIN, TX, WAS DISCIPLINED BY TEXAS ON AUGUST 20, 1992
DISCIPLINARY ACTION: 2-MONTH LICENSE SUSPENSION; 60-MONTH PROBATION
OFFENSE: SUBSTANCE ABUSE

NOTES: ADDITIONAL FIVE-YEAR SUSPENSION, STAYED. PROBATION UNDER TERMS AND CONDITIONS. ON 11/3/94 ORDER MODIFIED AS FOLLOWS: SEPARATE FROM PATIENT RECORDS, HE SHALL MAINTAIN A LOG CONSISTING OF A COPY OF EVERY PRESCRIPTION WRITTEN FOR CONTROLLED SUBSTANCES OR DANGEROUS DRUGS BY DATE ISSUED WHICH SHALL BE AVAILABLE TO BOARD FOR INSPECTION; MAY TELEPHONE PRESCRIPTIONS OR REFILLS FOR DANGEROUS DRUGS IN TO PHARMACIES BUT NOT FOR CONTROLLED SUBSTANCES; SHALL MAINTAIN A LOGBOOK FOR ALL PRESCRIPTIONS OR REFILLS TELEPHONED IN CHRONOLOGICAL ORDER BY DATE.

BANJO, CHAIM MD, LICENSE NUMBER G4442 OF DALLAS, TX, WAS DISCIPLINED BY TEXAS ON AUGUST 22, 1998
DISCIPLINARY ACTION: 60-MONTH PROBATION; FINE
OFFENSE: SUBSTANDARD CARE, INCOMPETENCE OR NEGLIGENCE

NOTES: SIXTEEN CHARTS OF PATIENTS SEEN BETWEEN 1992 AND 1996 WERE REVIEWED BY THE BOARD WITH THE FOLLOWING DEFICIENCIES: PATIENTS ON NUMEROUS OCCASIONS WERE PRESCRIBED DRUGS MULTIPLE TIMES WITH NO DOCUMENTATION AS TO WHY THE DRUGS WERE PRESCRIBED OR WITHOUT APPROPRIATE TESTS; POOR MEDICAL MANAGEMENT IN ONE CASE; IN ONE CASE HE CONTINUED TO PRESCRIBE TO A PATIENT AFTER BEING TOLD BY ANOTHER PHYSICIAN'S OFFICE THEY WERE PRESCRIBING DRUGS AT THE SAME TIME. SUSPENSION STAYED FOR PROBATION WITH FOLLOWING TERMS AND CONDITIONS: SHALL ATTEND 50 HOURS OF CONTINUING MEDICAL EDUCATION, WITH AT LEAST 1 HOUR IN RISK MANAGEMENT; SHALL MAINTAIN ADEQUATE MEDICAL RECORDS WHICH SHALL BE AVAILABLE FOR REVIEW; SHALL NOT PRESCRIBE OR ADMINISTER SCHEDULE II OR SCHEDULE III DRUGS TO ANY PATIENT OUTSIDE OF A HOSPITAL SETTING; SHALL NOT TREAT ANY PATIENT OUTSIDE OF THE HOSPITAL SETTING FOR INTRACTABLE PAIN; SEPARATE FROM PATIENT RECORDS, SHALL MAINTAIN A LOGBOOK OF EVERY PRESCRIPTION WRITTEN BY HIM FOR DANGEROUS DRUGS WITH ADDICTIVE POTENTIAL WHICH SHALL BE MADE AVAILABLE FOR REVIEW; HIS MEDICAL PRACTICE SHALL BE MONITORED BY A BOARD APPROVED TEXAS PHYSICIAN WHO SHALL PROVIDE QUARTERLY REPORTS TO THE BOARD; SHALL COOPERATE WITH THE BOARD IN VERIFYING COMPLIANCE; SHALL APPEAR BEFORE THE BOARD AT LEAST ONCE A YEAR; $1,000 FINE TO BE PAID WITHIN 90 DAYS; TIME SPENT OUT OF TEXAS DOES NOT COUNT TOWARD PROBATION; SHALL INFORM THE BOARD OF CHANGE OF ADDRESS WITHIN 10 DAYS OR IF HE LEAVES THE STATE; SHALL NOT SEEK MODIFICATION FOR ONE YEAR; SHALL GIVE A COPY OF THIS ORDER TO ANY HEALTH CARE ENTITY WHERE HE HAS PRIVILEGES.

BANTA, MIGUEL B JR MD, LICENSE NUMBER D6942 OF FORT WORTH, TX, WAS DISCIPLINED BY TEXAS ON AUGUST 22, 1998
DISCIPLINARY ACTION: 60-MONTH PROBATION; RESTRICTION PLACED ON LICENSE
OFFENSE: LOSS OR RESTRICTION OF HOSPITAL PRIVILEGES

NOTES: ON OR ABOUT 11/11/93 HE COMPLETED AN APPLICATION FOR REAPPOINTMENT AT HARRIS METHODIST HOSPITAL; WITH RESPECT TO THAT APPLICATION: HE ANSWERED "NO" TO THE QUESTION "HAVE YOU EVER VOLUNTARILY OR INVOLUNTARILY SURRENDERED ANY CLINICAL PRIVILEGES OR MEDICAL OR DENTAL STAFF MEMBERSHIPS?"; HE CONSULTED AN ATTORNEY AS TO HOW TO APPROPRIATELY RESPOND TO SUCH QUESTION, IN VIEW OF HIS APPLICATION FOR REAPPOINTMENT AT ST. JOSEPH HOSPITAL HAVING BEEN DECLINED, AND BASED HIS ANSWER ON THE ADVICE HE RECEIVED; ON OR ABOUT 4/25/94 HARRIS HOSPITAL SUMMARILY SUSPENDED HIS MEDICAL STAFF PRIVILEGES; ON OR ABOUT 3/6/96 COMPLAINT FILED ALLEGING THAT HE DID NOT ADEQUATELY DOCUMENT, MANAGE, OR EVALUATE PREOPERATIVE ANESTHESIA PATIENTS, THAT INTRA-OPERATIVE ANESTHESIA MANAGEMENT WAS NOT ADEQUATELY DOCUMENTED, AND THAT HIS PATIENTS EXPERIENCED COMPLICATIONS OF UNUSUAL OR UNEXPECTED SEVERITY; ON OR ABOUT 3/25/96 PLAZA MEDICAL CENTER DENIED HIS REQUEST FOR ELEVATION TO ACTIVE STAFF STATUS. SUSPENSION STAYED FOR PROBATION WITH FOLLOWING TERMS AND CONDITIONS: SHALL NOT PRACTICE ANESTHESIA IN A HOSPITAL SETTING UNTIL HE REQUESTS IN WRITING TO DO SO, AND PERSONALLY APPEARS BEFORE THE BOARD PROVIDING SUFFICIENT EVIDENCE OF HIS COMPETENCE TO PRACTICE SAFELY; SHALL MAINTAIN ADEQUATE MEDICAL RECORDS WHICH SHALL BE AVAILABLE FOR REVIEW; SHALL ATTEND 50 HOURS PER YEAR OF CONTINUING MEDICAL EDUCATION, WITH 5 HOURS IN RISK MANAGEMENT; SHALL APPEAR BEFORE THE BOARD AT LEAST ONCE A YEAR; WITHIN 6 MONTHS SHALL TAKE AND SUCCESSFULLY COMPLETE AN ADVANCED CARDIAC LIFE SUPPORT COURSE AND OBTAIN CERTIFICATION; SHALL COOPERATE WITH THE BOARD IN VERIFYING COMPLIANCE; SHALL GIVE A COPY OF THIS ORDER TO ANY HEALTH CARE ENTITY WHERE HE HAS PRIVILEGES; TIME SPENT OUT OF TEXAS DOES NOT COUNT TOWARD PROBATION; SHALL INFORM THE BOARD OF CHANGE OF ADDRESS WITHIN 10 DAYS OR IF HE LEAVES THE STATE; SHALL NOT SEEK MODIFICATION FOR ONE YEAR.

BANTA, MIGUEL B JR MD, LICENSE NUMBER D6942 OF FORT WORTH, TX, WAS DISCIPLINED BY TEXAS ON AUGUST 28, 1999
DISCIPLINARY ACTION: 60-MONTH PROBATION; FINE
OFFENSE: PROFESSIONAL MISCONDUCT

NOTES: AIDING OR ABETTING, DIRECTLY OR INDIRECTLY, THE PRACTICE OF MEDICINE BY ANY PERSON, PARTNERSHIP, ASSOCIATION, OR CORPORATION NO DULY LICENSED TO PRACTICE MEDICINE BY THE BOARD; HE WAS EMPLOYED BY THE OWNER OF THE CONTINUING MEDICAL CARE CLINIC IN DALLAS; PER THE CONTRACT, HE WAS TO BE PAID AN ANNUAL SALARY OF $150,000 PLUS BENEFITS; THE OWNER WOULD PROVIDE OFFICE SPACE, STAFF, BILLING, EQUIPMENT, SUPPLIES, ETC. SUSPENSION STAYED FOR PROBATION WITH FOLLOWING TERMS AND CONDITIONS: WITHIN 6 MONTHS SHALL TAKE AND PASS WITH A SCORE OF 75 OR ABOVE, WITHIN 3 ATTEMPTS, THE MEDICAL JURISPRUDENCE EXAM; SHALL OBTAIN 50 HOURS PER YEAR OF CONTINUING MEDICAL EDUCATION WITH 10 HOURS IN ETHICS AND 10 IN RISK MANAGEMENT; $1,500 FINE; SHALL APPEAR BEFORE THE BOARD UPON REQUEST; TIME SPENT OUT OF TEXAS DOES NOT COUNT TOWARD PROBATION; SHALL INFORM THE BOARD OF CHANGE OF ADDRESS WITHIN 10 DAYS OR IF HE LEAVES THE STATE; SHALL NOT SEEK MODIFICATION FOR ONE YEAR; TERMS OF 8/22/98 ORDER REMAIN IN EFFECT.

BARBA, PEDRO MD, LICENSE NUMBER 00F7695 OF PACUHCA, MEXICO, WAS DISCIPLINED BY TEXAS ON APRIL 15, 1994
DISCIPLINARY ACTION: LICENSE SUSPENSION
OFFENSE: SUBSTANCE ABUSE

NOTES: FAILED TO KEEP RECORDS OF PURCHASES AND DISPOSALS OF CONTROLLED DRUGS; STARTED SELF-PRESCRIBING DRUGS FOR BACK PAIN MANAGEMENT AFTER AN AUTO ACCIDENT IN 1989 LEADING TO HIS ADDICTION TO LORTAB AND DEMEROL; CLOSED HIS PRACTICE TO ADDRESS HIS DRUG PROBLEM IN 1/92 AND HAS BEEN TREATED; HAS BEEN LIVING IN MEXICO. SUSPENSION UNTIL HE OBTAINS AN IN-PATIENT PSYCHIATRIC EVALUATION AND APPEARS BEFORE THE BOARD PROVIDING SUFFICIENT INFORMATION THAT HE IS PHYSICALLY, MENTALLY AND OTHERWISE COMPETENT TO SAFELY PRACTICE.

BARON, JAY KENT MD OF PASADENA, TX, WAS DISCIPLINED BY ILLINOIS ON AUGUST 1, 1991
DISCIPLINARY ACTION: 60-MONTH LICENSE SUSPENSION
OFFENSE: DISCIPLINARY ACTION BY ANOTHER STATE OR AGENCY

NOTES: DISCIPLINED BY TEXAS FOR FAILING TO PROVIDE ACCEPTABLE MEDICAL TREATMENT TO A PATIENT CONSISTENT WITH PUBLIC HEALTH AND WELFARE. INDEFINITE SUSPENSION FOR A MINIMUM OF FIVE YEARS.

BARON, JAY KENT MD, LICENSE NUMBER 00D5675 OF HOUSTON, TX, WAS DISCIPLINED BY TEXAS ON MARCH 6, 1992
DISCIPLINARY ACTION: 84-MONTH PROBATION
OFFENSE: PROFESSIONAL MISCONDUCT

NOTES: AIDING OR ABETTING THE PRACTICE OF MEDICINE BY ANY PERSON, PARTNERSHIP, ASSOCIATION OR CORPORATION NOT DULY LICENSED TO PRACTICE MEDICINE BY THE BOARD. LICENSE REVOKED, REVOCATION STAYED; PROBATION UNDER TERMS AND CONDITIONS.

BARON, JAY KENT MD, LICENSE NUMBER 1020400 OF 1929 TEAKWOOD, RICHMOND, TX, WAS DISCIPLINED BY INDIANA ON DECEMBER 7, 1995
DISCIPLINARY ACTION: LICENSE REVOCATION; FINE
OFFENSE: DISCIPLINARY ACTION BY ANOTHER STATE OR AGENCY

NOTES: ON 3/30/89, HE WAS PUT ON A FIVE YEAR PROBATION BY TEXAS FOR ALLEGEDLY FAILING TO PROVIDE ACCEPTABLE MEDICAL TREATMENT FOR A PATIENT IN A NON-SMOKING TREATMENT PROGRAM, THAT HE OVERCHARGED HER FOR SUCH TREATMENT AND FAILED TO TELL HER THE DRUGS HE PRESCRIBED WERE EXPERIMENTAL; ON 3/6/91, THE ILLINOIS MEDICAL DISCIPLINARY BOARD RECOMMENDED DISCIPLINARY ACTIONS AGAINST HIM BASED ON THE TEXAS ACTION; HE FAILED TO RESPOND TO THE BOARD'S COMPLAINT, RESULTING IN THE SUSPENSION OF HIS ILLINOIS LICENSE FOR FIVE YEARS. ON 3/2/92, THE TEXAS BOARD SUPERSEDED THE ORDER OF 1989 AND TOOK DISCIPLINARY ACTION AGAINST HIS LICENSE FOR ENGAGING IN THE CORPORATE PRACTICE OF MEDICINE; ORDER FOR REVOCATION WAS STAYED AND HIS LICENSE WAS PLACED ON A SEVEN YEAR PROBATION. ON 5/3/93, HE MISSTATED THE EFFECT OF HIS TEXAS PROBATIONARY ORDER IN HIS INDIANA RENEWAL APPLICATION, INDICATING THAT THERE WERE NO LIMITATIONS PUT ON HIS LICENSE TO PRACTICE MEDICINE IN TEXAS; HE ALSO FAILED TO INDICATE THAT ILLINOIS TOOK DISCIPLINARY ACTION AGAINST HIM IN 1991. DEFAULT ORDER. $1,000 FINE; ORDERED TO PAY COSTS OF ACTION IN THE AMOUNT OF $318.52.

BARRADA, M ISMAIL MD, LICENSE NUMBER G6898 OF HOUSTON, TX, WAS DISCIPLINED BY TEXAS ON AUGUST 9, 1997
DISCIPLINARY ACTION: FINE; REPRIMAND
OFFENSE: NONCOMPLIANCE WITH A PROFESSIONAL RULE

NOTES: IN 1/96 AND 2/96 HE FAILED TO SUPPLY MEDICAL RECORDS FOR SEVERAL MONTHS DESPITE BOARD STAFF'S REPEATED VERBAL AND WRITTEN REQUESTS; DURING 1/97-3/97 HE FAILED AGAIN TO SUPPLY ANOTHER SET OF MEDICAL RECORDS THAT WERE AGAIN REQUESTED FROM HIM; IN 5/97 HE FAILED TO COMPLY WITH A SUBPOENA FOR HIS MEDICAL RECORDS; IN 1/97 A PATIENT REQUESTED HER MEDICAL RECORDS FROM HIM AND HE FAILED TO PROPERLY RESPOND WITHIN 30 DAYS WILL COMPLY WITH ALL WRITTEN REQUESTS FOR MEDICAL RECORDS; SHALL TAKE AND PASS THE MEDICAL JURISPRUDENCE EXAM WITHIN 90 DAYS; $10,000 FINE; SHALL COOPERATE WITH THE BOARD IN VERIFYING COMPLIANCE; WILL COMPLY WITH ALL WRITTEN REQUESTS FOR MEDICAL RECORDS; TIME SPENT OUT OF TEXAS DOES NOT COUNT TOWARD RESTRICTION; SHALL INFORM THE BOARD OF CHANGE OF ADDRESS WITHIN 10 DAYS OR IF HE LEAVES THE STATE; SHALL NOT SEEK MODIFICATION FOR ONE YEAR. ON 4/4/98 GRANTED AN EXTENSION OF TIME OR DEFERRAL OF NO MORE THAN 1 YEAR DUE TO BECOMING FINANCIALLY UNABLE TO PAY AN ADMINISTRATIVE PENALTY; SHALL PAY $10,000 FINE ON OR BEFORE 7/2/98 OR ALTERNATIVELY PRIOR TO 4/2/99 PERFORM AND PROVIDE DOCUMENTATION OF 300 HOURS OF COMMUNITY SERVICE FOR A BOARD-APPROVED NON-PROFIT ORGANIZATION.

BARRADA, M ISMAIL MD, LICENSE NUMBER G6898 OF HOUSTON, TX, WAS DISCIPLINED BY TEXAS ON AUGUST 22, 1998
DISCIPLINARY ACTION: 36-MONTH RESTRICTION PLACED ON LICENSE; REQUIRED TO TAKE ADDITIONAL MEDICAL EDUCATION
OFFENSE: NONCOMPLIANCE WITH A PROFESSIONAL RULE

NOTES: THE BOARD INVESTIGATED HIS CARE AND TREATMENT OF 10 OBSTETRICAL/GYNECOLOGICAL PATIENTS AND FOUND THAT HE FAILED TO ADEQUATELY DOCUMENT INDICATIONS FOR HYSTERECTOMIES WHICH HE PERFORMED, HIS ATTEMPTS AT CONSERVATIVE THERAPIES, AND THAT HE FAILED TO TIMELY NOTIFY ONE PATIENT OF AN ABNORMAL LABORATORY RESULT RELATED TO HER PREGNANCY; HE MAINTAINS THAT HE HAS UNDERTAKEN REVISIONS IN HIS DOCUMENTATION PROCESS IN ORDER TO ADEQUATELY DOCUMENT HIS CARE AND TREATMENT OF PATIENTS AND HE PRESENTED EXAMPLES OF THIS TO THE BOARD. LICENSE LIMITED AS FOLLOWS: WITHIN 1 YEAR SHALL OBTAIN 1 COURSE PER YEAR IN ETHICS; PRIOR TO PERFORMING HOSPITAL SURGERIES, SHALL OBTAIN A WRITTEN CONSULTATION FROM A LICENSED TEXAS PHYSICIAN; SHALL ATTEND 50 HOURS PER YEAR OF CONTINUING MEDICAL EDUCATION WITH ONE HOUR IN RISK MANAGEMENT; SHALL MAINTAIN ADEQUATE MEDICAL RECORDS WHICH SHALL BE AVAILABLE FOR REVIEW; HIS MEDICAL PRACTICE SHALL BE MONITORED BY A BOARD APPROVED TEXAS PHYSICIAN WHO SHALL PROVIDE QUARTERLY REPORTS TO THE BOARD; SHALL APPEAR BEFORE THE BOARD AT LEAST ONCE A YEAR; SHALL COOPERATE WITH THE BOARD IN VERIFYING COMPLIANCE; TIME SPENT OUT OF TEXAS DOES NOT COUNT TOWARD RESTRICTION; SHALL INFORM THE BOARD OF CHANGE OF ADDRESS WITHIN 10 DAYS OR IF HE LEAVES THE STATE; SHALL NOT SEEK MODIFICATION FOR ONE YEAR; SHALL GIVE A COPY OF THIS ORDER TO ANY HEALTH CARE ENTITY WHERE

HE HAS PRIVILEGES.

BARRADA, M ISMAIL MD, LICENSE NUMBER G6898 OF HOUSTON, TX, WAS DISCIPLINED BY TEXAS ON APRIL 8, 1999
DISCIPLINARY ACTION: LICENSE SUSPENSION
OFFENSE: FAILURE TO COMPLY WITH PREVIOUS BOARD ORDER

NOTES: VIOLATED 4/4/98 BOARD ORDER BY NEITHER PAYING THE ADMINISTRATIVE PENALTY BY 7/2/98, OR BY PERFORMING AND PROVIDING DOCUMENTATION OF THE PERFORMANCE OF COMMUNITY SERVICE PRIOR TO 4/2/99.

BARRERA, ADRIAN V MD, DATE OF BIRTH AUGUST 28, 1965 OF C/O 412 E BUSTAMANTEST, LAREDO, TX, WAS DISCIPLINED BY MEDICARE ON DECEMBER 30, 1996
DISCIPLINARY ACTION: EXCLUSION FROM THE MEDICARE AND/OR MEDICAID PROGRAM
OFFENSE: NONCOMPLIANCE WITH A PROFESSIONAL RULE

NOTES: DEFAULTED ON PUBLIC HEALTH SERVICE EDUCATION LOAN. INDEFINITE EXCLUSION.

BARRIER, ALVIS LAYTON MD, LICENSE NUMBER D9354 OF ROCK SPRINGS, WY, WAS DISCIPLINED BY TEXAS ON APRIL 4, 1998
OFFENSE: DISCIPLINARY ACTION BY ANOTHER STATE OR AGENCY

NOTES: VIOLATED 7/27/95 WYOMING BOARD ORDER TO CEASE SELF-PRESCRIPTION OF CONTROLLED SUBSTANCES IN THAT BETWEEN 2/96 AND 7/96 HE WROTE A NUMBER OF PRESCRIPTIONS TO HIMSELF FOR PHENTERMINE AND FENFLURAMINE CLAIMING HE WAAS UNAWARE THAT THESE DRUGS WERE AMONG THE TYPE HE WAS SUPPOSED TO REFRAIN FROM USING; ON 12/17/96 LICENSE SUSPENDED IN WYOMING FOLLOWED BY PROBATION. TEXAS LICENSE LIMITED AS FOLLOWS: SHALL NOT PRACTICE MEDICINE IN TEXAS UNTIL HE REQUESTS PERMISSION IN WRITING AND APPEARS BEFORE THE BOARD TO ORALLY PETITION FOR PERMISSION TO RESUME PRACTICE; SHALL COMPLY WITH HIS WYOMING BOARD ORDER; SHALL COOPERATE WITH THE BOARD IN VERIFYING COMPLIANCE INCLUDING PROVIDING COPIES OF DOCUMENTS SENT TO WYOMING; SHALL INFORM THE BOARD OF CHANGE OF ADDRESS WITHIN 10 DAYS; SHALL NOT SEEK MODIFICATION FOR ONE YEAR.

BARTH, THOMAS LESLIE MD, LICENSE NUMBER E0800 OF LEWISVILLE, TX, WAS DISCIPLINED BY TEXAS ON MAY 14, 1999
DISCIPLINARY ACTION: LICENSE SUSPENSION; REPRIMAND
OFFENSE: CRIMINAL CONVICTION OR PLEA OF GUILTY, NOLO CONTENDERE, OR NO CONTEST TO A CRIME

NOTES: IN 10/97 HE WAS CONVICTED OF FIRST DEGREE MURDER BY A JURY IN DENTON COUNTY, TEXAS; HE MAINTAINS HIS INNOCENCE AND REPORTS THAT HE IS APPEALING THE JURY'S VERDICT; IN ADDITION TO THE CONVICTION, HE HAS ALSO BEEN INVESTIGATED BY THE BOARD REGARDING HIS INABILITY TO FIT A PATIENT WITH THE CORRECT CONTACT LENS PRESCRIPTION IN 1994; WHEN MEDICAL RECORDS WERE REQUESTED OF HIM, HE FAILED TO PROVIDE COPIES. INDEFINITE SUSPENSION UNTIL HIS CONVICTION IS FINALLY ADJUDICATED; SHALL INFORM THE BOARD OF CHANGE OF ADDRESS WITHIN 10 DAYS; SHALL COOPERATE WITH THE BOARD IN VERIFYING COMPLIANCE.

BARTLEY, MICHAEL ALAN MD, LICENSE NUMBER 00H6033 OF HOUSTON, TX, WAS DISCIPLINED BY TEXAS ON MAY 15, 1992
DISCIPLINARY ACTION: EMERGENCY SUSPENSION

BARTLEY, MICHAEL ALAN MD, LICENSE NUMBER 00H6033 OF HOUSTON, TX, WAS DISCIPLINED BY TEXAS ON JUNE 17, 1992
DISCIPLINARY ACTION: 12-MONTH LICENSE SUSPENSION
OFFENSE: SUBSTANCE ABUSE

BARTLEY, MICHAEL ALAN MD, LICENSE NUMBER 00H6033, WAS DISCIPLINED BY TEXAS ON SEPTEMBER 10, 1993
DISCIPLINARY ACTION: 120-MONTH PROBATION; RESTRICTION PLACED ON LICENSE

NOTES: PURSUANT TO THE TERMS OF THE 6/17/92 SUSPENSION ORDER HE PROVIDED EVIDENCE TO SHOW THAT HE IS MENTALLY, PHYSICALLY AND OTHERWISE COMPETENT TO PRACTICE MEDICINE INCLUDING PROOF OF A DOCUMENTED AFTERCARE PROGRAM SATISFACTORY TO THE BOARD. SUSPENSION LIFTED AND STAYED. CONDITIONS OF PROBATION: PRACTICE LIMITED TO THAT ASSOCIATED WITH A FELLOWSHIP PROGRAM WITH QUARTERLY REPORTS; SHALL NOT APPLY FOR OR POSSESS ANY DEA OR TEXAS CONTROLLED SUBSTANCES REGISTRATION CERTIFICATES; SHALL ABSTAIN FROM THE CONSUMPTION OF ALCOHOL OR DRUGS IN ANY FORM UNLESS PRESCRIBED BY ANOTHER PHYSICIAN FOR A LEGITIMATE AND THERAPEUTIC PURPOSE; SHALL PARTICIPATE IN AA NOT LESS THAN TWICE A WEEK WITH QUARTERLY REPORTS TO THE BOARD; SHALL PARTICIPATE IN ACTIVITIES OF A PHYSICIAN COUNSELING COMMITTEE WITH QUARTERLY REPORTS; SHALL SUBMIT HIMSELF FOR APPROPRIATE EXAMS INCLUDING DRUG OR ALCOHOL SCREENS; SHALL GIVE A COPY OF THIS ORDER TO ANY HEALTH CARE ENTITY WHERE HE HAS PRIVILEGES; SHALL COOPERATE WITH THE BOARD IN VERIFYING COMPLIANCE; SHALL INFORM BOARD OF CHANGE OF ADDRESS WITHIN 10 DAYS OR IF HE LEAVES THE STATE; TIME SPENT OUT OF TEXAS DOES NOT COUNT TOWARD PROBATION. ON 11/24/93 THIS ORDER MODIFIED BECAUSE OF A LACK OF AVAILABILITY OF A FELLOWSHIP PROGRAM UNTIL 7/1/94; HIS MEDICAL PRACTICE WILL BE LIMITED TO THAT ASSOCIATED WITH TWO HOSPITALS WITH SUPERVISOR MAKING QUARTERLY REPORTS UNTIL FELLOWSHIP BECOMES AVAILABLE. ON 5/11/95 HIS REQUEST TO TERMINATE PROBATION DENIED BUT ORDER MODIFIED AS FOLLOWS: MAY PRACTICE IN AN INSTITUTIONAL OR GROUP SETTING; HIS PRACTICE SHALL BE MONITORED BY A LICENSED PHYSICIAN WHO SHALL COUNSEL HIM ON ANY PERCEIVED DEFICIENCIES AND PROVIDE QUARTERLY REPORTS; AUTHORIZED TO REAPPLY TO THE DEA AND TEXAS DEPARTMENT OF PUBLIC SAFETY TO OBTAIN AUTHORIZATION TO PRESCRIBE SCHEDULE IV; SHALL MAINTAIN A LOG OF ALL PRESCRIPTIONS WRITTEN FOR CONTROLLED SUBSTANCES OR DRUGS WITH ADDICTIVE POTENTIAL WHICH SHALL BE AVAILABLE FOR INSPECTION; SHALL APPEAR BEFORE THE BOARD AT LEAST ONE TIME EACH YEAR; SHALL PROVIDE COPIES OF ANY REPORTS, DOCUMENTS OR OTHER MATERIALS THAT HE HAS RECEIVED OR SUBMITTED TO OTHER STATE MEDICAL BOARDS; UPON BOARD REQUEST. ON 5/15/96 ORDER MODIFIED AS FOLLOWS: MAY REAPPLY TO THE DEA AND TEXAS DEPARTMENT OF PUBLIC SAFETY FOR FULL PRESCRIBING AUTHORITY FOR CONTROLLED SUBSTANCES; MUST PARTICIPATE IN AA AT LEAST THREE TIMES PER WEEK AND SHALL MAKE WRITTEN REPORTS QUARTERLY DIRECTLY TO THE BOARD; NO LONGER HAS TO PARTICIPATE IN PHYSICIAN COUNSELING COMMITTEE; ALL OTHER CONDITIONS REMAIN IN EFFECT. ON 5/10/97 PETITION TO TERMINATE ORDER DENIED; ORDER MODIFIED DELETING REQUIREMENT THAT HE PRACTICE ONLY IN A GROUP OR INSTITUTIONAL SETTING. ON 5/16/98

PETITION TO TERMINATE ORDER DENIED; ORDER MODIFIED DELETING REQUIREMENT THAT HIS OFFICE AND SURGICAL PRACTICE BE MONITORED. ON 5/14/99 PETITION TO TERMINATE ORDER DENIED; ORDER MODIFIED ALLOWING HIM TO PETITION FOR MODIFICATION OR TERMINATION OF ORDER ONCE EVERY SIX MONTHS. ON 12/11/99 ORDER TERMINATED.

BASKIN, TONEY W MD OF FORT BRAGG, NC, WAS DISCIPLINED BY LOUISIANA ON OCTOBER 22, 1992
DISCIPLINARY ACTION: 36-MONTH PROBATION
OFFENSE: DISCIPLINARY ACTION BY ANOTHER STATE OR AGENCY
NOTES: ADMINISTRATIVE ACTION TAKEN BY TEXAS; HABITUAL OR RECURRING ABUSE OF DRUGS, INCLUDING ALCOHOL. SUBJECT TO CONTINUING FULL COMPLIANCE WITH ORDER PREVIOUSLY ENTERED BY TEXAS; PRIOR NOTICE TO BOARD OF INTENT TO RELOCATE PRACTICE TO LOUISIANA; ABSTINENCE FROM THE USE OF ALCOHOL AND OTHER MOOD-ALTERING SUBSTANCES.

BASKIN, TONEY WILLIAM MD, LICENSE NUMBER 00D8502 OF FORT BRAGG, NC, WAS DISCIPLINED BY TEXAS ON MARCH 6, 1992
DISCIPLINARY ACTION: 36-MONTH PROBATION
OFFENSE: DISCIPLINARY ACTION BY ANOTHER STATE OR AGENCY
NOTES: DISCIPLINARY ACTION TAKEN BY ANOTHER STATE OR UNIFORMED SERVICES OF THE UNITED STATES FOR INTEMPERATE USE OF ALCOHOL OR DRUGS. LICENSE SUSPENDED, SUSPENSION STAYED; PROBATION UNDER TERMS AND CONDITIONS. PROBATION TERMINATED ON 6/22/94.

BASPED, BEAUFORD JR DO, LICENSE NUMBER E3813 OF FORT WORTH, TX, WAS DISCIPLINED BY TEXAS ON AUGUST 22, 1998
DISCIPLINARY ACTION: FINE; REPRIMAND
OFFENSE: OVERPRESCRIBING OR MISPRESCRIBING DRUGS
NOTES: ON 1/14/93 HE DIAGNOSED A PATIENT AS HAVING CHRONIC BACK PAIN SYNDROME FOR WHICH HE PRESCRIBED LORCET; NOTHING IN THE MEDICAL RECORDS REVEALED THAT HE DID ANY TYPE OF WORKUP TO SUPPORT THIS DIAGNOSIS; THIS PATIENT CONTINUED TO RECEIVE THE SCHEDULE III NARCOTIC THROUGH 12/11/97, WITH 1 OFFICE VISIT RECORDED ON 6/30/94; A BOARD CONSULTANT FOUND THAT THE CHART REVEALED NONTHERAPEUTIC PRESCRIBING AND POSSIBLY NONTHERAPEUTIC TREATMENT. $1,000 ADMINISTRATIVE PENALTY.

BASS, ROBERT K MD, LICENSE NUMBER 00C4230, WAS DISCIPLINED BY TEXAS ON AUGUST 17, 1996
DISCIPLINARY ACTION: SURRENDER OF LICENSE
OFFENSE: SEXUAL ABUSE OF OR SEXUAL MISCONDUCT WITH A PATIENT
NOTES: ALLEGEDLY INAPPROPRIATELY TOUCHED ONE ADULT FEMALE PATIENT DURING THE PERFORMANCE OF A MEDICAL EVALUATION AND WITHOUT A CHAPERONE BEING PRESENT. VOLUNTARY AND PERMANENT SURRENDER.

BATSON, RICHARD E MD OF ROUTE 1, BOX 195, FLATONIA, TX, WAS DISCIPLINED BY DEA ON NOVEMBER 13, 1998
DISCIPLINARY ACTION: SURRENDER OF CONTROLLED SUBSTANCE LICENSE
NOTES: IN LIEU OF PUBLIC INTEREST REVOCATION.

BATTLE, CLINTON CHARLES MD, LICENSE NUMBER 00F1368 OF FORT WORTH, TX, WAS DISCIPLINED BY TEXAS ON DECEMBER 3, 1990
DISCIPLINARY ACTION: RESTRICTION PLACED ON CONTROLLED SUBSTANCE LICENSE; REQUIRED TO TAKE ADDITIONAL MEDICAL EDUCATION
OFFENSE: NONCOMPLIANCE WITH A PROFESSIONAL RULE
NOTES: FAILED TO KEEP INVENTORIES AND RECORDS OF CONTROLLED SUBSTANCES DISPENSED; FAILED TO CREATE RECORDS ADEQUATE TO SUPPORT PRESCRIPTION DECISIONS. SHALL NOT PRESCRIBE, ORDER, ADMINISTER, OR DISPENSE SCHEDULE II CONTROLLED SUBSTANCES TO ANY PERSON EXCEPT FOR PATIENTS WHO ARE ADMITTED TO A HOSPITAL OR A HOSPITAL EMERGENCY ROOM; SHALL NOT PRESCRIBE, ADMINISTER, OR DISPENSE SEDATIVES OR STIMULANT MEDICATIONS FOR ANY PATIENT FOR LONGER THAN 90 DAYS IN ANY ONE-YEAR PERIOD; SHALL NOT PRESCRIBE, ADMINISTER, OR DISPENSE ANY NARCOTIC DRUG TO A PATIENT FOR RELIEF OF CHRONIC OR ACUTE PAIN FOR LONGER THAN 60 DAYS IN ANY ONE-YEAR PERIOD; SHALL MAINTAIN ADEQUATE MEDICAL RECORDS ON ALL PATIENT OFFICE VISITS AND MAKE PATIENT MEDICAL RECORDS AVAILABLE FOR COPYING AND EVALUATION BY INVESTIGATORS, CONSULTANTS OR MEMBERS OF THE BOARD; SHALL ENROLL IN, AND SUBSEQUENTLY COMPLETE WITHIN 12 MONTHS FROM THE DATE OF THIS ORDER, A 2 WEEK PRECEPTORSHIP ON THE PREVENTION AND TREATMENT OF DRUG ABUSE; SHALL MAINTAIN IN A FILE SEPARATE FROM PATIENT RECORDS, A COPY OF EVERY PRESCRIPTION WRITTEN FOR CONTROLLED SUBSTANCES AND DANGEROUS DRUGS, BY DATE ISSUED, AND SUCH FILE OF PRESCRIPTION COPIES SHALL BE AVAILABLE FOR INSPECTION BY INVESTIGATORS OR AGENTS OF THE BOARD DURING REGULAR OFFICE HOURS WITHOUT NOTICE; SHALL APPEAR BEFORE THE BOARD OR A COMMITTEE OF THE BOARD SEMIANNUALLY, WHEN REQUESTED IN WRITING. RESTRICTIONS TERMINATED EFFECTIVE 2/6/92; LICENSE FREE OF ANY RESTRICTION OR LIMITATION.

BATTLE, ROBERT MCREE MD, LICENSE NUMBER 00D2355 OF HOUSTON, TX, WAS DISCIPLINED BY TEXAS ON OCTOBER 26, 1990
DISCIPLINARY ACTION: 24-MONTH PROBATION; REPRIMAND
NOTES: MUST OBTAIN CONTINUING MEDICAL EDUCATION; PERFORM PHYSICAL EXAMINATIONS AND TAKE HISTORY BEFORE PERFORMING OTHER TESTS ON OR TREATING ANY PATIENT.

BAUMAN, DALE V MD OF SHREVEPORT, LA, WAS DISCIPLINED BY LOUISIANA ON JANUARY 29, 1992
DISCIPLINARY ACTION: 36-MONTH PROBATION; FINE
OFFENSE: PROVIDING FALSE INFORMATION TO THE BOARD OR OTHER HEALTH AGENCY
NOTES: FRAUD, DECEIT OR PERJURY IN OBTAINING A LICENSE; PROFESSIONAL OR MEDICAL INCOMPETENCY. PROBATION INCLUDES CONTINUING PROCTORING AND REVIEW OF ALL SURGICAL PROCEDURES WITH QUARTERLY REPORTS TO THE BOARD, SUCCESSFUL PASSAGE OF RECERTIFICATION EXAMINATION OF AMERICAN BOARD OF OBSTETRICS AND GYNECOLOGY, $3000 FINE.

BAUMAN, DALE VICTOR MD, LICENSE NUMBER 00E5348 OF SHREVEPORT, LA, WAS DISCIPLINED BY TEXAS ON AUGUST 20, 1992
DISCIPLINARY ACTION: 36-MONTH PROBATION
OFFENSE: DISCIPLINARY ACTION BY ANOTHER STATE OR AGENCY
NOTES: SUSPENSION, STAYED. PROBATION UNDER TERMS

AND CONDITIONS.

BAURER, MARTIN MD OF HEWITT, TX, WAS DISCIPLINED BY ILLINOIS ON OCTOBER 1, 1994
DISCIPLINARY ACTION: PROBATION
OFFENSE: DISCIPLINARY ACTION BY ANOTHER STATE OR AGENCY

NOTES: DISCIPLINED IN TEXAS. INDEFINITE PROBATION.

BAURER, MARTIN E MD, LICENSE NUMBER 00F5829 OF GATESVILLE, TX, WAS DISCIPLINED BY TEXAS ON AUGUST 20, 1992
DISCIPLINARY ACTION: 36-MONTH PROBATION
OFFENSE: NONCOMPLIANCE WITH A PROFESSIONAL RULE

NOTES: FAILURE TO KEEP COMPLETE AND ACCURATE RECORDS OF PURCHASES AND DISPOSALS OF CONTROLLED SUBSTANCES. ORDERED TO UNDERGO A PSYCHIATRIC EXAM. SUSPENSION, STAYED. PROBATION UNDER TERMS AND CONDITIONS. ON 1/14/94 ORDER MODIFIED SO THAT THE REQUIREMENT THAT HE PARTICIPATE IN ACTIVITIES OF THE CORYELL OR MCCLENNAN COUNTY MEDICAL SOCIETY ON PHYSICIAN HEALTH AND REHABILITATION IS DELETED; REQUIRED TO MAKE ANNUAL APPEARANCES BEFORE THE BOARD DURING EACH YEAR OF PROBATION.

BECK, KEITH DEXTER MD, LICENSE NUMBER 00G0607 OF SAN ANTONIO, TX, WAS DISCIPLINED BY TEXAS ON JUNE 10, 1991
DISCIPLINARY ACTION: 60-MONTH PROBATION; RESTRICTION PLACED ON CONTROLLED SUBSTANCE LICENSE
OFFENSE: SUBSTANCE ABUSE

NOTES: INTEMPERATE USE OF ALCOHOL OR DRUGS. CONDITIONS OF PROBATION: SHALL APPEAR BEFORE THE BOARD ONCE A YEAR; SHALL NOT PRESCRIBE TO OR TREAT IMMEDIATE FAMILY; MAY ADMINISTER TO SELF OR FAMILY ONLY DRUGS PRESCRIBED BY OTHER PHYSICIANS; DEA AND DPS REGISTRATIONS LIMITED TO SCHEDULES III, III-N, IV AND V; SHALL SURRENDER ALL UNUSED TRIPLICATE PRESCRIPTION FORMS; SHALL SUBMIT TO DRUG AND ALCOHOL SCREENS; SHALL PARTICIPATE IN IMPAIRED PHYSICIANS PROGRAM; SHALL PARTICIPATE IN AA NOT LESS THAN THREE TIMES PER WEEK.

BECK, KEITH DEXTER MD, LICENSE NUMBER 00G0607 OF SAN ANTONIO, TX, WAS DISCIPLINED BY TEXAS ON AUGUST 20, 1992
DISCIPLINARY ACTION: 45-MONTH PROBATION

NOTES: PROFESSIONAL FAILURE TO PRACTICE MEDICINE IN AN ACCEPTABLE MANNER CONSISTENT WITH PUBLIC HEALTH AND WELFARE. SUSPENSION, STAYED. PLACED ON PROBATION UNDER TERMS AND CONDITIONS UNTIL 6/10/96. IF HE IS NOT BOARD CERTIFIED BY THIS DATE, THE PROBATION CONTINUES INDEFINITELY UNTIL HE GETS CERTIFICATION.

BECK, KEITH DEXTER MD OF 11 DEVONWOOD, SAN ANTONIO, TX, WAS DISCIPLINED BY DEA ON OCTOBER 29, 1993
DISCIPLINARY ACTION: RESTRICTION PLACED ON CONTROLLED SUBSTANCE LICENSE
OFFENSE: DISCIPLINARY ACTION BY ANOTHER STATE OR AGENCY

NOTES: LICENSE RESTRICTED FOR SELF PRESCRIBING RITALIN AND DEVELOPING AN ADDICTION TO THE DRUG. RESTRICTED BY TEXAS STATE BOARD TO SCHEDULES III, IIIN, IV AND V.

BECK, KEITH DEXTER MD, LICENSE NUMBER 00G0607 OF SEGUIN, TX, WAS DISCIPLINED BY TEXAS ON AUGUST 18, 1995
DISCIPLINARY ACTION: 1-MONTH LICENSE REVOCATION; 58-MONTH PROBATION
OFFENSE: FAILURE TO COMPLY WITH PREVIOUS BOARD ORDER

NOTES: FAILED TO OBTAIN ADVANCED CARDIAC LIFE SUPPORT(ACLS) CERTIFICATION AND ADVANCED TRAUMA LIFE SUPPORT(ATLS) CERTIFICATION AS AN INSTRUCTOR BY 8/20/93 AS REQUIRED BY 8/20/92 ORDER; FROM 11/92 THROUGH 3/94 HE KNOWINGLY SUBMITTED FORGED COPIES OF A BASIC CARDIAC LIFE SUPPORT CERTIFICATE, AN ACLS CERTIFICATE AND AN ATLS CERTIFICATE TO THE BOARD AS PROOF THAT HE HAD BECOME CERTIFIED; ALSO SUBMITTED FORGED COPIES OF CERTIFICATES TO TWO FACILITIES, IN ONE CASE FOR PURPOSES OF REAPPOINTMENT OF HIS PRIVILEGES. REVOCATION STAYED. PROBATION WITH TERMS: ON 10/1/95 LICENSE SHALL BE CONSIDERED REVOKED FOR 30 DAYS; AFTER 30 DAYS REVOCATION WILL BE AUTOMATICALLY STAYED TO PROBATION; SHALL ABSTAIN FROM THE CONSUMPTION OF ALCOHOL/DRUGS IN ANY FORM UNLESS PRESCRIBED BY ANOTHER PHYSICIAN FOR A LEGITIMATE AND THERAPEUTIC PURPOSE; SHALL SUBMIT HIMSELF FOR APPROPRIATE EXAMS INCLUDING DRUG OR ALCOHOL SCREENS; SHALL CONTINUE TO PARTICIPATE IN AA'S PROGRAM NOT LESS THAN THREE TIMES A WEEK WITH QUARTERLY REPORTS TO THE BOARD; SHALL CONTINUE TO PARTICIPATE IN THE ACTIVITIES OF AN IMPAIRED PHYSICIAN'S GROUP AND ATTEND WEEKLY MEETINGS WITH QUARTERLY REPORTS; SHALL NOT TREAT OR OTHERWISE SERVE AS PHYSICIAN, PRESCRIBE, DISPENSE OR ADMINISTER DRUGS THAT MAY BE SUBJECT TO ABUSE TO HIMSELF OR TO ANY MEMBER OF HIS FAMILY; SHALL SUBMIT HIMSELF FOR EVALUATION AND TREATMENT BY A BOARD-APPROVED PSYCHIATRIST WHOM HE SHALL SEE AT LEAST ONCE A MONTH AND WHO SHALL SUBMIT REPORTS TO THE BOARD; HIS PRACTICE SHALL BE MONITORED BY A BOARD-APPROVED PHYSICIAN WHO SHALL SUBMIT QUARTERLY REPORTS TO THE BOARD; WITHIN SIX MONTHS SHALL TAKE AND COMPLETE ACLS AND ATLS COURSES WITH PROOF TO THE BOARD; SHALL OBTAIN AT LEAST 50 HOURS PER YEAR OF CONTINUING MEDICAL EDUCATION; SHALL OBTAIN 10 HOURS PER YEAR OF AN ETHICS COURSE; SHALL PERFORM AT LEAST 60 HOURS PER YEAR OF COMMUNITY SERVICE; SHALL APPEAR BEFORE BOARD AT LEAST TWICE A YEAR; SHALL COOPERATE WITH BOARD IN VERIFYING COMPLIANCE; SHALL GIVE A COPY OF THIS ORDER TO ANY HEALTH CARE ENTITY WHERE HE HAS PRIVILEGES; TIME PERIOD OUT OF TEXAS DOES NOT COUNT TOWARD PROBATION; SHALL INFORM BOARD OF ANY CHANGE IN ADDRESS WITHIN 10 DAYS OR IF HE LEAVES THE STATE. SHALL PAY FINE OF $10,000. SHALL NOT SEEK MODIFICATION FOR ONE YEAR. ON 10/5/96 ORDER MODIFIED SO HE IS NO LONGER REQUIRED TO SUBMIT HIMSELF FOR EVALUATION AND TREATMENT BY A BOARD CERTIFIED PSYCHIATRIST. ON 10/24/98 ORDER MODIFIED DELETING REQUIREMENT THAT HIS MEDICAL PRACTICE BE MONITORED. ON 4/10/99 PETITION TO TERMINATE ORDER DENIED.

BECKSTROM, HARRIETT M P DO, LICENSE NUMBER 00E4970, WAS DISCIPLINED BY TEXAS ON OCTOBER 5, 1991
DISCIPLINARY ACTION: 60-MONTH RESTRICTION PLACED ON LICENSE
OFFENSE: DISCIPLINARY ACTION BY ANOTHER STATE OR AGENCY

NOTES: A HOSPITAL REMOVED ANESTHESIA PRIVILEGES ON 2/4/87; SHE NEITHER ADMITS NOR DENIES VIOLATING MEDICAL PRACTICE ACT. TERMS AND CONDITIONS OF RESTRICTION ARE AS FOLLOWS: SHALL REFRAIN FROM PERFORMING GENERAL ANESTHESIA, AND

SHALL NOT PETITION THE BOARD FOR MODIFICATION OF THIS ORDER FOR A PERIOD OF AT LEAST ONE YEAR; SHALL COOPERATE WITH THE BOARD IN VERIFYING COMPLIANCE; SHALL ADVISE THE BOARD OF A CHANGE OF ADDRESS WITHIN 10 DAYS; TIME SPENT OUT OF TEXAS DOES NOT COUNT TOWARD RESTRICTION.

BEDNER, TOM DAVID MD, LICENSE NUMBER 00D3149 OF HOUSTON, TX, WAS DISCIPLINED BY TEXAS ON JANUARY 6, 1995
DISCIPLINARY ACTION: LICENSE SUSPENSION; MONITORING OF PHYSICIAN PERFORMANCE
OFFENSE: SUBSTANCE ABUSE
NOTES: HAS NOT PRACTICED FOR APPROXIMATELY THE LAST TWO YEARS DUE TO A REPORTED DISABILITY FROM DEPRESSION, ANXIETY, PANIC DISORDER AND ALCOHOLISM; HAS A HISTORY OF CHRONIC AND ACUTE ALCOHOLISM FOR WHICH HE RECEIVED TREATMENT IN 1987 AND 1991; RELAPSES IN 4/94, 9/94 AND 11/94 LED TO HOSPITAL ADMISSIONS; PARTICIPATING IN TREATMENT AND ATTENDS AA ON A REGULAR BASIS; IN LIEU OF FURTHER INVESTIGATION HE AGREES TO THIS ORDER. SUSPENSION UNTIL HE PERSONALLY APPEARS BEFORE THE BOARD AND PROVIDES SUFFICIENT EVIDENCE WHICH INDICATES HE IS PHYSICALLY, MENTALLY AND OTHERWISE COMPETENT TO SAFELY PRACTICE INCLUDING BUT NOT LIMITED TO COPIES OF MEDICAL RECORDS AND REPORTS OF PSYCHOLOGICAL AND NEUROPSYCHIATRIC EVALUATIONS.

BELUE, JOE BILL MD, LICENSE NUMBER 00D2088 OF TYLER, TX, WAS DISCIPLINED BY TEXAS ON JUNE 22, 1994
DISCIPLINARY ACTION: REPRIMAND; REQUIRED TO TAKE ADDITIONAL MEDICAL EDUCATION
OFFENSE: SUBSTANDARD CARE, INCOMPETENCE OR NEGLIGENCE
NOTES: MISTAKENLY ARTIFICIALLY INSEMINATED A FEMALE PATIENT DUE TO RELYING TOO MUCH ON THE CHART PLACED ON THE DOOR OF THE EXAMINING ROOM; PATIENT WENT TO ROOM WHEN NURSE CALLED A NAME THAT WAS SIMILAR TO BUT NOT HERS; WAS SCHEDULED FOR A VAGINAL EXAM; HE FAILED TO PROMPTLY INFORM PATIENT OF MISTAKE UNTIL SHE TELEPHONED THAT AFTERNOON; APOLOGIZED IN WRITING TO PATIENT AND INSERTED THAT LETTER IN FILE; DID NOT SPECIFICALLY MARK THE ERROR DOWN ON PATIENT CHART AS HE FELT THE LETTER WAS SUFFICIENT. CONDITIONS OF THREE YEAR RESTRICTION: SHALL ATTEND AT LEAST 50 HOURS PER YEAR OF CONTINUING MEDICAL EDUCATION WITH AT LEAST ONE COURSE IN RISK MANAGEMENT AND OFFICE PROCEDURE; SHALL APPEAR BEFORE THE BOARD ONCE A YEAR; SHALL MAINTAIN ADEQUATE RECORDS ON ALL PATIENT OFFICE VISITS WHICH SHALL BE AVAILABLE FOR INSPECTION; SHALL NOT SIGN ANY PATIENT CHARTS UNLESS HE HAS PERSONALLY EXAMINED THE PATIENT UNLESS THE CHART CLEARLY REFLECTS THAT HE DID NOT; SHALL UTILIZE AN ADEQUATE SYSTEM OF PATIENT RECORD KEEPING; SHALL GIVE A COPY OF THIS ORDER TO ANY HEALTH CARE ENTITY WHERE HE HAS PRIVILEGES; SHALL COOPERATE WITH THE BOARD IN VERIFYING COMPLIANCE; SHALL INFORM BOARD OF CHANGE OF ADDRESS WITHIN 10 DAYS OR IF HE LEAVES THE STATE; TIME SPENT OUT OF TEXAS DOES NOT COUNT TOWARD RESTRICTION. SHALL NOT SEEK MODIFICATION FOR ONE YEAR. ON 10/13/95 ORDER TERMINATED BASED ON COMPLIANCE WITH TERMS AND CHANGES HE HAS EFFECTED IN HIS OFFICE PRACTICE.

BENTLEY, GEORGE N MD, LICENSE NUMBER 00F6432 OF PALESTINE, TX, WAS DISCIPLINED BY TEXAS ON JUNE 28, 1995
DISCIPLINARY ACTION: 60-MONTH RESTRICTION PLACED ON CONTROLLED SUBSTANCE LICENSE; REQUIRED TO TAKE ADDITIONAL MEDICAL EDUCATION
OFFENSE: SUBSTANCE ABUSE
NOTES: IN 7/90, VOLUNTARILY ADMITTED HIMSELF TO A HOSPITAL FOR TREATMENT OF OPIATE DEPENDENCY PRESCRIBED TO HIM FOR PAIN MANAGEMENT RELATING TO SURGERIES HE HAD UNDERGONE IN 1985 AND 1990; IN 1991, HAD A THIRD OPERATION; IN 3/92, VOLUNTARILY ADMITTED HIMSELF TO HOSPITAL AND CONTINUED TREATMENT AT ANOTHER FACILITY; RETURNED TO SURGICAL PRACTICE IN 7/92; IN 1993, APPLIED FOR AND WAS GRANTED FULL PRIVILEGES AT A HOSPITAL; SINCE 11/93 HAS BEEN UNDER THE CARE OF A PSYCHIATRIST WHO STATES HE IS CAPABLE OF PRACTICING MEDICINE WITH REASONABLE SKILL AND SAFETY. LICENSE RESTRICTED FOR FIVE YEARS WITH TERMS: SHALL ABSTAIN FROM THE CONSUMPTION OF ALCOHOL/DRUGS IN ANY FORM UNLESS PRESCRIBED BY ANOTHER PHYSICIAN FOR A LEGITIMATE AND THERAPEUTIC PURPOSE; SHALL SUBMIT HIMSELF FOR APPROPRIATE EXAMS INCLUDING DRUG OR ALCOHOL SCREENS; SHALL SUBMIT TO EVALUATION AND TREATMENT BY BOARD-APPROVED PSYCHIATRIST WHOM HE SHALL SEE AT LEAST ONCE A MONTH AND WHO SHALL SUBMIT QUARTERLY REPORTS; SHALL PARTICIPATE IN THE ACTIVITIES OF AN IMPAIRED PHYSICIAN'S GROUP AND ATTEND WEEKLY MEETINGS WITH QUARTERLY REPORTS; IF AN IMPAIRED PHYSICIAN'S GROUP IS NOT AVAILABLE IN HIS COUNTY OF PRACTICE, SHALL PARTICIPATE IN NARCOTICS ANONYMOUS PROGRAM NOT LESS THAN THREE TIMES A WEEK WITH QUARTERLY REPORTS TO THE BOARD; SHALL NOT TREAT OR OTHERWISE SERVE AS A PHYSICIAN, PRESCRIBE, DISPENSE OR ADMINISTER DRUGS THAT MAY BE SUBJECT TO ABUSE TO HIMSELF OR TO ANY MEMBER OF HIS FAMILY; SHALL MAINTAIN A COPY OF EVERY PRESCRIPTION WRITTEN BY HIM FOR CONTROLLED SUBSTANCES OR DRUGS WITH ADDICTIVE POTENTIAL WHICH SHALL BE AVAILABLE FOR REVIEW; SHALL NOT TELEPHONE TO A PHARMACY ANY PRESCRIPTION OR REFILL OF SUCH DRUGS; SHALL OBTAIN AT LEAST 50 HOURS PER YEAR OF CONTINUING MEDICAL EDUCATION; SHALL APPEAR BEFORE THE BOARD AT LEAST ONCE A YEAR; SHALL COOPERATE WITH THE BOARD IN VERIFYING COMPLIANCE INCLUDING PROVIDING ANY MEDICAL RELEASES UPON REQUEST; SHALL GIVE A COPY OF THIS ORDER TO ANY HEALTH CARE ENTITY WHERE HE HAS PRIVILEGES; SHALL PROVIDE A COPY OF THIS ORDER TO ANYONE WHO REQUESTS IT WITHIN 10 DAYS; TIME PERIOD OUT OF TEXAS DOES NOT COUNT TOWARD PROBATION; SHALL INFORM BOARD OF CHANGE OF ADDRESS WITHIN 10 DAYS OR IF HE LEAVES THE STATE. SHALL NOT SEEK MODIFICATION FOR ONE YEAR. ON 8/17/95 ORDER AMENDED AS FOLLOWS: HE SHALL CONTINUE TO RECEIVE CARE AND TREATMENT FROM BOARD AUTHORIZED PHYSICIAN WHO HE SHALL SEE NO LESS THAN ONCE PER MONTH; SHALL AUTHORIZE THAT THIS PHYSICIAN PROVIDE WRITTEN QUARTERLY REPORTS AND MONITOR HIS ALCOHOL OR DRUG SCREENS. ON 10/24/98 ORDER TERMINATED.

BENZAQUEN, MATHEWS MD OF 3265 ROOSVELT AVE, SAN ANTONIO, TX, WAS DISCIPLINED BY DEA ON NOVEMBER 7, 1994
DISCIPLINARY ACTION: SURRENDER OF CONTROLLED SUBSTANCE LICENSE
OFFENSE: DISCIPLINARY ACTION BY ANOTHER STATE OR AGENCY

NOTES: STATE BOARD.

BENZAQUEN, MATHEWS MD, LICENSE NUMBER 00D3560 OF SAN ANTONIO, TX, WAS DISCIPLINED BY TEXAS ON NOVEMBER 11, 1994
DISCIPLINARY ACTION: SURRENDER OF CONTROLLED SUBSTANCE LICENSE; LICENSE SUSPENSION
OFFENSE: OVERPRESCRIBING OR MISPRESCRIBING DRUGS

NOTES: IN 1991 DEA INVESTIGATED HIM FOR NON-THERAPEUTIC PRESCRIBING; TWO AGENTS OBTAINED PHENTERMINE FROM HIM FROM 3/7/91 THROUGH 11/13/91 BY REPRESENTING THEMSELVES AS TRUCK DRIVERS WHO WANTED TO STAY AWAKE FOR LONG PERIODS OF TIME; THE DRUGS WERE DISPENSED BY DR. BENZAQUEN DIRECTLY FROM HIS OFFICE; SUBSEQUENTLY SURRENDERED HIS OFFICE SUPPLY OF PHENTERMINE TO DEA DIVERSION; HE INFORMED BOARD HE HAD ORDERED PHENTERMINE TO BEGIN A DIET PROGRAM IN THE AREA OF HIS OFFICE PRACTICE; ON 7/23/93 AN AGREED JUDGMENT ASSESSING A FINE OF $5,000 WAS ENTERED AGAINST HIM IN SETTLEMENT TO RESOLVE THE ALLEGATIONS; BOARD FOUND HIS MEDICAL RECORDS FAILED TO SUPPORT OR OTHERWISE PROVIDE A LEGITIMATE MEDICAL BASIS FOR DISPENSING AND THAT PRESCRIBING OF PAIN MEDICATIONS TO ONE PATIENT WAS EXCESSIVE. SUSPENSION STAYED AFTER SEVEN DAYS. CONDITIONS OF FIVE-YEAR PROBATION: SHALL SURRENDER DEA AND TEXAS CONTROLLED SUBSTANCES CERTIFICATES, ALL UNUSED TRIPLICATE PRESCRIPTION FORMS, AND ALL CONTROLLED SUBSTANCES IN HIS POSSESSION INCLUDING SAMPLES; SHALL NOT SEEK REREGISTRATION WITHOUT PERMISSION; SHALL MAINTAIN ADEQUATE MEDICAL RECORDS ON ALL PATIENT OFFICE VISITS WHICH SHALL BE AVAILABLE FOR INSPECTION; SEPARATE FROM PATIENT RECORDS SHALL MAINTAIN A LOG OF EVERY PRESCRIPTION FOR DANGEROUS DRUGS WHICH SHALL BE AVAILABLE FOR INSPECTION; SHALL NOT TELEPHONE PRESCRIPTIONS TO A PHARMACY FOR DANGEROUS DRUGS OR PERMIT OTHER PEOPLE TO DO SO ON HIS BEHALF; SHALL ATTEND AT LEAST 50 HOURS PER YEAR OF CONTINUING MEDICAL EDUCATION WITH AT LEAST 20 HOURS IN PHARMACOLOGY OR ADDICTIONOLOGY DURING THE FIRST YEAR; WITHIN ONE YEAR SHALL PASS THE SPEX EXAM AND THE MEDICAL JURISPRUDENCE EXAM; SHALL APPEAR BEFORE THE BOARD ONCE A YEAR; SHALL GIVE A COPY OF THIS ORDER TO ANY HEALTH CARE ENTITY WHERE HE HAS PRIVILEGES; SHALL COOPERATE WITH THE BOARD IN VERIFYING COMPLIANCE; SHALL INFORM BOARD OF CHANGE OF ADDRESS WITHIN 10 DAYS OR IF HE LEAVES THE STATE; TIME SPENT OUT OF TEXAS DOES NOT COUNT TOWARD PROBATION. SHALL NOT SEEK MODIFICATION FOR ONE YEAR. ON 5/8/97 PETITION TO LIFT SUSPENSION DENIED.

BENZAQUEN, MATHEWS MD, LICENSE NUMBER 0003144 OF SAN ANTONIO, TX, WAS DISCIPLINED BY VERMONT ON SEPTEMBER 8, 1995
DISCIPLINARY ACTION: SURRENDER OF LICENSE
OFFENSE: DISCIPLINARY ACTION BY ANOTHER STATE OR AGENCY

NOTES: ON 11/3/94 TEXAS BOARD TOOK ACTION AGAINST HIS LICENSE CHARGING THAT HE ILLEGALLY DISPENSED PHENTERMINE TO TWO UNDERCOVER POLICE OFFICERS. HIS RECORDS FAILED TO SUPPORT OR PROVIDE A LEGITIMATE MEDICAL BASIS FOR HIS DISPENSING OF PHENTERMINE TO THE UNDERCOVER AGENTS. VOLUNTARY AND PERMANENT SURRENDER.

BEREZOSKI, ROBERT N MD, LICENSE NUMBER 0C37375 OF DAYTON, OH, WAS DISCIPLINED BY CALIFORNIA ON MAY 21, 1990
DISCIPLINARY ACTION: SURRENDER OF LICENSE

NOTES: VOLUNTARY SURRENDER ACCEPTED WHILE CHARGES PENDING.

BEREZOSKI, ROBERT N MD, LICENSE NUMBER 00E0812 OF STAFFORD, TX, WAS DISCIPLINED BY TEXAS ON MAY 24, 1990
DISCIPLINARY ACTION: MONITORING OF PHYSICIAN PERFORMANCE
OFFENSE: DISCIPLINARY ACTION BY ANOTHER STATE OR AGENCY

NOTES: STIPULATED ORDER. MUST SUBMIT TO PSYCHIATRIST FOR EVALUATION/TREATMENT, APPEAR FOR ANNUAL REPORT TO BOARD, INFORM TEXAS BOARD OF ANY CHANGES IN OHIO MEDICAL LICENSURE STATUS OR CONCERNING FELONY CONVICTION IN OHIO RESULTING FROM PENDING LEGAL ACTION. ORDER EFFECTIVE FOR FIVE YEARS.

BEREZOSKI, ROBERT N MD, LICENSE NUMBER 00E0812, WAS DISCIPLINED BY TEXAS ON NOVEMBER 15, 1996
DISCIPLINARY ACTION: 24-MONTH LICENSE SUSPENSION; 96-MONTH PROBATION
OFFENSE: SUBSTANDARD CARE, INCOMPETENCE OR NEGLIGENCE

NOTES: ON 9/5/95 HE ADMINISTERED AN OVERDOSE OF KETALAR AND VALIUM TO AN OUTPATIENT SURGICAL PATIENT, PLACING HER UNDER GENERAL ANESTHESIA AND NOT CONSCIOUS SEDATION AS HE INTENDED; HE AND HIS STAFF FAILED TO PROPERLY MONITOR AND MANAGE HER ONCE SHE WAS PLACED UNDER GENERAL ANESTHESIA; THE OVERDOSE HE ADMINISTERED CAUSED HER TO GO INTO RESPIRATORY ARREST AND SHE SUFFERED SEVERE ANOXIC BRAIN INJURY AND DIED THREE DAYS LATER; NO ONE IN HIS OPERATING ROOM WAS ADVANCED CARDIAC LIFE SUPPORT (ACLS) CERTIFIED: THE NURSE HAD SOME LIMITED EXPERIENCE WITH CARDIAC AND RESPIRATORY ARREST BUT WAS NOT QUALIFIED TO HANDLE THE CRISIS SITUATION WHICH DEVELOPED AND THE SCRUB TECHNICIAN HAD NO FORMAL MEDICAL TRAINING AND WAS INCAPABLE OF PROVIDING MEANINGFUL MEDICAL ASSISTANCE IN THIS EMERGENCY; PHYSICIAN DID NOT HAVE ADEQUATE SURGICAL SUPPORT TO PERFORM THE LARYNGOSCOPY AND SEPTOPLASTY ON PATIENT; HE WAS NOT EXPERIENCED IN ADMINISTERING GENERAL ANESTHETICS AND SHOULD NOT HAVE ADMINISTERED KETALAR AND VALIUM TO PATIENT WITHOUT THE PRESENCE OF AN ANESTHESIOLOGIST OR NURSE ANESTHETIST; HE DID NOT HAVE SUFFICIENT KNOWLEDGE OF AND SKILL WITH ANESTHESIOLOGY TO ANTICIPATE THE LIFE-THREATENING COMPLICATIONS WHICH DEVELOPED DURING THIS SURGERY. SUSPENSION WILL BE STAYED AFTER TWO YEARS TO PROBATION. DURING BOTH SUSPENSION AND PROBATION HE SHALL BE SUBJECT TO THE FOLLOWING TERMS: SHALL OBTAIN AT LEAST 100 HOURS PER YEAR OF CONTINUING MEDICAL EDUCATION, AT LEAST 10 HOURS IN RISK MANAGEMENT, FIVE HOURS IN MEDICAL RECORD KEEPING AND 10 HOURS IN PHARMACOLOGY; IN ADDITION SHALL OBTAIN 10 HOURS OF AN ETHICS COURSE OR PROGRAM PER YEAR; WITHIN ONE YEAR SHALL TAKE AND PASS THE MEDICAL JURISPRUDENCE EXAM; WITHIN ONE YEAR SHALL TAKE AND COMPLETE AN ADVANCED CARDIAC LIFE SUPPORT COURSE AND AN ADVANCED TRAUMA LIFE SUPPORT COURSE AND SHALL MAINTAIN CERTIFICATION IN BOTH; SHALL PERFORM 125 HOURS PER YEAR OF COMMUNITY SERVICE; SHALL APPEAR BEFORE THE BOARD AT LEAST TWICE A YEAR OR AT BOARD REQUEST; SHALL GIVE A COPY OF THIS

ORDER TO ANY HEALTH CARE ENTITY WHERE HE HAS PRIVILEGES; SHALL PROVIDE A COPY OF THIS ORDER TO ANYONE REQUESTING IT WITHIN 10 DAYS; SHALL INFORM BOARD OF CHANGE OF ADDRESS WITHIN 10 DAYS OR IF HE LEAVES THE STATE. PROBATION WITH ADDITIONAL TERMS: HIS PRACTICE INCLUDING ANY OFFICE OR SURGICAL PRACTICE SHALL BE MONITORED BY A BOARD-APPROVED TEXAS PHYSICIAN WHO SHALL SUBMIT QUARTERLY REPORTS TO THE BOARD; SHALL MAINTAIN ADEQUATE MEDICAL RECORDS WHICH SHALL BE AVAILABLE FOR REVIEW; SHALL NOT SIGN OR INDICATE IN ANY MANNER IN PATIENT RECORDS THAT HE HAS SEEN PATIENTS UNLESS HE ACTUALLY HAS SEEN AND EXAMINED THE PATIENT UNLESS IT IS CLEARLY NOTED THAT HE DID NOT PERSONALLY EXAMINE THE PATIENT; SHALL OBTAIN AND MAINTAIN HOSPITAL PRIVILEGES AT A HOSPITAL WITHIN 25 MILES OF HIS OFFICE PRACTICE; SHALL NOT PERFORM ANY SURGERY REQUIRING ANY TYPE OF ANESTHESIA OR SEDATION WITHOUT A BOARD-CERTIFIED ANESTHESIOLOGIST PRESENT TO ADMINISTER THE ANESTHESIA AND MONITOR THE PATIENT; SHALL NOT PERFORM ANY SURGERY WITHOUT A TEXAS REGISTERED NURSE SERVING AS A CIRCULATING NURSE WHO HAS SUCCESSFULLY COMPLETED AN ACLS COURSE AND HAS ACLS CERTIFICATION; SHALL ADEQUATELY SUPERVISE THE ACTIVITIES OF ALL OF HIS EMPLOYEES AND OTHER INDIVIDUALS UNDER HIS SUPERVISION; SHALL ENSURE THAT THE SITE OF ANY SURGERY WHICH REQUIRES ANESTHESIA OR SEDATION INCLUDES ALL EQUIPMENT NECESSARY; TIME SPENT OUT OF TEXAS DOES NOT COUNT TOWARD PROBATION. SHALL NOT SEEK MODIFICATION FOR ONE YEAR. SHALL PAY $5,000 FINE.

BERGES, BENJAMIN MD, DATE OF BIRTH OCTOBER 10, 1937, LICENSE NUMBER 00G0356 OF 435 WEST MERRICK ROAD, FREEPORT, NY, WAS DISCIPLINED BY TEXAS ON SEPTEMBER 30, 1994
DISCIPLINARY ACTION: SURRENDER OF LICENSE
OFFENSE: DISCIPLINARY ACTION BY ANOTHER STATE OR AGENCY

NOTES: ON 12/23/92 PLED GUILTY TO AND WAS CONVICTED OF SEXUAL ABUSE IN THE SECOND DEGREE; THE PERSON INVOLVED WAS A PATIENT; HE WAS SENTENCED TO THREE YEARS PROBATION; ON 10/20/93 NEW YORK LICENSE WAS REVOKED BASED ON THE CRIMINAL CONVICTION. SHALL NOT PETITION THE BOARD FOR REINSTATEMENT OF HIS TEXAS LICENSE.

BERNATH, ALEXANDER S MD, LICENSE NUMBER 136076 OF 2308 MEADOWS LANE, SHERMAN, TX, WAS DISCIPLINED BY NEW YORK ON MARCH 27, 1997
DISCIPLINARY ACTION: REPRIMAND
OFFENSE: DISCIPLINARY ACTION BY ANOTHER STATE OR AGENCY

NOTES: DISCIPLINED BY THE TEXAS BOARD FOR INAPPROPRIATELY PRESCRIBING CONTROLLED SUBSTANCES TO TWO PATIENTS AND FAILING TO APPROPRIATELY MANAGE OR REFER TO MEDICAL SPECIALISTS CHRONIC PAIN PATIENTS.

BERNATH, ALEXANDER SANDOR MD, LICENSE NUMBER 00G4525, WAS DISCIPLINED BY TEXAS ON AUGUST 17, 1996
DISCIPLINARY ACTION: REPRIMAND; REQUIRED TO TAKE ADDITIONAL MEDICAL EDUCATION
OFFENSE: OVERPRESCRIBING OR MISPRESCRIBING DRUGS

NOTES: FROM 7/21/92 TO 4/04/95 PRESCRIBED LARGE QUANTITIES OF CONTROLLED SUBSTANCES, NAMELY VALIUM, TO AN ADULT FEMALE PATIENT WITHOUT ADEQUATE MEDICAL INDICATION AND WHOM HE KNEW OR SHOULD HAVE KNOWN WAS ABUSING PRESCRIPTION DRUGS; FROM 1/03/94 TO 2/21/95 PRESCRIBED LARGE QUANTITIES OF CONTROLLED SUBSTANCES, INCLUDING DARVON, CARISOPRODOL, XANAX, AND LORCET PLUS, TO AN ADULT FEMALE, WHOM HE KNEW OR SHOULD HAVE KNOWN WAS A HABITUAL ABUSER OF CONTROLLED SUBSTANCES; FAILED TO APPROPRIATELY MANAGE CHRONIC PATIENTS AND FAILED TO REFER CHRONIC PATIENTS TO APPROPRIATE MEDICAL SPECIALISTS. RESTRICTED UNDER TERMS AND CONDITIONS FOR THREE YEARS: SHALL MAINTAIN A LOGBOOK OF ALL PRESCRIPTIONS WRITTEN FOR CONTROLLED SUBSTANCES OR DANGEROUS DRUGS WITH ADDICTIVE POTENTIAL OR POTENTIAL FOR ABUSE AND SHALL MAKE IT AVAILABLE UPON BOARD REQUEST; SHALL REFRAIN FROM THE PRESCRIPTION OR ADMINISTRATION OF ANY DRUG FOR ANY PATIENT UNLESS THE DRUG IS MEDICALLY INDICATED AND IS PRESCRIBED IN THERAPEUTIC DOSES; SHALL CONDUCT ADEQUATE FOLLOW-UP EXAMINATIONS ON ALL PATIENTS TO DETERMINE WHETHER THE COURSE OF TREATMENT, INCLUDING THE PRESCRIPTION OF DRUGS, IS APPROPRIATE; SHALL MAINTAIN ADEQUATE MEDICAL RECORDS WHICH SHALL BE AVAILABLE UPON BOARD REQUEST; SHALL ATTEND AT LEAST 50 HOURS PER YEAR OF CONTINUING MEDICAL EDUCATION AT LEAST ONE COURSE SHALL BE IN THE AREA OF RISK MANAGEMENT AND ONE COURSE IN THE AREA OF PHARMACOLOGY/ADDICTIONOLOGY AND SUBMIT PROOF TO THE BOARD; WITHIN SIX MONTHS SHALL TAKE AND PASS THE MEDICAL JURISPRUDENCE EXAMINATION AND SUBMIT PROOF TO THE BOARD; SHALL APPEAR BEFORE THE BOARD AT LEAST TWICE PER YEAR AND UPON WRITTEN BOARD REQUEST; SHALL COOPERATE WITH THE BOARD IN VERIFYING COMPLIANCE INCLUDING PROVIDING COPIES OF PEER REVIEW RECORDS UPON REQUEST; SHALL GIVE A COPY OF THIS ORDER TO ANY HEALTH CARE ENTITY WHERE HE HAS PRIVILEGES; SHALL PROVIDE A COPY OF THIS ORDER TO ANYONE REQUESTING IT WITHIN 10 DAYS; TIME PERIOD OUT OF TEXAS DOES NOT COUNT TOWARD RESTRICTION; SHALL INFORM THE BOARD OF CHANGE OF ADDRESS WITHIN 10 DAYS OF IF HE LEAVES THE STATE; SHALL NOT SEEK MODIFICATION FOR ONE YEAR. ON 9/20/97 THE BOARD GRANTED HIS PETITION FOR TERMINATION OF THIS ORDER BASED ON COMPLIANCE WITH CONDITIONS.

BERNDT, JACK E MD OF 400 10TH AVE NW, WATERTOWN, SD, WAS DISCIPLINED BY DEA ON FEBRUARY 21, 1995
DISCIPLINARY ACTION: SURRENDER OF CONTROLLED SUBSTANCE LICENSE
OFFENSE: DISCIPLINARY ACTION BY ANOTHER STATE OR AGENCY

NOTES: STATE BOARD.

BERNDT, JACK EDWARD MD, LICENSE NUMBER 0003314, WAS DISCIPLINED BY SOUTH DAKOTA ON AUGUST 16, 1994
DISCIPLINARY ACTION: LICENSE REVOCATION
OFFENSE: SUBSTANCE ABUSE

NOTES: SUFFERS FROM A CHEMICAL DEPENDENCY. VOLUNTARY SURRENDER.

BERNDT, JACK EDWARD MD, DATE OF BIRTH FEBRUARY 24, 1959 OF 600 4TH STREET NE, WATERTOWN, SD, WAS DISCIPLINED BY MEDICARE ON MAY 4, 1995
DISCIPLINARY ACTION: EXCLUSION FROM THE MEDICARE AND/OR

MEDICAID PROGRAM
OFFENSE: DISCIPLINARY ACTION BY ANOTHER STATE OR AGENCY

NOTES: LICENSE SURRENDERED FOR REASONS BEARING ON PROFESSIONAL COMPETENCE. REINSTATED ON 1/7/99.

BERNDT, JACK EDWARD MD, LICENSE NUMBER 00H0177 OF WATERTOWN, SD, WAS DISCIPLINED BY TEXAS ON JUNE 28, 1995
DISCIPLINARY ACTION: 60-MONTH PROBATION; RESTRICTION PLACED ON LICENSE
OFFENSE: DISCIPLINARY ACTION BY ANOTHER STATE OR AGENCY

NOTES: ON 8/16/94 DUE TO HIS CHEMICAL DEPENDENCY, SOUTH DAKOTA ACCEPTED HIS VOLUNTARY SURRENDER AND INDEFINITELY REVOKED HIS LICENSE; HE RECEIVED TREATMENT FOR CHEMICAL DEPENDENCY IN 1987 AND REMAINED CLEAN UNTIL APPROXIMATELY 5/94; ENTERED INPATIENT TREATMENT ON 8/17/94 AND WAS DISCHARGED TO TALBOTT-MARSH RECOVERY CAMPUS ON 8/24/94 AND WAS DISCHARGED IN 1/95 WITH AN AFTERCARE PLAN; REPORTS SOBRIETY DATE OF 8/15/94; REPORTS ATTENDING ONE OR TWO AA MEETINGS EACH DAY; HAS RETURNED TO TALBOTT-MARSH FOR A ROUTINE RETURN VISIT OF FOUR DAYS; HIS DRUG OF CHOICE IS FENTANYL. SUSPENSION STAYED. PROBATION WITH TERMS: SHALL NOT PRACTICE MEDICINE IN TEXAS UNTIL HE TAKES AND PASSES THE SPECIAL PURPOSE EXAMINATION; SHALL ABSTAIN FROM THE CONSUMPTION OF ALCOHOL/DRUGS IN ANY FORM UNLESS PRESCRIBED BY ANOTHER PHYSICIAN FOR A LEGITIMATE AND THERAPEUTIC PURPOSE; SHALL SUBMIT HIMSELF FOR APPROPRIATE EXAMS INCLUDING DRUG OR ALCOHOL SCREENS; SHALL SUBMIT HIMSELF FOR EVALUATION AND TREATMENT BY A BOARD-APPROVED PSYCHIATRIST WHOM HE SHALL SEE AT LEAST ONCE A MONTH AND WHO SHALL SUBMIT REPORTS TO THE BOARD; SHALL PARTICIPATE IN AA'S PROGRAM NOT LESS THAN FIVE TIMES A WEEK WITH QUARTERLY REPORTS TO THE BOARD; SHALL PARTICIPATE IN THE ACTIVITIES OF AN IMPAIRED PHYSICIAN'S GROUP AND ATTEND WEEKLY MEETINGS WITH QUARTERLY REPORTS; SHALL COMPLY WITH THE TERMS OF ANY CONTINUING CARE CONTRACT ENTERED INTO AND SHALL SUBMIT QUARTERLY REPORTS TO THE BOARD; SHALL COMPLY WITH THE TERMS OF ANY CONTRACT FOR HOSPITAL PRIVILEGES AND SHALL REPORT ANY DISCIPLINARY ACTIONS TO THE BOARD; SHALL NOT POSSESS ALCOHOL, CONTROLLED SUBSTANCES OR DRUGS WITH POTENTIAL FOR ABUSE; SHALL NOT TREAT OR OTHERWISE SERVE AS PHYSICIAN, PRESCRIBE, DISPENSE OR ADMINISTER DRUGS THAT MAY BE SUBJECT TO ABUSE TO HIMSELF OR TO ANY MEMBER OF HIS FAMILY; SHALL NOT TELEPHONE PHARMACIES WITH PRESCRIPTIONS FOR CONTROLLED SUBSTANCES OR PERMIT ANYONE UNDER HIS SUPERVISION TO DO SO; SHALL IMMEDIATELY SURRENDER HIS CONTROLLED SUBSTANCES REGISTRATION CERTIFICATE TO THE DEA, ANY UNUSED TRIPLICATE PRESCRIPTION FORMS AND SHALL NOT ATTEMPT TO ORDER MORE, AND ANY CONTROLLED SUBSTANCES IN HIS POSSESSION INCLUDING SAMPLES; SHALL MAINTAIN A COPY OF PRESCRIPTIONS WRITTEN FOR DRUGS WITH POTENTIAL FOR ABUSE WHICH SHALL BE AVAILABLE FOR REVIEW; SHALL NOT PRACTICE ANESTHESIOLOGY AND SHALL PRACTICE MEDICINE ONLY IN A GROUP PRACTICE SETTING; HIS OFFICE AND SURGICAL PRACTICE SHALL BE MONITORED BY A BOARD-APPROVED PHYSICIAN WHO SHALL SUBMIT QUARTERLY REPORTS TO THE BOARD; SHALL MAINTAIN ADEQUATE MEDICAL RECORDS WHICH SHALL BE AVAILABLE FOR REVIEW; SHALL OBTAIN AT LEAST 50 HOURS PER YEAR OF CONTINUING MEDICAL EDUCATION; SHALL APPEAR BEFORE BOARD AT LEAST ONCE A YEAR OR AT BOARD REQUEST; SHALL COOPERATE WITH THE BOARD IN VERIFYING COMPLIANCE INCLUDING PROVIDING ANY COPIES OF MEDICAL RELEASES OR PEER REVIEW RECORDS UPON REQUEST; SHALL GIVE A COPY OF ORDER TO ANY HEALTH CARE ENTITY WHERE HE HAS PRIVILEGES; SHALL PROVIDE A COPY OF THE ORDER TO ANYONE WHO REQUESTS IT WITHIN 10 DAYS; TIME PERIOD OUT OF TEXAS DOES NOT COUNT TOWARD PROBATION; SHALL INFORM BOARD OF ANY CHANGE OF ADDRESS WITHIN 10 DAYS OR IF HE LEAVES THE STATE. SHALL NOT SEEK MODIFICATION FOR ONE YEAR. ON 8/9/97 PETITION TO MODIFY ORDER DENIED. ON 4/10/99 PETITION TO MODIFY ORDER DENIED.

BERNDT, JACK EDWARD MD, LICENSE NUMBER 0003314, WAS DISCIPLINED BY SOUTH DAKOTA ON MARCH 12, 1996
DISCIPLINARY ACTION: LICENSE REINSTATEMENT; PROBATION
OFFENSE: OVERPRESCRIBING OR MISPRESCRIBING DRUGS

NOTES: INDEFINITE SUSPENSION, STAYED AS INDEFINITE PROBATION UNDER TERMS AND CONDITIONS: SHALL PERMIT THE BOARD TO HAVE FREE ACCESS TO ALL RECORDS RELATING TO MEDICAL SERVICES PROVIDED BY HIM TO PATIENTS; SHALL COMPLY WITH BOARD REQUESTS; SHALL MAKE APPEARANCES BEFORE THE BOARD ANNUALLY AND/OR UPON REQUEST; SHALL NOT USE ALCOHOL OR ANY CONTROLLED SUBSTANCES UNLESS PRESCRIBED BY A LICENSED PHYSICIAN; SHALL PROVE TO THE BOARD THAT HE HAS NOT EXHIBITED HABITS OF ALCOHOL USE OR DRUG USE OR ALCOHOL OR DRUG ADDICTION; SHALL PROVIDE THE BOARD WITH VERIFICATION OF FIVE TIMES PER WEEK ATTENDANCE AT AA AND/OR NARCOTICS ANONYMOUS MEETINGS ON AT LEAST A MONTHLY BASIS; SHALL SUBMIT AT LEAST TWICE PER WEEK TO WITNESSED BLOOD AND/OR URINALYSIS UPON BOARD REQUEST; SHALL NOT HANDLE OR ADMINISTER NARCOTIC MEDICATIONS IN HIS PRACTICE OF MEDICINE; SHALL SUBMIT TO MONITORED ADMINISTRATIONS OF NALTREXONE BY A BOARD APPROVED PHYSICIAN; AND SHALL OBTAIN COUNSELING FROM A BOARD APPROVED PHYSICIAN OR COUNSELOR AND SHALL PROVIDE AUTHORIZATION TO THEM TO PROVIDE AN INITIAL REPORT AS WELL AS QUARTERLY REPORTS TO THE BOARD; SHALL NOT PRACTICE IN SOUTH DAKOTA.

BERNDT, JACK EDWARD MD, LICENSE NUMBER 3314, WAS DISCIPLINED BY SOUTH DAKOTA ON AUGUST 31, 1998
DISCIPLINARY ACTION: PROBATION; MONITORING OF PHYSICIAN PERFORMANCE

NOTES: SUSPENSION STAYED FOR PROBATION WITH FOLLOWING TERMS AND CONDITIONS: SHALL PERMIT THE BOARD ACCESS TO ALL HIS PATIENT MEDICAL RECORDS; SHALL MAKE APPEARANCES BEFORE THE BOARD UPON REQUEST; SHALL NOT ENGAGE IN THE USE OF ALCOHOL OR ANY CONTROLLED SUBSTANCE UNLESS PRESCRIBED BY A PHYSICIAN; SHALL PROVIDE VERIFICATION OF REGULAR ATTENDANCE OF TWO TIMES PER WEEK AT AA AND/OR NARCOTICS ANONYMOUS MEETINGS ON A MONTHLY BASIS; SHALL SUBMIT TO BLOOD AND/OR URINALYSIS TESTS; SHALL OBTAIN COUNSELING FROM A BOARD-APPROVED PHYSICIAN OR COUNSELOR WHO SHALL PROVIDE QUARTERLY REPORTS; SHALL NOTIFY THE BOARD OF ALL CHANGES OF EMPLOYMENT WITHIN 15 DAYS.

BERRY, G L DO, DATE OF BIRTH FEBRUARY 8, 1939, LICENSE NUMBER 00F3409 OF 130 DAFFODIL, LAKE JACKSON, TX, WAS DISCIPLINED BY TEXAS ON JUNE 15, 1993
DISCIPLINARY ACTION: EMERGENCY SUSPENSION
OFFENSE: SUBSTANCE ABUSE

NOTES: APPEARED ON 4/20/93 TO DISCUSS ALLEGATIONS OF INTEMPERATE USE OF DRUGS AND ALCOHOL; BOARD RECEIVED INFORMATION THAT HE OFTEN SMELLED OF ALCOHOL WHEN PERFORMING DUTIES AS PHYSICIAN; HAD RECEIVED TREATMENT IN 1992 IN CALIFORNIA FOR ALCOHOL ABUSE; BOARD CHOSE TO RECOMMEND CLOSING THAT INVESTIGATION DUE TO LACK OF EVIDENCE; ON 5/20/93 HE APPEARED FOR DUTY UNDER THE INFLUENCE OF ALCOHOL AND WAS DISCIPLINED BY EMPLOYER.

BERRY, G L DO, DATE OF BIRTH FEBRUARY 8, 1939, LICENSE NUMBER 00F3409 OF 130 DAFFODIL, LAKE JACKSON, TX, WAS DISCIPLINED BY TEXAS ON AUGUST 20, 1993
DISCIPLINARY ACTION: LICENSE SUSPENSION
OFFENSE: SUBSTANCE ABUSE

NOTES: UNABLE TO PRACTICE WITH REASONABLE SKILL AND SAFETY BECAUSE OF THE INTEMPERATE USE OF ALCOHOL. SUSPENSION UNTIL SUCH TIME AS HE PERSONALLY APPEARS BEFORE BOARD TO PROVIDE SUFFICIENT EVIDENCE TO SHOW HE IS COMPETENT TO PRACTICE INCLUDING A CURRENT PSYCHIATRIC EXAMINATION; SHALL GIVE A COPY OF THIS ORDER TO ANY HEALTH CARE ENTITY WHERE HE HAS PRIVILEGES; SHALL COOPERATE WITH THE BOARD IN VERIFYING COMPLIANCE; SHALL INFORM BOARD OF CHANGE OF ADDRESS WITHIN 10 DAYS.

BERRY, JAMES E MD, DATE OF BIRTH JULY 16, 1958 OF 5010 GROVE W BLVD, #810, STAFFORD, TX, WAS DISCIPLINED BY MEDICARE ON DECEMBER 30, 1996
DISCIPLINARY ACTION: EXCLUSION FROM THE MEDICARE AND/OR MEDICAID PROGRAM
OFFENSE: NONCOMPLIANCE WITH A PROFESSIONAL RULE

NOTES: DEFAULTED ON PUBLIC HEALTH SERVICE EDUCATION LOAN. INDEFINITE EXCLUSION.

BERRY, RICHARD WILLIAM MD, LICENSE NUMBER 00E0814 OF AUSTIN, TX, WAS DISCIPLINED BY TEXAS ON JUNE 22, 1994
DISCIPLINARY ACTION: REQUIRED TO TAKE ADDITIONAL MEDICAL EDUCATION; MONITORING OF PHYSICIAN PERFORMANCE
OFFENSE: SUBSTANCE ABUSE

NOTES: ADMITTED TO THE USE OF MARIJUANA ON A LIMITED BASIS PRIOR TO 3/91; IS CURRENTLY COUNSELED AND TREATED BY A PSYCHIATRIST; VOLUNTARILY ADMITTED HIMSELF FOR RECOVERY TREATMENT IN 2/91 AND SIGNED AN AFTERCARE AGREEMENT; REVIEW OF RECORDS REVEALED NO EVIDENCE OF IMPROPER PATIENT CARE; SELF-PRESCRIBED AND INGESTED FIORICET IN 9/92 DUE TO SEVERE HEADACHES; DENIES ANY VIOLATION OF THE RULE AGAINST INTEMPERATE USE OF ALCOHOL OR DRUGS THAT COULD ENDANGER THE LIVES OF PATIENTS BUT DESIRES TO RESOLVE THIS MATTER AND THUS SIGNED THE FOLLOWING AGREED ORDER. CONDITIONS OF FIVE YEAR RESTRICTION: SHALL CONTINUE COUNSELING WITH PRESENT PSYCHIATRIST WITH QUARTERLY REPORTS; SHALL OBTAIN SERVICES OF A PRIMARY CARE PHYSICIAN AND INFORM THE BOARD WHO THIS IS; SHALL ABSTAIN FROM THE CONSUMPTION OF ALCOHOL OR DRUGS WITH ADDICTIVE POTENTIAL IN ANY FORM UNLESS PRESCRIBED, DISPENSED OR AUTHORIZED BY ANOTHER PHYSICIAN FOR A LEGITIMATE OR THERAPEUTIC PURPOSE; SHALL SUBMIT HIMSELF FOR APPROPRIATE EXAMS INCLUDING DRUG OR ALCOHOL SCREENS; SHALL PARTICIPATE IN AA'S PROGRAM AT LEAST TWICE A WEEK WITH QUARTERLY REPORTS TO THE BOARD; SHALL NOT TREAT OR OTHERWISE SERVE AS PHYSICIAN, PRESCRIBE, DISPENSE OR ADMINISTER DRUGS THAT MAY BE SUBJECT TO ABUSE TO HIMSELF OR ANY MEMBER OF HIS FAMILY; SHALL ATTEND AT LEAST 50 HOURS PER YEAR OF CONTINUING MEDICAL EDUCATION; SHALL APPEAR BEFORE THE BOARD ONCE A YEAR; SHALL GIVE A COPY OF THIS ORDER TO ANY HEALTH CARE ENTITY WHERE HE HAS PRIVILEGES; SHALL COOPERATE WITH THE BOARD IN VERIFYING COMPLIANCE; SHALL INFORM BOARD OF CHANGE OF ADDRESS WITHIN 10 DAYS OR IF HE LEAVES THE STATE; TIME SPENT OUT OF TEXAS DOES NOT COUNT TOWARD RESTRICTION. SHALL NOT SEEK MODIFICATION FOR ONE YEAR. ON 8/9/97 BOARD GRANTED HIS PETITION FOR TERMINATION OF THIS ORDER BASED ON COMPLIANCE WITH CONDITIONS.

BERRY, SHELLIE J MD, LICENSE NUMBER 00H5222 OF CANTON, TX, WAS DISCIPLINED BY TEXAS ON AUGUST 18, 1995
DISCIPLINARY ACTION: FINE
OFFENSE: NONCOMPLIANCE WITH A PROFESSIONAL RULE

NOTES: ON 4/6/95 REQUESTED BY BOARD VERBALLY AND IN A SUBPOENA TO PROVIDE THE MEDICAL RECORDS OF 10 PATIENTS; TWO WEEKS LATER BOARD INVESTIGATOR CALLED TO INQUIRE ABOUT THE STATUS OF THE REQUESTED MEDICAL RECORDS AND ONE MONTH AFTER THE ORIGINAL REQUEST, PHYSICIAN HAD NOT YET PROVIDED RECORDS; ON 5/31/95, PROVIDED RECORDS AFTER HAVING BEEN NOTIFIED OF PROCEEDING SCHEDULED FOR 6/1/95. SHALL PAY $1,000 FINE; SHALL COOPERATE WITH THE BOARD IN VERIFYING COMPLIANCE.

BERRY, SHELLIE J MD, LICENSE NUMBER H5222 OF CANTON, TX, WAS DISCIPLINED BY TEXAS ON JULY 16, 1997
DISCIPLINARY ACTION: SURRENDER OF CONTROLLED SUBSTANCE LICENSE; LICENSE SUSPENSION
OFFENSE: OVERPRESCRIBING OR MISPRESCRIBING DRUGS

NOTES: IN 1994, SHE PRESCRIBED CONTROLLED SUBSTANCES, SUCH AS HYDROCODONE AND VICODIN, AND DANGEROUS DRUGS TO SEVERAL ADULT PATIENTS WITHOUT ADEQUATELY DOCUMENTING THE MEDICAL RATIONALE FOR THE PRESCRIBING IN THE PATIENTS' MEDICAL CHARTS. FROM 4/22/94 TO 11/24/94 SHE PRESCRIBED 1400 TABLETS OF VICODIN TO AN ADULT MALE PATIENT WITHOUT ADEQUATE DOCUMENTATION TO SUPPORT THIS AMOUNT. SHE CONTINUED TO PRESCRIBE SUCH LARGE AMOUNTS TO PATIENTS WHO WERE KNOWN SUBSTANCE ABUSERS. SHE FAILED TO ADEQUATELY TREAT CHRONIC PAIN PATIENTS BY EXCESSIVELY PRESCRIBING CONTROLLED SUBSTANCES AND NOT CONSIDERING OTHER TREATMENT MODALITIES. SHE FAILED TO DOCUMENT A HISTORY AND PHYSICAL IN NUMEROUS PATIENTS' CHARTS. SHE IS CURRENTLY SELF-PRESCRIBING PROZAC. SHE HAS PROVIDED SAMPLE MEDICATION TO HER OFFICE STAFF WITHOUT MAINTAINING ADEQUATE DOCUMENTATION OR TREATMENT RATIONALE. SUSPENSION UNTIL SHE REQUESTS TO HAVE HER SUSPENSION STAYED OR APPEARS BEFORE THE BOARD WITH SUFFICIENT EVIDENCE THAT SHE IS PHYSICALLY, MENTALLY AND OTHERWISE COMPETENT TO SAFELY PRACTICE MEDICINE INCLUDING AT A MINIMUM COMPLETE COPIES OF MEDICAL RECORDS AND REPORTS OF PSYCHOLOGICAL AND NEUROPSYCHIATRIC

EVALUATIONS, INCLUDING A 96 HOUR INPATIENT EVALUATION CONDUCTED BY A BOARD-APPROVED CERTIFIED PSYCHIATRIST; SHALL PASS WITH A SCORE OF 75 OR BETTER THE SPEX AND THE JURISPRUDENCE EXAM; SHALL SUCCESSFULLY COMPLETE A COURSE IN PHARMACOLOGY, ONE IN CHRONIC PAIN, AND ONE IN RISK MANAGEMENT; IF NOT ALREADY DONE SO, SHE SHALL IMMEDIATELY SURRENDER HER DRUG ENFORCEMENT ADMINISTRATION AND TEXAS DEPARTMENT OF PUBLIC SAFETY CONTROLLED SUBSTANCES REGISTRATION CERTIFICATES, AND ALL UNUSED TRIPLICATE PRESCRIPTION FORMS; SHALL GIVE A COPY OF THIS ORDER TO ANY HEALTH CARE ENTITY WHERE SHE HAS PRIVILEGES; SHALL INFORM THE BOARD OF CHANGE OF ADDRESS WITHIN 10 DAYS.

BERRY, SHELLIE J MD, DATE OF BIRTH DECEMBER 29, 1956 OF ROUTE 3, BOX 52, CANTON, TX, WAS DISCIPLINED BY MEDICARE ON DECEMBER 18, 1997
DISCIPLINARY ACTION: EXCLUSION FROM THE MEDICARE AND/OR MEDICAID PROGRAM
OFFENSE: NONCOMPLIANCE WITH A PROFESSIONAL RULE

NOTES: DEFAULTED ON PUBLIC HEALTH SERVICE EDUCATION LOAN.

BIBEAU, GUY R MD, LICENSE NUMBER 000T580 OF SAN ANGELO, TX, WAS DISCIPLINED BY SOUTH CAROLINA ON FEBRUARY 15, 1990
DISCIPLINARY ACTION: RESTRICTION PLACED ON LICENSE

NOTES: TEMPORARY LICENSE ISSUED WITH CONDITIONS.

BICKERS, PETER W MD, LICENSE NUMBER 00G6267 OF AMARILLO, TX, WAS DISCIPLINED BY TEXAS ON APRIL 15, 1994
DISCIPLINARY ACTION: SURRENDER OF LICENSE

NOTES: IN LIEU OF FURTHER INVESTIGATION OR A HEARING ON ALLEGATIONS. SHALL NOT PETITION FOR REINSTATEMENT.

BICKERS, PETER W MD OF 1901 MEDI-PARK PLACE #100, AMARILLO, TX, WAS DISCIPLINED BY DEA ON JUNE 30, 1994
DISCIPLINARY ACTION: SURRENDER OF CONTROLLED SUBSTANCE LICENSE
OFFENSE: DISCIPLINARY ACTION BY ANOTHER STATE OR AGENCY

NOTES: STATE BOARD.

BIDDIX, JERRY WAYNE MD, LICENSE NUMBER E3855, WAS DISCIPLINED BY TEXAS ON MAY 10, 1997
OFFENSE: LOSS OR RESTRICTION OF HOSPITAL PRIVILEGES

NOTES: ON 8/8/93 AN ADULT MALE PATIENT INJURED IN A MOTORCYCLE ACCIDENT WAS SEEN AND TREATED BY HIM IN THE ER FOR MULTIPLE ABRASIONS DESCRIBED AS DEEP AND EXTENSIVE. HE CLEANED AND DRESSED THE WOUNDS WITH SILVADENE AND DISCHARGED THE PATIENT WITH INSTRUCTIONS TO RETURN IN TWO DAYS FOR REDRESSING. UPON RETURN TO THE CLINIC, THE PATIENT WAS ADMITTED FOR INTENSIVE WOUND CARE WITH WHIRLPOOL TREATMENT AND PAIN CONTROL AND WAS SUBSEQUENTLY DISCHARGED SIX DAYS LATER WITH OUTPATIENT THERAPY AND CONVALESCENT LEAVE. HE DID NOT ADEQUATELY DOCUMENT THE PATIENT'S VITAL SIGNS OR CONDUCT ADEQUATE EVALUATION AND TESTING INCLUDING URINALYSIS TO RULE OUT HEMATURIA. HIS CLINICAL PRIVILEGES WERE SUBSEQUENTLY REVOKED BY THE US AIR FORCE DUE TO HIS ACTIONS OR OMISSIONS WITH REGARD TO HIS PATIENT. WITHIN SIX MONTHS SHALL PASS THE SPEX; SHALL COOPERATE WITH THE BOARD IN VERIFYING COMPLIANCE; SHALL GIVE A COPY OF THIS ORDER TO ANY HEALTH CARE ENTITY WHERE HE HAS PRIVILEGES.

BIGGERS, JEREL RAYMOND DO, LICENSE NUMBER 0004510 OF 3908 DALGREEN, DALLAS, TX, WAS DISCIPLINED BY FLORIDA ON JANUARY 12, 1990
DISCIPLINARY ACTION: FINE; REPRIMAND
OFFENSE: DISCIPLINARY ACTION BY ANOTHER STATE OR AGENCY

NOTES: ON OR ABOUT 6/12/87 THE TEXAS BOARD ACCEPTED HIS VOLUNTARY LIMITATION OF MEDICAL PRACTICE IN WHICH HIS DEA AND TEXAS CONTROLLED SUBSTANCES REGISTRATIONS WERE MODIFIED TO ELIMINATE SCHEDULES II AND II-N FOR FIVE YEARS. HE NEITHER ADMITS NOR DENIES ALLEGATIONS; $1,000 FINE; SHALL NOT PRACTICE OSTEOPATHIC MEDICINE UNTIL HE APPEARS BEFORE THE BOARD AND DEMONSTRATES HE IS CAPABLE OF PRACTICING WITH SKILL AND SAFETY TO PATIENTS AND HIS TEXAS LICENSE IS FREE AND CLEAR OF ANY RESTRICTIONS OR CONDITIONS; UPON REINSTATEMENT OF HIS LICENSE HE MAY BE PLACED ON PROBATION FOR THREE YEARS WITH CONDITIONS TO BE SET AT THAT TIME.

BIGGS, CHARLES R DO OF AUSTIN, TX, WAS DISCIPLINED BY MISSOURI ON FEBRUARY 28, 1990
DISCIPLINARY ACTION: RESTRICTION PLACED ON LICENSE
OFFENSE: DISCIPLINARY ACTION BY ANOTHER STATE OR AGENCY

NOTES: AGREEMENT NOT TO PERFORM SURGERY OR NON-SURGICAL INVASIVE PROCEDURES.

BILDERBACK, ROBERT DOUG MD, LICENSE NUMBER C032983 OF SAN ANTONIO, TX, WAS DISCIPLINED BY CALIFORNIA ON JANUARY 30, 1991
DISCIPLINARY ACTION: LICENSE REVOCATION
OFFENSE: DISCIPLINARY ACTION BY ANOTHER STATE OR AGENCY

NOTES: DISCIPLINED BY TEXAS BOARD AND MISSOURI BOARD FOR MENTAL ILLNESS. DEFAULT DECISION.

BILSING, WILLIAM ALBERT MD, LICENSE NUMBER 00C2986 OF NORMANGEE, TX, WAS DISCIPLINED BY TEXAS ON JANUARY 14, 1994
DISCIPLINARY ACTION: SURRENDER OF CONTROLLED SUBSTANCE LICENSE; 60-MONTH PROBATION
OFFENSE: OVERPRESCRIBING OR MISPRESCRIBING DRUGS

NOTES: ALLEGATIONS CONCERNING HIS NON-THERAPEUTIC PRESCRIBING OF CONTROLLED SUBSTANCES TO 11 PATIENTS, AT LEAST ONE OF WHICH WAS ALLEGED TO BE A SUBSTANCE ABUSER; FAILED TO KEEP ANY MEDICAL REPORTS ON ANY OF THESE PATIENTS. CONDITIONS OF PROBATION: SHALL MAINTAIN ADEQUATE MEDICAL RECORDS ON ALL PATIENT OFFICE VISITS AND SHALL MAKE THESE RECORDS AVAILABLE FOR REVIEW; SHALL SURRENDER DEA AND TEXAS CONTROLLED SUBSTANCES CERTIFICATIONS AND SHALL NOT ATTEMPT TO REREGISTER THESE WITHOUT PERMISSION; PUBLIC REPRIMAND; SHALL GIVE A COPY OF THIS ORDER TO ANY HEALTH CARE ENTITY WHERE HE HAS PRIVILEGES; SHALL COOPERATE WITH THE BOARD IN VERIFYING COMPLIANCE; SHALL INFORM BOARD OF CHANGE OF ADDRESS WITHIN 10 DAYS OR IF HE LEAVES THE STATE; TIME SPENT OUT OF TEXAS OR IN OFFICIAL RETIRED STATUS WITH THE BOARD DOES NOT COUNT TOWARD PROBATION. SHALL NOT SEEK MODIFICATION FOR ONE YEAR.

BILSING, WILLIAM ALBERT MD OF #1 WILSON NURSERY ROAD, NORMANGEE, TX, WAS DISCIPLINED BY DEA ON FEBRUARY 11, 1994
DISCIPLINARY ACTION: SURRENDER OF CONTROLLED SUBSTANCE LICENSE

NOTES: IN LIEU OF PUBLIC INTEREST REVOCATION.

BIRDWELL, LARRY RAY DO, LICENSE NUMBER 00F6445 OF HONEY GROVE, TX, WAS DISCIPLINED BY TEXAS ON NOVEMBER 9, 1991
DISCIPLINARY ACTION: LICENSE SUSPENSION
OFFENSE: SUBSTANCE ABUSE

NOTES: SUSPENDED INDEFINITELY.

BIRDWELL, LARRY RAY DO, LICENSE NUMBER 00F6445, WAS DISCIPLINED BY TEXAS ON DECEMBER 2, 1991
DISCIPLINARY ACTION: SURRENDER OF CONTROLLED SUBSTANCE LICENSE; LICENSE SUSPENSION
OFFENSE: SUBSTANCE ABUSE

NOTES: ENGAGED IN THE INTEMPERATE USE OF ALCOHOL OR DRUGS THAT COULD ENDANGER THE LIVES OF HIS PATIENTS. AS A RESULT OF THIS, ON 11/8/91 HE SIGNED AN INITIAL IMPAIRED PHYSICIANS CONTRACT WITH THE TEXAS OSTEOPATHIC MEDICAL ASSOCIATION, IN WHICH HE AGREED TO ENTER INTO A TREATMENT PROGRAM. CONDITIONS OF HIS SUSPENSION ARE AS FOLLOWS: SHALL SURRENDER HIS DEA AND TEXAS CONTROLLED SUBSTANCE REGISTRATION CERTIFICATES; SHALL SURRENDER ALL UNUSED TRIPLICATE PRESCRIPTION FORMS IN HIS POSSESSION, AND SHALL NOT ATTEMPT TO ORDER ANY MORE TRIPLICATE PRESCRIPTION FORMS UNTIL HE HAS WRITTEN AUTHORITY; SHALL SURRENDER ALL CONTROLLED SUBSTANCES, INCLUDING SAMPLES, PRESENTLY IN HIS POSSESSION, AND MAY NOT POSSESS ANY CONTROLLED SUBSTANCES IN THE FUTURE; SHALL GIVE A COPY OF THIS ORDER TO ALL HOSPITALS WHERE HE HAS PRIVILEGES; SHALL COOPERATE WITH THE BOARD IN VERIFYING COMPLIANCE; SHALL ADVISE THE BOARD OF ANY CHANGE OF ADDRESS WITHIN 10 DAYS.

BIRDWELL, LARRY RAY DO, LICENSE NUMBER 00F6445 OF SAN MARCOS, TX, WAS DISCIPLINED BY TEXAS ON JUNE 26, 1992
DISCIPLINARY ACTION: 60-MONTH PROBATION

NOTES: REQUEST FOR LIFTING OF SUSPENSION IMPOSED 11/9/91 GRANTED; LICENSE SUSPENDED, SUSPENSION STAYED. PROBATION UNDER TERMS AND CONDITIONS. ON 8/19/94 ORDER MODIFIED AS FOLLOWS: REQUIREMENT TO PARTICIPATE IN THE ACTIVITIES OF THE PHYSICIANS ASSISTANCE PROGRAM COMMITTEE AND TO ABIDE BY THE TERMS OF HIS 24 MONTH AFTERCARE PROGRAM CONTRACT IS DELETED. ON 3/2/96 PROBATION TERMINATED.

BISCHOFF, SCOTT BARRY MD, LICENSE NUMBER H6055 OF SUGARLAND, TX, WAS DISCIPLINED BY TEXAS ON AUGUST 28, 1999
DISCIPLINARY ACTION: FINE
OFFENSE: NONCOMPLIANCE WITH A PROFESSIONAL RULE

NOTES: FAILED TO FILL THE REQUESTS OF NUMEROUS PATIENTS FOR THEIR MEDICAL RECORDS WITHIN MANDATED TIME PERIODS. $5,000 FINE; SHALL COOPERATE WITH THE BOARD IN VERIFYING COMPLIANCE; SHALL GIVE A COPY OF THIS ORDER TO ANY HEALTH CARE ENTITY WHERE HE HAS PRIVILEGES; SHALL PROVIDE A COPY OF THIS ORDER TO ANYONE REQUESTING IT WITHIN 10 DAYS; SHALL INFORM THE BOARD OF CHANGE OF ADDRESS WITHIN 10 DAYS.

BITTLE, CHARLES CARROLL JR MD, LICENSE NUMBER 00H0184 OF SANGER, TX, WAS DISCIPLINED BY TEXAS ON APRIL 15, 1994
DISCIPLINARY ACTION: REQUIRED TO TAKE ADDITIONAL MEDICAL EDUCATION; MONITORING OF PHYSICIAN PERFORMANCE
OFFENSE: SUBSTANDARD CARE, INCOMPETENCE OR NEGLIGENCE

NOTES: FAILED TO PERFORM SUFFICIENT FOLLOW-UP VISITS ON NINE GERIATRIC PATIENTS ADMITTED TO A HOSPITAL; ONE WAS DISCHARGED WITH A HIGH FEVER; DR. BITTLE IS PRESENTLY WORKING IN PRIMARILY AN ADMINISTRATIVE CAPACITY. FOR THREE YEARS LICENSE UNDER THE FOLLOWING RESTRICTIONS: SHALL ATTEND AT LEAST 50 HOURS PER YEAR OF CONTINUING MEDICAL EDUCATION INCLUDING AT LEAST 10 HOURS IN RISK MANAGEMENT OR RECORD-KEEPING COURSES; SHALL MAINTAIN ADEQUATE MEDICAL RECORDS ON ALL PATIENT OFFICE VISITS WHICH SHALL BE AVAILABLE FOR INSPECTION; SHALL NOT SIGN ANY PATIENT RECORD UNLESS HE HAS PERSONALLY EXAMINED THE PATIENT OR CLEARLY NOTES IN THE RECORD THAT HE DID NOT; SHALL APPEAR BEFORE THE BOARD ONCE A YEAR; SHALL GIVE A COPY OF THIS ORDER TO ANY HEALTH CARE ENTITY WHERE HE HAS PRIVILEGES; SHALL COOPERATE WITH THE BOARD IN VERIFYING COMPLIANCE; SHALL INFORM BOARD OF CHANGE OF ADDRESS WITHIN 10 DAYS OR IF HE LEAVES THE STATE; TIME SPENT OUT OF TEXAS DOES NOT COUNT TOWARD RESTRICTION. SHALL NOT SEEK MODIFICATION FOR ONE YEAR. ORDER TERMINATED ON 5/15/96.

BLACK, JAMES WILLIAM JR MD, DATE OF BIRTH OCTOBER 2, 1936, LICENSE NUMBER 00D4036 OF 12854 SPURLING DRIVE, DALLAS, TX, WAS DISCIPLINED BY TEXAS ON APRIL 30, 1993
DISCIPLINARY ACTION: SURRENDER OF LICENSE
OFFENSE: PROFESSIONAL MISCONDUCT

NOTES: BOARD HAS INVESTIGATED ALLEGATIONS OF UNPROFESSIONAL CONDUCT WHICH HE DENIES; RETIRED FROM PRACTICE 1/92. SURRENDER IS PERMANENT; SHALL GIVE A COPY OF THIS ORDER TO ANY HEALTH CARE ENTITY WHERE HE HAS PRIVILEGES.

BLACKWELL, MICHAEL L MD OF 123 BARRACUDA AVENUE, GALVESTON, TX, WAS DISCIPLINED BY MEDICARE ON FEBRUARY 8, 1995
DISCIPLINARY ACTION: EXCLUSION FROM THE MEDICARE AND/OR MEDICAID PROGRAM

NOTES: REINSTATED ON 4/14/95.

BLAIR, DONALD LEVESTER JR MD, LICENSE NUMBER H4171 OF FORT WORTH, TX, WAS DISCIPLINED BY TEXAS ON AUGUST 9, 1997
DISCIPLINARY ACTION: REPRIMAND
OFFENSE: SUBSTANDARD CARE, INCOMPETENCE OR NEGLIGENCE

NOTES: DURING 1995, HE PERFORMED A HYSTEROSCOPY, LAPAROSCOPY, AND DILATATION AND CURETTAGE ON A 22-YEAR-OLD PATIENT. FOLLOWING SURGERY, THE PATIENT DEVELOPED HYPONATREMIC ENCEPHALOPATHY, SECONDARY TO IMPROPER INTRAVENOUS FLUID ADMINISTRATION GIVEN IN CONTRAVENTION TO HIS ORDERS. IT IS ALLEGED THAT HE FAILED TO TIMELY TREAT THE PATIENT'S HYPONATREMIA, ALTHOUGH DIFFERING QUALIFIED OPINIONS EXIST CONCERNING THE STANDARD OF CARE FOR THE RATE OF CORRECTION OF HYPONATREMIA. WHILE HE DID TIMELY RECOGNIZE THE NEED FOR AN INTERNAL MEDICINE CONSULTATION AND ORDERED IT IN A TIMELY MANNER, HE DID NOT ORDER A "STAT" INTERNAL

MEDICINE CONSULTATION. HE SHALL GIVE A COPY OF THIS ORDER TO ANY HEALTH CARE ENTITY WHERE HE HAS PRIVILEGES; SHALL PROVIDE A COPY OF THIS ORDER TO ANYONE REQUESTING IT WITHIN 10 DAYS.

BLAISDELL, GLENN D MD, LICENSE NUMBER 00C5606 OF COLLEGE STATION, TX, WAS DISCIPLINED BY TEXAS ON OCTOBER 9, 1992
DISCIPLINARY ACTION: SURRENDER OF LICENSE

NOTES: IN LIEU OF FURTHER DISCIPLINARY ACTION.

BLAISDELL, GLENN D MD OF MOSCOW, ID, WAS DISCIPLINED BY MISSOURI ON MARCH 24, 1994
DISCIPLINARY ACTION: LICENSE REVOCATION
OFFENSE: DISCIPLINARY ACTION BY ANOTHER STATE OR AGENCY

NOTES: TEXAS LICENSE WAS FINALLY AND UNCONDITIONALLY REVOKED FOR FELONY CONVICTION OF POSSESSION OF A FIREARM, TERMINAL MISCHIEF AND INTEMPERATE USE OF ALCOHOL OR DRUGS. NO REAPPLICATION FOR LICENSE FOR SEVEN YEARS.

BLANCHETT, LEO M III MD, LICENSE NUMBER 00E6240 OF EL PASO, TX, WAS DISCIPLINED BY TEXAS ON SEPTEMBER 28, 1990

NOTES: MAY NOT PRACTICE MEDICINE UNTIL HE RECEIVES BOARD APPROVAL TO REENTER SUCH PRACTICE OF MEDICINE UNDER TERMS AS BOARD MAY DETERMINE APPROPRIATE, PASSES SPECIAL PURPOSE EXAMINATION, AND PROVIDES BOARD WITH PSYCHIATRIC REPORT; CORRESPOND WITH BOARD REGARDING CURRENT MEDICAL AND OCCUPATIONAL STATUS.

BLEDIN, ANTHONY GERALD MD, LICENSE NUMBER C42124 OF THOUSAND OAKS, CA, WAS DISCIPLINED BY CALIFORNIA ON JULY 28, 1997
DISCIPLINARY ACTION: 36-MONTH PROBATION
OFFENSE: PROFESSIONAL MISCONDUCT

NOTES: UNLAWFUL PAYMENT OF PATIENT REFERRAL FEES AND FALSELY CONCEALING THOSE REFERRAL FEES AS RENTAL FEES. REVOCATION STAYED.

BLEDIN, ANTHONY GERALD MD, LICENSE NUMBER F7406 OF THOUSAND OAKS, CA, WAS DISCIPLINED BY TEXAS ON AUGUST 22, 1998
DISCIPLINARY ACTION: RESTRICTION PLACED ON LICENSE
OFFENSE: DISCIPLINARY ACTION BY ANOTHER STATE OR AGENCY

NOTES: ON 7/28/97 DISCIPLINED BY THE CALIFORNIA BOARD. LICENSE LIMITED AS FOLLOWS: SHALL NOT PRACTICE IN TEXAS UNTIL HE REQUESTS PERMISSION AND APPEARS BEFORE THE BOARD WITH SUFFICIENT EVIDENCE THAT HE IS PHYSICALLY, MENTALLY OR OTHERWISE COMPETENT TO PRACTICE SAFELY, INCLUDING AT A MINIMUM: SHALL PROVIDE EVIDENCE THAT ANY RESTRICTIONS IMPOSED BY CALIFORNIA BOARD HAVE BEEN REMOVED OR COMPLETED; SHALL TAKE AND PASS, WITHIN 3 MONTHS, THE MEDICAL JURISPRUDENCE EXAM; SHALL COOPERATE WITH THE BOARD IN VERIFYING COMPLIANCE; SHALL INFORM THE BOARD OF CHANGE OF ADDRESS WITHIN 10 DAYS; SHALL NOT SEEK MODIFICATION FOR ONE YEAR.

BLESIUS, CORNELIUS K MD, LICENSE NUMBER 00D4714 OF EL PASO, TX, WAS DISCIPLINED BY TEXAS ON AUGUST 20, 1992
DISCIPLINARY ACTION: REPRIMAND
OFFENSE: PROFESSIONAL MISCONDUCT

NOTES: CONDUCT LIKELY TO DECEIVE THE PUBLIC.

BLESIUS, CORNELIUS K MD, LICENSE NUMBER 00D4714 OF EL PASO, TX, WAS DISCIPLINED BY TEXAS ON AUGUST 18, 1995
DISCIPLINARY ACTION: REQUIRED TO TAKE ADDITIONAL MEDICAL EDUCATION; MONITORING OF PHYSICIAN PERFORMANCE
OFFENSE: PROFESSIONAL MISCONDUCT

NOTES: DURING 1991 HE INJECTED A PATIENT WITH A MEDICATION IN ORDER TO VACCINATE THE PATIENT AGAINST FUNGI WHICH WAS NONTHERAPEUTIC SINCE THERE IS NO DOCUMENTED VACCINATION FOR THE PREVENTION OF FUNGI; IN 9/91 DIAGNOSED A PATIENT WITH IRON DEFICIENCY AND INJECTED PATIENT WITH IMFERON DESPITE PATIENT'S NORMAL SERUM IRON VALUE AND LACK OF GASTROINTESTINAL COMPLAINTS. LICENSE RESTRICTED FOR THREE YEARS UNDER THE FOLLOWING TERMS: HIS PRACTICE SHALL BE MONITORED BY A BOARD-APPROVED PHYSICIAN WHO SHALL SUBMIT BIMONTHLY FOR THE FIRST YEAR AND THEN QUARTERLY REPORTS TO THE BOARD; SHALL OBTAIN AT LEAST 75 HOURS PER YEAR OF CONTINUING MEDICAL EDUCATION INCLUDING AT LEAST ONE EPIDEMIOLOGY OR INFECTIOUS DISEASE COURSE/SEMINAR; SHALL MAINTAIN ADEQUATE MEDICAL RECORDS WHICH SHALL BE AVAILABLE FOR REVIEW; SHALL ADOPT OR ESTABLISH A SYSTEM OF RECORD KEEPING AND BILLING; SHALL APPEAR BEFORE BOARD AT LEAST ONCE A YEAR OR AT BOARD REQUEST; SHALL COOPERATE WITH THE BOARD IN VERIFYING COMPLIANCE; SHALL GIVE A COPY OF THIS ORDER TO ANY HEALTH CARE ENTITY WHERE HE HAS PRIVILEGES; SHALL PROVIDE A COPY OF THIS ORDER TO ANYONE REQUESTING IT WITHIN 10 DAYS; TIME PERIOD OUT OF TEXAS DOES NOT COUNT TOWARD RESTRICTION; SHALL INFORM BOARD OF CHANGE OF ADDRESS WITHIN 10 DAYS OR IF HE LEAVES THE STATE. SHALL NOT SEEK MODIFICATION FOR ONE YEAR. ON 9/20/97 THE BOARD GRANTED HIS PETITION FOR TERMINATION OF THIS ORDER BASED ON COMPLIANCE WITH CONDITIONS.

BLISSARD, PAUL KING MD, LICENSE NUMBER 00F6453 OF HUNTSVILLE, TX, WAS DISCIPLINED BY TEXAS ON DECEMBER 3, 1990
DISCIPLINARY ACTION: 12-MONTH PROBATION; REQUIRED TO TAKE ADDITIONAL MEDICAL EDUCATION

NOTES: MUST MAINTAIN ADEQUATE MEDICAL RECORDS ON ALL PATIENT OFFICE VISITS; ATTEND AT LEAST 50 HOURS OF CONTINUING MEDICAL EDUCATION APPROVED FOR CREDITS, AND PROVIDE PROOF OF ATTENDANCE.

BLOCK, ROBERT JEROME MD, LICENSE NUMBER 00C6174 OF LINCOLNWOOD, IL, WAS DISCIPLINED BY TEXAS ON MARCH 6, 1992
DISCIPLINARY ACTION: SURRENDER OF LICENSE
OFFENSE: DISCIPLINARY ACTION BY ANOTHER STATE OR AGENCY

NOTES: ACTION TAKEN BY ANOTHER STATE BOARD. LICENSE VOLUNTARILY SURRENDERED IN LIEU OF FURTHER DISCIPLINARY ACTION.

BLOOM, BERNARD H MD OF 243 STANDFORD DRIVE, SAN ANTONIO, TX, WAS DISCIPLINED BY DEA ON OCTOBER 4, 1995
DISCIPLINARY ACTION: SURRENDER OF CONTROLLED SUBSTANCE LICENSE

NOTES: IN LIEU OF PUBLIC INTEREST REVOCATION.

BLOSSMAN, ROBERT CHARLES MD, LICENSE NUMBER 00D5591 OF HOUMA, LA, WAS DISCIPLINED BY TEXAS ON OCTOBER 26, 1990

NOTES: IF DESIRING TO PRACTICE MEDICINE IN TEXAS, MUST

DEMONSTRATE TO TEXAS BOARD HIS CAPACITY TO PRACTICE WITH REASONABLE SKILL AND SAFETY AND PROVIDE REPORT ON STATUS OF LOUISIANA LICENSE AND ANY OTHER MEDICAL LICENSE HELD AT THAT TIME; IF GRANTED PERMISSION TO PRACTICE, MAY HAVE IMPOSED PROBATIONARY TERMS AS BOARD MAY DETERMINE APPROPRIATE.

BLUM, JACK MD, DATE OF BIRTH JANUARY 9, 1934, LICENSE NUMBER 0C28144 OF FAIR OAKS, CA, WAS DISCIPLINED BY CALIFORNIA ON JUNE 22, 1990
DISCIPLINARY ACTION: SURRENDER OF LICENSE

NOTES: VOLUNTARY SURRENDER ACCEPTED WHILE CHARGES PENDING.

BLUM, JACK MD, LICENSE NUMBER 0006978 OF CONROE, TX, WAS DISCIPLINED BY MISSISSIPPI ON NOVEMBER 21, 1991
DISCIPLINARY ACTION: SURRENDER OF LICENSE
OFFENSE: DISCIPLINARY ACTION BY ANOTHER STATE OR AGENCY

NOTES: ACTION TAKEN IN CALIFORNIA.

BLUM, JACK MD, DATE OF BIRTH JANUARY 9, 1934, LICENSE NUMBER 0005293, WAS DISCIPLINED BY ARIZONA ON JANUARY 23, 1992
DISCIPLINARY ACTION: PROBATION
OFFENSE: DISCIPLINARY ACTION BY ANOTHER STATE OR AGENCY

NOTES: CALIFORNIA LICENSE SURRENDERED EFFECTIVE 6/22/90 IN CONJUNCTION WITH DISCIPLINARY PROCEEDINGS PENDING AGAINST HIM IN CALIFORNIA. ADMITTED THAT HE USED OR ADMINISTERED TO HIMSELF CONTROLLED SUBSTANCES AND DANGEROUS DRUGS WHICH CAUSED URINE SAMPLES TO TEST POSITIVE ON SIX TESTS DURING THE PERIOD FROM 4/18/88 THROUGH 6/22/89. DR. BLUM IS GUILTY OF UNPROFESSIONAL CONDUCT FOR USE OF CONTROLLED SUBSTANCES EXCEPT IF PRESCRIBED BY ANOTHER PHYSICIAN FOR USE DURING A PRESCRIBED COURSE OF TREATMENT. SHALL MEET WITH THE ARIZONA BOARD PRIOR TO PRACTICING MEDICINE IN ARIZONA AND SHALL BE SUBJECT TO ANY PSYCHIATRIC, PSYCHOMETRIC AND PHYSICAL EVALUATION OR COMPETENCY TESTS THAT THE BOARD MAY DEEM NECESSARY PRIOR TO PERMITTING HIM TO PRACTICE MEDICINE.

BLUM, JACK MD, DATE OF BIRTH JANUARY 9, 1934, LICENSE NUMBER 0003057 OF DALLAS, TX, WAS DISCIPLINED BY VERMONT ON OCTOBER 15, 1992
OFFENSE: DISCIPLINARY ACTION BY ANOTHER STATE OR AGENCY

NOTES: SURRENDERED LICENSE IN CALIFORNIA ON 3/29/90. DISCIPLINED FOR UNPROFESSIONAL CONDUCT, IN THAT HE ADMITTED HE USED OR ADMINISTERED TO HIMSELF CONTROLLED SUBSTANCES AND DANGEROUS DRUGS WHICH CAUSED URINE SAMPLES TO TEST POSITIVE BETWEEN 1/19/89 AND 6/22/89. IF HE SHOULD REAPPLY FOR LICENSURE IN CALIFORNIA, HIS APPLICATION SHALL BE TREATED AS AN ORIGINAL APPLICATION AND HE SHALL BE REQUIRED TO MEET ALL THE REQUIREMENTS OF A NEW APPLICANT. BEFORE PRACTICING IN VERMONT, WILL APPEAR BEFORE THE BOARD AND BE SUBJECT TO ANY COMPETENCY TESTS THEY DEEM NECESSARY.

BLUM, JACK MD, LICENSE NUMBER 0013563 OF DALLAS, TX, WAS DISCIPLINED BY WASHINGTON ON NOVEMBER 20, 1992
DISCIPLINARY ACTION: PROBATION
OFFENSE: DISCIPLINARY ACTION BY ANOTHER STATE OR AGENCY

NOTES: CHARGES OF SUSPENSION, REVOCATION, OR RESTRICTION OF THE LICENSE TO PRACTICE IN ANOTHER JURISDICTION. UNABLE TO PRACTICE IN WASHINGTON UNTIL CERTAIN CONDITIONS ARE MET.

BLUM, JACK MD, DATE OF BIRTH JANUARY 9, 1934, LICENSE NUMBER 00D2660 OF 10044 INWOOD ROAD, DALLAS, TX, WAS DISCIPLINED BY TEXAS ON JANUARY 29, 1993
DISCIPLINARY ACTION: 60-MONTH PROBATION; RESTRICTION PLACED ON CONTROLLED SUBSTANCE LICENSE
OFFENSE: DISCIPLINARY ACTION BY ANOTHER STATE OR AGENCY

NOTES: DISCIPLINED BY CALIFORNIA BOARD FOR SELF-ADMINISTRATION OF DANGEROUS OR CONTROLLED SUBSTANCES LEADING TO SURRENDER OF HIS LICENSE; MISSISSIPPI LICENSE ALSO SURRENDERED ALTHOUGH HE HAD NEVER PRACTICED THERE; DISCIPLINED BY ARIZONA BOARD ALTHOUGH HE NEVER PRACTICED THERE; SELF-ADMINISTERED DIAZEPAM, CODEINE, PHENERGAN, AND PROCARDIA; CURRENTLY PRACTICING IN GEORGIA. 5 YEAR SUSPENSION STAYED. CONDITIONS OF PROBATION: SHALL PARTICIPATE IN ACTIVITIES OF A PHYSICIAN HEALTH AND REHABILITATION COMMITTEE AND ATTEND WEEKLY MEETINGS WITH QUARTERLY REPORTS; SHALL PARTICIPATE IN AA'S 12 STEP PROGRAM NOT LESS THAN 2 TIMES A WEEK WITH QUARTERLY REPORTS; SHALL FURNISH THE BOARD WITH WRITTEN REPORTS ON HIS MEDICAL CONDITION AND COMPLIANCE WITH THIS ORDER WHEN REQUESTED; SHALL ABSTAIN FROM THE CONSUMPTION OF ALCOHOL/CONTROLLED SUBSTANCES IN ANY FORM; SHALL SUBMIT HIMSELF FOR APPROPRIATE EXAMS INCLUDING DRUG OR ALCOHOL SCREENS; SHALL NOT TREAT OR OTHERWISE SERVE AS THE PHYSICIAN, PRESCRIBE, DISPENSE OR ADMINISTER DRUGS THAT MAY BE SUBJECT TO ABUSE TO HIMSELF OR ANY MEMBER OF HIS FAMILY; SHALL NOT POSSESS, ADMINISTER, DISPENSE OR PRESCRIBE SCHEDULE II OR IIN CONTROLLED SUBSTANCES OUTSIDE OF A HOSPITAL SETTING; SHALL MAINTAIN A SEPARATE LOG OF ALL PRESCRIPTIONS WRITTEN FOR CONTROLLED SUBSTANCES WHICH SHALL BE AVAILABLE FOR INSPECTION; SHALL OBTAIN THE SERVICES OF A PRIMARY CARE PHYSICIAN WHO SHALL RELEASE INFORMATION TO THE BOARD; BOARD WILL BE INFORMED IF ANY DRUG HAVING ADDICTION-FORMING OR ADDICTION-SUSTAINING LIABILITY IS PRESCRIBED; SHALL OBTAIN NO PRESCRIPTIONS FROM ANY OTHER PHYSICIAN UNLESS IT IS APPROVED IN WRITING WITHIN 24 HOURS; ANY PRESCRIPTIONS WRITTEN CAN BE FILLED ONLY AT BOARD-APPROVED PHARMACIES; SHALL BE EVALUATED BY A BOARD-APPROVED PSYCHIATRIST TO WHOM HE WILL PROVIDE A COPY OF THE ORDER; SHALL COOPERATE WITH THE BOARD IN VERIFYING COMPLIANCE; SHALL INFORM BOARD OF CHANGE OF ADDRESS WITHIN 10 DAYS; TIME SPENT OUT OF TEXAS OR GEORGIA DOES NOT COUNT TOWARD PROBATION; SHALL APPEAR BEFORE THE BOARD ONCE A YEAR; SHALL APPEAR BEFORE THE BOARD PRIOR TO PRACTICING IN TEXAS. SHALL NOT SEEK MODIFICATION UNTIL FEBRUARY 6, 1994.

BLUM, JACK MD, DATE OF BIRTH JANUARY 9, 1934, LICENSE NUMBER 0016004 OF 101 BOWENS MILL ROAD, DOUGLAS, GA, WAS DISCIPLINED BY GEORGIA ON JUNE 28, 1993
DISCIPLINARY ACTION: EMERGENCY SUSPENSION

NOTES: IMPAIRMENT.

BLUM, JACK MD, DATE OF BIRTH JANUARY 9, 1934, LICENSE NUMBER 0016004 OF 10044 INWOOD ROAD, DALLAS, TX, WAS

DISCIPLINED BY GEORGIA ON OCTOBER 7, 1993
DISCIPLINARY ACTION: LICENSE SUSPENSION

NOTES: IMPAIRMENT; SHALL NOT ENGAGE IN OR RETURN TO PRACTICE OF MEDICINE IN GEORGIA UNTIL FURTHER ORDER OF THE BOARD.

BLUM, JACK MD, DATE OF BIRTH JANUARY 9, 1934, LICENSE NUMBER 00D2660 OF DALLAS, TX, WAS DISCIPLINED BY TEXAS ON OCTOBER 14, 1993
DISCIPLINARY ACTION: EMERGENCY SUSPENSION
OFFENSE: FAILURE TO COMPLY WITH PREVIOUS BOARD ORDER

NOTES: VIOLATED 1/29/93 ORDER IN THAT HE REFUSED TO SUPPLY A URINE SAMPLE IN 8/93 AND INGESTED CONTROLLED SUBSTANCES IN 9/93.

BLUM, JACK MD OF 10044 INWOOD ROAD, DALLAS, TX, WAS DISCIPLINED BY DEA ON NOVEMBER 24, 1993
DISCIPLINARY ACTION: SURRENDER OF CONTROLLED SUBSTANCE LICENSE

NOTES: CONTINUES TO ATTEMPT TO OBTAIN CONTROLLED SUBSTANCES BY CALL-IN PRESCRIPTIONS.

BLUM, JACK MD, DATE OF BIRTH JANUARY 9, 1934, LICENSE NUMBER 00D2660 OF DALLAS, TX, WAS DISCIPLINED BY TEXAS ON JUNE 22, 1994
DISCIPLINARY ACTION: PROBATION
OFFENSE: FAILURE TO COMPLY WITH PREVIOUS BOARD ORDER

NOTES: VIOLATED 1/29/93 TEXAS ORDER IN THAT HE REFUSED TO SUPPLY A URINE SAMPLE ON 8/26/93, INGESTED CONTROLLED SUBSTANCES THREE TIMES IN 9/93; SURRENDERED HIS DEA CONTROLLED SUBSTANCES REGISTRATION ON 11/22/93. SUSPENSION STAYED. CONDITIONS OF INDEFINITE PROBATION: SHALL NOT PRACTICE MEDICINE UNTIL HE HAS UNDERGONE A 72 HOUR INPATIENT EVALUATION FOR CHEMICAL DEPENDENCY, HAS OBTAINED A COMPLETE NEUROLOGIC EXAM FROM A BOARD APPROVED PSYCHIATRIST, CAN DEMONSTRATE COMPLIANCE WITH THIS PSYCHIATRIST'S RECOMMENDATIONS AND APPEARS BEFORE THE BOARD TO REQUEST PERMISSION TO PRACTICE. UPON AN ADEQUATE SHOWING BEFORE THE BOARD THAT HE IS ABLE TO SAFELY PRACTICE MEDICINE, HE SHALL BE ALLOWED TO RESUME THE PRACTICE OF MEDICINE UNDER VARIOUS TERMS AND CONDITIONS.

BLUM, JACK MD, DATE OF BIRTH JANUARY 9, 1934, LICENSE NUMBER 00D2660, WAS DISCIPLINED BY TEXAS ON JANUARY 5, 1995
DISCIPLINARY ACTION: 120-MONTH PROBATION; RESTRICTION PLACED ON CONTROLLED SUBSTANCE LICENSE
OFFENSE: FAILURE TO COMPLY WITH PREVIOUS BOARD ORDER

NOTES: SUSPENSION STAYED. CONDITIONS OF PROBATION: SHALL ABSTAIN FROM THE CONSUMPTION OR ALCOHOL OR CONTROLLED SUBSTANCES IN ANY FORM UNLESS PRESCRIBED BY ANOTHER PHYSICIAN FOR A LEGITIMATE AND THERAPEUTIC PURPOSE; SHALL SUBMIT HIMSELF FOR APPROPRIATE EXAMS INCLUDING DRUG OR ALCOHOL SCREENS; SHALL NOT TREAT OR OTHERWISE SERVE AS PHYSICIAN FOR HIMSELF OR ANY MEMBER OF HIS FAMILY AND SHALL NOT PRESCRIBE, DISPENSE OR ADMINISTER ANY DRUGS THAT MAY BE SUBJECT TO ABUSE TO HIMSELF OR ANY MEMBER OF HIS FAMILY; SHALL ONLY ORDER AND ADMINISTER CONTROLLED SUBSTANCES FOR PERSONS UNDERGOING INPATIENT PROCEDURES AND/OR TREATMENTS AT A HOSPITAL FOR PURPOSES OF INPATIENT CARE; SHALL SURRENDER ALL UNUSED TRIPLICATE PRESCRIPTION FORMS AND CONTROLLED SUBSTANCES IN HIS POSSESSION INCLUDING SAMPLES; SHALL BE MONITORED BY A BOARD-APPROVED PHYSICIAN WITH QUARTERLY REPORTS TO THE BOARD; SEPARATE FROM PATIENT RECORDS SHALL MAINTAIN A FILE OF EVERY PRESCRIPTION WRITTEN FOR DANGEROUS DRUGS WHICH SHALL BE AVAILABLE FOR REVIEW; SHALL NOT TELEPHONE ANY PRESCRIPTION TO A PHARMACY FOR DANGEROUS DRUGS THAT MAY BE HABIT-FORMING; SHALL PARTICIPATE IN THE ACTIVITIES OF A PHYSICIANS' HEALTH AND REHABILITATION COMMITTEE AND ABIDE BY TERMS OF AN AFTERCARE PROGRAM CONTRACT WITH QUARTERLY REPORTS; SHALL PARTICIPATE IN AA'S PROGRAMS NOT LESS THAN THREE TIMES A WEEK WITH QUARTERLY REPORTS TO THE BOARD; SHALL SUBMIT HIMSELF FOR EVALUATION AND TREATMENT TO A BOARD-APPROVED PSYCHIATRIST WITH QUARTERLY REPORTS; SHALL ATTEND AT LEAST 40 HOURS OF CONTINUING MEDICAL EDUCATION PER YEAR; SHALL APPEAR BEFORE THE BOARD TWICE A YEAR; SHALL GIVE A COPY OF THIS ORDER TO ANY HEALTH CARE ENTITY WHERE HE HAS PRIVILEGES; SHALL COOPERATE WITH THE BOARD IN VERIFYING COMPLIANCE; SHALL INFORM BOARD OF CHANGE OF ADDRESS WITHIN 10 DAYS OR IF HE LEAVES THE STATE; TIME SPENT OUT OF TEXAS DOES NOT COUNT TOWARD PROBATION. SHALL NOT SEEK MODIFICATION FOR ONE YEAR.

BLUM, JACK MD, DATE OF BIRTH JANUARY 9, 1934, LICENSE NUMBER 00D2660, WAS DISCIPLINED BY TEXAS ON JUNE 28, 1995
DISCIPLINARY ACTION: LICENSE REVOCATION
OFFENSE: FAILURE TO COMPLY WITH PREVIOUS BOARD ORDER

NOTES: BETWEEN 10/6/94 AND 1/5/95 DIAGNOSED, TREATED, AND PRESCRIBED TO PATIENTS IN VIOLATION OF ORDER; NONCOMPLIANCE TO 1/05/95 ORDER IN THAT HE FAILED TO CAUSE HIS TREATING PHYSICIAN TO REPORT THE INGESTION OF FIORCET AND DIRECTED A MEDICAL ASSISTANT OF HIS MONITORING PHYSICIAN TO PREPARE PRESCRIPTIONS OF CHLORAL HYDRATE AND DIAZEPAM IN HIS WIFE'S NAME WHICH HE TRIED TO FILL, NEITHER OF WHICH WERE AUTHORIZED OR DIRECTED BY HIS MONITORING PHYSICIAN. ON 1/29/99 PETITION TO REINSTATE LICENSE DENIED.

BLUM, JACK MD, DATE OF BIRTH JANUARY 9, 1934, LICENSE NUMBER 0003057 OF DALLAS, TX, WAS DISCIPLINED BY VERMONT ON NOVEMBER 3, 1995
DISCIPLINARY ACTION: LICENSE REVOCATION
OFFENSE: DISCIPLINARY ACTION BY ANOTHER STATE OR AGENCY

NOTES: TEXAS BOARD TOOK DISCIPLINARY ACTION AGAINST HIS MEDICAL LICENSE; ON HIS 1994-1996 LICENSE RENEWAL APPLICATION HE FALSELY ANSWERED "NO" TO A QUESTION REGARDING DISCIPLINARY ACTION TAKEN BY ANOTHER STATE WHEN HE HAD ACTIONS TAKEN BY SEVERAL STATES BETWEEN 1990 AND 1993; ALSO ANSWERED "NO" TO A QUESTION REGARDING REDUCTION, SUSPENSION OR REVOCATION OF STAFF PRIVILEGES, EMPLOYMENT OR APPOINTMENT IN A HOSPITAL OR OTHER HEALTH CARE INSTITUTION WHEN HE HAD RESIGNED FROM A HOSPITAL IN GEORGIA IN 4/93.

BLUM, JACK MD, DATE OF BIRTH JANUARY 9, 1934, LICENSE NUMBER 0005293, WAS DISCIPLINED BY ARIZONA ON JANUARY 19, 1996
DISCIPLINARY ACTION: LICENSE REVOCATION
OFFENSE: DISCIPLINARY ACTION BY ANOTHER STATE OR AGENCY

NOTES: VIOLATED TERMS OF TEXAS PROBATION OF 1/93 IN

THAT HE REFUSED TO SUPPLY A URINE SAMPLE AT THE REQUEST OF A COMPLIANCE OFFICER IN 8/93; IN 9/93, INGESTED CHLORAL HYDRATE, CODEINE, AND XANAX WITHOUT A PRESCRIPTION FROM HIS PRIMARY PHYSICIAN AS REQUIRED BY PROBATION TERMS; SURRENDERED HIS DEA CONTROLLED SUBSTANCES REGISTRATION ON 11/22/93; PLACED ON 10 YEAR PROBATION IN TEXAS IN 1/95 BASED ON NONCOMPLIANCE. IN 1993,1994 AND 1995 APPLICATIONS FOR LICENSE RENEWAL IN ARIZONA, HE DENIED ANY DISCIPLINARY ACTION TAKEN AGAINST HIS LICENSE DURING THE REGISTRATION PERIODS AND DENIED ANY DENIAL, RESTRICTION, SUSPENSION, OR LOSS/REVOCATION OF DEA OR PRESCRIPTION PERMIT, DESPITE ACTIONS BY ARIZONA, TEXAS AND SURRENDER OF HIS DEA REGISTRATION DURING THOSE PERIODS. PERMANENT REVOCATION; FINAL DECISION WITH NO OPPORTUNITY FOR REHEARING OR REVIEW.

BLUM, JACK MD, DATE OF BIRTH JANUARY 9, 1934, LICENSE NUMBER 18306, WAS DISCIPLINED BY COLORADO ON APRIL 10, 1997
DISCIPLINARY ACTION: SURRENDER OF LICENSE

NOTES: NO UNPROFESSIONAL CONDUCT IDENTIFIED.

BLUM, JACK MD, LICENSE NUMBER 13563 OF DALLAS, TX, WAS DISCIPLINED BY WASHINGTON ON MARCH 16, 1998
DISCIPLINARY ACTION: LICENSE SUSPENSION

NOTES: FAILED TO APPEAR AT A PREHEARING CONFERENCE.

BLUME, HORST G MD, DATE OF BIRTH MARCH 12, 1926, LICENSE NUMBER 0017208 OF SIOUX CITY, IA, WAS DISCIPLINED BY IOWA ON FEBRUARY 22, 1990
DISCIPLINARY ACTION: 60-MONTH PROBATION; 3-MONTH RESTRICTION PLACED ON CONTROLLED SUBSTANCE LICENSE

NOTES: MAY NOT PRESCRIBE ADMINISTER OR DISPENSE CONTROLLED SUBSTANCES EXCEPT IN HOSPITAL

BLUME, HORST G MD, WAS DISCIPLINED BY ARIZONA ON JUNE 21, 1991
OFFENSE: DISCIPLINARY ACTION BY ANOTHER STATE OR AGENCY

NOTES: PLACED ON PROBATION FOR 5 YEARS BY IOWA. BOARD ACCEPTED THE SIGNED STIPULATION AND ORDER SAYING THAT HE WILL NOT PRACTICE MEDICINE IN ARIZONA UNTIL HE HAS FIRST MET WITH THE BOARD.

BLUME, HORST G MD, WAS DISCIPLINED BY NEBRASKA ON NOVEMBER 21, 1991
DISCIPLINARY ACTION: PROBATION
OFFENSE: DISCIPLINARY ACTION BY ANOTHER STATE OR AGENCY

BLUME, HORST G MD OF SIOUX CITY, IA, WAS DISCIPLINED BY MISSOURI ON OCTOBER 1, 1992
DISCIPLINARY ACTION: 60-MONTH PROBATION
OFFENSE: DISCIPLINARY ACTION BY ANOTHER STATE OR AGENCY

NOTES: ALSO PRESCRIPTION VIOLATIONS.

BLUME, HORST GUNTHER MD, LICENSE NUMBER 00D1551 OF SIOUX CITY, IA, WAS DISCIPLINED BY TEXAS ON OCTOBER 26, 1990

NOTES: MUST COMPLY WITH IOWA RESTRICTIONS AND AUTHORIZE IOWA BOARD TO RELEASE INFORMATION AS TO STATUS AND PROBATIONARY COMPLIANCE; MUST RECEIVE APPROVAL FROM TEXAS BOARD PRIOR TO PRACTICING MEDICINE IN TEXAS.

BLUME, HORST GUNTHER MD, LICENSE NUMBER D1551 OF SIOUX CITY, IA, WAS DISCIPLINED BY TEXAS ON OCTOBER 24, 1998
DISCIPLINARY ACTION: FINE
OFFENSE: PROFESSIONAL MISCONDUCT

NOTES: IN 4/96 HE TESTIFIED AS AN EXPERT WITNESS IN A LAWSUIT IN ST. LOUIS, MISSOURI; IN A DEPOSITION HE TESTIFIED CONCERNING THE STATUS OF HIS TEXAS LICENSE; SINCE THE 1990 TEXAS ORDER HAD BEEN BASED UPON THE IOWA ORDER, HE BELIEVED THAT TERMINATION OF AN IOWA ORDER SIMILARLY SATISFIED THE TERM OF THE TEXAS ORDER; HE CONTENDS THAT HE DID NOT UNDERSTAND HIS TEXAS LICENSE TO BE IN A PROBATIONARY OR RESTRICTED STATUS, SINCE HE WAS NOT AND HAD NOT BEEN PRACTICING IN TEXAS; HE DENIES INTENTIONALLY OR KNOWINGLY TESTIFYING IN A FALSE OR MISLEADING MANNER; THE 1990 TEXAS ORDER REQUIRING HIM TO APPEAR BEFORE BOARD BEFORE PRACTICING REMAINS IN EFFECT TO DATE. $7,500 FINE.

BOERNER, MARK JAMES MD, LICENSE NUMBER 00H5751 OF SAN ANTONIO, TX, WAS DISCIPLINED BY TEXAS ON OCTOBER 13, 1995
DISCIPLINARY ACTION: FINE
OFFENSE: PROFESSIONAL MISCONDUCT

NOTES: AIDING AND ABETTING THE PRACTICE OF MEDICINE BY A PERSON, PARTNERSHIP, ASSOCIATION OR CORPORATION NOT DULY LICENSED BY THE BOARD TO PRACTICE MEDICINE IN THAT IN 5/93 HE ENTERED INTO A PROVIDER SERVICES AGREEMENT WITH A CORPORATION WHOLLY OWNED BY AN OPHTHALMOLOGY PRACTITIONER AND SURGEON WHO IS NOT A LICENSED TEXAS PHYSICIAN; HE MAINTAINS THAT HE WAS UNAWARE THAT THE AGREEMENT WOULD CONSTITUTE AIDING AND ABETTING THE UNLICENSED PRACTICE OR MEDICINE, THAT HIS VIOLATION OF THE LAW WAS UNINTENTIONAL AND THAT HE TERMINATED HIS RELATIONSHIP WITH THE CORPORATION IN 12/94 AS SOON AS HE WAS AWARE THAT THE AGREEMENT WAS PROHIBITED BY STATUTE; HE IS CURRENTLY PRACTICING MEDICINE IN CALIFORNIA. SHALL PAY $1,000 FINE.

BOGER, JAMES ROBERT MD, WAS DISCIPLINED BY TEXAS ON AUGUST 17, 1996
DISCIPLINARY ACTION: 36-MONTH RESTRICTION PLACED ON LICENSE; 36-MONTH MONITORING OF PHYSICIAN PERFORMANCE
OFFENSE: SUBSTANDARD CARE, INCOMPETENCE OR NEGLIGENCE

NOTES: IN PROCESSING HIS APPLICATION, THE BOARD FOUND INFORMATION INDICATING THAT WHILE HE PERFORMED HIS RESIDENCY HE HAD BEEN ABSENT FROM A NUMBER OF HIS ASSIGNED CLINICS, WHILE ON COMMUNITY SERVICE ROTATION; AND INFORMATION RECEIVED FROM THE RESIDENCY PROGRAM REVEALED A CONCERN WITH HIS ABILITY TO RESPOND IN A TIMELY MANNER TO THE PATIENT WHILE ON CALL. GRANTED A LICENSE UNDER TERMS AND CONDITIONS FOR THREE YEARS: HIS PRACTICE OF MEDICINE SHALL BE LIMITED AND CONFINED TO THE WICHITA STATE HOSPITAL SYSTEM AND ITS CLINICS; SHALL NOT ENGAGE IN THE PRACTICE OF MEDICINE IN ANY OTHER SETTING INCLUDING A PRIVATE MEDICAL PRACTICE SETTING; SHALL INFORM THE BOARD IF HE LEAVES HIS POSITION AT WICHITA STATE HOSPITAL SYSTEM FOR ANY REASON; HIS MEDICAL PRACTICE, INCLUDING ANY OFFICE, HOSPITAL AND SURGICAL PRACTICE, SHALL BE MONITORED BY A BOARD APPROVED TEXAS PHYSICIAN WHO SHALL SUBMIT QUARTERLY

REPORTS TO THE BOARD; SHALL PROVIDE ALL MEDICAL RELEASES AND PEER REVIEW RECORDS UPON REQUEST; SHALL GIVE A COPY OF THIS ORDER TO ANY HEALTH CARE ENTITY WHERE HE HAS PRIVILEGES; SHALL PROVIDE A COPY OF THIS ORDER TO ANYONE REQUESTING IT WITHIN 10 DAYS; TIME PERIOD OUT OF TEXAS DOES NOT COUNT TOWARD RESTRICTION; SHALL INFORM THE BOARD OF CHANGE OF ADDRESS WITHIN 10 DAYS OF IF HE LEAVES THE STATE; SHALL NOT SEEK MODIFICATION FOR ONE YEAR. ON 5/16/98 ORDER TERMINATED.

BOLAND, GREGORY H MD, DATE OF BIRTH JULY 8, 1953, LICENSE NUMBER 0032049 OF LOVELAND, CO, WAS DISCIPLINED BY COLORADO ON JULY 16, 1992
DISCIPLINARY ACTION: 60-MONTH PROBATION; MONITORING OF PHYSICIAN PERFORMANCE
OFFENSE: SUBSTANCE ABUSE

NOTES: HABITUAL INTEMPERANCE OR EXCESSIVE USE OF ANY HABIT-FORMING DRUG OR CONTROLLED SUBSTANCE (IN ABEYANCE). LICENSE GRANTED WITH PROBATION INCLUDING TREATMENT AND PRACTICE MONITORING. PROBATION DEEMED COMPLETED ON 2/16/95 AND LICENSE RESTORED TO UNENCUMBERED STATUS.

BOLAND, GREGORY H MD, DATE OF BIRTH JULY 8, 1953, LICENSE NUMBER 0032049, WAS DISCIPLINED BY COLORADO ON NOVEMBER 16, 1995
DISCIPLINARY ACTION: RESTRICTION PLACED ON LICENSE

NOTES: WILL PERFORM NO ACT REQUIRING A LICENSE TO PRACTICE MEDICINE IN COLORADO UNTIL FURTHER BOARD NOTICE. INTERIM CESSATION OF PRACTICE APPROVED; ORDER IN EFFECT UNTIL ADDITIONAL INFORMATION IS REVIEWED.

BOLAND, GREGORY H MD, DATE OF BIRTH JULY 8, 1953, LICENSE NUMBER 0032049, WAS DISCIPLINED BY COLORADO ON OCTOBER 17, 1996
DISCIPLINARY ACTION: SURRENDER OF LICENSE
OFFENSE: PHYSICAL OR MENTAL ILLNESS INHIBITING THE ABILITY TO PRACTICE WITH SKILL AND SAFETY

NOTES: MENTAL DISABILITY.

BOLAND, GREGORY H MD OF 4601 CORBETT DRIVE, FORT COLLINS, CO, WAS DISCIPLINED BY DEA ON DECEMBER 6, 1996
DISCIPLINARY ACTION: SURRENDER OF CONTROLLED SUBSTANCE LICENSE

BOLAND, GREGORY HAROLD MD, LICENSE NUMBER H7045 OF PUEBLO, CO, WAS DISCIPLINED BY TEXAS ON AUGUST 9, 1997
DISCIPLINARY ACTION: SURRENDER OF LICENSE
OFFENSE: DISCIPLINARY ACTION BY ANOTHER STATE OR AGENCY

NOTES: A 6/23/92 COLORADO BOARD ORDER INDICATES HIS ADMISSION AND AGREEMENT TO HAVING BEEN TREATED FOR EMOTIONAL PROBLEMS MANIFESTED BY MALADAPTIVE CHARATEROLOGICAL, DEPRESSIVE AND ANXIETY SYMPTOMS COMPLICATED BY POLYSUBSTANCE ABUSE IN 1975 AND 1976, AND HAVING BEEN HOSPITALIZED IN 1984 FOR SUBSTANCE ABUSE; ON 11/16/95 THE COLORADO BOARD SUSPENDED HIS LICENSE BECAUSE HE HAD RESUMED ALCOHOL AND DRUG USE AND HAD BEEN ARRESTED IN 10/95 FOR ASSAULT; ON 10/25/96 HE WAS CONVICTED OF TWO COUNTS: SECOND DEGREE ASSAULT, AND UNLAWFUL USE OF A CONTROLLED SUBSTANCE. VOLUNTARY SURRENDER; SHALL GIVE A COPY OF THIS ORDER TO ANY HEALTH CARE ENTITY WHERE HE HAS PRIVILEGES.

BOLAND, GREGORY HAROLD MD, DATE OF BIRTH JULY 8, 1953 OF PO BOX 300, UNIT A, 91573, CANYON CITY, CO, WAS DISCIPLINED BY MEDICARE ON DECEMBER 20, 1998
DISCIPLINARY ACTION: EXCLUSION FROM THE MEDICARE AND/OR MEDICAID PROGRAM
OFFENSE: DISCIPLINARY ACTION BY ANOTHER STATE OR AGENCY

NOTES: LICENSE REVOKED, SUSPENDED, SURRENDERED OR OTHERWISE LOST FOR REASONS BEARING ON PROFESSIONAL PERFORMANCE, PROFESSIONAL COMPETENCE OR FINANCIAL INTEGRITY.

BOLIN, DANIEL HUFFMAN MD, LICENSE NUMBER 00E6042 OF WICHITA FALLS, TX, WAS DISCIPLINED BY TEXAS ON OCTOBER 5, 1991
DISCIPLINARY ACTION: 120-MONTH PROBATION; MONITORING OF PHYSICIAN PERFORMANCE
OFFENSE: SUBSTANCE ABUSE

NOTES: INTEMPERATE USE OF HISTUSSIN FROM 9/90 UNTIL 7/91, WHEN HE ENTERED INPATIENT TREATMENT FOR HIS DRUG USE. REVOCATION STAYED AND PUT ON PROBATION WITH FOLLOWING TERMS AND CONDITIONS: SHALL ABSTAIN FROM THE CONSUMPTION OF ALCOHOL/CHEMICAL SUBSTANCES IN ANY FORM; SHALL PARTICIPATE IN THE ACTIVITIES OF THE IMPAIRED PHYSICIANS PROGRAM, INCLUDING WEEKLY MEETINGS, WITH QUARTERLY REPORTS TO THE BOARD; SHALL PARTICIPATE IN ALCOHOLICS ANONYMOUS ON A REGULAR BASIS, INCLUDING A 12-STEP PROGRAM, OF NOT LESS THAN FOUR TIMES A WEEK; SHALL SUBMIT HIMSELF FOR RANDOM SCREENS OF BIOLOGICAL FLUIDS; SHALL OBTAIN TREATMENT FROM A BOARD APPROVED PSYCHIATRIST, WITH QUARTERLY REPORTS TO BOARD; SHALL NOT TREAT OR OTHERWISE SERVE AS THE PHYSICIAN, PRESCRIBE, DISPENSE, OR ADMINISTER CONTROLLED SUBSTANCES, OR ANY OTHER DRUGS THAT MAY BE SUBJECT TO ABUSE, FOR HIMSELF OR ANY MEMBER OF HIS IMMEDIATE FAMILY; SHALL MAINTAIN A LOG BOOK FOR THE RECEIPT AND DISPENSING OF ALL DRUG SAMPLES AND SHALL PROVIDE THEM TO BOARD UPON REQUEST; SHALL APPEAR BEFORE THE BOARD TWICE A YEAR; SHALL COOPERATE WITH BOARD IN VERIFYING COMPLIANCE; SHALL ADVISE THE BOARD OF CHANGE OF ADDRESS WITHIN 10 DAYS; TIME SPENT OUT OF TEXAS DOES NOT COUNT TOWARDS PROBATION. ON 1/18/97 HIS PETITION FOR TERMINATION OF THIS ORDER GRANTED BASED ON COMPLIANCE WITH CONDITIONS.

BOLLING, DAVID R MD OF 2046 BABCOKC ROAD #2, SAN ANTONIO, TX, WAS DISCIPLINED BY DEA ON JUNE 15, 1994
DISCIPLINARY ACTION: SURRENDER OF CONTROLLED SUBSTANCE LICENSE

NOTES: IN LIEU OF PUBLIC INTEREST REVOCATION.

BOLLING, DAVID RANDOLPH JR MD, LICENSE NUMBER 00D4039 OF SAN ANTONIO, TX, WAS DISCIPLINED BY TEXAS ON APRIL 15, 1994
DISCIPLINARY ACTION: LICENSE SUSPENSION
OFFENSE: PHYSICAL OR MENTAL ILLNESS INHIBITING THE ABILITY TO PRACTICE WITH SKILL AND SAFETY

NOTES: ON 3/3/94 HE WAS ADJUDGED OF UNSOUND MIND BY A PROBATE COURT; CONSENTED TO THIS ORDER THROUGH HIS GUARDIAN. SUSPENSION UNTIL HE CAN APPEAR BEFORE THE BOARD AND PROVIDE INFORMATION TO PROVE HIS COMPETENCY. ON 8/16/96 REQUEST TO TERMINATE SUSPENSION

DENIED.

BOMMAKANTI, SWAMISARAN MD, LICENSE NUMBER 00G8532 OF OSHKOSH, WI, WAS DISCIPLINED BY TEXAS ON JUNE 10, 1991
DISCIPLINARY ACTION: 60-MONTH PROBATION; RESTRICTION PLACED ON LICENSE
OFFENSE: DISCIPLINARY ACTION BY ANOTHER STATE OR AGENCY

NOTES: DISCIPLINARY ACTION TAKEN BY ANOTHER STATE BOARD DUE TO PROFESSIONAL MISCONDUCT. LICENSE PARTIALLY SUSPENDED IN THE AREA OF SURGERY; UPON TERMINATION OF THE SUSPENSION OF NEW YORK LICENSE, TEXAS LICENSE SHALL BE PLACED ON PROBATION FOR FIVE YEARS; PRIOR TO PRACTICING MEDICINE IN TEXAS, SHALL APPEAR BEFORE AND RECEIVE APPROVAL FROM THE TEXAS BOARD.

BOND, WELDON EUGENE JR DO, LICENSE NUMBER 00E3210 OF ARLINGTON, TX, WAS DISCIPLINED BY TEXAS ON MARCH 4, 1995
DISCIPLINARY ACTION: 60-MONTH PROBATION; REQUIRED TO TAKE ADDITIONAL MEDICAL EDUCATION
OFFENSE: PROFESSIONAL MISCONDUCT

NOTES: FROM 1987 AND INTO 1991, ENGAGED IN NON-INVASIVE OVERTESTING OF VARIOUS PATIENTS WITHOUT ADEQUATE INDICATIONS, WHICH RESULTED IN EXCESSIVE BILLINGS. SUSPENSION STAYED. PROBATION WITH CONDITIONS: SHALL BE MONITORED BY A BOARD-APPROVED MONITORING PHYSICIAN WHO SHALL SUBMIT QUARTERLY REPORTS TO THE BOARD; SHALL MAINTAIN ADEQUATE MEDICAL RECORDS WHICH WILL BE AVAILABLE FOR INSPECTION; SHALL OBTAIN AT LEAST 50 HOURS PER YEAR OF CONTINUING MEDICAL EDUCATION; SHALL OBTAIN FIVE HOURS OF AN ETHICS COURSE PER YEAR; EACH YEAR SHALL PERFORM 100 HOURS OF COMMUNITY SERVICE FOR A NON-PROFIT CHARITABLE ORGANIZATION APPROVED BY THE BOARD; SHALL APPEAR BEFORE THE BOARD AT LEAST ONCE A YEAR; SHALL COOPERATE WITH BOARD IN VERIFYING COMPLIANCE; SHALL GIVE A COPY OF ORDER TO ANY HEALTH CARE ENTITIES WHERE HE HAS PRIVILEGES; TIME SPENT OUT OF TEXAS DOES NOT COUNT TOWARD PROBATION; SHALL INFORM BOARD OF ANY CHANGE OF ADDRESS WITHIN 10 DAYS OR IF LEAVES STATE; SHALL NOT SEEK MODIFICATION FOR ONE YEAR.

BONHAM, H E EUGENE MD OF 11803 SOUTH FREEWAY #215, FORT WORTH, TX, WAS DISCIPLINED BY DEA ON OCTOBER 5, 1998
DISCIPLINARY ACTION: SURRENDER OF CONTROLLED SUBSTANCE LICENSE

NOTES: IN LIEU OF PUBLIC INTEREST REVOCATION.

BONHAM, HENRY EDWARD MD, LICENSE NUMBER D4076 OF FORT WORTH, TX, WAS DISCIPLINED BY TEXAS ON MAY 16, 1998
DISCIPLINARY ACTION: LICENSE SUSPENSION
OFFENSE: CRIMINAL CONVICTION OR PLEA OF GUILTY, NOLO CONTENDERE, OR NO CONTEST TO A CRIME

NOTES: ON 7/14/97 CONVICTED OF MAIL FRAUD AND FALSE CLAIMS BY A JURY IN U.S. DISTRICT COURT IN FORT WORTH, TEXAS, AND WAS SENTENCED TO INCARCERATION FOR 87 MONTHS, PLUS AN ADDITIONAL 3 YEAR PROBATIONARY PERIOD; MAINTAINS HIS INNOCENCE OF THE CHARGES. INDEFINITE SUSPENSION UNTIL HIS CRIMINAL CONVICTION IS FINALLY ADJUDICATED; SHALL INFORM THE BOARD OF CHANGE OF ADDRESS WITHIN 10 DAYS; SHALL COOPERATE WITH THE BOARD IN VERIFYING COMPLIANCE.

BONHAM, HENRY EDWARD EUGENE MD, DATE OF BIRTH OCTOBER 15, 1941 OF 2113 N HWY 175, #29175-077FCI, SEAGOVILLE, TX, WAS DISCIPLINED BY MEDICARE ON AUGUST 20, 1998
DISCIPLINARY ACTION: 240-MONTH EXCLUSION FROM THE MEDICARE AND/OR MEDICAID PROGRAM
OFFENSE: CRIMINAL CONVICTION OR PLEA OF GUILTY, NOLO CONTENDERE, OR NO CONTEST TO A CRIME

NOTES: CONVICTED OF A CRIME INVOLVING THE MEDICARE, MEDICAID, MATERNAL AND CHILD HEALTH SERVICES BLOCK GRANT OR BLOCK GRANTS TO STATES FOR SOCIAL SERVICES PROGRAMS.

BONILLA, JAIME MD, LICENSE NUMBER E2416 OF HOUSTON, TX, WAS DISCIPLINED BY TEXAS ON AUGUST 28, 1999
DISCIPLINARY ACTION: FINE; REPRIMAND
OFFENSE: CRIMINAL CONVICTION OR PLEA OF GUILTY, NOLO CONTENDERE, OR NO CONTEST TO A CRIME

NOTES: ON 6/27/97 HE WAS IN POSSESSION OF $140,000 AND ATTEMPTED TO TRANSPORT THE MONEY OUTSIDE OF THE UNITED STATES WITHOUT FILING THE PRESCRIBED REPORT; AS A RESULT, HE WAS INDICTED AND SUBSEQUENTLY CONVICTED OF A FELONY; THE TERMS OF HIS PROBATION INCLUDED A DRUG AND ALCOHOL TREATMENT PROGRAM. LICENSE LIMITED AS FOLLOWS: SHALL PRODUCE A REPORT FROM HIS FEDERAL PROBATION OFFICER ON HIS CURRENT STATUS AND ONGOING STATUS EVERY SIX MONTHS; WITHIN 1 YEAR SHALL OBTAIN 10 HOURS OF ETHICS THROUGH BOARD-APPROVED COURSES OR PROGRAMS; $5,000 FINE; TIME SPENT OUT OF TEXAS DOES NOT COUNT TOWARD RESTRICTION; SHALL INFORM THE BOARD OF CHANGE OF ADDRESS WITHIN 10 DAYS OR IF HE LEAVES THE STATE; SHALL NOT SEEK MODIFICATION FOR ONE YEAR.

BOONE, GEORGE DANIEL MD, LICENSE NUMBER 00F6460 OF KERRVILLE, TX, WAS DISCIPLINED BY TEXAS ON JANUARY 14, 1994
DISCIPLINARY ACTION: REPRIMAND
OFFENSE: OVERPRESCRIBING OR MISPRESCRIBING DRUGS

NOTES: IN 1991 AFTER ADVISING THE PATIENTS OF THE RISKS OF STEROID USE AND DANGERS OF BLACK MARKET STEROIDS, HE PRESCRIBED ANABOLIC STEROIDS TO TWO PATIENTS FOR NON-MEDICAL PURPOSES RELATED TO WEIGHT GAIN AND BODY BUILDING; NO OTHER COMPLAINTS HAVE BEEN FILED AGAINST HIM WITH BOARD.

BOONE, MICHAEL K MD OF 1700 MURCHISON SUITE 200, EL PASO, TX, WAS DISCIPLINED BY DEA ON OCTOBER 3, 1994
DISCIPLINARY ACTION: SURRENDER OF CONTROLLED SUBSTANCE LICENSE

NOTES: IN LIEU OF PUBLIC INTEREST REVOCATION.

BOONE, MICHAEL KEVIN MD, LICENSE NUMBER 00H4177 OF EL PASO, TX, WAS DISCIPLINED BY TEXAS ON JUNE 28, 1995
DISCIPLINARY ACTION: 60-MONTH PROBATION; 60-MONTH RESTRICTION PLACED ON CONTROLLED SUBSTANCE LICENSE
OFFENSE: SUBSTANCE ABUSE

NOTES: WROTE FALSE PRESCRIPTIONS FOR DANGEROUS DRUGS OR CONTROLLED SUBSTANCES; BEGINNING IN 1991, BEGAN ABUSING VICODIN AND LATER LORCET AND LORTAB; SURRENDERED HIS DEA/DPS CONTROLLED SUBSTANCES REGISTRATION; RECEIVED INPATIENT SUBSTANCE ABUSE TREATMENT IN ARIZONA IN 11/94; REPORTS SOBRIETY DATE OF 9/28/94; REPORTS ATTENDING AA MEETINGS APPROXIMATELY THREE TIMES PER WEEK AND PARTICIPATING REGULARLY IN THE ACTIVITIES OF

THE COMMITTEE ON PHYSICIAN HEALTH AND REHABILITATION; IN 1/95, ENTERED INTO A TWO-YEAR CONTINUING CARE CONTRACT WITH COMMITTEE; UNDER THE CARE OF A PSYCHIATRIST. SUSPENSION STAYED. PROBATION WITH TERMS: SHALL ABSTAIN FROM THE CONSUMPTION OF ALCOHOL/DRUGS IN ANY FORM UNLESS PRESCRIBED BY ANOTHER PHYSICIAN FOR A LEGITIMATE AND THERAPEUTIC PURPOSE; SHALL SUBMIT HIMSELF FOR APPROPRIATE EXAMS INCLUDING DRUG OR ALCOHOL SCREENS; SHALL CONTINUE TO RECEIVE CARE AND TREATMENT OF PSYCHIATRIST AT LEAST ONCE A MONTH WHO SHALL SUBMIT QUARTERLY REPORTS; SHALL PARTICIPATE IN AA'S PROGRAM NOT LESS THAN FIVE TIMES A WEEK WITH QUARTERLY REPORTS; SHALL OBTAIN A MALE AA SPONSOR WHO IS NOT A PHYSICIAN; SHALL CONTINUE TO PARTICIPATE IN ACTIVITIES OF AN IMPAIRED PHYSICIAN'S GROUP AND ATTEND WEEKLY MEETINGS WITH QUARTERLY REPORTS; SHALL NOT POSSESS ALCOHOL, CONTROLLED SUBSTANCES OR DRUGS WITH ADDICTIVE POTENTIAL; SHALL NOT TREAT OR OTHERWISE SERVE AS PHYSICIAN, PRESCRIBE, DISPENSE OR ADMINISTER DRUGS THAT MAY BE SUBJECT TO ABUSE TO HIMSELF OR TO ANY MEMBER OF HIS FAMILY; SHALL SURRENDER HIS DEA/DPS CONTROLLED SUBSTANCES REGISTRATION CERTIFICATE; SHALL MAINTAIN A FILE WITH EVERY PRESCRIPTION WRITTEN FOR DRUGS WITH POTENTIAL FOR ABUSE WHICH SHALL BE AVAILABLE FOR REVIEW; SHALL NOT TELEPHONE PHARMACY WITH PRESCRIPTIONS FOR THESE DRUGS; SHALL OBTAIN AT LEAST 50 HOURS PER YEAR OF CONTINUING MEDICAL EDUCATION; SHALL APPEAR BEFORE BOARD AT LEAST TWO TIMES PER YEAR OR AT BOARD REQUEST; SHALL COOPERATE WITH BOARD IN VERIFYING COMPLIANCE INCLUDING PROVIDING ANY MEDICAL RELEASES UPON REQUEST; SHALL GIVE A COPY OF THIS ORDER TO ANY HEALTH CARE ENTITY WHERE HE HAS PRIVILEGES; SHALL PROVIDE A COPY OF THIS ORDER TO ANYONE WHO REQUESTS IT WITHIN 10 DAYS; TIME PERIOD OUT OF TEXAS DOES NOT COUNT TOWARD PROBATION; SHALL INFORM BOARD OF CHANGE OF ADDRESS WITHIN 10 DAYS OR IF HE LEAVES THE STATE. SHALL NOT SEEK MODIFICATION FOR ONE YEAR. ON 8/9/97 PETITION TO MODIFY ORDER GRANTED REDUCING AA PARTICIPATION FROM FIVE TIMES A WEEK TO THREE. ON 2/7/98 ORDER MODIFIED REDUCING APPEARANCES BEFORE THE BOARD FROM BIANNUAL TO ANNUAL.

BORCHERDING, HARLAN J DO OF HOUSTON, TX, WAS DISCIPLINED BY DEA ON JULY 3, 1995
DISCIPLINARY ACTION: REVOCATION OF CONTROLLED SUBSTANCE LICENSE
OFFENSE: OVERPRESCRIBING OR MISPRESCRIBING DRUGS

NOTES: PRESCRIPTIONS OF TRANXENE AND VALIUM ISSUED TO AN UNDERCOVER OFFICER ON 12/14/90, 1/25/91, AND 2/26/91 WERE NOT LEGITIMATELY DISPENSED OR PRESCRIBED IN REGARD TO THE TIME SPENT, AMOUNT OF FOLLOW UP, OR DISPENSING AFTER PATIENT SAID HE WAS TAKING LARGER AMOUNTS. HIS RECORDKEEPING PRACTICES IN 1992 WERE INADEQUATE INCLUDING FAILURE TO MAINTAIN COMPLETE AND ACCURATE RECORDS OF CONTROLLED SUBSTANCES RECEIVED AND DISPENSED; FAILURE TO TAKE AN INITIAL OR BIENNIAL INVENTORY OF ALL STOCKS OF CONTROLLED SUBSTANCES; AND FAILURE TO MAINTAIN DISPENSING RECORDS OF CONTROLLED SUBSTANCES IN A READILY RETRIEVABLE FORM.

BORCHERDING, HARLAN JAMES DO, LICENSE NUMBER 00D7531 OF HOUSTON, TX, WAS DISCIPLINED BY TEXAS ON AUGUST 19, 1994
DISCIPLINARY ACTION: 120-MONTH PROBATION; RESTRICTION PLACED ON CONTROLLED SUBSTANCE LICENSE
OFFENSE: OVERPRESCRIBING OR MISPRESCRIBING DRUGS

NOTES: ON 3/20/92 HE ENTERED A GUILTY PLEA TO FRAUD OF A CONTROLLED SUBSTANCE, A MISDEMEANOR, AND RECEIVED DEFERRED ADJUDICATION WITH TWO YEARS PROBATION; ON 5/25/94 HE GAVE TESTIMONY IN REGARD TO A DEA AUDIT OF HIS OFFICE ON 2/19/93 WHICH IDENTIFIED VARIOUS VIOLATIONS PERTAINING TO HIS PRESCRIBING PRACTICES AND RECORD KEEPING; ENTERED INTO A SETTLEMENT AGREEMENT WITH DEA WITH NO ADMISSION OF GUILT; ADMITS TO PREVIOUSLY POOR RECORD KEEPING AND ASSERTS HE IS WORKING TO IMPROVE THIS; DENIES EVER SELLING A PRESCRIPTION. SUSPENSION STAYED. CONDITIONS OF PROBATION: SHALL MAINTAIN ADEQUATE MEDICAL RECORDS ON ALL PATIENT OFFICE VISITS WHICH SHALL BE AVAILABLE FOR INSPECTION; SHALL NOT SIGN ANY PATIENT RECORD UNLESS HE HAS PERSONALLY EXAMINED THE PATIENT OR CLEARLY NOTES IN THE RECORD THAT HE DID NOT; SHALL REQUEST MODIFICATION OF DEA AND TEXAS CONTROLLED SUBSTANCES CERTIFICATES TO BE LIMITED TO SCHEDULES III, IV AND V; SHALL NOT ATTEMPT TO REREGISTER WITHOUT PERMISSION; SHALL PASS THE JURISPRUDENCE EXAM WITHIN ONE YEAR; SHALL COMPLETE A BOARD-APPROVED PHARMACOLOGY COURSE AND AN ETHICS COURSE; SHALL ATTEND AT LEAST 50 HOURS PER YEAR OF CONTINUING MEDICAL EDUCATION; SHALL APPEAR BEFORE THE BOARD TWICE A YEAR; SHALL GIVE A COPY OF THIS ORDER TO ANY HEALTH CARE ENTITY WHERE HE HAS PRIVILEGES; SHALL COOPERATE WITH THE BOARD IN VERIFYING COMPLIANCE; SHALL INFORM BOARD OF CHANGE OF ADDRESS WITHIN 10 DAYS OR IF HE LEAVES THE STATE; TIME SPENT OUT OF TEXAS DOES NOT COUNT TOWARD PROBATION. SHALL NOT SEEK MODIFICATION FOR THREE YEARS. ON 9/20/97 PETITION TO TERMINATE ORDER DENIED; ORDER MODIFIED REDUCING APPEARANCES BEFORE THE BOARD FROM BIANNUAL TO ANNUAL. ON 10/24/98 ORDER TERMINATED.

BORDELON, JERRY PHILLIP MD, LICENSE NUMBER 00D8998 OF AUSTIN, TX, WAS DISCIPLINED BY TEXAS ON NOVEMBER 3, 1994
DISCIPLINARY ACTION: REPRIMAND; REQUIRED TO TAKE ADDITIONAL MEDICAL EDUCATION
OFFENSE: SUBSTANDARD CARE, INCOMPETENCE OR NEGLIGENCE

NOTES: ON 11/1/93 HE PERFORMED LASER SURGERY ON A PATIENT TO REMOVE PAPILLOMAS FROM THE THROAT AREA; INDICATORS WERE THAT HELIOX WAS THE REQUIRED ANESTHESIA GAS, HOWEVER, THE ANESTHESIOLOGIST ADMINISTERED ESSENTIALLY PURE OXYGEN; DR. BORDELON WAS NOT AWARE OF THIS AND USED A LASER; AN ACCIDENT ENSUED AND THE PATIENT DIED NEARLY TWO MONTHS LATER FROM COMPLICATIONS; MAINTAINS THE ANESTHESIOLOGIST NEVER WARNED HIM THAT HE ADMINISTERED PURE OXYGEN; NEITHER ADMITS NOR DENIES ALLEGATIONS BUT CONSENTS TO THE ORDER TO REACH AN EXPEDITIOUS RESOLUTION. SHALL WITHIN SIX MONTHS OBTAIN A BOARD-APPROVED COURSE IN RISK MANAGEMENT; SHALL GIVE A COPY OF THIS ORDER TO ANY HEALTH CARE ENTITY WHERE HE HAS PRIVILEGES; SHALL COOPERATE WITH THE BOARD IN VERIFYING COMPLIANCE; SHALL INFORM CHANGE OF ADDRESS WITHIN 10 DAYS. SHALL NOT SEEK MODIFICATION FOR SIX MONTHS.

BORDEN, LARRY IGOR MD, LICENSE NUMBER 0C31710 OF LONG BEACH, CA, WAS DISCIPLINED BY CALIFORNIA ON MARCH 12, 1992
DISCIPLINARY ACTION: 120-MONTH PROBATION

NOTES: REVOCATION, STAYED. JUDICIAL REVIEW FILED - STAY ORDER ISSUED.

BORDEN, LARRY IGOR MD, LICENSE NUMBER 0C31710 OF LONG BEACH, CA, WAS DISCIPLINED BY CALIFORNIA ON AUGUST 7, 1992
DISCIPLINARY ACTION: LICENSE REVOCATION
OFFENSE: SUBSTANDARD CARE, INCOMPETENCE OR NEGLIGENCE

NOTES: GROSS NEGLIGENCE AND INCOMPETENCE IN ANESTHESIOLOGY PRACTICE RESULTING IN 2 DEATHS. REVOCATION, JUDICIAL REVIEW FILED, STAY ORDER ISSUED. ON 2/23/95 COURT APPEALS COMPLETED UPHOLDING THE REVOCATION.

BORDEN, LARRY IGOR MD, LICENSE NUMBER 00D5684 OF ARCADIA, CA, WAS DISCIPLINED BY TEXAS ON MAY 12, 1995
DISCIPLINARY ACTION: LICENSE REVOCATION
OFFENSE: DISCIPLINARY ACTION BY ANOTHER STATE OR AGENCY

NOTES: FOUND GUILTY OF GROSS NEGLIGENCE, REPEATED NEGLIGENT ACTS AND INCOMPETENCE IN HIS ADMINISTERING OF ANESTHESIA TO TWO PATIENTS WHO DIED AFTER BEING ANESTHETIZED FOR WHICH HIS CALIFORNIA LICENSE WAS REVOKED.

BORGE, ADOLF NORMAN MD, LICENSE NUMBER 00D1555 OF FORT WORTH, TX, WAS DISCIPLINED BY TEXAS ON MARCH 31, 1990
DISCIPLINARY ACTION: 60-MONTH PROBATION; REQUIRED TO TAKE ADDITIONAL MEDICAL EDUCATION

NOTES: STIPULATED ORDER. REVOCATION STAYED. MUST ATTEND CONTINUING MEDICAL EDUCATION, OBTAIN WRITTEN CONSULTATIONS ON HOSPITALIZATIONS AND HOSPITAL QUALITY ASSURANCE COMMITTEE. MUST SUBMIT QUARTERLY REPORTS TO BOARD. PROBATION TERMINATED EFFECTIVE 4/30/93; LICENSE FREE OF ANY RESTRICTION OR LIMITATION.

BOUDREAU, DANIEL ALEXANDER DO, LICENSE NUMBER 00D5354 OF MESQUITE, TX, WAS DISCIPLINED BY TEXAS ON JANUARY 6, 1995
DISCIPLINARY ACTION: 60-MONTH RESTRICTION PLACED ON LICENSE; REQUIRED TO TAKE ADDITIONAL MEDICAL EDUCATION
OFFENSE: SUBSTANDARD CARE, INCOMPETENCE OR NEGLIGENCE

NOTES: DURING 3/91 PERFORMED A MICRODISKECTOMY AT THE WRONG LEVEL ON A PATIENT DUE TO A MISCALCULATION; THE PATIENT FILED A MALPRACTICE ACTION WHICH WAS SETTLED FOR $200,000; SINCE THEN HE REPORTS REVISING HIS PROCEDURES TO BETTER IDENTIFY THE CORRECT SURGICAL LEVEL; NO LONGER PERFORMING BACK SURGERIES; HE AGREES TO THE ENTRY OF THE ORDER IN LIEU OF FURTHER INVESTIGATION. CONDITIONS OF RESTRICTION: SHALL NOT PERFORM BACK SURGERIES OF ANY KIND BUT MAY ASSIST AT BACK SURGERIES PERFORMED BY ANOTHER SURGEON; SHALL MAINTAIN ADEQUATE MEDICAL RECORDS ON ALL PATIENT OFFICE VISITS WHICH SHALL BE AVAILABLE FOR INSPECTION; SHALL OBTAIN AT LEAST 50 HOURS PER YEAR OF CONTINUING MEDICAL EDUCATION; SHALL APPEAR BEFORE THE BOARD ONCE A YEAR OR UPON REQUEST; SHALL COOPERATE WITH THE BOARD IN VERIFYING COMPLIANCE; SHALL PROVIDE AS NEEDED ALL MEDICAL RELEASES AND RELEASES OF PEER REVIEW RECORDS; SHALL GIVE A COPY OF THIS ORDER TO ANY HEALTH CARE ENTITY WHERE HE HAS OR APPLIES FOR PRIVILEGES AND ANYONE ELSE WHO ASKS FOR IT; SHALL ENSURE ANY INQUIRIES REGARDING HIS TEXAS LICENSURE STATUS ARE ANSWERED BY REFERENCE TO THIS ORDER; SHALL INFORM BOARD OF CHANGE OF ADDRESS WITHIN 10 DAYS OR IF HE LEAVES THE STATE; TIME SPENT OUT OF TEXAS DOES NOT COUNT TOWARD RESTRICTION. SHALL NOT SEEK MODIFICATION FOR ONE YEAR. ON 5/10/97 PETITION TO TERMINATE ORDER DENIED; ORDER MODIFIED ALLOWING HIM THE AUTHORITY TO REQUEST TERMINATION OR MODIFICATION ONCE EVERY SIX MONTHS. ON 2/7/98 ORDER TERMINATED.

BOWLER, DONALD L MD, LICENSE NUMBER 00D2928 OF HUNTSVILLE, TX, WAS DISCIPLINED BY TEXAS ON AUGUST 24, 1991
DISCIPLINARY ACTION: LICENSE SUSPENSION
OFFENSE: CRIMINAL CONVICTION OR PLEA OF GUILTY, NOLO CONTENDERE, OR NO CONTEST TO A CRIME

NOTES: FELONY CONVICTION OF FRAUD IN THE PRESCRIPTION AND DELIVERY OF A CONTROLLED SUBSTANCE.

BOWLES, THEODORE A JR DO, DATE OF BIRTH MARCH 22, 1952, LICENSE NUMBER 0H35804, WAS DISCIPLINED BY MARYLAND ON SEPTEMBER 23, 1992
DISCIPLINARY ACTION: REPRIMAND
OFFENSE: PROVIDING FALSE INFORMATION TO THE BOARD OR OTHER HEALTH AGENCY

NOTES: IN 1988 HE WAS ALLEGED TO HAVE USED A CONTROLLED SUBSTANCE, AND WAS THEN TERMINATED FROM HIS ANESTHESIOLOGY RESIDENCY PROGRAM AT BROOKE ARMY MEDICAL CENTER, BUT CONTINUED TO SERVE IN THEIR DEPARTMENT OF PRIMARY CARE. THE ARMY DROPPED ALL CHARGES, AND HE VOLUNTARILY RESIGNED FROM THE MILITARY IN 1990. ON THE RENEWAL APPLICATION FOR HIS MARYLAND LICENSE HE STATED THAT HIS PRIVILEGES HAD NEVER BEEN LIMITED, RESTRICTED, SUSPENDED, OR REVOKED. HE STATED LATER THAT HE DID NOT THINK HIS TERMINATION FELL INTO ANY OF THOSE CATEGORIES. HE PRACTICES IN TEXAS AND HAS NO PRESENT PLANS TO PRACTICE IN MARYLAND.

BOWLES, THEODORE A JR DO, LICENSE NUMBER 00H7392 OF SAN ANTONIO, TX, WAS DISCIPLINED BY TEXAS ON MAY 15, 1996
DISCIPLINARY ACTION: 120-MONTH PROBATION; RESTRICTION PLACED ON LICENSE
OFFENSE: SUBSTANCE ABUSE

NOTES: INTEMPERATE USE OF ALCOHOL AND DRUGS IN THAT IN 1/93, AFTER APPROXIMATELY FIVE YEARS OF SOBRIETY HE STOPPED ATTENDING AA MEETINGS; IN 7/93 HE BEGAN CONSUMING ALCOHOL AGAIN AND STARTED USING VICODIN WITHOUT A LEGITIMATE MEDICAL PURPOSE AND IN 11/93 HIS INTEMPERATE DRUG USE ESCALATED TO FENTANYL; IN 1/94 VOLUNTARILY ADMITTED HIMSELF INTO A CHEMICAL DEPENDENCY TREATMENT PROGRAM OF WHICH HE COMPLETED A MONTH PRIOR TO HIS RELEASE IN 2/94; REPORTS THAT SOON AFTER THE 2/94 DISCHARGE HE RESUMED CONSUMING FENTANYL AND OTHER CHEMICAL SUBSTANCES INCLUDING ALCOHOL, WITHOUT A LEGITIMATE MEDICAL PURPOSE; IN 4/94 HE VOLUNTARILY ADMITTED HIMSELF AS AN INPATIENT INTO A GEORGIA CHEMICAL DEPENDENCY TREATMENT FACILITY AT THE REQUEST OF HIS FAMILY AND OTHER INDIVIDUALS; FOLLOWING DISCHARGE HE RETURNED TO THE FULL-TIME PRACTICE OF EMERGENCY MEDICINE; ENTERED INTO A MONITORING AGREEMENT WITH THE PHYSICIAN HEALTH AND REHABILITATION COMMITTEE AND REMAINS COMPLIANT WITH THE AGREEMENT; BOARD

HAS RECEIVED A FAVORABLE LETTER IN HIS SUPPORT FROM A HOSPITAL; HE IS RECEIVING TREATMENT FROM A PSYCHIATRIST. SUSPENSION STAYED. PROBATION WITH TERMS AND CONDITIONS: SHALL ABSTAIN FROM THE CONSUMPTION OF ALCOHOL/DRUGS IN ANY FORM UNLESS PRESCRIBED BY ANOTHER PHYSICIAN FOR A LEGITIMATE AND THERAPEUTIC PURPOSE; SHALL SUBMIT HIMSELF FOR EVALUATION AND TREATMENT BY BOARD-APPROVED PSYCHIATRIST WHOM HE SHALL SEE AT LEAST ONCE A MONTH AND WHO SHALL SUBMIT REPORTS TO THE BOARD; SHALL PROVIDE REPORTS REGARDING ANY ASPECT OF HIS PHYSICAL OR MENTAL CONDITION AT BOARD REQUEST; SHALL SUBMIT TO ALCOHOL AND DRUG SCREENS; SHALL REQUEST A MEETING WITH THE PHYSICIAN HEALTH AND REHABILITATION COMMITTEE AND SHALL CONTINUE TO PARTICIPATE IN ACTIVITIES AND ATTEND WEEKLY MEETINGS WITH QUARTERLY REPORTS; SHALL COMPLY WITH TERMS AND CONDITIONS OF HIS CONTINUING CARE CONTRACT WITH THE PHYSICIAN HEALTH AND REHABILITATION COMMITTEE AND SHALL SUBMIT QUARTERLY REPORTS TO THE BOARD; SHALL CONTINUE TO PARTICIPATE IN AA'S PROGRAM NOT LESS THAN FIVE TIMES A WEEK WITH QUARTERLY REPORTS TO THE BOARD; SHALL NOT TREAT OR OTHERWISE SERVE AS PHYSICIAN, PRESCRIBE, DISPENSE OR ADMINISTER DRUGS THAT MAY BE SUBJECT TO ABUSE TO HIMSELF OR TO ANY MEMBER OF HIS FAMILY; SHALL MAINTAIN A LOG OF ALL PRESCRIPTIONS WRITTEN OR TELEPHONED FOR THESE DRUGS SUBJECT TO REVIEW; SHALL NOT PRACTICE ANESTHESIOLOGY; SHALL APPEAR BEFORE BOARD AT LEAST TWICE A YEAR OR UPON REQUEST; SHALL COOPERATE WITH THE BOARD IN VERIFYING COMPLIANCE INCLUDING PROVIDING COPIES OF MEDICAL RELEASES AND PEER REVIEW RECORDS UPON REQUEST; TIME SPENT OUT OF TEXAS DOES NOT COUNT TOWARD PROBATION; SHALL INFORM BOARD OF CHANGE OF ADDRESS WITHIN 10 DAYS OR IF HE LEAVES THE STATE. SHALL NOT SEEK MODIFICATION FOR ONE YEAR.

BOWLES, THEODORE A MD, DATE OF BIRTH MARCH 22, 1952, LICENSE NUMBER 025724 OF 19942 PARK RANCH, SAN ANTONIO, TX, WAS DISCIPLINED BY GEORGIA ON JUNE 5, 1997
DISCIPLINARY ACTION: 120-MONTH PROBATION
OFFENSE: DISCIPLINARY ACTION BY ANOTHER STATE OR AGENCY

NOTES: DISCIPLINARY ACTION IN TEXAS. MUST ABIDE BY TEXAS ORDER.

BOWLES, THEODORE A JR DO, LICENSE NUMBER H7392 OF SAN ANTONIO, TX, WAS DISCIPLINED BY TEXAS ON AUGUST 9, 1997
DISCIPLINARY ACTION: LICENSE SUSPENSION; REQUIRED TO ENTER AN IMPAIRED PHYSICIAN PROGRAM OR SUBSTANCE ABUSE TREATMENT
OFFENSE: SUBSTANCE ABUSE

NOTES: IN 1/89 HE WAS ISSUED A RESTRICTED TEXAS LICENSE THAT INCLUDED MONITORING HIS SOBRIETY; IN 7/93 HE BEGAN CONSUMING ALCOHOL AGAIN, AND BEGAN INGESTING VICODIN WITHOUT A LEGITIMATE MEDICAL PURPOSE; HIS INTEMPERATE DRUG USE ESCALATED TO THE USE OF FENTANYL IN 11/93; AFTER COMPLETING INPATIENT CHEMICAL DEPENDENCY TREATMENT AROUND 2/94 AND AGAIN IN 7/94, HE RELAPSED IN 12/95 WITH THE BOARD ISSUING A NEW ORDER ON 5/15/96; IN 10/96 HE RELAPSED AGAIN USING ULTRAM, VICODIN AND FENTANYL; ADMITTED FOR TREATMENT IN 4/97; SUSPENSION UNTIL HE REQUESTS TO HAVE IT STAYED OR APPEARS BEFORE THE BOARD AND PROVIDES SUFFICIENT EVIDENCE THAT INDICATES HE IS PHYSICALLY, MENTALLY AND OTHERWISE COMPETENT TO SAFELY PRACTICE MEDICINE, INCLUDING AT A MINIMUM COMPLETE COPIES OF MEDICAL RECORDS AND REPORTS OF SUCCESSFUL TREATMENT IN AN INPATIENT FACILITY FOR AT LEAST 30 DAYS; SHALL INFORM THE BOARD OF CHANGE OF ADDRESS WITHIN 10 DAYS.

BOWLES, THEODORE A JR DO, LICENSE NUMBER H7392, WAS DISCIPLINED BY TEXAS ON APRIL 4, 1998
DISCIPLINARY ACTION: 60-MONTH PROBATION; RESTRICTION PLACED ON CONTROLLED SUBSTANCE LICENSE

NOTES: PURSUANT TO 8/9/97 BOARD ORDER, REQUEST TO HAVE SUSPENSION STAYED IS GRANTED. CONDITIONS OF PROBATION AS FOLLOWS: SHALL NOT PRESCRIBE, DISPENSE OR ADMINISTER DRUGS THAT MAY BE SUBJECT TO ABUSE EXCEPT FOR PATIENTS IN AN EMERGENCY ROOM; SEPARATE FROM PATIENT RECORDS, SHALL MAINTAIN A FILE OF EVERY PRESCRIPTION WRITTEN BY HIM FOR DANGEROUS DRUGS WITH ADDICTIVE POTENTIAL WHICH SHALL BE MADE AVAILABLE FOR REVIEW; SHALL MAINTAIN ADEQUATE MEDICAL RECORDS WHICH SHALL BE AVAILABLE FOR REVIEW; SHALL COOPERATE WITH THE BOARD IN VERIFYING COMPLIANCE; SHALL ABSTAIN FROM THE CONSUMPTION OF ALCOHOL/DRUGS IN ANY FORM UNLESS PRESCRIBED BY ANOTHER PHYSICIAN FOR A LEGITIMATE AND THERAPEUTIC PURPOSE; SHALL SUBMIT HIMSELF FOR APPROPRIATE EXAMS INCLUDING DRUG OR ALCOHOL SCREENS; SHALL NOMINATE THREE CERTIFIED PSYCHIATRISTS FOR BOARD SELECTION OF A THERAPIST AND SHALL EXPEDITIOUSLY SUBMIT HIMSELF TO EVALUATION AND TREATMENT BY THE APPROVED PRACTITIONER; SHALL PARTICIPATE IN THE ACTIVITIES OF A PHYSICIAN HEALTH AND REHABILITATION COMMITTEE AND ATTEND WEEKLY MEETINGS WITH QUARTERLY REPORTS; SHALL PARTICIPATE IN AA'S PROGRAM NOT LESS THAN THREE TIMES A WEEK; SHALL REPORT ON HIS ATTENDANCE; SHALL COMPLY WITH THE TERMS AND CONDITIONS OF HIS CONTINUING CARE CONTRACT WITH SANTE CENTER FOR HEALING WITH QUARTERLY REPORTS; SHALL NOT TREAT OR OTHERWISE SERVE AS PHYSICIAN, PRESCRIBE, DISPENSE OR ADMINISTER DRUGS THAT MAY BE SUBJECT TO ABUSE TO HIMSELF OR TO ANY MEMBER OF HIS FAMILY; SHALL LIMIT PRACTICE TO THE SEGUIN HOSPITAL EMERGENCY ROOM, OR AN EMERGENCY ROOM SETTING APPROVED BY THE BOARD; HIS MEDICAL PRACTICE SHALL BE MONITORED BY A BOARD APPROVED TEXAS PHYSICIAN WHO SHALL PROVIDE QUARTERLY REPORTS TO THE BOARD; SHALL GIVE A COPY OF THIS ORDER TO ANY HEALTH CARE ENTITY WHERE HE HAS PRIVILEGES; TIME SPENT OUT OF TEXAS DOES NOT COUNT TOWARD PROBATION; SHALL INFORM THE BOARD OF CHANGE OF ADDRESS WITHIN 10 DAYS OR IF HE LEAVES THE STATE.

BOWLES, THEODORE A JR DO, LICENSE NUMBER H7392 OF SAN ANTONIO, TX, WAS DISCIPLINED BY TEXAS ON SEPTEMBER 16, 199Ɛ
DISCIPLINARY ACTION: EMERGENCY SUSPENSION
OFFENSE: FAILURE TO COMPLY WITH PREVIOUS BOARD ORDER

NOTES: VIOLATED 4/98 ORDER WHEN AN 8/13/98 DRUG SCREEN TESTED POSITIVE FOR FENTANYL.

BOWLES, THEODORE A JR DO, LICENSE NUMBER H7392 OF SAN ANTONIO, TX, WAS DISCIPLINED BY TEXAS ON JANUARY 29, 1999
DISCIPLINARY ACTION: PROBATION

OFFENSE: FAILURE TO COMPLY WITH PREVIOUS BOARD ORDER

NOTES: VIOLATED THE 4/4/98 ORDER IN THAT HE PRACTICED MEDICINE AT A PHYSICIAN'S OFFICE IN 5/98 & TESTED POSITIVE FOR FENTANYL ON 8/13/98; ON 9/16/98 TEXAS BOARD TEMPORARILY SUSPENDED HIS LICENSE; ON 12/16/98 THE BOARD RECEIVED CORRESPONDENCE DATED 11/19/98 FROM HIS DOCTOR STATING THAT PRIOR TO HIS MOVING TO GEORGIA, DR. BOWLES HAD A POSITIVE DRUG OF ABUSE SCREEN; DR. BOWLES CONTENDS THAT THE POSITIVE SCREENS WERE THE RESULT OF HIS COMING IN CONTACT WITH A DEFECTIVE DURAGESIC PATCH WHILE TREATING A PATIENT; HIS DOCTOR STATED HE SAW NO EVIDENCE OF DRUG USE. SUSPENSION STAYED, INDEFINITE PROBATION WITH THE FOLLOWING TERMS AND CONDITIONS: SHALL NOT PRACTICE IN TEXAS UNTIL HE REQUESTS IN WRITING TO RESUME PRACTICE, AND APPEARS BEFORE THE BOARD PROVIDING SUFFICIENT EVIDENCE OF HIS COMPETENCE TO PRACTICE SAFELY INCLUDING: SHALL HAVE COMPLETE LEGIBLE COPIES OF PSYCHOLOGICAL AND NEUROPSYCHIATRIC EVALUATIONS CONDUCTED WITHIN 60 DAYS PRIOR TO HIS REQUEST TO RESUME PRACTICE; DOCUMENTED EVIDENCE THAT, FOR NO LESS THAN 12 CONSECUTIVE MONTHS IMMEDIATELY PRECEDING HIS REQUEST FOR PERMISSION TO RESUME PRACTICE, HE HAS MAINTAINED SOBRIETY AND ABSTINENCE FROM ALCOHOL, DANGEROUS DRUGS, OR CONTROLLED SUBSTANCES IN ANY FORM UNLESS PRESCRIBED FOR A LEGITIMATE AND THERAPEUTIC PURPOSE; SHALL INFORM THE BOARD OF CHANGE OF ADDRESS WITHIN 10 DAYS.

BOWLES, THEODORE A DO, LICENSE NUMBER H35804 OF 219 PLANTATION CENTRE DRIVE #813, MACON, GA, WAS DISCIPLINED BY MARYLAND ON APRIL 14, 1999
DISCIPLINARY ACTION: LICENSE SUSPENSION
OFFENSE: DISCIPLINARY ACTION BY ANOTHER STATE OR AGENCY

NOTES: SANCTIONED BY THE TEXAS BOARD FOR SUBSTANCE ABUSE ISSUES.

BOYCE, ALFRED E DO, DATE OF BIRTH NOVEMBER 9, 1929, LICENSE NUMBER 002076L OF 7001 N.W. 91ST. TERRACE, TAMARAC, FL, WAS DISCIPLINED BY PENNSYLVANIA ON OCTOBER 11, 1995
DISCIPLINARY ACTION: LICENSE SUSPENSION
OFFENSE: DISCIPLINARY ACTION BY ANOTHER STATE OR AGENCY

NOTES: ON 12/21/92 IN TEXAS FIVE YEAR SUSPENSION, STAYED AS PROBATION SUBJECT TO VARIOUS TERMS INCLUDING PASSING THE SPEX EXAMINATION BASED ON THE FACTS THAT HE FAILED TO ADEQUATELY DOCUMENT THE HISTORY AND TREATMENT OF PATIENTS; FAILED TO DEMONSTRATE AND ADEQUATE KNOWLEDGE OF PHARMACOLOGY; FAILED TO DEMONSTRATE AN ABILITY TO CARE FOR PATIENTS IN ACUTE AND CRITICAL CARE EMERGENCIES; DID NOT RECOGNIZE CONGESTIVE HEART FAILURE AND DIABETIC KETOACIDOSIS; AND FAILED TO TRANSFER PATIENTS IN A TIMELY MANNER. ON 4/15/94 THE TEXAS BOARD ACCEPTED HIS PERMANENT SURRENDER AND CANCELLATION OF HIS TEXAS LICENSE TO PRACTICE MEDICINE FOR FAILING THE SPEX EXAMINATION AND NOT ATTEMPTING TO TAKE IT A SECOND TIME. SHALL NOT PRACTICE MEDICINE IN PENNSYLVANIA UNTIL TEXAS REINSTATES LICENSE.

BOYCE, ALFRED E DO, LICENSE NUMBER 0102501 OF 7001 NW 91ST TERRACE, TAMARAC, FL, WAS DISCIPLINED BY NEW YORK ON JANUARY 18, 1996
DISCIPLINARY ACTION: SURRENDER OF LICENSE
OFFENSE: DISCIPLINARY ACTION BY ANOTHER STATE OR AGENCY

NOTES: LICENSE SURRENDER IN TEXAS.

BOYCE, ALFRED EVERSLEY DO, DATE OF BIRTH NOVEMBER 8, 1929, LICENSE NUMBER 00F0898 OF 1007 15TH STREET, WELLINGTON, TX, WAS DISCIPLINED BY TEXAS ON JANUARY 29, 1993
DISCIPLINARY ACTION: 60-MONTH PROBATION; RESTRICTION PLACED ON LICENSE
OFFENSE: LOSS OR RESTRICTION OF HOSPITAL PRIVILEGES

NOTES: ON 1/16/91 HOSPITAL PRIVILEGES WERE RESTRICTED DUE TO INSUFFICIENT DOCUMENTATION OF QUALIFICATIONS TO DO SURGERY BY THE CHILLICOTHE HOSPITAL; THEY TERMINATED HIS CONTRACT 8/91 DUE TO AN UNACCEPTABLE COMPLICATION RATE DURING SURGERY. A BOARD REVIEW OF 20 PATIENT CHARTS REVEALED THE FOLLOWING DEFICIENCIES: FAILED TO ADEQUATELY DOCUMENT THE HISTORY AND TREATMENT OF PATIENTS; FAILED TO DEMONSTRATE AN ADEQUATE KNOWLEDGE OF PHARMACOLOGY OR AN ABILITY TO CARE FOR PATIENTS IN ACUTE AND CRITICAL CARE EMERGENCIES; DID NOT RECOGNIZE CONGESTIVE HEART FAILURE AND DIABETIC KETOACIDOSIS; FAILED TO TRANSFER PATIENTS IN A TIMELY MANNER. 5 YEAR SUSPENSION STAYED. CONDITIONS OF PROBATION: SHALL TAKE AND PASS THE SPEX EXAM; SHALL TAKE AT LEAST 50 CREDITS CONTINUING MEDICAL EDUCATION PER YEAR; SHALL BE MONITORED BY A BOARD-APPROVED PHYSICIAN WITH BI-MONTHLY REPORTS TO THE BOARD; WITHIN THREE MONTHS SHALL ENROLL IN A PHARMACOLOGY RETRAINING COURSE; SHALL COMPLETE AN INTENSIVE REVIEW COURSE OF AREAS RELEVANT TO FAMILY PRACTICE, INCLUDING HANDS-ON WORKSHOPS WITHIN 6 MONTHS; SHALL BE ACCEPTED IN A SPECIFIED PERSONALIZED CONTINUING MEDICAL EDUCATION ACUTE MINI-RESIDENCY WITHIN ONE MONTH WHICH SHALL BE APPROVED BY THE BOARD; SHALL MAINTAIN ADEQUATE MEDICAL RECORDS ON ALL PATIENT OFFICE VISITS; SHALL COMPLETE AN ADVANCED CARDIAC LIFE SUPPORT PROGRAM AND AN ADVANCED TRAUMA LIFE SUPPORT PROGRAM; IS RESTRICTED FROM PERFORMING ANY MAJOR SURGERY IN AN OUTPATIENT OR HOSPITAL SETTING; SHALL GIVE A COPY OF THIS ORDER TO ANY HEALTH CARE ENTITY WHERE HE HAS PRIVILEGES; SHALL COOPERATE WITH THE BOARD IN VERIFYING COMPLIANCE; SHALL INFORM BOARD OF CHANGE OF ADDRESS WITHIN 10 DAYS OR IF HE LEAVES THE STATE; TIME SPENT OUT OF TEXAS DOES NOT COUNT TOWARD PROBATION; SHALL NOT SEEK MODIFICATION OF THIS ORDER.

BOYCE, ALFRED EVERSLEY DO, DATE OF BIRTH NOVEMBER 8, 1929, LICENSE NUMBER 00F0898 OF 1007 15TH STREET, WELLINGTON, TX, WAS DISCIPLINED BY TEXAS ON MAY 21, 1993
DISCIPLINARY ACTION: EMERGENCY SUSPENSION
OFFENSE: FAILURE TO COMPLY WITH PREVIOUS BOARD ORDER

NOTES: AS A CONDITION OF 01/29/93 PROBATION HE WAS ORDERED TO TAKE AND PASS SPEX EXAM; HE DID NOT PASS EXAM 0N 3/18/93. LICENSE SUSPENDED UNTIL HE PASSES THE EXAM.

BOYCE, ALFRED EVERSLEY DO, DATE OF BIRTH NOVEMBER 8, 1929, LICENSE NUMBER 00F0898 OF WELLINGTON, TX, WAS DISCIPLINED BY TEXAS ON APRIL 15, 1994
DISCIPLINARY ACTION: SURRENDER OF LICENSE
OFFENSE: FAILURE TO COMPLY WITH PREVIOUS BOARD ORDER

NOTES: DID NOT TAKE THE SPEX EXAM IN 12/93 AS REQUIRED

BY A PREVIOUS ORDER; BOARD ALSO RECEIVED ALLEGATIONS OF OTHER VIOLATIONS WHICH HE DENIED. SURRENDER IN LIEU OF FURTHER INVESTIGATION OR A HEARING ON THE ALLEGATIONS. SHALL NOT APPLY FOR REINSTATEMENT OF LICENSE.

BRAMANTI, HENRY R MD, DATE OF BIRTH JUNE 8, 1940, LICENSE NUMBER 00E3214 OF 2512 HORNE STREET SUITE A, FORT WORTH, TX, WAS DISCIPLINED BY TEXAS ON APRIL 30, 1993
DISCIPLINARY ACTION: 24-MONTH PROBATION; REPRIMAND
OFFENSE: LOSS OR RESTRICTION OF HOSPITAL PRIVILEGES

NOTES: DURING THE COURSE OF A DELIVERY ON 9/23/91 HE INTERACTED WITH STAFF IN AN ABRASIVE AND ABUSIVE MANNER; MADE INSENSITIVE COMMENTS IN THE PRESENCE OF THE PATIENT AND HER HUSBAND; DUE TO COMPLICATIONS THE INFANT SUFFERED A PERIOD OF OXYGEN DEPRIVATION BUT APPARENTLY RECOVERED; AFTER THIS HE ENTERED INTO A CONTINUATION OF PRACTICE AGREEMENT WITH HOSPITAL REQUIRING HIM TO UNDERGO REGULAR COUNSELING WITH A PSYCHIATRIST. CONDITIONS OF PROBATION: SHALL COMPLY WITH ALL TERMS OF CONTINUATION OF PRACTICE AGREEMENT WITH HOSPITAL; SHALL CONTINUE TO RECEIVE COUNSELING WITH QUARTERLY REPORTS; SHALL ATTEND AT LEAST 50 HOURS PER YEAR OF CONTINUING MEDICAL EDUCATION; SHALL APPEAR BEFORE THE BOARD TWICE DURING THE FIRST YEAR OF PROBATION AND AT LEAST ONCE DURING THE SECOND; SHALL GIVE A COPY OF THIS ORDER TO ANY HEALTH CARE ENTITY WHERE HE HAS PRIVILEGES; SHALL COOPERATE WITH THE BOARD IN VERIFYING COMPLIANCE; SHALL INFORM BOARD OF ADDRESS CHANGE WITHIN 10 DAYS OR IF HE LEAVES THE STATE; TIME SPENT OUT OF TEXAS DOES NOT COUNT TOWARD PROBATION. SHALL NOT SEEK MODIFICATION FOR ONE YEAR.

BRANCH, THOMAS COE MD, DATE OF BIRTH AUGUST 26, 1961, LICENSE NUMBER 00C8909 OF PLAINVIEW, TX, WAS DISCIPLINED BY TEXAS ON JUNE 22, 1994
DISCIPLINARY ACTION: 120-MONTH PROBATION; REQUIRED TO TAKE ADDITIONAL MEDICAL EDUCATION
OFFENSE: CRIMINAL CONVICTION OR PLEA OF GUILTY, NOLO CONTENDERE, OR NO CONTEST TO A CRIME

NOTES: ON 5/15/92 DURING REGULAR BUSINESS HOURS ENGAGED IN SEXUAL INTERCOURSE WITH AN EMPLOYEE OF METHODIST HOSPITAL AT HIS MEDICAL OFFICE; ON 5/20/92 CONSUMED AN EXCESSIVE AMOUNT OF ALCOHOL AND BENZODIAZEPINES; IN 1993 ENTERED A PLEA OF NOLO CONTENDERE TO DRIVING WHILE INTOXICATED RELATED TO THIS AND CONSEQUENTLY WAS FINED AND PLACED ON TWO YEARS PROBATION; PRIVILEGES AT METHODIST HOSPITAL WERE SUMMARILY SUSPENDED WHICH HE DID NOT CONTEST OR APPEAL; HAS BEGUN A MONITORING PROGRAM WITH PHYSICIANS HEALTH AND REHABILITATION COMMITTEE AND BEGAN ATTENDING AA ON A REGULAR BASIS. SUSPENSION STAYED. CONDITIONS OF PROBATION: SHALL ABSTAIN FROM THE CONSUMPTION OF ALCOHOL/CHEMICAL SUBSTANCES IN ANY FORM UNLESS PRESCRIBED BY ANOTHER PHYSICIAN FOR A LEGITIMATE AND THERAPEUTIC PURPOSE; SHALL SUBMIT HIMSELF FOR APPROPRIATE EXAMS INCLUDING DRUG OR ALCOHOL SCREENS; SHALL NOT TREAT OR OTHERWISE SERVE AS PHYSICIAN, PRESCRIBE, DISPENSE OR ADMINISTER DRUGS THAT MAY BE SUBJECT TO ABUSE TO HIMSELF OR ANY MEMBER OF HIS FAMILY; SHALL PARTICIPATE IN AA'S PROGRAM NOT LESS THAN THREE TIMES A WEEK WITH QUARTERLY REPORTS TO THE BOARD; SHALL SUBMIT HIMSELF FOR EVALUATION AND TREATMENT TO A BOARD-APPROVED PSYCHIATRIST WITH QUARTERLY REPORTS; SHALL COMPLETE 10 HOURS OF ETHICS COURSES OR AN ETHICS PROGRAM WITHIN ONE YEAR AND 50 HOURS OF CONTINUING MEDICAL EDUCATION PER YEAR; SHALL APPEAR BEFORE THE BOARD TWICE A YEAR; SHALL GIVE A COPY OF THIS ORDER TO ANY HEALTH CARE ENTITY WHERE HE HAS PRIVILEGES; SHALL COOPERATE WITH THE BOARD IN VERIFYING COMPLIANCE; SHALL INFORM BOARD OF CHANGE OF ADDRESS WITHIN 10 DAYS OR IF HE LEAVES THE STATE; TIME SPENT OUT OF TEXAS DOES NOT COUNT TOWARD PROBATION. SHALL NOT SEEK MODIFICATION FOR ONE YEAR. ON 1/27/96 ORDER MODIFIED SO HE SHALL APPEAR BEFORE THE BOARD AT LEAST ONE TIME EACH YEAR; ALL OTHER CONDITIONS REMAIN IN EFFECT. ON 2/7/98 PETITION TO TERMINATE ORDER DENIED; ORDER MODIFIED REDUCING PSYCHIATRIC VISITS FROM MONTHLY TO QUARTERLY. ON 4/10/99 PETITION TO TERMINATE ORDER DENIED; ORDER MODIFIED DELETING MANDATED FREQUENCY OF AA PARTICIPATION, AND REQUIREMENTS OF ONGOING PSYCHIATRIC CARE, AND TEN HOURS OF ETHICS COURSES.

BRASWELL, ROY B II MD, LICENSE NUMBER 00G2915 OF SULPHUR, LA, WAS DISCIPLINED BY TEXAS ON JANUARY 12, 1991

NOTES: MUST SUBMIT TO PSYCHIATRIST FOR EVALUATION, IF APPLICABLE, UNDERGO RECOMMENDED TREATMENT.

BRASWELL, ROY B II MD OF MONTEREY, LA, WAS DISCIPLINED BY LOUISIANA ON AUGUST 30, 1991
DISCIPLINARY ACTION: 60-MONTH PROBATION; REQUIRED TO ENTER AN IMPAIRED PHYSICIAN PROGRAM OR SUBSTANCE ABUSE TREATMENT
OFFENSE: DISCIPLINARY ACTION BY ANOTHER STATE OR AGENCY

NOTES: ALSO CHARGED WITH EXCESSIVE USE OF ALCOHOL. PROBATION CONDITIONED ON CONTINUING PSYCHIATRIC TREATMENT AND MONITORING, EXECUTION OF TREATMENT CONTRACT WITH IMPAIRED PHYSICIANS PROGRAM, PERIODIC REPORTS TO BOARD BY SUPERVISING PHYSICIAN, AND OBTAIN SPECIFIED CONTINUING MEDICAL EDUCATION.

BRAUNSDORF, DELL HARKEY MD, LICENSE NUMBER J5548, WAS DISCIPLINED BY TEXAS ON MARCH 1, 1997
DISCIPLINARY ACTION: 60-MONTH PROBATION
OFFENSE: FAILURE TO COMPLY WITH PREVIOUS BOARD ORDER

NOTES: ON 4/15/94 SHE WAS GRANTED A MEDICAL LICENSE SUBJECT TO CERTAIN TERMS AND CONDITIONS, INCLUDING THAT SHE ABSTAIN FROM THE CONSUMPTION OF DRUGS OR ALCOHOL. IN 7/96 SUFFERED A RELAPSE INTO THE USE OF DRUGS IN THAT SHE INGESTED VICODIN, A SCHEDULE III CONTROLLED SUBSTANCE, AND STADOL NASAL SPRAY, A DANGEROUS DRUG, WHICH WAS CONFIRMED BY A DRUG SCREEN. SHE ATTRIBUTES HER RELAPSE TO AN ATTEMPT TO SELF-MEDICATE SEVERE NECK PAIN CAUSED BY AN OLD CERVICAL INJURY. SHE ENTERED AN INPATIENT TREATMENT PROGRAM FROM 8/20/96 TO 9/20/96. SUSPENSION STAYED FOR PROBATION UNDER THE FOLLOWING TERMS AND CONDITIONS: SHALL ABSTAIN FROM THE CONSUMPTION OF ALCOHOL/DRUGS IN ANY FORM UNLESS PRESCRIBED BY ANOTHER PHYSICIAN FOR A LEGITIMATE AND THERAPEUTIC PURPOSE; SHALL SUBMIT HERSELF FOR APPROPRIATE EXAMS INCLUDING DRUG OR ALCOHOL SCREENS; SHE SHALL CONTINUE TO RECEIVE TREATMENT AND CARE FROM

A SPECIFIED PHYSICIAN AT LEAST MONTHLY WITH QUARTERLY REPORTS; SHALL PARTICIPATE IN THE ACTIVITIES OF A PHYSICIAN HEALTH AND REHABILITATION COMMITTEE AND ATTEND WEEKLY MEETINGS WITH QUARTERLY REPORTS; SHALL PARTICIPATE IN AA'S PROGRAM NOT LESS THAN THREE TIMES A WEEK; SHALL REPORT ON HER ATTENDANCE; SEPARATE FROM PATIENT RECORDS, SHALL MAINTAIN A FILE OF EVERY PRESCRIPTION WRITTEN BY HER FOR DANGEROUS DRUGS WITH ADDICTIVE POTENTIAL WHICH SHALL BE MADE AVAILABLE FOR REVIEW; SHALL NOT TREAT OR OTHERWISE SERVE AS PHYSICIAN, PRESCRIBE, DISPENSE OR ADMINISTER DRUGS THAT MAY BE SUBJECT TO ABUSE TO HERSELF OR TO ANY MEMBER OF HER FAMILY; SHALL MAINTAIN ADEQUATE MEDICAL RECORDS WHICH SHALL BE AVAILABLE FOR REVIEW; SHALL OBTAIN AT LEAST 50 HOURS OF CONTINUING MEDICAL EDUCATION PER YEAR; SHALL PERSONALLY APPEAR BEFORE THE BOARD AT LEAST TWICE YEARLY; SHALL GIVE A COPY OF THIS ORDER TO ANY HEALTH CARE ENTITY WHERE SHE HAS PRIVILEGES; SHALL COOPERATE WITH THE BOARD IN VERIFYING COMPLIANCE; TIME SPENT OUT OF TEXAS DOES NOT COUNT TOWARD PROBATION; SHALL INFORM THE BOARD OF CHANGE OF ADDRESS WITHIN 10 DAYS OR IF SHE LEAVES THE STATE; SHALL NOT SEEK MODIFICATION FOR ONE YEAR.

BREITENSTEIN, LARRY J DO, DATE OF BIRTH OCTOBER 17, 1942, LICENSE NUMBER 0041326 OF 1110 KINGWOOD DRIVE, SUITE 201, KINGWOOD, TX, WAS DISCIPLINED BY NEW JERSEY ON DECEMBER 16, 1994
DISCIPLINARY ACTION: 120-MONTH PROBATION; RESTRICTION PLACED ON CONTROLLED SUBSTANCE LICENSE
OFFENSE: DISCIPLINARY ACTION BY ANOTHER STATE OR AGENCY

NOTES: BASED ON ACTION BY TEXAS. TEN YEAR SUSPENSION STAYED. CONDITIONS OF PROBATION: SHALL NOT WRITE ANY PRESCRIPTIONS FOR CONTROLLED SUBSTANCES; SHALL APPEAR BEFORE A COMMITTEE OF THE BOARD TO DISCUSS THE STATUS OF LICENSURE PRIVILEGES IN ALL OTHER JURISDICTIONS, HIS PARTICIPATION IN CONTINUING MEDICAL EDUCATION AND HIS PLANS FOR NEW JERSEY PRACTICE PRIOR TO PRACTICE IN NEW JERSEY.

BREITENSTEIN, LARRY JACK DO, LICENSE NUMBER 00D5923 OF 818 BURNING TREE, KINGWOOD, TX, WAS DISCIPLINED BY TEXAS ON OCTOBER 27, 1993
DISCIPLINARY ACTION: EMERGENCY SUSPENSION
OFFENSE: SUBSTANCE ABUSE

NOTES: BETWEEN 12/92 AND 8/93 ENGAGED IN THE INTEMPERATE USE OF DRUGS INCLUDING COCAINE, VICODIN AND XANAX WHICH COULD ENDANGER THE LIVES OF PATIENTS; ALSO DURING 1993 INJECTED OR OTHERWISE PROVIDED COCAINE TO AN ADULT FEMALE WHO SUBSEQUENTLY DIED OF ACUTE COCAINE TOXICITY ON 8/11/93.

BREITENSTEIN, LARRY JACK DO OF 1110 KINGWOOD DRIVE SUITE 201, KINGWOOD, TX, WAS DISCIPLINED BY DEA ON NOVEMBER 17, 1993
DISCIPLINARY ACTION: SURRENDER OF CONTROLLED SUBSTANCE LICENSE
OFFENSE: PROFESSIONAL MISCONDUCT

NOTES: SEIZURE OF COCAINE FROM RESIDENCE 08/11/93 IN KINGWOOD TEXAS DURING CONSENT TO SEARCH.

BREITENSTEIN, LARRY JACK DO, LICENSE NUMBER 00D5923 OF KINGWOOD, TX, WAS DISCIPLINED BY TEXAS ON NOVEMBER 19, 1993
DISCIPLINARY ACTION: LICENSE SUSPENSION; REQUIRED TO ENTER AN IMPAIRED PHYSICIAN PROGRAM OR TREATMENT
OFFENSE: SUBSTANCE ABUSE

NOTES: HAS ATTEMPTED TO GET INPATIENT TREATMENT SINCE EMERGENCY SUSPENSION; HOWEVER ECONOMIC PROBLEMS AND THE SCARCITY OF AVAILABLE BEDS HAS PREVENTED HIS ADMISSION INTO INPATIENT TREATMENT; MAINTAINS HE REMAINS DRUG-FREE SINCE 8/11/93. SUSPENSION UNTIL HE SUCCESSFULLY COMPLETES INPATIENT TREATMENT AND SHOWS THE BOARD HE IS PHYSICALLY, MENTALLY AND OTHERWISE COMPETENT TO SAFELY PRACTICE MEDICINE. SUSPENSION WILL THEN BE STAYED TO 10 YEAR PROBATION WITH CONDITIONS. SHALL NOT SEEK MODIFICATION FOR ONE YEAR.

BREITENSTEIN, LARRY JACK DO, LICENSE NUMBER D5923, WAS DISCIPLINED BY TEXAS ON MAY 9, 1997
DISCIPLINARY ACTION: EMERGENCY SUSPENSION
OFFENSE: FAILURE TO COMPLY WITH PREVIOUS BOARD ORDER

NOTES: ON 11/19/93 THE BOARD ENTERED INTO AN AGREEMENT WITH HIM SUSPENDING HIS LICENSE UNTIL THE SUCCESSFUL COMPLETION OF HIS TREATMENT AND HIS APPEARANCE BEFORE THE BOARD PROVIDING EVIDENCE OF HIS COMPETENCE TO PRACTICE MEDICINE. HE WAS SUBSEQUENTLY CHARGED WITH THE FIRST DEGREE FELONY OF "UNLAWFULLY, INTENTIONALLY, AND KNOWINGLY DELIVERING A CONTROLLED SUBSTANCE" IN CONNECTION WITH THE DEATH OF A PATIENT. ON 11/9/94 THE DOCTOR PLED NO CONTEST TO THE CHARGES, RECEIVED A SENTENCE OF DEFERRED ADJUDICATION, AND WAS PLACED ON PROBATION FOR TEN YEARS WITH TERMS. ON 3/27/96 HE REQUESTED THE STAY OF HIS SUSPENSION, WHICH WAS GRANTED WITH A TEN-YEAR TERM OF PROBATION, INCLUDING REQUIREMENTS THAT HE PASS THE SPEX AND OBTAIN A FAVORABLE PSYCHIATRIC EVALUATION PRIOR TO PRACTICING MEDICINE IN TEXAS. HE COMPLIED WITH THESE CONDITIONS AND RESUMED PRACTICE IN TEXAS; ON 3/16/97 HE INGESTED ALCOHOL IN VIOLATION OF THE 3/27/96 ORDER, CONFIRMED BY A BLOOD SPECIMEN TAKEN IMMEDIATELY FOLLOWING A ONE VEHICLE ACCIDENT, WHICH INDICATED A BLOOD ALCOHOL LEVEL OF 0.26.

BREITENSTEIN, LARRY JACK DO, LICENSE NUMBER D5923 OF HOUSTON, TX, WAS DISCIPLINED BY TEXAS ON FEBRUARY 7, 1998
DISCIPLINARY ACTION: LICENSE SUSPENSION
OFFENSE: FAILURE TO COMPLY WITH PREVIOUS BOARD ORDER

NOTES: ON 3/16/97 HE VIOLATED A 3/27/96 BOARD ORDER BY INGESTING ALCOHOL; HE WAS INVOLVED IN A CAR ACCIDENT WHILE DRIVING UNDER THE INFLUENCE OF ALCOHOL; HE MAINTAINS THAT HE WAS UNABLE TO CONTROL HIS CAR BECAUSE HE "PASSED OUT" AFTER BEING SUBJECTED TO SOLVENT FUMES WHICH HAD ACCUMULATED IN THE CAR, FUMES ACCUMULATED AFTER A HARSH SOLVENT WAS USED TO REMOVE THE CAR'S WINDOW TINTING; ON 5/9/97 THE BOARD TEMPORARILY SUSPENDED HIS LICENSE. SUSPENSION UNTIL HE REQUESTS TO HAVE HIS SUSPENSION STAYED OR APPEARS BEFORE THE BOARD WITH SUFFICIENT EVIDENCE THAT HE IS PHYSICALLY, MENTALLY AND OTHERWISE COMPETENT TO SAFELY PRACTICE MEDICINE INCLUDING AT A MINIMUM COMPLETE COPIES OF MEDICAL RECORDS AND REPORTS OF

PSYCHOLOGICAL AND NEUROPSYCHIATRIC EVALUATIONS, INCLUDING A 96 HOUR INPATIENT EVALUATION CONDUCTED BY A BOARD-APPROVED CERTIFIED PSYCHIATRIST; SHALL COOPERATE WITH THE BOARD IN VERIFYING COMPLIANCE INCLUDING PROVIDING COPIES OF MEDICAL RELEASES UPON REQUEST; SHALL GIVE A COPY OF THIS ORDER TO ANY HEALTH CARE ENTITY WHERE HE HAS PRIVILEGES; SHALL PROVIDE A COPY OF THIS ORDER TO ANYONE REQUESTING IT WITHIN 10 DAYS; SHALL INFORM THE BOARD OF CHANGE OF ADDRESS WITHIN 10 DAYS; SHALL NOT SEEK MODIFICATION FOR ONE YEAR.

BREITENSTEIN, LARRY JACK DO, DATE OF BIRTH OCTOBER 17, 1942 OF 2302 MAST COURT, KINGWOOD, TX, WAS DISCIPLINED BY MEDICARE ON OCTOBER 20, 1998
DISCIPLINARY ACTION: EXCLUSION FROM THE MEDICARE AND/OR MEDICAID PROGRAM
OFFENSE: DISCIPLINARY ACTION BY ANOTHER STATE OR AGENCY

NOTES: LICENSE REVOKED, SUSPENDED, SURRENDERED OR OTHERWISE LOST FOR REASONS BEARING ON PROFESSIONAL PERFORMANCE, PROFESSIONAL COMPETENCE OR FINANCIAL INTEGRITY.

BRENNER, JOHN FREDERICK DO, LICENSE NUMBER F6476 OF FORT WORTH, TX, WAS DISCIPLINED BY TEXAS ON AUGUST 9, 1997
DISCIPLINARY ACTION: FINE; 36-MONTH RESTRICTION PLACED ON LICENSE
OFFENSE: SUBSTANDARD CARE, INCOMPETENCE OR NEGLIGENCE

NOTES: DURING JULY AND AUGUST 1991, FAILED TO ADEQUATELY COMMUNICATE WITH OTHER PHYSICIANS INVOLVED IN THE CARE AND TREATMENT OF A PATIENT FOR SQUAMOUS CELL CARCINOMA IN HIS LEFT LUNG WHICH CONTRIBUTED TO THE INAPPROPRIATE TREATMENT OF THE PATIENT. $2,500 FINE; SHALL PERFORM 100 HOURS OF COMMUNITY SERVICE; SHALL TAKE 65 HOURS PER YEAR OF CONTINUING MEDICAL EDUCATION TO INCLUDE RISK MANAGEMENT; SHALL OBTAIN 10 HOURS OF AN ETHICS COURSE OR COURSES OR AN ETHICS PROGRAM PER YEAR FOR 3 YEARS; SHALL SUBMIT A GENERAL PLAN OF TREATMENT TO THE BOARD WITHIN 90 DAYS; SHALL MAINTAIN ADEQUATE MEDICAL RECORDS; SHALL APPEAR BEFORE THE BOARD ONCE A YEAR; SHALL PROVIDE A COPY OF THIS ORDER TO ANYONE REQUESTING IT WITHIN 10 DAYS; TIME SPENT OUT OF TEXAS DOES NOT COUNT TOWARD RESTRICTION; SHALL INFORM THE BOARD OF CHANGE OF ADDRESS WITHIN 10 DAYS OR IF HE LEAVES THE STATE; SHALL NOT SEEK MODIFICATION FOR ONE YEAR. ON 10/24/98 THE ORDER WAS TERMINATED.

BREWER, EUGENE ALLAN MD, LICENSE NUMBER 0045064 OF KANSAS CITY, MO, WAS DISCIPLINED BY OHIO ON JULY 11, 1996
DISCIPLINARY ACTION: LICENSE SUSPENSION; PROBATION
OFFENSE: SUBSTANDARD CARE, INCOMPETENCE OR NEGLIGENCE

NOTES: FAILURE TO EMPLOY ACCEPTABLE SCIENTIFIC METHODS IN THE SELECTION OF MODALITIES FOR TREATMENT OF DISEASE AND FAILURE TO CONFORM TO MINIMAL STANDARDS OF CARE WITH RESPECT TO TREATMENT OF PATIENTS IN THE COURSE OF HIS PRACTICE OF UROLOGY. INDEFINITELY SUSPENDED; MINIMUM OF THREE MONTHS; CONDITIONS FOR REINSTATEMENT; ON 9/3/96 THE FRANKLIN COUNTY COURT OF COMMON PLEAS GRANTED A STAY OF THIS ORDER. ON 10/30/97 FRANKLIN COURT OF COMMON PLEAS AFFIRMED BOARD'S SUSPENSION ORDER.

BREWER, EUGENE ALLAN MD, LICENSE NUMBER G59832 OF BIG SPRING, TX, WAS DISCIPLINED BY CALIFORNIA ON AUGUST 11, 1997
DISCIPLINARY ACTION: 36-MONTH PROBATION
OFFENSE: DISCIPLINARY ACTION BY ANOTHER STATE OR AGENCY

NOTES: DISCIPLINED BY OHIO FOR PERFORMING OPERATIONS, IN SEVERAL INSTANCES, WITHOUT SUFFICIENT INTERVAL TO ALLOW FOR HEALING, AND SELECTING SURGERY AS A TREATMENT BEFORE RULING OUT OTHER CAUSES FOR THE SYMPTOMS AND WITHOUT ATTEMPTING CONSERVATIVE THERAPY. REVOCATION STAYED.

BREWER, EUGENE ALLAN MD, DATE OF BIRTH SEPTEMBER 26, 1953, LICENSE NUMBER 055362L OF 300 VETERANS BLVD, BIG SPRINGS, TX, WAS DISCIPLINED BY PENNSYLVANIA ON MARCH 12, 1998
DISCIPLINARY ACTION: LICENSE SUSPENSION
OFFENSE: DISCIPLINARY ACTION BY ANOTHER STATE OR AGENCY

NOTES: RECIPROCAL ACTION FROM OHIO. LICENSE SUSPENDED UNTIL COMPLETION OF PROBATION IN OHIO AND LICENSE RETURNED TO UNRESTRICTED STATUS.

BRICE, NELSON MD, LICENSE NUMBER E6250 OF SNYDER, TX, WAS DISCIPLINED BY TEXAS ON DECEMBER 11, 1999
DISCIPLINARY ACTION: REPRIMAND; REQUIRED TO TAKE ADDITIONAL MEDICAL EDUCATION
OFFENSE: OVERPRESCRIBING OR MISPRESCRIBING DRUGS

NOTES: PRESCRIBED CONTROLLED SUBSTANCES TO A PATIENT FOR BACK PAIN FOR MORE THAN TWO YEARS WITHOUT REFERRAL TO A PAIN CLINIC OR A REFERRAL OR CONSULTATION WITH A NEUROSURGEON INCLUDING XANAX WITHOUT ANY DOCUMENTED EVIDENCE OF ANXIETY OR A FINDING OF ANXIETY DISORDER AND THE DOSAGE PRESCRIBED WAS SUBSTANTIALLY HIGHER THAN STANDARD PRACTICE GUIDELINES AND PRESCRIBED PLACIDYL WITHOUT A PHYSICAL EXAM AND WITHOUT A SLEEP STUDY; FOR ANOTHER PATIENT HE PRESCRIBED LODINE, LORCET AND VALIUM WITHOUT ATTEMPTING APPROPRIATE MEDICAL MANAGEMENT, PHYSICAL THERAPY, OR CONSULTATIONS AND FAILED TO OBTAIN ADEQUATE LABORATORY FINDINGS; FOR ANOTHER PATIENT HE TREATED FOR THIRTEEN YEARS, CHIEFLY FOR HEADACHES AND GASTRIC PAIN, HE GAVE INJECTIONS OF VARIOUS CONTROLLED SUBSTANCES, INCLUDING TALWIN, STADOL, NUBAIN, AND PHENERGAN; HE CLAIMS THE PATIENT WAS REFERRED TO A PAIN CLINIC BUT THERE IS NO DOCUMENTATION OF THIS; ANOTHER PATIENT DOCUMENTED WITH HIGH BLOOD PRESSURE WAS PRESCRIBED SEVERAL APPETITE SUPPRESSANTS WHICH WERE CONTRADICTED DUE TO THE PATIENT'S HIGH BLOOD PRESSURE; HE ALSO DIAGNOSED THE PATIENT WITH DEPRESSION WITHOUT DOCUMENTATION OF APPROPRIATE EXAMINATION AND CLINICAL STUDIES IN THE MEDICAL RECORDS AND PRESCRIBED XANAX AS TREATMENT; HE REPRESENTED THAT HE NO LONGER PRESCRIBES XANAX AND GREATLY IMPROVED HIS PROGRESS NOTES AND HIS INITIAL HISTORY AND PHYSICAL DOCUMENTATION. LICENSE LIMITED FOR TWO YEARS AS FOLLOWS: SHALL OBTAIN 50 HOURS PER YEAR OF CONTINUING MEDICAL EDUCATION; WITHIN 90 DAYS SHALL SUBMIT A CORRECTIVE PLAN OF ACTION; SHALL MAINTAIN A LOGBOOK OF ALL PRESCRIPTIONS WRITTEN BY HIM FOR DANGEROUS DRUGS WITH ADDICTIVE POTENTIAL OR POTENTIAL FOR ABUSE WHICH SHALL BE AVAILABLE FOR REVIEW; SHALL COOPERATE WITH THE BOARD IN VERIFYING

COMPLIANCE; SHALL GIVE A COPY OF THIS ORDER TO ANY HEALTH CARE ENTITY WHERE HE HAS PRIVILEGES; SHALL PROVIDE A COPY OF THIS ORDER TO ANYONE REQUESTING IT WITHIN 10 DAYS; TIME SPENT OUT OF TEXAS DOES NOT COUNT TOWARD RESTRICTION; SHALL INFORM THE BOARD OF CHANGE OF ADDRESS WITHIN 10 DAYS OR IF HE LEAVES THE STATE; SHALL NOT SEEK MODIFICATION FOR ONE YEAR.

BRINER, BARBARA H MD OF HOUSTON, TX, WAS DISCIPLINED BY DEA ON MARCH 17, 1997
DISCIPLINARY ACTION: DENIAL OF NEW LICENSE
OFFENSE: DISCIPLINARY ACTION BY ANOTHER STATE OR AGENCY

NOTES: ON 6/28/95 THE TEXAS BOARD PLACED HER LICENSE ON PROBATION FOR FIVE YEARS AND PROHIBITED HER FROM PRESCRIBING, ADMINISTERING OR DISPENSING CONTROLLED SUBSTANCES.

BRINER, BARBARA HADEN MD, LICENSE NUMBER 00H1346 OF HUMBLE, TX, WAS DISCIPLINED BY TEXAS ON JUNE 28, 1995
DISCIPLINARY ACTION: 60-MONTH PROBATION; RESTRICTION PLACED ON LICENSE
OFFENSE: SUBSTANCE ABUSE

NOTES: IN 1986, SHE WENT ON LEAVE OF ABSENCE FROM RESIDENCY TO SEEK OUTPATIENT DRUG ABUSE REHABILITATION; RETURNED TO RESIDENCY IN 7/87; BETWEEN 1990 AND 1993, ALLEGATIONS AROSE THAT SHE WAS DIVERTING CONTROLLED SUBSTANCES (LORTAB, SOMA AND VICODIN) FOR HER OWN NONTHERAPEUTIC USE; SURRENDERED HER DEA/DPS CONTROLLED SUBSTANCES REGISTRATIONS IN 4/93 WITHOUT ADMITTING MISCONDUCT; EVALUATED BY BOARD-APPROVED ADDICTIONOLOGIST IN 10/94 WHO FOUND SUBSTANCE ABUSE AS HER DIAGNOSIS; FROM 11/94 TO 12/94 WAS IN TREATMENT FOR SUBSTANCE ABUSE; REPORTS A SOBRIETY DATE OF 11/26/93; REPORTS A 25 YEAR HISTORY OF VERTEBRAL BASILAR MIGRAINES AND AN ILEOSTOMY AS A CHILD. CURRENTLY UNDER CARE OF PSYCHIATRIST FOR HEADACHE MANAGEMENT; ATTENDS AA THREE TIMES A WEEK. SUSPENSION STAYED. PROBATION WITH TERMS: SHALL ABSTAIN FROM THE CONSUMPTION OF ALCOHOL/DRUGS IN ANY FORM UNLESS PRESCRIBED BY ANOTHER PHYSICIAN FOR A LEGITIMATE AND THERAPEUTIC PURPOSE; SHALL SUBMIT HERSELF FOR APPROPRIATE EXAMS INCLUDING DRUG OR ALCOHOL SCREENS; SHALL CONTINUE TO RECEIVE CARE AND TREATMENT FROM PSYCHIATRIST NO LESS THAN ONCE A MONTH WHO SHALL SUBMIT QUARTERLY REPORTS TO THE BOARD; SHALL CONTINUE TO PARTICIPATE IN AA'S PROGRAM NOT LESS THAN THREE TIMES PER WEEK WITH QUARTERLY REPORTS TO THE BOARD; SHALL PARTICIPATE IN ACTIVITIES OF A PHYSICIAN'S COUNSELING COMMITTEE AND ATTEND WEEKLY MEETINGS WITH QUARTERLY REPORTS; SHALL COMPLY WITH THE TERMS OF ANY CONTINUING CARE CONTRACTS WITH QUARTERLY REPORTS; SHALL COMPLY WITH THE TERMS OF CONTRACTS FOR HOSPITAL PRIVILEGES AND INFORM BOARD OF ANY DISCIPLINARY ACTION TAKEN; SHALL NOT POSSESS ALCOHOL, CONTROLLED SUBSTANCES OR DRUGS WITH ADDICTIVE POTENTIAL OR POTENTIAL FOR ABUSE; SHALL NOT TREAT OR OTHERWISE SERVE AS PHYSICIAN, PRESCRIBE OR DISPENSE DRUGS THAT MAY BE SUBJECT TO ABUSE TO HERSELF OR TO ANY MEMBER OF HER FAMILY; SHALL NOT TELEPHONE A PHARMACY WITH PRESCRIPTIONS FOR THESE DRUGS OR PERMIT ANYONE UNDER HER SUPERVISION TO DO SO; MAY REAPPLY FOR DEA/DPS CONTROLLED SUBSTANCES REGISTRATIONS BUT SHALL NOT PRESCRIBE, ADMINISTER OR DISPENSE ANY CONTROLLED SUBSTANCES UNDER THE AUTHORITY OF THESE REGISTRATIONS; SHALL SURRENDER ALL UNUSED TRIPLICATE PRESCRIPTION FORMS AND SHALL NOT ATTEMPT TO ORDER MORE; SHALL MAINTAIN A FILE WITH COPIES OF EVERY PRESCRIPTION WRITTEN FOR DRUGS WITH ADDICTIVE POTENTIAL WHICH SHALL BE AVAILABLE FOR REVIEW; SHALL PRACTICE ONLY IN A FAMILY PRACTICE GROUP SETTING NO MORE THAN EIGHT HOURS PER DAY AND NO MORE THAN 40 HOURS PER WEEK AND SHALL EXAMINE, DIAGNOSE OR TREAT NO MORE THAN 15 PATIENTS PER DAY; EXCEPT IN AN EMERGENCY, SHE SHALL BE TREATED FOR MIGRAINE HEADACHES ONLY BY A BOARD-APPROVED NEUROLOGIST; HER MEDICAL PRACTICE SHALL BE MONITORED BY A BOARD-APPROVED PHYSICIAN WHO SHALL SUBMIT QUARTERLY REPORTS; SHALL MAINTAIN ADEQUATE MEDICAL RECORDS WHICH SHALL BE AVAILABLE FOR REVIEW; SHALL OBTAIN AT LEAST 50 HOURS PER YEAR OF CONTINUING MEDICAL EDUCATION; WITHIN SIX MONTHS, SHALL TAKE AND PASS THE SPECIAL PURPOSE EXAMINATION; SHALL APPEAR BEFORE BOARD AT LEAST TWICE A YEAR OR AT BOARD REQUEST; SHALL COOPERATE WITH BOARD IN VERIFYING COMPLIANCE INCLUDING PROVIDING COPIES OF MEDICAL RELEASES OR PEER REVIEW REPORTS UPON REQUEST; SHALL GIVE A COPY OF THIS ORDER TO ANY HEALTH CARE ENTITY WHERE SHE HAS PRIVILEGES; SHALL PROVIDE A COPY OF THE ORDER TO ANYONE REQUESTING IT WITHIN 10 DAYS; TIME PERIOD OUT OF TEXAS DOES NOT COUNT TOWARD PROBATION; SHALL INFORM BOARD OF CHANGE OF ADDRESS WITHIN 10 DAYS OR IF SHE LEAVES THE STATE. SHALL NOT SEEK MODIFICATION FOR ONE YEAR. ORDER MODIFIED ON 8/17/96 ALLOWING HER TO REAPPLY FOR FULL PRESCRIBING AUTHORITY TO THE DEA AND THE TEXAS DPS; ALL OTHER PROVISIONS OF THIS ORDER REMAIN IN FULL FORCE AND EFFECT. ON 8/22/98 PETITION TO TERMINATE ORDER DENIED; ORDER MODIFIED DELETING REQUIREMENT OF CONTINUING CARE BY HER TREATING PHYSICIAN, AND TO SURRENDER HER TRIPLICATE PRESCRIPTION FORMS AND NOT REAPPLY; REDUCTION OF APPEARANCES BEFORE THE BOARD FROM BIANNUAL TO ANNUAL. ON 10/15/99 ORDER TERMINATED.

BRINER, BARBARA HADEN MD OF 2818 TANGLEY, HOUSTON, TX, WAS DISCIPLINED BY DEA ON NOVEMBER 12, 1997
DISCIPLINARY ACTION: RESTRICTION PLACED ON CONTROLLED SUBSTANCE LICENSE

NOTES: MEMO OF UNDERSTANDING.

BRITTAIN, ROBERT D III MD, LICENSE NUMBER 00G4858 OF SAN ANTONIO, TX, WAS DISCIPLINED BY TEXAS ON AUGUST 24, 1991
DISCIPLINARY ACTION: 60-MONTH PROBATION; MONITORING OF PHYSICIAN PERFORMANCE
OFFENSE: SUBSTANCE ABUSE

NOTES: ALCOHOL ABUSE. LICENSE SUSPENDED, STAYED; SHALL PARTICIPATE IN AA; SHALL CONTINUE TREATMENT FROM DESIGNATED PHYSICIAN; SHALL SUBMIT TO DRUG OR ALCOHOL SCREENS; SHALL APPEAR BEFORE THE BOARD TWICE YEARLY DURING PROBATION.

BROOKS, JESSE M MD, DATE OF BIRTH MARCH 17, 1918 OF PO BOX 1069, ATLANTA, TX, WAS DISCIPLINED BY MEDICARE ON DECEMBER 10, 1997

DISCIPLINARY ACTION: 120-MONTH EXCLUSION FROM THE MEDICARE AND/OR MEDICAID PROGRAM
OFFENSE: NONCOMPLIANCE WITH A PROFESSIONAL RULE

NOTES: EXCLUDED BASED ON A RECOMMENDATION FROM A PEER REVIEW ORGANIZATION THAT THE SUBJECT VIOLATED STATUTORY OBLIGATIONS.

BROOKS, JESSE M MD, DATE OF BIRTH MARCH 17, 1918 OF 230 LOUISE STREET, ATLANTA, TX, WAS DISCIPLINED BY MEDICARE ON JUNE 9, 1998
DISCIPLINARY ACTION: 120-MONTH EXCLUSION FROM THE MEDICARE AND/OR MEDICAID PROGRAM
OFFENSE: NONCOMPLIANCE WITH A PROFESSIONAL RULE

NOTES: EXCLUDED BASED ON A RECOMMENDATION FROM A PEER REVIEW ORGANIZATION THAT THE SUBJECT VIOLATED STATUTORY OBLIGATIONS.

BROOKS, JESSE MILES MD, LICENSE NUMBER 00B5748 OF ATLANTA, TX, WAS DISCIPLINED BY TEXAS ON AUGUST 18, 1990
DISCIPLINARY ACTION: REQUIRED TO TAKE ADDITIONAL MEDICAL EDUCATION

NOTES: STIPULATED ORDER. MUST OBTAIN CONTINUING MEDICAL EDUCATION, PARTICIPATE IN PRECEPTORSHIP PROGRAM TO INCLUDE SPECIFIC CURRICULUM, CONCLUDE AGREEMENT REGARDING ACCEPTANCE OF CERTAIN PATIENTS, AND OBTAIN PHYSICIAN TO JOIN HOSPITAL STAFF WHO WILL BE AVAILABLE FOR BACKUP COVERAGE.

BROOKS, JESSE MILES MD, LICENSE NUMBER 00B5748 OF ATLANTA, TX, WAS DISCIPLINED BY TEXAS ON APRIL 15, 1994
DISCIPLINARY ACTION: MONITORING OF PHYSICIAN PERFORMANCE
OFFENSE: PROFESSIONAL MISCONDUCT

NOTES: DURING 1990 AND 1991 HE ORDERED EXCESSIVE LAB TESTS AND CHARGED FOR THEM IN THE CASE OF TWO PATIENTS; MADE DIAGNOSES FOR THESE PATIENTS THAT ARE NOT SUPPORTED BY MEDICAL RECORDS AND PRESCRIBED MEDICATIONS TO THEM THAT WERE NOT MEDICALLY INDICATED. CONDITIONS OF ORDER: HE SHALL SUBMIT ONE OUT OF EVERY FIVE PATIENT FILES HOSPITALIZED FOR A PERIOD OF 24 HOURS OR MORE TO A HOSPITAL REVIEW COMMITTEE EACH WEEK; COMMITTEE WILL SUBMIT REPORTS TO BOARD; THE NUMBER OF FILES CHOSEN FOR REVIEW WILL BE REDUCED IF NO PROBLEMS ARE SEEN FOR ONE YEAR; PROGRAM WILL DISCONTINUE IN TWO YEARS IF NO PROBLEMS ARE FOUND; SHALL MAINTAIN ADEQUATE MEDICAL RECORDS AND SHALL MAKE THESE RECORDS AVAILABLE FOR INSPECTION; SHALL REFRAIN FROM PRESCRIBING ANY DRUG THAT IS NOT MEDICALLY INDICATED; SHALL GIVE A COPY OF THIS ORDER TO ANY HEALTH CARE ENTITY WHERE HE HAS PRIVILEGES; SHALL COOPERATE WITH THE BOARD IN VERIFYING COMPLIANCE; SHALL INFORM BOARD OF CHANGE OF ADDRESS WITHIN 10 DAYS OR IF HE LEAVES THE STATE; TIME SPENT OUT OF TEXAS DOES NOT COUNT TOWARD RESTRICTIONS. SHALL NOT SEEK MODIFICATION FOR ONE YEAR.

BROOKS, JESSE MILES MD, LICENSE NUMBER 00B5748 OF ATLANTA, TX, WAS DISCIPLINED BY TEXAS ON AUGUST 18, 1995
DISCIPLINARY ACTION: RESTRICTION PLACED ON CONTROLLED SUBSTANCE LICENSE; REPRIMAND
OFFENSE: OVERPRESCRIBING OR MISPRESCRIBING DRUGS

NOTES: BETWEEN 1986 AND 1993, HE PRESCRIBED THYROID MEDICATION TO MULTIPLE PATIENTS WITHOUT MEDICAL INDICATION IN A MANNER INCONSISTENT WITH PUBLIC HEALTH AND WELFARE AND HE FAILED TO ADEQUATELY DOCUMENT EXAMINATIONS, FINDINGS AND PRESCRIPTIONS FOR MULTIPLE PATIENTS. NEITHER ADMITS NOR DENIES ALLEGATIONS. LICENSE RESTRICTED WITH TERMS: SHALL ORDER A COMPLETE BLOOD COUNT AND APPROPRIATE LAB WORK FOR EACH PATIENT RECEIVING WEIGHT MANAGEMENT MEDICATION OR ON A DIET PROGRAM AT INTERVALS TO INCLUDE THE INITIAL VISIT AND EVERY SIX MONTHS THEREAFTER; SHALL NOT PRESCRIBE, ADMINISTER OR DISPENSE THYROID MEDICATION OR DIURETICS FOR WEIGHT MANAGEMENT; SHALL PRESCRIBE ALL WEIGHT MANAGEMENT MEDICATIONS ONLY FOR A 40 DAY PERIOD; SHALL MAINTAIN ADEQUATE MEDICAL RECORDS WHICH SHALL BE AVAILABLE FOR REVIEW; WITHIN TWO YEARS, SHALL OBTAIN 20 HOURS OF CONTINUING MEDICAL EDUCATION IN PHARMACOLOGY AND 20 HOURS IN BARIATRICS AND SHALL COMPLETE AT LEAST ONE COURSE IN PHARMACOLOGY AND BARIATRICS WITHIN SIX MONTHS; SHALL RETAIN A BOARD-APPROVED OFFICE MANAGEMENT CONSULTANT; SHALL COOPERATE WITH THE BOARD IN VERIFYING COMPLIANCE INCLUDING PROVIDING COPIES OF MEDICAL RECORDS UPON REQUEST; SHALL APPEAR BEFORE BOARD AT LEAST TWO TIMES PER YEAR; SHALL GIVE A COPY OF THIS ORDER TO ANY HEALTH CARE ENTITY WHERE HE HAS PRIVILEGES; SHALL INFORM BOARD OF CHANGE OF ADDRESS WITHIN 10 DAYS OR IF HE LEAVES THE STATE; TIME SPENT OUT OF TEXAS DOES NOT COUNT TOWARD RESTRICTION. SHALL NOT SEEK MODIFICATION FOR ONE YEAR. ON 9/20/97 PETITION TO MODIFY ORDER GRANTED CHANGING REQUIREMENT TO OBTAIN CONTINUING MEDICAL EDUCATION IN SPECIFIED SUBJECTS TO REQUIRING FIFTY HOURS ONLY.

BROOKS, JESSE MILES MD, LICENSE NUMBER B5748 OF ATLANTA, TX, WAS DISCIPLINED BY TEXAS ON FEBRUARY 7, 1998
DISCIPLINARY ACTION: 60-MONTH PROBATION; REQUIRED TO TAKE ADDITIONAL MEDICAL EDUCATION
OFFENSE: FAILURE TO COMPLY WITH PREVIOUS BOARD ORDER

NOTES: FROM 1993-1996 HE TREATED AND PRESCRIBED CONTROLLED SUBSTANCES FOR CERTAIN PERSONS RELATED TO HIM WHO WERE KNOWN SUBSTANCE ABUSERS, FAILED TO KEEP ADEQUATE RECORDS AND DID NOT MEET STANDARDS OF CARE; HE MAINTAINS THAT HE TREATED THESE PATIENTS ONLY AFTER TWO ATTEMPTS AT INSTITUTIONAL TREATMENT HAD FAILED, HIS TREATMENT REGIMEN MIRRORED THAT OF THE INSTITUTIONAL TREATMENT, AND WITHOUT HIS HIGHLY CONTROLLED INTERVENTION, THE PATIENTS WOULD HAVE GONE TO THE "STREET" FOR DRUGS; A BOARD CONSULTANT EVALUATED THE RECORDS OF 9 PATIENTS TREATED BY HIM IN 1994 AND DETERMINED HIS TREATMENT FELL BELOW THE STANDARD OF CARE AND THAT HE FAILED TO KEEP ADEQUATE MEDICAL RECORDS; THE BELOW STANDARD CARE INVOLVED TREATMENT OF A BROAD RANGE OF DISEASES AND INCLUDED GROSSLY INAPPROPRIATE PRESCRIPTION OF MEDICATIONS; VIOLATED 1994 BOARD ORDER. SUSPENSION STAYED FOR PROBATION WITH FOLLOWING TERMS AND CONDITIONS: SHALL NOMINATE THREE CERTIFIED NEUROLOGISTS FOR BOARD SELECTION AND SHALL EXPEDITIOUSLY SUBMIT HIMSELF TO EVALUATION AND TREATMENT BY THE APPROVED PRACTITIONER; SHALL SUCCESSFULLY COMPLETE 18 SESSIONS OF THE GEORGIA ACADEMY OF FAMILY PHYSICIAN EDUCATIONAL FOUNDATION'S FAMILY MEDICINE REFRESHER COURSE; SHALL HAVE A PHYSICIAN WITH AN UNRESTRICTED TEXAS MEDICAL LICENSE CO-MANAGE EACH OF HIS OFFICE AND HOSPITAL PATIENTS; SHALL EMPLOY A MEDICAL RECORDS

TECHNICIAN WHO WILL REVIEW HIS RECORDS WITHIN 7 DAYS OF TREATMENT OF EACH PATIENT; HIS MEDICAL PRACTICE SHALL BE MONITORED BY A BOARD APPROVED TEXAS PHYSICIAN WHO SHALL PROVIDE QUARTERLY REPORTS TO THE BOARD; SHALL NOT TREAT OR OTHERWISE SERVE AS PHYSICIAN, PRESCRIBE, DISPENSE OR ADMINISTER DRUGS THAT MAY BE SUBJECT TO ABUSE TO HIMSELF OR TO ANY MEMBER OF HIS FAMILY; SEPARATE FROM PATIENT RECORDS, SHALL MAINTAIN A FILE OF EVERY PRESCRIPTION WRITTEN BY HIM FOR DANGEROUS DRUGS WITH ADDICTIVE POTENTIAL WHICH SHALL BE MADE AVAILABLE FOR REVIEW; SHALL NOT TREAT OR OTHERWISE SERVE AS PHYSICIAN, PRESCRIBE, DISPENSE OR ADMINISTER DRUGS THAT MAY BE SUBJECT TO ABUSE TO HIMSELF OR TO ANY MEMBER OF HIS FAMILY; SHALL MAINTAIN ADEQUATE MEDICAL RECORDS WHICH SHALL BE AVAILABLE FOR REVIEW; SHALL APPEAR BEFORE THE BOARD TWICE A YEAR; SHALL COOPERATE WITH THE BOARD IN VERIFYING COMPLIANCE INCLUDING PROVIDING COPIES OF MEDICAL RELEASES UPON REQUEST; SHALL GIVE A COPY OF THIS ORDER TO ANY HEALTH CARE ENTITY WHERE HE HAS PRIVILEGES; SHALL INFORM THE BOARD OF CHANGE OF ADDRESS WITHIN 10 DAYS. ON 4/10/99 THE BOARD ORDERED THAT HE SHALL TAKE AND PASS THE SPEX EXAM WITHIN 90 DAYS AS REQUIRED BY THE ORDER. ON 10/15/99 HIS PETITION TO MODIFY THE ORDER WAS DENIED IN PART AND GRANTED IN PART; DELETION OF THE REQUIREMENT OF TWO PERSONAL APPEARANCES PER YEAR BEFORE THE BOARD; AND, IT WAS ORDERED THAT HE TAKE AND PASS THE SPEX WITHIN 90 DAYS; OTHER REQUESTED CHANGES WERE DENIED. ALL OTHER PROVISIONS OF ORDER REMAIN IN EFFECT UNTIL SUPERSEDED BY A SUBSEQUENT BOARD ORDER.

BROOKS, MARSHALL JAMES JR MD, LICENSE NUMBER 00B5369 OF ATLANTA, TX, WAS DISCIPLINED BY TEXAS ON AUGUST 18, 1990
DISCIPLINARY ACTION: REQUIRED TO TAKE ADDITIONAL MEDICAL EDUCATION

NOTES: STIPULATED ORDER. MUST OBTAIN CONTINUING MEDICAL EDUCATION, PARTICIPATE IN PRECEPTORSHIP PROGRAM TO INCLUDE SPECIFIC CURRICULUM, CONCLUDE AGREEMENT REGARDING ACCEPTANCE OF CERTAIN PATIENTS, AND OBTAIN PHYSICIAN TO JOIN HOSPITAL STAFF WHO WILL BE AVAILABLE FOR BACKUP COVERAGE.

BROOKS, MARSHALL JAMES JR MD, LICENSE NUMBER 00B5369 OF ATLANTA, TX, WAS DISCIPLINED BY TEXAS ON AUGUST 18, 1995
DISCIPLINARY ACTION: RESTRICTION PLACED ON CONTROLLED SUBSTANCE LICENSE; REPRIMAND
OFFENSE: OVERPRESCRIBING OR MISPRESCRIBING DRUGS

NOTES: DURING 1986 TO 1993 PRESCRIBED THYROID MEDICATION TO MULTIPLE PATIENTS WITHOUT MEDICAL INDICATION IN A MANNER INCONSISTENT WITH PUBLIC HEALTH AND WELFARE. FAILED TO ADEQUATELY DOCUMENT EXAMINATIONS, FINDINGS AND PRESCRIPTIONS FOR MULTIPLE PATIENTS. LICENSE RESTRICTED WITH TERMS: SHALL ORDER A COMPLETE BLOOD COUNT AND APPROPRIATE LAB WORK FOR EACH PATIENT RECEIVING WEIGHT MANAGEMENT MEDICATION OR ON A DIET PROGRAM AT INTERVALS TO INCLUDE THE INITIAL VISIT AND EVERY SIX MONTHS THEREAFTER; SHALL NOT PRESCRIBE, ADMINISTER OR DISPENSE THYROID MEDICATION OR DIURETICS FOR WEIGHT MANAGEMENT; SHALL PRESCRIBE ALL WEIGHT MANAGEMENT MEDICATIONS ONLY FOR A 40 DAY PERIOD; SHALL MAINTAIN ADEQUATE MEDICAL RECORDS WHICH SHALL BE AVAILABLE FOR REVIEW; WITHIN TWO YEARS, SHALL OBTAIN 20 HOURS OF CONTINUING MEDICAL EDUCATION IN PHARMACOLOGY AND 20 HOURS IN BARIATRICS AND SHALL COMPLETE AT LEAST ONE COURSE IN PHARMACOLOGY AND BARIATRICS WITHIN SIX MONTHS; SHALL RETAIN A BOARD-APPROVED OFFICE MANAGEMENT CONSULTANT; WITHIN SIX MONTHS, SHALL EITHER ENTER A BOARD-APPROVED PRECEPTOR PROGRAM OR SHALL TAKE AND PASS THE SPECIAL PURPOSE EXAMINATION; SHALL PROVIDE ACCESS TO MEDICAL RECORDS BY BOARD; SHALL APPEAR BEFORE BOARD AT LEAST TWO TIMES PER YEAR; HIS PRACTICE SHALL BE MONITORED BY A BOARD- APPROVED PHYSICIAN WHO SHALL SUBMIT QUARTERLY REPORTS TO THE BOARD; SHALL GIVE A COPY OF THIS ORDER TO ANY HEALTH CARE ENTITY WHERE HE HAS PRIVILEGES; SHALL COOPERATE WITH BOARD IN VERIFYING COMPLIANCE; SHALL INFORM BOARD OF CHANGE OF ADDRESS WITHIN 10 DAYS OR IF HE LEAVES THE STATE; TIME SPENT OUT OF TEXAS DOES NOT COUNT TOWARD PROBATION. SHALL NOT SEEK MODIFICATION FOR ONE YEAR.

BROOKS, MARSHALL JAMES JR MD, LICENSE NUMBER 00B5369, WAS DISCIPLINED BY TEXAS ON MARCH 4, 1996
DISCIPLINARY ACTION: LICENSE SUSPENSION
OFFENSE: FAILURE TO COMPLY WITH PREVIOUS BOARD ORDER

NOTES: FAILED TO ENTER A PRECEPTORSHIP PROGRAM OR FAILURE TO TAKE AND PASS THE SPEX EXAMINATION AS ORDERED IN 8/18/95 BOARD ORDER. SUSPENSION UNTIL HE ENTERS A PRECEPTORSHIP PROGRAM OR TAKES AND PASSES THE SPEX EXAMINATION AND SUBSEQUENTLY APPEARS BEFORE THE BOARD AND PROVIDES EVIDENCE THAT HE POSSESSES THE SKILLS AND KNOWLEDGE TO SAFELY PRACTICE MEDICINE IN TEXAS AND IS OTHERWISE PHYSICALLY AND MENTALLY COMPETENT TO RESUME THE PRACTICE OF MEDICINE.

BROOKS, MARSHALL JAMES JR MD OF 111 LOUISE STREET P.O. BOX 967, ATLANTA, TX, WAS DISCIPLINED BY DEA ON APRIL 29, 199(
DISCIPLINARY ACTION: SURRENDER OF CONTROLLED SUBSTANCE LICENSE

NOTES: IN LIEU OF ORDER TO SHOW CAUSE.

BROOKS, QUENTIN T MD, LICENSE NUMBER C7261 OF RICHARDSON, TX, WAS DISCIPLINED BY TEXAS ON AUGUST 22, 1998
DISCIPLINARY ACTION: 60-MONTH RESTRICTION PLACED ON LICENSE; REQUIRED TO TAKE ADDITIONAL MEDICAL EDUCATION
OFFENSE: LOSS OR RESTRICTION OF HOSPITAL PRIVILEGES

NOTES: DURING 1996 A PEER REVIEW ACTION WAS TAKEN INVOLVING HIS MAMMOGRAM AND ULTRASOUND PRIVILEGES WHICH RESULTED IN THE RETENTION OF MAMMOGRAM PRIVILEGES SUBJECT TO OVER-READ BY ANOTHER RADIOLOGIST FOR THE FIRST 50 CASES AND REMOVAL OF HIS PRIVILEGES TO PERFORM ULTRASOUND PROCEDURES. CONDITIONS ON LICENSE: SHALL LIMIT HIS PRACTICE OF RADIOLOGY TO NOT ENGAGE IN ULTRASOUND PROCEDURES; SHALL OBTAIN 75 HOURS PER YEAR OF CONTINUING MEDICAL EDUCATION, WITH 25 HOURS IN CONTRAST MEDIUM INTERPRETATION, NUCLEAR MEDICINE, CT, OR MRI PROCEDURES AND THE BALANCE OF THE HOURS IN RADIOLOGY; SHALL APPEAR BEFORE THE BOARD AT LEAST ONCE A YEAR; SHALL COOPERATE WITH THE BOARD IN VERIFYING COMPLIANCE INCLUDING PROVIDING COPIES OF PEER REVIEW RECORDS UPON REQUEST; SHALL GIVE A COPY OF

THIS ORDER TO ANY HEALTH CARE ENTITY WHERE HE HAS PRIVILEGES; TIME SPENT OUT OF TEXAS DOES NOT COUNT TOWARD RESTRICTION; SHALL INFORM THE BOARD OF CHANGE OF ADDRESS WITHIN 10 DAYS OR IF HE LEAVES THE STATE; SHALL NOT SEEK MODIFICATION FOR ONE YEAR. ON 12/11/99 PETITION TO TERMINATE ORDER DENIED.

BROOKS, THOMAS C MD, LICENSE NUMBER 00B8251 OF DAYTON, TX, WAS DISCIPLINED BY TEXAS ON DECEMBER 1, 1990
DISCIPLINARY ACTION: LICENSE REVOCATION
OFFENSE: PROFESSIONAL MISCONDUCT

NOTES: IMPERSONATED A LICENSED PRACTITIONER OR PERMITTED OR ALLOWED ANOTHER TO USE LICENSE TO PRACTICE MEDICINE. AIDED OR ABETTED, DIRECTLY OR INDIRECTLY, THE PRACTICE OF MEDICINE BY ANY PERSON, PARTNERSHIP, ASSOCIATION, OR CORPORATION NOT LICENSED TO PRACTICE.

BROUGH, ROYCE D MD, LICENSE NUMBER 0025110 OF HOUSTON, TX, WAS DISCIPLINED BY VIRGINIA ON SEPTEMBER 12, 1995
DISCIPLINARY ACTION: PROBATION
OFFENSE: DISCIPLINARY ACTION BY ANOTHER STATE OR AGENCY

NOTES: PROBATION BY TEXAS BOARD FOR SUBSTANCE ABUSE. INDEFINITE PROBATION UNDER TERMS AND CONDITIONS. ON 9/5/97 PROBATION TERMINATED; FULL AND UNRESTRICTED LICENSE GRANTED.

BROUGH, ROYCE DONALD JR MD, DATE OF BIRTH MAY 7, 1943, LICENSE NUMBER 00E4808 OF 2020 NAOMI, HOUSTON, TX, WAS DISCIPLINED BY TEXAS ON JANUARY 29, 1993
DISCIPLINARY ACTION: 60-MONTH PROBATION; MONITORING OF PHYSICIAN PERFORMANCE
OFFENSE: SUBSTANCE ABUSE

NOTES: ON 9/14/92 VOLUNTARILY BEGAN A TREATMENT PROGRAM AND WAS SUCCESSFULLY DISCHARGED; HAS ENTERED AN AFTERCARE PROGRAM CONTRACT. 5 YEAR SUSPENSION STAYED. CONDITIONS OF PROBATION: SHALL APPEAR BEFORE THE BOARD ONCE A YEAR; SHALL NOT SELF-TREAT OR OTHERWISE SERVE AS PHYSICIAN, PRESCRIBE, DISPENSE OR ADMINISTER DRUGS THAT MAY BE SUBJECT TO ABUSE FOR HIMSELF OR ANY MEMBER OF HIS FAMILY; SHALL ABSTAIN FROM THE CONSUMPTION OF ALCOHOL/CHEMICAL SUBSTANCES IN ANY FORM UNLESS PRESCRIBED BY ANOTHER PHYSICIAN FOR A LEGITIMATE AND THERAPEUTIC PURPOSE; SHALL PARTICIPATE IN ACTIVITIES OF A PHYSICIAN COUNSELING COMMITTEE WITH QUARTERLY REPORTS; SHALL PARTICIPATE IN AA NOT LESS THAN 3 TIMES A WEEK WITH QUARTERLY REPORTS TO THE BOARD; SHALL SUBMIT HIMSELF FOR APPROPRIATE EXAMS INCLUDING DRUG OR ALCOHOL SCREENS; SHALL CONTINUE TO RECEIVE TREATMENT FROM THE ADDICTIONOLOGIST AND PSYCHIATRIST HE IS NOW SEEING; SHALL FURNISH THE BOARD WITH WRITTEN REPORTS ON HIS MEDICAL CONDITION AND COMPLIANCE WITH THIS ORDER WHEN REQUESTED; SHALL COMPLY WITH THE TERMS OF HIS AFTERCARE CONTRACT; SHALL GIVE A COPY OF THIS ORDER TO ANY HEALTH CARE ENTITY WHERE HE HAS PRIVILEGES; SHALL COOPERATE WITH THE BOARD IN VERIFYING COMPLIANCE; SHALL INFORM THE BOARD OF CHANGE OF ADDRESS OR IF HE LEAVES THE STATE; TIME SPENT OUT OF TEXAS DOES NOT COUNT TOWARD PROBATION. SHALL NOT SEEK MODIFICATION FOR 1 YEAR. ON 5/11/95 HIS PETITION FOR TERMINATION WAS DENIED. PROBATION TERMINATED ON 5/15/96.

BROUGH, ROYCE DONALD JR MD, DATE OF BIRTH MAY 7, 1943, LICENSE NUMBER 0006701 OF 400 SECOND AVE NORTH, AMORY, MS, WAS DISCIPLINED BY MISSISSIPPI ON JULY 15, 1993
DISCIPLINARY ACTION: PROBATION; MONITORING OF PHYSICIAN PERFORMANCE
OFFENSE: DISCIPLINARY ACTION BY ANOTHER STATE OR AGENCY

NOTES: BASED ON ACTIONS IN TEXAS. FIVE YEAR SUSPENSION STAYED; HE IS SUBJECT TO TERMS AND CONDITIONS INCLUDING RANDOM, UNANNOUNCED AND WITNESSED BLOOD AND URINE SCREENS. ON 7/18/96 REQUEST FOR REMOVAL OF RESTRICTIONS DENIED. ON 6/19/97 ALL RESTRICTIONS ON LICENSE REMOVED.

BROUGH, ROYCE DONALD JR MD, DATE OF BIRTH MAY 7, 1943, LICENSE NUMBER 0016780 OF 109 SUNSET, FOREST, MO, WAS DISCIPLINED BY GEORGIA ON MAY 5, 1995
DISCIPLINARY ACTION: 60-MONTH PROBATION

NOTES: IMPAIRED.

BROWN, BARRY M MD, LICENSE NUMBER D6234 OF HOUSTON, TX, WAS DISCIPLINED BY TEXAS ON AUGUST 22, 1998
DISCIPLINARY ACTION: 60-MONTH PROBATION; RESTRICTION PLACED ON LICENSE
OFFENSE: SEXUAL ABUSE OF OR SEXUAL MISCONDUCT WITH A PATIENT

NOTES: SELF-PRESCRIBED VARIOUS PRESCRIPTION DRUGS, INCLUDING MOOD ALTERING DRUGS; FAILED TO DOCUMENT THE RATIONALE FOR THE PRESCRIBING IN THAT HE FAILED TO MAKE AND MAINTAIN A MEDICAL RECORD FOR HIMSELF AS A PATIENT; IN 2/96 A DRUG AUDIT BY THE BOARD FOUND THE FOLLOWING DEFICIENCIES: CONTROLLED SUBSTANCES WERE STORED IN AN UNSECURED MANNER; TRIPLICATE PRESCRIPTION PADS WERE NOT PROPERLY SECURED; NO DOCUMENTATION WHICH WOULD TRACK HOW PHARMACEUTICAL SAMPLES WERE DISPENSED; ALLEGATIONS HAVE BEEN MADE THAT DURING THE COURSE OF HIS PRACTICE HE ENGAGED IN CONDUCT OF A SEXUAL NATURE WITH 2 ADULT FEMALE PATIENTS; HE DENIES THE SEXUAL MISCONDUCT. SUSPENSION STAYED FOR PROBATION WITH FOLLOWING TERMS AND CONDITIONS: SHALL NOT TREAT OR OTHERWISE SERVE AS PHYSICIAN, PRESCRIBE, DISPENSE OR ADMINISTER DRUGS THAT MAY BE SUBJECT TO ABUSE TO HIMSELF OR TO ANY MEMBER OF HIS FAMILY; SHALL NOMINATE THREE CERTIFIED PSYCHIATRISTS FOR BOARD SELECTION OF A THERAPIST AND SHALL EXPEDITIOUSLY SUBMIT HIMSELF TO EVALUATION AND TREATMENT BY THE APPROVED PRACTITIONER; SHALL ABSTAIN FROM THE CONSUMPTION OF ALCOHOL/DRUGS IN ANY FORM UNLESS PRESCRIBED BY ANOTHER PHYSICIAN FOR A LEGITIMATE AND THERAPEUTIC PURPOSE; SHALL SUBMIT HIMSELF FOR APPROPRIATE EXAMS INCLUDING DRUG OR ALCOHOL SCREENS; SEPARATE FROM PATIENT RECORDS, SHALL MAINTAIN A FILE OF EVERY PRESCRIPTION WRITTEN BY HIM FOR DANGEROUS DRUGS WITH ADDICTIVE POTENTIAL WHICH SHALL BE MADE AVAILABLE FOR REVIEW; SHALL MAINTAIN ADEQUATE MEDICAL RECORDS WHICH SHALL BE AVAILABLE FOR REVIEW; HIS MEDICAL PRACTICE SHALL BE MONITORED BY A BOARD APPROVED TEXAS PHYSICIAN WHO SHALL PROVIDE QUARTERLY REPORTS TO THE BOARD; SHALL HAVE A CHAPERONE PRESENT WHEN PERFORMING PHYSICAL EXAMS ON FEMALE PATIENTS; SHALL OBTAIN 10 HOURS OF AN ETHICS COURSE PER YEAR FOR 5 YEARS; WITHIN 3 MONTHS,

SHALL TAKE AND PASS THE MEDICAL JURISPRUDENCE EXAM; SHALL COOPERATE WITH THE BOARD IN VERIFYING COMPLIANCE INCLUDING PROVIDING COPIES OF MEDICAL RELEASES AND PEER REVIEW RECORDS UPON REQUEST; SHALL GIVE A COPY OF THIS ORDER TO ANY HEALTH CARE ENTITY WHERE HE HAS PRIVILEGES; SHALL PROVIDE A COPY OF THIS ORDER TO ANYONE REQUESTING IT WITHIN 10 DAYS; SHALL APPEAR BEFORE THE BOARD UPON REQUEST; TIME SPENT OUT OF TEXAS DOES NOT COUNT TOWARD PROBATION; SHALL INFORM THE BOARD OF CHANGE OF ADDRESS WITHIN 10 DAYS OR IF HE LEAVES THE STATE; SHALL NOT SEEK MODIFICATION FOR ONE YEAR.

BROWN, BARRY M MD, LICENSE NUMBER D6234 OF HOUSTON, TX, WAS DISCIPLINED BY TEXAS ON DECEMBER 4, 1998
DISCIPLINARY ACTION: LICENSE SUSPENSION
OFFENSE: FAILURE TO COMPLY WITH PREVIOUS BOARD ORDER

NOTES: VIOLATION OF PROBATION.

BROWN, CYNTHIA A MD, LICENSE NUMBER 0D26655 OF 16816 5TH AVENUE SE, BUTHELL, WA, WAS DISCIPLINED BY MARYLAND ON MARCH 12, 1990
DISCIPLINARY ACTION: SURRENDER OF LICENSE; SURRENDER OF CONTROLLED SUBSTANCE LICENSE
OFFENSE: SUBSTANDARD CARE, INCOMPETENCE OR NEGLIGENCE

NOTES: HAS NOT PRACTICED IN MARYLAND SINCE 10/26/88; LICENSED IN TEXAS AND HAS APPLIED IN WASHINGTON STATE; MAY APPLY FOR REINSTATEMENT UPON COMPLETION OF A BOARD-APPROVED TRAINING PROGRAM.

BROWN, CYNTHIA A MD, LICENSE NUMBER 00D8160 OF BOTHELL, WA, WAS DISCIPLINED BY TEXAS ON FEBRUARY 22, 1991

NOTES: MAY NOT PRACTICE IN TEXAS UNTIL THE MARYLAND BOARD HAS ACTED ON ANY PETITION SHE HAS FILED OR MAY FILE FOR REINSTATEMENT OF HER LICENSE; RECEIVE PERMISSION OF TEXAS BOARD BEFORE RETURNING TO PRACTICE MEDICINE IN TEXAS AND BE SUBJECT TO ANY TERMS IMPOSED.

BROWN, JONEL L II MD, LICENSE NUMBER 0C24881 OF ATLANTA, GA, WAS DISCIPLINED BY CALIFORNIA ON SEPTEMBER 18, 1996
DISCIPLINARY ACTION: LICENSE REVOCATION

NOTES: DEFAULT ACTION.

BROWN, JONEL LEONARD II MD, LICENSE NUMBER 00C9410 OF TEMPLE, TX, WAS DISCIPLINED BY TEXAS ON MAY 11, 1995
DISCIPLINARY ACTION: LICENSE REVOCATION
OFFENSE: CRIMINAL CONVICTION OR PLEA OF GUILTY, NOLO CONTENDERE, OR NO CONTEST TO A CRIME

NOTES: IN 1/94, FOUND GUILTY OF ONE COUNT OF AGGRAVATED ASSAULT AND SENTENCED TO CONFINEMENT IN THE GEORGIA DEPARTMENT OF CORRECTIONS, WHERE HE IS CURRENTLY INCARCERATED; HE REPORTS HAVING ENGAGED IN THE INTEMPERATE USE OF ALCOHOL PRIOR TO 12/91 AND HAS ADMITTED TO BEING AN ALCOHOLIC. VOLUNTARY REVOCATION.

BROWN, JONEL LEONARD MD, DATE OF BIRTH FEBRUARY 28, 1937, LICENSE NUMBER 0009443 OF 404 S. FREYERS CREEK CIRCLE #716, TEMPLE, TX, WAS DISCIPLINED BY GEORGIA ON JULY 12, 1996
DISCIPLINARY ACTION: SURRENDER OF LICENSE
OFFENSE: PROFESSIONAL MISCONDUCT

NOTES: UNPROFESSIONAL CONDUCT.

BROWN, STEVEN M MD, LICENSE NUMBER 0A49127 OF DALLAS, TX, WAS DISCIPLINED BY CALIFORNIA ON JULY 14, 1994
DISCIPLINARY ACTION: 60-MONTH PROBATION
OFFENSE: CRIMINAL CONVICTION OR PLEA OF GUILTY, NOLO CONTENDERE, OR NO CONTEST TO A CRIME

NOTES: THREE SUBSTANCE ABUSE CONVICTIONS IN TEXAS, 1985 TO 1988; FAILED TO DISCLOSE THEM IN HIS APPLICATION FOR CALIFORNIA LICENSE IN 1989. REVOCATION STAYED.

BROWN, STUART L MD OF 1258 PROSPECT STREET, LA JOLLA, CA, WAS DISCIPLINED BY DEA ON APRIL 12, 1990
DISCIPLINARY ACTION: SURRENDER OF CONTROLLED SUBSTANCE LICENSE
OFFENSE: SUBSTANDARD CARE, INCOMPETENCE OR NEGLIGENCE

NOTES: MEDICAL LICENSE REVOKED 09/21/89 FOR GROSS NEGLIGENCE, INCOMPETENCE AND SEXUAL MISCONDUCT.

BROWN, STUART L MD, DATE OF BIRTH JANUARY 10, 1933 OF 6687 LA JOLLA SCENIC DR, LA JOLLA, CA, WAS DISCIPLINED BY MEDICARE ON MAY 22, 1990
DISCIPLINARY ACTION: EXCLUSION FROM THE MEDICARE AND/OR MEDICAID PROGRAM
OFFENSE: DISCIPLINARY ACTION BY ANOTHER STATE OR AGENCY

NOTES: LICENSE REVOCATION OR SUSPENSION.

BROWN, STUART L MD, DATE OF BIRTH JANUARY 10, 1933, LICENSE NUMBER 0016045 OF 1258 PROSPECT, LA JOLLA, CA, WAS DISCIPLINED BY MINNESOTA ON NOVEMBER 14, 1992
DISCIPLINARY ACTION: SURRENDER OF LICENSE
OFFENSE: DISCIPLINARY ACTION BY ANOTHER STATE OR AGENCY

NOTES: DISCIPLINARY ACTION BY ANOTHER STATE; ENGAGING IN CONDUCT WITH A PATIENT WHICH IS SEXUAL OR MAY REASONABLY BE INTERPRETED BY THE PATIENT AS SEXUAL.

BROWN, STUART LEO MD, LICENSE NUMBER 00C7341 OF LA JOLLA, CA, WAS DISCIPLINED BY TEXAS ON MAY 24, 1990
DISCIPLINARY ACTION: SURRENDER OF LICENSE

NOTES: STIPULATED ORDER. MEDICAL LICENSE VOLUNTARILY SURRENDERED IN LIEU OF DISCIPLINARY HEARING.

BROWN, WILLIAM C MD, LICENSE NUMBER 00H3859, WAS DISCIPLINED BY TEXAS ON AUGUST 17, 1996
DISCIPLINARY ACTION: LICENSE SUSPENSION; REQUIRED TO TAKE ADDITIONAL MEDICAL EDUCATION
OFFENSE: CRIMINAL CONVICTION OR PLEA OF GUILTY, NOLO CONTENDERE, OR NO CONTEST TO A CRIME

NOTES: IN 1991 BEGAN USING DRUGS, NAMELY COCAINE, AND WAS USING THE DRUG REGULARLY AFTER HIS WIFE LEFT HIM AND HIS FINANCIAL SITUATION DETERIORATED; HAD PREVIOUSLY ENGAGED IN RECREATIONAL USE OF DRUGS AND ALCOHOL ON AN INTERMITTENT BASIS SINCE EARLY ADULTHOOD; IN FEBRUARY 1993 ENTERED A 30 DAY INPATIENT TREATMENT FACILITY; IN JUNE 1993 RELAPSED AND ENTERED INTO TREATMENT FOR AFTERCARE AND COMPLETED SIX WEEKS OF RESIDENTIAL FACILITY REHABILITATION CONTRACT WITH A COLLEGE OF MEDICINE NOT RENEWED IN 7/93; RELAPSED AGAIN WITH THE USE OF COCAINE AND METHAMPHETAMINE WHICH CONTINUED UNINTERRUPTED UNTIL 9/21/95; ON 1/11/95 ARRESTED FOR INTENT TO DELIVER COCAINE AND AMPHETAMINE, PLED GUILTY TO THESE CHARGES AND WAS PLACED ON DEFERRED

ADJUDICATION ON 9/21/95 FOR FIVE YEARS; COMPLETED A 30 DAY PROGRAM FOR SUBSTANCE ABUSE; SUBMITS TO WEEKLY AND RANDOM DRUG SCREENS AND PARTICIPATES IN AA AND SPONSORS OTHER SUBSTANCE ABUSERS; AND ON 7/15/96 ENTERED INTO A CONTRACT WITH AN IMPAIRED PHYSICIANS SUPERVISION PROGRAM. SUSPENSION UNTIL HE REQUESTS THE SUSPENSION TO BE STAYED OR LIFTED AND APPEARS BEFORE THE BOARD AND PROVIDES SUFFICIENT EVIDENCE THAT INDICATES THAT HE IS PHYSICALLY, MENTALLY, AND OTHERWISE COMPETENT TO SAFELY PRACTICE MEDICINE. INCLUDING AT A MINIMUM COMPLETE COPIES OF MEDICAL RECORDS AND REPORTS OF PSYCHOLOGICAL AND NEUROPSYCHIATRIC EVALUATIONS, INCLUDING A 96 HOUR INPATIENT EVALUATION, CONDUCTED BY A BOARD APPROVED CERTIFIED PSYCHIATRIST; SUCCESSFUL COMPLETION OR COMPLIANCE WITH ALL TERMS AND CONDITIONS OF HIS DEFERRED ADJUDICATION OF 9/21/95; AND COMPLETION OF 50 HOURS OF CONTINUING MEDICAL EDUCATION; EVIDENCE THAT HE IS NOT THE SUBJECT OF ANY OTHER COMPLAINTS.

BROWN, WILLIAM C MD, DATE OF BIRTH JULY 22, 1961 OF 14800 MEMORIAL #40, HOUSTON, TX, WAS DISCIPLINED BY MEDICARE ON DECEMBER 30, 1996
DISCIPLINARY ACTION: EXCLUSION FROM THE MEDICARE AND/OR MEDICAID PROGRAM
OFFENSE: NONCOMPLIANCE WITH A PROFESSIONAL RULE

NOTES: DEFAULTED ON PUBLIC HEALTH SERVICE EDUCATION LOAN. INDEFINITE EXCLUSION.

BROWNE, DUNCAN JAMES MD, LICENSE NUMBER 00H9193 OF HOUSTON, TX, WAS DISCIPLINED BY TEXAS ON JUNE 22, 1994
DISCIPLINARY ACTION: 60-MONTH RESTRICTION PLACED ON LICENSE; REQUIRED TO TAKE ADDITIONAL MEDICAL EDUCATION
OFFENSE: SUBSTANCE ABUSE

NOTES: HAS A HISTORY OF ABUSING THE DRUG NITROUS OXIDE SINCE 1991; DRUG USE SECONDARY TO DEPRESSION DUE TO FAMILY MATTERS; RECEIVED OUTPATIENT TREATMENT IN 1991 AND UNDERWENT PSYCHIATRIC CARE; SOBRIETY DATE IS 6/17/92; COMPLETED A ONE YEAR RECOVERY AND SUPERVISION PROGRAM WITH THE UNIVERSITY OF TEXAS; CURRENTLY MEETS WITH PSYCHIATRIST AND PSYCHOLOGIST ONCE A MONTH. LICENSE RESTRICTED FIVE YEARS WITH THE FOLLOWING CONDITIONS: SHALL ABSTAIN FROM THE CONSUMPTION OF ALCOHOL/CHEMICAL SUBSTANCES IN ANY FORM UNLESS PRESCRIBED BY ANOTHER PHYSICIAN FOR A LEGITIMATE AND THERAPEUTIC PURPOSE; SHALL NOT TREAT OR OTHERWISE SERVE AS PHYSICIAN, PRESCRIBE, DISPENSE, OR ADMINISTER DRUGS THAT MAY BE SUBJECT TO ABUSE TO HIMSELF OR ANY MEMBER OF HIS FAMILY; SHALL LIMIT MEDICAL PRACTICE SOLELY TO THE PRACTICE OF ANESTHESIOLOGY IN A HOSPITAL OR OUTPATIENT PAIN SETTING; SHALL NOT POSSESS, ADMINISTER, DISPENSE OR PRESCRIBE ANY CONTROLLED SUBSTANCES OR DANGEROUS DRUGS EXCEPT AS NECESSARY FOR TREATMENT OF INPATIENTS IN HOSPITAL OR OUTPATIENT PAIN SETTING; SHALL CONTINUE TO PARTICIPATE IN AA'S PROGRAM AT LEAST THREE TIMES A WEEK WITH QUARTERLY REPORTS TO THE BOARD; SHALL SUBMIT HIMSELF FOR APPROPRIATE EXAMS INCLUDING DRUG OR ALCOHOL SCREENS; SHALL CONTINUE TO MEET WITH PSYCHIATRIST AND PSYCHOLOGIST MONTHLY WITH QUARTERLY REPORTS; SHALL ATTEND AT LEAST 50 HOURS PER YEAR OF CONTINUING MEDICAL EDUCATION; SHALL APPEAR BEFORE THE BOARD ONCE A YEAR; SHALL GIVE A COPY OF THIS ORDER TO ANY HEALTH CARE ENTITY WHERE HE HAS PRIVILEGES; SHALL COOPERATE WITH THE BOARD IN VERIFYING COMPLIANCE; SHALL INFORM BOARD OF CHANGE OF ADDRESS WITHIN 10 DAYS OR IF HE LEAVES THE STATE; TIME SPENT OUT OF TEXAS DOES NOT COUNT TOWARD PROBATION. SHALL NOT SEEK MODIFICATION FOR ONE YEAR. ON 8/17/96 THE BOARD DENIED HIS PETITION FOR TERMINATION OF THIS ORDER. ON 8/9/97 THE BOARD GRANTED HIS PETITION FOR TERMINATION OF THIS ORDER BASED ON COMPLIANCE WITH CONDITIONS.

BROXTON, KYREL DARICE MD, DATE OF BIRTH JUNE 18, 1952, LICENSE NUMBER 00G2333 OF 17070 RED OAK DRIVE SUITE 101, HOUSTON, TX, WAS DISCIPLINED BY TEXAS ON AUGUST 20, 1993
DISCIPLINARY ACTION: REPRIMAND; REQUIRED TO TAKE ADDITIONAL MEDICAL EDUCATION
OFFENSE: SUBSTANDARD CARE, INCOMPETENCE OR NEGLIGENCE

NOTES: INAPPROPRIATELY HANDLED THE FLUID AND ELECTROLYTE BALANCE OF A 20 MONTH OLD CHILD AND INAPPROPRIATELY TREATED HIS HYPERGLYCEMIA ON 12/19/88 WHEN THE PATIENT APPEARED IN AN EMERGENCY ROOM IN RESPIRATORY DISTRESS; SHE OBTAINED CONSULTATION WHEN SHE RECOGNIZED THE CHILD'S CARE WAS BEYOND HER CAPABILITIES. FOR THREE YEARS SHE SHALL ATTEND AT LEAST 50 HOURS PER YEAR OF CONTINUING MEDICAL EDUCATION INCLUDING COURSES RELATING TO FLUID AND ELECTROLYTE MANAGEMENT AND METABOLIC AND ACUTE-CARE MANAGEMENT; SHALL GIVE A COPY OF THIS ORDER TO ANY HEALTH CARE ENTITY WHERE SHE HAS PRIVILEGES; SHALL COOPERATE WITH THE BOARD IN VERIFYING COMPLIANCE; SHALL INFORM BOARD OF CHANGE OF ADDRESS WITHIN 10 DAYS OR IF SHE LEAVES THE STATE; TIME SPENT OUT OF TEXAS DOES NOT COUNT TOWARDS ORDER. SHALL NOT SEEK MODIFICATION FOR ONE YEAR. ON 9/30/94 ORDER WAS TERMINATED.

BRUNKEN, ROBERT B MD, LICENSE NUMBER 00C3593 OF DALLAS, TX, WAS DISCIPLINED BY TEXAS ON AUGUST 19, 1994
DISCIPLINARY ACTION: 60-MONTH PROBATION; MONITORING OF PHYSICIAN PERFORMANCE
OFFENSE: SUBSTANCE ABUSE

NOTES: ENTERED TREATMENT AND PARTICIPATED WITH A PROFESSIONALS TREATMENT PROGRAM FOR LONG TERM TREATMENT OF ALCOHOL DEPENDENCE; SELF-REPORTED THIS TREATMENT TO THE BOARD; IS BEING TREATED BY A PSYCHIATRIST, ATTENDS AA AND HAS REGULAR URINE SCREENS. SUSPENSION STAYED. CONDITIONS OF PROBATION: SHALL ABSTAIN FROM THE CONSUMPTION OF ALCOHOL/CHEMICAL SUBSTANCES IN ANY FORM UNLESS PRESCRIBED BY ANOTHER PHYSICIAN FOR LEGITIMATE AND THERAPEUTIC PURPOSES; SHALL SUBMIT HIMSELF FOR APPROPRIATE EXAMS INCLUDING DRUG OR ALCOHOL SCREENS; SHALL PARTICIPATE IN AA'S PROGRAM NOT LESS THAN THREE TIMES A WEEK WITH QUARTERLY REPORTS TO THE BOARD; SHALL SUBMIT HIMSELF FOR EVALUATION AND TREATMENT TO A BOARD-APPROVED PSYCHIATRIST WITH REPORTS TO THE BOARD; SHALL NOT TREAT OR OTHERWISE SERVE AS PHYSICIAN, PRESCRIBE, DISPENSE OR ADMINISTER ANY DRUGS THAT MAY BE SUBJECT TO ABUSE TO HIMSELF OR ANY MEMBER OF HIS FAMILY; SHALL APPEAR BEFORE THE BOARD ONCE A YEAR; SHALL GIVE A COPY OF THIS ORDER TO ANY HEALTH CARE ENTITY WHERE HE HAS

PRIVILEGES; SHALL COOPERATE WITH THE BOARD IN VERIFYING COMPLIANCE; SHALL INFORM BOARD OF CHANGE OF ADDRESS WITHIN 1O DAYS OR IF HE LEAVES THE STATE; TIME SPENT OUT OF TEXAS DOES NOT COUNT TOWARD PROBATION. SHALL NOT SEEK MODIFICATION FOR ONE YEAR. ON 8/17/96 THE BOARD DENIED HIS PETITION FOR TERMINATION OF THIS ORDER. ON 4/4/98 PETITION TO MODIFY ORDER GRANTED REDUCING PSYCHIATRIC TREATMENTS FROM MONTHLY TO QUARTERLY.

BRUSENHAN, ROBERT LEE JR MD, LICENSE NUMBER C4961 OF SAN ANTONIO, TX, WAS DISCIPLINED BY TEXAS ON AUGUST 22, 1998
DISCIPLINARY ACTION: REQUIRED TO TAKE ADDITIONAL MEDICAL EDUCATION; REQUIRED TO ENTER AN IMPAIRED PHYSICIAN PROGRAM OR SUBSTANCE ABUSE TREATMENT
OFFENSE: LOSS OR RESTRICTION OF HOSPITAL PRIVILEGES

NOTES: ON 11/1/95 NURSES, STAFF, AND INMATES OF THE INSTITUTION COMPLAINED THAT HE SMELLED OF ALCOHOL, WALKED POORLY, AND APPEARED DRUNK; ON 11/2/95 THE STAFF DISCUSSED THE ALCOHOL PROBLEM WITH HIM; HE MAINTAINS THAT HE HAS NEVER BEEN IMPAIRED WHILE PRACTICING MEDICINE, THAT HE OFFERED HIS RESIGNATION ON 11/5/95 AND THAT THE RESIGNATION OFFER WAS DECLINED; ON 5/1/96 HE REGISTERED A 37 mg/Dl BLOOD ALCOHOL CONCENTRATION (LEGAL CONCENTRATION IS 100 mg/dL); ON 5/3/96 HE WAS TERMINATED DUE TO WORKING UNDER THE INFLUENCE OF ALCOHOL; HE MAINTAINS THAT HE WAS NOT UNDER THE INFLUENCE ON 5/1/96; IN 1996 A MEDICAL SOCIETY RECOMMENDED HE UNDERGO A 96 HOUR PSYCHIATRIC EVALUATION WHICH HE REFUSED; HE MAINTAINS THAT HE OFFERED THE MEDICAL SOCIETY THAT HE UNDERGO AN EVALUATION AT ANY FACILITY IN TEXAS WHICH THEY REFUSED; IN 12/97, UPON RECOMMENDATION BY THE BOARD, HE UNDERWENT A 96 HOUR PSYCHIATRIC EVALUATION AT COPAC, INC.; COPAC DIAGNOSED HIM WITH ALCOHOL ABUSE, RULE OUT DEPENDENCE, NICOTINE DEPENDENCE, AND OBSESSIVE-COMPULSIVE FEATURES. LICENSE LIMITED FOR FIVE YEARS AS FOLLOWS: SHALL FOLLOW COPAC RECOMMENDATIONS INCLUDING ATTENDING OUTPATIENT TREATMENT, AND A CONTRACT WITH RECOVERING PHYSICIAN'S COMMITTEE; SHALL NOMINATE THREE CERTIFIED PSYCHIATRISTS FOR BOARD SELECTION OF A THERAPIST AND SHALL EXPEDITIOUSLY SUBMIT HIMSELF TO EVALUATION AND TREATMENT BY THE APPROVED PRACTITIONER; SHALL PARTICIPATE IN AA'S PROGRAM NOT LESS THAN THREE TIMES A WEEK; SHALL REPORT ON HIS ATTENDANCE; SHALL ABSTAIN FROM THE CONSUMPTION OF ALCOHOL/DRUGS IN ANY FORM UNLESS PRESCRIBED BY ANOTHER PHYSICIAN FOR A LEGITIMATE AND THERAPEUTIC PURPOSE; SHALL SUBMIT HIMSELF FOR APPROPRIATE EXAMS INCLUDING DRUG OR ALCOHOL SCREENS; SHALL RECEIVE CARE AND TREATMENT FROM A BOARD CERTIFIED PHYSICIAN WHO SPECIALIZES IN INTERNAL MEDICINE OR FAMILY PRACTICE WITH QUARTERLY REPORTS; SHALL NOT TREAT OR OTHERWISE SERVE AS PHYSICIAN, PRESCRIBE, DISPENSE OR ADMINISTER DRUGS THAT MAY BE SUBJECT TO ABUSE TO HIMSELF; SHALL ATTEND 1 COURSE IN RISK MANAGEMENT DURING EACH YEAR OF THE ORDER; SHALL APPEAR BEFORE THE BOARD UPON REQUEST; SHALL COOPERATE WITH THE BOARD IN VERIFYING COMPLIANCE INCLUDING PROVIDING COPIES OF MEDICAL RELEASES UPON REQUEST; SHALL GIVE A COPY OF THIS ORDER TO ANY HEALTH CARE ENTITY WHERE HE HAS PRIVILEGES; SHALL PROVIDE A COPY OF THIS ORDER TO ANYONE REQUESTING IT WITHIN 10 DAYS; TIME SPENT OUT OF TEXAS DOES NOT COUNT TOWARD RESTRICTION; SHALL INFORM THE BOARD OF CHANGE OF ADDRESS WITHIN 10 DAYS OR IF HE LEAVES THE STATE; SHALL NOT SEEK MODIFICATION FOR ONE YEAR.

BRYANT, MARY M MD, LICENSE NUMBER 0033408 OF PUYALLUP, WA, WAS DISCIPLINED BY WASHINGTON ON AUGUST 23, 1996
DISCIPLINARY ACTION: SURRENDER OF LICENSE

BRYANT, MARY M MD, WAS DISCIPLINED BY NEBRASKA ON JUNE 6, 1997
DISCIPLINARY ACTION: LICENSE REVOCATION
OFFENSE: DISCIPLINARY ACTION BY ANOTHER STATE OR AGENCY

NOTES: OTHER STATE ACTION.

BRYANT, MARY M MD, DATE OF BIRTH APRIL 6, 1951 OF 14819 113TH AVENUE COURT E, PUYALLUP, WA, WAS DISCIPLINED BY MEDICARE ON NOVEMBER 20, 1997
DISCIPLINARY ACTION: EXCLUSION FROM THE MEDICARE AND/OR MEDICAID PROGRAM
OFFENSE: DISCIPLINARY ACTION BY ANOTHER STATE OR AGENCY

NOTES: LICENSE REVOKED, SUSPENDED, SURRENDERED OR OTHERWISE LOST FOR REASONS BEARING ON PROFESSIONAL PERFORMANCE, PROFESSIONAL COMPETENCE OR FINANCIAL INTEGRITY.

BRYANT, MARY M MD, LICENSE NUMBER H6786 OF PUYALLUP, WA, WAS DISCIPLINED BY TEXAS ON DECEMBER 10, 1998
DISCIPLINARY ACTION: LICENSE REVOCATION
OFFENSE: DISCIPLINARY ACTION BY ANOTHER STATE OR AGENCY

NOTES: ON 8/19/96 SHE VOLUNTARILY SURRENDERED HER WASHINGTON MEDICAL LICENSE AS A RESULT OF HER FAILURE TO COMPLETE TREATMENT FOR ALCOHOL ABUSE; IN 1/96 AND 2/96 ALCOHOL HAD BEEN SMELLED ON HER BREATH WHILE SHE WAS TREATING PATIENTS; ENTERED TREATMENT BUT LEFT AGAINST MEDICAL ADVICE; VIOLATED A 9/5/89 TEXAS AGREEMENT BY USING ALCOHOL, NOT PARTICIPATING IN AA, NOT MAKING WRITTEN REPORTS TO THE BOARD AND NOT INFORMING BOARD OF ADDRESS CHANGE. ACTION WILL NOT BE FINAL UNTIL ALL APPEALS EXHAUSTED.

BRYANT, MARY MADELINE MD, LICENSE NUMBER 0003899, WAS DISCIPLINED BY SOUTH DAKOTA ON DECEMBER 4, 1996
DISCIPLINARY ACTION: SURRENDER OF LICENSE
OFFENSE: SUBSTANCE ABUSE

NOTES: IN 1988 VOLUNTARILY UNDERWENT TREATMENT FOR ALCOHOL ABUSE; IN 1989 GRANTED A LICENSE TO PRACTICE IN TEXAS AND ENTERED INTO AN AGREEMENT TO ABSTAIN FROM ALCOHOL AND PARTICIPATE IN AA; IN JANUARY AND FEBRUARY 1996 A MEDICAL ASSISTANT SMELLED ALCOHOL ON HER BREATH WHILE SHE WAS TREATING PATIENTS ON FOUR OR FIVE OCCASIONS; ON 5/02/96 SEVERAL STAFF MEMBERS SMELLED ALCOHOL ON HER BREATH WHILE SHE WAS TREATING PATIENTS AND WHEN SHE UNDERWENT A BREATH-ALCOHOL TEST AND A BLOOD ALCOHOL TEST AND BOTH TEST RESULTS WERE POSITIVE FOR THE PRESENCE OF ALCOHOL; ON 7/10/96 SHE ENTERED SPRINGBROOK NORTHWEST FOR TREATMENT AND EVALUATION OF ALCOHOL ABUSE; SHE LEFT SPRINGBROOK NORTHWEST AGAINST MEDICAL ADVICE AND WITHOUT COMPLETING TREATMENT OR EVALUATION.

BUCKLEY, THOMAS P MD, LICENSE NUMBER F2571 OF DALLAS, TX, WAS DISCIPLINED BY TEXAS ON FEBRUARY 7, 1998
DISCIPLINARY ACTION: FINE; REPRIMAND
OFFENSE: OVERPRESCRIBING OR MISPRESCRIBING DRUGS

NOTES: FOR SEVERAL YEARS, CONCLUDING IN 1996, HE PRESCRIBED TO AN ADULT PATIENT ON A FREQUENT AND CONTINUOUS BASIS LARGE QUANTITIES OF CONTROLLED SUBSTANCES WITHOUT PERFORMING ADEQUATE SUBSEQUENT REASSESSMENTS OF THE PATIENT'S MEDICAL CONDITION, INCLUDING WHAT EFFECT THE PRESCRIBED MEDICATION WAS HAVING; HE DID NOT ADEQUATELY FOLLOW THE PATIENT, IN THAT HE INFREQUENTLY EXAMINED THEM IN LIGHT OF THE AMOUNT AND FREQUENCY OF THE PRESCRIPTIONS, MOST OF WHICH WERE TELEPHONE REFILLS AND WITHOUT TREATING THE PATIENT'S UNDERLYING MEDICAL CONDITION; PRESCRIBING WAS MEDICALLY EXCESSIVE AND WITHOUT LEGITIMATE RATIONALE; IN 1993 HE PRESCRIBED DRUGS FOR AN ADULT PATIENT DESPITE HIS NOTING THAT THE PATIENT SHOULD NO LONGER RECEIVE MEDICATION OF THE KIND PRESCRIBED BY HIM. $1,000 FINE; SHALL COOPERATE WITH THE BOARD IN VERIFYING COMPLIANCE.

BUNN, RUSSELL B DO, LICENSE NUMBER 00C5945 OF MT ENTERPRISE, TX, WAS DISCIPLINED BY TEXAS ON MARCH 1, 1990
DISCIPLINARY ACTION: 120-MONTH RESTRICTION PLACED ON CONTROLLED SUBSTANCE LICENSE

NOTES: STIPULATED ORDER. MUST CEASE PRESCRIBING, ADMINISTERING, SUPPLYING OR DISPENSING CONTROLLED SUBSTANCES AND DANGEROUS DRUGS. ORDER IN EFFECT FOR TEN YEARS BEGINNING 90 DAYS FROM 12/4/89.

BUNN, RUSSELL BURTON DO OF PO BOX 160, MOUNT ENTERPRISE, TX, WAS DISCIPLINED BY DEA ON MARCH 12, 1990
DISCIPLINARY ACTION: SURRENDER OF CONTROLLED SUBSTANCE LICENSE
OFFENSE: OVERPRESCRIBING OR MISPRESCRIBING DRUGS

NOTES: PRESCRIBED CONTROLLED SUBSTANCES FOR NONTHERAPEUTIC REASON AND FAILED TO KEEP PROPER RECORDS AND MAINTAIN INVENTORIES OF CONTROLLED SUBSTANCES DISPENSED TO PATIENTS.

BURGOS, HERNAN ENRIQUE MD, DATE OF BIRTH JULY 14, 1926 OF PO BOX 629, #29107-077, BASTROP, TX, WAS DISCIPLINED BY MEDICARE ON OCTOBER 5, 1997
DISCIPLINARY ACTION: 120-MONTH EXCLUSION FROM THE MEDICARE AND/OR MEDICAID PROGRAM
OFFENSE: CRIMINAL CONVICTION OR PLEA OF GUILTY, NOLO CONTENDERE, OR NO CONTEST TO A CRIME

NOTES: CONVICTED OF A CRIME RELATED TO THE DELIVERY OF HEALTH CARE OR FINANCIAL MISCONDUCT INVOLVING A GOVERNMENT-OPERATED PROGRAM.

BURGOS, HERNAN ENRIQUE MD, LICENSE NUMBER D2649 OF FORT WORTH, TX, WAS DISCIPLINED BY TEXAS ON JANUARY 28, 1999
DISCIPLINARY ACTION: LICENSE REVOCATION; FINE
OFFENSE: CRIMINAL CONVICTION OR PLEA OF GUILTY, NOLO CONTENDERE, OR NO CONTEST TO A CRIME

NOTES: ON OR ABOUT 11/7/96 AFTER ENTERING A PLEA OF "NOT GUILTY," HE WAS CONVICTED OF 14 COUNTS OF MAIL FRAUD AND AIDING AND ABETTING IN A SCHEME TO FACILITATE THE PAYMENT OF MORE THAN $1,000,000,00 TO THE PSYCHIATRIC INSTITUTE OF FORT WORTH GENERATED BY FALSE HEALTH INSURANCE CLAIMS. $15,000 FINE. ACTION WILL NOT BE FINAL UNTIL ALL APPEALS HAVE BEEN EXHAUSTED

BURKES, WALTER JOE MD, LICENSE NUMBER 00G6909 OF MEMPHIS, TN, WAS DISCIPLINED BY TEXAS ON JULY 1, 1990
DISCIPLINARY ACTION: LICENSE SUSPENSION
OFFENSE: LOSS OR RESTRICTION OF HOSPITAL PRIVILEGES

NOTES: FAILURE TO PRACTICE MEDICINE IN ACCEPTABLE MANNER CONSISTENT WITH PUBLIC HEALTH AND WELFARE. DISCIPLINED BY LICENSED HOSPITAL OR MEDICAL STAFF. LICENSE SUSPENDED INDEFINITELY UNTIL HE APPEARS BEFORE BOARD AND SHOWS GOOD CAUSE WHY LICENSE SHOULD BE REINSTATED.

BURKETT, DAVID G MD, LICENSE NUMBER 55163 OF 141 DESIARD STREET, MONROE, LA, WAS DISCIPLINED BY MASSACHUSETTS ON JULY 28, 1999
DISCIPLINARY ACTION: SURRENDER OF LICENSE
OFFENSE: DISCIPLINARY ACTION BY ANOTHER STATE OR AGENCY

NOTES: ALLEGATIONS THAT HE WAS DISCIPLINED IN LOUISIANA; RELAPSED INTO THE USE OF ALCOHOL AND LOST HIS CLINICAL PRIVILEGES AT THREE HOSPITALS AS A RESULT OF FABRICATING DATA AND RECORDING PROCEDURES THAT WERE NEVER PERFORMED. VOLUNTARY PERMANENT RESIGNATION WHILE INVESTIGATION PENDING.

BURKETT, DAVID GARY MD, LICENSE NUMBER 00E9555 OF MONROE, LA, WAS DISCIPLINED BY TEXAS ON OCTOBER 26, 1990
DISCIPLINARY ACTION: MONITORING OF PHYSICIAN PERFORMANCE

NOTES: MUST COMPLY WITH LOUISIANA RESTRICTIONS AND AUTHORIZE LOUISIANA BOARD TO RELEASE INFORMATION AS TO STATUS AND PROBATIONARY COMPLIANCE; RECEIVE APPROVAL FROM TEXAS BOARD PRIOR TO PRACTICING MEDICINE IN TEXAS.

BURKETT, DAVID GARY MD OF MONROE, LA, WAS DISCIPLINED BY LOUISIANA ON MAY 5, 1997
DISCIPLINARY ACTION: 6-MONTH LICENSE SUSPENSION; 36-MONTH PROBATION
OFFENSE: SUBSTANDARD CARE, INCOMPETENCE OR NEGLIGENCE

NOTES: RECURRING ABUSE OF ALCOHOL; INABILITY TO PRACTICE MEDICINE WITH REASONABLE SKILL AND SAFETY; EFFORTS TO DECEIVE OR DEFRAUD THE PUBLIC; MAKING OR SUBMITTING FALSE, DECEPTIVE OR UNFOUNDED CLAIMS OR REPORTS; PROFESSIONAL OR MEDICAL INCOMPETENCY; UNPROFESSIONAL CONDUCT; LICENSE SUBJECT TO GENERAL PROBATIONARY TERMS: MAINTENANCE OF COMPLETE ABSTINENCE FROM THE USE OF ALCOHOL AND MOOD-ALTERING DRUGS (INCLUDING STADOL, NUBANE AND DALGAN); PARTICIPATION IN PHYSICIANS' HEALTH PROGRAM OF THE LOUISIANA STATE MEDICAL SOCIETY; SUBMISSION TO PERIODIC, UNANNOUNCED DRUG AND ALCOHOL SCREENS; MONITORING FOR BIPOLAR DISORDER; WEEKLY CONSULTATION WITH COUNSELOR; PAYMENT OF $5,000 FINE. DECISION AMENDED BY ORDERS ISSUED 7/14/97 AND 8/21/97, VACATING SIX MONTH SUSPENSION, PERMITTING HIM TO RESUME NON-INVASIVE CARDIOLOGY FOR THREE MONTHS AND INVASIVE CARDIOLOGY THEREAFTER.

BURKETT, DAVID GARY MD, DATE OF BIRTH OCTOBER 19, 1950, LICENSE NUMBER 019791E OF 3 BUIE DRIVE, MONROE, LA, WAS DISCIPLINED BY PENNSYLVANIA ON NOVEMBER 18, 1997
DISCIPLINARY ACTION: 36-MONTH PROBATION
OFFENSE: DISCIPLINARY ACTION BY ANOTHER STATE OR AGENCY

NOTES: DISCIPLINARY ACTION TAKEN BY LOUISIANA. THREE-

YEAR SUSPENSION STAYED.

BURKETT, DAVID GARY MD, LICENSE NUMBER E9555 OF MONROE, LA, WAS DISCIPLINED BY TEXAS ON APRIL 4, 1998
DISCIPLINARY ACTION: 36-MONTH PROBATION; MONITORING OF PHYSICIAN PERFORMANCE
OFFENSE: DISCIPLINARY ACTION BY ANOTHER STATE OR AGENCY
NOTES: ON 5/5/97 LICENSE SUSPENDED THEN PLACED ON PROBATION BY LOUISIANA BOARD FOR ALCOHOL ABUSE AND A DIAGNOSIS OF BIPOLAR DISORDER; ALSO DISCIPLINED BY THE PENNSYLVANIA BOARD BASED ON THE LOUISIANA BOARD ORDERS. SUSPENSION STAYED FOR PROBATION WITH FOLLOWING TERMS AND CONDITIONS: SHALL ABSTAIN FROM THE CONSUMPTION OF ALCOHOL/DRUGS IN ANY FORM UNLESS PRESCRIBED BY ANOTHER PHYSICIAN FOR THERAPEUTIC PURPOSES; SHALL UNDERGO A COMPLETE EXAM BY A BOARD-APPROVED PHYSICIAN WITH MONTHLY REPORTS TO THE BOARD; SHALL SUBMIT HIMSELF FOR APPROPRIATE EXAMS INCLUDING DRUG OR ALCOHOL SCREENS; SHALL PARTICIPATE IN THE ACTIVITIES OF A PHYSICIAN HEALTH AND REHABILITATION COMMITTEE AND ATTEND WEEKLY MEETINGS WITH QUARTERLY REPORTS; SHALL PARTICIPATE IN AA'S PROGRAM NOT LESS THAN THREE TIMES A WEEK; SHALL REPORT ON HIS ATTENDANCE; SHALL NOT TREAT OR OTHERWISE SERVE AS PHYSICIAN, PRESCRIBE, DISPENSE OR ADMINISTER DRUGS THAT MAY BE SUBJECT TO ABUSE TO HIMSELF OR TO ANY MEMBER OF HIS FAMILY; SEPARATE FROM PATIENT RECORDS, SHALL MAINTAIN A LOGBOOK OF EVERY PRESCRIPTION WRITTEN BY HIM FOR DANGEROUS DRUGS WITH ADDICTIVE POTENTIAL WHICH SHALL BE MADE AVAILABLE FOR REVIEW; SHALL APPEAR BEFORE THE BOARD ONCE A YEAR; SHALL COOPERATE WITH THE BOARD IN VERIFYING COMPLIANCE INCLUDING PROVIDING COPIES OF MEDICAL RELEASES AND ANY REPORTS SENT TO LOUISIANA AND PENNSYLVANIA; SHALL GIVE A COPY OF THIS ORDER TO ANY HEALTH CARE ENTITY WHERE HE HAS PRIVILEGES; TIME SPENT OUT OF TEXAS DOES NOT COUNT TOWARD PROBATION; SHALL INFORM THE BOARD OF CHANGE OF ADDRESS WITHIN 10 DAYS OR IF HE LEAVES THE STATE; SHALL NOT SEEK MODIFICATION FOR ONE YEAR. ON 10/24/98 THE BOARD ORDERED THAT THE 4/4/98 BOARD ORDER BE CORRECTED TO INCLUDE THE FOLLOWING STATEMENT: "THIS ORDER SUPERSEDES ALL PREVIOUS ORDERS OF THE BOARD."

BURLESON, JAMES D MD, LICENSE NUMBER 00H1932 OF BIG SPRING, TX, WAS DISCIPLINED BY TEXAS ON AUGUST 19, 1994
DISCIPLINARY ACTION: 60-MONTH PROBATION; RESTRICTION PLACED ON CONTROLLED SUBSTANCE LICENSE
OFFENSE: OVERPRESCRIBING OR MISPRESCRIBING DRUGS
NOTES: ADMITTED THAT HE WROTE PRESCRIPTIONS FOR CONTROLLED SUBSTANCES, SPECIFICALLY DEMEROL, IN THE NAME OF A PATIENT AND THEN DIVERTED THE SUBSTANCES TO A RELATIVE; HAS BEEN UNDER SIGNIFICANT STRESS DUE TO HIS DAUGHTER'S ILLNESS; HAS RECEIVED TREATMENT REGARDING CO-DEPENDENCY PROBLEMS; IS CURRENTLY SEEING A PSYCHOLOGIST. SUSPENSION STAYED. CONDITIONS OF PROBATION: SHALL ABSTAIN FROM THE CONSUMPTION OF ALCOHOL/CHEMICAL SUBSTANCES IN ANY FORM UNLESS PRESCRIBED BY ANOTHER PHYSICIAN FOR A LEGITIMATE AND THERAPEUTIC PURPOSE; SHALL SUBMIT HIMSELF FOR APPROPRIATE EXAMS INCLUDING DRUG OR ALCOHOL SCREENS; WITHIN ONE YEAR SHALL PASS THE MEDICAL JURISPRUDENCE EXAM; SHALL ATTEND AT LEAST 50 HOURS PER YEAR OF CONTINUING MEDICAL EDUCATION; SHALL SURRENDER ALL UNUSED TRIPLICATE PRESCRIPTION FORMS AND 222 FORMS IN HIS POSSESSION OTHER THAN THOSE ASSOCIATED WITH HIS EMS DIRECTORSHIP; SEPARATE FROM PATIENT RECORDS, SHALL MAINTAIN A FILE OF EVERY PRESCRIPTION WRITTEN FOR DANGEROUS DRUGS WHICH SHALL BE AVAILABLE FOR INSPECTION; SHALL NOT CALL IN ANY PRESCRIPTIONS FOR CONTROLLED SUBSTANCES OR DANGEROUS DRUGS; SHALL NOT POSSESS, ADMINISTER, DISPENSE OR PRESCRIBE ANY CONTROLLED SUBSTANCES BUT MAY ORDER THEM TO BE ADMINISTERED TO HOSPITAL OR NURSING HOME PATIENTS; SHALL NOT TREAT OR OTHERWISE SERVE AS PHYSICIAN, PRESCRIBE, DISPENSE OR ADMINISTER DRUGS THAT MAY BE SUBJECT TO ABUSE TO HIMSELF OR ANY MEMBER OF HIS FAMILY; SHALL CONTINUE TO RECEIVE PSYCHIATRIC TREATMENT WITH QUARTERLY REPORTS; SHALL COMPLY WITH TERMS OF HIS CONTRACT WITH SCENIC MOUNTAIN MEDICAL CENTER; SHALL APPEAR BEFORE THE BOARD ONCE A YEAR; SHALL GIVE A COPY OF THIS ORDER TO ANY HEALTH CARE ENTITY WHERE HE HAS PRIVILEGES; SHALL COOPERATE WITH THE BOARD IN VERIFYING COMPLIANCE; SHALL INFORM BOARD OF CHANGE OF ADDRESS WITHIN 10 DAYS OR IF HE LEAVES THE STATE; TIME SPENT OUT OF TEXAS DOES NOT COUNT TOWARD PROBATION. SHALL NOT SEEK MODIFICATION FOR ONE YEAR. ON 3/27/95 ORDER MODIFIED AS FOLLOWS: HE ADMITTED ABUSING DEMEROL, LORCET, FIORCET AND ELAVIL DURING THE LAST TWO YEARS AND ETHYL CHLORIDE DURING THE LAST NINE MONTHS; PRIVILEGES IN A HOSPITAL WERE TERMINATED; HIS TREATING PSYCHIATRIST WAS SPECIFIED AND HE MUST COMPLY WITH THE TERMS OF ANY AFTERCARE CONTRACT HE MAY EXECUTE; SHALL PROVIDE MEDICAL RELEASES REQUIRED TO OBTAIN TREATMENT RECORDS. ON 8/9/97 PETITION TO MODIFY ORDER DENIED. ON 5/16/98 PETITION TO MODIFY ORDER GRANTED ALLOWING HIM TO PRESCRIBE CONTROLLED SUBSTANCES UNLESS OTHERWISE PROHIBITED BY THIS ORDER, AND TO RECEIVE TREATMENT FROM A PSYCHIATRIST APPROVED BY THE BOARD. ON 5/14/99 ORDER TERMINATED.

BURLTON, ROGERS C MD, LICENSE NUMBER 0D04506 OF 981 RUSSELL AVE, GAITHERSBURG, MD, WAS DISCIPLINED BY MARYLAND ON MAY 24, 1995
DISCIPLINARY ACTION: 24-MONTH PROBATION
OFFENSE: SUBSTANDARD CARE, INCOMPETENCE OR NEGLIGENCE
NOTES: FAILED TO MEET STANDARDS OF CARE IN HIS PRACTICE OF PSYCHIATRY IN REGARD TO ONE CASE THAT WAS SUBJECT TO PEER REVIEW. ON 7/31/96 PROBATION TERMINATED.

BURLTON, ROGERS C MD, LICENSE NUMBER 00D4055 OF GAITHERSBURG, TX, WAS DISCIPLINED BY TEXAS ON MAY 15, 1996
DISCIPLINARY ACTION: LICENSE SUSPENSION
OFFENSE: DISCIPLINARY ACTION BY ANOTHER STATE OR AGENCY
NOTES: DISCIPLINARY ACTION BY MARYLAND IN THAT ON 5/24/95 LICENSE PLACED ON TWO YEAR PROBATION WITH CONDITIONS BASED ON TREATMENT OF ONE PATIENT WHERE IT WAS FOUND HE HAD TAKEN SERIOUS POTENTIAL RISKS AND CROSSED APPROPRIATE BOUNDARIES; HAD A NAIVE AND THOUGHTLESS APPROACH TO THESE RISKS. SHALL NOT PRACTICE IN TEXAS UNTIL HE REQUESTS PERMISSION TO RESUME PRACTICE, APPEARS

BEFORE BOARD AND PROVIDES SUFFICIENT EVIDENCE WHICH INDICATES THAT HE IS PHYSICALLY, MENTALLY AND OTHERWISE COMPETENT TO SAFELY PRACTICE MEDICINE INCLUDING AT A MINIMUM EVIDENCE THAT HE IS IN COMPLIANCE WITH TERMS OF HIS MARYLAND ORDER AND EVIDENCE THAT HE IS NOT THE SUBJECT OF ANY OTHER FORMAL COMPLAINT OR DISCIPLINARY PROCEEDING WITH ANY STATE OR FEDERAL LICENSING ENTITY. SHALL NOT SEEK MODIFICATION FOR ONE YEAR.

BURLTON, ROGERS C MD, LICENSE NUMBER 00D4055, WAS DISCIPLINED BY TEXAS ON NOVEMBER 16, 1996
DISCIPLINARY ACTION: REQUIRED TO TAKE ADDITIONAL MEDICAL EDUCATION
OFFENSE: DISCIPLINARY ACTION BY ANOTHER STATE OR AGENCY

NOTES: DISCIPLINARY ACTION BY MARYLAND BOARD. ON 7/31/96 MARYLAND PROBATION TERMINATED. GRANTED PERMISSION TO PRACTICE IN TEXAS UPON THE FOLLOWING TERMS: MUST PASS THE TEXAS MEDICAL JURISPRUDENCE EXAMINATION; MUST COMPLETE AT LEAST ONE CONTINUING MEDICAL EDUCATION COURSE IN TRANSFERENCE/COUNTER-TRANSFERENCE OR PHYSICIAN-PATIENT BOUNDARIES WITHIN ONE YEAR; SHALL SUBMIT HIMSELF FOR EVALUATION AND TREATMENT BY A BOARD- APPROVED PSYCHIATRIST.

BUSHART, JAMES F MD OF DALLAS, TX, WAS DISCIPLINED BY LOUISIANA ON MAY 21, 1992
DISCIPLINARY ACTION: PROBATION
OFFENSE: DISCIPLINARY ACTION BY ANOTHER STATE OR AGENCY

NOTES: ADMINISTRATIVE ACTION BY TEXAS; HABITUAL OR RECURRING ABUSE OF ALCOHOL. PROBATION FOR PERIOD CONCURRENT WITH PROBATION IMPOSED BY TEXAS STATE BOARD OF MEDICAL EXAMINERS, SUBJECT TO CONTINUING COMPLETE COMPLIANCE WITH TERMS OF ORDER PREVIOUSLY ENTERED BY TEXAS BOARD, PRIOR NOTICE TO BOARD OF INTENT TO RELOCATE PRACTICE TO LOUISIANA, MAINTENANCE OF COMPLETE ABSTINENCE FROM THE USE OF ALCOHOL AND OTHER MOOD-ALTERING SUBSTANCES.

BUSHART, JAMES F MD OF 9406 DIXIE LANE, DALLAS, TX, WAS DISCIPLINED BY DEA ON SEPTEMBER 6, 1994
DISCIPLINARY ACTION: SURRENDER OF CONTROLLED SUBSTANCE LICENSE
OFFENSE: DISCIPLINARY ACTION BY ANOTHER STATE OR AGENCY

NOTES: STATE BOARD.

BUSHART, JAMES F MD OF JACKSON, MS, WAS DISCIPLINED BY LOUISIANA ON DECEMBER 8, 1994
DISCIPLINARY ACTION: LICENSE SUSPENSION; MONITORING OF PHYSICIAN PERFORMANCE
OFFENSE: DISCIPLINARY ACTION BY ANOTHER STATE OR AGENCY

NOTES: HABITUAL AND RECURRING ABUSE OF DRUGS, INCLUDING ALCOHOL; DISCIPLINARY ACTION BY TEXAS; VIOLATION OF PREVIOUS BOARD ORDER. REINSTATEMENT CONDITIONED UPON REINSTATEMENT OF UNRESTRICTED MEDICAL LICENSURE IN TEXAS; PERIODIC REPORTS ON TREATMENT DURING SUSPENSION; MAINTENANCE OF COMPLETE ABSTINENCE FROM THE USE OF ALCOHOL AND OTHER MOOD-ALTERING SUBSTANCES AND OTHER CONDITIONS AS DETERMINED BY THE BOARD.

BUSHART, JAMES FREDERICK MD, LICENSE NUMBER 00G5869 OF DALLAS, TX, WAS DISCIPLINED BY TEXAS ON AUGUST 24, 1991
DISCIPLINARY ACTION: 36-MONTH PROBATION; MONITORING OF PHYSICIAN PERFORMANCE
OFFENSE: FAILURE TO COMPLY WITH PREVIOUS BOARD ORDER

NOTES: VIOLATION OF PREVIOUS AGREED ORDER. SHALL PARTICIPATE IN AA; SHALL APPEAR BEFORE BOARD ONCE A YEAR; SHALL SUBMIT TO DRUG OR ALCOHOL SCREENS.

BUSHART, JAMES FREDERICK MD, LICENSE NUMBER 00G5869 OF RIDGELAND, MS, WAS DISCIPLINED BY TEXAS ON JUNE 22, 1994
DISCIPLINARY ACTION: LICENSE SUSPENSION
OFFENSE: LOSS OR RESTRICTION OF HOSPITAL PRIVILEGES

NOTES: LICENSE WAS PLACED ON PROBATION FOR FIVE YEARS ON 10/20/86; EXHIBITED A HISTORY OF ALCOHOL AND OPIATE ABUSE BETWEEN 1986 AND 1990 AND SUFFERED RELAPSES IN 8/88 AND 5/90; LICENSE AGAIN PLACED ON PROBATION ON 8/24/91; SUFFERED RELAPSES IN 9/92 AND 9/93 AFTER WHICH HE WAS ADMITTED FOR TREATMENT; IN OCTOBER 1993 AND DECEMBER 1993 HOSPITAL PRIVILEGES WERE TERMINATED AT TWO FACILITIES. BASED ON THE RELAPSE. SUSPENSION UNTIL SUCH TIME AS HE APPEARS BEFORE THE BOARD AND PROVIDES SUFFICIENT EVIDENCE THAT INDICATES HE IS PHYSICALLY, MENTALLY AND OTHERWISE COMPETENT TO SAFELY PRACTICE.

BUSHART, JAMES FREDERICK MD, DATE OF BIRTH JULY 31, 1950 OF 110 PINE KNOLL DRIVE #243, RIDGELAND, MS, WAS DISCIPLINED BY MEDICARE ON APRIL 23, 1996
DISCIPLINARY ACTION: EXCLUSION FROM THE MEDICARE AND/OR MEDICAID PROGRAM
OFFENSE: DISCIPLINARY ACTION BY ANOTHER STATE OR AGENCY

NOTES: LICENSE SUSPENDED FOR REASONS BEARING ON PROFESSIONAL PERFORMANCE.

BUTKA, GARY N MD, LICENSE NUMBER 00G6479 OF BROWNWOOD, TX, WAS DISCIPLINED BY TEXAS ON MAY 11, 1995
DISCIPLINARY ACTION: FINE
OFFENSE: NONCOMPLIANCE WITH A PROFESSIONAL RULE

NOTES: DURING 1993 AND 1994, DID NOT COMPLETE 16 DEATH CERTIFICATES IN A TIMELY MANNER AS REQUIRED BY THE TEXAS HEALTH AND SAFETY CODE; MAINTAINS THAT THE DELAYS WERE A RESULT OF A HIGH PATIENT CASE LOAD AND HAS REPORTED INITIATING CHANGES IN PROCEDURE TO ELIMINATE FUTURE DELAYS. SHALL PAY $3,200 FINE; SHALL FULLY COOPERATE WITH BOARD IN VERIFYING COMPLIANCE.

BUTLER, WELDON FRED MD, LICENSE NUMBER 00H0224 OF ODESSA, TX, WAS DISCIPLINED BY TEXAS ON MARCH 1, 1996
DISCIPLINARY ACTION: MONITORING OF PHYSICIAN PERFORMANCE
OFFENSE: SUBSTANCE ABUSE

NOTES: ON 1/07/96 ARRESTED IN ODESSA, TEXAS FOR PUBLIC INTOXICATION; ADMITTED THAT ON 5/10/93 ARRESTED IN MIDLAND TEXAS FOR PUBLIC INTOXICATION; AND ON 1/08/96 WAS ADMITTED FOR EVALUATION AND TREATMENT RELATED TO SUBSTANCE ABUSE. SHALL NOT PRACTICE MEDICINE IN TEXAS UNTIL HE PERSONALLY APPEARS BEFORE THE BOARD AND PROVIDES SUFFICIENT EVIDENCE AND INFORMATION WHICH ADEQUATELY INDICATES THAT HE IS PHYSICALLY, MENTALLY, AND OTHERWISE COMPETENT TO SAFELY PRACTICE MEDICINE INCLUDING AT A MINIMUM VERIFIED COPIES OF ALL RECORDS RELATING TO EVALUATION AND/OR TREATMENT FOR SUBSTANCE ABUSE FROM 1/01/93 THROUGH THE DATE HE REQUESTS PERMISSION TO

RESUME PRACTICE, DIARIES OF LOGS DEMONSTRATING HIS HISTORY OF ATTENDANCE AT AA, AND COPIES OF ANY AFTER TREATMENT OR MONITORING CONTRACTS ENTERED INTO; SHALL ABSTAIN FROM THE CONSUMPTION OF ALCOHOL/DRUGS IN ANY FORM UNLESS PRESCRIBED BY ANOTHER PHYSICIAN FOR A LEGITIMATE AND THERAPEUTIC PURPOSE; SHALL SUBMIT HIMSELF FOR APPROPRIATE EXAMS, INCLUDING DRUG OR ALCOHOL SCREENS; SHALL COOPERATE WITH THE BOARD IN VERIFYING COMPLIANCE INCLUDING PROVIDING COPIES OF MEDICAL RELEASES UPON REQUEST; SHALL GIVE A COPY OF THIS ORDER TO ANY HEALTH CARE ENTITY WHERE HE HAS PRIVILEGES; SHALL PROVIDE A COPY OF THIS ORDER TO ANYONE REQUESTING IT WITHIN 10 DAYS; SHALL INFORM THE BOARD OF CHANGE OF ADDRESS WITHIN 10 DAYS.

BUTLER, WELDON FRED MD, LICENSE NUMBER 00H0224 OF ODESSA, TX, WAS DISCIPLINED BY TEXAS ON MAY 15, 1996
DISCIPLINARY ACTION: 60-MONTH PROBATION; REQUIRED TO TAKE ADDITIONAL MEDICAL EDUCATION
OFFENSE: SUBSTANCE ABUSE

NOTES: BASED ON AN INPATIENT SUBSTANCE ABUSE EVALUATION OF HIM REQUESTED BY THE BOARD AND CONDUCTED DURING HOSPITALIZATION FROM 4/1/96 TO 4/4/96, IT WAS INDICATED THAT HE IS PHYSICALLY, MENTALLY AND OTHERWISE COMPETENT TO SAFELY PRACTICE MEDICINE. SUSPENSION STAYED. PROBATION WITH TERMS AND CONDITIONS: SHALL ABSTAIN FROM THE CONSUMPTION OF ALCOHOL/DRUGS IN ANY FORM UNLESS PRESCRIBED BY ANOTHER PHYSICIAN FOR A LEGITIMATE AND THERAPEUTIC PURPOSE; SHALL SUBMIT HIMSELF FOR APPROPRIATE EXAMS INCLUDING DRUG OR ALCOHOL SCREENS; SHALL SUBMIT HIMSELF FOR EVALUATION AND TREATMENT BY A BOARD-APPROVED PSYCHIATRIST WHOM HE SHALL SEE AT LEAST ONCE A MONTH AND WHO SHALL SUBMIT REPORTS TO THE BOARD; SHALL CONTINUE TO PARTICIPATE IN AA'S PROGRAM NOT LESS THAN THREE TIMES A WEEK WITH QUARTERLY REPORTS TO THE BOARD; SHALL PARTICIPATE IN THE ACTIVITIES OF A PHYSICIAN'S HEALTH AND REHABILITATION GROUP AND ATTEND WEEKLY MEETINGS WITH QUARTERLY REPORTS; SHALL COMPLY WITH TERMS OF THE CONTINUING CARE CONTRACT WITH THE HOSPITAL AND SHALL PROVIDE QUARTERLY REPORTS TO THE BOARD; SHALL NOT TREAT OR OTHERWISE SERVE AS PHYSICIAN, PRESCRIBE, DISPENSE OR ADMINISTER DRUGS THAT MAY BE SUBJECT TO ABUSE TO HIMSELF OR TO ANY MEMBER OF HIS FAMILY; SHALL OBTAIN AT LEAST 50 HOURS OF CONTINUING MEDICAL EDUCATION PER YEAR; SHALL APPEAR BEFORE BOARD AT LEAST TWO TIMES PER YEAR OR AT BOARD REQUEST; SHALL COOPERATE WITH THE BOARD IN VERIFYING COMPLIANCE INCLUDING PROVIDING COPIES OF MEDICAL RELEASES UPON REQUEST; SHALL GIVE A COPY OF THIS ORDER TO ANY HEALTH CARE ENTITY WHERE HE HAS PRIVILEGES; SHALL PROVIDE A COPY OF THIS ORDER TO ANYONE REQUESTING IT WITHIN 10 DAYS; TIME SPENT OUT OF TEXAS DOES NOT COUNT TOWARD PROBATION; SHALL INFORM BOARD OF CHANGE OF ADDRESS WITHIN 10 DAYS OR IF HE LEAVES THE STATE. SHALL NOT SEEK MODIFICATION FOR ONE YEAR. ON 11/22/97 PETITION TO MODIFY ORDER GRANTED REDUCING FOLLOW-UP PSYCHIATRIC CARE FROM MONTHLY TO QUARTERLY. ON 10/24/98 ORDER TERMINATED.

BUTTERY, HAROLD DONOP MD OF 1023 NIX PROF BLDG, SAN ANTONIO, TX, WAS DISCIPLINED BY DEA ON FEBRUARY 23, 1999
DISCIPLINARY ACTION: SURRENDER OF CONTROLLED SUBSTANCE LICENSE

NOTES: IN LIEU OF PUBLIC INTEREST REVOCATION.

BYRNE, MICHAEL EDWARD MD, LICENSE NUMBER 00E2495 OF HOUSTON, TX, WAS DISCIPLINED BY TEXAS ON AUGUST 18, 1995
DISCIPLINARY ACTION: REQUIRED TO TAKE ADDITIONAL MEDICAL EDUCATION; MONITORING OF PHYSICIAN PERFORMANCE
OFFENSE: OVERPRESCRIBING OR MISPRESCRIBING DRUGS

NOTES: BETWEEN 1/92 AND 8/94 ADMINISTERED OR ORDERED MULTIPLE INJECTIONS OF NUBAIN OR STADOL AND/OR PHENERGAN FOR A PATIENT WITHOUT ADEQUATELY DOCUMENTED INDICATIONS; FAILED TO ADEQUATELY DOCUMENT THE BASIS FOR THE DIAGNOSIS OF INTRACTABLE PAIN AND/OR OTHER EFFORTS ATTEMPTED TO RESOLVE THE PAIN IN THE CASE OF THE PATIENT; HE NEITHER ADMITS NOR DENIES THE ALLEGATIONS. LICENSE RESTRICTED FOR TWO YEARS WITH TERMS: SHALL MAINTAIN ADEQUATE MEDICAL RECORDS WHICH SHALL BE AVAILABLE FOR REVIEW; SHALL NOT PRESCRIBE OR ADMINISTER ANY DRUG FOR ANY PATIENT UNLESS IT IS MEDICALLY INDICATED AND IS PRESCRIBED IN THERAPEUTIC DOSES AND HE HAS CONDUCTED AN ADEQUATE EXAMINATION AND HISTORY; SHALL OBTAIN AT LEAST 50 HOURS PER YEAR OF CONTINUING MEDICAL EDUCATION; SHALL APPEAR BEFORE THE BOARD AT LEAST ONCE A YEAR OR UPON BOARD REQUEST; SHALL COOPERATE WITH THE BOARD IN VERIFYING COMPLIANCE; SHALL GIVE A COPY OF THIS ORDER TO ANY HEALTH CARE ENTITY WHERE HE HAS PRIVILEGES; SHALL PROVIDE A COPY OF THIS ORDER TO ANYONE REQUESTING IT WITHIN 10 DAYS; TIME SPENT OUT OF TEXAS DOES NOT COUNT TOWARD RESTRICTION; SHALL INFORM BOARD OF CHANGE OF ADDRESS WITHIN 10 DAYS OR IF HE LEAVES THE STATE. SHALL NOT SEEK MODIFICATION FOR ONE YEAR.

BYRNES, ROBERT J DO, LICENSE NUMBER J1904 OF JACKSONVILLE, TX, WAS DISCIPLINED BY TEXAS ON AUGUST 9, 1997
DISCIPLINARY ACTION: FINE
OFFENSE: OVERPRESCRIBING OR MISPRESCRIBING DRUGS

NOTES: IN 1/97 HE PRESCRIBED TYLENOL #4 , A CONTROLLED SUBSTANCE, TO AN INDIVIDUAL WHO HE DID NOT EXAMINE AND FOR WHOM HE DID NOT MAINTAIN MEDICAL RECORDS. $2,000 FINE.

CADDELL, JAMES DONALD DO, LICENSE NUMBER 00F6497 OF DALLAS, TX, WAS DISCIPLINED BY TEXAS ON APRIL 21, 1990

NOTES: STIPULATED ORDER. MUST MAINTAIN COMPLETE AND ACCURATE RECORDS OF PURCHASES AND DISPOSALS OF CONTROLLED SUBSTANCES. ORDER EFFECTIVE FOR THREE YEARS.

CAMMACK, JAMES THOMAS MD OF GRIGGS PROF BUILDING #300, KERRVILLE, TX, WAS DISCIPLINED BY DEA ON AUGUST 23, 1994
DISCIPLINARY ACTION: SURRENDER OF CONTROLLED SUBSTANCE LICENSE
OFFENSE: CRIMINAL CONVICTION OR PLEA OF GUILTY, NOLO CONTENDERE, OR NO CONTEST TO A CRIME

NOTES: CONVICTED OF OBTAINING CONTROLLED SUBSTANCE BY FRAUD.

CAMMACK, JAMES THOMAS MD, LICENSE NUMBER 00H5696 OF KERRVILLE, TX, WAS DISCIPLINED BY TEXAS ON MAY 11, 1995

DISCIPLINARY ACTION: 60-MONTH PROBATION; RESTRICTION PLACED ON CONTROLLED SUBSTANCE LICENSE
OFFENSE: SUBSTANCE ABUSE

NOTES: FROM APPROXIMATELY 8/93 TO 8/94, SELF-PRESCRIBED AND INGESTED TYLENOL WITH CODEINE WITHOUT A LEGITIMATE MEDICAL PURPOSE; IN 8/94, SURRENDERED HIS DEA AND DPS CONTROLLED SUBSTANCES REGISTRATION CERTIFICATES; WHILE UNDER BOARD INVESTIGATION IN 8/94, VOLUNTARILY ADMITTED HIMSELF AS AN INPATIENT TO A CHEMICAL SUBSTANCE ABUSE TREATMENT FACILITY; AFTER FOUR WEEKS, ENTERED OUTPATIENT AFTERCARE TREATMENT UNDER THE CARE OF A BOARD-CERTIFIED PSYCHIATRIST; REPORTS HIS CONTINUED PARTICIPATION IN OUTPATIENT PROGRAM; REPORTS HIS SOBRIETY DATE AS 8/25/94. SUSPENSION STAYED. PROBATION WITH TERMS: SHALL ABSTAIN FROM THE CONSUMPTION OF ALCOHOL/DRUGS IN ANY FORM UNLESS PRESCRIBED BY ANOTHER PHYSICIAN FOR A LEGITIMATE AND THERAPEUTIC PURPOSE; SHALL SUBMIT HIMSELF FOR APPROPRIATE EXAMS INCLUDING DRUG OR ALCOHOL SCREENS; SHALL CONTINUE TO RECEIVE CARE AND TREATMENT FROM THE BOARD-APPROVED PHYSICIAN AT LEAST ONCE A MONTH WHO SHALL SUBMIT QUARTERLY REPORTS TO THE BOARD; SHALL PARTICIPATE IN NARCOTICS ANONYMOUS PROGRAMS NOT LESS THAN THREE TIMES A WEEK WITH QUARTERLY REPORTS TO THE BOARD; SHALL CONTINUE TO PARTICIPATE IN ACTIVITIES OF AN IMPAIRED PHYSICIANS GROUP AND ATTEND WEEKLY MEETINGS WITH QUARTERLY REPORTS; MAY REAPPLY WITH THE PROPER GOVERNMENTAL AUTHORITIES FOR A PERMIT FOR SCHEDULE IV AND V CONTROLLED SUBSTANCES ONLY; SHALL NOT ATTEMPT TO REREGISTER OR OTHERWISE OBTAIN CONTROLLED SUBSTANCES REGISTRATIONS WITHOUT PRIOR AUTHORITY FROM THE BOARD; SHALL NOT TREAT OR OTHERWISE SERVE AS PHYSICIAN, PRESCRIBE, DISPENSE OR ADMINISTER DRUGS THAT MAY BE SUBJECT TO ABUSE TO HIMSELF OR A MEMBER OF HIS FAMILY; SHALL MAINTAIN A FILE OF EVERY PRESCRIPTION WRITTEN FOR DANGEROUS DRUGS WITH ADDICTIVE POTENTIAL WHICH SHALL BE AVAILABLE FOR REVIEW; SHALL NOT TELEPHONE IN PRESCRIPTIONS OR REFILL OF DRUGS; SHALL OBTAIN AT LEAST 50 HOURS PER YEAR OF CONTINUING MEDICAL EDUCATION; SHALL APPEAR BEFORE BOARD AT LEAST TWO TIMES PER YEAR AND AT BOARD REQUEST; SHALL INFORM BOARD OF CHANGE OF ADDRESS WITHIN 10 DAYS OR IF HE LEAVES THE STATE; SHALL COOPERATE WITH BOARD IN VERIFYING COMPLIANCE INCLUDING PROVIDING MEDICAL RELEASES AND PEER REVIEW RECORDS UPON REQUEST; SHALL GIVE A COPY OF THIS ORDER TO ANY HEALTH CARE ENTITY WHERE HE HAS PRIVILEGES; SHALL PROVIDE A COPY OF THIS ORDER TO ANYONE REQUESTING IT WITHIN 10 DAYS; TIME PERIOD OUT OF TEXAS DOES NOT COUNT TOWARD PROBATION. SHALL NOT SEEK MODIFICATION FOR ONE YEAR.

CAMMACK, JAMES THOMAS MD, LICENSE NUMBER H5696, WAS DISCIPLINED BY TEXAS ON MAY 10, 1997
DISCIPLINARY ACTION: 120-MONTH PROBATION; RESTRICTION PLACED ON CONTROLLED SUBSTANCE LICENSE
OFFENSE: FAILURE TO COMPLY WITH PREVIOUS BOARD ORDER

NOTES: ON 5/11/95 HE ENTERED INTO AN AGREED ORDER WITH THE BOARD WHICH SUSPENDED HIS LICENSE, STAYED THE SUSPENSION, AND PLACED IT ON PROBATION FOR FIVE YEARS. HE WAS PLACED ON ULTRAM, A DANGEROUS DRUG, BY HIS TREATING PHYSICIAN IN OCTOBER OR NOVEMBER 1995, FOR STRESS HEADACHES. HE ALSO OBTAINED THE DRUG THROUGH SAMPLES KEPT IN HIS OFFICE, AND ON 4/17/96 HE HAD A SEIZURE WHICH WAS PROBABLY DUE TO HIS EXTENSIVE USE OF ULTRAM (10-12 TABLETS A DAY). ON 4/29/96 HE ENTERED A SPECIFIED FACILITY FOR A 96-HOUR EVALUATION. HE DID NOT AGREE WITH THE ASSESSMENT OR RECOMMENDATIONS AND SOUGHT ANOTHER OPINION AND TREATMENT AT A SECOND FACILITY, WHERE HE WAS TREATED FROM 6/25/96 TO 8/17/96. HE REPORTS A SOBRIETY DATE OF 4/17/96. SUSPENSION STAYED FOR PROBATION UNDER THE FOLLOWING TERMS: SHALL ABSTAIN FROM THE CONSUMPTION OF ALCOHOL/DRUGS IN ANY FORM UNLESS PRESCRIBED BY ANOTHER PHYSICIAN FOR A LEGITIMATE AND THERAPEUTIC PURPOSE; SHALL SUBMIT HIMSELF FOR APPROPRIATE EXAMS INCLUDING DRUG OR ALCOHOL SCREENS; SHALL CONTINUE TO RECEIVE TREATMENT AND CARE FROM SPECIFIED PHYSICIAN NO LESS THAN MONTHLY WITH QUARTERLY REPORTS; SHALL PARTICIPATE IN THE ACTIVITIES OF A PHYSICIAN HEALTH AND REHABILITATION COMMITTEE AND ATTEND WEEKLY MEETINGS WITH QUARTERLY REPORTS; SHALL PARTICIPATE IN AA'S PROGRAM NOT LESS THAN THREE TIMES A WEEK; SHALL REPORT ON HIS ATTENDANCE; SHALL COMPLY WITH HIS CONTINUING CARE CONTRACT; HE IS AUTHORIZED TO REAPPLY TO THE DEA AND THE TEXAS DEPARTMENT OF SAFETY TO OBTAIN AUTHORIZATION TO PRESCRIBE SCHEDULES IV AND V CONTROLLED SUBSTANCES; EXCEPT AS OTHERWISE PROVIDED FOR IN THIS ORDER, HE SHALL NOT POSSESS ALCOHOL, CONTROLLED SUBSTANCES, OR DANGEROUS DRUGS; SHALL NOT TREAT OR OTHERWISE SERVE AS PHYSICIAN, PRESCRIBE, DISPENSE OR ADMINISTER DRUGS THAT MAY BE SUBJECT TO ABUSE TO HIMSELF OR TO ANY MEMBER OF HIS FAMILY; SEPARATE FROM PATIENT RECORDS, SHALL MAINTAIN A FILE OF EVERY PRESCRIPTION WRITTEN BY HIM FOR DANGEROUS DRUGS WITH ADDICTIVE POTENTIAL WHICH SHALL BE MADE AVAILABLE FOR REVIEW; SHALL MAINTAIN ADEQUATE MEDICAL RECORDS WHICH SHALL BE AVAILABLE FOR REVIEW; SHALL OBTAIN AT LEAST 50 HOURS CONTINUING MEDICAL EDUCATION PER YEAR; SHALL APPEAR BEFORE THE BOARD AT LEAST TWICE YEARLY; SHALL NOT HAVE PHYSICAL ACCESS TO SAMPLES OF CONTROLLED SUBSTANCES OR DANGEROUS DRUGS; SHALL COOPERATE WITH THE BOARD IN VERIFYING COMPLIANCE INCLUDING PROVIDING COPIES OF MEDICAL RELEASES UPON REQUEST; SHALL GIVE A COPY OF THIS ORDER TO ANY HEALTH CARE ENTITY WHERE HE HAS PRIVILEGES; SHALL PROVIDE A COPY OF THIS ORDER TO ANYONE REQUESTING IT WITHIN 10 DAYS; TIME SPENT OUT OF TEXAS DOES NOT COUNT TOWARD PROBATION; SHALL INFORM THE BOARD OF CHANGE OF ADDRESS WITHIN 10 DAYS OR IF HE LEAVES THE STATE; SHALL NOT SEEK MODIFICATION FOR ONE YEAR. ON 5/14/99 THE ORDER WAS MODIFIED AS FOLLOWS: HE IS AUTHORIZED TO REAPPLY TO THE DEA AND DPS TO OBTAIN CONTROLLED SUBSTANCE REGISTRATION FOR ALL SCHEDULES; REGISTRATIONS LIMITED TO PRESCRIBING OF THESE SUBSTANCES; ALL OTHER PROVISIONS OF THE ORDER REMAIN IN FULL EFFECT UNTIL SUPERSEDED BY A SUBSEQUENT ORDER.

CANNON, CARRIE S MD, LICENSE NUMBER H7277 OF HOUSTON, TX, WAS DISCIPLINED BY TEXAS ON NOVEMBER 10, 1998
DISCIPLINARY ACTION: EMERGENCY SUSPENSION

NOTES: EVIDENCE AND INFORMATION THAT HER

CONTINUATION IN THE PRACTICE OF MEDICINE WOULD CONSTITUTE A CONTINUING THREAT TO PUBLIC WELFARE.

CANNON, RICHARD A MD, LICENSE NUMBER C6271 OF RICHMOND, TX, WAS DISCIPLINED BY TEXAS ON AUGUST 28, 1999
DISCIPLINARY ACTION: 120-MONTH PROBATION; RESTRICTION PLACED ON CONTROLLED SUBSTANCE LICENSE
OFFENSE: OVERPRESCRIBING OR MISPRESCRIBING DRUGS

NOTES: FROM 1/94 - 12/95 HE PRESCRIBED LARGE AMOUNTS OF DEMEROL, ORALLY AND BY INTRAMUSCULAR INJECTION, TO A PATIENT REPEATEDLY FOR COMPLAINT OF SEVERE MIGRAINE HEADACHES WHO WAS SIMULTANEOUSLY UNDER THE CARE OF ANOTHER PHYSICIAN FOR HER MIGRAINE HEADACHES WHO WAS ALSO PROVIDING HER TREATMENT WITH DEMEROL, PROPOXYPHENE AND SEDATIVE-HYPNOTIC MEDICATIONS. LICENSE LIMITED AS FOLLOWS: WITHIN 30 DAYS SHALL TERMINATE, IN WRITING, HIS PHYSICIAN-PATIENT RELATIONSHIP AND TREATMENT OF PATIENT MENTIONED, AND PROVIDE A COPY OF THE TERMINATION LETTER FOR THE DIRECTOR OF COMPLIANCE; SHALL LIMIT HIS PRESCRIBING OR ADMINISTERING OF SCHEDULED II AND II-N CONTROLLED SUBSTANCES TO PATIENTS 18 YEARS OF AGE OR YOUNGER; SHALL APPEAR BEFORE THE BOARD AT LEAST ONCE A YEAR; SHALL COOPERATE WITH THE BOARD IN VERIFYING COMPLIANCE; TIME SPENT OUT OF TEXAS DOES NOT COUNT TOWARD PROBATION; SHALL INFORM THE BOARD OF CHANGE OF ADDRESS WITHIN 10 DAYS OR IF HE LEAVES THE STATE; SHALL NOT SEEK MODIFICATION FOR ONE YEAR.

CAPLAN, MISCHA MD, LICENSE NUMBER 00B9072 OF HOUSTON, TX, WAS DISCIPLINED BY TEXAS ON JUNE 28, 1995
DISCIPLINARY ACTION: SURRENDER OF LICENSE

NOTES: VOLUNTARY AND PERMANENT SURRENDER OF LICENSE IN LIEU OF FURTHER PROCEEDINGS ON ALLEGATIONS THAT HE VIOLATED THE MEDICAL PRACTICE ACT. DOES NOT ADMIT VIOLATION.

CARAM, PEDRO C MD, LICENSE NUMBER 00C5628 OF HOUSTON, TX, WAS DISCIPLINED BY TEXAS ON OCTOBER 13, 1995
DISCIPLINARY ACTION: RESTRICTION PLACED ON LICENSE; REQUIRED TO TAKE ADDITIONAL MEDICAL EDUCATION
OFFENSE: PHYSICAL OR MENTAL ILLNESS INHIBITING THE ABILITY TO PRACTICE WITH SKILL AND SAFETY

NOTES: REPORTS THAT HE HAS SUFFERED MULTIPLE CEREBRAL INFARCTIONS WHICH HAVE RESULTED IN HIS DISCONTINUING THE PRACTICE OF MEDICINE; HE REPORTS THAT DUE TO HIS PHYSICAL INABILITY TO PRACTICE HE VOLUNTARILY CLOSED HIS MEDICAL PRACTICE ON 12/31/94; SELF REPORTED THIS CONDITION TO THE BOARD; BOARD ALSO RECEIVED INFORMATION WHICH ALLEGES THAT HE VIOLATED THE MEDICAL PRACTICE ACT. DOES NOT ADMIT VIOLATION. LICENSE RESTRICTED SO THAT HE MAY NOT EXAMINE, DIAGNOSE, EVALUATE OR TREAT PATIENTS UNTIL HE REQUESTS TO HAVE RESTRICTION LIFTED AND APPEARS BEFORE BOARD WITH SUFFICIENT EVIDENCE WHICH INDICATES THAT HE IS PHYSICALLY, MENTALLY AND OTHERWISE COMPETENT TO SAFELY PRACTICE MEDICINE INCLUDING AT A MINIMUM PROVIDING COPIES OF MEDICAL RECORDS AND REPORTS OF COMPLETE PHYSICAL EXAMINATION AS WELL AS PSYCHOLOGICAL AND NEUROPSYCHIATRIC EVALUATIONS BY A BOARD-CERTIFIED PSYCHIATRIST AND NEUROLOGIST; PASSAGE OF THE SPECIAL PURPOSE EXAMINATION; AND PROOF THAT HE HAS OBTAINED AT LEAST 24 HOURS PER YEAR OF CONTINUING MEDICAL EDUCATION.

CARNINE, KENNETH S MD, LICENSE NUMBER 0010798 OF MT VERNON, WA, WAS DISCIPLINED BY WASHINGTON ON MARCH 11, 1993
DISCIPLINARY ACTION: EMERGENCY SUSPENSION
OFFENSE: SEXUAL ABUSE OF OR SEXUAL MISCONDUCT WITH A PATIENT

NOTES: ALLEGATIONS OF MORAL TURPITUDE, ABUSE AND/OR SEXUAL CONTACT WITH A PATIENT.

CARNINE, KENNETH S MD, LICENSE NUMBER 00D4946 OF MT VERNON, WA, WAS DISCIPLINED BY TEXAS ON SEPTEMBER 30, 1994
DISCIPLINARY ACTION: SURRENDER OF LICENSE
OFFENSE: DISCIPLINARY ACTION BY ANOTHER STATE OR AGENCY

NOTES: ALLEGATIONS OF DISCIPLINARY ACTION BY ANOTHER STATE OR BY THE UNIFORMED SERVICES OF THE U.S. SURRENDER IN LIEU OF FURTHER INVESTIGATION; SHALL NOT PETITION FOR REINSTATEMENT OF LICENSE.

CARNINE, KENNETH S MD, LICENSE NUMBER 0010798 OF MOUNT VERNON, WA, WAS DISCIPLINED BY WASHINGTON ON APRIL 21, 1995
DISCIPLINARY ACTION: SURRENDER OF LICENSE; FINE
OFFENSE: CRIMINAL CONVICTION OR PLEA OF GUILTY, NOLO CONTENDERE, OR NO CONTEST TO A CRIME

NOTES: PLED GUILTY TO ONE COUNT OF FOURTH DEGREE ASSAULT, DESCRIBED AS INTENTIONAL OR OFFENSIVE CONTACT WITH ANOTHER PERSON WITHOUT THE PERMISSION OF THAT PERSON AND NOT IN SELF DEFENSE; THE VICTIM WAS A FEMALE PATIENT; A JAIL SENTENCE AND FINE OF $2,500 WAS IMPOSED; FROM APPROXIMATELY 1975 UNTIL 1993, HE PERFORMED BREAST OR PELVIC EXAMINATIONS ON 25 FEMALE PATIENTS WHICH DID NOT MEET THE STANDARD OF A REASONABLY PRUDENT PHYSICIAN PRACTICING IN WASHINGTON. SHALL PERMANENTLY SURRENDER HIS WASHINGTON LICENSE, NEVER TO PRACTICE MEDICINE OR SURGERY IN THIS STATE; $1,000 FINE.

CARNINE, KENNETH S MD, DATE OF BIRTH DECEMBER 20, 1941 OF PO BOX 2662, RANCHO MIRAGE, CA, WAS DISCIPLINED BY MEDICARE ON APRIL 9, 1996
DISCIPLINARY ACTION: 60-MONTH EXCLUSION FROM THE MEDICARE AND/OR MEDICAID PROGRAM
OFFENSE: CRIMINAL CONVICTION OR PLEA OF GUILTY, NOLO CONTENDERE, OR NO CONTEST TO A CRIME

NOTES: CONVICTED OF A CRIME RELATED TO PATIENT ABUSE OR NEGLECT.

CARPENTER, CHARLES MD, LICENSE NUMBER 00F2585 OF MCALLEN, TX, WAS DISCIPLINED BY TEXAS ON MAY 15, 1996
DISCIPLINARY ACTION: SURRENDER OF LICENSE
OFFENSE: OVERPRESCRIBING OR MISPRESCRIBING DRUGS

NOTES: ALLEGATIONS THAT IN LATE 1994 HE AIDED AND ABETTED THE UNLICENSED PRACTICE OF MEDICINE IN TEXAS AND PRESCRIBED MEDICATIONS WITHOUT PERFORMING ADEQUATE PHYSICAL EXAMINATIONS. DOES NOT ADMIT VIOLATION. VOLUNTARY AND PERMANENT SURRENDER OF TEXAS LICENSE IN LIEU OF FURTHER PROCEEDINGS.

CARSTENSEN, HAROLD G MD, LICENSE NUMBER 0C17546 OF HARLINGEN, TX, WAS DISCIPLINED BY CALIFORNIA ON MAY 25, 1990
DISCIPLINARY ACTION: LICENSE REVOCATION
OFFENSE: DISCIPLINARY ACTION BY ANOTHER STATE OR AGENCY

NOTES: DISCIPLINED BY TEXAS BOARD FOR PROVOCATIVE TOUCHING OF FEMALE PATIENT. NO APPEARANCE BY DOCTOR.

CARTER, PETER JOSEPH MD, LICENSE NUMBER 00C4265 OF FORT WORTH, TX, WAS DISCIPLINED BY TEXAS ON JUNE 10, 1991
DISCIPLINARY ACTION: SURRENDER OF LICENSE

NOTES: LICENSE PLACED ON IRREVOCABLE RETIREMENT STATUS IN LIEU OF DISCIPLINARY ACTION.

CARTWRIGHT, GREGORY B MD, LICENSE NUMBER 00H7544 OF SILSBEE, TX, WAS DISCIPLINED BY TEXAS ON AUGUST 18, 1995
DISCIPLINARY ACTION: 60-MONTH PROBATION
OFFENSE: SUBSTANCE ABUSE

NOTES: INTEMPERATE USE OF ALCOHOL OR DRUGS AND DISCIPLINARY ACTION TAKEN BY HIS PEERS. SUSPENSION STAYED. PROBATION UNDER VARIOUS TERMS AND CONDITIONS.

CARTWRIGHT, GREGORY B MD, LICENSE NUMBER 00H7544, WAS DISCIPLINED BY TEXAS ON MAY 29, 1996
DISCIPLINARY ACTION: EMERGENCY SUSPENSION
OFFENSE: FAILURE TO COMPLY WITH PREVIOUS BOARD ORDER

NOTES: INTEMPERATE USE OF ALCOHOL AND DRUGS; AVAILABLE EVIDENCE AND INFORMATION INDICATE THE FOLLOWING VIOLATIONS OF 10/95 ORDER: IN 12/95, FAILED TO SUBMIT A URINE SAMPLE WHEN REQUESTED BY BOARD; IN 1/96, HE INGESTED ALCOHOL AND WAS ARRESTED AFTER BEING INVOLVED IN A ONE VEHICLE ACCIDENT AND ALCOHOL CONCENTRATION OF AN INTOXILYZER TEST WAS .12; SUBSEQUENTLY CHARGED WITH DRIVING WHILE INTOXICATED; IN 5/96, HE CONTACTED A PHARMACY BY TELEPHONE AND ATTEMPTED TO OBTAIN A PRESCRIPTION FOR SOMA, A DANGEROUS DRUG WITH ADDICTIVE POTENTIAL OR POTENTIAL FOR ABUSE.

CARTWRIGHT, GREGORY B MD, LICENSE NUMBER 00H7544, WAS DISCIPLINED BY TEXAS ON AUGUST 17, 1996
DISCIPLINARY ACTION: LICENSE SUSPENSION
OFFENSE: FAILURE TO COMPLY WITH PREVIOUS BOARD ORDER

NOTES: VIOLATED THE ORDER OF 10/09/95 WHEN ON 12/04/95 FAILED TO SUBMIT A URINE SAMPLE WHEN REQUESTED BY THE BOARD; ON 1/26/96 INGESTED ALCOHOL; ON 1/26/96 WAS ARRESTED AND CHARGED WITH DRIVING WHILE INTOXICATED; AND ON 5/10/96 ATTEMPTED TO OBTAIN A PRESCRIPTION FOR SOMA, A DANGEROUS DRUG WITH ADDICTIVE POTENTIAL OR POTENTIAL FOR ABUSE BY TELEPHONE. SUSPENSION UNTIL HE REQUESTS TO HAVE THE SUSPENSION STAYED OR APPEARS BEFORE THE BOARD WITH SUFFICIENT EVIDENCE THAT HIS PHYSICALLY, MENTALLY, AND OTHERWISE COMPETENT TO SAFELY PRACTICE MEDICINE INCLUDING AT A MINIMUM COMPLETE COPIES OF MEDICAL RECORDS AND REPORTS OF PSYCHOLOGICAL AND NEUROPSYCHIATRIC EVALUATIONS, INCLUDING A 96 HOUR INPATIENT EVALUATION, CONDUCTED BY A BOARD APPROVED CERTIFIED PSYCHIATRIST. SHALL NOT REQUEST TERMINATION OF THE SUSPENSION FOR AT LEAST SIX MONTHS AFTER COMPLETION OF A 96 HOUR INPATIENT EVALUATION.

CARTWRIGHT, GREGORY B MD, LICENSE NUMBER H7544, WAS DISCIPLINED BY TEXAS ON MARCH 1, 1997
DISCIPLINARY ACTION: 60-MONTH PROBATION; REQUIRED TO TAKE ADDITIONAL MEDICAL EDUCATION
OFFENSE: FAILURE TO COMPLY WITH PREVIOUS BOARD ORDER

NOTES: IN AN ORDER OF 8/17/96 HIS LICENSE WAS SUSPENDED UNTIL SUBMITTAL OF SATISFACTORY PROOF THAT HE IS PHYSICALLY, MENTALLY, AND OTHERWISE COMPETENT TO PRACTICE MEDICINE, AT WHICH TIME THE SUSPENSION WOULD BE STAYED FOR FIVE YEARS PROBATION. HE HAS REQUESTED THAT THE SUSPENSION OF HIS LICENSE BE LIFTED DUE TO HIS COMPLIANCE WITH THE MINIMUM REQUIREMENTS OF THE ORDER. HIS SUSPENSION IS STAYED AND HE IS PLACED ON PROBATION UNDER THE FOLLOWING TERMS: SHALL ABSTAIN FROM THE CONSUMPTION OF ALCOHOL/DRUGS IN ANY FORM UNLESS PRESCRIBED BY ANOTHER PHYSICIAN FOR A LEGITIMATE AND THERAPEUTIC PURPOSE; SHALL SUBMIT HIMSELF FOR APPROPRIATE EXAMS INCLUDING DRUG OR ALCOHOL SCREENS; SHALL NOMINATE THREE CERTIFIED PSYCHIATRISTS FOR BOARD SELECTION OF A THERAPIST AND SHALL EXPEDITIOUSLY SUBMIT HIMSELF TO EVALUATION AND TREATMENT BY THE APPROVED PRACTITIONER; SHALL COOPERATE WITH THE BOARD IN VERIFYING COMPLIANCE INCLUDING PROVIDING COPIES OF MEDICAL RELEASES UPON REQUEST; SHALL PARTICIPATE IN THE ACTIVITIES OF A PHYSICIAN HEALTH AND REHABILITATION COMMITTEE AND ATTEND WEEKLY MEETINGS WITH QUARTERLY REPORTS; SHALL PARTICIPATE IN AA'S PROGRAM NOT LESS THAN THREE TIMES A WEEK; SHALL REPORT ON HIS ATTENDANCE; SHALL APPEAR PERSONALLY BEFORE THE BOARD AT LEAST ANNUALLY; SHALL NOT TREAT OR OTHERWISE SERVE AS PHYSICIAN, PRESCRIBE, DISPENSE OR ADMINISTER DRUGS THAT MAY BE SUBJECT TO ABUSE TO HIMSELF OR TO ANY MEMBER OF HIS FAMILY; SHALL INFORM THE BOARD OF ANY RESTRICTIONS IMPOSED ON HIS HOSPITAL PRIVILEGES DURING HIS PROBATION AND SHALL COMPLY WITH SAID RESTRICTIONS; SEPARATE FROM PATIENT RECORDS, SHALL MAINTAIN A FILE OF EVERY PRESCRIPTION WRITTEN BY HIM FOR DANGEROUS DRUGS WITH ADDICTIVE POTENTIAL WHICH SHALL BE MADE AVAILABLE FOR REVIEW; SHALL OBTAIN AT LEAST 50 HOURS OF CONTINUING MEDICAL EDUCATION WITHIN ONE YEAR; SHALL GIVE A COPY OF THIS ORDER TO ANY HEALTH CARE ENTITY WHERE HE HAS PRIVILEGES; SHALL PROVIDE A COPY OF THIS ORDER TO ANYONE REQUESTING IT WITHIN 10 DAYS; TIME SPENT OUT OF TEXAS DOES NOT COUNT TOWARD PROBATION; SHALL INFORM THE BOARD OF CHANGE OF ADDRESS WITHIN 10 DAYS OR IF HE LEAVES THE STATE; SHALL NOT SEEK MODIFICATION FOR ONE YEAR.

CARTWRIGHT, GREGORY B MD, LICENSE NUMBER H7544 OF FORT WORTH, TX, WAS DISCIPLINED BY TEXAS ON APRIL 4, 1998
DISCIPLINARY ACTION: 60-MONTH PROBATION; FINE
OFFENSE: FAILURE TO COMPLY WITH PREVIOUS BOARD ORDER

NOTES: VIOLATED 3/1/97 ORDER IN THAT HE: FAILED TO OBTAIN AND/OR SUBMIT PROOF OF 50 HOURS OF CONTINUING MEDICAL EDUCATION; FAILED TO CAUSE HIS TREATING PHYSICIAN TO IMMEDIATELY REPORT THE MEDICAL CONDITION BEING TREATED. SUSPENSION STAYED; PROBATION STARTING ON 3/1/97; $2,500 FINE; SHALL OBTAIN COURSES IN ETHICS AND RISK MANAGEMENT AS PART OF REQUIREMENT OF 3/7/97 ORDER; ALL OTHER PROVISIONS OF PREVIOUS ORDER REMAIN IN EFFECT.

CASEY, JAMES GORDON MD, LICENSE NUMBER 00C6128 OF ABILENE, TX, WAS DISCIPLINED BY TEXAS ON OCTOBER 10, 1992
DISCIPLINARY ACTION: LICENSE REVOCATION
OFFENSE: PROFESSIONAL MISCONDUCT

NOTES: UNPROFESSIONAL AND DISHONORABLE CONDUCT LIKELY TO DECEIVE, DEFRAUD OR INJURE THE PUBLIC.

CASEY, JAMES GORDON MD, LICENSE NUMBER C6128, WAS DISCIPLINED BY TEXAS ON APRIL 10, 1999
DISCIPLINARY ACTION: LICENSE REINSTATEMENT
OFFENSE: SEXUAL ABUSE OF OR SEXUAL MISCONDUCT WITH A PATIENT

NOTES: LICENSE REVOKED ON 10/10/92 FOR ENGAGING IN A SEXUAL RELATIONSHIP WITH A PATIENT WHO HE TREATED FOR EMOTIONAL PROBLEMS AND DEPRESSION ALTHOUGH HE LACKED EXPERIENCE TO TREAT SUCH PROBLEMS; ON 5/26/98 HE WAS EVALUATED BY A PSYCHIATRIST WHO CONCLUDED THAT HE WAS COMPETENT AND ABLE TO SAFELY PRACTICE MEDICINE. APPLICATION FOR REINSTATEMENT IS CONDITIONALLY GRANTED UPON PASSING THE SPEX AND THE MEDICAL JURISPRUDENCE EXAM WITHIN 3 ATTEMPTS WITHIN 1 YEAR; WILL THEN BE PLACED ON PROBATION WITH STATED CONDITIONS.

CASO, WILLIAM D MD, DATE OF BIRTH FEBRUARY 25, 1934, LICENSE NUMBER 0013615 OF HARDIN CO., KY, WAS DISCIPLINED BY KENTUCKY ON JUNE 27, 1990
DISCIPLINARY ACTION: 60-MONTH PROBATION; RESTRICTION PLACED ON CONTROLLED SUBSTANCE LICENSE

NOTES: NO SCHEDULE II, IIN PRESCRIBING PRIVILEGES, SUCCESSFUL COMPLETION OF "THE PRESCRIBING AND USE OF CONTROLLED SUBSTANCES MINI-RESIDENCY". CASE CURRENTLY UNDER APPEAL.

CASO, WILLIAM D MD, WAS DISCIPLINED BY DEA ON OCTOBER 26, 1992
DISCIPLINARY ACTION: REVOCATION OF CONTROLLED SUBSTANCE LICENSE
OFFENSE: OVERPRESCRIBING OR MISPRESCRIBING DRUGS

NOTES: PRESCRIBED AND DISPENSED CONTROLLED SUBSTANCES TO PATIENTS FOR NO LEGITIMATE MEDICAL PURPOSE. ISSUED PRESCRIPTIONS WITHOUT PERFORMING PHYSICAL EXAMINATIONS, WITHOUT PROVIDING PSYCHIATRIC COUNSELING, AND WITHOUT KNOWLEDGE OF ANY OTHER SUBSTANCES WHICH THE PATIENTS MIGHT BE TAKING. HAS IGNORED STATE AND FEDERAL LAWS AND REGULATIONS REGARDING THE PRESCRIBING OF CONTROLLED SUBSTANCES FOR A LEGITIMATE MEDICAL NEED; KENTUCKY HAD SUSPENDED HIS PRIVILEGE TO HANDLE CONTROLLED SUBSTANCES.

CASO, WILLIAM D MD, DATE OF BIRTH FEBRUARY 25, 1934, LICENSE NUMBER 0013615 OF HARDIN COUNTY, KY, WAS DISCIPLINED BY KENTUCKY ON AUGUST 30, 1993
DISCIPLINARY ACTION: LICENSE SUSPENSION
OFFENSE: LOSS OR RESTRICTION OF HOSPITAL PRIVILEGES

NOTES: DISCIPLINARY ACTION TAKEN BY HOSPITAL. SUSPENSION NOT TO EXCEED 5 YEARS; MAY REQUEST REINSTATEMENT UPON COMPLETION OF NEUROLOGICAL AND PSYCHOLOGICAL EVALUATIONS AND SUCCESSFUL COMPLETION OF SPECIAL PURPOSE EXAMINATION.

CASO, WILLIAM D MD, LICENSE NUMBER 0082787 OF 14217 CHERRY AVENUE, FLUSHING, NY, WAS DISCIPLINED BY NEW YORK ON APRIL 20, 1994
DISCIPLINARY ACTION: LICENSE SUSPENSION
OFFENSE: DISCIPLINARY ACTION BY ANOTHER STATE OR AGENCY

NOTES: FOUND GUILTY OF IMPROPER PRACTICE BY THE KENTUCKY BOARD. INDEFINITE SUSPENSION.

CASO, WILLIAM D MD, DATE OF BIRTH FEBRUARY 25, 1934, LICENSE NUMBER 1021871 OF 1103 WOODLAND DRIVE, ELIZABETHTOWN, KY, WAS DISCIPLINED BY INDIANA ON JULY 28, 1994
DISCIPLINARY ACTION: LICENSE SUSPENSION
OFFENSE: DISCIPLINARY ACTION BY ANOTHER STATE OR AGENCY

NOTES: ON 5/5/93 LICENSE RENEWAL APPLICATION HE STATED HE HAD NOT HAD DISCIPLINARY ACTION TAKEN AGAINST HIS LICENSE BY ANOTHER STATE OR HOSPITAL OR HEALTH CARE FACILITY; KENTUCKY LICENSE WAS PLACED ON PROBATION FOR 5 YEARS ON 6/27/90 FOR IMPROPER PRESCRIBING OF CONTROLLED SUBSTANCES; FOR ADDITIONAL PRESCRIBING DEFICIENCIES KENTUCKY AGAIN PUT HIS LICENSE ON PROBATION ON 10/28/92 FOR 5 YEARS AND SUSPENDED HIS LICENSE ON 8/30/93. DR. CASO STATED HE DID NOT REPORT THIS IN 1993 BECAUSE HE BELIEVED HE HAD INFORMED THE BOARD OF PENDING DISCIPLINE IN 9/91 AND THAT ALL DISCIPLINES WERE BEING APPEALED. HE SHALL HAVE THE RIGHT TO APPLY FOR TERMINATION OF SUSPENSION AFTER 5 YEARS; PRIOR TO REINSTATEMENT SHALL PASS SPEX EXAM AND HAVE NEUROLOGICAL AND PSYCHOLOGICAL EXAMS BY BOARD CERTIFIED PHYSICIANS; SHALL PAY COSTS OF $415.

CASO, WILLIAM D MD, DATE OF BIRTH FEBRUARY 25, 1934, LICENSE NUMBER 00E5027 OF ELIZABETHTOWN, KY, WAS DISCIPLINED BY TEXAS ON MARCH 4, 1995
OFFENSE: DISCIPLINARY ACTION BY ANOTHER STATE OR AGENCY

NOTES: LICENSE PLACED ON PROBATION FOR FIVE YEARS BY KENTUCKY BOARD IN 6/90; LICENSE FURTHER RESTRICTED BY KENTUCKY IN 11/90 WITH THE PROVISION THAT HE NOT PRESCRIBE, DISPENSE OR ORDER ANY CONTROLLED SUBSTANCES; PLACED ON A FIVE YEAR PROBATION WITH RESTRICTIONS ON HIS KENTUCKY LICENSE IN 10/92, BASED ON NEW ALLEGATIONS OF EXCESSIVE PRESCRIBING OF CONTROLLED SUBSTANCES AND LACK OF DOCUMENTATION CONCERNING INDICATIONS FOR THE PRESCRIPTIONS; KENTUCKY LICENSE SUSPENDED FOR FIVE YEARS IN 8/93, BASED ON THE REVOCATION OF HIS HOSPITAL PRIVILEGES FOR UNPROFESSIONAL CONDUCT; HAS APPEALED THESE ACTIONS. INDEFINITE RESTRICTION FROM PRACTICING IN TEXAS; PRIOR TO PRACTICING IN TEXAS SHALL APPEAR BEFORE BOARD AND RECEIVE APPROVAL SUBJECT TO TERMS AND CONDITIONS; SHALL APPRISE BOARD EVERY THREE MONTHS OF THE STATUS OF HIS APPEAL OF THE KENTUCKY ACTION; SHALL INFORM BOARD OF ANY CHANGE OF ADDRESS WITHIN 10 DAYS.

CASO, WILLIAM D MD, DATE OF BIRTH FEBRUARY 25, 1934 OF 1103 WOODLAND DRIVE, ELIZABETH, KY, WAS DISCIPLINED BY MEDICARE ON MARCH 5, 1997
DISCIPLINARY ACTION: EXCLUSION FROM THE MEDICARE AND/OR MEDICAID PROGRAM
OFFENSE: DISCIPLINARY ACTION BY ANOTHER STATE OR AGENCY

NOTES: LICENSE SUSPENDED FOR REASONS BEARING ON PROFESSIONAL PERFORMANCE.

CASTANEDA, JOSE LUIS MD, LICENSE NUMBER F3818 OF BROWNSVILLE, TX, WAS DISCIPLINED BY TEXAS ON AUGUST 9, 1997
DISCIPLINARY ACTION: FINE; REPRIMAND
OFFENSE: PROFESSIONAL MISCONDUCT

NOTES: HE PERMITTED UNLICENSED PHYSICIANS TO ASSESS, DIAGNOSE, TREAT, AND PRESCRIBE FOR PATIENTS IN HIS CLINICS IN HIS ABSENCE WITHOUT ADEQUATE, OR AT TIMES ANY, SUPERVISION. $5,000 FINE.

CASTANEDA, MANUEL F MD, LICENSE NUMBER 31594 OF HOUSTON, TX, WAS DISCIPLINED BY OHIO ON MARCH 11, 1998
DISCIPLINARY ACTION: LICENSE REVOCATION
OFFENSE: DISCIPLINARY ACTION BY ANOTHER STATE OR AGENCY

NOTES: PRIOR ACTION BY TEXAS BOARD FOLLOWING ITS FINDINGS THAT HE HAD BEEN ARRESTED AND CHARGED WITH FOUR COUNTS OF INDECENCY WITH A CHILD AND ONE COUNT OF ASSAULT WITH INTENT TO CAUSE BODILY HARM; HAD INAPPROPRIATELY SELF-PRESCRIBED CONTROLLED SUBSTANCES AND DANGEROUS DRUGS; HAD INAPPROPRIATELY PRESCRIBED A CONTROLLED SUBSTANCE TO A PATIENT WITHOUT ADEQUATE MEDICAL INDICATION. TEXAS BOARD MODIFIED ITS ORDER ON 11/22/97 TO REFLECT THAT HE HAD NOT BEEN FOUND GUILTY OF AFOREMENTIONED CRIMINAL CHARGES AND DELETED REQUIREMENT THAT HE HAVA A THIRD PARTY PRESENT WHEN EXAMINING FEMALE AND MINOR PATIENTS.

CASTANEDA, MANUEL FRANCO MD, LICENSE NUMBER 00G6798, WAS DISCIPLINED BY TEXAS ON NOVEMBER 16, 1996
DISCIPLINARY ACTION: 60-MONTH PROBATION; RESTRICTION PLACED ON LICENSE
OFFENSE: OVERPRESCRIBING OR MISPRESCRIBING DRUGS

NOTES: IN 6/96, HE WAS ARRESTED FOR FOUR COUNTS OF INDECENCY WITH A CHILD AND ONE COUNT OF ASSAULT WITH INTENT TO CAUSE BODILY INJURY; ALLEGATIONS STEM FROM HIS RELATIONSHIP WITH HIS ESTRANGED WIFE AND TWO STEP-DAUGHTERS; HE DENIES THE ALLEGATIONS AND PLANS TO CONTEST THEM IN A FUTURE CRIMINAL TRIAL; HAS INAPPROPRIATELY SELF-PRESCRIBED CONTROLLED SUBSTANCES AND DANGEROUS DRUGS FOR PAIN CONTROL REGARDING HIS RIGHT LEG AND POLIO HE SUFFERED AS A CHILD; IN 1/94, HE INAPPROPRIATELY PRESCRIBED LORTAB, A CONTROLLED SUBSTANCE, TO AN EMERGENCY ROOM PATIENT WITHOUT ADEQUATE MEDICAL INDICATION. DOES NOT ADMIT VIOLATION. SUSPENSION STAYED. PROBATION WITH TERMS AND CONDITIONS: SHALL NOT TREAT OR OTHERWISE SERVE AS PHYSICIAN, PRESCRIBE, DISPENSE OR ADMINISTER DRUGS THAT MAY BE SUBJECT TO ABUSE TO HIMSELF OR TO ANY MEMBER OF HIS FAMILY; SHALL ABSTAIN FROM THE CONSUMPTION OF ALCOHOL/DRUGS IN ANY FORM UNLESS PRESCRIBED BY ANOTHER PHYSICIAN FOR A LEGITIMATE AND THERAPEUTIC PURPOSE; SHALL SUBMIT HIMSELF FOR APPROPRIATE EXAMS INCLUDING DRUG OR ALCOHOL SCREENS; SHALL SUBMIT HIMSELF FOR EVALUATION AND TREATMENT BY A BOARD-APPROVED PSYCHIATRIST WHOM HE SHALL SEE AT LEAST ONCE A MONTH AND WHO SHALL SUBMIT REPORTS TO THE BOARD; WITHIN SIX MONTHS SHALL TAKE AND PASS THE MEDICAL JURISPRUDENCE EXAMINATION; SHALL OBTAIN AT LEAST 50 HOURS PER YEAR OF CONTINUING MEDICAL EDUCATION; WITHIN SIX MONTHS SHALL SUCCESSFULLY COMPLETE A COURSE IN THE AREA OF CONFLICT RESOLUTION OR AN EQUIVALENT; SHALL HAVE A THIRD PARTY IN THE ROOM DURING THE EXAMINATION OF ANY FEMALE OR MINOR PATIENT AND SHALL NOTE THIS IN THE PATIENT'S CHART; SHALL COOPERATE WITH THE BOARD IN VERIFYING COMPLIANCE INCLUDING PROVIDING COPIES OF MEDICAL RELEASES UPON REQUEST. SHALL APPEAR BEFORE THE BOARD AT LEAST TWICE A YEAR; SHALL GIVE A COPY OF THIS ORDER TO ANY HEALTH CARE ENTITY WHERE HE HAS PRIVILEGES; TIME SPENT OUT OF TEXAS DOES NOT COUNT TOWARD PROBATION; SHALL INFORM BOARD OF CHANGE OF ADDRESS WITHIN 10 DAYS OR IF HE LEAVES THE STATE. SHALL NOT SEEK MODIFICATION FOR ONE YEAR. ON 11/22/97 PETITION TO TERMINATE ORDER DENIED; ORDER MODIFIED DELETING CHAPERONE REQUIREMENT, AND THE FOLLOWING FINDING OF FACT HAS BEEN ADDED: "HAS BEEN FOUND NOT GUILTY OF THE NOTED CRIMINAL CHARGES AND THE LAWSUIT FILED IN AN UNRELATED MATTER AGAINST HIM HAS BEEN DISMISSED". ON 5/16/98 ORDER MODIFIED REDUCING APPEARANCES BEFORE THE BOARD FROM BIANNUAL TO ANNUAL.

CASTANEDA, MANUEL FRANCO MD, LICENSE NUMBER G6798 OF GALVESTON, TX, WAS DISCIPLINED BY TEXAS ON AUGUST 28, 1999
DISCIPLINARY ACTION: PROBATION; REQUIRED TO TAKE ADDITIONAL MEDICAL EDUCATION
OFFENSE: FAILURE TO COMPLY WITH PREVIOUS BOARD ORDER

NOTES: FAILED TO COMPLETE A COURSE IN CONFLICT RESOLUTION AS REQUIRED BY A 11/16/96 BOARD ORDER. SUSPENSION STAYED FOR PROBATION UNDER THE FOLLOWING TERMS AND CONDITIONS: WITHIN 6 MONTHS SHALL SUCCESSFULLY COMPLETE A COURSE IN CONFLICT RESOLUTION, OR AN EQUIVALENT COURSE, APPROVED IN ADVANCE BY THE BOARD; ALL OTHER PROVISIONS OF THE 11/16/96 ORDER REMAIN IN FULL FORCE AND EFFECT.

CAVAZOS, MIGUEL A JR MD OF 1616 LOGAN, LAREDO, TX, WAS DISCIPLINED BY DEA ON MARCH 10, 1995
DISCIPLINARY ACTION: SURRENDER OF CONTROLLED SUBSTANCE LICENSE

NOTES: IN LIEU OF PUBLIC INTEREST REVOCATION.

CAVENDER, LUNDY E JR MD, LICENSE NUMBER 00H7711 OF FORT WORTH, TX, WAS DISCIPLINED BY TEXAS ON MAY 11, 1995
DISCIPLINARY ACTION: 60-MONTH PROBATION; RESTRICTION PLACED ON LICENSE
OFFENSE: LOSS OR RESTRICTION OF HOSPITAL PRIVILEGES

NOTES: BETWEEN APPROXIMATELY THE FALL OF 1990 AND 11/93, ENGAGED IN INAPPROPRIATE PHYSICAL CONTACT WITH THE MOTHERS OF VARIOUS PEDIATRIC PATIENTS WHICH INCLUDED IN SOME INSTANCES KISSING, HUGGING AND OTHER INAPPROPRIATE TOUCHING; IN 5/94, HOSPITAL PRIVILEGES WERE SUSPENDED AND HE WAS ADMITTED TO TREATMENT PROGRAM TO ADDRESS ISSUES OF SEXUAL COMPULSIVITY; SUSPENSION OF HOSPITAL PRIVILEGES WAS LIFTED UPON COMPLETION OF TREATMENT AND HE WAS PLACED ON A TWO YEAR PROBATION PERIOD WITH RESTRICTIONS INCLUDING A CHAPERONE REQUIREMENT; HAS ENTERED INTO A PROFESSIONAL RE-ENTRY PLAN WITH A TREATING PSYCHIATRIST INCLUDING PRACTICE REVIEW AND A 12-STEP RECOVERY PROGRAM FOR SEXUAL ADDICTION. SUSPENSION STAYED. PROBATION WITH TERMS: SHALL SUBMIT HIMSELF FOR EVALUATION AND TREATMENT BY A BOARD-APPROVED PSYCHIATRIST AT LEAST ONCE A MONTH WHO SHALL SUBMIT REPORTS TO THE BOARD; SHALL HAVE A CHAPERONE

PRESENT ANYTIME HE PERFORMS A PHYSICAL EXAMINATION ON ANY PATIENT; SHALL COMPLY WITH ALL TERMS OF THE PROFESSIONAL RE-ENTRY PLAN AND THE AGREEMENT FOR HOSPITAL PRIVILEGES; SHALL MAINTAIN ADEQUATE MEDICAL RECORDS WHICH SHALL BE AVAILABLE FOR REVIEW; SHALL APPEAR BEFORE BOARD AT LEAST ONCE EACH YEAR OR AT BOARD REQUEST; SHALL FULLY COOPERATE WITH BOARD IN VERIFYING COMPLIANCE INCLUDING PROVIDING ANY MEDICAL RELEASES AND PEER REVIEW RECORDS UPON REQUEST; SHALL GIVE A COPY OF THIS ORDER TO ANY HEALTH CARE ENTITY WHERE HE HAS PRIVILEGES; TIME PERIOD OUT OF TEXAS DOES NOT COUNT TOWARD PROBATION; SHALL INFORM BOARD OF CHANGE OF ADDRESS WITHIN 10 DAYS OR IF HE LEAVES THE STATE. SHALL NOT SEEK MODIFICATION FOR ONE YEAR. ON 8/22/98 ORDER TERMINATED.

CAVENDER, LUNDY E JR MD OF FORT WORTH, TX, WAS DISCIPLINED BY LOUISIANA ON DECEMBER 7, 1995
DISCIPLINARY ACTION: 60-MONTH PROBATION; RESTRICTION PLACED ON LICENSE
OFFENSE: DISCIPLINARY ACTION BY ANOTHER STATE OR AGENCY

NOTES: ACTION IN TEXAS. PROHIBITED FROM PRACTICING IN LOUISIANA DURING PROBATION; SHALL COMPLY WITH THE TEXAS PROBATIONARY ORDER; SHALL APPEAR BEFORE THE BOARD PRIOR TO PRACTICING IN LOUISIANA.

CAVENDER, LUNDY E JR MD, LICENSE NUMBER 0013744 OF 11803 S FREEWAY #204, FORT WORTH, TX, WAS DISCIPLINED BY OKLAHOMA ON DECEMBER 21, 1995
DISCIPLINARY ACTION: EMERGENCY SUSPENSION
OFFENSE: DISCIPLINARY ACTION BY ANOTHER STATE OR AGENCY

NOTES: ON 5/11/95 TEXAS BOARD PLACED LICENSE ON PROBATION BASED ON HIS ENGAGING IN INAPPROPRIATE PHYSICAL CONDUCT WITH MOTHERS OF PEDIATRIC PATIENTS; TWO HOSPITALS TEMPORARILY SUSPENDED PRIVILEGES AS A RESULT OF THIS CONDUCT.

CAVENDER, LUNDY E JR MD, LICENSE NUMBER 0013744 OF 11803 S. FREEWAY, SUITE 204, OKLAHOMA CITY, OK, WAS DISCIPLINED BY OKLAHOMA ON JANUARY 25, 1996
DISCIPLINARY ACTION: LICENSE REVOCATION
OFFENSE: DISCIPLINARY ACTION BY ANOTHER STATE OR AGENCY

NOTES: ACTION IN TEXAS ON 5/11/95 PLACING HIM ON FIVE YEAR PROBATION. THIS ORDER STATED THAT HE ENGAGED IN INAPPROPRIATE PHYSICAL CONTACT WITH MOTHERS OF VARIOUS PEDIATRIC PATIENTS. AS A RESULT OF HIS CONDUCT, HUGULEY HOSPITAL AND HARRIS SOUTHWEST HOSPITAL TEMPORARILY SUSPENDED HIS LICENSE.

CAYLOR, ARTHUR BERNARD JR MD OF 1600 UNIVERSITY DRIVE, COLLEGE STATION, TX, WAS DISCIPLINED BY DEA ON SEPTEMBER 27, 1993
DISCIPLINARY ACTION: SURRENDER OF CONTROLLED SUBSTANCE LICENSE

CAYLOR, ARTHUR BERNARD JR MD, LICENSE NUMBER 00F9287 OF COLLEGE STATION, TX, WAS DISCIPLINED BY TEXAS ON JUNE 22, 1994
DISCIPLINARY ACTION: SURRENDER OF CONTROLLED SUBSTANCE LICENSE; 60-MONTH PROBATION
OFFENSE: SUBSTANCE ABUSE

NOTES: ADMITS TO CHEMICAL DEPENDENCY, SPECIFICALLY HYDROCODONE, AND RECEIVED INPATIENT TREATMENT ONCE IN 1987 AND ONCE IN 1993; FAILED TO KEEP ACCURATE AND COMPLETE RECORDS OF THE CONTROLLED SUBSTANCE, VICODIN WHICH HE ORDERED IN LARGE QUANTITIES FROM A PHARMACEUTICAL SUPPLY HOUSE; DENIES USE OF ALCOHOL; SURRENDERED HIS DEA REGISTRATION IN 9/93; IS IN TREATMENT WITH A PSYCHOTHERAPIST AND UNDER THE CARE OF A PRIMARY CARE PHYSICIAN FOR HIS PHYSICAL CONDITION WHICH IS DESCRIBED AS AN AUTOIMMUNE DISEASE MANIFESTED BY GASTRITIS, DUODENITIS, NEUROSENSORY HEARING LOSS, AXONAL MOTOR DEGENERATION WITH PROXIMAL MYOPATHY, MYELODYSPLASIA AND BASEL CELL CARCINOMA OF THE FOREHEAD; HIS CONDITION IS PRESENTLY STABILIZED; PARTICIPATES IN AA AND HAS COMPLETED THE 12 STEPS. SUSPENSION STAYED. CONDITIONS OF PROBATION: SHALL APPEAR BEFORE THE BOARD ONCE A YEAR; SHALL ABSTAIN FROM THE CONSUMPTION OF ALCOHOL/CHEMICAL SUBSTANCES IN ANY FORM UNLESS PRESCRIBED BY ANOTHER PHYSICIAN FOR A LEGITIMATE AND THERAPEUTIC PURPOSE; SHALL NOT TREAT OR OTHERWISE SERVE AS PHYSICIAN, PRESCRIBE, DISPENSE OR ADMINISTER DRUGS THAT MAY BE SUBJECT TO ABUSE TO HIMSELF OR ANY MEMBER OF HIS FAMILY; SHALL SUBMIT HIMSELF FOR APPROPRIATE EXAMS INCLUDING DRUG OR ALCOHOL SCREENS; SHALL SUBMIT HIMSELF TO A BOARD-APPROVED PSYCHIATRIST FOR EVALUATION AND TREATMENT WITH REPORTS TO THE BOARD; SHALL PARTICIPATE IN AA'S PROGRAM NOT LESS THAN THREE TIMES A WEEK WITH QUARTERLY REPORTS TO THE BOARD; SHALL PARTICIPATE IN ACTIVITIES OF A PHYSICIAN'S HEALTH AND REHABILITATION COMMITTEE AND ATTEND WEEKLY MEETINGS WITH QUARTERLY REPORTS; SHALL ATTEND AT LEAST 50 HOURS PER YEAR OF CONTINUING MEDICAL EDUCATION; SHALL SURRENDER DEA AND TEXAS CONTROL SUBSTANCES REGISTRATION CERTIFICATES; SHALL NOT REAPPLY FOR THESE WITHOUT APPROVAL; SEPARATE FROM PATIENT RECORDS, SHALL MAINTAIN A FILE OF EVERY PRESCRIPTION WRITTEN FOR DANGEROUS DRUGS WHICH SHALL BE AVAILABLE FOR INSPECTION; SHALL GIVE A COPY OF THIS ORDER TO ANY HEALTH CARE ENTITY WHERE HE HAS PRIVILEGES; SHALL COOPERATE WITH THE BOARD IN VERIFYING COMPLIANCE; SHALL INFORM BOARD OF CHANGE OF ADDRESS WITHIN 10 DAYS OR IF HE LEAVES THE STATE; TIME SPENT OUT OF TEXAS DOES NOT COUNT TOWARD PROBATION. SHALL NOT SEEK MODIFICATION FOR ONE YEAR.

CERDAY, EDDIE LEON MD, LICENSE NUMBER F9289 OF SAN ANTONIO, TX, WAS DISCIPLINED BY TEXAS ON APRIL 10, 1999
DISCIPLINARY ACTION: REQUIRED TO TAKE ADDITIONAL MEDICAL EDUCATION; MONITORING OF PHYSICIAN PERFORMANCE
OFFENSE: NONCOMPLIANCE WITH A PROFESSIONAL RULE

NOTES: IN 9/97 AN INVESTIGATION WAS INITIATED REGARDING A PATIENT'S ATTEMPTS TO OBTAIN HER AND HER TWO CHILDREN'S MEDICAL RECORDS FROM HIM; HE RELEASED SPARSE BUT APPARENTLY COMPLETE MEDICAL RECORDS WITHIN 30 DAYS; ON OR ABOUT 1/23/98 MEDICAL RECORDS AND PATIENT APPOINTMENT BOOKS, FOR SIX RANDOMLY SELECTED PATIENTS, FOR THE LAST 3 YEARS WERE SUBPOENAED FROM HIM; ON 3/24/98 HE WROTE HE WAS UNABLE TO PROVIDE THE REQUESTED INFORMATION; HE DID NOT MAINTAIN RECORDS FOR THESE PATIENTS AS REQUIRED; ON OR ABOUT 5/19/98 MEDICAL RECORDS FOR THIS PATIENT'S CHILDREN AND CONTROLLED SUBSTANCE LOGS FOR THE PAST

YEAR WERE SUBPOENAED FROM HIM; HE RESPONDED BY AN UNDATED LETTER RECEIVED BY THE BOARD ON 6/19/98 THAT HE WAS UNABLE TO PROVIDE THESE RECORDS; HE DID NOT MAINTAIN THESE RECORDS AS REQUIRED; HE ALSO RESPONDED THAT HE DID NOT KEEP CONTROLLED SUBSTANCES OR ANY MEDICATION IN HIS OFFICE; HOWEVER, HE RECEIVED TESTOSTERONE AS OFFICE STOCK ON OR ABOUT 6/26, 8/1 & 10/4/97; IN ADDITION, GENOTROPIN AND OTHER MEDICATIONS WERE DISTRIBUTED AS OFFICE STOCK SEVERAL TIMES BETWEEN 3/26 & 10/20/97; THOUGH HIS OFFICE WAS CLOSED DURING THE LAST WEEK OF 9/97, PATIENTS CONTINUED TO RECEIVE PRESCRIPTIONS UNTIL 11/7/97 FOR POTENTIALLY DANGEROUS DRUGS; HOWEVER, HE COULD NOT PRODUCE MEDICAL RECORDS FOR THESE PATIENTS; HE STATES THAT AFTER HIS OFFICE CLOSED, HE CONDUCTED HOUSE CALLS; HOWEVER, HE CANNOT SUBSTANTIATE THIS CLAIM BECAUSE HE HAS NOT PROVIDED MEDICAL RECORDS NOR HAVE PATIENTS WHO RECEIVED LETTERS REQUESTING INFORMATION RESPONDED; HE STATED THAT MEDICAL RECORDS WERE INADVERTENTLY BURNED OR JUST THROWN OUT. LICENSE LIMITED FOR ONE YEAR AS FOLLOWS: SHALL, WITHIN A YEAR, TAKE AND PASS WITH A SCORE OF 75 OR ABOVE, WITHIN 3 ATTEMPTS, THE MEDICAL JURISPRUDENCE EXAM; SHALL ATTEND 50 HOURS PER YEAR OF CONTINUING MEDICAL EDUCATION WITH 1 COURSE IN RISK MANAGEMENT; SHALL MAINTAIN ADEQUATE MEDICAL RECORDS WHICH SHALL BE AVAILABLE FOR REVIEW; SHALL APPEAR BEFORE THE BOARD UPON REQUEST; SHALL COOPERATE WITH THE BOARD IN VERIFYING COMPLIANCE; TIME SPENT OUT OF TEXAS DOES NOT COUNT TOWARD RESTRICTION; SHALL INFORM THE BOARD OF CHANGE OF ADDRESS WITHIN 10 DAYS OR IF HE LEAVES THE STATE; SHALL NOT SEEK MODIFICATION FOR ONE YEAR.

CHALAIRE, FRANK M MD, LICENSE NUMBER 00D0375 OF SAN ANTONIO, TX, WAS DISCIPLINED BY TEXAS ON APRIL 21, 1990
DISCIPLINARY ACTION: 60-MONTH PROBATION; RESTRICTION PLACED ON CONTROLLED SUBSTANCE LICENSE

NOTES: STIPULATED ORDER. MUST NOT DISPENSE CONTROLLED SUBSTANCES EXCEPT TO MEET IMMEDIATE NEEDS OF PATIENT FOR TREATMENT OF ANY MEDICAL CONDITION, MUST PROVIDE PRESCRIPTIONS WHEN AND TO DEGREE CALLED FOR BY CURRENT MEDICAL PRACTICE, MUST NOT PRESCRIBE CONTROLLED SUBSTANCE OR DANGEROUS DRUG FOR OBESITY PATIENT EXCEPT AFTER COMPLETION OF DIAGNOSTIC WORK-UP AS SPECIFIED.

CHALAIRE, FRANK M MD OF SAN ANTONIO, TX, WAS DISCIPLINED BY LOUISIANA ON APRIL 11, 1991
DISCIPLINARY ACTION: PROBATION
OFFENSE: DISCIPLINARY ACTION BY ANOTHER STATE OR AGENCY

NOTES: CHARGED WITH ACTION TAKEN BY TEXAS STATE BOARD OF MEDICAL EXAMINERS. LICENSE ON PROBATION CONCURRENTLY WITH FIVE-YEAR PROBATION IMPOSED BY TEXAS, SUBJECT TO STRICT COMPLIANCE WITH PENDING ORDER OF TEXAS STATE BOARD OF MEDICAL EXAMINERS, PRIOR WRITTEN NOTICE TO BOARD OF INTENT TO RELOCATE TO LOUISIANA.

CHALAIRE, FRANK M MD, LICENSE NUMBER 0C24984 OF SAN ANTONIO, TX, WAS DISCIPLINED BY CALIFORNIA ON SEPTEMBER 5, 1992
DISCIPLINARY ACTION: SURRENDER OF LICENSE

NOTES: VOLUNTARY SURRENDER WHILE CHARGES PENDING.

CHAMBERLAIN, CHARLES D MD, LICENSE NUMBER 00C6886, WAS DISCIPLINED BY TEXAS ON NOVEMBER 16, 1996
DISCIPLINARY ACTION: LICENSE SUSPENSION; REQUIRED TO ENTER AN IMPAIRED PHYSICIAN PROGRAM OR SUBSTANCE ABUSE TREATMENT
OFFENSE: SUBSTANCE ABUSE

NOTES: IN 9/96, HE PERFORMED A SURGICAL PROCEDURE ON A MINOR PATIENT WHILE HE WAS UNDER THE INFLUENCE OF ALCOHOL AND DARVOCET; SUSPICIONS OF HIS IMPAIRMENT WERE REPORTED BY THE ANESTHESIOLOGIST AND NURSING STAFF AND HIS BLOOD AND URINE SAMPLES TAKEN FOLLOWING THE SURGERY REVEALED POSITIVE FINDINGS FOR ALCOHOL AND DARVOCET; HIS MEDICAL STAFF PRIVILEGES AT THE HOSPITAL WERE SUBSEQUENTLY SUMMARILY SUSPENDED; HE HAS REPORTED THAT HE IS PLANNING TO ENROLL HIMSELF IN AN ALCOHOL AND DRUG DEPENDENCE PROGRAM. DOES NOT ADMIT VIOLATION. WITHIN 30 DAYS, HE SHALL ENTER A BOARD-APPROVED INPATIENT DRUG REHABILITATION FACILITY WHOSE DIRECTOR OR PHYSICIAN SHALL SUBMIT MONTHLY REPORTS TO THE BOARD; SUSPENSION UNTIL HE REQUESTS TO HAVE SUSPENSION STAYED OR LIFTED AND APPEARS BEFORE THE BOARD WITH EVIDENCE THAT INDICATES THAT HE IS PHYSICALLY, MENTALLY AND OTHERWISE COMPETENT TO SAFELY PRACTICE MEDICINE INCLUDING AT A MINIMUM COPIES OF MEDICAL RECORDS AND REPORTS OF PSYCHOLOGICAL AND NEUROPSYCHIATRIC EVALUATIONS CONDUCTED BY A BOARD-APPROVED PSYCHIATRIST.

CHAMBERLAIN, CHARLES D MD, LICENSE NUMBER C6886, WAS DISCIPLINED BY TEXAS ON MARCH 1, 1997
DISCIPLINARY ACTION: 60-MONTH PROBATION; REQUIRED TO TAKE ADDITIONAL MEDICAL EDUCATION

NOTES: REINSTATED FROM SUSPENSION ON FOLLOWING CONDITIONS: SHALL ENTER A BOARD-APPROVED INPATIENT DRUG REHABILITATION FACILITY WITH MONTHLY REPORTS TO THE BOARD; SHALL ABSTAIN FROM THE CONSUMPTION OF ALCOHOL/DRUGS IN ANY FORM UNLESS PRESCRIBED BY ANOTHER PHYSICIAN FOR A LEGITIMATE AND THERAPEUTIC PURPOSE; SHALL NOT TREAT OR OTHERWISE SERVE AS PHYSICIAN, PRESCRIBE, DISPENSE OR ADMINISTER DRUGS THAT MAY BE SUBJECT TO ABUSE TO HIMSELF OR TO ANY MEMBER OF HIS FAMILY; SHALL NOMINATE THREE CERTIFIED PSYCHIATRISTS FOR BOARD SELECTION OF A THERAPIST AND SHALL EXPEDITIOUSLY SUBMIT HIMSELF TO EVALUATION AND TREATMENT BY THE APPROVED PRACTITIONER; SHALL PROVIDE REPORTS REGARDING COMPLIANCE TO THE BOARD; SHALL SUBMIT HIMSELF FOR APPROPRIATE EXAMS INCLUDING DRUG OR ALCOHOL SCREENS; SHALL PARTICIPATE IN THE ACTIVITIES OF A PHYSICIAN HEALTH AND REHABILITATION COMMITTEE AND ATTEND WEEKLY MEETINGS WITH QUARTERLY REPORTS; SHALL PARTICIPATE IN AA'S PROGRAM; SHALL REPORT ON HIS ATTENDANCE; SHALL COMPLY WITH ANY CONTINUING CARE CONTRACT WITH QUARTERLY REPORTS TO THE BOARD; SHALL MAINTAIN A LOGBOOK OF PRESCRIPTIONS WRITTEN WHICH SHALL BE MADE AVAILABLE FOR REVIEW; SHALL OBTAIN FIFTY HOURS PER YEAR OF CONTINUING MEDICAL EDUCATION; SHALL COOPERATE WITH THE BOARD IN VERIFYING COMPLIANCE INCLUDING PROVIDING COPIES OF

MEDICAL RELEASES AND PEER REVIEW RECORDS UPON REQUEST; SHALL APPEAR BEFORE THE BOARD TWICE A YEAR; SHALL GIVE A COPY OF THIS ORDER TO ANY HEALTH CARE ENTITY WHERE HE HAS PRIVILEGES; SHALL PROVIDE A COPY OF THIS ORDER TO ANYONE REQUESTING IT WITHIN 10 DAYS; TIME SPENT OUT OF TEXAS DOES NOT COUNT TOWARD PROBATION; SHALL INFORM THE BOARD OF CHANGE OF ADDRESS WITHIN 10 DAYS OR IF HE LEAVES THE STATE; SHALL NOT SEEK MODIFICATION FOR ONE YEAR. ON 4/10/99 PETITION TO TERMINATE ORDER DENIED BUT MODIFIED AS FOLLOWS: MONTHLY PSYCHIATRIC CARE REDUCED TO ONCE EVERY THREE MONTHS; TWO APPEARANCES PER YEAR BEFORE THE BOARD REDUCED TO ONE APPEARANCE PER YEAR. ON 4/4/98 PETITION TO TERMINATE ORDER DENIED.

CHAMBERLIN, DAN STEVEN DO, LICENSE NUMBER 00H2295 OF PORT ARANSAS, TX, WAS DISCIPLINED BY TEXAS ON SEPTEMBER 9, 1992
DISCIPLINARY ACTION: LICENSE REVOCATION
OFFENSE: PROFESSIONAL MISCONDUCT

NOTES: UNPROFESSIONAL OR DISHONORABLE CONDUCT LIKELY TO DECEIVE, DEFRAUD OR INJURE THE PUBLIC; AND PROFESSIONAL FAILURE TO PRACTICE MEDICINE IN AN ACCEPTABLE MANNER CONSISTENT WITH PUBLIC HEALTH AND WELFARE.

CHAN, KWOK WEI MD, LICENSE NUMBER 0043820 OF 119 BELMONT STREET, WORCESTER, MA, WAS DISCIPLINED BY MASSACHUSETTS ON NOVEMBER 17, 1993
DISCIPLINARY ACTION: FINE; MONITORING OF PHYSICIAN PERFORMANCE
OFFENSE: PROFESSIONAL MISCONDUCT

NOTES: VIOLATION OF A BOARD REGULATION. $10,000 FINE, ADMONISHMENT, PLAN FOR JOINT PSYCHOTHERAPY, REPORTS FROM DEPARTMENT HEAD.

CHAN, KWOK WEI MD, LICENSE NUMBER 0039381 OF 5 NORTHLAND ROAD, SHREWSBURY, MA, WAS DISCIPLINED BY VIRGINIA ON OCTOBER 13, 1994
DISCIPLINARY ACTION: REPRIMAND
OFFENSE: DISCIPLINARY ACTION BY ANOTHER STATE OR AGENCY

NOTES: ON 11/17/93 LICENSE TO PRACTICE MEDICINE WAS RESTRICTED BY THE MASSACHUSETTS BOARD, WAS FINED $10,000 AND REQUIRED TO ENGAGE IN PSYCHOTHERAPY AND SUBJECTED TO MONITORING OF HIS CLINICAL PRACTICE FOR ENGAGING IN A PHYSICAL ALTERCATION WITH A COLLEAGUE IN THE PRESENCE OF AN ANESTHETIZED PATIENT; HE WAS SANCTIONED BY THE HOSPITAL AND FAILED TO REPORT THIS SANCTION TO THE BOARD WITHIN 30 DAYS AS REQUIRED.

CHAN, KWOK WEI MD, LICENSE NUMBER 031972E OF SHREWSBURY, MA, WAS DISCIPLINED BY PENNSYLVANIA ON NOVEMBER 15, 1994
DISCIPLINARY ACTION: FINE; REPRIMAND
OFFENSE: DISCIPLINARY ACTION BY ANOTHER STATE OR AGENCY

NOTES: RECIPROCAL ACTION TAKEN IN MASSACHUSETTS. $500 CIVIL PENALTY.

CHAN, KWOK WEI MD, DATE OF BIRTH OCTOBER 18, 1950, LICENSE NUMBER 00G7184 OF WORCESTER, MA, WAS DISCIPLINED BY TEXAS ON FEBRUARY 1, 1995
DISCIPLINARY ACTION: SURRENDER OF LICENSE
OFFENSE: DISCIPLINARY ACTION BY ANOTHER STATE OR AGENCY

NOTES: LICENSE IN MASSACHUSETTS ADMONISHED AND FINED AFTER GETTING INTO A FIGHT WITH ANOTHER PHYSICIAN IN AN OPERATING ROOM; THE HOSPITAL PLACED HIM ON FIVE YEARS PROBATION WHICH HE DID NOT REPORT TO MASSACHUSETTS BOARD. SURRENDER IS PERMANENT.

CHAN, KWOK WEI MD, LICENSE NUMBER 0044763 OF SHREWSBURY, MA, WAS DISCIPLINED BY OHIO ON APRIL 21, 1995
DISCIPLINARY ACTION: PROBATION; RESTRICTION PLACED ON LICENSE
OFFENSE: DISCIPLINARY ACTION BY ANOTHER STATE OR AGENCY

NOTES: DISCIPLINED BY MASSACHUSETTS FOR ENGAGING IN AN ALTERCATION WITH ANOTHER PHYSICIAN IN THE HOSPITAL OPERATING ROOM. PROBATIONARY TERMS, CONDITIONS AND LIMITATIONS FOR AT LEAST FOUR YEARS.

CHAN, KWOK WEI MD, LICENSE NUMBER 0C42736 OF SHREWSBURY, MA, WAS DISCIPLINED BY CALIFORNIA ON AUGUST 25, 1995
DISCIPLINARY ACTION: SURRENDER OF LICENSE

NOTES: WHILE CHARGES PENDING.

CHAN, KWOK WEI MD, DATE OF BIRTH OCTOBER 18, 1950, LICENSE NUMBER 0027166 OF 5 NORTHLAND RD, SHREWSBURY, MA, WAS DISCIPLINED BY GEORGIA ON NOVEMBER 3, 1995
DISCIPLINARY ACTION: REPRIMAND
OFFENSE: DISCIPLINARY ACTION BY ANOTHER STATE OR AGENCY

NOTES: UNPROFESSIONAL CONDUCT. DISCIPLINARY ACTION IN MASSACHUSETTS.

CHANDLER, DONALD S MD, DATE OF BIRTH SEPTEMBER 30, 1941, LICENSE NUMBER 0030857 OF 1453 BAR HARBOR DRIVE, DALLAS, TX, WAS DISCIPLINED BY MICHIGAN ON MAY 19, 1993
DISCIPLINARY ACTION: 35-MONTH PROBATION; REPRIMAND
OFFENSE: SUBSTANDARD CARE, INCOMPETENCE OR NEGLIGENCE

NOTES: NEGLIGENCE AND INCOMPETENCE.

CHANDLER, DONALD S MD, DATE OF BIRTH AUGUST 3, 1941, LICENSE NUMBER 0013501 OF 900 N COKRELL HILL RD, DESOTO, TX, WAS DISCIPLINED BY GEORGIA ON SEPTEMBER 2, 1994
DISCIPLINARY ACTION: 60-MONTH PROBATION
OFFENSE: DISCIPLINARY ACTION BY ANOTHER STATE OR AGENCY

NOTES: DISCIPLINARY ACTION IN TEXAS AND MICHIGAN.

CHANDLER, DONALD STANLEY MD, LICENSE NUMBER 00G0967 OF DALLAS, TX, WAS DISCIPLINED BY TEXAS ON APRIL 20, 1991
DISCIPLINARY ACTION: 60-MONTH PROBATION; RESTRICTION PLACED ON LICENSE

NOTES: SUSPENSION STAYED. TERMS OF PROBATION: SHALL APPEAR BEFORE THE BOARD TWICE A YEAR; SHALL REFRAIN FROM ACCEPTING EMPLOYMENT OR ENTERING INTO CONTRACTUAL ARRANGEMENTS WHEREIN HE WOULD BE COMPENSATED TO DIAGNOSE AND/OR TREAT PATIENTS BY A LAY PERSON, CORPORATION, OR OTHER ENTITY NOT COMPRISED EXCLUSIVELY OF LICENSED PHYSICIANS; SHALL NOT PRACTICE BARIATRIC MEDICINE ON ANY PATIENT EXCEPT OVERWEIGHT PEDIATRIC PATIENTS WHO ARE APPROPRIATE CANDIDATES FOR WEIGHT CONTROL TREATMENT; SHALL ATTEND 50 HOURS CONTINUING MEDICAL EDUCATION PER YEAR; MUST COMPLETE COURSE IN MEDICAL ETHICS. ON 4/15/94 HIS REQUEST FOR TERMINATION OF ORDER DENIED. HOWEVER, ORDER IS MODIFIED AS FOLLOWS: HE

SHALL APPEAR BEFORE THE BOARD ONCE A YEAR DURING EACH YEAR OF PROBATION TO REPORT ON HIS COMPLIANCE. ALL OTHER PROVISIONS OF THIS ORDER REMAIN IN EFFECT. ON 10/13/95 ORDER TERMINATED.

CHANDLER, HAROLD MULLINS MD, LICENSE NUMBER 0007636 OF 11101 MAPLE GROVE, OKLAHOMA CITY, OK, WAS DISCIPLINED BY OKLAHOMA ON MAY 20, 1993
DISCIPLINARY ACTION: 12-MONTH LICENSE SUSPENSION
OFFENSE: SUBSTANCE ABUSE

NOTES: IN 1992 WAS USING ALCOHOL IN EXCESSIVE AMOUNTS AND IN 9/92 ADMITTED HIMSELF FOR ASSESSMENT AND TREATMENT; CONTINUED OUTPATIENT TREATMENT INCLUDING AA PARTICIPATION, PSYCHIATRIC TREATMENT AND ADDITIONAL HOSPITALIZATION; ALSO WAS DIAGNOSED WITH A BRAIN TUMOR AND UNDERWENT SURGERY FOR REMOVAL. WHEN HE APPLIES FOR REINSTATEMENT MUST PROVIDE COPIES OF ALL EVALUATIONS, REPORTS AND PROGNOSIS FROM RECOVERY CENTER AND EVALUATIONS OF RECOVERY FROM BRAIN SURGERY.

CHANDLER, HAROLD MULLINS MD, LICENSE NUMBER 0007636, WAS DISCIPLINED BY OKLAHOMA ON FEBRUARY 17, 1994
DISCIPLINARY ACTION: 60-MONTH PROBATION; RESTRICTION PLACED ON LICENSE

NOTES: IN COMPLIANCE WITH 5/14/93 SUSPENSION ORDER HAS COMPLETED IN-PATIENT EVALUATION AND TREATMENT AND PROVIDED DISCHARGE SUMMARY AND LETTERS OF SUPPORT AND AN MRI DATED 2/2/94. LICENSE REINSTATED FROM SUSPENSION. PROBATION TO BEGIN 2/11/94. CONDITIONS OF PROBATION: SHALL MEET REGULARLY WITH PHYSICIAN RECOVERY COMMITTEE; SHALL NOT PRESCRIBE, ADMINISTER OR DISPENSE ANY MEDICATIONS FOR HIS PERSONAL USE AND TAKE NO MEDICATION UNLESS IT IS AUTHORIZED BY ANOTHER PHYSICIAN FOR A LEGITIMATE MEDICAL NEED; SHALL ABSTAIN FROM THE CONSUMPTION OF ALCOHOL OR ANY SUBSTANCE WHICH WOULD ADVERSELY AFFECT HIS ABILITY TO PRACTICE MEDICINE; SHALL NOT INGEST ANY SUBSTANCE THAT WOULD TEST POSITIVE FOR ALCOHOL OR ANY CONTROLLED SUBSTANCE; SHALL SUBMIT BIOLOGICAL FLUID SPECIMENS; SHALL HAVE HIS PHYSICIAN MONITOR LITHIUM LEVELS AND PROVIDE QUARTERLY REPORTS; SHALL PRACTICE UNDER A BOARD-APPROVED MONITOR; SHALL HAVE HIS PATIENTS SIGN A PATIENT'S RIGHTS STATEMENT; SHALL FURNISH BOARD WITH ADDRESS AND/OR CHANGE OF ADDRESS; SHALL APPEAR BEFORE THE BOARD UPON REQUEST AND PROVIDE REQUIRED REPORTS; SHALL PAY COSTS; SHALL SUPPLY A COPY OF THIS ORDER TO ANY HEALTH CARE ENTITY WHERE HE HAS PRIVILEGES; SHALL NOT SUPERVISE A PHYSICIAN'S ASSISTANT.

CHANDLER, HAROLD MULLINS MD, LICENSE NUMBER 00H5382 OF BEAUMONT, TX, WAS DISCIPLINED BY TEXAS ON APRIL 15, 1994
DISCIPLINARY ACTION: 60-MONTH PROBATION; REQUIRED TO TAKE ADDITIONAL MEDICAL EDUCATION
OFFENSE: DISCIPLINARY ACTION BY ANOTHER STATE OR AGENCY

NOTES: ON 5/20/93 OKLAHOMA SUSPENDED HIS LICENSE FOR ONE YEAR BASED ON INTEMPERATE USE OF ALCOHOL; ADMITS HE IS AN ALCOHOLIC AND HAS SOUGHT IN-PATIENT TREATMENT ON HIS OWN INITIATIVE IN THE PAST; HAS BEEN SOBER SINCE 9/8/92; HE IS CURRENTLY PRACTICING PSYCHIATRY IN TEXAS AND BEING TREATED BY HIS PHYSICIAN IN OKLAHOMA; OKLAHOMA REINSTATED HIS LICENSE ON PROBATION ON 2/11/94. SUSPENSION STAYED. CONDITIONS OF PROBATION: SHALL ABSTAIN FROM THE CONSUMPTION OF ALCOHOL/CHEMICAL SUBSTANCES IN ANY FORM UNLESS PRESCRIBED BY ANOTHER PHYSICIAN FOR A LEGITIMATE AND THERAPEUTIC PURPOSE; SHALL NOT TREAT OR OTHERWISE SERVE AS PHYSICIAN, PRESCRIBE, DISPENSE OR ADMINISTER DRUGS THAT MAY BE SUBJECT TO ABUSE TO HIMSELF OR ANY MEMBER OF HIS FAMILY; SHALL SUBMIT HIMSELF FOR APPROPRIATE EXAMS INCLUDING DRUG AND ALCOHOL SCREENS; SHALL PARTICIPATE IN AA'S PROGRAM NOT LESS THAN TWO TIMES A WEEK WITH QUARTERLY REPORTS TO THE BOARD; SHALL CONTINUE TREATMENT WITH HIS PRESENT PHYSICIAN AND MONITORING WITH HIS PRESENT SUPERVISOR WITH QUARTERLY REPORTS; SHALL ATTEND AT LEAST 50 HOURS PER YEAR OF CONTINUING MEDICAL EDUCATION INCLUDING COURSES ADDRESSING ADDICTIONOLOGY, DRUG ABUSE, AND CO-DEPENDENCY; SHALL PERFORM TWO HOURS PER WEEK OF COMMUNITY SERVICE FOR FIVE YEARS; SHALL FOLLOW ALL TERMS OF OKLAHOMA ORDER AND PROVIDE TEXAS BOARD ALL DOCUMENTS SUBMITTED TO OKLAHOMA BOARD; SHALL APPEAR BEFORE THE BOARD TWICE A YEAR; SHALL GIVE A COPY OF THIS ORDER TO ANY HEALTH CARE ENTITY WHERE HE HAS PRIVILEGES; SHALL COOPERATE WITH THE BOARD IN VERIFYING COMPLIANCE; SHALL INFORM BOARD OF CHANGE OF ADDRESS WITHIN 10 DAYS OR IF HE LEAVES THE STATE; TIME SPENT OUT OF TEXAS DOES NOT COUNT TOWARD PROBATION. SHALL NOT SEEK MODIFICATION FOR ONE YEAR. ON 5/11/95 REQUEST FOR TERMINATION DENIED AND ORDER MODIFIED AS FOLLOWS: NO LONGER HAS TO CONTINUE TO RECEIVE TREATMENT FROM BOARD APPROVED PHYSICIAN; NO LONGER HAS TO PERFORM TWO HOURS PER WEEK OF COMMUNITY SERVICE; SHALL APPEAR BEFORE THE BOARD AT LEAST ONE TIME PER YEAR; ALL OTHER CONDITIONS REMAIN IN EFFECT.

CHANEY, MARTIN HESTER MD, LICENSE NUMBER 00C8220, WAS DISCIPLINED BY TEXAS ON DECEMBER 9, 1995
DISCIPLINARY ACTION: 60-MONTH RESTRICTION PLACED ON LICENSE; REQUIRED TO TAKE ADDITIONAL MEDICAL EDUCATION
OFFENSE: SUBSTANDARD CARE, INCOMPETENCE OR NEGLIGENCE

NOTES: BETWEEN 8/24/94 AND 9/07/94 FAILED TO ADEQUATELY EVALUATE AN ADULT MALE PATIENT IN A TIMELY MANNER, WHICH RESULTED IN MISSING A DIAGNOSIS OF MENINGITIS; THE PATIENT WAS LATER HOSPITALIZED WITH FULMINANT CRYPTOCOCCUS NEOFORMANS MENINGITIS; THE PATIENT'S HEALTH SUBSEQUENTLY DETERIORATED AND, AFTER BECOMING COMATOSE, PRONOUNCED BRAIN-DEAD ON 9/29/94. SHALL PRACTICE ONLY IN A FACILITY OF THE TEXAS DEPARTMENT OF CRIMINAL JUSTICE OR IN A BOARD APPROVED INSTITUTIONAL SETTING; SHALL MAINTAIN ADEQUATE MEDICAL RECORDS WHICH SHALL BE AVAILABLE FOR REVIEW; PRACTICE SHALL BE MONITORED BY A LICENSED BOARD APPROVED TEXAS PHYSICIAN WHO SHALL PROVIDE QUARTERLY REPORTS; SHALL OBTAIN AT LEAST 50 HOURS PER YEAR OF CONTINUING MEDICAL EDUCATION AND SHALL SUBMIT PROOF OF COMPLETION TO THE BOARD; SHALL PERSONALLY APPEAR BEFORE THE BOARD AT LEAST ONE TIME PER YEAR OR UPON REQUEST; SHALL COOPERATE WITH THE BOARD IN VERIFYING COMPLIANCE; SHALL ADEQUATELY SUPERVISE THE ACTIVITIES OF ALL INDIVIDUALS UNDER HIS SUPERVISION TO ENSURE THEY ARE

COMPLYING WITH THE LAWS RELATED TO HIS PRACTICE OF MEDICINE AND THEY ARE NOT CAUSING HIM TO BE IN VIOLATION OF THE LAWS RELATING TO HIS PRACTICE OF MEDICINE; SHALL GIVE A COPY OF THIS ORDER TO ANY HEALTH CARE ENTITY WHERE HE HAS PRIVILEGES; SHALL PROVIDE A COPY OF THIS ORDER TO ANYONE REQUESTING IT WITHIN 10 DAYS; TIME PERIOD OUT OF TEXAS DOES NOT COUNT TOWARD RESTRICTION; SHALL INFORM THE BOARD OF CHANGE OF ADDRESS WITHIN 10 DAYS OR IF HE LEAVES THE STATE; SHALL NOT SEEK MODIFICATION FOR ONE YEAR.

CHAPPELL, TIMOTHY RAE MD, LICENSE NUMBER 00E7029 OF PLANO, TX, WAS DISCIPLINED BY TEXAS ON JUNE 22, 1994
DISCIPLINARY ACTION: REPRIMAND; REQUIRED TO TAKE ADDITIONAL MEDICAL EDUCATION
OFFENSE: OVERPRESCRIBING OR MISPRESCRIBING DRUGS

NOTES: PRESCRIBED HYCODAN FOR ONE PATIENT FROM 11/89 TO 5/92 IN INCREASING QUANTITIES WHEN HE HAD REASON TO SUSPECT SHE WAS ADDICTED AS EARLY AS 8/90; TALKED WITH PATIENT ABOUT THIS CONCERN BUT DID NOT INSIST SHE SEEK TREATMENT. SHALL WITHIN SIX MONTHS COMPLETE A BOARD-APPROVED CLINICAL PHARMACOLOGY OR PAIN MANAGEMENT COURSE AND ETHICS COURSE OR PROGRAM; SHALL GIVE A COPY OF THIS ORDER TO ANY HEALTH CARE ENTITY WHERE HE HAS PRIVILEGES; SHALL COOPERATE WITH THE BOARD IN VERIFYING COMPLIANCE; SHALL INFORM BOARD OF CHANGE OF ADDRESS WITHIN 10 DAYS OR IF HE LEAVES THE STATE; TIME SPENT OUT OF TEXAS DOES NOT COUNT TOWARD ORDER. SHALL NOT SEEK MODIFICATION FOR ONE YEAR.

CHEARS, WILLIAM C JR MD, LICENSE NUMBER 00C7199, WAS DISCIPLINED BY TEXAS ON AUGUST 17, 1996
DISCIPLINARY ACTION: FINE; REPRIMAND
OFFENSE: NONCOMPLIANCE WITH A PROFESSIONAL RULE

NOTES: FAILED TO OBTAIN 24 HOURS OF CONTINUING MEDICAL EDUCATION BY 12/1/95 AS REQUIRED FOR RENEWAL OF HIS LICENSE; HE WAS GRANTED AN EXTENSION TO 2/29/96 WHICH HE ALSO FAILED TO MEET; STILL REQUIRED TO MEET CONTINUING MEDICAL EDUCATION REQUIREMENT. $100 ADMINISTRATIVE PENALTY. SHALL COOPERATE WITH THE BOARD IN VERIFYING COMPLIANCE.

CHEN, RAY HUANG TSANG MD, DATE OF BIRTH JANUARY 2, 1942, LICENSE NUMBER 00E5356 OF 6305 NEWCASTLE, BELLAIRE, TX, WAS DISCIPLINED BY TEXAS ON JANUARY 29, 1993
DISCIPLINARY ACTION: 60-MONTH PROBATION; RESTRICTION PLACED ON CONTROLLED SUBSTANCE LICENSE
OFFENSE: OVERPRESCRIBING OR MISPRESCRIBING DRUGS

NOTES: PRESCRIBED DEMEROL AND VALIUM TO HIS EX-WIFE IN EXCESSIVE AMOUNTS WHEN HE KNEW SHE WAS HABITUATED TO CONTROLLED SUBSTANCES. 5 YEAR SUSPENSION STAYED. CONDITIONS OF PROBATION: SHALL SURRENDER ALL UNUSED TRIPLICATE PRESCRIPTION FORMS AND NOT ORDER ANY MORE WITHOUT WRITTEN AUTHORITY; SHALL NOT POSSESS, ADMINISTER, DISPENSE OR PRESCRIBE ANY CONTROLLED SUBSTANCES OUTSIDE OF A HOSPITAL SETTING; SHALL NOT TREAT OR OTHERWISE SERVE AS PHYSICIAN, PRESCRIBE, DISPENSE OR ADMINISTER CONTROLLED SUBSTANCES THAT MAY BE SUBJECT TO ABUSE TO HIMSELF OR ANY MEMBER OF HIS FAMILY; SHALL MAINTAIN ADEQUATE MEDICAL RECORDS ON ALL OFFICE VISITS WHICH SHALL BE AVAILABLE FOR INSPECTION; SHALL APPEAR BEFORE THE BOARD ONCE A YEAR; SHALL GIVE A COPY OF THIS ORDER TO ANY HEALTH CARE ENTITY WHERE HE HAS PRIVILEGES; SHALL COOPERATE WITH THE BOARD IN VERIFYING COMPLIANCE; SHALL INFORM BOARD OF CHANGE OF ADDRESS WITHIN 10 DAYS OR IF HE LEAVES THE STATE; TIME SPENT OUT OF TEXAS DOES NOT COUNT TOWARD PROBATION. SHALL NOT SEEK MODIFICATION UNLESS HE LOCATES PRACTICE OUTSIDE OF TEXAS AND AT LEAST ONE YEAR HAS ELAPSED. PROBATION TERMINATED ON 5/15/96.

CHEPKO, JAMES DOUGLAS MD, LICENSE NUMBER F0931 OF HOUSTON, TX, WAS DISCIPLINED BY TEXAS ON FEBRUARY 7, 1998
DISCIPLINARY ACTION: REQUIRED TO TAKE ADDITIONAL MEDICAL EDUCATION; MONITORING OF PHYSICIAN PERFORMANCE
OFFENSE: PROFESSIONAL MISCONDUCT

NOTES: ON OR ABOUT 3/20/91 WHILE HE WAS WORKING AS THE EMERGENCY ROOM PHYSICIAN, A 23 YEAR OLD MALE PRESENTED COMPLAINING OF A HEADACHE WITH ACCOMPANYING DIZZINESS, WEAKNESS AND TINGLING IN HIS LEFT ARM AND LEG; INSTEAD OF PERSONALLY EVALUATING THE PATIENT, HE PERMITTED AN INADEQUATELY SUPERVISED MEDICAL STUDENT AND AN INTERN TO EXAMINE AND DICTATE CARE; HE SIGNED OFF ON THE PATIENT'S CHART WITHOUT HAVING PERSONALLY SEEN OR EXAMINED HIM; THE PATIENT WAS SUBSEQUENTLY DISCHARGED; ON OR ABOUT 3/21/91 THE PATIENT SUFFERED A RIGHT SUPERIOR CEREBELLAR INFARCT; THROUGH HIS FAILURE TO ACT AND THROUGH THE ACTIONS OF OTHERS FOR WHOM HE WAS DIRECTLY RESPONSIBLE, HE FAILED TO PERFORM AN ADEQUATE NEUROLOGICAL EXAMINATION AND FAILED TO ADEQUATELY RECOGNIZE THE SIGNS OF A STROKE-IN-EVOLUTION GIVEN THE NATURE OF THE PATIENT'S INJURY AND THE SYMPTOMS MANIFESTED BY IT. LICENSE LIMITED FOR THREE YEARS AS FOLLOWS: SHALL ATTEND 50 HOURS PER YEAR OF CONTINUING MEDICAL EDUCATION AT LEAST 25 HOURS OF WHICH SHALL BE IN EMERGENCY MEDICINE; SHALL ADEQUATELY SUPERVISE THE ACTIVITIES OF ALL HIS EMPLOYEES AND OTHERS UNDER HIS SUPERVISION; SHALL NOT SIGN OR INDICATE IN ANY MANNER IN PATIENT RECORDS THAT HE HAS SEEN PATIENTS UNLESS HE ACTUALLY HAS SEEN AND EXAMINED THE PATIENT UNLESS IT IS CLEARLY NOTED THAT HE DID NOT PERSONALLY EXAMINE THE PATIENT; SHALL SUCCESSFULLY COMPLETE AN ADVANCED CARDIAC LIFE SUPPORT COURSE AND OBTAIN CERTIFICATION IF HE HASN'T ALREADY DONE SO WITHIN THE PAST 12 MONTHS; SHALL SUCCESSFULLY COMPLETE AN ADVANCED TRAUMA LIFE SUPPORT COURSE AND OBTAIN CERTIFICATION WITHIN ONE YEAR; SHALL APPEAR BEFORE THE BOARD UPON REQUEST; SHALL COOPERATE WITH THE BOARD IN VERIFYING COMPLIANCE; SHALL GIVE A COPY OF THIS ORDER TO ANY HEALTH CARE ENTITY WHERE HE HAS PRIVILEGES; TIME SPENT OUT OF TEXAS DOES NOT COUNT TOWARD RESTRICTION; SHALL INFORM THE BOARD OF CHANGE OF ADDRESS WITHIN 10 DAYS OR IF HE LEAVES THE STATE; SHALL NOT SEEK MODIFICATION FOR ONE YEAR.

CHEPKO, JAMES DOUGLAS MD, LICENSE NUMBER F0931 OF HOUSTON, TX, WAS DISCIPLINED BY TEXAS ON APRIL 10, 1999
DISCIPLINARY ACTION: FINE; RESTRICTION PLACED ON LICENSE
OFFENSE: FAILURE TO COMPLY WITH PREVIOUS BOARD ORDER

NOTES: FAILED TO TAKE AND SUCCESSFULLY COMPLETE AN ADVANCED TRAUMA LIFE SUPPORT COURSE AND

OBTAIN CERTIFICATION AS REQUIRED BY THE 2/7/98 BOARD ORDER; ALSO FAILED TO COOPERATE WITH BOARD STAFF BY FAILING TO RESPOND TO TELEPHONE MESSAGES AND CORRESPONDENCE FROM HIS ASSIGNED COMPLIANCE OFFICER; HE DENIES THAT HE RECEIVED THE TELEPHONE MESSAGES BUT ADMITS THAT, ON AT LEAST 1 OCCASION, FAIL TO RESPOND TO A WRITTEN REQUEST OF HIS COMPLIANCE OFFICER; HE NO LONGER PRACTICES EMERGENCY MEDICINE AND CURRENTLY HAS A GENERAL PRACTICE. LICENSE LIMITED AS FOLLOWS: SHALL NOT PRACTICE EMERGENCY MEDICINE UNTIL SUCH TIME AS HE HAS PROVIDED TO THE BOARD EVIDENCE THAT HE HAS SUCCESSFULLY COMPLETED AN ADVANCED TRAUMA LIFE SUPPORT COURSE AND OBTAINED CERTIFICATION; ALL OTHER PROVISIONS OF 2/7/98 ORDER REMAIN IN FULL FORCE AND EFFECT UNTIL SUPERSEDED BY A SUBSEQUENT BOARD ORDER; $1,000 FINE.

CHERIAN, FRANCIS MD, LICENSE NUMBER 00F8052 OF COLLEGE STATION, TX, WAS DISCIPLINED BY TEXAS ON JANUARY 27, 1996
DISCIPLINARY ACTION: 60-MONTH RESTRICTION PLACED ON LICENSE; 60-MONTH RESTRICTION PLACED ON CONTROLLED SUBSTANCE LICENSE
OFFENSE: SUBSTANDARD CARE, INCOMPETENCE OR NEGLIGENCE

NOTES: DURING THE COURSE OF CARE AND TREATMENT OF TWO PATIENTS, SEEN OCCASIONALLY FROM 1991 THROUGH 1994, FAILED TO APPROPRIATELY DIAGNOSE, TREAT, AND ADEQUATELY DOCUMENT THE CARE RENDERED INCLUDING MULTIPLE INJECTIONS OF DANGEROUS DRUGS WHICH WERE ADMINISTERED DURING THE COURSE OF TREATMENT; FAILED TO ADEQUATELY ASSESS A PATIENT'S NEED FOR A PRESCRIPTION OF PHENTERMINE, FAILED TO ADEQUATELY MONITOR THE PATIENT, AND FAILED TO KEEP COMPLETE MEDICAL RECORDS ON THE CARE AND TREATMENT OF THE PATIENT. FIVE YEAR RESTRICTION: SHALL NOT ORDER, ADMINISTER, OR PRESCRIBE CONTROLLED SUBSTANCE OR DANGEROUS DRUGS WITH POTENTIAL FOR ABUSE TO ANY PATIENT FOR LONGER THAN 60 CONSECUTIVE DAYS OF TREATMENT, INCLUDING PATIENTS UNDERGOING TREATMENT FOR PROLONGED, CHRONIC, OR INTRACTABLE PAIN; SHALL NOT DISPENSE FROM HIS OFFICE OR ANY OTHER PRACTICE LOCATION, EITHER FOR IMMEDIATE NEEDS OR OTHERWISE, ANY CONTROLLED SUBSTANCES FOR DANGEROUS DRUGS WITH POTENTIAL FOR ABUSE; SHALL MAINTAIN A LOGBOOK FOR ALL PRESCRIPTIONS OR REFILLS TELEPHONED IN BY HIM OR AT HIS DIRECTION FOR CONTROLLED SUBSTANCES AND DANGEROUS DRUGS WITH ADDICTIVE POTENTIAL AVAILABLE FOR REVIEW; SEPARATE FROM PATIENT RECORDS, SHALL MAINTAIN A FILE WITH A COPY OF EVERY PRESCRIPTION WRITTEN FOR CONTROLLED SUBSTANCES AND DRUGS WITH ADDICTIVE POTENTIAL; SHALL MAINTAIN ADEQUATE MEDICAL RECORDS WHICH SHALL BE AVAILABLE FOR REVIEW; SHALL NOT TREAT ANY PATIENT FOR WEIGHT CONTROL OR OBESITY WITH ANY CONTROLLED SUBSTANCES, DANGEROUS DRUGS, OR OVER-THE-COUNTER DRUGS, WHETHER MARKETED NOW OR IN THE FUTURE, BY WHATEVER NAME; SHALL OBTAIN AT LEAST 50 HOURS PER YEAR OF CONTINUING MEDICAL EDUCATION; SHALL APPEAR BEFORE THE BOARD AT LEAST ONE TIME PER YEAR; SHALL GIVE A COPY OF THIS ORDER TO ANY HEALTH CARE ENTITY WHERE HE HAS PRIVILEGES; SHALL PROVIDE A COPY OF THIS ORDER TO ANYONE REQUESTING IT WITHIN 10 DAYS; TIME PERIOD OUT OF TEXAS DOES NOT COUNT TOWARD RESTRICTION; SHALL INFORM THE BOARD OF CHANGE OF ADDRESS WITHIN 10 DAYS OF IF HE LEAVES THE STATE; SHALL NOT SEEK MODIFICATION FOR ONE YEAR.

CHESTER, JEREMY DAVID MD, LICENSE NUMBER 00H4234 OF DUNCANVILLE, TX, WAS DISCIPLINED BY TEXAS ON SEPTEMBER 25, 1993
DISCIPLINARY ACTION: 60-MONTH RESTRICTION PLACED ON CONTROLLED SUBSTANCE LICENSE; MONITORING OF PHYSICIAN PERFORMANCE
OFFENSE: SUBSTANCE ABUSE

NOTES: HAS SUFFERED FROM DEPRESSION, POST-TRAUMATIC STRESS AND CHEMICAL DEPENDENCE INVOLVING ABUSE OF FENTANYL; UNDERWENT INPATIENT TREATMENT FOR CHEMICAL DEPENDENCE FROM 7/91 THROUGH 11/91 AND INPATIENT CARE FOR DEPRESSION AND POST-TRAUMATIC STRESS BEGINNING 12/92; PARTICIPATES IN AA AND IS IN THERAPY. CONDITIONS OF RESTRICTION: SHALL ABSTAIN FROM THE CONSUMPTION OF ALCOHOL/CHEMICAL SUBSTANCES IN ANY FORM UNLESS PRESCRIBED BY ANOTHER PHYSICIAN FOR A LEGITIMATE AND THERAPEUTIC PURPOSE; SHALL SUBMIT HIMSELF FOR APPROPRIATE EXAMS INCLUDING DRUG OR ALCOHOL SCREENS; SHALL CONTINUE TO RECEIVE TREATMENT FROM SPECIFIED PHYSICIANS WITH QUARTERLY REPORTS; SHALL PARTICIPATE IN AA'S PROGRAM NOT LESS THAN TWO TIMES A WEEK; SHALL PARTICIPATE IN ACTIVITIES OF A PHYSICIAN HEALTH AND REHABILITATION COMMITTEE AND ATTEND WEEKLY MEETINGS WITH QUARTERLY REPORTS; SHALL NOT POSSESS, ADMINISTER, OR PRESCRIBE CONTROLLED SUBSTANCES EXCEPT IN A HOSPITAL EMERGENCY ROOM; SEPARATE FROM PATIENT RECORDS, SHALL MAINTAIN A WRITTEN RECORD OF EVERY DANGEROUS DRUG ORDERED OR PRESCRIBED; SHALL NOT TELEPHONE IN ANY PRESCRIPTIONS; EMPLOYER SHALL SUBMIT REPORTS TO THE BOARD EVERY SIX MONTHS; SHALL GIVE A COPY OF THIS ORDER TO ANY HEALTH CARE ENTITY WHERE HE HAS PRIVILEGES; SHALL COOPERATE WITH THE BOARD IN VERIFYING COMPLIANCE; SHALL INFORM BOARD OF CHANGE OF ADDRESS WITHIN 10 DAYS OR IF HE LEAVES THE STATE; TIME SPENT OUT OF TEXAS DOES NOT COUNT TOWARD RESTRICTION. SHALL NOT SEEK MODIFICATION FOR ONE YEAR.

CHODOSH, THOMAS B DO OF CORPUS CHRISTI, TX, WAS DISCIPLINED BY MISSOURI ON SEPTEMBER 7, 1990
OFFENSE: DISCIPLINARY ACTION BY ANOTHER STATE OR AGENCY

NOTES: UNSUCCESSFULLY ATTEMPTED A NORMAL DELIVERY BY A 15-YEAR-OLD MOTHER USING FORCEPS IN A RECKLESS AND DANGEROUS MANNER; UNDUE DELAY IN OBTAINING A C-SECTION RESULTED IN BRAIN DAMAGE TO THE INFANT AND UNNECESSARY DAMAGE TO THE MOTHER AND CHILD IN GENERAL. AGREEMENT - MUST APPEAR BEFORE BOARD BEFORE RETURNING TO PRACTICE IN MISSOURI

CHONG, JUAN A MD, LICENSE NUMBER 00E0855 OF CLEVELAND, TX, WAS DISCIPLINED BY TEXAS ON OCTOBER 5, 1991
DISCIPLINARY ACTION: 48-MONTH RESTRICTION PLACED ON LICENSE; REQUIRED TO TAKE ADDITIONAL MEDICAL EDUCATION
OFFENSE: SUBSTANDARD CARE, INCOMPETENCE OR NEGLIGENCE

NOTES: INAPPROPRIATE OBSTETRICAL/ GYNECOLOGICAL TREATMENT OF NINE PATIENTS; VOLUNTARILY AGREED TO A HOSPITAL REVIEW OF RECORDS, TO GET SECOND OPINIONS ON ALL SURGERY CASES,

AND TO OBTAIN FURTHER EDUCATION; VOLUNTARILY RELINQUISHED HIS GYNECOLOGICAL PRIVILEGES AT CHARTER REGIONAL MEDICAL CENTER UNTIL THEY HIRED A QUALIFIED PHYSICIAN WHO COULD REVIEW HIS RECORDS, WHICH WAS ACCEPTED BY THE HOSPITAL ON 2/22/91; HAS NOT PRACTICED OBSTETRICS FOR MORE THAN A YEAR. LICENSE IS RESTRICTED UNDER THE FOLLOWING TERMS AND CONDITIONS: SHALL ATTEND AT LEAST 50 HOURS PER YEAR OF CONTINUING MEDICAL EDUCATION; SHALL NOT PRACTICE OBSTETRICS UNTIL SUCH TIME AS THE MEDICAL EXECUTIVE COMMITTEE OF AN ACCREDITED HOSPITAL IS PREPARED TO EXTEND HOSPITAL OBSTETRICS PRIVILEGES; SHALL REFRAIN FROM PERFORMING GYNECOLOGICAL SURGERY UNLESS PERFORMED IN A ACCREDITED HOSPITAL WHERE HE HAS PRIVILEGES TO PERFORM SUCH SURGERY; SHALL HAVE A BOARD APPROVED SUPERVISOR WITH QUARTERLY REPORTS TO THE BOARD; SHALL COOPERATE WITH THE BOARD IN VERIFYING COMPLIANCE; SHALL ADVISE THE BOARD OF ANY ADDRESS CHANGE WITHIN 10 DAYS; TIME SPENT OUT OF TEXAS DOES NOT COUNT TOWARD PROBATION; SHALL NOT SEEK MODIFICATION OF ORDER FOR AT LEAST ONE YEAR. ON 3/5/94 ORDER TERMINATED.

CHOUTEAU, ROBERT MICHAEL DO, LICENSE NUMBER 00E9578 OF DALLAS, TX, WAS DISCIPLINED BY TEXAS ON JANUARY 6, 1995
DISCIPLINARY ACTION: REPRIMAND
OFFENSE: NONCOMPLIANCE WITH A PROFESSIONAL RULE

NOTES: INADEQUATELY DOCUMENTED THE CARE AND TREATMENT OF A PATIENT. SHALL GIVE A COPY OF THIS ORDER TO ANY HEALTH CARE ENTITY WHERE HE HAS PRIVILEGES.

CHOUTEAU, ROBERT MICHAEL DO, LICENSE NUMBER 0001998, WAS DISCIPLINED BY OKLAHOMA ON APRIL 2, 1996
DISCIPLINARY ACTION: REPRIMAND
OFFENSE: DISCIPLINARY ACTION BY ANOTHER STATE OR AGENCY

NOTES: ON 1/06/95 THE TEXAS BOARD ORDERED A PUBLIC REPRIMAND FOR FAILING TO ADEQUATELY DOCUMENT CARE AND TREATMENT RENDERED. SHALL GIVE A COPY OF THIS ORDER TO ANY HEALTH CARE ENTITY WHERE HE HAS PRIVILEGES; SHALL APPEAR BEFORE THE BOARD BEFORE PRACTICING IN OKLAHOMA; $925 ADMINISTRATIVE COSTS.

CHRIST, JOHN MD, LICENSE NUMBER 0044427 OF BASTROP, TX, WAS DISCIPLINED BY FLORIDA ON AUGUST 31, 1995
DISCIPLINARY ACTION: SURRENDER OF LICENSE
OFFENSE: DISCIPLINARY ACTION BY ANOTHER STATE OR AGENCY

NOTES: LICENSE TO PRACTICE IN TEXAS WAS SUSPENDED; FAILING TO REPORT THIS TO THE BOARD WITHIN 30 DAYS. CONVICTED OF THE FELONY OFFENSE OF ATTEMPTED MURDER. VOLUNTARY RELINQUISHMENT OF LICENSE; AGREES NEVER AGAIN TO APPLY FOR LICENSURE UNLESS HE PRESENTS TO THE BOARD AND DEMONSTRATES THE CRIMINAL CHARGES HAVE BEEN OVERTURNED OR OTHERWISE INVALIDATED.

CHRIST, JOHN E MD, LICENSE NUMBER 0123047 OF BISHOP COUNTY JAIL, BASTROP, TX, WAS DISCIPLINED BY NEW YORK ON OCTOBER 24, 1994
DISCIPLINARY ACTION: LICENSE REVOCATION
OFFENSE: DISCIPLINARY ACTION BY ANOTHER STATE OR AGENCY

NOTES: CONVICTED OF ATTEMPTED MURDER AND FOUND GUILTY OF MISCONDUCT BY THE TEXAS BOARD.

CHRIST, JOHN E MD, LICENSE NUMBER 0055213 OF 6560 FANNIN STREET, HOUSTON, TX, WAS DISCIPLINED BY MASSACHUSETTS ON NOVEMBER 9, 1994
DISCIPLINARY ACTION: LICENSE REVOCATION
OFFENSE: DISCIPLINARY ACTION BY ANOTHER STATE OR AGENCY

NOTES: DISCIPLINE BY TEXAS; CRIMINAL CONVICTION.

CHRIST, JOHN ERNEST MD, LICENSE NUMBER 00E0856 OF HOUSTON, TX, WAS DISCIPLINED BY TEXAS ON JANUARY 14, 1994
DISCIPLINARY ACTION: LICENSE SUSPENSION
OFFENSE: CRIMINAL CONVICTION OR PLEA OF GUILTY, NOLO CONTENDERE, OR NO CONTEST TO A CRIME

NOTES: ON 9/16/93 JUDGMENT ENTERED WHICH FOUND HIM GUILTY OF ATTEMPTED MURDER; SENTENCED TO 20 YEARS IN PRISON AND A $10,000 FINE; IS PRESENTLY INCARCERATED; IS IN THE PROCESS OF APPEALING THIS CONVICTION. IF APPEAL OF CONVICTION IS SUCCESSFUL SUSPENSION SHALL BE LIFTED UNLESS LICENSE HAS BEEN SUSPENDED FOR MORE THAN 24 MONTHS; IN THAT CASE SUSPENSION SHALL REMAIN IN EFFECT UNTIL HE PASSES SPEX EXAM; IF CONVICTION IS UPHELD, LICENSE SHALL BE REVOKED.

CHRIST, JOHN ERNEST MD OF 6560 FANNIN STE 1144, HOUSTON, TX, WAS DISCIPLINED BY DEA ON MARCH 5, 1996
DISCIPLINARY ACTION: SURRENDER OF CONTROLLED SUBSTANCE LICENSE

NOTES: IN LIEU OF PUBLIC INTEREST REVOCATION.

CHRISTENSEN, DENNIS W MD, LICENSE NUMBER 0012595 OF CONWAY, SC, WAS DISCIPLINED BY SOUTH CAROLINA ON JULY 24, 1990
DISCIPLINARY ACTION: PROBATION; FINE
OFFENSE: PROVIDING FALSE INFORMATION TO THE BOARD OR OTHER HEALTH AGENCY

NOTES: SUBSTANCE ABUSE AND FALSE ANSWER ON REREGISTRATION. SUSPENSION STAYED; $1,000 FINE AND INDEFINITE PROBATION.

CHRISTENSEN, DENNIS W MD, LICENSE NUMBER 0012595 OF CONWAY, SC, WAS DISCIPLINED BY SOUTH CAROLINA ON DECEMBER 5, 1990
DISCIPLINARY ACTION: LICENSE REVOCATION
OFFENSE: FAILURE TO COMPLY WITH PREVIOUS BOARD ORDER

NOTES: VIOLATED CONDITIONS OF PROBATION.

CHRISTENSEN, DENNIS W MD, LICENSE NUMBER 00C8923 OF CONWAY, SC, WAS DISCIPLINED BY TEXAS ON APRIL 20, 1991
DISCIPLINARY ACTION: REQUIRED TO ENTER AN IMPAIRED PHYSICIAN PROGRAM OR SUBSTANCE ABUSE TREATMENT; MONITORING OF PHYSICIAN PERFORMANCE
OFFENSE: DISCIPLINARY ACTION BY ANOTHER STATE OR AGENCY

NOTES: PRIOR TO PRACTICING IN TEXAS MUST APPEAR BEFORE THE BOARD; CONTINUE TO PARTICIPATE IN A MAINTENANCE PROGRAM FOR RECOVERING ALCOHOLICS; MUST ABSTAIN FROM THE CONSUMPTION OF ALCOHOL/CHEMICAL SUBSTANCES; MUST SUBMIT TO ALCOHOL AND DRUG SCREENS.

CHRISTENSEN, DENNIS W MD OF CONWAY, SC, WAS DISCIPLINED BY NORTH CAROLINA ON SEPTEMBER 30, 1991
DISCIPLINARY ACTION: SURRENDER OF LICENSE

CHRISTENSEN, DENNIS W MD, LICENSE NUMBER 0C26098 OF ROHNERT PARK, CA, WAS DISCIPLINED BY CALIFORNIA ON JUNE 19, 1993

DISCIPLINARY ACTION: 96-MONTH PROBATION

NOTES: REVOCATION STAYED.

CHRISTIANSON, PAUL BARR MD, LICENSE NUMBER 00G6487 OF GRIFFISS AFB, NY, WAS DISCIPLINED BY TEXAS ON JANUARY 24, 1992
DISCIPLINARY ACTION: SURRENDER OF LICENSE

NOTES: PROFESSIONAL FAILURE TO PRACTICE MEDICINE IN AN ACCEPTABLE MANNER CONSISTENT WITH PUBLIC HEALTH AND WELFARE. LICENSE VOLUNTARILY SURRENDERED IN LIEU OF FURTHER DISCIPLINARY ACTION.

CHUMAK, BOGDAN ALBERTO MD, LICENSE NUMBER 038466 OF 218 WESTHILL DRIVE, HEWITT, TX, WAS DISCIPLINED BY VIRGINIA ON AUGUST 9, 1999
DISCIPLINARY ACTION: LICENSE SUSPENSION
OFFENSE: CRIMINAL CONVICTION OR PLEA OF GUILTY, NOLO CONTENDERE, OR NO CONTEST TO A CRIME

NOTES: ON 5/12/93 CONVICTED IN COLORADO FOR AIDING AND ABETTING THE USE OF A FALSE DOCUMENT. ON 10/21/99 PETITION FOR REINSTATEMENT GRANTED AND FULL AND UNRESTRICTED LICENSE ISSUED.

CLARK, CORDELL MD, LICENSE NUMBER F8827 OF DALLAS, TX, WAS DISCIPLINED BY TEXAS ON AUGUST 28, 1999
DISCIPLINARY ACTION: REPRIMAND; REQUIRED TO TAKE ADDITIONAL MEDICAL EDUCATION
OFFENSE: PROFESSIONAL MISCONDUCT

NOTES: FAILED TO SEE OR EVALUATE A PATIENT PRIOR TO ORDERING PHYSICAL THERAPY, ALONG WITH FAILING TO MAINTAIN RECORDS AND RELEASING PATIENT RECORDS TO DALLAS COUNTY COURT OR TO DEFENDANT'S ATTORNEY IN LAWSUIT IN WHICH A PATIENT WAS THE PLAINTIFF EVEN AFTER BEING SUBPOENAED; HE STATES THAT IT IS HIS OFFICE PRACTICE TO KEEP MEDICAL RECORDS OF PATIENTS TREATED FOR TRAUMATIC DISORDERS ONLY FOR 1 YEAR BEFORE RELEASING THE RECORDS TO THE PATIENT'S REPRESENTATIVE; HE MAINTAINS THAT HE MADE HIMSELF AVAILABLE ON THE TRIAL DATE BUT THAT PLAINTIFF'S ATTORNEY DID NOT SHOW UP AT COURT. LICENSE LIMITED FOR THREE YEARS AS FOLLOWS: SHALL ATTEND 50 HOURS PER YEAR OF CONTINUING MEDICAL EDUCATION WITH 1 COURSE IN THE AREA OF RISK MANAGEMENT AND 1 IN THE AREA OF ACCURATE RECORD KEEPING AND MAINTENANCE; SHALL MAINTAIN ADEQUATE MEDICAL RECORDS WHICH SHALL BE AVAILABLE FOR REVIEW; SHALL COMPLY WITH ONE OF THE FOLLOWING: BEGINNING NO LATER THAN 60 DAYS HIS MEDICAL PRACTICE SHALL BE MONITORED BY A BOARD APPROVED TEXAS PHYSICIAN WHO SHALL PROVIDE QUARTERLY REPORTS TO THE BOARD, OR WITHIN 1 YEAR TAKE AND PASS THE SPEX WITH A SCORE OF 75 OR BETTER, WITHIN 3 ATTEMPTS; SHALL APPEAR BEFORE THE BOARD AT LEAST ONCE A YEAR; SHALL COOPERATE WITH THE BOARD IN VERIFYING COMPLIANCE; TIME SPENT OUT OF TEXAS DOES NOT COUNT TOWARD RESTRICTION; SHALL INFORM THE BOARD OF CHANGE OF ADDRESS WITHIN 10 DAYS OR IF HE LEAVES THE STATE; SHALL NOT SEEK MODIFICATION FOR ONE YEAR.

CLARK, GARTH A A MD, LICENSE NUMBER 00H7005 OF SHERMAN, TX, WAS DISCIPLINED BY TEXAS ON JUNE 28, 1995
DISCIPLINARY ACTION: REPRIMAND; MONITORING OF PHYSICIAN PERFORMANCE
OFFENSE: LOSS OR RESTRICTION OF HOSPITAL PRIVILEGES

NOTES: ON 11/22/93, HOSPITAL PRIVILEGES WERE SUSPENDED DUE TO PROBLEMS COMPLETING MEDICAL RECORDS, FAILURE TO ADEQUATELY FOLLOW-UP ON PATIENTS AND PROBLEMS CONTACTING HIM BY HOSPITAL STAFF; IN 2/94, HIS PRIVILEGES AT A SECOND HOSPITAL WERE SUSPENDED BASED ON CARE AND TREATMENT OF A PATIENT FAILING TO TIMELY OBTAIN A NEUROLOGICAL OR INFECTIOUS DISEASE CONSULT AND HIS ALLEGED FAILURE TO NOTIFY HOSPITAL OF 11/93 SUSPENSION; IN A REVIEW OF 11 PATIENT RECORDS IT WAS DETERMINED THAT HE FAILED TO ADEQUATELY DOCUMENT AND FOLLOW UP ON PATIENTS; SUBSEQUENTLY SOUGHT PSYCHIATRIC TREATMENT FOR DEPRESSION. LICENSE RESTRICTED FOR FIVE YEARS WITH TERMS: SHALL UNDERGO A COMPLETE NEUROPSYCHIATRIC EXAMINATION BY A BOARD-APPROVED PHYSICIAN WITH ANY TREATMENT RECOMMENDED WHO SHALL SUBMIT MONTHLY REPORTS; HIS PRACTICE SHALL BE MONITORED BY A BOARD-APPROVED PHYSICIAN WHO SHALL SUBMIT QUARTERLY REPORTS TO THE BOARD; SHALL MAINTAIN ADEQUATE MEDICAL RECORDS WHICH SHALL BE AVAILABLE FOR REVIEW; SHALL TAKE AND PASS THE SPECIAL PURPOSE EXAMINATION WITHIN ONE YEAR; SHALL APPEAR BEFORE BOARD AT LEAST ONCE A YEAR; SHALL COOPERATE WITH THE BOARD IN VERIFYING COMPLIANCE INCLUDING PROVIDING COPIES OF MEDICAL RELEASES UPON REQUEST; SHALL GIVE A COPY OF THIS ORDER TO ANY HEALTH CARE ENTITY WHERE HE HAS PRIVILEGES; TIME PERIOD OUT OF TEXAS DOES NOT COUNT TOWARD RESTRICTION; SHALL INFORM BOARD OF CHANGE OF ADDRESS WITHIN 10 DAYS OR IF HE LEAVES THE STATE. SHALL NOT SEEK MODIFICATION FOR ONE YEAR.

CLARK, GARTH A A MD OF TX, WAS DISCIPLINED BY DEA ON NOVEMBER 12, 1998
DISCIPLINARY ACTION: REVOCATION OF CONTROLLED SUBSTANCE LICENSE
OFFENSE: DISCIPLINARY ACTION BY ANOTHER STATE OR AGENCY

NOTES: ON 2/11/97 THE TEXAS BOARD SUSPENDED HIS LICENSE AND ON 2/18/97 CANCELED HIS STATE CONTROLLED SUBSTANCE REGISTRATION.

CLARK, GEORGE B DO, LICENSE NUMBER 00D1400 OF DALLAS, TX, WAS DISCIPLINED BY TEXAS ON JANUARY 6, 1995
DISCIPLINARY ACTION: REPRIMAND
OFFENSE: OVERPRESCRIBING OR MISPRESCRIBING DRUGS

NOTES: FROM 1984 THROUGH 7/93 PRESCRIBED CONTROLLED SUBSTANCES TO AN ADULT FEMALE PATIENT WITHOUT ADEQUATE INDICATION OR APPROPRIATE DOCUMENTATION; KNEW OR SHOULD HAVE KNOWN SHE WAS AN ABUSER OF CONTROLLED SUBSTANCES; AGREES TO THE ENTRY OF THIS ORDER IN LIEU OF FURTHER INVESTIGATION.

CLARK, ROBERT ERNEST III MD, LICENSE NUMBER 00F6532 OF HEREFORD, TX, WAS DISCIPLINED BY TEXAS ON AUGUST 20, 1992
DISCIPLINARY ACTION: 60-MONTH PROBATION
OFFENSE: DISCIPLINARY ACTION BY ANOTHER STATE OR AGENCY

NOTES: UNPROFESSIONAL OR DISHONORABLE CONDUCT LIKELY TO DECEIVE, DEFRAUD OR INJURE THE PUBLIC; AND DISCIPLINARY ACTION BY A PEER REVIEW ENTITY. SUSPENSION, STAYED. PROBATION UNDER TERMS AND CONDITIONS.

CLAYTON, EUGENE N III MD, LICENSE NUMBER 00H7968 OF KERRVILLE, TX, WAS DISCIPLINED BY TEXAS ON MARCH 2, 1996

DISCIPLINARY ACTION: 120-MONTH PROBATION; REQUIRED TO TAKE ADDITIONAL MEDICAL EDUCATION
OFFENSE: SUBSTANDARD CARE, INCOMPETENCE OR NEGLIGENCE

NOTES: ON 7/14/95 HE INAPPROPRIATELY ADMINISTERED ANESTHESIA TO A CHILD AND THEN LEFT THE OPERATING ROOM WHILE THE CHILD WAS STILL UNDER ANESTHESIA WHICH IS BELOW THE STANDARD OF CARE; IN 6/95 INTUBATED AN ADULT FEMALE PATIENT AND FAILED TO RECOGNIZE A RIGHT MAIN STEM BRONCHUS INTUBATION; HIS MEDICAL RECORD DOCUMENTATION FOR THE TWO PATIENTS WAS INADEQUATE; AND ON 7/13/95 CRUMBLED A PATIENT ORDER SHEET AND THREW THE ORDER IN THE TRASH CAN WHICH IS THE DESTRUCTION OF MEDICAL RECORDS. SUSPENSION, STAYED AS PROBATION UNDER TERMS AND CONDITIONS: HIS MEDICAL PRACTICE, INCLUDING ANY OFFICE, ANESTHESIA, AND SURGICAL PRACTICE, SHALL BE MONITORED BY A BOARD APPROVED TEXAS PHYSICIAN WHO SHALL SUBMIT QUARTERLY REPORTS TO THE BOARD; WITHIN ONE YEAR SHALL COMPLETION OF A BOARD APPROVED COURSE IN ETHICS; SHALL OBTAIN AT LEAST 50 HOURS PER YEAR OF CONTINUING MEDICAL EDUCATION WHICH SHALL INCLUDE AT LEAST 25 HOURS IN ANESTHESIOLOGY; WITHIN ONE YEAR SHALL COMPLETE A PEDIATRIC ADVANCED LIFE SUPPORT COURSE AND AN ADVANCED TRAUMA LIFE SUPPORT COURSE (ATLS) AND FOR BOTH SHALL OBTAIN CERTIFICATION; SHALL APPEAR BEFORE THE BOARD AT LEAST TWO TIMES EACH YEAR; SHALL COOPERATE WITH THE BOARD IN VERIFYING COMPLIANCE; SHALL GIVE A COPY OF THIS ORDER TO ANY HEALTH CARE ENTITY WHERE HE HAS PRIVILEGES; TIME PERIOD OUT OF TEXAS DOES NOT COUNT TOWARD PROBATION; SHALL INFORM THE BOARD OF CHANGE OF ADDRESS WITHIN 10 DAYS OR IF HE LEAVES THE STATE; SHALL NOT SEEK MODIFICATION FOR ONE YEAR. ON 5/10/97 PETITION TO MODIFY ORDER GRANTED DELETING MONITORING OF HIS MEDICAL PRACTICE, AND REDUCING APPEARANCES BEFORE THE BOARD FROM BIANNUAL TO ANNUAL. ON 5/16/98 ORDER MODIFIED REPLACING BIANNUAL APPEARANCES BEFORE THE BOARD TO APPEARANCES UPON REQUEST.

CLYNCH, MICHAEL RICHARD MD, LICENSE NUMBER F1458, WAS DISCIPLINED BY TEXAS ON MARCH 1, 1997
DISCIPLINARY ACTION: SURRENDER OF CONTROLLED SUBSTANCE LICENSE; 60-MONTH PROBATION
OFFENSE: SUBSTANDARD CARE, INCOMPETENCE OR NEGLIGENCE

NOTES: FROM APPROXIMATELY 2/95 THROUGH 1996 HE PRESCRIBED ON A CONTINUOUS AND FREQUENT BASIS EXCESSIVE AMOUNTS OF POTENTIALLY ADDICTIVE DRUGS, SUCH AS BENZODIAZEPINES AND BARBITURATES, TO AN ADULT FEMALE PATIENT WITHOUT ADEQUATE MEDICAL INDICATION WHEN HE HAD PERSONAL KNOWLEDGE THAT THE PATIENT WAS ADDICTED TO CHEMICAL SUBSTANCES. ON VARIOUS OCCASIONS HE PRESCRIBED MULTIPLE KINDS OF CONTROLLED SUBSTANCES IN LARGE QUANTITIES TO THIS PATIENT ALTHOUGH HE KNEW OR SHOULD HAVE KNOWN THAT SHE HAD PREVIOUSLY ATTEMPTED SUICIDE; HE FAILED TO CREATE MEDICALLY ADEQUATE RECORDS CONCERNING HIS CARE OF THIS PATIENT OR TO TREAT HER SUICIDAL IDEATION AND ATTEMPTS. SUSPENSION STAYED FOR PROBATION UNDER THE FOLLOWING TERMS: SHALL NOT ENGAGE IN THE SOLO PRACTICE OF MEDICINE BUT ONLY PRACTICE WITHIN A GROUP OR INSTITUTIONAL SETTING APPROVED BY THE BOARD; HIS MEDICAL PRACTICE SHALL BE MONITORED BY A BOARD APPROVED TEXAS PHYSICIAN WHO SHALL PROVIDE QUARTERLY REPORTS TO THE BOARD; SHALL MAINTAIN ADEQUATE MEDICAL RECORDS WHICH SHALL BE AVAILABLE FOR REVIEW; SHALL SURRENDER HIS DEA AND TEXAS DEPARTMENT OF PUBLIC SAFETY CONTROLLED SUBSTANCES REGISTRATIONS, AND ANY TRIPLICATE PRESCRIPTION FORMS IN HIS POSSESSION; SHALL NOT ADMINISTER, DISPENSE, OR POSSESS ANY DANGEROUS DRUG TO ANY PERSON OUTSIDE OF THE GROUP OR INSTITUTION IN WHICH HE PRACTICES; SEPARATE FROM PATIENT RECORDS, SHALL MAINTAIN A FILE OF EVERY PRESCRIPTION WRITTEN BY HIM FOR DANGEROUS DRUGS WITH ADDICTIVE POTENTIAL WHICH SHALL BE MADE AVAILABLE FOR REVIEW; SHALL OBTAIN AT LEAST 50 HOURS PER YEAR OF CONTINUING MEDICAL EDUCATION; IN ADDITION, WITHIN SIX MONTHS SHALL SUCCESSFULLY COMPLETE AN APPROVED COURSE IN PHARMACOLOGY OR ADDICTIONOLOGY AND ONE IN TRANSFERENCE/COUNTER TRANSFERENCE ISSUES; SHALL COOPERATE WITH THE BOARD IN VERIFYING COMPLIANCE INCLUDING PROVIDING COPIES OF PEER REVIEW RECORDS UPON REQUEST; SHALL APPEAR PERSONALLY BEFORE THE BOARD AT LEAST TWICE YEARLY FOR THE FIRST YEAR AND ANNUALLY THEREAFTER; SHALL GIVE A COPY OF THIS ORDER TO ANY HEALTH CARE ENTITY WHERE HE HAS PRIVILEGES; SHALL PROVIDE A COPY OF THIS ORDER TO ANYONE REQUESTING IT WITHIN 10 DAYS; TIME SPENT OUT OF TEXAS DOES NOT COUNT TOWARD PROBATION; SHALL INFORM THE BOARD OF CHANGE OF ADDRESS WITHIN 10 DAYS OR IF HE LEAVES THE STATE; SHALL NOT SEEK MODIFICATION FOR ONE YEAR.

CLYNCH, MICHAEL RICHARD MD, LICENSE NUMBER F1458 OF PRINCETON, TX, WAS DISCIPLINED BY TEXAS ON AUGUST 22, 1998
DISCIPLINARY ACTION: SURRENDER OF LICENSE
OFFENSE: PHYSICAL OR MENTAL ILLNESS INHIBITING THE ABILITY TO PRACTICE WITH SKILL AND SAFETY

NOTES: ALLEGATIONS THAT HE IS UNABLE TO PRACTICE WITH REASONABLE SKILL AND SAFETY TO PATIENTS BY REASON OF A PSYCHIATRIC CONDITION WHICH COULD IMPAIR HIS MEDICAL JUDGMENT OR ABILITY TO PRACTICE AS A PHYSICIAN. VOLUNTARY AND PERMANENT SURRENDER.

COATS, ROBERT EUGENE JR DO, DATE OF BIRTH AUGUST 12, 1946, LICENSE NUMBER 00G7795 OF 103 E ADKINS, SEAGOVILLE, TX, WAS DISCIPLINED BY TEXAS ON MARCH 26, 1993
DISCIPLINARY ACTION: RESTRICTION PLACED ON LICENSE; RESTRICTION PLACED ON CONTROLLED SUBSTANCE LICENSE

NOTES: ALLEGATIONS MADE WHICH QUESTION HIS ABILITY TO SAFELY PRACTICE DUE TO MEDICAL PROBLEMS ASSOCIATED WITH A DAMAGED HIP AND POSSIBLE INTEMPERATE USE OF DRUGS; HE DOES NOT ADMIT THESE ALLEGATIONS. AFTER 3/31/93 SHALL NOT PRACTICE MEDICINE UNTIL HE IS EVALUATED BY A BOARD-APPROVED PSYCHIATRIST AND ORTHOPEDIST. SHALL NOT REQUEST RENEWAL OF DEA AND DPS CONTROLLED SUBSTANCES REGISTRATIONS WHICH EXPIRE ON 3/31/93; SHALL KEEP A SEPARATE LOG OF ALL SUCH PRESCRIPTIONS WRITTEN BETWEEN 3/13/93 AND 3/31/94 WHICH IS TO BE AVAILABLE FOR INSPECTION.

COATS, ROBERT EUGENE JR DO, DATE OF BIRTH AUGUST 12, 1946, LICENSE NUMBER 00G7795 OF ARLINGTON, TX, WAS DISCIPLINED BY TEXAS ON MARCH 5, 1994
DISCIPLINARY ACTION: 84-MONTH PROBATION; RESTRICTION PLACED ON CONTROLLED SUBSTANCE LICENSE

OFFENSE: PHYSICAL OR MENTAL ILLNESS INHIBITING THE ABILITY TO PRACTICE WITH SKILL AND SAFETY

NOTES: ADMITS THAT PHYSICAL AILMENTS INCLUDING TWO TOTAL HIP REPLACEMENTS AND MAJOR BACK SURGERY HAVE IMPAIRED HIS ABILITY TO PRACTICE; CONTENDS HE HAS NEVER ABUSED PAIN MEDICATIONS AND NEVER PRESCRIBED MEDICATIONS WITHOUT ADEQUATE INDICATION; HE BELIEVES HE NO LONGER HAS ANY IMPAIRMENT THAT WOULD AFFECT HIS ABILITY TO PRACTICE MEDICINE SAFELY; VOLUNTARILY SUBMITTED TO PSYCHIATRIC AND ORTHOPEDIC EVALUATIONS REQUIRED BY PREVIOUS ORDER; IN LIEU OF A CONTESTED HEARING, THE FOLLOWING ORDER WAS AGREED TO. SUSPENSION STAYED. CONDITIONS OF PROBATION: SHALL APPEAR BEFORE THE BOARD TWICE A YEAR; SHALL ATTEND AT LEAST 50 HOURS PER YEAR OF CONTINUING MEDICAL EDUCATION; SHALL MAINTAIN ADEQUATE MEDICAL RECORDS ON ALL PATIENT OFFICE VISITS AND SHALL MAKE SUCH RECORDS AVAILABLE FOR REVIEW; SHALL NOT SIGN ANYTHING ON A PATIENT RECORD UNLESS HE HAS PERSONALLY SEEN AND EXAMINED THE PATIENT UNLESS THE RECORD CLEARLY REFLECTS HE HAS NOT; SHALL ABSTAIN FROM THE CONSUMPTION OF ALCOHOL/CHEMICAL SUBSTANCES IN ANY FORM UNLESS PRESCRIBED BY ANOTHER PHYSICIAN FOR A LEGITIMATE AND THERAPEUTIC PURPOSE; SHALL NOT TREAT OR OTHERWISE SERVE AS PHYSICIAN, PRESCRIBE, DISPENSE OR ADMINISTER DRUGS THAT MAY BE SUBJECT TO ABUSE TO HIMSELF OR ANY MEMBER OF HIS FAMILY; SEPARATE FROM PATIENT RECORDS SHALL MAINTAIN A FILE OF EVERY PRESCRIPTION WRITTEN FOR DANGEROUS DRUGS WHICH SHALL BE AVAILABLE FOR INSPECTION; SHALL NOT PERMIT AN UNLICENSED PERSON TO PHONE IN A PRESCRIPTION ON HIS BEHALF UNLESS HE HAS FIRST PERFORMED AN EXAM AND MADE A DIAGNOSIS; SHALL SUBMIT HIMSELF FOR APPROPRIATE EXAMS INCLUDING DRUG OR ALCOHOL SCREENS; SHALL CONTINUE TO RECEIVE PSYCHIATRIC TREATMENT WITH QUARTERLY REPORTS; SHALL SUBMIT TO THE CARE AND TREATMENT OF A BOARD-APPROVED ORTHOPEDIC PHYSICIAN; SHALL PROVIDE WRITTEN REPORTS VERIFYING COMPLIANCE UPON REQUEST; MAY REAPPLY FOR DEA AND TEXAS CONTROLLED SUBSTANCES CERTIFICATES FOR SCHEDULES II AND III BUT SHALL LIMIT PRESCRIBING TO A HOSPITAL, EMERGENCY ROOM OR MINOR EMERGENCY CLINIC; SHALL GIVE A COPY OF THE ORDER TO ANY HEALTH CARE ENTITY WHERE HE HAS PRIVILEGES; SHALL COOPERATE WITH THE BOARD IN VERIFYING COMPLIANCE; SHALL INFORM BOARD OF ANY CHANGE OF ADDRESS WITHIN 10 DAYS OR IF HE LEAVES THE STATE; TIME PERIOD SPENT OUT OF TEXAS DOES NOT COUNT TOWARD PROBATION. SHALL NOT SEEK MODIFICATION FOR ONE YEAR. ON 10/10/94 THIS ORDER CORRECTED SUCH THAT HE WAS GIVEN PERMISSION TO APPLY FOR SCHEDULE IV AND V CONTROLLED SUBSTANCES CERTIFICATES.

COATS, ROBERT EUGENE JR DO, DATE OF BIRTH AUGUST 12, 1946, LICENSE NUMBER 00G7795, WAS DISCIPLINED BY TEXAS ON AUGUST 17, 1996
DISCIPLINARY ACTION: 72-MONTH PROBATION; RESTRICTION PLACED ON CONTROLLED SUBSTANCE LICENSE
OFFENSE: FAILURE TO COMPLY WITH PREVIOUS BOARD ORDER

NOTES: FAILED TO COMPLY WITH THE 3/5/94 ORDER IN THAT HE FAILED TO FULLY COOPERATE WITH HIS PSYCHIATRIST BY CANCELING OR MISSING APPOINTMENTS; FAILED TO ATTEND 50 HOURS OF CONTINUING MEDICAL EDUCATION OR TO SUBMIT PROOF OF ATTENDANCE FOR 1995 AND 1996; AND FAILED TO SUBMIT TO THE CARE AND TREATMENT OF AN ORTHOPEDIC PHYSICIAN. SUSPENSION, STAYED. CONDITIONS OF PROBATION: SHALL APPEAR BEFORE THE BOARD AT LEAST TWO TIMES PER YEAR; SHALL OBTAIN AT LEAST 50 HOURS PER YEAR OF CONTINUING MEDICAL EDUCATION AND SUBMIT PROOF TO THE BOARD; SHALL MAINTAIN ADEQUATE MEDICAL RECORDS WHICH SHALL BE AVAILABLE FOR REVIEW; SHALL NOT SIGN OR INDICATE IN ANY MANNER IN PATIENT RECORDS THAT HE HAS SEEN PATIENTS UNLESS HE ACTUALLY HAS SEEN AND EXAMINED THE PATIENT UNLESS IT'S CLEARLY NOTED THAT HE DID NOT EXAMINE THE PATIENT; SHALL REFRAIN FROM THE PRESCRIPTION OR ADMINISTRATION OF ANY DRUG FOR ANY PATIENT UNLESS THE DRUG IS MEDICALLY INDICATED AND IS PRESCRIBED IN THERAPEUTIC DOSES; SHALL CONDUCT ADEQUATE FOLLOW-UP EXAMINATIONS ON ALL PATIENTS TO DETERMINE WHETHER THE COURSE OF TREATMENT, INCLUDING THE PRESCRIPTION OF DRUGS, IS APPROPRIATE; SHALL ABSTAIN FROM THE CONSUMPTION OF ALCOHOL/ DRUGS IN ANY FORM UNLESS PRESCRIBED BY ANOTHER PHYSICIAN FOR A LEGITIMATE AND THERAPEUTIC PURPOSE; SHALL NOT TREAT OR OTHERWISE SERVE AS PHYSICIAN PRESCRIBE, DISPENSE, OR ADMINISTER DRUGS THAT MAY BE SUBJECT TO ABUSE TO HIMSELF OR ANY MEMBER OF HIS FAMILY; SEPARATE FROM PATIENT RECORDS, SHALL MAINTAIN A COPY OF EVERY PRESCRIPTION WRITTEN FOR CONTROLLED SUBSTANCES OR DANGEROUS DRUGS WITH ADDICTIVE POTENTIAL OR POTENTIAL FOR ABUSE AND MAKE IT AVAILABLE UPON BOARD REQUEST; SHALL NOT HIMSELF TELEPHONE OR PERMIT ANY PERSON WHO IS NOT BOARD LICENSED TO TELEPHONE A PRESCRIPTION TO ANY PHARMACY FOR ANY PATIENT UNLESS HE HAS FIRST PERFORMED A MEDICALLY APPROPRIATE EXAMINATION AND MADE A DIAGNOSIS; SHALL SUBMIT HIMSELF FOR APPROPRIATE EXAMS, INCLUDING DRUG OR ALCOHOL SCREENS; SHALL CONTINUE TO RECEIVE CARE AND TREATMENT FROM HIS TREATING PSYCHIATRIST WHO SHALL SUBMIT REPORTS QUARTERLY TO THE BOARD; SHALL SUBMIT TO THE CARE AND TREATMENT OF A BOARD APPROVED ORTHOPEDIC PHYSICIAN; SHALL LIMIT HIS SCHEDULE II, II-N, III, OR III-N PRESCRIBING TO THAT OF A HOSPITAL, EMERGENCY ROOM, OR MINOR EMERGENCY CLINIC; SHALL GIVE A COPY OF THIS ORDER TO ANY HEALTH CARE ENTITY WHERE HE HAS PRIVILEGES; SHALL COOPERATE WITH THE BOARD IN VERIFYING COMPLIANCE; TIME PERIOD OUT OF TEXAS DOES NOT COUNT TOWARD PROBATION; SHALL INFORM THE BOARD OF CHANGE OF ADDRESS WITHIN 10 DAYS OF IF HE LEAVES THE STATE; SHALL NOT SEEK MODIFICATION FOR ONE YEAR.

COE, RICHARD OREN JR MD, LICENSE NUMBER 00C5634 OF OLATHE, KS, WAS DISCIPLINED BY TEXAS ON MARCH 31, 1990
DISCIPLINARY ACTION: 60-MONTH PROBATION; MONITORING OF PHYSICIAN PERFORMANCE
OFFENSE: DISCIPLINARY ACTION BY ANOTHER STATE OR AGENCY

NOTES: STIPULATED ORDER. MUST COMPLY WITH STIPULATION ENTERED INTO WITH KANSAS BOARD AND TERMS OF KANSAS IMPAIRED PHYSICIAN MONITORING CONTRACT, FURNISH TEXAS BOARD REPORTS AND RECEIVE APPROVAL FROM BOARD PRIOR TO PRACTICING MEDICINE IN TEXAS.

COE, RICHARD OREN JR MD, LICENSE NUMBER 00C5634 OF OVERLAND PARK, KS, WAS DISCIPLINED BY TEXAS ON JUNE 10,

1991
DISCIPLINARY ACTION: LICENSE REVOCATION
OFFENSE: DISCIPLINARY ACTION BY ANOTHER STATE OR AGENCY

NOTES: ALCOHOL ABUSE LED TO DISCIPLINARY ACTION BY ANOTHER STATE.

COGBURN, CLARENCE G DO, LICENSE NUMBER 00C7270 OF HOUSTON, TX, WAS DISCIPLINED BY TEXAS ON JUNE 22, 1994
DISCIPLINARY ACTION: REPRIMAND; REQUIRED TO TAKE ADDITIONAL MEDICAL EDUCATION
OFFENSE: OVERPRESCRIBING OR MISPRESCRIBING DRUGS

NOTES: NON-THERAPEUTICALLY PRESCRIBED TO ONE PATIENT IN THAT ON 9/10/93 HE DISPENSED 200 SOMA TABLETS AND AT THE SAME TIME PRESCRIBED OR DISPENSED 60 ANEXSIA TABLETS; CLAIMED THE PATIENT REQUESTED THIS QUANTITY OF DRUGS DUE TO TRAVEL PLANS; WAS OPERATING AN UNLICENSED PHARMACY BY DISPENSING BEYOND THE PATIENT'S IMMEDIATE NEEDS. CONDITIONS OF LICENSE RESTRICTION: SHALL NOT ORDER OR MAINTAIN IN HIS POSSESSION ANY CONTROLLED SUBSTANCES OR DANGEROUS DRUGS, INCLUDING SAMPLES, UNLESS PRESCRIBED OR DISPENSED BY ANOTHER PHYSICIAN FOR A LEGITIMATE MEDICAL NEED; SEPARATE FROM PATIENT RECORDS, SHALL MAINTAIN A LOG OF ALL PRESCRIPTIONS HE WRITES FOR CONTROLLED SUBSTANCES OR DANGEROUS DRUGS WHICH SHALL BE AVAILABLE FOR INSPECTION; SHALL ATTEND AT LEAST 50 HOURS PER YEAR OF CONTINUING MEDICAL EDUCATION; SHALL APPEAR BEFORE THE BOARD ONCE A YEAR; SHALL GIVE A COPY OF THIS ORDER TO ANY HEALTH CARE ENTITY WHERE HE HAS PRIVILEGES; SHALL COOPERATE WITH THE BOARD IN VERIFYING COMPLIANCE; SHALL INFORM BOARD OF CHANGE OF ADDRESS WITHIN 10 DAYS OR IF HE LEAVES THE STATE; TIME SPENT OUT OF TEXAS SHALL NOT COUNT TOWARD RESTRICTION. SHALL NOT SEEK MODIFICATION FOR ONE YEAR. ON 8/22/98 PETITION TO TERMINATE ORDER DENIED.

COHEN, NATHANIEL M MD, DATE OF BIRTH AUGUST 24, 1922, LICENSE NUMBER 0028463 OF SALT LAKE CITY, UT, WAS DISCIPLINED BY KENTUCKY ON DECEMBER 1, 1992
DISCIPLINARY ACTION: FINE
OFFENSE: NONCOMPLIANCE WITH A PROFESSIONAL RULE

NOTES: FAILED TO COMPLETE REQUIRED CONTINUING MEDICAL EDUCATION IN THE AREA OF HIV/AIDS.

COHEN, NATHANIEL M MD, DATE OF BIRTH AUGUST 24, 1922, LICENSE NUMBER 0021299 OF 258 HARVARD ST #323, BROOKLINE, MA, WAS DISCIPLINED BY MASSACHUSETTS ON JULY 26, 1995
DISCIPLINARY ACTION: RESTRICTION PLACED ON LICENSE
OFFENSE: LOSS OR RESTRICTION OF HOSPITAL PRIVILEGES

NOTES: LOSS OF HOSPITAL PRIVILEGES.

COHEN, NATHANIEL M MD, DATE OF BIRTH AUGUST 24, 1922, LICENSE NUMBER 1062523 OF 5655 EAST RIVER RD, STE 101-207, TUCSON, AZ, WAS DISCIPLINED BY MICHIGAN ON APRIL 17, 1996
DISCIPLINARY ACTION: RESTRICTION PLACED ON LICENSE
OFFENSE: DISCIPLINARY ACTION BY ANOTHER STATE OR AGENCY

NOTES: FAILURE TO REPORT/COMPLY.

COHEN, NATHANIEL M MD, DATE OF BIRTH AUGUST 24, 1922, LICENSE NUMBER 0028463 OF TUCSON, AZ, WAS DISCIPLINED BY KENTUCKY ON MAY 20, 1996
DISCIPLINARY ACTION: RESTRICTION PLACED ON LICENSE
OFFENSE: DISCIPLINARY ACTION BY ANOTHER STATE OR AGENCY

NOTES: DISCIPLINARY ACTION TAKEN BY THE MASSACHUSETTS BOARD. MAY NOT ATTEND DELIVERIES, PRACTICE IN AN EMERGENCY ROOM, NEONATAL OR PEDIATRIC INTENSIVE CARE UNIT OR ANY CRITICAL CARE SETTING; PROHIBITED FROM PRACTICING MEDICINE EXCEPT IN A GROUP PRACTICE OR INSTITUTIONAL SETTING WHERE SUPERVISION AND BACKUP ARE READILY AVAILABLE.

COHEN, NATHANIEL M MD, LICENSE NUMBER 0425680 OF 5655 EAST RIVER RD SUITE 101-207, TUCSON, AZ, WAS DISCIPLINED BY KANSAS ON JULY 23, 1996
DISCIPLINARY ACTION: RESTRICTION PLACED ON LICENSE
OFFENSE: DISCIPLINARY ACTION BY ANOTHER STATE OR AGENCY

NOTES: ACTION IN MASSACHUSETTS ON 7/26/95 LIMITING HIS KANSAS LICENSE FOR AN INDEFINITE PERIOD, BUT AT LEAST AS LONG AS THE MASSACHUSETTS BOARD MAINTAINS ITS LIMITATIONS. KANSAS PROHIBITS HIM FROM: ATTENDING DELIVERIES; PRACTICING IN AN EMERGENCY ROOM, NEONATAL OR PEDIATRIC INTENSIVE CARE UNIT, OR ANY CRITICAL CARE SETTING; AND PRACTICING MEDICINE EXCEPT IN A GROUP PRACTICE OR INSTITUTIONAL SETTING WHERE SUPERVISION AND BACK-UP ARE READILY AVAILABLE.

COHEN, NATHANIEL M MD, DATE OF BIRTH AUGUST 24, 1922, LICENSE NUMBER 0032717 OF 5655 EAST RIVER ROAD #107-207, TUCSON, AZ, WAS DISCIPLINED BY WISCONSIN ON AUGUST 22, 1996
DISCIPLINARY ACTION: RESTRICTION PLACED ON LICENSE; MONITORING OF PHYSICIAN PERFORMANCE
OFFENSE: DISCIPLINARY ACTION BY ANOTHER STATE OR AGENCY

NOTES: ON 7/25/95 THE MASSACHUSETTS BOARD IMPOSED DISCIPLINE UPON HIS LICENSE TO PRACTICE MEDICINE. HIS WISCONSIN LICENSE IS LIMITED AS FOLLOWS: SHALL REFRAIN FROM PRACTICING OBSTETRICS, EMERGENCY MEDICINE, NEONATAL MEDICINE, SURGERY, PEDIATRIC INTENSIVE CARE OR IN ANY OTHER CRITICAL CARE SETTING; SHALL REFRAIN FROM THE PRACTICE OF MEDICINE IN WISCONSIN OR THE PRACTICE OF MEDICINE ELSEWHERE UNDER THE USE OF HIS WISCONSIN LICENSE EXCEPT IN A GROUP PRACTICE OR INSTITUTIONAL SETTING AND UNDER SUPERVISION BY OTHER LICENSED PHYSICIANS; PRIOR TO ENGAGING IN THE PRACTICE OF MEDICINE IN WISCONSIN, SHALL SUBMIT AND OBTAIN APPROVAL BY THE BOARD OF A PLAN OF SUPERVISION FOR HIS PRACTICE; SHALL IMMEDIATELY SURRENDER ALL INDICIA OF WISCONSIN REGISTRATION TO THE DEPARTMENT MONITOR WHO SHALL REISSUE CREDENTIALS MARKED "LIMITED."

COHEN, NATHANIEL M MD, LICENSE NUMBER 00G1904 OF TUCSON, AZ, WAS DISCIPLINED BY CALIFORNIA ON AUGUST 30, 1996
DISCIPLINARY ACTION: SURRENDER OF LICENSE

NOTES: WHILE CHARGES PENDING.

COHEN, NATHANIEL M MD, DATE OF BIRTH AUGUST 24, 1922, LICENSE NUMBER J5730, WAS DISCIPLINED BY TEXAS ON MAY 10, 1997
OFFENSE: DISCIPLINARY ACTION BY ANOTHER STATE OR AGENCY

NOTES: ON 7/26/95 ENTERED INTO AN AGREED ORDER WITH THE MASSACHUSETTS BOARD RESTRICTING HIS LICENSE BASED ON SOME HOSPITAL PRIVILEGES BEING WITHDRAWN FOLLOWING TWO INCIDENTS IN WHICH HIS RESPONSE TO TWO CESAREAN SECTIONS WAS DEEMED TO BE INSUFFICIENTLY AGGRESSIVE; FAILED TO REPORT RESTRICTION TO THE BOARD WITHIN 30 DAYS SHALL NOT PRACTICE MEDICINE IN

TEXAS UNTIL HE REQUESTS PERMISSION IN WRITING TO RESUME THE PRACTICE OF MEDICINE THERE, AND PERSONALLY APPEARS BEFORE THE BOARD TO PROVIDE SUFFICIENT EVIDENCE THAT HE IS OTHERWISE COMPETENT TO PRACTICE MEDICINE SAFELY INCLUDING AT A MINIMUM: EVIDENCE THAT THE 7/26/95 ORDER'S TERMS AND CONDITIONS HAVE BEEN TERMINATED/LIFTED OR MODIFIED; AND EVIDENCE THAT HE IS NOT THE SUBJECT OF ANY OTHER STATE DISCIPLINARY ACTION, INVESTIGATION, OR PROCEEDINGS; SHALL COOPERATE WITH THE BOARD IN VERIFYING COMPLIANCE INCLUDING PROVIDING COPIES OF ANY DOCUMENTS SUBMITTED TO MASSACHUSETTS UPON REQUEST; SHALL GIVE A COPY OF THIS ORDER TO ANY HEALTH CARE ENTITY WHERE HE HAS PRIVILEGES; SHALL INFORM THE BOARD OF CHANGE OF ADDRESS WITHIN 10 DAYS; SHALL NOT SEEK MODIFICATION FOR ONE YEAR.

COHEN, NATHANIEL MAURICE MD, DATE OF BIRTH AUGUST 24, 1922, LICENSE NUMBER 0003379 OF 5655 EAST RIVER ROAD NO. 101-207, TUCSON, AZ, WAS DISCIPLINED BY HAWAII ON OCTOBER 30, 1996
DISCIPLINARY ACTION: RESTRICTION PLACED ON LICENSE; MONITORING OF PHYSICIAN PERFORMANCE
OFFENSE: DISCIPLINARY ACTION BY ANOTHER STATE OR AGENCY

NOTES: RESTRICTIONS ON LICENSES IN MICHIGAN (4/17/96), KANSAS (7/23/96), AND KENTUCKY (5/17/96). HAWAII ORDER FOR INDEFINITE LIMITED LICENSE. TERMS AND CONDITIONS: SHALL COMPLY WITH MICHIGAN, KANSAS, AND KENTUCKY TERMS AND CONDITIONS: PROHIBITED FROM ATTENDING DELIVERIES OR PRACTICING IN AN EMERGENCY ROOM, NEONATAL, OR PEDIATRIC INTENSIVE CARE UNIT, OR ANY CRITICAL CARE SETTING; SHALL ONLY PRACTICE MEDICINE IN A GROUP PRACTICE OR INSTITUTIONAL SETTING WHERE SUPERVISION AND BACK-UP ARE READILY AVAILABLE; RESTRICTIONS IN HAWAII FOR AT LEAST AS LONG AS MASSACHUSETTS MAINTAINS LIMITATIONS.

COHN, JACQUELINE ELLEN MD OF 1521 S STAPLES #801, CORPUS CHRISTI, TX, WAS DISCIPLINED BY DEA ON SEPTEMBER 14, 1992
DISCIPLINARY ACTION: RESTRICTION PLACED ON CONTROLLED SUBSTANCE LICENSE
OFFENSE: DISCIPLINARY ACTION BY ANOTHER STATE OR AGENCY

NOTES: HAD SURRENDERED SCHEDULES II AND IIN IN 1983 ACCORDING TO ORDER BY THE TEXAS STATE BOARD OF MEDICAL EXAMINERS. IN 1985 SHE WAS GIVEN PERMISSION TO REAPPLY. SCHEDULES II AND IIN PRIVILEGES WERE REINSTATED 09/14/92. ALIAS: JACQUELINE COHN BUCK.

COLE, GEORGE MARTIN DO, LICENSE NUMBER 00F5175 OF AMARILLO, TX, WAS DISCIPLINED BY TEXAS ON NOVEMBER 13, 1992
DISCIPLINARY ACTION: 36-MONTH RESTRICTION PLACED ON LICENSE

NOTES: PROFESSIONAL FAILURE TO PRACTICE MEDICINE IN AN ACCEPTABLE MANNER CONSISTENT WITH PUBLIC HEALTH AND WELFARE. ON 6/28/95 HIS PETITION FOR TERMINATION WAS DENIED.

COLE, GEORGE MARTIN DO, LICENSE NUMBER 0002071, WAS DISCIPLINED BY OKLAHOMA ON JANUARY 11, 1994
DISCIPLINARY ACTION: RESTRICTION PLACED ON LICENSE; MONITORING OF PHYSICIAN PERFORMANCE
OFFENSE: DISCIPLINARY ACTION BY ANOTHER STATE OR AGENCY

NOTES: ON 11/13/92 HIS TEXAS LICENSE TO PRACTICE OSTEOPATHIC MEDICINE WAS RESTRICTED FOR THREE YEARS UNDER TERMS AND CONDITIONS. OKLAHOMA LICENSE PLACED ON INDEFINITE RESTRICTION UNDER THE FOLLOWING TERMS AND CONDITIONS: SHALL NOT PETITION THE BOARD FOR A MODIFICATION FOR AT LEAST ONE YEAR; SHALL NOT PERFORM CERVICAL SPINE SURGERY IN OKLAHOMA; SHALL NOTIFY AND PROVIDE A COPY OF THIS ORDER TO ALL HEALTH CARE ENTITIES WHERE HE HAS PRIVILEGES; SHALL NOTIFY THE BOARD IN WRITING OF ANY CHANGES IN ADDRESS, EMPLOYMENT, EMPLOYMENT TERMINATION OR HOSPITAL OR HEALTH CARE ENTITIES PRIVILEGE RESTRICTION OR ANY ADMINISTRATIVE PROCEEDING INITIATED AGAINST HIM BY ANY OTHER STATE OR FEDERAL REGULATORY BODY WITHIN 14 DAYS OF SUCH ACTION; SHALL COOPERATE WITH THE BOARD AND PROVIDE ANY REQUIRED REPORTS; MUST APPEAR BEFORE THE BOARD PRIOR TO PRACTICING IN OKLAHOMA WITH HIS PLANS AND HIS COMPLIANCE WITH THE TERMS AND CONDITIONS OF THE TEXAS ORDER; SHALL PAY THE COST OF ADMINISTRATIVE PROCEEDING OF $1,525.50.

COLE, GEORGE MARTIN DO, LICENSE NUMBER F5175 OF AMARILLO, TX, WAS DISCIPLINED BY TEXAS ON AUGUST 9, 1997
DISCIPLINARY ACTION: RESTRICTION PLACED ON LICENSE
OFFENSE: SUBSTANDARD CARE, INCOMPETENCE OR NEGLIGENCE

NOTES: FROM APPROXIMATELY 1991 THROUGH APPROXIMATELY 1995, HE PERFORMED VARIOUS BACK, KNEE AND ANKLE SURGERIES WHICH RESULTED IN ADVERSE MEDICAL OUTCOMES, INCLUDING REQUIRING SEVERAL PATIENTS TO UNDERGO ADDITIONAL SURGERIES BY OTHER PHYSICIANS TO CORRECT HIS ALLEGED SURGICAL DEFICIENCIES; HE REPORTS THAT HE VOLUNTARILY CEASED PERFORMING SURGERIES IN 6/95, DUE TO THE CHANGE IN HIS PRACTICE PHILOSOPHY AND HIS EMPHASIS ON PREVENTATIVE MEDICINE; HE DENIES THE CHARGES. HE SHALL NOT PERFORM ANY INVASIVE SURGICAL PROCEDURE AS DEFINED IN THE ORDER; SHALL COOPERATE WITH THE BOARD IN VERIFYING COMPLIANCE INCLUDING PROVIDING COPIES OF MEDICAL RELEASES UPON REQUEST; SHALL GIVE A COPY OF THIS ORDER TO ANY HEALTH CARE ENTITY WHERE HE HAS PRIVILEGES; SHALL PROVIDE A COPY OF THIS ORDER TO ANYONE REQUESTING IT WITHIN 10 DAYS; SHALL INFORM THE BOARD OF CHANGE OF ADDRESS WITHIN 10 DAYS; SHALL NOT SEEK MODIFICATION FOR ONE YEAR; SHALL APPEAR BEFORE THE BOARD UPON REQUEST.

COLEMAN, MILBURN LEE DO, LICENSE NUMBER 00D7549 OF DALLAS, TX, WAS DISCIPLINED BY TEXAS ON SEPTEMBER 8, 1992
DISCIPLINARY ACTION: RESTRICTION PLACED ON LICENSE
OFFENSE: PROFESSIONAL MISCONDUCT

NOTES: VIOLATION OF THE LAWS OF TEXAS CONNECTED WITH HIS PRACTICE OF MEDICINE.

CONDE, ARTHUR BAAY MD, LICENSE NUMBER D3766 OF HOUSTON, TX, WAS DISCIPLINED BY TEXAS ON DECEMBER 11, 1999
DISCIPLINARY ACTION: SURRENDER OF LICENSE
OFFENSE: PROFESSIONAL MISCONDUCT

NOTES: VOLUNTARY AND PERMANENT SURRENDER IN LIEU OF FURTHER PROCEEDINGS.

CONNER, PATRICK T MD, LICENSE NUMBER 0C41076 OF SPRINGFIELD, MO, WAS DISCIPLINED BY CALIFORNIA ON MAY 19, 1993
DISCIPLINARY ACTION: 60-MONTH PROBATION

NOTES: REVOCATION STAYED.

CONNER, PATRICK TRAVIS MD, LICENSE NUMBER 00G3243 OF SPRINGFIELD, MO, WAS DISCIPLINED BY TEXAS ON OCTOBER 26, 1990
DISCIPLINARY ACTION: MONITORING OF PHYSICIAN PERFORMANCE

NOTES: MUST COMPLY WITH MISSOURI RESTRICTIONS AND AUTHORIZE MISSOURI BOARD TO RELEASE INFORMATION AS TO STATUS AND PROBATIONARY COMPLIANCE; RECEIVE APPROVAL FROM TEXAS BOARD PRIOR TO PRACTICING MEDICINE IN TEXAS. ON 11/3/94 ORDER TERMINATED.

CONRAD, EDGAR DONALD DO, LICENSE NUMBER 00C7271 OF WEATHERFORD, TX, WAS DISCIPLINED BY TEXAS ON DECEMBER 3, 1990
DISCIPLINARY ACTION: LICENSE SUSPENSION; 120-MONTH PROBATION
OFFENSE: SUBSTANCE ABUSE

NOTES: LICENSE SUSPENDED FOR ADMISSION INTO A SUBSTANCE ABUSE TREATMENT PROGRAM. ON 4/19/91 REINSTATED AND PLACED ON PROBATION UNDER CONDITIONS INCLUDING: MUST APPEAR BEFORE THE BOARD OR A COMMITTEE OF THE BOARD TWO TIMES A YEAR DURING EACH YEAR OF PROBATION; CONTINUING PARTICIPATION IN THE ACTIVITIES OF THE TARRANT COUNTY MEDICAL SOCIETY COMMITTEE ON PHYSICIAN HEALTH AND REHABILITATION, INCLUDING PARTICIPATION IN THE WEEKLY MEETINGS; CONTINUING PARTICIPATION IN THE ACTIVITIES AND PROGRAMS OF ALCOHOLICS ANONYMOUS ON A REGULAR BASIS; MAINTENANCE OF ADEQUATE MEDICAL RECORDS ON ALL PATIENT OFFICE VISITS; SUBMISSION FOR APPROPRIATE CHEMICAL EXAMINATIONS AT THE REQUEST OF THE BOARD OR ITS REPRESENTATIVE.

CONRAD, EDGAR DONALD DO, LICENSE NUMBER 00C7271 OF WEATHERFORD, TX, WAS DISCIPLINED BY TEXAS ON OCTOBER 4, 1991
DISCIPLINARY ACTION: LICENSE REVOCATION
OFFENSE: NONCOMPLIANCE WITH A PROFESSIONAL RULE

NOTES: LICENSE SUSPENDED ON 12/3/90 UNTIL HE COMPLETED AN INPATIENT SUBSTANCE ABUSE PROGRAM; ON 4/19/91 LICENSE WAS REINSTATED ON 10 YEARS PROBATION SUBJECT TO TERMS AND CONDITIONS, INCLUDING RANDOM DRUG SCREENS; ON 5/23/91 TESTED POSITIVE FOR ALCOHOL ON A DRUG SCREEN.

CONTE, MAURICE S MD, DATE OF BIRTH SEPTEMBER 4, 1937, LICENSE NUMBER 00E7036 OF HOUSTON, TX, WAS DISCIPLINED BY TEXAS ON MAY 24, 1990
DISCIPLINARY ACTION: REQUIRED TO TAKE ADDITIONAL MEDICAL EDUCATION; MONITORING OF PHYSICIAN PERFORMANCE

NOTES: STIPULATED ORDER. SHALL ATTEND CONTINUING MEDICAL EDUCATION COURSES, UTILIZE PATIENT RECORD-KEEPING SYSTEM TO ACCURATELY REFLECT CERTAIN INFORMATION, AND MAKE ANNUAL APPEARANCES BEFORE BOARD OR BOARD COMMITTEE.

CONTE, MAURICE S MD, DATE OF BIRTH SEPTEMBER 4, 1937, LICENSE NUMBER 00E7036 OF HOUSTON, TX, WAS DISCIPLINED BY TEXAS ON MARCH 6, 1992
DISCIPLINARY ACTION: RESTRICTION PLACED ON LICENSE

NOTES: PROFESSIONAL FAILURE TO PRACTICE MEDICINE IN AN ACCEPTABLE MANNER CONSISTENT WITH PUBLIC HEALTH AND WELFARE.

CONTE, MAURICE S MD, DATE OF BIRTH SEPTEMBER 4, 1937, LICENSE NUMBER 00E7036 OF HENDERSON, NV, WAS DISCIPLINED BY TEXAS ON FEBRUARY 8, 1993
DISCIPLINARY ACTION: LICENSE SUSPENSION
OFFENSE: FAILURE TO COMPLY WITH PREVIOUS BOARD ORDER

NOTES: HE WAS REQUIRED BY AN ORDER OF 3/6/92 TO TAKE AND PASS THE SPEX EXAM; HE HAS TAKEN THE EXAM TWICE IN 9/92 AND 12/92 AND FAILED BOTH TIMES. LICENSE SUSPENDED UNTIL HE PASSES THE SPEX EXAM. ON 3/3/95 SUSPENSION TERMINATED.

CONTE, MAURICE S MD, DATE OF BIRTH SEPTEMBER 4, 1937, LICENSE NUMBER 0021080 OF 1313 SPYGLASS, AUSTIN, TX, WAS DISCIPLINED BY NEW JERSEY ON JUNE 27, 1994
DISCIPLINARY ACTION: LICENSE SUSPENSION

NOTES: MUST APPEAR BEFORE A COMMITTEE OF THIS BOARD FOR A STATUS CONFERENCE PRIOR TO RESUMING NEW JERSEY PRACTICE. LICENSE IS SUSPENDED UNTIL SUCH TIME THAT HE DEMONSTRATES TO THE BOARD THAT HIS LICENSE TO PRACTICE MEDICINE IN TEXAS IS REINSTATED.

CONTIN, JUAN U MD, LICENSE NUMBER 00D7815 OF EL PASO, TX, WAS DISCIPLINED BY TEXAS ON OCTOBER 5, 1991
DISCIPLINARY ACTION: 36-MONTH PROBATION; REQUIRED TO TAKE ADDITIONAL MEDICAL EDUCATION
OFFENSE: PROFESSIONAL MISCONDUCT

NOTES: WHILE ACTING AS MEDICAL DIRECTOR OF THE SOUTHWEST PAIN MANAGEMENT/BIOFEEDBACK CLINIC, HE AFFIXED HIS SIGNATURE TO INSURANCE CLAIM FORMS WITHOUT ADEQUATE KNOWLEDGE OF THE UNDERLYING BASIS FOR THE CLAIMS AND WITHOUT CONSIDERING THE REPRESENTATIONS TO INSURANCE CARRIERS WHICH WERE BEING MADE BY VIRTUE OF HIS SIGNATURES ON THESE CLAIM FORMS. SUSPENSION STAYED AND PLACED ON PROBATION WITH FOLLOWING TERMS AND CONDITIONS: SHALL OBTAIN 25 HOURS OF ETHICS CREDITS THROUGH SUCCESSFUL COMPLETION OF ETHICS COURSES OR PROGRAMS WITHIN ONE YEAR; DURING THE FIRST YEAR OF PROBATION, SHALL TAKE AND PASS THE MEDICAL JURISPRUDENCE EXAMINATION GIVEN BY THE TEXAS BOARD; SHALL APPEAR BEFORE THE BOARD ONCE A YEAR; SHALL COOPERATE WITH BOARD IN VERIFYING COMPLIANCE; SHALL ADVISE THE BOARD OF CHANGE OF ADDRESS WITHIN 10 DAYS; TIME SPENT OUT OF TEXAS DOES NOT COUNT TOWARDS PROBATION; SHALL NOT SEEK MODIFICATION OF ORDER FOR AT LEAST ONE YEAR.

CONTIN, JUAN U MD, DATE OF BIRTH APRIL 25, 1936, LICENSE NUMBER 0026570 OF 5728 KINGSFIELD AVENUE, EL PASO, TX, WAS DISCIPLINED BY NEW JERSEY ON FEBRUARY 9, 1993
DISCIPLINARY ACTION: 36-MONTH PROBATION
OFFENSE: DISCIPLINARY ACTION BY ANOTHER STATE OR AGENCY

NOTES: DISCIPLINED IN TEXAS FOR UNPROFESSIONAL CONDUCT. THREE YEAR SUSPENSION STAYED. PRIOR TO RESUMING PRACTICE IN NEW JERSEY, MUST DEMONSTRATE SATISFACTORY COMPLETION OF ALL REQUIREMENTS IN TEXAS AND APPEAR BEFORE A COMMITTEE OF THE BOARD FOR A STATUS CONFERENCE.

CONTIN, JUAN U MD, LICENSE NUMBER 0017694 OF EL PASO, TX, WAS DISCIPLINED BY FLORIDA ON APRIL 16, 1993
DISCIPLINARY ACTION: SURRENDER OF LICENSE

OFFENSE: DISCIPLINARY ACTION BY ANOTHER STATE OR AGENCY

NOTES: CHARGED WITH HAVING A LICENSE ACTED AGAINST, BY THE LICENSING AUTHORITY OF ANOTHER JURISDICTION AND FAILING TO REPORT TO THE BOARD, IN WRITING, WITHIN 30 DAYS OF THIS ACTION. IN LIEU OF FURTHER PROSECUTION, ACCEPTED A VOLUNTARY RELINQUISHMENT OF LICENSE WITH THE AGREEMENT NEVER AGAIN TO APPLY FOR LICENSURE AS A PHYSICIAN IN FLORIDA.

COOK, TED ALLEN MD, LICENSE NUMBER 0013047 OF PORTLAND, OR, WAS DISCIPLINED BY OREGON ON AUGUST 10, 1990
DISCIPLINARY ACTION: 3-MONTH PROBATION; FINE

NOTES: NO LONGER LISTED ON PROBATION AS OF 2/16/96.

COOK, TED ALLEN MD, LICENSE NUMBER 00D1589 OF PORTLAND, OR, WAS DISCIPLINED BY TEXAS ON APRIL 20, 1991
DISCIPLINARY ACTION: PROBATION
OFFENSE: DISCIPLINARY ACTION BY ANOTHER STATE OR AGENCY

NOTES: DISCIPLINARY ACTION TAKEN BY ANOTHER STATE FOR UNPROFESSIONAL CONDUCT. MUST COMPLY WITH ALL TERMS OF OREGON PROBATION; PRIOR TO PRACTICING IN TEXAS, MUST APPEAR BEFORE BOARD FOR APPROVAL. ON 10/5/96 PROBATION TERMINATED.

COOKE, THOMAS R DO, LICENSE NUMBER 00E6056 OF CHEHALIS, WA, WAS DISCIPLINED BY TEXAS ON FEBRUARY 22, 1991

NOTES: MUST COMPLY WITH WASHINGTON STATE BOARD ORDER; RECEIVE PERMISSION OF TEXAS BOARD BEFORE RETURNING TO PRACTICE OF OBSTETRICS IN TEXAS AND BE SUBJECT TO ANY TERMS IMPOSED. ON 2/7/98 ORDER TERMINATED.

COOMANSINGH, BELDEN J L MD, DATE OF BIRTH OCTOBER 14, 1937, LICENSE NUMBER 00F8446 OF 7213 HARRIS COURT, FORT WORTH, TX, WAS DISCIPLINED BY TEXAS ON JUNE 22, 1994
DISCIPLINARY ACTION: 120-MONTH PROBATION; RESTRICTION PLACED ON LICENSE
OFFENSE: LOSS OR RESTRICTION OF HOSPITAL PRIVILEGES

NOTES: BOARD INVESTIGATED ALLEGATIONS HE HAD MADE INAPPROPRIATE COMMENTS TO THREE PATIENTS INCLUDING ASKING THEM OUT ON DATES; ALSO OFFERED PAIN MEDICATIONS TO ONE PATIENT IN EXCHANGE FOR SEXUAL FAVORS; ALSO INAPPROPRIATELY TOLD A PATIENT SHE HAD AN URGENT NEED FOR SEXUAL GRATIFICATION; HE DENIES THESE ALLEGATIONS; IN 3/93 RESTRICTIONS PUT ON HOSPITAL PRIVILEGES BECAUSE HIS CARE AND TREATMENT OF EIGHT PATIENTS DEMONSTRATED A DEFICIENCY IN DEALING WITH HIGH RISK PREGNANCIES, INCLUDING TREATING PREGNANCY INDUCED HYPERTENSION WITH ALDOMET AND PHENOBARB; HOSPITAL SUBSEQUENTLY TERMINATED HIS PRIVILEGES WHEN HE DID NOT MEET ONE OF THE REQUIREMENTS, OBTAINING A RISK MANAGEMENT COURSE; SOUGHT DISTRICT COURT ACTION REGARDING THE TERMINATION WHICH WAS STILL PENDING AS OF THE ORDER DATE; IN 1/91 HE WAS NOT REAPPOINTED TO STAFF OF ANOTHER HOSPITAL BASED UPON SEVEN QUALITY OF CARE CASES REGARDING HIS MANAGEMENT OF PREGNANCY INDUCED HYPERTENSION, PITOCIN AUGMENTATION THERAPY, SUSPECTED SEPSIS, CLASS III PAP SMEARS AND HIS LACK OF APPRECIATION OF INDICATIONS FOR C-SECTIONS; HOSPITAL RECOMMENDED A RESIDENCY TYPE TRAINING PROGRAM; HE DID NOT APPEAL THIS DECISION; RECENTLY SUFFERED A MYOCARDIAL INFARCTION AND WISHES TO LIMIT HIS PRACTICE. SUSPENSION STAYED. CONDITIONS OF PROBATION: SHALL APPEAR BEFORE THE BOARD ONCE A YEAR; SHALL ATTEND AT LEAST 50 HOURS PER YEAR OF CONTINUING MEDICAL EDUCATION; SHALL BE SUPERVISED BY A BOARD-APPROVED PHYSICIAN WITH QUARTERLY REPORTS; SHALL MAINTAIN ADEQUATE MEDICAL RECORDS ON ALL PATIENT OFFICE VISITS WHICH SHALL BE AVAILABLE FOR INSPECTION; SHALL COMPLETE A SIX MONTH MINI-RESIDENCY IN OBSTETRICS/GYNECOLOGY PRIOR TO PRACTICING OB/GYN OTHER THAN IN A FAMILY PRACTICE SETTING; SHALL NOT PERFORM ANY PHYSICAL EXAM ON A FEMALE PATIENT WITHOUT THE PRESENCE OF A CHAPERONE AND THIS SHALL BE DOCUMENTED IN THE RECORD; SHALL GIVE A COPY OF THIS ORDER TO ANY HEALTH CARE ENTITY WHERE HE HAS PRIVILEGES; SHALL COOPERATE WITH THE BOARD IN VERIFYING COMPLIANCE; SHALL INFORM BOARD OF CHANGE OF ADDRESS WITHIN 10 DAYS OR IF HE LEAVES THE STATE; TIME SPENT OUT OF TEXAS DOES NOT COUNT TOWARD PROBATION. SHALL NOT SEEK MODIFICATION FOR ONE YEAR.

COOMANSINGH, BELDEN J MD, LICENSE NUMBER 0139893 OF 12 NORTH HILLS ESTATE, CLEVELAND, TX, WAS DISCIPLINED BY NEW YORK ON MAY 23, 1995
DISCIPLINARY ACTION: 120-MONTH PROBATION
OFFENSE: DISCIPLINARY ACTION BY ANOTHER STATE OR AGENCY

NOTES: ACTION IN TEXAS FOR NEGLIGENCE. HE NEGLIGENTLY TREATED HIGH RISK PREGNANCIES AND IMPROPERLY TREATED A PREGNANCY INDUCED HYPERTENSIVE PATIENT WITH ALDOMET AND PHENOBARBITAL. TEN YEAR SUSPENSION, STAYED WITH PROBATION UPON COMMENCING PRACTICE IN NEW YORK.

COOMANSINGH, BELDEN J L MD, DATE OF BIRTH OCTOBER 14, 1937, LICENSE NUMBER 00F8446 OF 7213 HARRIS COURT, FORT WORTH, TX, WAS DISCIPLINED BY TEXAS ON AUGUST 14, 1995
DISCIPLINARY ACTION: EMERGENCY SUSPENSION
OFFENSE: FAILURE TO COMPLY WITH PREVIOUS BOARD ORDER

NOTES: ON MULTIPLE OCCASIONS PRIOR TO 8/2/95 HE PROVIDED LORCET PLUS TABLETS, A SCHEDULE III CONTROLLED SUBSTANCE TO AN ADULT FEMALE IN EXCHANGE FOR MONEY AND CERTAIN SEXUAL FAVORS; IN 7/95 INFORMED HER THAT SHE WAS TOO OLD FOR HIM AND THAT HE WOULD NO LONGER SUPPLY THE TABLETS TO HER IN EXCHANGE FOR SEXUAL FAVORS AND REQUESTED THAT SHE ARRANGE TO HAVE AVAILABLE FOR HIM YOUNG GIRLS 12 TO 13 YEARS OF AGE; ON 8/2/95, DURING A TELEPHONE CONVERSATION BETWEEN PHYSICIAN AND A NARCOTICS INVESTIGATOR, WHO HAS NEVER BEEN A PATIENT OF HIS AND WHO HAS NO VALID MEDICAL REASON FOR RECEIVING DIAZEPAM (VALIUM), HE AGREED TO PROVIDE INVESTIGATOR WITH 50 DIAZEPAM TABLETS, A SCHEDULE IV CONTROLLED SUBSTANCE, IN EXCHANGE FOR ORAL SEX; ON 8/03/95 UPON DELIVERY OF THE DRUGS HE WAS ARRESTED BY ELEMENTS OF THE NARCOTICS UNIT; IN VIOLATION OF 6/22/94 ORDER, HE HAS FAILED OR REFUSED TO OBTAIN A MONITORING PHYSICIAN; HAS PROVIDED OBSTETRICAL/GYNECOLOGICAL CARE, OTHER THAN IN A FAMILY PRACTICE SETTING, TO FOUR PATIENTS; HAS FAILED TO DOCUMENT THE PRESENCE OF A CHAPERONE, OR TO HAVE A CHAPERONE PRESENT DURING PHYSICAL EXAMINATIONS OF FOUR PATIENTS; ABANDONED THREE OF THE FOUR PATIENTS IMMEDIATELY PRIOR TO THEIR EXPECTED DELIVERY DATE. TEMPORARY SUSPENSION SHALL REMAIN IN EFFECT UNTIL

SUPERSEDED BY A SUBSEQUENT ORDER OF THE BOARD.

COOMANSINGH, BELDEN J MD OF 7213 HARRIS COURT, FORT WORTH, TX, WAS DISCIPLINED BY DEA ON NOVEMBER 13, 1995
DISCIPLINARY ACTION: SURRENDER OF CONTROLLED SUBSTANCE LICENSE

NOTES: IN LIEU OF PUBLIC INTEREST REVOCATION.

COOMANSINGH, BELDEN J L MD, DATE OF BIRTH OCTOBER 14, 1937, LICENSE NUMBER 00F8446 OF 7213 HARRIS COURT, FORT WORTH, TX, WAS DISCIPLINED BY TEXAS ON OCTOBER 4, 1996
DISCIPLINARY ACTION: LICENSE REVOCATION; FINE
OFFENSE: FAILURE TO COMPLY WITH PREVIOUS BOARD ORDER

NOTES: NONCOMPLIANCE TO AN ORDER DATED 6/22/94: FAILED TO OBTAIN A MONITORING PHYSICIAN WHO WAS ACCEPTABLE TO THE BOARD; CONTINUED TO PROVIDE OBSTETRICAL AND GYNECOLOGICAL CARE TO PATIENTS, OTHER THAN IN A FAMILY PRACTICE SETTING, BUT HAS FAILED TO TAKE A MINI-RESIDENCY COURSE; AND FAILED TO HAVE A CHAPERONE PRESENT WHILE CONDUCTING EXAMINATIONS OF FEMALE PATIENTS. ON NUMEROUS OCCASIONS PROVIDED LORCET PLUS TABLETS, A SCHEDULE III CONTROLLED SUBSTANCE TO AN ADULT FEMALE IN EXCHANGE FOR SEXUAL FAVORS; ON 8/03/95 ARRESTED AND CHARGED WITH DELIVERY OF DIAZEPAM UNDER 28 GRAMS; ON 12/14/95 INDICTED FOR THE "DELIVERY OF A CONTROLLED SUBSTANCE"; AND IN AUGUST AND SEPTEMBER 1994 ABANDONED FOUR OBSTETRICAL PATIENTS IMMEDIATELY PRIOR TO THEIR EXPECTED DELIVERY DATES. $25,000 FINE.

COOPER, APRIL DENISE MD, DATE OF BIRTH APRIL 24, 1961 OF 7900 WESTHEIMER ROAD, HOUSTON, TX, WAS DISCIPLINED BY MEDICARE ON DECEMBER 30, 1996
DISCIPLINARY ACTION: EXCLUSION FROM THE MEDICARE AND/OR MEDICAID PROGRAM
OFFENSE: NONCOMPLIANCE WITH A PROFESSIONAL RULE

NOTES: DEFAULTED ON PUBLIC HEALTH SERVICE EDUCATION LOAN. INDEFINITE EXCLUSION.

COOPER, BRUCE T MD, LICENSE NUMBER H2317 OF HOUSTON, TX, WAS DISCIPLINED BY TEXAS ON MAY 16, 1998
DISCIPLINARY ACTION: FINE
OFFENSE: NONCOMPLIANCE WITH A PROFESSIONAL RULE

NOTES: IN REGARD TO A PATIENT'S BREAST AUGMENTATION TREATMENT IN 1995, HE FAILED TO ADEQUATELY DOCUMENT HIS POST-OPERATIVE CARE AND TREATMENT; POST-OP EVALUATION AND RECOMMENDATIONS AS WELL AS PATIENT INSTRUCTIONS WERE NOT DOCUMENTED IN ANY MANNER; HE REPORTS THAT HE HAS TAKEN REMEDIAL MEASURES IN REGARD TO HIS RECORD KEEPING. $2,500 FINE.

COPPOLA, JOSEPH C MD, LICENSE NUMBER E6290 OF HOUSTON, TX, WAS DISCIPLINED BY TEXAS ON AUGUST 28, 1999
DISCIPLINARY ACTION: 60-MONTH PROBATION; FINE
OFFENSE: PROVIDING FALSE INFORMATION TO THE BOARD OR OTHER HEALTH AGENCY

NOTES: IN 1983 - 85, 1987 - 88, 1990 & 1/30/97 HE CLAIMED HE WAS CERTIFIED BY THE AMERICAN BOARD OF INTERNAL MEDICINE WHEN APPLYING FOR APPOINTMENTS AND PRIVILEGES AT THREE HOSPITALS; AS EVIDENCE, HE SUBMITTED A FORGED LETTER FROM THE AMERICAN BOARD OF INTERNAL MEDICINE IN THE 1997 APPLICATION; HE STATES HE SUBMITTED THIS LETTER BECAUSE THE ORIGINAL LETTER WAS DESTROYED IN A MISHAP IN 1980; THE AMERICAN BOARD OF INTERNAL MEDICINE INVESTIGATED HIM AND REVOKED HIS ELIGIBILITY FOR ADMISSION TO THE EXAMINATION. SUSPENSION STAYED FOR PROBATION AND PUBLIC REPRIMAND WITH FOLLOWING TERMS AND CONDITIONS: SHALL OBTAIN 10 HOURS OF AN ETHICS COURSE PER YEAR FOR 5 YEARS; WITHIN 6 MONTHS SHALL TAKE AND PASS THE MEDICAL JURISPRUDENCE EXAM WITH A SCORE OF 75 OR BETTER, WITHIN 3 ATTEMPTS; SHALL PERFORM 96 HOURS OF COMMUNITY SERVICE PER YEAR FOR A BOARD-APPROVED NON-PROFIT; SHALL PAY $10,000 FINE WITHIN 90 DAYS; SHALL APPEAR BEFORE THE BOARD AT LEAST ONCE A YEAR; SHALL COOPERATE WITH THE BOARD IN VERIFYING COMPLIANCE; SHALL GIVE A COPY OF THIS ORDER TO ANY HEALTH CARE ENTITY WHERE HE HAS PRIVILEGES; TIME SPENT OUT OF TEXAS DOES NOT COUNT TOWARD PROBATION/RESTRICTION; SHALL INFORM THE BOARD OF CHANGE OF ADDRESS WITHIN 10 DAYS OR IF HE LEAVES THE STATE; SHALL NOT SEEK MODIFICATION FOR ONE YEAR.

CORMIA, FRANK E JR MD, WAS DISCIPLINED BY ALASKA ON JULY 11, 1997
DISCIPLINARY ACTION: DENIAL OF NEW LICENSE
OFFENSE: DISCIPLINARY ACTION BY ANOTHER STATE OR AGENCY

NOTES: SUSPENSION OF LICENSE IN TEXAS.

CORMIA, FRANK EDWARD JR MD, LICENSE NUMBER 00E3885, WAS DISCIPLINED BY TEXAS ON AUGUST 17, 1996
DISCIPLINARY ACTION: 60-MONTH PROBATION; REQUIRED TO TAKE ADDITIONAL MEDICAL EDUCATION
OFFENSE: SUBSTANDARD CARE, INCOMPETENCE OR NEGLIGENCE

NOTES: IN 4/91 FAILED TO ADEQUATELY TREAT A PATIENT IN REGARD TO THIS PATIENT'S DIABETES MANAGEMENT; AND THE MEDICAL RECORDS FAILED TO ADEQUATELY DOCUMENT THE PATIENT'S CARE, TREATMENT, AND RECOMMENDATIONS. SUSPENSION, STAYED AS PROBATION WITH TERMS AND CONDITIONS; WITHIN SIX MONTHS SHALL TAKE AND PASS THE SPEX EXAMINATION AND THE MEDICAL JURISPRUDENCE EXAMINATION; SHALL OBTAIN AT LEAST 50 HOURS PER YEAR OF CONTINUING MEDICAL EDUCATION INCLUDING AT LEAST ONE COURSE IN RISK MANAGEMENT AND THE REMAINING HOURS IN FAMILY PRACTICE; SHALL MAINTAIN ADEQUATE MEDICAL RECORDS WHICH SHALL BE AVAILABLE FOR REVIEW; HIS MEDICAL PRACTICE, INCLUDING ANY OFFICE AND SURGICAL PRACTICE, SHALL BE MONITORED BY A BOARD APPROVED TEXAS PHYSICIAN WHO SHALL PROVIDE QUARTERLY REPORTS TO THE BOARD; WITHIN ONE YEAR SHALL TAKE AN ADVANCED CARDIAC LIFE SUPPORT COURSE AND AN ADVANCED TRAUMA LIFE SUPPORT COURSE AND OBTAIN CERTIFICATION OF BOTH; SHALL COOPERATE WITH THE BOARD IN VERIFYING COMPLIANCE; SHALL APPEAR BEFORE THE BOARD AT LEAST TWICE A YEAR; SHALL GIVE A COPY OF THIS ORDER TO ANY HEALTH CARE ENTITY WHERE HE HAS PRIVILEGES; SHALL PROVIDE A COPY OF THIS ORDER TO ANYONE REQUESTING IT WITHIN 10 DAYS; TIME PERIOD OUT OF TEXAS DOES NOT COUNT TOWARD PROBATION; SHALL INFORM THE BOARD OF CHANGE OF ADDRESS WITHIN 10 DAYS OF IF HE LEAVES THE STATE; SHALL NOT SEEK MODIFICATION FOR ONE YEAR.

CORMIA, FRANK EDWARD JR MD, LICENSE NUMBER E3885 OF FORT COLLINS, CO, WAS DISCIPLINED BY TEXAS ON MAY 16, 1998
DISCIPLINARY ACTION: 54-MONTH PROBATION; REQUIRED TO

TAKE ADDITIONAL MEDICAL EDUCATION

NOTES: FAILED TO TAKE AND PASS SPEX, AND MEDICAL JURISPRUDENCE EXAM BY 2/17/97, IN VIOLATION OF 8/17/96 ORDER; LICENSE WAS SUSPENDED; ON 10/27/97 HE PASSED THE SPEX WITH A SCORE OF 80. SUSPENSION STAYED FOR PROBATION WITH FOLLOWING TERMS AND CONDITIONS: SHALL OBTAIN 50 HOURS PER YEAR OF CONTINUING MEDICAL EDUCATION WITH AT LEAST ONE COURSE IN RISK MANAGEMENT; SHALL MAINTAIN ADEQUATE MEDICAL RECORDS WHICH SHALL BE AVAILABLE FOR REVIEW; HIS MEDICAL PRACTICE SHALL BE MONITORED BY A BOARD APPROVED TEXAS PHYSICIAN WHO SHALL PROVIDE QUARTERLY REPORTS TO THE BOARD; WITHIN ONE YEAR SHALL TAKE AND SUCCESSFULLY COMPLETE AN ADVANCED CARDIAC LIFE SUPPORT COURSE AND AN ADVANCED TRAUMA LIFE SUPPORT COURSE AND OBTAIN CERTIFICATION; SHALL COOPERATE WITH THE BOARD IN VERIFYING COMPLIANCE; SHALL APPEAR BEFORE THE BOARD TWICE A YEAR; SHALL GIVE A COPY OF THIS ORDER TO ANY HEALTH CARE ENTITY WHERE HE HAS PRIVILEGES; SHALL PROVIDE A COPY OF THIS ORDER TO ANYONE REQUESTING IT WITHIN 10 DAYS; TIME SPENT OUT OF TEXAS DOES NOT COUNT TOWARD PROBATION; SHALL INFORM THE BOARD OF CHANGE OF ADDRESS WITHIN 10 DAYS OR IF HE LEAVES THE STATE; SHALL NOT SEEK MODIFICATION FOR ONE YEAR.

CORNITIUS, TIMOTHY GAVIN MD OF ROUTE 1, BOX 321, CADOO MILLS, TX, WAS DISCIPLINED BY KANSAS ON JUNE 14, 1993
DISCIPLINARY ACTION: MONITORING OF PHYSICIAN PERFORMANCE
OFFENSE: SUBSTANCE ABUSE

NOTES: PRIOR TO APPLYING FOR LICENSURE ON 3/26/93, SUFFERED FROM IMPAIRMENT DUE TO CHEMICAL ABUSE; WAS SUCCESSFULLY DISCHARGED FROM INPATIENT TREATMENT ON 4/23/93. RESTRICTIONS INCLUDE: ENTERING INTO A MONITORING CONTRACT WITH KANSAS MEDICAL SOCIETY AND IMPAIRED PROVIDER PROGRAM WHICH MAY DISCUSS OR OTHERWISE COMMUNICATE TO THE BOARD DETAILS OF HIS CASE AS NECESSARY; HE AGREES TO RELEASE ALL MATERIAL IN HIS PROGRAM FILE IN THE EVENT THAT HE IS TERMINATED FROM PROGRAM FOR NONCOMPLIANCE; PROGRAM LENGTH SHALL BE AT LEAST FOUR YEARS WITH OPTION TO RENEW PROGRAM FOR ADDITIONAL TIME AT THE DISCRETION OF PROGRAM OR THE BOARD; CONDITIONS OF PROGRAM INCLUDE: URINALYSIS TESTING THREE TIMES A WEEK AT RANDOM TIMES FOR SIX MONTHS. AGREES NOT TO USE ANY MIND ALTERING DRUG OR SUBSTANCE INCLUDING ALCOHOL, WILL NOT DO ANY SELF PRESCRIBING, ANY CHANGE OF ADDRESS OR NEED FOR MEDICATION WILL IMMEDIATELY BE COMMUNICATED TO PROGRAM.

CORNITIUS, TIMOTHY GAVIN MD, LICENSE NUMBER 00H0266 OF DODGE CITY, KS, WAS DISCIPLINED BY TEXAS ON JANUARY 6, 1995
DISCIPLINARY ACTION: SURRENDER OF LICENSE
OFFENSE: DISCIPLINARY ACTION BY ANOTHER STATE OR AGENCY

NOTES: IN 1992 AND FOR APPROXIMATELY A YEAR AND A HALF ENGAGED IN THE INTEMPERATE USE OF THE CONTROLLED SUBSTANCES XANAX AND DARVOCET; VOLUNTARILY ADMITTED HIMSELF FOR TREATMENT IN 3/93 AND SUCCESSFULLY COMPLETED INPATIENT TREATMENT; ENTERED AN AGREEMENT AND ENFORCEMENT ORDER WITH KANSAS BOARD ON 6/14/93 AND HAS REPORTED FULL COMPLIANCE WITH THIS ORDER TO TEXAS; IN LIEU OF FURTHER INVESTIGATION AGREES TO THIS ORDER. SHALL NOT PETITION FOR REINSTATEMENT.

COSTA, FELIX AUGUSTO MD, LICENSE NUMBER D9972 OF HOUSTON, TX, WAS DISCIPLINED BY TEXAS ON AUGUST 9, 1997
DISCIPLINARY ACTION: 60-MONTH RESTRICTION PLACED ON LICENSE; REQUIRED TO TAKE ADDITIONAL MEDICAL EDUCATION
OFFENSE: SUBSTANDARD CARE, INCOMPETENCE OR NEGLIGENCE

NOTES: IN 12/95 AFTER AN INVESTIGATION BY HIS EMPLOYER, THE MENTAL HEALTH MENTAL RETARDATION AUTHORITY; HE WAS PLACED ON PROBATION FOR: IMPROPERLY REFERRING PRIORITY POPULATION PATIENTS TO OTHER AGENCIES WITHOUT CLEAR DOCUMENTATION AS TO WHY; IMPROPERLY DIAGNOSING PATIENTS AND INAPPROPRIATELY PRESCRIBING AND/OR ADMINISTERING MEDICATIONS WHICH WERE CONTRAINDICATED OR NON THERAPEUTIC; HE FOLLOWED THE TERMS OF THIS PROBATION AND HAS PRESENTED INFORMATION THAT THE CRITICISMS WERE MOTIVATED BY FINANCIAL CONCERNS. MEDICAL PRACTICE SHALL BE LIMITED TO AN INSTITUTIONAL SETTING OR GROUP PRACTICE; SHALL NOT PRACTICE CRISIS PSYCHIATRY WHERE CRISES ARE HANDLED; SHALL MAINTAIN ADEQUATE MEDICAL RECORDS WHICH SHALL BE AVAILABLE FOR REVIEW; SHALL OBTAIN AT LEAST 50 HOURS PER YEAR OF CONTINUING MEDICAL EDUCATION; WITHIN 1 YEAR SHALL SUCCESSFULLY COMPLETE A COURSE IN PHARMACOLOGY; SHALL REFRAIN FROM THE PRESCRIPTION OR ADMINISTRATION OF ANY DRUG UNLESS THE DRUG IS MEDICALLY INDICATED AND IS PRESCRIBED IN THERAPEUTIC DOSES; SHALL APPEAR BEFORE THE BOARD UPON REQUEST; SHALL COOPERATE WITH THE BOARD IN VERIFYING COMPLIANCE INCLUDING PROVIDING COPIES OF PEER REVIEW RECORDS UPON REQUEST; TIME SPENT OUT OF TEXAS DOES NOT COUNT TOWARD RESTRICTION; SHALL INFORM THE BOARD OF CHANGE OF ADDRESS WITHIN 10 DAYS OR IF HE LEAVES THE STATE; SHALL NOT SEEK MODIFICATION FOR ONE YEAR.

COSTA, FELIX AUGUSTO MD, LICENSE NUMBER 31389 OF HOUSTON, TX, WAS DISCIPLINED BY OHIO ON SEPTEMBER 9, 1998
DISCIPLINARY ACTION: LICENSE REVOCATION
OFFENSE: DISCIPLINARY ACTION BY ANOTHER STATE OR AGENCY

NOTES: ACTION BY TEXAS MEDICAL BOARD FOLLOWING THAT BOARD'S FINDING THAT, WHILE EMPLOYED AS A CRISIS PSYCHIATRIST, HE HAD BEEN PLACED ON PROBATION BY CITY MENTAL HEALTH/MENTAL RETARDATION AUTHORITY FOLLOWING ALLEGATIONS OF IMPROPER REFERRALS, IMPROPER DIAGNOSES OF PATIENTS AND IMPROPER PRESCRIBING AND/OR ADMINISTRATION OF MEDICATION.

COSTA, FELIX AUGUSTO MD, LICENSE NUMBER 0003625 OF HOUSTON, TX, WAS DISCIPLINED BY VERMONT ON OCTOBER 7, 1998
DISCIPLINARY ACTION: CEASE AND DESIST ORDER

NOTES: HE AGREED NOT TO PRACTICE MEDICINE IN VERMONT UNLESS AND UNTIL HE SUBMITS A PETITION WHICH SHALL BE IN A MANNER AND FORM APPROVED BY THE BOARD.

COWDEN, WILLIAM L MD, LICENSE NUMBER 00F1483 OF DALLAS, TX, WAS DISCIPLINED BY TEXAS ON JANUARY 6, 1995
DISCIPLINARY ACTION: REPRIMAND; REQUIRED TO TAKE ADDITIONAL MEDICAL EDUCATION
OFFENSE: PROFESSIONAL MISCONDUCT

NOTES: ON FOUR OCCASIONS DURING 1992 HE ADMINISTERED

AN INJECTION OF A SUBSTANCE UNDER DEVELOPMENT IN ENGLAND TO A PATIENT SUFFERING FROM HODGKIN'S DISEASE WITHOUT KNOWING THE VARIOUS COMPONENTS, SIDE EFFECTS, TOXICITY OR CONTRAINDICATIONS OF THE DRUG; DRUG WAS FOR PALLIATION OF SYMPTOMS NOT CURE; SUBSTANCE NOT FDA APPROVED; ALSO DURING 1991 AND 1992 PRESCRIBED CYTOMEL TO A PATIENT WITHOUT APPROPRIATE INDICATION OR DOCUMENTATION; NEITHER ADMITS NOR DENIES THE ALLEGATIONS. CONDITIONS OF TWO YEAR RESTRICTION ON LICENSE INCLUDE: SHALL OBTAIN AT LEAST 50 HOURS PER YEAR OF CONTINUING MEDICAL EDUCATION INCLUDING AT LEAST ONE COURSE PER YEAR IN PHARMACOLOGY AND ENDOCRINOLOGY; SHALL APPEAR BEFORE THE BOARD ONCE A YEAR OR UPON REQUEST; SHALL COOPERATE WITH THE BOARD IN VERIFYING COMPLIANCE; SHALL GIVE A COPY OF THIS ORDER TO ANY HEALTH CARE ENTITY WHERE HE HAS OR APPLIES FOR PRIVILEGES OR ANYONE ELSE THAT REQUESTS IT; SHALL ENSURE ANY INQUIRIES REGARDING HIS TEXAS LICENSURE STATUS ARE ANSWERED BY REFERENCE TO THIS ORDER; SHALL INFORM BOARD OF CHANGE OF ADDRESS WITHIN 10 DAYS OR IF HE LEAVES THE STATE; TIME SPENT OUT OF TEXAS DOES NOT COUNT TOWARD RESTRICTION. SHALL NOT SEEK MODIFICATION FOR ONE YEAR.

COX, ANN KATHLEEN MD, LICENSE NUMBER H1359 OF DALLAS, TX, WAS DISCIPLINED BY TEXAS ON AUGUST 22, 1998
DISCIPLINARY ACTION: FINE; REPRIMAND
OFFENSE: NONCOMPLIANCE WITH A PROFESSIONAL RULE

NOTES: ON OR ABOUT 6/18/97 SHE CERTIFIED THAT SHE HAD COMPLETED 40 HOURS OF CONTINUING MEDICAL EDUCATION DURING THE REPORTING PERIOD BETWEEN 9/1/96 - 8/31/97; SHE WAS SUBJECT TO A RANDOM AUDIT AND WAS ABLE TO PROVIDE PROOF OF ATTENDING ONLY 4 HOURS OF CONTINUING MEDICAL EDUCATION DURING THE REFERENCED PERIOD; SHE MAINTAINS THAT THERE WAS NO INTENT TO MISLEAD THE BOARD; SHE INDICATES THAT SHE HAS TAKEN REMEDIAL MEASURES TO TRACK HER CONTINUING MEDICAL EDUCATION DOCUMENTATION. $100 FINE.

COX, BRUCE E MD, LICENSE NUMBER E4272 OF BIG SPRING, TX, WAS DISCIPLINED BY TEXAS ON APRIL 10, 1999
DISCIPLINARY ACTION: RESTRICTION PLACED ON CONTROLLED SUBSTANCE LICENSE; MONITORING OF PHYSICIAN PERFORMANCE
OFFENSE: NONCOMPLIANCE WITH A PROFESSIONAL RULE

NOTES: IN REGARD TO 9 PATIENTS REVIEWED BY THE BOARD, HE FAILED TO ADEQUATELY DOCUMENT INDICATIONS FOR PRESCRIPTIONS OF ANTI-ANXIETY AND PAIN MEDICATIONS; HE INDICATES THAT HE HAS IMPROVED HIS RECORD KEEPING AND NOW TRANSCRIBES PATIENT CHARTS. LICENSE LIMITED FOR THREE YEARS AS FOLLOWS: SHALL ATTEND 50 HOURS PER YEAR OF CONTINUING MEDICAL EDUCATION WITH 1 COURSE IN RISK MANAGEMENT; SHALL LIMIT PRESCRIBING OF SCHEDULE II DRUGS TO THE ORDERING OF SUCH DRUGS IN A HOSPITAL SETTING TO INPATIENTS ONLY; SEPARATE FROM PATIENT RECORDS, SHALL MAINTAIN A FILE OF EVERY PRESCRIPTION WRITTEN BY HIM FOR DANGEROUS DRUGS WITH ADDICTIVE POTENTIAL WHICH SHALL BE MADE AVAILABLE FOR REVIEW; SHALL IMMEDIATELY SURRENDER ANY UNUSED TRIPLICATE PRESCRIPTION FORMS; SHALL MAINTAIN ADEQUATE MEDICAL RECORDS WHICH SHALL BE AVAILABLE FOR REVIEW; SHALL APPEAR BEFORE THE BOARD AT LEAST ONCE A YEAR; SHALL COOPERATE WITH THE BOARD IN VERIFYING COMPLIANCE; TIME SPENT OUT OF TEXAS DOES NOT COUNT TOWARD RESTRICTION; SHALL INFORM THE BOARD OF CHANGE OF ADDRESS WITHIN 10 DAYS OR IF HE LEAVES THE STATE; SHALL NOT SEEK MODIFICATION FOR ONE YEAR.

COX, JOHNSTON S MD OF 601 EAST SAN ANTONIO SUITE #401, VICTORIA, TX, WAS DISCIPLINED BY DEA ON NOVEMBER 8, 1995
DISCIPLINARY ACTION: SURRENDER OF CONTROLLED SUBSTANCE LICENSE

NOTES: IN LIEU OF PUBLIC INTEREST REVOCATION.

COX, JOHNSTON STEWART MD, LICENSE NUMBER 00F6546 OF VICTORIA, TX, WAS DISCIPLINED BY TEXAS ON AUGUST 19, 1994
DISCIPLINARY ACTION: FINE; REQUIRED TO TAKE ADDITIONAL MEDICAL EDUCATION
OFFENSE: OVERPRESCRIBING OR MISPRESCRIBING DRUGS

NOTES: HE PRESCRIBED CONTROLLED SUBSTANCES TO A SINGLE PATIENT WHO EXHIBITED SIGNS OF HABITUATION WITHOUT ADEQUATE JUSTIFICATION AND DOCUMENTATION OF PHYSICAL EXAMS, REFERRALS OR CONSULTATIONS REGARDING POSSIBLE CHRONIC PAIN AND WITHOUT OBJECTIVE TESTING OR FINDINGS. CONDITIONS OF RESTRICTION: SHALL ATTEND AT LEAST 50 HOURS PER YEAR OF CONTINUING MEDICAL EDUCATION INCLUDING 10 HOURS IN RISK MANAGEMENT AND 25 HOURS IN PHARMACOLOGY/ADDICTIONOLOGY IN THE FIRST YEAR; SHALL NOT TREAT OR OTHERWISE SERVE AS PHYSICIAN, PRESCRIBE, DISPENSE OR ADMINISTER DRUGS THAT MAY BE SUBJECT TO ABUSE TO HIMSELF OR ANY MEMBER OF HIS FAMILY; SHALL MAINTAIN ADEQUATE MEDICAL RECORDS ON ALL PATIENT OFFICE VISITS WHICH SHALL BE AVAILABLE FOR INSPECTION; SHALL PERSONALLY EXAMINE PATIENTS WHENEVER ANY FORM CERTIFIES THAT A PERSONAL EXAM HAS BEEN PERFORMED BY A PHYSICIAN, WHERE STATE LAW REQUIRES THIS OR WHERE AN INITIAL DIAGNOSIS OF PROBABLE DISEASE OR INJURY HAS BEEN MADE; SHALL PERSONALLY EXAMINE THE PATIENT DURING THE FIRST VISIT; SHALL NOT SIGN ANY PATIENT RECORD UNLESS HE HAS PERSONALLY EXAMINED THE PATIENT OR CLEARLY NOTES IN THE RECORD THAT HE HAS NOT; $1,000 ADMINISTRATIVE PENALTY; SHALL APPEAR BEFORE THE BOARD ONCE A YEAR; SHALL GIVE A COPY OF THIS ORDER TO ANY HEALTH CARE ENTITY WHERE HE HAS PRIVILEGES; SHALL COOPERATE WITH THE BOARD IN VERIFYING COMPLIANCE; SHALL INFORM BOARD OF CHANGE OF ADDRESS WITHIN 10 DAYS OR IF HE LEAVES THE STATE; TIME SPENT OUT OF TEXAS DOES NOT COUNT TOWARD PROBATION. SHALL NOT SEEK MODIFICATION FOR ONE YEAR.

COX, JOHNSTON STEWART MD, LICENSE NUMBER 00F6546 OF VICTORIA, TX, WAS DISCIPLINED BY TEXAS ON OCTOBER 14, 1995
DISCIPLINARY ACTION: EMERGENCY SUSPENSION
OFFENSE: FAILURE TO COMPLY WITH PREVIOUS BOARD ORDER

NOTES: AVAILABLE EVIDENCE AND INFORMATION INDICATE THAT DURING THE PAST THREE YEARS HE HAS PRESCRIBED LORCET, A SCHEDULE III CONTROLLED SUBSTANCE, FLEXERIL, A DANGEROUS DRUG AND PHENTERMINE, A SCHEDULE IV CONTROLLED SUBSTANCE USING FICTITIOUS PATIENT NAMES WHICH WERE FOR HIS PERSONAL USE IN VIOLATION OF THE 8/94 ORDER; IN APPROXIMATELY 7/95 HE INGESTED LSD WHILE ATTENDING A MEDICAL CONVENTION IN FLORIDA; AVAILABLE EVIDENCE AND INFORMATION INDICATE THAT BETWEEN 1/95 AND 9/95

HE PRESCRIBED LARGE QUANTITIES OF MULTIPLE CONTROLLED SUBSTANCES TO A PATIENT WITHOUT A LEGITIMATE PURPOSE, IN DANGEROUS COMBINATIONS AND DESPITE HER PAST HISTORY OF DRUG ABUSE AND CONTINUED TO PRESCRIBE DEPRESSANT MEDICATIONS TO PATIENT DESPITE HER DIAGNOSIS OF DEPRESSION; MEDICAL RECORDS FOR THIS PATIENT INDICATE PROGRESS NOTES FOR 17 VISITS BETWEEN 1/95 AND 8/95 BUT CONTAIN NO DOCUMENTATION OF THE MEDICATIONS PRESCRIBED, NOR ANY JUSTIFICATION FOR THE QUANTITIES OF OPIATES AND BENZODIAZEPINES; AVAILABLE EVIDENCE AND INFORMATION INDICATE THAT IN 9/95 HE CEASED TO PROVIDE MEDICAL CARE FOR VARIOUS PATIENTS WHOM HE HAD ADMITTED TO A HOSPITAL AND FOR FOUR PATIENTS AT A NURSING HOME WITHOUT PRIOR OR ADEQUATE NOTICE; FAILED TO MAKE ANY OR ADEQUATE ARRANGEMENTS WITH ANOTHER PHYSICIAN FOR THE CONTINUING CARE OR TREATMENT OF THESE PATIENTS.

COX-TEEL, ANN K MD, LICENSE NUMBER 211619 OF 7118 LAKEWOOD BOULEVARD, DALLAS, TX, WAS DISCIPLINED BY NEW YORK ON JUNE 4, 1999
DISCIPLINARY ACTION: REPRIMAND
OFFENSE: DISCIPLINARY ACTION BY ANOTHER STATE OR AGENCY

NOTES: DISCIPLINED BY THE TEXAS BOARD FOR FAILING TO PROVIDE PROOF OF HER COMPLETION OF 40 HOURS OF CONTINUING MEDICAL EDUCATION.

COX-TEEL, ANN KATHLEEN MD OF 7118 LAKEWOOD BLVD., DALLAS, TX, WAS DISCIPLINED BY MARYLAND ON JULY 20, 1999
OFFENSE: NONCOMPLIANCE WITH A PROFESSIONAL RULE

NOTES: WAS NOT ABLE TO PROVIDE PROOF OF CONTINUING MEDICAL EDUCATION TO THE TEXAS BOARD, WAS INVESTIGATED FOR THIS AT THE TEXAS BOARD, AND DID NOT REPORT THIS TO THE MARYLAND BOARD. APPLICATION FOR LICENSURE TO BE GRANTED UPON COMPLETION OF CONDITION; IF GRANTED THEN LICENSE REPRIMANDED.

CRALL, H DOUGLAS MD, DATE OF BIRTH DECEMBER 27, 1954, LICENSE NUMBER 0027106 OF MCCRACKEN COUNTY, KY, WAS DISCIPLINED BY KENTUCKY ON JULY 21, 1994
DISCIPLINARY ACTION: LICENSE SUSPENSION; 60-MONTH PROBATION

NOTES: LICENSE SUSPENDED UNTIL CONFIRMATION RECEIVED THAT HE HAS COMPLETED APPROVED TREATMENT PROGRAM AND IS FIT TO RETURN TO PRACTICE; NOT TO EXCEED 2 YEARS. SUSPENSION TO BE FOLLOWED BY PROBATION. ON 3/16/98 ORDER MODIFIED TERMINATING SUSPENSION; TERMS OF PROBATION INCLUDE PRACTICE LOCATION RESTRICTION; USE OF CHAPERONE; AND MAINTAINING CONTRACTUAL RELATIONSHIP WITH IMPAIRED PHYSICIANS PROGRAM.

CRALL, H DOUGLAS MD, LICENSE NUMBER 00H0040 OF PADUCAH, KY, WAS DISCIPLINED BY TEXAS ON OCTOBER 13, 1995
DISCIPLINARY ACTION: LICENSE SUSPENSION; REQUIRED TO TAKE ADDITIONAL MEDICAL EDUCATION
OFFENSE: DISCIPLINARY ACTION BY ANOTHER STATE OR AGENCY

NOTES: FROM APPROXIMATELY 1988 TO 1994 HE ENGAGED IN THE INTEMPERATE USE OF PRESCRIPTION MEDICATIONS, NAMELY XANAX, A SCHEDULE IV CONTROLLED SUBSTANCE; PRIOR TO 1/94 AND WHILE PRACTICING OBSTETRICS AND GYNECOLOGY IN KENTUCKY, HE ENGAGED IN SEXUAL ACTS WITH APPROXIMATELY 10 OF HIS ADULT FEMALE PATIENTS AND HAS ALSO ENGAGED IN SEXUAL ACTS, INCLUDING SEXUAL INTERCOURSE, WITH FEMALE NURSES AND OFFICE STAFF MEMBERS; IN 1/94, VOLUNTARILY ADMITTED HIMSELF INTO A HOSPITAL COMPLAINING OF SEXUAL ADDICTION; DIAGNOSED WITH MAJOR DEPRESSION, OBSESSIVE COMPULSIVE DISORDER AND SEXUAL ADDICTION AND RECEIVED PSYCHIATRIC CARE AND COUNSELING; PRIOR TO COMPLETING THE TREATMENT PROGRAM, HE WAS DISCHARGED BY THE HOSPITAL IN 1/94 FOR FAILING TO COMPLY WITH THE REQUIREMENTS OF THE PROGRAM; IN 7/94 ENTERED INTO AN ORDER WITH KENTUCKY BOARD PLACING HIS LICENSE ON PROBATION BASED ON HIS INAPPROPRIATE SEXUAL CONTACT WITH ONE OR MORE OF HIS PATIENTS; IN 8/94, VOLUNTARILY ADMITTED HIMSELF INTO A DALLAS PSYCHIATRIC FACILITY FOR SEXUAL ADDICTION TREATMENT; REPORTS THAT HE COMPLETED INPATIENT PORTION OF THE TREATMENT PROGRAM AND IS CURRENTLY UNDERGOING FURTHER TREATMENT AS AN OUTPATIENT. SUSPENSION UNTIL HE REQUESTS TO HAVE SUSPENSION LIFTED AND APPEARS BEFORE BOARD WITH EVIDENCE WHICH ADEQUATELY INDICATES THAT HE IS PHYSICALLY, MENTALLY AND OTHERWISE COMPETENT TO SAFELY PRACTICE MEDICINE INCLUDING AT A MINIMUM EVIDENCE THAT HIS KENTUCKY LICENSE IS NO LONGER SUSPENDED AND HE IS AUTHORIZED TO PRACTICE IN KENTUCKY; EVIDENCE THAT HE HAS TAKEN AND PASSED THE SPECIAL PURPOSE EXAMINATION; EVIDENCE THAT HE HAS COMPLETED 150 HOURS OF CONTINUING MEDICAL EDUCATION OR COMPLETED A SIX-MONTH MINI-RESIDENCY IN INTERNAL MEDICINE OR FAMILY PRACTICE APPROVED BY THE BOARD.

CRALL, H DOUGLAS MD, LICENSE NUMBER 27106 OF OLDHAM COUNTY, KY, WAS DISCIPLINED BY KENTUCKY ON MAY 13, 1999
DISCIPLINARY ACTION: RESTRICTION PLACED ON LICENSE; MONITORING OF PHYSICIAN PERFORMANCE

NOTES: TERMS AND CONDITIONS INCLUDE: PRACTICE LOCATION RESTRICTION; USE OF CHAPERONE AND MAINTAINING CONTRACTUAL RELATIONSHIP WITH IMPAIRED PHYSICIANS PROGRAM.

CRAMER, ALAN T MD, LICENSE NUMBER 00D0839 OF HOUSTON, TX, WAS DISCIPLINED BY TEXAS ON AUGUST 18, 1995
DISCIPLINARY ACTION: FINE
OFFENSE: NONCOMPLIANCE WITH A PROFESSIONAL RULE

NOTES: IN 1994 ALLEGEDLY FAILED TO TIMELY FURNISH MEDICAL RECORDS TO A PATIENT WHO HAD MADE A PROPER REQUEST FOR THE RECORDS; HE MAINTAINS HE FURNISHED THE RECORDS. SHALL PAY $500 FINE; SHALL COOPERATE WITH THE BOARD IN VERIFYING COMPLIANCE.

CRAMER, ALAN THOMAS MD, LICENSE NUMBER D0839, WAS DISCIPLINED BY TEXAS ON MARCH 1, 1997
DISCIPLINARY ACTION: FINE; MONITORING OF PHYSICIAN PERFORMANCE
OFFENSE: NONCOMPLIANCE WITH A PROFESSIONAL RULE

NOTES: FAILED TO RELEASE PERSONAL MEDICAL RECORDS TO TWO FORMER PATIENTS FOLLOWING REQUESTS AND/OR AUTHORIZATIONS FOR THE RELEASE OF SUCH RECORDS; FAILED TO RESPOND WITHIN 30 DAYS AS TO WHY HE DID NOT PROVIDE RECORDS; HAD PREVIOUSLY ENTERED INTO AN AGREEMENT WITH THE BOARD ON 8/18/95 WHICH FOUND THAT HE DID NOT TIMELY FURNISH MEDICAL RECORDS TO A PATIENT ALTHOUGH THE PATIENT MADE A PROPER

REQUEST. SHALL PAY AN ADMINISTRATIVE PENALTY OF $3000; SHALL PASS THE MEDICAL JURISPRUDENCE EXAM WITHIN 6 MONTHS; SHALL COOPERATE WITH THE BOARD IN VERIFYING COMPLIANCE.

CRENWELGE, WILBUR E MD OF 710 EAST MAIN STREET, FREDERICKSBURG, TX, WAS DISCIPLINED BY DEA ON APRIL 3, 1995
DISCIPLINARY ACTION: SURRENDER OF CONTROLLED SUBSTANCE LICENSE

NOTES: IN LIEU OF PUBLIC INTEREST REVOCATION.

CRENWELGE, WILBUR E MD, LICENSE NUMBER 00C5016 OF FREDERICKSBURG, TX, WAS DISCIPLINED BY TEXAS ON AUGUST 18, 1995
DISCIPLINARY ACTION: SURRENDER OF LICENSE
OFFENSE: OVERPRESCRIBING OR MISPRESCRIBING DRUGS

NOTES: ALLEGEDLY PRESCRIBED LARGE AMOUNTS OF VARIOUS CONTROLLED SUBSTANCES AND DANGEROUS DRUGS TO SEVERAL ADULT PATIENTS WITHOUT ADEQUATE INDICATIONS OF THE LEGITIMATE MEDICAL PURPOSES; HAS VOLUNTARILY SURRENDERED HIS DEA CONTROLLED SUBSTANCES REGISTRATION CERTIFICATE. DOES NOT ADMIT VIOLATION. VOLUNTARY AND PERMANENT SURRENDER OF LICENSE IN LIEU OF FURTHER PROCEEDINGS SHALL NOT PETITION FOR REINSTATEMENT.

CROPPER, KENNETH R MD, LICENSE NUMBER 00D5948 OF LAKE JACKSON, TX, WAS DISCIPLINED BY TEXAS ON NOVEMBER 3, 1994
DISCIPLINARY ACTION: LICENSE SUSPENSION
OFFENSE: SUBSTANCE ABUSE

NOTES: ON 4/16/94 WENT TO A HOSPITAL EMERGENCY ROOM CLAIMING TO HAVE KIDNEY STONES AND ASKING FOR DEMEROL WHICH HE RECEIVED; HE RETURNED THE NEXT DAY AND WAS ADMITTED FOR PAIN; SPECIALIST FOUND NO EVIDENCE OF KIDNEY STONES AND WHEN THE HOSPITAL REFUSED TO INCREASE DEMEROL HE CHECKED OUT AGAINST MEDICAL ADVICE; ACTED INAPPROPRIATELY IN THE HOSPITAL INCLUDING CURSING AT THE STAFF; TOLD BOARD HE WAS UNDER THE CARE OF A PSYCHIATRIST DUE TO CHEMICAL DEPENDENCY AND THAT HE WAS HOSPITALIZED ON 5/20/94 FOR SUBSTANCE ABUSE AND DEPRESSION; REPORTEDLY RESPONDED WELL TO TREATMENT WITH MEDICATIONS AND PSYCHOTHERAPY; HE IS CURRENTLY SEEING A PSYCHIATRIST AND ATTENDS AA; REPORTED SOBRIETY DATE IS 4/19/94; IS CURRENTLY ON DISABILITY. SUSPENSION UNTIL HE PERSONALLY APPEARS BEFORE THE BOARD AND PROVIDES SUFFICIENT EVIDENCE AND INFORMATION WHICH ADEQUATELY INDICATES THAT HE IS PHYSICALLY, MENTALLY AND OTHERWISE COMPETENT TO SAFELY PRACTICE MEDICINE INCLUDING AT A MINIMUM COMPLETE LEGIBLE COPIES OF MEDICAL RECORDS AND REPORTS OF PSYCHOLOGICAL AND NEUROPSYCHIATRIC EVALUATIONS.

CROPPER, KENNETH ROSS MD, DATE OF BIRTH OCTOBER 10, 1944 OF PO BOX 1617, LAKE JACKSON, TX, WAS DISCIPLINED BY MEDICARE ON APRIL 9, 1996
DISCIPLINARY ACTION: EXCLUSION FROM THE MEDICARE AND/OR MEDICAID PROGRAM
OFFENSE: DISCIPLINARY ACTION BY ANOTHER STATE OR AGENCY

NOTES: LICENSE SUSPENDED FOR REASONS BEARING ON PROFESSIONAL PERFORMANCE.

CROSS, CRISS CONRAD MD, LICENSE NUMBER 00H7286 OF SAN ANTONIO, TX, WAS DISCIPLINED BY TEXAS ON OCTOBER 9, 1992
DISCIPLINARY ACTION: 120-MONTH PROBATION
OFFENSE: FAILURE TO COMPLY WITH PREVIOUS BOARD ORDER

NOTES: NONCOMPLIANCE WITH 4/20/90 ORDER. REVOCATION, STAYED. PROBATION UNDER TERMS AND CONDITIONS. ON 9/20/97 THE BOARD GRANTED HIS PETITION FOR TERMINATION OF THIS ORDER BASED ON COMPLIANCE WITH CONDITIONS.

CULBERSON, JOHN MD OF 1776 YORKTOWN #150, HOUSTON, TX, WAS DISCIPLINED BY DEA ON DECEMBER 14, 1999
DISCIPLINARY ACTION: SURRENDER OF CONTROLLED SUBSTANCE LICENSE

NOTES: IN LIEU OF ORDER TO SHOW CAUSE.

CULBERSON, JOHN WHITFIELD MD, LICENSE NUMBER J9653 OF SUGAR LAND, TX, WAS DISCIPLINED BY TEXAS ON AUGUST 22, 1998
DISCIPLINARY ACTION: LICENSE SUSPENSION
OFFENSE: FAILURE TO COMPLY WITH PREVIOUS BOARD ORDER

NOTES: ON 12/9/95 ENTERED INTO AN ORDER BASED ON HIS UNTRUTHFUL RESPONSE ON A LICENSE APPLICATION REGARDING CRIMINAL ARREST, INTEMPERATE USE OF ALCOHOL, AND SUBSTANCE ABUSE TREATMENT; VIOLATED THIS ORDER BY SELF-ADMITTING THAT ON 5/12/98, 6 HOURS PRIOR TO PROVIDING THE REQUESTED URINE SPECIMEN, HE HAD CONSUMED 2 QUARTS OF BEER AND BY HIS FAILURE TO REPORT BY TELEPHONE, FOLLOWED WITH A LETTER WITHIN 24 HOURS OF HIS INGESTION OF ALCOHOL ON 5/12/98 AND ON 7/9-12; HE AGREES TO REMAIN ON MEDICAL LEAVE OF ABSENCE, NOT TO RESUME THE PRACTICE OF MEDICINE UNTIL THE BOARD HAS AN OPPORTUNITY TO CONSIDER THE EXECUTION OF THIS ORDER, AND THENCEFORTH TO COMPLY WITH THE ORDER OF THE BOARD. SUSPENSION UNTIL HE REQUESTS TO HAVE HIS SUSPENSION STAYED OR APPEARS BEFORE THE BOARD WITH SUFFICIENT EVIDENCE THAT HE IS PHYSICALLY, MENTALLY AND OTHERWISE COMPETENT TO SAFELY PRACTICE MEDICINE INCLUDING AT A MINIMUM COMPLETE COPIES OF MEDICAL RECORDS AND REPORTS OF PSYCHOLOGICAL AND NEUROPSYCHIATRIC EVALUATIONS, INCLUDING A 96 HOUR INPATIENT EVALUATION CONDUCTED BY A BOARD-APPROVED CERTIFIED PSYCHIATRIST; SHALL COOPERATE WITH THE BOARD IN VERIFYING COMPLIANCE INCLUDING PROVIDING COPIES OF MEDICAL RELEASES AND PEER REVIEW RECORDS UPON REQUEST; SHALL PROVIDE A COPY OF THIS ORDER TO ANYONE REQUESTING IT WITHIN 10 DAYS; TIME SPENT OUT OF TEXAS DOES NOT COUNT TOWARD SUSPENSION; SHALL INFORM THE BOARD OF CHANGE OF ADDRESS WITHIN 10 DAYS OR IF HE LEAVES THE STATE.

CULBERSON, JOHN WHITFIELD MD OF 1315 CALHOUN #1404, HOUSTON, TX, WAS DISCIPLINED BY DEA ON OCTOBER 7, 1998
DISCIPLINARY ACTION: SURRENDER OF CONTROLLED SUBSTANCE LICENSE

NOTES: IN LIEU OF PUBLIC INTEREST REVOCATION.

CULBERSON, JOHN WHITFIELD MD, LICENSE NUMBER J9653 OF 4734 CAMBRIDGE STREET, SUGARLAND, TX, WAS DISCIPLINED BY TEXAS ON DECEMBER 8, 1999
DISCIPLINARY ACTION: LICENSE SUSPENSION
OFFENSE: FAILURE TO COMPLY WITH PREVIOUS BOARD ORDER

NOTES: VIOLATED 8/28/98 BOARD ORDER BY TESTING POSITIVE FOR ETHANOL ON 12/6/99; ON 12/8/99 HE ACKNOWLEDGED THAT HE RELAPSED INTO ALCOHOL

BY OCCASIONAL CONSUMPTION OF APPROXIMATELY TWO WEEKS PRIOR DUE TO STRESSES RELATED TO HIS ONGOING DIVORCE PROCEEDINGS.

CURVIN, THOMAS J MD, LICENSE NUMBER 00H8616, WAS DISCIPLINED BY TEXAS ON AUGUST 17, 1996
DISCIPLINARY ACTION: 36-MONTH PROBATION; MONITORING OF PHYSICIAN PERFORMANCE
OFFENSE: SUBSTANCE ABUSE

NOTES: ON 11/18/93 ENTERED INTO A REHABILITATION CONTRACT WITH THE PHYSICIANS HEALTH AND REHABILITATION COMMITTEE; HAS ENGAGED IN THE INTEMPERATE USE OF FASTIN, ATIVAN, HYDROCODONE, MARIJUANA, AND OTHER SUBSTANCES; HIS SUBSTANCE ABUSE PROBLEMS CULMINATED IN HIS FALLING ASLEEP WHILE EXAMINING A PATIENT; IN MARCH 1993 VOLUNTARILY ADMITTED HIMSELF TO CHARTER REAL HOSPITAL AND WAS DISCHARGED TO SELF-CARE WITH DIAGNOSIS OF MAJOR DEPRESSION AND POLY SUBSTANCE ABUSE; REPORTS REGULAR ATTENDANCE WITH AA AND THE PHYSICIAN HEALTH AND REHABILITATION GROUP. SUSPENSION, STAYED. CONDITIONS OF PROBATION: SHALL ABSTAIN FROM THE CONSUMPTION OF ALCOHOL/DRUGS, IN ANY FORM UNLESS PRESCRIBED BY ANOTHER PHYSICIAN FOR A LEGITIMATE AND THERAPEUTIC PURPOSE; SHALL SUBMIT HIMSELF FOR APPROPRIATE EXAMS INCLUDING DRUG OR ALCOHOL SCREENS; SHALL SUBMIT HIMSELF FOR EVALUATION AND TREATMENT TO A BOARD APPROVED PSYCHIATRIST AT LEAST ONCE A MONTH WHO SHALL SUBMIT REPORTS; SHALL CONTINUE TO PARTICIPATE IN AA'S PROGRAMS AT LEAST THREE TIMES A WEEK WITH QUARTERLY REPORTS; SHALL PARTICIPATE IN THE ACTIVITIES OF PHYSICIAN HEALTH AND REHABILITATION COMMITTEE AND WEEKLY MEETINGS WITH QUARTERLY REPORTS; SHALL NOT TREAT OR OTHERWISE SERVE AS PHYSICIAN, PRESCRIBE, DISPENSE, OR ADMINISTER DRUGS WITH POTENTIAL FOR ABUSE, OR ALCOHOL TO HIMSELF OR TO ANY MEMBER OF HIS FAMILY; SHALL APPEAR BEFORE THE BOARD AT LEAST TWO TIMES A YEAR; SHALL COOPERATE WITH THE BOARD IN VERIFYING COMPLIANCE INCLUDING PROVIDING COPIES OF MEDICAL RELEASES UPON REQUEST; TIME PERIOD OUT OF TEXAS DOES NOT COUNT TOWARD PROBATION; SHALL INFORM THE BOARD OF CHANGE OF ADDRESS WITHIN 10 DAYS OF IF HE LEAVES THE STATE; SHALL NOT SEEK MODIFICATION FOR ONE YEAR. ON 8/22/98 ORDER TERMINATED.

CZEKAJ, PHILIP STEPHEN MD OF 2418 KELSO, SAN ANTONIO, TX, WAS DISCIPLINED BY DEA ON MARCH 21, 1995
DISCIPLINARY ACTION: SURRENDER OF CONTROLLED SUBSTANCE LICENSE

NOTES: IN LIEU OF ORDER TO SHOW CAUSE.

CZEKAJ, PHILIP STEPHEN MD, LICENSE NUMBER 00G4946 OF SAN ANTONIO, TX, WAS DISCIPLINED BY TEXAS ON AUGUST 18, 1995
DISCIPLINARY ACTION: 60-MONTH PROBATION; MONITORING OF PHYSICIAN PERFORMANCE
OFFENSE: SUBSTANCE ABUSE

NOTES: ADMITS TO SELF-PRESCRIBING PHENDIMETRAZINE AND BENZODIAZEPINE; IN 3/95 VOLUNTARILY SURRENDERED HIS DEA REGISTRATIONS IN AN EFFORT TO ALLEVIATE CONCERNS INVOLVING HIS SELF-PRESCRIBING; REPORTS ATTENDING AA MEETINGS AN AVERAGE OF FIVE TIMES A WEEK AND REPORTS REGULAR PARTICIPATION IN THE ACTIVITIES OF THE COMMITTEE ON PHYSICIAN HEALTH AND REHABILITATION; HE IS UNDER THE CARE OF A PSYCHIATRIST AND AN ADDICTIONOLOGIST. SUSPENSION STAYED. PROBATION WITH TERMS: SHALL ABSTAIN FROM THE CONSUMPTION OF ALCOHOL/DRUGS IN ANY FORM UNLESS PRESCRIBED BY ANOTHER PHYSICIAN FOR A LEGITIMATE AND THERAPEUTIC PURPOSE; SHALL SUBMIT HIMSELF FOR APPROPRIATE EXAMS INCLUDING DRUG OR ALCOHOL SCREENS; SHALL CONTINUE TO SEE PSYCHIATRIST AT LEAST ONCE A MONTH WITH REPORTS; SHALL CONTINUE TO PARTICIPATE IN AA'S PROGRAM NOT LESS THAN FIVE TIMES A WEEK WITH QUARTERLY REPORTS TO THE BOARD; SHALL CONTINUE TO PARTICIPATE IN THE ACTIVITIES OF AN IMPAIRED PHYSICIAN GROUP AND ATTEND WEEKLY MEETINGS WITH QUARTERLY REPORTS; SHALL COMPLY WITH TERMS OF CONTINUING CARE CONTRACT WITH QUARTERLY REPORTS TO THE BOARD; SHALL APPEAR BEFORE BOARD AT LEAST ONCE A YEAR; SHALL COOPERATE WITH THE BOARD IN VERIFYING COMPLIANCE INCLUDING PROVIDING COPIES OF MEDICAL RELEASES UPON REQUEST; SHALL NOT TREAT OR OTHERWISE SERVE AS PHYSICIAN, PRESCRIBE, DISPENSE OR ADMINISTER DRUGS THAT MAY BE SUBJECT TO ABUSE TO HIMSELF OR TO ANY MEMBER OF HIS FAMILY; SHALL SURRENDER HIS DEA AND DPS CONTROLLED SUBSTANCES REGISTRATION CERTIFICATES; SHALL GIVE A COPY OF THIS ORDER TO ANY HEALTH CARE ENTITY WHERE HE HAS PRIVILEGES; TIME SPENT OUT OF TEXAS DOES NOT COUNT TOWARD PROBATION; SHALL INFORM BOARD OF CHANGE OF ADDRESS WITHIN 10 DAYS OR IF HE LEAVES THE STATE. SHALL NOT SEEK MODIFICATION FOR ONE YEAR. ON 10/5/96 ORDER AMENDED AS FOLLOWS: HE MAY REAPPLY TO DEA AND TEXAS DEPARTMENT OF PUBLIC SAFETY FOR AUTHORITY TO PRESCRIBE SCHEDULES III, IV AND V; MUST MAINTAIN A COPY OF ALL SUCH PRESCRIPTIONS WRITTEN WHICH SHALL BE AVAILABLE FOR REVIEW. ON 9/20/97 THE BOARD GRANTED HIS PETITION FOR TERMINATION OF THIS ORDER BASED ON COMPLIANCE WITH CONDITIONS.

DAIL, ROBERT W MD OF CHATTANOOGA, TN, WAS DISCIPLINED BY TENNESSEE ON MARCH 1, 1995
DISCIPLINARY ACTION: 6-MONTH LICENSE SUSPENSION; 30-MONTH PROBATION
OFFENSE: DISCIPLINARY ACTION BY ANOTHER STATE OR AGENCY

NOTES: DISCIPLINARY ACTION TAKEN BY TEXAS. REMAINDER OF THREE YEAR SUSPENSION STAYED; MUST APPEAR BEFORE BOARD TWICE A YEAR DURING PROBATION; MUST EXECUTE A CONTRACT WITH THE IMPAIRED PHYSICIANS PROGRAM; A RANDOM SAMPLING OF HIS MEDICAL CHARTS AND BILLING RECORDS WILL BE REVIEWED SEMIANNUALLY BY THE MEDICAL DIRECTOR OF THE BOARD OF MEDICAL EXAMINERS.

DAIL, ROBERT W MD, WAS DISCIPLINED BY NEW MEXICO ON JULY 17, 1995
DISCIPLINARY ACTION: LICENSE REVOCATION
OFFENSE: NONCOMPLIANCE WITH A PROFESSIONAL RULE

NOTES: FAILURE TO REPORT ACTION BY ANOTHER BOARD.

DAIL, ROBERT WOOD MD, LICENSE NUMBER 00E3244 OF CHATTANOOGA, TN, WAS DISCIPLINED BY TEXAS ON APRIL 15, 1994
DISCIPLINARY ACTION: SURRENDER OF LICENSE
OFFENSE: PROFESSIONAL MISCONDUCT

NOTES: ALLEGATIONS CONCERNING ORDERING OF MULTIPLE MODALITIES FOR AUTO ACCIDENT PATIENTS; BOARD

FINDS THAT VARIOUS PATIENTS RECEIVED UNNECESSARY TREATMENT; PRACTICES IN TENNESSEE AND DOES NOT PLAN ON PRACTICING IN TEXAS. SHALL NOT SEEK REINSTATEMENT OF LICENSE.

DANG, JOHN TAI MD, LICENSE NUMBER J4068 OF CLEBURNE, TX, WAS DISCIPLINED BY TEXAS ON APRIL 4, 1998
DISCIPLINARY ACTION: FINE
OFFENSE: PROFESSIONAL MISCONDUCT

NOTES: IN OR ABOUT 4/97 ENGAGED IN INAPPROPRIATE VERBAL CONVERSATION WITH A PATIENT. $2,500 FINE.

DANKS, KELLY RICHARD MD, LICENSE NUMBER E0433 OF FAYETTEVILLE, AR, WAS DISCIPLINED BY ARKANSAS ON SEPTEMBER 12, 1997
DISCIPLINARY ACTION: EMERGENCY SUSPENSION

DANKS, KELLY RICHARD MD, LICENSE NUMBER E0433 OF SPRINGDALE, AR, WAS DISCIPLINED BY ARKANSAS ON DECEMBER 12, 1997
DISCIPLINARY ACTION: LICENSE REVOCATION

DANKS, KELLY RICHARD MD, LICENSE NUMBER E0433 OF SPRINGDALE, AR, WAS DISCIPLINED BY ARKANSAS ON FEBRUARY 6, 1998
DISCIPLINARY ACTION: LICENSE REINSTATEMENT; 60-MONTH PROBATION

NOTES: ON 2/3/00 PROBATION LIFTED.

DANKS, KELLY RICHARD MD, LICENSE NUMBER H7718 OF FAYETTEVILLE, AR, WAS DISCIPLINED BY TEXAS ON AUGUST 28, 1999
DISCIPLINARY ACTION: LICENSE SUSPENSION
OFFENSE: DISCIPLINARY ACTION BY ANOTHER STATE OR AGENCY

NOTES: ON 11/7/97 THE ARKANSAS BOARD SUSPENDED HIS LICENSE ON AN EMERGENCY BASIS DUE TO ALLEGATIONS THAT HE HAD INGESTED NITROUS OXIDE AND THAT HE SUFFERED FROM BIPOLAR II, AXIS I SUBSTANCE ABUSE; ON 2/21/98 ARKANSAS BOARD PLACED HIS LICENSE ON PROBATION; HE ADMITS HE WAS FOUND ABUSING NITROUS OXIDE IN 1998; HE STATES THAT HE WAS OUT OF THE PRACTICE OF MEDICINE FROM 5/97 TO 2/98; HE ALSO ADMITS TO ABUSING ALCOHOL, BEING DIAGNOSED AS HAVING AN AFFECTIVE DISORDER AS WELL AS SUBSTANCE ABUSE DISORDER, AND TAKING PROZAC AT THE RECOMMENDATION OF A COLLEAGUE. SUSPENSION WITH THE FOLLOWING TERMS AND CONDITIONS: SHALL NOT PRACTICE IN TEXAS UNTIL HE APPEARS BEFORE THE BOARD WITH EVIDENCE THAT HE IS PHYSICALLY, MENTALLY, AND OTHERWISE COMPETENT TO PRACTICE SAFELY INCLUDING EVIDENCE THAT HE HAS COMPLIED WITH THE ARKANSAS ORDER; SHALL INFORM THE BOARD OF CHANGE OF ADDRESS WITHIN 10 DAYS; SHALL NOT SEEK MODIFICATION FOR ONE YEAR.

DARBY, CASTILLA ADOLPHUS JR MD, LICENSE NUMBER 00F8840 OF GARLAND, TX, WAS DISCIPLINED BY TEXAS ON MARCH 4, 1994
DISCIPLINARY ACTION: EMERGENCY SUSPENSION
OFFENSE: SUBSTANCE ABUSE

NOTES: EVIDENCE AND INFORMATION INDICATE THAT BETWEEN 1/7/91 AND 12/30/93 HE WAS HOSPITALIZED FOR SEVERE PSYCHIATRIC DISORDERS AND POLYSUBSTANCE ABUSE RELATED TO HIS USE OF ALCOHOL, STREET DRUGS AND PRESCRIPTION MEDICATIONS AT LEAST SEVEN TIMES. EVIDENCE ALSO INDICATES HE HAS FAILED TO COMPLY WITH REQUIREMENTS FOR OUTPATIENT THERAPY, PARTICIPATION IN AA AND IMPAIRED PHYSICIANS GROUP ACTIVITIES; HAS A LONG HISTORY OF SUBSTANCE ABUSE AND PSYCHOTIC SYMPTOMS.

DARBY, CASTILLA ADOLPHUS JR MD, LICENSE NUMBER 00F8840 OF GARLAND, TX, WAS DISCIPLINED BY TEXAS ON APRIL 15, 1994
DISCIPLINARY ACTION: LICENSE SUSPENSION
OFFENSE: SUBSTANCE ABUSE

NOTES: ON 3/4/94 PLACED HIS LICENSE ON A TEMPORARY SUSPENSION DUE TO ADMITTED ALCOHOL ABUSE FOR APPROXIMATELY 20 YEARS AND PROBLEMS WITH BENZODIAZEPINES; HAS BEEN IN THERAPY SINCE 3/11/94; CLAIMS A SOBRIETY DATE FROM ALCOHOL OF 1/2/93 AND BENZODIAZEPINES FROM 11/26/93. SUSPENSION UNTIL HE APPEARS BEFORE THE BOARD AND PROVIDES SUFFICIENT EVIDENCE THAT HE IS PHYSICALLY, MENTALLY AND OTHERWISE COMPETENT TO SAFELY PRACTICE. SHALL NOT SEEK MODIFICATION FOR ONE YEAR.

DARBY, CASTILLA ADOLPHUS JR MD OF 1400 MARTIN LUTHER KING, DALLAS, TX, WAS DISCIPLINED BY DEA ON JUNE 3, 1994
DISCIPLINARY ACTION: SURRENDER OF CONTROLLED SUBSTANCE LICENSE
OFFENSE: DISCIPLINARY ACTION BY ANOTHER STATE OR AGENCY

NOTES: STATE BOARD.

DARBY, CASTILLA ADOLPHUS JR MD, LICENSE NUMBER 00F8840, WAS DISCIPLINED BY TEXAS ON JUNE 28, 1995
DISCIPLINARY ACTION: 120-MONTH PROBATION; RESTRICTION PLACED ON CONTROLLED SUBSTANCE LICENSE
OFFENSE: SUBSTANCE ABUSE

NOTES: HAS MADE AN ADEQUATE SHOWING THAT HE IS PHYSICALLY, MENTALLY AND OTHERWISE COMPETENT TO SAFELY PRACTICE. SUSPENSION IMPOSED BY THE 4/15/94 ORDER LIFTED. PROBATION UNDER TERMS AND CONDITIONS; SHALL ABSTAIN FROM THE CONSUMPTION OF ALCOHOL/DRUGS IN ANY FORM UNLESS PRESCRIBED BY ANOTHER PHYSICIAN FOR A LEGITIMATE AND THERAPEUTIC PURPOSE; SHALL SUBMIT HIMSELF FOR APPROPRIATE EXAMS INCLUDING DRUG OR ALCOHOL SCREENS; SHALL NOT TREAT OR OTHERWISE SERVE AS PHYSICIAN, PRESCRIBE, DISPENSE OR ADMINISTER DRUGS THAT MAY BE SUBJECT TO ABUSE TO HIMSELF OR TO ANY MEMBER OF HIS FAMILY; SHALL SURRENDER TO THE DEA HIS CONTROLLED SUBSTANCE REGISTRATION CERTIFICATE AND TEXAS DEPARTMENT OF CONTROLLED SUBSTANCES REGISTRATION CERTIFICATE; SHALL SURRENDER TO THE BOARD ALL UNUSED TRIPLICATE PRESCRIPTION FORMS AND SHALL NOT ATTEMPT TO ORDER MORE; SHALL SURRENDER ALL CONTROLLED SUBSTANCES, INCLUDING SAMPLES; SEPARATE FROM PATIENT RECORDS, SHALL MAINTAIN A FILE CONSISTING OF EVERY PRESCRIPTION WRITTEN BY HIM FOR DANGEROUS DRUGS WHICH HAVE POTENTIAL FOR ABUSE WHICH SHALL BE AVAILABLE FOR REVIEW; SHALL NOT TELEPHONE ANY PRESCRIPTION TO A PHARMACY FOR DANGEROUS DRUGS WHICH MAY BE HABIT FORMING; SHALL PARTICIPATE IN THE ACTIVITIES OF A PHYSICIAN HEALTH AND REHABILITATION COMMITTEE, AND ATTEND WEEKLY MEETINGS WITH QUARTERLY REPORTS; SHALL PARTICIPATE IN AA'S PROGRAM NOT LESS THAN

THREE TIMES A WEEK WITH QUARTERLY REPORTS; SHALL SUBMIT HIMSELF FOR EVALUATION AND TREATMENT BY A BOARD PSYCHIATRIST WHO HE SHALL SEE AT LEAST ONCE A MONTH AND SHALL FURNISH QUARTERLY REPORTS TO THE BOARD; SHALL ATTEND AT LEAST 50 HOURS PER YEAR OF CONTINUING MEDICAL EDUCATION AND SHALL SUBMIT PROOF TO THE BOARD; SHALL APPEAR BEFORE THE BOARD TWO TIMES A YEAR; SHALL GIVE A COPY OF THIS ORDER TO ANY HEALTH CARE ENTITY WHERE HE HAS PRIVILEGES; SHALL COOPERATE WITH THE BOARD IN VERIFYING COMPLIANCE; HIS PRACTICE, INCLUDING ANY MEDICAL OR SURGICAL PRACTICE SHALL BE MONITORED BY A BOARD APPROVED TEXAS PHYSICIAN WHO SHALL SUBMIT QUARTERLY REPORTS TO THE BOARD; TIME PERIOD OUT OF TEXAS DOES NOT COUNT TOWARD PROBATION; SHALL INFORM THE BOARD OF CHANGE OF ADDRESS WITHIN 10 DAYS OF IF HE LEAVES THE STATE; SHALL NOT SEEK MODIFICATION FOR ONE YEAR. ON 8/17/96 ORDER MODIFIED SO THAT HE MAY REAPPLY FOR DEA AND DPS PRIVILEGES TO PRESCRIBE SCHEDULE IV SUBSTANCES FOR WHICH HE WILL KEEP A SEPARATE LOG. ON 8/22/98 PETITION TO MODIFY ORDER GRANTED DELETING PRACTICE MONITOR REQUIREMENT. ON 10/15/99 ORDER MODIFIED TO REQUIRE ONE APPEARANCE PER YEAR BEFORE THE BOARD, AND TO ALLOW FOR MODIFICATION REQUESTS AT SIX MONTH INTERVALS.

DARBY, FRANK JOSEPH JR MD, LICENSE NUMBER 00D3195 OF PASADENA, TX, WAS DISCIPLINED BY TEXAS ON AUGUST 24, 1991
DISCIPLINARY ACTION: LICENSE REVOCATION
OFFENSE: PROFESSIONAL MISCONDUCT

NOTES: UNPROFESSIONAL AND DISHONORABLE CONDUCT LIKELY TO INJURE THE PUBLIC.

DAVIS, ANTHONY A MD, LICENSE NUMBER 00H2329 OF BAYTOWN, TX, WAS DISCIPLINED BY TEXAS ON SEPTEMBER 30, 1994
DISCIPLINARY ACTION: REPRIMAND; MONITORING OF PHYSICIAN PERFORMANCE
OFFENSE: PROFESSIONAL MISCONDUCT

NOTES: ADMITTED THAT MISCOMMUNICATION BETWEEN HIMSELF AND OFFICE STAFF RESULTED IN A PATIENT RECEIVING DUPLICATE PRESCRIPTIONS WHICH THE PATIENT USED IN A SUICIDE ATTEMPT; REPORTS THAT HE HAS NOW INSTITUTED RECORD KEEPING PROCEDURES IN ORDER TO AVOID FUTURE MISCOMMUNICATIONS. CONDITIONS OF ORDER; SHALL MAINTAIN ADEQUATE MEDICAL RECORDS ON ALL PATIENT OFFICE VISITS WHICH SHALL BE AVAILABLE FOR INSPECTION; SHALL ADEQUATELY SUPERVISE THE ACTIVITIES OF ALL EMPLOYEES; SHALL GIVE A COPY OF THIS ORDER TO ANY HEALTH CARE ENTITY WHERE HE HAS PRIVILEGES; SHALL COOPERATE WITH THE BOARD IN VERIFYING COMPLIANCE; SHALL INFORM BOARD OF CHANGE OF ADDRESS WITHIN 10 DAYS.

DAVIS, ANTHONY A MD OF 4201 GARTH ROAD #119, BAYTOWN, TX, WAS DISCIPLINED BY DEA ON APRIL 19, 1999
DISCIPLINARY ACTION: SURRENDER OF CONTROLLED SUBSTANCE LICENSE

NOTES: IN LIEU OF PUBLIC INTEREST REVOCATION.

DAVIS, ANTHONY A MD, LICENSE NUMBER H2329 OF BAYTOWN, TX, WAS DISCIPLINED BY TEXAS ON AUGUST 28, 1999
DISCIPLINARY ACTION: LICENSE SUSPENSION
OFFENSE: CRIMINAL CONVICTION OR PLEA OF GUILTY, NOLO CONTENDERE, OR NO CONTEST TO A CRIME

NOTES: ON 1/28/99 PLED GUILTY TO DELIVERY OF A PRESCRIPTION FORM FOR OTHER THAN A VALID MEDICAL PURPOSE, A FELONY; ON 8/19/98 HE WAS ADMITTED TO A HOSPITAL FOR SUBSTANCE ABUSE AND DEPRESSION; HE WAS DISCHARGED ON 8/22/98 WHEN HE WAS TAKEN INTO CUSTODY BY LAW ENFORCEMENT; HIS FINAL DIAGNOSIS WAS MAJOR DEPRESSIVE AFFECTIVE DISORDER, BARBITURATE/SEDATIVE/HYPNOTIC DEPENDENCE, OPIOID TYPE DEPENDENCE, AND DRUG WITHDRAWAL SYNDROME; ON 8/14/98 HIS PRIVILEGES WERE SUSPENDED AT BAYCOAST MEDICAL CENTER AS HE HAD NOT COMPLIED WITH THE TERMS OF HIS TREATMENT PROGRAM AND THAT HE CHECKED INTO THE HOSPITAL; THIS WAS A DIRECT VIOLATION OF THE CONDITIONS OF THE RE-INSTATEMENT OF HIS PRIVILEGES IN 12/97, WHEN HIS PRIVILEGES WERE SUSPENDED FOR SIMILAR INCIDENTS. SUSPENSION UNTIL HE REQUESTS TO HAVE THE SUSPENSION STAYED OR APPEARS BEFORE THE BOARD WITH EVIDENCE THAT HE IS PHYSICALLY, MENTALLY OR OTHERWISE COMPETENT TO PRACTICE SAFELY INCLUDING AT A MINIMUM: COMPLETE COPIES OF MEDICAL RECORDS AND REPORTS OF PSYCHOLOGICAL AND NEUROPSYCHIATRIC EVALUATIONS; A COPY OF THIS ORDER SHALL BE PROVIDED BY HIM TO THE APPROVED PSYCHIATRIST AS A REFERENCE FOR THE EVALUATION, AND AS AUTHORIZATION FOR THE PSYCHIATRIST TO PROVIDE TO THE BOARD ANY AND ALL RECORDS AND REPORTS; TIME SPENT OUT OF TEXAS DOES NOT COUNT TOWARD RESTRICTION; SHALL INFORM THE BOARD OF CHANGE OF ADDRESS WITHIN 10 DAYS OR IF HE LEAVES THE STATE; SHALL NOT SEEK MODIFICATION FOR ONE YEAR.

DAVIS, CARL C JR MD, LICENSE NUMBER E9598 OF BAYTOWN, TX, WAS DISCIPLINED BY TEXAS ON AUGUST 28, 1999
DISCIPLINARY ACTION: 60-MONTH PROBATION; RESTRICTION PLACED ON LICENSE
OFFENSE: LOSS OR RESTRICTION OF HOSPITAL PRIVILEGES

NOTES: ON 8/27/97 HIS PRIVILEGES WERE REVOKED AT A HOSPITAL BASED ON HIS FAILURE TO MEET THE BASIC QUALIFICATIONS, STANDARDS, REQUIREMENTS, AND RESPONSIBILITIES REQUIRED FOR CLINICAL PRIVILEGES AND MEDICAL STAFF MEMBERSHIP; HE DID NOT INFORM THE BOARD OF HIS REVOCATION OF PRIVILEGES ON HIS ANNUAL RENEWAL FORM. IN THREE CASES THERE WERE INDICATIONS OF SUBSTANDARD CARE: IN THE FIRST CASE HE DID NOT ADDRESS A PATHOLOGY OR THE DISCREPANCY BETWEEN THE PATHOLOGY AND HIS IMPRESSION WHICH REPRESENTED SLOPPY RECORD KEEPING AND MOST LIKELY POOR CARE OF THE PATIENT; IN THE SECOND CASE THE PATIENT'S TREATMENT WAS POORLY MANAGED AND APPEARED TO BE BELOW THE STANDARD OF CARE IN THAT THE PATIENT APPEARED TO BE WELL CONTROLLED ON MEDICATIONS AND DID NOT NEED THE SURGERY HE PERFORMED AND WHEN HE PERFORMED A THYROID LOBECTOMY WHICH MAY NOT HAVE BEEN NECESSARY HE USED IODINE PREOPERATIVELY WHICH IS NOT ROUTINE; IN THE THIRD CASE HE INADEQUATELY MANAGED A PATIENT FOR SEPSIS AND A TOE INFECTION WHICH LED TO HER DEATH. SUSPENSION STAYED WITH THE FOLLOWING TERMS AND CONDITIONS: SHALL OBTAIN 50 HOURS PER YEAR FOR CONTINUING MEDICAL EDUCATION WITH 50 HOURS IN SURGERY; BEGINNING NO LATER THAN 60 DAYS, HIS MEDICAL PRACTICE SHALL BE MONITORED BY A BOARD APPROVED TEXAS PHYSICIAN WHO SHALL PROVIDE QUARTERLY REPORTS TO THE

BOARD; SHALL MAINTAIN ADEQUATE MEDICAL RECORDS WHICH SHALL BE AVAILABLE FOR REVIEW; SHALL NOMINATE THREE CERTIFIED PSYCHIATRISTS FOR BOARD SELECTION OF A THERAPIST AND SHALL EXPEDITIOUSLY SUBMIT HIMSELF TO EVALUATION AND TREATMENT BY THE APPROVED PRACTITIONER; SHALL OBTAIN AT LEAST ONE BOARD- APPROVED COURSE IN INTERPERSONAL SKILLS WITHIN 1 YEAR; SHALL NOT ENGAGE IN THE PRACTICE OF INPATIENT HOSPITAL SURGERIES FOR A MINIMUM OF 6 MONTHS; SHALL APPEAR BEFORE THE BOARD UPON REQUEST; SHALL COOPERATE WITH THE BOARD IN VERIFYING COMPLIANCE; TIME SPENT OUT OF TEXAS DOES NOT COUNT TOWARD PROBATION; SHALL INFORM THE BOARD OF CHANGE OF ADDRESS WITHIN 10 DAYS OR IF HE LEAVES THE STATE; SHALL NOT SEEK MODIFICATION FOR ONE YEAR.

DAVIS, DAVID W DO OF HOUSTON, TX, WAS DISCIPLINED BY DEA ON OCTOBER 2, 1995
DISCIPLINARY ACTION: REVOCATION OF CONTROLLED SUBSTANCE LICENSE
OFFENSE: OVERPRESCRIBING OR MISPRESCRIBING DRUGS

NOTES: ON 4/23/92, HE PLED NOLO CONTENDERE TO ONE COUNT OF PRESCRIBING A SCHEDULE III CONTROLLED SUBSTANCE (TYLENOL 4) TO AN UNDERCOVER OFFICER WITHOUT A VALID MEDICAL PURPOSE. PRESCRIBED CONTROLLED SUBSTANCES TO AN UNDERCOVER OFFICER ON THREE SEPARATE OCCASIONS, BETWEEN 5/91 - 7/91 WITHOUT A VALID MEDICAL PURPOSE.

DAVIS, HERBERT ALLEN MD, DATE OF BIRTH FEBRUARY 7, 1940, LICENSE NUMBER 0021196 OF TYLER, TX, WAS DISCIPLINED BY COLORADO ON SEPTEMBER 17, 1993
DISCIPLINARY ACTION: SURRENDER OF LICENSE
OFFENSE: SUBSTANDARD CARE, INCOMPETENCE OR NEGLIGENCE

NOTES: ALLEGATIONS OF SUBSTANDARD PATIENT CARE.

DAVIS, HERBERT ALLEN MD, DATE OF BIRTH FEBRUARY 7, 1940, LICENSE NUMBER 00D2408 OF TYLER, TX, WAS DISCIPLINED BY TEXAS ON AUGUST 19, 1994
DISCIPLINARY ACTION: REPRIMAND
OFFENSE: DISCIPLINARY ACTION BY ANOTHER STATE OR AGENCY

NOTES: ON 8/4/93 HE VOLUNTARILY SURRENDERED COLORADO LICENSE IN LIEU OF FURTHER PROCEEDINGS. HE TREATED A PATIENT BETWEEN 1985 AND 1988 AND TOWARDS THE END OF TREATMENT A SOCIAL AND LATER SEXUAL RELATIONSHIP DEVELOPED; HE CLAIMED THE SEXUAL RELATIONSHIP OCCURRED AFTER TERMINATION OF TREATMENT; HE UNDERSTANDS THE RELATIONSHIP WAS NON-THERAPEUTIC AND DETRIMENTAL TO THE PATIENT. NO OTHER COMPLAINTS ABOUT HIS PRACTICE IN TEXAS HAVE BEEN RECEIVED. SHALL SUBMIT TO A FULL EXAMINATION FOR SEXUAL DISORDERS/ADDICTION WITHIN 30 DAYS; SHALL GIVE A COPY OF THIS ORDER TO ANY HEALTH CARE ENTITY WHERE HE HAS PRIVILEGES; SHALL COOPERATE WITH THE BOARD IN VERIFYING COMPLIANCE. SHALL NOT SEEK MODIFICATION FOR ONE YEAR. THE BOARD RESERVES THE RIGHT TO SEEK OR IMPOSE ADDITIONAL DISCIPLINARY ACTION SHOULD AN UNFAVORABLE REPORT BE RECEIVED FROM THE AFOREMENTIONED EXAMINATION.

DAVIS, HERBERT ALLEN MD, DATE OF BIRTH FEBRUARY 7, 1940, LICENSE NUMBER 00D2408 OF 2323 W FRONT STREET, TYLER, TX, WAS DISCIPLINED BY TEXAS ON MARCH 4, 1995
DISCIPLINARY ACTION: RESTRICTION PLACED ON LICENSE; REQUIRED TO TAKE ADDITIONAL MEDICAL EDUCATION

NOTES: ON 11/7/94 BOARD RECEIVED REPORT ORDERED BY 8/19/94 AGREEMENT IN WHICH THE EVALUATOR STATED THAT DR. DAVIS WAS NOT IMPAIRED OR POTENTIALLY IMPAIRED IN HIS PRACTICE OF PSYCHIATRY, ALTHOUGH HE REMAINS VULNERABLE TO BOUNDARY VIOLATIONS AND ROLE BLURRING DUE TO LIMITED INSIGHT TO ENGAGE IN AND COMMIT TO THERAPEUTIC PROCESS; HE IS COMMITTED TO THE THERAPEUTIC PROCESS; THE EVALUATOR SUPPORTED CONTINUED EMPLOYMENT IN HIS CURRENT POSITION WITH APPROPRIATE SAFEGUARDS AND CONTINUED MEDICAL EDUCATION. SHALL NOT ENGAGE IN THE PRACTICE OF PSYCHOTHERAPY UNLESS APPROVED IN ADVANCE BY HIS THERAPIST; SHALL LIMIT HIS PRACTICE TO CRISIS INTERVENTION, MEDICATION MANAGEMENT, AND GROUP WORK WITH A CO-FACILITATOR PRESENT; SHALL SEE PATIENTS IN HIS OFFICE ALONE ONLY FOR BRIEF VISITS AND INITIAL EVALUATIONS WITH OFFICE DOOR OPEN AND OTHERS AT HIS WORKPLACE; SHALL USE A NURSE CHAPERONE IN ALL SITUATIONS WHERE A RISK OF MISINTERPRETATION EXISTS AND THIS WILL BE MARKED ON MEDICAL RECORDS; PRACTICE SHALL BE SUPERVISED BY A BOARD APPROVED MONITOR WHO SHALL HAVE RANDOM ACCESS TO HIS RECORDS AND PROVIDE QUARTERLY REPORTS; SHALL HAVE A BOARD APPROVED EXPERT REVIEW HIS THERAPEUTIC PROCESS; SHALL OBTAIN AT LEAST 30 HOURS PER YEAR OF CONTINUING MEDICAL EDUCATION, INCLUDING AT LEAST ONE COURSE IN MEDICAL ETHICS, SEXUAL ABUSE, OR TRANSFERENCE/COUNTERTRANSFERENCE/PROFESSIONAL BOUNDARIES PER YEAR; CONDITIONS SHALL REMAIN IN EFFECT FOR TWO YEARS; HE HAS A RIGHT TO PETITION FOR MODIFICATION YEARLY. ON 5/15/96 BOARD DENIED A REQUEST TO TERMINATE THIS ORDER. EFFECTIVE 3/4/97 THIS ORDER EXPIRED.

DE LOS SANTOS, RAMIRO MD, LICENSE NUMBER 00F5182 OF EAGLE PASS, TX, WAS DISCIPLINED BY TEXAS ON OCTOBER 1, 1993
DISCIPLINARY ACTION: 60-MONTH PROBATION; REQUIRED TO TAKE ADDITIONAL MEDICAL EDUCATION
OFFENSE: SUBSTANDARD CARE, INCOMPETENCE OR NEGLIGENCE

NOTES: FROM 3/10/89 THROUGH 6/30/89 PERFORMED REPEAT C-SECTIONS ON THREE PATIENTS WITHOUT MEDICAL INDICATIONS; EVEN THOUGH SONOGRAMS WERE NORMAL AND THERE WAS NO EVIDENCE OF FETAL DISTRESS, THE BABIES WERE DELIVERED AT 37 WEEKS GESTATION; ON 4/27/89 HE FAILED TO ADEQUATELY TREAT A PATIENT IN THE EMERGENCY ROOM AND PREMATURELY DISCHARGED HER PRIOR TO STABILIZING HER BLOOD PRESSURE; ON 8/5/89 HE PERFORMED AN ABORTION ON ONE PATIENT AND KNOWINGLY DISCHARGED HER WITH FETAL TISSUE REMAINING IN THE UTERUS; FROM 3/10/89 THROUGH 8/5/89 HE FAILED TO ACCURATELY DOCUMENT PATIENT MEDICAL RECORDS. SUSPENSION STAYED. CONDITIONS OF PROBATION: SHALL ATTEND AT LEAST 50 HOURS PER YEAR OF CONTINUING MEDICAL EDUCATION 60 PERCENT OF WHICH SHALL BE IN BOARD-APPROVED COURSES ON OBSTETRICS AND HIGH-RISK PREGNANCY; SHALL MAINTAIN ADEQUATE PATIENT MEDICAL RECORDS WHICH WILL BE MADE AVAILABLE FOR REVIEW; SHALL APPEAR BEFORE THE BOARD ONCE A YEAR; SHALL COOPERATE WITH THE BOARD IN VERIFYING COMPLIANCE; SHALL INFORM BOARD OF CHANGE OF ADDRESS WITHIN 10 DAYS OR IF HE LEAVES THE STATE; TIME SPENT OUT OF TEXAS DOES NOT COUNT TOWARD PROBATION. SHALL NOT SEEK MODIFICATION FOR ONE YEAR.

DE QUEVEDO, ANA J GARCIA MD, DATE OF BIRTH SEPTEMBER 13, 1945 OF 2151 S KIRKWOOD ROAD #256, HOUSTON, TX, WAS DISCIPLINED BY MEDICARE ON OCTOBER 10, 1994
DISCIPLINARY ACTION: EXCLUSION FROM THE MEDICARE AND/OR MEDICAID PROGRAM
OFFENSE: DISCIPLINARY ACTION BY ANOTHER STATE OR AGENCY

NOTES: LICENSE REVOKED FOR REASONS BEARING ON PROFESSIONAL COMPETENCE.

DECARVALHO, GUARACY F MD, LICENSE NUMBER 00E3677 OF GEORGE WEST, TX, WAS DISCIPLINED BY TEXAS ON DECEMBER 1, 1990
DISCIPLINARY ACTION: 60-MONTH PROBATION; RESTRICTION PLACED ON LICENSE
OFFENSE: LOSS OR RESTRICTION OF HOSPITAL PRIVILEGES

NOTES: UNPROFESSIONAL CONDUCT LIKELY TO DECEIVE, DEFRAUD, OR INJURE PUBLIC. DISCIPLINED BY HOSPITAL OR HOSPITAL MEDICAL STAFF INCLUDING REMOVAL, SUSPENSION OR LIMITATION OF HOSPITAL PRIVILEGES OR OTHER DISCIPLINARY ACTIONS. FAILURE TO PRACTICE MEDICINE IN ACCEPTABLE MANNER CONSISTENT WITH PUBLIC HEALTH AND WELFARE. SUSPENSION STAYED. PROBATIONARY CONDITIONS INCLUDE CHANGE IN OBSTETRICAL PRACTICE, COMPLETION OF CONTINUING MEDICAL EDUCATION, REQUIREMENT FOR FEMALE STAFF MEMBER OR CHAPERONE DURING CERTAIN EXAMINATIONS AND/OR TREATMENTS.

DELAFLOR, RICARDO MD, DATE OF BIRTH MARCH 30, 1908, LICENSE NUMBER 0021641 OF 423 SAN SABA, EL PASO, TX, WAS DISCIPLINED BY NEW JERSEY ON MAY 5, 1990
DISCIPLINARY ACTION: SURRENDER OF LICENSE
OFFENSE: DISCIPLINARY ACTION BY ANOTHER STATE OR AGENCY

NOTES: DISCIPLINED IN TEXAS DUE TO QUESTIONABLE CONTROLLED SUBSTANCE PRESCRIBING.

DELGADILLO, FRANCISCO PEDRO MD, LICENSE NUMBER E0233 OF HOUSTON, TX, WAS DISCIPLINED BY TEXAS ON OCTOBER 24, 1998
DISCIPLINARY ACTION: REQUIRED TO TAKE ADDITIONAL MEDICAL EDUCATION; MONITORING OF PHYSICIAN PERFORMANCE
OFFENSE: SUBSTANDARD CARE, INCOMPETENCE OR NEGLIGENCE

NOTES: FROM 1993 - 1994 HE DID NOT MAINTAIN ADEQUATE MEDICAL RECORDS ON TWO PATIENTS AND DID NOT ADEQUATELY DOCUMENT THE BASIS FOR CARE RENDERED AND MEDICATIONS PRESCRIBED; ALSO PROVIDED MEDICATIONS TO TWO PATIENTS WITHOUT MEDICAL INDICATIONS. LICENSE LIMITED FOR FIVE YEARS AS FOLLOWS: SHALL MAINTAIN ADEQUATE MEDICAL RECORDS WHICH SHALL BE AVAILABLE FOR REVIEW; SEPARATE FROM PATIENT RECORDS, SHALL MAINTAIN A LOGBOOK OF EVERY PRESCRIPTION WRITTEN BY HIM FOR DANGEROUS DRUGS WITH ADDICTIVE POTENTIAL AND ALL INJECTIONS EXCEPT VACCINATIONS; WHICH SHALL BE MADE AVAILABLE FOR REVIEW; SHALL OBTAIN 50 HOURS PER YEAR OF CONTINUING MEDICAL EDUCATION; IN ADDITION, SHALL OBTAIN 1 COURSE IN RISK MANAGEMENT PER YEAR; SHALL APPEAR BEFORE THE BOARD UPON REQUEST; SHALL COOPERATE WITH THE BOARD IN VERIFYING COMPLIANCE INCLUDING PROVIDING COPIES OF PEER REVIEW RECORDS UPON REQUEST; SHALL GIVE A COPY OF THIS ORDER TO ANY HEALTH CARE ENTITY WHERE HE HAS PRIVILEGES; SHALL PROVIDE A COPY OF THIS ORDER TO ANYONE REQUESTING IT WITHIN 10 DAYS; TIME SPENT OUT OF TEXAS DOES NOT COUNT TOWARD RESTRICTION; SHALL INFORM THE BOARD OF CHANGE OF ADDRESS WITHIN 10 DAYS OR IF HE LEAVES THE STATE; SHALL NOT SEEK MODIFICATION FOR ONE YEAR.

DELGADO, VICTOR MANUEL MD OF 1602 LORRAINE, HOUSTON, TX, WAS DISCIPLINED BY DEA ON JULY 5, 1990
DISCIPLINARY ACTION: RESTRICTION PLACED ON CONTROLLED SUBSTANCE LICENSE
OFFENSE: OVERPRESCRIBING OR MISPRESCRIBING DRUGS

NOTES: PURSUANT TO AN AGREEMENT WITH THE TEXAS MEDICAL BOARD, DR. DELGADO SURRENDERED SCHEDULES II AND IIN OF HIS DEA REGISTRATION, BASED ON AN APPEARANCE BEFORE THE BOARD ON 10/28/85 TO DISCUSS HIS ALLEGED NONTHERAPEUTIC PRESCRIBING OF CONTROLLED SUBSTANCES. THE AGREEMENT WITH THE BOARD INCLUDES THE FOLLOWING STIPULATIONS: MUST SURRENDER ALL UNUSED TRIPLICATE PRESCRIPTIONS; SHALL REFRAIN FROM TREATING ANY PATIENTS FOR WEIGHT CONTROL WITH CONTROLLED SUBSTANCES; SHALL NOT PETITION THE TEXAS STATE BOARD OF MEDICAL EXAMINERS FOR MODIFICATION OF THE AGREEMENT FOR ONE YEAR; THE AGREEMENT WILL BE IN EFFECT FOR FIVE YEARS.

DELL, ROBERT V MD, LICENSE NUMBER 0009654 OF SAN ANTONIO, TX, WAS DISCIPLINED BY SOUTH CAROLINA ON OCTOBER 31, 1990
DISCIPLINARY ACTION: SURRENDER OF LICENSE

NOTES: VOLUNTARY SURRENDER; NOT ELIGIBLE FOR REINSTATEMENT

DELL, ROBERT V MD OF POPLAR BLUFF, MO, WAS DISCIPLINED BY MISSOURI ON NOVEMBER 6, 1990
DISCIPLINARY ACTION: 24-MONTH LICENSE SUSPENSION; 60-MONTH PROBATION
OFFENSE: DISCIPLINARY ACTION BY ANOTHER STATE OR AGENCY

NOTES: DISCIPLINARY ACTION TAKEN IN KANSAS BASED ON PERSONAL IMPAIRMENT. TWO YEAR SUSPENSION RETROACTIVE TO 9/15/88.

DELL, ROBERT V MD OF HANNIBAL, MO, WAS DISCIPLINED BY MISSOURI ON JUNE 16, 1993
DISCIPLINARY ACTION: 84-MONTH PROBATION
OFFENSE: FAILURE TO COMPLY WITH PREVIOUS BOARD ORDER

NOTES: ALSO DRUG USE, SUBSTANDARD CARE, LIMITATION OF CONTROLLED SUBSTANCE AUTHORITY.

DEMETRI, LESLIE R SR MD, LICENSE NUMBER D9417 OF DALLAS, TX, WAS DISCIPLINED BY TEXAS ON AUGUST 9, 1997
DISCIPLINARY ACTION: REQUIRED TO TAKE ADDITIONAL MEDICAL EDUCATION; MONITORING OF PHYSICIAN PERFORMANCE
OFFENSE: PROFESSIONAL MISCONDUCT

NOTES: OVER THE COURSE OF SEVERAL YEARS, AND AS RECENTLY AS 1995, HE PROVIDED VARIOUS PATIENTS WITH CONTROLLED SUBSTANCES AND DANGEROUS POTENTIALLY ADDICTIVE DRUGS FOR PAIN TREATMENT; HE DID NOT ADEQUATELY DOCUMENT RELATED TREATMENT PLANS AND FOLLOW-UP ASSESSMENTS; DURING 1996 HE DID NOT ADEQUATELY STORE AND SECURE CONTROLLED SUBSTANCES AT HIS OFFICE AND DID NOT ADEQUATELY DOCUMENT PURCHASES OF CONTROLLED SUBSTANCES AND DISPOSAL OF SUCH DRUGS; HE HAS REPORTED THE IMPLEMENTATION OF REMEDIAL MEASURES TO ADDRESS THE DEFICIENCIES REFLECTED ABOVE. LICENSE LIMITED FOR FIVE YEARS AS FOLLOWS: SHALL OBTAIN AT LEAST 75 HOURS PER YEAR OF CONTINUING MEDICAL EDUCATION WITH AN ADDITIONAL 25 HOURS PER YEAR IN PAIN MANAGEMENT; SHALL MAINTAIN

ADEQUATE MEDICAL RECORDS WHICH SHALL BE AVAILABLE FOR REVIEW; SEPARATE FROM PATIENT RECORDS, SHALL MAINTAIN A LOGBOOK OF EVERY PRESCRIPTION WRITTEN OR TELEPHONED BY HIM FOR DANGEROUS DRUGS WITH ADDICTIVE POTENTIAL WHICH SHALL BE MADE AVAILABLE FOR REVIEW; SHALL APPEAR BEFORE THE BOARD UPON REQUEST; SHALL COOPERATE WITH THE BOARD IN VERIFYING COMPLIANCE INCLUDING PROVIDING COPIES OF MEDICAL RELEASES AND PEER REVIEW RECORDS UPON REQUEST; SHALL GIVE A COPY OF THIS ORDER TO ANY HEALTH CARE ENTITY WHERE HE HAS PRIVILEGES; SHALL PROVIDE A COPY OF THIS ORDER TO ANYONE REQUESTING IT WITHIN 10 DAYS; TIME SPENT OUT OF TEXAS DOES NOT COUNT TOWARD RESTRICTION; SHALL INFORM THE BOARD OF CHANGE OF ADDRESS WITHIN 10 DAYS OR IF HE LEAVES THE STATE; SHALL NOT SEEK MODIFICATION FOR ONE YEAR. ON 10/15/99 THE ORDER WAS MODIFIED BY DELETING THE ANNUAL PERSONAL APPEARANCES BEFORE THE BOARD REQUIREMENT.

DENNIS, MICHAEL H MD, LICENSE NUMBER 00G0612 OF TAYLOR, TX, WAS DISCIPLINED BY TEXAS ON JUNE 10, 1991
DISCIPLINARY ACTION: 60-MONTH PROBATION; MONITORING OF PHYSICIAN PERFORMANCE

NOTES: PROFESSIONAL FAILURE TO PRACTICE MEDICINE IN AN ACCEPTABLE MANNER CONSISTENT WITH PUBLIC HEALTH AND WELFARE. SHALL APPEAR BEFORE BOARD ONCE A YEAR; SHALL PARTICIPATE IN AA; SHALL HAVE A RECOVERING ABUSE SPONSOR; SHALL SUBMIT TO DRUG OR ALCOHOL SCREENS.

DENNIS, MICHAEL H MD, LICENSE NUMBER 00G0612 OF TAYLOR, TX, WAS DISCIPLINED BY TEXAS ON MARCH 6, 1992
DISCIPLINARY ACTION: 60-MONTH PROBATION

NOTES: PROFESSIONAL FAILURE TO PRACTICE MEDICINE IN AN ACCEPTABLE MANNER CONSISTENT WITH PUBLIC HEALTH AND WELFARE. LICENSE SUSPENDED, SUSPENSION STAYED; PROBATION UNDER TERMS AND CONDITIONS.

DENNIS, MICHAEL H MD, LICENSE NUMBER 00G0612 OF TAYLOR, TX, WAS DISCIPLINED BY TEXAS ON APRIL 29, 1992
DISCIPLINARY ACTION: EMERGENCY SUSPENSION

DENNIS, MICHAEL H MD, LICENSE NUMBER 00G0612 OF TAYLOR, TX, WAS DISCIPLINED BY TEXAS ON JUNE 17, 1992
DISCIPLINARY ACTION: SURRENDER OF LICENSE
OFFENSE: FAILURE TO COMPLY WITH PREVIOUS BOARD ORDER

NOTES: IN LIEU OF FURTHER DISCIPLINARY ACTION DUE TO VIOLATION OF PREVIOUS BOARD ORDER.

DESHEFY, ALAN N MD, LICENSE NUMBER 00G6163 OF FORT WORTH, TX, WAS DISCIPLINED BY TEXAS ON JULY 1, 1990
DISCIPLINARY ACTION: EMERGENCY SUSPENSION
OFFENSE: SUBSTANDARD CARE, INCOMPETENCE OR NEGLIGENCE

NOTES: DISCIPLINED BY HOSPITAL MEDICAL STAFFS FOR UNPROFESSIONAL CONDUCT OR PROFESSIONAL INCOMPETENCE LIKELY TO HARM PUBLIC. SHALL SUBMIT TO EXAMINATION TO DETERMINE IF HE IS UNABLE TO PRACTICE MEDICINE WITH REASONABLE SKILL AND SAFETY AND PENDING BOARD ACTION ON REPORT, LICENSE SHALL BE SUSPENDED.

DESHEFY, ALAN N MD OF 2823 NW 29TH ST, FORT WORTH, TX, WAS DISCIPLINED BY DEA ON AUGUST 16, 1990
DISCIPLINARY ACTION: SURRENDER OF CONTROLLED SUBSTANCE LICENSE

NOTES: MEDICAL LICENSE SUSPENDED 03/31/90.

DESHEFY, ALAN N MD, DATE OF BIRTH JANUARY 4, 1954 OF 6006 NW 70 AVE, TAMARAC, FL, WAS DISCIPLINED BY MEDICARE ON APRIL 10, 1992
DISCIPLINARY ACTION: EXCLUSION FROM THE MEDICARE AND/OR MEDICAID PROGRAM
OFFENSE: DISCIPLINARY ACTION BY ANOTHER STATE OR AGENCY

NOTES: LICENSE REVOCATION OR SUSPENSION.

DESHEFY, ALAN N MD, LICENSE NUMBER 00G6163 OF FORT WORTH, TX, WAS DISCIPLINED BY TEXAS ON MARCH 3, 1995
DISCIPLINARY ACTION: 60-MONTH PROBATION; RESTRICTION PLACED ON LICENSE

NOTES: HAS SATISFIED MINIMUM REQUIREMENTS SET OUT IN 4/20/90 ORDER. SUSPENSION STAYED. PROBATION WITH TERMS: PRIOR TO PRACTICING MEDICINE IN TEXAS AND WITHIN ONE YEAR OF ORDER, SHALL TAKE AND PASS THE SPECIAL PURPOSE EXAMINATION; SHALL NOT ENGAGE IN ANY HOSPITAL SURGERIES EXCEPT IN THE CAPACITY OF AN ASSISTANT; SHALL UNDERGO EVALUATION AND TREATMENT WITH A BOARD-APPROVED PSYCHIATRIST, WHOM HE SHALL SEE AT LEAST ONCE A MONTH FOR FOLLOW-UP CARE AND COUNSELING AND WHO SHALL SUBMIT REPORTS TO THE BOARD; HIS PRACTICE SHALL BE MONITORED BY A BOARD-APPROVED PHYSICIAN WHO SHALL PROVIDE QUARTERLY REPORTS TO THE BOARD; SHALL OBTAIN AT LEAST 50 HOURS OF CONTINUING MEDICAL EDUCATION EACH YEAR; SHALL APPEAR BEFORE THE BOARD AT LEAST ONCE EACH YEAR; SHALL COOPERATE WITH THE BOARD IN VERIFYING COMPLIANCE INCLUDING PROVIDING COPIES OF MEDICAL RELEASES UPON REQUEST; TIME PERIOD OUT OF TEXAS DOES NOT COUNT TOWARD PROBATION; SHALL NOT SEEK MODIFICATION FOR ONE YEAR.

DESHEFY, ALAN NICHOLAS MD OF CORAL SPRINGS, FL, WAS DISCIPLINED BY CALIFORNIA ON APRIL 5, 1999
DISCIPLINARY ACTION: DENIAL OF NEW LICENSE
OFFENSE: DISCIPLINARY ACTION BY ANOTHER STATE OR AGENCY

NOTES: TEXAS BOARD SUSPENDED HIS LICENSE ON 3/18/96.

DHESI, TARSEM S MD, LICENSE NUMBER 00F6575 OF HOUSTON, TX, WAS DISCIPLINED BY TEXAS ON JANUARY 6, 1995
DISCIPLINARY ACTION: FINE
OFFENSE: PROFESSIONAL MISCONDUCT

NOTES: DURING 1992 AND 1993 FAILED TO ADEQUATELY OVERSEE THE BILLING FOR PATIENT CARE RENDERED THROUGH PHYSICAL THERAPY CLINICS OWNED IN PART BY HIM AND FOR WHICH HE WAS A MEDICAL DIRECTOR WHICH RESULTED IN BILLING WHICH DID NOT ACCURATELY REFLECT THE HEALTH-CARE PROVIDER WHO RENDERED THE SERVICE; USED IN-HOUSE BILLING AND MANAGEMENT; REPORTS HE HAS SOLD THE CLINICS DUE TO THE DIFFICULTY INVOLVED WITH KEEPING UP WITH THE WORKLOAD; IN LIEU OF FURTHER INVESTIGATION AGREES TO THIS ORDER. $1,000 ADMINISTRATIVE PENALTY TO BE PAID WITHIN FOUR MONTHS.

DIAZ, GUSTAVO A MD, LICENSE NUMBER 0026064 OF GOLIAD, TX, WAS DISCIPLINED BY FLORIDA ON FEBRUARY 18, 1991
DISCIPLINARY ACTION: REQUIRED TO TAKE ADDITIONAL MEDICAL EDUCATION

OFFENSE: PROVIDING FALSE INFORMATION TO THE BOARD OR OTHER HEALTH AGENCY

NOTES: CHARGED WITH RENEWING A LICENSE BY FRAUDULENT MISREPRESENTATIONS IN THAT HE FALSELY CERTIFIED THAT HE COMPLETED THE CONTINUING MEDICAL EDUCATION REQUIREMENTS FOR LICENSURE RENEWAL; VIOLATED A BOARD RULE IN THAT HE FAILED TO SUBMIT DOCUMENTATION VERIFYING CONTINUING MEDICAL EDUCATION IN RESPONSE TO THE BOARD'S RANDOM AUDIT. IN LIEU OF FURTHER PROSECUTION, HE MUST PAY $1000 ADMINISTRATIVE COST AND APPEAR BEFORE THE BOARD AND DEMONSTRATE COMPLETION OF ALL CONTINUING MEDICAL EDUCATION REQUIREMENTS; MUST ALSO COMPLETE FIVE HOURS OF CONTINUING MEDICAL EDUCATION IN RISK MANAGEMENT WITHIN 180 DAYS OF 02/18/91; ATTACH TO SUBSEQUENT LICENSE RENEWAL APPLICATIONS DOCUMENTATION OF COMPLETION OF THE CONTINUING MEDICAL EDUCATION REQUIREMENTS.

DIAZ, J JESUS MD, LICENSE NUMBER 00E0882 OF HOUSTON, TX, WAS DISCIPLINED BY TEXAS ON OCTOBER 13, 1995
DISCIPLINARY ACTION: 60-MONTH PROBATION; FINE
OFFENSE: PROFESSIONAL MISCONDUCT

NOTES: DURING 1993 HE ALLOWED AN INDIVIDUAL NOT LICENSED TO PRACTICE MEDICINE IN TEXAS TO WORK IN HIS OFFICE AS A SURGICAL ASSISTANT; WHILE IN HIS OFFICE, THE INDIVIDUAL DIAGNOSED, TREATED AND PRESCRIBED FOR PATIENTS; DURING PHYSICIAN'S ABSENCE FROM HIS OFFICE FOR A VACATION OUT OF THE COUNTRY IN 12/93, UNLICENSED INDIVIDUAL ENGAGED IN THE CARE AND TREATMENT OF PATIENTS INCLUDING THE PRESCRIBING OF MEDICATIONS; DURING 1993, HE ALLOWED UNLICENSED INDIVIDUALS TO USE A SIGNATURE STAMP BEARING HIS NAME. SUSPENSION STAYED. PROBATION WITH TERMS: SHALL ADEQUATELY SUPERVISE THE ACTIVITIES OF ALL EMPLOYEES AND ALL OTHER INDIVIDUALS UNDER HIS SUPERVISION; SHALL ENSURE THAT ALL INDIVIDUALS TO WHOM HE DELEGATES MEDICAL TASKS SHALL BE ADEQUATELY QUALIFIED TO PERFORM SUCH TASKS; WITHIN ONE YEAR, SHALL TAKE AND PASS THE MEDICAL JURISPRUDENCE EXAMINATION; SHALL OBTAIN AT LEAST 50 HOURS PER YEAR OF CONTINUING MEDICAL EDUCATION, AT LEAST 10 HOURS OF WHICH SHALL BE IN ETHICS; SHALL MAINTAIN ADEQUATE MEDICAL RECORDS WHICH SHALL BE AVAILABLE FOR REVIEW; SHALL ADOPT OR ESTABLISH A SYSTEM OF PATIENT RECORD KEEPING AND BILLING; SHALL NOT SIGN OR INDICATE IN ANY MANNER IN PATIENTS RECORDS THAT HE HAS SEEN PATIENTS UNLESS HE ACTUALLY HAS SEEN AND EXAMINED THE PATIENT UNLESS IT IS CLEARLY NOTED THAT HE DID NOT PERSONALLY EXAMINE THE PATIENT; SHALL APPEAR BEFORE THE BOARD AT LEAST ONCE A YEAR OR AT BOARD REQUEST; SHALL COOPERATE WITH BOARD IN VERIFYING COMPLIANCE; SHALL GIVE A COPY OF THIS ORDER TO ANY HEALTH CARE ENTITY WHERE HE HAS PRIVILEGES; SHALL PROVIDE A COPY OF THIS ORDER TO ANYONE REQUESTING IT WITHIN 10 DAYS; TIME PERIOD OUT OF TEXAS DOES NOT COUNT TOWARD PROBATION; SHALL INFORM BOARD OF CHANGE OF ADDRESS WITHIN 10 DAYS OR IF HE LEAVES THE STATE. SHALL NOT SEEK MODIFICATION FOR ONE YEAR. SHALL PAY $15,000 FINE. ON 5/10/97 PETITION TO TERMINATE ORDER DENIED. ON 8/22/98 ORDER TERMINATED.

DICKEY, BILLY MELVIN MD, LICENSE NUMBER C8253 OF EL PASO, TX, WAS DISCIPLINED BY TEXAS ON FEBRUARY 7, 1998
DISCIPLINARY ACTION: FINE
OFFENSE: PROFESSIONAL MISCONDUCT

NOTES: A FAMILY MEMBER WHO IS AN OFFICE EMPLOYEE OF HIS CALLED IN PRESCRIPTIONS AND PERSONALLY RECEIVED CONTROLLED SUBSTANCES BY USING HIS NAME; HE LEARNED OF THE FAMILY MEMBER'S DIVERSION OF CONTROLLED SUBSTANCES FOR HER OWN USE IN 6/95 YET FAILED TO TIMELY INFORM THE BOARD. LICENSE LIMITED AS FOLLOWS: SHALL NOT PERMIT FAMILY MEMBERS TO TELEPHONE TO A PHARMACY A PRESCRIPTION OR REFILL FOR CONTROLLED SUBSTANCES OR DANGEROUS DRUGS WITH ADDICTIVE POTENTIAL; $5,000 FINE. ON 4/4/98 THE ORDER WAS TERMINATED.

DILLARD, HOWARD L JR MD, LICENSE NUMBER 00D9419 OF WEBSTER, TX, WAS DISCIPLINED BY TEXAS ON MARCH 4, 1995
DISCIPLINARY ACTION: 36-MONTH PROBATION; RESTRICTION PLACED ON LICENSE
OFFENSE: NONCOMPLIANCE WITH A PROFESSIONAL RULE

NOTES: FROM 1983 THROUGH 1987, FAILED TO KEEP ADEQUATE RECORDS ON HIS CARE AND TREATMENT OF A PATIENT, INCLUDING ADEQUATE DOCUMENTATION OF HIS PRESCRIBING OF PSYCHOTROPIC MEDICATIONS AND PATIENT'S RELATED PSYCHIATRIC PROBLEMS. SUSPENSION STAYED. PROBATION WITH TERMS: SHALL MAINTAIN ADEQUATE MEDICAL RECORDS WHICH SHALL BE AVAILABLE FOR INSPECTION BY THE BOARD; SHALL NOT SIGN OR INDICATE IN ANY MANNER IN PATIENT RECORDS THAT HE HAS SEEN PATIENTS UNLESS HE ACTUALLY HAS SEEN AND EXAMINED THE PATIENT; SHALL MAINTAIN A FILE OF EVERY PRESCRIPTION WRITTEN BY HIM FOR CONTROLLED SUBSTANCES OR DRUGS WITH ADDICTIVE POTENTIAL AND SHALL MAINTAIN A LOG OF ALL PRESCRIPTIONS OR REFILLS TELEPHONED IN FOR CONTROLLED SUBSTANCES OR DRUGS WITH ADDICTIVE POTENTIAL BOTH OF WHICH SHALL BE AVAILABLE FOR INSPECTION; SHALL NOT EXAMINE OR TREAT ANY PATIENT IN AN OFFICE SETTING WITHOUT BEING ACCOMPANIED BY A BOARD-APPROVED CHAPERONE, WHO SHALL SIGN ALL PATIENT CHARTS TO INDICATE ACCOMPANIMENT AND OBSERVATION OF PHYSICIAN; SHALL COOPERATE WITH THE BOARD IN VERIFYING COMPLIANCE INCLUDING PROVIDING COPIES OF MEDICAL RELEASES UPON REQUEST; SHALL GIVE A COPY OF THIS ORDER TO ANY HEALTH CARE ENTITY WHERE HE HAS PRIVILEGES; SHALL PROVIDE A COPY OF ORDER TO ANYONE REQUESTING IT WITHIN 30 DAYS; SHALL APPEAR BEFORE BOARD AT LEAST ONCE EACH YEAR OF PROBATION; SHALL INFORM BOARD OF ANY CHANGE OF HIS ADDRESS WITHIN 10 DAYS OR IF HE LEAVES THE STATE; TIME PERIOD OUT OF TEXAS DOES NOT COUNT TOWARD PROBATION. SHALL NOT SEEK MODIFICATION FOR ONE YEAR. ON 5/15/96 PROBATION TERMINATED.

DITTEMORE, HAROLD E MD OF 3400 ANDREWS HIGHWAY, MIDLAND, TX, WAS DISCIPLINED BY NEW MEXICO ON DECEMBER 22, 1993
DISCIPLINARY ACTION: SURRENDER OF LICENSE

NOTES: IN LIEU OF ACTION.

DITTEMORE, HAROLD E MD, LICENSE NUMBER 00E3897 OF MIDLAND, TX, WAS DISCIPLINED BY TEXAS ON MARCH 2, 1996
DISCIPLINARY ACTION: SURRENDER OF LICENSE

NOTES: VOLUNTARY AND PERMANENT SURRENDER; SHALL IMMEDIATELY RETIRE FROM THE PRACTICE OF

MEDICINE.

DITTEMORE, HAROLD E MD OF 3400 ANDREWS HIGHWAY, MIDLAND, TX, WAS DISCIPLINED BY DEA ON APRIL 29, 1996
DISCIPLINARY ACTION: SURRENDER OF CONTROLLED SUBSTANCE LICENSE
NOTES: IN LIEU OF ORDER TO SHOW CAUSE.

DITTEMORE, HAROLD EUGENE MD, LICENSE NUMBER C34845 OF MIDLAND, TX, WAS DISCIPLINED BY CALIFORNIA ON NOVEMBER 25, 1997
DISCIPLINARY ACTION: SURRENDER OF LICENSE
NOTES: WHILE CHARGES PENDING.

DIXON, JOSEPH ANDREW MD, DATE OF BIRTH JULY 31, 1959, LICENSE NUMBER 00H2342 OF 6300 HUMANA PLAZA SUITE 875, ABILENE, TX, WAS DISCIPLINED BY TEXAS ON JANUARY 29, 1993
DISCIPLINARY ACTION: REPRIMAND
OFFENSE: SUBSTANDARD CARE, INCOMPETENCE OR NEGLIGENCE
NOTES: WHILE ENROLLED IN A RESIDENCY PROGRAM IN 12/88 FAILED TO APPROPRIATELY READ A LUMBAR X-RAY OF A PATIENT WHILE HE WORKED UNSUPERVISED IN A HOSPITAL EMERGENCY ROOM AND TO MAKE AN APPROPRIATE DIAGNOSIS.

DOBSON, WALTER ALBERT DO, LICENSE NUMBER 00F2636 OF GRAND PRAIRIE, TX, WAS DISCIPLINED BY TEXAS ON OCTOBER 5, 1991
DISCIPLINARY ACTION: 60-MONTH PROBATION; REQUIRED TO TAKE ADDITIONAL MEDICAL EDUCATION
OFFENSE: OVERCHARGING
NOTES: FOR SERVICE PROVIDED TO EIGHT PATIENTS, HE OR HIS OFFICE PERSONNEL MADE ONE OR MORE OF THE FOLLOWING ERRORS: UPCODING; UNBUNDLED FEES; INCORRECTLY IDENTIFYING SERVICES; AND PERFORMING IV SEDATION AND MONITORING IN CASES NOT REQUIRING SAME, WHICH RESULTED IN THE UNNECESSARY USE OF AN OPERATING AND RECOVERY ROOM. ACTIONS CONSTITUTED PERSISTENT AND FLAGRANT OVERCHARGING AND OVERTREATING OF PATIENTS. SUSPENSION STAYED, TERMS AND CONDITIONS OF PROBATION ARE AS FOLLOWS: SHALL COMPLETE AT LEAST 50 HOURS PER YEAR OF CONTINUING MEDICAL EDUCATION, 25 HOURS OF WHICH SHALL BE IN GYNECOLOGY AND THE REMAINDER SHALL BE IN GENERAL MEDICAL COURSES AND IN ETHICS; SHALL UTILIZE THE BLUE CROSS/BLUE SHIELD, MCGRAW HILL, MEDICARE OR COMPARABLE GUIDELINES FOR ESTABLISHING HIS CHARGES FOR SERVICES RENDERED; SHALL ADEQUATELY SUPERVISE THE ACTIVITIES OF ALL OF HIS EMPLOYEES; SHALL HAVE COLPOSCOPY CASES REVIEWED BY BOARD APPROVED GYNECOLOGIC SURGEON; SHALL PERFORM COLPOSCOPIES ONLY AFTER THE PATIENT HAS OBTAINED A SECOND AGREEING OPINION FROM A BOARD CERTIFIED GYNECOLOGICAL SURGEON; SHALL APPEAR BEFORE THE BOARD TWICE A YEAR; SHALL COOPERATE WITH THE BOARD IN VERIFYING COMPLIANCE; SHALL INFORM THE BOARD OF CHANGE OF ADDRESS WITHIN 10 DAYS; TIME SPENT OUT OF TEXAS DOES NOT COUNT TOWARDS PROBATION; SHALL NOT PETITION FOR MODIFICATION FOR ONE YEAR. ON 11/19/93, ORDER MODIFIED TO DELETE THE PROVISION REQUIRING A SECOND OPINION FROM A BOARD CERTIFIED GYNECOLOGICAL SURGEON PRIOR TO PERFORMING COLPOSCOPIES.

DOBSON, WALTER ALBERT DO, LICENSE NUMBER 0002298 OF GRAND PRAIRIE, TX, WAS DISCIPLINED BY OHIO ON MARCH 14, 1996
DISCIPLINARY ACTION: PROBATION; RESTRICTION PLACED ON LICENSE
OFFENSE: DISCIPLINARY ACTION BY ANOTHER STATE OR AGENCY
NOTES: PRIOR ACTION BY TEXAS STATE BOARD BASED UPON INCIDENTS OF UPCODING, UNBUNDLING FEES, INCORRECTLY IDENTIFYING SERVICES AND PERFORMING I.V. SEDATION AND MONITORING IN CASES IN WHICH IT WAS NOT REQUIRED. AGREEMENT TO REMAIN IN EFFECT UNTIL AT LEAST 10/5/96 AND UNTIL HE IS RELEASED FROM TERMS AND CONDITIONS IMPOSED BY HIS 10/4/91 TEXAS ORDER. ON 4/10/97 HE WAS RELEASED FROM THE TERMS OF THE ORDER.

DOLENZ, BERNARD J MD, LICENSE NUMBER 00C7391 OF DALLAS, TX, WAS DISCIPLINED BY TEXAS ON NOVEMBER 12, 1990
DISCIPLINARY ACTION: PROBATION
OFFENSE: NONCOMPLIANCE WITH A PROFESSIONAL RULE
NOTES: FAILURE TO KEEP COMPLETE AND ACCURATE RECORDS OF PURCHASES AND DISPOSALS OF DRUGS LISTED IN THE TEXAS CONTROLLED SUBSTANCES ACT; FAILURE TO PRACTICE MEDICINE IN ACCEPTABLE MANNER CONSISTENT WITH PUBLIC HEALTH AND WELFARE. ONE YEAR SUSPENSION, SUSPENSION PROBATED WITH CONDITIONS. ON APPEAL TO TRAVIS COUNTY DISTRICT COURT.

DOOLITTLE, J B DO, LICENSE NUMBER 00C2451 OF MEXICO, MO, WAS DISCIPLINED BY TEXAS ON DECEMBER 1, 1990
DISCIPLINARY ACTION: LICENSE REVOCATION
OFFENSE: DISCIPLINARY ACTION BY ANOTHER STATE OR AGENCY
NOTES: DISCIPLINED BY MISSOURI, REQUESTED TEXAS ACCEPT SURRENDER. MAY SEEK REINSTATEMENT OF TEXAS LICENSE NO SOONER THAN ONE YEAR FROM ORDER DATE BY COMPLYING WITH CERTAIN PROVISIONS.

DOOLITTLE, J B DO OF MEXICO, MO, WAS DISCIPLINED BY MISSOURI ON MARCH 24, 1994
DISCIPLINARY ACTION: LICENSE REVOCATION
OFFENSE: CRIMINAL CONVICTION OR PLEA OF GUILTY, NOLO CONTENDERE, OR NO CONTEST TO A CRIME
NOTES: PLED GUILTY IN THE CIRCUIT COURT OF AUDRAIN COUNTY, MISSOURI TO UNLAWFUL POSSESSION OF A CONTROLLED SUBSTANCE. NO REAPPLICATION FOR LICENSE FOR SEVEN YEARS.

DOTSON, BEVERLY ANN MD, LICENSE NUMBER 00D3204 OF GRAHAM, TX, WAS DISCIPLINED BY TEXAS ON DECEMBER 1, 1990
DISCIPLINARY ACTION: LICENSE REVOCATION
OFFENSE: SUBSTANCE ABUSE
NOTES: INTEMPERATE USE OF ALCOHOL AND DRUGS, UNPROFESSIONAL OR DISHONORABLE CONDUCT LIKELY TO DECEIVE, DEFRAUD, OR INJURE PUBLIC, PROFESSIONAL FAILURE TO PRACTICE MEDICINE IN ACCEPTABLE MANNER CONSISTENT WITH PUBLIC HEALTH AND WELFARE. MOTION FOR REHEARING FILED.

DOTSON, DANIEL A MD, LICENSE NUMBER 00D4096 OF GRAHAM, TX, WAS DISCIPLINED BY TEXAS ON DECEMBER 1, 1990
DISCIPLINARY ACTION: LICENSE REVOCATION
OFFENSE: PROFESSIONAL MISCONDUCT
NOTES: UNPROFESSIONAL OR DISHONORABLE CONDUCT LIKELY TO DECEIVE, DEFRAUD OR INJURE PUBLIC, PROFESSIONAL FAILURE TO PRACTICE MEDICINE IN

ACCEPTABLE MANNER CONSISTENT WITH PUBLIC HEALTH AND WELFARE. FILED MOTION FOR REHEARING.

DOTSON, DANIEL A MD, DATE OF BIRTH NOVEMBER 14, 1941, LICENSE NUMBER 0025062 OF PUEBLO, CO, WAS DISCIPLINED BY COLORADO ON SEPTEMBER 11, 1992
DISCIPLINARY ACTION: SURRENDER OF CONTROLLED SUBSTANCE LICENSE
OFFENSE: SUBSTANDARD CARE, INCOMPETENCE OR NEGLIGENCE

NOTES: TWO OR MORE ACTS OR OMISSIONS WHICH FAILED TO MEET GENERALLY ACCEPTED STANDARDS OF MEDICAL PRACTICE. PERMANENT SURRENDER OF DRUG ENFORCEMENT ADMINISTRATION CERTIFICATE (ALL SCHEDULES). NOT TO SEEK CERTIFICATE REINSTATEMENT IN FUTURE.

DOTSON, HERMAN DO, DATE OF BIRTH MAY 27, 1947 OF 5733 OLD OX ROAD, DALLAS, TX, WAS DISCIPLINED BY MEDICARE ON NOVEMBER 19, 1998
DISCIPLINARY ACTION: EXCLUSION FROM THE MEDICARE AND/OR MEDICAID PROGRAM
OFFENSE: NONCOMPLIANCE WITH A PROFESSIONAL RULE

NOTES: DEFAULTED ON PUBLIC HEALTH SERVICE EDUCATION LOAN.

DOTSON, RODNEY N MD, WAS DISCIPLINED BY ARIZONA ON APRIL 10, 1991
DISCIPLINARY ACTION: DENIAL OF NEW LICENSE
OFFENSE: DISCIPLINARY ACTION BY ANOTHER STATE OR AGENCY

NOTES: ACTION BASED ON LICENSE RESTRICTION IN TEXAS.

DOTSON, RODNEY N MD, WAS DISCIPLINED BY ARIZONA ON JUNE 21, 1991
DISCIPLINARY ACTION: DENIAL OF NEW LICENSE

NOTES: FAILURE TO MEET STATUTORY REQUIREMENTS FOR LICENSURE.

DOTSON, RODNEY NORMAN MD, LICENSE NUMBER 00D9988 OF TEXARKANA, TX, WAS DISCIPLINED BY TEXAS ON JANUARY 12, 1991
DISCIPLINARY ACTION: 60-MONTH PROBATION; RESTRICTION PLACED ON LICENSE

NOTES: IMMEDIATE CESSATION OF CERVICAL CAUTERY EXCEPT UNDER DIRECT SUPERVISION OF A PHYSICIAN AS PART OF AN APPROVED FAMILY PRACTICE RESIDENCY OR PRECEPTORSHIP, PRESCRIBING OR ADMINISTERING CERTAIN DRUGS, OR PROVIDING ONGOING PRENATAL CARE, EXCEPT WITH PRIOR ARRANGEMENTS FOR DELIVERY AND FOLLOW-UP; LIMITATION OF MANAGEMENT OF YEAST INFECTION PATIENTS; NO TREATMENT OF ATTENTION DEFICIT DISORDER OR HYPERACTIVE PATIENTS WITHOUT ONGOING CONSULTATION WITH A PEDIATRICIAN; PERFORMANCE OF CIRCUMCISIONS LIMITED TO NEONATAL PATIENTS UNLESS UNDER DIRECT SUPERVISION OF A PHYSICIAN AS PART OF A FAMILY PRACTICE RESIDENCY OR PRECEPTORSHIP; OBTAINING AN ARIZONA LICENSE TO PRACTICE MEDICINE IMMEDIATELY, OR SURRENDER OF TEXAS MEDICAL LICENSE EFFECTIVE 7/1/91 UNLESS ENTERED INTO A ONE-YEAR PRECEPTORSHIP OR FAMILY PRACTICE RESIDENCY WITH TIMELY AND SUCCESSFUL COMPLETION.

DOTSON, RODNEY NORMAN MD, LICENSE NUMBER D9988 OF HEREFORD, TX, WAS DISCIPLINED BY TEXAS ON AUGUST 22, 1998
DISCIPLINARY ACTION: 60-MONTH PROBATION; REQUIRED TO TAKE ADDITIONAL MEDICAL EDUCATION
OFFENSE: OVERPRESCRIBING OR MISPRESCRIBING DRUGS

NOTES: IN 1983 HE SIGNED AN AFFIDAVIT WITH THE BOARD WHICH INVOLVED ALLEGATIONS OF NON-THERAPEUTIC PRESCRIBING AND FAILURE TO PRACTICE MEDICINE IN AN ACCEPTABLE MANNER; IN 1/91 THE BOARD AND HE ENTERED INTO AN AGREED ORDER OF PROVISIONS WHICH HE SUCCESSFULLY COMPLETED; A BOARD CONSULTANT DETERMINED THAT HIS ADMINISTRATION/PRESCRIPTION OF DONNAGEL PG WAS CONTRAINDICATED AND DANGEROUS; HE MAINTAINS THAT HE WITHDREW THE PRESCRIPTIONS AFTER HE WAS INFORMED BY A PHARMACIST THAT THE MEDICATION WAS NO LONGER AVAILABLE IN THE FORM HE WISHED TO USE IT AND, THEREFORE, USE AS PRESCRIBED WAS CONTRAINDICATED; HIS MEDICAL RECORDS FOR TREATMENT OF SEVERAL PATIENTS DID NOT CLEARLY INDICATE HIS ASSESSMENTS AND TREATMENT PLANS; DID NOT KEEP ADEQUATE RECORDS OF DRUGS; PHARMACY RECORDS INDICATE THAT HE ORDERED PRESCRIPTIONS FOR MEMBERS OF HIS FAMILY WITHOUT DOCUMENTING THESE PRESCRIPTIONS; HE HAS NO RECORDS FOR HIS TREATMENT OF FAMILY MEMBERS; UNTIL AT LEAST 4/97 HE HAD NOT CONTRACTED WITH A HAZARDOUS WASTE DISPOSAL COMPANY TO REMOVE HAZARDOUS WASTE FROM HIS OFFICE; CITY HEALTH INSPECTORS DETERMINED THAT HE WAS DISPOSING OF NEEDLES, USED SPECULUMS, BODY WASTE, AND SYRINGES, IN THE TRASH AND ALLEY BEHIND HIS OFFICE; HE HELD HIMSELF OUT TO BE A " BOARD TRAINED" PEDIATRICIAN; THIS VAGUE DISTINCTION IS INACCURATE AND HE MAINTAINS THAT HE NO LONGER HOLDS HIMSELF OUT TO BE "BOARD TRAINED"; HE MAINTAINS THAT HE HAS ENROLLED IN A COURSE OF STUDY OFFERED BY THE AMERICAN COLLEGE OF GENERAL MEDICINE, THROUGH THE COLLEGE OF WILLIAM AND MARY, WHICH WILL SUPPORT HIS CONTINUED RETRAINING; HE FURTHER MAINTAINS THAT THIS COURSE OF STUDY EVIDENCES HIS COMMITMENT TO EXCELLENCE IN HIS PRACTICE. SUSPENSION STAYED FOR PROBATION WITH FOLLOWING TERMS AND CONDITIONS: WITHIN 1 YEAR SHALL TAKE AND PASS THE SPEX WITHIN 3 ATTEMPTS; HIS MEDICAL PRACTICE SHALL BE MONITORED BY A BOARD APPROVED TEXAS PHYSICIAN WHO SHALL PROVIDE QUARTERLY REPORTS TO THE BOARD; SHALL OBTAIN 50 HOURS PER YEAR OF CONTINUING MEDICAL EDUCATION IN FAMILY PRACTICE AND/OR PEDIATRICS; SHALL BECOME FAMILIAR WITH AND COMPLY WITH THE LAWS OF THE TEXAS DEPARTMENT OF HEALTH AND OSHA PERTAINING TO BIO-HAZARDOUS WASTE DISPOSAL; SHALL MAINTAIN ADEQUATE MEDICAL RECORDS WHICH SHALL BE AVAILABLE FOR REVIEW; SHALL APPEAR BEFORE THE BOARD AT LEAST ONCE A YEAR; SHALL COOPERATE WITH THE BOARD IN VERIFYING COMPLIANCE; TIME SPENT OUT OF TEXAS DOES NOT COUNT TOWARD PROBATION; SHALL INFORM THE BOARD OF CHANGE OF ADDRESS WITHIN 10 DAYS OR IF HE LEAVES THE STATE; SHALL NOT SEEK MODIFICATION FOR ONE YEAR.

DOUGLAS, AUBRY CARTER MD OF 2000 CRAWFORD ST SUITE 860, HOUSTON, TX, WAS DISCIPLINED BY DEA ON SEPTEMBER 5, 1995
DISCIPLINARY ACTION: RESTRICTION PLACED ON CONTROLLED SUBSTANCE LICENSE

NOTES: MEMO OF UNDERSTANDING.

DOUGLAS, HOWARD T III MD, DATE OF BIRTH MARCH 31, 1949,

LICENSE NUMBER 24197, WAS DISCIPLINED BY COLORADO ON NOVEMBER 13, 1998
DISCIPLINARY ACTION: REPRIMAND; REQUIRED TO TAKE ADDITIONAL MEDICAL EDUCATION

NOTES: DISCIPLINE IN ANOTHER STATE. HE AGREES TO REEDUCATION ACTIVITIES.

DOUGLAS, HOWARD T III MD, DATE OF BIRTH MARCH 31, 1949, LICENSE NUMBER 24197, WAS DISCIPLINED BY COLORADO ON MAY 19, 1999

NOTES: ISSUE OF COMPLIANCE WITH INITIAL ORDER. LICENSE PLACED IN INACTIVE STATUS.

DOUGLAS, HOWARD THOMAS III MD, LICENSE NUMBER F1511, WAS DISCIPLINED BY TEXAS ON MAY 10, 1997
DISCIPLINARY ACTION: LICENSE SUSPENSION; FINE
OFFENSE: OVERPRESCRIBING OR MISPRESCRIBING DRUGS

NOTES: HE HAD A CONTRACT WITH SOUTHWEST MEDICAL ASSOCIATES, INC., INVOLVING HIS AGREEMENT TO PROVIDE CONTINUOUS PHYSICIAN COVERAGE, INCLUDING ER SERVICES, TO A SPECIFIED HOSPITAL IN SONORA, TEXAS BETWEEN 6 PM ON 7/6/94 AND 6 AM ON 7/11/94, INCLUSIVE. ON 7/10/94 HE BECAME ILL WITH A VIRUS, INCLUDING STOMACH CRAMPS, VOMITING, AND DIARRHEA, DROVE TO THE HOSPITAL ADMINISTRATOR'S HOUSE, AND TOLD HIM HE COULD NOT ADEQUATELY TREAT PATIENTS AND ASSUMED IT WAS ALL RIGHT TO LEAVE THE HOSPITAL WHILE IN FACT THE ADMINISTRATOR WAS SURPRISED AND UPSET THAT THE DOCTOR LEFT BEFORE THE REGULAR PHYSICIAN RETURNED OR A REPLACEMENT WAS SECURED. WITHOUT DEFINITELY TELLING THE NURSING STAFF HE WAS LEAVING, HE LEFT AND DID NOT CONTACT THE HOSPITAL AFTER HE LEFT. ON 7/9/94 HE HAD PRESCRIBED A CONTROLLED SUBSTANCE, VICODIN, TO A PATIENT HE NEVER EXAMINED AND WITHOUT CONSULTING ANY MEDICAL RECORDS ON THE BASIS OF HER TESTIMONY THAT SHE HAD A TOOTHACHE AND NEEDED A NEW SUPPLY OF HER PREVIOUS PRESCRIPTION FOR SAID SUBSTANCE. UNDER THE CIRCUMSTANCES THE PHYSICIAN HAD NO WAY OF KNOWING WHETHER THE DRUG WOULD BE THERAPEUTIC FOR THE PATIENT. LICENSE SUSPENDED UNTIL THE PHYSICIAN SATISFIES THE FOLLOWING: SHALL RECERTIFY IN ATLS AND ADVANCED CARDIAC LIFE SUPPORT; SHALL PASS 100 HOURS IN EMERGENCY ROOM MEDICINE AND CONTINUING MEDICAL EDUCATION; SHALL PASS AN APPROVED PHARMACOLOGY COURSE AND AN APPROVED RISK MANAGEMENT COURSE; SHALL PASS THE SPEX AND THE BOARD'S JURISPRUDENCE EXAM; SHALL SEND A BOARD-APPROVED WRITTEN APOLOGY TO THE CONCERNED HOSPITAL AND TO SOUTHWEST MEDICAL ASSOCIATES, INC.; SHALL INFORM ALL HOSPITALS WHERE HE HAS PRIVILEGES AND ALL ER COMPANIES WITH WHICH HE HAS OR HAS HAD CONTRACTS THAT HIS LICENSE IS SUSPENDED; SHALL SEND A COPY OF THIS ORDER TO ALL STATES WHERE HE IS LICENSED; AND SHALL FURNISH ACCEPTABLE PROOF TO THE BOARD THAT HE HAS NOTIFIED THE ABOVE ENTITIES. UPON FULFILLMENT OF THESE CONDITIONS, HE WILL BE SUSPENDED FOR ANOTHER FIVE YEARS; SUSPENSION STAYED AND LICENSE PLACED ON PROBATION WITH TERMS. $10,000 ADMINISTRATIVE FINE. ON 10/24/98 PETITION FOR REINSTATEMENT DENIED; THE FOLLOWING MODIFICATIONS WERE ORDERED HOWEVER: DELETION OF REQUIREMENT TO TAKE AND PASS A BOARD-APPROVED PHARMACOLOGY COURSE; MAY PASS THE AMERICAN BOARD OF EMERGENCY ROOM MEDICINE CERTIFICATION EXAM AS AN ALTERNATIVE TO PASSING THE SPEX EXAM; FINE REDUCED TO $5,000; LICENSE PLACED ON PROBATION AS SOON AS THESE CONDITIONS ARE MET; ALL OTHER PROVISIONS OF ORDER REMAIN IN EFFECT UNTIL SUPERSEDED BY A SUBSEQUENT BOARD ORDER. ON 5/14/99 REQUEST FOR REINSTATEMENT DENIED.

DOUGLAS, HOWARD THOMAS III MD, DATE OF BIRTH MARCH 31, 1949 OF 729 GRAPEVINE HIGHWAY, HURST, TX, WAS DISCIPLINED BY MEDICARE ON SEPTEMBER 20, 1998
DISCIPLINARY ACTION: EXCLUSION FROM THE MEDICARE AND/OR MEDICAID PROGRAM
OFFENSE: DISCIPLINARY ACTION BY ANOTHER STATE OR AGENCY

NOTES: LICENSE REVOKED, SUSPENDED, SURRENDERED OR OTHERWISE LOST FOR REASONS BEARING ON PROFESSIONAL PERFORMANCE, PROFESSIONAL COMPETENCE OR FINANCIAL INTEGRITY. REINSTATED ON 11/5/99.

DOUGLAS, JAKE S MD, LICENSE NUMBER 00B5654 OF BEAUMONT, TX, WAS DISCIPLINED BY TEXAS ON JANUARY 24, 1992
DISCIPLINARY ACTION: SURRENDER OF LICENSE
OFFENSE: PHYSICAL OR MENTAL ILLNESS INHIBITING THE ABILITY TO PRACTICE WITH SKILL AND SAFETY

NOTES: POSSIBLE INABILITY TO PRACTICE MEDICINE WITH REASONABLE SKILL AND SAFETY TO PATIENTS BY REASON OF ILLNESS. LICENSE VOLUNTARILY RETIRED IN LIEU OF DISCIPLINARY ACTION.

DOWD, DONNA CATHERINE MD, DATE OF BIRTH SEPTEMBER 4, 1952, LICENSE NUMBER 00F3913 OF 9147 POWHATAN, SAN ANTONIO, TX, WAS DISCIPLINED BY TEXAS ON JUNE 15, 1993
DISCIPLINARY ACTION: 60-MONTH PROBATION; MONITORING OF PHYSICIAN PERFORMANCE
OFFENSE: SUBSTANCE ABUSE

NOTES: HAS BEEN DIAGNOSED AS SUFFERING FROM AN ACUTE AND CHRONIC INFECTION BY THE EPSTEIN-BARR VIRUS SECONDARY TO A B CELL LYMPHOCYTIC DISORDER; DURING 1991 AND 1992 SELF-PRESCRIBED TYLENOL #3 FOR MUSCLE PAIN AND CONSUMED EXCESSIVE QUANTITIES WITHOUT A SUFFICIENT MEDICAL JUSTIFICATION; SHE VOLUNTARILY SOUGHT MEDICAL ASSISTANCE AND PSYCHIATRIC COUNSELING IN 10/92 AND TOOK A MEDICAL LEAVE OF ABSENCE; EVIDENCE DOES NOT INDICATE EXCESSIVE CONSUMPTION CAUSED PATIENT HARM. SUSPENSION STAYED. CONDITIONS OF PROBATION: SHALL NOT SELF-PRESCRIBE DANGEROUS DRUGS OR CONTROLLED SUBSTANCES; SHALL ABSTAIN FROM THE CONSUMPTION OF DANGEROUS DRUGS OR CONTROLLED SUBSTANCES IN ANY FORM UNLESS PRESCRIBED BY ANOTHER PHYSICIAN FOR A LEGITIMATE MEDICAL PURPOSE; SHALL SUBMIT HERSELF FOR APPROPRIATE EXAMS INCLUDING DRUG SCREENS; SHALL KEEP A SEPARATE RECORD OF EVERY PRESCRIPTION WRITTEN FOR CONTROLLED SUBSTANCES OR DANGEROUS DRUGS WHICH SHALL BE AVAILABLE FOR INSPECTION; SHALL CONTINUE TO RECEIVE TREATMENT WITH QUARTERLY REPORTS TO THE BOARD; SHALL APPEAR BEFORE THE BOARD ONCE A YEAR; SHALL GIVE A COPY OF THIS ORDER TO ANY HEALTH CARE ENTITY WHERE SHE HAS PRIVILEGES; SHALL COOPERATE WITH THE BOARD IN VERIFYING COMPLIANCE; SHALL INFORM BOARD OF CHANGE OF ADDRESS WITHIN 10 DAYS OR IF SHE LEAVES THE STATE; TIME SPENT OUT OF TEXAS DOES NOT COUNT TOWARD PROBATION. SHALL NOT SEEK MODIFICATION FOR ONE YEAR.

DOWD, DONNA CATHERINE MD, DATE OF BIRTH SEPTEMBER 4, 1952, LICENSE NUMBER 00F3913 OF SAN ANTONIO, TX, WAS DISCIPLINED BY TEXAS ON JANUARY 6, 1995
DISCIPLINARY ACTION: 48-MONTH PROBATION; MONITORING OF PHYSICIAN PERFORMANCE
OFFENSE: FAILURE TO COMPLY WITH PREVIOUS BOARD ORDER

NOTES: IN VIOLATION OF 06/15/93 ORDER BETWEEN 11/93 AND 3/94 SHE SELF-PRESCRIBED PRESCRIPTIONS FOR DIAZOXIDE, PYRIDIUM AND SEPTRA AND ON 6/20/94 INGESTED BARBITURATES AND BENZODIAZEPINES WHICH WERE PRESCRIBED BY TREATING PHYSICIAN BUT NOT REPORTED TO THE BOARD. SUSPENSION STAYED. CONDITIONS OF PROBATION: SHALL NOT SELF-PRESCRIBE DANGEROUS DRUGS; SHALL ABSTAIN FROM THE CONSUMPTION OF ALCOHOL/CHEMICAL SUBSTANCES IN ANY FORM UNLESS PRESCRIBED BY ANOTHER PHYSICIAN FOR A LEGITIMATE AND THERAPEUTIC PURPOSE; SHALL SUBMIT HERSELF FOR APPROPRIATE EXAMS INCLUDING DRUG OR ALCOHOL SCREENS; SEPARATE FROM PATIENT RECORDS, SHALL MAINTAIN A FILE OF EVERY PRESCRIPTION FOR CONTROLLED SUBSTANCES OR DANGEROUS DRUGS WHICH SHALL BE AVAILABLE FOR INSPECTION; SHALL NOT TELEPHONE ANY PRESCRIPTION TO A PHARMACY FOR THESE DRUGS; SHALL CONTINUE TO RECEIVE TREATMENT FROM SPECIFIED PHYSICIAN WITH QUARTERLY REPORTS; UPON VISIT TO ANY PHYSICIAN SHALL PROVIDE THEM WITH A REPORT OF MEDICATIONS SHE HAS BEEN PRESCRIBED OR IS CONSUMING WITH INITIALS OF THE PRESCRIBING PHYSICIAN; SHALL APPEAR BEFORE THE BOARD ONCE A YEAR; SHALL GIVE A COPY OF THIS ORDER TO ANY HEALTH CARE ENTITY WHERE SHE HAS PRIVILEGES; SHALL COOPERATE WITH THE BOARD IN VERIFYING COMPLIANCE; SHALL INFORM BOARD OF CHANGE OF ADDRESS WITHIN 10 DAYS OR IF SHE LEAVES THE STATE; TIME SPENT OUT OF TEXAS DOES NOT COUNT TOWARD PROBATION. SHALL NOT SEEK MODIFICATION FOR ONE YEAR. ALSO KNOWN AS DONNA C. CROMWELL.

DOWLING, GEORGE W MD, LICENSE NUMBER 0009159 OF ANDREWS, TX, WAS DISCIPLINED BY FLORIDA ON SEPTEMBER 25, 1991
DISCIPLINARY ACTION: SURRENDER OF LICENSE
OFFENSE: PROVIDING FALSE INFORMATION TO THE BOARD OR OTHER HEALTH AGENCY

NOTES: CHARGED WITH FRAUDULENT MISREPRESENTATION IN THAT HE FALSELY CERTIFIED THAT HE HAD COMPLETED CONTINUING MEDICAL EDUCATION REQUIREMENTS FOR LICENSE RENEWAL; FAILED TO SUBMIT DOCUMENTATION VERIFYING COMPLETION OF RISK MANAGEMENT AND HIV/AIDS CONTINUING MEDICAL EDUCATION IN RESPONSE TO THE BOARD'S RANDOM AUDIT. AGREES NEVER AGAIN TO APPLY FOR LICENSURE AS A PHYSICIAN IN FLORIDA.

DOYLE, PETER D MD, LICENSE NUMBER 00H6175 OF HOUSTON, TX, WAS DISCIPLINED BY TEXAS ON JANUARY 27, 1996
DISCIPLINARY ACTION: 60-MONTH PROBATION; REQUIRED TO TAKE ADDITIONAL MEDICAL EDUCATION
OFFENSE: LOSS OR RESTRICTION OF HOSPITAL PRIVILEGES

NOTES: ON 2/01/95 SUMMARILY SUSPENDED FROM METHODIST HOSPITAL FOR SUSPECTED SUBSTANCE ABUSE AND ABANDONMENT OF DUTY BECAUSE HE TOOK A NAP WHILE HE WAS SUPERVISING A NURSE ANESTHETIST; ON 2/02/95 ADMITTED TO THE PARTIAL DAY PROGRAM AT INTRACARE HOSPITAL AND WAS DISCHARGED ON 2/15/95 AND HAS BEEN UNDER FOLLOW-UP TREATMENT; ENTERED INTO AN AGREEMENT WITH METHODIST HOSPITAL WHICH INCLUDED REINSTATEMENT OF HIS PRIVILEGES, TWO YEAR PROBATION, PARTICIPATION IN THE HARRIS COUNTY PHYSICIAN'S COUNSELING COMMITTEE, A 12 STEP PROGRAM, RANDOM URINE SCREENS, AND REGULAR MEETINGS WITH A MONITOR, A PSYCHOTHERAPIST, AND A PSYCHIATRIST; REPORTS A SOBRIETY DATE OF 6/9/95. SUSPENSION, STAYED AS PROBATION WITH TERMS AND CONDITIONS: SHALL ABSTAIN FROM THE CONSUMPTION OF ALCOHOL/DRUGS IN ANY FORM UNLESS PRESCRIBED BY ANOTHER PHYSICIAN FOR A LEGITIMATE AND THERAPEUTIC PURPOSE; SHALL SUBMIT HIMSELF FOR APPROPRIATE EXAMS, INCLUDING DRUG OR ALCOHOL SCREENS; SHALL SUBMIT HIMSELF FOR EVALUATION AND TREATMENT BY A BOARD APPROVED PSYCHIATRIST WHOM HE SHALL SEE AT LEAST ONCE A MONTH AND WHO SHALL SUBMIT REPORTS TO THE BOARD; SHALL PROVIDE COMPLETE WRITTEN REPORTS REGARDING ANY ASPECT OF HIS PHYSICAL OR MENTAL CONDITION AND HIS COMPLIANCE WITH THE ORDER; SHALL PARTICIPATE IN AA'S PROGRAM NOT LESS THAN THREE TIMES PER WEEK WITH QUARTERLY REPORTS TO THE BOARD; SHALL PARTICIPATE IN THE ACTIVITIES OF AN IMPAIRED PHYSICIAN GROUP AND ATTEND WEEKLY MEETINGS WITH QUARTERLY REPORTS; SHALL COMPLY WITH THE METHODIST HOSPITAL CONTINUING CARE CONTRACT WITH QUARTERLY REPORTS TO THE BOARD; HIS MEDICAL PRACTICE INCLUDING ANY OFFICE AND SURGICAL PRACTICE, SHALL BE MONITORED BY A BOARD APPROVED TEXAS PHYSICIAN WHO SHALL SUBMIT QUARTERLY REPORTS; SHALL ATTEND A BOARD APPROVED ETHICS COURSE OR PROGRAM EACH YEAR FOR FIVE YEARS AND SHALL SUBMIT PROOF OF ATTENDANCE TO THE BOARD; SHALL APPEAR BEFORE THE BOARD AT LEAST TWO TIMES PER YEAR; SHALL COOPERATE WITH THE BOARD IN VERIFYING COMPLIANCE INCLUDING PROVIDING COPIES OF MEDICAL RELEASES UPON REQUEST.

DOYLE, PETER D MD, LICENSE NUMBER 00H6175 OF HOUSTON, TX, WAS DISCIPLINED BY TEXAS ON JUNE 1, 1996
DISCIPLINARY ACTION: LICENSE SUSPENSION; REQUIRED TO ENTER AN IMPAIRED PHYSICIAN PROGRAM OR SUBSTANCE ABUSE TREATMENT
OFFENSE: FAILURE TO COMPLY WITH PREVIOUS BOARD ORDER

NOTES: ON ABOUT 3/21/96 HE INGESTED COCAINE IN VIOLATION OF 1/27/96 ORDER; HIS INGESTION OF COCAINE WAS CONFIRMED BY A POSITIVE URINE SCREEN AND NOT PURSUANT TO A PRESCRIPTION FROM A TREATING PHYSICIAN; FAILED TO IMMEDIATELY REPORT HIS INGESTION OF COCAINE TO THE BOARD. SUSPENSION UNTIL HE REQUESTS TO HAVE SUSPENSION LIFTED OR STAYED AND APPEARS BEFORE BOARD WITH EVIDENCE THAT HE IS PHYSICALLY, MENTALLY AND OTHERWISE COMPETENT TO SAFELY PRACTICE MEDICINE INCLUDING, AT A MINIMUM, EVIDENCE OF COMPLETION OF INPATIENT DRUG REHABILITATION TREATMENT IN A BOARD-APPROVED FACILITY WITH MONTHLY REPORTS TO THE BOARD. ON 8/17/96 THE BOARD DENIED HIS REQUEST TO HAVE HIS SUSPENSION LIFTED AS HE DID NOT SATISFY THE MINIMUM REQUIREMENTS FOR STAYING THE SUSPENSION.

DOYLE, PETER D MD, LICENSE NUMBER H6175, WAS DISCIPLINED BY TEXAS ON SEPTEMBER 20, 1997
DISCIPLINARY ACTION: 120-MONTH PROBATION; RESTRICTION PLACED ON CONTROLLED SUBSTANCE LICENSE

OFFENSE: FAILURE TO COMPLY WITH PREVIOUS BOARD ORDER

NOTES: VIOLATED 1/27/96 BOARD ORDER BY INGESTING COCAINE ON OR ABOUT 3/21/96. SUSPENSION PLACED ON LICENSE IN 5/96 STAYED FOR PROBATION WITH FOLLOWING TERMS AND CONDITIONS: SHALL ABSTAIN FROM THE CONSUMPTION OF ALCOHOL/DRUGS IN ANY FORM UNLESS PRESCRIBED BY ANOTHER PHYSICIAN FOR A LEGITIMATE AND THERAPEUTIC PURPOSE; SHALL SUBMIT HIMSELF FOR APPROPRIATE EXAMS INCLUDING DRUG OR ALCOHOL SCREENS; SHALL CONTINUE CARE AND TREATMENT WITH A SPECIFIED PHYSICIAN AT LEAST MONTHLY WITH REPORTS TO THE BOARD UPON REQUEST; SHALL PARTICIPATE IN THE ACTIVITIES OF A PHYSICIAN HEALTH AND REHABILITATION COMMITTEE AND ATTEND WEEKLY MEETINGS WITH QUARTERLY REPORTS; SHALL PARTICIPATE IN AA'S PROGRAM NOT LESS THAN THREE TIMES A WEEK; SHALL REPORT ON HIS ATTENDANCE; SHALL NOT TREAT OR OTHERWISE SERVE AS PHYSICIAN, PRESCRIBE, DISPENSE OR ADMINISTER DRUGS THAT MAY BE SUBJECT TO ABUSE TO HIMSELF OR TO ANY MEMBER OF HIS FAMILY; SHALL SURRENDER ALL DRUGS WITH POTENTIAL FOR ABUSE IN HIS POSSESSION INCLUDING SAMPLES; SHALL NOT TELEPHONE, NOR PERMIT ANYONE UNDER HIS SUPERVISION TO TELEPHONE, TO A PHARMACY A PRESCRIPTION TO REFILL FOR CONTROLLED OR ADDICTIVE SUBSTANCES; HE IS AUTHORIZED TO REAPPLY FOR DEA AND TEXAS DEPARTMENT OF PUBLIC SAFETY FOR FULL PRESCRIBING AUTHORITY; SHALL NOT POSSESS, ADMINISTER, DISPENSE OR PRESCRIBE ANY DRUGS WITH POTENTIAL FOR ABUSE EXCEPT FOR INPATIENTS IN A HOSPITAL SETTING; SEPARATE FROM PATIENT RECORDS, SHALL MAINTAIN A FILE OF EVERY PRESCRIPTION WRITTEN BY HIM FOR DANGEROUS DRUGS WITH ADDICTIVE POTENTIAL WHICH SHALL BE MADE AVAILABLE FOR REVIEW; HIS MEDICAL PRACTICE SHALL BE MONITORED BY A BOARD APPROVED TEXAS PHYSICIAN WHO SHALL PROVIDE QUARTERLY REPORTS TO THE BOARD; SHALL MAINTAIN ADEQUATE MEDICAL RECORDS WHICH SHALL BE AVAILABLE FOR REVIEW; SHALL OBTAIN 50 HOURS PER YEAR OF CONTINUING MEDICAL EDUCATION; SHALL APPEAR BEFORE THE BOARD AT LEAST TWICE EACH YEAR; SHALL COOPERATE WITH THE BOARD IN VERIFYING COMPLIANCE INCLUDING PROVIDING COPIES OF MEDICAL RELEASES UPON REQUEST; SHALL GIVE A COPY OF THIS ORDER TO ANY HEALTH CARE ENTITY WHERE HE HAS PRIVILEGES; SHALL PROVIDE A COPY OF THIS ORDER TO ANYONE REQUESTING IT WITHIN 10 DAYS; TIME SPENT OUT OF TEXAS DOES NOT COUNT TOWARD RESTRICTION; SHALL INFORM THE BOARD OF CHANGE OF ADDRESS WITHIN 10 DAYS OR IF HE LEAVES THE STATE; SHALL NOT SEEK MODIFICATION FOR ONE YEAR. ON 10/15/99 PETITION TO TERMINATE ORDER IS DENIED WITH THE FOLLOWING MODIFICATION: SHALL PERSONALLY APPEAR BEFORE THE BOARD ONCE A YEAR RATHER THAN TWICE.

DRISCOLL, EDWARD T MD, LICENSE NUMBER 00C9498 OF ODESSA, TX, WAS DISCIPLINED BY CALIFORNIA ON MARCH 17, 1995
DISCIPLINARY ACTION: LICENSE REVOCATION
OFFENSE: DISCIPLINARY ACTION BY ANOTHER STATE OR AGENCY

NOTES: DISCIPLINE BY TEXAS BOARD DUE TO NEGLIGENT OR INCOMPETENT CARE PROVIDED TO SEVERAL PATIENTS. DEFAULT DECISION.

DRISCOLL, EDWARD THOMAS MD, LICENSE NUMBER 00B6008 OF ODESSA, TX, WAS DISCIPLINED BY TEXAS ON NOVEMBER 13, 1992
DISCIPLINARY ACTION: RESTRICTION PLACED ON LICENSE

NOTES: PRACTICE OF MEDICINE RESTRICTED TO NO MORE THAN EIGHT HOURS PER WEEK AND NO MORE THAN FOUR HOURS PER 24 HOUR PERIOD; PRACTICE LIMITED TO THE PHYSICAL CONFINES OF THE DRISCOLL CLINIC LOCATED IN ODESSA, TEXAS; SHALL NOT PERFORM SURGERY.

DRISCOLL, STEPHEN EDWARD MD, LICENSE NUMBER 00F1514 OF ODESSA, TX, WAS DISCIPLINED BY TEXAS ON APRIL 20, 1992
DISCIPLINARY ACTION: 24-MONTH PROBATION; REPRIMAND

NOTES: SEVERAL VIOLATIONS OF THE MEDICAL PRACTICE ACT, INCLUDING PROFESSIONAL FAILURE TO PRACTICE MEDICINE IN AN ACCEPTABLE MANNER CONSISTENT WITH PUBLIC HEALTH AND WELFARE. LICENSE SUSPENDED, SUSPENSION STAYED; PROBATION UNDER TERMS AND CONDITIONS.

DRISCOLL, STEPHEN EDWARD MD, LICENSE NUMBER 00F1514 OF ODESSA, TX, WAS DISCIPLINED BY TEXAS ON AUGUST 18, 1995
DISCIPLINARY ACTION: 48-MONTH PROBATION; RESTRICTION PLACED ON LICENSE
OFFENSE: SUBSTANDARD CARE, INCOMPETENCE OR NEGLIGENCE

NOTES: IN 9/86 HE PERFORMED SURGERY ON A PATIENT WITHOUT DOCUMENTED ADEQUATE MEDICAL INDICATION; FROM 1983 TO 1986 HE PERFORMED MULTIPLE BACK SURGERIES ON A SECOND PATIENT WITHOUT ADEQUATE MEDICAL INDICATION TO JUSTIFY SURGERIES DUE TO INCREASING LIKELIHOOD OF A POOR PROGNOSIS FOR EACH SUCCESSIVE SURGERY; FROM 11/89 TO 1/90 EXAMINED AND TREATED A THIRD PATIENT WITH BACK PAIN AND FAILED TO ADEQUATELY INTERVENE AND TREAT PATIENT DESPITE INDICATIONS THAT IMMEDIATE REFERRAL WAS NEEDED; HE NEITHER ADMITS NOR DENIES THESE FINDINGS. REVOCATION STAYED. PUBLIC REPRIMAND; PROBATION WITH TERMS: SHALL NOT PERFORM ANY BACK SURGERY OR SURGERY REQUIRING GENERAL ANESTHESIA WITHOUT OBTAINING A CONSULT FROM A BOARD-APPROVED PHYSICIAN; SHALL NOT PERFORM ANY BACK SURGERY OR SURGERY REQUIRING GENERAL ANESTHESIA WITHOUT A BOARD APPROVED ASSISTING SURGEON; SHALL OBTAIN AT LEAST 60 HOURS PER YEAR OF CONTINUING MEDICAL EDUCATION, AT LEAST 15 HOURS OF WHICH SHALL CONSIST OF SURGICAL COURSES OR SEMINARS; SHALL APPEAR BEFORE BOARD AT LEAST TWICE A YEAR; SHALL COOPERATE WITH THE BOARD IN VERIFYING COMPLIANCE; SHALL GIVE A COPY OF THIS ORDER TO ANY HEALTH CARE ENTITY WHERE HE HAS PRIVILEGES; SHALL PROVIDE A COPY OF THIS ORDER TO ANYONE REQUESTING IT WITHIN 10 DAYS; TIME SPENT OUT OF TEXAS DOES NOT COUNT TOWARD PROBATION; SHALL INFORM BOARD OF CHANGE OF ADDRESS WITHIN 10 DAYS OR IF HE LEAVES THE STATE. SHALL NOT SEEK MODIFICATION FOR ONE YEAR. ON 10/5/96 HIS REQUEST FOR MODIFICATION OF THIS ORDER WAS DENIED. ON 9/20/97 PETITION TO TERMINATE ORDER DENIED. ON 8/22/98 PETITION TO TERMINATE ORDER DENIED; ORDER MODIFIED ALLOWING HIM TO OBTAIN CONTINUING MEDICAL EDUCATION HOURS PRIOR TO THE BEGINNING OF THE ORDER'S YEAR, AND REDUCING APPEARANCES BEFORE THE BOARD FROM BIANNUAL TO UPON BOARD'S REQUEST.

DU, LIEM CHI MD, LICENSE NUMBER H9892 OF SAN ANTONIO, TX, WAS DISCIPLINED BY TEXAS ON AUGUST 9, 1997

DISCIPLINARY ACTION: FINE
OFFENSE: PROFESSIONAL MISCONDUCT

NOTES: ALLEGATIONS THAT HE IMPROPERLY USED HIS POSITION AS A PHYSICIAN BY CONTACTING SEVERAL OF HIS PATIENTS AND ATTEMPTING TO RECRUIT THEM INTO A BUSINESS VENTURE. $1,000 FINE; SHALL COOPERATE WITH THE BOARD IN VERIFYING COMPLIANCE.

DUBIN, JOSEPH DO, LICENSE NUMBER 00C2154 OF DALLAS, TX, WAS DISCIPLINED BY TEXAS ON JUNE 22, 1994
DISCIPLINARY ACTION: REPRIMAND
OFFENSE: OVERPRESCRIBING OR MISPRESCRIBING DRUGS

NOTES: ALLEGATIONS OF NON-THERAPEUTIC PRESCRIBING OF PHENMETRAZINE, PHENTERMINE HYDROCHLORIDE AND THYROID MEDICATIONS FOR WEIGHT LOSS; STAFF CONTENDS VIOLATION OF MEDICAL ACT; HE CONTENDS THAT THERE IS NO VIOLATION EXCEPT AS TO INADEQUATE RECORD-KEEPING; ALLEGATIONS RELATE TO EVENTS BETWEEN 1984 AND 1989; NO EVIDENCE THAT HE HAS TREATED PATIENTS FOR WEIGHT LOSS SINCE 1989; HE AGREED TO THIS ORDER IN LIEU OF A HEARING. SHALL GIVE A COPY OF THE ORDER TO ANY HEALTH CARE ENTITY WHERE HE HAS PRIVILEGES.

DUGGER, DAVID LEON MD, DATE OF BIRTH DECEMBER 26, 1944, LICENSE NUMBER 0006909 OF 3626 NORTH MACARTHUR, IRVING, TX, WAS DISCIPLINED BY MISSISSIPPI ON JANUARY 18, 1990
DISCIPLINARY ACTION: RESTRICTION PLACED ON LICENSE

NOTES: CONSENT ORDER RESTRICTED LICENSE.

DUNCAN, JOHN DAVID MD, LICENSE NUMBER 00D4980 OF DUMAS, TX, WAS DISCIPLINED BY TEXAS ON OCTOBER 1, 1993
DISCIPLINARY ACTION: SURRENDER OF CONTROLLED SUBSTANCE LICENSE; 84-MONTH PROBATION
OFFENSE: SUBSTANCE ABUSE

NOTES: HAS DEVELOPED AN ADMITTED ALCOHOL PROBLEM WHICH BECAME MORE ACUTE DURING 1992; HAS NOT CONSUMED ALCOHOL SINCE 10/92; HAS PERIODICALLY ATTENDED AA AND PARTICIPATED WITH PHYSICIANS HEALTH COMMITTEE; CHARGES WERE PENDING AS OF ORDER DATE FOR AN ALCOHOL-RELATED AUTOMOBILE-PEDESTRIAN ACCIDENT. SUSPENSION STAYED. CONDITIONS OF PROBATION: SHALL ABSTAIN FROM THE CONSUMPTION OF ALCOHOL/CHEMICAL SUBSTANCES UNLESS PRESCRIBED BY ANOTHER PHYSICIAN FOR A LEGITIMATE AND THERAPEUTIC PURPOSE; SHALL SUBMIT HIMSELF FOR APPROPRIATE EXAMS INCLUDING DRUG OR ALCOHOL SCREENS; SHALL SURRENDER HIS DEA AND TEXAS CONTROLLED SUBSTANCES CERTIFICATE AND ALL UNUSED TRIPLICATE PRESCRIPTION FORMS; SHALL NOT ATTEMPT TO REREGISTER THESE REGISTRATIONS WITHOUT PERMISSION; SHALL CONTINUE TO PARTICIPATE IN AA'S PROGRAM NOT LESS THAN ONCE A WEEK WITH QUARTERLY REPORTS; SHALL CONTINUE TO PARTICIPATE IN ACTIVITIES OF A PHYSICIAN HEALTH AND REHABILITATION COMMITTEE AND ATTEND WEEKLY MEETINGS WITH QUARTERLY REPORTS; SHALL SUBMIT HIMSELF FOR EVALUATION AND TREATMENT TO A BOARD-APPROVED PSYCHIATRIST; SHALL GIVE A COPY OF THIS ORDER TO ANY HEALTH CARE ENTITY WHERE HE HAS PRIVILEGES; SHALL COOPERATE WITH THE BOARD IN VERIFYING COMPLIANCE; SHALL INFORM THE BOARD OF CHANGE OF ADDRESS WITHIN 10 DAYS OR IF HE LEAVES THE STATE; TIME SPENT OUT OF TEXAS DOES NOT COUNT TOWARD PROBATION; SHALL APPEAR BEFORE THE BOARD ONCE A YEAR. SHALL NOT SEEK MODIFICATION FOR ONE YEAR.

DUNCAN, JOHN DAVID MD, DATE OF BIRTH NOVEMBER 5, 1942, LICENSE NUMBER 0024901 OF DEL RIO, TX, WAS DISCIPLINED BY NORTH CAROLINA ON JUNE 19, 1995

NOTES: SEVEN YEAR SUSPENSION, STAYED. MUST COMPLY WITH CONDITIONS OF CONSENT ORDER.

DUNCAN, JOHN DAVID MD, LICENSE NUMBER 00D4980, WAS DISCIPLINED BY TEXAS ON OCTOBER 5, 1996
DISCIPLINARY ACTION: LICENSE SUSPENSION; MONITORING OF PHYSICIAN PERFORMANCE
OFFENSE: FAILURE TO COMPLY WITH PREVIOUS BOARD ORDER

NOTES: NONCOMPLIANCE TO THE ORDER DATED 10/01/93: SUFFERED RELAPSE INTO THE USE OF ALCOHOL IN APRIL 1996; RECEIVED INPATIENT TREATMENT FROM 7/28/96 TO 8/25/96; AND REPORTS A SOBRIETY DATE OF 7/28/96. SCHEDULED TO STAND TRIAL ON 9/30/96 FOR INVOLUNTARY MANSLAUGHTER AND FAILURE TO RENDER AID IN CONNECTION WITH AN AUTOMOBILE ACCIDENT WHICH OCCURRED ON 10/16/92. SUSPENSION UNTIL HE REQUESTS TO HAVE THE SUSPENSION STAYED OR LIFTED AND APPEARS BEFORE THE BOARD WITH SUFFICIENT EVIDENCE THAT HE IS PHYSICALLY, MENTALLY, AND OTHERWISE COMPETENT TO SAFELY PRACTICE MEDICINE INCLUDING AT A MINIMUM EVIDENCE OF CONTINUED ABSTINENCE FROM ALCOHOL OR DRUGS; ADVOCACY OF A LOCAL COUNTY MEDICAL SOCIETY; COMPLETE COPIES OF MEDICAL RECORDS AND REPORTS OF HIS INPATIENT TREATMENT INDICATING HIS ABILITY TO SAFELY PRACTICE MEDICINE; AND MAINTENANCE OF CLINICAL COMPETENCY THROUGH APPROPRIATE CONTINUING MEDICAL EDUCATION. IF HE IS FOUND GUILTY OR CONVICTED OF A FELONY OR MISDEMEANOR INVOLVING MORAL TURPITUDE HIS LICENSE SHALL BE REVOKED; SHALL INFORM THE BOARD OF ANY CHANGES IN ADDRESS WITHIN 10 DAYS.

DUNCAN, RICHARD PERRY DO, LICENSE NUMBER 00D0452 OF HOUSTON, TX, WAS DISCIPLINED BY TEXAS ON JANUARY 12, 1991
DISCIPLINARY ACTION: SURRENDER OF CONTROLLED SUBSTANCE LICENSE; 120-MONTH CONTROLLED SUBSTANCE LICENSE PLACED ON PROBATION

NOTES: MUST SURRENDER ALL UNUSED TRIPLICATE PRESCRIPTION FORMS AND NOT ATTEMPT TO ORDER MORE UNTIL HE HAS BOARD PERMISSION; SURRENDER DEA AND TEXAS CONTROLLED SUBSTANCE REGISTRATION CERTIFICATES; NOT ATTEMPT TO REREGISTER OR OTHERWISE OBTAIN CONTROLLED SUBSTANCES REGISTRATIONS UNTIL HE HAS BOARD PERMISSION; SURRENDER ALL CONTROLLED SUBSTANCES, INCLUDING SAMPLES, IN HIS POSSESSION OR SUBJECT TO HIS CONTROL, NOR POSSESS ANY SUCH CONTROLLED SUBSTANCES; ABSTAIN FROM CONSUMPTION OF ALCOHOL/CHEMICAL SUBSTANCES; PARTICIPATE OR CONTINUE TO PARTICIPATE IN HARRIS COUNTY MEDICAL SOCIETY COMMITTEE ON PHYSICIAN HEALTH AND REHABILITATION, ALCOHOLICS ANONYMOUS, AND TEXAS OSTEOPATHIC MEDICAL ASSOCIATION PHYSICIAN ASSISTANCE PROGRAM; REPORT IMMEDIATELY ANY INCIDENT IN WHICH HE CONSUMES ALCOHOL OR USES CONTROLLED SUBSTANCE NOT PRESCRIBED BY ANOTHER PHYSICIAN; SUBMIT TO APPROPRIATE EXAMINATIONS TO DETERMINE FREEDOM FROM DRUGS AND ALCOHOL; MAINTAIN ADEQUATE MEDICAL RECORDS ON PATIENT OFFICE

VISITS TO INCLUDE SPECIFIC INFORMATION. ORDER TERMINATED ON 5/11/95.

DUNEGAN, MARK ALAN MD, LICENSE NUMBER H8013 OF HOUSTON, TX, WAS DISCIPLINED BY TEXAS ON DECEMBER 11, 1999
DISCIPLINARY ACTION: SURRENDER OF LICENSE
OFFENSE: SUBSTANCE ABUSE

NOTES: ALLEGED INTEMPERATE USE OF CONTROLLED SUBSTANCES. VOLUNTARY SURRENDER OF LICENSE.

DUNN, FRANK LANIER MD, LICENSE NUMBER 00B9641 OF KERRVILLE, TX, WAS DISCIPLINED BY TEXAS ON APRIL 26, 1991
DISCIPLINARY ACTION: LICENSE SUSPENSION
OFFENSE: OVERPRESCRIBING OR MISPRESCRIBING DRUGS

NOTES: NONTHERAPEUTIC PRESCRIBING AND INADEQUATE MEDICAL PRACTICES.

DUNN, FRANK LANIER MD, LICENSE NUMBER 00B9641 OF KERRVILLE, TX, WAS DISCIPLINED BY TEXAS ON JUNE 16, 1992
DISCIPLINARY ACTION: LICENSE REVOCATION
OFFENSE: DISCIPLINARY ACTION BY ANOTHER STATE OR AGENCY

NOTES: ALSO VIOLATIONS INVOLVING THE PRESCRIBING OF CONTROLLED SUBSTANCES. PROFESSIONAL FAILURE TO PRACTICE MEDICINE CONSISTENT WITH PUBLIC HEALTH AND WELFARE.

DUNN, JACK III MD, LICENSE NUMBER H6182 OF LUBBOCK, TX, WAS DISCIPLINED BY TEXAS ON SEPTEMBER 20, 1997
DISCIPLINARY ACTION: LICENSE SUSPENSION; REQUIRED TO TAKE ADDITIONAL MEDICAL EDUCATION
OFFENSE: LOSS OR RESTRICTION OF HOSPITAL PRIVILEGES

NOTES: IN 2/95 CONCERNS WERE RAISED THAT HE MAY HAVE BEEN IMPAIRED WHILE PERFORMING ANESTHESIOLOGY; IN APRIL/MAY 1995 HOSPITAL ADMINISTRATION RECEIVED COMPLAINTS OF HIS FAILING TO RESPOND TO PAGES, IF AT ALL, AND A LESS THAN PROFESSIONAL ATTITUDE TOWARDS ANESTHESIA AS HE FREQUENTLY ARRIVED LATE TO THE OPERATING ROOM; IN 5/95; A URINE SPECIMEN RESULTED IN A POSITIVE DRUG SCREEN FOR AMPHETAMINES; HE ATTRIBUTED THE RESULT TO ALLERGY MEDICATION; ON 7/3/95 RATHER THAN PROPERLY PLACING THE EPIDURAL'S CATHETER IN A PATIENT'S SPINAL CANAL, IN GROSS ERROR HE PLACED IT IN HER ABDOMEN; IN ADDITION, HE ALSO ADMINISTERED INAPPROPRIATE DOSAGES OF ANESTHESIA DRUGS; THE PATIENT WENT INTO SEIZURES, SUFFERED CARDIAC ARREST WHICH CAUSED HER AND HER UNBORN CHILD TO DIE; SETTLED A MALPRACTICE CLAIM WITH RESPECT TO THIS CASE FOR 1 MILLION DOLLARS; AS A RESULT OF THE SUBSTANDARD CARE OF THE PATIENT, HE WAS REMOVED AS A MEMBER OF THE PHYSICIAN GROUP; IN 10/95 THE NATURE OF THE COMPLAINTS ESCALATED: DISAPPEARING OR FALLING ASLEEP DURING SURGICAL CASES, HABITUALLY ARRIVING TO WORK LATE, ALONG WITH FAILING TO ADEQUATELY RESPOND TO CALLS; ON 10/13/95 HOSPITAL PRIVILEGES WERE SUMMARILY SUSPENDED; THE BOARD RECEIVED INFORMATION THAT HE HAD SELF-PRESCRIBED HALCION AND PROZAC WITHOUT LEGITIMATE MEDICAL PURPOSE; IN 1995/EARLY 1996 HE PRESCRIBED CONTROLLED SUBSTANCES AND DANGEROUS DRUGS TO AN ADULT FEMALE PATIENT WITHOUT A LEGITIMATE PURPOSE; HE WAS ROMANTICALLY INVOLVED WITH THE PATIENT WHO WAS UNDER THE CARE OF ANOTHER LICENSED TEXAS PHYSICIAN WHO HAD DIAGNOSED HER TO BE ADDICTED TO THE PAIN MEDICATION; HE HAS UNDERGONE MEDICAL EVALUATIONS BUT HAS NOT FOLLOWED RECOMMENDATIONS. SUSPENSION UNTIL HE REQUESTS TO HAVE THE SUSPENSION STAYED OR LIFTED AND APPEARS BEFORE THE BOARD WITH SUFFICIENT EVIDENCE THAT HE IS PHYSICALLY, MENTALLY AND OTHERWISE COMPETENT TO PRACTICE SAFELY INCLUDING AT A MINIMUM SATISFACTORILY COMPLETING AN INPATIENT EVALUATION WITH ALL MEDICAL RECORDS FURNISHED TO THE BOARD FOR CHEMICAL DEPENDENCY OF NOT LESS THAN 96 HOURS CONSECUTIVE DURATION; SHALL OBTAIN 50 HOURS OF CONTINUING MEDICAL EDUCATION PER YEAR. ON 10/15/99 REQUEST TO HAVE SUSPENSION STAYED DENIED.

DUNN, JACK III MD, DATE OF BIRTH SEPTEMBER 10, 1954 OF 4709 19TH STREET, LUBBOCK, TX, WAS DISCIPLINED BY MEDICARE ON JANUARY 20, 1999
DISCIPLINARY ACTION: EXCLUSION FROM THE MEDICARE AND/OR MEDICAID PROGRAM
OFFENSE: DISCIPLINARY ACTION BY ANOTHER STATE OR AGENCY

NOTES: LICENSE REVOKED, SUSPENDED, SURRENDERED OR OTHERWISE LOST FOR REASONS BEARING ON PROFESSIONAL PERFORMANCE, PROFESSIONAL COMPETENCE OR FINANCIAL INTEGRITY.

DWYER, EDWARD J MD, DATE OF BIRTH DECEMBER 18, 1943, LICENSE NUMBER 00D6582 OF AUSTIN, TX, WAS DISCIPLINED BY TEXAS ON AUGUST 24, 1991
DISCIPLINARY ACTION: 60-MONTH PROBATION; RESTRICTION PLACED ON LICENSE
OFFENSE: FAILURE TO COMPLY WITH PREVIOUS BOARD ORDER

NOTES: VIOLATED PREVIOUS BOARD ORDER. REVOCATION STAYED. TERMS OF PROBATION: SHALL ATTEND 10 HOURS PER YEAR OF AN ETHICS COURSE IN ADDITION TO 50 HOURS REQUIRED UNDER PREVIOUS ORDER; SHALL OBTAIN BLUE CROSS/BLUE SHIELD AND MEDICARE GUIDELINES FOR PHYSICIAN CHARGES; SHALL REFRAIN FROM PRESCRIBING OR ADMINISTERING TENS UNIT TREATMENT; SHALL MAKE REFUNDS TO PARTICULAR PATIENTS; SHALL APPEAR BEFORE BOARD TWICE A YEAR.

DWYER, EDWARD J MD, DATE OF BIRTH DECEMBER 18, 1943, LICENSE NUMBER 00D6582 OF 3410 FAR WEST BOULEVARD #145, AUSTIN, TX, WAS DISCIPLINED BY TEXAS ON AUGUST 20, 1993
DISCIPLINARY ACTION: SURRENDER OF LICENSE
OFFENSE: PHYSICAL OR MENTAL ILLNESS INHIBITING THE ABILITY TO PRACTICE WITH SKILL AND SAFETY

NOTES: HAS VOLUNTARILY CEASED PRACTICING MEDICINE DUE TO AN ILLNESS. SHALL SURRENDER HIS DEA AND TEXAS CONTROLLED SUBSTANCES REGISTRATION AND ALL UNUSED PRESCRIPTION AND TRIPLICATE PRESCRIPTION FORMS. LICENSE WILL BE REINSTATED UNDER THE FOLLOWING CONDITIONS: SHALL SUBMIT HIMSELF FOR EVALUATION TO TWO BOARD APPROVED PSYCHIATRISTS AND BOTH MUST CONCLUDE HIS HEALTH HAS BEEN RESTORED OR HIS ILLNESS IS CAPABLE OF BEING TREATED AND CONTROLLED ON A CONTINUING BASIS TO SUCH AN EXTENT THAT HE IS CAPABLE OF PRACTICING.

DWYER, EDWARD JOSEPH MD OF 3410 FAR WEST BLVD, AUSTIN, TX, WAS DISCIPLINED BY DEA ON SEPTEMBER 21, 1993
DISCIPLINARY ACTION: SURRENDER OF CONTROLLED SUBSTANCE LICENSE
OFFENSE: DISCIPLINARY ACTION BY ANOTHER STATE OR AGENCY

NOTES: SURRENDERED FOR CAUSE TO TEXAS STATE BOARD

OF MEDICAL EXAMINERS.

DWYER, PATRICK DAVID MD, LICENSE NUMBER 00E7393 OF SUGAR LAND, TX, WAS DISCIPLINED BY TEXAS ON APRIL 15, 1994
DISCIPLINARY ACTION: 60-MONTH PROBATION; REQUIRED TO TAKE ADDITIONAL MEDICAL EDUCATION
OFFENSE: OVERPRESCRIBING OR MISPRESCRIBING DRUGS

NOTES: PROVIDED MEDICATIONS TO HIS WIFE WITHOUT INDICATIONS OVER THE COURSE OF SEVERAL YEARS ENDING IN 1991; FAILED TO KEEP ADEQUATE RECORDS OF DRUGS AND THE QUANTITY OF THOSE DRUGS SUPPLIED TO HIS WIFE. SUSPENSION STAYED. CONDITIONS OF PROBATION: WITHIN ONE YEAR SHALL COMPLETE A TWO WEEK PRECEPTORSHIP ON THE PREVENTION AND TREATMENT OF DRUG ABUSE; SHALL REFRAIN FROM PRESCRIBING ANY DRUG THAT IS NOT MEDICALLY INDICATED; SHALL REFRAIN FROM THE USE OF AND SHALL NOT POSSESS, ADMINISTER OR PRESCRIBE ANY PRESCRIPTION DRUG UNLESS PRESCRIBED BY ANOTHER PHYSICIAN FOR A LEGITIMATE AND THERAPEUTIC PURPOSE; SHALL NOT TREAT OR OTHERWISE SERVE AS PHYSICIAN, PRESCRIBE, DISPENSE, OR ADMINISTER DRUGS THAT MAY BE SUBJECT TO ABUSE TO HIMSELF OR ANY MEMBER OF HIS FAMILY; HE SHALL MAINTAIN A FILE SEPARATE FROM PATIENT RECORDS OF EVERY PRESCRIPTION WRITTEN FOR CONTROLLED SUBSTANCES OR DANGEROUS DRUGS, A LOG OF ANY PRESCRIPTIONS CALLED INTO A PHARMACY. AND ADEQUATE MEDICAL RECORDS ON PATIENT OFFICE VISITS ALL OF WHICH SHALL BE AVAILABLE FOR INSPECTION; SHALL ATTEND AT LEAST 50 HOURS PER YEAR OF CONTINUING MEDICAL EDUCATION; SHALL APPEAR BEFORE THE BOARD ONCE A YEAR; SHALL GIVE A COPY OF THIS ORDER TO ANY HEALTH CARE ENTITY WHERE HE HAS PRIVILEGES; SHALL COOPERATE WITH THE BOARD IN VERIFYING COMPLIANCE; SHALL INFORM BOARD OF CHANGE OF ADDRESS WITHIN 10 DAYS OR IF HE LEAVES THE STATE; TIME SPENT OUT OF TEXAS DOES NOT COUNT TOWARD PROBATION. SHALL NOT SEEK MODIFICATION FOR ONE YEAR. ON 5/11/95 HIS REQUEST FOR TERMINATION DENIED. PROBATION TERMINATED ON 5/15/96.

DYKE, MARSHALL J MD OF 333 NORTH RIVERSIDE DR. STE 100, CONROE, TX, WAS DISCIPLINED BY DEA ON MAY 5, 1994
DISCIPLINARY ACTION: SURRENDER OF CONTROLLED SUBSTANCE LICENSE

NOTES: IN LIEU OF PUBLIC INTEREST REVOCATION.

DYKE, MARSHALL J MD, LICENSE NUMBER D1619, WAS DISCIPLINED BY TEXAS ON MARCH 1, 1997
DISCIPLINARY ACTION: LICENSE SUSPENSION
OFFENSE: FAILURE TO COMPLY WITH PREVIOUS BOARD ORDER

NOTES: VIOLATED TERMS OF 2/12/96 ORDER BY FAILING TO TAKE AND PASS THE SPEX BY 2/12/97. SUSPENDED UNTIL SUCH A TIME AS HE DOES PASS THE SPEX AND APPEARS BEFORE THE BOARD TO PROVIDE EVIDENCE OF SUFFICIENT SKILLS AND KNOWLEDGE TO SAFELY PRACTICE MEDICINE IN TEXAS AND OF PHYSICAL AND MENTAL COMPETENCE TO DO SO. ON 4/4/98 REQUEST TO HAVE SUSPENSION LIFTED DENIED.

DYKE, MARSHALL JAMES MD, LICENSE NUMBER 00D1619 OF CONROE, TX, WAS DISCIPLINED BY TEXAS ON DECEMBER 4, 1991
DISCIPLINARY ACTION: 60-MONTH PROBATION; RESTRICTION PLACED ON LICENSE
OFFENSE: SUBSTANCE ABUSE

NOTES: HAS ENGAGED IN THE INTEMPERATE USE OF COCAINE SINCE 4/91; VOLUNTARILY ADMITTED HIMSELF TO THE HOSPITAL ON 8/6/91. SUSPENSION STAYED; CONDITIONS OF PROBATION: SHALL SURRENDER SCHEDULE II AND IIN OF DEA AND TEXAS CONTROLLED SUBSTANCES REGISTRATIONS, AND SHALL NOT ATTEMPT TO REREGISTER OR OTHERWISE OBTAIN THESE LICENSES WITHOUT WRITTEN AUTHORITY OF THE BOARD; SHALL SURRENDER ALL UNUSED TRIPLICATE PRESCRIPTION FORMS; SHALL APPEAR BEFORE THE BOARD TWICE A YEAR; SHALL NOT TREAT OR PRESCRIBE DRUGS TO HIMSELF OR ANY MEMBER OF HIS IMMEDIATE FAMILY; SHALL ABSTAIN FROM THE CONSUMPTION OF ALCOHOL/CHEMICAL SUBSTANCES, WITH EXPLANATION TO THE BOARD WITHIN 24 HOURS IF HE DOES SO; SHALL PARTICIPATE IN IMPAIRED PHYSICIANS PROGRAM, WITH QUARTERLY REPORTS TO THE BOARD; SHALL PARTICIPATE IN AA OR NARCOTICS ANONYMOUS, INCLUDING A 12-STEP PROGRAM, AT LEAST 3 TIMES PER WEEK; SHALL SUBMIT TO RANDOM SCREENING OF BODILY FLUIDS, AND SHALL ALWAYS BE SCREENED TWICE ON DAYS HE PERFORMS SURGERY; SHALL CONTINUE IN EITHER INPATIENT OR OUTPATIENT CARE AS DETERMINED BY HIS TREATING PHYSICIAN, WITH QUARTERLY REPORTS TO THE BOARD; SHALL IMMEDIATELY NOTIFY THE BOARD IF HE DISCONTINUES TREATMENT; SHALL SUBMIT TO PSYCHIATRIC EVALUATION BY A BOARD APPROVED PSYCHIATRIST AND ABIDE BY RECOMMENDATIONS; SHALL NOT OPERATE ON ANY PATIENT UNLESS ANOTHER OTOLARYNGOLOGIST IS AVAILABLE IN THE BUILDING; SHALL GET BOARD PERMISSION TO CHANGE HIS SPECIALTY; SHALL COOPERATE WITH BOARD IN VERIFYING COMPLIANCE; SHALL ADVISE THE BOARD OF A CHANGE OF ADDRESS WITHIN 10 DAYS; TIME SPENT OUT OF TEXAS DOES NOT COUNT TOWARDS PROBATION; SHALL NOT SEEK MODIFICATION OF ORDER FOR AT LEAST ONE YEAR.

DYKE, MARSHALL JAMES MD, LICENSE NUMBER 00D1619 OF CONROE, TX, WAS DISCIPLINED BY TEXAS ON MARCH 4, 1994
DISCIPLINARY ACTION: EMERGENCY SUSPENSION
OFFENSE: FAILURE TO COMPLY WITH PREVIOUS BOARD ORDER

NOTES: ALLEGATIONS OF NONCOMPLIANCE WITH 12/4/91 ORDER INCLUDING INGESTING COCAINE AS INDICATED BY A POSITIVE REPORT OF A BLOOD SAMPLE TAKEN ON 2/17/94 NOT PURSUANT TO A PRESCRIPTION BY A PRIMARY CARE PHYSICIAN AND NOT REPORTED TO THE BOARD; HOSPITAL PRIVILEGES WERE TEMPORARILY SUSPENDED PENDING A HEARING ON HIS USE OF COCAINE.

DYKE, MARSHALL JAMES MD, LICENSE NUMBER 00D1619 OF CONROE, TX, WAS DISCIPLINED BY TEXAS ON MAY 11, 1995
DISCIPLINARY ACTION: LICENSE SUSPENSION; REQUIRED TO TAKE ADDITIONAL MEDICAL EDUCATION
OFFENSE: FAILURE TO COMPLY WITH PREVIOUS BOARD ORDER

NOTES: INABILITY TO PRACTICE MEDICINE WITH REASONABLE SKILL AND SAFETY DUE TO EXCESSIVE USE OF COCAINE; USED COCAINE IN 2/94 IN VIOLATION OF 12/04/91 ORDER; PRIVILEGES AT CLEVELAND REGIONAL MEDICAL CENTER SUBSEQUENTLY SUSPENDED; FOLLOWING 3/94 ORDER OF EMERGENCY SUSPENSION, HE RECEIVED INPATIENT TREATMENT FOR SUBSTANCE ABUSE FROM A RESIDENTIAL TREATMENT PROGRAM BETWEEN 5/16/94 AND 6/6/94; RECEIVED OUTPATIENT CARE AT A TRANSITIONAL LIVING FACILITY IN 6/94; HAS ATTENDED AA MEETINGS DAILY FOR 120 DAYS AND IS

NOW ATTENDING THREE TIMES PER WEEK AS REQUIRED BY HIS CONTRACT WITH THE COUNTY MEDICAL SOCIETY; HAS PARTICIPATED ON A REGULAR BASIS IN THE ACTIVITIES OF THE COMMITTEE ON PHYSICIAN HEALTH AND REHABILITATION; HAS ENTERED INTO A RECOVERY CONTRACT WITH AN IMPAIRED PHYSICIANS PROGRAM. SUSPENSION UNTIL HE REQUESTS TO HAVE SUSPENSION STAYED OR LIFTED AND APPEARS BEFORE BOARD WITH SUFFICIENT EVIDENCE THAT HE IS PHYSICALLY, MENTALLY AND OTHERWISE COMPETENT TO SAFELY PRACTICE MEDICINE INCLUDING AT A MINIMUM PROVIDING COPIES OF MEDICAL RECORDS AND REPORTS OF PSYCHOLOGICAL AND NEUROPSYCHIATRIC EVALUATIONS BY A BOARD-APPROVED PSYCHIATRIST. SHALL ABSTAIN FROM THE CONSUMPTION OF ALCOHOL/DRUGS IN ANY FORM UNLESS PRESCRIBED BY ANOTHER PHYSICIAN FOR A LEGITIMATE AND THERAPEUTIC PURPOSE; SHALL SUBMIT HIMSELF FOR APPROPRIATE EXAMS INCLUDING DRUG OR ALCOHOL SCREENS; SHALL SUBMIT HIMSELF FOR EVALUATION AND TREATMENT BY A BOARD APPROVED PSYCHIATRIST WHO SHALL REPORT TO THE BOARD; SHALL CONTINUE TO PARTICIPATE IN AA PROGRAMS NOT LESS THAN FIVE TIMES A WEEK WITH QUARTERLY REPORTS; SHALL PARTICIPATE IN THE ACTIVITIES OF A PHYSICIANS COUNSELING GROUP AND ATTEND WEEKLY MEETINGS WITH QUARTERLY REPORTS; SHALL OBTAIN AT LEAST 50 HOURS PER YEAR OF CONTINUING MEDICAL EDUCATION, WITH PROOF OF ATTENDANCE; SHALL INFORM BOARD OF CHANGE OF ADDRESS WITHIN 10 DAYS. SHALL NOT APPLY FOR TERMINATION OF ORDER FOR THREE MONTHS.

DYKE, MARSHALL JAMES MD, LICENSE NUMBER 00D1619, WAS DISCIPLINED BY TEXAS ON FEBRUARY 12, 1996
DISCIPLINARY ACTION: 120-MONTH PROBATION; RESTRICTION PLACED ON CONTROLLED SUBSTANCE LICENSE
OFFENSE: SUBSTANCE ABUSE

NOTES: SATISFIED THE MINIMUM REQUIREMENTS AS SET OUT IN THE 5/11/95 SUSPENSION. SUSPENSION STAYED, AS PROBATION WITH TERMS AND CONDITIONS: SHALL ABSTAIN FROM THE CONSUMPTION OF ALCOHOL/DRUGS IN ANY FORM UNLESS PRESCRIBED BY ANOTHER PHYSICIAN FOR A LEGITIMATE AND THERAPEUTIC PURPOSE; SHALL SUBMIT HIMSELF FOR APPROPRIATE EXAMS INCLUDING DRUG OR ALCOHOL SCREENS; SHALL CONTINUE TO RECEIVE CARE AND TREATMENT FROM A BOARD SPECIFIED PHYSICIAN WHOM HE SHALL SEE AT LEAST ONCE A MONTH AND WHO SHALL SUBMIT QUARTERLY REPORTS TO THE BOARD; SHALL CONTINUE TO PARTICIPATE IN AA'S PROGRAMS NOT LESS THAN THREE TIMES A WEEK WITH QUARTERLY REPORTS; SHALL PARTICIPATE IN THE ACTIVITIES OF A PHYSICIAN HEALTH AND REHABILITATION GROUP AND ATTEND WEEKLY MEETINGS WITH QUARTERLY REPORTS; SHALL COMPLY WITH THE TERMS AND CONDITIONS OF ANY CONTINUING CARE CONTRACT WITH QUARTERLY REPORTS TO THE BOARD EXCEPT AS OTHERWISE PROVIDED FOR IN THIS ORDER; SHALL NOT POSSESS ALCOHOL, CONTROLLED SUBSTANCES, OR DANGEROUS DRUGS WITH POTENTIAL FOR ABUSE; SHALL SURRENDER ALL CONTROLLED SUBSTANCES AND DANGEROUS DRUGS WITH ADDICTIVE POTENTIAL INCLUDING SAMPLES; SHALL NOT TREAT OR OTHERWISE SERVE AS PHYSICIAN, PRESCRIBE, DISPENSE OR ADMINISTER DRUGS WITH ADDICTIVE POTENTIAL TO HIMSELF OR ANY MEMBER OF HIS FAMILY; SHALL NOT TELEPHONE TO A PHARMACY A PRESCRIPTION OR REFILL FOR CONTROLLED SUBSTANCES OR DANGEROUS DRUGS WITH ADDICTIVE POTENTIAL AND SHALL NOT PERMIT ANY INDIVIDUAL UNDER HIS SUPERVISION TO DO SO; SHALL IMMEDIATELY SURRENDER HIS DEA CONTROLLED SUBSTANCE REGISTRATION CERTIFICATE AND TEXAS CONTROLLED SUBSTANCES REGISTRATION CERTIFICATE; SHALL IMMEDIATELY SURRENDER ALL UNUSED TRIPLICATE PRESCRIPTION FORMS; SEPARATE FROM PATIENT RECORDS, SHALL MAINTAIN A FILE OF EVERY PRESCRIPTION WRITTEN BY HIM FOR DANGEROUS DRUGS WITH ADDICTIVE POTENTIAL WHICH SHALL BE AVAILABLE FOR REVIEW; HIS MEDICAL PRACTICE, INCLUDING ANY OFFICE AND SURGICAL PRACTICE, SHALL BE MONITORED BY A BOARD APPROVED TEXAS PHYSICIAN WHO SHALL SUBMIT QUARTERLY REPORTS TO THE BOARD; SHALL MAINTAIN ADEQUATE MEDICAL RECORDS WHICH SHALL BE AVAILABLE FOR REVIEW; SHALL OBTAIN AT LEAST 50 HOURS PER YEAR OF CONTINUING MEDICAL EDUCATION; WITHIN ONE YEAR SHALL TAKE AND PASS THE SPEX EXAM; SHALL APPEAR BEFORE THE BOARD AT LEAST TWO TIMES EACH YEAR; SHALL COOPERATE WITH THE BOARD IN VERIFYING COMPLIANCE INCLUDING PROVIDING COPIES OF MEDICAL RELEASES UPON REQUEST; SHALL GIVE A COPY OF THIS ORDER TO ANY HEALTH CARE ENTITY WHERE HE HAS PRIVILEGES; SHALL PROVIDE A COPY OF THIS ORDER TO ANYONE REQUESTING IT WITHIN 10 DAYS; TIME PERIOD OUT OF TEXAS DOES NOT COUNT TOWARD PROBATION; SHALL INFORM THE BOARD OF CHANGE OF ADDRESS WITHIN 10 DAYS OR IF HE LEAVES THE STATE; SHALL NOT SEEK MODIFICATION FOR ONE YEAR. ON 10/5/96 ORDER AMENDED AS FOLLOWS: HE IS ALLOWED TO REAPPLY FOR SCHEDULES III, III-N, IV AND V; HE IS ONLY ALLOWED TO PRESCRIBE SCHEDULE III-N CONTROLLED SUBSTANCE IF THE SUBSTANCE CONTAINS CODEINE; MAY TELEPHONE TO A PHARMACY A PRESCRIPTION OR REFILL FOR CONTROLLED SUBSTANCES OR DANGEROUS DRUGS PROVIDED HE SUPPLIES A WRITTEN PRESCRIPTION WITHIN 72 HOURS AND MAINTAINS A LOGBOOK OF ALL SUCH PRESCRIPTIONS.

DYKE, MARSHALL JAMES MD, LICENSE NUMBER D1619, WAS DISCIPLINED BY TEXAS ON MARCH 1, 1997
DISCIPLINARY ACTION: LICENSE SUSPENSION
OFFENSE: FAILURE TO COMPLY WITH PREVIOUS BOARD ORDER

NOTES: ON 2/12/96 ENTERED AN ORDER WITH THE BOARD STIPULATING THAT HE WOULD PASS THE SPEX WITHIN ONE YEAR OR HAVE HIS LICENSE SUSPENDED; HE HAS TAKEN AND FAILED THE EXAM TWICE IN THE ONE-YEAR PERIOD ALLOWED. THE BOARD MODIFIED THE ORDER, MAINTAINING THE SUSPENSION BUT STIPULATING THAT IF AND WHEN HE OBTAINS A SCORE OF 75 OR GREATER ON THE SPEX, HIS SUSPENSION WILL BE IMMEDIATELY TERMINATED, GRANTED THAT HE IS IN COMPLIANCE WITH ALL OTHER TERMS AND CONDITIONS. ON 4/4/98 AND 12/12/98 REQUEST TO HAVE HIS SUSPENSION LIFTED DENIED.

DYKE, MARSHALL JAMES MD, DATE OF BIRTH SEPTEMBER 4, 1937 OF 201 TODD ROAD, MAGNOLIA, TX, WAS DISCIPLINED BY MEDICARE ON NOVEMBER 19, 1998
DISCIPLINARY ACTION: EXCLUSION FROM THE MEDICARE AND/OR MEDICAID PROGRAM
OFFENSE: DISCIPLINARY ACTION BY ANOTHER STATE OR AGENCY

NOTES: LICENSE REVOKED, SUSPENDED, SURRENDERED OR OTHERWISE LOST FOR REASONS BEARING ON PROFESSIONAL PERFORMANCE, PROFESSIONAL

COMPETENCE OR FINANCIAL INTEGRITY.

EAKIN, DARYL LEE MD OF 11044 RESEARCH BLVD. #B400, AUSTIN, TX, WAS DISCIPLINED BY DEA ON OCTOBER 15, 1998
DISCIPLINARY ACTION: SURRENDER OF CONTROLLED SUBSTANCE LICENSE

EARGLE, CANTRAL L JR MD, LICENSE NUMBER 00G0694 OF DALLAS, TX, WAS DISCIPLINED BY TEXAS ON JUNE 22, 1994
DISCIPLINARY ACTION: REPRIMAND
OFFENSE: CRIMINAL CONVICTION OR PLEA OF GUILTY, NOLO CONTENDERE, OR NO CONTEST TO A CRIME

NOTES: ON 4/23/90 WAS CONVICTED OF THREE COUNTS OF WILLFUL FAILURE TO FILE INCOME TAX RETURNS; ON 1/2/91 CONVICTION WAS AFFIRMED BY THE U.S. COURT OF APPEALS. SHALL GIVE A COPY OF THIS ORDER TO ANY HEALTH CARE ENTITY WHERE HE HAS PRIVILEGES.

EARL, GENE M MD OF 1315 DOCTORS DRIVE, TYLER, TX, WAS DISCIPLINED BY DEA ON MAY 25, 1994
DISCIPLINARY ACTION: SURRENDER OF CONTROLLED SUBSTANCE LICENSE
OFFENSE: DISCIPLINARY ACTION BY ANOTHER STATE OR AGENCY

NOTES: STATE BOARD.

EARL, GENE MARKLEY JR MD, LICENSE NUMBER 00D9991 OF TYLER, TX, WAS DISCIPLINED BY TEXAS ON APRIL 15, 1994
DISCIPLINARY ACTION: SURRENDER OF CONTROLLED SUBSTANCE LICENSE; 60-MONTH PROBATION
OFFENSE: SUBSTANCE ABUSE

NOTES: BEGINNING IN 1990 SELF-PRESCRIBED ADDICTIVE SCHEDULED CONTROLLED SUBSTANCES DUE TO PAIN ASSOCIATED WITH SURGERIES HE HAD UNDERGONE; SUBSEQUENTLY BECAME ADDICTED TO THESE SUBSTANCES; TO SUPPORT HIS ADDICTION HE WROTE AND CALLED IN PRESCRIPTIONS IN THE NAME OF FAMILY MEMBERS FROM 1/1/92 TO 6/1/93 WHEN HE ENTERED A TREATMENT PROGRAM; SOBRIETY DATE IS 6/10/93; PARTICIPATED IN AA MEETINGS; HOSPITAL PLACED CERTAIN RESTRICTIONS ON HIS PRACTICE; IS CURRENTLY UNDER THE CARE OF A PSYCHOTHERAPIST AND AN ADDICTIONOLOGIST. SUSPENSION STAYED. CONDITIONS OF PROBATION: SHALL COMPLY WITH RESTRICTIONS IMPOSED BY HOSPITAL WHICH INCLUDE SPECIFYING HIS PRIMARY PHYSICIAN AND HIS SUPERVISOR WITH THE IMPAIRED PHYSICIAN'S GROUP; PROVIDING COPIES OF AFTERCARE CONTRACT AND LETTERS DETAILING THE FINDINGS OF HIS PHYSICIAN REGARDING AFTERCARE; SHALL HAVE PRIMARY CARE PHYSICIAN PROVIDE REPORTS; SHALL SUBMIT TO RANDOM TESTS OF BODILY FLUIDS; REPORTS WILL BE OBTAINED FROM THE DIRECTOR OF NURSING; REVIEWS WILL BE MADE OF A RANDOM SELECTION OF HIS INPATIENT CHARTS; ADDITIONAL CONDITIONS IMPOSED BY THE BOARD: SHALL INFORM THE BOARD WITHIN 10 DAYS IF PRIVILEGES AT HOSPITAL ARE TERMINATED; SHALL COMPLY WITH THE AFOREMENTIONED REQUIREMENTS IMPOSED BY HOSPITAL AND FORWARD ALL REPORTS SUBMITTED TO THE HOSPITAL TO THE BOARD; SHALL BE SUPERVISED BY A BOARD-APPROVED PHYSICIAN WITH QUARTERLY REPORTS; SHALL ABSTAIN FROM THE CONSUMPTION OF ALCOHOL/CHEMICAL SUBSTANCES IN ANY FORM UNLESS PRESCRIBED BY ANOTHER PHYSICIAN FOR A LEGITIMATE AND THERAPEUTIC PURPOSE; SHALL NOT TREAT OR OTHERWISE SERVE AS PHYSICIAN, PRESCRIBE, DISPENSE OR ADMINISTER DRUGS THAT MAY BE SUBJECT TO ABUSE TO HIMSELF OR ANY MEMBER OF HIS FAMILY; SHALL SURRENDER HIS DEA AND TEXAS CONTROLLED SUBSTANCES CERTIFICATES, ALL UNUSED TRIPLICATE PRESCRIPTION FORMS, AND ALL CONTROLLED SUBSTANCES INCLUDING SAMPLES IN HIS POSSESSION; SHALL NOT ATTEMPT TO REREGISTER WITHOUT APPROVAL; SHALL CONTINUE TO PARTICIPATE IN AA'S PROGRAM NOT LESS THAN THREE TIMES A WEEK WITH QUARTERLY REPORTS TO THE BOARD; SHALL SUBMIT HIMSELF FOR APPROPRIATE EXAMS INCLUDING DRUG OR ALCOHOL SCREENS; SHALL CONTINUE TREATMENT WITH HIS PSYCHOTHERAPIST WITH QUARTERLY REPORTS; SHALL APPEAR BEFORE THE BOARD TWICE A YEAR; SHALL GIVE A COPY OF THIS ORDER TO ANY HEALTH CARE ENTITY WHERE HE HAS PRIVILEGES; SHALL COOPERATE WITH THE BOARD IN VERIFYING COMPLIANCE; SHALL INFORM BOARD OF CHANGE OF ADDRESS WITHIN 10 DAYS OR IF HE LEAVES THE STATE; TIME SPENT OUT OF TEXAS DOES NOT COUNT TOWARD PROBATION. SHALL NOT SEEK MODIFICATION FOR ONE YEAR. ON 5/11/95 ORDER MODIFIED AS FOLLOWS: HE IS AUTHORIZED TO REAPPLY TO THE DEA AND TEXAS DEPARTMENT OF PUBLIC SAFETY TO OBTAIN FULL PRESCRIBING AUTHORITY FOR CONTROLLED SUBSTANCES; REQUIREMENT TO SURRENDER UNUSED TRIPLICATE PRESCRIPTION FORMS DELETED; SHALL BECOME FAMILIAR WITH AND COMPLY WITH ALL STATUTES, RULES AND REGULATIONS PERTAINING TO THE PRESCRIBING, ADMINISTERING AND DISPENSING OF CONTROLLED SUBSTANCES AND DANGEROUS DRUGS WITH ADDICTIVE POTENTIAL FOR ABUSE; SEPARATE FROM PATIENT RECORDS, SHALL MAINTAIN A FILE OF EVERY PRESCRIPTION WRITTEN FOR CONTROLLED SUBSTANCES WHICH SHALL BE AVAILABLE UPON BOARD INSPECTION; SHALL MAINTAIN A LOG OF ALL PRESCRIPTIONS OR REFILLS TELEPHONED IN FOR CONTROLLED SUBSTANCES OR DRUGS WITH ADDICTIVE POTENTIAL WHICH SHALL BE AVAILABLE FOR INSPECTION; SHALL GIVE A COPY OF THIS ORDER TO ALL PHARMACIES WHICH ROUTINELY FILL HIS PRESCRIPTION ORDERS. ON 5/10/97 BOARD GRANTED HIS PETITION FOR TERMINATION OF THIS ORDER BASED ON COMPLIANCE WITH CONDITIONS.

EASTER, THOMAS G II MD, DATE OF BIRTH FEBRUARY 26, 1952, LICENSE NUMBER 27470, WAS DISCIPLINED BY COLORADO ON AUGUST 18, 1999
DISCIPLINARY ACTION: SURRENDER OF LICENSE
OFFENSE: DISCIPLINARY ACTION BY ANOTHER STATE OR AGENCY

NOTES: DISCIPLINED IN ANOTHER STATE.

EASTER, THOMAS G II MD, LICENSE NUMBER 049380 OF EL PASO, TX, WAS DISCIPLINED BY VIRGINIA ON NOVEMBER 15, 1999
DISCIPLINARY ACTION: PROBATION
OFFENSE: DISCIPLINARY ACTION BY ANOTHER STATE OR AGENCY

NOTES: DISCIPLINARY ACTION BY THE TEXAS BOARD FOR PRESCRIBING MEDICATIONS TO A PATIENT WITHOUT ADEQUATE MEDICAL INDICATION AND WITHOUT ADEQUATELY DOCUMENTING CARE AND TREATMENT.

EASTER, THOMAS GLENN II MD, LICENSE NUMBER G7801 OF EL PASO, TX, WAS DISCIPLINED BY TEXAS ON AUGUST 22, 1998
DISCIPLINARY ACTION: REPRIMAND; REQUIRED TO TAKE ADDITIONAL MEDICAL EDUCATION
OFFENSE: OVERPRESCRIBING OR MISPRESCRIBING DRUGS

NOTES: FOR SEVERAL YEARS AND UNTIL APPROXIMATELY 7/93, HE PRESCRIBED, DISPENSED AND/OR

ADMINISTERED INJECTABLE MORPHINE SULFATE AND DEMEROL TO AN ADULT FEMALE PATIENT, WITHOUT ADEQUATE MEDICATION INDICATION AND WITHOUT ADEQUATELY DOCUMENTING HIS CARE AND TREATMENT OF THIS PATIENT INCLUDING DOCUMENTATION OF THE DRUGS PRESCRIBED, DISPENSED OR ADMINISTERED; WHEN THE PATIENT DEVELOPED ABSCESSES, HE FAILED TO STOP PRESCRIBING MORPHINE AND FAILED TO PROVIDE ADEQUATE ALTERNATIVE TREATMENT IN LIEU OF NARCOTIC MEDICATIONS; HE HAS NOT MAINTAINED HIS UPDATED PRACTICE AND MAILING ADDRESSES WITH THE BOARD, AND HAS NOT RESPONDED TO BOARD'S REQUESTS FOR INFORMATION; CURRENTLY AND DURING THE PERIOD OF PRESCRIBING HE WAS COHABITING WITH THE PATIENT. LICENSE LIMITED FOR FIVE YEARS AS FOLLOWS: SHALL NOT TREAT OR OTHERWISE SERVE AS PHYSICIAN, PRESCRIBE, DISPENSE OR ADMINISTER DRUGS THAT MAY BE SUBJECT TO ABUSE TO HIMSELF OR TO ANY MEMBER OF HIS FAMILY; SEPARATE FROM PATIENT RECORDS, SHALL MAINTAIN A LOGBOOK OF EVERY PRESCRIPTION WRITTEN BY HIM FOR DANGEROUS DRUGS WITH ADDICTIVE POTENTIAL WHICH SHALL BE MADE AVAILABLE FOR REVIEW; SHALL MAINTAIN ADEQUATE MEDICAL RECORDS WHICH SHALL BE AVAILABLE FOR REVIEW; SHALL OBTAIN 50 HOURS PER YEAR OF CONTINUING MEDICAL EDUCATION; SHALL COOPERATE WITH THE BOARD IN VERIFYING COMPLIANCE INCLUDING PROVIDING COPIES OF PEER REVIEW RECORDS UPON REQUEST; SHALL GIVE A COPY OF THIS ORDER TO ANY HEALTH CARE ENTITY WHERE HE HAS PRIVILEGES; SHALL PROVIDE A COPY OF THIS ORDER TO ANYONE REQUESTING IT WITHIN 10 DAYS; SHALL APPEAR BEFORE THE BOARD UPON REQUEST; TIME SPENT OUT OF TEXAS DOES NOT COUNT TOWARD RESTRICTION; SHALL INFORM THE BOARD OF CHANGE OF ADDRESS WITHIN 10 DAYS OR IF HE LEAVES THE STATE; SHALL NOT SEEK MODIFICATION FOR ONE YEAR.

ECHOLS, BEN HARRIS MD, DATE OF BIRTH SEPTEMBER 20, 1949, LICENSE NUMBER 00F6227 OF 7400 FANNIN SUITE 1118, HOUSTON, TX, WAS DISCIPLINED BY TEXAS ON JANUARY 29, 1993
DISCIPLINARY ACTION: REPRIMAND
OFFENSE: PROFESSIONAL MISCONDUCT

NOTES: AIDED AND ABETTED THE UNLICENSED PRACTICE OF MEDICINE BY BEST RECOVERY HEALTH CARE, INC. A CONTRACT WITH WHICH AWARDED HIM 10% OF REVENUE COLLECTED FROM THE METHADONE CLINIC; HE NEVER COLLECTED THIS REVENUE. SHALL GIVE A COPY OF THIS ORDER TO ANY HEALTH CARE ENTITY WHERE HE HAS PRIVILEGES; SHALL INFORM THE BOARD OF CHANGE OF ADDRESS WITHIN 10 DAYS.

EDGEWORTH, LEWIS ANSON DAVID MD, LICENSE NUMBER 00E5743 OF BRIDGEPORT, TX, WAS DISCIPLINED BY TEXAS ON JANUARY 24, 1992
DISCIPLINARY ACTION: 24-MONTH PROBATION

NOTES: PROFESSIONAL FAILURE TO PRACTICE MEDICINE IN AN ACCEPTABLE MANNER CONSISTENT WITH PUBLIC HEALTH AND WELFARE. LICENSE SUSPENDED, SUSPENSION STAYED; PROBATION UNDER TERMS AND CONDITIONS.

EDWARDSON, DELBERT L MD, LICENSE NUMBER E2197, WAS DISCIPLINED BY TEXAS ON MAY 10, 1997
DISCIPLINARY ACTION: 60-MONTH REPRIMAND; REQUIRED TO TAKE ADDITIONAL MEDICAL EDUCATION
OFFENSE: OVERPRESCRIBING OR MISPRESCRIBING DRUGS

NOTES: FROM 1992 TO 1995, HE PRESCRIBED CONTROLLED SUBSTANCES TO NUMEROUS PATIENTS, PURPORTEDLY FOR "CHRONIC PAIN", WITHOUT ADEQUATE DIAGNOSTIC WORK-UP AND WITHOUT LEGITIMATE MEDICAL INDICATIONS, WHEN HE KNEW OR SHOULD HAVE KNOWN THAT MULTIPLE PATIENTS WERE ABUSERS OF SUCH DRUGS. HE FAILED TO MAINTAIN ADEQUATE MEDICAL RECORDS OF HIS CARE AND TREATMENT OF THESE PATIENTS, INCLUDING RECORDS OF MEDICATIONS PRESCRIBED. AN ADULT MALE PATIENT WHO WAS A CANDIDATE FOR SURGERY HAD TO BE TAPERED OFF HYDROCODONE MEDICATION PROVIDED PRIOR TO SURGERY BY ANOTHER PHYSICIAN. DESPITE RECOMMENDATIONS TO THE CONTRARY, HE SUBSEQUENTLY PROVIDED HYDROCODONE TO THE PATIENT AFTER SURGERY. HE REPORTS LIMITED CONTINUING EDUCATION IN CHRONIC PAIN MANAGEMENT AND HAS NO FORMAL TRAINING IN THIS AREA. BECAUSE OF CONCERNS REGARDING HIS INSIGHT, HE VOLUNTARILY SUBMITTED TO A PSYCHIATRIC EXAM AND THE SPEX. HIS PSYCHIATRIC EXAM RECOMMENDED PSYCHOTHERAPY TO ADDRESS INSIGHT ISSUES. HE PASSED THE SPEX WITH A SCORE OF 86. HIS LICENSE IS HEREBY RESTRICTED FOR FIVE YEARS AS FOLLOWS: SEPARATE FROM PATIENT RECORDS, SHALL MAINTAIN A FILE OF EVERY PRESCRIPTION WRITTEN BY HIM FOR DANGEROUS DRUGS WITH ADDICTIVE POTENTIAL WHICH SHALL BE MADE AVAILABLE FOR REVIEW; SHALL NOMINATE THREE CERTIFIED PSYCHIATRISTS FOR BOARD SELECTION OF A THERAPIST, AND SHALL EXPEDITIOUSLY SUBMIT HIMSELF TO EVALUATION AND TREATMENT BY THE APPROVED PRACTITIONER; SHALL COOPERATE WITH THE BOARD IN VERIFYING COMPLIANCE INCLUDING PROVIDING COPIES OF MEDICAL RELEASES AND PEER REVIEW RECORDS UPON REQUEST; HIS TREATMENT AND CARE OF PATIENTS WITH CHRONIC PAIN SHALL BE MONITORED BY A BOARD-APPROVED TEXAS PHYSICIAN WHO SHALL PROVIDE QUARTERLY REPORTS TO THE BOARD; SHALL OBTAIN AT LEAST 50 HOURS OF CONTINUING MEDICAL EDUCATION PER YEAR, INCLUDING AT LEAST 12 HOURS IN PHARMACOLOGY OR CHRONIC PAIN MANAGEMENT; SHALL ADEQUATELY SUPERVISE THE INDIVIDUALS UNDER HIS AUTHORITY TO ENSURE THAT THEY ARE COMPLYING WITH THE LAWS RELEVANT TO THE PRACTICE OF MEDICINE; SHALL GIVE A COPY OF THIS ORDER TO ANY HEALTH CARE ENTITY WHERE HE HAS PRIVILEGES; SHALL PROVIDE A COPY OF THIS ORDER TO ANYONE REQUESTING IT WITHIN 10 DAYS; SHALL INFORM THE BOARD OF CHANGE OF ADDRESS WITHIN 10 DAYS; SHALL NOT SEEK MODIFICATION FOR ONE YEAR.

EIBAND, JOHN M MD, LICENSE NUMBER 00C5037 OF HOUSTON, TX, WAS DISCIPLINED BY TEXAS ON DECEMBER 4, 1991
DISCIPLINARY ACTION: 60-MONTH PROBATION; REQUIRED TO ENTER AN IMPAIRED PHYSICIAN PROGRAM OR SUBSTANCE ABUSE TREATMENT
OFFENSE: SUBSTANCE ABUSE

NOTES: ABUSED DEMEROL AND ALCOHOL FROM 12/89 THROUGH 2/91; WAS SUSPENDED FROM HOSPITAL PRIVILEGES FROM 2/17/91 TO 4/91; HAS REACHED A MONITORING AGREEMENT WITH HOSPITAL; HAS NOT ABUSED DEMEROL OR ALCOHOL SINCE 2/91 AFTER COMPLETING INPATIENT HOSPITALIZATION. FIVE YEAR SUSPENSION STAYED; CONDITIONS OF PROBATION: SHALL ABSTAIN FROM THE CONSUMPTION OF ALCOHOL/CHEMICAL SUBSTANCES IN ANY FORM; SHALL CONTINUE TO MEET WITH IMPAIRED PHYSICIANS COMMITTEE, WITH QUARTERLY REPORTS

TO THE BOARD; SHALL PARTICIPATE IN AA, INCLUDING A 12-STEP PROGRAM, ATTENDING NOT LESS THAN 3 TIMES A WEEK, WITH QUARTERLY REPORTS TO THE BOARD; SHALL INITIATE TREATMENT, MONITORING, AND SUPERVISION, WITH THE STARTING POINT PROGRAM WITH QUARTERLY REPORTS TO THE BOARD; SHALL PARTICIPATE IN SCREENING OF BIOLOGICAL FLUIDS; SHALL IMMEDIATELY NOTIFY THE BOARD UPON DISCONTINUATION OF TREATMENT; SHALL MAINTAIN A LOG OF EVERY PRESCRIPTION WRITTEN FOR CONTROLLED SUBSTANCES OR DANGEROUS DRUGS, WHICH SHALL BE AVAILABLE FOR INSPECTION ON DEMAND; SHALL NOT PRESCRIBE FOR OR TREAT HIMSELF OR HIS IMMEDIATE FAMILY; SHALL APPEAR BEFORE THE BOARD TWICE A YEAR; SHALL SUPPLY WRITTEN REPORTS OF HIS MEDICAL CONDITION WHEN REQUESTED; MUST ADVISE THE BOARD OF ADDRESS CHANGE OR IF HE LEAVES THE STATE; TIME SPENT OUT OF TEXAS DOES NOT COUNT TOWARDS PROBATION; SHALL NOT PETITION FOR MODIFICATION OF ORDER AT LEAST UNTIL AFTER 10/1/93. ON 3/5/94 HIS REQUEST FOR TERMINATION OF ORDER DENIED. HOWEVER, ORDER MODIFIED AS FOLLOWS: WRITTEN REPORTS OF HIS PARTICIPATION IN THE PHYSICIANS COUNSELING COMMITTEE WILL BE REQUIRED EVERY SIX MONTHS INSTEAD OF EVERY THREE MONTHS; REQUIREMENT OF PARTICIPATION IN AA AND REQUIREMENT TO INITIATE TREATMENT, MONITORING AND SUPERVISION FROM THE STARTING POINT PROGRAM ARE DELETED; ALLOWED TO REQUEST TERMINATION OR MODIFICATION ONCE EVERY SIX MONTHS. ON 8/19/94 PROBATION TERMINATED.

EISAMAN, RALPH DR OF BEDFORD, TX, WAS DISCIPLINED BY ILLINOIS ON AUGUST 1, 1996
DISCIPLINARY ACTION: PROBATION
OFFENSE: PHYSICAL OR MENTAL ILLNESS INHIBITING THE ABILITY TO PRACTICE WITH SKILL AND SAFETY

NOTES: PHYSICAL AILMENT WHICH COULD PREVENT HIM FROM PRACTICING MEDICINE WITH A REASONABLE DEGREE OF SAFETY IF NOT PROPERLY TREATED. INDEFINITE PROBATION.

EITEL, JOHN BEN DO, LICENSE NUMBER 00B8453 OF PORT NECHES, TX, WAS DISCIPLINED BY TEXAS ON APRIL 15, 1994
DISCIPLINARY ACTION: SURRENDER OF CONTROLLED SUBSTANCE LICENSE
OFFENSE: NONCOMPLIANCE WITH A PROFESSIONAL RULE

NOTES: FAILED TO MAINTAIN ADEQUATE RECORDS RELATING TO CONTROLLED SUBSTANCES; PLED GUILTY TO A PORTION OF THE CHARGES AGAINST HIM, LEADING TO THE IMPOSITION OF A FINE AND SURRENDER OF DEA AND TEXAS CONTROLLED SUBSTANCES CERTIFICATES. SHALL NOT HOLD THESE CERTIFICATES AND SHALL NOT REAPPLY WITHOUT BOARD APPROVAL; SHALL GIVE A COPY OF THIS ORDER TO ANY HEALTH CARE ENTITY WHERE HE HAS PRIVILEGES; SHALL COOPERATE WITH THE BOARD IN VERIFYING COMPLIANCE; SHALL INFORM BOARD OF CHANGE OF ADDRESS WITHIN 10 DAYS. SHALL NOT SEEK MODIFICATION FOR ONE YEAR.

EITEL, JOHN BEN DO, LICENSE NUMBER 0000577, WAS DISCIPLINED BY OKLAHOMA ON MARCH 24, 1995
DISCIPLINARY ACTION: SURRENDER OF LICENSE
OFFENSE: DISCIPLINARY ACTION BY ANOTHER STATE OR AGENCY

NOTES: ALLEGATIONS OF ACTION IN TEXAS. HAD SURRENDERED HIS OKLAHOMA LICENSE AND CURRENT RENEWAL CERTIFICATE TO THE BOARD; LICENSE CANCELED.

ELKIN, SCOTT RICHARD DO, DATE OF BIRTH APRIL 8, 1950, LICENSE NUMBER 00G1644 OF 5806 MESA DRIVE SUITE 375, AUSTIN, TX, WAS DISCIPLINED BY TEXAS ON DECEMBER 4, 1991
DISCIPLINARY ACTION: 60-MONTH PROBATION; 60-MONTH REQUIRED TO TAKE ADDITIONAL MEDICAL EDUCATION
OFFENSE: PROFESSIONAL MISCONDUCT

NOTES: SEVERAL TIMES BETWEEN 11/6/89 AND 2/14/90 HE SIGNED INSURANCE FORMS FOR A PATIENT REPRESENTING HE HAD PROVIDED PSYCHOTHERAPY, WHEN IN FACT IT HAD BEEN PERFORMED BY AN UNLICENSED PSYCHOTHERAPIST. SUSPENSION STAYED. CONDITIONS OF PROBATION: SHALL COMPLETE FIVE HOURS PER YEAR OF AN ETHICS COURSE; SHALL REFRAIN FROM SIGNING INSURANCE FORMS AND/OR ATTENDING PHYSICIAN STATEMENTS FOR PATIENTS HE HAS NOT PERSONALLY TREATED; SHALL APPEAR BEFORE THE BOARD ONCE A YEAR; SHALL COOPERATE WITH BOARD IN VERIFYING COMPLIANCE; SHALL ADVISE THE BOARD OF CHANGE OF ADDRESS WITHIN 10 DAYS; TIME SPENT OUT OF TEXAS DOES NOT COUNT TOWARD PROBATION; MAY NOT PETITION FOR MODIFICATION FOR AT LEAST ONE YEAR. ON 8/20/93, ORDER TERMINATED AND LICENSE FREE AND CLEAR OF ANY PREVIOUS RESTRICTIONS.

ELKIN, SCOTT RICHARD DO, DATE OF BIRTH APRIL 8, 1950, LICENSE NUMBER 0023916 OF AUSTIN, TX, WAS DISCIPLINED BY COLORADO ON FEBRUARY 11, 1994
DISCIPLINARY ACTION: REPRIMAND
OFFENSE: DISCIPLINARY ACTION BY ANOTHER STATE OR AGENCY

NOTES: DISCIPLINARY ACTION TAKEN BY TEXAS.

ELLIOTT, PAUL T MD, LICENSE NUMBER D5979 OF RICHARDSON, TX, WAS DISCIPLINED BY TEXAS ON APRIL 10, 1999
DISCIPLINARY ACTION: REPRIMAND
OFFENSE: NONCOMPLIANCE WITH A PROFESSIONAL RULE

NOTES: DURING 1990 - 1996 HE INADEQUATELY DOCUMENTED HIS CARE, TREATMENT, AND EXAMINATION OF ONE PATIENT. SHALL GIVE A COPY OF THIS ORDER TO ANY HEALTH CARE ENTITY WHERE HE HAS PRIVILEGES.

ELLIS, CYNTHIA E MD, DATE OF BIRTH DECEMBER 5, 1959 OF 6428 OLD HARBOR LANE, AUSTIN, TX, WAS DISCIPLINED BY MEDICARE ON JUNE 1, 1995
DISCIPLINARY ACTION: EXCLUSION FROM THE MEDICARE AND/OR MEDICAID PROGRAM
OFFENSE: NONCOMPLIANCE WITH A PROFESSIONAL RULE

NOTES: DEFAULTED ON PUBLIC HEALTH SERVICE EDUCATION LOAN.

ELLIS, NEELY JOE MD, LICENSE NUMBER C3647 OF HOUSTON, TX, WAS DISCIPLINED BY TEXAS ON AUGUST 28, 1999
DISCIPLINARY ACTION: 60-MONTH PROBATION; MONITORING OF PHYSICIAN PERFORMANCE
OFFENSE: SUBSTANCE ABUSE

NOTES: FAILURE TO KEEP MEDICAL RECORDS REFLECTING HIS TREATMENT AND/OR PRESCRIBING TO A PATIENT AND HIMSELF; THE PATIENT WAS A RELATIVE TO WHOM HE PRESCRIBED PHENDIMETRAZINE TARTRATE FOR APPETITE CONTROL; THE RECOMMENDED DURATION IS A FEW WEEKS AND HE PRESCRIBED IT OVER A 10 MONTH PERIOD; IN 8/98 HE PARTICIPATED IN A 96 HOUR INPATIENT EVALUATION FOR SUBSTANCE ABUSE; HE REPORTED HIS LAST DRUG USE AS BEING IN 2/98; HE WAS DIAGNOSED AS BEING STIMULANT DEPENDENT WITH A DISCHARGE

RECOMMENDATION OF CONTINUING HIS PARTICIPATION IN A RECOVERY PLAN; HE SUBSEQUENTLY UNDERWENT CARDIAC SURGERY AND HAS REMAINED UNDER THE CARE OF A CARDIOLOGIST AND INTERNIST FOR SEVERAL MONTHS; HE IS PARTICIPATING IN THE HARRIS COUNTY MEDICAL SOCIETY COMMITTEE ON PHYSICIAN HEALTH AND REHABILITATION. SUSPENSION STAYED FOR PROBATION WITH THE FOLLOWING TERMS AND CONDITIONS: SHALL ABSTAIN FROM THE CONSUMPTION OF ALCOHOL/DRUGS IN ANY FORM UNLESS PRESCRIBED BY ANOTHER PHYSICIAN FOR A LEGITIMATE AND THERAPEUTIC PURPOSE; SHALL SUBMIT HIMSELF FOR APPROPRIATE EXAMS INCLUDING DRUG OR ALCOHOL SCREENS; SHALL NOMINATE THREE CERTIFIED PSYCHIATRISTS FOR BOARD SELECTION OF A THERAPIST AND SHALL EXPEDITIOUSLY SUBMIT HIMSELF TO EVALUATION AND TREATMENT BY THE APPROVED PRACTITIONER; SHALL CONTINUE TO RECEIVE CARE AND TREATMENT FROM HIS CARDIOLOGIST AND INTERNIST WITH QUARTERLY REPORTS TO THE BOARD; SHALL PARTICIPATE IN NARCOTICS ANONYMOUS NO LESS THAN ONCE A WEEK; SHALL PARTICIPATE IN THE ACTIVITIES OF A PHYSICIAN HEALTH AND REHABILITATION COMMITTEE AND ATTEND WEEKLY MEETINGS WITH QUARTERLY REPORTS; SHALL NOT TREAT OR OTHERWISE SERVE AS PHYSICIAN, PRESCRIBE, DISPENSE OR ADMINISTER DRUGS THAT MAY BE SUBJECT TO ABUSE TO HIMSELF OR TO ANY MEMBER OF HIS FAMILY; SEPARATE FROM PATIENT RECORDS, SHALL MAINTAIN A LOGBOOK OF EVERY PRESCRIPTION WRITTEN BY HIM FOR DANGEROUS DRUGS WITH ADDICTIVE POTENTIAL WHICH SHALL BE MADE AVAILABLE FOR REVIEW; SHALL MAINTAIN ADEQUATE MEDICAL RECORDS WHICH SHALL BE AVAILABLE FOR REVIEW; SHALL APPEAR BEFORE THE BOARD AT LEAST ONCE A YEAR; SHALL COOPERATE WITH THE BOARD IN VERIFYING COMPLIANCE INCLUDING PROVIDING COPIES OF MEDICAL RELEASES UPON REQUEST; TIME SPENT OUT OF TEXAS DOES NOT COUNT TOWARD PROBATION; SHALL INFORM THE BOARD OF CHANGE OF ADDRESS WITHIN 10 DAYS OR IF HE LEAVES THE STATE; SHALL NOT SEEK MODIFICATION FOR ONE YEAR.

ELOVITZ, STUART MD, LICENSE NUMBER 00E3906 OF CORPUS CHRISTI, TX, WAS DISCIPLINED BY TEXAS ON AUGUST 18, 1995
DISCIPLINARY ACTION: 1-MONTH LICENSE SUSPENSION; 60-MONTH PROBATION
OFFENSE: OVERCHARGING

NOTES: BETWEEN 11/92 AND 7/93 HE ALLEGEDLY PERFORMED UNNECESSARY TESTS OR PROCEDURES FOR A LARGE NUMBER OF PATIENTS WITHOUT ADEQUATE INDICATION AND/OR WITHOUT ADEQUATE DOCUMENTED INDICATIONS AND EXCESSIVELY BILLED A LARGE NUMBER OF PATIENTS BEING TREATED FOR A SIMILAR COMPLAINT. DOES NOT ADMIT VIOLATIONS. AFTER 30 DAYS OF SUSPENSION, SUSPENSION SHALL BE AUTOMATICALLY STAYED TO PROBATION WITH TERMS: HIS PRACTICE SHALL BE MONITORED BY A BOARD-APPROVED PHYSICIAN WHO SHALL SUBMIT QUARTERLY REPORTS TO THE BOARD; SHALL MAINTAIN ADEQUATE MEDICAL RECORDS WHICH SHALL BE MADE AVAILABLE FOR REVIEW; SHALL ADOPT OR ESTABLISH A SYSTEM OF PATIENT RECORD KEEPING AND BILLING; SHALL NOT SIGN OR INDICATE IN ANY MANNER IN PATIENT RECORDS THAT HE HAS SEEN PATIENTS UNLESS HE ACTUALLY HAS SEEN AND EXAMINED THE PATIENT UNLESS IT IS CLEARLY NOTED THAT HE DID NOT PERSONALLY EXAMINE THE PATIENT; SHALL OBTAIN AT LEAST 50 HOURS PER YEAR OF CONTINUING MEDICAL EDUCATION INCLUDING AT LEAST ONE COURSE PER YEAR IN ETHICS AND ONE COURSE PER YEAR IN RISK MANAGEMENT; SHALL PERFORM 120 HOURS OF COMMUNITY SERVICE EACH YEAR; SHALL APPEAR BEFORE BOARD AT LEAST ONCE A YEAR; SHALL COOPERATE WITH THE BOARD IN VERIFYING COMPLIANCE; SHALL GIVE A COPY OF THIS ORDER TO ANY HEALTH CARE ENTITY WHERE HE HAS PRIVILEGES; SHALL PROVIDE A COPY OF THIS ORDER TO ANYONE REQUESTING IT WITHIN 10 DAYS; TIME PERIOD OUT OF TEXAS DOES NOT COUNT TOWARD PROBATION; SHALL INFORM BOARD OF CHANGE OF ADDRESS WITHIN 10 DAYS OR IF HE LEAVES THE STATE. SHALL NOT SEEK MODIFICATION FOR ONE YEAR.

ELOVITZ, STUART MD, LICENSE NUMBER 00E3906, WAS DISCIPLINED BY TEXAS ON AUGUST 17, 1996
DISCIPLINARY ACTION: FINE; REPRIMAND
OFFENSE: NONCOMPLIANCE WITH A PROFESSIONAL RULE

NOTES: FAILED TO OBTAIN 24 HOURS OF CONTINUING MEDICAL EDUCATION BY 3/1/96 FOR THE RENEWAL OF HIS LICENSE; HE WAS GRANTED AN EXTENSION UNTIL 5/29/96 WHICH HE ALSO DID NOT MEET. STILL REQUIRED TO MEET CONTINUING MEDICAL EDUCATION REQUIREMENTS. $100 ADMINISTRATIVE PENALTY; SHALL COOPERATE WITH THE BOARD IN VERIFYING COMPLIANCE.

ELTERMAN, ROY D MD, LICENSE NUMBER 0G30587 OF DALLAS, TX, WAS DISCIPLINED BY CALIFORNIA ON JULY 5, 1993
DISCIPLINARY ACTION: 60-MONTH PROBATION

NOTES: REVOCATION STAYED; PROBATION WITH CONDITION PRECEDENT.

ELTERMAN, ROY D MD, LICENSE NUMBER 0026683 OF DALLAS, TX, WAS DISCIPLINED BY FLORIDA ON DECEMBER 22, 1994
DISCIPLINARY ACTION: FINE
OFFENSE: DISCIPLINARY ACTION BY ANOTHER STATE OR AGENCY

NOTES: LICENSE OR AUTHORITY TO PRACTICE MEDICINE REVOKED, SUSPENDED OR OTHERWISE ACTED AGAINST BY A LICENSING AUTHORITY OF ANY JURISDICTION. FAILED TO REPORT TO THE BOARD, IN WRITING AND WITHIN 30 DAYS, DISCIPLINARY ACTION TAKEN AGAINST LICENSE BY ANOTHER JURISDICTION. $500 FINE.

ELTERMAN, ROY DANA MD OF 12801 N CENTRAL EXPRESSWAY #580, DALLAS, TX, WAS DISCIPLINED BY DEA ON MARCH 7, 1990
DISCIPLINARY ACTION: SURRENDER OF CONTROLLED SUBSTANCE LICENSE
OFFENSE: SUBSTANCE ABUSE

NOTES: WROTE PRESCRIPTION FOR PERSONAL USE. ADMITTED TO SUBSTANCE ABUSE PROBLEM WITH PRESCRIPTION MEDICATION.

ELTERMAN, ROY DANA MD, LICENSE NUMBER 00E9188 OF DALLAS, TX, WAS DISCIPLINED BY TEXAS ON SEPTEMBER 28, 1990
DISCIPLINARY ACTION: 36-MONTH PROBATION; MONITORING OF PHYSICIAN PERFORMANCE

NOTES: MUST COMPLY WITH HIS AGREEMENT WITH HUMANA HOSPITAL-MEDICAL CITY DALLAS; CONTINUE PSYCHIATRIC TREATMENT; SUBMIT FOR APPROPRIATE EXAMINATIONS TO DETERMINE FREEDOM FROM DRUGS AND ALCOHOL; PARTICIPATE IN ALCOHOLICS ANONYMOUS; REPORT ANY INCIDENT IN WHICH HE PARTAKES OF ALCOHOL OR USES CONTROLLED SUBSTANCE NOT PRESCRIBED BY

ANOTHER PHYSICIAN FOR LEGITIMATE AND THERAPEUTIC CONDITION; NOT TREAT OR SERVE AS PHYSICIAN, PRESCRIBE, DISPENSE, OR ADMINISTER CONTROLLED SUBSTANCES OR ANY OTHER DRUGS THAT MAY BE SUBJECT TO ABUSE, OR WRITE PRESCRIPTIONS FOR CONTROLLED SUBSTANCES OR ANY OTHER DRUGS THAT MAY BE SUBJECT TO ABUSE FOR SELF OR IMMEDIATE FAMILY; ADMINISTER TO SELF OR IMMEDIATE FAMILY ONLY DRUGS AS PRESCRIBED BY OTHER PHYSICIANS; NOT TREAT HIMSELF FOR RECURRING MEDICAL CONDITION NOR ADMINISTER OR PRESCRIBE MOOD ELEVATORS OR CONTROLLED SUBSTANCES FOR PERSONAL USE; ABSTAIN FROM ALCOHOL CONSUMPTION; REFRAIN FROM USE OF, AND NOT POSSESS, ADMINISTER, OR PRESCRIBE CONTROLLED SUBSTANCES OR ANY DRUG OR MEDICATION REQUIRING PRESCRIPTION UNLESS SUCH IS PRESCRIBED, ADMINISTERED, OR DISPENSED BY PHYSICIAN TREATING HIM FOR LEGITIMATE MEDICAL NEED, AND SUCH TREATING PHYSICIAN REPORTS TO BOARD CONDITION BEING TREATED AND DRUG PRESCRIBED; APPEAR BEFORE BOARD WHEN REQUESTED.

EMANUEL, RAPHAEL JOHN MD, LICENSE NUMBER 00E7592 OF DALLAS, TX, WAS DISCIPLINED BY TEXAS ON OCTOBER 5, 1991
DISCIPLINARY ACTION: 24-MONTH PROBATION; REPRIMAND
OFFENSE: PROFESSIONAL MISCONDUCT

NOTES: INADVERTENTLY USED THE WRONG BILLING CODES FOR PULMONARY AND VASCULAR TESTING ON TWO PATIENTS IN MARCH AND AUGUST 1988. CONDITIONS OF PROBATION: SHALL ATTEND AT LEAST 20 HOURS OF CONTINUING MEDICAL EDUCATION IN RISK MANAGEMENT WITHIN ONE YEAR; SHALL APPEAR BEFORE THE BOARD ONCE A YEAR; SHALL COOPERATE WITH THE BOARD IN VERIFYING COMPLIANCE; SHALL ADVISE THE BOARD OF ANY CHANGE OF ADDRESS WITHIN 10 DAYS; TIME SPENT OUT OF STATE DOES NOT COUNT TOWARDS PROBATION.

EMERSON, TIMOTHY JOE MD, DATE OF BIRTH DECEMBER 28, 1956, LICENSE NUMBER 00G8831 OF 14 S JEFFERSON ST, SAN ANGELO, TX, WAS DISCIPLINED BY TEXAS ON DECEMBER 4, 1991
DISCIPLINARY ACTION: LICENSE SUSPENSION
OFFENSE: CRIMINAL CONVICTION OR PLEA OF GUILTY, NOLO CONTENDERE, OR NO CONTEST TO A CRIME

NOTES: SEVERAL TIMES DURING 1986 AND ON 3/25/87 HE ENGAGED IN SEXUAL CONTACT WITH A FEMALE CHILD YOUNGER THAN 17; PLED GUILTY TO SEXUAL ASSAULT OF A FEMALE CHILD YOUNGER THAN 17 ON 8/10/87; COURT PLACED HIM ON PROBATION FOR 10 YEARS WITH TERMS, INCLUDING THE REQUIREMENT THAT HE ATTEND PSYCHOLOGICAL COUNSELING SESSIONS. SUSPENSION UNTIL SUCH TIME AS HE SHOWS HE IS MENTALLY, PHYSICALLY AND OTHERWISE COMPETENT TO PRACTICE MEDICINE.

EMERSON, TIMOTHY JOE MD, DATE OF BIRTH DECEMBER 28, 1956, LICENSE NUMBER 00G8831 OF 14 S JEFFERSON ST, SAN ANGELO, TX, WAS DISCIPLINED BY TEXAS ON AUGUST 31, 1993
DISCIPLINARY ACTION: 84-MONTH PROBATION; RESTRICTION PLACED ON LICENSE

NOTES: PURSUANT TO TERMS OF 12/4/91 ORDER HE PROVIDED EVIDENCE TO SHOW HE IS MENTALLY, PHYSICALLY AND OTHERWISE COMPETENT TO PRACTICE MEDICINE. SUSPENSION LIFTED AND STAYED. CONDITIONS OF PROBATION: WITHIN ONE YEAR SHALL COMPLETE 50 HOURS OF CONTINUING MEDICAL EDUCATION IN FAMILY PRACTICE; WHEN PERFORMING PHYSICAL EXAMS ON CHILDREN AND FEMALE PATIENTS SHALL BE MONITORED AND CHAPERONED BY A FEMALE MONITOR WHO SHALL DOCUMENT HER PRESENCE; SHALL SUBMIT HIMSELF FOR EVALUATION AND TREATMENT TO A BOARD-APPROVED PSYCHIATRIST; UNTIL HE HAS SUCCESSFULLY COMPLETED THE AFOREMENTIONED 50 HOURS OF CONTINUING MEDICAL EDUCATION, SHALL BE MONITORED OR SUPERVISED BY A BOARD-APPROVED PHYSICIAN WHO WILL REPORT TO THE BOARD EVERY FOUR MONTHS; SHALL GIVE A COPY OF THIS ORDER TO ALL HEALTH CARE ENTITIES WHERE HE HAS PRIVILEGES; SHALL COOPERATE WITH BOARD IN VERIFYING COMPLIANCE; SHALL INFORM BOARD OF CHANGE OF ADDRESS WITHIN 10 DAYS OR IF HE LEAVES THE STATE; TIME SPENT OUT OF TEXAS DOES NOT COUNT TOWARD PROBATION. SHALL NOT SEEK MODIFICATION FOR ONE YEAR.

EMERSON, TIMOTHY JOE MD OF SAN ANGELO, TX, WAS DISCIPLINED BY NORTH CAROLINA ON FEBRUARY 1, 1994
DISCIPLINARY ACTION: LICENSE REVOCATION

EPPS, DEBRA KENNAMER MD, LICENSE NUMBER 00H2360 OF DALLAS, TX, WAS DISCIPLINED BY TEXAS ON DECEMBER 4, 1991
DISCIPLINARY ACTION: SURRENDER OF CONTROLLED SUBSTANCE LICENSE; 120-MONTH PROBATION
OFFENSE: SUBSTANCE ABUSE

NOTES: DURING THE PERIOD OF 7/86 TO 7/91 SHE ABUSED FIORICET, FIORINAL #3, LORCET PLUS, DARVOCET N-100, MORPHINE, AND INJECTABLE DEMEROL OBTAINED THROUGH THE USE OF SAMPLES AND PRESCRIPTIONS SHE WROTE USING OTHER PEOPLE'S NAMES; WAS UNABLE TO ADEQUATELY CARE FOR PATIENTS DUE TO IMPAIRMENT; HAS BEEN ENROLLED IN A TREATMENT PROGRAM FOR CHEMICAL DEPENDENCY SINCE 7/13/91. SUSPENSION STAYED; CONDITIONS OF PROBATIONS: SHALL REFRAIN FROM CONSUMING ALL MOOD ALTERING DRUGS INCLUDING ALCOHOL; MUST SUBMIT TO APPROPRIATE EXAMINATIONS INCLUDING SCREENS OF BODILY FLUIDS: MUST PARTICIPATE WITH IMPAIRED PHYSICIANS GROUP, INCLUDING WEEKLY MEETINGS, WITH QUARTERLY WRITTEN REPORTS TO THE BOARD; MUST PARTICIPATE IN AA, INCLUDING A 12-STEP PROGRAM, NOT LESS THAN TWICE A WEEK, WITH WRITTEN QUARTERLY REPORTS TO THE BOARD; TREATING PHYSICIAN SHALL ALSO SUBMIT REPORTS TO BOARD QUARTERLY; SHALL SURRENDER DEA AND TEXAS CONTROLLED SUBSTANCES REGISTRATIONS: SHALL NOT REAPPLY FOR THESE WITHOUT WRITTEN CONSENT FROM THE BOARD; SHALL SURRENDER ALL UNUSED TRIPLICATE PRESCRIPTION FORMS AND ALL CONTROLLED SUBSTANCES, INCLUDING SAMPLES; SHALL ENROLL IN AND COMPLETE, WITHIN SIX MONTHS, A REMEDIAL PHARMACOLOGY COURSE WITH PROOF OF COMPLETION SUBMITTED; SHALL APPEAR BEFORE THE BOARD TWICE A YEAR; SHALL COOPERATE WITH BOARD IN VERIFYING COMPLIANCE; SHALL ADVISE THE BOARD OF ANY ADDRESS CHANGE WITHIN 10 DAYS; TIME SPENT OUT OF TEXAS DOES NOT COUNT TOWARDS PROBATION; SHALL NOT PETITION FOR MODIFICATION OF ORDER FOR AT LEAST ON YEAR.

EPPS, DEBRA KENNAMER MD, LICENSE NUMBER 00H2360 OF DALLAS, TX, WAS DISCIPLINED BY TEXAS ON AUGUST 20, 1992
DISCIPLINARY ACTION: LICENSE SUSPENSION
OFFENSE: FAILURE TO COMPLY WITH PREVIOUS BOARD ORDER

NOTES: VIOLATION OF PREVIOUS BOARD ORDER.

EPPS, DEBRA KENNAMER MD, LICENSE NUMBER 00H2360, WAS DISCIPLINED BY TEXAS ON SEPTEMBER 7, 1993
DISCIPLINARY ACTION: 60-MONTH PROBATION; REQUIRED TO TAKE ADDITIONAL MEDICAL EDUCATION

NOTES: BASED ON HER PROGRESS AND PSYCHIATRIC EVALUATION BOARD GRANTED REQUEST TO TERMINATE SUSPENSION ENTERED ON 8/20/92. CONDITIONS OF PROBATION: SHALL ABSTAIN FROM THE CONSUMPTION OF ALCOHOL/CHEMICAL SUBSTANCES; SHALL SUBMIT HERSELF FOR APPROPRIATE EXAMS INCLUDING DRUG OR ALCOHOL SCREENS; SHALL CONTINUE TO PARTICIPATE IN THE ACTIVITIES OF THE BEXAR COUNTY MEDICAL SOCIETY AND ATTEND WEEKLY MEETINGS WITH QUARTERLY REPORTS; SHALL CONTINUE TO PARTICIPATE IN AA'S 12 STEP PROGRAM NOT LESS THAN THREE TIMES A WEEK WITH QUARTERLY REPORTS TO THE BOARD; SHALL CONTINUE TO RECEIVE PSYCHIATRIC COUNSELING WITH QUARTERLY REPORTS TO THE BOARD; SHALL ATTEND AT LEAST 50 HOURS PER YEAR OF CONTINUING MEDICAL EDUCATION; SHALL BE MONITORED BY A BOARD APPROVED PHYSICIAN WITH QUARTERLY REPORTS; SHALL APPEAR BEFORE THE BOARD TWICE A YEAR; SHALL COOPERATE WITH THE BOARD IN VERIFYING COMPLIANCE; SHALL INFORM BOARD OF CHANGE OF ADDRESS WITHIN 10 DAYS OR IF SHE LEAVES THE STATE; TIME SPENT OUT OF TEXAS DOES NOT COUNT TOWARD PROBATION. SHALL NOT SEEK MODIFICATION FOR ONE YEAR. ORDER MODIFIED ON 10/1/93 GRANTING HER PERMISSION TO REAPPLY TO THE DEA AND TEXAS DEPARTMENT OF PUBLIC SAFETY FOR SCHEDULES IV AND V CONTROLLED SUBSTANCE AUTHORITY; SHALL NOT POSSESS, ADMINISTER, DISPENSE OR PRESCRIBE ANY CONTROLLED SUBSTANCES BUT MAY ORDER THEM TO BE ADMINISTERED TO HOSPITALIZED PATIENTS IF THEY ARE COUNTERSIGNED. ORDER FURTHER MODIFIED ON 9/30/94 SUCH THAT SHE WOULD BE ABLE TO APPLY FOR SCHEDULE III SUBSTANCE AUTHORITY, THE REQUIREMENT THAT ALL PRESCRIPTIONS FOR CONTROLLED SUBSTANCES BE COUNTERSIGNED IS DROPPED AND THE CONDITION ADDED THAT SEPARATE FROM PATIENT RECORDS SHE SHALL MAINTAIN A FILE OF EVERY PRESCRIPTION WRITTEN FOR CONTROLLED SUBSTANCES OR DANGEROUS DRUGS WHICH SHALL BE AVAILABLE FOR INSPECTION.

ERDMANN, RALPH R MD, LICENSE NUMBER 00C7350 OF LUBBOCK, TX, WAS DISCIPLINED BY TEXAS ON AUGUST 20, 1992
DISCIPLINARY ACTION: SURRENDER OF LICENSE
OFFENSE: PROFESSIONAL MISCONDUCT

NOTES: UNPROFESSIONAL OR DISHONORABLE CONDUCT LIKELY TO DECEIVE, DEFRAUD OR INJURE THE PUBLIC; PROFESSIONAL FAILURE TO PRACTICE MEDICINE IN AN ACCEPTABLE MANNER CONSISTENT WITH PUBLIC HEALTH AND WELFARE; AND COMMITTING AN ACT THAT IS IN VIOLATION OF THE LAWS OF TEXAS. LICENSE RETIRED IN LIEU OF FURTHER DISCIPLINARY PROCEEDINGS.

ERICKSON, CARL F MD, LICENSE NUMBER 00H2361 OF SAN ANTONIO, TX, WAS DISCIPLINED BY TEXAS ON AUGUST 24, 1991
DISCIPLINARY ACTION: 60-MONTH PROBATION; MONITORING OF PHYSICIAN PERFORMANCE
OFFENSE: SUBSTANCE ABUSE

NOTES: INTEMPERATE USE OF ALCOHOL OR DRUGS. SUSPENSION STAYED. CONDITIONS OF PROBATION: MUST REFRAIN FROM ALCOHOL OR DRUG CONSUMPTION; MUST SUBMIT TO ALCOHOL OR DRUG SCREENS; MUST PARTICIPATE IN IMPAIRED PHYSICIANS PROGRAM; MUST PARTICIPATE IN AA; MUST APPEAR TWICE YEARLY BEFORE THE BOARD. ON 9/30/94 PROBATION TERMINATED.

ESCALER, BRUNO MD, LICENSE NUMBER J1241 OF MIAMI SPRINGS, FL, WAS DISCIPLINED BY TEXAS ON AUGUST 22, 1998
OFFENSE: LOSS OR RESTRICTION OF HOSPITAL PRIVILEGES

NOTES: IN 1/97 HIS PRIVILEGES AT THE VETERAN'S ADMINISTRATION MEDICAL CENTER ("VAMC") WERE TERMINATED DUE TO UNPROFESSIONAL CONDUCT BASED ON THE FOLLOWING EVENTS: ON 6/3/96 HE WAS COUNSELED AT THE VAMC REGARDING INAPPROPRIATE INVOLVEMENT WITH AN EMPLOYEE OF THE HOSPITAL; ON 7/10/96 HE WAS REPORTED FOR FAILURE TO RESPOND WHILE HE WAS ON CALL; REPORTS CONTINUED REGARDING HIS PERSONAL BEHAVIOR TOWARD A STAFF NURSE; IN 11/96 POLICE BECAME INVOLVED WHEN HE THREATENED ANOTHER PHYSICIAN ON STAFF AT VAMC; ON 1/2/97 HE FAILED TO RESPOND TO A CALL IN THE INTENSIVE CARE UNIT REGARDING A PATIENT. LICENSE LIMITED AS FOLLOWS: SHALL NOT PRACTICE MEDICINE IN TEXAS UNTIL HE REQUESTS TO RESUME PRACTICE, APPEARS BEFORE THE BOARD WITH SUFFICIENT EVIDENCE THAT HE IS PHYSICALLY, MENTALLY, OR OTHERWISE COMPETENT TO PRACTICE SAFELY INCLUDING AT A MINIMUM: SHALL HAVE A CURRENT PSYCHIATRIC EVALUATION FROM A BOARD CERTIFIED PSYCHIATRIST; SHALL COOPERATE WITH THE BOARD IN VERIFYING COMPLIANCE INCLUDING PROVIDING COPIES OF MEDICAL RELEASES UPON REQUEST; SHALL INFORM THE BOARD OF CHANGE OF ADDRESS WITHIN 10 DAYS.

ESPIRITU, EDGARDO T MD, DATE OF BIRTH FEBRUARY 23, 1940, LICENSE NUMBER 0031366 OF 2100 HIGHWAY 365, NEDERLAND, TX, WAS DISCIPLINED BY MICHIGAN ON MARCH 20, 1991
DISCIPLINARY ACTION: LICENSE REVOCATION; FINE
OFFENSE: SUBSTANDARD CARE, INCOMPETENCE OR NEGLIGENCE

NOTES: $250 FINE.

ESPIRITU, ERNESTO T MD, LICENSE NUMBER 00G0873 OF FANNETT, TX, WAS DISCIPLINED BY TEXAS ON MAY 24, 1990
DISCIPLINARY ACTION: 120-MONTH RESTRICTION PLACED ON CONTROLLED SUBSTANCE LICENSE; REQUIRED TO TAKE ADDITIONAL MEDICAL EDUCATION

NOTES: STIPULATED ORDER. MUST IMMEDIATELY DISPOSE OF CONTROLLED SUBSTANCES IN HIS POSSESSION OR SUBJECT TO HIS CONTROL, REFRAIN FROM PRESCRIBING, DISPENSING, OR ADMINISTERING CONTROLLED SUBSTANCES IN ALL SCHEDULES AND UNDER ALL CIRCUMSTANCES EXCEPT IN HOSPITAL EMERGENCY ROOMS, AND ATTEND CONTINUING MEDICAL EDUCATION COURSES. ORDER EFFECTIVE FOR TEN YEARS. ON 9/9/91 REQUEST FOR TERMINATION OF ORDER WAS DENIED WHEN BOARD FOUND INSUFFICIENT BASIS FOR GRANTING THE REQUEST. ON 8/18/95 HIS PETITION FOR TERMINATION WAS DENIED BUT ORDER MODIFIED AS FOLLOWS: REQUIREMENT THAT HE REFRAIN FROM PRESCRIBING, DISPENSING OR ADMINISTERING CONTROLLED SUBSTANCES EXCEPT IN EMERGENCY ROOMS IS DELETED; SEPARATE FROM PATIENT RECORDS, HE SHALL MAINTAIN A FILE OF EVERY PRESCRIPTION WRITTEN OUTSIDE OF AN EMERGENCY ROOM SETTING FOR CONTROLLED SUBSTANCES AND SHALL MAINTAIN A LOG FOR ALL PRESCRIPTIONS OR REFILLS TELEPHONED IN FOR CONTROLLED SUBSTANCES BOTH OF WHICH SHALL

BE AVAILABLE FOR REVIEW; ALL OTHER CONDITIONS REMAIN IN EFFECT. ON 10/5/96 ORDER TERMINATED.

ESQUIVEL, JULIO A MD, LICENSE NUMBER 00J1655, WAS DISCIPLINED BY TEXAS ON AUGUST 17, 1996
DISCIPLINARY ACTION: FINE; REPRIMAND
OFFENSE: NONCOMPLIANCE WITH A PROFESSIONAL RULE

NOTES: FAILED TO OBTAIN 24 HOURS OF CONTINUING MEDICAL EDUCATION AS REQUIRED BY 9/1/95 FOR THE RENEWAL OF HIS LICENSE; HE WAS GRANTED AN EXTENSION UNTIL 11/30/95 WHICH HE ALSO FAILED TO MEET; STILL REQUIRED TO MEET CONTINUING MEDICAL EDUCATION REQUIREMENTS. $100 ADMINISTRATIVE PENALTY; SHALL COOPERATE WITH THE BOARD IN VERIFYING COMPLIANCE.

EWING, CAROL T MD, LICENSE NUMBER 00E3260 OF PORT ARTHUR, TX, WAS DISCIPLINED BY TEXAS ON JANUARY 24, 1992
DISCIPLINARY ACTION: 60-MONTH PROBATION

NOTES: PROFESSIONAL FAILURE TO PRACTICE MEDICINE IN AN ACCEPTABLE MANNER CONSISTENT WITH PUBLIC HEALTH AND WELFARE. PROBATION UNDER TERMS AND CONDITIONS. ON 8/19/94 HER REQUEST FOR TERMINATION OF THIS ORDER DENIED.

FABIAN, HAROLD FRANK MD, DATE OF BIRTH DECEMBER 12, 1924, LICENSE NUMBER 00C3651 OF P.O. BOX 500, MCLEAN, TX, WAS DISCIPLINED BY TEXAS ON AUGUST 24, 1991
DISCIPLINARY ACTION: SURRENDER OF LICENSE
OFFENSE: OVERPRESCRIBING OR MISPRESCRIBING DRUGS

NOTES: NONTHERAPEUTIC PRESCRIBING. SHALL SURRENDER DEA AND DPS CONTROLLED SUBSTANCE REGISTRATION CERTIFICATE; SHALL NOT ATTEMPT TO REREGISTER OR OTHERWISE OBTAIN REGISTRATION WITHOUT PRIOR BOARD APPROVAL. ON 6/15/93 ORDER MODIFIED SO THAT HE MAY SEEK TO OBTAIN HIS DRUG ENFORCEMENT ADMINISTRATION AND TEXAS DEPARTMENT OF PUBLIC SAFETY CONTROLLED SUBSTANCES REGISTRATION CERTIFICATES; UPON OBTAINING THESE CERTIFICATES MAY ADMINISTER AND PRESCRIBE DRUGS WHICH ARE SUBJECT TO THESE REGISTRATIONS FOR LEGITIMATE THERAPEUTIC PURPOSES ONLY; SEPARATE FROM PATIENT RECORDS, HE SHALL MAINTAIN A FILE CONSISTING OF A COPY OF EVERY PRESCRIPTION WRITTEN BY HIM FOR CONTROLLED SUBSTANCES BY DATE ISSUED WHICH SHALL BE AVAILABLE FOR INSPECTION BY THE BOARD; HE SHALL NOT TELEPHONE ANY PRESCRIPTION TO A PHARMACY FOR CONTROLLED SUBSTANCES.

FALBEY, ROBERT JOSEPH DO, LICENSE NUMBER F4817 OF ARLINGTON, TX, WAS DISCIPLINED BY TEXAS ON DECEMBER 11, 1999
DISCIPLINARY ACTION: 60-MONTH PROBATION; RESTRICTION PLACED ON LICENSE
OFFENSE: SUBSTANCE ABUSE

NOTES: LONG HISTORY OF ALCOHOL USE AND ABUSE; IN 1988 ADMITTED FOR A SIX-WEEK INPATIENT PROGRAM; RELAPSED IN 1991 AFTER RETURN FROM GULF WAR; SUFFERED SEVERAL PERSONAL LOSSES AND LIFE CHANGES IN THE EARLY AND MID-90'S WHICH LED TO PERIODIC DRINKING BINGES; IN 5/97 TERMINATED FROM HIS EMPLOYMENT FOR COMING TO WORK AFTER CONSUMING ALCOHOL; ON 7/15/97 ENTERED INTO A CONTRACT WITH THE TEXAS OSTEOPATHIC MEDICAL ASSOCIATION (TOMA); IN 8/98 RELAPSED AND ADMITTED INTO A MEDICAL CENTER 8/6/98 AND DISCHARGED ON 8/8 AGREEING TO UNDERGO PSYCHOTHERAPY AND A PSYCHIATRIC EVALUATION; ON 9/6/98 ARRESTED FOR DRIVING WHILE INTOXICATED AND PLED GUILTY TO A LESSER CHARGE OF OBSTRUCTING A HIGHWAY PASSAGE BECAUSE HE WAS NOT DRIVING IN A SINGLE LANE; ON 9/18/98 THE TEXAS OSTEOPATHIC MEDICAL ASSOCIATION (TOMA) INCLUDED IN AGREEMENT THAT HE WOULD RECEIVE OUTPATIENT TREATMENT FIVE NIGHTS A WEEK; HE INFORMED TOMA THAT COULD NOT COMPLY WITH TERMS DUE TO ITS TIME COMMITMENT AND ON 11/9/98 TOMA WITHDREW ADVOCACY FOR HIM; MAINTAINS THAT HE HAS LONG ACKNOWLEDGED THAT ALCOHOL IS A PROBLEM FOR HIM AND STATES THAT HE ATTENDS AA FOUR TO FIVE TIMES A WEEK; HE STATES THAT HE DOES NOT PRESENTLY ATTEND CADUCEUS NOR RECEIVE PSYCHOTHERAPY; HE DENIES ANY RELAPSE; INFORMED THE BOARD THAT HE REMAINS UNEMPLOYED BUT HAS ATTENDED CONTINUING MEDICAL EDUCATION; STATES THAT HE HAS NOT ACTIVELY PRACTICED SINCE 10/98. FIVE YEAR SUSPENSION STAYED FOR PROBATION WITH FOLLOWING TERMS AND CONDITIONS: SHALL ABSTAIN FROM THE CONSUMPTION OF ALCOHOL/DRUGS IN ANY FORM UNLESS PRESCRIBED BY ANOTHER PHYSICIAN FOR A LEGITIMATE AND THERAPEUTIC PURPOSE; SHALL SUBMIT HIMSELF FOR APPROPRIATE EXAMS INCLUDING DRUG OR ALCOHOL SCREENS; SHALL NOMINATE THREE CERTIFIED PSYCHIATRISTS FOR BOARD SELECTION OF A THERAPIST AND SHALL EXPEDITIOUSLY SUBMIT HIMSELF TO EVALUATION AND TREATMENT BY THE APPROVED PRACTITIONER; SHALL PARTICIPATE IN THE ACTIVITIES OF A PHYSICIAN HEALTH AND REHABILITATION COMMITTEE WITH QUARTERLY REPORTS; SHALL PARTICIPATE IN AA'S PROGRAM NOT LESS THAN FOUR TIMES A WEEK; SHALL REPORT ON HIS ATTENDANCE; SHALL LIMIT MEDICAL PRACTICE TO A GROUP OR INSTITUTIONAL SETTING; HIS MEDICAL PRACTICE SHALL BE MONITORED BY A BOARD APPROVED TEXAS PHYSICIAN WHO SHALL PROVIDE QUARTERLY REPORTS TO THE BOARD; SHALL APPEAR BEFORE THE BOARD UPON REQUEST; SHALL COOPERATE WITH THE BOARD IN VERIFYING COMPLIANCE INCLUDING PROVIDING COPIES OF MEDICAL RELEASES AND PEER REVIEW RECORDS UPON REQUEST; SHALL OBTAIN 50 HOURS PER YEAR OF CONTINUING MEDICAL EDUCATION; SHALL GIVE A COPY OF THIS ORDER TO ANY HEALTH CARE ENTITY WHERE HE HAS PRIVILEGES; SHALL PROVIDE A COPY OF THIS ORDER TO ANYONE REQUESTING IT WITHIN 10 DAYS; TIME SPENT OUT OF TEXAS DOES NOT COUNT TOWARD PROBATION; SHALL INFORM THE BOARD OF CHANGE OF ADDRESS WITHIN 10 DAYS OR IF HE LEAVES THE STATE; SHALL NOT SEEK MODIFICATION FOR ONE YEAR.

FAM, FATHI MD, LICENSE NUMBER 00E7909 OF CORPUS CHRISTI, TX, WAS DISCIPLINED BY TEXAS ON MARCH 4, 1995
DISCIPLINARY ACTION: 36-MONTH PROBATION; RESTRICTION PLACED ON LICENSE
OFFENSE: SUBSTANDARD CARE, INCOMPETENCE OR NEGLIGENCE

NOTES: ALLEGEDLY FAILED TO ADEQUATELY TREAT FOUR PATIENTS BY FAILING TO ORDER OR PERFORM APPROPRIATE PROCEDURES, FAILING TO OBTAIN A SURGICAL CONSULTATION, PERFORMING PROCEDURES IN HIS OFFICE DESPITE EXTENSIVE DISEASE IN A PATIENT AND FAILING TO CONDUCT AN ADEQUATE EXAMINATION ON A PATIENT; HE DENIES THESE ALLEGATIONS. SUSPENSION STAYED. PROBATION WITH TERMS: SHALL APPEAR BEFORE BOARD ONCE A YEAR; SHALL ATTEND AT LEAST 30

HOURS PER YEAR OF CONTINUING MEDICAL EDUCATION, INCLUDING AT LEAST 20 HOURS IN GASTROENTEROLOGY; SHALL NOT ENGAGE IN LASER HEMORRHOIDECTOMY SURGERIES UNTIL FURTHER ORDER OF THE BOARD, IRRESPECTIVE OF PROBATIONARY TERMS; SHALL GIVE A COPY OF ORDER TO ANY HEALTH CARE ENTITY WHERE HE HAS PRIVILEGES; SHALL COOPERATE WITH THE BOARD IN VERIFYING COMPLIANCE; SHALL INFORM THE BOARD OF ANY CHANGE OF ADDRESS WITHIN 10 DAYS OR IF HE LEAVES THE STATE; TIME PERIOD OUT OF TEXAS DOES NOT COUNT TOWARD PROBATION. SHALL NOT SEEK MODIFICATION FOR ONE YEAR. ON 5/15/96 PROBATION TERMINATED.

FARHA, ABDUL-MASIH MD, LICENSE NUMBER G0698, WAS DISCIPLINED BY TEXAS ON MAY 10, 1997
DISCIPLINARY ACTION: 36-MONTH FINE; REQUIRED TO TAKE ADDITIONAL MEDICAL EDUCATION
OFFENSE: NONCOMPLIANCE WITH A PROFESSIONAL RULE

NOTES: THE MEDICAL RECORDS REGARDING HIS CARE AND TREATMENT OF ONE PATIENT FAIL TO DOCUMENT HIS RATIONALE FOR FAILING TO ORDER SUBCLAVIAN VENOUS ACCESS FOR THIS PATIENT'S CHEMOTHERAPY. THE PATIENT WAS ORDERED A PERIPHERAL INTRAVENOUS LINE WHICH LATER DEVELOPED TISSUE NECROSIS. HE FAILED TO ADEQUATELY DOCUMENT HIS MONITORING OF THIS PATIENT'S IV LINE. HE FAILED ALSO TO DOCUMENT A REFERRAL OF THE PATIENT TO A SURGEON AFTER THE PATIENT COMPLAINED OF BURNING AND PAIN. LICENSE IS RESTRICTED FOR THREE YEARS AS FOLLOWS: SHALL MAINTAIN ADEQUATE MEDICAL RECORDS WHICH SHALL BE MADE AVAILABLE FOR REVIEW; SHALL ATTEND AT LEAST 50 HOURS OF CONTINUING MEDICAL EDUCATION A YEAR, INCLUDING ONE COURSE IN RISK MANAGEMENT OR RECORD KEEPING; SHALL PAY AN ADMINISTRATIVE PENALTY OF $1,000; SHALL APPEAR BEFORE THE BOARD AT LEAST ANNUALLY; SHALL COOPERATE WITH THE BOARD IN VERIFYING COMPLIANCE; SHALL GIVE A COPY OF THIS ORDER TO ANY HEALTH CARE ENTITY WHERE HE HAS PRIVILEGES; TIME SPENT OUT OF TEXAS DOES NOT COUNT TOWARD RESTRICTION; SHALL INFORM THE BOARD OF CHANGE OF ADDRESS WITHIN 10 DAYS OR IF HE LEAVES THE STATE; SHALL NOT SEEK MODIFICATION FOR ONE YEAR. ON 5/16/98 THE ORDER WAS TERMINATED.

FARLEY, PATRICK CLARE MD, LICENSE NUMBER 0030541 OF SEATTLE, WA, WAS DISCIPLINED BY WASHINGTON ON JULY 27, 1994
DISCIPLINARY ACTION: EMERGENCY SUSPENSION
OFFENSE: PHYSICAL OR MENTAL ILLNESS INHIBITING THE ABILITY TO PRACTICE WITH SKILL AND SAFETY

NOTES: UNABLE TO PRACTICE WITH REASONABLE SKILL AND SAFETY DUE TO A MENTAL OR PHYSICAL CONDITION, HE HAS COMMITTED ACTS OF MORAL TURPITUDE AND HE MISREPRESENTED A FACT IN HIS APPLICATION FOR A LICENSE TO PRACTICE MEDICINE.

FARLEY, PATRICK CLARE MD, LICENSE NUMBER 00G2696 OF SEATTLE, WA, WAS DISCIPLINED BY TEXAS ON OCTOBER 27, 1994
DISCIPLINARY ACTION: EMERGENCY SUSPENSION
OFFENSE: DISCIPLINARY ACTION BY ANOTHER STATE OR AGENCY

NOTES: AVAILABLE EVIDENCE AND INFORMATION INDICATE THE FOLLOWING: HAS ENGAGED IN CONDUCT INDICATIVE OF A MENTAL CONDITION WHICH CAUSES HIM TO BE UNABLE TO PRACTICE WITH REASONABLE SKILL AND SAFETY; HAS UNDERGONE AN INDEPENDENT PSYCHIATRIC EXAM WHICH LED TO A DIAGNOSIS OF SUCH A MENTAL CONDITION; ON 7/27/94 WASHINGTON SUMMARILY SUSPENDED HIS LICENSE BASED ON THIS.

FARLEY, PATRICK CLARE MD, LICENSE NUMBER 0030541 OF EL PASO, TX, WAS DISCIPLINED BY WASHINGTON ON APRIL 19, 1996
DISCIPLINARY ACTION: LICENSE SUSPENSION

NOTES: INDEFINITE SUSPENSION PENDING THE COMPLETION OF A NUMBER OF CONDITIONS.

FARLEY, PATRICK CLARE MD, LICENSE NUMBER 00G2696, WAS DISCIPLINED BY TEXAS ON AUGUST 17, 1996
DISCIPLINARY ACTION: 60-MONTH PROBATION; REQUIRED TO TAKE ADDITIONAL MEDICAL EDUCATION
OFFENSE: PHYSICAL OR MENTAL ILLNESS INHIBITING THE ABILITY TO PRACTICE WITH SKILL AND SAFETY

NOTES: ON 10/27/94 TEMPORARILY SUSPENDED BY THE TEXAS BOARD BASED ON AN ASSAULT AND CRIMINAL TRESPASS CONVICTION IN SEATTLE IN 1994 AND INABILITY TO PRACTICE BY REASON OF A MENTAL CONDITION; AFTER 7/27/94 ENTERED TREATMENT FOR BI-POLAR DISORDER; THREE PHYSICIANS ON 4/05/96, 7/09/96, AND 7/22/96 EXPRESSED THEIR OPINION THAT HE IS ABLE TO PRACTICE MEDICINE; MET ALL REQUIREMENTS SET FOR THE LIFTING OF SUSPENSION OF WASHINGTON ACTION. SUSPENSION STAYED. CONDITIONS OF PROBATION: SHALL NOT PRACTICE MEDICINE IN TEXAS UNTIL HE REQUESTS IN WRITING TO THE BOARD TO RESUME THE PRACTICE OF MEDICINE IN TEXAS AND PROVIDES SUFFICIENT EVIDENCE AND INFORMATION WHICH INDICATES THAT THE SUSPENSION PREVIOUSLY IMPOSED ON HIS WASHINGTON LICENSE HAS BEEN STAYED OR LIFTED; SHALL CONTINUE TO RECEIVE CARE AND TREATMENT FROM A BOARD APPROVED PSYCHIATRIST NO LESS THAN ONCE PER MONTH WHO SHALL PROVIDE QUARTERLY REPORTS; SHALL PARTICIPATE IN ALCOHOL OR DRUG SCREENS; HIS MEDICAL PRACTICE, INCLUDING ANY OFFICE AND SURGICAL PRACTICE, SHALL BE MONITORED BY A BOARD APPROVED TEXAS PHYSICIAN WITH QUARTERLY REPORTS TO THE BOARD; SHALL OBTAIN AT LEAST 50 HOURS PER YEAR OF CONTINUING MEDICAL EDUCATION; SHALL APPEAR BEFORE THE BOARD AT LEAST ONE TIME PER YEAR OR UPON REQUEST; SHALL COOPERATE WITH THE BOARD IN VERIFYING COMPLIANCE INCLUDING PROVIDING COPIES OF MEDICAL RELEASES UPON REQUEST; SHALL COMPLY WITH THE WASHINGTON ORDER; SHALL GIVE A COPY OF THIS ORDER TO ANY HEALTH CARE ENTITY WHERE HE HAS PRIVILEGES; SHALL PROVIDE A COPY OF THIS ORDER TO ANYONE REQUESTING IT WITHIN 10 DAYS; TIME PERIOD OUT OF TEXAS DOES NOT COUNT TOWARD RESTRICTION; SHALL INFORM THE BOARD OF CHANGE OF ADDRESS WITHIN 10 DAYS OR IF HE LEAVES THE STATE; SHALL NOT SEEK MODIFICATION FOR ONE YEAR. ON 8/22/98 ORDER MODIFIED AS FOLLOWS: REQUIRED MONTHLY TREATMENTS REPLACED WITH TREATMENT AS DIRECTED BY TREATING PHYSICIAN, AND DELETION OF ANNUAL APPEARANCE BEFORE THE BOARD.

FARLEY, PATRICK CLARE MD, LICENSE NUMBER 0030541 OF EL PASO, TX, WAS DISCIPLINED BY WASHINGTON ON SEPTEMBER 25, 1996

NOTES: PREVIOUS SUSPENSION NOW RESTRICTED TO THE TERMS OF THE 4/96 CONSENT ORDER.

FARLEY, PATRICK CLARE MD, LICENSE NUMBER G2696 OF EL PASO, TX, WAS DISCIPLINED BY TEXAS ON JANUARY 13, 1999
DISCIPLINARY ACTION: EMERGENCY SUSPENSION

NOTES: DURING 10/98 AND 11/98 HIS MEDICAL RECORDS INDICATE HE BEGAN TO BECOME INCREASINGLY IRRITABLE, HAD POOR IMPULSE CONTROL AND DIFFICULTY IN PROFESSIONAL RELATIONSHIPS; HAD A VIOLENT INCIDENT IN A STORE, THROWING VIDEOCASSETTES AND SENT THREATENING LETTERS TO A FORMER EMPLOYEE; ON 11/17/98 ADMITTED HIMSELF FOR TREATMENT, DENIED HE WAS IN A MANIC PHASE OF HIS DISORDER AND LEFT ON HIS OWN ACCORD ON 11/30/98.

FARLEY, PATRICK CLARE MD, LICENSE NUMBER G2696 OF EL PASO, TX, WAS DISCIPLINED BY TEXAS ON APRIL 10, 1999
DISCIPLINARY ACTION: 120-MONTH PROBATION; REQUIRED TO TAKE ADDITIONAL MEDICAL EDUCATION

NOTES: HE WAS PREVIOUSLY UNDER A 8/17/96 BOARD ORDER WHICH WAS MODIFIED ON 6/3/98; ON OR ABOUT 11/17/98 VOLUNTARILY ADMITTED HIMSELF TO COLUMBIA BEHAVIORAL CENTER, BUT LEFT AGAINST RECOMMENDATIONS; ON 1/13/99 HIS LICENSE WAS TEMPORARILY SUSPENDED; IN A LETTER 3/1/99 THE BOARD CERTIFIED PSYCHIATRIST EXPRESSED THAT THE DOCTOR IS CLEARED TO RETURN TO CLINICAL DUTIES; HE HAS STATED HIS INTENTION TO RETURN TO PRACTICE IN A CONTROLLED PRACTICE SETTING. SUSPENSION PREVIOUSLY IMPOSED IS STAYED FOR PROBATION WITH THE FOLLOWING TERMS AND CONDITIONS: SHALL NOT PRACTICE UNTIL HE REQUESTS IN WRITING TO RESUME PRACTICE AND PROVIDES SUFFICIENT EVIDENCE AND INFORMATION INDICATING THAT THE SUSPENSION PREVIOUSLY IMPOSED BY THE WASHINGTON BOARD HAS BEEN STAYED OR LIFTED; SHALL CONTINUE TO RECEIVE CARE AND TREATMENT FROM HIS DOCTOR OR SHALL NOMINATE THREE CERTIFIED PSYCHIATRISTS FOR BOARD SELECTION OF A THERAPIST AND SHALL EXPEDITIOUSLY SUBMIT HIMSELF TO EVALUATION AND TREATMENT BY THE APPROVED PRACTITIONER; HIS MEDICAL PRACTICE SHALL BE MONITORED BY A BOARD APPROVED TEXAS PHYSICIAN WHO SHALL PROVIDE QUARTERLY REPORTS TO THE BOARD; SHALL OBTAIN 50 HOURS OF CONTINUING MEDICAL EDUCATION; SHALL APPEAR BEFORE THE BOARD UPON REQUEST; SHALL COMPLY WITH TERMS OF WASHINGTON BOARD ORDER; SHALL COOPERATE WITH THE BOARD IN VERIFYING COMPLIANCE INCLUDING PROVIDING COPIES OF MEDICAL RELEASES UPON REQUEST; SHALL GIVE A COPY OF THIS ORDER TO ANY HEALTH CARE ENTITY WHERE HE HAS PRIVILEGES; SHALL PROVIDE A COPY OF THIS ORDER TO ANYONE REQUESTING IT WITHIN 10 DAYS; TIME SPENT OUT OF TEXAS DOES NOT COUNT TOWARD PROBATION; SHALL INFORM THE BOARD OF CHANGE OF ADDRESS WITHIN 10 DAYS OR IF HE LEAVES THE STATE; SHALL NOT SEEK MODIFICATION FOR ONE YEAR.

FARLEY, PATRICK CLARE MD, LICENSE NUMBER 30541 OF EL PASO, TX, WAS DISCIPLINED BY WASHINGTON ON SEPTEMBER 23, 1999
DISCIPLINARY ACTION: 120-MONTH PROBATION

FAUST, HARRY LOUIS JR DO, LICENSE NUMBER 00E0905, WAS DISCIPLINED BY TEXAS ON AUGUST 17, 1996
DISCIPLINARY ACTION: REPRIMAND; REQUIRED TO TAKE ADDITIONAL MEDICAL EDUCATION
OFFENSE: SUBSTANCE ABUSE

NOTES: PRESCRIBED BENZODIAZEPINES TO A PATIENT FOR EIGHT YEARS WITHOUT ADEQUATE DOCUMENTATION TO SUPPORT CONTINUED USE; IN 4/94 INSTRUCTED THIS PATIENT TO CEASE TAKING BENZODIAZEPINES WITHOUT ADEQUATE DOCUMENTATION TO SUPPORT A SUDDEN CESSATION OF THIS MEDICATION; RECEIVED INPATIENT SUBSTANCE ABUSE TREATMENT FROM 5/08/92 TO 05/16/92; REPORTED A SOBRIETY DATE OF 5/08/92; AND NOT CURRENTLY UNDER THE CARE OF ANY PROFESSIONAL IN RELATION TO HIS SOBRIETY. FIVE YEAR RESTRICTIONS: SHALL ABSTAIN FROM THE CONSUMPTION OF ALCOHOL/DRUGS, IN ANY FORM UNLESS PRESCRIBED BY ANOTHER PHYSICIAN FOR A LEGITIMATE AND THERAPEUTIC PURPOSE; SHALL SUBMIT HIMSELF FOR APPROPRIATE EXAMS, INCLUDING DRUG AND ALCOHOL SCREENS; SHALL SUBMIT HIMSELF TO EVALUATION AND TREATMENT BY A BOARD APPROVED PSYCHIATRIST WHO HE SHALL SEE AT LEAST ONCE A MONTH AND WHO SHALL MAKE REPORTS TO THE BOARD; SHALL PARTICIPATE IN AA'S PROGRAM NOT LESS THAN THREE TIMES PER WEEK WITH QUARTERLY REPORTS TO THE BOARD; SHALL PARTICIPATE IN THE ACTIVITIES OF A PHYSICIAN HEALTH AND REHABILITATION PROGRAM AND ATTEND WEEKLY MEETINGS WITH QUARTERLY REPORTS; SHALL NOT TREAT OR OTHERWISE SERVE AS PHYSICIAN, PRESCRIBE, DISPENSE, OR ADMINISTER DRUGS WITH POTENTIAL FOR ABUSE TO HIMSELF OR ANY MEMBER OF HIS FAMILY; HIS MEDICAL PRACTICE, INCLUDING ANY OFFICE AND SURGICAL PRACTICE SHALL BE MONITORED BY A BOARD APPROVED TEXAS PHYSICIAN WHO SHALL SUBMIT QUARTERLY REPORTS; SHALL MAINTAIN ADEQUATE MEDICAL RECORDS WHICH SHALL BE AVAILABLE FOR REVIEW; SHALL OBTAIN AT LEAST 50 HOURS PER YEAR OF CONTINUING MEDICAL EDUCATION; SHALL APPEAR BEFORE THE BOARD AT LEAST TWO TIMES PER YEAR OR UPON REQUEST; SHALL COOPERATE WITH THE BOARD IN VERIFYING COMPLIANCE INCLUDING SUPPLYING REPORTS FROM BETTY FORD CENTER; SHALL GIVE A COPY OF THIS ORDER TO ANY HEALTH CARE ENTITY WHERE HE HAS PRIVILEGES; SHALL PROVIDE A COPY OF THIS ORDER TO ANYONE REQUESTING IT WITHIN 10 DAYS; TIME PERIOD OUT OF TEXAS DOES NOT COUNT TOWARD RESTRICTION; SHALL INFORM THE BOARD OF CHANGE OF ADDRESS WITHIN 10 DAYS OF IF HE LEAVES THE STATE; SHALL NOT SEEK MODIFICATION FOR ONE YEAR. ON 8/22/98 ORDER TERMINATED.

FERGUSON, JAMES W MD OF 3115 PINE STREET #304, WACO, TX, WAS DISCIPLINED BY DEA ON FEBRUARY 4, 1997
DISCIPLINARY ACTION: SURRENDER OF CONTROLLED SUBSTANCE LICENSE

FERGUSON, JAMES W MD, LICENSE NUMBER E4327 OF WACO, TX, WAS DISCIPLINED BY TEXAS ON NOVEMBER 22, 1997
DISCIPLINARY ACTION: 48-MONTH RESTRICTION PLACED ON LICENSE; RESTRICTION PLACED ON CONTROLLED SUBSTANCE LICENSE
OFFENSE: LOSS OR RESTRICTION OF HOSPITAL PRIVILEGES

NOTES: HE ORDERED-BY-MAIL AND DISTRIBUTED CONTROLLED SUBSTANCES TO HIS GIRLFRIEND, HER FAMILY AND OTHERS ALONG WITH HIMSELF; HE DID NOT MAINTAIN PROPER MEDICAL RECORDS REGARDING THESE DISTRIBUTIONS OR TREATMENTS; ON 2/3/97 THE DEA APPROACHED HIM REGARDING APPARENT PRESCRIPTION IRREGULARITIES WHICH HE ACKNOWLEDGED AND VOLUNTARILY SURRENDERED HIS DEA REGISTRATION; ON 2/12/97 HIS PRIVILEGES AT HILLCREST BAPTIST MEDICAL

CENTER WERE RESTRICTED BASED UPON THE DEA ACTION; ON 4/29/97 HIS PRESCRIBING/DISPENSING PRIVILEGES WERE SUSPENDED AT ANOTHER HEALTH CENTER ON AN INTERIM BASIS. LICENSE LIMITED AS FOLLOWS: SHALL NOMINATE THREE CERTIFIED PSYCHIATRISTS FOR BOARD SELECTION OF A THERAPIST AND SHALL EXPEDITIOUSLY SUBMIT HIMSELF TO EVALUATION AND TREATMENT BY THE APPROVED PRACTITIONER; SHALL NOT TREAT OR OTHERWISE SERVE AS PHYSICIAN, PRESCRIBE, DISPENSE OR ADMINISTER DRUGS THAT MAY BE SUBJECT TO ABUSE TO HIMSELF OR TO ANY MEMBER OF HIS FAMILY; SHALL NOT SERVE AS PHYSICIAN FOR ANY PATIENT OVER 21; SHALL NOT DISPENSE ANY DRUGS WITH POTENTIAL FOR ABUSE; SHALL REAPPLY TO THE DEA AND THE TEXAS DEPARTMENT OF PUBLIC SAFETY TO OBTAIN FULL PRESCRIBING AUTHORITY FOR CONTROLLED SUBSTANCES; SEPARATE FROM PATIENT RECORDS, SHALL MAINTAIN A LOGBOOK OF EVERY PRESCRIPTION WRITTEN BY HIM FOR DANGEROUS DRUGS WITH ADDICTIVE POTENTIAL WHICH SHALL BE MADE AVAILABLE FOR REVIEW; SHALL OBTAIN 12 HOURS PER YEAR OF AN ETHICS COURSE AND 50 HOURS PER YEAR OF CONTINUING MEDICAL EDUCATION; SHALL MAINTAIN ADEQUATE MEDICAL RECORDS WHICH SHALL BE AVAILABLE FOR REVIEW; SHALL APPEAR BEFORE THE BOARD AT LEAST ONCE A YEAR; SHALL COOPERATE WITH THE BOARD IN VERIFYING COMPLIANCE INCLUDING PROVIDING COPIES OF MEDICAL RELEASES; SHALL GIVE A COPY OF THIS ORDER TO ANY HEALTH CARE ENTITY WHERE HE HAS PRIVILEGES; TIME SPENT OUT OF TEXAS DOES NOT COUNT TOWARD RESTRICTION; SHALL INFORM THE BOARD OF CHANGE OF ADDRESS WITHIN 10 DAYS OR IF HE LEAVES THE STATE; SHALL NOT SEEK MODIFICATION FOR ONE YEAR. ON 1/29/99 THE ORDER WAS MODIFIED BY DELETING THE REQUIREMENTS RELATING TO ONGOING PSYCHIATRIC TREATMENT; ALL OTHER PROVISIONS OF BOARD ORDER REMAIN IN EFFECT UNTIL SUPERSEDED BY A SUBSEQUENT BOARD ORDER.

FERGUSON, JOHN MD, LICENSE NUMBER 00C2487 OF SHERMAN, TX, WAS DISCIPLINED BY ARKANSAS ON SEPTEMBER 1, 1996
DISCIPLINARY ACTION: LICENSE REVOCATION

FERNANDEZ, CARLOS ANTONIO MD, LICENSE NUMBER 00C2460 OF EL PASO, TX, WAS DISCIPLINED BY TEXAS ON FEBRUARY 22, 1991
DISCIPLINARY ACTION: 60-MONTH PROBATION; RESTRICTION PLACED ON LICENSE

NOTES: MUST SUBMIT TO PSYCHIATRIC EVALUATION AND UNDERGO RECOMMENDED TREATMENT; APPEAR FOR ANNUAL REPORT TO BOARD; EXAMINE NO FEMALE PATIENTS UNLESS A CHAPERONE IS PRESENT IN THE EXAMINATION ROOM. ON 1/24/92 REQUEST TO TERMINATE ORDER DENIED.

FERNANDEZ, CARLOS H MD, LICENSE NUMBER 00D9438, WAS DISCIPLINED BY TEXAS ON AUGUST 17, 1996
DISCIPLINARY ACTION: REPRIMAND
OFFENSE: PROFESSIONAL MISCONDUCT

NOTES: DURING 1995 DID NOT MAINTAIN ADEQUATE RECORDS OF PATIENT CARE DELIVERED INCLUDING CHARTING OF THERAPEUTIC RADIATION PROVIDED; AND WITHOUT LEGAL AUTHORITY, TOOK SOLE POSSESSION OF PATIENT RECORDS FROM A RADIATION TREATMENT CLINIC.

FERNANDEZ, CARLOS H MD, LICENSE NUMBER D9438 OF HOUSTON, TX, WAS DISCIPLINED BY TEXAS ON APRIL 7, 1998
DISCIPLINARY ACTION: EMERGENCY SUSPENSION
OFFENSE: SUBSTANDARD CARE, INCOMPETENCE OR NEGLIGENCE

NOTES: APPEARS TO HAVE USED TREATMENTS THAT WERE NONTHERAPEUTIC OR OVERUSED IN THE PROCEDURES IN SEVEN PATIENTS HE TREATED FOR CANCER AS FOLLOWS: ON 1/27/98 HE WAS ADVISED BY DOCTORS AND FELLOW RADIATION ONCOLOGISTS REGARDING ONE PATIENT THAT "NO TREATMENT SHOULD BE GIVEN UNLESS AN ADEQUATE REASON IS DOCUMENTED ON THE CHARTS" ; HE STILL SCHEDULED THIS PATIENT TO UNDERGO RADIATION THERAPY, CONTRIBUTED TO DELAY IN TREATMENT, AND REFUSED TO REFER THE PATIENT TO ANOTHER ONCOLOGIST FOR TREATMENT; ON OR ABOUT 1/6/98 HE DECLINED TO FOLLOW THE SUGGESTIONS OF THE OWNER AND CHAIRMAN OF THE BOARD OF THE CANCER CENTER IN REGARDS TO HIS USE OF PREOPERATIVE RADIATION THERAPY, ON A 10 YEAR OLD GIRL, WHICH WAS NOT THE CURRENT STANDARD OF CARE IN THAT CANCER CENTER'S COMMUNITY; HE WAS INFORMED THAT OTHER STAFF MEMBERS CONCURRED WITH THIS OPINION; HE DECLINED TO FOLLOW THE SUGGESTIONS AND SAID THAT HE WOULD CONTINUE WITH HIS ORIGINAL DECISION TO TREAT THE PATIENT WITH PRE-OPERATIVE AND POST-OPERATIVE RADIATION TREATMENTS; ON THE 5/14 SIMULATION OF AN IMPLANT WHICH HE INSERTED IN QUESTION WAS WELL OUTSIDE THE EXTERNAL BEAM TREATMENT FIELD WHERE IT SHOULD HAVE BEEN; REGARDING A 77 YEAR OLD FEMALE PATIENT DIAGNOSED WITH SQUAMOUS CELL CARCINOMA OF THE LEG AND HAVING RECEIVED GOLD SEED IMPLANT BY HIM ON 4/9/96, IT WAS INAPPROPRIATE FOR HIM TO BEGIN SO SOON AFTER THE IMPLANT SINCE THE MINIMUM WAIT SHOULD HAVE BEEN 3 WEEKS; THE PATIENT EVENTUALLY HAD TO HAVE HER LEG AMPUTATED DUE TO THE SEVERE ULCERATIONS; ON OR ABOUT 4/4/96, REGARDING A 73 YEAR OLD MALE PATIENT WITH A KNOWN DIAGNOSIS OF CARCINOMA OF THE PROSTATE DATING BACK TO 1994, 2 STRONTIUM 89 INJECTIONS HE ADMINISTERED WITHIN A SHORT PERIOD OF TIME LED TO BONE MARROW FAILURE AND MAY HAVE HASTENED THE PATIENT'S DEATH; IN 10/96 REGARDING A 75 YEAR OLD MALE PATIENT, HE INSERTED A BLOCK CLOSE TO A TUMOR THEN DELIVERED 6 TREATMENTS TO THE PATIENT; NUMEROUS ATTEMPTS WERE MADE BY THE CANCER CENTER STAFF TO BRING TO HIS ATTENTION THE QUESTIONABLE DOSAGE ADMINISTERED BY HIM; HE RELENTED AND REMOVED THE BLOCK THAT COVERED THE TUMOR; REGARDING A 91 YEAR OLD FEMALE PATIENT WITH CARCINOMA OF THE CERVIX, SHE DEVELOPED SEVERE ULCERATIONS TO HER PELVIC REGION AS A RESULT OF THE EXCESSIVE RADIATION SHE HAD RECEIVED FROM HIM DURING 1993-1995.

FERNANDEZ, CARLOS H MD, LICENSE NUMBER D9438 OF HOUSTON, TX, WAS DISCIPLINED BY TEXAS ON MAY 16, 1998
DISCIPLINARY ACTION: 84-MONTH PROBATION; RESTRICTION PLACED ON LICENSE
OFFENSE: SUBSTANDARD CARE, INCOMPETENCE OR NEGLIGENCE

NOTES: BASED ON OFFENSES LISTED IN 4/7/98 ORDER. SUSPENSION STAYED FOR PROBATION WITH FOLLOWING TERMS AND CONDITIONS: FOR ALL THERAPEUTIC DECISIONS IN THE AREA OF RADIATION ONCOLOGY, PRIOR TO INITIATING ANY TREATMENT OR THERAPY, SHALL OBTAIN A SECOND OPINION FROM A BOARD CERTIFIED RADIATION ONCOLOGIST; SHALL NOT PERFORM ANY INVASIVE RADIOTHERAPEUTIC PROCEDURE INCLUDING BUT NOT LIMITED TO GOLD SEED IMPLANTATION OR

INTRACAVITARY THERAPY; HIS MEDICAL PRACTICE SHALL BE MONITORED BY A BOARD APPROVED TEXAS PHYSICIAN WHO SHALL PROVIDE QUARTERLY REPORTS TO THE BOARD; SHALL MAINTAIN ADEQUATE MEDICAL RECORDS WHICH SHALL BE AVAILABLE FOR REVIEW; WITHIN 1 YEAR SHALL TAKE AND PASS THE SPEX; SHALL OBTAIN 75 HOURS PER YEAR OF CONTINUING MEDICAL EDUCATION; AND SHALL TAKE AND SUCCESSFULLY COMPLETE AN ADVANCED CARDIAC LIFE SUPPORT COURSE AND OBTAIN CERTIFICATION; SHALL PERFORM 100 HOURS OF COMMUNITY SERVICE; SHALL APPEAR BEFORE THE BOARD TWICE A YEAR; SHALL COOPERATE WITH THE BOARD IN VERIFYING COMPLIANCE; SHALL GIVE A COPY OF THIS ORDER TO ANY HEALTH CARE ENTITY WHERE HE HAS PRIVILEGES; TIME SPENT OUT OF TEXAS DOES NOT COUNT TOWARD PROBATION; SHALL INFORM THE BOARD OF CHANGE OF ADDRESS WITHIN 10 DAYS OR IF HE LEAVES THE STATE; SHALL NOT SEEK MODIFICATION FOR 6 MONTHS.

FERNANDEZ, CARLOS H MD, LICENSE NUMBER D9438 OF HOUSTON, TX, WAS DISCIPLINED BY TEXAS ON MAY 17, 1999
DISCIPLINARY ACTION: LICENSE SUSPENSION
OFFENSE: FAILURE TO COMPLY WITH PREVIOUS BOARD ORDER

NOTES: FAILED TO TAKE AND PASS THE SPEX, OR IN THE ALTERNATIVE HAS FAILED TO SUCCESSFULLY PASS THE CERTIFICATION OR RECERTIFICATION EXAM OF THE AMERICAN BOARD OF MEDICAL SPECIALTIES IN RADIOLOGY, AS REQUIRED BY THE 5/16/98 BOARD ORDER.

FERNANDEZ-VILA, WILFREDO MD, LICENSE NUMBER 0D03201 OF 1714 HOUSTON BOULEVARD, SOUTH HOUSTON, TX, WAS DISCIPLINED BY MARYLAND ON MAY 23, 1990
DISCIPLINARY ACTION: SURRENDER OF LICENSE
OFFENSE: DISCIPLINARY ACTION BY ANOTHER STATE OR AGENCY

NOTES: ON 9/4/87 HE ENTERED INTO A MEMORANDUM OF AGREEMENT WITH THE DEA IN WHICH HE AGREED NOT TO PRESCRIBE, ORDER, OR HANDLE SCHEDULE II, IIN, III OR IIIN CONTROLLED SUBSTANCES, OR ANY SCHEDULE V NARCOTIC SUBSTANCES, FOR FIVE YEARS. ORIGINALLY PLACED ON PROBATIONARY STATUS BY TEXAS BOARD UNTIL SEPTEMBER 3, 1992. AS PART OF HIS AGREED BOARD ORDER, HE WAS ALSO REQUIRED TO ENROLL AND COMPLETE A TWO WEEK PRECEPTORSHIP ON THE PREVENTION AND TREATMENT OF DRUG ABUSE.

FERNANDEZ-VILA, WILFREDO MD, DATE OF BIRTH JULY 1, 1916, LICENSE NUMBER 0012162 OF 1714 HOUSTON BLVD, SOUTH HOUSTON, TX, WAS DISCIPLINED BY GEORGIA ON NOVEMBER 15, 1990
DISCIPLINARY ACTION: LICENSE REVOCATION
OFFENSE: DISCIPLINARY ACTION BY ANOTHER STATE OR AGENCY

FERNANDEZ-VILA, WILFREDO MD, LICENSE NUMBER 0100494 OF 1714 HOUSTON BOULEVARD, SOUTH HOUSTON, TX, WAS DISCIPLINED BY NEW YORK ON AUGUST 2, 1993
DISCIPLINARY ACTION: LICENSE REVOCATION
OFFENSE: DISCIPLINARY ACTION BY ANOTHER STATE OR AGENCY

NOTES: FOUND GUILTY BY THE DRUG ENFORCEMENT ADMINISTRATION OF VIOLATING FEDERAL LAWS AND REGULATIONS RELATING TO THE PRESCRIBING OF CONTROLLED SUBSTANCES.

FILARDI, H H MD OF 300 OVERLOCK, GRANBURY, TX, WAS DISCIPLINED BY DEA ON SEPTEMBER 7, 1995
DISCIPLINARY ACTION: SURRENDER OF CONTROLLED SUBSTANCE LICENSE
OFFENSE: DISCIPLINARY ACTION BY ANOTHER STATE OR AGENCY

NOTES: STATE BOARD.

FILARDI, HECTOR HIRAM MD, DATE OF BIRTH MARCH 28, 1923, LICENSE NUMBER 00C5531 OF GRANBURY, TX, WAS DISCIPLINED BY TEXAS ON APRIL 15, 1994
DISCIPLINARY ACTION: RESTRICTION PLACED ON LICENSE
OFFENSE: SEXUAL ABUSE OF OR SEXUAL MISCONDUCT WITH A PATIENT

NOTES: CRIMINAL COMPLAINT HAS BEEN FILED AGAINST HIM ALLEGING THAT HE HAS ENGAGED IN BEHAVIOR CONSTITUTING SEXUAL INDECENCY WITH VARIOUS MINORS WHO WERE HIS PATIENTS; DENIES ALL OF THE ALLEGATIONS AND WHILE MAKING NO ADMISSION REGARDING ANY PENDING ACCUSATIONS VOLUNTARILY AGREED TO THE ENTRY OF THIS ORDER. PRACTICE RESTRICTED IN THAT HE SHALL NOT EXAMINE OR TREAT ANY PEDIATRIC PATIENT UNDER 16 YEARS OF AGE; IN THE EVENT THE CRIMINAL CHARGES ARE DISPOSED OF THROUGH DISMISSAL OR ACQUITTAL THIS RESTRICTION SHALL TERMINATE; SHALL COOPERATE WITH THE BOARD IN VERIFYING COMPLIANCE; SHALL INFORM BOARD OF CHANGE OF ADDRESS WITHIN 10 DAYS.

FILARDI, HECTOR HIRAM MD, DATE OF BIRTH MARCH 28, 1923, LICENSE NUMBER 00C5531 OF 4526 OVERLOOK DRIVE, ACTON, TX, WAS DISCIPLINED BY TEXAS ON JUNE 28, 1995
DISCIPLINARY ACTION: SURRENDER OF LICENSE

NOTES: ALLEGEDLY ENGAGED IN PRACTICE WHICH COULD CONSTITUTE PROFESSIONAL FAILURE TO PRACTICE IN AN ACCEPTABLE MANNER CONSISTENT WITH PUBLIC HEALTH AND WELFARE; DENIES ALLEGATIONS. VOLUNTARY AND PERMANENT SURRENDER OF LICENSE.

FINCH, ALBERT B MD, LICENSE NUMBER C3297 OF ODESSA, TX, WAS DISCIPLINED BY TEXAS ON AUGUST 22, 1998
DISCIPLINARY ACTION: RESTRICTION PLACED ON LICENSE; REQUIRED TO TAKE ADDITIONAL MEDICAL EDUCATION
OFFENSE: SUBSTANDARD CARE, INCOMPETENCE OR NEGLIGENCE

NOTES: DURING 1992-1995 HE ENGAGED IN INAPPROPRIATE ANTIBIOTIC TREATMENT OF VARIOUS PATIENTS AND FAILED TO ADEQUATELY DOCUMENT THE RATIONALE FOR HIS TREATMENTS; HIS MEDICAL RECORDS OF VARIOUS PATIENTS FAILED TO ADEQUATELY SUPPORT HIS CARE AND TREATMENT. LICENSE LIMITED FOR THREE YEARS AS FOLLOWS: SHALL OBTAIN 50 HOURS OF CONTINUING MEDICAL EDUCATION PER YEAR, WITH 1 COURSE IN ANTIBIOTIC THERAPY AND TREATMENT, PHARMACOLOGY, AND DIABETIC MANAGEMENT AND TREATMENT; SHALL MAINTAIN ADEQUATE MEDICAL RECORDS WHICH SHALL BE AVAILABLE FOR REVIEW; SEPARATE FROM PATIENT RECORDS, SHALL MAINTAIN A LOGBOOK OF EVERY PRESCRIPTION WRITTEN BY HIM FOR DANGEROUS DRUGS WITH ADDICTIVE POTENTIAL WHICH SHALL BE MADE AVAILABLE FOR REVIEW; SHALL APPEAR BEFORE THE BOARD AT LEAST ONCE A YEAR; SHALL NOT REFER ANY PATIENT TO A LAB IN WHICH HE OWNS A FINANCIAL INTEREST; SHALL COOPERATE WITH THE BOARD IN VERIFYING COMPLIANCE; TIME SPENT OUT OF TEXAS DOES NOT COUNT TOWARD RESTRICTION; SHALL INFORM THE BOARD OF CHANGE OF ADDRESS WITHIN 10 DAYS OR IF HE LEAVES THE STATE; SHALL NOT SEEK MODIFICATION FOR ONE YEAR.

FINCHER, MARK LYNN MD, LICENSE NUMBER 0014822 OF 1512 BARWICK, NORMAN, OK, WAS DISCIPLINED BY OKLAHOMA ON JUNE 22, 1991
DISCIPLINARY ACTION: 24-MONTH LICENSE SUSPENSION
OFFENSE: PROVIDING FALSE INFORMATION TO THE BOARD OR OTHER HEALTH AGENCY

NOTES: ON 5/31/90, ARRESTED IN STEPHENS COUNTY, OKLAHOMA, AND CHARGED WITH TWO COUNTS OF LARCENY OF DOMESTIC ANIMALS. FORMALLY CHARGED ON 6/1/90. ON 10/2/90, SUBMITTED AN APPLICATION FOR REINSTATEMENT OF LICENSE, AND FALSELY ANSWERED TWO QUESTIONS; SPECIFICALLY, ANSWERED "NO" TO "HAVE YOU EVER BEEN CHARGED WITH OR CONVICTED OF A FELONY OR MISDEMEANOR?" BEFORE NEXT BOARD APPEARANCE, SHALL PRESENT EVIDENCE FROM PSYCHIATRIST THAT HE IS FREE OF ANY MENTAL CONDITION THAT WOULD PREVENT HIM FROM PRACTICING WITH REASONABLE SKILL AND SAFETY.

FINCHER, MARK LYNN MD, LICENSE NUMBER 00H7413 OF NORMAN, OK, WAS DISCIPLINED BY TEXAS ON JUNE 17, 1992
DISCIPLINARY ACTION: SURRENDER OF LICENSE
OFFENSE: DISCIPLINARY ACTION BY ANOTHER STATE OR AGENCY

FINCHER, MARK LYNN MD OF 1512 BARWICK, NORMAN, OK, WAS DISCIPLINED BY DEA ON JUNE 22, 1992
DISCIPLINARY ACTION: REVOCATION OF CONTROLLED SUBSTANCE LICENSE
OFFENSE: DISCIPLINARY ACTION BY ANOTHER STATE OR AGENCY

NOTES: EFFECTIVE 06/22/91 OKLAHOMA SUSPENDED HIS MEDICAL LICENSE FOR TWO YEARS BASED ON HIS FRAUDULENT MISREPRESENTATION OF HIS PREVIOUS CRIMINAL RECORD IN AN APPLICATION THAT HE SUBMITTED FOR REINSTATEMENT OF HIS MEDICAL LICENSE. ALSO, AS OF 01/28/92 HE CONTINUED TO BE UNREGISTERED WITH THE CONTROLLED SUBSTANCES LICENSING AUTHORITY IN OKLAHOMA.

FINELY, OLIVIA ISABELLE MD OF 1436 SIDNEY BAKER STREET, KERRVILLE, TX, WAS DISCIPLINED BY DEA ON APRIL 26, 1994
DISCIPLINARY ACTION: SURRENDER OF CONTROLLED SUBSTANCE LICENSE

NOTES: IN LIEU OF PUBLIC INTEREST REVOCATION.

FINK, JOHN M MD, DATE OF BIRTH FEBRUARY 13, 1945, LICENSE NUMBER 1035367 OF 2100 REGIONAL MEDICAL DRIVE, WHARTON, TX, WAS DISCIPLINED BY MICHIGAN ON AUGUST 27, 1999
DISCIPLINARY ACTION: FINE; REPRIMAND
OFFENSE: DISCIPLINARY ACTION BY ANOTHER STATE OR AGENCY

NOTES: FAILURE TO REPORT/COMPLY; SISTER STATE DISCIPLINARY ACTION. $1,000 FINE.

FINK, JOHN MARK MD, LICENSE NUMBER G1896, WAS DISCIPLINED BY TEXAS ON MAY 9, 1997
DISCIPLINARY ACTION: REPRIMAND
OFFENSE: SEXUAL ABUSE OF OR SEXUAL MISCONDUCT WITH A PATIENT

NOTES: A PATIENT WAS FIRST SEEN BY HIM ON 1/10/92 AT WHICH TIME HE PERFORMED AN ANNUAL GYNECOLOGICAL EXAMINATION AS WELL AS OTHER TESTS. THE PATIENT HAD COMPLAINTS ABOUT NAUSEA ASSOCIATED WITH HER BIRTH CONTROL PILLS, AND IN AN EFFORT TO ALLEVIATE HER DISCOMFORT HE PROVIDED HER WITH SAMPLES AND A PRESCRIPTION FOR LOESTRIN AS A SUBSTITUTE BIRTH CONTROL PILL. IN OR AROUND APRIL OR MAY 1992 HE GAVE HER A YEAR-LONG SUPPLY. HE ATTEMPTED TO TREAT ONGOING PROBLEMS WITH THE PATIENT'S BIRTH CONTROL BY CHANGING THE PRESCRIPTION ON SEVERAL OCCASIONS THROUGH THE PROVISION OF SAMPLES WITHOUT INDICATION IN HER RECORDS BETWEEN JANUARY AND MAY 1992. IN 10/92 THE PATIENT WAS HOSPITALIZED FOR DEPRESSION. SUBSEQUENT TO THE CARE PROVIDED IN 5/92, AND WHILE STILL ON THE PILLS PRESCRIBED BY THE DOCTOR, KISSING AND SEXUAL INTERCOURSE TOOK PLACE BETWEEN THE TWO. BETWEEN LATE JULY AND EARLY AUGUST 1992, HE INITIATED THE FIRST SEXUAL CONTACT. THEY SUBSEQUENTLY ENGAGED IN INTERCOURSE ON 8/5/92 AND 8/27/92. HER MENTAL STATE AFTER THE DISCOVERY OF THE RELATIONSHIP LED TO SUICIDAL GESTURES AND AFOREMENTIONED HOSPITALIZATION. A LAWSUIT AGAINST HIM WAS SETTLED FOR $50,000. THE PATIENT DID NOT BELIEVE THERE HAD BEEN ANY TERMINATION OF A PHYSICIAN-PATIENT RELATIONSHIP DURING 1992, WHILE THE DOCTOR ARGUES THERE WAS NO ONGOING RELATIONSHIP UNLESS SHE HAD PROBLEMS WITH HER PILLS AND THAT SAID RELATIONSHIP EXTENDED ONLY FROM 1/92 TO 5/92.

FINK, JOHN MARK MD, DATE OF BIRTH FEBRUARY 13, 1945, LICENSE NUMBER 020545E OF 2100 REGIONAL MEDICAL DRIVE, WHARTON, TX, WAS DISCIPLINED BY PENNSYLVANIA ON JANUARY 20, 1999
DISCIPLINARY ACTION: REPRIMAND
OFFENSE: DISCIPLINARY ACTION BY ANOTHER STATE OR AGENCY

NOTES: DISCIPLINARY ACTION TAKEN BY TEXAS.

FINLEY, OLIVIA I MD, LICENSE NUMBER 00G6105 OF KERRVILLE, TX, WAS DISCIPLINED BY TEXAS ON MARCH 24, 1994
DISCIPLINARY ACTION: EMERGENCY SUSPENSION
OFFENSE: SUBSTANCE ABUSE

NOTES: ON TWO OCCASIONS IN 3/94 EVIDENCE AND INFORMATION INDICATE THAT SHE WAS UNDER THE INFLUENCE OF COCAINE WHILE TREATING PATIENTS AND THAT AS A RESULT OF THIS SUBSTANCE ABUSE SHE HAS FAILED TO SHOW UP AT WORK IN A TIMELY MANNER AND TO PROVIDE COVERAGE FOR HER PATIENTS DURING HER ABSENCE; THESE FAILURES CONSTITUTE ABANDONMENT OF PATIENTS.

FINLEY, OLIVIA I MD, LICENSE NUMBER 00G6105 OF KERRVILLE, TX, WAS DISCIPLINED BY TEXAS ON SEPTEMBER 30, 1994
DISCIPLINARY ACTION: LICENSE SUSPENSION; MONITORING OF PHYSICIAN PERFORMANCE
OFFENSE: SUBSTANCE ABUSE

NOTES: SHE HAS ADMITTED TO THE INTEMPERATE USE OF COCAINE ON VARIOUS OCCASIONS AFTER SUBSTANCE ABUSE TREATMENT INCLUDING USE AS RECENTLY AS 11/93. SUSPENSION UNTIL SHE PERSONALLY APPEARS BEFORE THE BOARD AND PROVIDES SUFFICIENT EVIDENCE THAT SHE IS PHYSICALLY, MENTALLY AND OTHERWISE COMPETENT TO PRACTICE; EVIDENCE SHALL INCLUDE BUT NOT BE LIMITED TO COMPLETE MEDICAL RECORDS AND REPORTS OF PSYCHOLOGICAL, NEUROPSYCHIATRIC AND PHYSICAL EVALUATIONS.

FINLEY, OLIVIA I MD, DATE OF BIRTH JUNE 12, 1955 OF 1344 SHEPHERD STREET, NE, WASHINGTON, DC, WAS DISCIPLINED BY MEDICARE ON SEPTEMBER 10, 1996
DISCIPLINARY ACTION: EXCLUSION FROM THE MEDICARE AND/OR MEDICAID PROGRAM
OFFENSE: DISCIPLINARY ACTION BY ANOTHER STATE OR AGENCY

NOTES: LICENSE REVOKED FOR REASONS BEARING ON PROFESSIONAL COMPETENCE.

FIORE, CHARLES N MD, LICENSE NUMBER B6894 OF HOUSTON, TX, WAS DISCIPLINED BY TEXAS ON APRIL 4, 1998
DISCIPLINARY ACTION: SURRENDER OF LICENSE

NOTES: VOLUNTARY AND PERMANENT SURRENDER.

FIORE, CHARLES N MD OF 6725 WESLAYAN, HOUSTON, TX, WAS DISCIPLINED BY DEA ON JUNE 2, 1998
DISCIPLINARY ACTION: SURRENDER OF CONTROLLED SUBSTANCE LICENSE

NOTES: IN LIEU OF PUBLIC INTEREST REVOCATION.

FISCHER, CONRAD ALEXANDER MD, LICENSE NUMBER 00E7071 OF HOUSTON, TX, WAS DISCIPLINED BY TEXAS ON MAY 15, 1996
DISCIPLINARY ACTION: FINE
OFFENSE: NONCOMPLIANCE WITH A PROFESSIONAL RULE

NOTES: IN 1/94, HIS 93-YEAR OLD FATHER INJURED HIMSELF WHILE VACATIONING IN ARIZONA AND WAS IN PAIN BUT REFUSED TO GO TO THE HOSPITAL; PHYSICIAN WAS CONTACTED BY VARIOUS FAMILY MEMBERS PLEADING WITH HIM TO CALL AN ARIZONA PHARMACY AND PRESCRIBE A PAIN MEDICATION FOR HIS FATHER; HE TELEPHONED A PHARMACY AND WAS INFORMED THAT IT WAS THE PHARMACIST'S UNDERSTANDING THAT ARIZONA LAW PROHIBITED THE PHARMACIST FROM FILLING A CONTROLLED SUBSTANCE PRESCRIPTION FOR A PHYSICIAN'S FAMILY MEMBER AND DID NOT FILL THE PRESCRIPTION; PHYSICIAN CALLED A SECOND PHARMACY WHICH FILLED A PRESCRIPTION FOR LORCET PLUS. DOES NOT ADMIT VIOLATING MEDICAL PRACTICE ACT. SHALL PAY $1,500 FINE; SHALL COOPERATE WITH THE BOARD IN VERIFYING COMPLIANCE.

FISCHER, ROY LEE DO, LICENSE NUMBER 00C4317 OF DALLAS, TX, WAS DISCIPLINED BY TEXAS ON JULY 1, 1990
DISCIPLINARY ACTION: LICENSE REVOCATION
OFFENSE: SUBSTANDARD CARE, INCOMPETENCE OR NEGLIGENCE

NOTES: ACTIONS CONSTITUTED PROFESSIONAL FAILURE TO PRACTICE MEDICINE IN ACCEPTABLE MANNER CONSISTENT WITH PUBLIC HEALTH AND WELFARE. RECURRING MERITORIOUS HEALTH CARE LIABILITY CLAIMS FILED AGAINST HIM EVIDENCE PROFESSIONAL INCOMPETENCE LIKELY TO INJURE PUBLIC.

FISCHER, ROY LEE DO, LICENSE NUMBER C4317, WAS DISCIPLINED BY TEXAS ON MAY 10, 1997
DISCIPLINARY ACTION: SURRENDER OF LICENSE

NOTES: ON 4/20/90 THE BOARD ISSUED AN ORDER REVOKING HIS TEXAS MEDICAL LICENSE. AFTER A MOTION FOR REHEARING, WHICH WAS DENIED, HE SOUGHT AND OBTAINED A STAY OF THE REVOCATION. THEREAFTER, PLEADINGS WERE FILED FOR AN APPEAL, WHICH IS STILL PENDING. HE IS NO LONGER PRACTICING MEDICINE AND DOES NOT WISH TO RETURN TO THE PRACTICE OF MEDICINE IN TEXAS. AGREES TO VOLUNTARY AND PERMANENT SURRENDER OF HIS TEXAS MEDICAL LICENSE, DUE TO HIS RETIREMENT. HIS LICENSE NUMBER IS PERMANENTLY CANCELED. HE SHALL IMMEDIATELY RETIRE FROM PRACTICE IN TEXAS AND SHALL NOT PETITION FOR REINSTATEMENT.

FISHER, ANNA L MD, LICENSE NUMBER 00F5423, WAS DISCIPLINED BY TEXAS ON AUGUST 17, 1996
DISCIPLINARY ACTION: FINE; REPRIMAND
OFFENSE: NONCOMPLIANCE WITH A PROFESSIONAL RULE

NOTES: FAILED TO OBTAIN 24 HOURS OF CONTINUING MEDICAL EDUCATION BY 3/1/96 AS REQUIRED FOR RENEWAL OF HER LICENSE; SHE WAS GRANTED AN EXTENSION UNTIL 5/29/96 WHICH SHE ALSO DID NOT MEET; STILL REQUIRED TO MEET CONTINUING MEDICAL EDUCATION REQUIREMENTS. $100 ADMINISTRATIVE PENALTY. SHALL COOPERATE WITH THE BOARD IN VERIFYING COMPLIANCE.

FISHER, PETER B MD OF 6560 FANIN #1836, HOUSTON, TX, WAS DISCIPLINED BY DEA ON JUNE 15, 1998
DISCIPLINARY ACTION: SURRENDER OF CONTROLLED SUBSTANCE LICENSE

NOTES: IN LIEU OF PUBLIC INTEREST REVOCATION.

FISHER, PETER BERNARD MD, LICENSE NUMBER C7448 OF HOUSTON, TX, WAS DISCIPLINED BY TEXAS ON FEBRUARY 7, 1998
DISCIPLINARY ACTION: SURRENDER OF LICENSE
OFFENSE: LOSS OR RESTRICTION OF HOSPITAL PRIVILEGES

NOTES: ON OR ABOUT 11/25/96 HE WAS SUSPENDED FROM A HOSPITAL FOLLOWING A DRUG SCREEN THAT INDICATED THE PRESENCE OF COCAINE; AN 11/27/96 INVESTIGATION DISCOVERED THAT HE HAD FALLEN ASLEEP DURING A PATIENT EXAM; HE ADMITTED TO THE BOARD THAT HE HAD A 9 YEAR HISTORY OF DRUG AND ALCOHOL ABUSE; HAD ATTEMPTED REHABILITATION FROM 11/95 TO 3/96. VOLUNTARY AND PERMANENT SURRENDER.

FISHER, PETER BERNARD MD, DATE OF BIRTH JUNE 15, 1932 OF 6560 FANNIN STREET SUITE 1836, HOUSTON, TX, WAS DISCIPLINED BY MEDICARE ON OCTOBER 20, 1998
DISCIPLINARY ACTION: EXCLUSION FROM THE MEDICARE AND/OR MEDICAID PROGRAM
OFFENSE: DISCIPLINARY ACTION BY ANOTHER STATE OR AGENCY

NOTES: LICENSE REVOKED, SUSPENDED, SURRENDERED OR OTHERWISE LOST FOR REASONS BEARING ON PROFESSIONAL PERFORMANCE, PROFESSIONAL COMPETENCE OR FINANCIAL INTEGRITY.

FISHER, ROY RAY DO, LICENSE NUMBER D7408 OF CHILLICOTHE, TX, WAS DISCIPLINED BY TEXAS ON AUGUST 22, 1998
DISCIPLINARY ACTION: RESTRICTION PLACED ON LICENSE; REPRIMAND
OFFENSE: SUBSTANDARD CARE, INCOMPETENCE OR NEGLIGENCE

NOTES: IN 2/97 & 5/97 HE FAILED TO ADEQUATELY DIAGNOSE AND TREAT MYOCARDIAL INFARCTIONS IN 2 PATIENTS; BOTH WERE DIAGNOSED INCORRECTLY WITH GASTRITIS AND SENT HOME. LICENSE LIMITED AS FOLLOWS: SHALL LIMIT PRACTICE TO A BOARD-APPROVED INSTITUTIONAL SETTING; SHALL APPEAR BEFORE THE BOARD AT LEAST ONCE A YEAR; SHALL COOPERATE WITH THE BOARD IN VERIFYING COMPLIANCE; TIME SPENT OUT OF TEXAS DOES NOT COUNT TOWARD RESTRICTION; SHALL INFORM THE BOARD OF CHANGE OF ADDRESS WITHIN 10 DAYS OR IF HE LEAVES THE STATE; SHALL NOT SEEK MODIFICATION FOR ONE YEAR. ON 12/11/99, THE ORDER WAS TERMINATED.

FLEMING, JAMES M DO, LICENSE NUMBER 0004511 OF SEABROOK, TX, WAS DISCIPLINED BY OHIO ON APRIL 12, 1991
DISCIPLINARY ACTION: LICENSE REVOCATION
OFFENSE: CRIMINAL CONVICTION OR PLEA OF GUILTY, NOLO CONTENDERE, OR NO CONTEST TO A CRIME

NOTES: CONVICTION OF SIX FELONY COUNTS OF MEDICAID FRAUD. PERMANENT REVOCATION.

FLEMING, JAMES M DO, DATE OF BIRTH DECEMBER 28, 1943, LICENSE NUMBER 0006308 OF 1087 DENNISON AVE, COLUMBUS, OH, WAS DISCIPLINED BY MICHIGAN ON JANUARY 21, 1992
DISCIPLINARY ACTION: LICENSE REVOCATION
OFFENSE: CRIMINAL CONVICTION OR PLEA OF GUILTY, NOLO CONTENDERE, OR NO CONTEST TO A CRIME

FLEMING, JAMES M DO, DATE OF BIRTH DECEMBER 28, 1943 OF 2711 LITTLE YORK ROAD SUITE 200, HOUSTON, TX, WAS DISCIPLINED BY MEDICARE ON JUNE 2, 1993
DISCIPLINARY ACTION: 60-MONTH EXCLUSION FROM THE MEDICARE AND/OR MEDICAID PROGRAM
OFFENSE: CRIMINAL CONVICTION OR PLEA OF GUILTY, NOLO CONTENDERE, OR NO CONTEST TO A CRIME

NOTES: CONVICTED OF SUBMITTING FALSE STATEMENTS TO THE MEDICAID PROGRAM FOR PHYSICIAN SERVICES.

FLEMING, JAMES MICHAEL DO, LICENSE NUMBER 00E0006 OF SEABROOK, TX, WAS DISCIPLINED BY TEXAS ON AUGUST 24, 1991
DISCIPLINARY ACTION: REPRIMAND
OFFENSE: CRIMINAL CONVICTION OR PLEA OF GUILTY, NOLO CONTENDERE, OR NO CONTEST TO A CRIME

NOTES: CONVICTED OF MEDICAID FRAUD.

FLEMING, JAMES MICHAEL DO, LICENSE NUMBER 00E0006, WAS DISCIPLINED BY TEXAS ON AUGUST 17, 1996
DISCIPLINARY ACTION: MONITORING OF PHYSICIAN PERFORMANCE
OFFENSE: PHYSICAL OR MENTAL ILLNESS INHIBITING THE ABILITY TO PRACTICE WITH SKILL AND SAFETY

NOTES: ALLEGED EXCESSIVE TESTING AND TREATMENT OF TWO MINOR FEMALE PATIENTS BETWEEN 12/93 AND 3/94; BASED ON HIS MEDICAL CONDITION, CORONARY ARTERY DISEASE, HE HAS DECIDED HE WILL NOT CONTINUE TO PRACTICE MEDICINE IN TEXAS AT THIS TIME. RESTRICTED UNDER THE FOLLOWING TERMS AND CONDITIONS: SHALL IMMEDIATELY CEASE THE PRACTICE OF MEDICINE IN TEXAS AND SHALL NOT PRACTICE UNTIL HE REQUESTS PERMISSION TO RESUME PRACTICE, APPEARS BEFORE THE BOARD, AND PROVIDE SUFFICIENT EVIDENCE AND INFORMATION THAT HE IS PHYSICALLY, MENTALLY, AND OTHERWISE COMPETENT TO SAFELY PRACTICE MEDICINE INCLUDING AT A MINIMUM COPIES OF MEDICAL RECORDS AND REPORTS OF PHYSICAL AND NEUROPSYCHIATRIC EVALUATIONS CONDUCTED UNDER THE DIRECTION OF A BOARD APPROVED CERTIFIED PHYSICIAN; SHALL PROVIDE DOCUMENTATION OF CONTINUING MEDICAL EDUCATION WHICH AT LEAST MEETS THE MINIMUM REQUIREMENTS FOR RENEWAL; SHALL PASS THE SPEX EXAM WITHIN THE THREE MONTHS PRIOR TO HIS REQUEST TO RESUME PRACTICE; SHALL SUBMIT A TYPED-WRITTEN NARRATIVE, REFERRING TO PATIENTS BY INITIAL ONLY, WHICH DESCRIBED WITH SPECIFICITY THE CARE RENDERED AND SETS FORTH A DETAILED CORRECTIVE ACTION PLAN TO AVOID SIMILAR DIFFICULTIES AND POSSIBLE ADVERSE OUTCOMES; SHALL COOPERATE WITH THE BOARD IN VERIFYING COMPLIANCE INCLUDING PROVIDING COPIES OF MEDICAL RELEASES AND PEER REVIEW RECORDS UPON REQUEST; SHALL PROVIDE A COPY OF THIS ORDER TO ANYONE REQUESTING IT WITHIN 10 DAYS; TIME PERIOD OUT OF TEXAS DOES NOT COUNT TOWARD RESTRICTION; SHALL INFORM THE BOARD OF CHANGE OF ADDRESS WITHIN 10 DAYS OF IF HE LEAVES THE STATE; SHALL NOT SEEK MODIFICATION FOR ONE YEAR.

FLORES, ALBERTO MD, DATE OF BIRTH FEBRUARY 7, 1955 OF 1611 ROCKDALE DRIVE, ARLINGTON, TX, WAS DISCIPLINED BY MEDICARE ON MARCH 6, 1994
DISCIPLINARY ACTION: EXCLUSION FROM THE MEDICARE AND/OR MEDICAID PROGRAM
OFFENSE: NONCOMPLIANCE WITH A PROFESSIONAL RULE

NOTES: DEFAULTED ON PUBLIC HEALTH SERVICE EDUCATION LOAN. REINSTATED ON 6/8/94.

FLYNN, STEPHEN EUGENE MD, LICENSE NUMBER 00C6937 OF PHOENIX, AZ, WAS DISCIPLINED BY TEXAS ON MARCH 6, 1992
DISCIPLINARY ACTION: 60-MONTH PROBATION
OFFENSE: DISCIPLINARY ACTION BY ANOTHER STATE OR AGENCY

NOTES: DISCIPLINARY ACTION TAKEN BY ANOTHER STATE BOARD AND INTEMPERATE USE OF ALCOHOL OR DRUGS. LICENSE SUSPENDED, SUSPENSION STAYED; PROBATION UNDER TERMS AND CONDITIONS.

FLYNN, STEPHEN EUGENE MD, LICENSE NUMBER 00C6937 OF PHOENIX, AZ, WAS DISCIPLINED BY TEXAS ON OCTOBER 9, 1992
DISCIPLINARY ACTION: SURRENDER OF LICENSE

NOTES: PERMANENTLY SURRENDERED.

FOLLETT, WILLIAM III MD, WAS DISCIPLINED BY NEW MEXICO ON MAY 31, 1995
DISCIPLINARY ACTION: SURRENDER OF LICENSE
OFFENSE: PROFESSIONAL MISCONDUCT

NOTES: SEXUAL MISCONDUCT.

FOLLETT, WILLIAM WALLACE III MD, LICENSE NUMBER 00D4118 OF EL PASO, TX, WAS DISCIPLINED BY TEXAS ON MARCH 5, 1994
DISCIPLINARY ACTION: 84-MONTH PROBATION; REQUIRED TO TAKE ADDITIONAL MEDICAL EDUCATION
OFFENSE: PROFESSIONAL MISCONDUCT

NOTES: FROM 5/27/92 THROUGH 6/2/92 MAINTAINED AN INAPPROPRIATE SOCIAL RELATIONSHIP WITH A FEMALE PATIENT; FAILED TO RECOGNIZE THE OCCURRENCE OF TRANSFERENCE AND COUNTERTRANSFERENCE WHILE TREATING THE PATIENT AND THAT SHE WAS IN A VULNERABLE POSITION RELATING TO THE DEATH OF HER HUSBAND; PATIENT BELIEVES SHE WAS EXPLOITED BY DR. FOLLETT; HE DOES NOT HAVE A PAST DISCIPLINARY HISTORY. SUSPENSION STAYED. CONDITIONS OF PROBATION: SHALL ATTEND AT LEAST 50 HOURS OF CONTINUING MEDICAL EDUCATION AND AN ADDITIONAL SIX HOURS OF ETHICS COURSES PER YEAR; SHALL SUBMIT HIMSELF TO A BOARD-APPROVED PSYCHIATRIST FOR EVALUATION AND FOLLOW RECOMMENDATIONS FOR CARE AND TREATMENT IF ANY; SHALL GIVE THIS PSYCHIATRIST A COPY OF THE BOARD ORDER; SHALL APPEAR BEFORE THE BOARD ONCE A YEAR; SHALL NOT MAINTAIN A PERSONAL OR SOCIAL RELATIONSHIP WITH PATIENTS; WITHIN ONE YEAR SHALL SUBMIT A PUBLISHABLE PAPER REGARDING DOCTOR-PATIENT BOUNDARIES; SHALL COOPERATE WITH THE BOARD IN VERIFYING COMPLIANCE; SHALL INFORM BOARD OF CHANGE OF ADDRESS WITHIN 10 DAYS OR IF HE LEAVES THE STATE; TIME SPENT OUT OF TEXAS DOES NOT COUNT TOWARD PROBATION. SHALL NOT SEEK MODIFICATION FOR ONE YEAR. ON 4/4/98 ORDER TERMINATED.

FONG, ROBERT Y DO, LICENSE NUMBER 00D3223 OF IRVING, TX,

WAS DISCIPLINED BY TEXAS ON MAY 15, 1996
DISCIPLINARY ACTION: 60-MONTH PROBATION; RESTRICTION PLACED ON CONTROLLED SUBSTANCE LICENSE
OFFENSE: SUBSTANDARD CARE, INCOMPETENCE OR NEGLIGENCE

NOTES: IN 10/95, THE DALLAS COUNTY DISTRICT COURT AWARDED A PATIENT $242,084 IN A LAWSUIT WHICH ALLEGED THAT PHYSICIAN INAPPROPRIATELY PRESCRIBED ANORECTIC MEDICATIONS AND FAILED TO ADEQUATELY MONITOR PATIENT; FAILED TO ADEQUATELY DOCUMENT THE CARE AND TREATMENT OF MULTIPLE PATIENTS DURING LONG-TERM CONTINUING CARE; FAILED TO ADEQUATELY EVALUATE AND CONDUCT APPROPRIATE FOLLOW-UP OF MULTIPLE PATIENTS RECEIVING ANORECTIC MEDICATIONS OVER PERIODS OF LONG-TERM CARE LASTING MONTHS OR YEARS; PROVIDED ANORECTIC STIMULANT MEDICATIONS FOR WEIGHT CONTROL FOR MULTIPLE PATIENTS WITHOUT ADEQUATE INDICATIONS AND WITHOUT ADEQUATELY DOCUMENTING A LEGITIMATE BASIS FOR THE PROVISION OF THE MEDICATIONS; FAILED TO PROVIDE ADEQUATE AND APPROPRIATE COVERAGE FOR HIS PRACTICE AND ADEQUATE SUPERVISION OF HIS OFFICE STAFF WHEN HE WAS OUT OF TOWN; FAILED TO ADEQUATELY SUPERVISE AND MONITOR THE PROVISION OF ANORECTIC MEDICATIONS TO PATIENTS BY HIS OFFICE STAFF AND ALLOWED HIS STAFF TO UTILIZE PRE-SIGNED PRESCRIPTIONS FOR THESE MEDICATIONS WITHOUT ADEQUATE SUPERVISION AND FOLLOW-UP EVALUATIONS OF MULTIPLE PATIENTS; FAILED TO KEEP COMPLETE AND ACCURATE RECORDS FOR SAMPLES OF LORTAB, A CONTROLLED SUBSTANCE; HE REPORTS THAT HE HAS IMPLEMENTED REMEDIAL MEASURES. SUSPENSION STAYED. PROBATION WITH TERMS AND CONDITIONS: SHALL MAINTAIN ADEQUATE MEDICAL RECORDS WHICH SHALL BE AVAILABLE FOR REVIEW; SHALL NOT PRESCRIBE OR ADMINISTER ANY DRUG UNLESS IT IS MEDICALLY INDICATED AND IS PRESCRIBED IN THERAPEUTIC DOSES; SHALL EVALUATE PATIENT'S HISTORY INCLUDING DIETARY STATUS AND PERFORM A PHYSICAL EXAM DURING INITIAL PATIENT EVALUATION FOR WEIGHT CONTROL OR OBESITY; SHALL PROVIDE COUNSELING REGARDING DIETARY MODIFICATION, EXERCISE AND THE RISKS AND BENEFITS OF TREATMENT PRIOR TO THE START OF THERAPY FOR WEIGHT CONTROL AND AT SIX MONTH INTERVALS; SHALL NOT PRESCRIBE ANY MEDICATION FOR WEIGHT CONTROL IN AMOUNTS GREATER THAN THAT WHICH WOULD BE USED DURING A TWO-MONTH PERIOD; HE SHALL EXAMINE AND EVALUATE EACH PATIENT RECEIVING WEIGHT CONTROL TREATMENT AT LEAST EVERY TWO MONTHS AND WHENEVER PATIENT IS PRESENTING FOR REFILLS; SHALL NOT TELEPHONE TO A PHARMACY A PRESCRIPTION OR REFILL FOR CONTROLLED SUBSTANCES OR DANGEROUS DRUGS WITH ADDICTIVE POTENTIAL OR POTENTIAL FOR ABUSE; SHALL MAINTAIN A FILE CONSISTING OF COPIES OF EVERY PRESCRIPTION WRITTEN BY HIM FOR DANGEROUS DRUGS WITH ADDICTIVE POTENTIAL OR POTENTIAL FOR ABUSE WHICH SHALL BE AVAILABLE FOR REVIEW; HIS PRACTICE INCLUDING ANY OFFICE AND SURGICAL PRACTICE SHALL BE MONITORED BY A BOARD-APPROVED TEXAS PHYSICIAN WHO SHALL SUBMIT QUARTERLY REPORTS TO THE BOARD; SHALL NOT SIGN OR INDICATE IN ANY MANNER IN PATIENT RECORDS THAT HE HAS SEEN PATIENTS UNLESS HE ACTUALLY HAS SEEN AND EXAMINED THE PATIENT UNLESS IT IS CLEARLY NOTED THAT HE DID NOT PERSONALLY EXAMINE THE PATIENT; SHALL OBTAIN AT LEAST 50 HOURS PER YEAR OF CONTINUING MEDICAL EDUCATION; WITHIN 18 MONTHS SHALL EITHER BECOME BOARD CERTIFIED IN A SPECIALTY RECOGNIZED BY THE BOARD OF SPECIALTIES OR SHALL TAKE AND PASS THE SPECIAL PURPOSE EXAMINATION; SHALL APPEAR BEFORE BOARD AT LEAST ONCE A YEAR OR AT BOARD REQUEST; SHALL COOPERATE WITH THE BOARD IN VERIFYING COMPLIANCE; SHALL ADEQUATELY SUPERVISE THE ACTIVITIES OF ALL EMPLOYEES OR OTHERS UNDER HIS SUPERVISION; SHALL EXAMINE AND/OR TREAT PATIENTS IN ANY SITUATION IN WHICH IT IS INDICATED THAT AN EXAMINATION OR TREATMENT HAS TAKEN PLACE; SHALL GIVE A COPY OF THIS ORDER TO ANY HEALTH CARE ENTITY WHERE HE HAS PRIVILEGES; SHALL PROVIDE A COPY OF THIS ORDER TO ANYONE REQUESTING IT WITHIN 10 DAYS; TIME SPENT OUT OF TEXAS DOES NOT COUNT TOWARD PROBATION; SHALL INFORM BOARD OF CHANGE OF ADDRESS WITHIN 10 DAYS OR IF HE LEAVES THE STATE. SHALL NOT SEEK MODIFICATION FOR ONE YEAR. ON 8/22/98 ORDER MODIFIED DELETING ANNUAL APPEARANCES BEFORE THE BOARD. ON 10/15/99 ORDER TERMINATED.

FONTANIER, CHARLES EUGENE DO, LICENSE NUMBER 00F3960 OF HOUSTON, TX, WAS DISCIPLINED BY TEXAS ON APRIL 15, 1994
DISCIPLINARY ACTION: 60-MONTH RESTRICTION PLACED ON LICENSE; REQUIRED TO TAKE ADDITIONAL MEDICAL EDUCATION
OFFENSE: OVERPRESCRIBING OR MISPRESCRIBING DRUGS

NOTES: AS RECENTLY AS 1991 HE HAS REGULARLY DISPENSED QUANTITIES OF FASTIN WHICH EXCEEDED AMOUNTS NECESSARY TO MEET PATIENTS' IMMEDIATE NEEDS; REGULARLY PRESCRIBED TO PATIENTS FOR WEIGHT CONTROL QUANTITIES OF FASTIN AND OTHER ANOREXICS FOR PERIODS OF TIME WHICH EXCEED THOSE RECOMMENDED BY THE MANUFACTURER. SHALL ATTEND AT LEAST 50 HOURS PER YEAR OF CONTINUING MEDICAL EDUCATION; SHALL MAINTAIN ADEQUATE MEDICAL RECORDS ON ALL PATIENT OFFICE VISITS AND SEPARATE FROM PATIENT RECORDS SHALL MAINTAIN A FILE OF EVERY PRESCRIPTION WRITTEN FOR CONTROLLED SUBSTANCES OR DANGEROUS DRUGS BOTH OF WHICH SHALL BE AVAILABLE FOR INSPECTION; SHALL REFRAIN FROM PRESCRIBING ANY DRUG UNLESS MEDICALLY INDICATED; SHALL NOT TREAT ANY PATIENT FOR WEIGHT CONTROL OR OBESITY WITH ANY DRUGS; MAY TREAT SUCH PATIENTS ONLY WITH COUNSELING, DIET AND EXERCISE; WITHIN TWO YEARS SHALL COMPLETE ADDITIONAL TRAINING IN PHARMACOLOGY AND FAMILY PRACTICE; SHALL APPEAR BEFORE THE BOARD ONCE A YEAR; SHALL GIVE A COPY OF THIS ORDER TO ANY HEALTH CARE ENTITY WHERE HE HAS PRIVILEGES; SHALL COOPERATE WITH THE BOARD IN VERIFYING COMPLIANCE; SHALL INFORM BOARD OF CHANGE OF ADDRESS WITHIN 10 DAYS OR IF HE LEAVES THE STATE; TIME SPENT OUT OF TEXAS DOES NOT COUNT TOWARD RESTRICTION. SHALL NOT SEEK MODIFICATION FOR ONE YEAR. ON 10/13/95 ORDER TERMINATED BASED ON COMPLIANCE WITH TERMS.

FONTANIER, CHARLES EUGENE DO, LICENSE NUMBER 0141552 OF 210 WEST GREENS ROAD SUITE C, HOUSTON, TX, WAS DISCIPLINED BY NEW YORK ON NOVEMBER 7, 1995
DISCIPLINARY ACTION: LICENSE REVOCATION
OFFENSE: DISCIPLINARY ACTION BY ANOTHER STATE OR AGENCY

NOTES: ACTION IN TEXAS FOR REGULARLY DISPENSING EXCESSIVE QUANTITIES OF FASTIN TO WEIGHT CONTROL PATIENTS.

FOREMAN, ADOLPHUS MD, LICENSE NUMBER D4997 OF HOUSTON, TX, WAS DISCIPLINED BY TEXAS ON AUGUST 9, 1997
DISCIPLINARY ACTION: REQUIRED TO TAKE ADDITIONAL MEDICAL EDUCATION; MONITORING OF PHYSICIAN PERFORMANCE
OFFENSE: PROFESSIONAL MISCONDUCT

NOTES: IN 1994 HE FAILED TO KEEP SCHEDULED APPOINTMENTS WITH SEVERAL OF HIS OBSTETRICAL PATIENTS AND INSTRUCTED HIS STAFF TO TRANSFER THEM TO OTHER PHYSICIANS WITHOUT HIS ADEQUATELY INFORMING THE PATIENTS; HE EFFECTIVELY ABANDONED HIS RESPONSIBILITIES TO SEVERAL ESTABLISHED PATIENTS; IN 4/94 FOR A PATIENT ON WHOM HE PERFORMED A CESAREAN SECTION HE FAILED TO PROVIDE POSTOPERATIVE CARE, NEVER SAW HER AFTER THE OPERATION, MADE NO ARRANGEMENTS FOR PHYSICIAN COVERAGE AND PROVIDED INSUFFICIENT ORDERS TO THE NURSING STAFF; REPORTS THAT HE WAS UNDERGOING DIVORCE AND THAT THE STRESS CARRIED OVER TO HIS PROFESSIONAL MEDICAL PRACTICE; HIS DIVORCE IS NOW FINAL; HE HAS RECEIVED AND CONTINUES TO RECEIVE COUNSELING; IN 6/94 HE VOLUNTARILY SUBMITTED TO A PSYCHIATRIC EVALUATION AND WAS DIAGNOSED AS HAVING AN ADJUSTMENT DISORDER WITH MIXED EMOTIONAL FEATURES SECONDARY TO IMPENDING DIVORCE. LICENSE LIMITED FOR THREE YEARS AS FOLLOWS: SHALL NOMINATE THREE CERTIFIED PSYCHIATRISTS FOR BOARD SELECTION OF A THERAPIST AND SHALL EXPEDITIOUSLY SUBMIT HIMSELF TO EVALUATION AND TREATMENT BY THE APPROVED PRACTITIONER; SHALL COOPERATE WITH THE BOARD IN VERIFYING COMPLIANCE INCLUDING PROVIDING COPIES OF MEDICAL RELEASES AND PEER REVIEW RECORDS UPON REQUEST; SHALL SUBMIT HIMSELF FOR APPROPRIATE EXAMS INCLUDING DRUG OR ALCOHOL SCREENS; HIS MEDICAL PRACTICE SHALL BE MONITORED BY A BOARD APPROVED TEXAS PHYSICIAN WHO SHALL PROVIDE QUARTERLY REPORTS TO THE BOARD; SHALL OBTAIN AT LEAST 50 HOURS PER YEAR OF CONTINUING MEDICAL EDUCATION AND 10 HOURS OF ETHICS THROUGH COURSES OR PROGRAMS, WITHIN ONE YEAR; SHALL APPEAR BEFORE THE BOARD UPON REQUEST; SHALL GIVE A COPY OF THIS ORDER TO ANY HEALTH CARE ENTITY WHERE HE HAS PRIVILEGES; SHALL PROVIDE A COPY OF THIS ORDER TO ANYONE REQUESTING IT WITHIN 10 DAYS; TIME SPENT OUT OF TEXAS DOES NOT COUNT TOWARD RESTRICTION; SHALL INFORM THE BOARD OF CHANGE OF ADDRESS WITHIN 10 DAYS OR IF HE LEAVES THE STATE; SHALL NOT SEEK MODIFICATION FOR ONE YEAR. ON 10/24/98 THE ORDER WAS MODIFIED BY DELETING REQUIREMENT TO SUBMIT FOR RANDOM DRUG SCREENS; AND, DELETION OF REQUIREMENT TO APPEAR BEFORE THE BOARD TWICE ANNUALLY; REQUEST FOR TERMINATION OF THE ORDER DENIED; ALL OTHER PROVISIONS OF ORDER REMAIN IN EFFECT UNTIL SUPERSEDED BY A SUBSEQUENT BOARD ORDER.

FOWLER, DONALD H MD, LICENSE NUMBER 0006769 OF MARION, SC, WAS DISCIPLINED BY SOUTH CAROLINA ON JUNE 12, 1990
DISCIPLINARY ACTION: 6-MONTH LICENSE SUSPENSION; PROBATION
OFFENSE: OVERPRESCRIBING OR MISPRESCRIBING DRUGS

NOTES: INAPPROPRIATE PRESCRIBING OF CONTROLLED SUBSTANCES. SUSPENSION STAYED AFTER 6 MONTHS, PAYMENT OF $10,000 FINE, PASSAGE OF SPEX AND SURRENDER OF SCHEDULES II AND III CONTROLLED SUBSTANCE REGISTRATION; INDEFINITE PROBATION.

FOWLER, DONALD H MD OF 1301 N MAIN ST, MARION, SC, WAS DISCIPLINED BY DEA ON NOVEMBER 6, 1990
DISCIPLINARY ACTION: SURRENDER OF CONTROLLED SUBSTANCE LICENSE
OFFENSE: OVERPRESCRIBING OR MISPRESCRIBING DRUGS

NOTES: OVERPRESCRIBING PERCODAN, DARVON, VALIUM AND TALWIN NX AND NOT KEEPING ADEQUATE RECORDS OF DRUGS. ON 06/12/90 LICENSE INDEFINITELY SUSPENDED WITH REINSTATEMENT STIPULATIONS TO PROBATIONARY STATUS AFTER SIX MONTHS, $10,000 FINE AND SURRENDER OF SOUTH CAROLINA REGISTRATION.

FOWLER, DONALD H MD, LICENSE NUMBER 00C6321 OF MARION, SC, WAS DISCIPLINED BY TEXAS ON APRIL 20, 1991
DISCIPLINARY ACTION: PROBATION
OFFENSE: DISCIPLINARY ACTION BY ANOTHER STATE OR AGENCY

NOTES: ACTION TAKEN BY ANOTHER STATE BOARD FOR PRESCRIBING CONTROLLED SUBSTANCES AND DANGEROUS DRUGS IN QUANTITIES THAT WERE WITHOUT VALID DOCUMENTED MEDICAL JUSTIFICATION AND FOR OTHER THAN DOCUMENTED LEGITIMATE PURPOSES. MUST RECEIVE APPROVAL FROM THE TEXAS BOARD PRIOR TO PRACTICING MEDICINE IN TEXAS.

FOWLER, DONALD H MD OF 210 EAST DOZIER P.O. BOX 875, MARION, SC, WAS DISCIPLINED BY DEA ON AUGUST 24, 1994
DISCIPLINARY ACTION: RESTRICTION PLACED ON CONTROLLED SUBSTANCE LICENSE
OFFENSE: DISCIPLINARY ACTION BY ANOTHER STATE OR AGENCY

NOTES: STATE BOARD.

FOWLER, JAMES H MD, LICENSE NUMBER F7755 OF DALLAS, TX, WAS DISCIPLINED BY TEXAS ON AUGUST 9, 1997
DISCIPLINARY ACTION: REPRIMAND
OFFENSE: PROFESSIONAL MISCONDUCT

NOTES: DURING 1995, PERFORMED LIPOSUCTION SURGERY ON A PATIENT AT AN OUT-PATIENT FACILITY. SEVERAL HOURS AFTER THE SURGERY THE PATIENT DEVELOPED ABDOMINAL PAIN, NAUSEA, HYPOTENSION, AND REMAINED WEAK AND PALE. HE HAD BY THEN LEFT THE FACILITY. THE PATIENT WAS LATER DISCOVERED TO HAVE DEVELOPED COMPLICATIONS OF THE SURGERY. HE CONTENDS THAT HIS FAILURE TO INFORM THE PATIENT AND THE ON-CALL PHYSICIAN THAT HE WOULD NOT BE PHYSICALLY PRESENT TO ATTEND TO THE PATIENT, AND HIS FAILURE TO RETURN TO ATTEND THE PATIENT WHEN HE KNEW OR SHOULD HAVE KNOWN THE PATIENT WAS DEVELOPING COMPLICATIONS DOES NOT CONSTITUTE UNPROFESSIONAL CONDUCT LIKELY TO DECEIVE, DEFRAUD, OR INJURE THE PUBLIC. SHALL COOPERATE WITH THE BOARD IN VERIFYING COMPLIANCE; SHALL GIVE A COPY OF THIS ORDER TO ANY HEALTH CARE ENTITY WHERE HE HAS PRIVILEGES.

FOWLER, STEPHEN MD OF 1000 EAST WILLIAMS, BRECKENRIDGE, TX, WAS DISCIPLINED BY DEA ON NOVEMBER 10, 1999
DISCIPLINARY ACTION: SURRENDER OF CONTROLLED SUBSTANCE LICENSE
OFFENSE: DISCIPLINARY ACTION BY ANOTHER STATE OR AGENCY

NOTES: STATE BOARD.

FOWLER, STEPHEN RICE MD, LICENSE NUMBER H9514 OF BRECKENRIDGE, TX, WAS DISCIPLINED BY TEXAS ON SEPTEMBER 3, 1998

DISCIPLINARY ACTION: EMERGENCY SUSPENSION
OFFENSE: LOSS OR RESTRICTION OF HOSPITAL PRIVILEGES

NOTES: ALLEGATIONS THAT: IN 1994 HE HAD A SEXUAL RELATIONSHIP WITH A PATIENT HE WAS TREATING FOR BIPOLAR DISORDER; HE DENIES HAVING A PERSONAL RELATIONSHIP WITH THE PATIENT; BETWEEN 10/95 AND 1/96 AN EMPLOYEE OF HIS SAW A BOTTLE OF LIQUOR IN HIS OFFICE; HE SMELLED OF ALCOHOL WHILE HE WAS ACTIVELY TREATING PATIENTS; HE CONSUMED VODKA AND THEN TRAVELED TO THE HOSPITAL AND EXAMINED PATIENTS; ON OR ABOUT 1/17/97 HE WAS ARRESTED FOR DRIVING WHILE INTOXICATED AND HIS DRIVERS LICENSE WAS SUSPENDED FOR 60 DAYS; ON OR ABOUT 9/2/98 HE ADMITTED TO THE BOARD THAT ON OCCASION HE HAS CONSUMED ALCOHOL AT LUNCH TIME AND TREATED PATIENTS SHORTLY THEREAFTER, AND THAT HE CURRENTLY CONSUMES 5-6 DRINKS OF ALCOHOL PER DAY; ON OR ABOUT 3/7/97 HE EXAMINED A PATIENT AND SMELLED OF ALCOHOL; ON 8/11/98 HE SMELLED OF ALCOHOL WHILE AT THE HOSPITAL; ON 8/26/98 WHILE ADMINISTERING A STRESS TEST ON A PATIENT HE LEFT THE ROOM TO ALLEGEDLY VOMIT, AND A WITNESS SMELLED THE ODOR OF ALCOHOL ON HIS BREATH; ON OR ABOUT 8/28/98 HIS PRIVILEGES AT STEPHENS MEMORIAL HOSPITAL WERE SUSPENDED FOR FAILURE TO COMPLETE MEDICAL RECORDS AFTER BEING WARNED OF THE DELINQUENCY OF HIS RECORDS; ONE OF THE HOSPITAL PATIENTS FOR WHICH HE WAS RESPONSIBLE ON HE DATE HIS PRIVILEGES WERE SUSPENDED WAS FOUND TO HAVE BEEN A PATIENT OF THE HOSPITAL FOR 9 DAYS WHILE UNDER HIS CARE; HE APPARENTLY FAILED TO RECORD ANY HISTORY AND PHYSICAL ON THE PATIENT RECORD, AND FAILED TO RECORD ANY PROGRESS NOTES; ON OR ABOUT 9/2/98 A DOCTOR WHO WORKS AT SAME HOSPITAL SMELLED ALCOHOL ON DOCTOR FOWLER'S BREATH AND HAD NOT RESPONDED TO REPEATED PAGES FROM THE HOSPITAL; HE MAINTAINS THAT HE NEVER FAILED TO RESPOND TO HOSPITAL PAGES.

FOWLER, STEPHEN RICE MD, LICENSE NUMBER H9514 OF BRECKENRIDGE, TX, WAS DISCIPLINED BY TEXAS ON OCTOBER 24, 1998
DISCIPLINARY ACTION: LICENSE SUSPENSION
OFFENSE: LOSS OR RESTRICTION OF HOSPITAL PRIVILEGES

NOTES: BASED ON CHARGES ENUMERATED IN 9/3/98 TEMPORARY SUSPENSION. SUSPENSION UNTIL HE REQUESTS TO HAVE HIS SUSPENSION STAYED OR APPEARS BEFORE THE BOARD WITH SUFFICIENT EVIDENCE THAT HE IS PHYSICALLY, MENTALLY AND OTHERWISE COMPETENT TO SAFELY PRACTICE MEDICINE INCLUDING AT A MINIMUM COMPLETE COPIES OF MEDICAL RECORDS AND REPORTS OF PSYCHOLOGICAL AND NEUROPSYCHIATRIC EVALUATIONS, INCLUDING A 96 HOUR INPATIENT EVALUATION CONDUCTED BY A BOARD-APPROVED CERTIFIED PSYCHIATRIST; SHALL COOPERATE WITH THE BOARD IN VERIFYING COMPLIANCE INCLUDING PROVIDING COPIES OF MEDICAL RELEASES UPON REQUEST; SHALL GIVE A COPY OF THIS ORDER TO ANY HEALTH CARE ENTITY WHERE HE HAS PRIVILEGES; SHALL INFORM THE BOARD OF CHANGE OF ADDRESS WITHIN 10 DAYS OR IF HE LEAVES THE STATE.

FOWLER, STEPHEN RICE MD, LICENSE NUMBER H9514, WAS DISCIPLINED BY TEXAS ON OCTOBER 15, 1999
DISCIPLINARY ACTION: 84-MONTH PROBATION; RESTRICTION PLACED ON LICENSE
OFFENSE: SUBSTANCE ABUSE

NOTES: THE 10/24/98 BOARD ORDER SUSPENDED HIS LICENSE UNTIL HE REQUESTED TO RESUME PRACTICE PROVIDING EVIDENCE OF HIS COMPETENCE TO PRACTICE SAFELY; HE HAS PROVIDED SUFFICIENT EVIDENCE AND INFORMATION WHICH IN THE DISCRETION OF THE BOARD ADEQUATELY INDICATES HIS COMPETENCE; HE HAS COMPLETED TREATMENT AND ATTENDS REGULAR AA MEETINGS. SUSPENSION STAYED FOR PROBATION WITH FOLLOWING TERMS AND CONDITIONS: SHALL NOT PRACTICE MEDICINE BEYOND 20 HOURS PER WEEK; SHALL LIMIT HIS PRACTICE, INCLUDING ANY OFFICE AND INPATIENT PRACTICE, TO A GROUP OR INSTITUTIONAL SETTING, APPROVED IN ADVANCE BY THE BOARD; SHALL ABSTAIN FROM THE CONSUMPTION OF ALCOHOL/DRUGS IN ANY FORM UNLESS PRESCRIBED BY ANOTHER PHYSICIAN FOR A LEGITIMATE AND THERAPEUTIC PURPOSE; SHALL SUBMIT HIMSELF FOR APPROPRIATE EXAMS INCLUDING DRUG OR ALCOHOL SCREENS; SHALL NOMINATE THREE CERTIFIED PSYCHIATRISTS FOR BOARD SELECTION OF A THERAPIST AND SHALL EXPEDITIOUSLY SUBMIT HIMSELF TO EVALUATION AND TREATMENT BY THE APPROVED PRACTITIONER; SHALL PARTICIPATE IN THE ACTIVITIES OF A PHYSICIAN HEALTH AND REHABILITATION COMMITTEE AND ATTEND WEEKLY MEETINGS WITH QUARTERLY REPORTS; SHALL PARTICIPATE IN AA'S PROGRAM NOT LESS THAN FIVE TIMES A WEEK; SHALL REPORT ON HIS ATTENDANCE; SHALL NOT TREAT OR OTHERWISE SERVE AS PHYSICIAN, PRESCRIBE, DISPENSE OR ADMINISTER DRUGS THAT MAY BE SUBJECT TO ABUSE TO HIMSELF OR TO ANY MEMBER OF HIS FAMILY; SHALL SURRENDER DEA AND TEXAS DEPARTMENT OF PUBLIC SAFETY CONTROLLED SUBSTANCE CERTIFICATES AND ANY DRUGS WITH POTENTIAL FOR ABUSE IN HIS POSSESSION INCLUDING SAMPLES; SEPARATE FROM PATIENT RECORDS, SHALL MAINTAIN A LOGBOOK OF EVERY PRESCRIPTION WRITTEN BY HIM FOR DANGEROUS DRUGS WITH ADDICTIVE POTENTIAL WHICH SHALL BE MADE AVAILABLE FOR REVIEW; SHALL NOT ENGAGE IN INPATIENT OR OUTPATIENT INVASIVE SURGERY OR ENDOSCOPIC SURGERY; WITHIN 60 DAYS HIS MEDICAL PRACTICE SHALL BE MONITORED BY A BOARD APPROVED TEXAS PHYSICIAN WHO SHALL PROVIDE QUARTERLY REPORTS TO THE BOARD; SHALL OBTAIN 50 HOURS PER YEAR OF CONTINUING MEDICAL EDUCATION; SHALL APPEAR BEFORE THE BOARD UPON REQUEST; SHALL COOPERATE WITH THE BOARD IN VERIFYING COMPLIANCE INCLUDING PROVIDING COPIES OF MEDICAL RELEASES AND PEER REVIEW RECORDS UPON REQUEST; SHALL GIVE A COPY OF THIS ORDER TO ANY HEALTH CARE ENTITY WHERE HE HAS PRIVILEGES; SHALL PROVIDE A COPY OF THIS ORDER TO ANYONE REQUESTING IT WITHIN 10 DAYS; TIME SPENT OUT OF TEXAS DOES NOT COUNT TOWARD PROBATION; SHALL INFORM THE BOARD OF CHANGE OF ADDRESS WITHIN 10 DAYS OR IF HE LEAVES THE STATE; SHALL NOT SEEK MODIFICATION FOR ONE YEAR.

FRANZ, F PERRY MD, LICENSE NUMBER K3193 OF AUSTIN, TX, WAS DISCIPLINED BY TEXAS ON DECEMBER 16, 1999
DISCIPLINARY ACTION: EMERGENCY SUSPENSION
OFFENSE: PHYSICAL OR MENTAL ILLNESS INHIBITING THE ABILITY TO PRACTICE WITH SKILL AND SAFETY

NOTES: ON 10/15/99 DETAINED BY AUSTIN AIRPORT POLICE FOR BIZARRE BEHAVIOR AND THREATS OF SUICIDE; MENTAL HEALTH OFFICERS WERE CALLED IN FROM

THE SHERIFF'S DEPARTMENT, BUT CRITERIA FOR INVOLUNTARY COMMITMENT WERE NOT MET, AND HE WAS RELEASED; ON 10/14/99 HIS EX-WIFE REPORTED HE HAD BEEN EXHIBITING BIZARRE BEHAVIOR, SPECIFICALLY, THAT HE HAD BEEN SEARCHING HIS HOUSE WITH A FLASHLIGHT FOR UP TO 20 PEOPLE WHO WERE SUPPOSEDLY IN HIS HOUSE; ON 11/22/99 HE CALLED POLICE TO HIS HOME AFTER HE NOTICED MULTIPLE PEOPLE THREATENING HIM WITH GUNS IN HIS HOUSE; POLICE FOUND NO ONE IN THE HOUSE; WAS TAKEN TO THE EMERGENCY ROOM OF A HOSPITAL WITH THE DIAGNOSIS OF ACUTE PSYCHOSIS; A TOXICOLOGY SCREEN TESTED POSITIVE FOR PCP; ON 11/24/99 DISCHARGED FROM HOSPITAL WITH DIAGNOSIS OF BIPOLAR DISORDER, HYPOMANIC, WITH PSYCHOTIC FEATURES; ON 12/7/99 DELIVERED TO THE BOARD A LETTER REPORTING HIMSELF AS POTENTIALLY IMPAIRED BY BIPOLAR DISORDER; PLANNED TO OPEN A NEW CLINIC IN THE FOLLOWING DAYS; HIS PSYCHIATRIST STATED THAT HIS DIAGNOSIS IS BIPOLAR DISEASE, DEPRESSIVE PHASE WITH PSYCHOTIC FEATURES, AND THAT HE WAS NON-COMPLIANT WITH THE TREATMENT PLAN AND IS AN IMMINENT DANGER TO THE PUBLIC.

FREDMAN, RAPHA P MD, LICENSE NUMBER 00G1397 OF ATLANTA, GA, WAS DISCIPLINED BY TEXAS ON DECEMBER 3, 1990
DISCIPLINARY ACTION: 60-MONTH PROBATION; REQUIRED TO ENTER AN IMPAIRED PHYSICIAN PROGRAM OR SUBSTANCE ABUSE TREATMENT

NOTES: CONTINUED PARTICIPATION IN ACTIVITIES AND PROGRAMS OF ALCOHOLICS ANONYMOUS OR COCAINE ANONYMOUS ON A REGULAR BASIS; SUBMISSION FOR APPROPRIATE CHEMICAL EXAMINATIONS AT THE REQUEST OF A REPRESENTATIVE OF THE BOARD; CONTINUATION OF COMPLIANCE WITH TERMS AND CONDITIONS OF AFTER CARE CONTRACT, AND CONTINUATION OF WORK WITH RECOVERING ABUSE SPONSOR.

FREDMAN, RAPHA P MD, LICENSE NUMBER 00G1397, WAS DISCIPLINED BY TEXAS ON JANUARY 14, 1994
DISCIPLINARY ACTION: 36-MONTH PROBATION; MONITORING OF PHYSICIAN PERFORMANCE
OFFENSE: FAILURE TO COMPLY WITH PREVIOUS BOARD ORDER

NOTES: DURING 1993 CONCERNS WERE RAISED ABOUT COMPLIANCE WITH 12/3/90 ORDER BECAUSE OF DIFFICULTIES OF MAINTAINING ADEQUATE COMMUNICATION BETWEEN DR. FREDMAN AND COMPLIANCE OFFICER; ALLEGATIONS OF UNTIMELY SUBMISSION OF AA REPORTS, FAILURE TO OBTAIN AN AA SPONSOR, AND A POSITIVE URINALYSIS FOR MARIJUANA METABOLITES; HE EXPLAINED COMMUNICATION PROBLEMS AS A PRODUCT OF HIS SURGICAL SCHEDULE; DENIES USING MARIJUANA AND SUBSEQUENT SCREENS DO NOT SHOW ANY EVIDENCE OF MARIJUANA USE. 1990 PROBATION EXTENDED WITH ADDITIONAL CONDITIONS: SHALL CONTACT THE BOARD COMPLIANCE OFFICER WITHIN EIGHT HOURS AFTER WHICH A MESSAGE IS LEFT; SHALL SUBMIT HIMSELF FOR APPROPRIATE EXAMS INCLUDING DRUG AND ALCOHOL SCREENS WITHIN 24 HOURS AFTER A REQUEST; ALL OTHER TERMS OF THE 1990 ORDER ARE STILL IN EFFECT; SHALL GIVE A COPY OF THIS ORDER TO ANY HEALTH CARE ENTITY WHERE HE HAS PRIVILEGES. SHALL NOT SEEK MODIFICATION FOR ONE YEAR.

FREIBERGER, JOHN J MD OF 830 KENMORE ROAD, CHAPEL HILL, NC, WAS DISCIPLINED BY DEA ON APRIL 25, 1996
DISCIPLINARY ACTION: SURRENDER OF CONTROLLED SUBSTANCE LICENSE

NOTES: IN LIEU OF PUBLIC INTEREST REVOCATION.

FREIBERGER, JOHN J MD OF 7407 STONECREST, DALLAS, TX, WAS DISCIPLINED BY DEA ON APRIL 25, 1996
DISCIPLINARY ACTION: SURRENDER OF CONTROLLED SUBSTANCE LICENSE

NOTES: IN LIEU OF PUBLIC INTEREST REVOCATION.

FREIBERGER, JOHN JACOB MD, LICENSE NUMBER F3968 OF CHAPEL HILL, NC, WAS DISCIPLINED BY TEXAS ON AUGUST 9, 1997
DISCIPLINARY ACTION: SURRENDER OF LICENSE
OFFENSE: DISCIPLINARY ACTION BY ANOTHER STATE OR AGENCY

NOTES: ENGAGED IN SUBSTANCE ABUSE AND DRUG DIVERSION, AND AS A RESULT HAS SURRENDERED HIS NORTH CAROLINA LICENSE. ON 3/4/96, HE WAS INDICTED BY NORTH CAROLINA FOR ACQUIRING AND OBTAINING POSSESSION OF CONTROLLED SUBSTANCES IN THAT HE DID BY DECEPTION AND SUBTERFUGE DIVERT DOSAGE UNITS OF SUFENTANIL AND FENTANYL FROM THE SURGICAL SUITE OF A HOSPITAL FROM JANUARY 1995 THROUGH NOVEMBER 1995 BY SIGNING OUT SAID DRUG FOR PATIENTS AND CONVERTING IT TO HIS OWN USE. VOLUNTARY SURRENDER; SHALL IMMEDIATELY RETIRE FROM THE PRACTICE OF MEDICINE IN TEXAS.

FREMMING, BRET GORDON MD, LICENSE NUMBER 00C8361 OF 1500 MCLAIN ST, NEWPORT, AR, WAS DISCIPLINED BY ARKANSAS ON JULY 1, 1995
DISCIPLINARY ACTION: 24-MONTH PROBATION
OFFENSE: SUBSTANCE ABUSE

NOTES: HABITUAL INDULGENCE AND USE OF ALCOHOL WHICH RENDERS HIM INCAPABLE OF EXERCISING THE SKILL AND JUDGMENT NECESSARY TO TREAT HIS PATIENTS. ON 6/9/97 PROBATION COMPLETED.

FREMMING, BRET GORDON MD, LICENSE NUMBER 00H4333 OF NEWPORT, AR, WAS DISCIPLINED BY TEXAS ON OCTOBER 13, 1995
DISCIPLINARY ACTION: REQUIRED TO ENTER AN IMPAIRED PHYSICIAN PROGRAM OR SUBSTANCE ABUSE TREATMENT
OFFENSE: DISCIPLINARY ACTION BY ANOTHER STATE OR AGENCY

NOTES: IN 7/95, PLACED ON PROBATION BY ARKANSAS BOARD BASED ON HIS ACKNOWLEDGED HABITUAL ABUSE OF ALCOHOL; PRIOR TO ARKANSAS BOARD ACTION, HE VOLUNTARILY ADMITTED HIMSELF INTO A CHEMICAL DEPENDENCY TREATMENT FACILITY; REPORTS HAVING SUCCESSFULLY COMPLETED THE INPATIENT PORTION OF TREATMENT PROGRAM AND THAT HE IS AND HAS BEEN REGULARLY ATTENDING AA AND SIMILAR PROGRAMS AN AVERAGE OF FOUR TIMES A WEEK; REPORTS A SOBRIETY DATE OF 12/8/94; ENTERED INTO AN AFTERCARE CONTRACT WITH THE PHYSICIAN'S HEALTH COMMITTEE ON 3/7/95. LICENSE RESTRICTED SUCH THAT HE WILL NOT PRACTICE IN TEXAS UNTIL HE REQUESTS PERMISSION TO RESUME PRACTICE AND APPEARS BEFORE BOARD WITH SUFFICIENT EVIDENCE WHICH INDICATES THAT HE IS PHYSICALLY, MENTALLY AND OTHERWISE COMPETENT TO SAFELY PRACTICE MEDICINE IN TEXAS INCLUDING AT A MINIMUM COMPLIANCE WITH ALL TERMS OF ARKANSAS ORDER; COMPLIANCE WITH ALL TERMS OF AFTERCARE CONTRACT; EVIDENCE THAT HE HAS CONTINUED TO REMAIN ALCOHOL-FREE; SHALL PROVIDE COPIES OF ANY REPORTS HE HAS SUBMITTED TO OR RECEIVED FROM THE ARKANSAS BOARD AT BOARD REQUEST; TERMS OF THIS ORDER ARE INDEPENDENT OF ANY OTHER ORDER. SHALL NOT SEEK MODIFICATION FOR ONE YEAR.

FROELICH, JAMES EUGENE III DO, LICENSE NUMBER 00F9452 OF BONHAM, TX, WAS DISCIPLINED BY TEXAS ON AUGUST 18, 1995
DISCIPLINARY ACTION: 60-MONTH PROBATION; RESTRICTION PLACED ON LICENSE
OFFENSE: OVERPRESCRIBING OR MISPRESCRIBING DRUGS

NOTES: PRESCRIBING OR ADMINISTERING A DRUG IN A NONTHERAPEUTIC MANNER IN THAT BETWEEN 1990 AND 1994 HE MAINTAINED VARIOUS PATIENTS ON COURSES OF MEDICATION FOR WEIGHT LOSS TREATMENT INCLUDING THYROID SUPPLEMENTS, PHENTERMINE, PHENDIMETRAZINE, HYDROCHLOROTHIAZIDE AND LASIX, IN SOME INSTANCES WITHOUT ADEQUATE ASSESSMENT OR DOCUMENTATION. PROBATION WITH TERMS: SHALL NOT TREAT ANY PATIENT FOR WEIGHT CONTROL OR OBESITY WITH ANY CONTROLLED SUBSTANCES, DANGEROUS DRUGS OR OVER-THE-COUNTER DRUGS; SHALL NOT PRESCRIBE, DISPENSE, ADMINISTER OR POSSESS SYMPATHOMIMETIC DRUGS INCLUDING BUT NOT LIMITED TO ANORECTIC DRUGS; SHALL MAINTAIN ADEQUATE MEDICAL RECORDS WHICH SHALL BE AVAILABLE FOR REVIEW; SHALL OBTAIN AT LEAST 50 HOURS PER YEAR OF CONTINUING MEDICAL EDUCATION; SHALL APPEAR BEFORE THE BOARD AT LEAST ONCE A YEAR OR AT BOARD REQUEST; SHALL PERFORM 100 HOURS OF COMMUNITY SERVICE; SHALL COOPERATE WITH BOARD IN VERIFYING COMPLIANCE; SHALL GIVE A COPY OF THIS ORDER TO ANY HEALTH CARE ENTITY WHERE HE HAS PRIVILEGES; SHALL PROVIDE A COPY OF THIS ORDER TO ANYONE REQUESTING IT WITHIN 10 DAYS; TIME PERIOD OUT OF TEXAS DOES NOT COUNT TOWARD PROBATION; SHALL INFORM BOARD OF CHANGE OF ADDRESS WITHIN 10 DAYS OR IF HE LEAVES THE STATE. SHALL NOT SEEK MODIFICATION FOR ONE YEAR. ON 10/5/96 THE BOARD DENIED HIS REQUEST FOR TERMINATION OF THIS ORDER. ON 9/20/97 ORDER TERMINATED.

FRY, LEE PAUL MD, LICENSE NUMBER D1639 OF SAN ANGELO, TX, WAS DISCIPLINED BY TEXAS ON MAY 14, 1999
DISCIPLINARY ACTION: FINE; 48-MONTH RESTRICTION PLACED ON LICENSE
OFFENSE: SUBSTANDARD CARE, INCOMPETENCE OR NEGLIGENCE

NOTES: ON 4/2/93 HE PERFORMED A TONSILLECTOMY AND ADENOIDECTOMY ON A PATIENT; A BOARD CONSULTANT DETERMINED THAT THE CHART LACKED A DETAILED PHYSICAL AND HISTORY, AND THERE WAS NO DOCUMENTATION OF THE DISCUSSION OF DIAGNOSIS WITH THE FAMILY AND NO DISCUSSION OF THE DETAILS OF THE SURGERY; A BOARD CONSULTANT DETERMINED THAT FOR A TONSILLECTOMY PERFORMED ON 12/17/92 RECORDS WERE RELATIVELY SCANTY REGARDING THE RISKS OF TONSILLECTOMY, PRE-OPERATIVE DIAGNOSIS, INDICATIONS FOR SURGERY AND POSTOPERATIVE FOLLOWUP; ON 11/3/92 AFTER PERFORMING ENDOSCOPIC SINUS SURGERY, A POST-OPERATIVE CT SCAN ORDERED BY ANOTHER PHYSICIAN REVEALED A LARGE RIGHT FRONTOTEMPOROPARIETAL ACUTE SUBDURAL HEMATOMA; HE WAS NOTED TO BE LETHARGIC AND UNRESPONSIVE IN THE RECOVERY ROOM; ON 8/12/87 HE PERFORMED A SEPTORHINOPLASTY ON A PATIENT AND HAD NO SURGICAL RECORDS OF THAT PROCEDURE; HIS DEPOSED TESTIMONY ON 7/24/90 COVERED HIS LACK OF RECORDS, PROGRESS NOTES, AND INFORMED CONSENT; THE BOARD CONSULTANT CRITICIZED THE LACK OF DETAIL IN PRE-OPERATIVE HISTORY; ON 10/5/94 REGARDING HIS HAVING PERFORMED A FULL-FACE DERMABRASION ON A PATIENT, THE BOARD CONSULTANT DETERMINED THAT THERE WAS NO HISTORY OR PHYSICAL EXAM FORMATTED IN A STANDARD FASHION, NO DOCUMENTATION OF THE FUNDAMENTAL DIAGNOSIS WHICH LED TO THE PROCEDURE AND NO DETAILED FORMAL OPERATIVE REPORT; HE VOLUNTARILY RESIGNED HIS HOSPITAL AND SURGICAL PRIVILEGES. LICENSE LIMITED FOR FOUR YEARS AS FOLLOWS: SHALL ATTEND 50 HOURS PER YEAR OF CONTINUING MEDICAL EDUCATION WITH 1 COURSE IN THE AREA OF RISK MANAGEMENT; SHALL HAVE NO HOSPITAL SURGICAL PRIVILEGES, OR AMBULATORY SURGICAL CENTER PRIVILEGES; SHALL OBTAIN ONE ETHICS COURSE OR AN ETHICS PROGRAM PER YEAR; SHALL MAINTAIN ADEQUATE MEDICAL RECORDS WHICH SHALL BE AVAILABLE FOR REVIEW; WITHIN 60 DAYS HIS MEDICAL PRACTICE SHALL BE MONITORED BY A BOARD APPROVED TEXAS PHYSICIAN WHO SHALL PROVIDE QUARTERLY REPORTS TO THE BOARD; $3,000 FINE; SHALL APPEAR BEFORE THE BOARD ONCE A YEAR; SHALL COOPERATE WITH THE BOARD IN VERIFYING COMPLIANCE; TIME SPENT OUT OF TEXAS DOES NOT COUNT TOWARD RESTRICTION; SHALL INFORM THE BOARD OF CHANGE OF ADDRESS WITHIN 10 DAYS OR IF HE LEAVES THE STATE; SHALL NOT SEEK MODIFICATION FOR ONE YEAR.

FULLER, CHARLES H III MD, LICENSE NUMBER C5056, WAS DISCIPLINED BY TEXAS ON FEBRUARY 27, 1997
DISCIPLINARY ACTION: LICENSE REVOCATION
OFFENSE: DISCIPLINARY ACTION BY ANOTHER STATE OR AGENCY

NOTES: LICENSE EXPIRED ON 8/31/96 BECAUSE HE FAILED TO PAY THE ANNUAL LICENSING FEE. ON 7/7/95 THE CALIFORNIA BOARD FOUND HE PERFORMED LIP AUGMENTATIONS USING LIQUID SILICONE IN VIOLATION OF FEDERAL LAW AND TO THE HARM OF HIS PATIENTS; ON 12/15/92, HE TOLD THE FOOD AND DRUG ADMINISTRATION THAT HE NO LONGER USED SILICONE INJECTIONS FOR TREATMENT OF ANY CONDITIONS WHEN IN FACT HE CONTINUED TO RECOMMEND IT FOR LIP AUGMENTATIONS. INVESTIGATIONS YIELDED EVIDENCE OF GROSS NEGLIGENCE AND INCOMPETENCE IN THE TREATMENT OF AT LEAST TWO PATIENTS AND DISHONEST AND CORRUPT ACTS IN VIOLATION OF THE CALIFORNIA BUSINESS AND PROFESSIONS CODE. HIS CALIFORNIA LICENSE WAS REVOKED; REVOCATION SUBSEQUENTLY STAYED FOR FIVE YEARS PROBATION.

FUSTOK, ABDEL KADER MD, LICENSE NUMBER F4727 OF HOUSTON, TX, WAS DISCIPLINED BY TEXAS ON AUGUST 9, 1997
DISCIPLINARY ACTION: FINE
OFFENSE: NONCOMPLIANCE WITH A PROFESSIONAL RULE

NOTES: IN 5/94, REMOVED SILICONE BREAST IMPLANTS OF A PATIENT AND REPLACED THEM WITH SALINE IMPLANTS. HIS BILLING RECORDS DO NOT ADEQUATELY DEMONSTRATE THE CHARGES TO THE PATIENT AND THE AMOUNT BILLED TO HER INSURANCE COMPANY. ADMINISTRATIVE PENALTY OF $5000.

GAGLIANO, ANGELO V MD, LICENSE NUMBER 0G49526 OF SAN ANTONIO, TX, WAS DISCIPLINED BY CALIFORNIA ON NOVEMBER 16, 1995
DISCIPLINARY ACTION: REPRIMAND
OFFENSE: DISCIPLINARY ACTION BY ANOTHER STATE OR AGENCY

NOTES: ACTION IN TEXAS FOR ADMINISTERING ANESTHESIA ON A NON-EMERGENT, CRITICALLY ILL SURGICAL PATIENT WITHOUT FIRST ESTABLISHING

APPROPRIATE MONITORING.

GAGLIANO, ANGELO V MD, DATE OF BIRTH SEPTEMBER 24, 1938, LICENSE NUMBER 0013876 OF 16903 HIDDEN TIMBERWOOD, SAN ANTONIO, TX, WAS DISCIPLINED BY SOUTH CAROLINA ON OCTOBER 21, 1996
DISCIPLINARY ACTION: REPRIMAND
OFFENSE: SUBSTANDARD CARE, INCOMPETENCE OR NEGLIGENCE
NOTES: ADMINISTERED ANESTHESIA ON A NON-EMERGENCY, CRITICALLY ILL SURGICAL PATIENT WITHOUT FIRST ESTABLISHING PROPER MONITORING.

GAGLIANO, ANGELO V MD OF SAN ANTONIO, TX, WAS DISCIPLINED BY ILLINOIS ON DECEMBER 1, 1996
DISCIPLINARY ACTION: FINE; REPRIMAND
OFFENSE: DISCIPLINARY ACTION BY ANOTHER STATE OR AGENCY
NOTES: DISCIPLINED IN TEXAS. FINE $250.

GAGLIANO, ANGELO V MD, LICENSE NUMBER 34556 OF 16903 HIDDEN TIMBER WOOD, SAN ANTONIO, TX, WAS DISCIPLINED BY MASSACHUSETTS ON JUNE 4, 1997
DISCIPLINARY ACTION: REPRIMAND
OFFENSE: DISCIPLINARY ACTION BY ANOTHER STATE OR AGENCY
NOTES: DISCIPLINED BY TEXAS.

GAGLIANO, ANGELO VINCENT MD, LICENSE NUMBER 00H6820 OF SAN ANTONIO, TX, WAS DISCIPLINED BY TEXAS ON JANUARY 6, 1995
DISCIPLINARY ACTION: REPRIMAND
OFFENSE: SUBSTANDARD CARE, INCOMPETENCE OR NEGLIGENCE
NOTES: IN 8/92 HE ADMINISTERED ANESTHESIA ON A NON-EMERGENT CRITICALLY ILL SURGICAL PATIENT WITHOUT FIRST ESTABLISHING APPROPRIATE MONITORING; AGREED TO THIS ORDER IN LIEU OF FURTHER INVESTIGATION.

GAGLIANO, ANGELO VINCENT MD, LICENSE NUMBER 53569 OF SAN ANTONIO, TX, WAS DISCIPLINED BY OHIO ON MARCH 11, 1998
DISCIPLINARY ACTION: REPRIMAND
OFFENSE: DISCIPLINARY ACTION BY ANOTHER STATE OR AGENCY
NOTES: HE ADMINISTERED ANESTHESIA ON A NON-EMERGENT CRITICALLY ILL SURGICAL PATIENT WITHOUT FIRST ESTABLISHING APPROPRIATE MONITORING, AND HE HAS BEEN REPRIMANDED BY ILLINOIS, MASSACHUSETTS, AND SOUTH CAROLINA ON THE BASIS OF THIS CONDUCT.

GALINDO, CONRADO G III MD, DATE OF BIRTH JANUARY 9, 1947, LICENSE NUMBER 00F0189 OF 1300 BEDELL, DEL RIO, TX, WAS DISCIPLINED BY TEXAS ON DECEMBER 3, 1990
DISCIPLINARY ACTION: 60-MONTH PROBATION; RESTRICTION PLACED ON CONTROLLED SUBSTANCE LICENSE
NOTES: PARTICIPATION IN PRECEPTORSHIP PROGRAM TO INCLUDE SPECIFIC CURRICULUM; ATTENDANCE AT CONTINUING MEDICAL EDUCATION COURSES; NOT PRESCRIBING ANY SCHEDULE II CONTROLLED DRUG EXCEPT FOR HOSPITALIZED PATIENTS; CONTINUATION OF TREATMENT FROM A PSYCHIATRIST; APPEARANCE BEFORE BOARD TWICE ANNUALLY; SUBMIT HIMSELF FOR APPROPRIATE EXAMINATIONS AND SCREENINGS TO DETERMINE FREEDOM FROM DRUGS OR ALCOHOL; PARTICIPATION IN ACTIVITIES AND PROGRAMS OF ALCOHOLICS ANONYMOUS ON A REGULAR BASIS. ON 8/20/93 BOARD DENIED HIS REQUEST FOR TERMINATION AND MODIFIED THIS ORDER SO THAT HE IS REQUIRED TO MAKE ANNUAL RATHER THAN SEMI-ANNUAL APPEARANCES BEFORE THE BOARD. ALL OTHER PROVISIONS OF THIS ORDER REMAIN IN EFFECT. ON 8/19/94 HIS REQUEST FOR TERMINATION OF THIS ORDER DENIED.

GALINDO, CONRADO G III MD OF 1300 BEDELL AVENUE, DEL RIO, TX, WAS DISCIPLINED BY DEA ON JANUARY 24, 1997
DISCIPLINARY ACTION: SURRENDER OF CONTROLLED SUBSTANCE LICENSE
NOTES: IN LIEU OF PUBLIC INTEREST REVOCATION.

GALINDO, CONRADO G III MD, LICENSE NUMBER F0189 OF DEL RIO, TX, WAS DISCIPLINED BY TEXAS ON APRIL 4, 1998
DISCIPLINARY ACTION: 120-MONTH PROBATION; RESTRICTION PLACED ON LICENSE
OFFENSE: LOSS OR RESTRICTION OF HOSPITAL PRIVILEGES
NOTES: ON 12/3/90 THE BOARD DISCIPLINED HIM FOR ABUSE OF DEMEROL IN 1988 AND 1989; THIS ORDER EXPIRED ON 12/3/95; ON 1/21/97 HE SELF-REPORTED THAT HE AGAIN USED DEMEROL; IN 1/97 HE ENTERED A TREATMENT PROGRAM AND WAS DISCHARGED IN 6/97; IN 8/97 HE WAS INDICTED IN U.S. DISTRICT COURT FOR CLAIMING IN HIS 1995 DEA REGISTRATION RENEWAL THAT HE HAD NEVER BEEN PLACED ON PROBATION BY THE TEXAS BOARD; IN 2/97 HOSPITAL PRIVILEGES SUSPENDED; HE HAS ENTERED INTO A 5 YEAR AFTERCARE RECOVERY CONTRACT WITH A MEDICAL SOCIETY AND MAINTAINS THAT HE HAS BEEN IN FULL COMPLIANCE WITH THE CONTRACT. SUSPENSION STAYED FOR PROBATION WITH TERMS AS FOLLOWS: SHALL LIMIT PRACTICE OF OBSTETRICS AND GYNECOLOGY TO NO MORE THAN 40 DELIVERIES AND 18 GYNECOLOGICAL SURGERIES DURING THE FIRST 6 MONTHS THAT THIS ORDER IS IN EFFECT; SHALL NOT EMPLOY HIS SPOUSE OR ALLOW HER TO VOLUNTEER TO ASSIST HIM IN HIS PRACTICE OR THE ADMINISTRATION OF THAT PRACTICE; SHALL ABSTAIN FROM THE CONSUMPTION OF ALCOHOL/DRUGS IN ANY FORM UNLESS PRESCRIBED BY ANOTHER PHYSICIAN FOR A LEGITIMATE AND THERAPEUTIC PURPOSE; SHALL SUBMIT HIMSELF FOR APPROPRIATE EXAMS INCLUDING DRUG OR ALCOHOL SCREENS; SHALL CONTINUE TO RECEIVE CARE AND TREATMENT FROM HIS PHYSICIAN NO LESS THAN ONCE A MONTH WITH QUARTERLY REPORTS TO THE BOARD; SHALL PARTICIPATE IN THE ACTIVITIES OF A PHYSICIAN HEALTH AND REHABILITATION COMMITTEE AND ATTEND WEEKLY MEETINGS WITH QUARTERLY REPORTS; SHALL PARTICIPATE IN AA'S PROGRAM NOT LESS THAN THREE TIMES A WEEK; SHALL REPORT ON HIS ATTENDANCE; SHALL COMPLY WITH HIS CONTINUING CARE CONTRACTS WITH QUARTERLY REPORTS TO THE BOARD; SHALL NOT POSSESS ALCOHOL, CONTROLLED SUBSTANCES OR DRUGS WITH POTENTIAL FOR ABUSE AND SHALL SURRENDER ANY SUCH SUBSTANCES STILL IN HIS POSSESSION INCLUDING SAMPLES; SHALL OBTAIN 50 HOURS PER YEAR OF CONTINUING MEDICAL EDUCATION; SHALL APPEAR BEFORE THE BOARD AT LEAST ONCE A YEAR; SHALL COOPERATE WITH THE BOARD IN VERIFYING COMPLIANCE; SHALL PROVIDE A COPY OF THIS ORDER TO ANYONE REQUESTING IT WITHIN 10 DAYS; TIME SPENT OUT OF TEXAS DOES NOT COUNT TOWARD PROBATION; SHALL INFORM THE BOARD OF CHANGE OF ADDRESS WITHIN 10 DAYS OR IF HE LEAVES THE STATE; SHALL NOT SEEK MODIFICATION FOR ONE YEAR. ON 4/10/99 THE ORDER WAS MODIFIED AS FOLLOWS: DELETION OF RESTRICTION ON OBSTETRICS AND GYNECOLOGY PRACTICE; HE MAY EMPLOY HIS SPOUSE OR ALLOW HER TO VOLUNTEER TO ASSIST HIM IN ADMINISTRATIVE

DUTIES ONLY; DELETION OF REQUIREMENT TO PARTICIPATE WITH THE COUNTY MEDICAL SOCIETY COMMITTEE ON PHYSICIAN HEALTH AND REHABILITATION; AND, DELETION OF COMPLIANCE REQUIREMENT WITH HIS MEDICAL SOCIETY PHYSICIANS COMMITTEE CONTRACT; ALL OTHER PROVISIONS OF ORDER REMAIN IN FULL EFFECT UNTIL SUPERSEDED BY A SUBSEQUENT BOARD ORDER.

GALLMAN, DOYLE F JR DO, LICENSE NUMBER 00H2391 OF MANSFIELD, TX, WAS DISCIPLINED BY TEXAS ON AUGUST 19, 1994
DISCIPLINARY ACTION: 60-MONTH PROBATION; RESTRICTION PLACED ON CONTROLLED SUBSTANCE LICENSE
OFFENSE: SUBSTANCE ABUSE

NOTES: AFTER UNDERGOING KNEE SURGERY IN 1989 HE BECAME ADDICTED TO THE VICODIN HE WAS TAKING FOR PAIN RELIEF; OCCASIONALLY USED IM INJECTABLE MEDICINE SUCH AS NUBAIN, TALWIN AND DEMEROL; INITIATED HIS OWN TREATMENT AND WAS HOSPITALIZED FROM 8/16/93 THROUGH 9/16/93; IS PRESENTLY IN OUTPATIENT THERAPY. SUSPENSION STAYED. CONDITIONS OF PROBATION: SHALL APPEAR BEFORE BOARD TWICE A YEAR; SHALL NOT TREAT OR OTHERWISE SERVE AS PHYSICIAN, PRESCRIBE, DISPENSE OR ADMINISTER DRUGS THAT MAY BE SUBJECT TO ABUSE TO HIMSELF OR ANY MEMBER OF HIS FAMILY; SHALL NOT POSSESS, ADMINISTER, DISPENSE OR PRESCRIBE ANY CONTROLLED SUBSTANCES BUT MAY ORDER THEM TO BE ADMINISTERED TO HOSPITAL OR NURSING HOME PATIENTS AND MAY WRITE PRESCRIPTIONS FOR CONTROLLED SUBSTANCES FOR PATIENTS SEEN IN OTHER PHYSICIAN'S OFFICES IN THE COURSE OF HIS LOCUM TENENS WORK; SHALL SUBMIT HIMSELF FOR APPROPRIATE EXAMS INCLUDING DRUG OR ALCOHOL SCREENS; SHALL CONTINUE TO PARTICIPATE IN AA'S PROGRAM NOT LESS THAN THREE TIMES A WEEK WITH MONTHLY REPORTS; SHALL ABSTAIN FROM THE CONSUMPTION OF ALCOHOL/CHEMICAL SUBSTANCES IN ANY FORM UNLESS PRESCRIBED BY ANOTHER PHYSICIAN FOR A LEGITIMATE AND THERAPEUTIC PURPOSE; SHALL CONTINUE TO PARTICIPATE IN ACTIVITIES OF THE TEXAS OSTEOPATHIC MEDICAL ASSOCIATION AND ATTEND WEEKLY MEETINGS WITH QUARTERLY REPORTS; SHALL CONTINUE TO RECEIVE TREATMENT FROM SPECIFIED PHYSICIAN WITH QUARTERLY REPORTS; WITHIN ONE YEAR SHALL TAKE A BOARD-APPROVED COURSE IN ADDICTIONOLOGY; SEPARATE FROM PATIENT RECORDS SHALL MAINTAIN A FILE OF EVERY PRESCRIPTION WRITTEN FOR DANGEROUS DRUGS WHICH SHALL BE AVAILABLE FOR INSPECTION; SHALL GIVE A COPY OF THIS ORDER TO ANY HEALTH CARE ENTITY WHERE HE HAS PRIVILEGES; SHALL COOPERATE WITH THE BOARD IN VERIFYING COMPLIANCE; SHALL INFORM BOARD OF CHANGE OF ADDRESS WITHIN 10 DAYS OR IF HE LEAVES THE STATE; TIME SPENT OUT OF TEXAS DOES NOT COUNT TOWARD PROBATION. SHALL NOT SEEK MODIFICATION FOR ONE YEAR. ON 1/18/97 PETITION TO TERMINATE ORDER DENIED. ON 3/1/97 PETITION TO TERMINATE ORDER DENIED. ON 8/9/97 BOARD GRANTED HIS PETITION FOR TERMINATION OF THIS ORDER BASED ON COMPLIANCE WITH CONDITIONS.

GALLOWAY, ROBERT E MD, LICENSE NUMBER 00E9198 OF HOUSTON, TX, WAS DISCIPLINED BY TEXAS ON MARCH 5, 1994
DISCIPLINARY ACTION: 60-MONTH PROBATION; REQUIRED TO TAKE ADDITIONAL MEDICAL EDUCATION
OFFENSE: PROVIDING FALSE INFORMATION TO THE BOARD OR OTHER HEALTH AGENCY

NOTES: SINCE 1978 HE HAS SUBMITTED OR ALLOWED OFFICE STAFF TO SUBMIT INFORMATION TO 10 HOSPITALS THAT HE IS AMERICAN BOARD OF INTERNAL MEDICINE CERTIFIED WHEN HE IS NOT; VOLUNTARILY AGREED TO A PSYCHIATRIC EXAM; HAS NOT BEEN THE SUBJECT OF HOSPITAL OR PATIENT COMPLAINTS. ONE YEAR SUSPENSION STAYED. CONDITIONS OF PROBATION: SHALL APPEAR BEFORE THE BOARD TWICE A YEAR; SHALL ATTEND AT LEAST 50 HOURS PER YEAR OF CONTINUING EDUCATION; SHALL ALSO ATTEND SIX HOURS OF AN ETHICS COURSE OR PROGRAM PER YEAR FOR FIVE YEARS; WITHIN ONE YEAR SHALL PASS THE BOARD'S JURISPRUDENCE EXAM; SHALL PERFORM EIGHT HOURS PER MONTH OF COMMUNITY SERVICE FOR THREE YEARS; SHALL CONTINUE TO RECEIVE PSYCHIATRIC TREATMENT WITH QUARTERLY REPORTS; SHALL COOPERATE WITH THE BOARD IN VERIFYING COMPLIANCE; SHALL INFORM BOARD OF CHANGE OF ADDRESS WITHIN 10 DAYS OR IF HE LEAVES THE STATE; TIME SPENT OUT OF TEXAS DOES NOT COUNT TOWARD PROBATION. SHALL NOT SEEK MODIFICATION FOR ONE YEAR.

GALLOWAY, ROBERT E MD, LICENSE NUMBER 00E9198 OF HOUSTON, TX, WAS DISCIPLINED BY TEXAS ON JUNE 22, 1994
DISCIPLINARY ACTION: 60-MONTH PROBATION; REQUIRED TO TAKE ADDITIONAL MEDICAL EDUCATION
OFFENSE: SUBSTANDARD CARE, INCOMPETENCE OR NEGLIGENCE

NOTES: FAILED TO ADEQUATELY SUPERVISE THE ACTIVITIES OF HIS ASSISTANT WHO WAS NOT REGISTERED AS A PHYSICIAN'S ASSISTANT; IN 4/90 FAILED TO FOLLOW UP ON LAB WORK OF ONE PATIENT WHO WAS LATER FOUND TO HAVE CANCER OF THE DUODENUM. ON 3/5/94 HE ENTERED INTO AN AGREED ORDER WHICH IS INCORPORATED WITH THIS ORDER. ONE YEAR SUSPENSION STAYED. CONDITIONS OF PROBATION: SHALL OBTAIN AT LEAST EIGHT HOURS OF CONTINUING MEDICAL EDUCATION IN RISK MANAGEMENT WITHIN ONE YEAR FROM THE DATE OF THIS ORDER; SHALL SUBMIT WRITTEN PROTOCOL OF SUPERVISION OF HIS PHYSICIAN ASSISTANT WITHIN 30 DAYS; SHALL NOT PRESIGN PRESCRIPTIONS FOR CONTROLLED SUBSTANCES OR DANGEROUS DRUGS; SHALL DOCUMENT ON EACH RECORD THAT HE HAS PERSONALLY SEEN OR REVIEWED EACH PATIENT CHART; SHALL KEEP A SEPARATE LIST OF PATIENTS SEEN BY THE PHYSICIAN'S ASSISTANT WHICH SHALL BE AVAILABLE FOR REVIEW; SHALL MAINTAIN A COMPLETE CREDENTIALS/PERSONNEL FILE ON EACH EMPLOYEE AND ENSURE THAT ALL NECESSARY DOCUMENTATION HAS BEEN OBTAINED; SHALL MAINTAIN RESPONSIBILITY FOR THE ACTS OR OMISSIONS OF HIS EMPLOYEES; SHALL GIVE A COPY OF THIS ORDER TO ANY HEALTH CARE ENTITY WHERE HE HAS PRIVILEGES; SHALL COOPERATE WITH THE BOARD IN VERIFYING COMPLIANCE; SHALL INFORM BOARD OF CHANGE OF ADDRESS WITHIN 10 DAYS OR IF HE LEAVES THE STATE. TIME SPENT OUT OF TEXAS DOES NOT COUNT TOWARD PROBATION. SHALL NOT SEEK MODIFICATION FOR ONE YEAR. ON 5/10/97 BOARD GRANTED HIS PETITION FOR TERMINATION OF THIS ORDER BASED ON COMPLIANCE WITH CONDITIONS.

GALLOWAY, ROBERT E MD OF CHICAGO, IL, WAS DISCIPLINED BY ILLINOIS ON NOVEMBER 1, 1995
DISCIPLINARY ACTION: PROBATION
OFFENSE: DISCIPLINARY ACTION BY ANOTHER STATE OR AGENCY

NOTES: DISCIPLINED IN TEXAS. INDEFINITE SUSPENSION.

GANACIAS, ADELA RAMIREZ OF 1619 KINGSPOINT DRIVE,

CARROLLTON, TX, WAS DISCIPLINED BY OKLAHOMA ON JULY 1, 1993
DISCIPLINARY ACTION: DENIAL OF NEW LICENSE
NOTES: HAS FAILED THE FLEX EXAM 10 TIMES, WHICH RAISES SERIOUS ISSUES AS TO CLINICAL COMPETENCY AND FITNESS TO PRACTICE. DENIAL REAFFIRMED ON 12/2/93.

GARCIA, CLOTILDE P MD OF HOSPITAL BLVD SUITE 118, CORPUS CHRISTI, TX, WAS DISCIPLINED BY DEA ON JANUARY 24, 1994
DISCIPLINARY ACTION: SURRENDER OF CONTROLLED SUBSTANCE LICENSE
NOTES: IN LIEU OF PUBLIC INTEREST REVOCATION.

GARCIA, EDUARDO A MD, LICENSE NUMBER J6446 OF HOUSTON, TX, WAS DISCIPLINED BY TEXAS ON AUGUST 28, 1999
DISCIPLINARY ACTION: RESTRICTION PLACED ON LICENSE; REPRIMAND
OFFENSE: PROFESSIONAL MISCONDUCT
NOTES: ABETTING THE UNLICENSED PRACTICE OF MEDICINE AND FAILURE TO SUPERVISE DELEGATES.

GARCIA, EDUARDO I MD, LICENSE NUMBER 00F3978 OF HOUSTON, TX, WAS DISCIPLINED BY TEXAS ON JANUARY 24, 1992
DISCIPLINARY ACTION: 24-MONTH PROBATION
OFFENSE: SUBSTANDARD CARE, INCOMPETENCE OR NEGLIGENCE
NOTES: PROFESSIONAL FAILURE TO PRACTICE MEDICINE IN AN ACCEPTABLE MANNER CONSISTENT WITH PUBLIC HEALTH AND WELFARE. LICENSE SUSPENDED, SUSPENSION STAYED; PROBATION UNDER TERMS AND CONDITIONS.

GARCIA, EDUARDO IGNACIO MD, LICENSE NUMBER F3978 OF THE WOODLANDS, TX, WAS DISCIPLINED BY TEXAS ON AUGUST 22, 1998
DISCIPLINARY ACTION: REPRIMAND
OFFENSE: NONCOMPLIANCE WITH A PROFESSIONAL RULE
NOTES: THE MEDICAL RECORDS OF 24 PATIENTS, CONSISTING OF APPROXIMATELY 3000 PAGES, WERE REVIEWED BY A BOARD CONSULTANT; THE RECORDS WERE, WITHOUT EXCEPTION, COMPLETELY ILLEGIBLE; BECAUSE OF THE ILLEGIBLE RECORDS, THE BOARD WAS UNABLE TO DETERMINE WHETHER THE RECORDS SUPPORTED THE CARE AND TREATMENT OF THE REFERENCED PATIENTS.

GARCIA, FRANCISCO J MD, LICENSE NUMBER 00G8846 OF SAN ANTONIO, TX, WAS DISCIPLINED BY TEXAS ON AUGUST 18, 1995
DISCIPLINARY ACTION: REPRIMAND
OFFENSE: PROFESSIONAL MISCONDUCT
NOTES: AIDING OR ABETTING, DIRECTLY OR INDIRECTLY, THE PRACTICE OF MEDICINE BY ANY PERSON NOT DULY LICENSED TO PRACTICE MEDICINE IN THAT HE HAD BEEN EMPLOYED ON A SALARIED BASIS BY AN INDIVIDUAL NOT LICENSED TO PRACTICE MEDICINE IN TEXAS. SHALL GIVE A COPY OF THIS ORDER TO ANY HEALTH CARE ENTITY WHERE HE HAS PRIVILEGES; SHALL PROVIDE A COPY OF THIS ORDER TO ANYONE REQUESTING IT WITHIN 10 DAYS.

GARCIA, JOSE GERARDO MD, DATE OF BIRTH NOVEMBER 21, 1935, LICENSE NUMBER 00D1310 OF LAREDO, TX, WAS DISCIPLINED BY TEXAS ON AUGUST 24, 1991
DISCIPLINARY ACTION: 36-MONTH PROBATION; REQUIRED TO TAKE ADDITIONAL MEDICAL EDUCATION
OFFENSE: PROFESSIONAL MISCONDUCT
NOTES: UNPROFESSIONAL AND/OR DISHONORABLE CONDUCT LIKELY TO DECEIVE, DEFRAUD, OR INJURE THE PUBLIC. LICENSE SUSPENDED, STAYED; CONDITIONS OF PROBATION INCLUDE: COMPLETION OF TEN HOURS OF AN ETHICS COURSE PER YEAR FOR THREE YEARS; SUBMITTING TO PSYCHIATRIC EVALUATION AND TREATMENT BY A PSYCHIATRIST APPROVED BY THE BOARD ONCE A YEAR; SHALL APPEAR BEFORE THE BOARD ONCE ANNUALLY DURING EACH YEAR OF PROBATION. ORDER TERMINATED ON 6/21/93; LICENSE FREE AND CLEAR OF RESTRICTIONS.

GARCIA, ROBERT WILLIAM MD, DATE OF BIRTH SEPTEMBER 20, 1959 OF C/O 840 W CLEMENTS AVE, ODESSA, TX, WAS DISCIPLINED BY MEDICARE ON SEPTEMBER 15, 1996
DISCIPLINARY ACTION: EXCLUSION FROM THE MEDICARE AND/OR MEDICAID PROGRAM
OFFENSE: NONCOMPLIANCE WITH A PROFESSIONAL RULE
NOTES: DEFAULTED ON PUBLIC HEALTH SERVICE EDUCATION LOAN. REINSTATED ON 9/27/96.

GARCIAARECHA, LUIS A MD, LICENSE NUMBER 00D9140 OF SAN ANTONIO, TX, WAS DISCIPLINED BY TEXAS ON JANUARY 12, 1991
DISCIPLINARY ACTION: REPRIMAND

GARDINER, HENRY GEORGE MD, LICENSE NUMBER 00C4120 OF FORT WORTH, TX, WAS DISCIPLINED BY TEXAS ON AUGUST 24, 1991
DISCIPLINARY ACTION: 60-MONTH PROBATION; RESTRICTION PLACED ON CONTROLLED SUBSTANCE LICENSE
OFFENSE: PROFESSIONAL MISCONDUCT
NOTES: UNPROFESSIONAL OR DISHONORABLE CONDUCT LIKELY TO DECEIVE, DEFRAUD, OR INJURE THE PUBLIC; PROFESSIONAL FAILURE TO PRACTICE MEDICINE IN AN ACCEPTABLE MANNER CONSISTENT WITH PUBLIC HEALTH AND WELFARE. REVOCATION STAYED. CONDITIONS OF PROBATION: SHALL SURRENDER SCHEDULE II AND II-N DEA AND DPS CONTROLLED SUBSTANCES REGISTRATIONS; SHALL NOT ATTEMPT TO REREGISTER WITHOUT PRIOR BOARD APPROVAL; SHALL SURRENDER ALL UNUSED TRIPLICATE PRESCRIPTION FORMS AND NOT ATTEMPT TO ORDER MORE WITHOUT PRIOR APPROVAL OF THE BOARD; SHALL NOT PRESCRIBE, ADMINISTER, OR POSSESS ANY SCHEDULE III, IV, OR V CONTROLLED SUBSTANCES EXCEPT FOR HOSPITALIZED PATIENTS; SHALL ATTEND AT LEAST 50 HOURS PER YEAR FOR THREE YEARS CONTINUING MEDICAL EDUCATION, TO INCLUDE AT LEAST FIVE HOURS IN RISK MANAGEMENT.

GARDNER, ROBERT L MD, LICENSE NUMBER 00D7045 OF LANCASTER, TX, WAS DISCIPLINED BY TEXAS ON OCTOBER 26, 1990
DISCIPLINARY ACTION: REPRIMAND; REQUIRED TO TAKE ADDITIONAL MEDICAL EDUCATION
NOTES: MUST OBTAIN MONITOR FOR CASES; UNDERGO PHYSICAL EXAMINATION AND FOLLOW ANY RECOMMENDED TREATMENT; SUBMIT FOR PSYCHIATRIC EVALUATION AND FOLLOW ANY RECOMMENDED TREATMENT; OBTAIN CONTINUING MEDICAL EDUCATION; VISIT BOARD ANNUALLY FOR NEXT FIVE YEARS.

GARDNER, ROBERT L MD, LICENSE NUMBER D7045 OF DUNCANVILLE, TX, WAS DISCIPLINED BY TEXAS ON OCTOBER 15, 1999
DISCIPLINARY ACTION: 36-MONTH RESTRICTION PLACED ON CONTROLLED SUBSTANCE LICENSE; REPRIMAND

OFFENSE: OVERPRESCRIBING OR MISPRESCRIBING DRUGS

NOTES: EXCESSIVELY PRESCRIBED CONTROLLED SUBSTANCES TO A PATIENT AND MAINTAINED INADEQUATE DOCUMENTATION FOR PRESCRIBING; HIS ACTIONS DO NOT CONFORM TO THE GUIDELINES REGARDING PRESCRIBING FOR THE TREATMENT OF PAIN. LICENSE LIMITED AS FOLLOWS: SHALL REQUEST MODIFICATION OF DEA AND TEXAS DEPARTMENT OF PUBLIC SAFETY CONTROLLED SUBSTANCES REGISTRATION CERTIFICATES TO ELIMINATE HIS ABILITY TO PRESCRIBE SCHEDULES II, IIN, III AND IIIN; SHALL SURRENDER ALL UNUSED TRIPLICATE PRESCRIPTION FORMS; SEPARATE FROM PATIENT RECORDS, SHALL MAINTAIN A LOGBOOK OF EVERY PRESCRIPTION WRITTEN BY HIM FOR DANGEROUS DRUGS WITH ADDICTIVE POTENTIAL WHICH SHALL BE MADE AVAILABLE FOR REVIEW; WITHIN 60 DAYS HIS MEDICAL PRACTICE SHALL BE MONITORED BY A BOARD APPROVED TEXAS PHYSICIAN WHO SHALL PROVIDE QUARTERLY REPORTS TO THE BOARD; SHALL MAINTAIN ADEQUATE MEDICAL RECORDS WHICH SHALL BE AVAILABLE FOR REVIEW; SHALL OBTAIN 50 HOURS PER YEAR OF CONTINUING MEDICAL EDUCATION; SHALL APPEAR BEFORE THE BOARD UPON REQUEST; TIME SPENT OUT OF TEXAS DOES NOT COUNT TOWARD RESTRICTION; SHALL INFORM THE BOARD OF CHANGE OF ADDRESS WITHIN 10 DAYS OR IF HE LEAVES THE STATE; SHALL GIVE A COPY OF THIS ORDER TO ANY HEALTH CARE ENTITY WHERE HE HAS PRIVILEGES; SHALL PROVIDE A COPY OF THIS ORDER TO ANYONE REQUESTING IT WITHIN 10 DAYS; SHALL COOPERATE WITH THE BOARD IN VERIFYING COMPLIANCE INCLUDING PROVIDING COPIES OF MEDICAL RELEASES AND PEER REVIEW RECORDS UPON REQUEST; SHALL NOT SEEK MODIFICATION FOR ONE YEAR.

GARNER, JAMES FRANCIS MD, DATE OF BIRTH NOVEMBER 3, 1950, LICENSE NUMBER 00E6363 OF 1606 MORSE STREET, HOUSTON, TX, WAS DISCIPLINED BY TEXAS ON JANUARY 29, 1993
DISCIPLINARY ACTION: 120-MONTH PROBATION; RESTRICTION PLACED ON LICENSE
OFFENSE: SUBSTANCE ABUSE

NOTES: ON 2/3/91 HE FAILED TO DIAGNOSE A FOUR-YEAR-OLD'S PNEUMONIA AND PRESCRIBED CHLORDIAZEPOXIDE FOR WHICH THERE WAS NO VALID MEDICAL REASON; HAD PREVIOUSLY INGESTED CODEINE ON MULTIPLE OCCASIONS WITHOUT A LEGITIMATE MEDICAL PURPOSE; IN JULY 1991 ADMITTED HIMSELF FOR INPATIENT TREATMENT AND THEN ENTERED INTO A MONITORING CONTRACT WITH A PHYSICIAN'S COUNSELING COMMITTEE; NOW PRACTICES ONLY AT INDIGENT CLINICS. SUSPENSION STAYED. CONDITIONS OF PROBATION: SHALL NOT WORK IN AN EMERGENCY ROOM SETTING, URGENT CARE FACILITY OR SIMILAR CLINIC AND SHALL RESTRICT PRACTICE TO THE TWO INDIGENT CLINICS WHERE HE CURRENTLY PRACTICES; SHALL OBTAIN WRITTEN APPROVAL OF THE BOARD BEFORE CHANGING HIS PRACTICE; ANY CHANGE WILL BE LIMITED TO A GROUP OR CLINIC PRACTICE; SHALL SUBMIT HIMSELF FOR EVALUATION AND TREATMENT TO A BOARD-APPROVED PSYCHIATRIST WHO WILL HAVE A COPY OF THIS ORDER; SHALL PARTICIPATE IN ACTIVITIES OF A PHYSICIAN HEALTH AND REHABILITATION COMMITTEE AND SHALL ATTEND WEEKLY MEETINGS WITH QUARTERLY REPORTS; SHALL ABSTAIN FROM THE CONSUMPTION OF ALCOHOL/DRUGS IN ANY FORM UNLESS PRESCRIBED BY ANOTHER PHYSICIAN FOR A LEGITIMATE AND THERAPEUTIC PURPOSE; SHALL SUBMIT HIMSELF FOR APPROPRIATE EXAMS INCLUDING DRUG OR ALCOHOL SCREENS; SHALL NOT ADMINISTER, PRESCRIBE, DISPENSE ANY CONTROLLED SUBSTANCES EXCEPT AS IS MEDICALLY NECESSARY TO TREAT HIV/AIDS PATIENTS AT THE CLINICS WHERE HE WORKS AND LIMITED TO ENUMERATED SUBSTANCES; SHALL MAINTAIN A SEPARATE WRITTEN LOG OF THESE PRESCRIPTIONS WHICH SHALL BE AVAILABLE FOR INSPECTION; SHALL ATTEND AT LEAST 50 HOURS PER YEAR OF CONTINUING MEDICAL EDUCATION; SHALL APPEAR BEFORE THE BOARD TWICE A YEAR; SHALL GIVE A COPY OF THIS ORDER TO ANY HEALTH CARE ENTITY WHERE HE HAS PRIVILEGES; SHALL COOPERATE WITH THE BOARD IN VERIFYING COMPLIANCE; SHALL INFORM BOARD OF CHANGE OF ADDRESS WITHIN 10 DAYS AND IF HE LEAVES THE STATE; TIME SPENT OUT OF TEXAS DOES NOT COUNT TOWARD PROBATION; SHALL NOT SEEK MODIFICATION FOR ONE YEAR. ON 8/9/97 BOARD GRANTED HIS PETITION FOR TERMINATION OF THIS ORDER BASED ON COMPLIANCE WITH CONDITIONS.

GARZA, JUAN JOEL MD, WAS DISCIPLINED BY TEXAS ON OCTOBER 24, 1998
DISCIPLINARY ACTION: MONITORING OF PHYSICIAN PERFORMANCE
OFFENSE: CRIMINAL CONVICTION OR PLEA OF GUILTY, NOLO CONTENDERE, OR NO CONTEST TO A CRIME

NOTES: IN 1992 HE WAS ARRESTED ON CHARGES OF DWI, WHICH WERE ULTIMATELY REDUCED TO SEVERAL MOVING VIOLATIONS; ON 7/28/93 HE WAS INVOLVED IN AN AUTOMOBILE ACCIDENT THAT RESULTED IN THE DEATH OF A 22 YEAR OLD; AT THE TIME OF THE ACCIDENT, HE WAS LEGALLY INTOXICATED; HE WAS CONVICTED OF INVOLUNTARY MANSLAUGHTER AND SENTENCED TO 10 YEARS PROBATION; IN 6/98 HE WAS DISCHARGED FROM PROBATION; THE FINDING OF GUILT WAS SET ASIDE; HE ASSERTS THAT HE NO LONGER DRINKS ALCOHOL NOR DOES HE PLAN TO DO SO IN THE FUTURE; HE WAS EVALUATED BY A PSYCHOLOGIST WHO FOUND NO EVIDENCE OF ANY PSYCHIATRIC PROBLEMS OR SUBSTANCE ABUSE; HIS EVALUATIONS HAVE BEEN CONSISTENTLY SATISFACTORY TO ABOVE AVERAGE; OVERALL HE HAS PERFORMED WELL AT THE PROGRAM. LICENSE LIMITED FOR TEN YEARS AS FOLLOWS: SHALL ABSTAIN FROM THE CONSUMPTION OF ALCOHOL/DRUGS IN ANY FORM UNLESS PRESCRIBED BY ANOTHER PHYSICIAN FOR A LEGITIMATE AND THERAPEUTIC PURPOSE; SHALL SUBMIT HIMSELF FOR APPROPRIATE EXAMS INCLUDING DRUG OR ALCOHOL SCREENS; SHALL NOMINATE THREE CERTIFIED PSYCHIATRISTS FOR BOARD SELECTION OF A THERAPIST AND SHALL EXPEDITIOUSLY SUBMIT HIMSELF TO EVALUATION AND TREATMENT BY THE APPROVED PRACTITIONER; SHALL PARTICIPATE IN THE ACTIVITIES OF A PHYSICIAN HEALTH AND REHABILITATION COMMITTEE AND ATTEND WEEKLY MEETINGS WITH QUARTERLY REPORTS; SHALL PARTICIPATE IN AA'S PROGRAM NOT LESS THAN THREE TIMES A WEEK; SHALL REPORT ON HIS ATTENDANCE; SHALL COOPERATE WITH THE BOARD IN VERIFYING COMPLIANCE INCLUDING PROVIDING COPIES OF MEDICAL RELEASES UPON REQUEST; SHALL APPEAR BEFORE THE BOARD AT LEAST TWICE A YEAR; TIME SPENT OUT OF TEXAS DOES NOT COUNT TOWARD RESTRICTION; SHALL INFORM THE BOARD OF CHANGE OF ADDRESS WITHIN 10 DAYS OR IF HE LEAVES THE STATE; SHALL NOT SEEK MODIFICATION FOR ONE YEAR.

GARZA, RAUL MD, LICENSE NUMBER 00F3134, WAS DISCIPLINED BY TEXAS ON AUGUST 17, 1996

DISCIPLINARY ACTION: FINE; RESTRICTION PLACED ON LICENSE
OFFENSE: PROFESSIONAL MISCONDUCT

NOTES: FROM 1/94 TO 9/95 DELEGATED ACTS REQUIRING INDEPENDENT MEDICAL JUDGMENT TO AN INDIVIDUAL NOT LICENSED TO PRACTICE MEDICINE IN TEXAS WHO REPRESENTED HIMSELF AS A PHYSICIANS ASSISTANT WHEN IN FACT HE WASN'T. RESTRICTED UNDER TERMS AND CONDITIONS FOR FIVE YEARS: SHALL ADEQUATELY SUPERVISE THE ACTIVITIES OF ALL HIS EMPLOYEES AND ALL OTHER INDIVIDUALS UNDER HIS SUPERVISION TO ENSURE SUCH INDIVIDUALS ARE COMPLYING WITH THE LAWS RELATED TO HIS PRACTICE OF MEDICINE AND ARE NOT CAUSING HIM TO BE IN VIOLATION OF THESE LAWS; SHALL NOT SERVE AS A SUPERVISOR FOR A PHYSICIAN ASSISTANT; SHALL MAINTAIN ADEQUATE MEDICAL RECORDS WHICH SHALL BE AVAILABLE UPON BOARD REQUEST; DURING THE FIRST YEAR, SHALL OBTAIN AT LEAST 50 HOURS PER YEAR OF CONTINUING MEDICAL EDUCATION IN RISK MANAGEMENT AND SHALL SUBMIT PROOF TO THE BOARD; WITHIN ONE YEAR SHALL TAKE AND PASS THE MEDICAL JURISPRUDENCE EXAMINATION; EVERY YEAR SHALL PERFORM 100 HOURS OF COMMUNITY SERVICE, NO LESS THAN EIGHT HOURS PER MONTH, FOR A BOARD APPROVED NON-PROFIT CHARITABLE ORGANIZATION AND SUBMIT PROOF TO THE BOARD; SHALL APPEAR BEFORE THE BOARD AT LEAST ONCE PER YEAR OR UPON BOARD REQUEST; SHALL COOPERATE WITH THE BOARD IN VERIFYING COMPLIANCE; SHALL GIVE A COPY OF THIS ORDER TO ANY HEALTH CARE ENTITY WHERE HE HAS PRIVILEGES; SHALL PROVIDE A COPY OF THIS ORDER TO ANYONE REQUESTING IT WITHIN 10 DAYS; TIME PERIOD OUT OF TEXAS DOES NOT COUNT TOWARD RESTRICTION; SHALL INFORM THE BOARD OF CHANGE OF ADDRESS WITHIN 10 DAYS OF IF HE LEAVES THE STATE; SHALL NOT SEEK MODIFICATION FOR ONE YEAR. $10,000 ADMINISTRATIVE FINE; REPRIMAND. ON 8/22/98 ORDER TERMINATED.

GEMOETS, THOMAS H MD OF 6620 HARWIN SUITE 300, HOUSTON, TX, WAS DISCIPLINED BY DEA ON OCTOBER 11, 1994
DISCIPLINARY ACTION: SURRENDER OF CONTROLLED SUBSTANCE LICENSE

NOTES: IMPAIRED PHYSICIAN. IN LIEU OF PUBLIC INTEREST REVOCATION.

GEMOETS, THOMAS HENRY MD, LICENSE NUMBER 00C5678 OF HOUSTON, TX, WAS DISCIPLINED BY TEXAS ON JANUARY 27, 1996
DISCIPLINARY ACTION: LICENSE SUSPENSION
OFFENSE: SUBSTANCE ABUSE

NOTES: HAS A HISTORY OF SUBSTANCE ABUSE OVER THE LAST 30 YEARS, HAS RECEIVED TREATMENT ON VARIOUS OCCASIONS, AND HAS PARTICIPATED IN RECOVERY GROUPS; BETWEEN 7/93 AND 8/94 SELF-PRESCRIBED VARIOUS MEDICATIONS WITHOUT A LEGITIMATE MEDICAL PURPOSE INCLUDING TUSSIONEX SYRUP, HYCODAN SYRUP, HYDROCODONE SYRUP, HYCODAN TABLETS, TYLENOL #4, HYDROCODONE TABLETS, VICODIN, AND VALIUM; AND WROTE PRESCRIPTIONS FOR TUSSIONEX SYRUP IN THE NAME OF A FAMILY MEMBER AND DIVERTED IT TO HIS OWN USE; CURRENTLY FACING CRIMINAL CHARGES FOR INSURANCE FRAUD. SUSPENSION UNTIL HE APPEARS BEFORE THE BOARD AND PROVIDES SUFFICIENT EVIDENCE TO SHOW THAT HE IS PHYSICALLY, MENTALLY, AND OTHERWISE COMPETENT TO SAFELY PRACTICE MEDICINE INCLUDING AT A MINIMUM COPIES OF MEDICAL RECORDS AND REPORTS OF PSYCHOLOGICAL AND NEUROPSYCHIATRIC EVALUATIONS, INCLUDING A 96 HOUR INPATIENT EVALUATION, CONDUCTED BY A BOARD APPROVED PSYCHIATRIST; AND SHALL TAKE AND PASS THE SPEX EXAM.

GEMOETS, THOMAS HENRY MD, LICENSE NUMBER C5678 OF HOUSTON, TX, WAS DISCIPLINED BY TEXAS ON APRIL 4, 1998
DISCIPLINARY ACTION: SURRENDER OF LICENSE
OFFENSE: DISCIPLINARY ACTION BY ANOTHER STATE OR AGENCY

NOTES: ON OR ABOUT 2/5/97 HE WAS FOUND GUILTY OF ENGAGING IN ORGANIZED CRIMINAL ACTIVITY; HE IS CURRENTLY APPEALING THE CONVICTION; HE HAS BEEN PREVIOUSLY DISCIPLINED BY THE BOARD ON 10/27/89 AND 1/24/96. VOLUNTARY AND PERMANENT SURRENDER; SHALL GIVE A COPY OF THIS ORDER TO ANY HEALTH CARE ENTITY WHERE HE HAS PRIVILEGES.

GEMOETS, THOMAS HENRY MD, DATE OF BIRTH SEPTEMBER 30, 1930 OF 11410 PEPPERDINE LANE, HOUSTON, TX, WAS DISCIPLINED BY MEDICARE ON NOVEMBER 19, 1998
DISCIPLINARY ACTION: EXCLUSION FROM THE MEDICARE AND/OR MEDICAID PROGRAM
OFFENSE: DISCIPLINARY ACTION BY ANOTHER STATE OR AGENCY

NOTES: LICENSE REVOKED, SUSPENDED, SURRENDERED OR OTHERWISE LOST FOR REASONS BEARING ON PROFESSIONAL PERFORMANCE, PROFESSIONAL COMPETENCE OR FINANCIAL INTEGRITY.

GEORGE, PHILIP N MD, DATE OF BIRTH SEPTEMBER 5, 1955, LICENSE NUMBER 0026283 OF 13311 INNSHIRE, HOUSTON, TX, WAS DISCIPLINED BY IOWA ON AUGUST 20, 1993
DISCIPLINARY ACTION: LICENSE REVOCATION
OFFENSE: SUBSTANDARD CARE, INCOMPETENCE OR NEGLIGENCE

NOTES: CHARGES OF SUBSTANDARD MEDICAL CARE. ALSO CHARGES OF VIOLATING MISDEMEANOR STATUTE RELATED TO PRACTICE OF MEDICINE.

GEORGE, PHILIP N MD, LICENSE NUMBER 0A50027 OF HOUSTON, TX, WAS DISCIPLINED BY CALIFORNIA ON FEBRUARY 24, 1995
DISCIPLINARY ACTION: LICENSE REVOCATION
OFFENSE: DISCIPLINARY ACTION BY ANOTHER STATE OR AGENCY

NOTES: DISCIPLINE BY IOWA BOARD FOR SUBSTANDARD PRACTICES IN A BLOOD PLASMA CENTER, AND FOR A CONVICTION FOR RESISTING ARREST WHEN HE REFUSED TO BE REMOVED FROM THE CENTER. DEFAULT DECISION.

GERSHON, JULIAN R JR DO, DATE OF BIRTH MAY 1, 1953, LICENSE NUMBER 1007967 OF 1100 DALLAS DRIVE SUITE 106, DENTON, TX, WAS DISCIPLINED BY MICHIGAN ON MAY 1, 1999
DISCIPLINARY ACTION: FINE
OFFENSE: DISCIPLINARY ACTION BY ANOTHER STATE OR AGENCY

NOTES: FAILURE TO REPORT/COMPLY. $1000 FINE.

GERSHON, JULIAN ROBERT DO, LICENSE NUMBER G9462 OF DENTON, TX, WAS DISCIPLINED BY TEXAS ON FEBRUARY 7, 1998
DISCIPLINARY ACTION: FINE
OFFENSE: NONCOMPLIANCE WITH A PROFESSIONAL RULE

NOTES: BETWEEN 1990-1991 OUTSIDE HIS MEDICAL PRACTICE, HE OWNED A COMPANY ENGAGED IN PERIPHERAL/VASCULAR TESTING WHICH, MANAGED AND OPERATED BY OTHERS, FAILED TO INSURE ADEQUATE DOCUMENTATION OF PATIENT CHARTS FOR PATIENTS WHO RECEIVED THE TESTING. $1,000 FINE; SHALL GIVE A COPY OF THIS ORDER TO ANY

HEALTH CARE ENTITY WHERE HE HAS PRIVILEGES.

GERSON, BENJAMIN MD, DATE OF BIRTH DECEMBER 14, 1947, LICENSE NUMBER 045168E OF 200 TEMPLE STREET, NEWTON, MA, WAS DISCIPLINED BY PENNSYLVANIA ON JUNE 24, 1997
DISCIPLINARY ACTION: FINE; REPRIMAND
OFFENSE: DISCIPLINARY ACTION BY ANOTHER STATE OR AGENCY

NOTES: DISCIPLINARY ACTION TAKEN BY MASSACHUSETTS. $1000 CIVIL PENALTY.

GERSON, BENJAMIN MD, DATE OF BIRTH DECEMBER 14, 1947, LICENSE NUMBER G7650 OF NEWTON, MA, WAS DISCIPLINED BY TEXAS ON MAY 16, 1998
DISCIPLINARY ACTION: REPRIMAND
OFFENSE: DISCIPLINARY ACTION BY ANOTHER STATE OR AGENCY

NOTES: ON 10/25/95 DISCIPLINED BY THE MASSACHUSETTS BOARD FOR DISPENSING CONTROLLED SUBSTANCES TO HIMSELF AND TO FAMILY MEMBERS; FAILED TO MAINTAIN ADEQUATE DRUG RECORDS; HE WAS ALSO DISCIPLINED BY CONNECTICUT AND MARYLAND BOARDS; HE SELF-REPORTED THE DISCIPLINARY ACTION TO THE TEXAS BOARD; SHALL INFORM THE BOARD OF ANY CHANGE OF ADDRESS WITHIN 10 DAYS.

GEST, ALFRED LOUIS MD OF ONE BAYLOR PLAZA, HOUSTON, TX, WAS DISCIPLINED BY DEA ON OCTOBER 23, 1996
DISCIPLINARY ACTION: SURRENDER OF CONTROLLED SUBSTANCE LICENSE

NOTES: IN LIEU OF PUBLIC INTEREST REVOCATION.

GEYER, WALTER LESLIE MD, LICENSE NUMBER D2226 OF FORT WORTH, TX, WAS DISCIPLINED BY TEXAS ON NOVEMBER 22, 1997
DISCIPLINARY ACTION: 36-MONTH PROBATION; RESTRICTION PLACED ON CONTROLLED SUBSTANCE LICENSE
OFFENSE: NONCOMPLIANCE WITH A PROFESSIONAL RULE

NOTES: ON 2/5/97 A DRUG AUDIT REVEALED DEFICIENCIES REGARDING BOTH THE MANNER IN WHICH THE CONTROLLED SUBSTANCES WERE STORED IN HIS OFFICE AND THE RECORD KEEPING ASSOCIATED WITH THE RECEIPT MAINTENANCE, AND DISPENSING OF DANGEROUS DRUGS AND/OR CONTROLLED SUBSTANCES; SEVERAL CASES WERE LISTED WHERE RECORD KEEPING WAS INADEQUATE OR SUBSTANDARD; SINCE 2/97 HE MAINTAINS THAT HIS SCHEDULED DRUG RECORD KEEPING HAS BEEN UPDATED AND CORRECTED. SUSPENSION STAYED FOR PROBATION WITH FOLLOWING TERMS AND CONDITIONS: SHALL IMMEDIATELY REQUEST MODIFICATION OF HIS DEA CONTROLLED SUBSTANCES REGISTRATION AND TEXAS DEPARTMENT OF PUBLIC SAFETY CERTIFICATES TO ALLOW HIM TO PRESCRIBE SCHEDULES I, II, III; HIS MEDICAL PRACTICE SHALL BE MONITORED BY A BOARD APPROVED TEXAS PHYSICIAN WHO SHALL PROVIDE QUARTERLY REPORTS TO THE BOARD; SHALL MAINTAIN ADEQUATE MEDICAL RECORDS WHICH SHALL BE AVAILABLE FOR REVIEW; SHALL OBTAIN AT LEAST 50 HOURS PER YEAR OF CONTINUING MEDICAL EDUCATION; SHALL APPEAR BEFORE THE BOARD AT LEAST ONCE A YEAR; SHALL COOPERATE WITH THE BOARD IN VERIFYING COMPLIANCE; TIME SPENT OUT OF TEXAS DOES NOT COUNT TOWARD PROBATION; SHALL INFORM THE BOARD OF CHANGE OF ADDRESS WITHIN 10 DAYS OR IF HE LEAVES THE STATE; SHALL NOT SEEK MODIFICATION FOR ONE YEAR. ON 10/24/98 REQUEST TO TERMINATE THE ORDER WAS DENIED. ON 12/11/99 THE ORDER WAS TERMINATED.

GHEN, MITCHELL J DO, LICENSE NUMBER 0004280 OF HILLSBORO BEACH, FL, WAS DISCIPLINED BY FLORIDA ON OCTOBER 8, 1993
DISCIPLINARY ACTION: FINE; MONITORING OF PHYSICIAN PERFORMANCE
OFFENSE: SUBSTANDARD CARE, INCOMPETENCE OR NEGLIGENCE

NOTES: CHARGED WITH FAILING TO PRACTICE MEDICINE WITH AN ACCEPTABLE LEVEL OF CARE AND SKILL. $2,500 FINE; SHALL HAVE EVALUATION OF PRACTICE BY A CERTIFIED RISK MANAGER.

GHEN, MITCHELL J DO, LICENSE NUMBER 004996L OF 1167 HILLSBORO MILE APT 616, HILLSBORO BEACH, FL, WAS DISCIPLINED BY PENNSYLVANIA ON MAY 10, 1995
DISCIPLINARY ACTION: FINE
OFFENSE: DISCIPLINARY ACTION BY ANOTHER STATE OR AGENCY

NOTES: ON 10/05/93 ENTERED INTO A CONSENT AGREEMENT IN FLORIDA ACCEPTING A FINE, LETTER OF CONCERN, AND ORDER TO UNDERGO A QUALITY ASSURANCE CONSULTATION RESULTING FROM PRACTICING MEDICINE BELOW A STANDARD OF REASONABLE CARE. $1,000 CIVIL PENALTY.

GHEN, MITCHELL J DO, LICENSE NUMBER 00J1669 OF HILLSBORO BEACH, FL, WAS DISCIPLINED BY TEXAS ON AUGUST 18, 1995
DISCIPLINARY ACTION: REPRIMAND
OFFENSE: DISCIPLINARY ACTION BY ANOTHER STATE OR AGENCY

NOTES: DISCIPLINARY ACTION TAKEN BY FLORIDA IN 8/93 WHEN HE WAS FINED $2,500 AND REQUIRED TO HAVE HIS PRACTICE REVIEWED BY A CERTIFIED RISK MANAGER BASED ON SUBSTANDARD CARE OF ONE PATIENT.

GHEN, MITCHELL J DO, DATE OF BIRTH FEBRUARY 19, 1950, LICENSE NUMBER 0058654 OF 1167 HILLSBORO MILE #616F, HILLSBORO BEACH, FL, WAS DISCIPLINED BY NEW JERSEY ON JUNE 21, 1996
OFFENSE: DISCIPLINARY ACTION BY ANOTHER STATE OR AGENCY

NOTES: ACTION IN FLORIDA CONCERNING ALLEGATIONS OF GROSS MALPRACTICE. SHALL COMPLY WITH THE TERMS AND CONDITIONS OF THE FLORIDA BOARD OF OSTEOPATHIC MEDICINE ORDER AND THOSE OF ANY OTHER JURISDICTION; SHALL NOTIFY THE BOARD OF ANY CHANGES IN THOSE TERMS; SHALL APPEAR BEFORE THE BOARD PRIOR TO ACTIVE PRACTICE IN NEW JERSEY.

GIBBONS, WILLIAM EDWIN MD, LICENSE NUMBER 00C0719 OF DALLAS, TX, WAS DISCIPLINED BY TEXAS ON JUNE 28, 1995
DISCIPLINARY ACTION: RESTRICTION PLACED ON LICENSE; REQUIRED TO TAKE ADDITIONAL MEDICAL EDUCATION
OFFENSE: PROFESSIONAL MISCONDUCT

NOTES: HAS BEEN THE SUBJECT OF TWO MERITORIOUS HEALTH CARE LIABILITY CLAIMS: IN 1993 SETTLEMENT OF $400,000 WAS REACHED AS A RESULT OF HIS FAILURE TO DETECT, DIAGNOSE AND ADEQUATELY TREAT A PERIRECTAL ABSCESS WHICH SHOULD HAVE BEEN EVIDENT DURING AN EIGHT-YEAR COURSE OF TREATMENT OF THIS PATIENT; IN 9/90 CASE SETTLED WHERE HE PERFORMED A LYMPH NODE REMOVAL AND SEVERED A NERVE. SHALL NOT PERFORM ANY INVASIVE PROCEDURE UNTIL HE PROVIDES EVIDENCE TO THE BOARD THAT HE HAS TAKEN AND PASSED THE SPECIAL PURPOSE EXAMINATION AND OBTAINED RECERTIFICATION IN GENERAL SURGERY; SHALL OBTAIN AT LEAST 50 HOURS PER YEAR OF CONTINUING MEDICAL EDUCATION; SHALL COOPERATE WITH THE BOARD IN VERIFYING COMPLIANCE; SHALL GIVE A COPY OF THIS ORDER TO

ANY HEALTH CARE ENTITY WHERE HE HAS PRIVILEGES; SHALL PROVIDE A COPY OF THIS ORDER TO ANYONE REQUESTING IT WITHIN 10 DAYS; TIME PERIOD OUT OF TEXAS DOES NOT COUNT TOWARD PROBATION; SHALL INFORM THE BOARD OF CHANGE OF ADDRESS WITHIN 10 DAYS OR IF HE LEAVES THE STATE. SHALL NOT SEEK MODIFICATION FOR ONE YEAR.

GIBSON, JOSEPH V JR MD, LICENSE NUMBER 00C3381 OF CORSICANA, TX, WAS DISCIPLINED BY TEXAS ON JANUARY 30, 1990
DISCIPLINARY ACTION: SURRENDER OF LICENSE

NOTES: STIPULATED ORDER. LICENSE RETIRED.

GIFFORD, L ARDEN MD OF 1300 MURCHISON DRIVE #390, EL PASO, TX, WAS DISCIPLINED BY DEA ON JULY 16, 1996
DISCIPLINARY ACTION: SURRENDER OF CONTROLLED SUBSTANCE LICENSE

GIFFORD, LORING A MD, LICENSE NUMBER D2888, WAS DISCIPLINED BY TEXAS ON JANUARY 18, 1997
DISCIPLINARY ACTION: SURRENDER OF LICENSE
OFFENSE: CRIMINAL CONVICTION OR PLEA OF GUILTY, NOLO CONTENDERE, OR NO CONTEST TO A CRIME

NOTES: IN 9/96 HE WAS FOUND GUILTY ON TEN CRIMINAL COUNTS INVOLVING MAIL FRAUD, AIDING AND ABETTING FRAUD, CONSPIRACY AND DEFRAUDING HEALTH CARE INSURERS, TAMPERING WITH A GOVERNMENT WITNESS, AND ENGAGING IN MONETARY TRANSACTIONS IN PROPERTY DERIVED FROM UNLAWFUL ACTIVITY. HE HAS A HISTORY OF SUCH CONVICTIONS AND HAS SERVED TIME FOR SUCH. HIS LICENSE HAS BEEN CANCELED AND, SUBSEQUENT TO RELEASE FROM CUSTODY, REINSTATED WITH RESTRICTIONS. ALLEGATIONS THAT HE OVER/MISPRESCRIBED DRUGS AND ALLOWED UNLICENSED OFFICE STAFF TO PERFORM MEDICAL SERVICES; HE DENIES THE ALLEGATIONS; HE CLAIMS TO BE IN POOR HEALTH AND HAS THEREFORE PERMANENTLY, VOLUNTARILY SURRENDERED HIS LICENSE TO PRACTICE MEDICINE.

GILLILAND, MARK B MD, LICENSE NUMBER G2088 OF HOUSTON, TX, WAS DISCIPLINED BY TEXAS ON AUGUST 22, 1998
DISCIPLINARY ACTION: 48-MONTH PROBATION; MONITORING OF PHYSICIAN PERFORMANCE
OFFENSE: SUBSTANCE ABUSE

NOTES: HE WROTE PRESCRIPTIONS FOR CONTROLLED SUBSTANCES FOR FAMILY MEMBERS; THE PRESCRIPTIONS WERE CALLED INTO A PHARMACY LOCATED IN THE BUILDING LOBBY OF HIS OFFICE AND LATER PICKED UP AND PAID FOR IN CASH BY AN EMPLOYEE OF HIS; BETWEEN 1/94 AND 10/96 CONTROLLED SUBSTANCES WERE PRESCRIBED TO HIS WIFE, WHO STATED SHE RECEIVED SOME BUT NOT ALL OF THE CONTROLLED SUBSTANCES; HE RECEIVED AN INPATIENT SUBSTANCE ABUSE EVALUATION FROM 3/27/97 - 3/31/97 WITH A DISCHARGE DIAGNOSIS OF OPIATE DEPENDENCE; THE TREATING PHYSICIAN NOTED THAT HE WAS NOT PRESENTLY IMPAIRED AND HAS INSIGHT INTO THE PROBLEMS; BETWEEN 7/97 AND 7/98 HE RECEIVED TREATMENT AND WAS MONITORED BY A BOARD-CERTIFIED ADDICTIONOLOGIST. PROBATION WITH FOLLOWING TERMS AND CONDITIONS: SHALL ABSTAIN FROM THE CONSUMPTION OF ALCOHOL/DRUGS IN ANY FORM UNLESS PRESCRIBED BY ANOTHER PHYSICIAN FOR A LEGITIMATE AND THERAPEUTIC PURPOSE; SHALL SUBMIT HIMSELF FOR APPROPRIATE EXAMS INCLUDING DRUG OR ALCOHOL SCREENS; SHALL NOMINATE THREE CERTIFIED PSYCHIATRISTS FOR BOARD SELECTION OF A THERAPIST AND SHALL EXPEDITIOUSLY SUBMIT HIMSELF TO EVALUATION AND TREATMENT BY THE APPROVED PRACTITIONER; SHALL NOT TREAT OR OTHERWISE SERVE AS PHYSICIAN, PRESCRIBE, DISPENSE OR ADMINISTER DRUGS THAT MAY BE SUBJECT TO ABUSE TO HIMSELF OR TO ANY MEMBER OF HIS FAMILY; SEPARATE FROM PATIENT RECORDS, SHALL MAINTAIN A FILE OF EVERY PRESCRIPTION WRITTEN BY HIM FOR DANGEROUS DRUGS WITH ADDICTIVE POTENTIAL WHICH SHALL BE MADE AVAILABLE FOR REVIEW; SHALL APPEAR BEFORE THE BOARD AT LEAST TWICE A YEAR; SHALL COOPERATE WITH THE BOARD IN VERIFYING COMPLIANCE INCLUDING PROVIDING COPIES OF MEDICAL RELEASES UPON REQUEST; SHALL INFORM THE BOARD OF CHANGE OF ADDRESS WITHIN 10 DAYS; SHALL NOT SEEK MODIFICATION FOR ONE YEAR. ON 10/15/99 REQUEST FOR TERMINATION OF THE ORDER DENIED.

GILNER, LEON I MD OF 115 MEDICAL DRIVE SUITE 208, VICTORIA, TX, WAS DISCIPLINED BY DEA ON OCTOBER 26, 1994
DISCIPLINARY ACTION: RESTRICTION PLACED ON CONTROLLED SUBSTANCE LICENSE

NOTES: IMPAIRED PRACTITIONER.

GILNER, LEON I MD OF 115 MEDICAL DRIVE #208, VICTORIA, TX, WAS DISCIPLINED BY DEA ON SEPTEMBER 11, 1997
DISCIPLINARY ACTION: RESTRICTION PLACED ON CONTROLLED SUBSTANCE LICENSE

NOTES: MEMO OF AGREEMENT.

GINTHER, CLARK E MD, LICENSE NUMBER 00C1099 OF BISHOP, TX, WAS DISCIPLINED BY TEXAS ON AUGUST 19, 1994
OFFENSE: CRIMINAL CONVICTION OR PLEA OF GUILTY, NOLO CONTENDERE, OR NO CONTEST TO A CRIME

NOTES: ON 4/5/93 HE WAS CONVICTED OF AIDING AND ABETTING THE ATTEMPTED ILLEGAL POSSESSION OF PHENTERMINE AND DIAZEPAM TO TWO PATIENTS WHO WERE UNDERCOVER DEA AGENTS, A MISDEMEANOR OFFENSE; WAS PLACED ON PROBATION FOR ONE YEAR WITH A FINE OF $5,000 AND REQUIRED COMMUNITY SERVICE; SURRENDERED DEA REGISTRATION AS A RESULT OF CONVICTION. HE DENIES ANY MISCONDUCT IN PRESCRIBING TO THE TWO DEA AGENTS. SHALL RETIRE FROM PRACTICE EFFECTIVE 12/31/94 AND MEDICAL LICENSE SHALL BE CANCELED; SHALL GIVE A COPY OF THIS ORDER TO ANY HEALTH CARE ENTITY WHERE HE HAS PRIVILEGES; SHALL COOPERATE WITH THE BOARD IN VERIFYING COMPLIANCE; SHALL INFORM BOARD OF CHANGE OF ADDRESS WITHIN 10 DAYS.

GIPSON, EDDIE MACK MD, LICENSE NUMBER 00C8982 OF DALLAS, TX, WAS DISCIPLINED BY TEXAS ON JANUARY 24, 1992
DISCIPLINARY ACTION: 60-MONTH PROBATION
OFFENSE: OVERPRESCRIBING OR MISPRESCRIBING DRUGS

NOTES: SEVERAL VIOLATIONS OF THE MEDICAL PRACTICE ACT, INCLUDING NONTHERAPEUTIC PRESCRIBING AND INABILITY TO PRACTICE MEDICINE WITH REASONABLE SKILL AND SAFETY TO PATIENTS BY REASON OF ILLNESS, DRUNKENNESS, EXCESSIVE USE OF DRUGS, NARCOTICS, CHEMICALS, OR ANY OTHER TYPE OF MATERIAL OR AS A RESULT OF ANY MENTAL OR PHYSICAL CONDITION. LICENSE SUSPENDED, SUSPENSION STAYED; PROBATION UNDER TERMS AND CONDITIONS.

GIPSON, EDDIE MACK MD, LICENSE NUMBER 00C8982 OF WHITNEY, TX, WAS DISCIPLINED BY TEXAS ON AUGUST 28, 1992
DISCIPLINARY ACTION: EMERGENCY SUSPENSION
OFFENSE: FAILURE TO COMPLY WITH PREVIOUS BOARD ORDER

NOTES: FAILURE TO COMPLY WITH TERMS OF JANUARY 1992 ORDER.

GIPSON, EDDIE MACK MD, LICENSE NUMBER 00C8982 OF WHITNEY, TX, WAS DISCIPLINED BY TEXAS ON NOVEMBER 13, 1992
DISCIPLINARY ACTION: LICENSE SUSPENSION

NOTES: SUSPENDED UNTIL SUCH TIME AS HE PERSONALLY APPEARS BEFORE THE BOARD AND PROVIDES EVIDENCE WHICH IN THE JUDGMENT OF THE BOARD IS SUFFICIENT TO SHOW THAT HE IS PHYSICALLY, MENTALLY, AND OTHERWISE COMPETENT TO SAFELY PRACTICE MEDICINE.

GIPSON, EDDIE MACK MD, LICENSE NUMBER 0030840 OF 2042 SOUTH BUCKNER BOULEVARD, DALLAS, TX, WAS DISCIPLINED BY MASSACHUSETTS ON MAY 11, 1994
DISCIPLINARY ACTION: NONRENEWAL OF LICENSE
OFFENSE: DISCIPLINARY ACTION BY ANOTHER STATE OR AGENCY

NOTES: DISCIPLINE BY TEXAS; MENTAL IMPAIRMENT. SUSPENSION OF INCHOATE RIGHT TO RENEW LICENSE.

GIRTANNER, ROBERT EDWARD MD, LICENSE NUMBER 00D7983 OF HOUSTON, TX, WAS DISCIPLINED BY TEXAS ON SEPTEMBER 30, 1994
DISCIPLINARY ACTION: LICENSE SUSPENSION; 60-MONTH PROBATION
OFFENSE: OVERPRESCRIBING OR MISPRESCRIBING DRUGS

NOTES: FROM 4/88 THROUGH 4/92 ON MULTIPLE OCCASIONS ORDERED OR PRESCRIBED CONTROLLED SUBSTANCES TO THREE PATIENTS WITHOUT ADEQUATELY DOCUMENTING A SUFFICIENT MEDICAL BASIS FOR THIS ONE OF WHOM IS A FAMILY MEMBER WHO HAD A DRUG ADDICTION PROBLEM WHICH HE KNEW ABOUT; ON MULTIPLE OCCASIONS FROM 6/88 THROUGH 2/91 HE ORDERED OR PRESCRIBED CONTROLLED SUBSTANCES IN THE NAMES OF INDIVIDUALS WHO HE DID NOT INTEND TO RECEIVE THE MEDICATIONS AND WHICH HE SUBSEQUENTLY DIVERTED FOR THE USE OF THE FAMILY MEMBER REFERENCED ABOVE; DURING 1991 AND 1992 HE SELF-PRESCRIBED TYLENOL #4 WITHOUT MAINTAINING DOCUMENTATION OF THE BASIS FOR THE PRESCRIBING. SUSPENSION STAYED AFTER SEVEN DAYS. CONDITIONS OF PROBATION: SHALL NOT TREAT OR OTHERWISE SERVE AS PHYSICIAN, PRESCRIBE, DISPENSE OR ADMINISTER DRUGS THAT MAY BE SUBJECT TO ABUSE TO HIMSELF OR ANY MEMBER OF HIS IMMEDIATE FAMILY; SHALL ABSTAIN FROM THE CONSUMPTION OF CONTROLLED SUBSTANCES OR DANGEROUS DRUGS WITH POTENTIAL FOR ABUSE IN ANY FORM UNLESS PRESCRIBED BY ANOTHER PHYSICIAN FOR A LEGITIMATE AND THERAPEUTIC PURPOSE; SHALL ENSURE ANY PRESCRIPTION WRITTEN FOR SCHEDULE II OR III CONTROLLED SUBSTANCES SHALL BE COUNTERSIGNED BY ANOTHER LICENSED TEXAS PHYSICIAN WORKING WITHIN HIS PLACE OF EMPLOYMENT; PRESCRIBING, DISPENSING, ORDERING OR ADMINISTERING OF CONTROLLED SUBSTANCES AND DANGEROUS DRUGS LIMITED TO PATIENTS RECEIVING CARE WITHIN THE HEALTH CARE DELIVERY SYSTEM OF THE BAYLOR COLLEGE OF MEDICINE; SHALL SUBMIT HIMSELF FOR APPROPRIATE EXAMS INCLUDING DRUG OR ALCOHOL SCREENS; SHALL SUBMIT HIMSELF FOR EVALUATION AND TREATMENT TO A BOARD-APPROVED PSYCHIATRIST WITH REPORTS TO THE BOARD; SHALL BE SUPERVISED BY A BOARD-APPROVED PHYSICIAN WITH QUARTERLY REPORTS; SHALL ATTEND AT LEAST 50 HOURS PER YEAR OF CONTINUING MEDICAL EDUCATION; SHALL MAINTAIN ADEQUATE MEDICAL RECORDS ON ALL PATIENT OFFICE VISITS WHICH SHALL BE AVAILABLE FOR INSPECTION; SHALL APPEAR BEFORE THE BOARD ONCE A YEAR; SHALL GIVE A COPY OF THIS ORDER TO ANY HEALTH CARE ENTITY WHERE HE HAS PRIVILEGES; SHALL COOPERATE WITH THE BOARD IN VERIFYING COMPLIANCE; SHALL INFORM BOARD OF CHANGE OF ADDRESS WITHIN 10 DAYS OR IF HE LEAVES THE STATE; TIME SPENT OUT OF TEXAS DOES NOT COUNT TOWARD PROBATION. SHALL NOT SEEK MODIFICATION FOR ONE YEAR.

GIRTANNER, ROBERT EDWARD MD, LICENSE NUMBER 00D7983 OF HOUSTON, TX, WAS DISCIPLINED BY TEXAS ON JANUARY 25, 1995
DISCIPLINARY ACTION: EMERGENCY SUSPENSION
OFFENSE: FAILURE TO COMPLY WITH PREVIOUS BOARD ORDER

NOTES: WAS IN NONCOMPLIANCE WITH 10/94 ORDER IN THAT IN 1/95, HE INGESTED COCAINE, A SCHEDULE II CONTROLLED SUBSTANCE WITHOUT A PRESCRIPTION FROM ANOTHER PHYSICIAN FOR A LEGITIMATE AND THERAPEUTIC PURPOSE; FAILED TO IMMEDIATELY REPORT HIS INGESTION OF COCAINE TO THE BOARD.

GIRTANNER, ROBERT EDWARD MD, LICENSE NUMBER 00D7983 OF HOUSTON, TX, WAS DISCIPLINED BY TEXAS ON MARCH 4, 1995
DISCIPLINARY ACTION: LICENSE SUSPENSION
OFFENSE: FAILURE TO COMPLY WITH PREVIOUS BOARD ORDER

NOTES: SUSPENSION UNTIL HE REQUESTS IN WRITING TO HAVE SUSPENSION STAYED OR LIFTED, AND APPEARS BEFORE BOARD WITH SUFFICIENT EVIDENCE WHICH ADEQUATELY INDICATES THAT HE IS PHYSICALLY, MENTALLY AND OTHERWISE COMPETENT TO SAFELY PRACTICE MEDICINE, INCLUDING BUT NOT LIMITED TO COPIES OF MEDICAL RECORDS AND REPORTS OF PSYCHOLOGICAL AND NEUROPSYCHIATRIC EVALUATIONS CONDUCTED BY A BOARD-CERTIFIED PSYCHIATRIST.

GIRTANNER, ROBERT EDWARD MD, DATE OF BIRTH JULY 24, 1935 OF 3000 MURWORTH DRIVE APT 511, HOUSTON, TX, WAS DISCIPLINED BY MEDICARE ON APRIL 23, 1996
DISCIPLINARY ACTION: EXCLUSION FROM THE MEDICARE AND/OR MEDICAID PROGRAM
OFFENSE: DISCIPLINARY ACTION BY ANOTHER STATE OR AGENCY

NOTES: LICENSE SUSPENDED FOR REASONS BEARING ON PROFESSIONAL PERFORMANCE.

GLIDDEN, WELDON EDWARD DO, LICENSE NUMBER 00G3397 OF QUANAH, TX, WAS DISCIPLINED BY TEXAS ON NOVEMBER 3, 1994
DISCIPLINARY ACTION: 60-MONTH PROBATION; RESTRICTION PLACED ON CONTROLLED SUBSTANCE LICENSE
OFFENSE: SUBSTANCE ABUSE

NOTES: FROM 1/92 THROUGH 3/94 INGESTED LARGE NUMBERS OF TYLENOL #4 WITHOUT A LEGITIMATE MEDICAL PURPOSE; CALLED FICTITIOUS PRESCRIPTIONS TO SEVERAL PHARMACIES IN VARIOUS NAMES AND DIVERTED THESE FOR HIS OWN USE; HAD NO PATIENT RECORDS CORRESPONDING TO THE NAMES HE USED TO OBTAIN THE CONTROLLED SUBSTANCES; ON 3/10/94 HE CONTACTED IMPAIRED PHYSICIANS PROGRAM AND SIGNED A CONTRACT WITH THEM; ON 3/15/94 HE NOTIFIED THE BOARD THAT HE WAS RECEIVING INPATIENT TREATMENT; STATES

SOBRIETY DATE AS 3/12/94; HAS ATTENDED AA MEETINGS REGULARLY AFTER DISCHARGE FROM INPATIENT TREATMENT. SUSPENSION STAYED. CONDITIONS OF PROBATION: SHALL ABSTAIN FROM THE CONSUMPTION OF ALCOHOL/CHEMICAL SUBSTANCES WITH ADDICTIVE POTENTIAL UNLESS PRESCRIBED, DISPENSED OR AUTHORIZED BY ANOTHER PHYSICIAN FOR A LEGITIMATE THERAPEUTIC PURPOSE; WITHIN 30 DAYS SHALL SUBMIT TO A PSYCHIATRIC EVALUATION TO INCLUDE A COMPLETE NEUROPSYCHIATRIC EVALUATION BY A BOARD-APPROVED PSYCHIATRIST; SHALL FOLLOW THE PSYCHIATRIST'S RECOMMENDATIONS REGARDING TREATMENT THAT AT A MINIMUM WILL INCLUDE FOLLOW-UP CARE AND COUNSELING AT LEAST ONCE PER MONTH; SHALL NOT TREAT OR OTHERWISE SERVE AS PHYSICIAN, PRESCRIBE, DISPENSE OR ADMINISTER DRUGS THAT MAY BE SUBJECT TO ABUSE TO HIMSELF OR ANY MEMBER OF HIS FAMILY; SHALL CONTINUE TO PARTICIPATE IN AA'S PROGRAM NOT LESS THAN THREE TIMES A WEEK WITH QUARTERLY REPORTS TO THE BOARD; SHALL ADHERE TO THE TERMS OF 24 MONTH AFTERCARE CONTRACT WITH IMPAIRED PHYSICIANS PROGRAM; SHALL SUBMIT HIMSELF FOR APPROPRIATE EXAMS INCLUDING DRUG OR ALCOHOL SCREENS; SHALL SURRENDER ALL CONTROLLED SUBSTANCES AND DANGEROUS DRUGS IN HIS POSSESSION INCLUDING SAMPLES; SHALL NOT TELEPHONE PRESCRIPTIONS FOR CONTROLLED SUBSTANCES OR DANGEROUS DRUGS TO A PHARMACY OR PERMIT ANYONE TO DO SO ON HIS BEHALF; SEPARATE FROM PATIENT RECORDS, SHALL MAINTAIN A FILE OF EVERY PRESCRIPTION WRITTEN FOR CONTROLLED SUBSTANCES OR DANGEROUS DRUGS WHICH SHALL BE AVAILABLE FOR INSPECTION; MAY ORDER ALL SCHEDULED DRUGS AND DANGEROUS DRUGS FOR INPATIENTS IN HOSPITAL AND NURSING HOME SETTINGS, BUT MAY NOT OTHERWISE PRESCRIBE, ADMINISTER, DISPENSE OR POSSESS SUCH DRUGS WITH THE FOLLOWING EXCEPTIONS -- MAY PRESCRIBE ALL SCHEDULED AND DANGEROUS DRUGS FOR OUTPATIENTS SUFFERING FROM ATTENTION DEFICIT DISORDER AND MAY PRESCRIBE SCHEDULE IV DRUGS AND THOSE DANGEROUS DRUGS WHICH ARE NOT GENERALLY CONSIDERED TO HAVE ADDICTIVE POTENTIAL TO ALL OTHER OUTPATIENTS. SHALL ATTEND AT LEAST 50 HOURS PER YEAR OF CONTINUING MEDICAL EDUCATION; SHALL APPEAR BEFORE THE BOARD ONCE A YEAR; SHALL GIVE A COPY OF THIS ORDER TO ANY HEALTH CARE ENTITY WHERE HE HAS PRIVILEGES; SHALL COOPERATE WITH THE BOARD IN VERIFYING COMPLIANCE; SHALL INFORM BOARD OF CHANGE OF ADDRESS WITHIN 10 DAYS OR IF HE LEAVES THE STATE; TIME SPENT OUT OF TEXAS DOES NOT COUNT TOWARD PROBATION. SHALL NOT SEEK MODIFICATION FOR ONE YEAR. ON 1/18/97 PETITION TO TERMINATE ORDER DENIED; ORDER MODIFIED DELETING MONTHLY FOLLOW-UP CARE AND COUNSELING FROM A CERTIFIED PSYCHIATRIST.

GLIDDEN, WELDON EDWARD DO, LICENSE NUMBER G3397 OF QUANAH, TX, WAS DISCIPLINED BY TEXAS ON AUGUST 9, 1997
DISCIPLINARY ACTION: 60-MONTH PROBATION; RESTRICTION PLACED ON LICENSE
OFFENSE: FAILURE TO COMPLY WITH PREVIOUS BOARD ORDER

NOTES: ON OR ABOUT 4/28/97, HE INGESTED TRANXENE, A SCHEDULE IV CONTROLLED SUBSTANCE, IN VIOLATION OF HIS 11/3/94 AGREED ORDER; ON 4/29/97, HE INGESTED MIDOL AND TELEPHONED IN TO A PHARMACY A PRESCRIPTION FOR AND LATER INGESTED ESGIC PLUS, A DANGEROUS DRUG, ALSO IN VIOLATION OF THE 11/3/94 ORDER. ON 5/1/97 HE SELF-REPORTED HIS INGESTION OF DRUGS. SUSPENSION STAYED FOR PROBATION UNDER THE FOLLOWING TERMS: SHALL ABSTAIN FROM THE CONSUMPTION OF ALCOHOL/DRUGS IN ANY FORM UNLESS PRESCRIBED BY ANOTHER PHYSICIAN FOR A LEGITIMATE AND THERAPEUTIC PURPOSE; SHALL SUBMIT HIMSELF FOR APPROPRIATE EXAMS INCLUDING DRUG OR ALCOHOL SCREENS; SHALL NOMINATE THREE CERTIFIED PSYCHIATRISTS FOR BOARD SELECTION OF A THERAPIST AND SHALL EXPEDITIOUSLY SUBMIT HIMSELF TO EVALUATION AND TREATMENT BY THE APPROVED PRACTITIONER; SHALL PARTICIPATE IN AA OR A SIMILAR PROGRAM WHICH HAS BEEN APPROVED IN WRITING BY THE BOARD NO LESS THAN THREE TIMES A WEEK; SHALL REPORT ON HIS ATTENDANCE; SHALL COMPLY WITH HIS CONTINUING CARE CONTRACT; SHALL APPEAR BEFORE THE BOARD AT LEAST TWICE YEARLY; SHALL NOT POSSESS ALCOHOL, CONTROLLED, SUBSTANCES, OR DRUGS AND SHALL SURRENDER ANY IN HIS POSSESSION INCLUDING SAMPLES; SHALL NOT TREAT OR OTHERWISE SERVE AS PHYSICIAN, PRESCRIBE, DISPENSE OR ADMINISTER DRUGS THAT MAY BE SUBJECT TO ABUSE TO HIMSELF OR TO ANY MEMBER OF HIS FAMILY; SHALL NOT TELEPHONE TO A PHARMACY A PRESCRIPTION OR REFILL FOR CONTROLLED SUBSTANCES OR DANGEROUS DRUGS OR PERMIT ANY INDIVIDUAL UNDER HIS SUPERVISION TO DO SO; SEPARATE FROM PATIENT RECORDS, SHALL MAINTAIN A FILE OF EVERY PRESCRIPTION WRITTEN BY HIM FOR DANGEROUS DRUGS WITH ADDICTIVE POTENTIAL WHICH SHALL BE MADE AVAILABLE FOR REVIEW; SHALL MAINTAIN ADEQUATE MEDICAL RECORDS WHICH SHALL BE AVAILABLE FOR REVIEW; SHALL OBTAIN AT LEAST 50 HOURS PER YEAR OF CONTINUING MEDICAL EDUCATION; SHALL COOPERATE WITH THE BOARD IN VERIFYING COMPLIANCE INCLUDING PROVIDING COPIES OF MEDICAL RELEASES UPON REQUEST; SHALL GIVE A COPY OF THIS ORDER TO ANY HEALTH CARE ENTITY WHERE HE HAS PRIVILEGES; SHALL PROVIDE A COPY OF THIS ORDER TO ANYONE REQUESTING IT WITHIN 10 DAYS; TIME SPENT OUT OF TEXAS DOES NOT COUNT TOWARD PROBATION; SHALL INFORM THE BOARD OF CHANGE OF ADDRESS WITHIN 10 DAYS OR IF HE LEAVES THE STATE; SHALL NOT SEEK MODIFICATION FOR ONE YEAR.

GLIDDEN, WELDON EDWARD DO, LICENSE NUMBER G3397 OF QUANAH, TX, WAS DISCIPLINED BY TEXAS ON FEBRUARY 17, 1998
DISCIPLINARY ACTION: LICENSE SUSPENSION
OFFENSE: FAILURE TO COMPLY WITH PREVIOUS BOARD ORDER

NOTES: VIOLATED 8/9/97 ORDER IN THAT HE INGESTED HYDROCODONE AND BARBITURATES ON OR ABOUT 10/15/97; ON 10/21/97 HE NOTIFIED THE DIRECTOR OF COMPLIANCE THAT HE INGESTED FIORICET AND VICODIN ON 10/15/97 AND THAT THESE DRUGS HAD NOT BEEN PRESCRIBED TO HIM BY ANOTHER PHYSICIAN; ON OR ABOUT 10/29/97 HE INGESTED BARBITURATES; FAILED TO MAINTAIN A MINIMUM AVERAGE ATTENDANCE OF 3 AA MEETING PER WEEK. SUSPENSION UNTIL HE REQUESTS TO HAVE HIS SUSPENSION STAYED OR APPEARS BEFORE THE BOARD WITH SUFFICIENT EVIDENCE THAT HE IS PHYSICALLY, MENTALLY AND OTHERWISE COMPETENT TO SAFELY PRACTICE MEDICINE INCLUDING AT A MINIMUM COMPLETE COPIES OF MEDICAL RECORDS AND REPORTS OF PSYCHOLOGICAL AND NEUROPSYCHIATRIC EVALUATIONS, INCLUDING A 96 HOUR INPATIENT EVALUATION CONDUCTED BY A BOARD-APPROVED CERTIFIED PSYCHIATRIST.

GLIDDEN, WELDON EDWARD DO, LICENSE NUMBER G3397 OF QUANAH, TX, WAS DISCIPLINED BY TEXAS ON MAY 16, 1998
DISCIPLINARY ACTION: SURRENDER OF CONTROLLED SUBSTANCE LICENSE; 120-MONTH PROBATION
OFFENSE: SUBSTANCE ABUSE

NOTES: VIOLATED 11/3/94, 8/9/97, AND 1/14/98 BOARD ORDERS BY INTEMPERATE USE OF DRUGS, AND UNPROFESSIONAL OR DISHONORABLE CONDUCT THAT IS LIKELY TO DECEIVE, DEFRAUD, OR INJURE THE PUBLIC; ON 2/21/98 HE WAS HOSPITALIZED UNDER EMERGENCY CONDITIONS SUBSEQUENT TO AN INTENTIONAL OVERDOSE OF CONTROLLED SUBSTANCES; ON 3/23/98 HE ENTERED INTO AN INTERIM AGREEMENT WITH THE PHYSICIAN HEALTH AND REHABILITATION COMMITTEE OF THE TEXAS OSTEOPATHIC MEDICAL ASSOCIATION; HE HAS PROVIDED SUFFICIENT EVIDENCE AND INFORMATION TO INDICATE THAT HE IS PHYSICALLY, MENTALLY, AND OTHERWISE COMPETENT TO SAFELY PRACTICE MEDICINE SUBJECT TO TERMS AND CONDITIONS. SUSPENSION STAYED FOR PROBATION UNDER THE FOLLOWING TERMS; SHALL SUBMIT IN WRITING A PROPOSED PRACTICE OF MEDICINE ARRANGEMENT AND SETTING, INVOLVING PRACTICE OF NO MORE THAN 175 HOURS PER MONTH; SUCH ARRANGEMENT AND SETTING MAY NOT INCLUDE THE SOLO PRACTICE OF MEDICINE; HIS MEDICAL PRACTICE SHALL BE MONITORED BY A BOARD APPROVED TEXAS PHYSICIAN WHO SHALL PROVIDE QUARTERLY REPORTS TO THE BOARD; SHALL ABSTAIN FROM THE CONSUMPTION OF ALCOHOL/DRUGS IN ANY FORM UNLESS PRESCRIBED BY ANOTHER PHYSICIAN FOR A LEGITIMATE AND THERAPEUTIC PURPOSE; SHALL SUBMIT HIMSELF FOR APPROPRIATE EXAMS INCLUDING DRUG OR ALCOHOL SCREENS; SHALL NOMINATE THREE CERTIFIED PSYCHIATRISTS FOR BOARD SELECTION OF A THERAPIST AND SHALL EXPEDITIOUSLY SUBMIT HIMSELF TO EVALUATION AND TREATMENT BY THE APPROVED PRACTITIONER; SHALL PARTICIPATE IN THE ACTIVITIES OF A PHYSICIAN HEALTH AND REHABILITATION COMMITTEE AND ATTEND WEEKLY MEETINGS WITH QUARTERLY REPORTS; SHALL PARTICIPATE IN AA'S PROGRAM NOT LESS THAN FIVE TIMES A WEEK; SHALL REPORT ON HIS ATTENDANCE; SHALL IMMEDIATELY SURRENDER DEA AND TEXAS DEPARTMENT OF PUBLIC SAFETY CONTROLLED SUBSTANCES REGISTRATIONS AND ANY DRUGS WITH POTENTIAL FOR ABUSE IN HIS POSSESSION INCLUDING SAMPLES; SHALL APPEAR BEFORE THE BOARD UPON REQUEST; SEPARATE FROM PATIENT RECORDS, SHALL MAINTAIN A FILE OF EVERY PRESCRIPTION WRITTEN BY HIM FOR DANGEROUS DRUGS WITH ADDICTIVE POTENTIAL WHICH SHALL BE MADE AVAILABLE FOR REVIEW; SHALL NOT TREAT OR OTHERWISE SERVE AS PHYSICIAN, PRESCRIBE, DISPENSE OR ADMINISTER DRUGS THAT MAY BE SUBJECT TO ABUSE TO HIMSELF OR TO ANY MEMBER OF HIS FAMILY; SHALL OBTAIN 50 HOURS PER YEAR OF CONTINUING MEDICAL EDUCATION; SHALL APPEAR BEFORE THE BOARD UPON REQUEST; SHALL COOPERATE WITH THE BOARD IN VERIFYING COMPLIANCE INCLUDING PROVIDING COPIES OF MEDICAL RELEASES AND PEER REVIEW RECORDS UPON REQUEST; SHALL GIVE A COPY OF THIS ORDER TO ANY HEALTH CARE ENTITY WHERE HE HAS PRIVILEGES; SHALL PROVIDE A COPY OF THIS ORDER TO ANYONE REQUESTING IT WITHIN 10 DAYS; TIME SPENT OUT OF TEXAS DOES NOT COUNT TOWARD PROBATION; SHALL INFORM THE BOARD OF CHANGE OF ADDRESS WITHIN 10 DAYS OR IF HE LEAVES THE STATE; SHALL NOT SEEK MODIFICATION FOR ONE YEAR. ON 5/14/99 THE ORDER WAS MODIFIED AS FOLLOWS: FREQUENCY OF VISITS WITH PSYCHIATRIST DECREASED; HE IS AUTHORIZED TO REAPPLY TO THE DEA AND TEXAS DEPARTMENT OF PUBLIC SAFETY TO OBTAIN CONTROLLED SUBSTANCE REGISTRATIONS; WHEN RECEIVED HIS USE OF CONTROLLED SUBSTANCES SHALL BE LIMITED TO INPATIENT ORDERING ONLY; ALL OTHER PROVISIONS OF THE ORDER REMAIN IN EFFECT UNTIL SUPERSEDED BY A SUBSEQUENT ORDER.

GOAL, JAY C MD, LICENSE NUMBER 00H7306, WAS DISCIPLINED BY TEXAS ON AUGUST 17, 1996
DISCIPLINARY ACTION: REQUIRED TO TAKE ADDITIONAL MEDICAL EDUCATION; MONITORING OF PHYSICIAN PERFORMANCE
OFFENSE: SUBSTANDARD CARE, INCOMPETENCE OR NEGLIGENCE

NOTES: ON 7/14/94 FAILED TO CORRECTLY DIAGNOSE ATRIAL FIBRILLATION IN A 62 YEAR OLD PATIENT AS INDICATED BY A CURRENT ELECTROCARDIOGRAM READING AVAILABLE TO HIM; AND AS A RESULT OF HIS FAILURE, ADMINISTERED ADENOCARD, VERAPAMIL, AND INDERAL, NONE OF WHICH WERE INDICATED FOR TREATMENT OF THE PATIENT'S ACTUAL CONDITION. RESTRICTED UNDER TERMS AND CONDITIONS FOR ONE YEAR: WITHIN ONE YEAR SHALL OBTAIN 50 HOURS OF CONTINUING MEDICAL EDUCATION WITH AT LEAST 25 HOURS IN THE AREA OF CARDIOLOGY IN THE ACUTE CARE SETTING AND SUBMIT PROOF TO THE BOARD; WITHIN ONE YEAR SHALL TAKE AND SUCCESSFULLY COMPLETE AN ADVANCED CARDIAC LIFE SUPPORT COURSE, OBTAIN CERTIFICATION AND SUBMIT PROOF TO THE BOARD; HIS MEDICAL PRACTICE, INCLUDING ANY OFFICE AND SURGICAL PRACTICE, SHALL BE MONITORED BY A BOARD APPROVED TEXAS PHYSICIAN WHO SHALL SUBMIT QUARTERLY REPORTS; WITHIN TWO MONTHS SHALL SUBMIT TO THE BOARD A WRITTEN CORRECTIVE ACTION PLAN WHICH PROVIDES FOR A METHOD OR SYSTEM TO ELIMINATE OR DECREASE THE MISDIAGNOSING OF ATRIAL FIBRILLATION; SHALL PERSONALLY APPEAR BEFORE THE BOARD AT LEAST TWO TIMES PER YEAR OR UPON REQUEST; SHALL COOPERATE WITH THE BOARD IN VERIFYING COMPLIANCE; SHALL GIVE A COPY OF THIS ORDER TO ANY HEALTH CARE ENTITY WHERE HE HAS PRIVILEGES; SHALL PROVIDE A COPY OF THIS ORDER TO ANYONE REQUESTING IT WITHIN 10 DAYS; TIME PERIOD OUT OF TEXAS DOES NOT COUNT TOWARD RESTRICTION; SHALL INFORM THE BOARD OF CHANGE OF ADDRESS WITHIN 10 DAYS OF IF HE LEAVES THE STATE.

GOH, BENJAMIN WO-SHUN DO, LICENSE NUMBER 20A6533 OF ORANGE PARK, FL, WAS DISCIPLINED BY CALIFORNIA ON JUNE 18, 1996
DISCIPLINARY ACTION: 36-MONTH PROBATION
OFFENSE: DISCIPLINARY ACTION BY ANOTHER STATE OR AGENCY

NOTES: ACTION IN FLORIDA FOR GROSS OR REPEATED MALPRACTICE. PROBATION UPON ENTERING CALIFORNIA.

GOH, BENJAMIN WO-SHUN DO, LICENSE NUMBER 00H3386 OF 609 KINGSLEY AVENUE, ORANGE PARK, FL, WAS DISCIPLINED BY TEXAS ON AUGUST 17, 1996
DISCIPLINARY ACTION: FINE
OFFENSE: DISCIPLINARY ACTION BY ANOTHER STATE OR AGENCY

NOTES: IN 10/95 FINED AND PLACED ON TWO YEAR PROBATION IN FLORIDA BASED ON TWO HEALTH CARE LIABILITY CLAIMS: ONE INVOLVED A HOSPITAL PATIENT WITH AN ABNORMAL PAP SMEAR, WHO WAS

NOT NOTIFIED IN A TIMELY MANNER; AND THE OTHER INVOLVED PRESCRIBING A MEDICATION TO A PATIENT WHICH WAS CONTRAINDICATED DUE TO THE PATIENT'S HISTORY AND OTHER MEDICATIONS BEING PRESCRIBED. $2,500 FINE AND SHALL COMPLY WITH THE TERMS OF THE FLORIDA ORDER.

GOH, EWE GHEE MD, LICENSE NUMBER F4842 OF DALLAS, TX, WAS DISCIPLINED BY TEXAS ON AUGUST 9, 1997
DISCIPLINARY ACTION: FINE
OFFENSE: SUBSTANDARD CARE, INCOMPETENCE OR NEGLIGENCE

NOTES: IN 11/95 HE ORDERED 25 MG. OF PHENERGAN TO A TWO YEAR OLD PATIENT, AN EXCESSIVE AMOUNT. A DOSAGE OF 6.6 MG. WOULD BE APPROPRIATE FOR THIS CHILD'S WEIGHT; HE FAILED TO ADEQUATELY COMMUNICATE THIS ERROR TO THE PATIENT'S MOTHER. $1,200 FINE.

GOLD, JACOB CHARLES MD OF 5411 NORDLING, HOUSTON, TX, WAS DISCIPLINED BY DEA ON MARCH 12, 1990
DISCIPLINARY ACTION: SURRENDER OF CONTROLLED SUBSTANCE LICENSE
OFFENSE: CRIMINAL CONVICTION OR PLEA OF GUILTY, NOLO CONTENDERE, OR NO CONTEST TO A CRIME

NOTES: CONVICTED 05/03/89 IN HOUSTON, TEXAS FOR DISTRIBUTING METHAMPHETAMINE, PHENTERMINE, ETHCHLORVYNOL, PHENDIMETRAZINE AND DEXTROAMPHETAMINE AND SENTENCED 08/21/89 TO SIX MONTHS PRISON, FIVE YEARS PROBATION AND $4950 SPECIAL ASSESSMENT FEE.

GOLD, JACOB CHARLES MD, LICENSE NUMBER 00C5685 OF HOUSTON, TX, WAS DISCIPLINED BY TEXAS ON JULY 1, 1990
DISCIPLINARY ACTION: SURRENDER OF CONTROLLED SUBSTANCE LICENSE
OFFENSE: CRIMINAL CONVICTION OR PLEA OF GUILTY, NOLO CONTENDERE, OR NO CONTEST TO A CRIME

NOTES: CONVICTED OF FELONY. SUSPENSION STAYED PENDING OUTCOME OF APPEAL, MUST SURRENDER ALL NARCOTIC LICENSES, PERMITS, AND REGISTRATIONS. LICENSE TO BE AUTOMATICALLY RESTORED IF APPEAL UPHELD.

GOLD, JACOB CHARLES MD, DATE OF BIRTH FEBRUARY 26, 1925 OF 15922 MILLER RD #1, HOUSTON, TX, WAS DISCIPLINED BY MEDICARE ON MAY 24, 1991
DISCIPLINARY ACTION: 120-MONTH EXCLUSION FROM THE MEDICARE AND/OR MEDICAID PROGRAM
OFFENSE: CRIMINAL CONVICTION OR PLEA OF GUILTY, NOLO CONTENDERE, OR NO CONTEST TO A CRIME

NOTES: CONVICTION RELATING TO CONTROLLED SUBSTANCES.

GOLD, JACOB CHARLES MD, LICENSE NUMBER 00C5685 OF HOUSTON, TX, WAS DISCIPLINED BY TEXAS ON DECEMBER 4, 1991
DISCIPLINARY ACTION: LICENSE REVOCATION
OFFENSE: CRIMINAL CONVICTION OR PLEA OF GUILTY, NOLO CONTENDERE, OR NO CONTEST TO A CRIME

NOTES: ON 5/3/89 HE WAS CONVICTED ON SIX COUNTS FOR KNOWINGLY AND UNLAWFULLY DISPENSING BY PRESCRIPTION TO ONE PATIENT DESOXYN, FASTIN, AND PLACIDYL NOT IN THE USUAL COURSE OF PROFESSIONAL PRACTICE AND NOT FOR A LEGITIMATE MEDICAL PURPOSE; WAS ALSO CONVICTED OF 93 COUNTS OF DISPENSING BY PRESCRIPTION TO ANOTHER PATIENT THESE SAME DRUGS AND ALSO PRELU-2 AND DEXEDRINE NOT FOR A LEGITIMATE MEDICAL PURPOSE. ON 8/21/89 HE WAS SENTENCED TO SIX MONTHS IMPRISONMENT, FOLLOWED BY A FIVE YEAR PROBATION; PRESENTLY INCARCERATED. VOLUNTARILY SURRENDERED HIS LICENSE. SHALL SURRENDER DEA AND TEXAS CONTROLLED SUBSTANCES REGISTRATION CERTIFICATES, ALL UNUSED TRIPLICATE PRESCRIPTION FORMS, AND ALL CONTROLLED SUBSTANCES PRESENTLY IN HIS OFFICE, INCLUDING SAMPLES.

GOLDBERG, IRA B MD, DATE OF BIRTH NOVEMBER 8, 1940, LICENSE NUMBER 0023889 OF WHITLEY COUNTY, KY, WAS DISCIPLINED BY KENTUCKY ON JANUARY 19, 1996
DISCIPLINARY ACTION: SURRENDER OF CONTROLLED SUBSTANCE LICENSE

NOTES: MUST SURRENDER DEA PERMIT. ON 9/3/96 ORDER AMENDED SO HE WAS ALLOWED TO APPLY FOR REINSTATEMENT OF DEA PERMIT WITH RESTRICTION THAT HE MAY PRESCRIBE OR DISPENSE CONTROLLED SUBSTANCES ONLY FOR IN-HOSPITAL PATIENTS.

GOLDBERG, IRA B MD, LICENSE NUMBER 0104926 OF 1007 18TH ST PO BOX 850, CORBIN, KY, WAS DISCIPLINED BY NEW YORK ON NOVEMBER 21, 1996
DISCIPLINARY ACTION: 24-MONTH LICENSE SUSPENSION; 36-MONTH PROBATION
OFFENSE: DISCIPLINARY ACTION BY ANOTHER STATE OR AGENCY

NOTES: ACTION IN KENTUCKY FOR PRESCRIBING CONTROLLED SUBSTANCES WITHOUT ADEQUATE MEDICAL JUSTIFICATION AND WITHOUT SEEKING ALTERNATIVE MEDICAL TREATMENTS. REMAINDER OF THREE YEAR SUSPENSION, LAST YEAR STAYED WITH PROBATION COMMENCING UPON PRACTICING IN NEW YORK.

GOLDBERG, IRA B MD, LICENSE NUMBER G6517 OF LONDON, KY, WAS DISCIPLINED BY TEXAS ON MAY 16, 1998
OFFENSE: DISCIPLINARY ACTION BY ANOTHER STATE OR AGENCY

NOTES: ON OR ABOUT 1/1/96 ENTERED INTO A CONSENT ORDER WITH THE KENTUCKY BOARD BASED ON OVER PRESCRIBING OF CONTROLLED SUBSTANCES TO 11 PATIENTS. LICENSE LIMITED AS FOLLOWS: SHALL NOT PRACTICE IN TEXAS UNTIL HE APPEARS BEFORE THE BOARD WITH SUFFICIENT EVIDENCE THAT HE IS PHYSICALLY, MENTALLY AND OTHERWISE COMPETENT TO PRACTICE SAFELY; SHOWS THAT THERE ARE NO CURRENT RESTRICTIONS ON HIS KENTUCKY LICENSE AND NO PENDING KENTUCKY OR OTHER STATE LICENSURE ACTIONS OR PROCEEDINGS; SHALL COOPERATE WITH THE BOARD IN VERIFYING COMPLIANCE; SHALL INFORM THE BOARD OF CHANGE OF ADDRESS WITHIN 10 DAYS OR IF HE LEAVES THE STATE; SHALL NOT SEEK MODIFICATION FOR ONE YEAR.

GOLDBERG, IRA BARRY MD OF 1007 18TH STREET, CORBIN, KY, WAS DISCIPLINED BY DEA ON FEBRUARY 16, 1996
DISCIPLINARY ACTION: SURRENDER OF CONTROLLED SUBSTANCE LICENSE
OFFENSE: DISCIPLINARY ACTION BY ANOTHER STATE OR AGENCY

NOTES: STATE BOARD.

GOLDEN, MITCHELL KEITH MD, LICENSE NUMBER H7151 OF MOUNT VERNON, TX, WAS DISCIPLINED BY TEXAS ON AUGUST 28, 1999
DISCIPLINARY ACTION: REPRIMAND
OFFENSE: SUBSTANDARD CARE, INCOMPETENCE OR NEGLIGENCE

NOTES: FROM 9/16/96 - 10/14/97 HE SAW A PATIENT FOR MIGRAINES AND ULCERS; ON 6/25/97 THE PHARMACY

CALLED HIM REPORTING THAT THE PATIENT WAS REQUESTING HER 11TH REFILL FROM A PRESCRIPTION WRITTEN ON 3/20/97; THE PHARMACIST WAS CONCERNED THAT THE PATIENT WAS EITHER ADDICTED OR SELLING THE MEDICATION; THE DOCTOR DECLINED TO APPROVE THE REFILL AND DOCUMENTED IN THE PATIENT'S CHART THAT HE WOULD REFER HER TO A NEUROLOGIST OR A CHRONIC PAIN CENTER; HE INDICATED IN THE PATIENT'S CHART THAT THE PRESCRIPTION WAS INTENDED TO LAST 1 YEAR WITH REFILLS ONCE A MONTH, BUT DUE TO AN ERROR AT THE PHARMACY THE INDICATION THAT REFILLS WERE TO BE ONCE A MONTH WAS LEFT OFF THE LABEL; ON 2/17/98 HE NOTIFIED THE PATIENT THAT HE WAS TERMINATING THE PHYSICIAN-PATIENT RELATIONSHIP; THE BOARD DETERMINED THAT THE MEDICAL RECORDS OF THE PATIENT FAILED TO INCLUDE A WRITTEN TREATMENT PLAN TAILORED FOR THE PATIENT'S NEEDS BY WHICH TREATMENT PROGRESS AND SUCCESS CAN BE EVALUATED WITH STATED OBJECTIVES SUCH AS PAIN RELIEF AND/OR IMPROVED PHYSICAL AND PSYCHOSOCIAL FUNCTION; THE BOARD DETERMINED THAT HE FAILED TO TIMELY REFER THE PATIENT TO A CHRONIC PAIN SPECIALIST, AND IN ADDITION, HE CONTINUED TO TREAT THE PATIENT WITHOUT MODIFICATION OF THERAPY FOR AN ADDITIONAL 7 MONTHS AFTER THE PATIENT'S REFUSAL TO SEE A CHRONIC PAIN SPECIALIST.

GOLDMAN, EUGENE J MD, LICENSE NUMBER 081311 OF 7500 BEACHNUT #388, HOUSTON, TX, WAS DISCIPLINED BY NEW YORK ON JULY 30, 1997
DISCIPLINARY ACTION: SURRENDER OF LICENSE
OFFENSE: DISCIPLINARY ACTION BY ANOTHER STATE OR AGENCY

NOTES: PERMANENTLY SURRENDERED HIS TEXAS LICENSE AS A RESULT OF ALLEGATIONS OF SEXUAL MISCONDUCT WITH HIS PATIENTS.

GOLDMAN, EUGENE J MD, LICENSE NUMBER GFE8640 OF HOUSTON, TX, WAS DISCIPLINED BY CALIFORNIA ON AUGUST 12, 1997
DISCIPLINARY ACTION: SURRENDER OF LICENSE

NOTES: WHILE CHARGES PENDING.

GOLDMAN, EUGENE JEROME MD, LICENSE NUMBER 00D1426, WAS DISCIPLINED BY TEXAS ON AUGUST 31, 1996
DISCIPLINARY ACTION: SURRENDER OF LICENSE
OFFENSE: SEXUAL ABUSE OF OR SEXUAL MISCONDUCT WITH A PATIENT

NOTES: ALLEGED INAPPROPRIATE SEXUAL MISCONDUCT WITH PATIENTS; EXPRESSLY DENIES ANY AND ALL ALLEGATIONS. VOLUNTARY AND PERMANENT SURRENDER.

GONZALES, RICCARDO H MD, DATE OF BIRTH FEBRUARY 16, 1950 OF 315O HORTON ROAD #06662-078, FORT WORTH, TX, WAS DISCIPLINED BY MEDICARE ON APRIL 20, 1998
DISCIPLINARY ACTION: 10-MONTH EXCLUSION FROM THE MEDICARE AND/OR MEDICAID PROGRAM
OFFENSE: CRIMINAL CONVICTION OR PLEA OF GUILTY, NOLO CONTENDERE, OR NO CONTEST TO A CRIME

NOTES: CONVICTED OF A CRIME INVOLVING THE MEDICARE, MEDICAID, MATERNAL AND CHILD HEALTH SERVICES BLOCK GRANT OR BLOCK GRANTS TO STATES FOR SOCIAL SERVICES PROGRAMS.

GONZALEZ, ALFONSO MD OF 4821 COUNTRY CLUB VIEW, BAYTOWN, TX, WAS DISCIPLINED BY DEA ON SEPTEMBER 8, 1997
DISCIPLINARY ACTION: SURRENDER OF CONTROLLED SUBSTANCE LICENSE

NOTES: IN LIEU OF PUBLIC INTEREST REVOCATION.

GONZALEZ, ALPHONSO MD, LICENSE NUMBER C9360, WAS DISCIPLINED BY TEXAS ON MAY 10, 1997
DISCIPLINARY ACTION: LICENSE SUSPENSION
OFFENSE: CRIMINAL CONVICTION OR PLEA OF GUILTY, NOLO CONTENDERE, OR NO CONTEST TO A CRIME

NOTES: ON 12/5/94 WAS INDICTED FOR INTENTIONALLY AND KNOWINGLY PARTICIPATING IN AN INSURANCE FRAUD SCHEME INVOLVING STAGED AUTOMOBILE ACCIDENTS. THE CRIMINAL INDICTMENT INDICATES THAT HE DEFRAUDED EIGHT INSURANCE COMPANIES AND COMMITTED THEFT FROM THOSE COMPANIES BY FILING FALSE CLAIMS BETWEEN 11/1/93 AND 8/31/94. ON 2/5/97 HE WAS CONVICTED BY A JURY OF ENGAGING IN ORGANIZED CRIMINAL ACTIVITY, A FIRST DEGREE FELONY. HE WAS SENTENCED TO 20 YEARS IN A STATE PRISON AND FINED $10,000. SUSPENSION UNTIL HE REQUESTS IN WRITING TO HAVE THE SUSPENSION STAYED OR LIFTED, AND PERSONALLY APPEARS BEFORE THE BOARD TO PROVIDE SUFFICIENT EVIDENCE THAT HE IS PHYSICALLY, MENTALLY, AND OTHERWISE COMPETENT TO SAFELY PRACTICE. SUCH EVIDENCE SHALL INCLUDE AT A MINIMUM: SUCCESSFUL COMPLETION OF HIS PRISON SENTENCE AND OF ANY TERMS OR CONDITIONS OF PROBATION AND/OR PAROLE; OR SUCCESSFUL APPEAL OF HIS CONVICTION.

GOOD, EDWARD F MD, LICENSE NUMBER 0014447 OF WEBSTER, TX, WAS DISCIPLINED BY FLORIDA ON APRIL 20, 1992
DISCIPLINARY ACTION: FINE
OFFENSE: NONCOMPLIANCE WITH A PROFESSIONAL RULE

NOTES: CHARGED WITH FAILING TO MAINTAIN AND SUBMIT DOCUMENTATION VERIFYING COMPLETION OF HIV/AIDS AND RISK MANAGEMENT CONTINUING MEDICAL EDUCATION IN RESPONSE TO THE BOARD'S RANDOM AUDIT. $1,000 FINE.

GORDON, GENE STEPHEN MD, DATE OF BIRTH JANUARY 15, 1947, LICENSE NUMBER 0020171 OF FARMINGTON, CT, WAS DISCIPLINED BY CONNECTICUT ON JUNE 18, 1991
DISCIPLINARY ACTION: 84-MONTH PROBATION; MONITORING OF PHYSICIAN PERFORMANCE
OFFENSE: SUBSTANDARD CARE, INCOMPETENCE OR NEGLIGENCE

NOTES: INCOMPETENCE/NEGLIGENCE. MODIFICATION OF CONSENT ORDER ON 2/21/95: FREQUENCY OF MONITORING SHALL BE REDUCED IN 5TH YEAR OF PROBATION. TERMS OF PROBATION COMPLETED EFFECTIVE 6/01/95.

GORDON, GENE STEPHEN MD, DATE OF BIRTH JANUARY 15, 1947, LICENSE NUMBER 00F1033 OF 6 PEMBROKE HILL DEVONWOOD, FARMINGTON, CT, WAS DISCIPLINED BY TEXAS ON JANUARY 29, 1993
DISCIPLINARY ACTION: 60-MONTH PROBATION; RESTRICTION PLACED ON LICENSE
OFFENSE: DISCIPLINARY ACTION BY ANOTHER STATE OR AGENCY

NOTES: CONNECTICUT LICENSE PUT ON PROBATION 6/18/91 BASED ON HIS MISHANDLING MEDICATION REGIMES FOR PATIENTS; FAILED TO ESTABLISH AND MAINTAIN APPROPRIATE BOUNDARIES FOR HIS PATIENTS; BREACHED PATIENT CONFIDENTIALITY ON NUMEROUS OCCASIONS; FAILED TO MAINTAIN ADEQUATE AND COMPLETE MEDICAL RECORDS; TESTIFIED FALSELY UNDER OATH AS TO AUTHORSHIP

OF CERTAIN DOCUMENTS RELATING TO HIS ROLE AS AN EXPERT WITNESS. 5 YEAR SUSPENSION STAYED. CONDITIONS OF PROBATION: SAME AS THOSE OF CONNECTICUT ORDER INCLUDING CONSULTING A BOARD-APPROVED PSYCHIATRIST WEEKLY, HAVING A PSYCHIATRIST MONITOR HIS PRACTICE -- BOTH OF WHOM SHALL SUBMIT REPORTS, SHALL NOT CONDUCT GROUP THERAPY SESSIONS WITHOUT A CO-FACILITATOR, AND SHALL NOT SERVE AS AN EXPERT WITNESS; PRIOR TO PRACTICING IN TEXAS SHALL APPEAR BEFORE THE BOARD; SHALL INFORM THE BOARD IF HE LEAVES TEXAS OR CONNECTICUT; TIME SPENT OUT OF THESE TWO STATES DOES NOT COUNT TOWARD PROBATION. SHALL NOT SEEK MODIFICATION FOR ONE YEAR.

GORDON, GENE STEPHEN MD OF FARMINGTON, CT, WAS DISCIPLINED BY NORTH CAROLINA ON OCTOBER 9, 1994

NOTES: CONSENT ORDER, UNSPECIFIED. ON 12/20/99 ORDER TERMINATED.

GORDON, GENE STEPHEN MD, DATE OF BIRTH JANUARY 15, 1947, LICENSE NUMBER 0020171 OF FARMINGTON, CT, WAS DISCIPLINED BY CONNECTICUT ON OCTOBER 16, 1996
DISCIPLINARY ACTION: 21-MONTH PROBATION; MONITORING OF PHYSICIAN PERFORMANCE
OFFENSE: SUBSTANDARD CARE, INCOMPETENCE OR NEGLIGENCE

NOTES: INCOMPETENCE/NEGLIGENCE. PROBATION UNTIL 6/30/98. SUPERVISION OF PRACTICE; AND THERAPY. ON 6/30/98 COMPLETED PROBATION; NO FURTHER LICENSURE RESTRICTIONS.

GORMAN, MARY G MD OF 5414 MOUNTAIN CEDAR COVE, AUSTIN, TX, WAS DISCIPLINED BY DEA ON OCTOBER 28, 1996
DISCIPLINARY ACTION: SURRENDER OF CONTROLLED SUBSTANCE LICENSE

NOTES: IN LIEU OF PUBLIC INTEREST REVOCATION.

GORMAN, MARY GWEN MD, LICENSE NUMBER 00H3249, WAS DISCIPLINED BY TEXAS ON AUGUST 17, 1996
DISCIPLINARY ACTION: LICENSE SUSPENSION; REQUIRED TO ENTER AN IMPAIRED PHYSICIAN PROGRAM OR SUBSTANCE ABUSE TREATMENT
OFFENSE: SUBSTANCE ABUSE

NOTES: IN OCTOBER 1995 SHE SELF-REPORTED TO THE BOARD HER PROBLEM WITH ALCOHOL AND DRUGS, NAMELY AMBIEN AND LORCET; RECEIVED OUTPATIENT TREATMENT FROM OCTOBER 1995 TO JANUARY 1996 FOR CHEMICAL DEPENDENCY, CONTINUES UNDER THE CARE OF A PSYCHIATRIST AND AN ADDICTIONOLOGIST, PARTICIPATES IN AA ON AVERAGE THREE TO FOUR TIMES PER WEEK, AND PARTICIPATES IN THE PHYSICIAN HEALTH AND REHABILITATION COMMITTEE; DURING OCTOBER, NOVEMBER, AND DECEMBER OF 1995 WROTE SEVERAL PRESCRIPTIONS FOR LORCET, TUSSIONEX, AMBIEN, AND PROMETHAZINE TO HER MOTHER AND TWO FORMER PATIENTS WITHOUT ADEQUATE EXAMINATION OR INDICATION AND WITHOUT MAINTAINING MEDICAL RECORDS; SUBSEQUENT TO AN INFORMAL SETTLEMENT CONFERENCE HELD ON 7/02/96 WROTE SEVERAL PRESCRIPTIONS PRIMARILY FOR LORCET, AMBIEN, AND SOMA FOR FORMER PATIENTS AND/OR FICTITIOUS PATIENTS; SOME OF THE PRESCRIPTIONS WERE WRITTEN ON A PRESCRIPTION PAD FROM A CLINIC WHERE SHE WAS NO LONGER EMPLOYED AT THE TIME SHE WROTE THEM; SHE PICKED UP THE PRESCRIPTIONS HERSELF FOR THE PURPOSE OF DIVERTING THE DRUGS TO HERSELF; ADMITTED TO INGESTING HYDROCODONE ON OR ABOUT 8/01/96. SUSPENSION UNTIL REQUESTS PERMISSION TO RESUME PRACTICE AND PROVIDES SUFFICIENT EVIDENCE INDICATING THAT SHE IS PHYSICALLY, MENTALLY, AND OTHERWISE COMPETENT TO SAFELY PRACTICE MEDICINE. WITHIN 30 DAYS SHALL ENTER A BOARD APPROVED INPATIENT REHABILITATION FACILITY FOR AT LEAST 30 DAYS; SHALL AUTHORIZE THAT THE PROGRAM DIRECTOR OR PHYSICIAN IN CHARGE OF HER CARE PROVIDE THE BOARD WITH WRITTEN REPORTS NO LESS THAN ONCE EACH MONTH; EVIDENCE AND INFORMATION OF FITNESS TO PRACTICE SHALL INCLUDE AT A MINIMUM: COPIES OF MEDICAL RECORDS AND REPORTS OF PSYCHOLOGICAL AND NEUROPSYCHIATRIC EVALUATIONS, INCLUDING A 96 HOUR INPATIENT EVALUATION, CONDUCTED BY A BOARD APPROVED PSYCHIATRIST; EVIDENCE OF ONGOING PARTICIPATION IN AA OR ANY OTHER BOARD APPROVED SUBSTANTIALLY SIMILAR PROGRAM; EVIDENCE OF ONGOING PARTICIPATION WITH A PHYSICIAN HEALTH AND REHABILITATION PROGRAM; AND EVIDENCE OF HER COMPLIANCE WITH ALL TREATMENT RECOMMENDATIONS MADE BY HEALTH CARE INDIVIDUALS.

GORMAN, MARY GWEN MD, LICENSE NUMBER H3249, WAS DISCIPLINED BY TEXAS ON APRIL 4, 1998
DISCIPLINARY ACTION: 60-MONTH PROBATION; RESTRICTION PLACED ON LICENSE
OFFENSE: SUBSTANCE ABUSE

NOTES: IN 10/95 SHE SELF-REPORTED TO THE BOARD THAT SHE HAD A PROBLEM WITH ALCOHOL AND DRUGS; ON 8/17/96 HER LICENSE WAS SUSPENDED AND SHE WAS ADMITTED TO A REHABILITATION CENTER FOR EXTENDED TREATMENT; ON 3/27/98 SHE REQUESTED LIFTING THE SUSPENSION FROM HER LICENSE; SHE HAS PRESENTED EVIDENCE OF COMPLIANCE WITH ALL TERMS OF HER 8/17/96 ORDER AND WAS SUCCESSFULLY REEVALUATED AT THE REHABILITATION CENTER ON 3/9/98 DURING A 96 HOUR INPATIENT EVALUATION; SHE REPORTED ATTENDING AA MEETINGS 4-5 TIMES A WEEK. SUSPENSION STAYED FOR PROBATION WITH FOLLOWING TERMS AND CONDITIONS: SHALL NOT PRACTICE MEDICINE FOR MORE THAN 20 HOURS A WEEK; SHALL ABSTAIN FROM THE CONSUMPTION OF ALCOHOL/DRUGS IN ANY FORM UNLESS PRESCRIBED BY ANOTHER PHYSICIAN FOR A LEGITIMATE AND THERAPEUTIC PURPOSE; SHALL SUBMIT HERSELF FOR APPROPRIATE EXAMS INCLUDING DRUG OR ALCOHOL SCREENS; SHALL NOMINATE THREE CERTIFIED PSYCHIATRISTS FOR BOARD SELECTION OF A THERAPIST AND SHALL EXPEDITIOUSLY SUBMIT HERSELF TO EVALUATION AND TREATMENT BY THE APPROVED PRACTITIONER; SHALL CONTINUE TO PARTICIPATE IN THE ACTIVITIES OF A PHYSICIAN HEALTH AND REHABILITATION COMMITTEE AND ATTEND WEEKLY MEETINGS WITH QUARTERLY REPORTS; SHALL PARTICIPATE IN AA'S PROGRAM NOT LESS THAN FIVE TIMES A WEEK FOR THE FIRST 6 MONTHS, AND THEN THREE TIMES PER WEEK THEREAFTER; SHALL REPORT ON HER ATTENDANCE; HER PRACTICE SHALL BE LIMITED TO A CRITICAL CARE OR EMERGENCY ROOM SETTING, BOARD APPROVED; SHALL NOT PRACTICE IN A SOLO PRACTICE SETTING; SHALL NOT POSSESS, ADMINISTER, DISPENSE OR PRESCRIBE EXCEPT FOR TREATING PATIENTS IN AN EMERGENCY ROOM; SHALL OBTAIN 50 HOURS PER YEAR OF CONTINUING MEDICAL EDUCATION; SEPARATE FROM PATIENT RECORDS, SHALL MAINTAIN A LOGBOOK OF EVERY PRESCRIPTION WRITTEN BY HIM FOR DANGEROUS

DRUGS WITH ADDICTIVE POTENTIAL WHICH SHALL BE MADE AVAILABLE FOR REVIEW; SHALL APPEAR BEFORE THE BOARD UPON REQUEST; SHALL COOPERATE WITH THE BOARD IN VERIFYING COMPLIANCE; SHALL GIVE A COPY OF THIS ORDER TO ANY HEALTH CARE ENTITY WHERE HE HAS PRIVILEGES; TIME SPENT OUT OF TEXAS DOES NOT COUNT TOWARD PROBATION; SHALL INFORM THE BOARD OF CHANGE OF ADDRESS WITHIN 10 DAYS OR IF SHE LEAVES THE STATE; SHALL NOT SEEK MODIFICATION FOR 6 MONTHS. ON 10/24/98 THE ORDER WAS MODIFIED AS FOLLOWS: SHALL NOT ENGAGE IN THE PRACTICE OF MEDICINE FOR MORE THAN 20 HOURS PER WEEK EXCEPT IF HER PRACTICE IS LIMITED TO A BOARD-APPROVED TRAINING PROGRAM, OF WHICH SHE MAY PRACTICE FOR A MAXIMUM OF 40 HOURS PER WEEK; SHALL NOT PRACTICE IN A SOLO PRACTICE SETTING; ALL OTHER PROVISIONS OF THE ORDER REMAIN IN FULL EFFECT UNTIL SUPERSEDED BY A SUBSEQUENT BOARD ORDER. ON 12/11/99 THE ORDER WAS MODIFIED BY DELETING THE FOLLOWING REQUIREMENTS: THAT HER PRACTICE BE RESTRICTED TO 20 HOURS PER WEEK OR 40 HOURS PER WEEK, IF IN A TRAINING PROGRAM; THE RESTRICTION TO PRACTICE IN A SOLO PRACTICE; AND THE RESTRICTION OF USING CONTROLLED SUBSTANCES TO TREAT PATIENTS IN AN EMERGENCY ROOM SETTING.

GOSWAMI, ANILKUMAR P MD, LICENSE NUMBER 00E7095 OF ODESSA, TX, WAS DISCIPLINED BY TEXAS ON OCTOBER 13, 1995
DISCIPLINARY ACTION: 48-MONTH RESTRICTION PLACED ON LICENSE; REQUIRED TO TAKE ADDITIONAL MEDICAL EDUCATION
OFFENSE: SUBSTANDARD CARE, INCOMPETENCE OR NEGLIGENCE

NOTES: IN 4/93 FAILED TO ADEQUATELY EVALUATE AND ADDRESS SYMPTOMS REPORTED BY A PATIENT AND DIAGNOSED HER AS HAVING AN UPPER RESPIRATORY INFECTION WITHOUT ADEQUATE INDICATIONS; ALLEGATIONS THAT IN 1986 AND 1987, HE HAD INAPPROPRIATE PHYSICAL CONTACT WITH THREE DIFFERENT ADULT FEMALES. DOES NOT ADMIT ALLEGATIONS. LICENSE RESTRICTION WITH TERMS: SHALL OBTAIN AT LEAST 80 HOURS PER YEAR OF CONTINUING MEDICAL EDUCATION; WITHIN ONE YEAR SHALL OBTAIN 10 HOURS OF ETHICS THROUGH BOARD-APPROVED COURSES OR PROGRAMS; SHALL HAVE A CHAPERONE PRESENT DURING ANY PHYSICAL EXAMINATION ON A FEMALE PATIENT; SHALL MAINTAIN ADEQUATE MEDICAL RECORDS WHICH SHALL BE AVAILABLE FOR REVIEW; SHALL SUBMIT HIMSELF FOR EVALUATION AND TREATMENT BY A BOARD-APPROVED PSYCHIATRIST WHO SHALL SUBMIT REPORTS TO THE BOARD; SHALL APPEAR BEFORE THE BOARD AT LEAST ONCE A YEAR; SHALL COOPERATE WITH THE BOARD IN VERIFYING COMPLIANCE; SHALL GIVE A COPY OF THIS ORDER TO ANY HEALTH CARE ENTITY WHERE HE HAS PRIVILEGES; TIME SPENT OUT OF TEXAS DOES NOT COUNT TOWARD PROBATION; SHALL INFORM BOARD OF CHANGE OF ADDRESS WITHIN 10 DAYS OR IF HE LEAVES THE STATE. SHALL NOT SEEK MODIFICATION FOR ONE YEAR.

GOSWAMI, ANILKUMAR P MD, LICENSE NUMBER 37170 OF ODESSA, TX, WAS DISCIPLINED BY OHIO ON MARCH 11, 1998
DISCIPLINARY ACTION: LICENSE REVOCATION
OFFENSE: DISCIPLINARY ACTION BY ANOTHER STATE OR AGENCY

NOTES: ACTION BY TEXAS MEDICAL BOARD FOLLOWING THAT BOARD'S FINDING THAT HE FAILED TO ADEQUATELY EVALUATE AND DIAGNOSE A PATIENT AND THAT HE HAD INAPPROPRIATE PHYSICAL CONTACT WITH THREE ADULT FEMALES; PRIOR ACTION BY MICHIGAN'S MEDICAL BOARD BASED ON HIS FAILURE TO NOTIFY MICHIGAN BOARD OF TEXAS ACTION WITHIN 30 DAYS AS REQUIRED BY LAW. PERMANENT REVOCATION.

GOSWAMI, ANILKUMAR P MD, LICENSE NUMBER E7095 OF ODESSA, TX, WAS DISCIPLINED BY TEXAS ON DECEMBER 4, 1998
DISCIPLINARY ACTION: EMERGENCY SUSPENSION

NOTES: EVIDENCE AND INFORMATION THAT HIS CONTINUATION IN THE PRACTICE OF MEDICINE WOULD CONSTITUTE A CONTINUING THREAT TO PUBLIC WELFARE.

GOSWAMI, ANILKUMAR P MD, LICENSE NUMBER E7095 OF ODESSA, TX, WAS DISCIPLINED BY TEXAS ON AUGUST 28, 1999
DISCIPLINARY ACTION: SURRENDER OF LICENSE

NOTES: IN LIEU OF FURTHER INVESTIGATION VOLUNTARY AND PERMANENT SURRENDER.

GRAHAM, DAVID L DO OF 922 WEST I-30 HIGHWAY APT. 404, GARLAND, TX, WAS DISCIPLINED BY PENNSYLVANIA ON JULY 12, 1996
DISCIPLINARY ACTION: REQUIRED TO TAKE ADDITIONAL MEDICAL EDUCATION; REQUIRED TO ENTER AN IMPAIRED PHYSICIAN PROGRAM OR SUBSTANCE ABUSE TREATMENT
OFFENSE: SUBSTANCE ABUSE

NOTES: ABUSED CONTROLLED SUBSTANCES INTERMITTENTLY BETWEEN 1965 AND 1988; AND SOUGHT TREATMENT ON SEVERAL OCCASIONS; ON 3/15/87 AND 3/14/88 ON AN APPLICATION FOR TEMPORARY LICENSE AND AN UNRESTRICTED LICENSE TO PRACTICE MEDICINE IN MISSOURI FALSELY ANSWERED THAT HE HAD NOT BEEN CONVICTED OF A CRIME AND HAD NEVER BEEN TREATED FOR A MENTAL OR EMOTIONAL ILLNESS; WHILE SERVING AS AN INTERN IN JOPLIN, MISSOURI, IN 1988, CONTRARY TO HIS LIMITED PRESCRIBING AUTHORITY, PRESCRIBED A SCHEDULE III CONTROLLED SUBSTANCE FOR SOMEONE WHO WAS NO LONGER A HOSPITAL PATIENT AND ON TWO OCCASIONS THAT YEAR, ABUSED A DECONGESTANT CONTAINING DILUTE COCAINE WHICH HAD BEEN LEGITIMATELY PRESCRIBED FOR HIM FOR THE TREATMENT OF HIS RESPIRATORY ALLERGIES; THE MISSOURI BOARD REVOKED HIS TEMPORARY LICENSE IN THE 10TH MONTH OF THE PROGRAM AND REFUSED TO PERMIT HIM TO SIT FOR THE FLEX EXAMINATION BECAUSE HE HAD LIED ON HIS APPLICATION; IN 1988 VOLUNTARILY ENTERED TREATMENT FOR DRUG ABUSE AT THE VA HOSPITAL IN TOPEKA AND DIAGNOSED AS SUFFERING FROM CHRONIC POST TRAUMATIC STRESS DISORDER RESULTING FROM MILITARY SERVICE IN VIETNAM; SUCCESSFULLY COMPLETED A 90 DAY INPATIENT TREATMENT PROGRAM AT THE VIRGINIA HOSPITAL; SINCE 10/07/91 HAS BEEN UNDER TREATMENT AND MONITORING CONTRACT WITH IMPAIRED PHYSICIANS PROGRAM EITHER IN MISSOURI OR TEXAS; HAS NOT ABUSED DRUGS OR ALCOHOL SINCE 1988. GRANTED A TEMPORARY TRAINING LICENSE UNDER THE FOLLOWING CONDITIONS: SHALL UNDERTAKE A TWO YEAR RESIDENCY IN AN APPROVED GRADUATE OSTEOPATHIC OR MEDICAL TRAINING PROGRAM T0 BEGIN NO LATER THAN IN ONE YEAR; PRIOR TO OBTAINING THE TEMPORARY LICENSE AND BEGINNING THE RESIDENCY, SHALL EXECUTE A TREATMENT AND MONITORING CONTRACT WITH THE PROFESSIONAL HEALTH MONITORING PROGRAM (PHMP) OF THE BUREAU OF PROFESSIONAL AND

OCCUPATIONAL AFFAIRS WHICH SHALL REQUIRE SCREENING FOR CONTROLLED SUBSTANCES FOR AT LEAST THREE YEARS; SHALL FULLY COOPERATE WITH THE PHMP AND REQUEST THAT THEY SUBMIT A REPORT TO THE BOARD ON HIS STATUS IN THE PROGRAM EVERY SIX MONTHS; DURING HIS RESIDENCY SHALL REQUEST THAT THE HEAD OF THE RESIDENCY SUBMIT A REPORT TO THE BOARD ON HIS STATUS IN THE RESIDENCY EVERY SIX MONTHS; SHALL PROVIDE A COPY OF THIS ORDER TO THE HEAD OF THE RESIDENCY PROGRAM TO WHICH HE APPLIES.

GRAHAM, NORMAN EUGENE MD OF 402 HOLDERRIETH, TOMBALL, TX, WAS DISCIPLINED BY DEA ON NOVEMBER 6, 1996
DISCIPLINARY ACTION: SURRENDER OF CONTROLLED SUBSTANCE LICENSE

NOTES: IN LIEU OF PUBLIC INTEREST REVOCATION.

GREEN, DEMETRIS A MD OF HOUSTON, TX, WAS DISCIPLINED BY DEA ON DECEMBER 30, 1996
DISCIPLINARY ACTION: REVOCATION OF CONTROLLED SUBSTANCE LICENSE
OFFENSE: DISCIPLINARY ACTION BY ANOTHER STATE OR AGENCY

NOTES: ON 11/03/94 THE TEXAS BOARD SUSPENDED HIS LICENSE TO PRACTICE MEDICINE BASED ON HIS USE OF ALCOHOL OR DRUGS AND THE FINDING THAT HE WAS INVOLUNTARILY ADMITTED TO A TREATMENT PROGRAM FOR SYMPTOMS RELATED TO COCAINE ADDICTION. HE WAS ORDERED TO SURRENDER HIS DEA REGISTRATION, AND HIS STATE CONTROLLED SUBSTANCE LICENSE. IN 3/95 HE ISSUED CONTROLLED SUBSTANCE PRESCRIPTIONS WHICH RESULTED IN THE TWO YEAR CONTINUATION OF HIS SUSPENSION.

GREEN, DEMETRIS ALLEN MD, LICENSE NUMBER 00J4168 OF HOUSTON, TX, WAS DISCIPLINED BY TEXAS ON NOVEMBER 3, 1994
DISCIPLINARY ACTION: LICENSE SUSPENSION; MONITORING OF PHYSICIAN PERFORMANCE
OFFENSE: SUBSTANCE ABUSE

NOTES: ON 10/7/94 WAS INVOLUNTARILY ADMITTED TO AN ADDICTION TREATMENT PROGRAM FOR SYMPTOMS RELATED TO COCAINE ADDICTION; DURING 1994 INGESTED COCAINE WITHOUT A LEGITIMATE MEDICAL PURPOSE. SUSPENSION UNTIL HE PERSONALLY APPEARS BEFORE THE BOARD AND PROVIDES SUFFICIENT EVIDENCE THAT HE IS PHYSICALLY, MENTALLY AND OTHERWISE COMPETENT TO PRACTICE SAFELY INCLUDING BUT NOT LIMITED TO COMPLETE LEGIBLE COPIES OF MEDICAL RECORDS AND REPORTS OF PSYCHOLOGICAL AND NEUROPSYCHIATRIC EVALUATIONS.

GREEN, DEMETRIS ALLEN MD, LICENSE NUMBER J4168, WAS DISCIPLINED BY TEXAS ON MAY 14, 1999
DISCIPLINARY ACTION: 120-MONTH PROBATION; RESTRICTION PLACED ON CONTROLLED SUBSTANCE LICENSE
OFFENSE: PRACTICING WITHOUT A VALID CONTROLLED SUBSTANCE LICENSE

NOTES: ON 11/3/94 HIS LICENSE WAS SUSPENDED REGARDING HIS DRUG ABUSE; ON 3/15/95 HE WROTE A PRESCRIPTION FOR AMPICILLIN AND PHENERGAN WITH CODEINE UNDER AN INDIVIDUAL'S NAME, WHICH HE TRIED TO PERSONALLY FILL; ON 3/14/95 HE WROTE 2 PRESCRIPTIONS FOR ANOTHER PATIENT FOR THE SAME DRUGS; HE ADMITS TO WRITING BOTH PRESCRIPTIONS FOR FRIENDS OF HIS, AND DENIES THAT THE PRESCRIPTIONS WERE FOR SELF-USE; HE REPORTS A SOBRIETY DATE OF 12/28/94; HIS AA MEETING ATTENDANCE HAS BEEN REPORTED BY HIM TO BE ON AN AVERAGE OF 2 TIMES PER WEEK; HE IS UNDER THE CARE OF A PSYCHIATRIST, FOR SUBSTANCE ABUSE. SUSPENSION STAYED FOR PROBATION WITH FOLLOWING TERMS AND CONDITIONS: SHALL LIMIT HIS PRACTICE TO A RESIDENCY PROGRAM APPROVED IN ADVANCE BY THE BOARD; SHALL ABSTAIN FROM THE CONSUMPTION OF ALCOHOL/DRUGS IN ANY FORM UNLESS PRESCRIBED BY ANOTHER PHYSICIAN FOR A LEGITIMATE AND THERAPEUTIC PURPOSE; SHALL SUBMIT HIMSELF FOR APPROPRIATE EXAMS INCLUDING DRUG OR ALCOHOL SCREENS; SHALL NOMINATE THREE CERTIFIED PSYCHIATRISTS FOR BOARD SELECTION OF A THERAPIST AND SHALL EXPEDITIOUSLY SUBMIT HIMSELF TO EVALUATION AND TREATMENT BY THE APPROVED PRACTITIONER; SHALL PARTICIPATE IN THE ACTIVITIES OF A PHYSICIAN HEALTH AND REHABILITATION COMMITTEE AND ATTEND WEEKLY MEETINGS WITH QUARTERLY REPORTS; SHALL PARTICIPATE IN AA'S PROGRAM NOT LESS THAN THREE TIMES A WEEK; SHALL REPORT ON HIS ATTENDANCE; SHALL NOT TREAT OR OTHERWISE SERVE AS PHYSICIAN, PRESCRIBE, DISPENSE OR ADMINISTER DRUGS THAT MAY BE SUBJECT TO ABUSE TO HIMSELF OR TO ANY MEMBER OF HIS FAMILY; SHALL NOT POSSESS, ADMINISTER, DISPENSE OR PRESCRIBE ANY DRUGS WITH POTENTIAL FOR ABUSE EXCEPT FOR INPATIENTS IN A HOSPITAL SETTING; SEPARATE FROM PATIENT RECORDS, SHALL MAINTAIN A LOGBOOK OF EVERY PRESCRIPTION WRITTEN BY HIM FOR DANGEROUS DRUGS WITH ADDICTIVE POTENTIAL AND FOR ALL PRESCRIPTIONS OR REFILLS TELEPHONED IN BY HIM OR AT HIS DIRECTION FOR CONTROLLED SUBSTANCES OR DANGEROUS DRUGS WITH ADDICTIVE POTENTIAL OR POTENTIAL FOR ABUSE WHICH SHALL BE MADE AVAILABLE FOR REVIEW; BEGINNING IN NO LATER THAN 60 DAYS, HIS MEDICAL PRACTICE SHALL BE MONITORED BY A BOARD APPROVED TEXAS PHYSICIAN WHO SHALL PROVIDE QUARTERLY REPORTS TO THE BOARD; TIME SPENT OUT OF TEXAS DOES NOT COUNT TOWARD PROBATION; SHALL INFORM THE BOARD OF CHANGE OF ADDRESS WITHIN 10 DAYS OR IF HE LEAVES THE STATE; SHALL NOT SEEK MODIFICATION FOR ONE YEAR.

GREEN, KENNETH W JR MD, DATE OF BIRTH APRIL 27, 1957 OF 2728 OAKLAWN AVENUE, DALLAS, TX, WAS DISCIPLINED BY MEDICARE ON JUNE 30, 1994
DISCIPLINARY ACTION: EXCLUSION FROM THE MEDICARE AND/OR MEDICAID PROGRAM
OFFENSE: NONCOMPLIANCE WITH A PROFESSIONAL RULE

NOTES: DEFAULTED ON PUBLIC HEALTH SERVICE EDUCATION LOAN.

GREEN, KENNETH WAYNE JR MD, LICENSE NUMBER 00H2414 OF DALLAS, TX, WAS DISCIPLINED BY TEXAS ON APRIL 10, 1992
DISCIPLINARY ACTION: 120-MONTH PROBATION
OFFENSE: SUBSTANCE ABUSE

NOTES: SEVERAL VIOLATIONS OF THE MEDICAL PRACTICE ACT, INCLUDING INTEMPERATE USE OF ALCOHOL OR DRUGS AND INABILITY TO PRACTICE MEDICINE WITH REASONABLE SKILL AND SAFETY TO PATIENTS. LICENSE SUSPENDED, SUSPENSION STAYED; PROBATION UNDER TERMS AND CONDITIONS.

GREEN, KENNETH WAYNE JR MD, LICENSE NUMBER 00H2414 OF DALLAS, TX, WAS DISCIPLINED BY TEXAS ON NOVEMBER 13, 1992

DISCIPLINARY ACTION: EMERGENCY SUSPENSION
OFFENSE: FAILURE TO COMPLY WITH PREVIOUS BOARD ORDER

NOTES: INTEMPERATE USE OF DRUGS AND VIOLATION OF PROBATION. TEMPORARILY SUSPENDED UNTIL A HEARING BEFORE THE STATE OFFICE OF ADMINISTRATIVE HEARINGS CAN BE CONDUCTED.

GREEN, KENNETH WAYNE JR MD, LICENSE NUMBER 00H2414, WAS DISCIPLINED BY TEXAS ON AUGUST 28, 1993
DISCIPLINARY ACTION: PROBATION; MONITORING OF PHYSICIAN PERFORMANCE
OFFENSE: FAILURE TO COMPLY WITH PREVIOUS BOARD ORDER

NOTES: IN SPITE OF DISCREPANCIES IN PROCEDURES TESTING A URINE SAMPLE HE GAVE ON 6/5/92 AND HIS CLAIM THAT A VITAMIN HE WAS TAKING TRIGGERED A POSITIVE RESULT ON THE DRUG SCREEN, THE BOARD DETERMINED THAT EMPIRICAL, SCIENTIFIC EVIDENCE SHOWED HE HAD INGESTED COCAINE ON OR ABOUT 6/5/92 IN VIOLATION OF THE 4/10/92 ORDER. TEN YEAR SUSPENSION STAYED. CONDITIONS OF 4/10/92 PROBATION MODIFIED: SHALL CONTINUE TREATMENT WITH COUNSELORS AND SHALL PARTICIPATE IN SCREENS AS DIRECTED BY THEM WITH REPORTS TO THE BOARD UPON REQUEST OR IMMEDIATELY IF ANY SCREEN IS POSITIVE; IF HE RECEIVED A DRUG FROM A PHYSICIAN FOR A LEGITIMATE AND THERAPEUTIC PURPOSE THE PHYSICIAN SHALL IMMEDIATELY REPORT THIS TO THE BOARD WITH DETAILS; TREATING PHYSICIAN SHALL BE GIVEN A COPY OF THIS ORDER; SHALL IN ADDITION TO DRUG SCREENS REQUESTED BY BOARD SUBMIT TO 12 PER YEAR TO BE ORDERED BY THE PHYSICIAN REHABILITATION COMMITTEE WITH RESULTS PROVIDED TO THE BOARD. SHALL NOT SEEK MODIFICATION FOR ONE YEAR.

GREEN, KENNETH WAYNE JR MD, LICENSE NUMBER 00H2414 OF DALLAS, TX, WAS DISCIPLINED BY TEXAS ON AUGUST 19, 1994
DISCIPLINARY ACTION: LICENSE REVOCATION
OFFENSE: FAILURE TO COMPLY WITH PREVIOUS BOARD ORDER

NOTES: IN VIOLATION OF 4/10/92 AND 8/20/93 ORDERS, ON 11/2/93 HE REFUSED TO PROVIDE A REQUESTED URINE SAMPLE; HE DID COMPLY THREE HOURS LATER; THIS SAMPLE TESTED POSITIVE FOR AMPHETAMINES AND METHAMPHETAMINES WHICH HAD NOT BEEN PRESCRIBED BY HIS ATTENDING PHYSICIAN; CONTINUED DRUG USAGE AND RELAPSES DO NOT PRESENT A FAVORABLE PICTURE IN TERMS OF POTENTIAL FOR REHABILITATION. ORDER WILL BECOME FINAL WHEN ADMINISTRATIVE APPEALS HAVE BEEN EXHAUSTED; HE HAS 20 DAYS TO FILE FOR A REHEARING.

GREEN, KENNETH WAYNE JR MD OF 729 GRAPEVINE HIGHWAY, HURST, TX, WAS DISCIPLINED BY DEA ON NOVEMBER 10, 1994
DISCIPLINARY ACTION: REVOCATION OF CONTROLLED SUBSTANCE LICENSE
OFFENSE: DISCIPLINARY ACTION BY ANOTHER STATE OR AGENCY

NOTES: TEXAS MEDICAL BOARD PLACED HIS LICENSE ON PROBATION IN 4/92 FOR TEN YEARS BASED UPON HIS ABUSE OF DEMEROL AND VICODIN WHICH RESULTED IN HIM LOSING HIS CLINICAL PRIVILEGES AT A MEDICAL CENTER IN 4/91. ON 6/5/92 URINE SAMPLE COLLECTED FROM HIM TESTED POSITIVE FOR COCAINE WHICH WAS AGAINST THE TERMS OF THE PREVIOUS ORDER AND HIS LICENSE WAS SUSPENDED FOR TEN YEARS WITH SUSPENSION STAYED. VIOLATED PROVISIONS OF BOTH BOARD ORDERS AND CONSEQUENTLY HAD HIS TEXAS LICENSE REVOKED ON 08/19/94.

GREGORIO, CESAR P JR MD, LICENSE NUMBER 00E7611 OF ROCKWALL, TX, WAS DISCIPLINED BY TEXAS ON JUNE 10, 1991
DISCIPLINARY ACTION: 36-MONTH PROBATION; REQUIRED TO TAKE ADDITIONAL MEDICAL EDUCATION
OFFENSE: PROFESSIONAL MISCONDUCT

NOTES: PROFESSIONAL FAILURE TO PRACTICE IN AN ACCEPTABLE MANNER CONSISTENT WITH PUBLIC HEALTH AND WELFARE. CONDITIONS OF PROBATION INCLUDE: 50 HOURS PER YEAR OF CONTINUING MEDICAL EDUCATION CLASSES APPROVED BY THE EXECUTIVE DIRECTOR; MUST APPEAR BEFORE THE BOARD ONCE A YEAR; MUST MAINTAIN SEPARATE FILES OF THOSE RECORDS THAT INDICATE A NEED TO DO PLETHYSMOGRAPHIC TESTS.

GREGORIO, CESAR P JR MD, LICENSE NUMBER 00E7611, WAS DISCIPLINED BY TEXAS ON AUGUST 17, 1996
DISCIPLINARY ACTION: 60-MONTH PROBATION; RESTRICTION PLACED ON CONTROLLED SUBSTANCE LICENSE
OFFENSE: PROFESSIONAL MISCONDUCT

NOTES: AS THE RESULT OF A DRUG AUDIT CONDUCTED BY THE BOARD, IT WAS FOUND THAT HE FAILED TO KEEP ADEQUATE RECORDS REGARDING DISPENSING AND RETENTION OF CONTROLLED SUBSTANCES AND DANGEROUS DRUGS; AND FAILED TO MAINTAIN ADEQUATE SECURITY FOR AND PERFORM PROPER DISPOSAL OF DANGEROUS DRUGS AND CONTROLLED SUBSTANCES. SUSPENSION, STAYED. CONDITIONS OF PROBATION: SHALL OBTAIN AT LEAST 50 HOURS OF CONTINUING MEDICAL EDUCATION CONSISTING OF AT LEAST ONE COURSE IN RISK MANAGEMENT AND ONE COURSE IN ADDICTION AND SHALL SUBMIT PROOF TO THE BOARD; WITHIN ONE YEAR SHALL TAKE AND PASS THE MEDICAL JURISPRUDENCE EXAMINATION; SHALL MAINTAIN A LOGBOOK OF ALL PRESCRIPTIONS FOR CONTROLLED SUBSTANCES OR DANGEROUS DRUGS WITH ADDICTIVE POTENTIAL OR POTENTIAL FOR ABUSE AND MAKE IT AVAILABLE UPON BOARD REQUEST; SHALL NOT POSSESS, ORDER, OR ACCEPT SAMPLES OF ANY CONTROLLED SUBSTANCES OR DANGEROUS DRUGS WITH ADDICTIVE POTENTIAL OR POTENTIAL FOR ABUSE; SHALL APPEAR BEFORE THE BOARD AT LEAST TWICE PER YEAR; SHALL COOPERATE WITH THE BOARD IN VERIFYING COMPLIANCE; SHALL MAINTAIN ADEQUATE MEDICAL RECORDS WHICH SHALL BE MADE AVAILABLE UPON BOARD REQUEST; SHALL GIVE A COPY OF THIS ORDER TO ANY HEALTH CARE ENTITY WHERE HE HAS PRIVILEGES; TIME PERIOD OUT OF TEXAS DOES NOT COUNT TOWARD PROBATION; SHALL INFORM THE BOARD OF CHANGE OF ADDRESS WITHIN 10 DAYS OF IF HE LEAVES THE STATE; SHALL NOT SEEK MODIFICATION FOR ONE YEAR. ON 10/15/99 ORDER MODIFIED DELETING REQUIREMENT OF TWO PERSONAL APPEARANCES PER YEAR BEFORE THE BOARD.

GRIFFIN, STEVEN WAYNE MD, LICENSE NUMBER 00E2587 OF MINEOLA, TX, WAS DISCIPLINED BY TEXAS ON AUGUST 24, 1991
DISCIPLINARY ACTION: SURRENDER OF LICENSE
OFFENSE: CRIMINAL CONVICTION OR PLEA OF GUILTY, NOLO CONTENDERE, OR NO CONTEST TO A CRIME

NOTES: LICENSE VOLUNTARILY SURRENDERED IN LIEU OF FURTHER DISCIPLINARY ACTION DUE TO FELONY CONVICTION OF CONSPIRACY TO OBTAIN A CONTROLLED SUBSTANCE.

GRIFFITH, KARL EDWARD MD, DATE OF BIRTH JULY 11, 1950, LICENSE NUMBER 00G5121 OF 6816 MCCALLUM, DALLAS, TX, WAS

DISCIPLINED BY TEXAS ON AUGUST 20, 1993
DISCIPLINARY ACTION: 120-MONTH PROBATION; RESTRICTION PLACED ON LICENSE
OFFENSE: LOSS OR RESTRICTION OF HOSPITAL PRIVILEGES

NOTES: IN 11/90 WAS ADMITTED FOR POLYSUBSTANCE ABUSE TREATMENT; THEN ENTERED RECOVERY RESIDENCE PROGRAM AT A HOSPITAL; EXPERIENCED DRUG-RELATED WORK DIFFICULTIES DUE TO A RELAPSE IN RECOVERY; HOSPITAL REQUIRED RANDOM DRUG SCREENS; TESTED POSITIVE FOR BENZODIAZEPINES IN 6/91; ALSO ABUSED SUFENTA, FENTANYL AND FORANE ANESTHETIC GAS; WAS REPLACED ON A SURGICAL CASE IN 12/91 WHEN HE WAS NOTED TO BE UNRESPONSIVE, SPONGES SOAKED IN FORANE WERE DISCOVERED IN THE SURGICAL MASK HE WAS WEARING; ANESTHESIA PRIVILEGES WERE SUSPENDED; WAS DISCHARGED FROM A TREATMENT PROGRAM ON 3/27/92 AND HAS CONTINUED AFTERCARE TREATMENT INCLUDING REGULAR AA ATTENDANCE AND THERAPY. REVOCATION STAYED. CONDITIONS OF PROBATION: SHALL ABSTAIN FROM THE CONSUMPTION OF ALCOHOL/DRUGS IN ANY FORM UNLESS PRESCRIBED BY ANOTHER PHYSICIAN FOR A LEGITIMATE AND THERAPEUTIC PURPOSE; SHALL SUBMIT HIMSELF FOR APPROPRIATE EXAMS INCLUDING DRUG OR ALCOHOL SCREENS; UPON BOARD REQUEST SHALL SUBMIT HIMSELF TO SARA CAPNOGRAPH TESTS; SHALL NOT POSSESS, ADMINISTER, DISPENSE OR PRESCRIBE ANY CONTROLLED SUBSTANCES EXCEPT FOR TREATMENT OF INPATIENTS AS A CLINICAL INSTRUCTOR IN ANESTHESIOLOGY; SHALL LIMIT PRACTICE SOLELY TO THE DUTIES OF CLINICAL INSTRUCTOR OF ANESTHESIOLOGY; SHALL BE UNDER THE OBSERVATION OF A PHYSICIAN OR CERTIFIED REGISTERED NURSE ANESTHESIOLOGIST WHILE ADMINISTERING OR SUPERVISING THE ADMINISTRATION OF ANESTHESIA; SHALL CONTINUE TREATMENT BY AN ADDICTIONOLOGIST WITH QUARTERLY REPORTS; SHALL SUBMIT HIMSELF FOR EVALUATION AND TREATMENT TO A BOARD-APPROVED PSYCHIATRIST; SHALL PARTICIPATE IN ACTIVITIES OF A PHYSICIAN HEALTH AND REHABILITATION COMMITTEE AND ATTEND WEEKLY MEETINGS WITH QUARTERLY REPORTS; SHALL PARTICIPATE IN AA'S PROGRAM NOT LESS THAN THREE TIMES A WEEK WITH QUARTERLY REPORTS TO THE BOARD; SHALL ATTEND AT LEAST 50 HOURS PER YEAR OF CONTINUING MEDICAL EDUCATION; SHALL PERFORM 12 HOURS PER MONTH OF COMMUNITY SERVICE WITH QUARTERLY REPORTS TO THE BOARD; SHALL GIVE A COPY OF THIS ORDER TO ANY HEALTH CARE ENTITY WHERE HE HAS PRIVILEGES; SHALL COOPERATE WITH THE BOARD IN VERIFYING COMPLIANCE; SHALL INFORM BOARD OF CHANGE OF ADDRESS WITHIN 10 DAYS OR IF HE LEAVES THE STATE; TIME SPENT OUT OF TEXAS DOES NOT COUNT TOWARD PROBATION. SHALL NOT SEEK MODIFICATION FOR ONE YEAR. ON 1/6/95 ORDER MODIFIED SUCH THAT HE MAY ALSO PRACTICE AS ASSISTANT OR ASSOCIATE PROFESSOR OF ANESTHESIOLOGY; SHALL BE UNDER THE SUPERVISION OF THE HOSPITAL RATHER THAN A SPECIFIED PERSON; COMMUNITY SERVICE REQUIREMENT IS DELETED. ON 8/17/96 THE BOARD DENIED HIS PETITION FOR TERMINATION OF THIS ORDER. ON 10/24/98 ORDER TERMINATED.

GROSS, GEORGE E DO, DATE OF BIRTH AUGUST 13, 1948 OF 400 S. ZANG BOULEVARD #518, DALLAS, TX, WAS DISCIPLINED BY MEDICARE ON JANUARY 5, 1997
DISCIPLINARY ACTION: EXCLUSION FROM THE MEDICARE AND/OR MEDICAID PROGRAM
OFFENSE: NONCOMPLIANCE WITH A PROFESSIONAL RULE

NOTES: DEFAULTED ON PUBLIC HEALTH SERVICE EDUCATION LOAN. REINSTATED ON 2/03/97.

GROSSMAN, MAURICE SIDNEY MD, DATE OF BIRTH JUNE 1, 1927, LICENSE NUMBER 00C3062 OF 1001 LOUISIANA PARKWAY SUITE 307, CORPUS CHRISTI, TX, WAS DISCIPLINED BY TEXAS ON JANUARY 29, 1993
DISCIPLINARY ACTION: REPRIMAND
OFFENSE: SUBSTANDARD CARE, INCOMPETENCE OR NEGLIGENCE

NOTES: ON 4/22/87 A PATIENT CAME TO HIS OFFICE WITH ABDOMINAL PAINS; PRIOR TO AND DURING A PLANNED COLONOSCOPY, A COMBINATION OF VALIUM, DEMEROL IV AND DEMEROL IM AND PHENERGAN WAS ADMINISTERED; THE PATIENT SUFFERED RESPIRATORY AND CARDIAC ARREST, BECAME NEUROLOGICALLY UNRESPONSIVE AND WAS TRANSPORTED TO A HOSPITAL WHERE RESUSCITATION WAS ATTEMPTED; SHE DIED ONE WEEK LATER. SHALL GIVE A COPY OF THIS ORDER TO ANY HEALTH CARE ENTITY WHERE HE HAS PRIVILEGES; SHALL INFORM THE BOARD OF CHANGE OF ADDRESS WITHIN 10 DAYS.

GUERRERO, JORGE MD, LICENSE NUMBER G8154 OF HOUSTON, TX, WAS DISCIPLINED BY TEXAS ON AUGUST 22, 1998
DISCIPLINARY ACTION: MONITORING OF PHYSICIAN PERFORMANCE
OFFENSE: CRIMINAL CONVICTION OR PLEA OF GUILTY, NOLO CONTENDERE, OR NO CONTEST TO A CRIME

NOTES: ARRESTED FOR DRIVING WHILE INTOXICATED ON 3 OCCASIONS: 6/3/93, 6/16/94 & 10/27/95; HE PLED NO CONTEST TO EACH CHARGE. LICENSE LIMITED FOR FIVE YEARS AS FOLLOWS: SHALL ABSTAIN FROM THE CONSUMPTION OF ALCOHOL/DRUGS IN ANY FORM UNLESS PRESCRIBED BY ANOTHER PHYSICIAN FOR A LEGITIMATE AND THERAPEUTIC PURPOSE; SHALL SUBMIT HIMSELF FOR APPROPRIATE EXAMS INCLUDING DRUG OR ALCOHOL SCREENS; SHALL CONTINUE TO RECEIVE CARE AND TREATMENT FROM SPECIFIED DOCTOR EVERY 3 MONTHS WITH QUARTERLY REPORTS; SHALL APPEAR BEFORE THE BOARD UPON REQUEST; SHALL COOPERATE WITH THE BOARD IN VERIFYING COMPLIANCE INCLUDING PROVIDING COPIES OF MEDICAL RELEASES AND PEER REVIEW RECORDS UPON REQUEST; SHALL GIVE A COPY OF THIS ORDER TO ANY HEALTH CARE ENTITY WHERE HE HAS PRIVILEGES; TIME SPENT OUT OF TEXAS DOES NOT COUNT TOWARD RESTRICTION; SHALL INFORM THE BOARD OF CHANGE OF ADDRESS WITHIN 10 DAYS OR IF HE LEAVES THE STATE; SHALL NOT SEEK MODIFICATION FOR ONE YEAR.

GUERRERORAMIREZ, LUIS MD, LICENSE NUMBER 00E0946 OF HOUSTON, TX, WAS DISCIPLINED BY TEXAS ON APRIL 9, 1992
DISCIPLINARY ACTION: LICENSE REVOCATION
OFFENSE: PROFESSIONAL MISCONDUCT

NOTES: SEVERAL VIOLATIONS OF THE MEDICAL PRACTICE ACT, INCLUDING PROFESSIONAL FAILURE TO PRACTICE MEDICINE IN AN ACCEPTABLE MANNER CONSISTENT WITH PUBLIC HEALTH AND WELFARE. HE HAS FILED A MOTION FOR REHEARING WHICH HAD NOT BEEN RULED ON AS OF SUMMER 1992.

GUILLERMO, ROMEO DUNGCA MD, LICENSE NUMBER E9678 OF RICHARDSON, TX, WAS DISCIPLINED BY TEXAS ON AUGUST 22, 1998
DISCIPLINARY ACTION: REPRIMAND
OFFENSE: SUBSTANDARD CARE, INCOMPETENCE OR NEGLIGENCE

NOTES: GAVE RADIOLOGICAL IMPRESSIONS OF SUBSEQUENT

X-RAY FILMS OF RESOLVED "PNEUMONITIS" WHEN THE REVIEWING RADIOLOGIST BELIEVED THAT NO SIGNIFICANT RADIOLOGIC CHANGE HAD TAKEN PLACE IN THE PRESENCE OF CHRONIC INTERSTITIAL FIBROSIS; HE HAS NEVER HAD A MEDICAL LIABILITY CLAIM OR OTHER ADVERSE PEER REVIEW ACTION; SINCE THE EVENTS, HE HAS OBTAINED 80 HOURS OF CONTINUING MEDICAL EDUCATION IN CHEST RADIOLOGY AND HAS ENROLLED IN AN ADDITIONAL 80 HOUR PROGRAM IN GENERAL RADIOLOGY. SHALL GIVE A COPY OF THIS ORDER TO ANY HEALTH CARE ENTITY WHERE HE HAS PRIVILEGES.

GUIMBARDA, LUIS A MD, LICENSE NUMBER 00D2945 OF SAN ANTONIO, TX, WAS DISCIPLINED BY TEXAS ON OCTOBER 5, 1991
DISCIPLINARY ACTION: 24-MONTH PROBATION; REQUIRED TO TAKE ADDITIONAL MEDICAL EDUCATION
OFFENSE: SUBSTANDARD CARE, INCOMPETENCE OR NEGLIGENCE

NOTES: INADEQUATE TREATMENT AND RECORDKEEPING REGARDING THREE PATIENTS SHOWED FAILURE TO PRACTICE MEDICINE IN AN ACCEPTABLE MANNER. CONDITIONS OF PROBATION: SHALL ATTEND AT LEAST 50 HOURS OF CONTINUING MEDICAL EDUCATION WITH 10 HOURS OF DIABETES MANAGEMENT PER YEAR; SHALL OBTAIN CONSULTATION WITH ANOTHER PHYSICIAN WITHIN 48 HOURS OF ADMITTING ANY PATIENT; SHALL NOT PETITION FOR MODIFICATION FOR AT LEAST ONE YEAR; SHALL COOPERATE WITH BOARD IN VERIFYING COMPLIANCE; SHALL ADVISE THE BOARD OF ANY CHANGE OF ADDRESS; TIME SPENT OUT OF STATE DOESN'T COUNT TOWARDS PROBATION.

GUINN, EDWARD WILLIAM MD, LICENSE NUMBER C5701, WAS DISCIPLINED BY TEXAS ON MAY 19, 1997
DISCIPLINARY ACTION: FINE
OFFENSE: NONCOMPLIANCE WITH A PROFESSIONAL RULE

NOTES: DID NOT RESPOND TO A REQUEST FOR MEDICAL RECORDS FROM A PATIENT APPLYING FOR DISABILITY BENEFITS UNDER THE SOCIAL SECURITY ACT. SINCE HE DID NOT RESPOND TO THE REQUEST, A HEARING WAS HELD AND A JUDGE WAS FORCED TO MAKE A DECISION REGARDING THE PATIENT'S DISABILITY WITHOUT THE BENEFIT OF SEEING HER MEDICAL RECORDS. ON 7/22/96 ANOTHER PATIENT SUBMITTED A REQUEST FOR HER MEDICAL RECORDS IN CONNECTION WITH A CLAIM FOR DISABILITY BENEFITS AND AGAIN HE DID NOT RESPOND. AFTER NUMEROUS ATTEMPTS TO OBTAIN THE RECORDS, HE FINALLY RELEASED THE RECORDS WHEN A COURT SUBPOENA WAS ISSUED ON 8/27/96. ADMINISTRATIVE FINE OF $1000; SHALL COOPERATE WITH THE BOARD IN VERIFYING COMPLIANCE; SHALL GIVE A COPY OF THIS ORDER TO ANY HEALTH CARE ENTITY WHERE HE HAS PRIVILEGES; SHALL INFORM THE BOARD OF CHANGE OF ADDRESS WITHIN 10 DAYS.

GULLION, JERRY C MD, LICENSE NUMBER 00C9001 OF MARSHALL, TX, WAS DISCIPLINED BY TEXAS ON JANUARY 26, 1990
DISCIPLINARY ACTION: 36-MONTH REPRIMAND; REQUIRED TO TAKE ADDITIONAL MEDICAL EDUCATION

NOTES: STIPULATED ORDER.

GUNDERSON, ERIK WATERS MD, LICENSE NUMBER J3111 OF PLANO, TX, WAS DISCIPLINED BY TEXAS ON APRIL 10, 1999
DISCIPLINARY ACTION: FINE
OFFENSE: PROFESSIONAL MISCONDUCT

NOTES: USED ADVERTISING THAT IS MISLEADING AND DOES NOT PROVIDE THE NAME OF THE CERTIFYING BOARD; HE INDICATED THAT HE FELT THAT THE ADVERTISEMENT IS A MATTER OF INTERPRETATION AND IS NOT MISLEADING; EVEN THOUGH HE ACKNOWLEDGES THAT THE PERSON PICTURED IN HIS AD IS NOT A PATIENT AND HAS NOT BEEN TO HIS OFFICE; HE ACKNOWLEDGED THAT THE CERTIFYING BOARD IS NOT IDENTIFIED AND STATED THAT HE WAS NOT AWARE OF THIS REQUIREMENT; HE DISCONTINUED THE AD IN THE FALL OF 1997 AND DENIES HE HAS VIOLATED THE MEDICAL PRACTICE ACT. $250 FINE; SHALL COOPERATE WITH THE BOARD IN VERIFYING COMPLIANCE.

GUO, GEORGE S MD, DATE OF BIRTH JUNE 19, 1961, LICENSE NUMBER 00H4368 OF 11123 ASHCOTT, HOUSTON, TX, WAS DISCIPLINED BY TEXAS ON JANUARY 29, 1993
DISCIPLINARY ACTION: LICENSE REVOCATION
OFFENSE: CRIMINAL CONVICTION OR PLEA OF GUILTY, NOLO CONTENDERE, OR NO CONTEST TO A CRIME

NOTES: CONVICTED OF THE FELONY OFFENSE OF BURGLARY OF A HABITATION AND SENTENCED TO 10 YEARS CONFINEMENT WITH SHOCK PROBATION AFTER 90 DAYS AND A FINE; HAS PRACTICED NO MEDICINE SINCE HIS ARREST ON 11/23/90. ORDER WILL BECOME FINAL WHEN ALL APPEALS HAVE BEEN EXHAUSTED.

GURAV, RAMCHANDRA S MD, DATE OF BIRTH MARCH 27, 1935, LICENSE NUMBER 0030126 OF 520 HOSPITAL DRIVE #2, NEW BOSTON, TX, WAS DISCIPLINED BY NEW JERSEY ON MARCH 22, 1991
DISCIPLINARY ACTION: SURRENDER OF LICENSE

NOTES: SHOULD DR. GURAV SEEK TO PRACTICE IN NEW JERSEY IN THE FUTURE, MUST APPEAR BEFORE THE BOARD FOR A STATUS CONFERENCE. THIS MATTER IS RESOLVED WITHOUT ANY FORMAL FINDING BEING MADE BY THE BOARD OF MEDICAL EXAMINERS. THIS DOES NOT CONSTITUTE A SUSPENSION OR REVOCATION.

GURAV, RAMCHANDRA S MD, LICENSE NUMBER 0025523 OF NEW BOSTON, TX, WAS DISCIPLINED BY VIRGINIA ON DECEMBER 16, 1993
DISCIPLINARY ACTION: LICENSE SUSPENSION
OFFENSE: CRIMINAL CONVICTION OR PLEA OF GUILTY, NOLO CONTENDERE, OR NO CONTEST TO A CRIME

NOTES: CRIMINAL CONVICTION OF UNLAWFUL DISPENSING OF SCHEDULE IV CONTROLLED SUBSTANCES.

GURAV, RANCHANDRA S MD, LICENSE NUMBER 0025523 OF 520 HOSPITAL DRIVE, SUITE 2, NEW BOSTON, TX, WAS DISCIPLINED BY VIRGINIA ON JUNE 16, 1994
DISCIPLINARY ACTION: PROBATION; RESTRICTION PLACED ON CONTROLLED SUBSTANCE LICENSE
OFFENSE: CRIMINAL CONVICTION OR PLEA OF GUILTY, NOLO CONTENDERE, OR NO CONTEST TO A CRIME

NOTES: ON 6/8/91 CONVICTED IN TEXAS FOR KNOWINGLY, INTENTIONALLY AND UNLAWFULLY DISPENSING AND CAUSING TO BE DISPENSED A SCHEDULE IV CONTROLLED SUBSTANCE NOT IN THE USUAL COURSE OF PROFESSIONAL PRACTICE FOR A LEGITIMATE MEDICAL PURPOSE. LICENSE REINSTATED FROM SUSPENSION. PROBATION WITH FOLLOWING TERMS AND CONDITIONS: SHALL BE PROHIBITED FROM PRESCRIBING SCHEDULE II CONTROLLED SUBSTANCES IN VIRGINIA EXCEPT IN A HOSPITAL SETTING. ON 5/4/99 PROBATION TERMINATED; FULL, UNRESTRICTED LICENSE ISSUED.

GUSTAFSON, W C JR MD OF 7500 BEECHNUT, HOUSTON, TX, WAS DISCIPLINED BY DEA ON NOVEMBER 19, 1993
DISCIPLINARY ACTION: SURRENDER OF CONTROLLED SUBSTANCE LICENSE
OFFENSE: NONCOMPLIANCE WITH A PROFESSIONAL RULE
NOTES: VIOLATIONS OF THE CONTROLLED SUBSTANCE ACT.

GUSTAFSON, WESLEY C JR MD, LICENSE NUMBER 00C9002 OF SEMINOLE, TX, WAS DISCIPLINED BY TEXAS ON JUNE 22, 1994
DISCIPLINARY ACTION: SURRENDER OF CONTROLLED SUBSTANCE LICENSE; 60-MONTH PROBATION
OFFENSE: OVERPRESCRIBING OR MISPRESCRIBING DRUGS
NOTES: BETWEEN 1/93 AND 12/93 PRESCRIBED LARGE QUANTITIES OF PROPOXYPHENE, HYDROCODONE, SOMA, RESTORIL, PHENERGAN WITH CODEINE, PENTAZOCINE, DIAZEPAM AND TEGRETOL TO TWO PATIENTS WITHOUT ANY LEGITIMATE MEDICAL REASON AND FOR A PERIOD AND IN QUANTITIES FAR IN EXCESS OF THAT INDICATED BY THE PATIENTS' MEDICAL CONDITIONS; THESE PERSONS WERE KNOWN TO HAVE A HISTORY OF SUBSTANCE ABUSE AND HE SHOULD HAVE KNOWN THEY WERE HABITUAL USERS OF DANGEROUS DRUGS; SURRENDERED HIS DEA AND TEXAS CONTROLLED SUBSTANCES CERTIFICATES ON 11/18/93. SUSPENSION STAYED. CONDITIONS OF PROBATION: SHALL APPEAR BEFORE THE BOARD ONCE A YEAR; SHALL ATTEND AT LEAST 50 HOURS PER YEAR OF CONTINUING MEDICAL EDUCATION AT LEAST FIVE HOURS OF WHICH SHALL BE IN THE AREA OF RECORD KEEPING AND/OR RISK MANAGEMENT AND 20 HOURS OF WHICH SHALL BE IN THE AREA OF ADDICTIONOLOGY AND/OR SUBSTANCE ABUSE; SHALL MAINTAIN ADEQUATE MEDICAL RECORDS ON ALL PATIENT OFFICE VISITS WHICH SHALL BE AVAILABLE FOR INSPECTION; SHALL PERSONALLY EXAMINE PATIENTS WHENEVER ANY FORM CERTIFIES THAT A PERSONAL EXAMINATION HAS BEEN PERFORMED AND ALWAYS ON A FIRST VISIT; SHALL NOT TREAT OR OTHERWISE SERVE AS PHYSICIAN, PRESCRIBE, DISPENSE OR ADMINISTER DRUGS THAT MAY BE SUBJECT TO ABUSE TO HIMSELF OR ANY MEMBER OF HIS IMMEDIATE FAMILY; SHALL SURRENDER DEA AND TEXAS CONTROLLED SUBSTANCES CERTIFICATES IF HE HAS NOT ALREADY DONE SO AS WELL AS ALL UNUSED TRIPLICATE PRESCRIPTION FORMS AND ALL CONTROLLED SUBSTANCES IN HIS POSSESSION INCLUDING SAMPLES; SHALL NOT REAPPLY WITHOUT PERMISSION; SEPARATE FROM PATIENT RECORDS, SHALL MAINTAIN A FILE OF ALL PRESCRIPTIONS WRITTEN FOR DANGEROUS DRUGS WHICH SHALL BE AVAILABLE FOR INSPECTION; SHALL NOT TELEPHONE IN ANY PRESCRIPTIONS FOR DANGEROUS DRUGS OR PERMIT ANY PERSON WHO IS NOT LICENSED TO DO SO ON HIS BEHALF; SHALL NOT SERVE AS PHYSICIAN TO CHRONIC PAIN PATIENTS; SHALL GIVE A COPY OF THIS ORDER TO ANY HEALTH CARE ENTITY WHERE HE HAS PRIVILEGES; SHALL COOPERATE WITH THE BOARD IN VERIFYING COMPLIANCE; SHALL INFORM BOARD OF CHANGE OF ADDRESS OR IF HE LEAVES THE STATE; TIME SPENT OUT OF TEXAS DOES NOT COUNT TOWARD PROBATION. SHALL NOT SEEK MODIFICATION FOR ONE YEAR. ON 8/18/95 ORDER MODIFIED AS FOLLOWS: HE IS AUTHORIZED TO REAPPLY TO THE DEA AND THE TEXAS DEPARTMENT OF PUBLIC SAFETY TO OBTAIN FULL PRESCRIBING AUTHORITY FOR CONTROLLED SUBSTANCES; SHALL NOT POSSESS, ADMINISTER, DISPENSE, OR PRESCRIBE ANY CONTROLLED SUBSTANCES EXCEPT AS ARE MEDICALLY NECESSARY FOR THE IMMEDIATE NEEDS OF PATIENTS IN A HOSPITAL EMERGENCY ROOM; SHALL MAINTAIN A LOG OF ALL PRESCRIPTIONS WRITTEN FOR CONTROLLED SUBSTANCES WHICH SHALL BE AVAILABLE FOR REVIEW; HIS ORDERING, ADMINISTERING, AND DISPENSING OF CONTROLLED SUBSTANCES SHALL BE MONITORED BY A LICENSED PHYSICIAN APPROVED BY THE BOARD WHO SHALL COUNSEL HIM ON PERCEIVED DEFICIENCIES AND SUBMIT QUARTERLY REPORTS; ALL OTHER CONDITIONS REMAIN IN EFFECT.

GUTIERREZ, OSCAR V MD, DATE OF BIRTH JANUARY 22, 1958 OF 1502 LOGAN, SUITE 104, LAREDO, TX, WAS DISCIPLINED BY MEDICARE ON DECEMBER 20, 1999
DISCIPLINARY ACTION: EXCLUSION FROM THE MEDICARE AND/OR MEDICAID PROGRAM
OFFENSE: NONCOMPLIANCE WITH A PROFESSIONAL RULE
NOTES: DEFAULTED ON PUBLIC HEALTH SERVICE EDUCATION LOAN. REINSTATED ON 12/21/99.

HAFFKE, OSCAR WILLIAM MD, LICENSE NUMBER 00B8894 OF FORT WORTH, TX, WAS DISCIPLINED BY TEXAS ON MARCH 31, 1994
DISCIPLINARY ACTION: SURRENDER OF LICENSE
NOTES: HAS NOT ADMITTED VIOLATIONS OF MEDICAL PRACTICE ACT; SURRENDER IN LIEU OF FURTHER INVESTIGATION; SHALL NOT PETITION FOR REINSTATEMENT OF LICENSE.

HAGER, JEROME P MD OF COON VALLEY, WI, WAS DISCIPLINED BY IOWA ON MARCH 28, 1997
DISCIPLINARY ACTION: LICENSE REVOCATION
OFFENSE: DISCIPLINARY ACTION BY ANOTHER STATE OR AGENCY
NOTES: TEXAS LICENSE HAD BEEN REVOKED BASED UPON FINDINGS THAT HE WAS GUILTY OF SEXUAL MISCONDUCT AND GENERAL PROFESSIONAL MISCONDUCT.

HAGER, JEROME PETER MD, DATE OF BIRTH JULY 15, 1923, LICENSE NUMBER 0G39489 OF RIVERSIDE, CA, WAS DISCIPLINED BY CALIFORNIA ON DECEMBER 19, 1992
DISCIPLINARY ACTION: SURRENDER OF LICENSE
NOTES: VOLUNTARY SURRENDER WHILE CHARGES PENDING.

HAGER, JEROME PETER MD, DATE OF BIRTH JULY 15, 1923 OF 7101 MAGNOLIA AVENUE SUITE A, RIVERSIDE, CA, WAS DISCIPLINED BY MEDICARE ON AUGUST 2, 1993
DISCIPLINARY ACTION: 60-MONTH EXCLUSION FROM THE MEDICARE AND/OR MEDICAID PROGRAM
OFFENSE: CRIMINAL CONVICTION OR PLEA OF GUILTY, NOLO CONTENDERE, OR NO CONTEST TO A CRIME
NOTES: CONVICTED OF A CRIME RELATED TO THE MEDI-CAL PROGRAM.

HAGER, JEROME PETER MD, DATE OF BIRTH JULY 15, 1923, LICENSE NUMBER 00D2233 OF 5645 VIA CEREZO, RIVERSIDE, CA, WAS DISCIPLINED BY TEXAS ON APRIL 16, 1994
DISCIPLINARY ACTION: LICENSE REVOCATION
OFFENSE: DISCIPLINARY ACTION BY ANOTHER STATE OR AGENCY
NOTES: ON 12/19/92 CALIFORNIA BOARD ACCEPTED SURRENDER OF HIS LICENSE BASED ON FINDINGS THAT HE WAS GUILTY OF SEXUAL MISCONDUCT AND SEXUAL RELATIONS WITH TWO CASES WHO WERE PSYCHIATRIC PATIENTS, GROSS NEGLIGENCE AND GENERAL UNPROFESSIONAL CONDUCT. ORDER WILL BECOME FINAL WHEN APPEALS HAVE BEEN EXHAUSTED. HE HAS 20 DAYS TO FILE A MOTION FOR REHEARING.

HALBERT, HORACE BURNARD JR MD, LICENSE NUMBER 00C6965 OF FRANKSTON, TX, WAS DISCIPLINED BY TEXAS ON JANUARY 14, 1994
DISCIPLINARY ACTION: 60-MONTH PROBATION; REQUIRED TO TAKE ADDITIONAL MEDICAL EDUCATION
OFFENSE: NONCOMPLIANCE WITH A PROFESSIONAL RULE

NOTES: INVESTIGATED ALLEGATIONS RELATED TO ALLEGED ACTION TAKEN BY TEXAS MEDICAL FOUNDATION; FOUND THAT MANY, IF NOT ALL OF HIS PROBLEMS AROSE FROM HIS FAILURE TO ADEQUATELY DOCUMENT PATIENT RECORDS DUE TO HIS EXTREMELY HEAVY PATIENT LOAD; HE DENIES ANY WRONGDOING. IN LIEU OF A CONTESTED CASE HEARING THIS AGREEMENT WAS REACHED. FIVE YEAR SUSPENSION STAYED. CONDITIONS OF PROBATION: SHALL APPEAR BEFORE THE BOARD ONCE A YEAR; SHALL ATTEND AT LEAST 50 HOURS PER YEAR OF CONTINUING MEDICAL EDUCATION; SHALL BE SUPERVISED BY A BOARD-APPROVED PHYSICIAN WITH REPORTS TO THE BOARD THREE TIMES A YEAR; SHALL MAINTAIN ADEQUATE MEDICAL RECORDS ON ALL PATIENT OFFICE VISITS WHICH SHALL BE AVAILABLE FOR REVIEW; SHALL COOPERATE WITH THE BOARD IN VERIFYING COMPLIANCE; SHALL INFORM BOARD OF CHANGE OF ADDRESS WITHIN 10 DAYS OR IF HE LEAVES THE STATE; TIME SPENT OUT OF TEXAS DOES NOT COUNT TOWARD PROBATION. SHALL NOT SEEK MODIFICATION FOR ONE YEAR. ON 3/4/95 ORDER MODIFIED SO THAT IF HE PRACTICES OUTSIDE THE INSTITUTIONAL SETTING OF THE TEXAS DEPARTMENT OF CRIMINAL JUSTICE, HIS MEDICAL PRACTICE SHALL BE SUPERVISED BY A BOARD APPROVED PHYSICIAN WHO SHALL COUNSEL HIM WITH REGARD TO PERCEIVED DEFICIENCIES AND WHO SHALL MAKE REPORTS TO THE BOARD EVERY FOUR MONTHS; ALL OTHER CONDITIONS REMAIN IN EFFECT. ON 3/1/97 PETITION TO TERMINATE ORDER DENIED; ORDER MODIFIED TO ALLOW HIM TO REQUEST MODIFICATION OR TERMINATION ONCE EVERY SIX MONTHS. ON 11/22/97 ORDER TERMINATED.

HALCOMB, WILLIAM W DO, LICENSE NUMBER 00E5774 OF MESA, AZ, WAS DISCIPLINED BY TEXAS ON SEPTEMBER 28, 1990
DISCIPLINARY ACTION: SURRENDER OF LICENSE

HALCOMB, WILLIAM W MD, LICENSE NUMBER 0A27934 OF MESA, AZ, WAS DISCIPLINED BY CALIFORNIA ON JANUARY 17, 1995
DISCIPLINARY ACTION: 60-MONTH PROBATION
OFFENSE: DISCIPLINARY ACTION BY ANOTHER STATE OR AGENCY

NOTES: SURRENDER OF LICENSE TO TEXAS BOARD WHILE UNDER INVESTIGATION. REVOCATION STAYED.

HALEY, RICHARD K DO, LICENSE NUMBER 00C9286 OF WESTERVILLE, OH, WAS DISCIPLINED BY TEXAS ON JANUARY 24, 1992
DISCIPLINARY ACTION: LICENSE REVOCATION
OFFENSE: CRIMINAL CONVICTION OR PLEA OF GUILTY, NOLO CONTENDERE, OR NO CONTEST TO A CRIME

NOTES: CONVICTION OF FELONY.

HALFON, VICTOR J MD, DATE OF BIRTH DECEMBER 5, 1916, LICENSE NUMBER 00D1664 OF 6521 HARRISBURG, HOUSTON, TX, WAS DISCIPLINED BY TEXAS ON JUNE 15, 1993
DISCIPLINARY ACTION: 60-MONTH RESTRICTION PLACED ON CONTROLLED SUBSTANCE LICENSE; REQUIRED TO TAKE ADDITIONAL MEDICAL EDUCATION
OFFENSE: DISCIPLINARY ACTION BY ANOTHER STATE OR AGENCY

NOTES: ON 7/19/91 DEA ISSUED AN ORDER TO SHOW CAUSE PROPOSING TO REVOKE HIS DEA CERTIFICATE ALLEGING THAT FROM 8/89 TO 1/90 HE SOLD AND DISPENSED PHENTERMINE, A SCHEDULE IV CONTROLLED SUBSTANCE TO DEA UNDERCOVER OFFICERS WITHOUT A LEGITIMATE MEDICAL PURPOSE; IN LIEU OF A HEARING AND WITHOUT ADMITTING TO CHARGES HE ENTERED INTO A MEMO OF AGREEMENT WITH THE DEA WITH VARIOUS CONDITIONS. LICENSE RESTRICTED FOR FIVE YEARS WITH THE FOLLOWING CONDITIONS: SHALL NOT DISPENSE ANY CONTROLLED SUBSTANCES OR SHALL NOT ORDER, REQUEST, PURCHASE OR RECEIVE ANY FOR OFFICE USE; SHALL PRESCRIBE NO MORE THAN A 14 A DAY SUPPLY OF CONTROLLED SUBSTANCES PER PATIENT FOR WEIGHT REDUCTION; SHALL MAINTAIN A SEPARATE FILE CONSISTING OF A COPY OF EVERY PRESCRIPTION WRITTEN FOR CONTROLLED SUBSTANCES WHICH SHALL BE AVAILABLE FOR INSPECTION; SHALL COMPLY WITH ALL TERMS OF DEA MEMORANDUM OF AGREEMENT; SHALL COMPLETE WITHIN ONE YEAR A CONTINUING MEDICAL EDUCATION PHARMACOLOGY COURSE OR COURSES FOR A TOTAL OF 20 HOURS; IN ADDITION SHALL COMPLETE 50 HOURS PER YEAR; SHALL APPEAR BEFORE THE BOARD ONCE A YEAR UPON REQUEST; SHALL GIVE A COPY OF THIS ORDER TO ANY HEALTH CARE ENTITY WHERE HE HAS PRIVILEGES; SHALL COOPERATE WITH THE BOARD IN VERIFYING COMPLIANCE; SHALL INFORM BOARD OF CHANGE OF ADDRESS WITHIN 10 DAYS OR IF HE LEAVES THE STATE; TIME SPENT OUT OF TEXAS DOES NOT COUNT TOWARD RESTRICTION. SHALL NOT SEEK MODIFICATION FOR ONE YEAR. ON 1/6/95 BOARD DENIED REQUEST TO TERMINATE THE ORDER; HOWEVER IT WAS MODIFIED SUCH THAT THE TIME ALLOWED FOR COMPLETION OF 20 HOURS OF A PHARMACOLOGY COURSE WAS EXTENDED TO WITHIN ONE YEAR OF THE MODIFICATION ORDER. ON 1/18/97 BOARD GRANTED HIS PETITION FOR TERMINATION OF THIS ORDER BASED ON COMPLIANCE WITH CONDITIONS.

HALFON, VICTOR J MD OF 6521 HARRISBURG, HOUSTON, TX, WAS DISCIPLINED BY DEA ON NOVEMBER 16, 1993
DISCIPLINARY ACTION: RESTRICTION PLACED ON CONTROLLED SUBSTANCE LICENSE

NOTES: MEMORANDUM OF AGREEMENT SIGNED ON 08/29/91.

HALFON, VICTOR J MD OF 6521 HARRISBURG, HOUSTON, TX, WAS DISCIPLINED BY DEA ON OCTOBER 10, 1996
DISCIPLINARY ACTION: RESTRICTION PLACED ON CONTROLLED SUBSTANCE LICENSE

NOTES: MEMO OF AGREEMENT IN LIEU OF PUBLIC INTEREST REVOCATION.

HALL, JAMES A MD, LICENSE NUMBER 0007604 OF ORMOND BEACH, FL, WAS DISCIPLINED BY FLORIDA ON DECEMBER 19, 1990
DISCIPLINARY ACTION: SURRENDER OF LICENSE

NOTES: IN LIEU OF FURTHER PROSECUTION, AGREED TO NEVER AGAIN APPLY FOR LICENSURE IN FLORIDA.

HALL, JAMES A MD, LICENSE NUMBER 00C9003 OF DALLAS, TX, WAS DISCIPLINED BY TEXAS ON FEBRUARY 22, 1991
DISCIPLINARY ACTION: REPRIMAND
OFFENSE: PROFESSIONAL MISCONDUCT

NOTES: ENGAGED IN INAPPROPRIATE PHYSICAL CONTACT WITH A PATIENT.

HAMAMCY, THARWAT DR OF MILLSAP, TX, WAS DISCIPLINED BY ILLINOIS ON OCTOBER 1, 1994
DISCIPLINARY ACTION: LICENSE REVOCATION
OFFENSE: DISCIPLINARY ACTION BY ANOTHER STATE OR AGENCY

NOTES: DISCIPLINED IN TEXAS.

HAMAMCY, THARWAT MD, LICENSE NUMBER 0117908 OF 925 SANTA ISABEL, LAGUNA VISTA, TX, WAS DISCIPLINED BY NEW YORK ON APRIL 17, 1995
DISCIPLINARY ACTION: LICENSE REVOCATION
OFFENSE: DISCIPLINARY ACTION BY ANOTHER STATE OR AGENCY

NOTES: CONVICTED OF THE BRIBERY OF A BANK OFFICIAL AND DISCIPLINED BY TEXAS FOR NEGLIGENCE AND FAILURE TO MAINTAIN ACCURATE PATIENT RECORDS.

HAMAMCY, THARWAT M MD, DATE OF BIRTH SEPTEMBER 20, 1943, LICENSE NUMBER 00G2715 OF 925 SANTA ISABEL, LAGUNA VISTA, TX, WAS DISCIPLINED BY TEXAS ON JUNE 25, 1993
DISCIPLINARY ACTION: LICENSE REVOCATION
OFFENSE: SUBSTANDARD CARE, INCOMPETENCE OR NEGLIGENCE

NOTES: PRACTICE INCONSISTENT WITH PUBLIC HEALTH AND WELFARE INCLUDING: CHARGING A PATIENT 3 TIMES FOR THE SAME TREATMENT; DID NOT USE, AT THE PATIENT'S REQUEST, AN IV DURING A HERNIA OPERATION PERFORMED IN HIS OFFICE WHICH WAS IMPORTANT FOR THE PATIENT'S SAFETY; WROTE HIS OPERATIVE REPORT FOR THIS SURGERY TWO YEARS LATER TO SUBMIT TO THE BOARD WITH REPORT FALSELY DATED WITH THE DATE OF SURGERY; IN SEVERAL INSTANCES FAILED TO DOCUMENT IN MEDICAL RECORDS SUFFICIENT INFORMATION OF PATIENTS TO WHOM HE HAD GIVEN PRENATAL CARE; TREATED A PATIENT WITH FLAGYL DURING HER FIRST TRIMESTER EVEN THOUGH FLAGYL IS CONTRAINDICATED UNLESS OTHER TREATMENTS HAVE BEEN TRIED; FAILED TO ORDER PRENATAL LAB TESTS FOR ONE PATIENT; FAILED TO ARRANGE MEDICAL COVERAGE WITH ANOTHER DOCTOR IN HIS ABSENCE FOR THIS PATIENT; DID NOT TRANSFER THIS PATIENT TO A MORE APPROPRIATELY EQUIPPED HOSPITAL; FAILED TO ADEQUATELY TREAT THE HIGH BLOOD PRESSURE OF ANOTHER PATIENT. ORDER WILL BECOME FINAL WHEN ALL APPEALS HAVE BEEN EXHAUSTED.

HAMAMCY, THARWAT M MD OF 925 SANTA ISABEL BOULEVARD, LAGUNA VISTA, TX, WAS DISCIPLINED BY DEA ON APRIL 28, 1994
DISCIPLINARY ACTION: SURRENDER OF CONTROLLED SUBSTANCE LICENSE
OFFENSE: DISCIPLINARY ACTION BY ANOTHER STATE OR AGENCY

NOTES: STATE BOARD.

HAMPTON, RAYMOND MADISON MD, LICENSE NUMBER B9647 OF PAMPA, TX, WAS DISCIPLINED BY TEXAS ON DECEMBER 12, 1998
DISCIPLINARY ACTION: FINE; REPRIMAND
OFFENSE: SUBSTANDARD CARE, INCOMPETENCE OR NEGLIGENCE

NOTES: BETWEEN 6/1/93 - 6/5/93 HE TREATED A PATIENT WHOSE PARENTS HAD PREVIOUSLY CONSULTED 2 OTHER PHYSICIANS AT 2 DIFFERENT HOSPITALS REGARDING HER SORE THROAT AND ELEVATED TEMPERATURE; THE 2 PHYSICIANS TREATED HER AS HAVING STREP THROAT; ON 6/1 HE ADMITTED PATIENT TO THE HOSPITAL WITH A DIAGNOSIS OF STREP THROAT; THE NEXT DAY HE CALLED A PEDIATRIC CONSULTANT AND THOUGHT A BLOOD CULTURE HAD BEEN ORDERED; HOWEVER, THE MEDICAL RECORD DOES NOT REFLECT THAT HE OR THE PEDIATRICIAN ORDERED A BLOOD CULTURE; HE FAILED TO FOLLOW-UP ON THE LACK OF BLOOD CULTURE EVEN THOUGH HE DISCUSSED THE POSSIBILITY OF SEPTICEMIA WITH CONSULTING PHYSICIANS; ON 6/3 HE SAW THE PATIENT AND REPORTED THAT THE CHILD "APPEARED WELL" AND "NON-TOXIC" AND LAB STUDIES HAD IMPROVED AS TO THE INFECTION; ON 6/4 THE PATIENT CONTINUED TO COMPLAIN OF ABDOMINAL SORENESS AND NAUSEA BUT THERE WERE "GOOD BOWEL SOUNDS"; BY 6/5 HER CONDITION WORSENED WITH SWELLING OF HER FACE AND OTHER INDICATIONS OF CENTRAL NERVOUS SYSTEM INVOLVEMENT; ON 6/5 HE TRANSFERRED HER TO A LARGER AND TERTIARY CARE FACILITY; ON 6/6 THE PATIENT DIED IN THAT FACILITY; UNTIL 6/6 NONE OF THE SEVEN PHYSICIANS WHO HAD SEEN HER, INCLUDING 2 PHYSICIANS RECEIVING HER AT THE TRANSFER FACILITY, CONSIDERED ROCKY MOUNTAIN SPOTTED FEVER ("RMSF") UNTIL A RELATIVE OF THE PATIENT INFORMED THE CARE TEAM THAT THE PATIENT HAD RECENTLY SUFFERED A TICK BITE; NO AUTOPSY WAS PERFORMED TO CONFIRM THE PRESENCE OF RMSF, AND THE CAUSE OF DEATH WAS LISTED AS SEPSIS; RMSF IS DIFFICULT TO DIAGNOSE IN ITS EARLY STAGES AND IS IMPOSSIBLE TO DISTINGUISH SEVERE CASES FROM OTHER POTENTIAL FATAL INFECTIONS THAT CAN MIMIC IT TO A REMARKABLE DEGREE; HE INITIALLY FAILED TO CONFIRM OR REFUTE THE ADMITTING DIAGNOSIS OF STREP THROAT AND FAILED TO TIMELY TRANSFER THE PATIENT ON 6/3 OR 6/4 WHEN SHE CONTINUED TO FARE POORLY;$2,000 FINE.

HANNA, CONSTANCE I MD, LICENSE NUMBER 00D9480 OF AUSTIN, TX, WAS DISCIPLINED BY TEXAS ON MAY 11, 1995
DISCIPLINARY ACTION: FINE
OFFENSE: NONCOMPLIANCE WITH A PROFESSIONAL RULE

NOTES: IN 6/94, FAILED TO TIMELY FURNISH COPIES OF MEDICAL RECORDS TO THE BOARD AS REQUESTED. SHALL PAY $1,500 FINE; SHALL COOPERATE WITH BOARD IN VERIFYING COMPLIANCE.

HANTON, EDWARD M MD, LICENSE NUMBER 0D33063 OF 5103 OVERHILL DR, COLLEYVILLE, TX, WAS DISCIPLINED BY MARYLAND ON DECEMBER 13, 1995
DISCIPLINARY ACTION: FINE
OFFENSE: NONCOMPLIANCE WITH A PROFESSIONAL RULE

NOTES: FAILED TO NOTIFY THE BOARD OF HIS CHANGE OF ADDRESS. $100 FINE.

HARDEY, CARLTON E MD, LICENSE NUMBER 00C3071 OF ARLINGTON, TX, WAS DISCIPLINED BY TEXAS ON FEBRUARY 26, 1990
DISCIPLINARY ACTION: RESTRICTION PLACED ON LICENSE; REPRIMAND
OFFENSE: PROFESSIONAL MISCONDUCT

NOTES: PROFESSIONAL FAILURE TO PRACTICE MEDICINE IN ACCEPTABLE MANNER CONSISTENT WITH PUBLIC HEALTH AND WELFARE. REQUIRED TO ATTEND RISK MANAGEMENT COURSE. MUST HAVE ATTENDANT PRESENT WHEN PERFORMING CERTAIN EXAMINATIONS. ON 6/22/94 THIS ORDER WAS TERMINATED.

HARDY, ROBERT HOWARD MD, LICENSE NUMBER 00E6401 OF COLLEYVILLE, TX, WAS DISCIPLINED BY TEXAS ON APRIL 20, 1991
DISCIPLINARY ACTION: 60-MONTH PROBATION; MONITORING OF PHYSICIAN PERFORMANCE

NOTES: CONDITIONS OF PROBATION INCLUDE: MUST APPEAR ANNUALLY BEFORE THE BOARD; MUST PARTICIPATE

IN AA; MUST SUBMIT TO ALCOHOL OR DRUG SCREENS; MUST CONTINUE TREATMENT WITH SPECIFIED PHYSICIAN WHO WILL SUBMIT QUARTERLY REPORTS TO THE BOARD. ON 4/15/94 ORDER MODIFIED AS FOLLOWS: PARTICIPATION IN AA REDUCED TO ONCE A WEEK; REQUIREMENT OF QUARTERLY REPORTS TO THE BOARD FROM HIS TREATING PHYSICIAN MODIFIED TO BIANNUAL REPORTS.

HARGETT, JOHN M MD, LICENSE NUMBER G3430 OF MCKINNEY, TX, WAS DISCIPLINED BY TEXAS ON AUGUST 9, 1997
DISCIPLINARY ACTION: LICENSE SUSPENSION
OFFENSE: SUBSTANCE ABUSE

NOTES: IN 1967 WAS CONVICTED FOR DRIVING WHILE INTOXICATED; IN 1977 WAS CONVICTED FOR PUBLIC INTOXICATION; IN 1992 HE WAS DIAGNOSED WITH AND TREATED FOR ALCOHOL DEPENDENCY; HE REPORTS A SOBRIETY DATE OF 6/3/97 AND MAINTAINS THAT HE MAY NOT BE AN ALCOHOLIC. SUSPENSION UNTIL HE REQUESTS TO HAVE HIS SUSPENSION STAYED OR APPEARS BEFORE THE BOARD WITH SUFFICIENT EVIDENCE THAT HE IS PHYSICALLY, MENTALLY AND OTHERWISE COMPETENT TO SAFELY PRACTICE MEDICINE INCLUDING AT A MINIMUM COMPLETE COPIES OF MEDICAL RECORDS AND REPORTS OF PSYCHOLOGICAL AND NEUROPSYCHIATRIC EVALUATIONS, INCLUDING A 96 HOUR INPATIENT EVALUATION CONDUCTED BY A BOARD-APPROVED CERTIFIED PSYCHIATRIST; SHALL COOPERATE WITH THE BOARD IN VERIFYING COMPLIANCE INCLUDING PROVIDING COPIES OF MEDICAL RELEASES UPON REQUEST; SHALL INFORM THE BOARD OF CHANGE OF ADDRESS WITHIN 10 DAYS; SHALL NOT SEEK MODIFICATION FOR ONE YEAR.

HARGETT, JOHN M MD, LICENSE NUMBER G3430 OF MCKINNEY, TX, WAS DISCIPLINED BY TEXAS ON DECEMBER 12, 1998
DISCIPLINARY ACTION: 60-MONTH PROBATION; MONITORING OF PHYSICIAN PERFORMANCE
OFFENSE: SUBSTANCE ABUSE

NOTES: ON 8/9/97 THE BOARD DISCIPLINED HIM BASED UPON INTEMPERATE USE OF ALCOHOL WHICH PROVIDED THAT HIS LICENSE WAS SUSPENDED UNTIL HE PROVIDES SUFFICIENT EVIDENCE THAT HE IS COMPETENT TO PRACTICE; IN 7 & 8/97 HE SUBMITTED HIMSELF FOR AN EVALUATION; HE IS CURRENTLY UNDER THE CARE OF A CHEMICAL DEPENDENCY COUNSELOR. SUSPENSION STAYED FOR PROBATION WITH FOLLOWING TERMS AND CONDITIONS: SHALL ABSTAIN FROM THE CONSUMPTION OF ALCOHOL/DRUGS IN ANY FORM UNLESS PRESCRIBED BY ANOTHER PHYSICIAN FOR A LEGITIMATE AND THERAPEUTIC PURPOSE; SHALL SUBMIT HIMSELF FOR APPROPRIATE EXAMS INCLUDING DRUG OR ALCOHOL SCREENS; SHALL NOMINATE THREE CERTIFIED PSYCHIATRISTS FOR BOARD SELECTION OF A THERAPIST AND SHALL EXPEDITIOUSLY SUBMIT HIMSELF TO EVALUATION AND TREATMENT BY THE APPROVED PRACTITIONER; SHALL PARTICIPATE IN THE ACTIVITIES OF A PHYSICIAN HEALTH AND REHABILITATION COMMITTEE AND ATTEND WEEKLY MEETINGS WITH QUARTERLY REPORTS; SHALL PARTICIPATE IN AA'S PROGRAM NOT LESS THAN THREE TIMES A WEEK; SHALL REPORT ON HIS ATTENDANCE; SHALL NOT TREAT OR OTHERWISE SERVE AS PHYSICIAN, PRESCRIBE, DISPENSE OR ADMINISTER DRUGS THAT MAY BE SUBJECT TO ABUSE TO HIMSELF OR TO ANY MEMBER OF HIS FAMILY; SHALL APPEAR BEFORE THE BOARD AT LEAST ONCE A YEAR; SHALL COOPERATE WITH THE BOARD IN VERIFYING COMPLIANCE INCLUDING PROVIDING COPIES OF MEDICAL RELEASES UPON REQUEST; TIME SPENT OUT OF TEXAS DOES NOT COUNT TOWARD PROBATION; SHALL INFORM THE BOARD OF CHANGE OF ADDRESS WITHIN 10 DAYS OR IF HE LEAVES THE STATE; SHALL NOT SEEK MODIFICATION FOR ONE YEAR.

HARGETT, JOHN M MD, DATE OF BIRTH DECEMBER 10, 1948 OF PO BOX 1954, VAN ALSTYNE, TX, WAS DISCIPLINED BY MEDICARE ON DECEMBER 20, 1998
DISCIPLINARY ACTION: EXCLUSION FROM THE MEDICARE AND/OR MEDICAID PROGRAM
OFFENSE: DISCIPLINARY ACTION BY ANOTHER STATE OR AGENCY

NOTES: LICENSE REVOKED, SUSPENDED, SURRENDERED OR OTHERWISE LOST FOR REASONS BEARING ON PROFESSIONAL PERFORMANCE, PROFESSIONAL COMPETENCE OR FINANCIAL INTEGRITY.

HARMON, DAVID R DO, DATE OF BIRTH DECEMBER 6, 1947, LICENSE NUMBER 0020974, WAS DISCIPLINED BY COLORADO ON JANUARY 12, 1996
DISCIPLINARY ACTION: EMERGENCY SUSPENSION
OFFENSE: PHYSICAL OR MENTAL ILLNESS INHIBITING THE ABILITY TO PRACTICE WITH SKILL AND SAFETY

NOTES: PHYSICAL OR MENTAL DISABILITY WHICH RENDERS HIM UNABLE TO PERFORM MEDICAL SERVICES WITH REASONABLE SKILL AND SAFETY.

HARMON, DAVID R DO OF 595 OBSERVATORY DRIVE, COLORADO SPRINGS, CO, WAS DISCIPLINED BY DEA ON APRIL 9, 1996
DISCIPLINARY ACTION: SURRENDER OF CONTROLLED SUBSTANCE LICENSE

NOTES: IN LIEU OF ORDER TO SHOW CAUSE.

HARMON, DAVID R DO, DATE OF BIRTH DECEMBER 6, 1947, LICENSE NUMBER 0020974, WAS DISCIPLINED BY COLORADO ON AUGUST 14, 1996
DISCIPLINARY ACTION: LICENSE REVOCATION
OFFENSE: CRIMINAL CONVICTION OR PLEA OF GUILTY, NOLO CONTENDERE, OR NO CONTEST TO A CRIME

NOTES: CONVICTION OF A LAW REGULATING CONTROLLED SUBSTANCES, HABITUAL INTEMPERANCE OR EXCESSIVE USE OF HABIT FORMING DRUG; FRAUD, MISREPRESENTATION OR DECEPTION IN APPLYING FOR A LICENSE; PHYSICAL OR MENTAL DISABILITY; FAILURE TO ACCURATELY ANSWER THE QUESTIONNAIRE ACCOMPANYING THE RENEWAL FORM AND FAILURE TO RESPOND IN A TIMELY MANNER TO A COMPLAINT.

HARMON, DAVID R DO, LICENSE NUMBER E9684 OF GRAND JUNCTION, CO, WAS DISCIPLINED BY TEXAS ON AUGUST 9, 1997
DISCIPLINARY ACTION: LICENSE SUSPENSION; REQUIRED TO ENTER AN IMPAIRED PHYSICIAN PROGRAM OR SUBSTANCE ABUSE TREATMENT
OFFENSE: DISCIPLINARY ACTION BY ANOTHER STATE OR AGENCY

NOTES: IN 8/93, HE WAS NONJUDICIALLY PUNISHED BY THE US NAVY CONCERNING ALLEGATIONS THAT HE WAS ALLEGEDLY UNABLE TO PERFORM HIS MEDICAL DUTIES, WHILE SERVING AS A RESIDENT IN THE NAVAL RESIDENCY PROGRAM, DUE TO ALLEGEDLY BEING UNDER THE INFLUENCE OF A MOOD ALTERING CHEMICAL SUBSTANCE ON A SPECIFIC DATE IN 6/93. IN 5/94, HE WAS TERMINATED FROM THE NAVAL RESIDENCY PROGRAM; FROM SEPTEMBER THROUGH DECEMBER 1995 HE WAS EVALUATED BY THE COLORADO PHYSICIAN HEALTH PROGRAM; HE FAILED

TO ENGAGE IN THEIR RECOMMENDED TREATMENT PROGRAM. IN 1/96 THE COLORADO BOARD SUMMARILY SUSPENDED HIS LICENSE AND IN 8/96, REVOKED HIS COLORADO LICENSE. HE DID NOT SELF-REPORT HIS INTEMPERANCE. SUSPENSION UNTIL HE REQUESTS TO HAVE THE SUSPENSION STAYED AND APPEARS BEFORE THE BOARD TO PROVIDE SUFFICIENT EVIDENCE THAT HE IS PHYSICALLY, MENTALLY, AND OTHERWISE COMPETENT TO SAFELY PRACTICE. SUCH EVIDENCE SHALL INCLUDE AT A MINIMUM, A CERTIFIED ORDER OF THE COLORADO BOARD REINSTATING HIS COLORADO LICENSE WITHOUT ANY RESTRICTIONS OR SUBSEQUENT DISCIPLINARY ACTION; COMPLETE MEDICAL RECORDS AND REPORTS OF PSYCHOLOGICAL AND NEUROPSYCHIATRIC EVALUATIONS CONDUCTED BY CERTIFIED PSYCHIATRIST(S); ALL PRIOR MEDICAL RECORDS FROM ANY TREATING PHYSICIAN OR FACILITY INCLUDING CHEMICAL DEPENDENCY TREATMENT FACILITIES, SATISFACTORY EVIDENCE THAT HE IS UNDER AN AFTERCARE MONITORING CONTRACT AND PARTICIPATING IN AA WITH A SPONSOR; COMPLETION OF ALL CONTINUING MEDICAL EDUCATION REQUIREMENTS DURING THE PERIOD OF SUSPENSION. UPON SUCH PROOF HE SHALL BE PLACED ON PROBATION WITH TERMS AND CONDITIONS. HE SHALL COOPERATE WITH THE BOARD IN VERIFYING COMPLIANCE INCLUDING PROVIDING COPIES OF MEDICAL RELEASES AND REPORTS SUBMITTED TO COLORADO UPON REQUEST; SHALL GIVE A COPY OF THIS ORDER TO ANY HEALTH CARE ENTITY WHERE HE HAS PRIVILEGES; SHALL PROVIDE A COPY OF THIS ORDER TO ANYONE REQUESTING IT WITHIN 10 DAYS; SHALL INFORM THE BOARD OF CHANGE OF ADDRESS WITHIN 10 DAYS.

HARMON, JOHN B JR MD OF 14585 ROBERT I WALKER, AUSTIN, TX, WAS DISCIPLINED BY DEA ON MAY 26, 1998
DISCIPLINARY ACTION: SURRENDER OF CONTROLLED SUBSTANCE LICENSE
NOTES: IN LIEU OF PUBLIC INTEREST REVOCATION.

HARRISON, JACK WINFRED MD, DATE OF BIRTH SEPTEMBER 10, 1935, LICENSE NUMBER 00D4777 OF 217 AVALON, DE SOTO, TX, WAS DISCIPLINED BY TEXAS ON JUNE 10, 1991
DISCIPLINARY ACTION: 60-MONTH PROBATION; RESTRICTION PLACED ON LICENSE
OFFENSE: SUBSTANDARD CARE, INCOMPETENCE OR NEGLIGENCE
NOTES: PROFESSIONAL INCOMPETENCE LIKELY TO INJURE THE PUBLIC, INABILITY TO PRACTICE MEDICINE WITH REASONABLE SKILL AND SAFETY TO PATIENTS, AND INTEMPERATE USE OF ALCOHOL OR DRUGS. SHALL NOT PERFORM ANY SURGERY; MUST SUBMIT TO ALCOHOL OR DRUG SCREENS. ON 8/20/93 ORDER TERMINATED AND LICENSE FREE AND CLEAR OF ANY PREVIOUS RESTRICTIONS.

HARRISON, MARK L MD, LICENSE NUMBER G4598 OF KEY BISCAYNE, FL, WAS DISCIPLINED BY TEXAS ON AUGUST 9, 1997
DISCIPLINARY ACTION: FINE; REPRIMAND
OFFENSE: PROFESSIONAL MISCONDUCT
NOTES: HE OPERATED A CLINIC IN HOUSTON, TEXAS, WHICH SPECIALIZED IN THE REMOVAL OF TATTOOS, BIRTHMARKS, AND OTHER SKIN DISCOLORATIONS. HIS ADVERTISEMENTS INDICATED THAT LASER TREATMENTS WERE PERFORMED BY A DELEGATE ASSOCIATE OF A LICENSED PHYSICIAN. HE SERVED AS THE SUPERVISING PHYSICIAN OF THIS FACILITY, HOWEVER, HE DID NOT EXAMINE ANY PATIENT OR REVIEW PATIENT CHARTS. HE ALLOWED UNLICENSED OFFICE STAFF TO SEE PATIENTS AND MAKE ALL TREATMENT DECISIONS. SHALL PAY A $1000 ADMINISTRATIVE PENALTY; SHALL GIVE A COPY OF THIS ORDER TO ANY HEALTH CARE ENTITY WHERE HE HAS PRIVILEGES; SHALL COOPERATE WITH THE BOARD IN VERIFYING COMPLIANCE.

HARRISON, MARK L MD, LICENSE NUMBER C42910 OF KEY BISCAYNE, FL, WAS DISCIPLINED BY CALIFORNIA ON JANUARY 13, 1998
DISCIPLINARY ACTION: REPRIMAND
OFFENSE: DISCIPLINARY ACTION BY ANOTHER STATE OR AGENCY
NOTES: DISCIPLINED BY TEXAS FOR INADEQUATE SUPERVISION OF MEDICAL ACTIVITIES AND FOR AIDING AND ABETTING THE UNLICENSED PRACTICE OF MEDICINE.

HARRISON, MARK L MD, LICENSE NUMBER 47889 OF KEY BISCAYNE, OH, WAS DISCIPLINED BY OHIO ON OCTOBER 14, 1998
DISCIPLINARY ACTION: LICENSE REVOCATION
OFFENSE: DISCIPLINARY ACTION BY ANOTHER STATE OR AGENCY
NOTES: PRIOR ACTION BY TEXAS MEDICAL BOARD BASED ON FINDINGS THAT HE HAD FAILED TO EXAMINE ANY PATIENT OR REVIEW PATIENT CHARTS, AND HAD ALLOWED UNLICENSED OFFICE STAFF TO SEE PATIENTS AND MAKE TREATMENT DECISIONS.

HARRISON, MARK L MD, DATE OF BIRTH JUNE 12, 1957, LICENSE NUMBER 11678 OF 101 OCEAN LANE DRIVE #407, KEY BISCAYNE, FL, WAS DISCIPLINED BY MISSISSIPPI ON NOVEMBER 19, 1998
DISCIPLINARY ACTION: REPRIMAND

HARTHCOCK, KERRY ALFRED MD, LICENSE NUMBER 00G1428 OF SEATTLE, WA, WAS DISCIPLINED BY TEXAS ON JANUARY 26, 1990
OFFENSE: DISCIPLINARY ACTION BY ANOTHER STATE OR AGENCY
NOTES: STIPULATED ORDER. SHALL COMPLY WITH PROBATIONARY REQUIREMENTS OF WASHINGTON BOARD ORDER, TEXAS BOARD TO HAVE ACCESS TO WASHINGTON BOARD DOCUMENTS, MUST OBTAIN APPROVAL FROM TEXAS BOARD PRIOR TO PRACTICING IN TEXAS. AS OF 4/20/91 PROBATION TERMINATED; LICENSE FREE OF ANY RESTRICTION OR LIMITATION.

HARTIN, RICHARD B JR MD, DATE OF BIRTH NOVEMBER 29, 1952, LICENSE NUMBER 00G6524 OF 2506 GRANDRIDGE TRAIL, CEDAR PARK, TX, WAS DISCIPLINED BY TEXAS ON JUNE 10, 1991
DISCIPLINARY ACTION: 60-MONTH PROBATION; MONITORING OF PHYSICIAN PERFORMANCE
OFFENSE: LOSS OR RESTRICTION OF HOSPITAL PRIVILEGES
NOTES: INABILITY TO PRACTICE MEDICINE WITH REASONABLE SKILL AND SAFETY, LOSS OF HOSPITAL PRIVILEGES, AND UNPROFESSIONAL CONDUCT OR PROFESSIONAL INCOMPETENCE LIKELY TO HARM THE PUBLIC. SHALL SUBMIT TO ALCOHOL OR DRUG SCREENS; SHALL CONTINUE TO PARTICIPATE IN ACTIVITIES OF IMPAIRED PHYSICIANS PROGRAM. ON 8/20/93 ORDER TERMINATED AND LICENSE FREE AND CLEAR OF ANY PREVIOUS RESTRICTIONS.

HARTLEY, LAWRENCE J MD OF 100 MEDICAL DR, LAKE JACKSON, TX, WAS DISCIPLINED BY DEA ON JULY 3, 1990
DISCIPLINARY ACTION: SURRENDER OF CONTROLLED SUBSTANCE LICENSE
NOTES: PLACED ON FIVE YEARS PROBATION BY TEXAS STATE BOARD OF MEDICAL EXAMINERS.

HARTLEY, LAWRENCE JUSTICE MD, LICENSE NUMBER 00C8117 OF LAKE JACKSON, TX, WAS DISCIPLINED BY TEXAS ON MAY 24, 1990
DISCIPLINARY ACTION: SURRENDER OF CONTROLLED SUBSTANCE LICENSE; 60-MONTH PROBATION

NOTES: STIPULATED ORDER. MUST APPEAR BEFORE BOARD TWICE YEARLY, SURRENDER CONTROLLED SUBSTANCES REGISTRATION CERTIFICATES AND ALL UNUSED TRIPLICATE PRESCRIPTION FORMS AND NOT ATTEMPT TO ORDER MORE, COMPLETE PRECEPTORSHIP ON PREVENTION AND TREATMENT OF DRUG ABUSE, NOT TREAT OR OFFER TO TREAT ANY DISEASE OR DISORDER OR ANY PHYSICAL DEFORMITY OR INJURY BY ANY SYSTEM OR METHOD OR TO EFFECT CURES THEREOF, AND NOT PRESCRIBE FOR OR TREAT ANY PATIENTS EXCEPT IN EMERGENCY SITUATIONS. ON 10/1/93, ORDER TERMINATED.

HARTMAN, TED E MD OF WILLIAMSTON, SC, WAS DISCIPLINED BY SOUTH CAROLINA ON OCTOBER 20, 1998
DISCIPLINARY ACTION: LICENSE REVOCATION
OFFENSE: SEXUAL ABUSE OF OR SEXUAL MISCONDUCT WITH A PATIENT

NOTES: HAD A SEXUAL RELATIONSHIP WITH A PATIENT ENTRUSTED TO HIS CARE.

HARTMAN, TED E MD, LICENSE NUMBER 0009605 OF MARSHFIELD, VT, WAS DISCIPLINED BY VERMONT ON MARCH 5, 1999
DISCIPLINARY ACTION: EMERGENCY SUSPENSION
OFFENSE: DISCIPLINARY ACTION BY ANOTHER STATE OR AGENCY

NOTES: ON 10/20/98 THE SOUTH CAROLINA BOARD OF MEDICAL EXAMINERS REVOKED HIS MEDICAL LICENSE. HE HAD ENGAGED IN UNPROFESSIONAL CONDUCT AS EVIDENCED BY HIS SEXUAL RELATIONSHIP WITH A PATIENT ENTRUSTED TO HIS CARE.

HARTMAN, TED E MD, LICENSE NUMBER 170849 OF 9411A WIER LOOP, AUSTIN, TX, WAS DISCIPLINED BY NEW YORK ON JULY 8, 1999
DISCIPLINARY ACTION: SURRENDER OF LICENSE
OFFENSE: DISCIPLINARY ACTION BY ANOTHER STATE OR AGENCY

NOTES: DISCIPLINED BY THE SOUTH CAROLINA BOARD FOR SEXUAL MISCONDUCT WITH A PATIENT.

HARTMAN, TED E MD OF MARSHFIELD, VT, WAS DISCIPLINED BY VERMONT ON AUGUST 17, 1999
DISCIPLINARY ACTION: LICENSE REVOCATION
OFFENSE: DISCIPLINARY ACTION BY ANOTHER STATE OR AGENCY

NOTES: SOUTH CAROLINA REVOKED HIS LICENSE AFTER THEY FOUND HE DATED AND ENGAGED IN SEXUAL INTERCOURSE WITH A PATIENT. SHALL NOT APPLY FOR REINSTATEMENT, AND THE BOARD SHALL NOT CONSIDER ANY LICENSE APPLICATION FOR THREE YEARS.

HARVEY, HEIDI LYNNE MD, LICENSE NUMBER K1464 OF LANCASTER, TX, WAS DISCIPLINED BY TEXAS ON AUGUST 22, 1998
DISCIPLINARY ACTION: FINE; REPRIMAND
OFFENSE: NONCOMPLIANCE WITH A PROFESSIONAL RULE

NOTES: FAILED TO PROVIDE SUFFICIENT PROOF OF HER CONTINUING MEDICAL EDUCATION ON HER ANNUAL REGISTRATION FOR 9/1/96 - 8/ 31/97. $1,000 FINE.

HASKELL, ROBERT DO, LICENSE NUMBER 00D2787 OF SAN RAFAEL, CA, WAS DISCIPLINED BY TEXAS ON MARCH 5, 1994
DISCIPLINARY ACTION: SURRENDER OF LICENSE
OFFENSE: DISCIPLINARY ACTION BY ANOTHER STATE OR AGENCY

NOTES: ON 12/9/91 LICENSE WAS SANCTIONED BY CALIFORNIA BOARD FOR REPEATED NEGLIGENT ACTS IN THE CARE AND TREATMENT OF ONE PATIENT. HE DOES NOT WISH TO MAINTAIN A TEXAS LICENSE OR CONTEST THE CALIFORNIA PROCEEDINGS. LICENSE IS SURRENDERED IN LIEU OF FURTHER DISCIPLINARY ACTION.

HATCHETT, ROBERT KEVIN MD, LICENSE NUMBER J0518, WAS DISCIPLINED BY TEXAS ON APRIL 9, 1997
DISCIPLINARY ACTION: EMERGENCY SUSPENSION
OFFENSE: LOSS OR RESTRICTION OF HOSPITAL PRIVILEGES

NOTES: ALLEGATIONS OF SUBSTANCE ABUSE. THE BOARD DEFERRED A DECISION PENDING THE RESULTS OF A 96-HOUR INPATIENT EVALUATION CONDUCTED AT AN APPROVED FACILITY. ON 7/29/96 HE ENTERED SUBSTANCE ABUSE TREATMENT. ON 9/9/96 HE LEFT AGAINST MEDICAL ADVICE. DURING 1996, HE WAS SUSPENDED FROM THREE HOSPITAL MEDICAL STAFFS. AVAILABLE EVIDENCE INDICATES THAT HE REFRAINED FROM PRACTICE FROM 8/96 TO 1/97 AND NUMEROUS DRUG SCREENS HAVE BEEN NEGATIVE SINCE THEN.

HAUSER, BILL OLIVER MD, LICENSE NUMBER 00D0158 OF SAN ANTONIO, TX, WAS DISCIPLINED BY TEXAS ON JANUARY 24, 1992
DISCIPLINARY ACTION: 36-MONTH PROBATION
OFFENSE: PROFESSIONAL MISCONDUCT

NOTES: AIDING OR ABETTING, DIRECTLY OR INDIRECTLY, THE PRACTICE OF MEDICINE BY ANY PERSON, PARTNERSHIP, ASSOCIATION, OR CORPORATION NOT DULY LICENSED TO PRACTICE MEDICINE BY THE BOARD. LICENSE SUSPENDED, SUSPENSION STAYED; PROBATION UNDER TERMS AND CONDITIONS.

HAVARD, THOMAS J III DO, LICENSE NUMBER 00E5103 OF INGRAM, TX, WAS DISCIPLINED BY TEXAS ON MAY 11, 1995
DISCIPLINARY ACTION: FINE
OFFENSE: NONCOMPLIANCE WITH A PROFESSIONAL RULE

NOTES: DURING HIS CARE OF VARIOUS PATIENTS IN 1992, FAILED TO KEEP ADEQUATE MEDICAL RECORDS OF EVALUATIONS CONDUCTED AND TREATMENT RENDERED. SHALL PAY $2,000 FINE.

HAWKINS, MICHAEL MURPHY MD, WAS DISCIPLINED BY TEXAS ON SEPTEMBER 20, 1997
DISCIPLINARY ACTION: RESTRICTION PLACED ON LICENSE

NOTES: LICENSE GRANTED CONTIGENT UPON PASSING THE MEDICAL JURISPRUDENCE EXAMINATION WITHIN A MAXIMUM OF THREE ATTEMPTS AND WITHIN 12 MONTHS AND WITH THE FOLLOWING TERMS AND CONDITIONS: SHALL LIMIT HIS PRACTICE IN TEXAS TO ADMINISTRATIVE MEDICINE IN THE CAPACITY OF A MEDICAL DIRECTOR; SHALL NOT CLINICALLY DIAGNOSE AND/OR TREAT ANY PATIENTS; SHALL COOPERATE WITH THE BOARD IN VERIFYING COMPLIANCE; SHALL PROVIDE A COPY OF THIS ORDER TO ANYONE REQUESTING IT WITHIN 10 DAYS; SHALL INFORM THE BOARD OF CHANGE OF ADDRESS WITHIN 10 DAYS OR IF HE LEAVES THE STATE; SHALL APPEAR BEFORE THE BOARD UPON REQUEST; SHALL NOT SEEK MODIFICATION FOR ONE YEAR.

HAYS, HARVEY JR MD, LICENSE NUMBER 00C2491 OF BORGER, TX, WAS DISCIPLINED BY TEXAS ON APRIL 10, 1992
DISCIPLINARY ACTION: 36-MONTH PROBATION

OFFENSE: PROFESSIONAL MISCONDUCT

NOTES: PROFESSIONAL FAILURE TO PRACTICE MEDICINE IN AN ACCEPTABLE MANNER CONSISTENT WITH PUBLIC HEALTH AND WELFARE. LICENSE SUSPENDED, SUSPENSION STAYED; PROBATION UNDER TERMS AND CONDITIONS.

HAYS, HARVEY JR MD, LICENSE NUMBER 00C2491 OF BORGER, TX, WAS DISCIPLINED BY TEXAS ON JUNE 22, 1994
DISCIPLINARY ACTION: RESTRICTION PLACED ON LICENSE; RESTRICTION PLACED ON CONTROLLED SUBSTANCE LICENSE
OFFENSE: FAILURE TO COMPLY WITH PREVIOUS BOARD ORDER

NOTES: HE ENTERED AN AGREED ORDER ON 4/10/92 BASED ON FINDINGS THAT HE HAD PRESCRIBED METHADONE TO A PATIENT WITHOUT BEING REGISTERED AS A METHADONE CLINIC AND HAD PRESCRIBED CONTROLLED SUBSTANCES TO ADDICTED INDIVIDUALS; ONE OF THE CONDITIONS OF THE ORDER WAS THAT HE COMPLETE A PHARMACOLOGY RETRAINING COURSE WITHIN SIX MONTHS; HAS FAILED TO COMPLETE SUCH A COURSE; HIS FAILURE TO COMPLY HAS BEEN CONTRIBUTED TO BY TEMPORARY HEALTH PROBLEMS WHICH HE HAS EXPERIENCED; HAS SURRENDERED HIS DEA AND TEXAS CONTROLLED SUBSTANCES CERTIFICATES, ALL UNUSED TRIPLICATE PRESCRIPTION FORMS AND ALL CONTROLLED SUBSTANCES; HAS CEASED PRIVATE PRACTICE AND IS NOT INVOLVED IN DIRECT PATIENT SERVICES. SHALL NOT ATTEMPT TO REENTER PRIVATE PRACTICE OR BE INVOLVED IN DIRECT PATIENT SERVICES; SHALL NOT ATTEMPT TO REREGISTER CONTROLLED SUBSTANCES CERTIFICATES WITHOUT BOARD PERMISSION; SHALL GIVE A COPY OF THIS ORDER TO ANY HEALTH CARE ENTITY WHERE HE HAS PRIVILEGES; SHALL COOPERATE WITH THE BOARD IN VERIFYING COMPLIANCE; SHALL INFORM BOARD OF CHANGE OF ADDRESS WITHIN 10 DAYS. SHALL NOT SEEK MODIFICATION FOR ONE YEAR. ON 11/16/96 ORDER MODIFIED AS FOLLOWS: SHALL NOT REENTER THE PRACTICE OF MEDICINE UNTIL HE SUCCESSFULLY PASSES THE SPECIAL PURPOSE EXAMINATION AND SHALL BE RESTRICTED FOR A PERIOD OF THREE YEARS UPON SUCCESSFUL PASSAGE; HE IS AUTHORIZED TO REAPPLY TO THE DEA AND THE TEXAS DEPARTMENT OF PUBLIC SAFETY TO OBTAIN AUTHORIZATION TO PRESCRIBE SCHEDULES III, III-N, IV AND V; SHALL REFRAIN FROM THE PRESCRIPTION OR ADMINISTRATION OF ANY DRUG FOR ANY PATIENT UNLESS THE DRUG IS MEDICALLY INDICATED AND PRESCRIBED IN THERAPEUTIC DOSES; SHALL NOT PRESCRIBE, ADMINISTER OR DISPENSE ANY DRUG WITH POTENTIAL FOR ABUSE UNLESS THERE IS A LEGITIMATE MEDICAL AND THERAPEUTIC NEED; SHALL CONDUCT ADEQUATE FOLLOW-UP EXAMINATIONS ON ALL PATIENTS TO DETERMINE THE COURSE OF TREATMENT, INCLUDING THE PRESCRIBING OF DRUGS; PRACTICE SHALL BE MONITORED BY A LICENSED PHYSICIAN WHO SHALL COUNSEL HIM ON ANY PERCEIVED DEFICIENCIES AND PROVIDE MONTHLY REPORTS; IF HE WORKS WITH A PHYSICIAN ASSISTANT SHALL ENSURE THAT THE PHYSICIAN ASSISTANT SUBMITS MONTHLY REPORTS TO THE BOARD DESIGNATING TASKS PERFORMED; SHALL PERSONALLY APPEAR BEFORE THE BOARD AT LEAST ONE TIME EACH YEAR; ALL OTHER CONDITIONS REMAIN IN EFFECT. ON 4/4/98 PETITION FOR MODIFICATION OF ORDER DENIED.

HEAD, WILLIAM J III MD, DATE OF BIRTH JANUARY 29, 1954, LICENSE NUMBER 0033365 OF 4126 SOUTHWEST FREEWAY, STE 500, HOUSTON, TX, WAS DISCIPLINED BY MINNESOTA ON SEPTEMBER 12, 1992
OFFENSE: DISCIPLINARY ACTION BY ANOTHER STATE OR AGENCY

NOTES: SUSPENSION STAYED UPON COMPLIANCE WITH THE FOLLOWING: SHALL COMPLY WITH ALL TERMS AND CONDITIONS IMPOSED ON TEXAS LICENSE. SHALL CAUSE COMPLIANCE REPORT TO BE SENT FROM TEXAS BOARD. IF HE MOVES TO MINNESOTA TO PRACTICE, SHALL MEET WITH COMPLAINT REVIEW COMMITTEE WHICH MAY THEN CONDITION OR RESTRICT HIS LICENSE AS DEEMED NECESSARY.

HEAD, WILLIAM JUSTUS III MD, LICENSE NUMBER 00F6730 OF HOUSTON, TX, WAS DISCIPLINED BY TEXAS ON SEPTEMBER 5, 1991
DISCIPLINARY ACTION: 60-MONTH PROBATION; RESTRICTION PLACED ON LICENSE
OFFENSE: SUBSTANDARD CARE, INCOMPETENCE OR NEGLIGENCE

NOTES: PERFORMED A CATARACT EXTRACTION AND AN INTRAOCULAR LENS IMPLANT IN A PATIENT ON 1/26/88; THE SURGERY WAS UNNECESSARY. REVOCATION STAYED; TERMS OF PROBATION INCLUDE; ATTENDING AT LEAST 40 HOURS APPROVED CONTINUING MEDICAL EDUCATION PER YEAR; MUST ATTEND 10 HOURS OF AN ETHICS COURSE OR PROGRAM PER YEAR FOR FIVE YEARS; SHALL PERFORM NO PROCEDURE INVOLVING SURGERY ON THE ADNEXA OF THE EYE UNLESS HE FIRST OBTAINS A SECOND OPINION FROM AN OPHTHALMOLOGIST WHO CONCURS WITH THE DECISION TO PERFORM THE SURGERY; MUST PERFORM 50 HOURS PER MONTH OF COMMUNITY SERVICE; MUST APPEAR BEFORE THE BOARD TWO TIMES A YEAR; TIME SPENT OUT OF TEXAS DOES NOT COUNT TOWARDS PROBATION. ON 11/19/93 PROBATION MODIFIED: HE MAY PERFORM MEDICALLY NECESSARY SURGERY ON THE ADNEXA OF THE EYE WITHOUT OBTAINING A CONCURRING SECOND OPINION FROM ANOTHER OPHTHALMOLOGIST; SHALL NOT, HOWEVER, PERFORM INTRAOCULAR PROCEDURES REQUIRING AN INCISION INTO THE EYE OF ANY KIND UNLESS HE FIRST OBTAINS A SECOND OPINION FROM AN OPHTHALMOLOGIST WHO CONCURS WITH HIS DECISION TO PERFORM THE PROCEDURE. PHYSICIANS WHO PROVIDE SUCH A SECOND OPINION SHALL HAVE NO BUSINESS RELATIONSHIP WITH HIM. ON 11/3/94 ORDER MODIFIED AS FOLLOWS: REQUIREMENT THAT HE NOT PERFORM INTRAOCULAR PROCEDURES REQUIRING AN INCISION INTO THE EYE UNLESS HE FIRST OBTAINS A SECOND OPINION FROM AN OPHTHALMOLOGIST IS DELETED AND HIS RECORDS OF ANY SURGERY PERFORMED SHALL BE SUBJECT TO RANDOM REVIEW. AS OF 11/16/96, THIS ORDER WAS CONSIDERED TO HAVE EXPIRED.

HEAD, WILLIAM JUSTUS III MD, LICENSE NUMBER 00F6730, WAS DISCIPLINED BY TEXAS ON NOVEMBER 16, 1996
DISCIPLINARY ACTION: LICENSE REVOCATION; 120-MONTH PROBATION
OFFENSE: SUBSTANCE ABUSE

NOTES: USED COCAINE IN A BINGE FASHION IN THE EARLY 1980S AND IN A RECREATIONAL FASHION ALONG WITH ECSTASY AND MARIJUANA DURING THE MID 1980S UNTIL 8/93; WAS TREATED AT TALBOT-MARSH RECOVERY CAMPUS FROM 3/28/96 TO 8/10/96; REPORTS SOBRIETY DATE OF 3/19/96; IS PARTICIPATING IN AA; HE HAS BEEN UNDERGOING CONTINUING CARE AND TREATMENT SINCE HIS DISCHARGE AND IS CURRENTLY MONITORED BY A BOARD-CERTIFIED PSYCHIATRIST PRACTICING ADDICTIONOLOGY. REVOCATION STAYED AFTER 15

DAYS. PROBATION WITH TERMS AND CONDITIONS: SHALL ABSTAIN FROM THE CONSUMPTION OF ALCOHOL/DRUGS IN ANY FORM UNLESS PRESCRIBED BY ANOTHER PHYSICIAN FOR A LEGITIMATE AND THERAPEUTIC PURPOSE; SHALL SUBMIT HIMSELF FOR APPROPRIATE EXAMS INCLUDING DRUG OR ALCOHOL SCREENS; SHALL CONTINUE TO RECEIVE CARE AND TREATMENT FROM HIS PHYSICIAN WHOM HE SHALL SEE AT LEAST ONCE A MONTH AND WHO SHALL SUBMIT QUARTERLY REPORTS TO THE BOARD; SHALL CONTINUE TO PARTICIPATE IN AA'S PROGRAM NOT LESS THAN FIVE TIMES PER WEEK WITH QUARTERLY REPORTS TO THE BOARD; SHALL PARTICIPATE IN THE ACTIVITIES OF A PHYSICIAN'S HEALTH AND REHABILITATION COMMITTEE AND ATTEND WEEKLY MEETINGS WITH QUARTERLY REPORTS; SHALL COMPLY WITH THE TERMS OF HIS CONTINUING CARE CONTRACT WITH TALBOTT MARSH AND SHALL REQUEST THAT REPORTS BE SUBMITTED TO THE BOARD; SHALL NOT POSSESS ALCOHOL, CONTROLLED SUBSTANCES OR DANGEROUS DRUGS WITH ADDICTIVE POTENTIAL OR POTENTIAL FOR ABUSE AND SHALL SURRENDER ANY SUCH DRUGS INCLUDING SAMPLES; SHALL NOT TREAT OR OTHERWISE SERVE AS PHYSICIAN, PRESCRIBE, DISPENSE OR ADMINISTER DRUGS THAT MAY BE SUBJECT TO ABUSE TO HIMSELF OR TO ANY MEMBER OF HIS FAMILY; SHALL NOT TELEPHONE TO A PHARMACY A PRESCRIPTION OR REFILL FOR CONTROLLED SUBSTANCES OR DANGEROUS DRUGS WITH ADDICTIVE POTENTIAL OR POTENTIAL FOR ABUSE OR ALLOW ANYONE UNDER HIS SUPERVISION TO DO SO; SHALL MAINTAIN A FILE OF EVERY PRESCRIPTION FOR THESE SUBSTANCES; SHALL MAINTAIN ADEQUATE MEDICAL RECORDS WHICH SHALL BE AVAILABLE FOR REVIEW; SHALL OBTAIN AT LEAST 50 HOURS PER YEAR OF CONTINUING MEDICAL EDUCATION; SHALL APPEAR BEFORE BOARD AT LEAST TWICE A YEAR; SHALL COOPERATE WITH THE BOARD IN VERIFYING COMPLIANCE INCLUDING PROVIDING COPIES OF MEDICAL RELEASES AND PEER REVIEW RECORDS UPON REQUEST; SHALL GIVE A COPY OF THIS ORDER TO ANY HEALTH CARE ENTITY WHERE HE HAS PRIVILEGES; SHALL PROVIDE A COPY OF THIS ORDER TO ANYONE REQUESTING IT WITHIN 10 DAYS; TIME SPENT OUT OF TEXAS DOES NOT COUNT TOWARD PROBATION; SHALL INFORM BOARD OF CHANGE OF ADDRESS WITHIN 10 DAYS OR IF HE LEAVES THE STATE. SHALL NOT SEEK MODIFICATION FOR ONE YEAR. ON 12/11/99 PETITION TO MODIFY ORDER GRANTED ALLOWING QUARTERLY RATHER THAN MONTHLY PSYCHIATRIC VISITS.

HEADLEY, DAVID M MD, LICENSE NUMBER 00G0724 OF PORT GIBSON, MS, WAS DISCIPLINED BY TEXAS ON AUGUST 18, 1990
OFFENSE: DISCIPLINARY ACTION BY ANOTHER STATE OR AGENCY

NOTES: STIPULATED ORDER. MUST COMPLY WITH MISSISSIPPI BOARD ORDER AND OBTAIN PERMISSION OF BOARD BEFORE PRACTICING IN TEXAS AND COMPLY WITH ANY PROBATIONARY TERMS WHICH MAY BE IMPOSED.

HEADLEY, DAVID M MD OF PORT GIBSON, MS, WAS DISCIPLINED BY DEA ON OCTOBER 29, 1993
DISCIPLINARY ACTION: DENIAL OF LICENSE REINSTATEMENT
OFFENSE: SUBSTANCE ABUSE

NOTES: IN 7/88 THE MISSISSIPPI BOARD RECEIVED COMPLAINTS REGARDING HIS ALLEGED POOR HANDLING OF OBSTETRICS AND GYNECOLOGICAL PATIENTS, HIS ALLEGED PERSONAL ABUSE OF NON-CONTROLLED SUBSTANCES, AS WELL AS PROBLEMS INVOLVING HIS ASSAULT AND BATTERY ON HIS WIFE. BOARD'S INVESTIGATION REVEALED THAT BETWEEN EARLY 1987 AND LATE 1988 HE PRESCRIBED LARGE QUANTITIES OF FIORINAL, HALCION, DARVON AND DARVOCET FOR HIS WIFE'S PERSONAL USE AND FAILED TO MAINTAIN AN INVENTORY OF THE NON-CONTROLLED SUBSTANCES THAT HE DISPENSED AND ADMINISTERED. HE ENTERED INTO A CONSENT AGREEMENT WITH THE MISSISSIPPI MEDICAL BOARD ON 9/28/88 IN WHICH HE WAS ORDERED NOT TO DISPENSE, ADMINISTER OR PRESCRIBE TO HIMSELF OR FAMILY MEMBERS ANY ADDICTIVE DRUGS, AND TO SUBMIT TO RANDOM URINE AND/OR BLOOD SCREENS. TESTED POSITIVE ON TWO OCCASIONS FOR CONTROLLED SUBSTANCES USE. AS A RESULT, THE BOARD ISSUED AN ORDER EFFECTIVE 8/11/89 PROHIBITING HIM FROM PRACTICING MEDICINE IN MISSISSIPPI UNTIL HE UNDERGOES AN EVALUATION FOR CHEMICAL DEPENDENCY AND IS DEEMED CAPABLE OF RETURNING TO PRACTICE. ON 10/24/89, HE ENTERED INTO A SECOND CONSENT AGREEMENT WHERE HE WAS ORDERED TO SUBMIT TO RANDOM, UNANNOUNCED URINE AND/OR BLOOD SCREENS FOR A PERIOD OF AT LEAST FIVE YEARS AND MUST SUCCESSFULLY COMPLETE ALL REQUIRED PHASES OF TREATMENT AT MISSISSIPPI IMPAIRED PROFESSIONALS PROGRAM; HE WAS ALSO ORDERED TO SURRENDER HIS DEA CERTIFICATE OF REGISTRATION.

HEADLEY, DAVID M MD OF PORT GIBSON, MS, WAS DISCIPLINED BY DEA ON AUGUST 22, 1996
DISCIPLINARY ACTION: RESTRICTION PLACED ON CONTROLLED SUBSTANCE LICENSE; MONITORING OF PHYSICIAN PERFORMANCE
OFFENSE: DISCIPLINARY ACTION BY ANOTHER STATE OR AGENCY

NOTES: IN 1987, AFTER MULTIPHASE REHABILITATION, HIS DEA REGISTRATION WAS REISSUED WITH RESTRICTIONS; ON 12/15/93 HE WAS STILL SUBJECT TO TERMS OF MISSISSIPPI AGREEMENT AND HAS REAPPLIED FOR DEA REGISTRATION IN SCHEDULES IV AND V. HE HAS NOT ABUSED CONTROLLED SUBSTANCES SINCE 8/16/89 AND THERE HAVE BEEN NO FURTHER COMPLAINTS TO THE BOARD REGARDING HIS DRUG ABUSE PROBLEM. DEA REGISTRATION IS GRANTED UNDER THE FOLLOWING RESTRICTIONS: SHALL SUBMIT ON A MONTHLY BASIS TO THE DEA A COPY OF HIS URINE SCREENING RESULTS; MUST CONTINUE TO ATTEND WEEKLY ALCOHOLICS ANONYMOUS MEETINGS OR OTHER SUPPORT GROUP MEETINGS FOR ONE YEAR.

HEALING, ROBERT DYSON MD, LICENSE NUMBER 00G2986 OF HAMLIN, TX, WAS DISCIPLINED BY TEXAS ON JUNE 17, 1992
DISCIPLINARY ACTION: 36-MONTH RESTRICTION PLACED ON LICENSE
OFFENSE: OVERPRESCRIBING OR MISPRESCRIBING DRUGS

NOTES: NONTHERAPEUTIC PRESCRIBING AND PROFESSIONAL FAILURE TO PRACTICE MEDICINE IN AN ACCEPTABLE MANNER CONSISTENT WITH PUBLIC HEALTH AND WELFARE. ON 8/19/94 ORDER TERMINATED.

HEDGES, DON W DO, DATE OF BIRTH OCTOBER 2, 1940 OF 6463 FOURTH STREET NW, ALBUQUERQUE, NM, WAS DISCIPLINED BY MEDICARE ON JUNE 14, 1991
DISCIPLINARY ACTION: 60-MONTH EXCLUSION FROM THE MEDICARE AND/OR MEDICAID PROGRAM
OFFENSE: CRIMINAL CONVICTION OR PLEA OF GUILTY, NOLO CONTENDERE, OR NO CONTEST TO A CRIME

NOTES: PROGRAM-RELATED CONVICTION. REINSTATED ON 11/22/96.

HEDGES, DON WALTER DO, LICENSE NUMBER 00E3303 OF ALBUQUERQUE, NM, WAS DISCIPLINED BY TEXAS ON MARCH 5, 1994
DISCIPLINARY ACTION: REPRIMAND
OFFENSE: INSURANCE, MEDICARE OR MEDICAID FRAUD

NOTES: WHILE PRACTICING IN NEW MEXICO HE INTENTIONALLY SUBMITTED INACCURATE DIAGNOSES TO MEDICARE FOR FIVE PATIENTS HE WAS TREATING WITH A DIET PLAN SO THAT HE WOULD RECEIVE REIMBURSEMENT SINCE THE DIET PLAN WAS NOT A COVERED BENEFIT.

HEMEYER, MARK M MD OF 13211 RIDGEHAVEN ROAD, LITTLE ROCK, AR, WAS DISCIPLINED BY DEA ON JUNE 5, 1998
DISCIPLINARY ACTION: SURRENDER OF CONTROLLED SUBSTANCE LICENSE

HEMEYER, MARK M MD, LICENSE NUMBER G0725 OF LITTLE ROCK, AR, WAS DISCIPLINED BY TEXAS ON OCTOBER 15, 1999
DISCIPLINARY ACTION: PROBATION
OFFENSE: DISCIPLINARY ACTION BY ANOTHER STATE OR AGENCY

NOTES: ON 6/29/97 THE ARKANSAS BOARD REVOKED HIS LICENSE, STAYED THE REVOCATION AND PLACED HIM ON 5 YEARS PROBATION; BASED ON HIS EXHIBITING THE HABITUAL OR EXCESSIVE USE OF SCHEDULED DRUGS FROM 1993 TO THE PRESENT, RESULTING IN AT LEAST 2 ENROLLMENTS IN DRUG REHABILITATION PROGRAMS; HE TESTED POSITIVE FOR HYDROCODONE ON 12/24/97; OBTAINED HYDROCODONE FOR HIS OWN USE BY TAKING SAMPLES FROM THE CLINIC; AND WROTE PRESCRIPTIONS FOR A SUBSTANCE CONTAINING HYDROCODONE FOR FICTITIOUS PATIENTS IN ORDER TO OBTAIN FOR HIS OWN USE. SUSPENSION STAYED FOR PROBATION WITH FOLLOWING TERMS AND CONDITIONS: SHALL NOT PRACTICE UNTIL HE REQUESTS PERMISSION IN WRITING TO RESUME PRACTICE AND APPEARS BEFORE THE BOARD TO ORALLY PETITION FOR PERMISSION TO RESUME PRACTICE, PROVIDING EVIDENCE OF HIS COMPETENCE TO PRACTICE SAFELY; SHALL INFORM THE BOARD OF CHANGE OF ADDRESS WITHIN 10 DAYS; SHALL NOT SEEK MODIFICATION FOR ONE YEAR.

HEMEYER, MARK MICHAEL MD, LICENSE NUMBER R3197 OF LITTLE ROCK, AR, WAS DISCIPLINED BY ARKANSAS ON JUNE 5, 1998
DISCIPLINARY ACTION: 60-MONTH PROBATION

NOTES: FIVE YEAR REVOCATION STAYED.

HENNESSY, ROBERT MD, LICENSE NUMBER E8547, WAS DISCIPLINED BY TEXAS ON APRIL 10, 1999
DISCIPLINARY ACTION: LICENSE REINSTATEMENT

NOTES: LICENSE HAD BEEN REVOKED ON 1/7/98 FOR PRESCRIBING DILAUDID AND PRELUDIN TO KNOWN DRUG ABUSERS IN A NONTHERAPEUTIC MANNER; APPEARS TO HAVE BEEN REHABILITATED. LICENSE LIMITED AS FOLLOWS: SHALL NOT PRACTICE UNTIL HE APPEARS BEFORE THE BOARD AND PROVIDES SUFFICIENT EVIDENCE THAT HE WILL BE DIRECTLY CONTRIBUTING TO THE HEALTH AND WELFARE OF THE CITIZENS OF TEXAS; SUCH EVIDENCE AND INFORMATION MAY INCLUDE THE ACCEPTANCE OF A POSITION TO PRACTICE IN A MEDICALLY UNDERSERVED AREA OR A MEDICALLY UNDERSERVED POPULATION; SHALL COOPERATE WITH THE BOARD IN VERIFYING COMPLIANCE; SHALL INFORM THE BOARD OF CHANGE OF ADDRESS WITHIN 10 DAYS; SHALL NOT SEEK MODIFICATION FOR ONE YEAR.

HERBERMAN, HARVEY G MD, LICENSE NUMBER D4664 OF EL PASO, TX, WAS DISCIPLINED BY TEXAS ON MAY 16, 1998
DISCIPLINARY ACTION: SURRENDER OF LICENSE

NOTES: DUE TO RETIREMENT, HE HAS CHOSEN TO VOLUNTARILY AND PERMANENTLY SURRENDER HIS LICENSE.

HERLIHY, DANIEL JAMES DO, LICENSE NUMBER 00H8125, WAS DISCIPLINED BY TEXAS ON NOVEMBER 16, 1996
DISCIPLINARY ACTION: LICENSE SUSPENSION
OFFENSE: CRIMINAL CONVICTION OR PLEA OF GUILTY, NOLO CONTENDERE, OR NO CONTEST TO A CRIME

NOTES: FROM APPROXIMATELY 1992 THROUGH APPROXIMATELY 1993 HE ENGAGED IN POTENTIALLY MISLEADING ADVERTISING, INADEQUATELY MANAGED AND TREATED THE MEDICAL CONDITION OF BARIATRIC PATIENTS AND PROVIDED SUBSTANDARD MEDICAL CARE TO SEVERAL PATIENTS INCLUDING, BUT NOT LIMITED TO ORDERING TESTS WITHOUT ADEQUATE INDICATION, FAILING TO PROVIDE ADEQUATE FOLLOW-UP CARE BASED ON TEST RESULTS, FAILING TO ADEQUATELY INFORM PATIENTS OF THEIR MEDICAL CONDITIONS AND FAILING TO FORMULATE AN APPROPRIATE ASSESSMENT AND TREATMENT PLAN FOR SEVERAL PATIENTS; IN 1/96, HE WAS ARRESTED BY FEDERAL LAW ENFORCEMENT AGENTS ON CHARGES OF VIOLATING SEVERAL FEDERAL LAWS DIRECTLY CONNECTED TO HIS PRACTICE; FOUND GUILTY ON CRIMINAL CHARGES OF CONSPIRACY, FALSE STATEMENTS AND MAIL FRAUD RELATED TO THEFT OF MONIES FROM A FEDERAL HEALTH CARE PROGRAM AND PRIVATE BUSINESSES AND INSURERS; MAINTAINS HIS INNOCENCE AND PLANS TO APPEAL THE VERDICT. INDEFINITE SUSPENSION UNTIL HIS CRIMINAL CONVICTION IS ADJUDICATED; SHALL INFORM THE BOARD OF CHANGE OF ADDRESS WITHIN 10 DAYS.

HERLIHY, DANIEL JAMES DO, DATE OF BIRTH APRIL 3, 1957 OF PO BOX 9300-5 #279750077, TEXARKANA, TX, WAS DISCIPLINED BY MEDICARE ON SEPTEMBER 4, 1997
DISCIPLINARY ACTION: 180-MONTH EXCLUSION FROM THE MEDICARE AND/OR MEDICAID PROGRAM
OFFENSE: CRIMINAL CONVICTION OR PLEA OF GUILTY, NOLO CONTENDERE, OR NO CONTEST TO A CRIME

NOTES: CONVICTED OF A CRIME RELATED TO THE DELIVERY OF HEALTH CARE OR FINANCIAL MISCONDUCT INVOLVING A GOVERNMENT-OPERATED PROGRAM.

HERNAL, PETER L JR MD, LICENSE NUMBER D0910 OF UNIVERSAL CITY, TX, WAS DISCIPLINED BY TEXAS ON MAY 16, 1998
DISCIPLINARY ACTION: 36-MONTH RESTRICTION PLACED ON LICENSE; REQUIRED TO TAKE ADDITIONAL MEDICAL EDUCATION
OFFENSE: OVERPRESCRIBING OR MISPRESCRIBING DRUGS

NOTES: PRESCRIBED EXCESSIVE AMOUNTS OF DARVON OR PROPOXYPHENE TO AN ADULT PATIENT REPORTEDLY SUFFERING FROM MODERATE TO SEVERE BACK PAIN WITH A HISTORY OF AN ASSAULT-RELATED INJURY AND A SUBSEQUENT SURGERY; HIS RECORDS OF THE PATIENT DID NOT CONTAIN SUFFICIENTLY SPECIFIC INFORMATION REGARDING THE PATIENT'S PRIOR INJURY AND TREATMENT, AND DID NOT ADEQUATELY REFLECT EXAMS, TESTING, AND REFERRALS; FROM ON OR ABOUT 7/3/96 - 9/6/97 HE PRESCRIBED CONTROLLED SUBSTANCES, FROM HIS HOME OFFICE, TO ANOTHER ADULT PATIENT REPORTEDLY

SUFFERING FROM SEVERE HEADACHES; DID NOT PROVIDE RECORDS REQUESTED FROM HIM BY BOARD STAFF; HE MAINTAINS THAT RECORDS WERE CONTEMPORANEOUSLY MADE AT THE TIME OF TREATMENT, BUT WERE EITHER MISFILED, MISPLACED, OR INADVERTENTLY DESTROYED; HE CANNOT DEMONSTRATE THAT ADEQUATE INDICATIONS EXISTED FOR THE PRESCRIBING OF PAIN MEDICATIONS TO THE PATIENT. LICENSE LIMITED AS FOLLOWS: SHALL OBTAIN 50 HOURS PER YEAR OF CONTINUING MEDICAL EDUCATION; SHALL OBTAIN 10 HOURS OF AN ETHICS COURSE OR AN ETHICS PROGRAM PER YEAR; SHALL BE IN AN APPROPRIATE MEDICAL OFFICE OR HOSPITAL SETTING, AND SHALL NOT BE OUT OF HIS HOME OR ANY OTHER RESIDENCE; SHALL MAINTAIN ADEQUATE MEDICAL RECORDS WHICH SHALL BE AVAILABLE FOR REVIEW; SEPARATE FROM PATIENT RECORDS, SHALL MAINTAIN A LOGBOOK OF EVERY PRESCRIPTION WRITTEN BY HIM FOR DANGEROUS DRUGS WITH ADDICTIVE POTENTIAL WHICH SHALL BE MADE AVAILABLE FOR REVIEW; SHALL TERMINATE PATIENT-PHYSICIAN RELATIONSHIP WITH TWO PATIENTS WHO WERE THE SUBJECT OF THIS ACTION; SHALL APPEAR BEFORE THE BOARD AT LEAST ONCE A YEAR; SHALL COOPERATE WITH THE BOARD IN VERIFYING COMPLIANCE; TIME SPENT OUT OF TEXAS DOES NOT COUNT TOWARD RESTRICTION; SHALL INFORM THE BOARD OF CHANGE OF ADDRESS WITHIN 10 DAYS OR IF HE LEAVES THE STATE; SHALL NOT SEEK MODIFICATION FOR ONE YEAR.

HERNANDEZ, ARTHUR MD, LICENSE NUMBER 00G1674 OF SAN ANTONIO, TX, WAS DISCIPLINED BY TEXAS ON OCTOBER 5, 1991
DISCIPLINARY ACTION: REPRIMAND
OFFENSE: SUBSTANDARD CARE, INCOMPETENCE OR NEGLIGENCE

NOTES: ON 8/14/87 HE INFUSED A PATIENT WITH APPROPRIATE ANESTHETIC MEDICATIONS FOR SURGERY; AFTER DRUGS WERE ADMINISTERED THE SURGERY WAS CANCELED; HE REVERSED, TO THE EXTENT POSSIBLE, THE NARCOTIC PREVIOUSLY ADMINISTERED, AND CHOSE NOT TO REVERSE THE MUSCLE RELAXANT SINCE THE DOSE WAS SMALL; PATIENT SUFFERED A SEIZURE AND BRAIN DAMAGE DUE TO DEPRIVATION OF OXYGEN; FAILED TO TAKE ADEQUATE PRECAUTIONS TO SAFEGUARD PATIENT'S HEALTH DESPITE AVAILABLE INFORMATION WHICH MAY HAVE SUGGESTED POOR OXYGEN EXCHANGE; HOSPITAL REPRIMANDED HIM FOR ERRORS IN JUDGMENT; REVIEWED 100 PERCENT OF HIS CASES FOR SIX MONTHS; FOUND THAT HIS PROFESSIONAL CONDUCT USUALLY FOLLOWS ACCEPTABLE STANDARDS OF CARE AND THAT THIS INCIDENT DID NOT REPRESENT HIS TYPICAL CARE; HAS SUCCESSFULLY COMPLETED THE SIX MONTH REVIEW AND HAS HAD NO SUBSEQUENT PROBLEMS.

HICKS, RAYMOND D MD, DATE OF BIRTH NOVEMBER 11, 1933, LICENSE NUMBER 00D9495 OF 5137 COLTER WAY, DALLAS, TX, WAS DISCIPLINED BY TEXAS ON AUGUST 19, 1994
DISCIPLINARY ACTION: LICENSE SUSPENSION; 120-MONTH PROBATION
OFFENSE: SEXUAL ABUSE OF OR SEXUAL MISCONDUCT WITH A PATIENT

NOTES: IN 10/93 STAFF AT A CLINIC REPORTED ALCOHOL ON HIS BREATH; ADMITTED TO IMPAIRED PHYSICIAN'S COMMITTEE THAT HE HAD BEEN DRINKING REGULARLY DURING OFFICE HOURS; PRIVILEGES WERE SUSPENDED AND HE ENTERED ALCOHOL TREATMENT; NOTIFIED THE BOARD OF THIS ON 11/17/93; TREATMENT RECORDS REVEALED A LENGTHY HISTORY OF DEPRESSIVE SYMPTOMS BECOMING MORE SEVERE FOLLOWING A MYOCARDIAL INFARCTION IN 1985; ADMITTED TO DRINKING REGULARLY THROUGHOUT THE DAY SINCE 1986; DURING TREATMENT REVEALED A HISTORY OF SEXUAL ACTIVITY WITH PATIENTS AND PROSTITUTES AS LATE AS 7/93; IN 11/92 HE PLED NO CONTEST TO CHARGES OF SOLICITATION OF PROSTITUTION; REQUESTED EVALUATION NOTED HE MET THE CRITERIA FOR PSYCHOSEXUAL DISORDER WITH ADDICTIVE FEATURES; COMPLETED TREATMENT AND IS UNDER THE CARE OF AN ADDICTIONOLOGIST; SOBRIETY DATE IS 9/29/93. SUSPENSION STAYED TO PROBATION AFTER 14 DAYS. CONDITIONS OF PROBATION: SHALL APPEAR BEFORE THE BOARD TWICE A YEAR; SHALL ABSTAIN FROM THE CONSUMPTION OF ALCOHOL/CHEMICAL SUBSTANCES IN ANY FORM UNLESS PRESCRIBED BY ANOTHER PHYSICIAN FOR A LEGITIMATE AND THERAPEUTIC PURPOSE; SHALL PARTICIPATE IN THE ACTIVITIES OF A PHYSICIAN HEALTH AND REHABILITATION COMMITTEE AND ATTEND WEEKLY MEETINGS WITH QUARTERLY REPORTS; SHALL PARTICIPATE IN AA'S PROGRAM AND SEXUAL ADDICTION ANONYMOUS NOT LESS THAN THREE TIMES A WEEK FOR EACH PROGRAM WITH QUARTERLY REPORTS TO THE BOARD; SHALL SUBMIT HIMSELF FOR APPROPRIATE EXAMS INCLUDING DRUG OR ALCOHOL SCREENS; SHALL CONTINUE TREATMENT WITH PRESENT ADDICTIONOLOGIST AT LEAST ONCE A MONTH WITH QUARTERLY REPORTS; SHALL NOT TREAT OR OTHERWISE SERVE AS PHYSICIAN, PRESCRIBE, DISPENSE OR ADMINISTER DRUGS THAT MAY BE SUBJECT TO ABUSE TO HIMSELF OR TO ANY MEMBER OF HIS FAMILY; SHALL BE SUPERVISED BY A BOARD-APPROVED PHYSICIAN WITH QUARTERLY REPORTS; SHALL LIMIT PRACTICE TO A BOARD-APPROVED INSTITUTIONAL SETTING WITH SUFFICIENT PROTOCOLS TO ENSURE HIS PRACTICE IS SUFFICIENTLY MONITORED; SHALL HAVE A CHAPERONE PRESENT FOR THE EXAMINATION OF ALL FEMALE PATIENTS WHICH SHALL BE DOCUMENTED IN THEIR RECORDS; SHALL FOLLOW TERMS OF ALL AFTERCARE CONTRACTS; SHALL EXECUTE RELEASES FOR TREATMENT RECORDS WITHIN 10 DAYS OF A REQUEST FROM THE BOARD; SHALL GIVE A COPY OF THIS ORDER TO ANY HEALTH CARE ENTITY WHERE HE HAS PRIVILEGES; SHALL COOPERATE WITH THE BOARD IN VERIFYING COMPLIANCE; SHALL INFORM BOARD OF CHANGE OF ADDRESS WITHIN 10 DAYS OR IF HE LEAVES THE STATE; TIME SPENT OUT OF TEXAS DOES NOT COUNT TOWARD PROBATION. SHALL NOT SEEK MODIFICATION FOR ONE YEAR. ON 10/13/95 ORDER MODIFIED LOOSENING RESTRICTIONS ON WHICH PHYSICIAN HEALTH COMMITTEE HE MAY PARTICIPATE WITH AND HOW OFTEN HE MUST ATTEND AA AND SEXUAL ADDICTION ANONYMOUS MEETINGS; ALL OTHER CONDITIONS REMAIN IN EFFECT.

HIDALGO, CARLOS H MD OF 427 WEST 20TH 403, HOUSTON, TX, WAS DISCIPLINED BY DEA ON SEPTEMBER 19, 1995
DISCIPLINARY ACTION: SURRENDER OF CONTROLLED SUBSTANCE LICENSE

NOTES: IN LIEU OF PUBLIC INTEREST REVOCATION.

HIDALGO, CARLOS H MD, LICENSE NUMBER 00F7782 OF 427 WEST 20TH STREET, HOUSTON, TX, WAS DISCIPLINED BY TEXAS ON OCTOBER 14, 1995
DISCIPLINARY ACTION: EMERGENCY SUSPENSION
OFFENSE: SEXUAL ABUSE OF OR SEXUAL MISCONDUCT WITH A PATIENT

NOTES: AVAILABLE EVIDENCE AND INFORMATION INDICATE THE FOLLOWING: IN OR ABOUT 8/95, LAW ENFORCEMENT AGENCIES RECEIVED INFORMATION THAT HE MAY HAVE ENGAGED IN ILLEGAL ACTS CONNECTED TO HIS PRACTICE; DURING THREE VISITS TO PHYSICIAN IN 8/95 AND 9/95 A FEMALE VICE OFFICER WITH THE POLICE DEPARTMENT PRESENTED AS A PATIENT REQUESTING PRESCRIPTIONS FOR FASTIN SO THAT SHE COULD STAY AWAKE AT HER WAITRESS AND ESCORT JOBS AND STATING THAT SHE LIKED TO GET HIGH ON FASTIN; ON THE FIRST VISIT HE ASKED TO SEE HER BREASTS AND BUTTOCKS WHICH SHE REFUSED AND HE GAVE HER A PRESCRIPTION FOR 20 UNITS OF FASTIN WHICH HE ADVISED HER NEVER TO FILL AT THE SAME PHARMACY; ON THE SECOND VISIT HE INFORMED HER THAT HE WOULD GIVE HER 10 MORE FASTIN DESPITE HIS KNOWLEDGE THAT HER REQUEST FOR MORE FASTIN WAS TOO SOON AND THAT HE WOULD GET IN TROUBLE; OFFERED THE OFFICER MONEY FOR SEXUAL FAVORS BUT THE OFFERS WERE DECLINED; ON THE THIRD VISIT, HE PERSISTENTLY REPEATED THE REQUEST THAT SHE EXPOSE HER BREASTS, WHICH SHE DECLINED TO DO; BUT DID GIVE HER A PRESCRIPTION FOR 20 UNITS OF FASTIN AFTER EXPOSING HIMSELF TO HER AND MASTURBATING; DURING THIS VISIT HE INFORMED THE OFFICER THAT HE HAD RECENTLY ENGAGED IN THE USE OF HERBAL ECSTASY, AN ILLICIT DRUG AND DESCRIBED TO HER THE EFFECT THE DRUG HAD ON HIM; HE HAS SURRENDERED HIS DEA/DPS CONTROLLED SUBSTANCE REGISTRATION CERTIFICATES AND HAS BEEN INDICTED BY A GRAND JURY FOR THE ALLEGED CRIMINAL OFFENSES OF DELIVERING CONTROLLED SUBSTANCES FOR OTHER THAN A VALID MEDICAL PURPOSE.

HIDALGO, CARLOS H MD, LICENSE NUMBER 00F7782 OF HOUSTON, TX, WAS DISCIPLINED BY TEXAS ON MAY 15, 1996
DISCIPLINARY ACTION: LICENSE REVOCATION
OFFENSE: CRIMINAL CONVICTION OR PLEA OF GUILTY, NOLO CONTENDERE, OR NO CONTEST TO A CRIME

NOTES: ON 11/9/95, HE ENTERED A PLEA OF GUILTY TO FRAUDULENT DELIVERY OF A CONTROLLED SUBSTANCE, A FELONY; THE DISTRICT COURT DEFERRED THE ADJUDICATION OF HIS GUILTY PLEA AND PLACED HIM ON PROBATION FOR SEVEN YEARS.

HILL, ROBERT D MD, LICENSE NUMBER 00C6143 OF ODESSA, TX, WAS DISCIPLINED BY TEXAS ON JANUARY 6, 1995
DISCIPLINARY ACTION: 60-MONTH PROBATION; REQUIRED TO TAKE ADDITIONAL MEDICAL EDUCATION
OFFENSE: LOSS OR RESTRICTION OF HOSPITAL PRIVILEGES

NOTES: ON 4/7/92 A HOSPITAL SUMMARILY SUSPENDED HIS PRIVILEGES DUE TO THE FOLLOWING: HE EXAMINED A NEWBORN INFANT WHO HIS NOTES REFLECTED WAS NORMAL, A POOR EATER, AND STATED "WATCH"; NURSES' NOTES REFLECT THE BABY WAS SPITTING UP EMESIS, REFUSING TO NURSE, WAS NOT STOOLING AND WAS NOT AROUSABLE; IN SPITE OF THIS DR. HILL DISCHARGED PATIENT AND ADVISED PARENTS TO CALL IF EATING DID NOT IMPROVE; THEY DID CALL LATER THAT DAY AND HE REFUSED TO SEE THE CHILD AS HE BELIEVED THE PROBLEM WOULD RESOLVE ITSELF; ANOTHER PHYSICIAN HOSPITALIZED THE INFANT THAT SAME DAY; THE INFANT WAS DIAGNOSED WITH CYSTIC FIBROSIS. HE RESIGNED FROM THE HOSPITAL AFTER BEING ADVISED THAT THE HOSPITAL'S EXECUTIVE COMMITTEE WOULD RECOMMEND A PERMANENT SUSPENSION. SUSPENSION STAYED. CONDITIONS OF PROBATION: SHALL HAVE A BOARD-APPROVED MONITORING PHYSICIAN WITH MONTHLY REPORTS; SHALL ATTEND AT LEAST 50 HOURS PER YEAR OF CONTINUING MEDICAL EDUCATION; SHALL APPEAR BEFORE THE BOARD ONCE A YEAR; SHALL COOPERATE WITH THE BOARD IN VERIFYING COMPLIANCE; SHALL INFORM BOARD OF CHANGE OF ADDRESS WITHIN 10 DAYS OR IF HE LEAVES THE STATE; TIME SPENT OUT OF TEXAS DOES NOT COUNT TOWARD PROBATION. SHALL NOT SEEK MODIFICATION FOR ONE YEAR. ON 3/2/96 REQUEST TO TERMINATE ORDER DENIED BUT ORDER MODIFIED SO HE SHALL PROVIDE WRITTEN REPORTS TO STAFF WHICH REFLECT THE LEVEL OF HIS PRACTICE SKILLS FROM ALL FACILITIES WHERE HE PRACTICES UPON BOARD REQUEST IN LIEU OF PREVIOUS REQUIREMENT FOR A MONITOR; MAY REQUEST MODIFICATION EVERY SIX MONTHS. PROBATION TERMINATED ON 8/17/96.

HILL, ROBERT DIXON MD, LICENSE NUMBER MD16554 OF CRESWELL, OR, WAS DISCIPLINED BY OREGON ON NOVEMBER 1, 1993
DISCIPLINARY ACTION: 24-MONTH RESTRICTION PLACED ON LICENSE; 24-MONTH RESTRICTION PLACED ON CONTROLLED SUBSTANCE LICENSE

NOTES: NO SCHEDULE II DRUGS EXCEPT FOR HOSPITAL PATIENTS; TRIPLICATE COPIES OF CONTROLLED SUBSTANCE PRESCRIPTIONS MUST BE PROVIDED FOR SCHEDULE III DRUGS; BOTH CONDITIONS SUBJECT TO REVIEW. VOLUNTARY LIMITATION SUBJECT TO REVIEW ON 11/1/95. NO LONGER LISTED ON PROBATION AS OF 11/27/95.

HILL, ROBERT DIXON MD, LICENSE NUMBER 0027422 OF CRESWELL, OR, WAS DISCIPLINED BY WASHINGTON ON JUNE 2, 1995
DISCIPLINARY ACTION: RESTRICTION PLACED ON CONTROLLED SUBSTANCE LICENSE

NOTES: AGREED ORDER RESTRICTING HIS PRESCRIBING OF CONTROLLED SUBSTANCES.

HILL, ROBERT DIXON MD, LICENSE NUMBER 0G13809 OF CREWELL, OR, WAS DISCIPLINED BY CALIFORNIA ON MARCH 4, 1996
DISCIPLINARY ACTION: LICENSE REVOCATION
OFFENSE: DISCIPLINARY ACTION BY ANOTHER STATE OR AGENCY

NOTES: ACTION IN OREGON. VOLUNTARY LIMITATION FILED LIMITING LICENSE TO PRACTICE MEDICINE WITH RESPECT TO SCHEDULES II AND III CONTROLLED SUBSTANCES. DEFAULT ACTION.

HILL, WELTON E MD, LICENSE NUMBER 00F6746, WAS DISCIPLINED BY TEXAS ON AUGUST 17, 1996
DISCIPLINARY ACTION: 60-MONTH PROBATION; RESTRICTION PLACED ON CONTROLLED SUBSTANCE LICENSE
OFFENSE: SUBSTANDARD CARE, INCOMPETENCE OR NEGLIGENCE

NOTES: BETWEEN 5/93 AND 9/93 PRESCRIBED MEDICATION WITHOUT ADEQUATE MONITORING AND ADMINISTERED MEDICATIONS WITHOUT KEEPING ADEQUATE PATIENT RECORDS IN ONE CASE; ALSO FAILED TO ADEQUATELY EVALUATE PATIENT AFTER POOR RESPONSE. ADMINISTERED VARIOUS MEDICATIONS TO HIS WIFE, A FORMER PATIENT WITHOUT KEEPING MEDICAL RECORDS WHICH MADE IT DIFFICULT TO ASCERTAIN THE FREQUENCY AND DOSAGES WITH WHICH THE MEDICATIONS PRESCRIBED WERE ADMINISTERED. SUSPENSION, STAYED AS PROBATION WITH TERMS AND CONDITIONS: SHALL MAINTAIN ADEQUATE MEDICAL RECORDS WHICH SHALL BE AVAILABLE FOR REVIEW;

SHALL OBTAIN AT LEAST 50 HOURS PER YEAR OF CONTINUING MEDICAL EDUCATION 10 HOURS OF WHICH SHALL BE IN PSYCHOTROPIC PRESCRIBING OR THE TREATMENT OF SUBSTANCE ABUSE OR PAIN MANAGEMENT; SHALL OBTAIN SIX HOURS OF AN ETHICS COURSE OR PROGRAM PER YEAR FOR FIVE YEARS; SHALL SUBMIT HIMSELF TO A BOARD APPROVED PSYCHIATRIST FOR EVALUATION AND TREATMENT WHO HE SHALL SEE AT LEAST ONCE A MONTH AND WHO SHALL SUBMIT REPORTS; SHALL PROVIDE ANY MEDICAL RELEASES UPON BOARD REQUEST; EXCEPT IN LIFE THREATENING EMERGENCY WHILE AWAITING OTHER DEFINITE CARE, SHALL NOT TREAT OR OTHERWISE SERVE AS PHYSICIAN, PRESCRIBE, DISPENSE, OR ADMINISTER DRUGS WITH POTENTIAL FOR ABUSE TO HIMSELF OR ANY MEMBER OF HIS FAMILY; SEPARATE FROM MEDICAL RECORDS, SHALL MAINTAIN A COPY OF EVERY PRESCRIPTION WRITTEN FOR DRUGS WITH POTENTIAL FOR ABUSE BY DATE WHICH SHALL BE AVAILABLE FOR INSPECTION UPON BOARD REQUEST; SHALL NOT TELEPHONE TO A PHARMACY ANY PRESCRIPTION OR REFILL OF SUCH DRUGS; HIS MEDICAL PRACTICE, INCLUDING ANY OFFICE AND SURGICAL PRACTICE, SHALL BE MONITORED BY A BOARD APPROVED TEXAS PHYSICIAN WHO SHALL PROVIDE QUARTERLY REPORTS; SHALL APPEAR BEFORE THE BOARD TWICE A YEAR FOR THE FIRST YEAR AND ONCE EACH YEAR THEREAFTER; SHALL COOPERATE WITH THE BOARD IN VERIFYING COMPLIANCE; SHALL GIVE A COPY OF THIS ORDER TO ANY HEALTH CARE ENTITY WHERE HE HAS PRIVILEGES; SHALL PROVIDE A COPY OF THIS ORDER TO ANYONE REQUESTING IT WITHIN 10 DAYS; TIME PERIOD OUT OF TEXAS DOES NOT COUNT TOWARD PROBATION; SHALL INFORM THE BOARD OF CHANGE OF ADDRESS WITHIN 14 DAYS OF IF HE LEAVES THE STATE; SHALL NOT SEEK MODIFICATION FOR ONE YEAR. ON 9/20/97 PETITION TO TERMINATE ORDER DENIED. ON 8/22/98 ORDER TERMINATED.

HINKLEY, BRUCE MD OF 1521 NORTH COOPER STREET #700, ARLINGTON, TX, WAS DISCIPLINED BY DEA ON OCTOBER 13, 1999
DISCIPLINARY ACTION: SURRENDER OF CONTROLLED SUBSTANCE LICENSE
OFFENSE: DISCIPLINARY ACTION BY ANOTHER STATE OR AGENCY

NOTES: STATE BOARD.

HINKLEY, BRUCE STANTON MD, LICENSE NUMBER D9497 OF ARLINGTON, TX, WAS DISCIPLINED BY TEXAS ON FEBRUARY 7, 1998
DISCIPLINARY ACTION: RESTRICTION PLACED ON LICENSE
OFFENSE: FAILURE TO COMPLY WITH PREVIOUS BOARD ORDER

NOTES: VIOLATED 8/25/89 BOARD ORDER BY TESTING POSITIVE FOR COCAINE METABOLITES OR BENZODIAZEPINES ON 1/12/98, 1/26/98 AND AGAIN ON 2/2/98; MAINTAINS THAT THE TESTS WERE INACCURATE SINCE HE HAS NOT INGESTED COCAINE SINCE 1988 AND HAS NOT INGESTED BENZODIAZEPINES OTHER THAN IN ACCORDANCE WITH HIS BOARD ORDER. LICENSE LIMITED AS FOLLOWS: SHALL NOT EXAMINE AND/OR TREAT PATIENTS UNTIL SUCH TIME AS HE REQUESTS IN WRITING TO HAVE THIS RESTRICTION MODIFIED OR TERMINATED, AND APPEARS BEFORE THE BOARD PROVIDING EVIDENCE OF HIS COMPETENCE; SHALL COOPERATE WITH THE BOARD IN VERIFYING COMPLIANCE INCLUDING PROVIDING COPIES OF MEDICAL RELEASES UPON REQUEST; SHALL INFORM THE BOARD OF CHANGE OF ADDRESS WITHIN 10 DAYS; SHALL NOT SEEK MODIFICATION FOR ONE YEAR.

HINKLEY, BRUCE STANTON MD, LICENSE NUMBER D9497 OF ARLINGTON, TX, WAS DISCIPLINED BY TEXAS ON APRIL 4, 1998
DISCIPLINARY ACTION: 60-MONTH PROBATION

NOTES: RESTRICTIONS PLACED ON HIS LICENSE ON 2/7/98 ARE RESCINDED; 8/25/89 REVOCATION IS TO REMAIN STAYED AND HE IS PLACED ON 60 MONTH PROBATION WITH FOLLOWING TERMS AND CONDITIONS: SHALL ABSTAIN FROM THE CONSUMPTION OF ALCOHOL/DRUGS IN ANY FORM UNLESS PRESCRIBED BY ANOTHER PHYSICIAN FOR A LEGITIMATE AND THERAPEUTIC PURPOSE; SHALL SUBMIT HIMSELF FOR APPROPRIATE EXAMS INCLUDING DRUG OR ALCOHOL SCREENS; SHALL CONTINUE TO RECEIVE CARE AND TREATMENT FROM HIS PHYSICIAN NO LESS THAN ONCE A WEEK AND SHALL ARRANGE FOR SAID PHYSICIAN TO PROVIDE QUARTERLY REPORTS TO THE BOARD; SHALL PARTICIPATE IN THE ACTIVITIES OF A PHYSICIAN HEALTH AND REHABILITATION COMMITTEE AND ATTEND WEEKLY MEETINGS WITH QUARTERLY REPORTS; SHALL PARTICIPATE IN AA'S PROGRAM NOT LESS THAN THREE TIMES A WEEK; SHALL REPORT ON HIS ATTENDANCE; SHALL APPEAR BEFORE THE BOARD TWICE A YEAR TO ADDRESS ISSUES RELATED TO COMPLIANCE WITH ORDER; SHALL GIVE A COPY OF THIS ORDER TO ANY HEALTH CARE ENTITY WHERE HE HAS PRIVILEGES; SHALL PROVIDE A COPY OF THIS ORDER TO ANYONE REQUESTING IT WITHIN 10 DAYS; TIME SPENT OUT OF TEXAS DOES NOT COUNT TOWARD PROBATION; SHALL INFORM THE BOARD OF CHANGE OF ADDRESS WITHIN 10 DAYS OR IF HE LEAVES THE STATE; SHALL NOT SEEK MODIFICATION FOR ONE YEAR; SHALL COOPERATE WITH THE BOARD IN VERIFYING COMPLIANCE INCLUDING PROVIDING COPIES OF MEDICAL RELEASES AND PEER REVIEW RECORDS UPON REQUEST.

HINKLEY, BRUCE STANTON MD, LICENSE NUMBER D9497 OF ARLINGTON, TX, WAS DISCIPLINED BY TEXAS ON JULY 26, 1999
DISCIPLINARY ACTION: EMERGENCY SUSPENSION
OFFENSE: SUBSTANCE ABUSE

NOTES: ON OR ABOUT 3/30/99 AND 6/28/99 HE VIOLATED 2/7/98 BOARD ORDER (SUBSEQUENTLY SUPERSEDED BY THE 4/4/98 ORDER) BY INGESTING COCAINE AS EVIDENCED BY URINE SAMPLES.

HIRSCH, EDWARD MD, LICENSE NUMBER 00F3499 OF EL PASO, TX, WAS DISCIPLINED BY TEXAS ON OCTOBER 9, 1992
DISCIPLINARY ACTION: RESTRICTION PLACED ON LICENSE
OFFENSE: PROFESSIONAL MISCONDUCT

NOTES: AIDING THE UNLICENSED PRACTICE OF MEDICINE BY AN ASSOCIATION OR CORPORATION. SHALL REFRAIN FROM PRACTICING MEDICINE UNTIL PASSAGE OF SPEX.

HIRSCH, EDWARD MD, LICENSE NUMBER 00F3499 OF EL PASO, TX, WAS DISCIPLINED BY TEXAS ON NOVEMBER 19, 1993
DISCIPLINARY ACTION: SURRENDER OF LICENSE

NOTES: LICENSE IS PERMANENTLY CANCELED; SHALL NOT PETITION THE BOARD FOR REINSTATEMENT.

HO, RICHARD KAY-YIN MD, LICENSE NUMBER 0G38504 OF SANTA CLARA, CA, WAS DISCIPLINED BY CALIFORNIA ON MAY 26, 1994
DISCIPLINARY ACTION: 6-MONTH LICENSE SUSPENSION; 54-MONTH PROBATION
OFFENSE: SUBSTANDARD CARE, INCOMPETENCE OR NEGLIGENCE

NOTES: GROSS NEGLIGENCE AND REPEATED NEGLIGENT ACTS IN OPHTHALMOLOGY PRACTICE. REVOCATION

STAYED.

HO, RICHARD KAY-YIN MD, LICENSE NUMBER 00F6254 OF SANTA CLARA, CA, WAS DISCIPLINED BY TEXAS ON MARCH 4, 1995
DISCIPLINARY ACTION: FINE
OFFENSE: DISCIPLINARY ACTION BY ANOTHER STATE OR AGENCY

NOTES: ON 5/26/94, PLACED ON PROBATION FOR FIVE YEARS BY CALIFORNIA BOARD, INCLUDING A SIX MONTH SUSPENSION, CONTINUING MEDICAL EDUCATION, COMMUNITY SERVICE, AND COSTS FOR NEGLIGENT ACTS WITH RESPECT TO FIVE PATIENTS TREATED BETWEEN 1984 AND 1990. SHALL NOT PRACTICE MEDICINE IN TEXAS UNTIL HE REQUESTS PERMISSION IN WRITING TO RESUME PRACTICE IN TEXAS AND APPEARS BEFORE THE BOARD AND PRESENTS SUFFICIENT EVIDENCE WHICH INDICATES THAT HE IS PHYSICALLY, MENTALLY AND OTHERWISE COMPETENT TO SAFELY PRACTICE MEDICINE; EVIDENCE SHALL INCLUDE INFORMATION INDICATING THAT HE HAS COMPLIED WITH THE TERMS AND CONDITIONS OF THE CALIFORNIA ORDER; SHALL PAY $1,000 FINE; SHALL GIVE A COPY OF THIS ORDER TO ANY HEALTH CARE ENTITY WHERE HE HAS PRIVILEGES; SHALL COOPERATE WITH THE BOARD IN VERIFYING COMPLIANCE; SHALL INFORM BOARD OF ANY CHANGE OF ADDRESS WITHIN 10 DAYS. SHALL NOT SEEK MODIFICATION FOR ONE YEAR.

HO, RICHARD KAY-YIN MD, LICENSE NUMBER G38504 OF SANTA CLARA, CA, WAS DISCIPLINED BY CALIFORNIA ON MARCH 15, 1997
DISCIPLINARY ACTION: SURRENDER OF LICENSE

NOTES: WHILE CHARGES PENDING.

HO, RICHARD KAY-YIN MD, DATE OF BIRTH JUNE 21, 1947 OF 4585 STEVENS CREEK BLVD, STE 200, SANTA CLARA, CA, WAS DISCIPLINED BY MEDICARE ON OCTOBER 7, 1997
DISCIPLINARY ACTION: EXCLUSION FROM THE MEDICARE AND/OR MEDICAID PROGRAM
OFFENSE: DISCIPLINARY ACTION BY ANOTHER STATE OR AGENCY

NOTES: LICENSE REVOKED, SUSPENDED, SURRENDERED OR OTHERWISE LOST FOR REASONS BEARING ON PROFESSIONAL PERFORMANCE, PROFESSIONAL COMPETENCE OR FINANCIAL INTEGRITY.

HOBBS, BOBBY R MD, LICENSE NUMBER F8511 OF DUNCANVILLE, TX, WAS DISCIPLINED BY TEXAS ON MAY 16, 1998
DISCIPLINARY ACTION: FINE; REPRIMAND
OFFENSE: SUBSTANDARD CARE, INCOMPETENCE OR NEGLIGENCE

NOTES: IN 1996 FAILED TO ADEQUATELY DIAGNOSE AND TREAT A PATIENT WHO WAS PRESENTED TO THE EMERGENCY ROOM WITH APPENDICITIS; MEDICAL TEST WERE PERFORMED AND HE EXAMINED THE PATIENT, BUT HE DID NOT OBTAIN A SURGICAL CONSULTATION ON THE PATIENT AND DISCHARGED THE PATIENT AFTER PRESCRIBING PAIN MEDICATION AND ANTIBIOTICS; THE PATIENT SUBSEQUENTLY SUFFERED A PERFORATED APPENDIX AND PERITONITIS, NECESSITATING AN 8 DAY HOSPITAL STAY. $1,000 FINE.

HOLLADAY, ROBERT E IV MD OF SHREVEPORT, LA, WAS DISCIPLINED BY LOUISIANA ON OCTOBER 26, 1995
DISCIPLINARY ACTION: 3-MONTH LICENSE SUSPENSION; 36-MONTH PROBATION
OFFENSE: PROVIDING FALSE INFORMATION TO THE BOARD OR OTHER HEALTH AGENCY

NOTES: FRAUD, DECEIT OR PERJURY IN OBTAINING ANY LICENSE ISSUED BY THE BOARD; PROFESSIONAL OR MEDICAL INCOMPETENCY; PRESCRIBING, DISPENSING OR ADMINISTERING CONTROLLED SUBSTANCES WITHOUT LEGITIMATE MEDICAL JUSTIFICATION. SHALL COMPLETE A COURSE IN PAIN MANAGEMENT AND SPECIFIED CONTINUING MEDICAL EDUCATION; $5,000 FINE. DECISION STAYED PENDING JUDICIAL REVIEW WHICH ULTIMATELY UPHELD THE DECISION ON 3/12/97. ON 6/12/97 LICENSE REINSTATED ON PROBATION SUBJECT TO TERMS AND CONDITIONS OF THIS DECISION.

HOLLADAY, ROBERT E IV MD, LICENSE NUMBER E3708 OF SHREVEPORT, LA, WAS DISCIPLINED BY TEXAS ON AUGUST 22, 1998
DISCIPLINARY ACTION: REQUIRED TO TAKE ADDITIONAL MEDICAL EDUCATION
OFFENSE: DISCIPLINARY ACTION BY ANOTHER STATE OR AGENCY

NOTES: ON 10/26/95 HE WAS DISCIPLINED BY THE LOUISIANA BOARD BASED UPON HIS FAILING TO NOTIFY THE BOARD OF A TEXAS BOARD INVESTIGATION AND ALSO BASED ON HIS QUALITY OF PATIENT CARE. LICENSE LIMITED FOR THREE YEARS AS FOLLOWS: SHALL OBTAIN 50 HOURS PER YEAR OF CONTINUING MEDICAL EDUCATION, WITH 1 COURSE IN PAIN MANAGEMENT; SHALL MAINTAIN ADEQUATE MEDICAL RECORDS WHICH SHALL BE AVAILABLE FOR REVIEW; SHALL APPEAR BEFORE THE BOARD AT LEAST ONCE A YEAR; SHALL COOPERATE WITH THE BOARD IN VERIFYING COMPLIANCE; SHALL COMPLY WITH LOUISIANA BOARD ORDER; SHALL GIVE A COPY OF THIS ORDER TO ANY HEALTH CARE ENTITY WHERE HE HAS PRIVILEGES; SHALL INFORM THE BOARD OF CHANGE OF ADDRESS WITHIN 10 DAYS; SHALL NOT SEEK MODIFICATION FOR ONE YEAR.

HOLLEN, JAKE THOMAS MD, DATE OF BIRTH AUGUST 8, 1951, LICENSE NUMBER 00G5926 OF LAKE CHARLES, LA, WAS DISCIPLINED BY TEXAS ON AUGUST 28, 1992
DISCIPLINARY ACTION: EMERGENCY SUSPENSION
OFFENSE: FAILURE TO COMPLY WITH PREVIOUS BOARD ORDER

NOTES: NONCOMPLIANCE WITH PREVIOUS BOARD ORDER.

HOLLEN, JAKE THOMAS MD, DATE OF BIRTH AUGUST 8, 1951, LICENSE NUMBER 00G5926 OF 701 CRICKETT ROAD, LAKE CHARLES, LA, WAS DISCIPLINED BY TEXAS ON JANUARY 30, 1993
DISCIPLINARY ACTION: 120-MONTH PROBATION; RESTRICTION PLACED ON CONTROLLED SUBSTANCE LICENSE
OFFENSE: FAILURE TO COMPLY WITH PREVIOUS BOARD ORDER

NOTES: FAILED TO COMPLY WITH 1988 BOARD ORDER IN THAT HE: FAILED TO SUBMIT SPECIMENS OF BODILY FLUIDS; FAILED TO SUBMIT PROOF OF ATTENDANCE OF AA MEETINGS OR ATTENDANCE AND PARTICIPATION WITH AN IMPAIRED PHYSICIANS GROUP AND FAILED TO COOPERATE WITH THE BOARD; TEN YEAR SUSPENSION STAYED, PROBATION ISSUED WITH FOLLOWING CONDITIONS: SHALL PARTICIPATE IN ACTIVITIES OF A PHYSICIAN HEALTH AND REHABILITATION COMMITTEE AND ATTEND WEEKLY MEETINGS WITH QUARTERLY REPORTS; SHALL PARTICIPATE IN AA'S 12 STEP PROGRAM NOT LESS THAN 3 TIMES A WEEK WITH QUARTERLY REPORTS TO THE BOARD; SHALL FURNISH THE BOARD WITH WRITTEN REPORTS ON HIS MEDICAL CONDITION AND COMPLIANCE WITH THIS ORDER WHEN REQUESTED; SHALL ABSTAIN FROM THE CONSUMPTION OF ALCOHOL/CHEMICAL SUBSTANCES IN ANY FORM; SHALL SUBMIT HIMSELF FOR APPROPRIATE EXAMS INCLUDING DRUG OR ALCOHOL SCREENS; SHALL NOT TREAT OR OTHERWISE SERVE AS THE PHYSICIAN, PRESCRIBE, DISPENSE OR ADMINISTER DRUGS THAT

MAY BE SUBJECT TO ABUSE FOR HIMSELF OR ANY MEMBER OF HIS FAMILY; DEA AND CONTROLLED SUBSTANCES REGISTRATION LIMITED TO SCHEDULES III THROUGH V; SHALL NOT ATTEMPT TO REREGISTER WITHOUT BOARD AUTHORIZATION; SHALL MAINTAIN A COPY OF EVERY PRESCRIPTION WRITTEN FOR CONTROLLED SUBSTANCES OR DANGEROUS DRUGS WHICH SHALL BE AVAILABLE FOR INSPECTION; SHALL NOT TELEPHONE IN ANY PRESCRIPTION FOR SUCH DRUGS; SHALL OBTAIN THE SERVICES OF A PRIMARY CARE PHYSICIAN WHO SHALL RELEASE INFORMATION TO THE BOARD AND NOTIFY THEM IF ANY DRUG HAVING ADDICTION-FORMING OR ADDICTION-SUSTAINING LIABILITY IS PRESCRIBED; SHALL OBTAIN NO PRESCRIPTIONS FROM ANY OTHER PHYSICIAN UNLESS IT IS APPROVED IN WRITING WITHIN 24 HOURS; ANY PRESCRIPTIONS WRITTEN BY PRIMARY CARE PHYSICIAN CAN BE FILLED ONLY AT BOARD-APPROVED PHARMACIES; SHALL BE EVALUATED BY A BOARD-APPROVED PSYCHIATRIST TO WHOM HE WILL PROVIDE A COPY OF THE ORDER; SHALL COOPERATE WITH THE BOARD IN VERIFYING COMPLIANCE; SHALL INFORM BOARD OF CHANGE OF ADDRESS WITHIN 10 DAYS OR IF HE LEAVES THE STATE; TIME SPENT OUT OF TEXAS OR LOUISIANA DOES NOT COUNT TOWARD PROBATION; SHALL APPEAR BEFORE THE BOARD ONCE A YEAR; SHALL MEET WITH PROBATION OFFICER 3 TIMES PER YEAR; SHALL APPEAR BEFORE THE BOARD PRIOR TO PRACTICING IN TEXAS. SHALL NOT SEEK MODIFICATION UNTIL DECEMBER 1, 1996.

HOLLEN, JAKE THOMAS MD OF LAKE CHARLES, LA, WAS DISCIPLINED BY LOUISIANA ON JUNE 24, 1993
DISCIPLINARY ACTION: 120-MONTH PROBATION; RESTRICTION PLACED ON CONTROLLED SUBSTANCE LICENSE
OFFENSE: DISCIPLINARY ACTION BY ANOTHER STATE OR AGENCY

NOTES: ACTION TAKEN BY TEXAS. SUBJECT TO FULL COMPLIANCE WITH TERMS OF CONSENT AGREEMENT WITH TEXAS BOARD, PROHIBITION ON PRESCRIPTION OF SCHEDULE II CONTROLLED SUBSTANCES, BOARD AUDITING OF RECORDS OF CONTROLLED SUBSTANCE PRESCRIPTIONS.

HOLLEN, JAKE THOMAS MD OF ELTON ROAD, JENNINGS, LA, WAS DISCIPLINED BY DEA ON AUGUST 25, 1993
DISCIPLINARY ACTION: RESTRICTION PLACED ON CONTROLLED SUBSTANCE LICENSE
OFFENSE: DISCIPLINARY ACTION BY ANOTHER STATE OR AGENCY

NOTES: TEXAS MEDICAL LICENSE PUT ON PROBATION 08/28/92. LOUISIANA AND TEXAS MEDICAL BOARDS REVOKED SCHEDULE II.

HOLMES, MICHAEL WESLEY MD, LICENSE NUMBER E7118 OF BEAUMONT, TX, WAS DISCIPLINED BY TEXAS ON APRIL 4, 1998
DISCIPLINARY ACTION: FINE
OFFENSE: SUBSTANDARD CARE, INCOMPETENCE OR NEGLIGENCE

NOTES: ON OR ABOUT 7/24/97 HE DID NOT CORRECTLY ASSESS AND TIMELY INTERVENE ON A PEDIATRIC PATIENT WITH A DIABETIC CRISIS IN THAT HE DID NOT ADMINISTER INSULIN OR UNDERTAKE HOSPITAL ADMISSION OF THE PATIENT UNTIL A RETURN APPOINTMENT THE NEXT DAY. $1,000 FINE; SHALL COOPERATE WITH THE BOARD IN VERIFYING COMPLIANCE.

HOLT, CECIL ZENO MD, LICENSE NUMBER 00B8784 OF WAXAHACHIE, TX, WAS DISCIPLINED BY TEXAS ON APRIL 10, 1992
DISCIPLINARY ACTION: 60-MONTH PROBATION
OFFENSE: SUBSTANDARD CARE, INCOMPETENCE OR NEGLIGENCE

NOTES: PROFESSIONAL FAILURE TO PRACTICE MEDICINE IN AN ACCEPTABLE MANNER CONSISTENT WITH PUBLIC HEALTH AND WELFARE. LICENSE SUSPENDED, SUSPENSION STAYED; PROBATION UNDER TERMS AND CONDITIONS.

HONG, SEUNG K MD, LICENSE NUMBER 009288, WAS DISCIPLINED BY MAINE ON MARCH 11, 1997
DISCIPLINARY ACTION: SURRENDER OF LICENSE
OFFENSE: DISCIPLINARY ACTION BY ANOTHER STATE OR AGENCY

NOTES: RECIPROCAL ACTION BASED ON ACTION TAKEN IN TEXAS. VOLUNTARY SURRENDER.

HONG, SEUNG KOOK MD, LICENSE NUMBER 00F5950 OF RICHARDSON, TX, WAS DISCIPLINED BY TEXAS ON JANUARY 12, 1991
DISCIPLINARY ACTION: 60-MONTH PROBATION; RESTRICTION PLACED ON LICENSE

NOTES: SHALL NOT PRACTICE OBSTETRICS OR SURGERY, EXCEPT FOR MINOR OFFICE PRACTICE SURGERY, WITHOUT MEETING ALL QUALIFICATIONS FOR BOARD CERTIFICATION IN GENERAL SURGERY, WHICH WOULD THEN BE PERMITTED; SHALL TREAT NO PATIENTS UNDER FOUR YEARS OF AGE EXCEPT TO PROVIDE IMMUNIZATIONS; OBTAIN CONTINUING MEDICAL EDUCATION; TAKE AND PASS THE SPECIAL PURPOSE EXAM (SPEX) WITHIN SIX MONTHS OF APPROVAL OF THIS ORDER.

HONG, SEUNG KOOK MD, LICENSE NUMBER 00F5950 OF RICHARDSON, TX, WAS DISCIPLINED BY TEXAS ON OCTOBER 17, 1994
DISCIPLINARY ACTION: 9-MONTH PROBATION; REQUIRED TO TAKE ADDITIONAL MEDICAL EDUCATION
OFFENSE: FAILURE TO COMPLY WITH PREVIOUS BOARD ORDER

NOTES: ON 1/12/91 HE ENTERED INTO AN AGREEMENT WITH BOARD DUE TO THE FINDING THAT HE HAD MERITORIOUS MEDICAL LIABILITY CLAIMS AGAINST HIM FOR TREATMENT RENDERED IN 1980. 1981, 1983 AND 1985 INVOLVING BOTH OBSTETRICS AND SURGERY; ONE OF THE TERMS OF THIS AGREEMENT WAS THAT HE WOULD PASS THE SPEX EXAM WITHIN 6 MONTHS; HE TOOK THE EXAM TWICE ONCE IN 9/91 AND ONCE IN 6/92 AND DID NOT PASS NOR DID HE COMPLETE THE EXAM ON BOTH OCCASIONS; CLAIMED HE HAD FAMILY PROBLEMS WHICH MADE IT DIFFICULT TO STUDY AND IT WAS DIFFICULT FOR HIM TO FINISH THE EXAM IN THE ALLOTTED TIME BECAUSE ENGLISH IS NOT HIS FIRST LANGUAGE. SUSPENSION STAYED. CONDITIONS OF PROBATION: SHALL PASS THE SPEX EXAM WITHIN TWO YEARS; SHALL BE GIVEN ONE AND A HALF NORMAL TIME ALLOTMENT TO TAKE THE EXAM; SHALL COMPLETE A 150 HOUR PRACTICAL REVIEW COURSE APPROVED BY THE BOARD WITHIN ONE YEAR; ALL OTHER TERMS OF 1/12/91 ORDER REMAIN IN EFFECT FOR TWO YEARS FROM THE DATE OF THIS ORDER. THE BOARD ORDER WILL BECOME FINAL WHEN ADMINISTRATIVE APPEALS HAVE BEEN EXHAUSTED; HE HAS 20 DAYS TO FILE A MOTION FOR REHEARING.

HOOPER, LAWRENCE H JR MD, LICENSE NUMBER 00G1293 OF EL PASO, TX, WAS DISCIPLINED BY TEXAS ON DECEMBER 3, 1990
DISCIPLINARY ACTION: PROBATION

NOTES: PLACED ON TEMPORARY PROBATION PENDING THE OUTCOME OF CRIMINAL TRIAL. PROBATION TERMINATED EFFECTIVE 6/17/92; LICENSE FREE OF ANY RESTRICTION OR LIMITATION.

HORSLEY, HEIDI CHARLOTTE MD, LICENSE NUMBER F4096 OF LUBBOCK, TX, WAS DISCIPLINED BY TEXAS ON APRIL 4, 1998
DISCIPLINARY ACTION: LICENSE SUSPENSION
OFFENSE: FAILURE TO COMPLY WITH PREVIOUS BOARD ORDER

NOTES: VIOLATED 6/22/96 BOARD ORDER IN THAT SHE PRESCRIBED DRUGS TO HER FAMILY AND FAILED TO KEEP ANY MEDICAL RECORDS REGARDING THESE TREATMENTS; SHE MAINTAINS THAT THE PRESCRIPTIONS WHICH SHE WROTE FOR HER FAMILY WERE LIMITED TO 4 PRESCRIPTIONS AND CONSTITUTED ONLY CONTINUING TREATMENT; SHE HAS BEEN DIAGNOSED WITH CERTAIN PHYSICAL AND PSYCHIATRIC DISORDERS WHICH HAVE CAUSED HER TO EXHIBIT UNPREDICTABLE, AND SOMETIMES DANGEROUS BEHAVIOR; SHE HAS BEEN DISABLED SINCE 1994 AND MAINTAINS THAT THE REASON FOR HER DISABILITY HAS BEEN ASCENDING CHOLANGITIS, BILIOUS GASTRITIS, AND CEREBELLAR DYSFUNCTION; TAKES SEVERAL MEDICATIONS AND ADMITS NO SINGLE TREATING PHYSICIAN IS AWARE OF ALL OF THEM; SHE HAS ADMINISTERED THYROID MEDICATION TO HER CHILDREN WHICH WAS ACQUIRED AS A PRESCRIPTION WRITTEN FOR HER USE ONLY. SUSPENSION UNTIL SHE REQUESTS TO HAVE HER SUSPENSION STAYED OR APPEARS BEFORE THE BOARD WITH SUFFICIENT EVIDENCE THAT HE IS PHYSICALLY, MENTALLY AND OTHERWISE COMPETENT TO SAFELY PRACTICE MEDICINE INCLUDING AT A MINIMUM COMPLETE COPIES OF MEDICAL RECORDS AND REPORTS OF PSYCHOLOGICAL AND NEUROPSYCHIATRIC EVALUATIONS, INCLUDING A 96 HOUR INPATIENT EVALUATION CONDUCTED BY A BOARD-APPROVED CERTIFIED PSYCHIATRIST; SHALL COOPERATE WITH THE BOARD IN VERIFYING COMPLIANCE INCLUDING PROVIDING COPIES OF MEDICAL RELEASES UPON REQUEST; SHALL PROVIDE A COPY OF THIS ORDER TO ANYONE REQUESTING IT WITHIN 10 DAYS; SHALL INFORM THE BOARD OF CHANGE OF ADDRESS WITHIN 10 DAYS OR IF SHE LEAVES THE STATE.

HORSLEY, HEIDI CHARLOTTE MD, DATE OF BIRTH AUGUST 15, 1954 OF 2604 MANIOCA ROAD, LUBBOCK, TX, WAS DISCIPLINED BY MEDICARE ON DECEMBER 20, 1998
DISCIPLINARY ACTION: EXCLUSION FROM THE MEDICARE AND/OR MEDICAID PROGRAM
OFFENSE: DISCIPLINARY ACTION BY ANOTHER STATE OR AGENCY

NOTES: LICENSE REVOKED, SUSPENDED, SURRENDERED OR OTHERWISE LOST FOR REASONS BEARING ON PROFESSIONAL PERFORMANCE, PROFESSIONAL COMPETENCE OR FINANCIAL INTEGRITY.

HOUSE, CHARLES HAROLD MD, LICENSE NUMBER 00D0390 OF KILLEEN, TX, WAS DISCIPLINED BY TEXAS ON JUNE 22, 1994
DISCIPLINARY ACTION: 60-MONTH PROBATION; RESTRICTION PLACED ON LICENSE
OFFENSE: SUBSTANDARD CARE, INCOMPETENCE OR NEGLIGENCE

NOTES: BETWEEN 8/19/91 AND 11/93 IN REGARD TO MULTIPLE PATIENTS, FAILED TO ADEQUATELY FOLLOW-UP GYNECOLOGICAL PROBLEMS, FAILED TO APPROPRIATELY INSTITUTE TREATMENT IN RESPONSE TO ABNORMAL PAP SMEARS, FAILED TO PROPERLY UTILIZE COLPOSCOPY AND CAUTERY AND FAILED TO OBTAIN A DEFINITE DIAGNOSIS OR KNOW PATIENT PATHOLOGY FROM PAP SMEAR OR BIOPSY REPORT BEFORE INITIATING TREATMENT; FAILED TO USE A PROGESTATIONAL AGENT IN CONJUNCTION WITH ESTROGEN THEREBY PUTTING PATIENTS AT RISK FOR ENDOMETRIAL CANCER; PATIENT CHART REVIEW REVEALED NUMEROUS SUCH DEFICIENCIES; IS NOT AMERICAN BOARD CERTIFIED BUT ADVERTISES THAT HE IS A FAMILY PRACTICE SPECIALIST WITH A SUBSPECIALTY IN OBSTETRICS/GYNECOLOGY. SUSPENSION STAYED. CONDITIONS OF PROBATION: SHALL NOT PRACTICE GYNECOLOGY UNTIL HE HAS OBTAINED 25 HOURS OF OUT- PATIENT GYNECOLOGICAL TRAINING INCLUDING A BOARD-APPROVED COLPOSCOPY COURSE; UPON COMPLETION OF THIS TRAINING SHALL BE SUPERVISED BY A BOARD-APPROVED PHYSICIAN FOR ALL GYNECOLOGIC CASES WITH REPORTS THREE TIMES A YEAR; SHALL REFER ALL ABNORMAL PAP SMEARS BEYOND CLASS II FOR A SECOND OPINION TO A BOARD-APPROVED PHYSICIAN; SHALL ATTEND AT LEAST 50 HOURS PER YEAR OF CONTINUING MEDICAL EDUCATION 25 HOURS OF WHICH SHALL BE IN OUT-PATIENT GYNECOLOGY; SHALL GIVE A COPY OF THIS ORDER TO ANY HEALTH CARE ENTITY WHERE HE HAS PRIVILEGES; SHALL COOPERATE WITH THE BOARD IN VERIFYING COMPLIANCE; SHALL INFORM BOARD OF ADDRESS CHANGE WITHIN 10 DAYS OR IF HE LEAVES THE STATE; TIME SPENT OUT OF TEXAS DOES NOT COUNT TOWARD PROBATION. SHALL NOT SEEK MODIFICATION FOR ONE YEAR.

HOUSE, FLOYD LEON MD, DATE OF BIRTH FEBRUARY 22, 1944, LICENSE NUMBER 00D9501 OF VICTORIA, TX, WAS DISCIPLINED BY TEXAS ON JULY 1, 1990
DISCIPLINARY ACTION: LICENSE REVOCATION
OFFENSE: SUBSTANCE ABUSE

NOTES: INTEMPERATE USE OF ALCOHOL WHICH IN BOARD'S OPINION COULD ENDANGER LIVES OF PATIENTS, UNPROFESSIONAL CONDUCT LIKELY TO DECEIVE, DEFRAUD, OR INJURE PUBLIC. REVOCATION STAYED PENDING JUDICIAL REVIEW. JUDGE UPHELD BOARD'S DECISION.

HOUSE, FLOYD LEON MD, DATE OF BIRTH FEBRUARY 22, 1944, LICENSE NUMBER 00D9501 OF 5603 EL CAMINO REAL, HARLINGEN, TX, WAS DISCIPLINED BY TEXAS ON MAY 14, 1993
DISCIPLINARY ACTION: LICENSE REINSTATEMENT; 120-MONTH PROBATION

NOTES: REINSTATEMENT FROM REVOCATION OF 10/12/90. TEN YEAR SUSPENSION STAYED. CONDITIONS OF PROBATION: RESTRICTED TO THE PRACTICE OF PSYCHIATRY AT ONE OF TWO FACILITIES; SHALL SUBMIT HIMSELF TO EVALUATION AND TREATMENT BY A BOARD-APPROVED PSYCHIATRIST TO WHOM HE SHALL PROVIDE A COPY OF THIS ORDER AND WHO SHALL MAKE MONTHLY REPORTS TO THE BOARD; SHALL BE SUPERVISED BY A BOARD-APPROVED PHYSICIAN WHO SHALL SUBMIT QUARTERLY REPORTS TO THE BOARD; SHALL ATTEND AT LEAST 50 HOURS OF CONTINUING MEDICAL EDUCATION AND SIX HOURS OF AN ETHICS COURSE PER YEAR; SHALL ABSTAIN FROM THE CONSUMPTION OF ALCOHOL/CHEMICAL SUBSTANCES IN ANY FORM; SHALL PARTICIPATE IN ACTIVITIES OF A PHYSICIAN HEALTH AND REHABILITATION COMMITTEE AND ATTEND WEEKLY MEETINGS WITH QUARTERLY REPORTS; THIS CONDITION MODIFIED ON 8/20/93 SUCH THAT HE SHALL PARTICIPATE IN AND BE SUBJECT TO REVIEW BY ANY PEER REVIEW COMMITTEE OF ANY STATE OF TEXAS MENTAL HEALTH AND MENTAL RETARDATION FACILITY WHERE HE PRACTICES WITH QUARTERLY REPORTS; SHALL PARTICIPATE IN AA'S PROGRAM NOT LESS THAN THREE TIMES A WEEK WITH QUARTERLY REPORTS TO THE BOARD; SHALL SUBMIT HIMSELF FOR APPROPRIATE EXAMS INCLUDING DRUG AND ALCOHOL SCREENS; SHALL FURNISH WRITTEN REPORTS TO THE BOARD UPON REQUEST TO VERIFY

COMPLIANCE; ANY CHANGE IN EMPLOYMENT SHALL BE REPORTED TO THE BOARD; SHALL NOT HAVE ANY PERSONAL RELATIONSHIP WITH ANY PATIENT; SHALL NOT TREAT OR OTHERWISE SERVE AS PHYSICIAN, PRESCRIBE, DISPENSE OR ADMINISTER DRUGS THAT MAY BE SUBJECT TO ABUSE FOR HIMSELF OR ANY MEMBER OF HIS FAMILY; SHALL APPEAR BEFORE THE BOARD TWICE A YEAR; SHALL ARRANGE A PAYMENT PLAN TO PAY COURT COSTS ASSOCIATED WITH THE ORIGINAL REVOCATION ACTION TAKEN AGAINST HIS LICENSE; SHALL GIVE A COPY OF THIS ORDER TO ANY HEALTH CARE ENTITY WHERE HE HAS PRIVILEGES; SHALL COOPERATE WITH THE BOARD IN VERIFYING COMPLIANCE; SHALL INFORM THE BOARD OF CHANGE OF ADDRESS WITHIN 10 DAYS OR IF HE LEAVES THE STATE; TIME SPENT OUT OF TEXAS DOES NOT COUNT TOWARD PROBATION. ON 6/22/94 A REQUEST TO ALLOW HIM TO ENGAGE IN PART-TIME PRIVATE PRACTICE WAS DENIED. ON 6/28/95 ORDER MODIFIED ALLOWING HIM TO PROVIDE PSYCHIATRIC CARE, EVALUATION AND CONSULTATION FOR EMERGENT PATIENTS FOR PURPOSES OF SHORT-TERM CARE ONLY. ON 5/15/96 REQUEST TO TERMINATE ORDER DENIED BUT ORDER MODIFIED AS FOLLOWS: REQUIREMENT RESTRICTING HIS PRACTICE TO A TEXAS MENTAL HEALTH FACILITY AND TO PROVIDING PSYCHIATRIC CARE, EVALUATION AND CONSULTATION TO EMERGENT PATIENTS IS DELETED; HE IS NO LONGER REQUIRED TO OBTAIN SIX HOURS OF AN ETHICS COURSE OR PROGRAM PER YEAR; ALL OTHER PROVISIONS REMAIN IN EFFECT. ON 2/7/98 ORDER MODIFIED AS FOLLOWS: SHALL NOT PRACTICE UNTIL HE APPEARS BEFORE THE PANEL AND SHOWS HE IS PHYSICALLY ABLE TO SAFELY PRACTICE MEDICINE AND COMPLY WITH TERMS OF ORDER; ANY TIME HE IS NOT AUTHORIZED TO PRACTICE MEDICINE THE ORDER WILL BE TOLLED; MAY PETITION FOR MODIFICATION OR TERMINATION REQUESTS ONLY ONCE EVERY TWELVE MONTHS.

HOUSE, FLOYD LEON MD OF 1901 S 24TH STREET, EDINBURG, TX, WAS DISCIPLINED BY DEA ON JULY 28, 1993
DISCIPLINARY ACTION: RESTRICTION PLACED ON CONTROLLED SUBSTANCE LICENSE
OFFENSE: DISCIPLINARY ACTION BY ANOTHER STATE OR AGENCY

NOTES: REGISTRATION REVOKED 10/12/90 IN TEXAS FOR INTEMPERATE USE OF ALCOHOL OR DRUGS AND UNPROFESSIONAL CONDUCT.

HOWARD, ANNETTE M MD, DATE OF BIRTH AUGUST 24, 1958 OF 3221 MILBURN STREET, HOUSTON, TX, WAS DISCIPLINED BY MEDICARE ON MARCH 6, 1994
DISCIPLINARY ACTION: EXCLUSION FROM THE MEDICARE AND/OR MEDICAID PROGRAM
OFFENSE: NONCOMPLIANCE WITH A PROFESSIONAL RULE

NOTES: DEFAULTED ON PUBLIC HEALTH SERVICE EDUCATION LOAN. REINSTATED ON 3/2/95.

HOWARD, JAMES MARSHALL MD, LICENSE NUMBER G5186 OF DALLAS, TX, WAS DISCIPLINED BY TEXAS ON AUGUST 22, 1998
DISCIPLINARY ACTION: LICENSE SUSPENSION
OFFENSE: SUBSTANCE ABUSE

NOTES: ON OR ABOUT 1 -2/98 HE WROTE FALSE AND FICTITIOUS PRESCRIPTIONS AND DIVERTED CONTROLLED SUBSTANCES FOR HIS OWN CONSUMPTION; HE IS CURRENTLY IN TREATMENT FOR SUBSTANCE ABUSE/DEPENDENCE; HE IS NOT CURRENTLY EMPLOYED IN THE PRACTICE OF MEDICINE, AND DOES NOT PLAN TO RETURN. SUSPENSION UNTIL HE REQUESTS TO HAVE HIS SUSPENSION STAYED OR APPEARS BEFORE THE BOARD WITH SUFFICIENT EVIDENCE THAT HE IS PHYSICALLY, MENTALLY AND OTHERWISE COMPETENT TO SAFELY PRACTICE MEDICINE INCLUDING AT A MINIMUM COMPLETE COPIES OF MEDICAL RECORDS AND REPORTS OF PSYCHOLOGICAL AND NEUROPSYCHIATRIC EVALUATIONS, INCLUDING A 96 HOUR INPATIENT EVALUATION CONDUCTED BY A BOARD-APPROVED CERTIFIED PSYCHIATRIST; SHALL COOPERATE WITH THE BOARD IN VERIFYING COMPLIANCE INCLUDING PROVIDING COPIES OF MEDICAL RELEASES UPON REQUEST; SHALL INFORM THE BOARD OF CHANGE OF ADDRESS WITHIN 10 DAYS; SHALL NOT SEEK MODIFICATION FOR ONE YEAR.

HOWELL, SHELLEY M DO, LICENSE NUMBER 00E3310, WAS DISCIPLINED BY TEXAS ON AUGUST 17, 1996
DISCIPLINARY ACTION: REPRIMAND; REQUIRED TO TAKE ADDITIONAL MEDICAL EDUCATION
OFFENSE: SUBSTANDARD CARE, INCOMPETENCE OR NEGLIGENCE

NOTES: BETWEEN 6/89 AND 11/89 TREATED AN ADULT FEMALE PATIENT FOR WEIGHT LOSS AND FAILED TO DOCUMENT AN ADEQUATE RESPONSE TO ABNORMAL LABORATORY STUDIES CONDUCTED DURING THIS PERIOD; AFTER COMPLAINTS FROM THE PATIENT OF BACK PAIN, PERFORMED OSTEOPATHIC MANIPULATION AND PROVIDED PAIN MEDICATION PRIOR TO PERFORMING DIAGNOSTIC TESTING INCLUDING X-RAYS; IN 12/89 THE PATIENT WAS DIAGNOSED BY ANOTHER PHYSICIAN AS SUFFERING FROM MULTIPLE MYELOMA AND HER PAIN WAS DETERMINED TO HAVE BEEN ASSOCIATED WITH RIB AND VERTEBRAL FRACTURES; IN REGARDS TO VARIOUS PATIENTS TREATED BETWEEN 1987 AND 1994 FAILED TO ADEQUATELY DOCUMENT EXAMINATIONS AND FAILED TO DOCUMENT APPROPRIATE TESTING PRIOR TO REACHING A DIAGNOSIS AND RENDERING TREATMENT; IN SOME INSTANCES INVOLVING PATIENTS BEING TREATED FOR WEIGHT LOSS, PROVIDED MEDICATIONS WHICH WERE NOT INDICATED BY ANY DOCUMENTED MEDICAL CONDITION AND FAILED TO ADEQUATELY DOCUMENT APPROPRIATE FOLLOW-UP THROUGH MONITORING AND TESTING WHICH WAS INDICATED; AND IN SOME INSTANCES, PRESCRIBED MEDICATIONS FOR PAIN, ANXIETY, OR WEIGHT LOSS, WITHOUT ADEQUATE AND APPROPRIATELY DOCUMENTED INDICATIONS. THREE YEAR RESTRICTION WITH TERMS AND CONDITIONS: SHALL REFRAIN FROM THE PRESCRIPTION OR ADMINISTRATION OF ANY DRUG FOR ANY PATIENT UNLESS THE DRUG IS MEDICALLY INDICATED AND IS PRESCRIBED IN THERAPEUTIC DOSES AND AFTER WHICH HAS TAKEN AN APPROPRIATE MEDICAL HISTORY AND CONDUCTED AN EXAMINATION WHICH IS CLINICALLY ADEQUATE TO DETERMINE A PROPER DIAGNOSIS AND COURSE OF TREATMENT; SHALL CONDUCT ADEQUATE FOLLOW-UP EXAMINATIONS ON ALL PATIENTS TO DETERMINE WHETHER THE COURSE OF TREATMENT, INCLUDING THE PRESCRIBING OF DRUGS, IS APPROPRIATE; SHALL MAINTAIN ADEQUATE MEDICAL RECORDS WHICH SHALL BE AVAILABLE FOR REVIEW; SHALL ATTEND AT LEAST 50 HOURS PER YEAR OF CONTINUING MEDICAL EDUCATION AT LEAST 10 HOURS OF WHICH SHALL BE IN RISK MANAGEMENT, AND SUBMIT PROOF TO THE BOARD; SHALL APPEAR BEFORE THE BOARD AT LEAST ONCE A YEAR OR UPON REQUEST; SHALL COOPERATE WITH THE BOARD IN VERIFYING COMPLIANCE; SHALL GIVE A COPY OF THIS ORDER TO ANY HEALTH CARE ENTITY WHERE HE HAS PRIVILEGES; TIME PERIOD OUT OF TEXAS DOES NOT COUNT TOWARD RESTRICTION;

SHALL INFORM THE BOARD OF CHANGE OF ADDRESS WITHIN 10 DAYS OF IF SHE LEAVES THE STATE; SHALL NOT SEEK MODIFICATION FOR ONE YEAR. ON 10/22/98 ORDER TERMINATED.

HOWELL, WYATT ALLEN MD, LICENSE NUMBER 00D8276 OF SEMINOLE, TX, WAS DISCIPLINED BY TEXAS ON AUGUST 20, 1992
DISCIPLINARY ACTION: 60-MONTH PROBATION
OFFENSE: SUBSTANCE ABUSE

NOTES: INTEMPERATE USE OF ALCOHOL OR DRUGS AND DISCIPLINARY ACTION TAKEN BY HIS PEERS. SUSPENSION, STAYED. PROBATION UNDER TERMS AND CONDITIONS.

HOWELL, WYATT ALLEN MD, LICENSE NUMBER 00D8276 OF BRADY, TX, WAS DISCIPLINED BY TEXAS ON AUGUST 18, 1995
DISCIPLINARY ACTION: 60-MONTH PROBATION; REQUIRED TO TAKE ADDITIONAL MEDICAL EDUCATION
OFFENSE: FAILURE TO COMPLY WITH PREVIOUS BOARD ORDER

NOTES: IN 3/94, A POSITIVE RANDOM BLOOD SCREEN REVEALED THAT HE INGESTED ALCOHOL WHICH WAS IN VIOLATION OF 8/92 BOARD ORDER; SUBSEQUENTLY RESIGNED FROM THE STAFF OF A HOSPITAL IN 4/94; RECEIVED INPATIENT SUBSTANCE ABUSE TREATMENT FROM 4/5/94 TO 4/28/94; REPORTS ATTENDING AN AVERAGE OF THREE AA MEETINGS PER WEEK. SUSPENSION STAYED. PROBATION WITH TERMS: SHALL ABSTAIN FROM THE CONSUMPTION OF ALCOHOL/DRUGS IN ANY FORM UNLESS PRESCRIBED BY ANOTHER PHYSICIAN FOR A LEGITIMATE AND THERAPEUTIC PURPOSE; SHALL SUBMIT HIMSELF FOR APPROPRIATE EXAMS INCLUDING DRUG OR ALCOHOL SCREENS; SHALL SUBMIT HIMSELF FOR EVALUATION AND TREATMENT BY A BOARD-APPROVED PSYCHIATRIST WHOM HE SHALL SEE AT LEAST ONCE A MONTH AND WHO SHALL SUBMIT REPORTS TO THE BOARD; SHALL CONTINUE TO PARTICIPATE IN AA'S PROGRAM NO LESS THAN THREE TIMES A WEEK WITH QUARTERLY REPORTS TO THE BOARD; SHALL PARTICIPATE IN THE ACTIVITIES OF AN IMPAIRED PHYSICIAN'S GROUP AND ATTEND WEEKLY MEETINGS WITH QUARTERLY REPORTS; SHALL COMPLY WITH THE TERMS AND CONDITIONS OF ANY CONTRACT FOR HOSPITAL PRIVILEGES AND SHALL REPORT ANY DISCIPLINARY ACTIONS TO THE BOARD; SHALL NOT TREAT OR OTHERWISE SERVE AS PHYSICIAN, PRESCRIBE, DISPENSE OR ADMINISTER DRUGS THAT MAY BE SUBJECT TO ABUSE TO HIMSELF OR TO ANY MEMBER OF HIS FAMILY; SHALL MAINTAIN A LOG WITH A COPY OF EVERY PRESCRIPTION WRITTEN FOR THESE DRUGS WHICH SHALL BE AVAILABLE FOR REVIEW; SHALL MAINTAIN ADEQUATE MEDICAL RECORDS WHICH ALSO SHALL BE AVAILABLE FOR REVIEW; SHALL NOT SIGN OR INDICATE IN ANY MANNER IN PATIENT RECORDS THAT HE HAS SEEN PATIENTS UNLESS HE ACTUALLY HAS SEEN AND EXAMINED THE PATIENT UNLESS IT IS CLEARLY NOTED THAT HE DID NOT PERSONALLY EXAMINE THE PATIENT; SHALL OBTAIN AT LEAST 50 HOURS PER YEAR OF CONTINUING MEDICAL EDUCATION; SHALL APPEAR BEFORE BOARD AT LEAST TWICE A YEAR OR AT BOARD REQUEST; SHALL COOPERATE WITH THE BOARD IN VERIFYING COMPLIANCE INCLUDING PROVIDING COPIES OF MEDICAL RELEASES OR PEER REVIEW RECORDS UPON REQUEST; SHALL GIVE A COPY OF THIS ORDER TO ANY HEALTH CARE ENTITY WHERE HE HAS PRIVILEGES; SHALL PROVIDE A COPY OF THIS ORDER TO ANYONE REQUESTING IT WITHIN 10 DAYS; TIME PERIOD OUT OF TEXAS DOES NOT COUNT TOWARD PROBATION; SHALL INFORM BOARD OF CHANGE OF ADDRESS WITHIN 10 DAYS OR IF HE LEAVES THE STATE. SHALL NOT SEEK MODIFICATION FOR ONE YEAR. ON 8/22/98 ORDER TERMINATED.

HSU, YU-TO MD OF HOUSTON, TX, WAS DISCIPLINED BY DEA ON APRIL 17, 1997
DISCIPLINARY ACTION: DENIAL OF LICENSE REINSTATEMENT
OFFENSE: CRIMINAL CONVICTION OR PLEA OF GUILTY, NOLO CONTENDERE, OR NO CONTEST TO A CRIME

NOTES: ON 7/23/93 PLED GUILTY TO SEVEN COUNTS OF UNLAWFUL PRESCRIBING OF CONTROLLED SUBSTANCES TO UNDERCOVER OFFICERS STEMMING FROM AN INVESTIGATION WHERE FIVE AGENTS CAME TO HIS OFFICE BETWEEN 2/28/91 AND 11/4/92 STATED THAT THEY USED CRACK COCAINE AN NEEDED SOMETHING TO COME DOWN FROM IT; HE PRESCRIBED THEM TYLENOL 4 OR VALIUM, SOME ON MORE THAN ONE OCCASION; ON 12/4/92 HE SURRENDERED HIS TEXAS CONTROLLED SUBSTANCE REGISTRATION AND HIS DEA REGISTRATION; HAS COMPLETED ALL TERMS OF DEFERRED ADJUDICATION AND HIS TEXAS PROBATION HAS BEEN TERMINATED.

HSU, YU-TO MD, LICENSE NUMBER F1065 OF HOUSTON, TX, WAS DISCIPLINED BY TEXAS ON SEPTEMBER 20, 1997
DISCIPLINARY ACTION: REPRIMAND
OFFENSE: CRIMINAL CONVICTION OR PLEA OF GUILTY, NOLO CONTENDERE, OR NO CONTEST TO A CRIME

NOTES: ON OR ABOUT 12/23/91, 1/29/92, 3/3/92, 4/23/92, AND 11/4/92 HE DELIVERED PRESCRIPTIONS TO TWO PATIENTS WITHOUT A VALID THERAPEUTIC MEDICAL PURPOSE; IN 1993 HE PLED GUILTY TO 7 CHARGES OF UNLAWFUL PRESCRIPTION IN THE DISTRICT COURT OF HARRIS COUNTY, TEXAS.

HUBBARD, GREGORY DO OF 1717 NORTH GARETT AVENUE, DALLAS, TX, WAS DISCIPLINED BY DEA ON OCTOBER 20, 1999
DISCIPLINARY ACTION: SURRENDER OF CONTROLLED SUBSTANCE LICENSE
OFFENSE: PROFESSIONAL MISCONDUCT

NOTES: OBTAINING CONTROLLED SUBSTANCES BY FRAUD.

HUBBARD, GREGORY GERARD DO, LICENSE NUMBER 00G3480 OF ARLINGTON, TX, WAS DISCIPLINED BY TEXAS ON MARCH 6, 1992
DISCIPLINARY ACTION: 120-MONTH PROBATION
OFFENSE: SUBSTANCE ABUSE

NOTES: ALSO WRITING FALSE OR FICTITIOUS PRESCRIPTIONS FOR DANGEROUS DRUGS. LICENSE REVOKED, REVOCATION STAYED; PROBATION UNDER TERMS AND CONDITIONS.

HUBBARD, GREGORY GERARD DO, LICENSE NUMBER 00G3480 OF BEDFORD, TX, WAS DISCIPLINED BY TEXAS ON JANUARY 14, 1994
DISCIPLINARY ACTION: 120-MONTH PROBATION; RESTRICTION PLACED ON CONTROLLED SUBSTANCE LICENSE
OFFENSE: FAILURE TO COMPLY WITH PREVIOUS BOARD ORDER

NOTES: IN VIOLATION OF THE 3/92 BOARD ORDER HE ABUSED STADOL NASAL SPRAY FROM 8/93 THROUGH 10/93 BY INGESTING IT WITHOUT A LEGITIMATE MEDICAL REASON; SELF-REPORTED THIS TO THE BOARD, HIS MONITORING PHYSICIAN AND THE PHYSICIAN HEALTH AND REHABILITATION COMMITTEE; ENTERED A SIX WEEK OUTPATIENT TREATMENT PROGRAM; IS UNDER THE CONTINUING CARE OF A PSYCHIATRIST. REVOCATION STAYED. CONDITIONS OF PROBATION: SHALL CONTINUE PSYCHIATRIC TREATMENT WITH QUARTERLY REPORTS; SHALL FURNISH WRITTEN REPORTS UPON REQUEST VERIFYING COMPLIANCE;

SHALL ABSTAIN FROM THE CONSUMPTION OF ALCOHOL/CHEMICAL SUBSTANCES IN ANY FORM UNLESS PRESCRIBED BY ANOTHER PHYSICIAN FOR A LEGITIMATE AND THERAPEUTIC PURPOSE; SHALL SUBMIT HIMSELF FOR APPROPRIATE EXAMS INCLUDING DRUG AND ALCOHOL SCREENS; SHALL SURRENDER DEA AND TEXAS CONTROLLED SUBSTANCES CERTIFICATES AND UNUSED TRIPLICATE PRESCRIPTION FORMS; SHALL NOT REREGISTER WITHOUT PERMISSION; SHALL NOT PRESCRIBE, DISPENSE, ADMINISTER OR POSSESS ANY CONTROLLED SUBSTANCE UNLESS PRESCRIBED TO HIM BY A TREATING PHYSICIAN; SHALL NOT TREAT OR OTHERWISE SERVE AS PHYSICIAN, PRESCRIBE, DISPENSE OR ADMINISTER DRUGS THAT MAY BE SUBJECT TO ABUSE TO HIMSELF OR ANY MEMBER OF HIS FAMILY; SHALL PARTICIPATE IN ACTIVITIES OF A PHYSICIAN HEALTH AND REHABILITATION COMMITTEE AND ATTEND WEEKLY MEETINGS WITH QUARTERLY REPORTS; SHALL BE SUPERVISED BY A BOARD-APPROVED PHYSICIAN WITH REPORTS THREE TIMES A YEAR; SHALL APPEAR BEFORE THE BOARD TWICE A YEAR; SHALL GIVE A COPY OF THIS ORDER TO ANY HEALTH CARE ENTITY WHERE HE HAS PRIVILEGES; SHALL COOPERATE WITH THE BOARD IN VERIFYING COMPLIANCE; SHALL INFORM BOARD OF CHANGE OF ADDRESS WITHIN 10 DAYS OR IF HE LEAVES THE STATE; TIME SPENT OUT OF TEXAS DOES NOT COUNT TOWARD PROBATION. SHALL NOT SEEK MODIFICATION FOR ONE YEAR.

HUBBARD, GREGORY GERARD DO, LICENSE NUMBER 00G3480 OF BEDFORD, TX, WAS DISCIPLINED BY TEXAS ON OCTOBER 27, 1994
DISCIPLINARY ACTION: EMERGENCY SUSPENSION
OFFENSE: FAILURE TO COMPLY WITH PREVIOUS BOARD ORDER

NOTES: AVAILABLE EVIDENCE AND INFORMATION INDICATE THE FOLLOWING: THAT ON 3/17/94 HE INGESTED AN UNSPECIFIED BARBITURATE AND ON 3/17/94 AND 9/13/94 HE INGESTED STADOL NOT PURSUANT TO A PRESCRIPTION FROM ANOTHER PHYSICIAN FOR A LEGITIMATE MEDICAL REASON AND IN VIOLATION OF A 1/14/94 AGREED ORDER; DID NOT SELF-REPORT THE SECOND INCIDENT; THIS WAS DETECTED BY A URINE SCREEN IN BOTH CASES; BETWEEN 9/23/94 AND 10/18/94 HE OBTAINED FOUR PRESCRIPTIONS FOR STADOL BY FRAUDULENT MEANS IN THAT PRESCRIPTIONS WERE WRITTEN FOR AN INDIVIDUAL WHO WAS NOT A PATIENT ON PREPRINTED FORMS WHICH HE SIGNED; HE PERSONALLY PRESENTED THE LAST PRESCRIPTION ON 10/18/94, ATTEMPTED TO LEAVE THE STORE WITHOUT PAYING AND WAS ARRESTED.

HUBBARD, GREGORY GERARD DO, LICENSE NUMBER 00G3480 OF BEDFORD, TX, WAS DISCIPLINED BY TEXAS ON MAY 11, 1995
DISCIPLINARY ACTION: LICENSE SUSPENSION; MONITORING OF PHYSICIAN PERFORMANCE
OFFENSE: FAILURE TO COMPLY WITH PREVIOUS BOARD ORDER

NOTES: IN VIOLATION OF 1/94 ORDER BETWEEN 3/17/94 AND 10/18/94 INGESTED CONTROLLED SUBSTANCES WITHOUT A LEGITIMATE MEDICAL REASON IN SOME CASES WRITING FICTITIOUS PRESCRIPTIONS TO OBTAIN THE DRUGS. LICENSE PLACED ON EMERGENCY SUSPENSION IN 10/94. SINCE 10/94 ORDER HE REPORTS REGULAR PARTICIPATION IN THE ACTIVITIES OF THE PHYSICIAN HEALTH AND REHABILITATION COMMITTEE; ENTERED INTO A TWO YEAR TREATMENT CONTRACT WITH THEM ON 11/29/94; RECEIVED INPATIENT SUBSTANCE ABUSE TREATMENT FROM 10/31/94 TO 11/27/94; ENTERED INTO A ONE YEAR AFTERCARE TREATMENT CONTRACT WITH THE HOSPITAL ON 11/22/94. SUSPENSION UNTIL HE REQUESTS TO HAVE SUSPENSION STAYED OR LIFTED AND APPEARS BEFORE BOARD WITH SUFFICIENT EVIDENCE THAT HE IS PHYSICALLY, MENTALLY OR OTHERWISE COMPETENT TO SAFELY PRACTICE MEDICINE WHICH SHALL INCLUDE AT A MINIMUM COPIES OF MEDICAL RECORDS AND REPORTS OF PSYCHOLOGICAL AND NEUROPSYCHIATRIC EVALUATIONS CONDUCTED BY A BOARD-APPROVED PSYCHIATRIST. SHALL NOT SEEK MODIFICATION FOR ONE YEAR.

HUBBARD, GREGORY GERARD DO, LICENSE NUMBER 00G3480, WAS DISCIPLINED BY TEXAS ON OCTOBER 13, 1995
DISCIPLINARY ACTION: PROBATION; 120-MONTH RESTRICTION PLACED ON CONTROLLED SUBSTANCE LICENSE
OFFENSE: SUBSTANCE ABUSE

NOTES: HAS SATISFIED THE MINIMUM REQUIREMENTS OF 5/95 ORDER AS PREREQUISITE FOR STAYING THE SUSPENSION IN THAT HE REPORTS REGULAR PARTICIPATION IN THE ACTIVITIES OF A PHYSICIAN HEALTH AND REHABILITATION COMMITTEE; ENTERED INTO A TWO YEAR TREATMENT CONTRACT WITH TEXAS OSTEOPATHIC MEDICAL ASSOCIATION ON 11/29/94; RECEIVED INPATIENT SUBSTANCE ABUSE TREATMENT FROM 10/31/94 TO 11/27/94; ENTERED INTO A ONE YEAR AFTERCARE TREATMENT CONTRACT WITH A HOSPITAL ON 11/22/94; 5/95 SUSPENSION STAYED. PROBATION WITH TERMS: SHALL ABSTAIN FROM THE CONSUMPTION OF ALCOHOL/DRUGS OF ANY FORM UNLESS PRESCRIBED BY ANOTHER PHYSICIAN FOR A LEGITIMATE AND THERAPEUTIC PURPOSE; SHALL SUBMIT HIMSELF FOR APPROPRIATE EXAMS INCLUDING DRUG OR ALCOHOL SCREENS; SHALL SUBMIT HIMSELF FOR EVALUATION AND TREATMENT BY A BOARD-APPROVED PSYCHIATRIST WHOM HE SHALL SEE FOR FOLLOW-UP CARE AND COUNSELING AT LEAST ONCE A MONTH AND WHO SHALL SUBMIT REPORTS TO THE BOARD; SHALL CONTINUE TO PARTICIPATE IN AA'S PROGRAM NOT LESS THAN THREE TIMES A WEEK WITH QUARTERLY REPORTS TO THE BOARD; SHALL PARTICIPATE IN THE ACTIVITIES OF AN IMPAIRED PHYSICIAN'S GROUP AND ATTEND WEEKLY MEETINGS WITH QUARTERLY REPORTS; SHALL COMPLY WITH THE TERMS OF ANY CONTINUING CARE CONTRACT AND SUBMIT QUARTERLY REPORTS TO THE BOARD; SHALL NOT POSSESS ALCOHOL, CONTROLLED SUBSTANCES OR DANGEROUS DRUGS WITH ADDICTIVE POTENTIAL OR POTENTIAL FOR ABUSE; SHALL SURRENDER ANY SUCH DRUGS IN HIS POSSESSION; SHALL NOT TREAT OR SERVE AS PHYSICIAN, PRESCRIBE, DISPENSE OR ADMINISTER DRUGS THAT MAY BE SUBJECT TO ABUSE TO HIMSELF OR TO ANY MEMBER OF HIS FAMILY; SHALL NOT TELEPHONE TO A PHARMACY A PRESCRIPTION OR REFILL FOR THESE DRUGS AND SHALL NOT PERMIT ANYONE UNDER HIS SUPERVISION TO DO SO; SHALL SURRENDER HIS DEA/DPS CONTROLLED SUBSTANCES REGISTRATION CERTIFICATES; SHALL SURRENDER ALL UNUSED TRIPLICATE PRESCRIPTIONS FORMS AND SHALL NOT ATTEMPT TO ORDER MORE; SHALL MAINTAIN A FILE WITH COPIES OF EVERY PRESCRIPTION WRITTEN BY HIM FOR DANGEROUS DRUGS WITH ADDICTIVE POTENTIAL OR POTENTIAL FOR ABUSE WHICH SHALL BE AVAILABLE FOR REVIEW; HIS PRACTICE SHALL BE MONITORED BY A BOARD-APPROVED PHYSICIAN WHO SHALL SUBMIT QUARTERLY REPORTS; SHALL MAINTAIN ADEQUATE MEDICAL RECORDS WHICH SHALL BE AVAILABLE FOR REVIEW; SHALL OBTAIN AT LEAST 50 HOURS PER YEAR OF CONTINUING MEDICAL EDUCATION; SHALL APPEAR BEFORE THE BOARD AT LEAST TWO TIMES A

YEAR; SHALL COOPERATE WITH BOARD IN VERIFYING COMPLIANCE INCLUDING PROVIDING MEDICAL RELEASES UPON REQUEST; SHALL GIVE A COPY OF THIS ORDER TO ANY HEALTH CARE ENTITY WHERE HE HAS PRIVILEGES; SHALL PROVIDE COPY OF THIS ORDER TO ANYONE REQUESTING IT WITHIN 10 DAYS; TIME SPENT OUT OF TEXAS DOES NOT COUNT TOWARD PROBATION; SHALL INFORM BOARD OF CHANGE OF ADDRESS WITHIN 10 DAYS OR IF HE LEAVES THE STATE. SHALL NOT SEEK MODIFICATION FOR ONE YEAR. ON 8/22/98 ORDER MODIFIED AS FOLLOWS: MAY REAPPLY FOR REGISTRATIONS FOR CONTROLLED SUBSTANCES IN SCHEDULES IV AND V; SHALL APPEAR BEFORE THE BOARD UPON REQUEST.

HUBBARD, GREGORY GERARD DO, LICENSE NUMBER G3480 OF DALLAS, TX, WAS DISCIPLINED BY TEXAS ON DECEMBER 11, 1999
DISCIPLINARY ACTION: LICENSE SUSPENSION
OFFENSE: FAILURE TO COMPLY WITH PREVIOUS BOARD ORDER

NOTES: VIOLATED 10/13/95 ORDER BY RELAPSING INTO NONTHERAPEUTIC USE OF VICODIN ON 10/15/99; HE REPORTS THAT HE INTENTIONALLY PROVIDED URINE OTHER THAN HIS OWN TO AVOID DETECTION OF HIS RELAPSE; HE IS CURRENTLY UNDER THE CARE OF A PHYSICIAN AND PARTICIPATING IN AN OUT-PATIENT PROGRAM. SUSPENSION UNTIL HE REQUESTS TO HAVE HIS SUSPENSION STAYED OR APPEARS BEFORE THE BOARD WITH SUFFICIENT EVIDENCE THAT HE IS PHYSICALLY, MENTALLY AND OTHERWISE COMPETENT TO SAFELY PRACTICE MEDICINE INCLUDING AT A MINIMUM COMPLETE COPIES OF MEDICAL RECORDS AND REPORTS OF PSYCHOLOGICAL AND NEUROPSYCHIATRIC EVALUATIONS; DOCUMENTED EVIDENCE OF 24 MONTHS OF SOBRIETY AND ABSTINENCE FROM ALCOHOL, DANGEROUS DRUGS, OR CONTROLLED SUBSTANCES IN ANY FORM UNLESS PRESCRIBED BY A TREATING PHYSICIAN; SHALL COOPERATE WITH THE BOARD IN VERIFYING COMPLIANCE; SHALL PROVIDE A COPY OF THIS ORDER TO ANYONE REQUESTING IT WITHIN 10 DAYS; SHALL INFORM THE BOARD OF CHANGE OF ADDRESS WITHIN 10 DAYS.

HUCKABY, HENRY L MD, LICENSE NUMBER 0010966 OF PO BOX 130687, HOUSTON, TX, WAS DISCIPLINED BY GEORGIA ON AUGUST 10, 1990
DISCIPLINARY ACTION: LICENSE REVOCATION
OFFENSE: DISCIPLINARY ACTION BY ANOTHER STATE OR AGENCY

NOTES: ON 10/29/88 THE TEXAS BOARD SUSPENDED HIS LICENSE, STAYED THE SUSPENSION, AND PLACED HIM ON PROBATION FOR 10 YEARS AFTER HE PLED GUILTY TO MAKING FALSE CLAIMS IN MEDICARE STATEMENTS. ON 12/13/89 ON GEORGIA LICENSE RENEWAL FORM HE SAID NO STATE BOARD HAD TAKEN DISCIPLINARY ACTION AGAINST HIM AND THAT HE HAD NOT BEEN CONVICTED OF ANY FEDERAL, STATE, OR LOCAL STATUTES.

HUCKABY, HENRY L MD, LICENSE NUMBER 0102519 OF 2619 HOLMAN, HOUSTON, TX, WAS DISCIPLINED BY NEW YORK ON MARCH 7, 1996
DISCIPLINARY ACTION: LICENSE REVOCATION
OFFENSE: DISCIPLINARY ACTION BY ANOTHER STATE OR AGENCY

NOTES: ACTION IN TEXAS FOR MAKING FALSE MEDICARE STATEMENTS. CONVICTED IN TEXAS FOR KNOWINGLY AND UNLAWFULLY MAKING FALSE MEDICARE CLAIMS.

HUDDLESTON, WILLIAM E MD, LICENSE NUMBER 00C5501 OF BRIDGEPORT, TX, WAS DISCIPLINED BY TEXAS ON AUGUST 19, 1994
DISCIPLINARY ACTION: MONITORING OF PHYSICIAN PERFORMANCE
OFFENSE: OVERPRESCRIBING OR MISPRESCRIBING DRUGS

NOTES: PRESCRIBED CONTROLLED SUBSTANCES FOR WHICH THERE WAS LITTLE DOCUMENTATION SUPPORTING THE NECESSITY OF THE PRESCRIPTION; DID NOT ADEQUATELY DOCUMENT TREATMENTS OR WHETHER CONSULTANTS WERE OBTAINED; DOES NOT ADMIT TO THE SPECIFIC ALLEGATIONS BUT AGREES TO THE ORDER. SEPARATE FROM PATIENT RECORDS SHALL MAINTAIN A FILE OF EVERY PRESCRIPTION WRITTEN FOR CONTROLLED SUBSTANCES OR DANGEROUS DRUGS WHICH SHALL BE AVAILABLE FOR INSPECTION; SHALL MAINTAIN ADEQUATE MEDICAL RECORDS ON ALL PATIENT OFFICE VISITS WHICH SHALL BE AVAILABLE FOR INSPECTION; SHALL COOPERATE WITH THE BOARD IN VERIFYING COMPLIANCE; SHALL INFORM BOARD OF CHANGE OF ADDRESS WITHIN 10 DAYS OR IF HE LEAVES THE STATE; TIME SPENT OUT OF TEXAS DOES NOT COUNT TOWARD ORDER. SHALL NOT SEEK MODIFICATION FOR ONE YEAR.

HUDDLESTON, WILLIAM ENNIS MD, LICENSE NUMBER 00C2402 OF 26 ROBINHOOD LN, BRIDGEPORT, TX, WAS DISCIPLINED BY ARKANSAS ON JULY 1, 1995
OFFENSE: DISCIPLINARY ACTION BY ANOTHER STATE OR AGENCY

NOTES: AGREED ORDER, BOARD WILL PASS CHARGES UNTIL TEXAS BOARD ORDER RESTRICTION PERIOD OF 2 YEARS IS COMPLETED.

HUDSON, RICHARD C DO, DATE OF BIRTH OCTOBER 22, 1946, LICENSE NUMBER 00E9485 OF BRIDGEPORT, TX, WAS DISCIPLINED BY TEXAS ON AUGUST 24, 1991
DISCIPLINARY ACTION: 60-MONTH PROBATION; RESTRICTION PLACED ON LICENSE
OFFENSE: DISCIPLINARY ACTION BY ANOTHER STATE OR AGENCY

NOTES: DISCIPLINARY ACTION TAKEN BY THE U.S. AIR FORCE. CONDITIONS OF PROBATION: SHALL APPEAR BEFORE THE BOARD ONCE A YEAR; SUBMIT FOR EVALUATION AND TREATMENT OF A PSYCHIATRIST APPROVED BY THE BOARD; MUST NOT CONDUCT ANY EXAMINATION UPON ANY FEMALE PATIENT UNLESS A THIRD PARTY IS PRESENT DURING EXAMINATION.

HUDSON, RICHARD C DO, DATE OF BIRTH OCTOBER 22, 1946, LICENSE NUMBER 0001802, WAS DISCIPLINED BY OKLAHOMA ON MARCH 18, 1993
DISCIPLINARY ACTION: 48-MONTH RESTRICTION PLACED ON LICENSE; MONITORING OF PHYSICIAN PERFORMANCE
OFFENSE: DISCIPLINARY ACTION BY ANOTHER STATE OR AGENCY

NOTES: ON 8/24/91 TEXAS LICENSE PLACED ON FIVE YEAR PROBATION UNDER TERMS AND CONDITIONS. SHALL NOT PETITION FOR MODIFICATION FOR AT LEAST ONE YEAR; SHALL COMPLY WITH PSYCHIATRIC EVALUATION, TREATMENT, AND RECOMMENDATIONS AS REQUIRED BY THE TEXAS BOARD AND SHALL SUBMIT A COPY OF SAID PSYCHIATRIST REPORTS TO THE OKLAHOMA BOARD; SHALL NOT CONDUCT ANY EXAMINATION UPON ANY FEMALE PATIENT UNLESS A FEMALE NURSE OR EMPLOYEE IS PRESENT DURING THE EXAMINATION; AND THIS SHALL BE ENTERED IN THE MEDICAL RECORDS; SHALL FURNISH WRITTEN REPORTS TO THE BOARD REGARDING HIS MEDICAL CONDITION AND COMPLIANCE WITH THIS ORDER UPON REQUEST; SHALL NOTIFY THE BOARD IN WRITING, OF ANY CHANGE IN ADDRESS, EMPLOYMENT, EMPLOYMENT TERMINATION OR HOSPITAL PRIVILEGE RESTRICTION AND ANY ADMINISTRATIVE PROCEEDING INITIATED AGAINST

HIM BY ANY OTHER STATE OR FEDERAL REGULATORY BODY WITHIN 14 DAYS; SHALL APPEAR BEFORE THE BOARD UPON REQUEST; AGREES TO RANDOM, UNANNOUNCED VISITS FROM THE BOARD AT HIS PLACE OF BUSINESS FOR OBSERVATION AND ACCESS TO ANY APPROPRIATE RECORDS, PROVIDED HOWEVER THAT THESE VISITS WILL NOT INTERRUPT HIS MEDICAL SERVICES; THE TIME PERIOD OF MONITORING THE RESTRICTIONS, LIMITATIONS, OR CONDITIONS ASSESSED SHALL NOT INCLUDE ANY PERIODS OF RESIDENCE OR PRACTICE OUTSIDE OF OKLAHOMA; $2,460.75 ADMINISTRATIVE COSTS. ON 3/17/94 PROVISION REQUESTING THAT HE NOT PETITION FOR MODIFICATION FOR ONE YEAR DROPPED; ON 6/20/96 ALL RESTRICTIONS ON LICENSE TERMINATED.

HUDSON, RICHARD C DO, DATE OF BIRTH OCTOBER 22, 1946, LICENSE NUMBER 00E9485 OF 4001 NW OZMUN, LAWTON, OK, WAS DISCIPLINED BY TEXAS ON JUNE 15, 1993
DISCIPLINARY ACTION: SURRENDER OF LICENSE
OFFENSE: NONCOMPLIANCE WITH A PROFESSIONAL RULE

NOTES: BOARD HAS RECEIVED ALLEGATIONS CONCERNING POSSIBLE VIOLATIONS OF THE MEDICAL PRACTICE ACT; WHILE NOT ADMITTING THESE HE VOLUNTARILY SURRENDERS HIS LICENSE IN LIEU OF FURTHER INVESTIGATION OR A HEARING. SHALL NOT PETITION THE BOARD FOR REINSTATEMENT.

HUDSON, RICHARD C DO, LICENSE NUMBER 1802, WAS DISCIPLINED BY OKLAHOMA ON JUNE 19, 1997
DISCIPLINARY ACTION: SURRENDER OF LICENSE

HUEY, RODNEY L MD, LICENSE NUMBER 00E6104, WAS DISCIPLINED BY TEXAS ON AUGUST 17, 1996
DISCIPLINARY ACTION: FINE; REPRIMAND
OFFENSE: NONCOMPLIANCE WITH A PROFESSIONAL RULE

NOTES: FAILED TO OBTAIN 24 CREDIT HOURS OF CONTINUING MEDICAL EDUCATION BY 3/1/96 AS REQUIRED FOR RENEWAL OF HIS LICENSE; HE WAS GRANTED AN EXTENSION UNTIL 5/29/96 WHICH HE ALSO DID NOT MEET; STILL REQUIRED TO MEET CONTINUING MEDICAL EDUCATION REQUIREMENT. $100 ADMINISTRATIVE PENALTY. SHALL COOPERATE WITH THE BOARD IN VERIFYING COMPLIANCE.

HUFF, JOHN D SR MD, LICENSE NUMBER 00D7993 OF SUGARLAND, TX, WAS DISCIPLINED BY TEXAS ON MAY 15, 1996
DISCIPLINARY ACTION: FINE
OFFENSE: SUBSTANDARD CARE, INCOMPETENCE OR NEGLIGENCE

NOTES: DURING 6/94, ALLEGEDLY FAILED TO ADEQUATELY DOCUMENT THE CARE AND TREATMENT OF A SURGICAL PATIENT INCLUDING APPROPRIATE INSTRUCTIONS FOR ADEQUATE FOLLOW-UP CARE; MAINTAINS THAT HE ADEQUATELY DOCUMENTED THE CARE AND TREATMENT OF THE PATIENT. SHALL PAY $1,000 FINE.

HULL, JAIME J MD, LICENSE NUMBER 00G3487, WAS DISCIPLINED BY TEXAS ON AUGUST 17, 1996
DISCIPLINARY ACTION: 60-MONTH PROBATION; FINE
OFFENSE: SEXUAL ABUSE OF OR SEXUAL MISCONDUCT WITH A PATIENT

NOTES: DURING 1993 ENGAGED IN CONSENSUAL CONTACT OF A SEXUAL NATURE WITH AN ADULT FEMALE PATIENT AND EMPLOYEE WHICH INCLUDED KISSING AND MUTUAL FONDLING; AROUND 1993 AND INTO 1994 ENGAGED IN A MUTUALLY CONSENSUAL SEXUAL RELATIONSHIP, INCLUDING SEXUAL INTERCOURSE, WITH AN EMPLOYEE WHO HE ALSO TREATED FOR MINOR MEDICAL PROBLEMS; ACKNOWLEDGED THAT HE HAS PROBLEMS WITH BOUNDARY ISSUES INVOLVING THE PHYSICIAN-PATIENT RELATIONSHIP AND CONCEDES THAT HIS CONDUCT VIOLATED THE BOUNDARIES; HAS INITIATED THERAPY AND IS ENGAGED IN ONGOING COUNSELING. SUSPENSION, STAYED. CONDITIONS OF PROBATION: SHALL SUBMIT HIMSELF FOR EVALUATION AND TREATMENT TO A BOARD APPROVED PSYCHIATRIST WHO HE SHALL SEE AT LEAST ONCE EACH MONTH AND WHO SHALL SUBMIT REPORTS; SHALL HAVE A CHAPERONE PRESENT IN THE ROOM DURING THE EXAMINATION OF FEMALE PATIENTS AND SHALL MAKE A NOTATION ON THE PATIENT'S CHART THAT THE CHAPERONE WAS PRESENT; SHALL MAINTAIN ADEQUATE MEDICAL RECORDS WHICH SHALL BE AVAILABLE UPON BOARD REQUEST; SHALL OBTAIN AT LEAST 50 HOURS PER YEAR OF CONTINUING MEDICAL EDUCATION CREDITS AND SHALL SUBMIT PROOF TO THE BOARD; SHALL OBTAIN 10 HOURS OF AN ETHICS COURSE OR PROGRAM PER YEAR EACH YEAR AND SUBMIT PROOF TO THE BOARD; WITHIN ONE YEAR SHALL TAKE AND PASS THE MEDICAL JURISPRUDENCE EXAMINATION (JP EXAM) AND PROVIDE PROOF TO THE BOARD; SHALL APPEAR BEFORE THE BOARD AT LEAST ONCE PER YEAR OR UPON BOARD REQUEST; SHALL COOPERATE WITH THE BOARD IN VERIFYING COMPLIANCE INCLUDING PROVIDING COPIES OF MEDICAL RELEASES AND PEER REVIEW RECORDS UPON REQUEST; SHALL GIVE A COPY OF THIS ORDER TO ANY HEALTH CARE ENTITY WHERE HE HAS PRIVILEGES; SHALL PROVIDE A COPY OF THIS ORDER TO ANYONE REQUESTING IT WITHIN 10 DAYS; TIME PERIOD OUT OF TEXAS DOES NOT COUNT TOWARD PROBATION; SHALL INFORM THE BOARD OF CHANGE OF ADDRESS WITHIN 10 DAYS OF IF HE LEAVES THE STATE; SHALL NOT SEEK MODIFICATION FOR ONE YEAR. $5,000 FINE.

HUMMER, MICHAEL GORMAN MD, LICENSE NUMBER 00G7827 OF AUSTIN, TX, WAS DISCIPLINED BY TEXAS ON JUNE 22, 1994
DISCIPLINARY ACTION: 120-MONTH PROBATION; MONITORING OF PHYSICIAN PERFORMANCE
OFFENSE: SUBSTANCE ABUSE

NOTES: HE SELF-REPORTED THE INTEMPERATE USE OF VICODIN DURING THE TIME PERIOD OF 1989 TO 1993; HAS A HISTORY OF ONE PRIOR SUBSTANCE ABUSE TREATMENT; DEVELOPED CHRONIC SHOULDER PAIN IN 1989 TO 1990; DURING 1993 WAS TAKING 10 TO 16 VICODIN TABLETS PER DAY; ENTERED RECOVERY PROGRAM IN 10/93; SOBRIETY DATE IS 10/13/93; IS ATTENDING AA DAILY AND RECEIVING TREATMENT FROM A PSYCHIATRIST AND A PRIMARY CARE PHYSICIAN. SUSPENSION STAYED. CONDITIONS OF PROBATION: SHALL ABSTAIN FROM THE CONSUMPTION OF ALCOHOL/CHEMICAL SUBSTANCES IN ANY FORM UNLESS PRESCRIBED BY ANOTHER PHYSICIAN FOR A LEGITIMATE AND THERAPEUTIC PURPOSE; SHALL NOT TREAT OR OTHERWISE SERVE AS PHYSICIAN, PRESCRIBE, DISPENSE OR ADMINISTER DRUGS THAT MAY BE SUBJECT TO ABUSE TO HIMSELF OR ANY MEMBER OF HIS FAMILY; SHALL CONTINUE TO PARTICIPATE IN THE ACTIVITIES OF A PHYSICIAN HEALTH AND REHABILITATION COMMITTEE AND ATTEND WEEKLY MEETINGS WITH QUARTERLY REPORTS. SHALL FOLLOW THE TERMS OF HIS AFTERCARE CONTRACT; SHALL CONTINUE TREATMENT WITH HIS PRIMARY CARE PHYSICIAN; SHALL SUBMIT HIMSELF FOR APPROPRIATE EXAMS INCLUDING DRUG OR ALCOHOL SCREENS; SHALL PARTICIPATE IN AA'S PROGRAM NOT LESS THAN

THREE TIMES A WEEK WITH QUARTERLY REPORTS TO THE BOARD; SHALL SUBMIT HIMSELF FOR EVALUATION AND TREATMENT BY A BOARD-APPROVED PSYCHIATRIST; UPON DEMAND HE SHALL SUBMIT TO AN EXAMINATION BY A PHYSICIAN SPECIALIST; SHALL APPEAR BEFORE THE BOARD TWICE A YEAR; SHALL GIVE A COPY OF THIS ORDER TO ANY HEALTH CARE ENTITY WHERE HE HAS PRIVILEGES; SHALL COOPERATE WITH THE BOARD IN VERIFYING COMPLIANCE; SHALL INFORM BOARD OF CHANGE OF ADDRESS WITHIN 10 DAYS OR IF HE LEAVES THE STATE; TIME SPENT OUT OF TEXAS DOES NOT COUNT TOWARD PROBATION. SHALL NOT SEEK MODIFICATION FOR ONE YEAR. ON 8/22/98 ORDER TERMINATED.

HUNT, JACKIE HANSEN MD, LICENSE NUMBER 00C1908 OF MASON, TX, WAS DISCIPLINED BY TEXAS ON JUNE 17, 1992
DISCIPLINARY ACTION: SURRENDER OF LICENSE
OFFENSE: PHYSICAL OR MENTAL ILLNESS INHIBITING THE ABILITY TO PRACTICE WITH SKILL AND SAFETY

NOTES: HEALTH REASONS. PERMANENT RETIREMENT.

HUNT, JOHN D MD, LICENSE NUMBER 00G4476 OF SAN ANGELO, TX, WAS DISCIPLINED BY TEXAS ON OCTOBER 9, 1992
DISCIPLINARY ACTION: 36-MONTH PROBATION
OFFENSE: OVERPRESCRIBING OR MISPRESCRIBING DRUGS

NOTES: NONTHERAPEUTIC PRESCRIBING. SUSPENSION, STAYED. PROBATION UNDER TERMS AND CONDITIONS. ON 1/6/95 PROBATION TERMINATED.

HUNT, JOHN D MD, LICENSE NUMBER 0021478 OF SAN ANGELO, TX, WAS DISCIPLINED BY CONNECTICUT ON OCTOBER 19, 1993
DISCIPLINARY ACTION: 24-MONTH PROBATION; MONITORING OF PHYSICIAN PERFORMANCE
OFFENSE: SUBSTANDARD CARE, INCOMPETENCE OR NEGLIGENCE

NOTES: INCOMPETENCE/NEGLIGENCE. IF PRACTICING IN CONNECTICUT, PROBATION TO INCLUDE MONTHLY SUPERVISION BY CONNECTICUT MEDICAL DOCTOR WITH QUARTERLY REPORTS.

HUNT, JOHN D MD, LICENSE NUMBER 0G43205 OF SAN ANGELO, TX, WAS DISCIPLINED BY CALIFORNIA ON APRIL 24, 1995
DISCIPLINARY ACTION: SURRENDER OF LICENSE

NOTES: VOLUNTARY SURRENDER WHILE CHARGES PENDING.

HUNTER, RICHARD BROOKSHIRE MD, DATE OF BIRTH AUGUST 22, 1925, LICENSE NUMBER 00C2062 OF DALLAS, TX, WAS DISCIPLINED BY TEXAS ON MARCH 6, 1992
DISCIPLINARY ACTION: EMERGENCY SUSPENSION
OFFENSE: FAILURE TO COMPLY WITH PREVIOUS BOARD ORDER

NOTES: VIOLATION OF PREVIOUS BOARD ORDER DUE TO INTEMPERATE USE OF ALCOHOL OR DRUGS. LICENSE TEMPORARILY SUSPENDED.

HUNTER, RICHARD BROOKSHIRE MD, DATE OF BIRTH AUGUST 22, 1925, LICENSE NUMBER 00C2062 OF DALLAS, TX, WAS DISCIPLINED BY TEXAS ON AUGUST 22, 1992
DISCIPLINARY ACTION: 120-MONTH PROBATION
OFFENSE: SUBSTANCE ABUSE

NOTES: UNPROFESSIONAL OR DISHONORABLE CONDUCT LIKELY TO DECEIVE, DEFRAUD OR INJURE THE PUBLIC. SUSPENSION STAYED. PROBATION UNDER TERMS AND CONDITIONS.

HUNTER, RICHARD BROOKSHIRE MD, DATE OF BIRTH AUGUST 22, 1925, LICENSE NUMBER 00C2062 OF 3600 GASTON 1006 BARNETT TOWER, DALLAS, TX, WAS DISCIPLINED BY TEXAS ON MARCH 26, 1993
DISCIPLINARY ACTION: SURRENDER OF LICENSE
OFFENSE: FAILURE TO COMPLY WITH PREVIOUS BOARD ORDER

NOTES: AN 8/22/92 ORDER PLACED TERMS AND CONDITIONS ON HIS CONTINUED PRACTICE; IN LIGHT OF HIS LONG CAREER AND PRACTICAL DIFFICULTIES IN COMPLYING WITH THESE TERMS, THE BOARD ALLOWED HIM TO PERMANENTLY RETIRE.

HURDIS-GRANT, HELEN LINDA MD, DATE OF BIRTH APRIL 2, 1947 OF PO BOX 1708, DENVER CITY, TX, WAS DISCIPLINED BY MEDICARE ON APRIL 16, 1994
DISCIPLINARY ACTION: EXCLUSION FROM THE MEDICARE AND/OR MEDICAID PROGRAM
OFFENSE: NONCOMPLIANCE WITH A PROFESSIONAL RULE

NOTES: DEFAULTED ON PUBLIC HEALTH SERVICE EDUCATION LOAN. REINSTATED ON 8/5/94.

HUSSAIN, RUQAIYA MD, DATE OF BIRTH JANUARY 1, 1947 OF 2701 FARMLAND DRIVE, PLANO, TX, WAS DISCIPLINED BY MEDICARE ON AUGUST 19, 1999
DISCIPLINARY ACTION: EXCLUSION FROM THE MEDICARE AND/OR MEDICAID PROGRAM
OFFENSE: CRIMINAL CONVICTION OR PLEA OF GUILTY, NOLO CONTENDERE, OR NO CONTEST TO A CRIME

NOTES: CONVICTED OF A CRIME INVOLVING THE MEDICARE, MEDICAID, MATERNAL AND CHILD HEALTH SERVICES BLOCK GRANT OR BLOCK GRANTS TO STATES FOR SOCIAL SERVICES PROGRAMS.

HUSSEIN, RUQAIYA MD, LICENSE NUMBER G1679 OF PLANO, TX, WAS DISCIPLINED BY TEXAS ON AUGUST 22, 1998
DISCIPLINARY ACTION: RESTRICTION PLACED ON LICENSE; REPRIMAND
OFFENSE: CRIMINAL CONVICTION OR PLEA OF GUILTY, NOLO CONTENDERE, OR NO CONTEST TO A CRIME

NOTES: ON 8/31/97 SHE PLED GUILTY TO ONE COUNT FOR ILLEGAL PATIENT ADMITTANCE AND RETENTION, SPECIFICALLY RELATED TO BILLING MEDICAID FOR SERVICES PREVIOUSLY PAID FOR BY 15 PATIENTS; SHE WAS SENTENCED TO 5 YEARS PROBATION AND PLACED ON HOME DETENTION FOR 180 DAYS (HOME AND WORK ONLY); SHE WAS ALSO ORDERED TO PAY $12,920.00 IN RESTITUTION TO THE PATIENTS INVOLVED, A $3,000 FINE, AND 200 HOURS OF COMMUNITY SERVICE; SHE ALSO SETTLED A CONCURRENT CIVIL CASE FOR $38,000; ASSERTS THAT THERE WAS CONFUSION OVER BILLING. AGREED NOT TO ACCEPT ANY NEW MEDICAID PATIENTS FOR SEVEN YEARS AND TO TREAT WITHOUT CHARGE ANY EMERGENCIES THAT PRESENT WHILE SHE IS ON CALL.

HUTCHENS, JEROME ENOS MD OF BIG SPRING STATE HOSP BOX 231, BIG SPRING, TX, WAS DISCIPLINED BY DEA ON SEPTEMBER 23, 1992
DISCIPLINARY ACTION: RESTRICTION PLACED ON CONTROLLED SUBSTANCE LICENSE
OFFENSE: CRIMINAL CONVICTION OR PLEA OF GUILTY, NOLO CONTENDERE, OR NO CONTEST TO A CRIME

NOTES: STATE MEDICAL LICENSE REVOKED 06/16/81; SURRENDERED DEA REGISTRATION CERTIFICATE 10/26/81. WROTE PRESCRIPTIONS FOR DILAUDID TABS. CONVICTED 04/12/82 OF KNOWINGLY AND INTENTIONALLY DISPENSING HYDROMORPHONE WITHOUT VALID MEDICAL PURPOSE AND NOT IN THE COURSE OF PROFESSIONAL PRACTICE. SENTENCED

TO FIVE YEARS IN PRISON. ALIAS: JEROME HUTCHINS.

HUTCHENS, JEROME ENOS MD, LICENSE NUMBER 1040961 OF 8510 KENPREDGE, HOUSTON, TX, WAS DISCIPLINED BY INDIANA ON DECEMBER 10, 1992
DISCIPLINARY ACTION: PROBATION

NOTES: PROBATIONARY LICENSE ISSUED. PROBATION WITHDRAWN ON 12/13/93.

HUTCHENS, JEROME ENOS MD OF HOUSTON, TX, WAS DISCIPLINED BY OHIO ON AUGUST 11, 1993
DISCIPLINARY ACTION: DENIAL OF NEW LICENSE
OFFENSE: DISCIPLINARY ACTION BY ANOTHER STATE OR AGENCY

NOTES: PRIOR REVOCATION OF HIS TEXAS MEDICAL LICENSE BY THE TEXAS BOARD; FELONY DRUG CONVICTION.

ILAHI, MOHAMMAD ARIF MD, LICENSE NUMBER 00D8885 OF BAYTOWN, TX, WAS DISCIPLINED BY TEXAS ON MAY 12, 1995
DISCIPLINARY ACTION: 60-MONTH PROBATION; REPRIMAND
OFFENSE: SUBSTANDARD CARE, INCOMPETENCE OR NEGLIGENCE

NOTES: PROVIDED CARE BELOW THE MINIMUM STANDARD IN THAT HE INCORRECTLY DIAGNOSED FIVE PATIENTS IN 1989 AND 1990; PERSISTENT AND FLAGRANT OVERCHARGING OF THESE FIVE PATIENTS IN THAT HE LISTED EXCESSIVE DIAGNOSES ON INSURANCE FORM, BILLED FOR UNNECESSARY TESTS AND IN THREE OF THE FIVE CASES BILLED FOR COMPLETE PHYSICAL EXAMINATIONS WHICH HE DID NOT PERFORM; FAILED TO ADEQUATELY DOCUMENT IN MEDICAL RECORDS FOR THREE PATIENTS FAILED TO OFFER TREATMENT IN FOUR INSTANCES; NO PROOF ANY OF THE FIVE PATIENTS WERE HARMED. SUSPENSION STAYED. PROBATION WITH TERMS: SHALL ATTEND AT LEAST 50 HOURS PER YEAR OF CONTINUING MEDICAL EDUCATION, AT LEAST 25 OF WHICH WILL BE IN RISK MANAGEMENT, ETHICS, RECORD KEEPING AND BILLING PRACTICES; SHALL MAINTAIN ADEQUATE MEDICAL RECORDS WHICH SHALL BE AVAILABLE FOR REVIEW; SHALL PERFORM 20 HOURS PER MONTH OF COMMUNITY SERVICE FOR A NON-PROFIT CHARITABLE ORGANIZATION; SHALL COOPERATE WITH BOARD IN VERIFYING COMPLIANCE; SHALL BE MONITORED BY A BOARD-APPROVED PHYSICIAN WHO WILL SUBMIT QUARTERLY REPORTS TO THE BOARD; SHALL APPEAR BEFORE THE BOARD AT LEAST ONCE A YEAR; SHALL INFORM THE BOARD OF ANY CHANGE OF ADDRESS WITHIN 10 DAYS OR IF HE LEAVES THE STATE; TIME PERIOD OUT OF TEXAS DOES NOT COUNT TOWARD PROBATION; SHALL GIVE A COPY OF ORDER TO ANY HEALTH CARE ENTITY WHERE HE HAS PRIVILEGES. SHALL NOT SEEK MODIFICATION FOR ONE YEAR. ON 8/8/95 THE BOARD WAS IMMEDIATELY RESTRAINED BY THE DISTRICT COURT FROM IMPLEMENTING THIS ORDER UNTIL THE COURT MADE ITS FINAL DECISION.

ILAHI, MOHAMMAD ARIF MD, LICENSE NUMBER 00D8885 OF HOUSTON, TX, WAS DISCIPLINED BY TEXAS ON MAY 15, 1996
DISCIPLINARY ACTION: SURRENDER OF LICENSE
OFFENSE: FAILURE TO COMPLY WITH PREVIOUS BOARD ORDER

NOTES: ON 1/6/96, THE DISTRICT COURT AFFIRMED THE BOARD'S 5/12/95 ORDER FINDING A VIOLATION OF THE MEDICAL PRACTICE ACT. ALLEGATIONS THAT HE VIOLATED THIS ORDER. DOES NOT ADMIT ALLEGATIONS. VOLUNTARY AND PERMANENT SURRENDER OF TEXAS LICENSE IN LIEU OF FURTHER PROCEEDINGS.

INGRAM, CHESTER WILLIAM JR MD, LICENSE NUMBER 00G1048 OF LIVINGSTON, TX, WAS DISCIPLINED BY TEXAS ON FEBRUARY 23, 1991
DISCIPLINARY ACTION: RESTRICTION PLACED ON LICENSE

NOTES: HEARING CONTINUED BECAUSE OF PENDING CRIMINAL TRIAL, TO RESUME ON OR BEFORE 5/31/91 IF SAID TRIAL HAS NOT BEEN COMMENCED BY 5/20/91; LIMITATION OF GYNECOLOGICAL PRACTICE TO HAVING TWO ADULTS PRESENT THROUGHOUT THE TIME OF EXAMINATION, WITH THE WITNESSES WRITING THEIR NAMES IN PATIENTS' CHARTS.

INGRAM, CHESTER WILLIAM JR MD, LICENSE NUMBER 00G1048, WAS DISCIPLINED BY TEXAS ON SEPTEMBER 17, 1991
DISCIPLINARY ACTION: LICENSE SUSPENSION
OFFENSE: CRIMINAL CONVICTION OR PLEA OF GUILTY, NOLO CONTENDERE, OR NO CONTEST TO A CRIME

NOTES: ON 9/12/91 HE WAS SENTENCED TO 40 YEARS IN PRISON FOR CONVICTION OF AGGRAVATED KIDNAPPING.

INGRAM, CHESTER WILLIAM JR MD, LICENSE NUMBER 0007526 OF TX, WAS DISCIPLINED BY ALABAMA ON MARCH 25, 1992
DISCIPLINARY ACTION: LICENSE REVOCATION
OFFENSE: DISCIPLINARY ACTION BY ANOTHER STATE OR AGENCY

NOTES: CONVICTED IN THE STATE COURT OF TEXAS OF THE OFFENSE OF AGGRAVATED KIDNAPPING AND SENTENCED TO A TERM OF IMPRISONMENT OF 40 YEARS; LICENSE TO PRACTICE MEDICINE IN TEXAS SUSPENDED DUE TO FELONY CONVICTION.

INGRAM, CHESTER WILLIAM JR MD, DATE OF BIRTH DECEMBER 20, 1949, LICENSE NUMBER 0021525 OF 3114 3RD ST NE, BIRMINGHAM, AL, WAS DISCIPLINED BY GEORGIA ON NOVEMBER 5, 1992
DISCIPLINARY ACTION: LICENSE SUSPENSION
OFFENSE: CRIMINAL CONVICTION OR PLEA OF GUILTY, NOLO CONTENDERE, OR NO CONTEST TO A CRIME

NOTES: CONVICTION OF A FELONY IN TEXAS. SUSPENSION INDEFINITE.

IVERSEN, MICHAEL GELLATLY MD, LICENSE NUMBER H8992 OF FORT WORTH, TX, WAS DISCIPLINED BY TEXAS ON AUGUST 28, 1999
DISCIPLINARY ACTION: 60-MONTH PROBATION; RESTRICTION PLACED ON CONTROLLED SUBSTANCE LICENSE
OFFENSE: PROFESSIONAL MISCONDUCT

NOTES: EXCESSIVELY PRESCRIBED CONTROLLED SUBSTANCES TO HIS WIFE; HE INADEQUATELY DOCUMENTED THIS PRESCRIBING TO HER, AND CONTINUED PRESCRIBING TO HER WITH KNOWN BEHAVIORS OF ABUSE OF NARCOTICS AND NARCOTIC DEPENDENCE; A DRUG AUDIT REVEALED SEVERAL VIOLATIONS; HE CURRENTLY ACKNOWLEDGES THAT HIS ACTIONS WERE INAPPROPRIATE AND DUE TO CODEPENDENCY ON HIS WIFE. SUSPENSION STAYED FOR PROBATION WITH FOLLOWING TERMS AND CONDITIONS: SHALL NOMINATE THREE CERTIFIED PSYCHIATRISTS FOR BOARD SELECTION OF A THERAPIST AND SHALL EXPEDITIOUSLY SUBMIT HIMSELF TO EVALUATION AND TREATMENT BY THE APPROVED PRACTITIONER; SHALL SUBMIT HIMSELF FOR APPROPRIATE EXAMS INCLUDING DRUG OR ALCOHOL SCREENS; WITHIN 1 YEAR SHALL SUCCESSFULLY COMPLETE A COURSE IN PAIN MANAGEMENT OF AT LEAST 10 HOURS DURATION AND A COURSE IN PHARMACOLOGY OF AT LEAST 10 HOURS IN DURATION; SHALL IMMEDIATELY REQUEST MODIFICATION OF HIS DEA AND TEXAS DEPARTMENT OF PUBLIC SAFETY CONTROLLED SUBSTANCES

REGISTRATION CERTIFICATES TO ELIMINATE SCHEDULE II DRUGS; SHALL NOT TREAT OR OTHERWISE SERVE AS PHYSICIAN, PRESCRIBE, DISPENSE OR ADMINISTER DRUGS THAT MAY BE SUBJECT TO ABUSE TO HIMSELF OR TO ANY MEMBER OF HIS FAMILY; SHALL NOT TELEPHONE TO A PHARMACY A PRESCRIPTION OR REFILL FOR CONTROLLED SUBSTANCES OR DANGEROUS DRUGS WITH ADDICTIVE POTENTIAL OR POTENTIAL FOR ABUSE AND SHALL NOT PERMIT ANY INDIVIDUAL HE IS SUPERVISING TO DO SO; SEPARATE FROM PATIENT RECORDS, SHALL MAINTAIN A LOGBOOK OF EVERY PRESCRIPTION WRITTEN BY HIM FOR DANGEROUS DRUGS WITH ADDICTIVE POTENTIAL WHICH SHALL BE MADE AVAILABLE FOR REVIEW; SHALL MAINTAIN ADEQUATE MEDICAL RECORDS WHICH SHALL BE AVAILABLE FOR REVIEW; SHALL OBTAIN AT LEAST 50 HOURS PER YEAR OF CONTINUING MEDICAL EDUCATION; SHALL APPEAR BEFORE THE BOARD UPON REQUEST; ANY PRESCRIPTION FOR SCHEDULE IIN DRUGS SHALL ONLY BE ISSUED IN THE COURSE OF TREATMENT OF ATTENTION DEFICIT DISORDER AND SHALL BE LIMITED TO RITALIN OR ADERAL; SHALL COOPERATE WITH THE BOARD IN VERIFYING COMPLIANCE; SHALL GIVE A COPY OF THIS ORDER TO ANY HEALTH CARE ENTITY WHERE HE HAS PRIVILEGES; SHALL PROVIDE A COPY OF THIS ORDER TO ANYONE REQUESTING IT WITHIN 10 DAYS; TIME SPENT OUT OF TEXAS DOES NOT COUNT TOWARD PROBATION; SHALL INFORM THE BOARD OF CHANGE OF ADDRESS WITHIN 10 DAYS OR IF HE LEAVES THE STATE; SHALL NOT SEEK MODIFICATION FOR ONE YEAR.

IVERSON, DALE ARTHUR MD, DATE OF BIRTH NOVEMBER 11, 1936 OF THE WOODLANDS, TX, WAS DISCIPLINED BY NORTH DAKOTA ON DECEMBER 11, 1992
DISCIPLINARY ACTION: RESTRICTION PLACED ON LICENSE
OFFENSE: SUBSTANDARD CARE, INCOMPETENCE OR NEGLIGENCE

NOTES: QUALITY OF CARE ISSUES. CONDITIONS MET AND ON 11/17/95 HE WAS ISSUED UNRESTRICTED LICENSE.

IVERSON, DALE ARTHUR MD, DATE OF BIRTH NOVEMBER 11, 1936, LICENSE NUMBER 00D0180 OF THE WOODLANDS, TX, WAS DISCIPLINED BY TEXAS ON MARCH 5, 1994
DISCIPLINARY ACTION: 60-MONTH PROBATION
OFFENSE: DISCIPLINARY ACTION BY ANOTHER STATE OR AGENCY

NOTES: LICENSE DISCIPLINED IN NORTH DAKOTA 12/10/92 FOR A CONSISTENT FAILURE TO DOCUMENT AN ADEQUATE HISTORY OR PHYSICAL EXAM; PATIENT CARE WAS SUBSTANDARD. SUSPENSION STAYED. CONDITIONS OF PROBATION: SHALL FULLY COMPLY WITH TERMS OF NORTH DAKOTA STIPULATION; SHALL PROVIDE TO TEXAS COPIES OF ALL DOCUMENTS SENT TO NORTH DAKOTA BOARD INCLUDING CONTINUING MEDICAL EDUCATION VERIFICATION; SHALL GIVE A COPY OF THIS ORDER TO ANY HEALTH CARE ENTITY WHERE HE HAS PRIVILEGES; SHALL COOPERATE WITH THE BOARD IN VERIFYING COMPLIANCE; SHALL INFORM BOARD OF CHANGE OF ADDRESS WITHIN 10 DAYS OR IF HE LEAVES THE STATE; TIME SPENT OUT OF TEXAS DOES NOT COUNT TOWARD PROBATION. SHALL NOT SEEK MODIFICATION FOR ONE YEAR. PROBATION TERMINATED ON 5/15/96.

JACKSON, JOSEPH J MD OF 8138 SAN LEANDRO, DALLAS, TX, WAS DISCIPLINED BY DEA ON MARCH 10, 1995
DISCIPLINARY ACTION: SURRENDER OF CONTROLLED SUBSTANCE LICENSE
OFFENSE: DISCIPLINARY ACTION BY ANOTHER STATE OR AGENCY

NOTES: STATE BOARD.

JACKSON, JOSEPH JORDAN MD, LICENSE NUMBER 00F9614 OF DALLAS, TX, WAS DISCIPLINED BY TEXAS ON SEPTEMBER 30, 1994
DISCIPLINARY ACTION: LICENSE REVOCATION
OFFENSE: SUBSTANDARD CARE, INCOMPETENCE OR NEGLIGENCE

NOTES: ON 5/22/93 WHILE HE WAS THE ONLY PHYSICIAN AT AN EMERGENCY ROOM HE BECAME ANGRY WITH THE NURSING STAFF AND TELEPHONED ANOTHER PHYSICIAN TO SAY HE WAS LEAVING; LEFT BEFORE THE OTHER DOCTOR COULD GET THERE TO RELIEVE HIM; IT IS STANDARD PRACTICE FOR DOCTORS LEAVING AN EMERGENCY ROOM TO BRIEF INCOMING DOCTORS ABOUT PATIENTS, PARTICULARLY CRITICAL CONDITION PATIENTS; HIS CONDUCT CONSTITUTES ABANDONING PATIENTS AND IS BELOW THE STANDARD OF CARE; ON THE SAME NIGHT ANOTHER PATIENT CAME TO EMERGENCY ROOM COMPLAINING OF CHEST PAIN, DIZZINESS, SHORTNESS OF BREATH AND BEING CLOSE TO PASSING OUT; DR. JACKSON BERATED THIS PATIENT FOR COMING TO THE HOSPITAL AND SAID HE WAS NOT HAVING A HEART ATTACK; HE THEN SENT THE PATIENT HOME WITHOUT CHECKING HIS CARDIAC ENZYMES, IV ACCESS, RECHECKING HIS BLOOD PRESSURE AND WATCHING HIM LONGER, CONDUCT WHICH WAS BELOW THE STANDARD OF CARE; THE PATIENT WAS ADMITTED TO THE HOSPITAL THE NEXT DAY FOR HYPERTENSION AND STAYED FIVE DAYS; ANOTHER PATIENT THAT NIGHT WAS IN CRITICAL CONDITION SUFFERING FROM HEAD TRAUMA AS A RESULT OF AN AUTO ACCIDENT AND HIS FAILURE TO RENDER RAPID AND IMMEDIATE ATTENTION WAS BELOW THE STANDARD OF CARE AS WAS HIS LEAVING THE HOSPITAL WITHOUT BRIEFING HIS REPLACEMENT ABOUT THIS PATIENT; FAILED TO DOCUMENT FINDINGS REGARDING FIVE PATIENTS HE SAW THAT NIGHT IN HOSPITAL RECORDS WHICH COULD CAUSE INJURY OR STRESS TO PATIENTS BECAUSE THE ONCOMING PHYSICIANS WOULD NOT BE INFORMED OF THE PATIENT'S HISTORY; LOUDLY AND RUDELY ACCUSED THE NURSING STAFF OF FRAUDULENT AND CRIMINAL ACTIVITIES RELATING TO MEDICARE AND ADMISSION POLICIES; HIS CONTINUED PRACTICE IS AN IMMINENT PERIL TO THE PUBLIC HEALTH.

JACKSON, JOSEPH JORDAN MD, DATE OF BIRTH SEPTEMBER 20, 1945 OF 8138 SAN LEANDRO DRIVE, DALLAS, TX, WAS DISCIPLINED BY MEDICARE ON MARCH 3, 1996
DISCIPLINARY ACTION: EXCLUSION FROM THE MEDICARE AND/OR MEDICAID PROGRAM
OFFENSE: DISCIPLINARY ACTION BY ANOTHER STATE OR AGENCY

NOTES: LICENSE REVOKED FOR REASONS BEARING ON PROFESSIONAL PERFORMANCE.

JACKSON, NICHOLAS M MD, LICENSE NUMBER 00E2632, WAS DISCIPLINED BY TEXAS ON JUNE 22, 1994
DISCIPLINARY ACTION: 84-MONTH PROBATION; RESTRICTION PLACED ON CONTROLLED SUBSTANCE LICENSE
OFFENSE: SUBSTANCE ABUSE

NOTES: HE HAS ENGAGED IN THE INTEMPERATE USE OF DALGAN AND DEVELOPED AN ADDICTION TO THE DRUG; WAS TREATED IN 1991, SUFFERED A RELAPSE AND ENTERED TREATMENT IN 6/93; HAS ADMITTED TO EXPERIMENTING WITH LSD, METHAMPHETAMINES AND MARIJUANA IN COLLEGE AND OCCASIONALLY USING MARIJUANA AND ALCOHOL DURING MEDICAL SCHOOL; ADMITS ALLOWING DALGAN ACCESS TO ONE PERSON WHO EVENTUALLY NEEDED TREATMENT FOR ADDICTION TO THE DRUG; HAS MAINTAINED

SOBRIETY SINCE 6/29/93; CURRENTLY UNDER THE CARE OF A PSYCHIATRIST AND ENTERED A REHABILITATION CONTRACT WITH PHYSICIANS HEALTH AND REHABILITATION COMMITTEE. SUSPENSION STAYED. CONDITIONS OF PROBATION: SHALL APPEAR BEFORE THE BOARD TWICE A YEAR; SHALL ABSTAIN FROM THE CONSUMPTION OF ALCOHOL/CHEMICAL SUBSTANCES IN ANY FORM UNLESS PRESCRIBED BY ANOTHER PHYSICIAN FOR A LEGITIMATE AND THERAPEUTIC PURPOSE; SHALL PARTICIPATE IN AA'S PROGRAM NOT LESS THAN THREE TIMES A WEEK WITH QUARTERLY REPORTS TO THE BOARD; SHALL SUBMIT HIMSELF FOR APPROPRIATE EXAMS INCLUDING DRUG AND ALCOHOL SCREENS; SHALL SUBMIT HIMSELF FOR EVALUATION AND TREATMENT TO A BOARD-APPROVED PSYCHIATRIST; SHALL NOT TREAT OR OTHERWISE SERVE AS PHYSICIAN, PRESCRIBE OR DISPENSE DRUGS THAT MAY BE SUBJECT TO ABUSE TO HIMSELF OR ANY MEMBER OF HIS FAMILY; SHALL SURRENDER HIS DEA AND TEXAS CONTROLLED SUBSTANCES CERTIFICATES AND NOT REAPPLY WITH PERMISSION; SHALL ATTEND AT LEAST 50 HOURS PER YEAR OF CONTINUING MEDICAL EDUCATION; SHALL COMPLY WITH TERMS OF CONTRACT WITH THE PHYSICIANS HEALTH AND REHABILITATION COMMITTEE AND PROVIDE A COPY OF THIS CONTRACT; SHALL GIVE A COPY OF THIS ORDER TO ANY HEALTH CARE ENTITY WHERE HE HAS PRIVILEGES; SHALL COOPERATE WITH THE BOARD IN VERIFYING COMPLIANCE; SHALL INFORM BOARD OF CHANGE OF ADDRESS OR IF HE LEAVES THE STATE; TIME SPENT OUT OF TEXAS DOES NOT COUNT TOWARD PROBATION. SHALL NOT SEEK MODIFICATION FOR ONE YEAR. ON 8/9/97 PETITION TO TERMINATE ORDER DENIED. ON 8/22/98 ORDER TERMINATED.

JACKSON, NICHOLAS M MD OF 1301 KAMIRA, KERRVILLE, TX, WAS DISCIPLINED BY DEA ON AUGUST 19, 1994
DISCIPLINARY ACTION: SURRENDER OF CONTROLLED SUBSTANCE LICENSE

NOTES: IMPAIRED DOCTOR.

JACKSON, NICHOLAS MAXWELL MD, LICENSE NUMBER 0C38425 OF KERRVILLE, TX, WAS DISCIPLINED BY CALIFORNIA ON NOVEMBER 5, 1995
DISCIPLINARY ACTION: 84-MONTH PROBATION
OFFENSE: DISCIPLINARY ACTION BY ANOTHER STATE OR AGENCY

NOTES: ACTION IN TEXAS FOR SELF SUPPLYING DALGAN, A NON-CONTROLLED DRUG, RESULTING IN ADDICTION FOR HIMSELF AND HIS WIFE. REVOCATION, STAYED.

JACOBI, RUDOLPH E MD, LICENSE NUMBER 00C2269 OF HOUSTON, TX, WAS DISCIPLINED BY TEXAS ON APRIL 10, 1992
DISCIPLINARY ACTION: SURRENDER OF LICENSE

NOTES: LICENSE PERMANENTLY RETIRED IN LIEU OF FURTHER DISCIPLINARY ACTION.

JACOBSON, KAREN S MD, LICENSE NUMBER 00F9615 OF AUSTIN, TX, WAS DISCIPLINED BY TEXAS ON JUNE 22, 1994
DISCIPLINARY ACTION: REPRIMAND
OFFENSE: PROFESSIONAL MISCONDUCT

NOTES: IN 1991 SHE ORDERED NUBAIN FOR A PATIENT WITH WHOM SHE BECAME PERSONALLY ACQUAINTED WHO HAD BEEN DIAGNOSED WITH CANCER; ALLEGES THAT SHE TOOK A HISTORY AND PHYSICAL OF THE PATIENT AND THAT THE PATIENT TOLD HER THAT OTHER PAIN MEDICATIONS WERE NOT BEING TAKEN; FAILED TO CONFER WITH PATIENT'S TREATING PHYSICIAN; ALLEGES THAT FOR TWO YEARS SHE KEPT THE APPROPRIATE RECORDS BUT DOES NOT KNOW WHERE THOSE RECORDS ARE; ALLEGES SHE DID NOT CHARGE THE PATIENT; THIS ORDER IS A SETTLEMENT IN LIEU OF A CONTESTED HEARING. SHALL GIVE A COPY OF THIS ORDER TO ANY HEALTH CARE ENTITY WHERE SHE HAS PRIVILEGES.

JAIKARAN, JACQUES S MD, LICENSE NUMBER 00F2731 OF HUMBLE, TX, WAS DISCIPLINED BY TEXAS ON OCTOBER 9, 1992
DISCIPLINARY ACTION: REPRIMAND
OFFENSE: NONCOMPLIANCE WITH A PROFESSIONAL RULE

NOTES: FALSE ADVERTISING.

JAIN, PREM L MD, LICENSE NUMBER 4128 OF DICKINSON, TX, WAS DISCIPLINED BY NEW HAMPSHIRE ON MARCH 4, 1999
DISCIPLINARY ACTION: RESTRICTION PLACED ON LICENSE
OFFENSE: DISCIPLINARY ACTION BY ANOTHER STATE OR AGENCY

NOTES: ACTION TAKEN BY TEXAS.

JAIN, PREM LATA MD, LICENSE NUMBER D3899 OF DICKINSON, TX, WAS DISCIPLINED BY TEXAS ON AUGUST 22, 1998
DISCIPLINARY ACTION: REQUIRED TO TAKE ADDITIONAL MEDICAL EDUCATION; MONITORING OF PHYSICIAN PERFORMANCE
OFFENSE: PROFESSIONAL MISCONDUCT

NOTES: PRIOR TO 1993, SHE PREPARED, REPACKAGED, AND DISPENSED FROM HER OFFICE MEDICATIONS THAT WERE LABELED INAPPROPRIATELY AND IN VIOLATION OF THE TEXAS PHARMACY ACT AND SHE PROVIDED 8 PATIENTS WITH MEDICATION IN A FREQUENT, EXCESSIVE AND NON-THERAPEUTIC MANNER; SHE MAINTAINS THAT IN 1993 SHE REFORMED HER PRACTICE, BECAME AFFILIATED WITH 5 HEALTH MAINTENANCE ORGANIZATIONS, AND ENTERED INTO AN AGREEMENT WITH THE DEPARTMENT OF DEFENSE TO SERVE AS THE PRIMARY CARE PHYSICIAN FOR SOME 500 ASSIGNED PATIENTS; SHE FURTHER MAINTAINS THAT IN 1993 SHE BEGAN PHASING OUT SOME NON-HMO PATIENTS IN ORDER TO TAKE CARE OF HMO SUBSCRIBERS AND THE DEPARTMENT OF DEFENSE PERSONNEL. LICENSE LIMITED FOR THREE YEARS AS FOLLOWS: SEPARATE FROM PATIENT RECORDS, SHALL MAINTAIN A LOGBOOK OF EVERY PRESCRIPTION WRITTEN BY HIM FOR DANGEROUS DRUGS WITH ADDICTIVE POTENTIAL WHICH SHALL BE MADE AVAILABLE FOR REVIEW; SHALL PROPERLY LABEL ALL DRUGS DISPENSED FROM HER OFFICE, INCLUDING SAMPLES; SHALL MAINTAIN ADEQUATE MEDICAL RECORDS WHICH SHALL BE AVAILABLE FOR REVIEW; SHALL ATTEND 100 HOURS PER YEAR OF CONTINUING MEDICAL EDUCATION, WITH 1 COURSE IN PREVENTION AND TREATMENT OF DRUG ABUSE AND 1 COURSE IN PRESCRIBING MEDICATIONS; SHALL APPEAR BEFORE THE BOARD AT LEAST ONCE A YEAR; SHALL COOPERATE WITH THE BOARD IN VERIFYING COMPLIANCE; SHALL GIVE A COPY OF THIS ORDER TO ANY HEALTH CARE ENTITY WHERE HE HAS PRIVILEGES; TIME SPENT OUT OF TEXAS DOES NOT COUNT TOWARD RESTRICTION; SHALL INFORM THE BOARD OF CHANGE OF ADDRESS WITHIN 10 DAYS OR IF SHE LEAVES THE STATE; SHALL NOT SEEK MODIFICATION FOR ONE YEAR. ON 12/11/99 THE ORDER WAS TERMINATED.

JAIN, PREM LATA MD, DATE OF BIRTH JULY 5, 1935, LICENSE NUMBER 24182 OF 2909 MAIN STREET, DICKINSON, TX, WAS DISCIPLINED BY WISCONSIN ON NOVEMBER 17, 1999
DISCIPLINARY ACTION: LICENSE SUSPENSION
OFFENSE: DISCIPLINARY ACTION BY ANOTHER STATE OR AGENCY

NOTES: ON 8/22/98 THE TEXAS BOARD ISSUED A LIMITED LICENSE DUE TO ACTS PRIOR TO 1993: PREPARING, REPACKAGING AND DISPENSING FROM HER OFFICE MEDICATIONS THAT WERE LABELED INAPPROPRIATELY; AND PROVIDING PATIENTS WITH MEDICATION IN A FREQUENT, EXCESSIVE AND NON-THERAPEUTIC MANNER; ON 3/1/99 THE NEW HAMPSHIRE BOARD ISSUED A RESTRICTED LICENSE BASED ON THE TEXAS ACTION; ON 10/12/99 SHE INDICATED THAT SHE WOULD BE VOLUNTARILY NOT RENEWING HER LICENSE TO PRACTICE MEDICINE AND SURGERY IN WISCONSIN.

JAIN, ROSHAN L MD, LICENSE NUMBER 0220079 OF 18339 CAPE BAHAMAS, HOUSTON, TX, WAS DISCIPLINED BY WISCONSIN ON MARCH 21, 1990
DISCIPLINARY ACTION: LICENSE REVOCATION
OFFENSE: DISCIPLINARY ACTION BY ANOTHER STATE OR AGENCY

NOTES: LICENSE WAS REVOKED IN NEW YORK IN 1986 BECAUSE OF 7 COUNTS OF UNPROFESSIONAL CONDUCT.

JAIN, ROSHAN L MD, DATE OF BIRTH SEPTEMBER 21, 1936 OF 18339 CAPE BAHAMAS, HOUSTON, TX, WAS DISCIPLINED BY MEDICARE ON JULY 23, 1991
DISCIPLINARY ACTION: EXCLUSION FROM THE MEDICARE AND/OR MEDICAID PROGRAM
OFFENSE: DISCIPLINARY ACTION BY ANOTHER STATE OR AGENCY

NOTES: LICENSE REVOCATION OR SUSPENSION.

JAKUBOWICZ, ISAAC E MD, LICENSE NUMBER F5962 OF LOS ANGELES, CA, WAS DISCIPLINED BY TEXAS ON AUGUST 9, 1997
DISCIPLINARY ACTION: REPRIMAND
OFFENSE: DISCIPLINARY ACTION BY ANOTHER STATE OR AGENCY

NOTES: ON OR ABOUT 7/1/94 HE WAS CONVICTED OF 3 COUNTS OF FILING OF FALSE TAX RETURN IN THE U.S. DISTRICT COURT, NORTHERN DISTRICT OF CALIFORNIA, SAN JOSE DIVISION FOR THE TAX YEARS 1986 - 1988; CALIFORNIA LICENSE SUSPENDED AFTER CONVICTION AND PRIVILEGES WERE RESTORED ON 2/20/97.

JAKUBOWICZ, ISAAC E MD, LICENSE NUMBER 44465 OF PO BOX 25287, LOS ANGELES, CA, WAS DISCIPLINED BY MASSACHUSETTS ON JULY 1, 1998
DISCIPLINARY ACTION: REPRIMAND
OFFENSE: PROFESSIONAL MISCONDUCT

NOTES: FEDERAL TAX VIOLATION.

JAMES, JOCELYN LEAH MD, LICENSE NUMBER 00G6668 OF SAN ANTONIO, TX, WAS DISCIPLINED BY TEXAS ON OCTOBER 9, 1992
DISCIPLINARY ACTION: 60-MONTH PROBATION
OFFENSE: SUBSTANDARD CARE, INCOMPETENCE OR NEGLIGENCE

NOTES: PROFESSIONAL FAILURE TO PRACTICE MEDICINE IN AN ACCEPTABLE MANNER CONSISTENT WITH PUBLIC HEALTH AND WELFARE. SUSPENSION STAYED. PROBATION UNDER TERMS AND CONDITIONS. ON 11/3/94 PROBATION TERMINATED.

JAREM, BOHDAN J MD, WAS DISCIPLINED BY ARIZONA ON DECEMBER 2, 1993
OFFENSE: DISCIPLINARY ACTION BY ANOTHER STATE OR AGENCY

NOTES: TEXAS ISSUED AN ORDER IN 01/93 SUSPENDING HIS LICENSE FOR FIVE YEARS. HE SIGNED AND ENTERED INTO A STIPULATION AND ORDER NOT TO PRACTICE MEDICINE IN ARIZONA.

JAREM, BOHDAN JOHN MD, DATE OF BIRTH JULY 22, 1941, LICENSE NUMBER 00D9829 OF 5400 PRESTON OAKS #2003, DALLAS, TX, WAS DISCIPLINED BY TEXAS ON JANUARY 30, 1993
DISCIPLINARY ACTION: EMERGENCY SUSPENSION
OFFENSE: PHYSICAL OR MENTAL ILLNESS INHIBITING THE ABILITY TO PRACTICE WITH SKILL AND SAFETY

NOTES: SUFFERS FROM A BIPOLAR DISORDER IN THE MANIC PHASE AND IS IN NEED OF PSYCHIATRIC COUNSELING.

JAREM, BOHDAN JOHN MD, DATE OF BIRTH JULY 22, 1941, LICENSE NUMBER 00D9829 OF 4118 KEYSTONE, GARLAND, TX, WAS DISCIPLINED BY TEXAS ON JUNE 15, 1993
DISCIPLINARY ACTION: 60-MONTH PROBATION; MONITORING OF PHYSICIAN PERFORMANCE
OFFENSE: PHYSICAL OR MENTAL ILLNESS INHIBITING THE ABILITY TO PRACTICE WITH SKILL AND SAFETY

NOTES: FROM 1/7/93-2/22/93 HE RECEIVED INPATIENT PSYCHIATRIC TREATMENT FOR A BIPOLAR DISORDER IN THE MANIC PHASE; DISORDER IS CURRENTLY IN REMISSION AND HE IS RECEIVING PSYCHIATRIC COUNSELING. FIVE YEAR SUSPENSION STAYED. CONDITIONS OF PROBATION: SHALL CONTINUE TO RECEIVE PSYCHIATRIC TREATMENT WITH QUARTERLY REPORTS TO THE BOARD; SHALL OBTAIN A BOARD-APPROVED PSYCHIATRIST AND CONTINUE TREATMENT IF HE RELOCATES; SHALL SUBMIT HIMSELF FOR RANDOM LAB TESTING OF HIS LITHIUM LEVEL; SHALL APPEAR BEFORE THE BOARD TWICE A YEAR; SHALL GIVE A COPY OF THIS ORDER TO ANY HEALTH CARE ENTITY WHERE HE HAS PRIVILEGES; SHALL COOPERATE WITH THE BOARD IN VERIFYING COMPLIANCE; SHALL INFORM BOARD OF CHANGE OF ADDRESS WITHIN 10 DAYS OR IF HE LEAVES TEXAS; TIME SPENT OUT OF TEXAS DOES NOT COUNT TOWARD PROBATION. SHALL NOT SEEK MODIFICATION FOR ONE YEAR. ON 6/28/95 HIS PETITION FOR TERMINATION OF THIS ORDER DENIED.

JAREM, BOHDAN JOHN MD, LICENSE NUMBER 0029241 OF GARLAND, TX, WAS DISCIPLINED BY OHIO ON MARCH 16, 1994
DISCIPLINARY ACTION: LICENSE SUSPENSION; PROBATION
OFFENSE: DISCIPLINARY ACTION BY ANOTHER STATE OR AGENCY

NOTES: PRIOR ACTION BY TEXAS BOARD DUE TO HIS BIPOLAR DISORDER. INDEFINITE SUSPENSION. CONDITIONS FOR REINSTATEMENT ESTABLISHED; PROBATION FOR AT LEAST TWO YEARS.

JAVIER, RICARDO R MD, LICENSE NUMBER 00D9186 OF HUBBARD, TX, WAS DISCIPLINED BY TEXAS ON MARCH 5, 1994
DISCIPLINARY ACTION: 36-MONTH RESTRICTION PLACED ON LICENSE; REQUIRED TO TAKE ADDITIONAL MEDICAL EDUCATION
OFFENSE: SUBSTANDARD CARE, INCOMPETENCE OR NEGLIGENCE

NOTES: IN 5/84 HE INITIATED A SURGICAL PROCEDURE AT A HOSPITAL INSUFFICIENTLY EQUIPPED TO HANDLE IT AND FAILED TO REFER THE PATIENT TO A SURGEON AND FACILITY BETTER ABLE TO CARE FOR THE PATIENT IN A TIMELY MANNER; IN 8/94 FAILED TO ADDRESS THE ACUTE ABDOMEN OF A PATIENT IN A TIMELY MANNER ALTHOUGH THERE WERE CLINICAL INDICATIONS FOR SURGERY; IN 1990 FAILED TO ADEQUATELY EVALUATE A NURSING HOME PATIENT ON A SUFFICIENTLY REGULAR BASIS OR TO ADEQUATELY DOCUMENT SUCH EVALUATIONS; HE NO LONGER PERFORMS SURGERY AND HAS NOT SEEN NURSING HOME PATIENTS FOR TWO YEARS. SHALL MAINTAIN A CURRENT ADVANCED CARDIAC LIFE SUPPORT AND ADVANCED TRAUMA LIFE SUPPORT CERTIFICATION; SHALL NOT ACT AS A PRIMARY SURGEON ON ANY SURGICAL CASE EXCEPT FOR

OFFICE PROCEDURES REQUIRING ONLY LOCAL ANESTHESIA; SHALL ATTEND AT LEAST 50 HOURS CONTINUING MEDICAL EDUCATION PER YEAR; DURING THE FIRST YEAR SHALL PROVIDE AT LEAST ONE LETTER OF RECOMMENDATION FROM A PHYSICIAN AT EACH HOSPITAL WHERE HE WORKS; SHALL GIVE A COPY OF THIS ORDER TO ANY HEALTH CARE ENTITY WHERE HE HAS PRIVILEGES; SHALL COOPERATE WITH THE BOARD IN VERIFYING COMPLIANCE; SHALL INFORM BOARD OF CHANGE OF ADDRESS WITHIN 10 DAYS OR IF HE LEAVES THE STATE; TIME SPENT OUT OF TEXAS DOES NOT COUNT TOWARD RESTRICTION. SHALL NOT SEEK MODIFICATION FOR ONE YEAR.

JAVIER, RICARDO R MD, LICENSE NUMBER 26885 OF HUBBARD, TX, WAS DISCIPLINED BY WASHINGTON ON JANUARY 9, 1997
DISCIPLINARY ACTION: LICENSE REVOCATION
OFFENSE: NONCOMPLIANCE WITH A PROFESSIONAL RULE

NOTES: FAILED TO RESPOND TO A STATEMENT OF CHARGES ALLEGING THAT HE HAD HIS LICENSE TO PRACTICE MEDICINE RESTRICTED IN TEXAS.

JESNECK, RICHARD J JR MD OF 5231 SPELLMAN ROAD, HOUSTON, TX, WAS DISCIPLINED BY DEA ON MAY 5, 1994
DISCIPLINARY ACTION: SURRENDER OF CONTROLLED SUBSTANCE LICENSE

NOTES: IN LIEU OF PUBLIC INTEREST REVOCATION.

JOHNSON, GERALD W MD, LICENSE NUMBER 3513A, WAS DISCIPLINED BY WYOMING ON JULY 9, 1999
OFFENSE: DISCIPLINARY ACTION BY ANOTHER STATE OR AGENCY

NOTES: BASED UPON A 1991 REPRIMAND ISSUED BY THE TEXAS BOARD ON 12/19/91 HE AGREED TO NOTIFY THE WYOMING BOARD AT LEAST 30 DAYS PRIOR TO MOVING TO WYOMING IF HE EVER INTENDED TO PRACTICE MEDICINE THERE; AN 8/22/98 AGREED ORDER BY THE TEXAS BOARD RESTRICTS AND IMPOSES CONDITIONS ON HIS TEXAS LICENSE. WYOMING PROCEEDINGS SHALL BE STAYED WITH FOLLOWING TERMS: SHALL INFORM THE BOARD OF ANY ACTIONS TAKEN OR ORDERS ENTERED BY THE TEXAS BOARD RELATIVE TO HIS TEXAS LICENSE; SHALL NOT PRACTICE MEDICINE OR SURGERY IN WYOMING; AND, SHALL NOT APPLY TO THE BOARD FOR REMOVAL OF THE CONDITIONS AND RESTRICTIONS UNTIL ALL RESTRICTIONS AND CONDITIONS HAVE BEEN REMOVED BY TEXAS.

JOHNSON, GERALD WAYNE MD, DATE OF BIRTH MARCH 11, 1940, LICENSE NUMBER 00D6462 OF 17115 RED OAK DRIVE #211, HOUSTON, TX, WAS DISCIPLINED BY TEXAS ON AUGUST 24, 1991
DISCIPLINARY ACTION: RESTRICTION PLACED ON LICENSE

NOTES: AGREES TO LIMIT HIMSELF TO REMOVING NO MORE THAN 2000 CCS. OF FAT DURING A LIPOSUCTION DAY SURGERY PROCEDURE; NO MORE THAN 4000 CCS. OF FAT IN A HOSPITAL SETTING; IF NECESSARY, MUST TRANSFUSE ONE UNIT OF BLOOD WHEN 2000 CCS. ARE REMOVED, WITH ANOTHER UNIT OF BLOOD WHEN 3000-4000 CCS. OF FAT ARE REMOVED. ALSO AGREES TO ENSURE THAT BEFORE BEGINNING ANY PLASTIC SURGERY PROCEDURE, TRANSPORTATION IS AVAILABLE TO A HOSPITAL FACILITY WITHIN A FIVE-MILE RADIUS FROM THE SURGICAL SITE FOR ANY PATIENT WHO EXPERIENCES COMPLICATIONS. ON 8/20/93 ORDER TERMINATED AND LICENSE FREE AND CLEAR OF ANY PREVIOUS RESTRICTIONS.

JOHNSON, GERALD WAYNE MD, LICENSE NUMBER D6462 OF HOUSTON, TX, WAS DISCIPLINED BY TEXAS ON AUGUST 22, 1998
DISCIPLINARY ACTION: REQUIRED TO TAKE ADDITIONAL MEDICAL EDUCATION; MONITORING OF PHYSICIAN PERFORMANCE
OFFENSE: SUBSTANDARD CARE, INCOMPETENCE OR NEGLIGENCE

NOTES: ON 7/12/94 PERFORMED A BREAST REDUCTION AND LIPOSUCTION; FAILED TO HAVE A BLOOD SUPPLY ON HAND; FAILED TO ADEQUATELY FOLLOW-UP ON A PATIENT FOLLOWING SIGNIFICANT BLOOD LOSS BY NOT PERSONALLY ENSURING THAT THE NURSING STAFF ACTUALLY GAVE THE PATIENT BLOOD PRODUCTS IN A TIMELY FASHION AS SOON AS THEY WERE AVAILABLE; DOCUMENTATION FAILS TO REFLECT THAT THE PATIENT GAVE INFORMED CONSENT FOR HAVING LIPOSUCTION PERFORMED ON HER; HE ASSERTS THAT THE INCLUSION OF LIPOSUCTION WAS SPECIFICALLY DISCUSSED WITH THE PATIENT. LICENSE LIMITED FOR FIVE YEARS AS FOLLOWS: HIS MEDICAL PRACTICE SHALL BE MONITORED BY A BOARD APPROVED TEXAS PHYSICIAN WHO SHALL PROVIDE QUARTERLY REPORTS TO THE BOARD; SHALL OBTAIN 50 HOURS PER YEAR OF CONTINUING MEDICAL EDUCATION, WITH 25 HOURS IN CRITICAL CARE AND POST-OPERATIVE CARE, BLOOD AND BLOOD PRODUCTS, AND RESUSCITATION INFECTION, AND 5 HOURS IN RISK MANAGEMENT AND RECORD KEEPING; WITHIN 1 YEAR SHALL TAKE ADDITIONAL HOURS OF CONTINUING MEDICAL EDUCATION AS FOLLOWS: 48 HOURS IN SURGERY AND 48 HOURS IN ANESTHESIOLOGY; SHALL TAKE A PLASTIC SURGERY REVIEW COURSE AND SHALL TAKE AND SUCCESSFULLY COMPLETE AN ADVANCED CARDIAC LIFE SUPPORT COURSE AND OBTAIN CERTIFICATION; SHALL MAINTAIN ADEQUATE MEDICAL RECORDS WHICH SHALL BE AVAILABLE FOR REVIEW; SHALL APPEAR BEFORE THE BOARD TWICE A YEAR; SHALL COOPERATE WITH THE BOARD IN VERIFYING COMPLIANCE; SHALL COOPERATE WITH THE BOARD IN VERIFYING COMPLIANCE; SHALL GIVE A COPY OF THIS ORDER TO ANY HEALTH CARE ENTITY WHERE HE HAS PRIVILEGES; TIME SPENT OUT OF TEXAS DOES NOT COUNT TOWARD RESTRICTION; SHALL INFORM THE BOARD OF CHANGE OF ADDRESS WITHIN 10 DAYS OR IF HE LEAVES THE STATE; SHALL NOT SEEK MODIFICATION FOR ONE YEAR.

JOHNSON, HAROLD Z MD, LICENSE NUMBER 00D0926 OF ADA, OK, WAS DISCIPLINED BY TEXAS ON JUNE 10, 1991
OFFENSE: DISCIPLINARY ACTION BY ANOTHER STATE OR AGENCY

NOTES: SHOULD HE DESIRE TO PRACTICE MEDICINE IN TEXAS, MUST DEMONSTRATE TO BOARD HIS CAPACITY TO PRACTICE WITH REASONABLE SKILL AND SAFETY AND PROVIDE STATUS REPORT OF WASHINGTON LICENSE; IF TEXAS GRANTS HIM PERMISSION TO PRACTICE, TEXAS BOARD MAY IMPOSE ADDITIONAL PROBATIONARY TERMS.

JOHNSON, HAROLD ZAY MD, LICENSE NUMBER 0G18683 OF LONG BEACH, CA, WAS DISCIPLINED BY CALIFORNIA ON MAY 1, 1994
DISCIPLINARY ACTION: LICENSE REVOCATION
OFFENSE: DISCIPLINARY ACTION BY ANOTHER STATE OR AGENCY

NOTES: DISCIPLINED BY WASHINGTON STATE BOARD BASED ON ALLEGED IMPAIRMENT DUE TO ALCOHOLISM. TEXAS DISCIPLINE BASED ON ABOVE ACTION. DEFAULT DECISION.

JOHNSON, HOOPER D MD, LICENSE NUMBER D7605 OF HARLINGEN, TX, WAS DISCIPLINED BY TEXAS ON NOVEMBER 22, 1997
DISCIPLINARY ACTION: 24-MONTH LICENSE SUSPENSION

OFFENSE: SUBSTANDARD CARE, INCOMPETENCE OR NEGLIGENCE

NOTES: ON 1/8/93 FAILED TO TIGHTLY SUTURE A SUPERFICIAL SEMI-PENETRATING WOUND; PATIENT DIED TWO DAYS LATER; FAILED TO RECOMMEND A RETURN VISIT IN ONE OR TWO DAYS TO INSPECT THE WOUND; FAILED TO DOCUMENT IN THE MEDICAL RECORDS WHETHER HE GAVE THE PATIENT A TETANUS SHOT; FAILED TO DOCUMENT IN THE MEDICAL RECORDS THE SPECIFIC INSTRUCTIONS HE GAVE REGARDING UNDER WHAT CONDITIONS THE PATIENT SHOULD RETURN TO THE HOSPITAL FOR FURTHER CARE. ACTION WILL NOT BECOME FINAL UNTIL ALL APPEALS HAVE BEEN EXHAUSTED.

JOHNSON, HOOPER D MD, DATE OF BIRTH APRIL 4, 1925 OF PO BOX 530121, HARLINGEN, TX, WAS DISCIPLINED BY MEDICARE ON JUNE 18, 1998
DISCIPLINARY ACTION: EXCLUSION FROM THE MEDICARE AND/OR MEDICAID PROGRAM
OFFENSE: DISCIPLINARY ACTION BY ANOTHER STATE OR AGENCY

NOTES: LICENSE REVOKED, SUSPENDED, SURRENDERED OR OTHERWISE LOST FOR REASONS BEARING ON PROFESSIONAL PERFORMANCE, PROFESSIONAL COMPETENCE OR FINANCIAL INTEGRITY.

JOHNSON, KENNETH W MD, LICENSE NUMBER 00J5794, WAS DISCIPLINED BY TEXAS ON AUGUST 17, 1996
DISCIPLINARY ACTION: FINE
OFFENSE: PROFESSIONAL MISCONDUCT

NOTES: IN 1/95 ENTERED INTO A BUSINESS RELATIONSHIP AT CLINIC SOLELY OWNED BY NON-PHYSICIANS THUS AIDING OR ABETTING, DIRECTLY OR INDIRECTLY, THE PRACTICE OF MEDICINE BY ANY PARTNERSHIP, NOT DULY LICENSED TO PRACTICE MEDICINE BY THE BOARD; TERMINATED THE RELATIONSHIP IMMEDIATELY UPON FINDING IT WAS A VIOLATION. DOES NOT ADMIT VIOLATION. $500 ADMINISTRATIVE PENALTY.

JOHNSON, NANCY JEAN MD OF SHREVEPORT, LA, WAS DISCIPLINED BY LOUISIANA ON JUNE 20, 1996
DISCIPLINARY ACTION: REVOCATION OF CONTROLLED SUBSTANCE LICENSE; 60-MONTH REQUIRED TO ENTER AN IMPAIRED PHYSICIAN PROGRAM OR SUBSTANCE ABUSE TREATMENT
OFFENSE: SUBSTANCE ABUSE

NOTES: HABITUAL AND RECURRING USE OF ALCOHOL AND DRUGS WHICH AFFECT THE CENTRAL NERVOUS SYSTEM AND ARE CAPABLE OF PRODUCING PHYSIOLOGICAL OR PSYCHOLOGICAL DEPENDENCE. ORDERED TO ENTER INTO A FIVE YEAR TREATMENT CONTRACT WITH THE PHYSICIANS' HEALTH PROGRAM; PROHIBITED FROM PRESCRIBING, DISPENSING, OR ADMINISTERING CONTROLLED SUBSTANCES DURING HER LIFETIME; AND ORDERED TO PAY ALL COSTS OF THE PROCEEDINGS.

JOHNSON, NANCY JEAN MD, LICENSE NUMBER G2403, WAS DISCIPLINED BY TEXAS ON MAY 10, 1997
OFFENSE: DISCIPLINARY ACTION BY ANOTHER STATE OR AGENCY

NOTES: ON 6/20/96 DISCIPLINARY ACTION WAS TAKEN BY THE LOUISIANA BOARD BASED ON HER HABITUAL AND RECURRING ABUSE OF DRUGS AND HER INABILITY TO PRACTICE WITH REASONABLE SKILL AND SAFETY DUE TO IMPAIRMENT. THE ORDER NECESSITATED A FIVE-YEAR CONTRACT WITH THE PHYSICIANS HEALTH PROGRAM AND PERMANENTLY RESTRICTED HER FROM PRESCRIBING, DISPENSING, OR ADMINISTERING CONTROLLED SUBSTANCES FOR THE DURATION OF HER MEDICAL CAREER; SHE WAS ALSO REQUIRED TO SURRENDER HER DEA REGISTRATION. SHALL NOT PRACTICE MEDICINE IN TEXAS UNTIL SHE REQUESTS PERMISSION TO DO SO AND PERSONALLY APPEARS BEFORE THE BOARD AND PROVIDES SUFFICIENT EVIDENCE WHICH ADEQUATELY INDICATES THAT SHE IS PHYSICALLY, MENTALLY, AND OTHERWISE COMPETENT TO ENGAGE IN THE PRACTICE OF MEDICINE. SUCH EVIDENCE SHALL INCLUDE AT A MINIMUM: CONTINUED MAINTENANCE OF SOBRIETY AND NO FURTHER ACTION TAKEN BY ANY OTHER STATE'S MEDICAL BOARD.

JOHNSON, NEAL D MD, LICENSE NUMBER 00G3500 OF AUSTIN, TX, WAS DISCIPLINED BY TEXAS ON JUNE 22, 1994
DISCIPLINARY ACTION: REQUIRED TO TAKE ADDITIONAL MEDICAL EDUCATION
OFFENSE: SUBSTANDARD CARE, INCOMPETENCE OR NEGLIGENCE

NOTES: FAILED TO CONSIDER AND/OR DIAGNOSE APPENDICITIS IN ONE PATIENT EVEN AFTER SERIAL PRESENTATIONS. SHALL WITHIN ONE YEAR ATTEND AT LEAST 50 HOURS OF CONTINUING MEDICAL EDUCATION WITH SIX HOURS IN RISK MANAGEMENT AND NINE HOURS IN AREAS DEALING WITH THE DIAGNOSIS OF ACUTE ABDOMINAL PAIN; SHALL GIVE A COPY OF THIS ORDER TO ANY HEALTH CARE ENTITY WHERE HE HAS PRIVILEGES; SHALL COOPERATE WITH THE BOARD IN VERIFYING COMPLIANCE; SHALL INFORM BOARD OF ADDRESS CHANGE WITHIN 10 DAYS. SHALL NOT SEEK MODIFICATION FOR SIX MONTHS. ON 6/28/95, BOARD GRANTED HIS PETITION FOR TERMINATION OF ORDER BASED ON HIS COMPLIANCE WITH ALL CONDITIONS.

JOHNSON, SHEILA M MD OF 11512 SPRINGHILL DRIVE, AUSTIN, TX, WAS DISCIPLINED BY DEA ON MARCH 27, 1995
DISCIPLINARY ACTION: SURRENDER OF CONTROLLED SUBSTANCE LICENSE
OFFENSE: DISCIPLINARY ACTION BY ANOTHER STATE OR AGENCY

NOTES: STATE BOARD.

JOHNSON, SHEILA M MD, LICENSE NUMBER 0047853 OF RADFORD, VA, WAS DISCIPLINED BY VIRGINIA ON JUNE 9, 1995
DISCIPLINARY ACTION: LICENSE SUSPENSION
OFFENSE: DISCIPLINARY ACTION BY ANOTHER STATE OR AGENCY

NOTES: SUSPENSION BY TEXAS FOR INTEMPERATE USE OF ALCOHOL OR DRUGS.

JOHNSON, SHEILA M MD, LICENSE NUMBER 0160759 OF 11512 SPRINGHILL DRIVE, AUSTIN, TX, WAS DISCIPLINED BY NEW YORK ON DECEMBER 7, 1995
DISCIPLINARY ACTION: SURRENDER OF LICENSE
OFFENSE: DISCIPLINARY ACTION BY ANOTHER STATE OR AGENCY

NOTES: ACTION IN TEXAS FOR HER INTEMPERATE USE OF ALCOHOL OR DRUGS.

JOHNSON, SHEILA MOLLY MD, LICENSE NUMBER 00G2069 OF AUSTIN, TX, WAS DISCIPLINED BY TEXAS ON MARCH 4, 1995
DISCIPLINARY ACTION: LICENSE SUSPENSION
OFFENSE: SUBSTANCE ABUSE

NOTES: RECEIVED INPATIENT SUBSTANCE ABUSE TREATMENT ON FOUR OCCASIONS BETWEEN 1/12/94 AND 3/26/94; REPORTS A SOBRIETY DATE OF 5/1/94; RECEIVED OUTPATIENT SUBSTANCE ABUSE TREATMENT FROM 5/94 TO 9/94; HAS BEEN ATTENDING AA ON A REGULAR BASIS SINCE 5/94; UNDER THE CARE OF A PSYCHIATRIST FOR MOOD DISORDER AND SUBSTANCE ABUSE. SUSPENSION

UNTIL SHE REQUESTS TO HAVE SUSPENSION STAYED OR LIFTED AND APPEARS BEFORE THE BOARD AND PROVIDES SUFFICIENT EVIDENCE WHICH ADEQUATELY INDICATES THAT SHE IS PHYSICALLY, MENTALLY AND OTHERWISE COMPETENT TO SAFELY PRACTICE MEDICINE. SUCH EVIDENCE SHALL INCLUDE AT A MINIMUM, COPIES OF MEDICAL RECORDS AND REPORTS OF PSYCHOLOGICAL AND NEUROPSYCHIATRIC EVALUATIONS CONDUCTED BY A BOARD-CERTIFIED PSYCHIATRIST WHO SHALL PROVIDE REPORTS.

JOHNSON, TONE JR MD, LICENSE NUMBER G6946 OF CORPUS CHRISTI, TX, WAS DISCIPLINED BY TEXAS ON APRIL 10, 1999
DISCIPLINARY ACTION: REPRIMAND
OFFENSE: PROFESSIONAL MISCONDUCT

NOTES: THE BOARD INVESTIGATED ALLEGATIONS REGARDING HIS PRACTICE AT BAY AREA CARE CENTER WHERE SEVERAL VIOLATIONS WERE FOUND REGARDING IMPROPER MANAGEMENT OF THE CENTER; HE HELD 55% OWNERSHIP OF THE CENTER AND WAS THE MEDICAL DIRECTOR AND PROGRAM SPONSOR; ON 10/17/97 THE FOLLOWING VIOLATIONS WERE FOUND: PATIENTS' DOSAGES OF METHADONE AND PATIENTS' FREQUENCY OF CLINIC ATTENDANCE WERE BEING CHANGED WITHOUT A PHYSICIAN'S ORDER AND/OR NOT BEING COUNTERSIGNED WITHIN 72 HOURS; ADMISSION MEDICAL EVALUATIONS WERE NOT BEING REVIEWED AND COUNTERSIGNED BY THE PROGRAM PHYSICIAN OR MEDICAL DIRECTOR WITHIN 72 HOURS TO SIGNIFY REVIEW OF AND CONCURRENCE WITH THE HISTORY AND PHYSICAL FINDINGS; A PATIENT' S FILE FAILED TO CONTAIN DOCUMENTATION OF A PERIODIC TREATMENT PLAN EVERY 90 DAYS THE FIRST YEAR OF THE PATIENT'S TREATMENT; PATIENTS' FILES FAILED TO CONTAIN A COPY OF A CURRENT STATE ISSUED IDENTIFICATION UPON ADMISSION; NON-PHYSICIANS PREDATED PHYSICIANS' ORDERS, AND SIGNED PHYSICIAN ORDERS; NON-PHYSICIANS INSTITUTED DETOXIFICATION ORDERS FOR PATIENTS WHO DID NOT PAY; THE CLINIC CLOSED ON 11/2/97.

JOHNSON, WILLIAM R MD, LICENSE NUMBER 00DO573 OF AUSTIN, TX, WAS DISCIPLINED BY TEXAS ON AUGUST 18, 1990
DISCIPLINARY ACTION: LICENSE REVOCATION
OFFENSE: OVERPRESCRIBING OR MISPRESCRIBING DRUGS

NOTES: STIPULATED ORDER. LICENSE IMMEDIATELY AND PERMANENTLY RETIRED IN LIEU OF CONTINUING CONTESTED CASE HEARING CONCERNING ALLEGATIONS OF NONTHERAPEUTIC PRESCRIBING OF CONTROLLED SUBSTANCES.

JOHNSON, WILLIAM RICHARD MD OF BOX 1507 BUNA, BUNA, TX, WAS DISCIPLINED BY DEA ON OCTOBER 18, 1990
DISCIPLINARY ACTION: SURRENDER OF CONTROLLED SUBSTANCE LICENSE
OFFENSE: OVERPRESCRIBING OR MISPRESCRIBING DRUGS

NOTES: NON-THERAPEUTIC PRESCRIBING.

JOHNSTON, JAMES C MD, LICENSE NUMBER 0022573, WAS DISCIPLINED BY ARIZONA ON OCTOBER 18, 1995

NOTES: SHALL NOT PRACTICE MEDICINE IN ARIZONA PRIOR TO MEETING WITH THE BOARD.

JOHNSTON, JAMES C MD, LICENSE NUMBER 25337 OF SAN ANTONIO, TX, WAS DISCIPLINED BY WASHINGTON ON JANUARY 24, 1997

NOTES: AGREED ORDER TO APPEAR BEFORE THE COMMISSION PRIOR TO PRACTICING MEDICINE IN WASHINGTON. ON 1/21/99 REQUEST TO TERMINATE THE CONDITIONS OF THIS ORDER GRANTED AND LICENSE IS NOW UNRESTRICTED.

JOHNSTON, JAMES C MD, DATE OF BIRTH NOVEMBER 20, 1954, LICENSE NUMBER 33573, WAS DISCIPLINED BY COLORADO ON APRIL 17, 1997
DISCIPLINARY ACTION: SURRENDER OF LICENSE

NOTES: NO UNPROFESSIONAL CONDUCT IDENTIFIED.

JOHNSTON, JAMES CHRISTOPHER MD, DATE OF BIRTH NOVEMBER 20, 1959, LICENSE NUMBER 00G8880 OF NACOGDOCHES, TX, WAS DISCIPLINED BY TEXAS ON JUNE 22, 1994
DISCIPLINARY ACTION: RESTRICTION PLACED ON LICENSE
OFFENSE: SEXUAL ABUSE OF OR SEXUAL MISCONDUCT WITH A PATIENT

NOTES: AS RECENTLY AS 6/8/94 CRIMINAL COMPLAINTS WERE FILED AGAINST HIM ALLEGING HE ENGAGED IN BEHAVIOR CONSTITUTING ATTEMPTED SEXUAL ASSAULT AGAINST INDIVIDUALS WHO WERE PATIENTS; DENIES ALLEGATIONS; BECAUSE HE DESIRES TO FOCUS RESOURCES AND TIME ON DEFENSE OF THE CRIMINAL CASE. AGREES TO THIS ORDER WITH THE BOARD. LICENSE IS RESTRICTED AS FOLLOWS: SHALL NOT EXAMINE OR TREAT PATIENTS AFTER THE ORDER DATE; WITHIN 30 DAYS SHALL SUBMIT HIMSELF FOR ASSESSMENT THROUGH THE BEHAVIOR CARE NETWORK PROGRAM OR OTHER BOARD-APPROVED PROGRAM WHICH WILL FOCUS ON THE DISPARITY BETWEEN THE COMPLAINTS AGAINST HIM AND HIS OWN VERSION OF EVENTS AND ATTEMPT TO DETERMINE THE DEGREE OF RISK TO THE PUBLIC INVOLVED IN HIS CONTINUED PRACTICE; SHOULD THIS EVALUATION INDICATE HIS PRACTICE CONSTITUTES NO THREAT TO THE PUBLIC HEALTH HE SHALL BE PERMITTED TO RESUME PRACTICE PENDING FURTHER ORDER OF THE BOARD PROVIDED HE SEES PATIENTS ONLY WHEN ACCOMPANIED BY A CHAPERONE APPROVED IN ADVANCE WHO WILL SIGN ALL CHARTS TO INDICATE PRESENCE; SHALL COOPERATE WITH THE BOARD IN VERIFYING COMPLIANCE; SHALL INFORM BOARD OF CHANGE OF ADDRESS WITHIN 10 DAYS.

JOHNSTON, JAMES CHRISTOPHER MD, DATE OF BIRTH NOVEMBER 20, 1959, LICENSE NUMBER 00G8880 OF 5601 BANDERA ROAD SUITE 416, SAN ANTONIO, TX, WAS DISCIPLINED BY TEXAS ON SEPTEMBER 30, 1994
DISCIPLINARY ACTION: RESTRICTION PLACED ON LICENSE
OFFENSE: SEXUAL ABUSE OF OR SEXUAL MISCONDUCT WITH A PATIENT

NOTES: CRIMINAL COMPLAINTS HAVE BEEN FILED AGAINST HIM ALLEGING THAT HE HAS ENGAGED IN BEHAVIOR CONSTITUTING ATTEMPTED SEXUAL ASSAULT AGAINST INDIVIDUALS WHO WERE PATIENTS; HE DENIES ALL OF THESE ALLEGATIONS; AS A CONDITION OF 6/22/94 AGREEMENT HAS UNDERGONE AN EXTENSIVE EVALUATION WHICH CONCLUDED THAT THERE WAS NOTHING TO SUGGEST THAT HE WOULD BE UNABLE TO PROVIDE CLINICAL SERVICES UNDER CERTAIN RESTRICTIONS AND SUPERVISION. CONDITIONS OF RESTRICTION WHICH SUPERSEDE PREVIOUS ORDER: SHALL NOT EXAMINE OR TREAT ANY PATIENT WITHOUT BEING ACCOMPANIED BY A BOARD APPROVED CHAPERONE WHO SHALL VERIFY PRESENCE BY SIGNING ALL CHARTS; SHALL OBTAIN AN EXAM TABLE WITH SPECIFICATIONS; SHALL REPOSITION THIS TABLE SO HE MAY WALK BEHIND

PATIENTS TO EXAMINE THE SHOULDER AND PROXIMAL AREAS; SHALL NOT PLACE A PAGER OR INSTRUMENTS IN HIS POCKETS DURING EXAMS; PATIENTS SHALL ONLY BE REPOSITIONED BY A NURSE OR TECHNICIAN; SHALL EXPLAIN TO ALL PATIENTS PROCEDURES WHICH INVOLVE CONTACT AND ASK THEM IN DETAIL REGARDING ANY PROBLEMS OR CONCERNS REGARDING HIS EXAM; WITHIN 60 DAYS SHALL UNDERGO ADDITIONAL PHALLOMETRIC TESTING; SHALL COOPERATE WITH THE BOARD IN VERIFYING COMPLIANCE; SHALL INFORM THE BOARD OF CHANGE OF ADDRESS WITHIN 10 DAYS; SHALL HAVE THE RIGHT TO PETITION FOR AMENDMENT OR TERMINATION UPON DISMISSAL OR ACQUITTAL ON THE CRIMINAL CHARGES; OTHERWISE MAY SEEK MODIFICATIONS ONCE A YEAR. ON 1/29/99 ORDER TERMINATED.

JOHNSTON, JAMES CHRISTOPHER MD, LICENSE NUMBER 00M5411, WAS DISCIPLINED BY IDAHO ON DECEMBER 14, 1994
DISCIPLINARY ACTION: RESTRICTION PLACED ON LICENSE; MONITORING OF PHYSICIAN PERFORMANCE
OFFENSE: DISCIPLINARY ACTION BY ANOTHER STATE OR AGENCY

NOTES: ON 9/30/94 TEXAS RESTRICTED HIS LICENSE BASED ON CRIMINAL ALLEGATIONS THAT HE HAD ENGAGED IN BEHAVIOR CONSTITUTING ATTEMPTED SEXUAL ASSAULT AGAINST PATIENTS. IDAHO BOARD ADOPTS AND INCORPORATES ALL TERMS AND CONDITIONS OF THE TEXAS ORDER WHICH INCLUDE: SHALL NOT EXAMINE OR TREAT ANY PATIENTS WITHOUT BEING ACCOMPANIED AT ALL TIMES BY A PROCTOR OR CHAPERONE APPROVED BY THE BOARD; SHALL OBTAIN AN EXAM TABLE THAT IS SPECIFICALLY DESIGNED FOR THE PERFORMANCE OF ELECTROMYOGRAPHY WITH A STANDARD ARM BOARD AND THE ABILITY TO ELEVATE THE HEAD OF THE PATIENT; SHALL REPOSITION HIS EXAMINATION TABLE SO THAT HE MAY WALK BEHIND PATIENTS TO EXAMINE THE SHOULDER AND PROXIMAL AREAS; SHALL NOT PLACE A PAGER OR INSTRUMENTS IN HIS POCKETS DURING EXAMINATION OF PATIENTS; PATIENTS SHALL BE REPOSITIONED DURING EVALUATIONS ONLY BY A NURSE OR TECHNICIAN; SHALL EXPLAIN TO ALL PATIENTS THOSE PROCEDURES WHICH INVOLVE CONTACT WITH HIM PRIOR TO SUCH CONTACT; SHALL ASK PATIENTS IN DETAIL REGARDING ANY PROBLEMS OR CONCERNS WHICH THEY MIGHT HAVE CONCERNING HIS EXAMINATIONS OR ANY PROCEDURES PERFORMED; SHALL UNDERGO ADDITIONAL PHALLOMETRIC TESTING WITHIN 60 DAYS. ON 1/13/99 ORDER TERMINATED.

JOHNSTON, JAMES CHRISTOPHER MD, LICENSE NUMBER 0A44527 OF NACOGDOCHES, TX, WAS DISCIPLINED BY CALIFORNIA ON DECEMBER 30, 1995
DISCIPLINARY ACTION: SURRENDER OF LICENSE

NOTES: WHILE CHARGES PENDING.

JOHNSTON, JAMES CHRISTOPHER MD, LICENSE NUMBER 0018716 OF SAN ANTONIO, TX, WAS DISCIPLINED BY OREGON ON NOVEMBER 4, 1996
DISCIPLINARY ACTION: SURRENDER OF LICENSE

NOTES: VOLUNTARY SURRENDER.

JONES, GARY ROY MD, LICENSE NUMBER 00D0928 OF AUSTIN, TX, WAS DISCIPLINED BY TEXAS ON OCTOBER 26, 1990
DISCIPLINARY ACTION: 24-MONTH PROBATION; RESTRICTION PLACED ON LICENSE

NOTES: MUST SUBMIT FOR PSYCHIATRIC EVALUATION AND FOLLOW ANY RECOMMENDED TREATMENT; HAVE NURSE/ASSISTANT PRESENT DURING CERTAIN EXAMINATIONS.

JONES, JAMES H MD OF 519 BRYAN ST. JHJ MEDICAL CLINIC, DENTON, TX, WAS DISCIPLINED BY DEA ON MARCH 30, 1994
DISCIPLINARY ACTION: SURRENDER OF CONTROLLED SUBSTANCE LICENSE
OFFENSE: DISCIPLINARY ACTION BY ANOTHER STATE OR AGENCY

NOTES: STATE BOARD.

JONES, JAMES HOLLIS MD, LICENSE NUMBER 00C2516 OF DENTON, TX, WAS DISCIPLINED BY TEXAS ON MARCH 5, 1994
DISCIPLINARY ACTION: SURRENDER OF CONTROLLED SUBSTANCE LICENSE; 60-MONTH PROBATION
OFFENSE: OVERPRESCRIBING OR MISPRESCRIBING DRUGS

NOTES: BETWEEN JUNE 1989 AND APRIL 1993 HE COMMITTED NUMEROUS PRESCRIPTION VIOLATIONS INCLUDING PRESCRIBING CONTROLLED SUBSTANCES SUCH AS LORTAB AND HYDROCODONE TO PATIENTS HE KNEW OR SHOULD HAVE KNOWN WERE HABITUAL USERS OF NARCOTIC DRUGS; PRESCRIBED VARIOUS CONTROLLED SUBSTANCES SUCH AS HYDROCODONE, XANAX, ANEXSIA, DARVOCET, FIORINAL, VALIUM, MOTRIN, AND TUSSIONEX TO PATIENTS WHO HAD NO EXAMINATIONS OR REASON FOR THE PRESCRIPTION NOTED IN THEIR RECORDS. FIVE YEAR SUSPENSION STAYED. CONDITIONS OF PROBATION: SHALL APPEAR BEFORE THE BOARD TWICE A YEAR; SHALL SURRENDER DEA AND TEXAS CONTROLLED SUBSTANCES REGISTRATION CERTIFICATES AND SHALL NOT REREGISTER WITHOUT THE BOARDS APPROVAL; SHALL NOT SIGN OR INDICATE IN ANY MANNER IN PATIENT RECORDS THAT HE HAS SEEN PATIENTS UNLESS HE ACTUALLY HAS SEEN AND EXAMINED THE PATIENT UNLESS IT IS CLEARLY NOTED THAT HE DID NOT PERSONALLY EXAMINE THE PATIENT; SHALL PERSONALLY EXAMINE PATIENT ON THE FIRST VISIT; SHALL ATTEND 50 HOURS PER YEAR OF CONTINUING MEDICAL EDUCATION; SHALL WITHIN SIX MONTHS COMPLETE A BOARD APPROVED ADDICTIONOLOGY COURSE; SHALL GIVE A COPY OF THIS ORDER TO ANY HEALTH CARE ENTITY WHERE HE HAS PRIVILEGES; SHALL COOPERATE WITH THE BOARD IN VERIFYING COMPLIANCE; SHALL INFORM BOARD OF CHANGE OF ADDRESS WITHIN 10 DAYS OR IF HE LEAVES THE STATE; TIME SPENT OUT OF TEXAS DOES NOT COUNT TOWARD PROBATION. SHALL NOT SEEK MODIFICATION FOR ONE YEAR.

JONES, JAMES HOLLIS MD, LICENSE NUMBER C2516, WAS DISCIPLINED BY TEXAS ON MAY 10, 1997
DISCIPLINARY ACTION: SURRENDER OF LICENSE

NOTES: THE BOARD HAS RECEIVED ALLEGATIONS WHICH, IF PROVEN, COULD CONSTITUTE VIOLATIONS OF THE MEDICAL PRACTICE ACT. WHILE NOT ADMITTING ANY WRONGDOING, HE AGREES TO PERMANENTLY AND VOLUNTARILY RETIRE FROM THE PRACTICE OF MEDICINE IN TEXAS AND SHALL NOT PETITION FOR REINSTATEMENT OF HIS LICENSE.

JONES, JAMES W DO, LICENSE NUMBER 0120716 OF 10545 MAYLEE, DALLAS, TX, WAS DISCIPLINED BY NEW YORK ON SEPTEMBER 30, 1993
DISCIPLINARY ACTION: 36-MONTH PROBATION
OFFENSE: DISCIPLINARY ACTION BY ANOTHER STATE OR AGENCY

NOTES: DISCIPLINED BY THE TEXAS BOARD. 3 YEAR

SUSPENSION STAYED.

JONES, JAMES WENDELL DO, LICENSE NUMBER 00E2032 OF DALLAS, TX, WAS DISCIPLINED BY TEXAS ON APRIL 21, 1990
DISCIPLINARY ACTION: REQUIRED TO TAKE ADDITIONAL MEDICAL EDUCATION; MONITORING OF PHYSICIAN PERFORMANCE

NOTES: STIPULATED ORDER. MUST MAINTAIN LIST OF ALL PATIENTS SEEN DURING EACH CALENDAR QUARTER AND AUTHORIZE PHYSICIAN TO REPORT TO BOARD CONCERNING QUALITY AND APPROPRIATENESS OF PHYSICIAN'S DIAGNOSTIC AND TREATMENT DECISIONS, OBTAIN CONTINUING MEDICAL EDUCATION, ATTEND RISK MANAGEMENT COURSE, COMPLETE FAMILY PRACTICE REVIEW OR REFRESHER COURSE, AND APPEAR ANNUALLY BEFORE BOARD.

JONES, JAMES WENDELL DO, LICENSE NUMBER 00E2032 OF DALLAS, TX, WAS DISCIPLINED BY TEXAS ON MARCH 6, 1992
DISCIPLINARY ACTION: 36-MONTH PROBATION

NOTES: PROFESSIONAL FAILURE TO PRACTICE MEDICINE IN AN ACCEPTABLE MANNER CONSISTENT WITH PUBLIC HEALTH AND WELFARE. LICENSE SUSPENDED, SUSPENSION STAYED; PROBATION UNDER TERMS AND CONDITIONS. EFFECTIVE 4/30/93 LICENSE FREE OF ANY RESTRICTION OR LIMITATION.

JONES, JAMES WILSON MD OF 275 O'CONNOR DR SUITE B, SAN JOSE, CA, WAS DISCIPLINED BY DEA ON DECEMBER 17, 1990
DISCIPLINARY ACTION: RESTRICTION PLACED ON CONTROLLED SUBSTANCE LICENSE
OFFENSE: OVERPRESCRIBING OR MISPRESCRIBING DRUGS

NOTES: EXCESSIVE PURCHASES OF PHENDIMETRAZINE AND PHENTERMINE. PLACED ON FIVE YEAR PROBATION EFFECTIVE 07/10/89 FOR EXCESSIVE PRESCRIBING OR ADMINISTERING PHENDIMETRAZINE.

JONES, JAMES WILSON MD OF 275 O'CONNOR DRIVE SUITE B, SAN JOSE, CA, WAS DISCIPLINED BY DEA ON MAY 1, 1994
DISCIPLINARY ACTION: RESTRICTION PLACED ON CONTROLLED SUBSTANCE LICENSE
OFFENSE: DISCIPLINARY ACTION BY ANOTHER STATE OR AGENCY

NOTES: STATE BOARD.

JONES, ROLAND WARD III MD, LICENSE NUMBER 00E9726 OF ORANGE, TX, WAS DISCIPLINED BY TEXAS ON OCTOBER 26, 1990
DISCIPLINARY ACTION: 120-MONTH PROBATION; RESTRICTION PLACED ON LICENSE
OFFENSE: LOSS OR RESTRICTION OF HOSPITAL PRIVILEGES

NOTES: DISCIPLINED BY LICENSED HOSPITAL OR MEDICAL STAFF OF HOSPITAL, INCLUDING REMOVAL, SUSPENSION, LIMITATION OF HOSPITAL PRIVILEGES OR OTHER DISCIPLINARY ACTION; FAILURE TO KEEP COMPLETE AND ACCURATE RECORDS OF PURCHASES AND DISPOSALS OF DRUGS OR CONTROLLED SUBSTANCES; INTEMPERANCE IN USE OF ALCOHOL OR DRUGS THAT COULD ENDANGER LIVES OF PATIENTS; INABILITY TO PRACTICE MEDICINE WITH REASONABLE SKILL AND SAFETY TO PATIENTS BY REASON OF ILLNESS, DRUNKENNESS, EXCESSIVE USE OF DRUGS, NARCOTICS, CHEMICALS, OR OTHER TYPE OF MATERIAL OR AS RESULT OF MENTAL OR PHYSICAL CONDITION.

JONES, ROLAND WARD III MD, LICENSE NUMBER 00E9726 OF ORANGE, TX, WAS DISCIPLINED BY TEXAS ON MAY 21, 1992
DISCIPLINARY ACTION: EMERGENCY SUSPENSION

JONES, ROLAND WARD III MD, LICENSE NUMBER 00E9726 OF ORANGE, TX, WAS DISCIPLINED BY TEXAS ON AUGUST 20, 1992
DISCIPLINARY ACTION: 12-MONTH LICENSE SUSPENSION
OFFENSE: SUBSTANCE ABUSE

NOTES: UNPROFESSIONAL OR DISHONORABLE CONDUCT LIKELY TO DECEIVE, DEFRAUD OR INJURE THE PUBLIC; AND INABILITY TO PRACTICE MEDICINE WITH REASONABLE SKILL AND SAFETY TO PATIENTS. SUSPENSION UNDER TERMS AND CONDITIONS. ON 4/16/94 HIS REQUEST FOR REINSTATEMENT OF HIS LICENSE WAS DENIED.

JONES, ROLAND WARD III MD OF ORANGE, TX, WAS DISCIPLINED BY DEA ON AUGUST 24, 1994
DISCIPLINARY ACTION: REVOCATION OF CONTROLLED SUBSTANCE LICENSE
OFFENSE: DISCIPLINARY ACTION BY ANOTHER STATE OR AGENCY

NOTES: ON 11/9/90 TEXAS BOARD PLACED HIS LICENSE ON PROBATION FOR TEN YEARS WITH SEVERAL TERMS AND CONDITIONS BECAUSE IT FOUND HE HAD ENGAGED IN THE INTEMPERATE USE OF ALCOHOL. HAD BEEN DISCIPLINED BY A HOSPITAL AND FAILED TO KEEP ACCURATE RECORDS OF PURCHASES AND DISPOSALS OF CONTROLLED SUBSTANCES. ON 6/26/92 HIS STATE REGISTRATION TO HANDLE CONTROLLED SUBSTANCES WAS CANCELED. ON 8/20/92 BOARD SUSPENDED HIS LICENSE FOR FAILURE TO FOLLOW TERMS OF THIS PROBATION. THEREFORE HE LACKS STATE AUTHORIZATION TO PRESCRIBE CONTROLLED SUBSTANCES.

JONES, SHELLIE J JR MD, LICENSE NUMBER 00C4383 OF LEESVILLE, LA, WAS DISCIPLINED BY TEXAS ON AUGUST 18, 1990
OFFENSE: DISCIPLINARY ACTION BY ANOTHER STATE OR AGENCY

NOTES: STIPULATED ORDER. MUST COMPLY WITH LOUISIANA ORDER, PROVIDE TEXAS BOARD WITH ANY REQUESTED REPORTS AND OBTAIN PERMISSION OF BOARD BEFORE PRACTICING IN TEXAS.

JOSEY, WILLIE L MD OF 18480 W 5TH STREET, BELOIT, OH, WAS DISCIPLINED BY DEA ON MARCH 20, 1990
DISCIPLINARY ACTION: SURRENDER OF CONTROLLED SUBSTANCE LICENSE
OFFENSE: DISCIPLINARY ACTION BY ANOTHER STATE OR AGENCY

NOTES: OHIO STATE MEDICAL BOARD HAS PLACED RESTRICTIONS ON HIS MEDICAL LICENSE. ONE OF THE CONDITIONS IMPOSED WAS THAT HE COULD NO LONGER POSSESS A DEA CERTIFICATE OF REGISTRATION.

JOSEY, WILLIE L MD, DATE OF BIRTH NOVEMBER 18, 1946, LICENSE NUMBER 0023878 OF 815 MAIN STREET, SOUTH SHORE, KY, WAS DISCIPLINED BY KENTUCKY ON JUNE 21, 1990
DISCIPLINARY ACTION: 60-MONTH PROBATION; RESTRICTION PLACED ON CONTROLLED SUBSTANCE LICENSE

NOTES: IMPLEMENTATION OF ORDER STAYED UNTIL HE RELOCATES TO PRACTICE IN KENTUCKY. CONDITIONS OF PROBATION: SHALL SUBMIT QUARTERLY DECLARATIONS OF COMPLIANCE WITH ORDER; SHALL SURRENDER HIS DEA CERTIFICATE AND SHALL NOT APPLY FOR REGISTRATION WITH DEA WITHOUT PRIOR BOARD APPROVAL AND NOT FOR A MINIMUM OF SIX MONTHS; UPON REINSTATEMENT SHALL KEEP A LOG OF ALL CONTROLLED SUBSTANCES PRESCRIBED, DISPENSED OR ADMINISTERED; SHALL ABSTAIN COMPLETELY FROM THE POSSESSION OR PERSONAL USE OF DRUGS EXCEPT AS DISPENSED BY ANOTHER PERSON WITH SUCH AUTHORITY WHO KNOWS OF HIS

HISTORY OF CHEMICAL DEPENDENCY; SHALL ABSTAIN FROM CONSUMING ALCOHOL; SHALL SUBMIT URINE OR BLOOD SPECIMENS UPON REQUEST; SHALL HAVE A BOARD-APPROVED MONITORING PHYSICIAN WITH QUARTERLY REPORTS TO THE BOARD; SHALL PROVIDE ALL HOSPITALS WHERE HE HAS PRIVILEGES WITH A COPY OF THE ORDER; SHALL COOPERATE WITH THE KENTUCKY IMPAIRED PHYSICIANS COMMITTEE WITH QUARTERLY REPORTS. ON 2/9/93 AN AMENDED ORDER PLACED HIS LICENSE ON PROBATION FOR FIVE YEARS WITH THE CONDITION THAT HE SHALL KEEP A LOG OF ALL CONTROLLED SUBSTANCES PRESCRIBED, DISPENSED OR ADMINISTERED; ALL OTHER TERMS OF THE ORIGINAL ORDER REMAIN IN FORCE.

JOSEY, WILLIE L MD, LICENSE NUMBER 00G6076 OF ALLIANCE, OH, WAS DISCIPLINED BY TEXAS ON AUGUST 18, 1990
OFFENSE: DISCIPLINARY ACTION BY ANOTHER STATE OR AGENCY

NOTES: STIPULATED ORDER. MUST COMPLY WITH OHIO BOARD ORDER, OBTAIN PERMISSION OF BOARD BEFORE PRACTICING IN TEXAS AND COMPLY WITH ANY ADDITIONAL PROBATIONARY TERMS WHICH MAY BE IMPOSED.

JUDICE, DONALD JOSEPH MD OF HOUMA, LA, WAS DISCIPLINED BY LOUISIANA ON MARCH 3, 1994
DISCIPLINARY ACTION: EMERGENCY SUSPENSION

JUDICE, DONALD JOSEPH MD OF HOUMA, LA, WAS DISCIPLINED BY LOUISIANA ON OCTOBER 13, 1994
DISCIPLINARY ACTION: 60-MONTH PROBATION; 60-MONTH RESTRICTION PLACED ON LICENSE
OFFENSE: SUBSTANCE ABUSE

NOTES: HABITUAL OR RECURRING ABUSE OF DRUGS, INCLUDING ALCOHOL. ORDER AMENDED 12/22/94. PROBATION SUBJECT TO CONTINUING TREATMENT AND PARTICIPATION IN PHYSICIANS HEALTH PROGRAM WITH PERIODIC REPORTS TO THE BOARD; MAINTENANCE OF COMPLETE ABSTINENCE FROM THE USE OF ALCOHOL AND OTHER MOOD-ALTERING SUBSTANCES; AND VARIOUS PRESCRIBED RESTRICTIONS ON PRACTICE AND PROFESSIONAL ACTIVITIES.

JUDICE, DONALD JOSEPH MD, LICENSE NUMBER 0C36089 OF HOUMA, TX, WAS DISCIPLINED BY CALIFORNIA ON NOVEMBER 16, 1995
DISCIPLINARY ACTION: LICENSE REVOCATION
OFFENSE: DISCIPLINARY ACTION BY ANOTHER STATE OR AGENCY

NOTES: ACTION IN LOUISIANA FOR HABITUAL OR RECURRING ABUSE OF ALCOHOL. DEFAULT ACTION.

JUNG, ANTHONY CHARLES MD, LICENSE NUMBER E8604 OF LANCASTER, TX, WAS DISCIPLINED BY TEXAS ON MAY 16, 1998
DISCIPLINARY ACTION: 60-MONTH PROBATION; REQUIRED TO TAKE ADDITIONAL MEDICAL EDUCATION
OFFENSE: OVERPRESCRIBING OR MISPRESCRIBING DRUGS

NOTES: ENGAGED IN THE NONTHERAPEUTIC PRESCRIBING OF CONTROLLED SUBSTANCES TO AT LEAST 5 PATIENTS; MOST OF THE PATIENTS WERE PRESCRIBED THESE DRUGS DESPITE INFORMATION WHICH HE KNEW OR SHOULD HAVE KNOWN THAT THEY WERE ABUSING THE DRUGS; HIS MEDICAL RECORDS FAIL TO SUPPORT ADEQUATELY HIS CARE AND TREATMENT OF THESE PATIENTS; HE REPORTS RECEIVING 20 HOURS OF CHRONIC PAIN MANAGEMENT THROUGH CONTINUING MEDICAL EDUCATION OVER THE LAST YEAR. SUSPENSION STAYED FOR PROBATION WITH FOLLOWING TERMS AND CONDITIONS: SHALL OBTAIN 50 HOURS PER YEAR OF CONTINUING MEDICAL EDUCATION, WITH 25 HOURS IN CHRONIC PAIN MANAGEMENT AND 1 COURSE IN CO-DEPENDENCY; SEPARATE FROM PATIENT RECORDS, SHALL MAINTAIN A LOGBOOK OF EVERY PRESCRIPTION WRITTEN BY HIM FOR DANGEROUS DRUGS WITH ADDICTIVE POTENTIAL WHICH SHALL BE MADE AVAILABLE FOR REVIEW; SHALL MAINTAIN ADEQUATE MEDICAL RECORDS WHICH SHALL BE AVAILABLE FOR REVIEW; SHALL SUCCESSFULLY COMPLETE ONCE COURSE IN ETHICS FOR 1 YEAR; SHALL TERMINATE RELATIONSHIP WITH SPECIFIED PATIENT; SHALL APPEAR BEFORE THE BOARD AT LEAST ONCE A YEAR; SHALL COOPERATE WITH THE BOARD IN VERIFYING COMPLIANCE; SHALL GIVE A COPY OF THIS ORDER TO ANY HEALTH CARE ENTITY WHERE HE HAS PRIVILEGES; TIME SPENT OUT OF TEXAS DOES NOT COUNT TOWARD PROBATION; SHALL INFORM THE BOARD OF CHANGE OF ADDRESS WITHIN 10 DAYS OR IF HE LEAVES THE STATE; SHALL NOT SEEK MODIFICATION FOR ONE YEAR.

JUST, ROBERT JOSEPH MD, LICENSE NUMBER K0850 OF ROUND ROCK, TX, WAS DISCIPLINED BY TEXAS ON AUGUST 28, 1999
DISCIPLINARY ACTION: FINE; RESTRICTION PLACED ON LICENSE
OFFENSE: CRIMINAL CONVICTION OR PLEA OF GUILTY, NOLO CONTENDERE, OR NO CONTEST TO A CRIME

NOTES: SUBMITTED FALSE STATEMENTS ON HIS APPLICATION FOR LICENSURE AND APPLICATION FOR LICENSURE RENEWAL; ON 12/11/94 HE WAS ARRESTED IN NEW JERSEY FOR DRIVING WHILE INTOXICATED; ON 5/8/96 HE ANSWERED NO TO QUESTION WHICH ASKED HAVE YOU EVER BEEN ARRESTED, FINED, CHARGED WITH A MISDEMEANOR, DWI, CONVICTED OF A CRIME, INDICTED, IMPRISONED, OR PLACED ON PROBATION?; ON 1/15/97 HE PLED GUILTY TO DRIVING WHILE INTOXICATED; ON 8/6/98 HE ANSWERED NO TO QUESTION ON TEXAS LICENSURE RENEWAL FORM WHICH ASKED SINCE YOUR LAST REGISTRATION OR SUBMISSION OF YOUR LICENSE APPLICATION, HAVE YOU BEEN ARRESTED, FINED (OVER $100), CHARGED WITH OR CONVICTED OF A CRIME, INDICTED, IMPRISONED, PLACED ON PROBATION, OR RECEIVED DEFERRED ADJUDICATION? PUBLIC REPRIMAND WITH FOLLOWING TERMS AND CONDITIONS FOR FIVE YEARS: SHALL APPEAR BEFORE THE BOARD AT LEAST TWICE A YEAR; SHALL PAY $10,000 FINE; SHALL OBTAIN AT LEAST 50 HOURS PER YEAR OF CONTINUING MEDICAL EDUCATION; SHALL OBTAIN 10 HOURS OF AN ETHICS COURSE OR PROGRAM PER YEAR; SHALL TAKE AND PASS WITH A SCORE OF 75 OR ABOVE, WITHIN 3 ATTEMPTS, THE MEDICAL JURISPRUDENCE EXAM; TIME SPENT OUT OF TEXAS DOES NOT COUNT TOWARD RESTRICTION; SHALL INFORM THE BOARD OF CHANGE OF ADDRESS WITHIN 10 DAYS OR IF HE LEAVES THE STATE; SHALL NOT SEEK MODIFICATION FOR ONE YEAR.

KAIN, THOMAS R MD, LICENSE NUMBER 00E3966, WAS DISCIPLINED BY TEXAS ON OCTOBER 5, 1991
DISCIPLINARY ACTION: EMERGENCY SUSPENSION
OFFENSE: LOSS OR RESTRICTION OF HOSPITAL PRIVILEGES

NOTES: HOSPITAL PRIVILEGES WERE SUSPENDED BY DEPARTMENT OF THE ARMY, UNITED STATES ARMY MEDICAL DEPARTMENT ACTIVITY, FORT HOOD, TEXAS, DUE TO INCOMPETENCY IN PERFORMING ANESTHETIC SERVICES.

KAN, DANIEL MD, LICENSE NUMBER 0041683 OF SAN ANTONIO, TX,

WAS DISCIPLINED BY FLORIDA ON OCTOBER 11, 1991
DISCIPLINARY ACTION: FINE
OFFENSE: PROFESSIONAL MISCONDUCT

NOTES: AIDING, ASSISTING, PROCURING, OR ADVISING AN UNLICENSED PERSON TO PRACTICE MEDICINE IN THAT HE ACTED AS A SUPERVISOR FOR AN UNLICENSED PHYSICIAN ASSISTANT; DELEGATING PROFESSIONAL RESPONSIBILITIES TO A PERSON HE KNEW OR HAD REASON TO KNOW WAS NOT QUALIFIED BY TRAINING, EXPERIENCE, OR LICENSURE TO PERFORM THEM, IN THAT AN UNLICENSED PERSON FUNCTIONED AS A PHYSICIAN ASSISTANT WHILE UNDER HIS SUPERVISION. $250 FINE, LETTER OF CONCERN.

KANTOR, JOHN R MD, LICENSE NUMBER 00C4667 OF ANDREWS, TX, WAS DISCIPLINED BY TEXAS ON AUGUST 18, 1995
DISCIPLINARY ACTION: 60-MONTH RESTRICTION PLACED ON LICENSE; 60-MONTH RESTRICTION PLACED ON CONTROLLED SUBSTANCE LICENSE
OFFENSE: OVERPRESCRIBING OR MISPRESCRIBING DRUGS

NOTES: DURING 1992 AND 1993, HE PRESCRIBED DIETHYLPROPION, A CONTROLLED SUBSTANCE, TO FAMILY MEMBERS WITHOUT AN APPROPRIATE EVALUATION, AN ADEQUATE DIAGNOSIS AND ADEQUATE DOCUMENTATION; DURING 1993, PRESCRIBED RITALIN, A CONTROLLED SUBSTANCE, TO FAMILY MEMBERS WITHOUT AN APPROPRIATE EVALUATION, AN ADEQUATE DIAGNOSIS AND ADEQUATE DOCUMENTATION. RESTRICTION FOR FIVE YEARS WITH TERMS: SHALL NOT TREAT OR OTHERWISE SERVE AS PHYSICIAN, PRESCRIBE, DISPENSE OR ADMINISTER DRUGS THAT MAY BE SUBJECT TO ABUSE TO HIMSELF OR TO ANY MEMBER OF HIS FAMILY; SHALL NOT TELEPHONE TO A PHARMACY A PRESCRIPTION OR REFILL FOR THESE DRUGS NOR PERMIT ANYONE HE IS SUPERVISING TO DO SO; SHALL MAINTAIN A FILE WITH COPIES OF EVERY PRESCRIPTION WRITTEN BY HIM FOR CONTROLLED SUBSTANCES OR DRUGS WITH ADDICTIVE POTENTIAL OR POTENTIAL FOR ABUSE AND SHALL MAINTAIN ADEQUATE MEDICAL RECORDS BOTH OF WHICH SHALL BE AVAILABLE FOR REVIEW; SHALL NOT PRACTICE EMERGENCY ROOM MEDICINE UNTIL HE OBTAINS ADVANCED TRAUMA LIFE SUPPORT (ATLS) AND ADVANCED CARDIAC LIFE SUPPORT (ACLS) CERTIFICATIONS; SHALL OBTAIN AT LEAST 50 HOURS PER YEAR OF CONTINUING MEDICAL EDUCATION; SHALL APPEAR BEFORE THE BOARD AT LEAST ONCE A YEAR OR AT BOARD REQUEST; SHALL COOPERATE WITH BOARD IN VERIFYING COMPLIANCE INCLUDING PROVIDING COPIES OF MEDICAL RELEASES AND PEER REVIEW RECORDS UPON REQUEST; SHALL GIVE A COPY OF THIS ORDER TO ANY HEALTH CARE ENTITY WHERE HE HAS PRIVILEGES; SHALL PROVIDE A COPY OF THIS ORDER TO ANYONE REQUESTING IT WITHIN 10 DAYS; TIME PERIOD OUT OF TEXAS DOES NOT COUNT TOWARD PROBATION; SHALL INFORM BOARD OF CHANGE OF ADDRESS WITHIN 10 DAYS OR IF HE LEAVES THE STATE. SHALL NOT SEEK MODIFICATION FOR ONE YEAR. ON 9/20/97 PETITION TO TERMINATE ORDER DENIED; ORDER MODIFIED DELETING FIFTY HOUR CONTINUING MEDICAL EDUCATION REQUIREMENT EACH YEAR. ON 8/22/98 ORDER TERMINATED.

KANTOR, JOHN R MD, DATE OF BIRTH NOVEMBER 12, 1924, LICENSE NUMBER 15719, WAS DISCIPLINED BY COLORADO ON MARCH 20, 1997
DISCIPLINARY ACTION: REPRIMAND

KASNER, MARTIN MD, LICENSE NUMBER 00F5251 OF FT LAUDERDALE, FL, WAS DISCIPLINED BY TEXAS ON AUGUST 24, 1991
DISCIPLINARY ACTION: SURRENDER OF LICENSE
OFFENSE: DISCIPLINARY ACTION BY ANOTHER STATE OR AGENCY

NOTES: ACTION TAKEN BY ANOTHER STATE BOARD FOR NONTHERAPEUTIC PRESCRIBING. SURRENDER IN LIEU OF FURTHER DISCIPLINARY ACTION.

KASNETZ, HERBERT ROY MD, DATE OF BIRTH JULY 22, 1935, LICENSE NUMBER 00D3908 OF 1420 N MACARTHUR BLVD, IRVING, TX, WAS DISCIPLINED BY TEXAS ON AUGUST 20, 1993
DISCIPLINARY ACTION: REPRIMAND
OFFENSE: SUBSTANDARD CARE, INCOMPETENCE OR NEGLIGENCE

NOTES: ADMINISTERED GAMMA GLOBULIN SHOTS TO A PATIENT WITH A TOTAL SERUM IGG LEVEL OF 1210 WITHOUT SUFFICIENT OBJECTIVE AND CLINICAL INDICATIONS REFLECTED IN THE PATIENT'S CHART. SHALL GIVE A COPY OF THIS ORDER TO ANY HEALTH CARE ENTITY WHERE HE HAS PRIVILEGES.

KASSAB, WAFIK M MD, LICENSE NUMBER 00E1213 OF GARLAND, TX, WAS DISCIPLINED BY TEXAS ON AUGUST 18, 1995
DISCIPLINARY ACTION: FINE; REPRIMAND
OFFENSE: NONCOMPLIANCE WITH A PROFESSIONAL RULE

NOTES: FAILED TO KEEP ADEQUATE MEDICAL RECORDS CONCERNING HIS CARE AND TREATMENT OF A PATIENT. SHALL PAY $1,000 FINE.

KASTNER, AARON MD, LICENSE NUMBER 00E7133 OF GARLAND, TX, WAS DISCIPLINED BY TEXAS ON APRIL 10, 1992
DISCIPLINARY ACTION: 48-MONTH PROBATION
OFFENSE: PROFESSIONAL MISCONDUCT

NOTES: UNPROFESSIONAL OR DISHONORABLE CONDUCT LIKELY TO DECEIVE, DEFRAUD OR INJURE THE PUBLIC; AND PROFESSIONAL FAILURE TO PRACTICE MEDICINE IN AN ACCEPTABLE MANNER CONSISTENT WITH PUBLIC HEALTH AND WELFARE. LICENSE REVOKED, REVOCATION STAYED; PROBATION UNDER TERMS AND CONDITIONS.

KASTNER, AARON MD, LICENSE NUMBER E7133, WAS DISCIPLINED BY TEXAS ON MARCH 1, 1997
DISCIPLINARY ACTION: SURRENDER OF LICENSE

NOTES: BY VIRTUE OF A PLEA AGREEMENT ENTERED INTO WITH THE U.S. DISTRICT COURT HE AGREED TO SURRENDER HIS TEXAS MEDICAL LICENSE AND NEVER TO PRACTICE MEDICINE AGAIN. THE BOARD HAS RECEIVED ALLEGATIONS INVOLVING ACTIONS ON HIS PART WHICH, IF PROVEN, COULD POSSIBLY CONSTITUTE VIOLATIONS OF THE MEDICAL PRACTICE ACT. HE DOES NOT ADMIT VIOLATIONS; VOLUNTARILY AND PERMANENTLY SURRENDERS HIS TEXAS LICENSE.

KASTNER, AARON MD, DATE OF BIRTH JULY 8, 1924 OF 16511 LOCH MAREE LANE, DALLAS, TX, WAS DISCIPLINED BY MEDICARE ON APRIL 27, 1997
DISCIPLINARY ACTION: 120-MONTH EXCLUSION FROM THE MEDICARE AND/OR MEDICAID PROGRAM
OFFENSE: CRIMINAL CONVICTION OR PLEA OF GUILTY, NOLO CONTENDERE, OR NO CONTEST TO A CRIME

NOTES: CONVICTED OF A CRIME RELATED TO THE DELIVERY OF HEALTH CARE OR FINANCIAL MISCONDUCT INVOLVING A GOVERNMENT-OPERATED PROGRAM.

KATERNDAHL, DAVID A MD, DATE OF BIRTH NOVEMBER 20, 1950, LICENSE NUMBER 00H2144 OF DEPT. FAMILY PRACTICE UTHSC,

SAN ANTONIO, TX, WAS DISCIPLINED BY TEXAS ON DECEMBER 4, 1991
DISCIPLINARY ACTION: 36-MONTH PROBATION; RESTRICTION PLACED ON CONTROLLED SUBSTANCE LICENSE
OFFENSE: OVERPRESCRIBING OR MISPRESCRIBING DRUGS

NOTES: PROVIDED CONTROLLED SUBSTANCES, IN A NONTHERAPEUTIC MANNER, TO A FAMILY MEMBER DURING 1988 AND 1989. ENTERED INTO IMPAIRED PHYSICIANS PROGRAM IN 9/89 AND HAS COMPLIED WITH REQUIREMENTS OF THAT CONTRACT. THREE YEAR SUSPENSION STAYED, PROBATION ISSUED WITH FOLLOWING CONDITIONS: SHALL APPEAR BEFORE BOARD TWICE A YEAR FOR COMPLIANCE REVIEW; SHALL WITHIN SIX MONTHS SUCCESSFULLY COMPLETE A MEDICAL PHARMACOLOGY COURSE; SHALL BE MONITORED BY A BOARD APPROVED PHYSICIAN WITH QUARTERLY REPORTS; SHALL REFRAIN FROM THE PRESCRIPTION OR ADMINISTRATION OF ANY DRUG FOR ANY PATIENT UNLESS THE DRUG IS MEDICALLY INDICATED AND PRESCRIBED IN THERAPEUTIC DOSES; SHALL REFRAIN FROM THE USE OF AND POSSESSION, ADMINISTERING, OR PRESCRIBING OF ANY CONTROLLED SUBSTANCES OR ANY OTHER DRUG OR MEDICATION REQUIRING A PRESCRIPTION, OR PRESCRIBING SAME TO FAMILY; REGISTRATIONS ARE LIMITED TO SCHEDULES III, III-N, IV, AND V IF DEA APPROVES; SHALL SUBMIT HIMSELF FOR APPROPRIATE EXAMINATIONS, INCLUDING DRUG OR ALCOHOL SCREENINGS; SHALL CONTINUE TREATMENT WITH QUARTERLY REPORTS TO THE BOARD; SHALL PROVIDE A COPY OF THE ORDER TO EMPLOYER; SHALL COOPERATE WITH BOARD IN VERIFYING COMPLIANCE; SHALL INFORM BOARD OF CHANGE OF ADDRESS WITHIN 10 DAYS OR IF HE LEAVES TEXAS; TIME SPENT OUT OF TEXAS DOES NOT COUNT TOWARD PROBATION; MAY NOT SEEK MODIFICATION OF ORDER FOR ONE YEAR. ON 1/29/93 MODIFICATION OF ORDER GRANTING HIM PERMISSION TO APPLY FOR ISSUANCE OF TEXAS DEPARTMENT OF PUBLIC SAFETY AND DRUG ENFORCEMENT ADMINISTRATION CONTROLLED SUBSTANCE REGISTRATION CERTIFICATES. ALL OTHER TERMS OF THIS ORDER REMAIN IN EFFECT. ON 1/14/94 PROBATION TERMINATED.

KATERNDAHL, DAVID ARTHUR MD, DATE OF BIRTH NOVEMBER 20, 1950, LICENSE NUMBER 0042398 OF SAN ANTONIO, TX, WAS DISCIPLINED BY OHIO ON JANUARY 13, 1993
DISCIPLINARY ACTION: 36-MONTH PROBATION
OFFENSE: DISCIPLINARY ACTION BY ANOTHER STATE OR AGENCY

NOTES: TEXAS SANCTION IMPOSED BECAUSE OF HIS PROVISION OF CONTROLLED SUBSTANCES IN A NON-THERAPEUTIC MANNER TO A FAMILY MEMBER. PROBATION CALCULATED FROM 12/4/91 AND TO RUN CONCURRENTLY WITH PROBATION IMPOSED BY TEXAS.

KATZ, STANLEY ALLEN MD, DATE OF BIRTH APRIL 30, 1960, LICENSE NUMBER 0014144 OF 13330 BLANCO RD. APT. 204, SAN ANTONIO, TX, WAS DISCIPLINED BY MISSISSIPPI ON SEPTEMBER 21, 1995
DISCIPLINARY ACTION: RESTRICTION PLACED ON LICENSE

NOTES: LICENSE RESTRICTIONS RUN FOR AN INDEFINITE TIME PERIOD.

KATZ, STANLEY ALLEN MD, DATE OF BIRTH APRIL 30, 1960, LICENSE NUMBER 0039629 OF SAN ANTONIO, TX, WAS DISCIPLINED BY NORTH CAROLINA ON MARCH 27, 1997
DISCIPLINARY ACTION: LICENSE SUSPENSION
OFFENSE: DISCIPLINARY ACTION BY ANOTHER STATE OR AGENCY

NOTES: ENTERED INTO A CONSENT ORDER WITH MISSISSIPPI AGREEING NOT TO PRACTICE OR RENEW HIS LICENSE UNTIL HE HAS SUBMITTED TO COMPREHENSIVE PSYCHIATRIC AND PSYCHOLOGICAL EVALUATIONS; HE DOES NOT DESIRE TO PRACTICE IN NORTH CAROLINA BUT WISHES TO ASSURE THE BOARD THAT IF HE EVER RETURNS, STEPS WILL BE TAKEN TO ENSURE HE CAN PRACTICE WITH REASONABLE SKILL AND SAFETY. HE SHALL RETURN HIS LICENSE CERTIFICATE TO THE BOARD WITHIN TEN DAYS.

KATZEN, KENNETH LEE DO, LICENSE NUMBER 00G6733 OF GRAND PRAIRIE, TX, WAS DISCIPLINED BY TEXAS ON MAY 15, 1996
DISCIPLINARY ACTION: 36-MONTH RESTRICTION PLACED ON LICENSE; REPRIMAND
OFFENSE: SEXUAL ABUSE OF OR SEXUAL MISCONDUCT WITH A PATIENT

NOTES: PRIOR TO 11/93, HE ENGAGED IN A SEXUAL RELATIONSHIP WITH AN ADULT FEMALE PATIENT WITHOUT PRIOR PROPER TERMINATION OF PHYSICIAN-PATIENT RELATIONSHIP. RESTRICTION OF LICENSE WITH TERMS: SHALL SUBMIT HIMSELF FOR EVALUATION AND TREATMENT BY A BOARD-APPROVED PSYCHIATRIST WHOM HE SHALL SEE AT LEAST ONCE A MONTH AND WHO SHALL SUBMIT REPORTS TO THE BOARD; SHALL OBTAIN 10 HOURS OF AN ETHICS COURSE OR PROGRAM PER YEAR; SHALL HAVE A CHAPERONE PRESENT ANY TIME HE PERFORMS A PHYSICAL EXAMINATION OF A FEMALE PATIENT AND SHALL NOTE THIS IN THE PATIENT'S CHART; SHALL APPEAR BEFORE BOARD AT LEAST ONCE A YEAR OR AT BOARD REQUEST; SHALL COOPERATE WITH THE BOARD IN VERIFYING COMPLIANCE INCLUDING PROVIDING COPIES OF PEER REVIEW RECORDS UPON REQUEST; SHALL GIVE A COPY OF THIS ORDER TO ANY HEALTH CARE ENTITY WHERE HE HAS PRIVILEGES; SHALL PROVIDE A COPY OF THIS ORDER TO ANYONE REQUESTING IT WITHIN 10 DAYS; TIME SPENT OUT OF TEXAS DOES NOT COUNT TOWARD RESTRICTION; SHALL INFORM BOARD OF CHANGE OF ADDRESS WITHIN 10 DAYS OR IF HE LEAVES THE STATE. SHALL NOT SEEK MODIFICATION FOR ONE YEAR. ON 5/10/97 PETITION TO MODIFY ORDER GRANTED, DELETING THE REQUIREMENT OF MONTHLY PSYCHIATRIC VISITS. ON 8/22/98 ORDER TERMINATED.

KAUFFMAN, ROBERT P MD, LICENSE NUMBER 00F4147 OF DALLAS, TX, WAS DISCIPLINED BY TEXAS ON APRIL 14, 1995
DISCIPLINARY ACTION: EMERGENCY SUSPENSION
OFFENSE: SUBSTANCE ABUSE

NOTES: HISTORY OF INTEMPERATE USE OF DRUGS BEGINNING IN APPROXIMATELY 1988 OR 1989 AND CONTINUING TO AS RECENTLY AS 3/95; CONSUMED VARIOUS CONTROLLED SUBSTANCES, INCLUDING LORCET, WITHOUT A LEGITIMATE MEDICAL REASON; IN 3/95, SUBMITTED URINE SAMPLES TO HOSPITALS WHERE HE HAD PRIVILEGES; URINE SAMPLES SHOWED THE PRESENCE OF HYDROCODONE OR ITS METABOLITES; HIS PRIVILEGES AT ONE OF THE HOSPITALS WERE SUSPENDED AS A RESULT OF THE URINE SCREEN. SUSPENSION EFFECTIVE 4/6/95.

KAUFFMAN, ROBERT P MD, LICENSE NUMBER 00F4147 OF DALLAS, TX, WAS DISCIPLINED BY TEXAS ON JUNE 28, 1995
DISCIPLINARY ACTION: LICENSE SUSPENSION
OFFENSE: SUBSTANCE ABUSE

NOTES: RECEIVED INPATIENT SUBSTANCE ABUSE TREATMENT FROM 5/27/94 TO 8/4/94; RECEIVED

OUTPATIENT SUBSTANCE ABUSE TREATMENT FROM 8/9/94 TO 11/5/94; IN APPROXIMATELY 1989, HE BEGAN DIVERTING DRUG SAMPLES FROM OFFICE STOCK FOR HIS OWN USE WITHOUT KEEPING COMPLETE AND ACCURATE RECORDS OF THE DISPOSAL OF THOSE SAMPLES; SIGNED A CONTINUING CARE CONTRACT WITH A HOSPITAL; UNDER THE CARE OF A PSYCHIATRIST FOR DEPRESSION AND DRUG ABUSE; IN 3/95 DRUG SCREEN HE SUBMITTED TO HOSPITAL SHOWED DETECTABLE AMOUNTS OF HYDROCODONE AND HIS HOSPITAL PRIVILEGES WERE SUSPENDED; ON 4/6/95 LICENSE TEMPORARILY SUSPENDED BY BOARD. SUSPENSION UNTIL HE APPEARS BEFORE BOARD WITH SUFFICIENT EVIDENCE TO SHOW THAT HE IS PHYSICALLY, MENTALLY AND OTHERWISE COMPETENT TO SAFELY PRACTICE MEDICINE INCLUDING AT A MINIMUM MEDICAL REPORTS AND RECORDS OF PSYCHOLOGICAL AND NEUROPSYCHIATRIC EVALUATIONS INCLUDING A 96 HOUR INPATIENT EVALUATION.

KAUFFMAN, ROBERT P MD, LICENSE NUMBER 00F4147 OF DALLAS, TX, WAS DISCIPLINED BY TEXAS ON JULY 7, 1995
DISCIPLINARY ACTION: 60-MONTH PROBATION; RESTRICTION PLACED ON CONTROLLED SUBSTANCE LICENSE
OFFENSE: SUBSTANCE ABUSE

NOTES: HE MET CONDITIONS REQUESTED BY PREVIOUS ORDER. SUSPENSION LIFTED. CONDITIONS OF PROBATION AS FOLLOWS: SHALL ABSTAIN FROM THE CONSUMPTION OF ALCOHOL/DRUGS IN ANY FORM UNLESS PRESCRIBED BY ANOTHER PHYSICIAN FOR A LEGITIMATE AND THERAPEUTIC PURPOSE; SHALL SUBMIT HIMSELF FOR APPROPRIATE EXAMS INCLUDING DRUG OR ALCOHOL SCREENS; SHALL SUBMIT HIMSELF FOR EVALUATION AND TREATMENT BY A BOARD-APPROVED PSYCHIATRIST AT LEAST ONCE A MONTH AND WHO SHALL SUBMIT REPORTS TO THE BOARD; SHALL CONTINUE TO PARTICIPATE IN AA'S PROGRAM NOT LESS THAN FIVE TIMES A WEEK WITH QUARTERLY REPORTS TO THE BOARD; SHALL PARTICIPATE IN THE ACTIVITIES OF AN IMPAIRED PHYSICIAN'S GROUP AND ATTEND WEEKLY MEETINGS WITH QUARTERLY REPORTS; SHALL COMPLY WITH THE TERMS OF CONTINUING CARE CONTRACT WITH QUARTERLY REPORTS; SHALL COMPLY WITH TERMS OF CONTRACT ENTERED INTO FOR HOSPITAL PRIVILEGES AND SHALL REPORT ANY DISCIPLINARY ACTION TO THE BOARD; SHALL NOT POSSESS ALCOHOL, CONTROLLED SUBSTANCES OR DRUGS WITH ADDICTIVE POTENTIAL AND SHALL SURRENDER ANY IN HIS POSSESSION; SHALL NOT TREAT OR OTHERWISE SERVE AS PHYSICIAN, PRESCRIBE, DISPENSE OR ADMINISTER DRUGS THAT MAY BE SUBJECT TO ABUSE TO HIMSELF OR TO ANY MEMBER OF HIS FAMILY; SHALL NOT TELEPHONE A PHARMACY WITH PRESCRIPTIONS FOR THESE DRUGS OR PERMIT ANYONE UNDER HIS SUPERVISION TO DO SO; MAY ORDER CONTROLLED SUBSTANCES FOR HIS HOSPITAL INPATIENTS AND MAY PRESCRIBE NO MORE THAN A 14 DAY SUPPLY OF SUCH DRUGS TO POST-SURGICAL PATIENTS AND GYNECOLOGICAL PATIENTS WHO HAVE UNDERGONE INVASIVE OFFICE PROCEDURES; SHALL KEEP A LOG OF ALL OF THESE WHICH SHALL BE AVAILABLE FOR REVIEW; HIS PRACTICE SHALL BE MONITORED BY A BOARD-APPROVED PHYSICIAN WHO SHALL SUBMIT QUARTERLY REPORTS TO THE BOARD; SHALL MAINTAIN A FILE WITH COPIES OF EVERY PRESCRIPTION WRITTEN FOR CONTROLLED SUBSTANCES OR DRUGS WITH ADDICTIVE POTENTIAL AND SHALL MAINTAIN ADEQUATE MEDICAL RECORDS BOTH OF WHICH SHALL BE AVAILABLE FOR REVIEW; SHALL NOT SIGN OR INDICATE IN ANY MANNER IN PATIENT RECORDS THAT HE HAS SEEN PATIENTS UNLESS HE ACTUALLY HAS SEEN AND EXAMINED THE PATIENT UNLESS IT IS CLEARLY NOTED THAT HE DID NOT PERSONALLY EXAMINE THE PATIENT; SHALL OBTAIN AT LEAST 50 HOURS PER YEAR OF CONTINUING MEDICAL EDUCATION; SHALL APPEAR BEFORE THE BOARD AT LEAST TWO TIMES PER YEAR OR AT BOARD REQUEST; SHALL COOPERATE WITH THE BOARD IN VERIFYING COMPLIANCE INCLUDING PROVIDING COPIES OF MEDICAL RELEASES AND PEER REVIEW RECORDS UPON REQUEST; SHALL GIVE A COPY OF THIS ORDER TO ANY HEALTH CARE ENTITY WHERE HE HAS PRIVILEGES; SHALL PROVIDE A COPY OF THIS ORDER TO ANYONE REQUESTING IT WITHIN 10 DAYS; TIME PERIOD OUT OF TEXAS DOES NOT COUNT TOWARD PROBATION/RESTRICTION; SHALL INFORM THE BOARD OF CHANGE OF ADDRESS WITHIN 10 DAYS OF IF HE LEAVES THE STATE; SHALL NOT SEEK MODIFICATION FOR ONE YEAR.

KAUFFMAN, ROBERT P MD, LICENSE NUMBER F4147 OF DALLAS, TX, WAS DISCIPLINED BY TEXAS ON AUGUST 9, 1997
DISCIPLINARY ACTION: LICENSE SUSPENSION
OFFENSE: FAILURE TO COMPLY WITH PREVIOUS BOARD ORDER

NOTES: ON 9/19/96 HE INGESTED HYDROCODONE, A SCHEDULE III CONTROLLED SUBSTANCE, IN VIOLATION OF HIS 7/7/95 ORDER. IT WAS A NON-THERAPEUTIC USE IN THAT IT WAS NOT PRESCRIBED BY A TREATING PHYSICIAN. HE RECEIVED RESIDENTIAL IN-PATIENT TREATMENT FROM 12/7/96 TO 3/27/97. ON 1/27/97 HE RESIGNED OR SURRENDERED HIS MEDICAL PRIVILEGES AT A SPECIFIED HOSPITAL. SUSPENSION UNTIL HE REQUESTS TO HAVE HIS SUSPENSION STAYED OR APPEARS BEFORE THE BOARD WITH EVIDENCE THAT HE IS PHYSICALLY, MENTALLY AND OTHERWISE COMPETENT TO SAFELY PRACTICE MEDICINE INCLUDING AT A MINIMUM: A FINAL DISCHARGE DIAGNOSIS FROM A SPECIFIED CENTER ADDRESSING HIS CURRENT MENTAL AND PHYSICAL STATUS AND CLEARLY INDICATING HIS COMPETENCY, AND COMPLETE MEDICAL RECORDS AND REPORTS OF PSYCHOLOGICAL AND NEUROPSYCHIATRIC EVALUATIONS CONDUCTED BY AN APPROVED, BOARD CERTIFIED PSYCHIATRIST. UPON ADEQUATE SHOWING, HIS LICENSE WILL BE REINSTATED TO PROBATION UNDER SPECIFIED TERMS. ON 9/20/97 REQUEST FOR TERMINATION DENIED.

KAUFFMAN, ROBERT P MD, LICENSE NUMBER F4147 OF DALLAS, TX, WAS DISCIPLINED BY TEXAS ON NOVEMBER 22, 1997
DISCIPLINARY ACTION: SURRENDER OF CONTROLLED SUBSTANCE LICENSE; 120-MONTH PROBATION
OFFENSE: FAILURE TO COMPLY WITH PREVIOUS BOARD ORDER

NOTES: ON 9/19/96 VIOLATED 7/7/95 ORDER BY INGESTING HYDROCODONE, HIS PRIMARY DRUG OF ABUSE; RECEIVED INPATIENT SUBSTANCE ABUSE TREATMENT FROM 12/7/96 UNTIL 3/27/97; ON OR ABOUT 1/27/97 HE RESIGNED OR SURRENDERED HIS MEDICAL PRIVILEGES AT COLUMBIA HOSPITAL. SUSPENSION STAYED WITH PROBATION ON FOLLOWING TERMS AND CONDITIONS: SHALL LIMIT HIS PRACTICE TO ACADEMIC MEDICINE; SHALL ABSTAIN FROM THE CONSUMPTION OF ALCOHOL/DRUGS IN ANY FORM UNLESS PRESCRIBED BY ANOTHER PHYSICIAN FOR A LEGITIMATE AND THERAPEUTIC PURPOSE; SHALL SUBMIT HIMSELF FOR APPROPRIATE EXAMS INCLUDING DRUG OR ALCOHOL SCREENS; SHALL NOMINATE THREE CERTIFIED PSYCHIATRISTS FOR BOARD SELECTION OF A THERAPIST AND SHALL EXPEDITIOUSLY SUBMIT

HIMSELF TO EVALUATION AND TREATMENT BY THE APPROVED PRACTITIONER; SHALL PARTICIPATE IN THE ACTIVITIES OF A PHYSICIAN HEALTH AND REHABILITATION COMMITTEE AND ATTEND WEEKLY MEETINGS WITH QUARTERLY REPORTS; SHALL PARTICIPATE IN AA'S PROGRAM NOT LESS THAN FIVE TIMES A WEEK; SHALL REPORT ON HIS ATTENDANCE; SHALL COMPLY WITH TERMS OF CONTINUING CARE CONTRACT WITH QUARTERLY REPORTS; SHALL NOT TREAT OR OTHERWISE SERVE AS PHYSICIAN, PRESCRIBE, DISPENSE OR ADMINISTER DRUGS THAT MAY BE SUBJECT TO ABUSE TO HIMSELF OR TO ANY MEMBER OF HIS FAMILY; SHALL NOT TELEPHONE, NOR PERMIT ANY INDIVIDUAL UNDER HIS SUPERVISION TELEPHONE, TO A PHARMACY A PRESCRIPTION OR REFILL FOR CONTROLLED SUBSTANCES OR POTENTIALLY ADDICTIVE DRUGS; SHALL IMMEDIATELY SURRENDER HIS DEA AND TEXAS DEPARTMENT OF PUBLIC SAFETY CONTROLLED SUBSTANCE CERTIFICATES; SHALL IMMEDIATELY SURRENDER ALL AND ANY UNUSED TRIPLICATE PRESCRIPTION FORMS; SEPARATE FROM PATIENT RECORDS, SHALL MAINTAIN A FILE OF EVERY PRESCRIPTION WRITTEN BY HIM FOR DANGEROUS DRUGS WITH ADDICTIVE POTENTIAL WHICH SHALL BE MADE AVAILABLE FOR REVIEW; HIS MEDICAL PRACTICE SHALL BE MONITORED BY A BOARD APPROVED TEXAS PHYSICIAN WHO SHALL PROVIDE QUARTERLY REPORTS TO THE BOARD; SHALL MAINTAIN ADEQUATE MEDICAL RECORDS WHICH SHALL BE AVAILABLE FOR REVIEW; SHALL OBTAIN 50 HOURS PER YEAR OF CONTINUING MEDICAL EDUCATION; SHALL APPEAR BEFORE THE BOARD TWICE A YEAR; SHALL COOPERATE WITH THE BOARD IN VERIFYING COMPLIANCE INCLUDING PROVIDING COPIES OF MEDICAL RELEASES UPON REQUEST; SHALL GIVE A COPY OF THIS ORDER TO ANY HEALTH CARE ENTITY WHERE HE HAS PRIVILEGES; SHALL PROVIDE A COPY OF THIS ORDER TO ANYONE REQUESTING IT WITHIN 10 DAYS; TIME SPENT OUT OF TEXAS DOES NOT COUNT TOWARD PROBATION; SHALL INFORM THE BOARD OF CHANGE OF ADDRESS WITHIN 10 DAYS OR IF HE LEAVES THE STATE; SHALL NOT SEEK MODIFICATION FOR ONE YEAR. ON 10/24/98 REQUEST TO MODIFY THIS ORDER DENIED. ON 12/11/99 THE FOLLOWING MODIFICATIONS WERE MADE TO THE ORDER: ACADEMIC MEDICINE MORE FULLY DEFINED BY THE BOARD; PSYCHIATRIC CARE REQUIREMENT REDUCED FROM MONTHLY TO QUARTERLY; AA PARTICIPATION REDUCED FROM FIVE TIMES A WEEK TO THREE TIMES A WEEK.

KAUFFMANN, ADOLPH FREDERICK III MD, LICENSE NUMBER 00B6910 OF FORT WORTH, TX, WAS DISCIPLINED BY TEXAS ON FEBRUARY 22, 1991
DISCIPLINARY ACTION: 60-MONTH PROBATION; RESTRICTION PLACED ON LICENSE

NOTES: MUST MAINTAIN ADEQUATE MEDICAL RECORDS ON ALL PATIENTS; OBTAIN SECOND OPINION FROM A BOARD CERTIFIED GENERAL SURGEON FOR ANY POSSIBLE BREAST SURGERY OR BREAST BIOPSY; APPEAR FOR ANNUAL REPORT TO BOARD. ON 6/22/94 REQUEST FOR TERMINATION OF THIS ORDER DENIED.

KAUFFMANN, ROBERT PORTER MD OF 7777 FOREST LANE #C-236, DALLAS, TX, WAS DISCIPLINED BY DEA ON AUGUST 16, 1995
DISCIPLINARY ACTION: RESTRICTION PLACED ON CONTROLLED SUBSTANCE LICENSE

KAUFMAN, IRA S MD, LICENSE NUMBER 00E9731 OF HOUSTON, TX, WAS DISCIPLINED BY TEXAS ON AUGUST 19, 1994
DISCIPLINARY ACTION: SURRENDER OF CONTROLLED SUBSTANCE LICENSE; 120-MONTH PROBATION
OFFENSE: CRIMINAL CONVICTION OR PLEA OF GUILTY, NOLO CONTENDERE, OR NO CONTEST TO A CRIME

NOTES: ON 6/30/93 HE PLED NOLO CONTENDERE TO TWO SECOND DEGREE FELONY CHARGES OF OBTAINING DRUGS BY FRAUD; THE CASES INVOLVED TWO PRESCRIPTIONS HE ISSUED ONE ON 2/7/92 AND ONE ON 9/24/92 FOR MEPERIDINE IN THE NAMES OF TWO PEOPLE WHO WERE NOT HIS PATIENTS; THERE WAS NO MEDICAL PURPOSE FOR PRESCRIBING THE DRUG; HE PRESENTED THESE PRESCRIPTIONS TO PHARMACISTS HIMSELF; ALSO PLED NOLO CONTENDERE TO A MISDEMEANOR OFFENSE OF CARRYING A WEAPON; BEGINNING ON 2/7/92 CONSUMED DRUGS INCLUDING MEPERIDINE FOR NO VALID MEDICAL PRACTICE SOME OF WHICH HE OBTAINED PRESCRIPTIONS FOR IN THE MANNER PREVIOUSLY DESCRIBED; WAS IMPAIRED BY THE USE OF DRUGS AND ALCOHOL PRIOR TO RECEIVING INPATIENT TREATMENT FROM 1/18/93 THROUGH 2/12/93. PROBATION REQUIRES HIM TO RECEIVE PSYCHIATRIC COUNSELING. SUSPENSION STAYED. CONDITIONS OF PROBATION: SHALL ABSTAIN FROM THE CONSUMPTION OF ALCOHOL/CHEMICAL SUBSTANCES IN ANY FORM UNLESS PRESCRIBED BY ANOTHER PHYSICIAN FOR A LEGITIMATE AND THERAPEUTIC PURPOSE; SHALL SUBMIT HIMSELF FOR APPROPRIATE EXAMS INCLUDING DRUG OR ALCOHOL SCREENS; SHALL PARTICIPATE IN ACTIVITIES OF A PHYSICIAN HEALTH AND REHABILITATION COMMITTEE AND ATTEND WEEKLY MEETINGS WITH QUARTERLY REPORTS; SHALL PARTICIPATE IN AA'S PROGRAM NOT LESS THAN THREE TIMES A WEEK WITH QUARTERLY REPORTS TO THE BOARD; SHALL SURRENDER DEA AND TEXAS CONTROLLED SUBSTANCES CERTIFICATES, UNUSED TRIPLICATE PRESCRIPTION FORMS AND ALL CONTROLLED SUBSTANCES IN HIS POSSESSION INCLUDING SAMPLES; SHALL NOT ATTEMPT TO REREGISTER WITHOUT PERMISSION; SHALL NOT TELEPHONE A PRESCRIPTION TO ANY PHARMACY; SHALL SUBMIT HIMSELF TO A BOARD-APPROVED PSYCHIATRIST FOR EXAMINATION AND TREATMENT AND SEE THIS PSYCHIATRIST AT LEAST ONCE A MONTH; SHALL ATTEND AT LEAST 50 HOURS PER YEAR OF CONTINUING MEDICAL EDUCATION; WITHIN ONE YEAR SHALL PASS THE MEDICAL JURISPRUDENCE EXAM; SHALL GIVE A COPY OF THIS ORDER TO ANY HEALTH CARE ENTITY WHERE HE HAS PRIVILEGES; SHALL COOPERATE WITH THE BOARD IN VERIFYING COMPLIANCE; SHALL INFORM BOARD OF CHANGE OF ADDRESS WITHIN 10 DAYS OR IF HE LEAVES THE STATE; TIME SPENT OUT OF TEXAS DOES NOT COUNT TOWARD PROBATION. SHALL NOT SEEK MODIFICATION FOR ONE YEAR.

KAUFMAN, IRA S MD, LICENSE NUMBER 0108953 OF 5757 WESTHEIMER, HOUSTON, TX, WAS DISCIPLINED BY NEW YORK ON NOVEMBER 20, 1995
DISCIPLINARY ACTION: 120-MONTH PROBATION
OFFENSE: DISCIPLINARY ACTION BY ANOTHER STATE OR AGENCY

NOTES: ACTION IN TEXAS FOR FRAUDULENTLY PRESCRIBING CONTROLLED SUBSTANCES AND PRACTICING MEDICINE WHILE IMPAIRED BY DRUGS AND ALCOHOL. TWO YEAR SUSPENSION, STAYED. PROBATION UPON COMMENCEMENT OF PRACTICE IN NEW YORK.

KAY, BILLY F MD, DATE OF BIRTH FEBRUARY 12, 1934, LICENSE NUMBER 00E9260 OF 6960 BELLAIRE BLVD APT 2214, HOUSTON, TX, WAS DISCIPLINED BY TEXAS ON APRIL 30, 1993
DISCIPLINARY ACTION: LICENSE SUSPENSION

OFFENSE: PHYSICAL OR MENTAL ILLNESS INHIBITING THE ABILITY TO PRACTICE WITH SKILL AND SAFETY

NOTES: UNABLE TO PRACTICE WITH REASONABLE SKILL AND SAFETY DUE TO INSUFFICIENT INTELLECTUAL FUNCTIONING. SUSPENSION A MINIMUM OF 1 YEAR; BEFORE MAKING AN APPLICATION FOR REINSTATEMENT HE SHALL SUBMIT HIMSELF FOR AN INDEPENDENT MENTAL AND PHYSICAL EXAM; SHALL PROVIDE PROOF OF A DOCUMENTED AFTERCARE PROGRAM; SHALL INFORM THE BOARD OF CHANGE OF ADDRESS WITHIN 10 DAYS OR IF HE LEAVES THE STATE; TIME SPENT OUT OF TEXAS DOES NOT COUNT TOWARD SUSPENSION.

KAY, BILLY F MD, DATE OF BIRTH FEBRUARY 12, 1934, LICENSE NUMBER 0013277 OF 6960 BELLAIRE BLVD, SUITE 2214, HOUSTON, TX, WAS DISCIPLINED BY KANSAS ON JUNE 20, 1994
DISCIPLINARY ACTION: DENIAL OF LICENSE REINSTATEMENT
OFFENSE: DISCIPLINARY ACTION BY ANOTHER STATE OR AGENCY

NOTES: ON 04/09/92, TEXAS BOARD TEMPORARILY SUSPENDED HIS TEXAS MEDICAL LICENSE DUE TO LONG-TERM ALCOHOL ABUSE AND MENTAL ILLNESS. ON 04/30/93 LICENSE WAS INDEFINITELY SUSPENDED BY TEXAS. HE HAS THE INABILITY TO PRACTICE MEDICINE WITH REASONABLE SKILL AND SAFETY TO PATIENTS BY REASON OF BIPOLAR DISORDER, ALCOHOL DEPENDENCY AND DEMENTIA ASSOCIATED WITH ALCOHOLISM. HE IS UNWILLING TO ENTER INTO A MONITORING CONTRACT WITH THE KANSAS MEDICAL SOCIETY WHICH WOULD INCLUDE ATTENDANCE OF AA MEETINGS AND RANDOM URINE SCREENING. APPLICATION FOR STATUS CHANGE FROM INACTIVE TO ACTIVE IS THEREFORE DENIED.

KAZA, SUDHEER MD, LICENSE NUMBER H9656 OF BEAUMONT, TX, WAS DISCIPLINED BY TEXAS ON AUGUST 22, 1998
DISCIPLINARY ACTION: FINE; REPRIMAND
OFFENSE: PROFESSIONAL MISCONDUCT

NOTES: IN A PATIENT HE STARTED SEEING IN 4/95 HE FAILED TO MAKE ADEQUATE MEDICAL ENTRIES INTO THEIR RECORD AND FAILED TO MAINTAIN PROPER PHYSICIAN-PATIENT BOUNDARIES BY MAKING A LOAN TO THE PATIENT INSTEAD OF APPROPRIATELY ADDRESSING PATIENTS SUICIDAL MENTAL STATE; FAILED TO TERMINATE PHYSICIAN-PATIENT RELATIONSHIP; IN A PATIENT HE SAW FROM 1/93 THROUGH 8/96, HE FAILED TO DOCUMENT IN THE MEDICAL RECORD, ALL THE DRUGS WHICH HE PRESCRIBED, AND AFTER ENTERING INTO A BUSINESS RELATIONSHIP WITH HER, FAILED TO TERMINATE THE PHYSICIAN-PATIENT RELATIONSHIP, AND FAILED TO REFER HER TO ANOTHER PHYSICIAN; SEPARATE AND APART FROM HIS TREATMENT OF THE ABOVE PATIENTS, HE WROTE PRESCRIPTIONS WITHOUT PROPER DOCUMENTATION. LICENSE LIMITED FOR THREE YEARS AS FOLLOWS: SEPARATE FROM PATIENT RECORDS, SHALL MAINTAIN A LOGBOOK OF EVERY PRESCRIPTION WRITTEN BY HIM FOR DANGEROUS DRUGS WITH ADDICTIVE POTENTIAL WHICH SHALL BE MADE AVAILABLE FOR REVIEW; SHALL MAINTAIN ADEQUATE MEDICAL RECORDS WHICH SHALL BE AVAILABLE FOR REVIEW; SHALL OBTAIN 50 HOURS PER YEAR OF CONTINUING MEDICAL EDUCATION, WITH A COURSE ADDRESSING PHYSICIAN-PATIENT BOUNDARIES AND A COURSE ADDRESSING PSYCHIATRIC TRANSFERENCE ISSUES; SHALL OBTAIN 10 HOURS OF AN ETHICS COURSE; SHALL PAY $5,000 FINE; SHALL COOPERATE WITH THE BOARD IN VERIFYING COMPLIANCE INCLUDING PROVIDING COPIES OF PEER REVIEW RECORDS UPON REQUEST; SHALL GIVE A COPY OF THIS ORDER TO ANY HEALTH CARE ENTITY WHERE HE HAS PRIVILEGES; SHALL PROVIDE A COPY OF THIS ORDER TO ANYONE REQUESTING IT WITHIN 10 DAYS; SHALL APPEAR BEFORE THE BOARD UPON REQUEST; TIME SPENT OUT OF TEXAS DOES NOT COUNT TOWARD RESTRICTION; SHALL INFORM THE BOARD OF CHANGE OF ADDRESS WITHIN 10 DAYS OR IF HE LEAVES THE STATE; SHALL NOT SEEK MODIFICATION FOR ONE YEAR. ON 10/15/99 THE ORDER WAS MODIFIED TO REDUCE HIS BOARD APPEARANCES TO ONCE A YEAR; HIS REQUEST TO TERMINATE THE ORDER WAS DENIED.

KAZA, SUDHEER MD, LICENSE NUMBER 28933 OF BEAUMONT, TX, WAS DISCIPLINED BY KENTUCKY ON DECEMBER 18, 1998
DISCIPLINARY ACTION: 36-MONTH RESTRICTION PLACED ON LICENSE; REPRIMAND

NOTES: ADDITIONAL TERMS AND CONDITIONS AS SPECIFIED IN ORDER.

KAZA, SUDHEER MD, DATE OF BIRTH SEPTEMBER 24, 1950, LICENSE NUMBER 1047113 OF 6430 WINDSOR PARKWAY, BEAUMONT, TX, WAS DISCIPLINED BY MICHIGAN ON MAY 5, 1999
DISCIPLINARY ACTION: LICENSE SUSPENSION
OFFENSE: DISCIPLINARY ACTION BY ANOTHER STATE OR AGENCY

NOTES: LICENSE SUSPENDED FOR A MINIMUM OF SIX MONTHS AND ONE DAY.

KEATTS, JAMES G MD OF 12970 EAST FREEWAY, HOUSTON, TX, WAS DISCIPLINED BY DEA ON MARCH 14, 1995
DISCIPLINARY ACTION: SURRENDER OF CONTROLLED SUBSTANCE LICENSE

NOTES: IN LIEU OF ORDER TO SHOW CAUSE.

KEATTS, JAMES G MD, DATE OF BIRTH AUGUST 1, 1937 OF PO BOX 16300, EL PASO, TX, WAS DISCIPLINED BY MEDICARE ON FEBRUARY 12, 1996
DISCIPLINARY ACTION: 84-MONTH EXCLUSION FROM THE MEDICARE AND/OR MEDICAID PROGRAM
OFFENSE: CRIMINAL CONVICTION OR PLEA OF GUILTY, NOLO CONTENDERE, OR NO CONTEST TO A CRIME

NOTES: CONVICTED OF A CRIME INVOLVING THE MEDICARE, MEDICAID, MATERNAL AND CHILD HEALTH SERVICES BLOCK GRANT OR BLOCK GRANTS TO STATES FOR SOCIAL SERVICES PROGRAMS.

KEATTS, JAMES G MD, DATE OF BIRTH AUGUST 1, 1937, LICENSE NUMBER 00D6285, WAS DISCIPLINED BY TEXAS ON AUGUST 17, 1996
DISCIPLINARY ACTION: LICENSE SUSPENSION
OFFENSE: CRIMINAL CONVICTION OR PLEA OF GUILTY, NOLO CONTENDERE, OR NO CONTEST TO A CRIME

NOTES: IN 1995 SENTENCED TO 18 MONTHS INCARCERATION AFTER PLEADING GUILTY TO THREE FELONY COUNTS FOR ENGAGING IN A SCHEME TO DEFRAUD VARIOUS HEALTH INSURERS BY MAKING FALSE STATEMENTS REGARDING THE MEDICAL SERVICES PROVIDED; NOW RESIDES IN A HALFWAY HOUSE UNDER CUSTODY UNTIL 9/9/96. BOARD ALSO INVESTIGATED A STANDARD OF CARE CASE IN AN ADULT FEMALE PATIENT WHO SUSTAINED BLINDNESS TO HER RIGHT EYE DURING A LASER PROCEDURE; HE MADE A MAJOR MISTAKE IN THAT WHEN PATIENT MOVED HER EYE, WAS NOT ABLE TO PREVENT A LASER APPLICATION WITHIN THE FOUCA; HE MAINTAINED IT WAS AN ACCIDENT; INDEPENDENT CONSULTANT RECOMMENDED HE NOT PERFORM THESE PROCEDURES IN THE FUTURE. SUSPENSION UNTIL HE

APPEARS BEFORE THE BOARD AND PROVIDES SUFFICIENT EVIDENCE INDICATING THAT HE IS PHYSICALLY, MENTALLY, AND OTHERWISE COMPETENT TO SAFELY PRACTICE MEDICINE INCLUDING THE FOLLOWING: CERTIFIED COPY OF A DOCUMENT FROM THE U.S. BUREAU OF PRISONS THAT HE HAS BEEN RELEASED FROM ITS INCARCERATED CUSTODY AND IN FULL COMPLIANCE WITH HIS TERMS OF CRIMINAL PROBATION; COPIES OF MEDICAL RECORDS AND REPORTS OF NEUROLOGICAL AND NEUROPSYCHOLOGICAL EVALUATIONS CONDUCTED BY A BOARD APPROVED CERTIFIED PHYSICIAN.

KELLER, WAYNE F MD OF 909 FROSTWOOD STE 362, HOUSTON, TX, WAS DISCIPLINED BY DEA ON DECEMBER 28, 1992
DISCIPLINARY ACTION: RESTRICTION PLACED ON CONTROLLED SUBSTANCE LICENSE
OFFENSE: OVERPRESCRIBING OR MISPRESCRIBING DRUGS

NOTES: AGREED TO THE RESTRICTIONS DUE TO ALLEGATIONS THAT HE WAS PRESCRIBING EXCESSIVE AMOUNTS OF SCHEDULE II CONTROLLED SUBSTANCES TO PATIENTS. REGISTRATION MODIFIED ON 03/15/89. SHALL NOT PRESCRIBE, ADMINISTER, POSSESS OR DISPENSE ANY DRUG IN SCHEDULES II, IIN, III OR IIIN CONTROLLED SUBSTANCES, WITH THE EXCEPTION THAT HE MAY ORDER SUCH MEDICATIONS FOR PATIENTS WHO ARE IN THE HOSPITAL.

KELLOGG, EUGENE L MD, LICENSE NUMBER 00E9737 OF AIEA, HI, WAS DISCIPLINED BY TEXAS ON JUNE 28, 1995
DISCIPLINARY ACTION: REQUIRED TO TAKE ADDITIONAL MEDICAL EDUCATION
OFFENSE: DISCIPLINARY ACTION BY ANOTHER STATE OR AGENCY

NOTES: ON 8/5/94, HIS PRIVILEGES IN ANATOMIC PATHOLOGY AT AN ARMY MEDICAL CENTER IN HAWAII WERE REVOKED BASED ON A ROUTINE QUALITY ASSURANCE REVIEW WHICH PROMPTED AN INTENSIVE REVIEW OF HIS PERFORMANCE IN SURGICAL PATHOLOGY AND CYTOPATHOLOGY. SHALL NOT PRACTICE MEDICINE IN TEXAS UNTIL HE APPEARS BEFORE BOARD WITH SUFFICIENT EVIDENCE THAT HE IS PHYSICALLY, MENTALLY AND OTHERWISE COMPETENT TO SAFELY PRACTICE MEDICINE INCLUDING AT A MINIMUM AT LEAST 50 HOURS PER YEAR OF CONTINUING MEDICAL EDUCATION; COOPERATION WITH THE BOARD IN VERIFYING COMPLIANCE; PROVIDING A COPY OF THIS ORDER TO ANY HEALTH CARE ENTITY WHERE HE HAS PRIVILEGES; PROVIDING A COPY OF THIS ORDER TO ANYONE REQUESTING IT WITHIN 10 DAYS; INFORMING THE BOARD OF CHANGE OF ADDRESS WITHIN 10 DAYS. SHALL NOT SEEK MODIFICATION FOR ONE YEAR.

KELLUM, DANIEL H SR DO, LICENSE NUMBER E2252, WAS DISCIPLINED BY TEXAS ON FEBRUARY 28, 1997
DISCIPLINARY ACTION: REPRIMAND
OFFENSE: SEXUAL ABUSE OF OR SEXUAL MISCONDUCT WITH A PATIENT

NOTES: ALLEGATIONS OF INAPPROPRIATE PHYSICAL EXAMINATIONS ON ONE OR MORE ADULT FEMALE PATIENTS WITH THE DOOR CLOSED AND NO CHAPERONE PRESENT; THE EXAMS WERE NOT CLINICALLY INAPPROPRIATE, BUT HE DISPLAYED BAD JUDGMENT BY EXAMINING PATIENTS WHO HAD PARTIALLY DISROBED WITHOUT A CHAPERONE.

KELLY, MICHAEL V II MD, LICENSE NUMBER D8302 OF HOUSTON, TX, WAS DISCIPLINED BY TEXAS ON AUGUST 22, 1998
DISCIPLINARY ACTION: FINE
OFFENSE: PROFESSIONAL MISCONDUCT

NOTES: IN 1997 FAILED TO PROPERLY TERMINATE THE PHYSICIAN-PATIENT RELATIONSHIP PRIOR TO ENGAGING IN A PERSONAL RELATIONSHIP WITH A PATIENT. $2,500 FINE.

KELLY, PATRICK M DO, LICENSE NUMBER 00D6653 OF CEDAR PARK, TX, WAS DISCIPLINED BY TEXAS ON SEPTEMBER 1, 1992
DISCIPLINARY ACTION: SURRENDER OF LICENSE

NOTES: PERMANENTLY SURRENDERED.

KENNADY, DONALD SCOTT MD, LICENSE NUMBER 00C4389 OF NEW BRAUNFELS, TX, WAS DISCIPLINED BY TEXAS ON JANUARY 6, 1995
DISCIPLINARY ACTION: 60-MONTH RESTRICTION PLACED ON LICENSE; REQUIRED TO TAKE ADDITIONAL MEDICAL EDUCATION
OFFENSE: SUBSTANDARD CARE, INCOMPETENCE OR NEGLIGENCE

NOTES: FROM 1987 THROUGH 1992 HE FAILED TO CONDUCT ADEQUATE EXAMS OF ONE PATIENT WHILE PRESCRIBING THYROID MEDICATION AND ESTINYL; PATIENT HAD BEEN SUBSEQUENTLY DIAGNOSED BY ANOTHER PHYSICIAN AS HAVING A TONSILLAR TUMOR; AGREED TO THIS ORDER IN LIEU OF FURTHER INVESTIGATION. CONDITIONS OF FIVE YEAR RESTRICTION: PRACTICE SHALL BE MONITORED BY A BOARD-APPROVED PHYSICIAN WITH QUARTERLY REPORTS; SHALL MAINTAIN ADEQUATE MEDICAL RECORDS ON ALL PATIENT OFFICE VISITS WHICH SHALL BE AVAILABLE FOR INSPECTION; SHALL OBTAIN AT LEAST 50 HOURS PER YEAR OF CONTINUING MEDICAL EDUCATION INCLUDING IN THE FIRST YEAR 15 HOURS IN DIAGNOSIS AND MANAGEMENT OF DISORDERS IN THE HEAD AND NECK AND FIVE HOURS IN RISK MANAGEMENT; WITHIN ONE YEAR SHALL PASS THE SPEX EXAM; SHALL APPEAR BEFORE THE BOARD ONCE A YEAR OR UPON REQUEST; SHALL COOPERATE WITH THE BOARD IN VERIFYING COMPLIANCE; SHALL EXECUTE ANY RELEASES NECESSARY FOR BOARD TO OBTAIN RECORDS PERTAINING TO HIS PRIVILEGES AT HOSPITALS OR HEALTH CARE FACILITIES; SHALL GIVE A COPY OF THIS ORDER TO ANY HEALTH CARE ENTITY WHERE HE HAS OR APPLIES FOR PRIVILEGES OR ANYONE ELSE WHO REQUESTS THEM; SHALL ENSURE ANY INQUIRIES REGARDING HIS TEXAS LICENSURE STATUS ARE ANSWERED BY REFERENCE TO THIS ORDER; SHALL INFORM BOARD OF CHANGE OF ADDRESS WITHIN 1O DAYS OR IF HE LEAVES THE STATE; TIME SPENT OUT OF TEXAS DOES NOT COUNT TOWARD RESTRICTION. SHALL NOT SEEK MODIFICATION FOR ONE YEAR.

KENNADY, DONALD SCOTT MD, LICENSE NUMBER 00C4389, WAS DISCIPLINED BY TEXAS ON MARCH 4, 1996
DISCIPLINARY ACTION: LICENSE SUSPENSION
OFFENSE: FAILURE TO COMPLY WITH PREVIOUS BOARD ORDER

NOTES: FAILED TO TAKE AND PASS THE SPEX EXAMINATION AS ORDERED IN 1/06/95 BOARD ORDER. SUSPENSION UNTIL HE TAKES AND PASSES THE SPEX AND SUBSEQUENTLY APPEARS BEFORE THE BOARD AND PROVIDES SUFFICIENT EVIDENCE THAT HE POSSESSES THE SKILLS AND KNOWLEDGE TO SAFELY PRACTICE MEDICINE IN TEXAS AND IS PHYSICALLY AND MENTALLY COMPETENT TO RESUME THE PRACTICE OF MEDICINE. ON 8/17/96 BOARD DENIED HIS REQUEST TO HAVE THE SUSPENSION LIFTED.

KENNEDY, JERETTA IRENE MD, LICENSE NUMBER 00C5745 OF HITCHCOCK, TX, WAS DISCIPLINED BY TEXAS ON APRIL 24, 1991
DISCIPLINARY ACTION: LICENSE REVOCATION
OFFENSE: SUBSTANCE ABUSE

NOTES: INTEMPERATE USE OF ALCOHOL OR DRUGS AND INABILITY TO PRACTICE WITH REASONABLE SKILL AND SAFETY TO PATIENTS. ON APPEAL.

KENNEDY, JERETTA IRENE MD OF 1172 SAILFISH DR, HITCHCOCK, TX, WAS DISCIPLINED BY DEA ON JUNE 6, 1991
DISCIPLINARY ACTION: SURRENDER OF CONTROLLED SUBSTANCE LICENSE
OFFENSE: PROFESSIONAL MISCONDUCT

NOTES: VOLUNTARY SURRENDER 05/15/90 IN HITCHCOCK, TEXAS DUE TO DIVERSION OF DEMEROL.

KENNEDY, KEVIN MEERS MD OF EL PASO, TX, WAS DISCIPLINED BY LOUISIANA ON MARCH 2, 1995
DISCIPLINARY ACTION: RESTRICTION PLACED ON LICENSE; REQUIRED TO TAKE ADDITIONAL MEDICAL EDUCATION
OFFENSE: OVERPRESCRIBING OR MISPRESCRIBING DRUGS

NOTES: PROFESSIONAL OR MEDICAL INCOMPETENCY; PRESCRIBING, DISPENSING OR ADMINISTERING CONTROLLED SUBSTANCES IN OTHER THAN A LEGAL OR LEGITIMATE MANNER. MUST SUCCESSFULLY PASS THE SPEX EXAMINATION AND SPECIFIED CONTINUING MEDICAL EDUCATION WITHIN ONE YEAR; SHALL NOT PRACTICE AT INDEPENDENT EMERGENCY MEDICAL CLINICS AND IMMEDIATE REPORTING OF MALPRACTICE CLAIMS ARISING DURING SPECIFIED PERIOD.

KENNEDY, KEVIN MEERS MD, DATE OF BIRTH DECEMBER 28, 1959, LICENSE NUMBER 0041150 OF PO BOX 12805, EL PASO, TX, WAS DISCIPLINED BY GEORGIA ON NOVEMBER 2, 1995
DISCIPLINARY ACTION: PROBATION

NOTES: IMPAIRMENT. LICENSE BY CONSENT ORDER. EFFECTIVE 10/4/96 PROBATION TERMINATED.

KEPPLER, JOHN PAUL MD, DATE OF BIRTH NOVEMBER 14, 1950, LICENSE NUMBER 0029482 OF 1669 PHOENIX PKWY #102, ATLANTA, GA, WAS DISCIPLINED BY GEORGIA ON MARCH 23, 1990
DISCIPLINARY ACTION: EMERGENCY SUSPENSION
OFFENSE: SUBSTANCE ABUSE

NOTES: IN 1982 HE VOLUNTARILY ENTERED AND COMPLETED A TREATMENT PROGRAM FOR DEPENDENCY ON ALCOHOL AND DRUGS. AN APRIL 1987 CONSENT ORDER PUTTING KEPPLER ON PROBATION WAS TERMINATED 4/24/89. BOARD RECEIVED RELIABLE INFORMATION THAT HE HAD SUFFERED RELAPSE. HE IS ALSO REQUIRED TO SUBMIT TO A 72-HOUR INPATIENT MENTAL/PHYSICAL EVALUATION.

KEPPLER, JOHN PAUL MD, DATE OF BIRTH NOVEMBER 14, 1950 OF 4015 SOUTH COBB DR STE 100, SMYRNA, GA, WAS DISCIPLINED BY DEA ON AUGUST 17, 1990
DISCIPLINARY ACTION: SURRENDER OF CONTROLLED SUBSTANCE LICENSE
OFFENSE: SUBSTANCE ABUSE

NOTES: SUSPENSION OF LICENSE TO PRACTICE MEDICINE 03/23/90 IN GEORGIA FOR ADDICTION TO LORACET AND HYDROCODONE.

KEPPLER, JOHN PAUL MD, LICENSE NUMBER 00F9100 OF ATLANTA, GA, WAS DISCIPLINED BY TEXAS ON DECEMBER 3, 1990
DISCIPLINARY ACTION: SURRENDER OF LICENSE

NOTES: SURRENDERED LICENSE IN LIEU OF DISCIPLINARY HEARING.

KEPPLER, JOHN PAUL MD, DATE OF BIRTH NOVEMBER 14, 1950, LICENSE NUMBER 0029482 OF 1669 PHOENIX PKWY #102, ATLANTA, GA, WAS DISCIPLINED BY GEORGIA ON APRIL 3, 1991
DISCIPLINARY ACTION: PROBATION; MONITORING OF PHYSICIAN PERFORMANCE

NOTES: SUSPENSION LIFTED. MAY RESUME PRACTICE UNDER TERMS AND CONDITIONS OF A CONSENT ORDER, INCLUDING SUPERVISED PROBATION. MAY PETITION FOR TERMINATION OF PROBATION AFTER DOCUMENTING SEVEN YEARS OF CONTINUOUS SOBRIETY OR UNTIL 3/10/87, WHICHEVER IS LATER. ON 10/7/92 ORDER MODIFYING THIS ORDER ISSUED. MAY UTILIZE DEA PERMIT FOR SCHEDULE IV TO BE FILLED IN CLINIC. SUPPLY TWO SPECIMENS MONTHLY AS OPPOSED TO THREE TIMES WEEKLY, AND QUARTERLY REPORTS AS OPPOSED TO MONTHLY REPORTS.

KEPPLER, JOHN PAUL MD, DATE OF BIRTH NOVEMBER 14, 1950, LICENSE NUMBER 0029482 OF 141 WEST SOLOMON STREET, GRIFFIN, GA, WAS DISCIPLINED BY GEORGIA ON JANUARY 12, 1994
DISCIPLINARY ACTION: EMERGENCY SUSPENSION

NOTES: IMPAIRMENT.

KEPPLER, JOHN PAUL MD, DATE OF BIRTH NOVEMBER 14, 1950, LICENSE NUMBER 0029482 OF 141 W SOLOMON STREET, GRIFFIN, GA, WAS DISCIPLINED BY GEORGIA ON MAY 16, 1994
DISCIPLINARY ACTION: PROBATION

NOTES: IMPAIRMENT. SUSPENSION LIFTED WITH INDEFINITE PROBATION.

KEPPLER, JOHN PAUL MD, DATE OF BIRTH NOVEMBER 14, 1950, LICENSE NUMBER 0029482 OF 141 W SOLOMON STREET, GRIFFIN, GA, WAS DISCIPLINED BY GEORGIA ON JUNE 9, 1994
DISCIPLINARY ACTION: EMERGENCY SUSPENSION

NOTES: IMPAIRMENT; RELAPSE.

KEPPLER, JOHN PAUL MD, DATE OF BIRTH NOVEMBER 14, 1950, LICENSE NUMBER 0029482 OF 141 W SOLOMAN STREET, GRIFFIN, GA, WAS DISCIPLINED BY GEORGIA ON SEPTEMBER 23, 1994
DISCIPLINARY ACTION: LICENSE REVOCATION
OFFENSE: SUBSTANCE ABUSE

NOTES: DRUG ADDICTION.

KEPPLER, JOHN PAUL MD, DATE OF BIRTH NOVEMBER 14, 1950 OF 141 WEST SOLOMAN STREET, GRIFFIN, GA, WAS DISCIPLINED BY MEDICARE ON JULY 3, 1997
DISCIPLINARY ACTION: EXCLUSION FROM THE MEDICARE AND/OR MEDICAID PROGRAM
OFFENSE: DISCIPLINARY ACTION BY ANOTHER STATE OR AGENCY

NOTES: LICENSE REVOKED, SUSPENDED, SURRENDERED OR OTHERWISE LOST FOR REASONS BEARING ON PROFESSIONAL PERFORMANCE, PROFESSIONAL COMPETENCE OR FINANCIAL INTEGRITY.

KERR, BRYANT A MD, DATE OF BIRTH JUNE 10, 1958 OF 4270 OCEAN DRIVE #15, CORPUS CHRISTI, TX, WAS DISCIPLINED BY MEDICARE ON APRIL 14, 1997
DISCIPLINARY ACTION: EXCLUSION FROM THE MEDICARE AND/OR MEDICAID PROGRAM
OFFENSE: NONCOMPLIANCE WITH A PROFESSIONAL RULE

NOTES: DEFAULTED ON PUBLIC HEALTH SERVICE EDUCATION LOAN.

KESLER, KEITH E MD, LICENSE NUMBER 00C8220 OF 5105 QUAIL RUN, AUSTIN, TX, WAS DISCIPLINED BY ARKANSAS ON DECEMBER 1, 1994
DISCIPLINARY ACTION: SURRENDER OF LICENSE

KESLER, KEITH ELDON DO, LICENSE NUMBER 00G9758 OF AUSTIN, TX, WAS DISCIPLINED BY TEXAS ON JANUARY 14, 1994
DISCIPLINARY ACTION: SURRENDER OF CONTROLLED SUBSTANCE LICENSE; 60-MONTH PROBATION
OFFENSE: LOSS OR RESTRICTION OF HOSPITAL PRIVILEGES
NOTES: ON 7/27/93 DIVERTED DEMEROL FOR HIS OWN USE FROM THE EMERGENCY ROOM OF HOSPITAL WHERE HE WAS EMPLOYED; PRIVILEGES WERE THEN SUSPENDED AT THIS HOSPITAL BECAUSE OF SUSPECTED IMPAIRMENT; ON 7/28/93 ENTERED TREATMENT FOR CHEMICAL DEPENDENCY AND THEN AN AFTERCARE CONTRACT AND A CONTRACT WITH IMPAIRED PHYSICIANS COMMITTEE. SUSPENSION STAYED. CONDITIONS OF PROBATION: SHALL ABSTAIN FROM THE CONSUMPTION OF ALCOHOL/CHEMICAL SUBSTANCES IN ANY FORM UNLESS PRESCRIBED BY ANOTHER PHYSICIAN FOR A LEGITIMATE AND THERAPEUTIC PURPOSE; SHALL SUBMIT HIMSELF FOR APPROPRIATE EXAMS INCLUDING DRUG OR ALCOHOL SCREENS; SHALL CONTINUE TO PARTICIPATE IN AA'S PROGRAM NOT LESS THAN THREE TIMES A WEEK WITH QUARTERLY REPORTS TO THE BOARD; SHALL SURRENDER DEA AND TEXAS CONTROLLED SUBSTANCES REGISTRATION AND SHALL NOT REREGISTER WITHOUT PERMISSION; SHALL PARTICIPATE IN ACTIVITIES OF A PHYSICIAN HEALTH AND REHABILITATION COMMITTEE AND ATTEND WEEKLY MEETINGS WITH QUARTERLY REPORTS; SHALL PARTICIPATE IN ALL ACTIVITIES AS REQUIRED BY HIS AFTERCARE CONTRACT; SHALL ATTEND AT LEAST 50 HOURS PER YEAR OF CONTINUING MEDICAL EDUCATION; SHALL GIVE A COPY OF THIS ORDER TO ANY HEALTH CARE ENTITY WHERE HE HAS PRIVILEGES; SHALL COOPERATE WITH THE BOARD IN VERIFYING COMPLIANCE; SHALL INFORM BOARD OF CHANGE OF ADDRESS WITHIN 10 DAYS OR IF HE LEAVES THE STATE; TIME SPENT OUT OF TEXAS DOES NOT COUNT TOWARD PROBATION; SHALL APPEAR BEFORE THE BOARD ONCE A YEAR. SHALL NOT SEEK MODIFICATION FOR ONE YEAR UNLESS HE IS ADMITTED TO A RESIDENCY TRAINING PROGRAM IN WHICH CASE HE MAY REQUEST PERMISSION TO REAPPLY FOR CONTROLLED SUBSTANCES CERTIFICATES. HE WAS ACCEPTED INTO A PSYCHIATRIC RESIDENCY PROGRAM AND ON 6/22/94 HE WAS GRANTED PERMISSION TO REAPPLY FOR SCHEDULE IV AND V CONTROLLED SUBSTANCES REGISTRATION. IF THESE CERTIFICATES ARE REISSUED THE FOLLOWING CONDITIONS ALSO APPLY: SHALL NOT POSSESS, ADMINISTER, DISPENSE OR PRESCRIBE CONTROLLED SUBSTANCES EXCEPT FOR PURPOSES OF TREATMENT OF PATIENTS IN THE CONTEXT OF HIS PSYCHIATRIC RESIDENCY PROGRAM; SHALL NOT TREAT OR OTHERWISE SERVE AS PHYSICIAN, PRESCRIBE, DISPENSE OR ADMINISTER DRUGS THAT MAY BE SUBJECT TO ABUSE TO HIMSELF OR ANY MEMBER OF HIS FAMILY; SEPARATE FROM PATIENT RECORDS, SHALL MAINTAIN A FILE OF EVERY PRESCRIPTION WRITTEN FOR CONTROLLED SUBSTANCES OR DANGEROUS DRUGS WHICH SHALL BE AVAILABLE FOR REVIEW; SHALL BE SUPERVISED BY THE DIRECTOR OF HIS PROGRAM WITH QUARTERLY REPORTS. ALL OTHER PROVISIONS OF THE ORDER REMAIN IN EFFECT. ON 10/5/96 ORDER MODIFIED AS FOLLOWS: HE IS AUTHORIZED TO REAPPLY TO THE DEA AND THE TEXAS DEPARTMENT OF PUBLIC SAFETY TO OBTAIN FULL PRESCRIBING AUTHORITY FOR CONTROLLED SUBSTANCES; ALL OTHER CONDITIONS REMAIN IN EFFECT. ON 11/22/97 ORDER TERMINATED.

KESLER, KEITH ELDON DO OF 2701 CLEARVIEW DRIVE, AUSTIN, TX, WAS DISCIPLINED BY DEA ON MARCH 14, 1994
DISCIPLINARY ACTION: SURRENDER OF CONTROLLED SUBSTANCE LICENSE
OFFENSE: DISCIPLINARY ACTION BY ANOTHER STATE OR AGENCY
NOTES: INVOLVED IN DEMEROL DIVERSION FROM HOSPITAL. MEDICAL LICENSE SUSPENDED 01/14/94. SUSPENSION STAYED AND PLACED ON PROBATION.

KESZLER, BERNEY R MD, DATE OF BIRTH JULY 18, 1942 OF PO BOX 151706, LUFKIN, TX, WAS DISCIPLINED BY MEDICARE ON NOVEMBER 1, 1990
DISCIPLINARY ACTION: 120-MONTH EXCLUSION FROM THE MEDICARE AND/OR MEDICAID PROGRAM; FINE
NOTES: IMPOSITION OF A CIVIL MONEY PENALTY OR ASSESSMENT. NO LONGER LISTED AS EXCLUDED AS OF 9/30/92.

KETTERER, CYNTHIA L MD, DATE OF BIRTH JANUARY 24, 1960 OF 1901 SANSOM STREET, PHILADELPHIA, PA, WAS DISCIPLINED BY MEDICARE ON SEPTEMBER 10, 1996
DISCIPLINARY ACTION: EXCLUSION FROM THE MEDICARE AND/OR MEDICAID PROGRAM
OFFENSE: NONCOMPLIANCE WITH A PROFESSIONAL RULE
NOTES: DEFAULTED ON PUBLIC HEALTH SERVICE EDUCATION LOAN. REINSTATED ON 4/14/97.

KETTERER, CYNTHIA LEE MD, LICENSE NUMBER K3771 OF EL CAMPO, TX, WAS DISCIPLINED BY TEXAS ON AUGUST 28, 1999
DISCIPLINARY ACTION: MONITORING OF PHYSICIAN PERFORMANCE
OFFENSE: SUBSTANCE ABUSE
NOTES: ON 4/7/98 HE ENTERED TREATMENT AT HAZELDEN FOUNDATION; ON 9/12/98 HE WAS ARRESTED FOR PUBLIC INTOXICATION; HE REPORTS A SOBRIETY DATE OF 9/14/98; HIS AA MEETING ATTENDANCE HAS BEEN REPORTED BY HIM TO BE ON AN AVERAGE OF 3 TIMES PER WEEK; HE REPORTS REGULAR PARTICIPATION IN THE ACTIVITIES OF THE HARRIS COUNTY MEDICAL SOCIETY COMMITTEE ON PHYSICIAN HEALTH AND REHABILITATION; HE SELF-REPORTED INTEMPERATE USE OF ALCOHOL ON 10/2/98. LICENSE LIMITED FOR FIVE YEARS AS FOLLOWS: SHALL ABSTAIN FROM THE CONSUMPTION OF ALCOHOL/DRUGS IN ANY FORM UNLESS PRESCRIBED BY ANOTHER PHYSICIAN FOR A LEGITIMATE AND THERAPEUTIC PURPOSE; SHALL SUBMIT HERSELF FOR APPROPRIATE EXAMS INCLUDING DRUG OR ALCOHOL SCREENS; SHALL PARTICIPATE IN THE ACTIVITIES OF A PHYSICIAN HEALTH AND REHABILITATION COMMITTEE AND ATTEND WEEKLY MEETINGS WITH QUARTERLY REPORTS; SHALL PARTICIPATE IN AA'S PROGRAM NOT LESS THAN FOUR TIMES A WEEK; SHALL REPORT ON HIS ATTENDANCE; SHALL NOMINATE THREE CERTIFIED PSYCHIATRISTS FOR BOARD SELECTION OF A THERAPIST AND SHALL EXPEDITIOUSLY SUBMIT HIMSELF TO EVALUATION AND TREATMENT BY THE APPROVED PRACTITIONER; SHALL APPEAR BEFORE THE BOARD UPON REQUEST; TIME SPENT OUT OF TEXAS DOES NOT COUNT TOWARD RESTRICTION; SHALL INFORM THE BOARD OF CHANGE OF ADDRESS WITHIN 10 DAYS OR IF SHE LEAVES THE STATE; SHALL NOT SEEK MODIFICATION FOR ONE YEAR.

KEY, LUTHER S MD, LICENSE NUMBER B9658 OF ALBANY, TX, WAS DISCIPLINED BY TEXAS ON AUGUST 22, 1998
DISCIPLINARY ACTION: 60-MONTH PROBATION; RESTRICTION PLACED ON LICENSE
OFFENSE: SUBSTANDARD CARE, INCOMPETENCE OR NEGLIGENCE

NOTES: THE BOARD FOUND THAT THE TEXAS MEDICAL FOUNDATION PLACED HIM ON A CORRECTIVE ACTION PLAN AS A RESULT OF HIS CARE AND TREATMENT OF: ONE PATIENT WHOM HE FAILED TO ADMINISTER IV FLUIDS IN AN APPROPRIATE MANNER IN RESPONSE TO EPISODES OF VOMITING AND THAT HE FAILED TO EVALUATE THE PATIENT'S RENAL STATUS AND OBTAIN A CULTURE OF THE SURGICAL WOUND DRAINAGE; REGARDING ANOTHER PATIENT, HE DID NOT MAKE APPROPRIATE DIAGNOSES AND ASSESSMENTS OF AND FAILED TO PERFORM A DIAGNOSTIC EVALUATION TO DETERMINE THE ETIOLOGY OF THE PATIENT'S SYMPTOMS; AND ANOTHER DIABETIC PATIENT FOR WHOM HE ADMINISTERED LENTE INSULIN WHEN REGULAR INSULIN WOULD HAVE BEEN MORE APPROPRIATE; ADDITIONALLY HE FAILED TO ADEQUATELY DOCUMENT HIS CARE AND TREATMENT OF A FOURTH PATIENT. SUSPENSION STAYED FOR PROBATION WITH FOLLOWING TERMS AND CONDITIONS: WITHIN 6 MONTHS SHALL TAKE AND PASS THE SPEX WITHIN 3 ATTEMPTS; SHALL NOT PRACTICE MEDICINE IN A HOSPITAL SETTING; HIS MEDICAL PRACTICE SHALL BE MONITORED BY A BOARD APPROVED TEXAS PHYSICIAN WHO SHALL PROVIDE QUARTERLY REPORTS TO THE BOARD; SHALL OBTAIN 50 HOURS PER YEAR OF CONTINUING MEDICAL EDUCATION; SHALL APPEAR BEFORE THE BOARD ONCE A YEAR; SHALL COOPERATE WITH THE BOARD IN VERIFYING COMPLIANCE; TIME SPENT OUT OF TEXAS DOES NOT COUNT TOWARD PROBATION; SHALL INFORM THE BOARD OF CHANGE OF ADDRESS WITHIN 10 DAYS OR IF HE LEAVES THE STATE; SHALL NOT SEEK MODIFICATION FOR ONE YEAR.

KEY, LUTHER S MD, LICENSE NUMBER B9658 OF ALBANY, TX, WAS DISCIPLINED BY TEXAS ON MARCH 24, 1999
DISCIPLINARY ACTION: LICENSE SUSPENSION
OFFENSE: FAILURE TO COMPLY WITH PREVIOUS BOARD ORDER

NOTES: FAILED TO TAKE AND PASS THE SPEX WITHIN 6 MONTHS AS REQUIRED BY THE 8/22/98 BOARD ORDER.

KHAN, AHMED I MD, LICENSE NUMBER H0073 OF BOONEVILLE, AR, WAS DISCIPLINED BY TEXAS ON AUGUST 22, 1998
DISCIPLINARY ACTION: 36-MONTH PROBATION; REQUIRED TO TAKE ADDITIONAL MEDICAL EDUCATION
OFFENSE: LOSS OR RESTRICTION OF HOSPITAL PRIVILEGES

NOTES: ON 6/25/95 HE WAS CONSULTED AND AGREED TO ADMIT A PATIENT PRESENTED IN AN EMERGENCY ROOM WITH ACUTE ABDOMINAL PAIN; AFTER WAITING 18 HOURS, THE PATIENT'S FAMILY CALLED IN ANOTHER PHYSICIAN TO TAKE OVER THE PATIENT'S CARE AND DECLINED TO PERMIT DOCTOR KHAN TO EXAMINE THE PATIENT; THE MEDICAL RECORD DOES NOT REFLECT HIS VISIT TO THE PATIENT; HE ASSERTS THAT HE COULD NOT SEE THE PATIENT BECAUSE HE WAS INVOLVED IN A SURGERY PROCEDURE AS AN ASSISTING SURGEON AT ANOTHER HOSPITAL; HE HAS BEEN UNABLE TO PRODUCE THE SURGICAL LOG FROM ANOTHER HOSPITAL WHICH LISTS HIM, AND MAINTAINS THAT SUCH LOGS ONLY LIST THE PRIMARY SURGEON; IN 1996 HIS EMERGENCY ROOM PRIVILEGES WERE SUSPENDED THEN RESTORED; HE RELOCATED HIS PRACTICE TO ARKANSAS; A BOARD CONSULTANT CRITICIZED HIS FAILURE TO TIMELY SEEK A THORACIC SURGEON CONSULTATION AND ALSO HIS USE OF A CHEST TUBE THAT WAS TOO SMALL; THE CONSULTANT DETERMINED THAT THE PATIENT'S DEMISE COULD HAVE BEEN AVOIDED IF THE PATIENT HAD RECEIVED PROMPT TREATMENT; THE HOSPITAL QUALITY ASSURANCE REVIEW FOUND NO FAULT IN HIS HANDLING THE CASE. SUSPENSION STAYED FOR PROBATION WITH FOLLOWING TERMS AND CONDITIONS: WITHIN 1 YEAR SHALL SUCCESSFULLY COMPLETE AN ADVANCED TRAUMA LIFE SUPPORT COURSE AND AN ADVANCED CARDIAC LIFE SUPPORT COURSE AND OBTAIN CERTIFICATION; SHALL CONTINUE TO ATTEND AT LEAST 50 HOURS PER YEAR OF CONTINUING MEDICAL EDUCATION IN RISK MANAGEMENT, SURGERY, TRAUMA, CRITICAL CARE AND EMERGENCY MEDICINE; SHALL OBTAIN 1 ETHICS COURSE PER YEAR; SHALL PERFORM 100 HOURS OF COMMUNITY SERVICE; SHALL APPEAR BEFORE THE BOARD ONCE A YEAR; SHALL COOPERATE WITH THE BOARD IN VERIFYING COMPLIANCE; TIME SPENT OUT OF TEXAS DOES NOT COUNT TOWARD PROBATION; SHALL INFORM THE BOARD OF CHANGE OF ADDRESS WITHIN 10 DAYS OR IF HE LEAVES THE STATE; SHALL NOT SEEK MODIFICATION FOR ONE YEAR. ON 10/15/99 THE ORDER WAS TERMINATED.

KHAN, AHMED I MD, LICENSE NUMBER 149941 OF 300 NORTH CLIFTON, FORDYCE, AR, WAS DISCIPLINED BY NEW YORK ON JULY 28, 1999
DISCIPLINARY ACTION: LICENSE SUSPENSION
OFFENSE: DISCIPLINARY ACTION BY ANOTHER STATE OR AGENCY

NOTES: DISCIPLINED BY THE TEXAS BOARD FOR FAILING TO PRACTICE MEDICINE IN AN ACCEPTABLE MANNER DURING HIS TREATMENT OF ONE PATIENT. SUSPENSION UNTIL THE COMPLETION OF ALL TERMS AND CONDITIONS IMPOSED BY THE TEXAS BOARD.

KHAN, AHMED IQBAL MD, DATE OF BIRTH JUNE 13, 1946, LICENSE NUMBER 039580E OF 18000 DAVENPORT ROAD, DALLAS, TX, WAS DISCIPLINED BY PENNSYLVANIA ON MARCH 23, 1999
DISCIPLINARY ACTION: SURRENDER OF LICENSE
OFFENSE: DISCIPLINARY ACTION BY ANOTHER STATE OR AGENCY

NOTES: DISCIPLINARY ACTION TAKEN BY TEXAS. LICENSE PERMANENTLY AND VOLUNTARILY SURRENDERED.

KHOLEIF, ALI A R MD, DATE OF BIRTH OCTOBER 20, 1938, LICENSE NUMBER 0021542 OF OTTUMWA, IA, WAS DISCIPLINED BY IOWA ON MAY 11, 1990
DISCIPLINARY ACTION: EMERGENCY SUSPENSION

NOTES: ON 6/5/90 SUSPENSION WAS LIFTED.

KHOLEIF, ALI A R MD, DATE OF BIRTH OCTOBER 20, 1938, LICENSE NUMBER 0021542 OF OTTUMWA, IA, WAS DISCIPLINED BY IOWA ON DECEMBER 6, 1990
DISCIPLINARY ACTION: LICENSE REVOCATION
OFFENSE: SUBSTANDARD CARE, INCOMPETENCE OR NEGLIGENCE

NOTES: ALSO ETHICAL VIOLATIONS.

KHOLEIF, ALI A R MD, DATE OF BIRTH OCTOBER 20, 1938 OF RR 7 BOX 188A, OTTUMWA, IA, WAS DISCIPLINED BY MEDICARE ON MAY 10, 1991
DISCIPLINARY ACTION: EXCLUSION FROM THE MEDICARE AND/OR MEDICAID PROGRAM
OFFENSE: DISCIPLINARY ACTION BY ANOTHER STATE OR AGENCY

NOTES: LICENSE REVOCATION OR SUSPENSION.

KHOLEIF, ALI ABDEL RAHIM MD OF WOODLAND, TX, WAS

DISCIPLINED BY MISSOURI ON FEBRUARY 22, 1993
DISCIPLINARY ACTION: LICENSE REVOCATION
OFFENSE: DISCIPLINARY ACTION BY ANOTHER STATE OR AGENCY

NOTES: SUBSTANDARD CARE AND MISCONDUCT. NO REINSTATEMENT OF LICENSE FOR SEVEN YEARS.

KIEPFER, RICHARD F MD OF 208 WOLLSCHLAGER DRIVE, BOERNE, TX, WAS DISCIPLINED BY DEA ON SEPTEMBER 29, 1993
DISCIPLINARY ACTION: SURRENDER OF CONTROLLED SUBSTANCE LICENSE
OFFENSE: CRIMINAL CONVICTION OR PLEA OF GUILTY, NOLO CONTENDERE, OR NO CONTEST TO A CRIME

NOTES: CONVICTED OF FAILURE TO MAKE, KEEP AND FURNISH CONTROLLED SUBSTANCES RECORDS ON PENTOBARBITAL. SENTENCED 6/25/93 TO PROBATION, FINE AND COMMUNITY SERVICE; LICENSE SUSPENDED 8/20/93.

KIEPFER, RICHARD F MD, LICENSE NUMBER 0092927 OF 208 WOLLSCHLAEGER DRIVE, BOERNE, TX, WAS DISCIPLINED BY NEW YORK ON MAY 22, 1995
DISCIPLINARY ACTION: LICENSE REVOCATION
OFFENSE: DISCIPLINARY ACTION BY ANOTHER STATE OR AGENCY

NOTES: ACTION IN NEW JERSEY AND TEXAS FOR CONVICTION OF A CRIME. CRIMINALLY CONVICTED OF FAILURE TO MAKE, KEEP AND FURNISH CONTROLLED SUBSTANCE RECORDS ON PENTOBARBITAL IN THE SECOND DEGREE.

KIEPFER, RICHARD F MD, DATE OF BIRTH APRIL 12, 1937 OF C/O 1 ST JOSEPH'S TERRACE, WOODBRIDGE, NJ, WAS DISCIPLINED BY MEDICARE ON MARCH 14, 1996
DISCIPLINARY ACTION: EXCLUSION FROM THE MEDICARE AND/OR MEDICAID PROGRAM
OFFENSE: DISCIPLINARY ACTION BY ANOTHER STATE OR AGENCY

NOTES: LICENSE SURRENDERED FOR REASONS BEARING ON PROFESSIONAL COMPETENCE.

KIEPFER, RICHARD FRANCIS MD, DATE OF BIRTH APRIL 12, 1937, LICENSE NUMBER 00F7503 OF 208 WOLLSCHLAEGER, BOERNE, TX, WAS DISCIPLINED BY TEXAS ON AUGUST 20, 1993
DISCIPLINARY ACTION: LICENSE SUSPENSION
OFFENSE: CRIMINAL CONVICTION OR PLEA OF GUILTY, NOLO CONTENDERE, OR NO CONTEST TO A CRIME

NOTES: ON 6/25/93 HE WAS FOUND GUILTY IN KENDALL COUNTY TEXAS OF THE FELONY OFFENSE OF FAILURE TO MAKE, KEEP AND FURNISH CONTROLLED SUBSTANCE RECORDS OF THE SCHEDULE II CONTROLLED SUBSTANCE PENTOBARBITAL; PLACED ON PROBATION FOR SIX YEARS AND FINED $10,000; IS IN THE PROCESS OF APPEALING THE CONVICTION. IF CONVICTION IS OVERTURNED WITHIN TWO YEARS BOARD WILL LIFT SUSPENSION; IF LONGER THAN TWO YEARS HE SHALL PASS SPEX EXAM BEFORE THE SUSPENSION IS LIFTED; IF CONVICTION IS UPHELD LICENSE WILL AUTOMATICALLY BE REVOKED.

KIEPFER, RICHARD FRANCIS MD, DATE OF BIRTH APRIL 12, 1937, LICENSE NUMBER 0021180 OF 1 ST. JOSEPH TERRACE, WOODBRIDGE, NJ, WAS DISCIPLINED BY NEW JERSEY ON JUNE 2, 1994
DISCIPLINARY ACTION: LICENSE REVOCATION
OFFENSE: CRIMINAL CONVICTION OR PLEA OF GUILTY, NOLO CONTENDERE, OR NO CONTEST TO A CRIME

NOTES: FINDING OF GUILT IN TEXAS ON THE FELONY OFFENSE OF FAILURE TO MAKE, KEEP AND FURNISH CONTROLLED SUBSTANCE RECORDS FOR SCHEDULE II CONTROLLED DANGEROUS SUBSTANCES MEDICATION. SENTENCING OF A SIX-YEAR PRISON SENTENCE WAS STAYED AND HE WAS PLACED ON SIX YEARS PROBATION AND FINED $10,000.

KILGORE, N A MD OF 4119 MONTROSE BLVD, HOUSTON, TX, WAS DISCIPLINED BY DEA ON FEBRUARY 15, 1995
DISCIPLINARY ACTION: SURRENDER OF CONTROLLED SUBSTANCE LICENSE

NOTES: IN LIEU OF PUBLIC INTEREST REVOCATION.

KILIAN, ROBERT JACK MD, LICENSE NUMBER 00D9333 OF LAKE JACKSON, TX, WAS DISCIPLINED BY TEXAS ON NOVEMBER 19, 1993
DISCIPLINARY ACTION: 60-MONTH PROBATION; REPRIMAND
OFFENSE: OVERPRESCRIBING OR MISPRESCRIBING DRUGS

NOTES: FROM 6/28/84 THROUGH 3/92 PRESCRIBED VARIOUS NARCOTIC DRUGS TO 15 PATIENTS FOR CHRONIC PAIN MANAGEMENT FOR WHICH HE FAILED TO TAKE ADEQUATE HISTORIES, TO ORDER FURTHER DIAGNOSTIC STUDIES AS INDICATED, MAINTAIN A COMPREHENSIVE PAIN AND DRUG ABUSE MANAGEMENT PLAN, APPROPRIATELY DOCUMENT MEDICAL RECORDS TO JUSTIFY TREATMENT AND PERFORM PERIODIC PHYSICAL EXAMS; WITHOUT HIS KNOWLEDGE SOME OF THE DRUGS WERE SOLD BY TWO PATIENTS WHICH RESULTED IN THEIR ARREST. CONDITIONS OF PROBATION: SHALL MAINTAIN ADEQUATE MEDICAL RECORDS ON ALL PATIENT OFFICE VISITS AND MAKE THESE RECORDS AVAILABLE FOR REVIEW; SHALL HAVE HIS PRACTICE MONITORED BY A BOARD APPROVED PHYSICIAN WITH QUARTERLY REPORTS; SHALL CONSULT WITH HIS MONITORING PHYSICIAN REGARDING APPROPRIATE MANAGEMENT OF ALL PATIENTS HE MAINTAINS ON CONTROLLED SUBSTANCES FOR LONGER THAN SIX MONTHS; WITHIN SIX MONTHS WILL ENROLL IN A REMEDIAL PHARMACOLOGY COURSE AND SHALL ATTEND 50 HOURS PER YEAR OF CONTINUING MEDICAL EDUCATION WITH AT LEAST ONE COURSE PER YEAR ON THE POTENTIAL FOR ABUSE OF CONTROLLED SUBSTANCES AND OTHER PRESCRIPTION DRUGS; DUPLICATE COPIES OF ALL PRESCRIPTIONS FOR CONTROLLED SUBSTANCES SHALL BE MAINTAINED AND AVAILABLE FOR REVIEW; SHALL APPEAR BEFORE THE BOARD TWICE A YEAR; SHALL GIVE A COPY OF THIS ORDER TO ANY HEALTH CARE ENTITY WHERE HE HAS PRIVILEGES; SHALL COOPERATE WITH THE BOARD IN VERIFYING COMPLIANCE; SHALL INFORM BOARD OF CHANGE OF ADDRESS WITHIN 10 DAYS OR IF HE LEAVES THE STATE; TIME SPENT OUT OF TEXAS DOES NOT COUNT TOWARD PROBATION. SHALL NOT SEEK MODIFICATION FOR ONE YEAR. ON 1/18/97 PETITION TO TERMINATE ORDER DELETED; ORDER MODIFIED TO ALLOW PETITIONS FOR MODIFICATION OR TERMINATION TO BE FILED ONCE EVERY SIX MONTHS. ON 8/9/97 BOARD GRANTED HIS PETITION FOR TERMINATION OF THIS ORDER BASED ON COMPLIANCE WITH CONDITIONS.

KIM, MYUNG JIN MD, LICENSE NUMBER 00F5978, WAS DISCIPLINED BY TEXAS ON MAY 14, 1996
DISCIPLINARY ACTION: REQUIRED TO TAKE ADDITIONAL MEDICAL EDUCATION; MONITORING OF PHYSICIAN PERFORMANCE
OFFENSE: SUBSTANDARD CARE, INCOMPETENCE OR NEGLIGENCE

NOTES: DURING 1990, HE PERFORMED A LIVER BIOPSY FOR A PATIENT WHICH WAS NOT INDICATED BASED ON THE RESULTS OF THE TESTS HE ADMINISTERED TO THE PATIENT AND THE AVAILABILITY OF NONINVASIVE TESTS THAT WERE NOT PERFORMED. SHALL ATTEND AT LEAST 100 HOURS PER YEAR FOR THREE YEARS

OF CONTINUING MEDICAL EDUCATION, AT LEAST 25 HOURS OF WHICH SHALL BE IN THE AREA OF INTERPRETING LABORATORY DATA AND AT LEAST 25 HOURS OF WHICH SHALL BE IN THE AREA OF RISK MANAGEMENT; SHALL COOPERATE WITH BOARD IN VERIFYING COMPLIANCE; SHALL GIVE A COPY OF THIS ORDER TO ANY HEALTH CARE ENTITY WHERE HE HAS PRIVILEGES; SHALL PROVIDE A COPY OF THIS ORDER TO ANYONE REQUESTING IT WITHIN 10 DAYS; SHALL INFORM BOARD OF CHANGE OF ADDRESS WITHIN 10 DAYS. SHALL NOT SEEK MODIFICATION FOR ONE YEAR. ON 10/24/98 ORDER TERMINATED.

KIM, YOUNGHOO MD, LICENSE NUMBER 00H7442 OF LOVELAND, CO, WAS DISCIPLINED BY TEXAS ON JUNE 17, 1992
DISCIPLINARY ACTION: SURRENDER OF LICENSE

KIMMONS, JOHN HENRY JR MD, LICENSE NUMBER 00D4799 OF COPPELL, TX, WAS DISCIPLINED BY TEXAS ON MAY 15, 1996
DISCIPLINARY ACTION: PROBATION; 60-MONTH RESTRICTION PLACED ON CONTROLLED SUBSTANCE LICENSE
OFFENSE: SUBSTANCE ABUSE

NOTES: HAS A HISTORY OF EXCESSIVE USE OF ALCOHOL AND SELF-PRESCRIPTION OF DRUGS WITHOUT ADEQUATE MEDICAL INDICATIONS; IN 1974, HE WAS HOSPITALIZED FOR CHEMICAL DEPENDENCY TREATMENT FOR 30 DAYS AFTER A PERIOD OF HEAVY ALCOHOL USE AND EXCESSIVE SELF-PRESCRIBING OF BARBITURATES WITHOUT A LEGITIMATE MEDICAL PURPOSE; IN 1982, HE WAS HOSPITALIZED FOR CHEMICAL DEPENDENCY TREATMENT FOR 34 DAYS AFTER BEING CONFRONTED BY HIS CHIEF OF SERVICE REGARDING HEAVY ALCOHOL USE AND EXCESSIVE USE OF DALMANE WITHOUT A LEGITIMATE MEDICAL PURPOSE; IN 1995, HE RESIGNED FROM A PRACTICE POSITION AND WAS VOLUNTARILY HOSPITALIZED FOR CHEMICAL DEPENDENCY TREATMENT FOR NINE DAYS; FROM 10/95 TO 2/96, WAS TREATED FOR INPATIENT CHEMICAL DEPENDENCY TREATMENT; DISCHARGE DIAGNOSIS NOTED BENZODIAZEPINE AND ALCOHOL DEPENDENCE; REPORTS SOBRIETY DATE OF 10/4/95; HAS MET WITH THE PHYSICIAN'S RECOVERY COMMITTEE AFTER DISCHARGE FROM INPATIENT TREATMENT; AFTER DISCHARGE FROM TREATMENT AND PRIOR TO 3/14/96 INFORMAL SETTLEMENT CONFERENCE/SHOW COMPLIANCE PROCEEDING, HE VOLUNTARILY REFRAINED FROM PRACTICING MEDICINE; REPORTS ATTENDING APPROXIMATELY FIVE AA MEETINGS PER WEEK AND HAS ENTERED INTO AN AFTERCARE RECOVERY CONTRACT. SUSPENSION STAYED. PROBATION WITH TERMS AND CONDITIONS: SHALL ABSTAIN FROM THE CONSUMPTION OF ALCOHOL/DRUGS IN ANY FORM UNLESS PRESCRIBED BY ANOTHER PHYSICIAN FOR A LEGITIMATE AND THERAPEUTIC PURPOSE; SHALL SUBMIT HIMSELF FOR APPROPRIATE EXAMS INCLUDING DRUG OR ALCOHOL SCREENS; SHALL SUBMIT HIMSELF FOR EVALUATION AND TREATMENT BY A BOARD-APPROVED PSYCHIATRIST WHOM HE SHALL SEE AT LEAST ONCE A MONTH AND WHO SHALL SUBMIT REPORTS TO THE BOARD; SHALL CONTINUE TO PARTICIPATE IN AA'S PROGRAM AT LEAST FOUR TIMES A WEEK WITH QUARTERLY REPORTS TO THE BOARD; SHALL PARTICIPATE IN THE ACTIVITIES OF A PHYSICIAN' S HEALTH AND REHABILITATION PROGRAM AND ATTEND WEEKLY MEETINGS WITH QUARTERLY REPORTS; SHALL COMPLY WITH THE TERMS OF CONTINUING CARE CONTRACT AND ANY CONTRACT ENTERED INTO BY HIM FOR HOSPITAL PRIVILEGES; SHALL NOT POSSESS ALCOHOL, CONTROLLED SUBSTANCES OR DANGEROUS DRUGS WITH ADDICTIVE POTENTIAL OR POTENTIAL FOR ABUSE AND SHALL SURRENDER ALL SUCH DRUGS INCLUDING SAMPLES; SHALL NOT TREAT OR OTHERWISE SERVE AS PHYSICIAN, PRESCRIBE, DISPENSE OR ADMINISTER DRUGS THAT MAY BE SUBJECT TO ABUSE TO HIMSELF OR TO ANY MEMBER OF HIS FAMILY; SHALL SURRENDER HIS DEA/DPS CONTROLLED SUBSTANCES REGISTRATION CERTIFICATES AND SHALL NOT ATTEMPT TO REREGISTER WITHOUT PRIOR AUTHORITY FROM THE BOARD; SHALL SURRENDER ALL UNUSED TRIPLICATE PRESCRIPTION FORMS AND SHALL NOT ATTEMPT TO ORDER MORE; SEPARATE FROM PATIENT RECORDS SHALL MAINTAIN A FILE OF EVERY PRESCRIPTION WRITTEN FOR DANGEROUS DRUGS WITH ADDICTIVE POTENTIAL OR POTENTIAL FOR ABUSE WHICH SHALL BE AVAILABLE FOR REVIEW; SHALL MAINTAIN ADEQUATE MEDICAL RECORDS WHICH SHALL BE AVAILABLE FOR REVIEW; SHALL OBTAIN AT LEAST 50 HOURS PER YEAR OF CONTINUING MEDICAL EDUCATION; SHALL APPEAR BEFORE BOARD AT LEAST TWICE A YEAR OR AT BOARD REQUEST; SHALL COOPERATE WITH BOARD IN VERIFYING COMPLIANCE; SHALL GIVE A COPY OF THIS ORDER TO ANY HEALTH CARE ENTITY WHERE HE HAS PRIVILEGES; SHALL PROVIDE A COPY OF THIS ORDER TO ANYONE REQUESTING IT WITHIN 10 DAYS; TIME SPENT OUT OF TEXAS DOES NOT COUNT TOWARD PROBATION; SHALL INFORM BOARD OF CHANGE OF ADDRESS WITHIN 10 DAYS OR IF HE LEAVES THE STATE. SHALL NOT SEEK MODIFICATION FOR ONE YEAR.

KIMMONS, JOHN HENRY MD, LICENSE NUMBER 3434 OF DALLAS, TX, WAS DISCIPLINED BY ALABAMA ON MARCH 12, 1997
DISCIPLINARY ACTION: RESTRICTION PLACED ON LICENSE
OFFENSE: DISCIPLINARY ACTION BY ANOTHER STATE OR AGENCY

NOTES: RESTRICTION AGAINST HIS MEDICAL LICENSE IN TEXAS; RESTRICTIONS IN BOTH STATES IN CONNECTION WITH HIS TREATMENT FOR CHEMICAL DEPENDENCY. VOLUNTARY RESTRICTION IN ALABAMA

KIMMONS, JOHN HENRY JR MD, LICENSE NUMBER D4799 OF COPPELL, TX, WAS DISCIPLINED BY TEXAS ON APRIL 4, 1998
DISCIPLINARY ACTION: 84-MONTH PROBATION; REQUIRED TO ENTER AN IMPAIRED PHYSICIAN PROGRAM OR SUBSTANCE ABUSE TREATMENT
OFFENSE: FAILURE TO COMPLY WITH PREVIOUS BOARD ORDER

NOTES: VIOLATED 5/15/96 BOARD ORDER BY TESTING POSITIVE FOR BENZODIAZEPINES ON OR ABOUT 12/9/97 AND FAILING TO MAKE NOTIFICATION OF THE INGESTION AS REQUIRED. SUSPENSION STAYED FOR PROBATION WITH FOLLOWING TERMS AND CONDITIONS: SHALL ABSTAIN FROM THE CONSUMPTION OF ALCOHOL/DRUGS IN ANY FORM UNLESS PRESCRIBED BY ANOTHER PHYSICIAN FOR A LEGITIMATE AND THERAPEUTIC PURPOSE; SHALL NOMINATE THREE CERTIFIED PSYCHIATRISTS FOR BOARD SELECTION OF A THERAPIST AND SHALL EXPEDITIOUSLY SUBMIT HIMSELF TO EVALUATION AND TREATMENT BY THE APPROVED PRACTITIONER; SHALL SUBMIT HIMSELF FOR APPROPRIATE EXAMS INCLUDING DRUG OR ALCOHOL SCREENS; SHALL PARTICIPATE IN THE ACTIVITIES OF A PHYSICIAN HEALTH AND REHABILITATION COMMITTEE AND ATTEND WEEKLY MEETINGS WITH QUARTERLY REPORTS; SHALL PARTICIPATE IN AA'S PROGRAM NOT LESS THAN FOUR TIMES A WEEK; SHALL REPORT ON HIS ATTENDANCE; SHALL COMPLY WITH TERMS OF HIS CONTINUING CARE CONTRACT WITH QUARTERLY REPORTS; SHALL NOT TREAT OR OTHERWISE SERVE AS PHYSICIAN, PRESCRIBE, DISPENSE OR

ADMINISTER DRUGS THAT MAY BE SUBJECT TO ABUSE TO HIMSELF OR TO ANY MEMBER OF HIS FAMILY; SHALL SURRENDER CONTROLLED SUBSTANCE CERTIFICATES AND ANY TRIPLICATE PRESCRIPTION FORMS OR SAMPLES IN HIS POSSESSION; SEPARATE FROM PATIENT RECORDS, SHALL MAINTAIN A FILE OF EVERY PRESCRIPTION WRITTEN BY HIM FOR DANGEROUS DRUGS WITH ADDICTIVE POTENTIAL WHICH SHALL BE MADE AVAILABLE FOR REVIEW; SHALL MAINTAIN ADEQUATE MEDICAL RECORDS WHICH SHALL BE AVAILABLE FOR REVIEW; SHALL OBTAIN 50 HOURS PER YEAR OF CONTINUING MEDICAL EDUCATION; SHALL APPEAR BEFORE THE BOARD UPON REQUEST; SHALL COOPERATE WITH THE BOARD IN VERIFYING COMPLIANCE; SHALL GIVE A COPY OF THIS ORDER TO ANY HEALTH CARE ENTITY WHERE HE HAS PRIVILEGES; SHALL PROVIDE A COPY OF THIS ORDER TO ANYONE REQUESTING IT WITHIN 10 DAYS; TIME SPENT OUT OF TEXAS DOES NOT COUNT TOWARD PROBATION; SHALL INFORM THE BOARD OF CHANGE OF ADDRESS WITHIN 10 DAYS OR IF HE LEAVES THE STATE; SHALL NOT SEEK MODIFICATION FOR ONE YEAR. ON 4/10/99 THE ORDER WAS MODIFIED DELETING THE REQUIREMENT THAT HE PARTICIPATE IN THE PHYSICIAN'S HEALTH AND REHABILITATION COMMITTEE'S RANDOM DRUG SCREENS PROGRAM AND REDUCING THE NUMBER OF APPEARANCES BEFORE THE BOARD FROM TWICE TO ONCE A YEAR; ALL OTHER PROVISIONS OF THE ORDER REMAIN IN FULL EFFECT UNTIL SUPERSEDED BY A SUBSEQUENT BOARD ORDER.

KINDRICK, JAMES W MD, LICENSE NUMBER 00H5181 OF ODESSA, TX, WAS DISCIPLINED BY TEXAS ON SEPTEMBER 28, 1990
DISCIPLINARY ACTION: 36-MONTH PROBATION; MONITORING OF PHYSICIAN PERFORMANCE

NOTES: MUST CONTINUE PSYCHIATRIC TREATMENT; CONFER WITH BOARD APPROVED LOCAL PHYSICIAN TO MONITOR OFFICE MEDICAL PRACTICE AND PROCEDURES; APPEAR BEFORE BOARD YEARLY.

KINDRICK, JAMES W MD, DATE OF BIRTH JUNE 21, 1958 OF FALLS CHURCH, VA, WAS DISCIPLINED BY VIRGINIA ON DECEMBER 4, 1990
DISCIPLINARY ACTION: LICENSE REVOCATION
OFFENSE: PROVIDING FALSE INFORMATION TO THE BOARD OR OTHER HEALTH AGENCY

NOTES: INTERN/RESIDENT LICENSE REVOKED FOR SUBMITTING A FALSE APPLICATION TO BOARD.

KINDRICK, JAMES W MD, DATE OF BIRTH JUNE 21, 1958, LICENSE NUMBER 0056108 OF ABILENE, TX, WAS DISCIPLINED BY OHIO ON FEBRUARY 13, 1991
DISCIPLINARY ACTION: LICENSE REVOCATION
OFFENSE: DISCIPLINARY ACTION BY ANOTHER STATE OR AGENCY

NOTES: SUSPENSION OF CLINICAL PRIVILEGES BY AIR FORCE; PRIOR DISCIPLINARY ACTION AGAINST LICENSE IN NEW JERSEY. PERMANENT REVOCATION.

KINDRICK, JAMES W MD, DATE OF BIRTH JUNE 21, 1958 OF 6200 WILSON BLVD #306, FALLS CHURCH, VA, WAS DISCIPLINED BY MEDICARE ON DECEMBER 4, 1991
DISCIPLINARY ACTION: EXCLUSION FROM THE MEDICARE AND/OR MEDICAID PROGRAM
OFFENSE: DISCIPLINARY ACTION BY ANOTHER STATE OR AGENCY

NOTES: LICENSE REVOCATION OR SUSPENSION.

KINDRICK, JAMES W MD, LICENSE NUMBER 00H5181 OF ROCKVILLE, MD, WAS DISCIPLINED BY TEXAS ON JANUARY 24, 1992
DISCIPLINARY ACTION: LICENSE REVOCATION
OFFENSE: DISCIPLINARY ACTION BY ANOTHER STATE OR AGENCY

NOTES: UNPROFESSIONAL OR DISHONORABLE CONDUCT LIKELY TO DECEIVE, DEFRAUD OR INJURE THE PUBLIC

KINDRICK, JAMES W MD, DATE OF BIRTH JUNE 21, 1958, WAS DISCIPLINED BY MARYLAND ON SEPTEMBER 7, 1993
DISCIPLINARY ACTION: DENIAL OF NEW LICENSE
OFFENSE: DISCIPLINARY ACTION BY ANOTHER STATE OR AGENCY

NOTES: ON 10/31/88 HE WAS DISCIPLINED BY THE AIR FORCE FOR INAPPROPRIATE PATIENT CARE; ON 6/15/90 WAS ASKED TO RESIGN FROM A FAMILY PRACTICE RESIDENCY IN TEXAS DUE TO MEDICAL REASONS AND SUBSEQUENTLY HAD HIS TEXAS LICENSE PLACED ON PROBATION; ON 12/4/90 HAD HIS LICENSE REVOKED IN VIRGINIA BASED ON THE TEXAS ACTION AND FALSE STATEMENTS ON HIS VIRGINIA LICENSE APPLICATION REGARDING PREVIOUS DISCIPLINE; ON 2/3/91 OHIO REVOKED HIS LICENSE BASED ON THE AIR FORCE AND TEXAS ACTIONS; IN HIS 7/91 APPLICATION IN MARYLAND DID NOT DISCLOSE THE OHIO AND TEXAS ACTIONS. AKA JAMEY LEE WEST.

KING, CLARENCE GORDON JR MD, LICENSE NUMBER 00E1883 OF SAN ANTONIO, TX, WAS DISCIPLINED BY TEXAS ON AUGUST 18, 1990
DISCIPLINARY ACTION: 60-MONTH RESTRICTION PLACED ON CONTROLLED SUBSTANCE LICENSE; MONITORING OF PHYSICIAN PERFORMANCE
OFFENSE: SUBSTANCE ABUSE

NOTES: STIPULATED ORDER. SHALL NOT POSSESS, ADMINISTER OR DISPENSE ANY SCHEDULE II OR II-N CONTROLLED SUBSTANCES BUT MAY ORDER SUCH TO BE ADMINISTERED BY STAFF MEMBER TO PATIENT IN HOSPITAL, HOSPITAL EMERGENCY ROOM, OR NURSING HOME. SHALL NOT ORDER TRIPLICATE PRESCRIPTION FORMS. SHALL NOT TREAT OR SERVE AS PHYSICIAN, DISPENSE, OR ADMINISTER CONTROLLED SUBSTANCES OR OTHER DRUGS THAT MAY BE SUBJECT TO ABUSE FOR ANY MEMBER OF IMMEDIATE FAMILY OR SELF, AND ADMINISTER TO SELF OR IMMEDIATE FAMILY ONLY SUCH DRUGS AS PRESCRIBED BY OTHER PHYSICIANS. MUST PARTICIPATE IN AA AND BEXAR COUNTY MEDICAL SOCIETY COMMITTEE ON PHYSICIAN HEALTH AND REHABILITATION, SUBMIT TO PSYCHIATRIC EVALUATION AND FOLLOW RECOMMENDATIONS, PROVIDE URINE OR BLOOD SAMPLES ON NO-NOTICE BASIS, NOT TREAT ANY PATIENT WHILE UNDER INFLUENCE OF CONTROLLED SUBSTANCE OR ALCOHOL, DISPOSE OF CONTROLLED SUBSTANCE SAMPLES IN POSSESSION AND NOT ACCEPT OR RECEIVE SUCH SAMPLES, SUBMIT HIMSELF FOR APPROPRIATE EXAMINATIONS AND SCREENINGS TO DETERMINE FREEDOM FROM DRUGS AND ALCOHOL, AND APPEAR BEFORE BOARD TWICE ANNUALLY. ON 4/15/94 ORDER TERMINATED.

KING, CLARENCE GORDON JR MD OF 1303 MCCULLOUGH SUITE 600, SAN ANTONIO, TX, WAS DISCIPLINED BY DEA ON NOVEMBER 9, 1995
DISCIPLINARY ACTION: SURRENDER OF CONTROLLED SUBSTANCE LICENSE
OFFENSE: PROFESSIONAL MISCONDUCT

NOTES: PLED GUILTY TO OBTAINING CONTROLLED SUBSTANCES BY FRAUD OR FORGERY.

KING, CLARENCE GORDON JR MD, LICENSE NUMBER 00E1883 OF

ATLANTA, GA, WAS DISCIPLINED BY TEXAS ON JANUARY 27, 1996
DISCIPLINARY ACTION: SURRENDER OF CONTROLLED SUBSTANCE LICENSE; LICENSE SUSPENSION
OFFENSE: SUBSTANCE ABUSE

NOTES: IN 4/95 THE BEXAR COUNTY MEDICAL SOCIETY PHYSICIAN REHABILITATION COMMITTEE INTERVENED ON HIM AND RECOMMENDED INPATIENT TREATMENT FOR HIS RELAPSE; ENTERED TREATMENT FOR OPIATE DEPENDENCY AND DEPRESSION; HE CONTINUES TO PARTICIPATE IN THE PROGRAM. SUSPENSION UNTIL HE APPEARS BEFORE THE BOARD AND PROVIDES SUFFICIENT EVIDENCE TO SHOW THAT HE IS PHYSICALLY, MENTALLY, AND OTHERWISE COMPETENT TO SAFELY PRACTICE MEDICINE INCLUDING AT A MINIMUM COMPLETE COPIES OF MEDICAL RECORDS AND REPORTS OF PSYCHOLOGICAL AND NEUROPSYCHIATRIC EVALUATIONS CONDUCTED BY A BOARD APPROVED PSYCHIATRIST. SHALL IMMEDIATELY SURRENDER TO THE APPROPRIATE AGENCY HIS DEA CONTROLLED SUBSTANCES REGISTRATION CERTIFICATE AND TEXAS CONTROLLED SUBSTANCE REGISTRATION CERTIFICATE; SHALL COOPERATE WITH THE BOARD IN VERIFYING COMPLIANCE INCLUDING PROVIDING COPIES OF MEDICAL RELEASES UPON REQUEST.

KING, CLARENCE GORDON JR MD, LICENSE NUMBER 00E1883, WAS DISCIPLINED BY TEXAS ON NOVEMBER 16, 1996
DISCIPLINARY ACTION: 120-MONTH PROBATION; RESTRICTION PLACED ON LICENSE
OFFENSE: SUBSTANCE ABUSE

NOTES: IN 4/96 HE VOLUNTARILY ENTERED A SUBSTANCE ABUSE TREATMENT PROGRAM AND WAS DIAGNOSED WITH OPIATE DEPENDENCY AND PERSONALITY DISORDER WITH NARCISSISTIC AND HISTRIONIC TRAITS; HIS PHYSICIAN RECOMMENDS THAT HE BE ALLOWED TO RETURN TO THE PRACTICE OF MEDICINE, OUTSIDE OF ADDICTION MEDICINE, AND THAT HIS PRACTICE BE LIMITED TO NO MORE THAN 40 HOURS PER WEEK AT AN INSTITUTIONAL SETTING; REPORTS ACTIVITY IN AA'S 12-STEP PROGRAM AND TREATMENT BY A PSYCHIATRIST FOR DEPRESSION WITH ZOLOFT; REPORTS A SOBRIETY DATE OF 4/13/95 DOCUMENTED BY RANDOM DRUG SCREENS BY THE COUNTY MEDICAL SOCIETY. 1/27/96 SUSPENSION STAYED TO PROBATION WITH TERMS AND CONDITIONS: SHALL LIMIT HIS PRACTICE TO A HOSPITAL OR INSTITUTIONAL SETTING APPROVED BY THE BOARD; SHALL NOT PRACTICE FOR MORE THAN 40 HOURS PER WEEK; SHALL NOT PRACTICE ADDICTION MEDICINE; SHALL ABSTAIN FROM THE CONSUMPTION OF DRUGS/ALCOHOL IN ANY FORM UNLESS PRESCRIBED BY ANOTHER PHYSICIAN FOR A LEGITIMATE AND THERAPEUTIC PURPOSE; SHALL SUBMIT HIMSELF FOR APPROPRIATE EXAMS INCLUDING DRUG OR ALCOHOL SCREENS; SHALL SUBMIT HIMSELF FOR EVALUATION AND TREATMENT BY A BOARD-APPROVED PSYCHIATRIST WHOM HE SHALL SEE AT LEAST ONCE A MONTH AND WHO SHALL SUBMIT REPORTS TO THE BOARD; SHALL CONTINUE TO PARTICIPATE IN AA'S PROGRAM NOT LESS THAN THREE TIMES A WEEK WITH QUARTERLY REPORTS TO THE BOARD; SHALL PARTICIPATE IN THE ACTIVITIES OF A PHYSICIAN'S HEALTH AND REHABILITATION GROUP AND ATTEND WEEKLY MEETINGS WITH QUARTERLY REPORTS; SHALL COMPLY WITH TERMS OF ANY CONTINUING CARE CONTRACT HE ENTERS INTO WITH QUARTERLY REPORTS; SHALL NOT POSSESS ALCOHOL, CONTROLLED SUBSTANCES OR DANGEROUS DRUGS WITH ADDICTIVE POTENTIAL OR POTENTIAL FOR ABUSE AND SHALL SURRENDER ALL SUCH DRUGS INCLUDING SAMPLES; SHALL NOT TREAT OR OTHERWISE SERVE AS PHYSICIAN, PRESCRIBE, DISPENSE OR ADMINISTER DRUGS THAT MAY BE SUBJECT TO ABUSE TO HIMSELF OR TO ANY MEMBER OF HIS FAMILY; SHALL NOT TELEPHONE TO A PHARMACY A PRESCRIPTION OR REFILL FOR THESE SUBSTANCES AND SHALL NOT PERMIT ANYONE UNDER HIS SUPERVISION TO DO SO; SHALL SURRENDER HIS DEA/DPS CONTROLLED SUBSTANCES REGISTRATION CERTIFICATES AND SHALL NOT ATTEMPT TO REREGISTER WITHOUT AUTHORITY FROM THE BOARD; SHALL SURRENDER ALL UNUSED TRIPLICATE PRESCRIPTION FORMS AND SHALL NOT ATTEMPT TO ORDER MORE; SHALL MAINTAIN A FILE WITH COPIES OF EVERY PRESCRIPTION WRITTEN FOR DANGEROUS DRUGS WITH ADDICTIVE POTENTIAL OR POTENTIAL FOR ABUSE WHICH SHALL BE AVAILABLE FOR REVIEW; HIS PRACTICE INCLUDING ANY OFFICE AND SURGICAL PRACTICE; SHALL BE MONITORED BY A BOARD-APPROVED TEXAS PHYSICIAN WHO SHALL SUBMIT QUARTERLY REPORTS TO THE BOARD; SHALL MAINTAIN ADEQUATE MEDICAL RECORDS WHICH SHALL BE AVAILABLE FOR REVIEW; SHALL OBTAIN AT LEAST 50 HOURS PER YEAR OF CONTINUING MEDICAL EDUCATION; SHALL APPEAR BEFORE BOARD AT LEAST TWO TIMES A YEAR; SHALL COOPERATE WITH BOARD IN VERIFYING COMPLIANCE INCLUDING PROVIDING ANY MEDICAL RELEASES UPON REQUEST; SHALL GIVE A COPY OF THIS ORDER TO ANY HEALTH CARE ENTITY WHERE HE HAS PRIVILEGES; SHALL PROVIDE A COPY OF THIS ORDER TO ANYONE REQUESTING IT WITHIN 10 DAYS; TIME SPENT OUT OF TEXAS DOES NOT COUNT TOWARD PROBATION; SHALL INFORM THE BOARD OF CHANGE OF ADDRESS WITHIN 10 DAYS OR IF HE LEAVES THE STATE. SHALL NOT SEEK MODIFICATION FOR ONE YEAR. ON 11/22/97 PETITION TO MODIFY ORDER GRANTED LIMITING HIS PRACTICE OF MEDICINE TO 200 HOURS PER CALENDAR MONTH. ON 10/24/98 ORDER MODIFIED TO ALLOW FOR QUARTERLY PSYCHIATRIC VISITS AND DELETION OF REQUIREMENT TO MONITOR HIS PRACTICE.

KING, DANIEL A MD OF 12622 WEST BUENA VISTA DRIVE, GALVESTON, TX, WAS DISCIPLINED BY DEA ON FEBRUARY 27, 1996
DISCIPLINARY ACTION: RESTRICTION PLACED ON CONTROLLED SUBSTANCE LICENSE
OFFENSE: PROFESSIONAL MISCONDUCT

NOTES: PAST CONTROLLED SUBSTANCE VIOLATIONS.

KING, DENNIS MAURICE MD, LICENSE NUMBER 00D7122 OF AUSTIN, TX, WAS DISCIPLINED BY TEXAS ON JANUARY 14, 1994
DISCIPLINARY ACTION: 60-MONTH PROBATION; MONITORING OF PHYSICIAN PERFORMANCE
OFFENSE: SUBSTANCE ABUSE

NOTES: HAS HAD ALCOHOL, MARIJUANA AND COCAINE PROBLEMS (INCLUDING IV COCAINE USAGE); TREATED IN GEORGIA; TREATING PHYSICIANS DO NOT RECOMMEND RE-ENTRY INTO MEDICAL PROFESSION. FIVE YEAR SUSPENSION STAYED. CONDITIONS OF PROBATION: PRIOR TO PRACTICING MEDICINE IN TEXAS SHALL APPEAR BEFORE BOARD AND DEMONSTRATE THAT HE IS PHYSICALLY, MENTALLY AND OTHERWISE COMPETENT TO PRACTICE AND OBTAIN APPROVAL AS TO ABILITY TO PRESCRIBE, DISPENSE OR ADMINISTER CONTROLLED SUBSTANCE DRUGS II-V; SHALL APPEAR BEFORE THE BOARD TWICE A YEAR; SHALL NOT TREAT OR OTHERWISE SERVE AS PHYSICIAN, PRESCRIBE, DISPENSE OR ADMINISTER DRUGS THAT MAY BE SUBJECT TO

ABUSE TO HIMSELF OR ANY MEMBER OF HIS FAMILY; SHALL ABSTAIN FROM THE CONSUMPTION OF ALCOHOL/CHEMICAL SUBSTANCES IN ANY FORM UNLESS PRESCRIBED BY ANOTHER PHYSICIAN FOR A LEGITIMATE AND THERAPEUTIC PURPOSE; SHALL PARTICIPATE IN ACTIVITIES OF A PHYSICIAN HEALTH AND REHABILITATION COMMITTEE AND ATTEND WEEKLY MEETINGS WITH QUARTERLY REPORTS; SHALL PARTICIPATE IN AA'S PROGRAM NOT LESS THAN THREE TIMES A WEEK WITH QUARTERLY REPORTS TO THE BOARD; SHALL SUBMIT HIMSELF FOR APPROPRIATE EXAMS INCLUDING DRUG OR ALCOHOL SCREENS; SHALL CONTINUE TREATMENT WITH SPECIFIED PHYSICIAN WITH QUARTERLY REPORTS; SHALL GIVE A COPY OF THIS ORDER TO ANY HEALTH CARE ENTITY WHERE HE HAS PRIVILEGES; SHALL COOPERATE WITH THE BOARD IN VERIFYING COMPLIANCE; SHALL INFORM BOARD OF CHANGE OF ADDRESS WITHIN 10 DAYS OR IF HE LEAVES THE STATE; TIME SPENT OUT OF TEXAS DOES NOT COUNT TOWARD PROBATION. SHALL NOT SEEK MODIFICATION FOR ONE YEAR.

KING, DENNIS MAURICE MD, LICENSE NUMBER 00D7122 OF AUSTIN, TX, WAS DISCIPLINED BY TEXAS ON MARCH 4, 1995
DISCIPLINARY ACTION: LICENSE SUSPENSION
OFFENSE: FAILURE TO COMPLY WITH PREVIOUS BOARD ORDER

NOTES: FAILED TO COMPLY WITH 1/14/94 BOARD ORDER IN THAT IN 10/94, HE INGESTED COCAINE AND ON 2/26/95 HE INGESTED MARIJUANA; HE SELF-REPORTED INGESTION OF COCAINE AND MARIJUANA TO THE BOARD ON 2/27/95. SUSPENSION UNTIL HE REQUESTS TO HAVE SUSPENSION STAYED OR LIFTED AND APPEARS BEFORE THE BOARD AND PROVIDES SUFFICIENT EVIDENCE WHICH ADEQUATELY INDICATES THAT HE IS PHYSICALLY, MENTALLY AND OTHERWISE COMPETENT TO SAFELY PRACTICE MEDICINE INCLUDING AT A MINIMUM COPIES OF MEDICAL RECORDS AND REPORTS OF PSYCHOLOGICAL AND NEUROPSYCHIATRIC EVALUATIONS, INCLUDING A 96-HOUR INPATIENT EVALUATION, CONDUCTED BY A BOARD-CERTIFIED PSYCHIATRIST WHO SHALL PROVIDE REPORTS.

KING, DENNIS MAURICE MD, LICENSE NUMBER D7122, WAS DISCIPLINED BY TEXAS ON FEBRUARY 7, 1998
DISCIPLINARY ACTION: 120-MONTH PROBATION; RESTRICTION PLACED ON LICENSE
OFFENSE: FAILURE TO COMPLY WITH PREVIOUS BOARD ORDER

NOTES: HAS BEEN DIAGNOSED WITH POLYDRUG DEPENDENCE (ALCOHOL, MARIJUANA, HALLUCINOGENS, LSD AND COCAINE), MAJOR DEPRESSION (RECURRENT), AND GENERALIZED ANXIETY DISORDER; IN 1992 TREATED AT A RECOVERY CENTER FOR 7 MONTHS; RELAPSED IN 1994 AND WENT BACK INTO TREATMENT FOR A MONTH; ON 2/27/95 SELF-REPORTED THAT HE INGESTED COCAINE AND MARIJUANA, VIOLATING THE 1/14/94 BOARD ORDER; ON 3/4/95 LICENSE WAS SUSPENDED; ON 4/29/97 SUBMITTED HIMSELF TO A TREATMENT CENTER FOR AN OUTPATIENT EVALUATION; CURRENTLY UNDER PSYCHIATRIC CARE FOR MAJOR DEPRESSION, RECURRENT WITH PSYCHOSIS, MILD TO MODERATE ATTENTION DEFICIT DISORDER, AND MIXED CHEMICAL DEPENDENCY. SUSPENSION STAYED FOR PROBATION WITH THE FOLLOWING TERMS: SHALL BE LIMITED TO THE PRACTICE OF PSYCHIATRIC MEDICINE, BUT SHALL NOT INCLUDE THE PRACTICE OF ELECTROCONVULSIVE THERAPY; SHALL LIMIT PRACTICE TO A GROUP OR BOARD-APPROVED INSTITUTIONAL SETTING; AS AN ALTERNATIVE, HIS MEDICAL PRACTICE SHALL BE MONITORED BY A BOARD APPROVED TEXAS PHYSICIAN WHO SHALL PROVIDE QUARTERLY REPORTS TO THE BOARD; SHALL ABSTAIN FROM THE CONSUMPTION OF ALCOHOL/DRUGS IN ANY FORM UNLESS PRESCRIBED BY ANOTHER PHYSICIAN FOR A LEGITIMATE AND THERAPEUTIC PURPOSE; SHALL SUBMIT HIMSELF FOR APPROPRIATE EXAMS INCLUDING DRUG OR ALCOHOL SCREENS; SHALL CONTINUE PSYCHIATRIC TREATMENT NO LESS THAN ONCE A MONTH WITH QUARTERLY REPORTS TO THE BOARD; SHALL PARTICIPATE IN THE ACTIVITIES OF A PHYSICIAN HEALTH AND REHABILITATION COMMITTEE AND ATTEND WEEKLY MEETINGS WITH QUARTERLY REPORTS; SHALL PARTICIPATE IN AA'S PROGRAM NOT LESS THAN THREE TIMES A WEEK; SHALL REPORT ON HIS ATTENDANCE; SHALL NOT TREAT OR OTHERWISE SERVE AS PHYSICIAN, PRESCRIBE, DISPENSE OR ADMINISTER DRUGS THAT MAY BE SUBJECT TO ABUSE TO HIMSELF OR TO ANY MEMBER OF HIS FAMILY; SHALL COOPERATE WITH THE BOARD IN VERIFYING COMPLIANCE; SHALL OBTAIN 50 HOURS PER YEAR OF CONTINUING MEDICAL EDUCATION; SHALL APPEAR BEFORE THE BOARD ONCE A YEAR; SHALL GIVE A COPY OF THIS ORDER TO ANY HEALTH CARE ENTITY WHERE HE HAS PRIVILEGES; TIME SPENT OUT OF TEXAS DOES NOT COUNT TOWARD PROBATION; SHALL INFORM THE BOARD OF CHANGE OF ADDRESS WITHIN 10 DAYS OR IF HE LEAVES THE STATE; SHALL NOT SEEK MODIFICATION FOR ONE YEAR.

KING, LEWIS R MD, DATE OF BIRTH SEPTEMBER 9, 1961 OF 3810 INWOOD ROAD, APT 107, DALLAS, TX, WAS DISCIPLINED BY MEDICARE ON JULY 6, 1995
DISCIPLINARY ACTION: EXCLUSION FROM THE MEDICARE AND/OR MEDICAID PROGRAM
OFFENSE: NONCOMPLIANCE WITH A PROFESSIONAL RULE

NOTES: DEFAULTED ON PUBLIC HEALTH SERVICE EDUCATION LOAN. REINSTATED ON 9/29/95.

KINNARD, PAUL MD, LICENSE NUMBER D3911 OF WICHITA FALLS, TX, WAS DISCIPLINED BY TEXAS ON AUGUST 22, 1998
DISCIPLINARY ACTION: FINE
OFFENSE: LOSS OR RESTRICTION OF HOSPITAL PRIVILEGES

NOTES: IN 1993 HIS PRIVILEGES WERE SUMMARILY SUSPENDED AT A HOSPITAL DUE TO PATIENT CARE, BUT IN 1994 PRIVILEGES WERE REINSTATED WITH RESTRICTIONS FOR A 6 MONTH PERIOD; IN OR ABOUT 6/94 THE RESTRICTIONS IMPOSED WERE LIFTED. $1,000 FINE.

KINZIE, DANIEL H IV MD, LICENSE NUMBER 0G11801 OF SAN ANTONIO, TX, WAS DISCIPLINED BY CALIFORNIA ON APRIL 28, 1995
DISCIPLINARY ACTION: REPRIMAND
OFFENSE: DISCIPLINARY ACTION BY ANOTHER STATE OR AGENCY

NOTES: DISCIPLINE BY TEXAS BOARD FOR FAILING TO PROPERLY SUPERVISE THE ACTIVITIES OF AN EMPLOYEE WHO HELD HIMSELF OUT AS A PHYSICIAN'S ASSISTANT WHEN HE WAS NOT REGISTERED AS SUCH.

KINZIE, DANIEL HARPINE IV MD, DATE OF BIRTH JULY 8, 1935, LICENSE NUMBER 00G8562 OF 6302 CYPRESS CREEK ROAD, SAN ANTONIO, TX, WAS DISCIPLINED BY TEXAS ON JANUARY 29, 1993
DISCIPLINARY ACTION: RESTRICTION PLACED ON LICENSE; REPRIMAND
OFFENSE: PROFESSIONAL MISCONDUCT

NOTES: FAILED TO SUPERVISE THE ACTIVITIES OF ONE OF HIS EMPLOYEES WHO REPRESENTED HIMSELF AS A PHYSICIAN'S ASSISTANT WHEN HE WAS NOT REGISTERED AS ONE; THIS PERSON ENGAGED IN THE EXAMINATION AND TREATMENT OF PATIENTS; DR. KINZIE WAS UNAWARE OF THIS DECEPTION OR THAT HE WAS ENGAGING IN THE TREATMENT OF PATIENTS. SHALL APPEAR BEFORE THE BOARD TWICE A YEAR; SHALL NOT SIGN ANY PATIENT RECORDS UNLESS HE HAS PERSONALLY SEEN AND EXAMINED THE PATIENT UNLESS IT IS CLEARLY SPELLED OUT IN THE CHART THAT HE DID NOT SEE THE PATIENT; SHALL ADEQUATELY SUPERVISE THE ACTIVITIES OF ALL HIS EMPLOYEES; SHALL PROVIDE BOARD WITH ANNUAL REPORTS REGARDING EMPLOYMENT DETAILS ON HIS EMPLOYEES, ASSOCIATES OR ANY PHYSICIANS WHO COVER FOR HIM; SHALL GIVE A COPY OF THIS ORDER TO ANY HEALTH CARE ENTITY WHERE HE HAS PRIVILEGES; SHALL COOPERATE WITH THE BOARD IN VERIFYING COMPLIANCE; SHALL INFORM BOARD OF ANY ADDRESS CHANGE WITHIN 10 DAYS; SHALL NOT SEEK MODIFICATION FOR ONE YEAR. ON 8/19/94 BASED ON HIS SUCCESSFULLY MEETING AND COMPLYING WITH ALL TERMS OF THE ORDER, THE ORDER WAS TERMINATED.

KIRKPATRICK, JAMES L MD, LICENSE NUMBER 00E2658 OF LUBBOCK, TX, WAS DISCIPLINED BY TEXAS ON MAY 15, 1996
DISCIPLINARY ACTION: 36-MONTH RESTRICTION PLACED ON CONTROLLED SUBSTANCE LICENSE; REPRIMAND
OFFENSE: SUBSTANDARD CARE, INCOMPETENCE OR NEGLIGENCE

NOTES: FOR APPROXIMATELY THE PAST FIVE YEARS, HE HAS PRESCRIBED LARGE AMOUNTS OF CONTROLLED SUBSTANCES AND DANGEROUS DRUGS TO FOUR OR MORE ADULT PATIENTS WITHOUT ADEQUATE MEDICAL EXAMS AND INDICATIONS; ON MULTIPLE OCCASIONS HE PRESCRIBED CONTROLLED SUBSTANCES, SUCH AS DARVOCET AND VALIUM, TO ONE PATIENT WHO HAD NOT PRESENTED TO HIM FOR ANY MEDICAL EVALUATION AND WITHOUT MEDICAL DOCUMENTATION TO SUPPORT THE EFFICACY OF THE PRESCRIPTIONS; HE DOCUMENTED THE PRESCRIPTIONS FOR ONE PATIENT IN ANOTHER PATIENT'S RECORD; FOR AT LEAST FOUR PATIENTS, HE FAILED TO KEEP ADEQUATE MEDICAL DOCUMENTATION AND FAILED TO ADEQUATELY DIAGNOSE, TREAT AND MANAGE THE PATIENTS' MEDICAL CONDITIONS; FOR ONE PATIENT, HE PRESCRIBED DESOXYN, AN AMPHETAMINE, FOR A CONDITION FOR WHICH THE DRUG WAS NOT MEDICALLY INDICATED AND FOR AN UNACCEPTABLE DURATION. RESTRICTION FOR THREE YEARS WITH TERMS AND CONDITIONS: SHALL NOT PRESCRIBE OR ADMINISTER ANY DRUG FOR ANY PATIENT UNLESS THE DRUG IS MEDICALLY INDICATED AND IS PRESCRIBED IN THERAPEUTIC DOSES; SHALL CONDUCT ADEQUATE FOLLOW-UP EXAMS TO DETERMINE WHETHER THE COURSE OF TREATMENT IS APPROPRIATE; SHALL NOT TELEPHONE TO A PHARMACY A PRESCRIPTION OR REFILL FOR CONTROLLED SUBSTANCES OR DANGEROUS DRUGS WITH ADDICTIVE POTENTIAL OR POTENTIAL FOR ABUSE AND SHALL NOT PERMIT ANYONE UNDER HIS SUPERVISION TO DO SO; SHALL IMMEDIATELY REQUEST MODIFICATION OF DEA/DPS CONTROLLED SUBSTANCES REGISTRATION CERTIFICATES TO ELIMINATE HIS AUTHORITY TO PRESCRIBE AND DISPENSE SCHEDULES II AND II-N AND SHALL NOT ATTEMPT TO REREGISTER WITHOUT AUTHORITY FROM THE BOARD; SHALL MAINTAIN A LOG OF ALL PRESCRIPTIONS WRITTEN FOR CONTROLLED SUBSTANCES OR DANGEROUS DRUGS WITH ADDICTIVE POTENTIAL OR POTENTIAL FOR ABUSE WHICH SHALL BE AVAILABLE FOR REVIEW; SHALL MAINTAIN ADEQUATE MEDICAL RECORDS WHICH SHALL BE AVAILABLE FOR REVIEW; SHALL ENROLL IN AND SUCCESSFULLY COMPLETE A BOARD-APPROVED PHARMACOLOGY COURSE AND A COURSE IN EITHER RISK MANAGEMENT OR MEDICAL RECORDS DOCUMENTATION WITHIN ONE YEAR; SHALL OBTAIN AT LEAST 50 HOURS OF CONTINUING MEDICAL EDUCATION; PRIOR TO PRESCRIBING MEDICATION FOR THE TREATMENT OF PAIN, HE SHALL CONDUCT A THOROUGH PHYSICAL EXAMINATION, SHALL PROVIDE THE PATIENT WITH A DETAILED PLAN OF TREATMENT WITH EXPLANATION AND SHALL DISCUSS THE RISKS AND BENEFITS OF THE PLAN WITH THE PATIENT; SHALL COOPERATE WITH THE BOARD IN VERIFYING COMPLIANCE INCLUDING PROVIDING COPIES OF PEER REVIEW RECORDS UPON REQUEST; SHALL GIVE A COPY OF THIS ORDER TO ANY HEALTH CARE ENTITY WHERE HE HAS PRIVILEGES; SHALL PROVIDE A COPY OF THIS ORDER TO ANYONE REQUESTING IT WITHIN 10 DAYS; SHALL APPEAR BEFORE BOARD AT LEAST TWO TIMES PER YEAR OR AT BOARD REQUEST; TIME SPENT OUT OF TEXAS DOES NOT COUNT TOWARD PROBATION; SHALL INFORM BOARD OF CHANGE OF ADDRESS WITHIN 10 DAYS OR IF HE LEAVES THE STATE. SHALL NOT SEEK MODIFICATION FOR ONE YEAR. ON 10/24/98 ORDER TERMINATED.

KIRLIN, PATRICK JOSEPH DO, LICENSE NUMBER 00C9448 OF GRAND PRAIRIE, TX, WAS DISCIPLINED BY TEXAS ON NOVEMBER 19, 1993
DISCIPLINARY ACTION: REPRIMAND
OFFENSE: NONCOMPLIANCE WITH A PROFESSIONAL RULE

NOTES: FAILED TO ADEQUATELY DOCUMENT THE EXAMINATION OF A PATIENT WHO IS ALSO ONE OF HIS EMPLOYEES. SHALL GIVE A COPY OF THIS ORDER TO ALL HEALTH CARE ENTITIES WHERE HE HAS PRIVILEGES.

KLAVON, AZIZ A MD, LICENSE NUMBER J4879 OF GRAPEVINE, TX, WAS DISCIPLINED BY TEXAS ON AUGUST 22, 1998
DISCIPLINARY ACTION: REPRIMAND; REQUIRED TO TAKE ADDITIONAL MEDICAL EDUCATION
OFFENSE: LOSS OR RESTRICTION OF HOSPITAL PRIVILEGES

NOTES: IRVING HEALTHCARE SYSTEMS RENEWED BUT RESTRICTED, WITH A QUALITY IMPROVEMENT PLAN, HIS HOSPITAL PRIVILEGES BASED UPON 2 CASES FOLLOWING A REVIEW OF 881 OF HIS PATIENT CHARTS: THE FIRST PATIENT WAS ADMITTED WITH PNEUMONIA AND SEPSIS; HE WAS UNABLE TO INTUBATE THE PATIENT WITHIN 2 ATTEMPTS AND THE PATIENT WAS SUCCESSFULLY INTUBATED ON THE THIRD ATTEMPT BY A COLLEAGUE FROM THE EMERGENCY ROOM; THE SECOND PATIENT WAS ADMITTED AFTER SUFFERING AN IRREVERSIBLE BRAIN HEMORRHAGE; FOLLOWING INTUBATION BY AN EMERGENCY ROOM PHYSICIAN, A NEUROSURGEON DEEMED THE PATIENT INOPERABLE; HE FOLLOWED THE PATIENT WITH PULSE-OXIMETRY WHILE WEANING HER DOWN ON THE VENTILATOR SETTINGS; HE STATES THAT HE DID NOT MONITOR THE PATIENT WITH A RADIAL ARTERIAL LINE BECAUSE HE HAD BEEN RESTRICTED FROM PERFORMING SUCH PROCEDURES DUE TO HIS CARE AND TREATMENT OF THE PREVIOUSLY MENTIONED PATIENT; HIS CARE AND TREATMENT DID NOT CONFORM TO THE INTENSIVE CARE UNIT'S STANDARD CRITERIA FOR WEANING A PATIENT OFF OF VENTILATOR SETTING, NOR DID HE SEEK ASSISTANCE FROM A COLLEAGUE SO THAT THE GASES COULD BE MONITORED IN ACCORDANCE WITH THE POLICY. LICENSE LIMITED

FOR THREE YEARS AS FOLLOWS: SHALL COMPLY WITH ANY RESTRICTIONS PLACED UPON HIM BY ANY HOSPITAL AT WHICH HE HOLDS PRIVILEGES; HIS INVASIVE PROCEDURES SHALL BE MONITORED BY A BOARD APPROVED TEXAS PHYSICIAN WHO SHALL PROVIDE QUARTERLY REPORTS TO THE BOARD; SHALL OBTAIN 50 HOURS PER YEAR OF CONTINUING MEDICAL EDUCATION, WITH AT LEAST 1 COURSE IN PHARMACOLOGY FOR EACH OF THE 5 YEARS; SHALL APPEAR BEFORE THE BOARD ONCE A YEAR; SHALL COOPERATE WITH THE BOARD IN VERIFYING COMPLIANCE; SHALL GIVE A COPY OF THIS ORDER TO ANY HEALTH CARE ENTITY WHERE HE HAS PRIVILEGES; TIME SPENT OUT OF TEXAS DOES NOT COUNT TOWARD RESTRICTION; SHALL INFORM THE BOARD OF CHANGE OF ADDRESS WITHIN 10 DAYS OR IF HE LEAVES THE STATE.

KNIGHT, KYLER SCOTT MD, LICENSE NUMBER J6005 OF PASADENA, TX, WAS DISCIPLINED BY TEXAS ON APRIL 10, 1999
DISCIPLINARY ACTION: REQUIRED TO TAKE ADDITIONAL MEDICAL EDUCATION; MONITORING OF PHYSICIAN PERFORMANCE
OFFENSE: PROFESSIONAL MISCONDUCT

NOTES: IN 11/96 HE ENGAGED IN UNPROFESSIONAL CONDUCT IN HIS USING INAPPROPRIATE LANGUAGE WITH A PATIENT AND A PATIENT'S FAMILY; HE EXPRESSLY DENIES WRONG DOING. LICENSE LIMITED FOR THREE YEARS AS FOLLOWS: SHALL NOMINATE THREE CERTIFIED PSYCHIATRISTS FOR BOARD SELECTION OF A THERAPIST AND SHALL EXPEDITIOUSLY SUBMIT HIMSELF TO EVALUATION AND TREATMENT BY THE APPROVED PRACTITIONER; SHALL OBTAIN 10 HOURS OF AN ETHICS COURSE PER YEAR FOR 3 YEARS; SHALL APPEAR BEFORE THE BOARD AT LEAST ONCE A YEAR; SHALL COOPERATE WITH THE BOARD IN VERIFYING COMPLIANCE INCLUDING PROVIDING COPIES OF MEDICAL RELEASES UPON REQUEST; TIME SPENT OUT OF TEXAS DOES NOT COUNT TOWARD RESTRICTION; SHALL INFORM THE BOARD OF CHANGE OF ADDRESS WITHIN 10 DAYS OR IF HE LEAVES THE STATE; SHALL NOT SEEK MODIFICATION FOR ONE YEAR.

KNIGHT, PATRICK L MD, LICENSE NUMBER 00E7638 OF PHOENIX, AZ, WAS DISCIPLINED BY TEXAS ON AUGUST 18, 1990
OFFENSE: DISCIPLINARY ACTION BY ANOTHER STATE OR AGENCY

NOTES: STIPULATED ORDER. MUST COMPLY WITH ARIZONA BOARD ORDER, OBTAIN PERMISSION OF BOARD BEFORE PRACTICING IN TEXAS, AND FOLLOW SUCH TERM AS MAY BE IMPOSED.

KODSY, RAOUF ABDALLAH TWEFIK DR, DATE OF BIRTH DECEMBER 19, 1955 OF 12126 CARRIAGE HILL, HOUSTON, TX, WAS DISCIPLINED BY IOWA ON APRIL 29, 1993
DISCIPLINARY ACTION: DENIAL OF NEW LICENSE
OFFENSE: PROVIDING FALSE INFORMATION TO THE BOARD OR OTHER HEALTH AGENCY

NOTES: BASED ON FALSIFIED MEDICAL APPLICATION. PERMANENT MEDICAL LICENSE DENIED.

KODSY, RAOUF ABDALLAH MD, LICENSE NUMBER 00E0029 OF ONEIDA CASTLE, NY, WAS DISCIPLINED BY ARKANSAS ON SEPTEMBER 1, 1996
DISCIPLINARY ACTION: LICENSE REVOCATION

KOMER, ROBERT A DO, LICENSE NUMBER 1005414, WAS DISCIPLINED BY MICHIGAN ON JUNE 7, 1990
DISCIPLINARY ACTION: LICENSE REVOCATION

KOMER, ROBERT A DO, DATE OF BIRTH NOVEMBER 30, 1938 OF 12600 MELVILLE, APT 219, MONTGOMERY, TX, WAS DISCIPLINED BY MEDICARE ON OCTOBER 1, 1990
DISCIPLINARY ACTION: EXCLUSION FROM THE MEDICARE AND/OR MEDICAID PROGRAM
OFFENSE: DISCIPLINARY ACTION BY ANOTHER STATE OR AGENCY

NOTES: LICENSE REVOCATION OR SUSPENSION. REINSTATED ON 2/26/99.

KOMER, ROBERT A DO, LICENSE NUMBER 20A3725 OF SAGINAW, MI, WAS DISCIPLINED BY CALIFORNIA ON SEPTEMBER 21, 1991
DISCIPLINARY ACTION: LICENSE REVOCATION
OFFENSE: DISCIPLINARY ACTION BY ANOTHER STATE OR AGENCY

NOTES: ACTION TAKEN BY ANOTHER STATE FOR ENGAGING IN LEWD CONDUCTS.

KOMER, ROBERT A DO OF MONTGOMERY, TX, WAS DISCIPLINED BY MISSOURI ON FEBRUARY 11, 1993
DISCIPLINARY ACTION: LICENSE REVOCATION
OFFENSE: DISCIPLINARY ACTION BY ANOTHER STATE OR AGENCY

NOTES: SEX ABUSE AND PRESCRIPTION VIOLATION. NO REINSTATEMENT OF LICENSE FOR SEVEN YEARS.

KOMER, ROBERT A DO OF SAGINAW, MI, WAS DISCIPLINED BY IOWA ON DECEMBER 4, 1995
DISCIPLINARY ACTION: LICENSE REVOCATION
OFFENSE: DISCIPLINARY ACTION BY ANOTHER STATE OR AGENCY

NOTES: MICHIGAN LICENSE REVOKED BASED UPON ALLEGATIONS WHICH INCLUDED THAT HE HAD ENGAGED IN SEXUAL ACTS WITH SIX PATIENTS. PERMANENT REVOCATION.

KOMER, ROBERT ALLAN DO, LICENSE NUMBER 00E5553 OF HUNTSVILLE, TX, WAS DISCIPLINED BY TEXAS ON JANUARY 12, 1991
DISCIPLINARY ACTION: 36-MONTH PROBATION; MONITORING OF PHYSICIAN PERFORMANCE
OFFENSE: DISCIPLINARY ACTION BY ANOTHER STATE OR AGENCY

NOTES: MICHIGAN MEDICAL LICENSE SUMMARILY SUSPENDED BY THE MICHIGAN BOARD. CONTINUED TREATMENT BY A SPECIFIC PSYCHIATRIST FOR NO LESS THAN THREE YEARS, WITH REGULAR REPORTS FROM THAT PSYCHIATRIST.

KOMER, ROBERT ALLAN DO, DATE OF BIRTH NOVEMBER 30, 1938, LICENSE NUMBER 0002512 OF 12600 MELVILLE #219, MONTGOMERY, TX, WAS DISCIPLINED BY OHIO ON JANUARY 13, 1992
DISCIPLINARY ACTION: LICENSE REVOCATION
OFFENSE: DISCIPLINARY ACTION BY ANOTHER STATE OR AGENCY

NOTES: MICHIGAN DISCIPLINARY ACTION FOR INAPPROPRIATE SEXUAL ACTIVITIES WITH PATIENTS AND IMPROPER PRESCRIBING PRACTICES; FRAUD, MISREPRESENTATION, OR DECEPTION IN RENEWING OHIO LICENSE. PERMANENT REVOCATION.

KOMER, ROBERT ALLAN DO, LICENSE NUMBER 00R2435 OF PO BOX 485, MONTGOMERY, TX, WAS DISCIPLINED BY ARKANSAS ON DECEMBER 10, 1992
DISCIPLINARY ACTION: EMERGENCY SUSPENSION
OFFENSE: DISCIPLINARY ACTION BY ANOTHER STATE OR AGENCY

NOTES: MICHIGAN BOARD FOUND HIM IN VIOLATION DUE TO SEXUAL MISCONDUCT. INCOMPETENCY IN PRESCRIBING MEDICATIONS WITHOUT MEDICAL INDICATIONS. CALIFORNIA AND OHIO LICENSES

REVOKED FOR THESE REASONS.

KOMER, ROBERT ALLAN DO, LICENSE NUMBER 00R2435 OF PO BOX 485, MONTGOMERY, TX, WAS DISCIPLINED BY ARKANSAS ON MAY 19, 1993
DISCIPLINARY ACTION: LICENSE REVOCATION
OFFENSE: SEXUAL ABUSE OF OR SEXUAL MISCONDUCT WITH A PATIENT

NOTES: MICHIGAN LICENSE REVOKED FOR ADMINISTERING MEDICATION WITHOUT MEDICAL INDICATIONS AND BEING GUILTY OF SEXUAL MISCONDUCT WITH SIX PATIENTS. CALIFORNIA AND OHIO ALSO REVOKED HIS LICENSE BASED ON THE MICHIGAN ACTION.

KOMER, ROBERT ALLAN DO, LICENSE NUMBER 0003640 OF MONTGOMERY, TX, WAS DISCIPLINED BY FLORIDA ON OCTOBER 5, 1993
DISCIPLINARY ACTION: LICENSE REVOCATION
OFFENSE: DISCIPLINARY ACTION BY ANOTHER STATE OR AGENCY

KONDEJEWSKI, RICHARD JOSEPH MD, DATE OF BIRTH FEBRUARY 25, 1946, LICENSE NUMBER 00F0548 OF PO BOX 1608, LEAGUE CITY, TX, WAS DISCIPLINED BY TEXAS ON JANUARY 14, 1994
DISCIPLINARY ACTION: 60-MONTH PROBATION; RESTRICTION PLACED ON LICENSE
OFFENSE: PROFESSIONAL MISCONDUCT

NOTES: IN 1981 WHILE TREATING A PATIENT FOR WEIGHT LOSS HE MAINTAINED A PERSONAL RELATIONSHIP WITH HER THAT WAS NOT TERMINATED UNTIL 1984 INCLUDING ALLOWING HER TO STAY AT HIS HOME WITH HIS FAMILY; FAILING TO OBTAIN PROFESSIONAL PSYCHIATRIC CARE WHEN SHE OBVIOUSLY NEEDED IT; TRIED TO TREAT HER PSYCHIATRIC PROBLEMS WHEN HE WAS NOT QUALIFIED TO DO SO; PURCHASING ONE OR MORE GIFTS FOR HER; PATIENT ALLEGES THAT SHE HAD SEX WITH HIM ON AT LEAST TWO OCCASIONS AND WAS GIVEN SEXUALLY EXPLICIT MATERIAL TO READ; HE ACKNOWLEDGES POOR JUDGMENT BUT DENIES HAVING SEX WITH HER OR EXHIBITING ANY ROMANTIC OVERTURES. SUSPENSION STAYED. CONDITIONS OF PROBATION: SHALL COMPLETE SIX HOURS OF ETHICS COURSES EACH YEAR; SHALL SUBMIT HIMSELF TO A BOARD-APPROVED PSYCHIATRIST FOR EVALUATION AND FOLLOW RECOMMENDATIONS REGARDING CARE AND TREATMENT; SHALL GIVE PSYCHIATRIST A COPY OF THIS ORDER AND HAVE HIM SUBMIT REPORTS THREE TIMES A YEAR IN THE EVENT TREATMENT IS NECESSARY; SHALL APPEAR BEFORE THE BOARD TWICE A YEAR; SHALL REFRAIN FROM TREATING ANY PATIENTS FOR PSYCHIATRIC PROBLEMS AND DEPRESSION; SHALL NOT EXAMINE ANY FEMALE PATIENT WITHOUT A CHAPERONE IN EXAMINING ROOM AND SUCH PRESENCE WILL BE DOCUMENTED IN THE PATIENT'S RECORD; SHALL COOPERATE WITH THE BOARD IN VERIFYING COMPLIANCE; SHALL INFORM BOARD OF CHANGE OF ADDRESS WITHIN 10 DAYS OR IF HE LEAVES THE STATE; TIME SPENT OUT OF TEXAS DOES NOT COUNT TOWARD PROBATION. SHALL NOT SEEK MODIFICATION FOR ONE YEAR. ON 8/9/97 BOARD GRANTED HIS PETITION FOR TERMINATION OF THIS ORDER BASED ON COMPLIANCE WITH CONDITIONS.

KOPPERSMITH, DANIEL LEONCE MD, LICENSE NUMBER H3691 OF HOUSTON, TX, WAS DISCIPLINED BY TEXAS ON AUGUST 28, 1999
DISCIPLINARY ACTION: FINE; REPRIMAND
OFFENSE: PROFESSIONAL MISCONDUCT

NOTES: TOLD HIS PATIENT'S HUSBAND (ALSO A PATIENT) THAT SHE WAS SEEING SOMEONE OUT OF STATE; HE ADMITTED THAT HE VIOLATED HIS PATIENT'S CONFIDENTIALITY. WITHIN 90 DAYS SHALL TAKE AND PASS WITH A SCORE OF 75 OR ABOVE, WITHIN 3 ATTEMPTS, THE MEDICAL JURISPRUDENCE EXAM AND PAY A $5,000 FINE; TIME SPENT OUT OF TEXAS DOES NOT COUNT TOWARD RESTRICTION; SHALL INFORM THE BOARD OF CHANGE OF ADDRESS WITHIN 10 DAYS OR IF HE LEAVES THE STATE; SHALL NOT SEEK MODIFICATION FOR ONE YEAR.

KORMAN, DAVID JOEL MD, LICENSE NUMBER 00G5263 OF MESQUITE, TX, WAS DISCIPLINED BY TEXAS ON AUGUST 18, 1995
DISCIPLINARY ACTION: 60-MONTH RESTRICTION PLACED ON LICENSE; REPRIMAND
OFFENSE: SEXUAL ABUSE OF OR SEXUAL MISCONDUCT WITH A PATIENT

NOTES: FROM THE FALL OF 1990 UNTIL 12/90, ENGAGED IN A SEXUAL RELATIONSHIP WITH A PATIENT WHICH HE REPORTED TO THE BOARD IN 1/95; SUBSEQUENT TO THIS RELATIONSHIP HE BEGAN MAKING FINANCIAL PAYMENTS TO PATIENT; DUE TO RELATIONSHIP HE SUBMITTED HIMSELF TO PSYCHOTHERAPY IN 1994 AND HAS DISCONTINUED HIS PSYCHOTHERAPY OF PATIENTS. RESTRICTION WITH TERMS: SHALL NOT ENGAGE IN PSYCHOTHERAPY OF FEMALE PATIENTS EXCEPT FOR SHORT-TERM ACUTE CARE IN A HOSPITAL SETTING; WITHIN ONE YEAR SHALL OBTAIN SIX HOURS OF ETHICS THROUGH BOARD-APPROVED COURSES OR PROGRAMS; SHALL SUBMIT HIMSELF FOR EVALUATION AND TREATMENT BY A BOARD-APPROVED PSYCHIATRIST WHOM HE SHALL SEE AT LEAST ONCE A MONTH AND WHO SHALL SUBMIT REPORTS TO THE BOARD; SHALL APPEAR BEFORE BOARD AT LEAST ONCE A YEAR OR AT BOARD REQUEST; SHALL COOPERATE WITH BOARD IN VERIFYING COMPLIANCE INCLUDING PROVIDING COPIES OF MEDICAL RELEASES OR PEER REVIEW RECORDS UPON REQUEST; SHALL GIVE A COPY OF THIS ORDER TO ANY HEALTH CARE ENTITY WHERE HE HAS PRIVILEGES; SHALL PROVIDE A COPY OF THIS ORDER TO ANYONE REQUESTING IT WITHIN 10 DAYS; TIME PERIOD OUT OF TEXAS WILL NOT COUNT TOWARD PROBATION; SHALL INFORM BOARD OF CHANGE OF ADDRESS WITHIN 10 DAYS OR IF HE LEAVES THE STATE. SHALL NOT SEEK MODIFICATION FOR ONE YEAR. ON 8/17/96 REQUEST FOR TERMINATION OF ORDER DENIED. ON 9/20/97 THE BOARD GRANTED HIS PETITION FOR TERMINATION OF THIS ORDER BASED ON COMPLIANCE WITH CONDITIONS.

KOROMPAI, FERENC L MD, LICENSE NUMBER 00D0936 OF PECS, HU, WAS DISCIPLINED BY TEXAS ON JANUARY 6, 1995
DISCIPLINARY ACTION: FINE; 60-MONTH RESTRICTION PLACED ON LICENSE
OFFENSE: SUBSTANDARD CARE, INCOMPETENCE OR NEGLIGENCE

NOTES: ON 7/19/91 REMOVED WHAT HE THOUGHT WAS A PATIENT'S NON-FUNCTIONING KIDNEY ALTHOUGH HE DID NOT OBTAIN CONSENT TO REMOVE IT UNDER THE BELIEF THAT IT WAS A POTENTIAL SOURCE OF INCREASED BLOOD PRESSURE; REMOVED THE SOLE FUNCTIONING KIDNEY INSTEAD; AGREED TO THIS ORDER IN LIEU OF FURTHER INVESTIGATION. CONDITIONS OF FIVE YEAR RESTRICTION: SHALL ATTEND AT LEAST 50 HOURS PER YEAR OF CONTINUING MEDICAL EDUCATION INCLUDING AT LEAST 10 HOURS IN RISK MANAGEMENT AND 25 IN CARDIOVASCULAR SURGERY; SHALL MAINTAIN ADEQUATE MEDICAL RECORDS ON ALL PATIENT OFFICE VISITS WHICH SHALL BE AVAILABLE FOR

INSPECTION; SHALL NOT SIGN ANY PATIENT RECORD UNLESS HE HAS PERSONALLY EXAMINED THE PATIENT OR CLEARLY NOTES IN THE RECORD THAT HE DID NOT; SHALL PAY $5,000 ADMINISTRATIVE PENALTY; SHALL PERFORM 75 HOURS PER YEAR OF COMMUNITY SERVICE; SHALL APPEAR BEFORE THE BOARD ONCE A YEAR OR UPON REQUEST; SHALL COOPERATE WITH THE BOARD IN VERIFYING COMPLIANCE; SHALL GIVE A COPY OF THIS ORDER TO ANY HEALTH CARE ENTITY WHERE HE HAS OR APPLIES FOR PRIVILEGES OR ANYONE WHO REQUESTS IT; SHALL ENSURE ANY INQUIRIES REGARDING HIS TEXAS LICENSURE STATUS ARE ANSWERED BY REFERENCING THIS ORDER; SHALL INFORM BOARD OF CHANGE OF ADDRESS WITHIN 10 DAYS OR IF HE LEAVES THE STATE; TIME SPENT OUT OF TEXAS DOES NOT COUNT TOWARD RESTRICTION. SHALL NOT SEEK MODIFICATION FOR ONE YEAR. PUBLIC REPRIMAND. ON 1/29/99 ORDER TERMINATED.

KOUSSAYER, TAREK MD, DATE OF BIRTH MARCH 27, 1961, LICENSE NUMBER 0054620 OF 1606 FALCON DRIVE, ABSECON, NJ, WAS DISCIPLINED BY NEW JERSEY ON MARCH 29, 1990
DISCIPLINARY ACTION: FINE; REPRIMAND
OFFENSE: PROVIDING FALSE INFORMATION TO THE BOARD OR OTHER HEALTH AGENCY

NOTES: PROVIDED FALSE INFORMATION ON LICENSURE APPLICATION. $500 PENALTY; REQUIRED TO SUCCESSFULLY COMPLETE A COURSE IN ETHICS WITHIN 1 YEAR.

KOUSSAYER, TAREK MD, DATE OF BIRTH MARCH 27, 1961, LICENSE NUMBER 0015824 OF 1606 FALCON DRIVE, ABSECON, NJ, WAS DISCIPLINED BY WEST VIRGINIA ON JULY 19, 1996
DISCIPLINARY ACTION: DENIAL OF NEW LICENSE
OFFENSE: PROVIDING FALSE INFORMATION TO THE BOARD OR OTHER HEALTH AGENCY

NOTES: HE WAS EJECTED FROM CALIFORNIA FLEX EXAM FOR EXAMINATION IRREGULARITIES; IN 1985 IN WEST VIRGINIA THEREAFTER ON SIX SUBMITTED APPLICATIONS FROM 1985 TO 1989 AND IN AN INTERVIEW WITH A BOARD MEMBER IN 1989 HE HAD SUBMITTED FALSE INFORMATION REGARDING THE CALIFORNIA INCIDENT; AFTER BEING QUESTIONED ABOUT THIS BY BOARD HE SURRENDERED WEST VIRGINIA LICENSE ON 2/15/91 AND WAS REPRIMANDED BY NEW JERSEY BOARD IN 1990 FOR PROVIDING FALSE INFORMATION WHICH HE LIED ABOUT IN A 10/23/94 APPLICATION.

KOUSSAYER, TAREK MD, DATE OF BIRTH MARCH 27, 1961, LICENSE NUMBER 043031E OF 4100 GREENBRIAR ROAD #119, HOUSTON, TX, WAS DISCIPLINED BY PENNSYLVANIA ON FEBRUARY 18, 1997
DISCIPLINARY ACTION: REPRIMAND
OFFENSE: DISCIPLINARY ACTION BY ANOTHER STATE OR AGENCY

NOTES: DISCIPLINARY ACTION TAKEN BY WEST VIRGINIA-DENIAL OF LICENSE.

KOVAL, ROBERT JOHN MD, LICENSE NUMBER G1694 OF DALLAS, TX, WAS DISCIPLINED BY TEXAS ON AUGUST 9, 1997
DISCIPLINARY ACTION: FINE; REQUIRED TO TAKE ADDITIONAL MEDICAL EDUCATION
OFFENSE: PROFESSIONAL MISCONDUCT

NOTES: ADMINISTERED A SCIENTIFICALLY UNPROVEN SMOKING CESSATION TREATMENT TO NUMEROUS ADULT PATIENTS WITHOUT OBTAINING ADEQUATE INFORMED CONSENT OR ADEQUATELY DOCUMENTING THE TREATMENT PROVIDED. HE FAILED TO ADEQUATELY DOCUMENT A HISTORY AND PHYSICAL EXAMINATION ON PATIENTS BEFORE ADMINISTERING THE TREATMENT OR TO DOCUMENT PROGRESS OF PATIENTS RECEIVING THE TREATMENT. HE BILLED PATIENTS FOR EXTENSIVE OFFICE VISITS WITHOUT ADEQUATELY DOCUMENTING THE NATURE OF THE EXTENDED OFFICE VISIT. HE HAS STATED HE WILL CEASE UTILIZING THE SMOKING CESSATION TREATMENT. CONDITIONS ON LICENSE FOR FIVE YEARS: SHALL MAINTAIN ADEQUATE MEDICAL RECORDS WHICH SHALL BE AVAILABLE FOR REVIEW; HE SHALL NOT UTILIZE ANY ACUPUNCTURE PRINCIPLES IN SMOKING CESSATION WITH HIS PRACTICE OR TREATMENT WHICH IS INCONSISTENT WITH PHYSICIAN GUIDELINES FOR MANAGING NICOTINE ADDICTION; SHALL PAY AN ADMINISTRATIVE PENALTY OF $2500; SHALL COOPERATE WITH THE BOARD IN VERIFYING COMPLIANCE; SHALL APPEAR BEFORE THE BOARD AT LEAST ANNUALLY; SHALL INFORM THE BOARD OF CHANGE OF ADDRESS WITHIN 10 DAYS OR IF HE LEAVES THE STATE; SHALL NOT SEEK MODIFICATION FOR ONE YEAR. ON 10/24/98 THE ORDER WAS MODIFIED DELETING THE REQUIREMENT TO TAKE A PHARMACOLOGY COURSE AS PART OF CONTINUING MEDICAL EDUCATION REQUIREMENT; ALL OTHER PROVISIONS OF THE ORDER REMAIN IN FULL EFFECT UNTIL SUPERSEDED BY A SUBSEQUENT BOARD ORDER. ON 10/15/99 THE ORDER WAS TERMINATED.

KRATZ, ARTHUR W DO, LICENSE NUMBER 0000526 OF DALLAS, TX, WAS DISCIPLINED BY OHIO ON APRIL 18, 1996
DISCIPLINARY ACTION: SURRENDER OF LICENSE

NOTES: PERMANENT VOLUNTARY SURRENDER OF LICENSE; HE IS INELIGIBLE FOR REINSTATEMENT IN FUTURE.

KRATZ, ARTHUR WILLIAM DO, LICENSE NUMBER 00C3950 OF DALLAS, TX, WAS DISCIPLINED BY TEXAS ON AUGUST 19, 1994
DISCIPLINARY ACTION: 60-MONTH RESTRICTION PLACED ON CONTROLLED SUBSTANCE LICENSE; REQUIRED TO TAKE ADDITIONAL MEDICAL EDUCATION
OFFENSE: DISCIPLINARY ACTION BY ANOTHER STATE OR AGENCY

NOTES: IN 9/92 SURRENDERED HIS DEA CONTROLLED SUBSTANCE CERTIFICATE IN THE FACE OF ALLEGATIONS THAT HE FAILED TO COMPLETELY ACCOUNT FOR 7,000 TABLETS OF ACETAMINOPHEN WITH CODEINE; IN 4/93 ENTERED INTO A MEMO OF UNDERSTANDING WITH DEA WHICH GRANTED HIM AUTHORITY TO PRESCRIBE ONLY SCHEDULE IV AND V CONTROLLED SUBSTANCES; THESE ACTIONS WERE IN LARGE PART PROMPTED BY HIS FAILURE TO COMPLETELY ACCOUNT FOR CONTROLLED SUBSTANCES WHICH WERE ORDERED BY HIS WIFE AND DISPENSED BY HER TO FAMILY MEMBERS; HE MAINTAINS HE WAS UNAWARE THAT HIS WIFE HAD BEEN DOING THIS; ENTERED INTO THIS AGREEMENT WITH DEA TO AVOID THE PURSUIT OF CRIMINAL CHARGES CONTEMPLATED WITH REGARD TO HIS WIFE. CONDITIONS OF FIVE YEAR RESTRICTION: SHALL REQUEST MODIFICATION OF DEA AND TEXAS CONTROLLED SUBSTANCES CERTIFICATES SUCH THAT HE CANNOT PRESCRIBE SCHEDULES II AND III AND SHALL NOT SEEK REREGISTRATION WITHOUT PERMISSION; SHALL SURRENDER ALL UNUSED TRIPLICATE PRESCRIPTION FORMS; SEPARATE FROM PATIENT RECORDS SHALL MAINTAIN A FILE OF EVERY PRESCRIPTION WRITTEN FOR CONTROLLED SUBSTANCES OR DANGEROUS DRUGS WHICH SHALL BE AVAILABLE FOR INSPECTION; SHALL NOT TELEPHONE ANY PRESCRIPTION TO A PHARMACY FOR CONTROLLED SUBSTANCES OR DANGEROUS DRUGS; SHALL NOT EMPLOY HIS WIFE AS A MEMBER

OF HIS MEDICAL STAFF; SHALL NOT PRESCRIBE, ADMINISTER OR DISPENSE DRUGS THAT MAY BE SUBJECT TO ABUSE TO HIMSELF OR ANY MEMBER OF HIS FAMILY; SHALL ATTEND AT LEAST 50 HOURS PER YEAR OF CONTINUING MEDICAL EDUCATION; SHALL GIVE A COPY OF THIS ORDER TO ANY HEALTH CARE ENTITY WHERE HE HAS PRIVILEGES; SHALL COOPERATE WITH THE BOARD IN VERIFYING COMPLIANCE; SHALL INFORM BOARD OF CHANGE OF ADDRESS WITHIN 10 DAYS OR IF HE LEAVES THE STATE; TIME SPENT OUT OF TEXAS DOES NOT COUNT TOWARD RESTRICTION. SHALL NOT SEEK MODIFICATION FOR ONE YEAR. ON 11/22/97 PETITION TO TERMINATE ORDER DENIED.

KRATZ, ARTHUR WILLIAM DO OF 7203 WEST LAKE, DALLAS, TX, WAS DISCIPLINED BY DEA ON MARCH 29, 1996
DISCIPLINARY ACTION: RESTRICTION PLACED ON CONTROLLED SUBSTANCE LICENSE
OFFENSE: PROFESSIONAL MISCONDUCT

NOTES: EXCESSIVE PURCHASES.

KRAUS, VERNON J MD, DATE OF BIRTH SEPTEMBER 25, 1940, LICENSE NUMBER 00D8747 OF FORT WORTH, TX, WAS DISCIPLINED BY TEXAS ON APRIL 21, 1990
DISCIPLINARY ACTION: REQUIRED TO ENTER AN IMPAIRED PHYSICIAN PROGRAM OR SUBSTANCE ABUSE TREATMENT; MONITORING OF PHYSICIAN PERFORMANCE
OFFENSE: SUBSTANCE ABUSE

NOTES: STIPULATED ORDER. MUST SUBMIT TO TESTS TO DETERMINE PRESENCE OF DRUGS OR ALCOHOL (CONSISTENT WITH HIS AFTERCARE AGREEMENT REQUIREMENTS), CONTINUE ATTENDING IMPAIRED PHYSICIAN COMMITTEE MEETINGS AND AA OR NARCOTICS ANONYMOUS MEETINGS, HAVE CONTACT WITH TARRANT COUNTY MEDICAL SOCIETY'S PHYSICIAN HEALTH AND REHABILITATION COMMITTEE, MEET WITH SPECIFIC PHYSICIAN AS PART OF HIS CONTINUED REHABILITATION PROGRAM, AND APPEAR BEFORE BOARD ANNUALLY. RESTRICTIONS MODIFIED EFFECTIVE 6/17/92. RESTRICTIONS ON LICENSE TERMINATED EFFECTIVE 4/30/93.

KRAUS, VERNON J MD, LICENSE NUMBER 0C29717 OF FORT WORTH, TX, WAS DISCIPLINED BY CALIFORNIA ON SEPTEMBER 11, 1992
DISCIPLINARY ACTION: 60-MONTH PROBATION
OFFENSE: DISCIPLINARY ACTION BY ANOTHER STATE OR AGENCY

NOTES: DISCIPLINED BY TEXAS BOARD FOR IMPAIRMENT DUE TO SUBSTANCE ABUSE. REVOCATION STAYED. PROBATION WITH TERMS AND CONDITIONS.

KRESH, HERBERT MD, LICENSE NUMBER C4671 OF DALLAS, TX, WAS DISCIPLINED BY TEXAS ON AUGUST 22, 1998
DISCIPLINARY ACTION: 36-MONTH PROBATION; REPRIMAND
OFFENSE: PROFESSIONAL MISCONDUCT

NOTES: FAILED TO ADEQUATELY SUPERVISE NON-PHYSICIANS AT A WEIGHT LOSS CENTER WHERE HE WAS EMPLOYED; THESE NON-PHYSICIANS ASSESSED AND TREATED PATIENTS AND HE SIGNED OFF ON THE PATIENT CHARTS AT A LATER DATE; THEY ALSO CALLED IN PRESCRIPTIONS FOR CONTROLLED SUBSTANCES USING HIS DEA NUMBER ON OCCASIONS HE WAS NOT PRESENT. SUSPENSION STAYED FOR PROBATION WITH FOLLOWING TERMS AND CONDITIONS: HIS MEDICAL PRACTICE SHALL BE MONITORED BY A BOARD APPROVED TEXAS PHYSICIAN WHO SHALL PROVIDE QUARTERLY REPORTS TO THE BOARD; WITHIN 1 YEAR SHALL TAKE AND PASS THE SPEX; SHALL OBTAIN 50 HOURS PER YEAR OF CONTINUING MEDICAL EDUCATION, WITH 1 COURSE IN RISK MANAGEMENT; SHALL APPEAR BEFORE THE BOARD ONCE A YEAR; SHALL MAINTAIN ADEQUATE MEDICAL RECORDS WHICH SHALL BE AVAILABLE FOR REVIEW; SHALL SUPERVISE THE ACTIVITIES OF ALL HIS EMPLOYEES AND ALL OTHER INDIVIDUALS UNDER HIS SUPERVISION TO ENSURE THEIR COMPLIANCE; SHALL PERSONALLY EXAMINE AND/OR TREAT PATIENTS IN ANY SITUATION WHICH INDICATES THAT A PERSONAL EXAM OR TREATMENT OF A PATIENT BY HIM HAS TAKEN PLACE; SEPARATE FROM PATIENT RECORDS, SHALL MAINTAIN A LOGBOOK OF EVERY PRESCRIPTION WRITTEN BY HIM FOR DANGEROUS DRUGS WITH ADDICTIVE POTENTIAL WHICH SHALL BE MADE AVAILABLE FOR REVIEW; SHALL COOPERATE WITH THE BOARD IN VERIFYING COMPLIANCE; SHALL GIVE A COPY OF THIS ORDER TO ANY HEALTH CARE ENTITY WHERE HE HAS PRIVILEGES; TIME SPENT OUT OF TEXAS DOES NOT COUNT TOWARD PROBATION; SHALL INFORM THE BOARD OF CHANGE OF ADDRESS WITHIN 10 DAYS OR IF HE LEAVES THE STATE; SHALL NOT SEEK MODIFICATION FOR ONE YEAR. ON 10/15/99 PETITION TO TERMINATE THE ORDER DENIED.

KROHN, DOUGLAS RUSSELL MD, DATE OF BIRTH MARCH 21, 1953, LICENSE NUMBER 0048383 OF 74 SHELTON ROAD, PISCATAWAY, NJ, WAS DISCIPLINED BY NEW JERSEY ON SEPTEMBER 28, 1990
DISCIPLINARY ACTION: FINE; REPRIMAND
OFFENSE: SEXUAL ABUSE OF OR SEXUAL MISCONDUCT WITH A PATIENT

NOTES: ACTION BASED UPON THE MAKING OF SEXUALLY INAPPROPRIATE COMMENTS TO PATIENTS AND A FEMALE COLLEAGUE. ASSESSED PENALTY OF $2500 AND COSTS OF $2539. ON 5/23/94 THE RESTRICTIONS PLACED ON HIS LICENSE BY THIS ORDER WERE VACATED RETROACTIVE TO 4/13/94.

KROHN, DOUGLAS RUSSELL MD, DATE OF BIRTH MARCH 21, 1953, LICENSE NUMBER 00H8713 OF SOMERSET, NJ, WAS DISCIPLINED BY TEXAS ON AUGUST 24, 1991
DISCIPLINARY ACTION: REPRIMAND
OFFENSE: DISCIPLINARY ACTION BY ANOTHER STATE OR AGENCY

NOTES: ACTION TAKEN BY ANOTHER STATE BOARD FOR SEXUAL MISCONDUCT. PRIOR TO PRACTICING MEDICINE IN TEXAS, MUST APPEAR BEFORE AND RECEIVE APPROVAL FROM THE TEXAS BOARD. ON 10/24/98 ORDER TERMINATED.

KRUEGER, PHILIP MICHAEL MD, LICENSE NUMBER 00D4187 OF BOISE, ID, WAS DISCIPLINED BY TEXAS ON APRIL 20, 1991
DISCIPLINARY ACTION: PROBATION
OFFENSE: DISCIPLINARY ACTION BY ANOTHER STATE OR AGENCY

NOTES: MUST INFORM BOARD IN WRITING OF INTENT TO RESUME PRACTICING MEDICINE IN TEXAS.

KRUK, KATHLEEN ADELE DR, LICENSE NUMBER 0017571 OF 10 HAPPY HILL, WICHITA FALLS, TX, WAS DISCIPLINED BY OKLAHOMA ON JANUARY 12, 1991
DISCIPLINARY ACTION: 60-MONTH PROBATION; MONITORING OF PHYSICIAN PERFORMANCE
OFFENSE: PHYSICAL OR MENTAL ILLNESS INHIBITING THE ABILITY TO PRACTICE WITH SKILL AND SAFETY

NOTES: HISTORY OF TREATMENT FOR DEPRESSION STARTING IN 1989. CURRENTLY UNDERGOING OUT-PATIENT TREATMENT. ISSUES RAISED AS TO HER PHYSICAL AND MENTAL FITNESS TO PRACTICE. LICENSE GRANTED UNDER PROBATIONARY TERMS AND

CONDITIONS: SHALL CONTINUE PSYCHIATRIC/PSYCHOLOGICAL CARE AND MAKE RECORDS AVAILABLE TO BOARD; SHALL SUBMIT BIOLOGICAL FLUID SPECIMENS FOR ANALYSIS; SHALL NOTIFY ANY HOSPITAL WHERE SHE HOLDS STAFF PRIVILEGES, OR CLINIC OR GROUP OF THE TERMS AND CONDITIONS; SHALL FURNISH BOARD WITH ADDRESS AND/OR CHANGE OF ADDRESS; SHALL APPEAR BEFORE BOARD UPON REQUEST.

KRUSEN, DONNA MD OF 5232 VILLAGE CREEK DRIVE #200, PLANO, TX, WAS DISCIPLINED BY DEA ON JUNE 28, 1999
DISCIPLINARY ACTION: SURRENDER OF CONTROLLED SUBSTANCE LICENSE
OFFENSE: DISCIPLINARY ACTION BY ANOTHER STATE OR AGENCY
NOTES: STATE BOARD.

KRUSEN, DONNA INGLE MD, LICENSE NUMBER H4474 OF 3941 LEGACY DRIVE #204-194A, PLANO, TX, WAS DISCIPLINED BY TEXAS ON JUNE 25, 1999
DISCIPLINARY ACTION: EMERGENCY SUSPENSION
OFFENSE: PHYSICAL OR MENTAL ILLNESS INHIBITING THE ABILITY TO PRACTICE WITH SKILL AND SAFETY
NOTES: SHE HAS EXPERIENCED DEPRESSION AND SUICIDAL IDEATION AS DOCUMENTED BY HER TREATING PSYCHIATRIST AND MARITAL THERAPIST; ON 3/4/98 SHE WAS ARRESTED FOR PRESCRIPTION FRAUD FOR ATTEMPTING ON 12/22/97 TO FILL A PRESCRIPTION FOR ADDERAL WRITTEN FOR ONE OF HER PATIENTS; ON 2/11/98 SHE WAS ARRESTED FOR SHOPLIFTING ITEMS FROM A DEPARTMENT STORE; ON 5/12/98 SHE FALSELY REPORTED THAT SHE HAD BEEN ASSAULTED BY A SECURITY OFFICER ON THE NIGHT OF 2/11/98 INCIDENT FOR WHICH SHE WAS SUBSEQUENTLY CHARGED; ON 2/9/99 HER HUSBAND REPORTED TO THE PLANO POLICE THAT HIS HOME HAD BEEN BURGLARIZED AND ITEMS VALUED IN EXCESS OF $159,000 HAD BEEN REMOVED; THE INCIDENT REPORT DOCUMENTED THAT A NEIGHBOR WITNESSED HER REMOVING ITEMS FROM THE RESIDENCE WHILE SHE WAS SUBJECT TO A RESTRAINING ORDER; ON 6/17/99 SHE WAS ARRESTED FOR DISORDERLY CONDUCT FOLLOWING AN INCIDENT AT HER CHILDREN'S DAY CARE CENTER WHERE SHE ATTEMPTED TO REMOVE HER TWO CHILDREN FROM THE CENTER; SHE WAS SUBJECT TO A 4/15/99 COURT ORDER INSTRUCTING HER TO HAVE NO FURTHER CONTACT WITH HER CHILDREN; RECENTLY, SHE HAS BEEN EXPERIENCING INCREASING DIFFICULTIES IN HER PERSONAL LIFE AND HAS BEEN HOSPITALIZED IN ORDER TO ADDRESS HER MENTAL STATUS.

KRUSEN, DONNA INGLE MD, LICENSE NUMBER H4474 OF PLANO, TX, WAS DISCIPLINED BY TEXAS ON DECEMBER 11, 1999
DISCIPLINARY ACTION: LICENSE SUSPENSION
OFFENSE: PHYSICAL OR MENTAL ILLNESS INHIBITING THE ABILITY TO PRACTICE WITH SKILL AND SAFETY
NOTES: HAS EXPERIENCED DEPRESSION AND SUICIDAL IDEATION; ARRESTED ON 3/4/98 FOR ALLEGEDLY ATTEMPTING TO FILL A PRESCRIPTION FOR ADDERAL WRITTEN FOR ONE OF HER PATIENTS; ON 2/11/98 FOR ALLEGEDLY SHOPLIFTING AND ON 6/17/99 FOR DISORDERLY CONDUCT; ALSO CHARGED WITH FILING A FALSE POLICE REPORT. SUSPENSION UNTIL SHE REQUESTS TO HAVE HER SUSPENSION STAYED OR APPEARS BEFORE THE BOARD WITH SUFFICIENT EVIDENCE THAT SHE IS PHYSICALLY, MENTALLY AND OTHERWISE COMPETENT TO SAFELY PRACTICE MEDICINE INCLUDING AT A MINIMUM COMPLETE COPIES OF MEDICAL RECORDS AND REPORTS OF PSYCHOLOGICAL AND NEUROPSYCHIATRIC EVALUATIONS, INCLUDING A 96 HOUR INPATIENT EVALUATION CONDUCTED BY A BOARD-APPROVED CERTIFIED PSYCHIATRIST; SHALL COOPERATE WITH THE BOARD IN VERIFYING COMPLIANCE; SHALL GIVE A COPY OF THIS ORDER TO ANY HEALTH CARE ENTITY WHERE SHE HAS PRIVILEGES; SHALL PROVIDE A COPY OF THIS ORDER TO ANYONE REQUESTING IT WITHIN 10 DAYS; SHALL INFORM THE BOARD OF CHANGE OF ADDRESS WITHIN 10 DAYS.

KUHL, IVAN WALTER MD, DATE OF BIRTH DECEMBER 2, 1920, LICENSE NUMBER 00C4396 OF 1111 N 10TH, MCALLEN, TX, WAS DISCIPLINED BY TEXAS ON APRIL 30, 1993
OFFENSE: PROFESSIONAL MISCONDUCT
NOTES: THROUGH 1990 HE PRESCRIBED ASIATIC CAPSULES CONTAINING ARSENIC TRIOXIDE FOR THE TREATMENT OF PSORIASIS; NOT IN THE PURVIEW OF ACCEPTABLE CURRENT MEDICAL PRACTICE. SHALL NOT PRESCRIBE, ADMINISTER OR DISPENSE ARSENIC TRIOXIDE; SHALL GIVE A COPY OF THIS ORDER TO ANY HEALTH CARE ENTITY WHERE HE HAS PRIVILEGES; SHALL COOPERATE WITH THE BOARD IN VERIFYING COMPLIANCE; SHALL INFORM BOARD OF CHANGE OF ADDRESS WITHIN 10 DAYS.

KUHL, PETER VAN DOREN MD OF 2829 BABCOCK ROAD #540, SAN ANTONIO, TX, WAS DISCIPLINED BY DEA ON AUGUST 6, 1996
DISCIPLINARY ACTION: SURRENDER OF CONTROLLED SUBSTANCE LICENSE

KUHL, PETER VAN DOREN MD, LICENSE NUMBER E6462, WAS DISCIPLINED BY TEXAS ON MARCH 1, 1997
DISCIPLINARY ACTION: 60-MONTH PROBATION; RESTRICTION PLACED ON CONTROLLED SUBSTANCE LICENSE
OFFENSE: SUBSTANCE ABUSE
NOTES: HAS ENGAGED IN THE ABUSE OF CODEINE AND HYDROCODONE OVER THE PAST ELEVEN YEARS. HE ORIGINALLY BEGAN TAKING THESE DRUGS FOR A KNEE INJURY, BUT THIS CULMINATED IN HIS DRUG ABUSE. IN 2/96 HE BEGAN SEEING A SPECIFIED PSYCHIATRIST; INITIATED A FIVE-YEAR OUTPATIENT CARE CONTRACT BEGINNING ON 10/10/96. HIS REPORTED SOBRIETY DATE IS 2/27/96. DRUG SCREENS HAVE BEEN NEGATIVE AND THE COMMITTEE REPORTS COMPLIANCE. HE HAS VOLUNTARILY SURRENDERED HIS CONTROLLED SUBSTANCE REGISTRATIONS. SUSPENSION STAYED FOR PROBATION UNDER THE FOLLOWING TERMS AND CONDITIONS: SHALL UNDERGO A 96-HOUR INPATIENT EVALUATION FOR SUBSTANCE ABUSE WITHIN 60 DAYS, WITH RESULTS REPORTED TO THE BOARD; SHALL FOLLOW ALL RECOMMENDATIONS; SHALL NOMINATE THREE CERTIFIED PSYCHIATRISTS FOR BOARD SELECTION OF A THERAPIST AND SHALL EXPEDITIOUSLY SUBMIT HIMSELF TO EVALUATION AND TREATMENT BY THE APPROVED PRACTITIONER; SHALL ABSTAIN FROM THE CONSUMPTION OF ALCOHOL/DRUGS IN ANY FORM UNLESS PRESCRIBED BY ANOTHER PHYSICIAN FOR A LEGITIMATE AND THERAPEUTIC PURPOSE; SHALL SUBMIT HIMSELF FOR APPROPRIATE EXAMS INCLUDING DRUG OR ALCOHOL SCREENS; SHALL PARTICIPATE IN THE ACTIVITIES OF A PHYSICIAN HEALTH AND REHABILITATION COMMITTEE AND ATTEND WEEKLY MEETINGS WITH QUARTERLY REPORTS; SHALL PARTICIPATE IN AA'S PROGRAM NOT LESS THAN THREE TIMES A WEEK; SHALL REPORT ON HIS ATTENDANCE; SHALL COMPLY WITH HIS CONTINUING CARE CONTRACT WITH QUARTERLY REPORTS; SHALL NOT TREAT OR

OTHERWISE SERVE AS PHYSICIAN, PRESCRIBE, DISPENSE OR ADMINISTER DRUGS THAT MAY BE SUBJECT TO ABUSE TO HIMSELF OR TO ANY MEMBER OF HIS FAMILY; SHALL NOT POSSESS, ADMINISTER, DISPENSE, OR PRESCRIBE ANY CONTROLLED SUBSTANCES EXCEPT AS MEDICALLY NECESSARY FOR TREATMENT OF INPATIENTS IN A HOSPITAL SETTING WHERE HE HAS PRIVILEGES; SEPARATE FROM PATIENT RECORDS, SHALL MAINTAIN A FILE OF EVERY PRESCRIPTION WRITTEN BY HIM FOR DANGEROUS DRUGS WITH ADDICTIVE POTENTIAL WHICH SHALL BE MADE AVAILABLE FOR REVIEW; SHALL APPEAR BEFORE THE BOARD AT LEAST TWICE YEARLY FOR THE FIRST YEAR AND ANNUALLY THEREAFTER; SHALL COOPERATE WITH THE BOARD IN VERIFYING COMPLIANCE INCLUDING PROVIDING COPIES OF MEDICAL RELEASES; SHALL GIVE A COPY OF THIS ORDER TO ANY HEALTH CARE ENTITY WHERE HE HAS PRIVILEGES; TIME SPENT OUT OF TEXAS DOES NOT COUNT TOWARD PROBATION; SHALL INFORM THE BOARD OF CHANGE OF ADDRESS WITHIN 10 DAYS OR IF HE LEAVES THE STATE; SHALL NOT SEEK MODIFICATION FOR SIX MONTHS. ON 4/10/99 THE ORDER WAS MODIFIED CHANGING THE REQUIREMENT FOR MONTHLY PSYCHIATRIC CARE TO CARE AS RECOMMENDED BY APPROVED PSYCHIATRIST; ALL OTHER PROVISIONS OF THE ORDER REMAIN IN FULL EFFECT UNTIL SUPERSEDED BY A SUBSEQUENT BOARD ORDER.

KULKARNI, NARAYAN R MD, LICENSE NUMBER 0008165 OF BRENT, AL, WAS DISCIPLINED BY ALABAMA ON DECEMBER 2, 1994
DISCIPLINARY ACTION: SURRENDER OF LICENSE
OFFENSE: PROFESSIONAL MISCONDUCT

NOTES: UNDER INVESTIGATION FOR ALLEGED VIOLATIONS RELATING TO UNPROFESSIONAL CONDUCT, PRACTICING MEDICINE IN SUCH A MANNER TO ENDANGER THE HEALTH OF PATIENTS, AND THE PERFORMANCE OF UNNECESSARY DIAGNOSTIC TESTS OR MEDICAL OR SURGICAL SERVICES. VOLUNTARY SURRENDER.

KULKARNI, NARAYAN R MD, DATE OF BIRTH JUNE 4, 1933 OF 2525 HIGHWAY 25, BOX 509, BRENT, AL, WAS DISCIPLINED BY MEDICARE ON MARCH 5, 1996
DISCIPLINARY ACTION: EXCLUSION FROM THE MEDICARE AND/OR MEDICAID PROGRAM
OFFENSE: DISCIPLINARY ACTION BY ANOTHER STATE OR AGENCY

NOTES: LICENSE SURRENDERED FOR REASONS BEARING ON PROFESSIONAL COMPETENCE.

KULKARNI, NARAYAN R MD, LICENSE NUMBER E9275, WAS DISCIPLINED BY TEXAS ON MARCH 1, 1997
DISCIPLINARY ACTION: SURRENDER OF LICENSE

NOTES: ON 12/2/94 THE DOCTOR SURRENDERED HIS ALABAMA LICENSE; HE DOES NOT PLAN TO PRACTICE IN TEXAS AND CURRENTLY SUFFERS HEALTH PROBLEMS. HE DENIES ALLEGATIONS. PERMANENT AND VOLUNTARY SURRENDER OF HIS LICENSE.

KULKARNI, NARAYAN RAGHAVENDRAR MD OF 2525 HIGHWAY 25, BRENT, AL, WAS DISCIPLINED BY DEA ON JANUARY 18, 1995
DISCIPLINARY ACTION: SURRENDER OF CONTROLLED SUBSTANCE LICENSE
OFFENSE: DISCIPLINARY ACTION BY ANOTHER STATE OR AGENCY

NOTES: STATE BOARD.

KUO, LIMEI MD, LICENSE NUMBER 00F5811 OF BELLAIRE, TX, WAS DISCIPLINED BY TEXAS ON JULY 23, 1992
DISCIPLINARY ACTION: EMERGENCY SUSPENSION
OFFENSE: SUBSTANCE ABUSE

NOTES: INTEMPERATE USE OF DRUGS.

KUO, LIMEI MD, LICENSE NUMBER 00F5811 OF BELLAIRE, TX, WAS DISCIPLINED BY TEXAS ON NOVEMBER 13, 1992
DISCIPLINARY ACTION: 12-MONTH LICENSE SUSPENSION

NOTES: MAY MAKE APPLICATION FOR REINSTATEMENT AFTER ONE YEAR.

KURTZ, IRWIN MD, LICENSE NUMBER 00C7021 OF 4402 VANCE JACKSON, SAN ANTONIO, TX, WAS DISCIPLINED BY TEXAS ON JULY 14, 1994
DISCIPLINARY ACTION: EMERGENCY SUSPENSION
OFFENSE: SUBSTANCE ABUSE

NOTES:

KURTZ, IRWIN MD, LICENSE NUMBER 00C7021 OF SAN ANTONIO, TX, WAS DISCIPLINED BY TEXAS ON AUGUST 19, 1994
DISCIPLINARY ACTION: LICENSE SUSPENSION
OFFENSE: SUBSTANCE ABUSE

NOTES: LICENSE WAS TEMPORARILY SUSPENDED ON 7/14/94 AFTER HE WAS DIAGNOSED AS POLYSUBSTANCE DEPENDENT, HYPOMANIC, AND HAVING BIPOLAR DISEASE; HE TESTED POSITIVE FOR BENZODIAZEPINES AND METHADONE ON 7/1/94; HAS ENGAGED IN THE INTEMPERATE USE OF PRESCRIPTION DRUGS; HAS ADMITTED TO A HISTORY OF POLYSUBSTANCE DEPENDENCE AND INTEMPERATE USE OF DRUGS, AS RECENTLY AS JULY 1994. SUSPENDED UNTIL SUCH TIME AS HE APPEARS BEFORE THE BOARD AND PROVIDES SUFFICIENT EVIDENCE THAT HE IS PHYSICALLY, MENTALLY AND OTHERWISE COMPETENT TO SAFELY PRACTICE MEDICINE. UPON SHOWING HE IS ABLE TO SAFELY PRACTICE, THE SUSPENSION WILL BE STAYED AND HIS LICENSE WILL BE PLACED ON PROBATION WITH VARIOUS TERMS AND CONDITIONS.

KURTZ, IRWIN MD OF 4402 VAMCE JACKSON, SAN ANTONIO, TX, WAS DISCIPLINED BY DEA ON NOVEMBER 16, 1994
DISCIPLINARY ACTION: SURRENDER OF CONTROLLED SUBSTANCE LICENSE
OFFENSE: DISCIPLINARY ACTION BY ANOTHER STATE OR AGENCY

NOTES: STATE BOARD.

KURTZ, IRWIN MD, DATE OF BIRTH NOVEMBER 1, 1928 OF PO BOX 1087, COMFORT, TX, WAS DISCIPLINED BY MEDICARE ON MARCH 3, 1996
DISCIPLINARY ACTION: EXCLUSION FROM THE MEDICARE AND/OR MEDICAID PROGRAM
OFFENSE: DISCIPLINARY ACTION BY ANOTHER STATE OR AGENCY

NOTES: LICENSE SUSPENDED FOR REASONS BEARING ON PROFESSIONAL COMPETENCE.

LADLEY, DAVID M MD, DATE OF BIRTH JUNE 19, 1953 OF 202 FM 1960 EAST BYPASS, HUMBLE, TX, WAS DISCIPLINED BY MEDICARE ON FEBRUARY 28, 1994
DISCIPLINARY ACTION: EXCLUSION FROM THE MEDICARE AND/OR MEDICAID PROGRAM
OFFENSE: DISCIPLINARY ACTION BY ANOTHER STATE OR AGENCY

NOTES: LICENSE REVOKED FOR REASONS BEARING ON PROFESSIONAL PERFORMANCE AND COMPETENCE.

LADLEY, DAVID MARK MD, LICENSE NUMBER 0025455 OF 105 N

HIGH ST, HENDERSON, TX, WAS DISCIPLINED BY GEORGIA ON AUGUST 28, 1991
DISCIPLINARY ACTION: NONRENEWAL OF LICENSE
OFFENSE: DISCIPLINARY ACTION BY ANOTHER STATE OR AGENCY

NOTES: DISCIPLINARY ACTION IN TEXAS. ADMINISTRATIVE REVOCATION FOR FAILURE TO RENEW.

LADLEY, DAVID MARK MD, LICENSE NUMBER 00G7839 OF HUMBLE, TX, WAS DISCIPLINED BY TEXAS ON DECEMBER 7, 1992
OFFENSE: OVERPRESCRIBING OR MISPRESCRIBING DRUGS

NOTES: SEVERAL VIOLATIONS OF THE MEDICAL PRACTICE ACT, INCLUDING NONTHERAPEUTIC PRESCRIBING, PRACTICE INCONSISTENT WITH PUBLIC HEALTH AND WELFARE, AND IMPAIRMENT DUE TO ILLNESS OR CHEMICAL ABUSE. ORDER OF REVOCATION. ON 12/30/92, HE FILED MOTION FOR REHEARING WHICH WAS DENIED ON 1/11/93. ON 1/28/93, HE FILED AN APPEAL IN TRAVIS COUNTY AND A DECISION IS CURRENTLY PENDING. ORDER WILL BECOME FINAL WHEN ALL APPEALS HAVE BEEN EXHAUSTED.

LAFLEUR, MELANIE KOHOUT MD, LICENSE NUMBER 00H3482 OF MESA, AZ, WAS DISCIPLINED BY TEXAS ON JANUARY 6, 1995
DISCIPLINARY ACTION: MONITORING OF PHYSICIAN PERFORMANCE
OFFENSE: DISCIPLINARY ACTION BY ANOTHER STATE OR AGENCY

NOTES: ENTERED INTO A REHABILITATION STIPULATION AND ORDER WITH THE ARIZONA BOARD ON 5/25/93 WHICH PLACED HER UNDER TERMS AND CONDITIONS BUT DOES NOT CONSTITUTE A DISCIPLINARY ORDER. SHALL NOT PRACTICE IN TEXAS UNTIL SHE PERSONALLY APPEARS BEFORE THE BOARD AND PROVIDES SUFFICIENT EVIDENCE THAT SHE IS PHYSICALLY, MENTALLY AND OTHERWISE COMPETENT TO SAFELY PRACTICE INCLUDING AT A MINIMUM REPORTS FROM TREATING PHYSICIAN, COMPETENCY EXAMS OR ANY THERAPIST; SHALL COMPLY WITH TERMS OF ARIZONA ORDER; SHALL PROVIDE COPIES OF REPORTS SENT TO OR RECEIVED FROM ARIZONA BOARD UPON REQUEST; SHALL SURRENDER TEXAS CONTROLLED SUBSTANCES CERTIFICATES AND UNUSED TRIPLICATE PRESCRIPTION FORMS; SHALL NOT SEEK REREGISTRATION WITHOUT PERMISSION.

LAMURE, DAVID S SR MD, LICENSE NUMBER 00D6695 OF DEXTER, NM, WAS DISCIPLINED BY TEXAS ON OCTOBER 9, 1992
DISCIPLINARY ACTION: LICENSE REVOCATION
OFFENSE: CRIMINAL CONVICTION OR PLEA OF GUILTY, NOLO CONTENDERE, OR NO CONTEST TO A CRIME

NOTES: CONVICTION OF A FELONY.

LANDGREBE, BERNHARD HANS MD, LICENSE NUMBER D2895 OF SAN ANTONIO, TX, WAS DISCIPLINED BY TEXAS ON AUGUST 22, 1998
DISCIPLINARY ACTION: REPRIMAND
OFFENSE: PROFESSIONAL MISCONDUCT

NOTES: TREATED 2 PATIENTS PROPHYLACTICALLY FOR PAIN ASSOCIATED WITH EPILEPSY WITH STELLATE GANGLION BLOCK (SGB); THESE TREATMENTS WERE ADMINISTERED EVEN THOUGH HE NOTED THAT THE PATIENTS WERE NOT SYMPTOMATIC AT THE TIME OF THE TREATMENT; ALTHOUGH HE MAINTAINS THAT THE PROPHYLACTIC USE OF SGB IS ACCEPTABLE PRACTICE IN GERMANY, HE IS NOT ABLE TO CITE TO ANY AUTHORITY IN THE UNITED STATES FOR THE PRACTICE. SHALL GIVE A COPY OF THIS ORDER TO ANY HEALTH CARE ENTITY WHERE HE HAS PRIVILEGES.

LANGLEY, LAURA LYNN MD, WAS DISCIPLINED BY TEXAS ON AUGUST 18, 1995
DISCIPLINARY ACTION: MONITORING OF PHYSICIAN PERFORMANCE
OFFENSE: SUBSTANDARD CARE, INCOMPETENCE OR NEGLIGENCE

NOTES: DURING 1995 ALLEGATIONS THAT SHE HAD RENDERED SUBSTANDARD CARE TO FIVE ADULT FEMALE PATIENTS; HAD COUNTERED A PEDIATRICIAN'S ORDERS FOR SUPPLEMENTAL FEEDINGS OF A NEWBORN INFANT; AND WANTED TO INDUCE LABOR IN FOUR PATIENTS WHEN THE NEED WAS ALLEGED NOT TO BE MEDICALLY INDICATED. SHE DENIES ALLEGATIONS. CONDITIONS FOR A PERIOD OF FIVE YEARS AS FOLLOWS: SHALL SUBMIT HERSELF FOR EVALUATION BY BOARD APPROVED PSYCHIATRIST FOR TREATMENT AND COUNSELING AT LEAST ONCE A MONTH AND SUBMIT REPORTS. SHALL ABSTAIN FROM THE CONSUMPTION OF ALCOHOL/DRUGS IN ANY FORM UNLESS PRESCRIBED BY ANOTHER PHYSICIAN FOR A LEGITIMATE AND THERAPEUTIC PURPOSE; SHALL SUBMIT FOR APPROPRIATE EXAMS INCLUDING ALCOHOL AND DRUG SCREENS; SHALL NOT TREAT OR OTHERWISE SERVE AS PHYSICIAN AND SHALL NOT PRESCRIBE, DISPENSE OR ADMINISTER CONTROLLED SUBSTANCES OR DANGEROUS DRUGS WITH ADDICTIVE POTENTIAL TO HER IMMEDIATE FAMILY; PRACTICE SHALL BE MONITORED BY A LICENSED PHYSICIAN WHO SHALL SUBMIT QUARTERLY REPORTS; SHALL COOPERATE WITH THE BOARD IN VERIFYING COMPLIANCE INCLUDING PROVIDING MEDICAL RELEASES AND PEER REVIEW RECORDS; WILL ENTER INTO AN AGREEMENT ANYWHERE SHE HAS PRIVILEGES TO NOTIFY BOARD OF ANY COMPLAINTS WITHIN 72 HOURS AND TO SUBMIT QUARTERLY A PROFESSIONAL EVALUATION; SHALL APPEAR BEFORE THE BOARD ONCE A YEAR OR UPON REQUEST; SHALL PROVIDE A COPY OF THIS ORDER TO ANYONE REQUESTING IT WITHIN 10 DAYS; SHALL PROVIDE A COPY OF THIS ORDER TO ANY HEALTH CARE ENTITY WHERE SHE HAS PRIVILEGES; TIME PERIOD SHALL BE EXTENDED FOR ANY PERIOD OF TIME SHE RESIDES OR PRACTICES MEDICINE OUT OF TEXAS; SHALL INFORM THE BOARD OF CHANGE OF ADDRESS WITHIN 10 DAYS OR IF SHE LEAVES THE STATE; SHALL NOT SEEK MODIFICATION FOR ONE YEAR. ON 11/22/97 ORDER TERMINATED.

LANIER, ANDREW JACKSON JR MD OF DALLAS, TX, WAS DISCIPLINED BY LOUISIANA ON JUNE 23, 1994

NOTES: INABILITY TO PRACTICE WITH REASONABLE SKILL AND SAFETY. PRACTICE OF MEDICINE IN LOUISIANA PRECLUDED UNTIL ORDERED BY THE BOARD.

LARA, FERNAN MD, LICENSE NUMBER 00E0251, WAS DISCIPLINED BY TEXAS ON AUGUST 17, 1996
DISCIPLINARY ACTION: FINE; 24-MONTH RESTRICTION PLACED ON CONTROLLED SUBSTANCE LICENSE
OFFENSE: SUBSTANDARD CARE, INCOMPETENCE OR NEGLIGENCE

NOTES: FROM AUGUST 1992 THROUGH MARCH 1994, PRESCRIBED DARVOCET N-100 AND ITS GENERIC EQUIVALENTS TO AN ADULT FEMALE PATIENT, PREVIOUSLY DIAGNOSED AS HAVING CHRONIC HEADACHES, WITHOUT CONDUCTING A FOLLOW-UP EXAMINATION. SUBJECT TO TERMS AND CONDITIONS FOR TWO YEARS: SHALL NOT PRESCRIBE CONTROLLED SUBSTANCES AND/OR DANGEROUS DRUGS TO ANY PATIENT FOR LONGER THAN THREE MONTHS WITHOUT HAVING THE PATIENT PERSONALLY PRESENT FOR A MEDICALLY APPROPRIATE REEVALUATION, INCLUDING TESTING,

AND/OR OTHER MEDICALLY APPROPRIATE FOLLOW-UP EXAMINATION; SHALL ESTABLISH AND UTILIZE A SYSTEM OF MEDICAL RECORD KEEPING AND CHARTING IN WHICH HE DICTATES AND/OR RECORDS THE CARE AND TREATMENT BEING RENDERED; EACH PRESCRIBED DRUG, INCLUDING REFILLS, SHALL BE RECORDED IN THE RESPECTIVE PATIENT'S MEDICAL RECORD IRREGARDLESS AS TO WHETHER THE DRUG IS RECORDED IN ANY OTHER RECORD, LOG OR DOCUMENT ALONG WITH THE MEDICAL RATIONALE TO SUPPORT THE PRESCRIBING OF THE DRUG; PRESCRIBING HABITS, RATIONALE, AND PRACTICE, SHALL BE MONITORED BY A BOARD APPROVED TEXAS PHYSICIAN WHO SHALL SUBMIT QUARTERLY REPORTS TO THE BOARD; WITHIN ONE YEAR SHALL ENROLL IN AND SUCCESSFULLY COMPLETE BOARD APPROVED COURSES IN RISK MANAGEMENT AND ADDICTIONOLOGY/PHARMACOLOGY AND SUBMIT DOCUMENTATION OF ATTENDANCE TO THE BOARD; SHALL COOPERATE WIT THE BOARD IN VERIFYING COMPLIANCE; SHALL APPEAR BEFORE THE BOARD AT LEAST TWO TIMES PER YEAR OR UPON REQUEST; SHALL GIVE A COPY OF THIS ORDER TO ANY HEALTH CARE ENTITY WHERE HE HAS PRIVILEGES; SHALL PROVIDE A COPY OF THIS ORDER TO ANYONE REQUESTING IT WITHIN 10 DAYS; TIME PERIOD OUT OF TEXAS DOES NOT COUNT TOWARD RESTRICTION; SHALL INFORM THE BOARD OF CHANGE OF ADDRESS WITHIN 10 DAYS OF IF HE LEAVES THE STATE; SHALL NOT SEEK MODIFICATION FOR ONE YEAR. $2,250 ADMINISTRATIVE PENALTY. REPRIMAND ON 9/20/97 THE BOARD GRANTED HIS PETITION FOR TERMINATION OF THIS ORDER BASED ON COMPLIANCE WITH CONDITIONS.

LATONN, EDWARD D MD, LICENSE NUMBER 0G15030 OF WILMINGTON, DE, WAS DISCIPLINED BY CALIFORNIA ON JULY 15, 1994
DISCIPLINARY ACTION: LICENSE REVOCATION
OFFENSE: DISCIPLINARY ACTION BY ANOTHER STATE OR AGENCY

NOTES: DISCIPLINED BY DELAWARE BOARD FOR OVERPRESCRIBING OR INAPPROPRIATE PRESCRIBING TO 24 PATIENTS. DEFAULT DECISION.

LATONN, EDWARD DALE MD, WAS DISCIPLINED BY DELAWARE ON JUNE 12, 1991
DISCIPLINARY ACTION: 1-MONTH LICENSE SUSPENSION; REQUIRED TO TAKE ADDITIONAL MEDICAL EDUCATION
OFFENSE: PROFESSIONAL MISCONDUCT

NOTES: GROSS MISCONDUCT, NEGLIGENCE, OR INCOMPETENCE IN THE PRACTICE OF MEDICINE. REQUIRED TO ATTEND A MINI-RESIDENCY IN PRESCRIBING CONTROLLED DANGEROUS SUBSTANCES; MAY NOT APPLY FOR REINSTATEMENT OF HIS FEDERAL OR STATE CONTROLLED SUBSTANCES REGISTRATIONS FOR ONE YEAR FROM THE DATE OF HIS STIPULATION WITH THE BOARD'S INVESTIGATIVE COMMITTEE; UPON REINSTATEMENT HIS PRACTICE SHALL BE MONITORED BY THE BOARD OR ITS DESIGNEE FOR A PERIOD OF TWO YEARS.

LATONN, EDWARD DALE MD, LICENSE NUMBER 00E1647 OF WILMINGTON, DE, WAS DISCIPLINED BY TEXAS ON DECEMBER 4, 1991
DISCIPLINARY ACTION: 1-MONTH LICENSE SUSPENSION; 24-MONTH PROBATION
OFFENSE: DISCIPLINARY ACTION BY ANOTHER STATE OR AGENCY

NOTES: DISCIPLINARY ACTION TAKEN BY DELAWARE BOARD ON 1/12/91. TWO YEAR SUSPENSION STAYED, PROBATION INCLUDES FOLLOWING CONDITIONS: MUST SUCCESSFULLY COMPLETE "MINI-RESIDENCY IN PRESCRIBING CONTROLLED DANGEROUS SUBSTANCES"; SHALL NOT APPLY FOR REINSTATEMENT OF FEDERAL CONTROLLED SUBSTANCES REGISTRATION FOR ONE YEAR FROM 4/2/91; MEDICAL PRACTICE SHALL BE MONITORED, INCLUDING BUT NOT LIMITED TO, THE REVIEW OF ANY AND ALL PATIENT RECORDS; SHALL APPEAR BEFORE BOARD ONCE A YEAR; SHALL PROVIDE COPIES OF REPORTS SENT TO DELAWARE TO TEXAS BOARD; SHALL APPEAR BEFORE BOARD PRIOR TO PRACTICING IN TEXAS; TIME SPENT OUT OF TEXAS OR DELAWARE DOES NOT COUNT TOWARD PROBATION; SHALL COOPERATE WITH BOTH BOARDS IN MONITORING COMPLIANCE; SHALL ADVISE BOARD OF ANY CHANGE OF ADDRESS WITHIN 10 DAYS.

LAWRENCE, LORRY DAVIS DO, LICENSE NUMBER 00H8193, WAS DISCIPLINED BY TEXAS ON AUGUST 17, 1996
DISCIPLINARY ACTION: REPRIMAND
OFFENSE: PROFESSIONAL MISCONDUCT

NOTES: FAILED TO ADEQUATELY SUPERVISE A MEDICAL STUDENT AS TO THE STUDENT'S CARE, TREATMENT, AND ASSESSMENT OF A PATIENT IN 8/94 IN THAT FAILED TO COMMUNICATE REGARDING WHETHER A PHYSICAL EXAMINATION HAD BEEN PERFORMED WHICH IT HAD NOT. SHALL GIVE A COPY OF THIS ORDER TO ALL HEALTH CARE ENTITIES WHERE HE HOLDS PRIVILEGES.

LAWRENCE, RICHARD BURNETT III MD, DATE OF BIRTH FEBRUARY 22, 1948, LICENSE NUMBER 00E2671 OF 1925 DARTMOOR COURT, FORT WORTH, TX, WAS DISCIPLINED BY TEXAS ON JUNE 17, 1992
DISCIPLINARY ACTION: RESTRICTION PLACED ON LICENSE; REPRIMAND
OFFENSE: PROFESSIONAL MISCONDUCT

NOTES: FAILING TO SUPERVISE ADEQUATELY THE ACTIVITIES OF THOSE ACTING UNDER THE SUPERVISION OF THE PHYSICIAN, AND PROFESSIONAL FAILURE TO PRACTICE MEDICINE IN AN ACCEPTABLE MANNER CONSISTENT WITH PUBLIC HEALTH AND WELFARE. ON 8/20/93 ORDER TERMINATED AND LICENSE FREE AND CLEAR OF ANY PREVIOUS RESTRICTIONS.

LEAMON, ROY L MD OF 711 WEST 38TH ST SUITE E4, AUSTIN, TX, WAS DISCIPLINED BY DEA ON OCTOBER 9, 1990
DISCIPLINARY ACTION: RESTRICTION PLACED ON CONTROLLED SUBSTANCE LICENSE
OFFENSE: OVERPRESCRIBING OR MISPRESCRIBING DRUGS

NOTES: OVERPRESCRIBED TO KNOWN ADDICT.

LEAMON, ROY LESLIE MD, LICENSE NUMBER 00C5140 OF AUSTIN, TX, WAS DISCIPLINED BY TEXAS ON SEPTEMBER 28, 1990
DISCIPLINARY ACTION: 60-MONTH PROBATION; RESTRICTION PLACED ON LICENSE

NOTES: MAY ASSIST BUT MAY NOT PERFORM SURGERY BY HIMSELF OR AS PRIMARY SURGEON; HAVE REGISTRATION CERTIFICATES TO BE AMENDED TO DELETE SCHEDULES II, II-N, III-N AND V AND SHALL NOT REREGISTER WITHOUT PRIOR BOARD AUTHORITY; MAINTAIN FILE COPY OF CERTAIN PRESCRIPTIONS; NOT TELEPHONE ANY CONTROLLED SUBSTANCE OR DANGEROUS DRUG PRESCRIPTION TO PHARMACY; SUBMIT FOR PSYCHIATRIC EVALUATION AND FOLLOW ANY RECOMMENDATIONS REGARDING CONTINUING CARE AND TREATMENT; IF CHOOSING TO PRACTICE IN FIELD OF MEDICINE OTHER THAN ORTHOPEDICS, SHALL FIRST OBTAIN APPROVAL OF COURSE OR PROGRAM

HE PROPOSES TO ATTEND TO DEVELOP PROFICIENCY OR CURRENCY IN PROPOSED NEW SPECIALTY. ON 9/30/94 PROBATION TERMINATED.

LEATH, MICHAEL CARTER MD, LICENSE NUMBER E2672 OF LONGVIEW, TX, WAS DISCIPLINED BY TEXAS ON AUGUST 22, 1998
DISCIPLINARY ACTION: 60-MONTH PROBATION; RESTRICTION PLACED ON LICENSE
OFFENSE: SEXUAL ABUSE OF OR SEXUAL MISCONDUCT WITH A PATIENT
NOTES: ENGAGED IN A SEXUAL RELATIONSHIP WITH 4 PATIENTS AND ALSO ADMITS THAT HE HAS A HISTORY OF ALCOHOLISM; HE REPRESENTS THAT HE HAS NEVER TREATED PATIENTS WHILE UNDER THE INFLUENCE OF ALCOHOL; IN 6/95 HE BEGAN ATTENDING AA MEETINGS AND SEX ADDICTS ANONYMOUS AND REPORTS THAT HE CONTINUES TO ATTEND THOSE MEETINGS ON A REGULAR BASIS; HE REPORTS A SOBRIETY DATE OF 5/25/95. SUSPENSION STAYED FOR PROBATION WITH FOLLOWING TERMS AND CONDITIONS: SHALL ABSTAIN FROM THE CONSUMPTION OF ALCOHOL/DRUGS IN ANY FORM UNLESS PRESCRIBED BY ANOTHER PHYSICIAN FOR A LEGITIMATE AND THERAPEUTIC PURPOSE; SHALL SUBMIT HIMSELF FOR APPROPRIATE EXAMS INCLUDING DRUG OR ALCOHOL SCREENS; SHALL NOMINATE THREE CERTIFIED PSYCHIATRISTS FOR BOARD SELECTION OF A THERAPIST AND SHALL EXPEDITIOUSLY SUBMIT HIMSELF TO EVALUATION AND TREATMENT BY THE APPROVED PRACTITIONER; SHALL PARTICIPATE IN THE ACTIVITIES OF A PHYSICIAN HEALTH AND REHABILITATION COMMITTEE AND ATTEND WEEKLY MEETINGS WITH QUARTERLY REPORTS; SHALL CONTINUE TO PARTICIPATE IN AA'S PROGRAM NOT LESS THAN THREE TIMES A WEEK AND SEX ADDICTS ANONYMOUS NOT LESS THAN ONCE A WEEK; SHALL REPORT ON HIS ATTENDANCE; SHALL COOPERATE WITH THE BOARD IN VERIFYING COMPLIANCE INCLUDING PROVIDING COPIES OF MEDICAL RELEASES UPON REQUEST; SHALL NOT TREAT OR OTHERWISE SERVE AS PHYSICIAN, PRESCRIBE, DISPENSE OR ADMINISTER DRUGS THAT MAY BE SUBJECT TO ABUSE TO HIMSELF OR TO ANY MEMBER OF HIS FAMILY; SHALL HAVE A CHAPERONE WHENEVER HE PERFORMS A PHYSICAL EXAM ON A FEMALE PATIENT; SHALL PERFORM 100 HOURS OF COMMUNITY SERVICE PER YEAR; SHALL OBTAIN 1 ETHICS COURSE PER YEAR FOR EACH YEAR OF THE ORDER; WITHIN 60 DAYS SHALL NOTIFY THE BOARD OF THE IDENTITY OF 3 PATIENTS WITH WHOM HE HAS ENGAGED IN SEXUAL RELATIONS; SHALL APPEAR BEFORE THE BOARD ONCE A YEAR; SHALL GIVE A COPY OF THIS ORDER TO ANY HEALTH CARE ENTITY WHERE HE HAS PRIVILEGES; TIME SPENT OUT OF TEXAS DOES NOT COUNT TOWARD PROBATION; SHALL INFORM THE BOARD OF CHANGE OF ADDRESS WITHIN 10 DAYS OR IF HE LEAVES THE STATE; SHALL NOT SEEK MODIFICATION FOR ONE YEAR.

LECONEY, THOMAS RATCLIFF MD, LICENSE NUMBER 00H0552 OF FORT WORTH, TX, WAS DISCIPLINED BY TEXAS ON AUGUST 19, 1994
DISCIPLINARY ACTION: REQUIRED TO TAKE ADDITIONAL MEDICAL EDUCATION; MONITORING OF PHYSICIAN PERFORMANCE
OFFENSE: SUBSTANCE ABUSE
NOTES: HE HAS HAD THREE SINUS SURGERIES TRYING TO CORRECT A MEDICAL CONDITION THAT PRODUCED SEVERE HEADACHES; HIS PHYSICIAN PRESCRIBED CERTAIN DRUGS FOR HIM INCLUDING DALGAN FOR A LEGITIMATE MEDICAL CONDITION; BECAME HABITUATED TO DALGAN; REALIZED THIS AND HAS SOUGHT ASSISTANCE; IS FOLLOWING AN AFTERCARE PROGRAM INCLUDING ATTENDING AA, A WEEKLY CADUCEUS MEETING AND ASSISTANCE FROM AN IMPAIRED PHYSICIANS GROUP AND MEETING WITH PSYCHIATRISTS. CONDITIONS OF FIVE YEAR RESTRICTION: SHALL ABSTAIN FROM THE CONSUMPTION OF ALCOHOL/CHEMICAL SUBSTANCES IN ANY FORM UNLESS PRESCRIBED BY ANOTHER PHYSICIAN FOR LEGITIMATE AND THERAPEUTIC PURPOSES; SHALL NOT TREAT OR OTHERWISE SERVE AS PHYSICIAN, PRESCRIBE, DISPENSE OR ADMINISTER DRUGS THAT MAY BE SUBJECT TO ABUSE TO HIMSELF OR ANY MEMBER OF HIS FAMILY; SHALL SUBMIT HIMSELF FOR APPROPRIATE EXAMS INCLUDING DRUG OR ALCOHOL SCREENS; SHALL CONTINUE TREATMENT WITH PRESENT PSYCHIATRIST WITH QUARTERLY REPORTS; SHALL PARTICIPATE IN AA'S PROGRAM NOT LESS THAN THREE TIMES A WEEK WITH QUARTERLY REPORTS TO THE BOARD; SHALL PARTICIPATE IN ACTIVITIES OF A PHYSICIAN HEALTH AND REHABILITATION COMMITTEE AND ATTEND WEEKLY MEETINGS WITH QUARTERLY REPORTS; SHALL ATTEND AT LEAST 50 HOURS PER YEAR OF CONTINUING MEDICAL EDUCATION; SHALL APPEAR BEFORE THE BOARD TWICE A YEAR; SHALL GIVE A COPY OF THIS ORDER TO ANY HEALTH CARE ENTITY WHERE HE HAS PRIVILEGES; SHALL COOPERATE WITH THE BOARD IN VERIFYING COMPLIANCE; SHALL INFORM BOARD OF CHANGE OF ADDRESS WITHIN 10 DAYS OR IF HE LEAVES THE STATE; TIME SPENT OUT OF TEXAS DOES NOT COUNT TOWARD RESTRICTION. SHALL NOT SEEK MODIFICATION FOR ONE YEAR. ON 9/20/97 PETITION TO TERMINATE ORDER DENIED. ON 8/22/98 ORDER TERMINATED.

LEDLIE, WILLIAM BOYER MD, DATE OF BIRTH JANUARY 4, 1950, LICENSE NUMBER 00E4475 OF 9218 MONTFORD, HOUSTON, TX, WAS DISCIPLINED BY TEXAS ON AUGUST 24, 1991
DISCIPLINARY ACTION: SURRENDER OF CONTROLLED SUBSTANCE LICENSE; 36-MONTH PROBATION
OFFENSE: SUBSTANCE ABUSE
NOTES: LICENSE SUSPENDED, STAYED; PROBATION TERMS ARE AS FOLLOWS: SHALL APPEAR BEFORE THE BOARD TWICE A YEAR; SHALL SURRENDER DEA AND DPS CONTROLLED SUBSTANCES REGISTRATION CERTIFICATES AND NOT ATTEMPT TO REREGISTER WITHOUT BOARD APPROVAL; SHALL SURRENDER ALL UNUSED TRIPLICATE PRESCRIPTION FORMS AND NOT ATTEMPT TO ORDER MORE WITHOUT BOARD APPROVAL; SHALL SURRENDER ALL CONTROLLED SUBSTANCES, INCLUDING SAMPLES; SHALL NOT TREAT OR OTHERWISE SERVE AS THE PHYSICIAN, PRESCRIBE, DISPENSE, OR ADMINISTER CONTROLLED SUBSTANCES, OR ANY OTHER DRUGS THAT MAY BE SUBJECT TO ABUSE, FOR SELF OR ANY MEMBER OF IMMEDIATE FAMILY; MAY ADMINISTER TO SELF OR IMMEDIATE FAMILY ONLY SUCH DRUGS AS ARE PRESCRIBED BY OTHER PHYSICIANS; SHALL ABSTAIN FROM CONSUMPTION OF ALCOHOL, CONTROLLED SUBSTANCES, DANGEROUS DRUGS, OR PRESCRIPTION DRUGS IN ANY FORM; SHALL PARTICIPATE WITH IMPAIRED PHYSICIANS PROGRAM; SHALL SUBMIT FOR ALCOHOL OR DRUG SCREENING; SHALL CONTINUE TREATMENT FROM TALBOTT-MARSH RECOVERY PROGRAM; SHALL FURNISH WRITTEN REPORTS WHEN REQUESTED; SHALL PARTICIPATE IN AA. ON 1/29/93 MODIFICATION OF ORDER GIVING HIM PERMISSION TO REAPPLY TO THE DRUG ENFORCEMENT ADMINISTRATION AND THE TEXAS DEPARTMENT OF PUBLIC SAFETY FOR SCHEDULES II, IIN, III, IIIN, IV OR V CONTROLLED SUBSTANCE AUTHORITY. ALL OTHER TERMS AND CONDITIONS

REMAIN IN EFFECT.

LEDLIE, WILLIAM BOYER MD OF HOUSTON, TX, WAS DISCIPLINED BY UTAH ON MAY 7, 1992
DISCIPLINARY ACTION: SURRENDER OF LICENSE; SURRENDER OF CONTROLLED SUBSTANCE LICENSE
OFFENSE: DISCIPLINARY ACTION BY ANOTHER STATE OR AGENCY

NOTES: ENGAGING IN THE INTEMPERATE USE OF A CONTROLLED SUBSTANCE RESULTING IN DISCIPLINARY ACTION AGAINST HIS LICENSE IN TEXAS. AGREED NOT TO REAPPLY FOR LICENSURE FOR 2 1/2 YEARS.

LEE, CHUN SHON MD, LICENSE NUMBER E3991 OF PECOS, TX, WAS DISCIPLINED BY TEXAS ON AUGUST 22, 1998
DISCIPLINARY ACTION: FINE; REPRIMAND
OFFENSE: SEXUAL ABUSE OF OR SEXUAL MISCONDUCT WITH A PATIENT

NOTES: IN 1994 - 1996 HE ALLEGEDLY ENGAGED IN INAPPROPRIATE VERBAL MISCONDUCT OF A SEXUAL NATURE WITH 3 PATIENTS; HE CONTENDS THAT HIS VERBAL COMMENTS WERE MISUNDERSTOOD; IN 7/97 HE VOLUNTARILY SUBMITTED TO A 96 HOUR INPATIENT EVALUATION TO DETERMINE WHETHER HE SUFFERS FROM ANY PHYSICAL/PSYCHIATRIC CONDITION WHICH MAY AFFECT HIS ABILITY TO SAFELY PRACTICE MEDICINE; THE EVALUATION FAILED TO DETERMINE ANY PROBLEM. $1,000 FINE.

LEE, HOWARD MONROE JR MD, LICENSE NUMBER 00F1738 OF EL PASO, TX, WAS DISCIPLINED BY TEXAS ON OCTOBER 5, 1991
DISCIPLINARY ACTION: 60-MONTH PROBATION; REQUIRED TO TAKE ADDITIONAL MEDICAL EDUCATION
OFFENSE: SUBSTANDARD CARE, INCOMPETENCE OR NEGLIGENCE

NOTES: ON OR ABOUT 12/20/88 MADE AN ERROR IN PERFORMING LUMBAR SURGERY FOR A HERNIATED DISC, WHICH RESULTED IN A DURAL LEAK AND OTHER COMPLICATIONS, CAUSING THE PATIENT TO HAVE SEVERAL ADDITIONAL OPERATIONS TO CORRECT HIS MISTAKE; DID NOT RELEASE HER MEDICAL RECORDS IN A TIMELY MANNER BECAUSE HE WAS EMBARRASSED ABOUT HIS MISTAKE. CONDITIONS OF PROBATION INCLUDE: COMPLETION OF AT LEAST 50 HOURS PER EACH YEAR OF CONTINUING MEDICAL EDUCATION; MUST APPEAR BEFORE THE BOARD ONCE A YEAR; SHALL COOPERATE WITH BOARD IN VERIFYING COMPLIANCE; SHALL ADVISE BOARD OF ANY ADDRESS CHANGE WITHIN 10 DAYS; TIME SPENT OUT OF TEXAS DOES NOT COUNT TOWARD PROBATION. ON 11/3/94 PROBATION TERMINATED.

LEE, JOHN H DO, DATE OF BIRTH AUGUST 30, 1957 OF 5885 W PORT ARTHUR ROAD, PORT ARTHUR, TX, WAS DISCIPLINED BY MEDICARE ON MAY 9, 1995
DISCIPLINARY ACTION: EXCLUSION FROM THE MEDICARE AND/OR MEDICAID PROGRAM
OFFENSE: NONCOMPLIANCE WITH A PROFESSIONAL RULE

NOTES: DEFAULTED ON PUBLIC HEALTH SERVICE EDUCATION LOAN. REINSTATED ON 5/16/95.

LEGGETT, JOSEPH E MD OF 815 11TH STREET, HUNTSVILLE, TX, WAS DISCIPLINED BY DEA ON NOVEMBER 18, 1994
DISCIPLINARY ACTION: SURRENDER OF CONTROLLED SUBSTANCE LICENSE

NOTES: IN LIEU OF PUBLIC INTEREST REVOCATION.

LEGGETT, JOSEPH EDWARD MD, DATE OF BIRTH JULY 10, 1943, LICENSE NUMBER 00E2676 OF 575 ELKINS LANE, HUNTSVILLE, TX, WAS DISCIPLINED BY TEXAS ON JUNE 17, 1992
DISCIPLINARY ACTION: RESTRICTION PLACED ON LICENSE

NOTES: RESTRICTED TO THE TREATMENT OF MALE PATIENTS WITHIN THE DEPARTMENT OF CORRECTIONS UNTIL SUCH TIME THAT THE IDAHO BOARD'S ACTION IS RESOLVED.

LEGGETT, JOSEPH EDWARD MD, DATE OF BIRTH JULY 10, 1943, LICENSE NUMBER 00M5108 OF COEUR D'ALENE, ID, WAS DISCIPLINED BY IDAHO ON SEPTEMBER 11, 1992
DISCIPLINARY ACTION: SURRENDER OF LICENSE
OFFENSE: SEXUAL ABUSE OF OR SEXUAL MISCONDUCT WITH A PATIENT

NOTES: CHARGED WITH HAVING SEX WITH TWO PATIENTS. HAS APPEALED A 9/28/89 ORDER OF THE BOARD REVOKING HIS LICENSE TO THE IDAHO SUPREME COURT. IN 11/91 DISTRICT COURT REJECTED AN APPEAL TO THE COURT. THE EARLIER APPEAL RESULTED IN A STAY OF THE REVOCATION ORDER. JUDGE CALLED FOR ADDITIONAL CONSIDERATION BY BOARD. A SECOND HEARING WAS CONDUCTED MAY 8-9 1990. ON 1/15/91 THE BOARD AFFIRMED THE 9/29/89 REVOCATION. ON 9/11/92, HE AGREED TO VOLUNTARILY SURRENDER HIS LICENSE AND NEVER AGAIN APPLY FOR REINSTATEMENT; THE REVOCATION WAS WITHDRAWN.

LEGGETT, JOSEPH EDWARD MD, DATE OF BIRTH JULY 10, 1943, LICENSE NUMBER 00E2676 OF 575 ELKINS LAKE, HUNTSVILLE, TX, WAS DISCIPLINED BY TEXAS ON NOVEMBER 19, 1993
DISCIPLINARY ACTION: 120-MONTH PROBATION; RESTRICTION PLACED ON LICENSE
OFFENSE: DISCIPLINARY ACTION BY ANOTHER STATE OR AGENCY

NOTES: ON 9/29/89 IDAHO BOARD REVOKED HIS MEDICAL LICENSE AFTER FINDING HE HAD ENGAGED IN IMPROPER SEXUAL CONDUCT WITH TWO PATIENTS; HE DENIED THESE CHARGES AND APPEALED THE RULING; THE DISTRICT COURT AFFIRMED THE BOARD'S RULING ON 11/22/91; HE APPEALED TO THE IDAHO SUPREME COURT; PRIOR TO A RULING BY THE COURT HE AND THE IDAHO BOARD ENTERED INTO A STIPULATION FOR DISMISSAL WITH PREJUDICE WHEREBY THE APPEAL WAS DISMISSED AND HE WAS ALLOWED TO SURRENDER HIS LICENSE IN LIEU OF REVOCATION; WAS ALSO INDICTED IN WYOMING FOR ALLEGED SEXUAL MISCONDUCT INVOLVING FEMALE PATIENTS; IS CONTESTING THESE ALLEGATIONS AND A TRIAL WAS PENDING AS OF THE ORDER DATE; HIS EMPLOYER IN TEXAS HAS PLACED HIM IN A PURELY ADMINISTRATIVE ROLE. TEXAS LICENSE SUSPENDED. SUSPENSION STAYED. CONDITIONS OF PROBATION: RESTRICTED FROM THE TREATMENT OF ANY PATIENT PENDING THE OUTCOME OF THE CRIMINAL MATTERS IN WYOMING; IF THIS DOES NOT RESULT IN A FINDING OF GUILT OR A CONVICTION MAY RETURN TO THE PRACTICE OF MEDICINE BUT MAY ONLY TREAT MALE PRISONERS. OTHER CONDITIONS INCLUDE: SHALL APPEAR BEFORE THE BOARD ONCE A YEAR; SHALL ATTEND AT LEAST 50 HOURS OF CONTINUING MEDICAL EDUCATION PER YEAR; SHALL GIVE A COPY OF THIS ORDER TO ANY HEALTH CARE ENTITY WHERE HE HAS PRIVILEGES; SHALL COOPERATE WITH THE BOARD IN VERIFYING COMPLIANCE; SHALL INFORM BOARD OF CHANGE OF ADDRESS WITHIN 10 DAYS OR IF HE LEAVES THE STATE; TIME SPENT OUT OF TEXAS DOES NOT COUNT TOWARD PROBATION. IF HE IS FOUND GUILTY OF THE PENDING CHARGES IN WYOMING, TEXAS LICENSE WILL BE REVOKED. SHALL NOT SEEK MODIFICATION FOR ONE YEAR.

LEGGETT, JOSEPH EDWARD MD, DATE OF BIRTH JULY 10, 1943, LICENSE NUMBER 00E2676 OF 575 ELKINS LAKE, HUNTSVILLE, TX, WAS DISCIPLINED BY TEXAS ON SEPTEMBER 20, 1994
DISCIPLINARY ACTION: LICENSE REVOCATION
OFFENSE: CRIMINAL CONVICTION OR PLEA OF GUILTY, NOLO CONTENDERE, OR NO CONTEST TO A CRIME

NOTES: ON 9/14/94 IN WYOMING HE ENTERED PLEAS OF NOLO CONTENDERE TO CHARGES OF SECOND DEGREE SEXUAL ASSAULT; THE COURT ORDERED HIM PLACED ON FIVE YEARS OF SUPERVISED PROBATION UNDER CONDITIONS.

LEGGETT, JOSEPH EDWARD MD, DATE OF BIRTH JULY 10, 1943 OF 575 ELKINS LAKE, HUNTSVILLE, TX, WAS DISCIPLINED BY MEDICARE ON MAY 4, 1995
DISCIPLINARY ACTION: 60-MONTH EXCLUSION FROM THE MEDICARE AND/OR MEDICAID PROGRAM
OFFENSE: CRIMINAL CONVICTION OR PLEA OF GUILTY, NOLO CONTENDERE, OR NO CONTEST TO A CRIME

NOTES: CONVICTED OF A CRIME RELATED TO PATIENT ABUSE OR NEGLECT.

LEHMILLER, JOHN ERICH MD, LICENSE NUMBER 00J3340 OF GALVESTON, TX, WAS DISCIPLINED BY TEXAS ON MAY 26, 1994
DISCIPLINARY ACTION: EMERGENCY SUSPENSION
OFFENSE: SUBSTANCE ABUSE

NOTES: AVAILABLE EVIDENCE AND INFORMATION INDICATE THAT BETWEEN 12/3/93 AND 4/18/94 CONSUMED COCAINE THREE TIMES AND ENGAGED IN INTEMPERATE USE OF ALCOHOL.

LEHMILLER, JOHN ERICH MD, LICENSE NUMBER 00J3340 OF GALVESTON, TX, WAS DISCIPLINED BY TEXAS ON AUGUST 19, 1994
DISCIPLINARY ACTION: LICENSE SUSPENSION
OFFENSE: SUBSTANCE ABUSE

NOTES: HE HAS ADMITTED TO A HISTORY OF POLYSUBSTANCE ABUSE AS RECENTLY AS 7/94 AND DATING BACK A NUMBER OF YEARS; HE CLAIMS A SOBRIETY DATE OF 7/10/94. LICENSE SUSPENDED UNTIL HE APPEARS BEFORE THE BOARD AND PROVIDES SUFFICIENT EVIDENCE THAT HE IS PHYSICALLY, MENTALLY AND OTHERWISE COMPETENT TO SAFELY PRACTICE.

LEHMILLER, JOHN ERICH MD, DATE OF BIRTH APRIL 25, 1965 OF 3500 E SIMCOE STREET, #67, LAFAYETTE, LA, WAS DISCIPLINED BY MEDICARE ON APRIL 23, 1996
DISCIPLINARY ACTION: EXCLUSION FROM THE MEDICARE AND/OR MEDICAID PROGRAM
OFFENSE: DISCIPLINARY ACTION BY ANOTHER STATE OR AGENCY

NOTES: LICENSE SUSPENDED FOR REASONS BEARING ON PROFESSIONAL COMPETENCE.

LEHRER, LLOYD MICHAEL MD, LICENSE NUMBER 00G4025 OF HOUSTON, TX, WAS DISCIPLINED BY TEXAS ON DECEMBER 3, 1990
DISCIPLINARY ACTION: 36-MONTH PROBATION; REQUIRED TO TAKE ADDITIONAL MEDICAL EDUCATION

NOTES: MUST MAINTAIN COMPLETE AND ACCURATE RECORDS OF PURCHASES AND DISPOSALS OF CONTROLLED SUBSTANCES.

LEHRER, LLOYD MICHAEL MD, LICENSE NUMBER 00G4025 OF HOUSTON, TX, WAS DISCIPLINED BY TEXAS ON AUGUST 20, 1992
DISCIPLINARY ACTION: SURRENDER OF LICENSE
OFFENSE: PHYSICAL OR MENTAL ILLNESS INHIBITING THE ABILITY TO PRACTICE WITH SKILL AND SAFETY

NOTES: INABILITY TO PRACTICE MEDICINE WITH REASONABLE SKILL AND SAFETY TO PATIENTS BY REASON OF ILLNESS. RETIREMENT UNDER TERMS AND CONDITIONS.

LEININGER, JAMES R MD, LICENSE NUMBER 00E1653, WAS DISCIPLINED BY TEXAS ON AUGUST 17, 1996
DISCIPLINARY ACTION: FINE; REPRIMAND
OFFENSE: NONCOMPLIANCE WITH A PROFESSIONAL RULE

NOTES: FAILED TO OBTAIN 24 HOURS OF CONTINUING MEDICAL EDUCATION AS REQUIRED BY 9/1/95 FOR THE RENEWAL OF HIS LICENSE; HE WAS GRANTED AN EXTENSION TO 11/30/95 WHICH HE ALSO DID NOT MEET; STILL REQUIRED TO MEET CONTINUING MEDICAL EDUCATION REQUIREMENTS; $100 ADMINISTRATIVE PENALTY; SHALL COOPERATE WITH THE BOARD IN VERIFYING COMPLIANCE.

LENGYEL, MIRCEA IAON MD, LICENSE NUMBER 00D2805 OF HOUSTON, TX, WAS DISCIPLINED BY TEXAS ON JANUARY 12, 1991
DISCIPLINARY ACTION: 12-MONTH PROBATION

NOTES: SHALL NOT TREAT OR SERVE AS PHYSICIAN, PRESCRIBE, DISPENSE, OR ADMINISTER CONTROLLED SUBSTANCES OR OTHER DRUGS THAT MAY BE SUBJECT TO ABUSE, OR WRITE PRESCRIPTIONS FOR CONTROLLED SUBSTANCES OR OTHER DRUGS THAT MAY BE SUBJECT TO ABUSE, FOR ANY MEMBER OF IMMEDIATE FAMILY OR SELF, AND ADMINISTER TO SELF OR IMMEDIATE FAMILY ONLY SUCH DRUGS AS PRESCRIBED BY OTHER PHYSICIANS.

LENTINO, EDUARDO P MD, LICENSE NUMBER 00E7649 OF HOUSTON, TX, WAS DISCIPLINED BY TEXAS ON DECEMBER 1, 1990
DISCIPLINARY ACTION: REPRIMAND

NOTES: STIPULATED ORDER.

LENTINO, JORGE A MD, LICENSE NUMBER 00E3994 OF HOUSTON, TX, WAS DISCIPLINED BY TEXAS ON DECEMBER 1, 1990
DISCIPLINARY ACTION: REPRIMAND

NOTES: STIPULATED ORDER. ON 1/18/97 BOARD GRANTED HIS PETITION FOR TERMINATION OF THIS ORDER BASED ON COMPLIANCE WITH CONDITIONS. ON 3/1/97 TERMINATION CONFIRMED.

LEONG, DANIEL K DO, LICENSE NUMBER 00G1462 OF DALLAS, TX, WAS DISCIPLINED BY TEXAS ON SEPTEMBER 28, 1990
DISCIPLINARY ACTION: 120-MONTH PROBATION; RESTRICTION PLACED ON CONTROLLED SUBSTANCE LICENSE

NOTES: MUST SUBMIT FOR PSYCHIATRIC EVALUATION AND FOLLOW ANY RECOMMENDATIONS REGARDING CARE; NOT SERVE AS PHYSICIAN, PRESCRIBE, DISPENSE, OR ADMINISTER CONTROLLED SUBSTANCES OR OTHER DRUGS THAT MAY BE SUBJECT TO ABUSE OR WRITE PRESCRIPTIONS FOR CONTROLLED SUBSTANCES OR OTHER DRUGS THAT MAY BE SUBJECT TO ABUSE FOR SELF OR IMMEDIATE FAMILY MEMBERS; ADMINISTER TO SELF OR IMMEDIATE FAMILY ONLY SUCH DRUGS AS PRESCRIBED BY OTHER PHYSICIANS; REFRAIN FROM PRESCRIBING OR UTILIZING HALCION IN HIS MEDICAL PRACTICE FOR SELF, FAMILY, OR PATIENTS; COMPLETE PRECEPTORSHIP ON PREVENTION AND TREATMENT OF DRUG ABUSE; ATTEND CONTINUING MEDICAL EDUCATION; REFRAIN FROM ORDERING MEDICATIONS FROM PHARMACEUTICAL SUPPLIER OR WHOLESALER FOR DISPENSING OR SUPPLYING TO PATIENTS; IF EMPLOYED IN HOSPITAL EMERGENCY ROOMS OR UNDER OTHER CIRCUMSTANCES REQUIRING

FREQUENT TRAVEL, SHALL PROVIDE TRAVEL OR WORK SCHEDULE TO THE BOARD; IF ORDERING ADMINISTRATION OF CONTROLLED SUBSTANCES FOR EMERGENCY ROOM OR HOSPITAL IN-PATIENTS OR PRESCRIBING CONTROLLED SUBSTANCES IN WRITING OR BY TELEPHONE FOR SAID PATIENTS, HE SHALL RECORD SAID PRESCRIPTIONS OR MEDICATION ORDERS IN LOG, SPECIFYING CERTAIN DATA, AND HAVE LOG AVAILABLE FOR INSPECTION; IF PRESCRIBING CONTROLLED SUBSTANCES IN OFFICE OR CLINIC SETTING, SHALL OBTAIN AND UTILIZE DUPLICATE, SERIALLY-NUMBERED PRESCRIPTIONS AND RETAIN DUPLICATES OF CONTROLLED SUBSTANCES FOR INSPECTION BY BOARD REPRESENTATIVES; APPEAR BEFORE BOARD OR BOARD COMMITTEE TWICE YEARLY. ON 6/28/95 HIS PETITION FOR TERMINATION DENIED BUT ORDER MODIFIED SO HE SHALL BE ABLE TO PETITION THE BOARD FOR MODIFICATION OR TERMINATION OF THIS ORDER EVERY SIX MONTHS. ON 1/18/97 HIS PETITION FOR TERMINATION OF THIS ORDER GRANTED BASED ON HIS COMPLIANCE WITH CONDITIONS.

LESHNOWER, ALAN C MD, LICENSE NUMBER 00G0756 OF ODESSA, TX, WAS DISCIPLINED BY TEXAS ON NOVEMBER 19, 1993
DISCIPLINARY ACTION: 36-MONTH PROBATION; RESTRICTION PLACED ON LICENSE
OFFENSE: SUBSTANDARD CARE, INCOMPETENCE OR NEGLIGENCE

NOTES: DURING 1991 IN THE COURSE OF TREATING THREE PATIENTS HE FAILED TO ADEQUATELY DOCUMENT THEIR RECORDS AND TO ENSURE THAT PROPER FOLLOW-UP CARE WAS PROVIDED FOLLOWING BYPASS SURGERY; TREATMENT WAS SUBSTANDARD AND CONTRIBUTED TO THE COMBINATION OF FACTORS WHICH LED TO THEIR DEATHS; AT THE TIME WAS PRACTICING AT A FACILITY WHICH DID NOT HAVE A CARDIOLOGIST READILY AVAILABLE AND WHICH WAS NOT ADEQUATELY SUITED TO PROVIDE SUFFICIENT SUPPORT FOR HIGH-RISK CARDIAC SURGERIES. SUSPENSION STAYED. CONDITIONS OF PROBATION: SHALL ATTEND AT LEAST 50 HOURS PER YEAR OF CONTINUING MEDICAL EDUCATION TO INCLUDE AT LEAST ONE COURSE IN CARDIOVASCULAR SURGERY AND ONE IN PHARMACOLOGY; SHALL REFER ALL HIGH-RISK CARDIOVASCULAR SURGERY CANDIDATES TO OTHER PHYSICIANS AND FACILITIES WHICH ARE ADEQUATELY SUITED AND EQUIPPED TO PERFORM HIGH-RISK CARDIOVASCULAR SURGERY; SHALL ENSURE AND DOCUMENT THAT EACH OF HIS SURGICAL PATIENTS RECEIVES ADEQUATE HOSPITAL CARE DURING THE 48 HOURS FOLLOWING SURGERY; SHALL MAINTAIN AN UP-TO-DATE LIST OF ALL HIS SURGICAL CASES AVAILABLE FOR REVIEW; SHALL SUBMIT A REPORT THREE TIMES A YEAR REFLECTING THE MORTALITY RATE FOR PATIENTS UNDER HIS CARE; SHALL APPEAR BEFORE THE BOARD TWICE A YEAR; SHALL GIVE A COPY OF THIS ORDER TO ANY HEALTH CARE ENTITY WHERE HE HAS PRIVILEGES; SHALL COOPERATE WITH THE BOARD IN VERIFYING COMPLIANCE; SHALL INFORM BOARD OF CHANGE OF ADDRESS WITHIN 10 DAYS OR IF HE LEAVES THE STATE; TIME SPENT OUT OF TEXAS DOES NOT COUNT TOWARD PROBATION. SHALL NOT SEEK MODIFICATION FOR ONE YEAR. ON 6/28/95 BOARD GRANTED TERMINATION OF THIS ORDER BASED ON HIS HISTORY OF COMPLIANCE, HIS COOPERATION WITH BOARD REPRESENTATIVES, AND BECAUSE THE HOSPITAL FACILITY WHERE HE PRACTICES HAS BEEN UPGRADED AND NOW PROVIDES SUPPORT FOR HIGH-RISK CARDIAC SURGERIES.

LESHNOWER, ALAN CHARLES MD, LICENSE NUMBER 0G35798 OF ODESSA, TX, WAS DISCIPLINED BY CALIFORNIA ON JUNE 19, 1996
DISCIPLINARY ACTION: 60-MONTH PROBATION
OFFENSE: DISCIPLINARY ACTION BY ANOTHER STATE OR AGENCY

NOTES: DISCIPLINARY ACTION IN TEXAS FOR FAILURE TO PRACTICE MEDICINE IN AN ACCEPTABLE MANNER CONSISTENT WITH PUBLIC HEALTH AND WELFARE. REVOCATION, STAYED.

LETT, CHARLES R MD, LICENSE NUMBER 0009543 OF 3938 SOUTH FRANKLIN, DALLAS, TX, WAS DISCIPLINED BY GEORGIA ON JULY 1, 1990
DISCIPLINARY ACTION: LICENSE REVOCATION
OFFENSE: DISCIPLINARY ACTION BY ANOTHER STATE OR AGENCY

NOTES: FAILURE TO RENEW AND DISCIPLINARY ACTION IN ANOTHER STATE. ADMINISTRATIVE REVOCATION.

LETT, CHARLES REGINALD MD, DATE OF BIRTH MAY 31, 1936, LICENSE NUMBER 00D3635 OF TENNESSEE COLONY, TX, WAS DISCIPLINED BY TEXAS ON MARCH 31, 1990
DISCIPLINARY ACTION: 60-MONTH RESTRICTION PLACED ON CONTROLLED SUBSTANCE LICENSE; REQUIRED TO TAKE ADDITIONAL MEDICAL EDUCATION
OFFENSE: SUBSTANCE ABUSE

NOTES: STIPULATED ORDER. MUST SUBMIT FOR PSYCHIATRIC EVALUATION AND ANY RECOMMENDED TREATMENT, PARTICIPATE IN AA OR NARCOTICS ANONYMOUS, OBTAIN CONTINUING MEDICAL EDUCATION, REQUEST MODIFICATION OF CONTROLLED SUBSTANCES REGISTRATIONS TO ELIMINATE SCHEDULES II, II-N, III AND III-N AND NOT REREGISTER WITHOUT BOARD AUTHORITY, SURRENDER UNUSED TRIPLICATE PRESCRIPTION FORMS AND NOT ORDER MORE UNTIL BOARD WILL PERMIT, NOT TREAT SELF FOR RECURRING MEDICAL CONDITIONS OR ADMINISTER OR PRESCRIBE CONTROLLED SUBSTANCES FOR SELF, PARTICIPATE IN ACTIVITIES OF COUNTY MEDICAL SOCIETY'S COMMITTEE ON PHYSICIAN HEALTH AND REHABILITATION, COMPLETE PRECEPTORSHIP ON PREVENTION AND TREATMENT OF DRUG ABUSE, AND SUBMIT FOR APPROPRIATE EXAMINATIONS TO DETERMINE FREEDOM FROM ALCOHOL AND DRUGS EXCEPT THOSE PRESCRIBED BY ANOTHER PHYSICIAN FOR VALID MEDICAL PURPOSE.

LETT, CHARLES REGINALD MD, DATE OF BIRTH MAY 31, 1936, LICENSE NUMBER 00D3635 OF 131 MEMORY LANE #912, PALESTINE, TX, WAS DISCIPLINED BY TEXAS ON OCTOBER 5, 1991
DISCIPLINARY ACTION: LICENSE SUSPENSION; 60-MONTH PROBATION
OFFENSE: FAILURE TO COMPLY WITH PREVIOUS BOARD ORDER

NOTES: FAILED TO COMPLY WITH 3/31/90 BOARD ORDER CONCERNING RECOMMENDATIONS OF BOARD APPROVED PSYCHIATRIST, INCLUDING: ENROLLING AND PARTICIPATING IN AN OUT-OF-STATE DRUG TREATMENT PROGRAM, ATTENDING WEEKLY MEETINGS WITH THE IMPAIRED PHYSICIANS GROUP IN DALLAS UPON COMPLETION OF THE ABOVE PROGRAM, SUBMITTING TO FOUR RANDOM URINE DRUG SCREENS PER YEAR, PARTICIPATING IN WEEKLY OUT-PATIENT PSYCHOTHERAPY FOR TWO YEARS, ATTENDING AA MEETINGS FIVE TIMES A WEEK; ALSO FAILED TO SUBMIT PROOF OF COMPLETION OF 50 HOURS OF CONTINUING MEDICAL EDUCATION BY 1/31/91, AND FAILED TO ENROLL IN A TWO-WEEK PRECEPTORSHIP ON THE PREVENTION AND TREATMENT OF DRUG ABUSE. REVOCATION STAYED, PROBATION WITH FOLLOWING CONDITIONS: LICENSE SUSPENDED UNTIL HE COMPLETES OUT-OF-

STATE DRUG TREATMENT PROGRAM; SHALL COMPLETE A TWO-WEEK PRECEPTORSHIP ON THE PREVENTION AND TREATMENT OF DRUG ABUSE WITHIN 14 MONTHS OF FINISHING THAT PROGRAM; SHALL PARTICIPATE IN THE FOLLOWING ACTIVITIES FOR A COMBINED TOTAL OF FIVE TIMES A WEEK DURING THE FIRST SIX MONTHS FROM THE DATE OF THIS ORDER: AA OR NARCOTICS ANONYMOUS, INCLUDING A 12-STEP PROGRAM; ANY COUNTY MEDICAL SOCIETY'S IMPAIRED PHYSICIAN PROGRAM, INCLUDING PARTICIPATION IN WEEKLY MEETINGS WITH QUARTERLY REPORTS TO THE BOARD; MUST CONTINUE PSYCHIATRIC TREATMENT WITH QUARTERLY REPORTS; SHALL OBTAIN AT LEAST 50 HOURS OF CONTINUING MEDICAL EDUCATION IN GENERAL MEDICAL COURSES, WHERE AT LEAST TEN HOURS SHALL INCLUDE TOPICS RELATED TO PSYCHOPHARMACOLOGY; SHALL LIMIT HIS CONTROLLED SUBSTANCE SCHEDULES TO IV AND V; SHALL SURRENDER ALL UNUSED TRIPLICATE PRESCRIPTION FORMS; SHALL NOT TREAT HIMSELF FOR ANY RECURRING MEDICAL CONDITION, AND SHALL NOT UNDER ANY CIRCUMSTANCES ADMINISTER OR PRESCRIBE CONTROLLED SUBSTANCES FOR HIMSELF; SHALL SUBMIT HIMSELF FOR EXAMINATIONS, INCLUDING SCREENING FOR ALCOHOL OR DRUGS; SHALL COOPERATE WITH BOARD IN VERIFYING COMPLIANCE; SHALL ADVISE THE BOARD IF HE CHANGES ADDRESS WITHIN 10 DAYS; TIME SPENT OUT OF TEXAS DOES NOT COUNT TOWARDS PROBATION; SHALL NOT PETITION FOR REINSTATEMENT FOR AT LEAST ONE YEAR. ON 1/29/93, THIS ORDER AMENDED SO THAT HE APPEAR BEFORE THE BOARD OR A COMMITTEE OF THE BOARD TWICE A YEAR DURING EACH YEAR OF PROBATION.

LETT, CHARLES REGINALD MD OF 131 MEMORY LANE #912, PALESTINE, TX, WAS DISCIPLINED BY DEA ON APRIL 27, 1992
DISCIPLINARY ACTION: RESTRICTION PLACED ON CONTROLLED SUBSTANCE LICENSE
OFFENSE: PROFESSIONAL MISCONDUCT

NOTES: BOARD NUMBER RETIRED 11/01/86 AND 11/01/88 AS DELINQUENT. RESTRICTION PLACED ON REGISTRATION DUE TO HIS PRESCRIBING 7,162 DOSAGE UNITS FIORINAL FOR HIMSELF BETWEEN 10/27/87 AND 04/12/89. VOLUNTARY SURRENDER OF CONTROLLED SUBSTANCES PRIVILEGES.

LEVENSON, ALVIN J MD, WAS DISCIPLINED BY WYOMING ON NOVEMBER 8, 1995
DISCIPLINARY ACTION: DENIAL OF NEW LICENSE
OFFENSE: PROFESSIONAL MISCONDUCT

NOTES: DURING HIS PERSONAL INTERVIEW WITH THE BOARD WHEN DISCUSSING HIS PRESENT MEDICAL, PERSONAL, AND PROFESSIONAL CIRCUMSTANCES, HE FREQUENTLY EXHIBITED INAPPROPRIATE ANGER, HOSTILITY, AND VERBAL COMBATIVENESS AND AN INABILITY TO THINK AND EXPRESS HIMSELF IN A RATIONAL AND COHERENT MANNER. THIS DEMONSTRATION FURTHER CORROBORATED THE CONCERNS EXPRESSED IN A REFERENCE LETTER THAT HE HAS DIFFICULTY IN INTERPERSONAL RELATIONSHIPS WHICH, COULD BE REASONABLY VIEWED AS POSING A DANGER TO THE HEALTH AND SAFETY OF THE PATIENTS AT THE WYOMING STATE HOSPITAL.

LEVENSON, ALVIN J MD, LICENSE NUMBER 174212 OF 3801 O'MEARA DRIVE APT 366, HOUSTON, TX, WAS DISCIPLINED BY NEW YORK ON JULY 13, 1998
DISCIPLINARY ACTION: LICENSE SUSPENSION
OFFENSE: FAILURE TO COMPLY WITH PREVIOUS BOARD ORDER

NOTES: FAILED TO COMPLY WITH AN ORDER OF THE BOARD ORDERING HIM TO SUBMIT TO AN EVALUATION. SUSPENSION UNTIL HE HAS COMPLIED WITH AN ORDER OF THE BOARD.

LEVENSON, ALVIN J MD, LICENSE NUMBER E1022 OF SUGAR LAND, TX, WAS DISCIPLINED BY TEXAS ON JANUARY 29, 1999
DISCIPLINARY ACTION: LICENSE SUSPENSION
OFFENSE: PROFESSIONAL MISCONDUCT

NOTES: FAILURE TO PAY CHILD SUPPORT.

LEVIE, CHARLES A MD OF 307 WILLIFORD ROAD, JONESBORO, IL, WAS DISCIPLINED BY DEA ON AUGUST 19, 1996
DISCIPLINARY ACTION: SURRENDER OF CONTROLLED SUBSTANCE LICENSE

LEVIE, CHARLES A MD, LICENSE NUMBER H7455 OF JONESBORO, IL, WAS DISCIPLINED BY TEXAS ON AUGUST 9, 1997
DISCIPLINARY ACTION: SURRENDER OF LICENSE
OFFENSE: DISCIPLINARY ACTION BY ANOTHER STATE OR AGENCY

NOTES: ON 3/13/96 THE ILLINOIS BOARD INDEFINITELY SUSPENDED HIS LICENSE; HE SELF-REPORTED HIS SUBSTANCE ABUSE PROBLEM, WHICH INVOLVED SELF-PRESCRIPTION AND SELF-ADMINISTRATION OF CONTROLLED SUBSTANCES IN ORDER TO TREAT HIS DEPRESSION AND MIGRAINE HEADACHES, TO ILLINOIS; HE REPORTS A SOBRIETY DATE OF 2/96 AND MAINTAINS THAT HE HAS NOT PRACTICED MEDICINE SINCE 7/94. VOLUNTARY SURRENDER.

LEVIN, IRA MD OF 504 WEST 24TH STREET, AUSTIN, TX, WAS DISCIPLINED BY DEA ON MAY 10, 1994
DISCIPLINARY ACTION: SURRENDER OF CONTROLLED SUBSTANCE LICENSE

NOTES: IN LIEU OF PUBLIC INTEREST REVOCATION.

LEVIN, IRA M MD, LICENSE NUMBER 0186535 OF 3614 BILL PRICE ROAD, DEL VALLEY, TX, WAS DISCIPLINED BY NEW YORK ON MARCH 14, 1995
DISCIPLINARY ACTION: LICENSE REVOCATION
OFFENSE: DISCIPLINARY ACTION BY ANOTHER STATE OR AGENCY

NOTES: ACTION IN TEXAS FOR INAPPROPRIATE PRESCRIBING OF CONTROLLED DANGEROUS SUBSTANCES. CONVICTED OF UNLAWFUL POSSESSION OF CONTROLLED SUBSTANCES.

LEVIN, IRA MARK MD, LICENSE NUMBER 00J3142 OF AUSTIN, TX, WAS DISCIPLINED BY TEXAS ON MAY 5, 1994
DISCIPLINARY ACTION: EMERGENCY SUSPENSION
OFFENSE: SUBSTANCE ABUSE

NOTES: AVAILABLE EVIDENCE AND INFORMATION INDICATE THE FOLLOWING: ON 3/11/94 AND 4/20/94 HE PURCHASED LARGE QUANTITIES OF SCHEDULE II NARCOTICS; MEDICAL PRACTICE IS LIMITED TO SERVING AS A LOCUM TENENS PHYSICIAN WITH NO NECESSITY FOR HIM TO POSSESS THE LARGE QUANTITIES OF DRUGS PURCHASED; HAS A HISTORY OF SUBSTANCE ABUSE AND TREATMENT; ACQUIRED THE DRUGS EITHER FOR SELF-USE OR TO DIVERT FOR USE BY ANOTHER INDIVIDUAL(S) OR FOR BOTH PURPOSES.

LEVIN, IRA MARK MD, LICENSE NUMBER 00J3142 OF AUSTIN, TX, WAS DISCIPLINED BY TEXAS ON SEPTEMBER 30, 1994
DISCIPLINARY ACTION: LICENSE SUSPENSION

OFFENSE: CRIMINAL CONVICTION OR PLEA OF GUILTY, NOLO CONTENDERE, OR NO CONTEST TO A CRIME

NOTES: WROTE PRESCRIPTIONS FOR CONTROLLED SUBSTANCES FOR HIS OWN USE AND WAS SUBSEQUENTLY ARRESTED BY DEA AGENTS FOR POSSESSION WITH INTENT TO DISTRIBUTE; CHARGE WAS REDUCED TO A MISDEMEANOR TO WHICH HE PLED GUILTY; ATTENDED A 28 DAY INPATIENT TREATMENT PROGRAM AND WAS AT A HALF-WAY HOUSE FOR SUBSTANCE ABUSERS AS OF THE DATE OF THIS ORDER. SUSPENSION UNTIL SUCH TIME AS HE APPEARS BEFORE THE BOARD AND PROVIDES SUFFICIENT EVIDENCE THAT HE IS PHYSICALLY, MENTALLY AND OTHERWISE COMPETENT TO SAFELY PRACTICE INCLUDING BUT NOT LIMITED TO A COMPLETE MEDICAL ASSESSMENT WITH PSYCHOLOGICAL AND NEUROPSYCHIATRIC EVALUATIONS.

LEVIN, IRA MARK MD, LICENSE NUMBER 00J3142, WAS DISCIPLINED BY TEXAS ON MAY 16, 1995
DISCIPLINARY ACTION: SURRENDER OF CONTROLLED SUBSTANCE LICENSE; 120-MONTH PROBATION
OFFENSE: CRIMINAL CONVICTION OR PLEA OF GUILTY, NOLO CONTENDERE, OR NO CONTEST TO A CRIME

NOTES: SUSPENSION TERMINATED. CONDITIONS OF PROBATION: SHALL PRACTICE ONLY IN A GROUP PRACTICE SETTING OR BOARD-APPROVED INSTITUTIONAL SETTING; PRACTICE SHALL BE MONITORED BY A BOARD-APPROVED TEXAS PHYSICIAN WHO SHALL SUBMIT QUARTERLY REPORTS; SHALL ABSTAIN FROM THE CONSUMPTION OF ALCOHOL/DRUGS IN ANY FORM UNLESS PRESCRIBED BY ANOTHER PHYSICIAN FOR A LEGITIMATE AND THERAPEUTIC PURPOSE; SHALL SUBMIT HIMSELF FOR APPROPRIATE EXAMS INCLUDING DRUG OR ALCOHOL SCREENS; SHALL NOT TREAT OR OTHERWISE SERVE AS PHYSICIAN, PRESCRIBE, DISPENSE OR ADMINISTER DRUGS THAT MAY BE SUBJECT TO ABUSE TO HIMSELF OR ANY MEMBER OF HIS FAMILY; SHALL SURRENDER ALL UNUSED TRIPLICATE PRESCRIPTIONS FORMS AND SHALL NOT ATTEMPT TO ORDER MORE; SHALL SURRENDER ALL CONTROLLED SUBSTANCES IN HIS OFFICE OR POSSESSION; SHALL KEEP A SEPARATE LOG OF PRESCRIPTIONS FOR DANGEROUS DRUGS WITH ADDICTIVE POTENTIAL SUBJECT TO REVIEW; SHALL PARTICIPATE IN ACTIVITIES OF AN IMPAIRED PHYSICIAN'S GROUP WITH QUARTERLY REPORTS; SHALL PARTICIPATE IN AA'S PROGRAM NOT LESS THAN THREE TIMES A WEEK WITH QUARTERLY REPORTS TO THE BOARD; SHALL SUBMIT HIMSELF FOR EVALUATION AND TREATMENT BY A BOARD-APPROVED PSYCHIATRIST WHOM HE SHALL SEE AT LEAST ONCE A MONTH AND WHO SHALL PROVIDE REPORTS; SHALL ATTEND AT LEAST 50 HOURS PER YEAR OF CONTINUING MEDICAL EDUCATION; SHALL APPEAR BEFORE THE BOARD TWO TIMES A YEAR; SHALL GIVE A COPY OF THIS ORDER TO ANY HEALTH CARE ENTITY WHERE HE HAS PRIVILEGES; SHALL FOLLOW RESTRICTIONS IMPOSED BY AUTHORITIES IN RELATION TO ANY CRIMINAL CHARGES; SHALL FOLLOW THE RESTRICTIONS IMPOSED BY THE NEW YORK AUTHORITIES; SHALL COOPERATE WITH THE BOARD IN VERIFYING COMPLIANCE; SHALL INFORM BOARD OF CHANGE OF ADDRESS WITHIN 10 DAYS OR IF HE LEAVES THE STATE; IF HE FAILS TO ACTIVELY PARTICIPATE IN THE PRACTICE OF MEDICINE FOR LONGER THAN 12 MONTHS, ADDITIONAL TERMS OR CONDITIONS MAY BE APPLIED; TIME PERIOD OUT OF TEXAS DOES NOT COUNT TOWARD PROBATION. SHALL NOT SEEK MODIFICATION FOR ONE YEAR. ON 5/15/96, ORDER AMENDED AS FOLLOWS: MAY REAPPLY TO DEA OR DPS FOR PERMISSION TO PRESCRIBE SCHEDULES IV AND V CONTROLLED SUBSTANCES; HE IS REQUIRED TO MAINTAIN A FILE OF ALL PRESCRIPTIONS WRITTEN FOR THESE SUBSTANCES WHICH SHALL BE AVAILABLE FOR REVIEW. ON 5/10/97 PETITION TO MODIFY ORDER GRANTED, GRANTING HIM AUTHORITY TO REAPPLY FOR SCHEDULE III, IV AND V CONTROLLED SUBSTANCES, AND ALLOWING HIM THE AUTHORITY TO TELEPHONE PRESCRIPTIONS OR REFILLS TO PHARMACIES.

LEVIN, IRA MARK MD, LICENSE NUMBER 1040841 OF 504 W 24TH ST, AUSTIN, TX, WAS DISCIPLINED BY INDIANA ON JULY 12, 1995
DISCIPLINARY ACTION: LICENSE REVOCATION; FINE
OFFENSE: DISCIPLINARY ACTION BY ANOTHER STATE OR AGENCY

NOTES: ON 9/30/94, THE TEXAS BOARD INDEFINITELY SUSPENDED HIS LICENSE ON THE GROUNDS THAT HE WROTE PRESCRIPTIONS FOR CONTROLLED SUBSTANCES FOR HIS OWN USE AND WAS SUBSEQUENTLY ARRESTED BY DEA FOR POSSESSION WITH THE INTENT TO DISTRIBUTE; HE PLEADED GUILTY TO A REDUCED MISDEMEANOR CHARGE; AND HE ATTENDED A 28 DAY INPATIENT TREATMENT PROGRAM AND WAS AT A HALF-WAY HOUSE FOR SUBSTANCE ABUSERS AS OF THE DATE OF THE TEXAS ACTION. DEFAULT DECISION. $1,000 FINE. ASSESSED PROCEEDINGS COSTS OF $377.

LEVIN, IRA MARK MD, LICENSE NUMBER J3142 OF AUSTIN, TX, WAS DISCIPLINED BY TEXAS ON APRIL 4, 1998
DISCIPLINARY ACTION: 120-MONTH PROBATION; REQUIRED TO TAKE ADDITIONAL MEDICAL EDUCATION
OFFENSE: FAILURE TO COMPLY WITH PREVIOUS BOARD ORDER

NOTES: VIOLATED PREVIOUS BOARD ORDERS IN THAT ON 2/27/98 HE REPORTED THAT HE INGESTED CONTROLLED SUBSTANCES; ON 3/2/98 HE SUBMITTED WRITTEN CORRESPONDENCE REPORTING THAT FROM 12/97 - 2/98 HE HAD INGESTED CONTROLLED SUBSTANCES INCLUDING VICOPROFEN, HYDROCODONE COUGH MEDICINE, AND NORCO, AND THAT HE HAD FRAUDULENTLY ISSUED A PRESCRIPTION IN HIS WIFE'S NAME AND OBTAINED THE CONTROLLED SUBSTANCE NORCO, #50 ON 2/20/98 FOR HIS OWN USE. REVOCATION STAYED FOR PROBATION WITH FOLLOWING TERMS AND CONDITIONS: SHALL ABSTAIN FROM THE CONSUMPTION OF ALCOHOL/DRUGS IN ANY FORM UNLESS PRESCRIBED BY ANOTHER PHYSICIAN FOR A LEGITIMATE AND THERAPEUTIC PURPOSE; SHALL SUBMIT HIMSELF FOR APPROPRIATE EXAMS INCLUDING DRUG OR ALCOHOL SCREENS; SHALL NOMINATE THREE CERTIFIED PSYCHIATRISTS FOR BOARD SELECTION OF A THERAPIST AND SHALL EXPEDITIOUSLY SUBMIT HIMSELF TO EVALUATION AND TREATMENT BY THE APPROVED PRACTITIONER; SHALL COOPERATE WITH THE BOARD IN VERIFYING COMPLIANCE INCLUDING PROVIDING COPIES OF MEDICAL RELEASES UPON REQUEST; SHALL PARTICIPATE IN THE ACTIVITIES OF A PHYSICIAN HEALTH AND REHABILITATION COMMITTEE AND ATTEND WEEKLY MEETINGS WITH QUARTERLY REPORTS; SHALL PARTICIPATE IN AA'S PROGRAM NOT LESS THAN FOUR TIMES A WEEK; SHALL REPORT ON HIS ATTENDANCE; SHALL NOT TREAT OR OTHERWISE SERVE AS PHYSICIAN, PRESCRIBE, DISPENSE OR ADMINISTER DRUGS THAT MAY BE SUBJECT TO ABUSE TO HIMSELF OR TO ANY MEMBER OF HIS FAMILY; IS AUTHORIZED TO REAPPLY FOR DEA AND TEXAS DEPARTMENT OF PUBLIC SAFETY TO REAPPLY

FOR SCHEDULES III - V DRUGS; SEPARATE FROM PATIENT RECORDS, SHALL MAINTAIN A LOGBOOK OF EVERY PRESCRIPTION WRITTEN BY HIM FOR DANGEROUS DRUGS WITH ADDICTIVE POTENTIAL WHICH SHALL BE MADE AVAILABLE FOR REVIEW; HIS MEDICAL PRACTICE SHALL BE MONITORED BY A BOARD APPROVED TEXAS PHYSICIAN WHO SHALL PROVIDE QUARTERLY REPORTS TO THE BOARD; SHALL OBTAIN 50 HOURS PER YEAR OF CONTINUING MEDICAL EDUCATION; WITHIN ONE YEAR, SHALL OBTAIN 20 HOURS OF TRAINING IN ADDICTIONOLOGY; SHALL APPEAR BEFORE THE BOARD UPON REQUEST; SHALL GIVE A COPY OF THIS ORDER TO ANY HEALTH CARE ENTITY WHERE HE HAS PRIVILEGES; SHALL PROVIDE A COPY OF THIS ORDER TO ANYONE REQUESTING IT WITHIN 10 DAYS; TIME SPENT OUT OF TEXAS DOES NOT COUNT TOWARD PROBATION; SHALL INFORM THE BOARD OF CHANGE OF ADDRESS WITHIN 10 DAYS OR IF HE LEAVES THE STATE; SHALL NOT SEEK MODIFICATION FOR 36 MONTHS.

LEVIN, IRA MARK MD OF 1204A A LAKEWAY DRIVE, AUSTIN, TX, WAS DISCIPLINED BY DEA ON MAY 14, 1998
DISCIPLINARY ACTION: SURRENDER OF CONTROLLED SUBSTANCE LICENSE

NOTES: IN LIEU OF PUBLIC INTEREST REVOCATION.

LEVIN, IRA MARK MD, LICENSE NUMBER J3142 OF AUSTIN, TX, WAS DISCIPLINED BY TEXAS ON SEPTEMBER 3, 1998
DISCIPLINARY ACTION: EMERGENCY SUSPENSION
OFFENSE: FAILURE TO COMPLY WITH PREVIOUS BOARD ORDER

NOTES: VIOLATED 4/4/98 ORDER WHEN URINE SAMPLES TESTED POSITIVE FOR BARBITURATES ON 8/20/98 AND 8/25/98.

LEVIN, IRA MARK MD, LICENSE NUMBER J3142 OF AUSTIN, TX, WAS DISCIPLINED BY TEXAS ON NOVEMBER 9, 1998
DISCIPLINARY ACTION: 120-MONTH PROBATION; RESTRICTION PLACED ON CONTROLLED SUBSTANCE LICENSE

NOTES: VIOLATED TERMS OF 4/4/98 ORDER BY TESTING POSITIVE FOR BARBITURATES; MAINTAINS HE HAS NOT RELAPSED AND INADVERTENTLY INGESTED HIS WIFE'S MEDICINE, MISTAKING IT FOR ADVIL. REVOCATION STAYED FOR PROBATION WITH FOLLOWING TERMS AND CONDITIONS: SHALL ABSTAIN FROM THE CONSUMPTION OF ALCOHOL/DRUGS IN ANY FORM UNLESS PRESCRIBED BY ANOTHER PHYSICIAN FOR A LEGITIMATE AND THERAPEUTIC PURPOSE; SHALL SUBMIT HIMSELF FOR APPROPRIATE EXAMS INCLUDING DRUG OR ALCOHOL SCREENS; SHALL NOMINATE THREE CERTIFIED PSYCHIATRISTS FOR BOARD SELECTION OF A THERAPIST AND SHALL EXPEDITIOUSLY SUBMIT HIMSELF TO EVALUATION AND TREATMENT BY THE APPROVED PRACTITIONER; SHALL PARTICIPATE IN THE ACTIVITIES OF A PHYSICIAN HEALTH AND REHABILITATION COMMITTEE AND ATTEND WEEKLY MEETINGS WITH QUARTERLY REPORTS; SHALL PARTICIPATE IN AA'S PROGRAM OR SUBSTANTIALLY SIMILAR PROGRAM NOT LESS THAN FOUR TIMES A WEEK; SHALL REPORT ON HIS ATTENDANCE; SHALL NOT TREAT OR OTHERWISE SERVE AS PHYSICIAN, PRESCRIBE, DISPENSE OR ADMINISTER DRUGS THAT MAY BE SUBJECT TO ABUSE TO HIMSELF OR TO ANY MEMBER OF HIS FAMILY; SHALL SURRENDER ANY DRUGS WITH POTENTIAL FOR ABUSE IN HIS POSSESSION INCLUDING SAMPLES AND SHALL ONLY DISPOSE THEM IN AN INPATIENT HOSPITAL SETTING; SEPARATE FROM PATIENT RECORDS, SHALL MAINTAIN A LOGBOOK OF EVERY PRESCRIPTION WRITTEN BY HIM OR TELEPHONED IN BY HIM FOR DANGEROUS DRUGS WITH ADDICTIVE POTENTIAL WHICH SHALL BE MADE AVAILABLE FOR REVIEW; HIS MEDICAL PRACTICE SHALL BE MONITORED BY A BOARD APPROVED TEXAS PHYSICIAN WHO SHALL PROVIDE QUARTERLY REPORTS TO THE BOARD; SHALL OBTAIN 50 HOURS PER YEAR OF CONTINUING MEDICAL EDUCATION; WITHIN 1 YEAR SHALL OBTAIN 20 HOURS OF TRAINING IN BOARD-APPROVED ADDICTIONOLOGY; SHALL APPEAR BEFORE THE BOARD UPON REQUEST; SHALL COOPERATE WITH THE BOARD IN VERIFYING COMPLIANCE INCLUDING PROVIDING COPIES OF MEDICAL RELEASES UPON REQUEST; SHALL GIVE A COPY OF THIS ORDER TO ANY HEALTH CARE ENTITY WHERE HE HAS PRIVILEGES; TIME SPENT OUT OF TEXAS DOES NOT COUNT TOWARD PROBATION; SHALL INFORM THE BOARD OF CHANGE OF ADDRESS WITHIN 10 DAYS OR IF HE LEAVES THE STATE; SHALL NOT SEEK MODIFICATION FOR 36 MONTHS.

LEVIN, MITCHELL L MD, LICENSE NUMBER 0049508 OF KISSIMMEE, FL, WAS DISCIPLINED BY FLORIDA ON APRIL 11, 1990
DISCIPLINARY ACTION: FINE; REPRIMAND
OFFENSE: PROFESSIONAL MISCONDUCT

NOTES: CHARGED WITH PAYING OR RECEIVING A COMMISSION, BONUS, KICKBACK, OR REBATE, OR ENGAGING IN A SPLIT FEE ARRANGEMENT WITH A PHYSICIAN, ORGANIZATION, AGENCY OR PERSON, EITHER DIRECTLY OR INDIRECTLY FOR PATIENTS REFERRED TO PROVIDERS OF HEALTH CARE GOODS AND SERVICES, INCLUDING BUT NOT LIMITED TO HOSPITALS, NURSING HOMES, CLINICAL LABORATORIES, AMBULATORY SURGICAL CENTERS OR PHARMACIES; SOLICITING PATIENTS, EITHER PERSONALLY OR THROUGH AN AGENT, THROUGH THE USE OF FRAUD, INTIMIDATION, UNDUE INFLUENCE, OR A FORM OF OVERREACHING OR VEXATIOUS CONDUCT. MUST PAY $5000 FINE; REPRIMAND; MUST REVIEW APPLICABLE LAWS AND RULES AND PROVIDE AFFIDAVIT DETAILING SAME IN LIEU OF FURTHER PROSECUTION.

LEVIN, MITCHELL L MD, LICENSE NUMBER 0049508 OF ST CLOUD, FL, WAS DISCIPLINED BY FLORIDA ON APRIL 8, 1992
DISCIPLINARY ACTION: 24-MONTH PROBATION; FINE
OFFENSE: SUBSTANDARD CARE, INCOMPETENCE OR NEGLIGENCE

NOTES: FAILING TO PRACTICE MEDICINE WITH AN ACCEPTABLE LEVEL OF CARE AND SKILL. $1,000 FINE.

LEVIN, MITCHELL L MD, LICENSE NUMBER 0049508 OF KISSIMMEE, FL, WAS DISCIPLINED BY FLORIDA ON AUGUST 10, 1993
DISCIPLINARY ACTION: FINE
OFFENSE: FAILURE TO COMPLY WITH PREVIOUS BOARD ORDER

NOTES: CHARGED WITH VIOLATING A PREVIOUS BOARD ORDER; FAILING TO INCLUDE IN HIS ADVERTISEMENT LETTER THE DISCLAIMER REQUIRED. IN LIEU OF FURTHER PROSECUTION, CONSENTED TO $1,500 FINE; SHALL APPEAR BEFORE THE BOARD AND EXPLAIN CIRCUMSTANCES OF THIS CASE AND HOW SUBSEQUENT TRAINING AND PRESENT APPROACH HAVE AND WILL PREVENT FUTURE OCCURRENCES.

LEVIN, MITCHELL LEE MD, DATE OF BIRTH JANUARY 16, 1954, LICENSE NUMBER 00G5819 OF 921 N MAIN STREET SUITE 201, KISSIMMEE, FL, WAS DISCIPLINED BY TEXAS ON JUNE 15, 1993
DISCIPLINARY ACTION: SURRENDER OF LICENSE

NOTES: DOES NOT WISH TO PRACTICE IN TEXAS; SURRENDER IS PERMANENT.

LEVIN, MITCHELL LEE MD OF OTTAWA, IL, WAS DISCIPLINED BY ILLINOIS ON JULY 1, 1994
DISCIPLINARY ACTION: LICENSE SUSPENSION
OFFENSE: DISCIPLINARY ACTION BY ANOTHER STATE OR AGENCY

NOTES: DISCIPLINED IN FLORIDA. SUSPENSION FOR A MINIMUM OF 5 YEARS.

LEVIN, MITCHELL LEE MD, DATE OF BIRTH JANUARY 16, 1954, LICENSE NUMBER 0048830 OF 921 NORTH MAIN ST SUITE 102, KISSIMMEE, FL, WAS DISCIPLINED BY NEW JERSEY ON JANUARY 9, 1995
DISCIPLINARY ACTION: 24-MONTH PROBATION
OFFENSE: DISCIPLINARY ACTION BY ANOTHER STATE OR AGENCY

NOTES: ACTION IN FLORIDA. 24 MONTH SUSPENSION, STAYED. SHALL APPEAR BEFORE COMMITTEE OF THE BOARD PRIOR TO PRACTICE IN NEW JERSEY.

LEVINSON, CARL MD, LICENSE NUMBER 00E1361, WAS DISCIPLINED BY TEXAS ON AUGUST 17, 1996
DISCIPLINARY ACTION: FINE
OFFENSE: DISCIPLINARY ACTION BY ANOTHER STATE OR AGENCY

NOTES: ON 8/09/95 PUBLICLY REPRIMANDED IN CALIFORNIA FOR HIS WRITING OF PRESCRIPTIONS FOR DANGEROUS DRUGS AND CONTROLLED SUBSTANCES FOR HIMSELF AND THREE MEMBERS OF HIS FAMILY WITHOUT ADEQUATE EXAMINATION, INDICATIONS AND SUPPORTING DOCUMENTATION. DOES NOT ADMIT NOR DENY FINDINGS; HAS COMPLIED WITH ALL OF THE CALIFORNIA TERMS. $5,000 ADMINISTRATIVE PENALTY.

LEVY, JAIME MD, LICENSE NUMBER 00C5773, WAS DISCIPLINED BY TEXAS ON OCTOBER 4, 1996
DISCIPLINARY ACTION: 60-MONTH REQUIRED TO TAKE ADDITIONAL MEDICAL EDUCATION; MONITORING OF PHYSICIAN PERFORMANCE
OFFENSE: SUBSTANDARD CARE, INCOMPETENCE OR NEGLIGENCE

NOTES: ON 5/18/93 FAILED TO ADEQUATELY DOCUMENT HIS CARE AND TREATMENT OF A PATIENT AND THERE IS NO INDICATION THAT HE PERFORMED A HISTORY AND PHYSICAL EXAMINATION; ON 7/19/93 HE FAILED TO PERFORM AN ADEQUATE EYE EXAMINATION, FAILED TO ADEQUATELY DOCUMENT HIS CARE AND TREATMENT AND PRESCRIBED TOBRADEX AND LINCOCIN BELOW THE RECOMMENDED DOSAGE AMOUNTS AND THUS WERE NONTHERAPEUTIC; ADMINISTERED LINCOCIN AS A FIRST LINE ANTIBIOTIC WHEN OTHER LESS TOXIC ANTIMICROBIAL AGENTS WERE MORE APPROPRIATE; ON 7/20, 21, AND 24/93 ADMINISTERED INJECTIONS BUT FAILED TO ADEQUATELY DOCUMENT THE PATIENT'S OFFICE VISIT ON EACH DAY AND THERE IS NO INDICATION THAT HE PERFORMED A PHYSICAL EXAMINATION OF THE PATIENT; AND ON 8/02/93 REFERRED THE PATIENT TO AN OPHTHALMOLOGIST, BUT THERE IS NOTHING DOCUMENTED IN THE MEDICAL RECORDS TO INDICATE THE REASON FOR REFERRAL. LICENSE RESTRICTED UNDER TERMS AND CONDITIONS FOR FIVE YEARS: SHALL OBTAIN AT LEAST 50 HOURS PER YEAR OF CONTINUING MEDICAL EDUCATION AT LEAST 10 HOURS IN RISK MANAGEMENT AND 10 HOURS IN PHARMACOLOGY AND SUBMIT PROOF TO THE BOARD; SHALL MAINTAIN ADEQUATE MEDICAL RECORDS AND MAKE THEM AVAILABLE UPON BOARD REQUEST; HIS MEDICAL PRACTICE, INCLUDING ANY OFFICE AND SURGICAL PRACTICE SHALL BE MONITORED BY A BOARD APPROVED LICENSED PHYSICIAN WHO SHALL SUBMIT QUARTERLY REPORTS TO THE BOARD; WITHIN ONE YEAR SHALL TAKE AND PASS THE SPEX WITH A SCORE OF 75 OR HIGHER AND SUBMIT PROOF TO THE BOARD; SHALL APPEAR BEFORE THE BOARD AT LEAST ONCE A YEAR; SHALL COOPERATE WITH THE BOARD IN VERIFYING COMPLIANCE; SHALL GIVE A COPY OF THIS ORDER TO ANY HEALTH CARE ENTITY WHERE HE HAS PRIVILEGES; TIME PERIOD OUT OF TEXAS DOES NOT COUNT TOWARD RESTRICTION; SHALL INFORM THE BOARD OF CHANGE OF ADDRESS WITHIN 10 DAYS OF IF HE LEAVES THE STATE; SHALL NOT SEEK MODIFICATION FOR ONE YEAR.

LEWIS, ADOLPHUS RAY DO, LICENSE NUMBER H2532 OF FORT WORTH, TX, WAS DISCIPLINED BY TEXAS ON AUGUST 22, 1998
DISCIPLINARY ACTION: RESTRICTION PLACED ON CONTROLLED SUBSTANCE LICENSE; REPRIMAND
OFFENSE: NONCOMPLIANCE WITH A PROFESSIONAL RULE

NOTES: THE BOARD REVIEWED 9 PATIENT CHARTS AND FOUND THE FOLLOWING DEFICIENCIES: FAILURE TO PROPERLY CHART THE PERFORMANCE OF AND RESULTS OF PHYSICAL EXAMS; FAILURE TO INDICATE IN THE CHART THE RATIONALE AND REASONS FOR PRESCRIBING NARCOTIC MEDICATIONS; INADEQUATE CHARTING OF TREATMENT PLANNING; PRESCRIBING OF LARGE QUANTITIES OF CONTROLLED SUBSTANCES WITHOUT REFLECTING ADEQUATE INITIAL AND INTERVAL MEDICAL HISTORIES, ADEQUATE MEDICAL EXAMS, OR MEDICALLY APPROPRIATE DIAGNOSTIC TESTING/STUDIES; INADEQUATE CHARTING TO REFLECT PROPER MEDICAL INDICATION FOR THE PRESCRIBING OF VALIUM AND VICODIN. LICENSE LIMITED FOR THREE YEARS AS FOLLOWS: SHALL ATTEND 50 HOURS PER YEAR OF CONTINUING MEDICAL EDUCATION WITH AT LEAST 20 HOURS IN PAIN MANAGEMENT; HIS MEDICAL PRACTICE SHALL BE MONITORED BY A BOARD APPROVED TEXAS PHYSICIAN WHO SHALL PROVIDE QUARTERLY REPORTS TO THE BOARD; SHALL MAINTAIN ADEQUATE MEDICAL RECORDS WHICH SHALL BE AVAILABLE FOR REVIEW; SHALL ONLY PRESCRIBE SCHEDULE II MEDICATIONS FOR HOSPICE AND LONG-TERM NURSING HOME PATIENTS, AS APPROPRIATE; SEPARATE FROM PATIENT RECORDS, SHALL MAINTAIN A LOGBOOK OF EVERY PRESCRIPTION WRITTEN BY HIM FOR DANGEROUS DRUGS WITH ADDICTIVE POTENTIAL WHICH SHALL BE MADE AVAILABLE FOR REVIEW; SHALL APPEAR BEFORE THE BOARD UPON REQUEST; SHALL GIVE A COPY OF THIS ORDER TO ANY HEALTH CARE ENTITY WHERE HE HAS PRIVILEGES; SHALL PROVIDE A COPY OF THIS ORDER TO ANYONE REQUESTING IT WITHIN 10 DAYS; TIME SPENT OUT OF TEXAS DOES NOT COUNT TOWARD RESTRICTION; SHALL INFORM THE BOARD OF CHANGE OF ADDRESS WITHIN 10 DAYS OR IF HE LEAVES THE STATE; SHALL NOT SEEK MODIFICATION FOR ONE YEAR. ON 10/15/99 THE ORDER TERMINATED UPON THE BOARD'S RECEIPT OF DOCUMENTED EVIDENCE THAT HE HAS SUCCESSFULLY COMPLETED THE GERIATRIC FELLOWSHIP PROGRAM AT THE UNIVERSITY OF NORTH TEXAS HEALTH SCIENCE CENTER.

LEWIS, EDWARD A MD, LICENSE NUMBER 00G8242 OF HOUSTON, TX, WAS DISCIPLINED BY TEXAS ON MARCH 4, 1995
DISCIPLINARY ACTION: 60-MONTH PROBATION; RESTRICTION PLACED ON CONTROLLED SUBSTANCE LICENSE
OFFENSE: SUBSTANCE ABUSE

NOTES: HAS HAD A SUBSTANCE ABUSE PROBLEM FOR APPROXIMATELY 10 YEARS; IN 4/92, WHILE ON DUTY AT A HOSPITAL, EXPERIENCED A LOSS OF CONSCIOUSNESS AND RESPIRATORY DIFFICULTIES RELATED TO SUBSTANCE ABUSE; HOSPITAL

SUMMARILY SUSPENDED HIS PRIVILEGES AND HE SUBSEQUENTLY RESIGNED FROM THE HOSPITAL STAFF; THEN HE VOLUNTARILY ENTERED AN INPATIENT SUBSTANCE ABUSE TREATMENT PROGRAM WHICH HE SUCCESSFULLY COMPLETED IN 9/92; SINCE COMPLETION OF INPATIENT TREATMENT, HE REPORTS REGULAR ATTENDANCE AT AA MEETINGS AND THE MEETINGS OF THE PHYSICIAN'S HEALTH AND REHABILITATION COMMITTEE AND ENROLLMENT IN A TWO-YEAR PHYSICIAN COUNSELING COMMITTEE MONITORING PROGRAM; HE REPORTS A SOBRIETY DATE OF 4/01/92. SUSPENSION STAYED. PROBATION WITH TERMS: SHALL ABSTAIN FROM THE CONSUMPTION OF ALCOHOL/DRUGS IN ANY FORM UNLESS PRESCRIBED BY ANOTHER PHYSICIAN FOR A LEGITIMATE AND THERAPEUTIC PURPOSE; SHALL SUBMIT HIMSELF FOR APPROPRIATE EXAMS INCLUDING DRUG OR ALCOHOL SCREENS; SHALL SUBMIT HIMSELF FOR EVALUATION AND TREATMENT BY A BOARD-APPROVED PSYCHIATRIST WHOM HE SHALL SEE AT LEAST ONCE A MONTH AND WHO SHALL SUBMIT REPORTS TO THE BOARD; SHALL PARTICIPATE IN AA'S PROGRAM NOT LESS THAN THREE TIMES A WEEK WITH QUARTERLY REPORTS TO THE BOARD; SHALL PARTICIPATE IN THE ACTIVITIES OF A PHYSICIAN HEALTH AND REHABILITATION COMMITTEE AND ATTEND WEEKLY MEETINGS WITH QUARTERLY REPORTS; SHALL COMPLY WITH TERMS OF ANY CONTRACT ENTERED INTO BY HIM FOR HOSPITAL PRIVILEGES AND SHALL REPORT TO THE BOARD ANY RESTRICTIONS OR LIMITATIONS OF HOSPITAL PRIVILEGES; SHALL NOT TREAT OR OTHERWISE SERVE AS A PHYSICIAN, PRESCRIBE, DISPENSE OR ADMINISTER DRUGS THAT MAY BE SUBJECT TO ABUSE TO HIMSELF OR ANY MEMBERS OF HIS FAMILY; SHALL NOT TELEPHONE TO A PHARMACY A PRESCRIPTION FOR CONTROLLED SUBSTANCES OR DRUGS WITH POTENTIAL FOR ABUSE; SHALL NOT POSSESS, ADMINISTER, DISPENSE OR PRESCRIBE CONTROLLED SUBSTANCES EXCEPT TO PATIENTS REQUIRING ANESTHESIA AND SHALL KEEP A LOG OF THESE PRESCRIPTIONS SUBJECT TO REVIEW; SHALL MAINTAIN ADEQUATE MEDICAL RECORDS WHICH SHALL BE AVAILABLE FOR BOARD INSPECTION; SHALL OBTAIN AT LEAST 50 HOURS PER YEAR OF CONTINUING MEDICAL EDUCATION; SHALL APPEAR BEFORE THE BOARD AT LEAST TWO TIMES EACH YEAR OR UPON BOARD REQUEST; SHALL COOPERATE WITH THE BOARD IN VERIFYING COMPLIANCE INCLUDING PROVIDING COPIES OF MEDICAL RELEASES UPON REQUEST; SHALL GIVE A COPY OF THIS ORDER TO ANY HEALTH CARE ENTITY WHERE HE HAS PRIVILEGES; SHALL INFORM BOARD OF CHANGE OF ADDRESS WITHIN 10 DAYS OR IF HE LEAVES THE STATE; TIME PERIOD OUT OF TEXAS DOES NOT COUNT TOWARD PROBATION. SHALL NOT SEEK MODIFICATION FOR ONE YEAR. ON 5/15/96 PROBATION TERMINATED.

LEWIS, ELBERT HAMPTON MD, DATE OF BIRTH JANUARY 2, 1929, LICENSE NUMBER 00C3124 OF DALLAS, TX, WAS DISCIPLINED BY TEXAS ON DECEMBER 4, 1991
DISCIPLINARY ACTION: 120-MONTH PROBATION; RESTRICTION PLACED ON CONTROLLED SUBSTANCE LICENSE
OFFENSE: SUBSTANCE ABUSE

NOTES: USING ALCOHOL, DEMEROL, AND HALCION, PROVIDED DEMEROL TO HIS MOTHER FOR SELF-ADMINISTRATION WHICH WAS PRESCRIBED IN THE NAME OF A PATIENT, FAILED TO KEEP RECORDS OF CONTROLLED SUBSTANCES ON HAND ON THE DATE INVENTORY IS TAKEN, AND FAILED TO KEEP RECORDS FOR RECEIVING AND DISPOSING OF CONTROLLED SUBSTANCES. TEN YEAR SUSPENSION STAYED, PROBATION ISSUED WITH FOLLOWING CONDITIONS: SHALL PARTICIPATE IN DALLAS COUNTY MEDICAL SOCIETY COMMITTEE ON PHYSICIAN HEALTH AND REHABILITATION, INCLUDING PARTICIPATION IN THE WEEKLY MEETINGS; SHALL PARTICIPATE IN THE ACTIVITIES AND PROGRAMS OF ALCOHOLICS ANONYMOUS, INCLUDING A 12-STEP PROGRAM NOT LESS THAN THREE TIMES PER WEEK, WITH QUARTERLY REPORTS TO THE BOARD; SHALL ABSTAIN FROM THE CONSUMPTION OF ALCOHOL/CHEMICAL SUBSTANCES IN ANY FORM; SHALL SUBMIT HIMSELF FOR ALCOHOL AND DRUG SCREENING EXAMINATIONS; DEA AND TEXAS CONTROLLED SUBSTANCES REGISTRATIONS SHALL REMAIN LIMITED TO SCHEDULES III, III-N, IV, AND V; SHALL NOT TREAT OR SERVE AS PHYSICIAN, PRESCRIBE, DISPENSE, OR ADMINISTER CONTROLLED SUBSTANCES OR ANY OTHER DRUGS THAT MAY BE SUBJECT TO ABUSE FOR HIMSELF OR HIS FAMILY; SHALL MAINTAIN A FILE CONSISTING OF A COPY OF EVERY PRESCRIPTION WRITTEN FOR CONTROLLED SUBSTANCES OR DANGEROUS DRUGS BY DATE ISSUED; SHALL NOT TELEPHONE ANY PRESCRIPTION TO A PHARMACY FOR CONTROLLED SUBSTANCES OR DANGEROUS DRUGS; SHALL COOPERATE WITH BOARD IN VERIFYING COMPLIANCE; SHALL ADVISE THE BOARD IF HE CHANGES ADDRESS WITHIN 10 DAYS; TIME SPENT OUT OF TEXAS DOES NOT COUNT TOWARDS PROBATION; SHALL NOT PETITION FOR MODIFICATION OF ORDER FOR FIVE YEARS; SHALL APPEAR BEFORE BOARD TWO TIMES A YEAR.

LEWIS, ELBERT HAMPTON MD, DATE OF BIRTH JANUARY 2, 1929, LICENSE NUMBER 00C3124 OF DALLAS, TX, WAS DISCIPLINED BY TEXAS ON AUGUST 20, 1992
DISCIPLINARY ACTION: 120-MONTH PROBATION
OFFENSE: SUBSTANCE ABUSE

NOTES: INABILITY TO PRACTICE MEDICINE WITH REASONABLE SKILL AND SAFETY TO PATIENTS BY REASON OF ILLNESS, DRUNKENNESS, EXCESSIVE USE OF DRUGS, NARCOTICS, CHEMICALS, OR ANY OTHER TYPE OF MATERIAL OR AS A RESULT OF ANY MENTAL OR PHYSICAL CONDITION. LICENSE SUSPENDED, SUSPENSION STAYED.

LEWIS, ELBERT HAMPTON MD, DATE OF BIRTH JANUARY 2, 1929, LICENSE NUMBER 00C3124 OF DALLAS, TX, WAS DISCIPLINED BY TEXAS ON NOVEMBER 13, 1992
DISCIPLINARY ACTION: EMERGENCY SUSPENSION
OFFENSE: FAILURE TO COMPLY WITH PREVIOUS BOARD ORDER

NOTES: VIOLATION OF 8/20/92 AGREED ORDER.

LEWIS, ELBERT HAMPTON MD, DATE OF BIRTH JANUARY 2, 1929, LICENSE NUMBER 00C3124 OF 7137 LAKEHURST AVENUE, DALLAS, TX, WAS DISCIPLINED BY TEXAS ON JANUARY 29, 1993
DISCIPLINARY ACTION: SURRENDER OF LICENSE
OFFENSE: PHYSICAL OR MENTAL ILLNESS INHIBITING THE ABILITY TO PRACTICE WITH SKILL AND SAFETY

NOTES: INABILITY TO PRACTICE MEDICINE WITH REASONABLE SKILL AND SAFETY BY REASON OF ILLNESS. HE HAS CHOSEN TO PERMANENTLY RETIRE; SHALL SURRENDER HIS TEXAS AND DEA CONTROLLED SUBSTANCES REGISTRATIONS.

LEWIS, HAROLD D DO, LICENSE NUMBER 00E6126 OF AUSTIN, TX, WAS DISCIPLINED BY TEXAS ON FEBRUARY 16, 1990
DISCIPLINARY ACTION: 12-MONTH RESTRICTION PLACED ON LICENSE

NOTES: STIPULATED ORDER. FOR PATIENTS LEWIS TREATS

FOR ALLERGY SYMPTOMS BY USE OF MEDICATIONS CONTAINING STEROIDS, MUST SEEK CONSULTATION OR REFER PATIENTS IF RELIEF OF SYMPTOMS NOT SHOWN WITHIN THREE MONTHS.

LEWIS, KENNETH D MD, DATE OF BIRTH OCTOBER 24, 1957 OF 7905 BORIXA STREET, HOUSTON, TX, WAS DISCIPLINED BY MEDICARE ON MAY 23, 1993
DISCIPLINARY ACTION: EXCLUSION FROM THE MEDICARE AND/OR MEDICAID PROGRAM
OFFENSE: NONCOMPLIANCE WITH A PROFESSIONAL RULE
NOTES: DEFAULTED ON HEALTH EDUCATION ASSISTANCE LOAN. REINSTATED ON 9/2/93.

LEWIS, MICHAEL L MD, DATE OF BIRTH DECEMBER 1, 1953 OF 3106 SOUTHMORE, HOUSTON, TX, WAS DISCIPLINED BY MEDICARE ON APRIL 16, 1994
DISCIPLINARY ACTION: EXCLUSION FROM THE MEDICARE AND/OR MEDICAID PROGRAM
OFFENSE: NONCOMPLIANCE WITH A PROFESSIONAL RULE
NOTES: DEFAULTED ON PUBLIC HEALTH SERVICE EDUCATION LOAN.

LEWIS, MICHAEL L MD OF TAMPA, FL, WAS DISCIPLINED BY MISSOURI ON AUGUST 30, 1995
DISCIPLINARY ACTION: REPRIMAND
OFFENSE: DISCIPLINARY ACTION BY ANOTHER STATE OR AGENCY
NOTES: FLORIDA FINED AND REQUIRED ADDITIONAL CONTINUING MEDICAL EDUCATION ALLEGING THAT HE INJECTED A CONTRAINDICATED CONTRAST MATERIAL IN A PATIENT IN THE PERFORMANCE OF LUMBAR MYELOGROUS CAUSING AN ADVERSE REACTION AND SERIOUS IMPAIRMENT.

LEWIS, MICHAEL L MD, LICENSE NUMBER 0139505 OF 4802 CULBREATH ISLES WAYS, TAMPA, FL, WAS DISCIPLINED BY NEW YORK ON NOVEMBER 7, 1996
DISCIPLINARY ACTION: FINE; REPRIMAND
OFFENSE: DISCIPLINARY ACTION BY ANOTHER STATE OR AGENCY
NOTES: ACTION IN FLORIDA FOR NEGLIGENCE INVOLVING THE INJECTION OF CONROY 60 INTO THE SPINE OF A PATIENT PRIOR TO PERFORMING A MYELOGRAM.

LEWIS, MICHAEL LLOYD MD, DATE OF BIRTH MARCH 12, 1947, LICENSE NUMBER 0050782 OF TAMPA, FL, WAS DISCIPLINED BY FLORIDA ON AUGUST 17, 1994
DISCIPLINARY ACTION: FINE; REQUIRED TO TAKE ADDITIONAL MEDICAL EDUCATION
OFFENSE: SUBSTANDARD CARE, INCOMPETENCE OR NEGLIGENCE
NOTES: CHARGED WITH FAILING TO PRACTICE MEDICINE WITH AN ACCEPTABLE LEVEL OF CARE AND SKILL; ADMINISTERING A LEGEND DRUG. $1,000 FINE; LETTER OF CONCERN; SHALL COMPLETE 20 HOURS OF CONTINUING MEDICAL EDUCATION IN RISK MANAGEMENT WITHIN ONE YEAR.

LEWIS, MICHAEL LLOYD MD, DATE OF BIRTH MARCH 12, 1947, LICENSE NUMBER 0017339 OF 4802 CULBREATH ISLES WAY, TAMPA, FL, WAS DISCIPLINED BY WEST VIRGINIA ON APRIL 12, 1995
DISCIPLINARY ACTION: REQUIRED TO TAKE ADDITIONAL MEDICAL EDUCATION
OFFENSE: DISCIPLINARY ACTION BY ANOTHER STATE OR AGENCY
NOTES: IN 8/94 FLORIDA BOARD REQUIRED HIM TO ATTEND CONTINUING MEDICAL EDUCATION IN RISK MANAGEMENT. WITHIN ONE YEAR HE SHALL PROVIDE EVIDENCE THAT HE HAS ATTENDED 20 HOURS OF CONTINUING MEDICAL EDUCATION IN RISK MANAGEMENT.

LEWIS, MICHAEL LLOYD MD, DATE OF BIRTH MARCH 12, 1947, LICENSE NUMBER 00G6848 OF LAKE HAVASU CITY, AR, WAS DISCIPLINED BY TEXAS ON AUGUST 18, 1995
DISCIPLINARY ACTION: REQUIRED TO TAKE ADDITIONAL MEDICAL EDUCATION
OFFENSE: DISCIPLINARY ACTION BY ANOTHER STATE OR AGENCY
NOTES: IN 8/94 ENTERED INTO A CONSENT AGREEMENT WITH THE FLORIDA BOARD REQUIRING HIM TO PAY $1,000 FINE, OBTAIN 20 HOURS OF CONTINUING MEDICAL EDUCATION IN RISK MANAGEMENT AND RECEIVE A LETTER OF CONCERN FROM THE BOARD BASED ON ALLEGATIONS OF THE SUBSTANDARD CARE OF ONE PATIENT. SHALL NOT PRACTICE MEDICINE IN TEXAS UNTIL HE APPEARS BEFORE BOARD WITH SUFFICIENT EVIDENCE AND INFORMATION WHICH ADEQUATELY INDICATES THAT HE IS PHYSICALLY, MENTALLY AND OTHERWISE COMPETENT TO SAFELY PRACTICE MEDICINE INCLUDING AT A MINIMUM A STATEMENT DESCRIBING INCIDENT LEADING TO DISCIPLINARY ACTION IN FLORIDA AND MEASURES TAKEN TO PREVENT A RECURRENCE, SUFFICIENT HOURS OF CONTINUING MEDICAL EDUCATION FOR LICENSE RENEWAL AND 10 HOURS IN RISK MANAGEMENT AND AN UP-TO-DATE CURRICULUM VITAE; SHALL PROVIDE A COPY OF ORDER TO ANYONE REQUESTING IT WITHIN 10 DAYS; TIME PERIOD OF THIS ORDER SHALL BE TOLLED UNTIL HE RETURNS TO TEXAS; SHALL INFORM BOARD OF CHANGE OF ADDRESS WITHIN 10 DAYS. SHALL NOT SEEK MODIFICATION FOR ONE YEAR.

LEWIS, MICHAEL LLOYD MD, DATE OF BIRTH MARCH 12, 1947, LICENSE NUMBER 0032938 OF 4802 CULBREATH ISLES WAY, TAMPA, FL, WAS DISCIPLINED BY GEORGIA ON SEPTEMBER 8, 1995
DISCIPLINARY ACTION: REPRIMAND
OFFENSE: DISCIPLINARY ACTION BY ANOTHER STATE OR AGENCY
NOTES: DISCIPLINARY ACTION IN FLORIDA.

LEWY, ROBERT IRA MD, LICENSE NUMBER F4931 OF HOUSTON, TX, WAS DISCIPLINED BY TEXAS ON AUGUST 9, 1997
DISCIPLINARY ACTION: FINE; REPRIMAND
OFFENSE: LOSS OR RESTRICTION OF HOSPITAL PRIVILEGES
NOTES: ON 8/1/95 HE PREMATURELY ISSUED A PRESS RELEASE TO PROSPECTIVE PATIENTS WHICH WAS CONFUSING AND INCORRECTLY CHARACTERIZED HIS PARTICIPATION STATUS REGARDING TWO RESEARCH STUDIES; HE CORRECTED THIS ON 8/3/95; IN 1994 HE CHARGED REFERRING AGENCIES A SURCHARGE FOR EVALUATING PATIENTS ON EVENINGS AND WEEKENDS; IN 1993 HE WAS EXCLUDED FROM THE MEDICAL STAFF AT THE METHODIST HOSPITAL FOR INADEQUATE MEDICAL RECORD KEEPING. $2,000 FINE; SHALL GIVE A COPY OF THIS ORDER TO ANY HEALTH CARE ENTITY WHERE HE HAS PRIVILEGES.

LEWY, ROBERT IRA MD, LICENSE NUMBER G30070 OF HOUSTON, TX, WAS DISCIPLINED BY CALIFORNIA ON JANUARY 14, 1998
DISCIPLINARY ACTION: REPRIMAND
OFFENSE: DISCIPLINARY ACTION BY ANOTHER STATE OR AGENCY
NOTES: DISCIPLINED BY TEXAS FOR ISSUING A PRESS RELEASE TO PROSPECTIVE PATIENTS THAT WAS CONFUSING AND MISLEADING AND FOR EXCLUSION FROM THE MEDICAL STAFF OF A HOSPITAL FOR INADEQUATE MEDICAL RECORD KEEPING.

LEWY, ROBERT IRA MD, DATE OF BIRTH OCTOBER 16, 1943,

LICENSE NUMBER 016586E OF 8181 NORTH STADIUM DRIVE, HOUSTON, TX, WAS DISCIPLINED BY PENNSYLVANIA ON JANUARY 26, 1999
DISCIPLINARY ACTION: FINE; REPRIMAND
OFFENSE: DISCIPLINARY ACTION BY ANOTHER STATE OR AGENCY

NOTES: DISCIPLINARY ACTION TAKEN BY TEXAS. CIVIL PENALTY OF $2000.

LIBERMAN, ALBERTO J MD, DATE OF BIRTH JANUARY 5, 1942 OF 513 EAST BROADWAY, PORTLAND, TX, WAS DISCIPLINED BY MEDICARE ON MARCH 16, 1995
DISCIPLINARY ACTION: 120-MONTH EXCLUSION FROM THE MEDICARE AND/OR MEDICAID PROGRAM
OFFENSE: CRIMINAL CONVICTION OR PLEA OF GUILTY, NOLO CONTENDERE, OR NO CONTEST TO A CRIME

NOTES: CONVICTED OF A CRIME INVOLVING THE MEDICARE, MEDICAID, MATERNAL AND CHILD HEALTH SERVICES BLOCK GRANT OR BLOCK GRANTS TO STATES FOR SOCIAL SERVICES PROGRAMS.

LIBERMAN, ALBERTO J MD, LICENSE NUMBER 00G8722 OF PORTLAND, TX, WAS DISCIPLINED BY TEXAS ON OCTOBER 13, 1995
DISCIPLINARY ACTION: SURRENDER OF LICENSE
OFFENSE: CRIMINAL CONVICTION OR PLEA OF GUILTY, NOLO CONTENDERE, OR NO CONTEST TO A CRIME

NOTES: IN 10/94 HE WAS FOUND GUILTY OF FIVE COUNTS OF TAMPERING WITH GOVERNMENT RECORDS; HE IS CURRENTLY ON TWO YEARS PROBATION WITH TERMS AS IMPOSED IN FIVE CRIMINAL JUDGMENTS DATED 10/11/94, INCLUDING FINES TOTALING $10,000 AND 500 HOURS OF COMMUNITY SERVICE OF WHICH 200 HOURS HAD BEEN SERVED AS OF 4/7/95. DOES NOT ADMIT VIOLATION. VOLUNTARY AND PERMANENT SURRENDER OF LICENSE IS ACCEPTED BY BOARD. SHALL NOT PETITION FOR REINSTATEMENT.

LIBERMAN, ALBERTO J MD OF 1700 WILDCAT DRIVE, PORTLAND, TX, WAS DISCIPLINED BY DEA ON DECEMBER 19, 1995
DISCIPLINARY ACTION: SURRENDER OF CONTROLLED SUBSTANCE LICENSE

NOTES: IN LIEU OF PUBLIC INTEREST REVOCATION.

LIDSTONE, JOHN DAVID MD, LICENSE NUMBER 00G7411 OF MADISON, TN, WAS DISCIPLINED BY TEXAS ON AUGUST 18, 1990
OFFENSE: DISCIPLINARY ACTION BY ANOTHER STATE OR AGENCY

NOTES: STIPULATED ORDER. MUST COMPLY WITH TENNESSEE BOARD RESTRICTIONS AND RECEIVE APPROVAL OF TEXAS BOARD PRIOR TO PRACTICING MEDICINE IN TEXAS. HAS FULLY COMPLIED WITH THE CONDITIONS OF TENNESSEE ORDER AND ON 10/20/94 TEXAS ORDER TERMINATED.

LIEGEL, JOYCE M MD, DATE OF BIRTH MARCH 14, 1946 OF 3217 DURHILL STREET, HOUSTON, TX, WAS DISCIPLINED BY MEDICARE ON MAY 23, 1993
DISCIPLINARY ACTION: EXCLUSION FROM THE MEDICARE AND/OR MEDICAID PROGRAM
OFFENSE: NONCOMPLIANCE WITH A PROFESSIONAL RULE

NOTES: DEFAULTED ON HEALTH EDUCATION ASSISTANCE LOAN. REINSTATED ON 12/13/96.

LIGHTFOOT, STANLEY AUGUSTUS MD, LICENSE NUMBER 00D0946 OF TYLER, TX, WAS DISCIPLINED BY TEXAS ON DECEMBER 1, 1990
DISCIPLINARY ACTION: LICENSE SUSPENSION
OFFENSE: CRIMINAL CONVICTION OR PLEA OF GUILTY, NOLO CONTENDERE, OR NO CONTEST TO A CRIME

NOTES: LICENSE SUSPENDED WHILE PHYSICIAN SERVES PRISON TERM IN PENITENTIARY.

LIGHTFOOT, STANLEY AUGUSTUS MD, LICENSE NUMBER 00D0946, WAS DISCIPLINED BY TEXAS ON SEPTEMBER 16, 1991
DISCIPLINARY ACTION: 60-MONTH PROBATION; RESTRICTION PLACED ON LICENSE

NOTES: SUSPENSION OF LICENSE TERMINATED. CONDITIONS OF PROBATION: SHALL APPEAR BEFORE THE BOARD TWICE A YEAR; SHALL NOT PETITION FOR MODIFICATION FOR AT LEAST ONE YEAR; PRACTICE LIMITED TO PATHOLOGY; SHALL COMPLY WITH TERMS OF PROBATION UNDER THE U.S. DISTRICT COURT OR FEDERAL CORRECTIONAL SYSTEM; SHALL GIVE A COPY OF ORDER TO ALL INSTITUTIONS WHERE HE HAS PRIVILEGES; SHALL COOPERATE WITH BOARD IN VERIFYING COMPLIANCE; SHALL ADVISE THE BOARD OF CHANGE OF ADDRESS WITHIN 10 DAYS; TIME SPENT OUT OF TEXAS DOES NOT COUNT TOWARDS PROBATION.

LIGHTFOOT, STANLEY AUGUSTUS MD OF 119 EAST HOUSTON, TYLER, TX, WAS DISCIPLINED BY OKLAHOMA ON MAY 9, 1992
DISCIPLINARY ACTION: 60-MONTH PROBATION; RESTRICTION PLACED ON LICENSE
OFFENSE: DISCIPLINARY ACTION BY ANOTHER STATE OR AGENCY

NOTES: ON 2/25/78, LICENSE REVOKED BY TEXAS, REVOCATION STAYED, PLACED ON FIVE YEARS PROBATION; FULLY REINSTATED 3/83. ON 5/15/90, PLED GUILTY TO FOUR COUNTS OF MAKING FALSE STATEMENTS TO BANKS FOR LOANS, SENTENCED TO TWO YEARS IN PRISON AND FIVE YEARS PROBATION; TEXAS LICENSE SUSPENDED 8/18/90. ON 8/23/91, TEXAS LICENSE REINSTATED UNDER FIVE YEARS PROBATION. OKLAHOMA LICENSE GRANTED WITH TEXAS TERMS AND CONDITIONS IMPOSED. SHALL APPEAR BEFORE BOARD TWICE A YEAR; SHALL NOT PETITION FOR MODIFICATION FOR ONE YEAR; PRACTICE LIMITED TO PATHOLOGY; SHALL NOT SUPERVISE A PHYSICIAN ASSISTANT; SHALL FURNISH BOARD WITH ADDRESS AND/OR CHANGE OF ADDRESS; SHALL APPEAR BEFORE BOARD UPON REQUEST; SHALL NOTIFY ANY HOSPITAL WHERE HE HOLDS STAFF PRIVILEGES, OR CLINIC OR GROUP OF THE TERMS AND CONDITIONS. ON 3/29/96 PROBATION TERMINATED.

LINSTRUM, THOMAS E MD, DATE OF BIRTH MARCH 23, 1925, LICENSE NUMBER 0031390 OF MCKINNEY, TX, WAS DISCIPLINED BY COLORADO ON FEBRUARY 9, 1995
DISCIPLINARY ACTION: LICENSE REVOCATION
OFFENSE: CRIMINAL CONVICTION OR PLEA OF GUILTY, NOLO CONTENDERE, OR NO CONTEST TO A CRIME

NOTES: FELONY CONVICTION.

LINSTRUM, TOM ELTON MD, DATE OF BIRTH MARCH 20, 1925, LICENSE NUMBER 00C4411 OF 310 BROOK LANE, MCKINNEY, TX, WAS DISCIPLINED BY TEXAS ON JUNE 15, 1993
DISCIPLINARY ACTION: RESTRICTION PLACED ON LICENSE
OFFENSE: PROFESSIONAL MISCONDUCT

NOTES: PENDING INVESTIGATION CHARGING HIM WITH SEXUAL IMPROPRIETIES WITH A CHILD NOT HIS PATIENT AND IMPROPER MEDICAL TREATMENT OF AN ADULT PATIENT; HE HAS REQUESTED THAT THE BOARD'S PROCEEDINGS BE DEFERRED PENDING FINAL RESOLUTION OF FELONY CRIMINAL CHARGES FILED AGAINST HIM IN TEXAS AND COLORADO; HAS AGREED TO REFRAIN FROM PRACTICING IN TEXAS AND ALL OTHER STATES UNTIL THE BOARD'S

PENDING PROCEEDINGS HAVE BEEN RESOLVED. SHALL NOTIFY BOARD IN WRITING WITHIN 10 DAYS OF EACH COURT DECISION; SHALL GIVE A COPY OF THIS ORDER TO ANY HEALTH CARE ENTITY WHERE HE HAS PRIVILEGES; SHALL COOPERATE WITH THE BOARD IN VERIFYING COMPLIANCE.

LINSTRUM, TOM ELTON MD, DATE OF BIRTH MARCH 20, 1925, LICENSE NUMBER 00C4411 OF 310 BROOK LANE, MCKINNEY, TX, WAS DISCIPLINED BY TEXAS ON APRIL 15, 1994
DISCIPLINARY ACTION: SURRENDER OF LICENSE
OFFENSE: CRIMINAL CONVICTION OR PLEA OF GUILTY, NOLO CONTENDERE, OR NO CONTEST TO A CRIME

NOTES: ON 12/9/93 HE WAS FOUND GUILTY OF THE FELONY OFFENSE OF INDECENCY WITH A CHILD; WHILE NOT ADMITTING HE HAS VIOLATED THE MEDICAL PRACTICE ACT HE SURRENDERED HIS LICENSE IN LIEU OF FURTHER INVESTIGATION. SHALL NOT PETITION FOR REINSTATEMENT OF LICENSE.

LINSTRUM, TOM ELTON MD OF PROFESSIONAL BUILDING, MC KINNEY, TX, WAS DISCIPLINED BY DEA ON JUNE 3, 1994
DISCIPLINARY ACTION: SURRENDER OF CONTROLLED SUBSTANCE LICENSE
OFFENSE: DISCIPLINARY ACTION BY ANOTHER STATE OR AGENCY

NOTES: STATE BOARD.

LIU, KUO TAI MD, LICENSE NUMBER 00E3047 OF MARLIN, TX, WAS DISCIPLINED BY TEXAS ON DECEMBER 4, 1991
DISCIPLINARY ACTION: 60-MONTH PROBATION; RESTRICTION PLACED ON LICENSE
OFFENSE: SUBSTANDARD CARE, INCOMPETENCE OR NEGLIGENCE

NOTES: FAILED TO DEMONSTRATE ADEQUATE KNOWLEDGE AND SKILLS IN TREATING FOUR PATIENTS AND PREPARING THEIR MEDICAL RECORDS. SUSPENSION STAYED; CONDITIONS OF PROBATION: SHALL LIMIT PRACTICE TO TREATING PATIENTS AT GOLDEN YEARS AND ELMWOOD NURSING HOMES ONLY; SHALL OBTAIN A BOARD APPROVED MONITORING PHYSICIAN WHO SHALL REPORT TO THE BOARD EVERY SIX MONTHS; A COPY OF THIS ORDER SHALL BE PROVIDED TO THE MONITOR AND ALL INSTITUTIONS WHERE HE HAS PRIVILEGES; SHALL REFRAIN FROM PRESCRIBING ANY DRUG UNLESS MEDICALLY INDICATED AND IN THERAPEUTIC DOSES, AND WITH AN APPROPRIATE MEDICAL HISTORY AND EXAM; SHALL CONDUCT FOLLOW-UP EXAMS TO DETERMINE IF DRUG REGIMEN IS WORKING AND IF IT SHOULD BE ALTERED; WITHIN THREE MONTHS SHALL COMPLETE A TWO WEEK MINIRESIDENCY COURSE; WITHIN NINE MONTHS MUST PASS THE SPEX EXAM; WITHIN SIX MONTHS SHALL COMPLETE A REMEDIAL PHARMACOLOGY COURSE; SHALL COOPERATE WITH BOARD IN VERIFYING COMPLIANCE; SHALL ADVISE THE BOARD OF A CHANGE OF ADDRESS WITHIN 10 DAYS; TIME SPENT OUT OF TEXAS DOES NOT COUNT TOWARDS PROBATION; SHALL APPEAR BEFORE THE BOARD TWICE A YEAR; SHALL NOT APPLY FOR MODIFICATION OF ORDER FOR ONE YEAR.

LIU, KUO TAI MD, LICENSE NUMBER 0010449, WAS DISCIPLINED BY OKLAHOMA ON JANUARY 15, 1993

NOTES: IN LIEU OF ANY FURTHER FORMAL PROCEEDINGS BOARD AGREED TO ACCEPT APPLICATION FOR PHYSICIAN EMERITUS STATUS (RETIRED STATUS, NOT ACTIVE TO PRACTICE) WITH THE PROVISION THAT HE FILES WITHIN 10 DAYS.

LOCKHART, ALBERT BELVILLE MD, LICENSE NUMBER 0034111 OF RICHARDSON, TX, WAS DISCIPLINED BY FLORIDA ON OCTOBER 29, 1990
DISCIPLINARY ACTION: LICENSE SUSPENSION
OFFENSE: FAILURE TO COMPLY WITH PREVIOUS BOARD ORDER

NOTES: FOUND GUILTY OF VIOLATING A LAWFUL ORDER OF THE BOARD PREVIOUSLY ENTERED IN A DISCIPLINARY HEARING BY FAILING TO PAY THE FINE. LICENSE SUSPENDED UNTIL SUCH TIME AS HE COMPLIES WITH THE ORDER OF 12/16/88 BY PAYING THE ADMINISTRATIVE FINE IMPOSED BY THAT ORDER AND UNTIL HE APPEARS BEFORE THE BOARD AND ESTABLISHES HIS ABILITY TO PRACTICE MEDICINE WITH SKILL AND SAFETY.

LOCKHART, ALBERT BELVILLE MD, LICENSE NUMBER 0034111 OF RICHARDSON, TX, WAS DISCIPLINED BY FLORIDA ON SEPTEMBER 23, 1991
DISCIPLINARY ACTION: LICENSE SUSPENSION; FINE
OFFENSE: NONCOMPLIANCE WITH A PROFESSIONAL RULE

NOTES: FAILED TO SUBMIT DOCUMENTATION VERIFYING CONTINUING MEDICAL EDUCATION IN RESPONSE TO THE BOARD'S RANDOM AUDIT. $5,000 FINE; LICENSE SUSPENDED UNTIL FINE IS PAID AND HE HAS COMPLETED AN ADDITIONAL 35 HOURS CONTINUING MEDICAL EDUCATION, AND FIVE HOURS OF RISK MANAGEMENT.

LOCKWOOD, RICHARD MD OF 1404 MISSOURI, HOUSTON, TX, WAS DISCIPLINED BY DEA ON OCTOBER 31, 1997
DISCIPLINARY ACTION: SURRENDER OF CONTROLLED SUBSTANCE LICENSE

NOTES: IN LIEU OF PUBLIC INTEREST REVOCATION.

LOCKWOOD, RICHARD L MD, LICENSE NUMBER 0017165 OF 1404 MISSOURI, HOUSTON, TX, WAS DISCIPLINED BY OKLAHOMA ON JUNE 21, 1990
DISCIPLINARY ACTION: LICENSE REVOCATION
OFFENSE: SUBSTANCE ABUSE

NOTES: GUILTY OF HABITUAL INTEMPERANCE OR THE HABITUAL USE OF HABIT-FORMING DRUGS WHICH IMPAIRS THE ABILITY TO PRACTICE MEDICINE WITH REASONABLE SKILL AND SAFETY TO THE PATIENT. ON 2/8/90 HOSPITAL WHERE HE WORKED AS AN ANESTHESIOLOGIST REQUESTED HIM TO STOP DELIVERING ANESTHETICS TO PATIENTS AND TO UNDERGO A MEDICAL EVALUATION; EVALUATOR AT HIS REQUEST WOULD NOT REVEAL RESULTS BUT SAID AT THAT TIME SHOULD NOT BE GIVING ANESTHESIA; AT ANOTHER HOSPITAL IN TEXAS HE EXPERIENCED SIMILAR PROBLEMS. HE RESIGNED WHEN ASKED TO UNDERGO A PHYSICAL EXAM INCLUDING TESTING FOR SUBSTANCE ABUSE.

LOCKWOOD, RICHARD L MD, LICENSE NUMBER 00G7083 OF HOUSTON, TX, WAS DISCIPLINED BY TEXAS ON AUGUST 18, 1990
DISCIPLINARY ACTION: LICENSE SUSPENSION; REQUIRED TO TAKE ADDITIONAL MEDICAL EDUCATION
OFFENSE: SUBSTANCE ABUSE

NOTES: STIPULATED ORDER. LICENSE INDEFINITELY SUSPENDED COMMENCING UPON BOARD VERBAL APPROVAL OF ORDER (8/17/90). MUST SUBMIT FOR PSYCHIATRIC EVALUATIONS AND RECOMMENDED TREATMENTS, PARTICIPATE IN HARRIS COUNTY MEDICAL SOCIETY COMMITTEE ON PHYSICIAN HEALTH AND REHABILITATION AND AA, SUBMIT FOR APPROPRIATE EXAMINATIONS TO DETERMINE FREEDOM FROM DRUGS AND ALCOHOL, AND OBTAIN CONTINUING MEDICAL EDUCATION.

LOCKWOOD, RICHARD L MD OF 1404 MISSOURI ST, HOUSTON, TX, WAS DISCIPLINED BY DEA ON OCTOBER 2, 1990
DISCIPLINARY ACTION: SURRENDER OF CONTROLLED SUBSTANCE LICENSE
OFFENSE: SUBSTANCE ABUSE

NOTES: OKLAHOMA MEDICAL LICENSE REVOKED 06/08/90; TESTED POSITIVE ON URINE DRUG SCREEN FOR BENZODIAZEPINE METABOLITES 11/10/89 AND 04/04/90; TREATED FOR ABUSE OF FENTANYL AND SODIUM PENTOTHAL 12/87.

LOCKWOOD, RICHARD L MD, LICENSE NUMBER 00G7083 OF IRVING, TX, WAS DISCIPLINED BY TEXAS ON APRIL 29, 1991
DISCIPLINARY ACTION: PROBATION; REQUIRED TO TAKE ADDITIONAL MEDICAL EDUCATION

NOTES: REINSTATED FROM SUSPENSION; PROBATION CONDITIONS INCLUDE: PARTICIPATION IN IMPAIRED PHYSICIANS PROGRAM; MUST PARTICIPATE IN AA; MUST SUBMIT TO ALCOHOL OR DRUG SCREENS; SHALL ATTEND AT LEAST 50 HOURS OF CONTINUING MEDICAL EDUCATION IN FAMILY PRACTICE.

LOCKWOOD, RICHARD L MD, LICENSE NUMBER G7083 OF HOUSTON, TX, WAS DISCIPLINED BY TEXAS ON AUGUST 9, 1997
DISCIPLINARY ACTION: LICENSE SUSPENSION
OFFENSE: FAILURE TO COMPLY WITH PREVIOUS BOARD ORDER

NOTES: HE VIOLATED 8/18/90 AND 4/29/91 BOARD ORDERS IN THAT HE FAILED TO PARTICIPATE IN ACTIVITIES OF A PHYSICIANS HEALTH AND REHABILITATION COMMITTEE OR IN AA; FAILED TO PROVIDE REQUIRED QUARTERLY REPORTS; FAILED TO ATTEND OR SHOW PROOF OF ATTENDANCE AT REQUIRED CONTINUING MEDICAL EDUCATION COURSES. SUSPENSION UNTIL HE REQUESTS TO HAVE THE SUSPENSION STAYED OR APPEARS BEFORE THE BOARD WITH SUFFICIENT EVIDENCE THAT HE IS PHYSICALLY, MENTALLY AND OTHERWISE COMPETENT TO SAFELY PRACTICE MEDICINE INCLUDING AT A MINIMUM: COMPLETE COPIES OF MEDICAL RECORDS AND REPORTS OF PSYCHOLOGICAL AND NEUROPSYCHIATRIC EVALUATIONS, INCLUDING A 96-HOUR INPATIENT EVALUATION CONDUCTED BY A BOARD-APPROVED CERTIFIED PSYCHIATRIST; SHALL INFORM THE BOARD OF CHANGE OF ADDRESS WITHIN 10 DAYS OR IF HE LEAVES THE STATE; SHALL NOT SEEK MODIFICATION FOR ONE YEAR.

LOCKWOOD, RICHARD L MD, LICENSE NUMBER G7083, WAS DISCIPLINED BY TEXAS ON AUGUST 22, 1998
DISCIPLINARY ACTION: 120-MONTH PROBATION; RESTRICTION PLACED ON LICENSE
OFFENSE: SUBSTANCE ABUSE

NOTES: SUCCESSFULLY COMPLETED A 96 HOUR INPATIENT EVALUATION AS REQUIRED BY 8/9/97 ORDER WHICH INDICATED THAT HIS OPIATE DEPENDENCE IS IN COMPLETE REMISSION; HE ATTENDS AA FOUR TIMES A WEEK AND HAS A SPONSOR; HE REPORTS A SOBRIETY DATE OF 3/3/93. SUSPENSION STAYED FOR PROBATION WITH FOLLOWING TERMS AND CONDITIONS AS SOON AS HE PASSES THE SPEX AND JURISPRUDENCE EXAM WITH A SCORE OF 75 OR ABOVE, WITHIN 3 ATTEMPTS. SHALL BE RESTRICTED TO A BOARD-APPROVED OUTPATIENT PRACTICE AND/OR CLINICAL SETTING; SHALL NOT PRACTICE IN A HOSPITAL SETTING; SHALL ABSTAIN FROM THE CONSUMPTION OF ALCOHOL/DRUGS IN ANY FORM UNLESS PRESCRIBED BY ANOTHER PHYSICIAN FOR A LEGITIMATE AND THERAPEUTIC PURPOSE; SHALL SUBMIT HIMSELF FOR APPROPRIATE EXAMS INCLUDING DRUG OR ALCOHOL SCREENS; SHALL PARTICIPATE IN THE ACTIVITIES OF A PHYSICIAN HEALTH AND REHABILITATION COMMITTEE AND ATTEND WEEKLY MEETINGS WITH QUARTERLY REPORTS; SHALL PARTICIPATE IN AA'S PROGRAM NOT LESS THAN THREE TIMES A WEEK; SHALL REPORT ON HIS ATTENDANCE; SHALL NOT TREAT OR OTHERWISE SERVE AS PHYSICIAN, PRESCRIBE, DISPENSE OR ADMINISTER DRUGS THAT MAY BE SUBJECT TO ABUSE TO HIMSELF OR TO ANY MEMBER OF HIS FAMILY; SHALL SURRENDER DEA AND TEXAS DEPARTMENT OF PUBLIC SAFETY CONTROLLED SUBSTANCE CERTIFICATES AND ANY DRUGS REMAINING IN HIS POSSESSION INCLUDING SAMPLES; SEPARATE FROM PATIENT RECORDS, SHALL MAINTAIN A LOGBOOK OF EVERY PRESCRIPTION WRITTEN BY HIM FOR DANGEROUS DRUGS WITH ADDICTIVE POTENTIAL WHICH SHALL BE MADE AVAILABLE FOR REVIEW; HIS MEDICAL PRACTICE SHALL BE MONITORED BY A BOARD APPROVED TEXAS PHYSICIAN WHO SHALL PROVIDE QUARTERLY REPORTS TO THE BOARD; SHALL MAINTAIN ADEQUATE MEDICAL RECORDS WHICH SHALL BE AVAILABLE FOR REVIEW; SHALL OBTAIN 50 HOURS PER YEAR OF CONTINUING MEDICAL EDUCATION WITH 1 COURSE IN GENERAL MEDICINE AND 1 COURSE IN PRIMARY CARE; SHALL APPEAR BEFORE THE BOARD UPON REQUEST; SHALL COOPERATE WITH THE BOARD IN VERIFYING COMPLIANCE INCLUDING PROVIDING COPIES OF MEDICAL RELEASES UPON REQUEST; SHALL GIVE A COPY OF THIS ORDER TO ANY HEALTH CARE ENTITY WHERE HE HAS PRIVILEGES; SHALL PROVIDE A COPY OF THIS ORDER TO ANYONE REQUESTING IT WITHIN 10 DAYS; TIME SPENT OUT OF TEXAS DOES NOT COUNT TOWARD PROBATION; SHALL INFORM THE BOARD OF CHANGE OF ADDRESS WITHIN 10 DAYS OR IF HE LEAVES THE STATE; SHALL NOT SEEK MODIFICATION FOR ONE YEAR.

LOFTIS, M DEAN MD, LICENSE NUMBER 00E2274 OF LUBBOCK, TX, WAS DISCIPLINED BY TEXAS ON JANUARY 14, 1994
DISCIPLINARY ACTION: LICENSE REVOCATION
OFFENSE: CRIMINAL CONVICTION OR PLEA OF GUILTY, NOLO CONTENDERE, OR NO CONTEST TO A CRIME

NOTES: ON 5/28/93 WAS SENTENCED TO 151 MONTHS OF IMPRISONMENT AFTER BEING CONVICTED IN THE U.S. DISTRICT COURT EASTERN DISTRICT OF TEXAS FOR ONE COUNT OF POSSESSION AND RECEIPT OF FIREARMS; TWO COUNTS OF RECEIVING AND CONCEALING STOLEN FIREARMS AND TWO COUNTS OF POSSESSION OF UNREGISTERED FIREARMS; INCARCERATED AS OF THE ORDER DATE. ORDER WILL BECOME FINAL WHEN ALL APPEALS HAVE BEEN EXHAUSTED.

LOGAN, WILLIAM M MD, LICENSE NUMBER 00H0573 OF DALLAS, TX, WAS DISCIPLINED BY TEXAS ON MAY 15, 1996
DISCIPLINARY ACTION: REPRIMAND; MONITORING OF PHYSICIAN PERFORMANCE
OFFENSE: SEXUAL ABUSE OF OR SEXUAL MISCONDUCT WITH A PATIENT

NOTES: IN 4/91, HE BEGAN PSYCHOANALYSIS WITH AN ADULT FEMALE PATIENT AND CONTINUED TO TREAT HER UNTIL 4/95; DURING THE COURSE OF TREATMENT AND IN APPROXIMATELY 4/95 AND 5/95, HE ENGAGED IN SEXUAL ACTS, INCLUDING SEXUAL INTERCOURSE, WITH THIS PATIENT AND FAILED TO RECOGNIZE AND APPROPRIATELY AND PROFESSIONALLY HANDLE AS A PSYCHIATRIST ISSUES OF TRANSFERENCE AND COUNTER-TRANSFERENCE; IN 11/95, HE REPORTED

THIS RELATIONSHIP TO THE BOARD; REPORTS THAT HE IS NOT CURRENTLY ENGAGED IN THE PRIVATE PRACTICE OF PSYCHIATRY BUT PRACTICES IN A PROGRAM RUN BY THE COUNTY AND UNIVERSITY, WHERE IT IS REPORTED HE HAS NO ONE-ON-ONE MEDICAL MANAGEMENT OF ANY PATIENT. THREE-YEAR LICENSE RESTRICTION WITH TERMS AND CONDITIONS: SHALL SUBMIT HIMSELF FOR EVALUATION AND TREATMENT BY A BOARD-APPROVED PSYCHIATRIST WHOM HE SHALL SEE AT LEAST ONCE A MONTH AND WHO SHALL SUBMIT REPORTS TO THE BOARD; SHALL COOPERATE WITH THE BOARD IN VERIFYING COMPLIANCE INCLUDING PROVIDING COPIES OF MEDICAL RELEASES OR PEER REVIEW RECORDS UPON REQUEST; SHALL GIVE A COPY OF THIS ORDER TO ANY HEALTH CARE ENTITY WHERE HE HAS PRIVILEGES; SHALL GIVE A COPY OF ORDER TO ANYONE REQUESTING IT WITHIN 10 DAYS; SHALL APPEAR BEFORE BOARD AT LEAST ONCE A YEAR OR AT BOARD REQUEST; TIME SPENT OUT OF TEXAS DOES NOT COUNT TOWARD PROBATION; SHALL INFORM BOARD OF CHANGE OF ADDRESS WITHIN 10 DAYS OR IF HE LEAVES THE STATE. SHALL NOT SEEK MODIFICATION FOR ONE YEAR. ON 8/22/98 ORDER TERMINATED.

LONG, JOSEPH M MD OF 2700 CITIZENS PLAZA #101, VICTORIA, TX, WAS DISCIPLINED BY DEA ON MARCH 27, 1996
DISCIPLINARY ACTION: RESTRICTION PLACED ON CONTROLLED SUBSTANCE LICENSE
OFFENSE: PROFESSIONAL MISCONDUCT

NOTES: PAST CONTROLLED SUBSTANCE VIOLATIONS.

LONG, JOSEPH MERL MD, DATE OF BIRTH JANUARY 31, 1945, LICENSE NUMBER 00E0095 OF 2710 HOSPITAL DRIVE #104, VICTORIA, TX, WAS DISCIPLINED BY TEXAS ON JANUARY 29, 1993
DISCIPLINARY ACTION: 36-MONTH PROBATION; RESTRICTION PLACED ON CONTROLLED SUBSTANCE LICENSE
OFFENSE: OVERPRESCRIBING OR MISPRESCRIBING DRUGS

NOTES: TREATED A PATIENT FOR A LONG HISTORY OF BACK PAIN, ULCERS, ESOPHAGEAL RUPTURE AND DEPRESSION BEGINNING IN 1982; FAILED TO DOCUMENT REASONS FOR PRESCRIBING CONTROLLED SUBSTANCES; WAS AWARE PATIENT WAS RECEIVING PERCODAN FROM OTHER PHYSICIANS; ATIVAN AND HALCION; DR. LONG WROTE PRESCRIPTIONS FOR DALMANE, VALIUM, FASTIN AND ALUPENT; FROM 1989 THROUGH 3/91 EXCESSIVE AMOUNTS OF DRUGS WERE PRESCRIBED. 3 YEAR SUSPENSION STAYED. CONDITIONS OF PROBATION: SHALL ATTEND AT LEAST 50 HOURS PER YEAR OF CONTINUING MEDICAL EDUCATION, 25 OF WHICH SHALL BE ASSOCIATED WITH INSTRUCTION IN PAIN MANAGEMENT; SHALL LEARN AND UNDERSTAND THE POTENTIAL FOR ABUSE OF CONTROLLED SUBSTANCES AND OTHER PRESCRIPTION DRUGS; SHALL SURRENDER ALL UNUSED TRIPLICATE PRESCRIPTION FORMS; SHALL NOT POSSESS, ADMINISTER, DISPENSE OR PRESCRIBE ANY CONTROLLED SUBSTANCES, BUT MAY ORDER SUCH TO BE ADMINISTERED TO HOSPITAL PATIENTS; SHALL APPEAR BEFORE THE BOARD ONCE A YEAR; SHALL GIVE A COPY OF THIS ORDER TO ANY HEALTH CARE ENTITY WHERE HE HAS PRIVILEGES; SHALL COOPERATE WITH THE BOARD IN VERIFYING COMPLIANCE; SHALL INFORM BOARD OF CHANGE OF ADDRESS WITHIN 10 DAYS OR IF HE LEAVES THE STATE; TIME SPENT OUT OF TEXAS DOES NOT COUNT TOWARD PROBATION. SHALL NOT SEEK MODIFICATION FOR 1 YEAR. ON 6/22/94 BASED ON HISTORY OF COMPLIANCE, AND COMPLETION OF CONTINUING MEDICAL EDUCATION THE ORDER WAS TERMINATED.

LONG, WALTER K MD, LICENSE NUMBER 0C28907 OF KINGWOOD, TX, WAS DISCIPLINED BY CALIFORNIA ON SEPTEMBER 3, 1995
DISCIPLINARY ACTION: LICENSE REVOCATION
OFFENSE: DISCIPLINARY ACTION BY ANOTHER STATE OR AGENCY

NOTES: ACTION IN TEXAS FOR FAILURE TO PRACTICE MEDICINE IN AN ACCEPTABLE MANNER CONSISTENT WITH PUBLIC HEALTH AND WELFARE. RESTRICTIONS INCLUDED NO GASTRIC REDUCTION SURGERY FOR OBESITY. DEFAULT ACTION.

LONG, WALTER K JR MD, LICENSE NUMBER 0015287 OF KINGWOOD, TX, WAS DISCIPLINED BY WASHINGTON ON NOVEMBER 17, 1995

NOTES: SHALL NOT PRACTICE IN WASHINGTON UNTIL HE APPEARS BEFORE THE BOARD AND PRESENTS EVIDENCE THAT HE CAN PRACTICE MEDICINE WITH REASONABLE SKILL AND SAFETY.

LONG, WALTER KEIRN JR MD, LICENSE NUMBER 00C4177 OF KINGWOOD, TX, WAS DISCIPLINED BY TEXAS ON APRIL 15, 1994
DISCIPLINARY ACTION: RESTRICTION PLACED ON LICENSE
OFFENSE: SUBSTANDARD CARE, INCOMPETENCE OR NEGLIGENCE

NOTES: ADMITTED THAT PATIENTS UNDER HIS TREATMENT HAD DEVELOPED COMPLICATIONS RELATED TO GASTRIC STAPLING PROCEDURES; SUCH COMPLICATIONS ARE COMMON AND ARE NOT INDICATIVE OF NEGLIGENCE PER SE; PROFESSIONAL FAILURE TO PRACTICE MEDICINE IN AN ACCEPTABLE MANNER CONSISTENT WITH PUBLIC HEALTH AND WELFARE. SHALL NOT PERFORM ANY GASTRIC REDUCTION SURGERY FOR OBESITY; SHALL GIVE A COPY OF THIS ORDER TO ANY HEALTH CARE ENTITY WHERE HE HAS PRIVILEGES; SHALL COOPERATE WITH THE BOARD IN VERIFYING COMPLIANCE; SHALL INFORM BOARD OF CHANGE OF ADDRESS WITHIN 10 DAYS. SHALL NOT SEEK MODIFICATION FOR ONE YEAR. ON 1/29/99 ORDER TERMINATED.

LOPEZ, DAVID NARANJO MD, DATE OF BIRTH JUNE 25, 1958 OF 1720 PLEASANTON ROAD, SAN ANTONIO, TX, WAS DISCIPLINED BY MEDICARE ON OCTOBER 20, 1998
DISCIPLINARY ACTION: EXCLUSION FROM THE MEDICARE AND/OR MEDICAID PROGRAM
OFFENSE: NONCOMPLIANCE WITH A PROFESSIONAL RULE

NOTES: DEFAULTED ON PUBLIC HEALTH SERVICE EDUCATION LOAN. REINSTATED ON 10/26/98.

LOPEZ, LOUIS ALFRED MD, LICENSE NUMBER 00H9538 OF GALVESTON, TX, WAS DISCIPLINED BY TEXAS ON AUGUST 18, 1995
DISCIPLINARY ACTION: 60-MONTH PROBATION; RESTRICTION PLACED ON LICENSE
OFFENSE: SEXUAL ABUSE OF OR SEXUAL MISCONDUCT WITH A PATIENT

NOTES: SUBSEQUENT TO THE LAST OCCASION ON WHICH HE TREATED HER, HE BECAME INVOLVED IN A ROMANTIC AND SEXUAL RELATIONSHIP WITH A FEMALE PATIENT WHOM HE HAD BEEN TREATING BETWEEN 5/93 AND 7/93; CLAIMED TO HAVE TERMINATED THE PHYSICIAN-PATIENT RELATIONSHIP BETWEEN HIMSELF AND PATIENT PRIOR TO BEGINNING THEIR SOCIAL RELATIONSHIP; DURING THE SEVERAL MONTHS OF THEIR SOCIAL RELATIONSHIP HE WROTE A NUMBER OF PRESCRIPTIONS FOR HER; HAS NOT ADMITTED TO CHARGES. SUSPENSION STAYED. PROBATION WITH TERMS: HIS PRACTICE SHALL BE MONITORED BY A

BOARD-APPROVED PHYSICIAN WHO SHALL SUBMIT QUARTERLY REPORTS TO THE BOARD; SHALL HAVE A CHAPERONE PRESENT IN THE ROOM DURING ANY PHYSICAL EXAMINATION OF A FEMALE PATIENT; SHALL OBTAIN 10 HOURS PER YEAR OF AN ETHICS PROGRAM; SHALL APPEAR BEFORE BOARD AT LEAST TWO TIMES PER YEAR; SHALL COOPERATE WITH BOARD IN VERIFYING COMPLIANCE; SHALL GIVE A COPY OF THIS ORDER TO ANY HEALTH CARE ENTITY WHERE HE HAS PRIVILEGES; SHALL PROVIDE A COPY OF THIS ORDER TO ANYONE REQUESTING IT WITHIN 10 DAYS; TIME PERIOD OUT OF TEXAS DOES NOT COUNT TOWARD PROBATION; SHALL INFORM BOARD OF CHANGE OF ADDRESS WITHIN 10 DAYS OR IF HE LEAVES THE STATE. SHALL NOT SEEK MODIFICATION FOR ONE YEAR. ON 10/5/96 REQUEST TO TERMINATE PROBATION DENIED; ORDER MODIFIED TO REDUCE REQUIRED APPEARANCES BEFORE THE BOARD TO ONCE A YEAR. ON 4/4/98 ORDER TERMINATED.

LOPEZ, LOUIS ALFRED MD, LICENSE NUMBER 1045695 OF 500 WEST BERRY, FT. WAYNE, IN, WAS DISCIPLINED BY INDIANA ON AUGUST 29, 1996
DISCIPLINARY ACTION: PROBATION; RESTRICTION PLACED ON LICENSE
OFFENSE: DISCIPLINARY ACTION BY ANOTHER STATE OR AGENCY

NOTES: ON 8/18/95 HIS LICENSE IN TEXAS WAS RESTRICTED FOR ALLEGED VIOLATIONS OF THE PROHIBITIONS AGAINST UNPROFESSIONAL OR DISHONORABLE CONDUCT UNDER THE TEXAS MEDICAL PRACTICE ACT. CURRENTLY RESIDES IN INDIANA AND HAS HAD NO VIOLATION OF ANY KIND EITHER IN TEXAS OR INDIANA SINCE THE ORDER WAS ENTERED; REVEALED TEXAS ACTION ON HIS 7/10/96 APPLICATION FOR INDIANA LICENSURE. CONDITIONS OF INDIANA LICENSURE: HIS MEDICAL PRACTICE, INCLUDING ANY OFFICE AND SURGICAL PRACTICE, SHALL BE MONITORED BY A BOARD APPROVED LICENSED PHYSICIAN WHO SHALL REVIEW HIS MEDICAL PRACTICE AND COUNSEL HIM ON ANY PERCEIVED DEFICIENCIES AND PROVIDE QUARTERLY REPORTS TO THE BOARD; SHALL HAVE A CHAPERONE PRESENT IN THE ROOM ANYTIME HE PERFORMS A PHYSICAL EXAMINATION ON A FEMALE PATIENT AND SHALL MAKE A NOTATION ON THE PATIENT'S CHART INDICATING THE CHAPERONE WAS PRESENT; SHALL OBTAIN 10 HOURS OF AN ETHICS COURSE OR AN ETHICS PROGRAM PER YEAR FOR FOUR YEARS AND SHALL SUBMIT TO THE BOARD DOCUMENTATION OF ATTENDANCE AND SUCCESSFUL COMPLETION; SHALL PERSONALLY APPEAR BEFORE THE BOARD AT LEAST TWO TIMES EACH YEAR; SHALL FULLY COOPERATE WITH THE BOARD IN VERIFYING COMPLIANCE; SHALL GIVE A COPY OF THIS ORDER TO ANY HEALTH CARE ENTITY WHERE HE HAS PRIVILEGES; SHALL PROVIDE A COPY OF THIS ORDER TO ANYONE REQUESTING IT WITHIN 10 DAYS; SHALL NOTIFY THE BOARD IN WRITING IF HE LEAVES INDIANA TO LIVE OR PRACTICE; SHALL INFORM THE BOARD OF CHANGE OF ADDRESS; TIME PERIOD OUT OF INDIANA MAY EXTEND TIME OF RESTRICTIONS; SHALL INFORM THE BOARD OF ANY CHANGE OF IF HE LEAVES THE STATE; MAY NOT PETITION FOR MODIFICATION FOR ONE YEAR UNLESS TEXAS ORDER MODIFIED; SHALL PROVIDE DOCUMENTATION REFLECTING COMPLIANCE; AND UPON THE SOONER OF THE REMAINING FOUR YEARS OF THE TERM OF THE ORDER OR THE LIFTING OF THE TEXAS ORDER, SHALL BE ELIGIBLE FOR CONSIDERATION FOR FULL, UNLIMITED LICENSURE. ON 11/24/98 PETITION FOR WITHDRAWAL OF PROBATION GRANTED.

LOPEZ, VICTOR M MD, LICENSE NUMBER G9684 OF LAREDO, TX, WAS DISCIPLINED BY TEXAS ON APRIL 4, 1998
DISCIPLINARY ACTION: FINE
OFFENSE: SUBSTANDARD CARE, INCOMPETENCE OR NEGLIGENCE

NOTES: ON 5/6/90 AN EMERGENCY ROOM PHYSICIAN, WHILE IN THE PROCESS OF PLACING A CENTRAL LINE FOR THE PURPOSE OF LIFE SUPPORTIVE MEASURES, INADVERTENTLY LEFT A GUIDE WIRE FROM THE CENTRAL LINE IN A PATIENT WHICH HE DISCOVERED; DID NOT DOCUMENT THIS IN HIS PROGRESS NOTE; DID NOT INFORM PATIENT OR PATIENT'S FAMILY OF ITS EXISTENCE ALTHOUGH PATIENT'S ATTENDING PHYSICIAN WAS INFORMED. $2,500 FINE; SHALL COOPERATE WITH THE BOARD IN VERIFYING COMPLIANCE.

LOSTETTER, ALVIN CHARLES MD, LICENSE NUMBER 00D6070 OF KILGORE, TX, WAS DISCIPLINED BY TEXAS ON MAY 15, 1996
DISCIPLINARY ACTION: REPRIMAND; REQUIRED TO TAKE ADDITIONAL MEDICAL EDUCATION
OFFENSE: LOSS OR RESTRICTION OF HOSPITAL PRIVILEGES

NOTES: IN 8/90, HE WAS REPRIMANDED BY A HOSPITAL FOR KICKING A NURSE IN THE BUTTOCKS; DURING 1992 HE PRESENTED TO THE OPERATING ROOM WITHOUT PROPER ATTIRE AND DUE TO PREVIOUS INCIDENTS HE WAS URGED TO CORRECT THE PROBLEM; ON ABOUT 3/6/95, HE SHOOK OXYGEN TUBING WHICH ALLEGEDLY CONTAINED BODY FLUIDS AT A NURSE, CAUSING FLUID TO SPLASH ON NURSE'S FACE; ON ABOUT 3/7/95, HE WAS SUMMARILY SUSPENDED FROM THE HOSPITAL FOR EXPOSING A NURSE TO POTENTIAL HARM, FOR DISRUPTING THE OPERATION OF THE HOSPITAL AND FOR NONCOMPLIANCE WITH POLICY. THREE YEAR LICENSE RESTRICTION WITH TERMS: SHALL SUBMIT HIMSELF FOR EVALUATION AND TREATMENT BY A BOARD-APPROVED PSYCHIATRIST WHOM HE SHALL SEE AT LEAST ONCE A MONTH AND WHO SHALL SUBMIT REPORTS TO THE BOARD; SHALL OBTAIN AT LEAST 50 HOURS PER YEAR OF CONTINUING MEDICAL EDUCATION, AT LEAST 10 OF WHICH SHALL BE IN INFECTION CONTROL; SHALL OBTAIN 10 HOURS OF AN ETHICS COURSE OR ETHICS PROGRAM PER YEAR FOR THREE YEARS; SHALL APPEAR BEFORE BOARD AT LEAST ONCE A YEAR; SHALL COOPERATE WITH THE BOARD IN VERIFYING COMPLIANCE INCLUDING PROVIDING MEDICAL RELEASES UPON REQUEST; SHALL PROVIDE ANY MEDICAL RELEASES AT BOARD REQUEST; SHALL GIVE A COPY OF THIS ORDER TO ANY HEALTH CARE ENTITY WHERE HE HAS PRIVILEGES; TIME SPENT OUT OF TEXAS DOES NOT COUNT TOWARD RESTRICTION; SHALL INFORM BOARD OF CHANGE OF ADDRESS WITHIN 10 DAYS OR IF HE LEAVES THE STATE. SHALL NOT SEEK MODIFICATION FOR ONE YEAR.

LOSTETTER, ALVIN CHARLES MD, LICENSE NUMBER D6070 OF RICHARDSON, TX, WAS DISCIPLINED BY TEXAS ON NOVEMBER 22, 1997
DISCIPLINARY ACTION: 36-MONTH PROBATION; REQUIRED TO TAKE ADDITIONAL MEDICAL EDUCATION
OFFENSE: FAILURE TO COMPLY WITH PREVIOUS BOARD ORDER

NOTES: VIOLATED 5/15/96 BOARD ORDER IN THAT ON 5/5/97 HE FAILED TO MAKE REQUIRED PERSONAL APPEARANCES AND FAILED TO COOPERATE WITH THE BOARD IN VERIFYING COMPLIANCE; REPORTS HE DID NOT RECEIVE NOTICE OF APPEARANCE. SUSPENSION STAYED WITH FOLLOWING TERMS AND CONDITIONS OF PROBATION: SHALL CONTINUE TO RECEIVE CARE AND TREATMENT FROM HIS PSYCHIATRIST AT LEAST MONTHLY; SHALL OBTAIN 50 HOURS PER YEAR OF CONTINUING MEDICAL

EDUCATION WITH 10 HOURS IN INFECTION CONTROL; SHALL OBTAIN 10 HOURS OF AN ETHICS COURSE PER YEAR FOR 3 YEARS; SHALL APPEAR BEFORE THE BOARD ONCE A YEAR; SHALL COOPERATE WITH THE BOARD IN VERIFYING COMPLIANCE INCLUDING PROVIDING COPIES OF MEDICAL RELEASES UPON REQUEST; SHALL GIVE A COPY OF THIS ORDER TO ANY HEALTH CARE ENTITY WHERE HE HAS PRIVILEGES; TIME SPENT OUT OF TEXAS DOES NOT COUNT TOWARD PROBATION; SHALL INFORM THE BOARD OF CHANGE OF ADDRESS WITHIN 10 DAYS OR IF HE LEAVES THE STATE; SHALL NOT SEEK MODIFICATION FOR ONE YEAR.

LOSTETTER, ALVIN CHARLES MD, LICENSE NUMBER D6070 OF LAREDO, TX, WAS DISCIPLINED BY TEXAS ON OCTOBER 24, 1998
DISCIPLINARY ACTION: 84-MONTH PROBATION; REQUIRED TO TAKE ADDITIONAL MEDICAL EDUCATION
OFFENSE: INSURANCE, MEDICARE OR MEDICAID FRAUD

NOTES: ALLEGATIONS OF FRAUDULENT BILLING, SPECIFICALLY THAT PATIENTS' INSURANCE COMPANIES WERE BILLED FOR SERVICES THAT WERE NEVER PROVIDED; HE WAS EMPLOYED BY ULT-I-MED CLINIC WHERE CHIROPRACTIC CARE WAS PROVIDED FOR MEMBERS OF A FITNESS CLUB LOCATED IN THE SAME BUILDING; MEMBERS OF THE CLUB WERE TOLD THAT IF THEY WENT TO THE HEALTH CLINIC, THEIR FITNESS CLUB MEMBERSHIP WOULD COVER ANY COPAYMENTS OR DEDUCTIBLES THAT THEIR INSURANCE DID NOT COVER; SIX PATIENTS INFORMED THE BOARD THAT THEIR INSURANCE COMPANIES WERE BILLED FOR SERVICES THAT WERE NEVER PROVIDED; THE BILLS WERE SUBMITTED UNDER HIS NAME; IN SOME CASES, THE PATIENTS NEVER MET HIM; AN INSURANCE COMPANY RECEIVING CLAIMS SUBMITTED UNDER HIS NAME REPORTS THAT CLAIMS BEARING THE SAME PATIENT NAME, WITH THE SAME DATE OF SERVICE AND USING THE SAME CPT CODES WERE ALSO SUBMITTED UNDER ANOTHER PHYSICIAN'S NAME RESULTING IN THE INSURANCE COMPANY BEING BILLED TWICE FOR THE SAME SERVICE; REPRESENTS THAT BILLING WAS SUBMITTED WITH HIS NAME ON INT WITHOUT HIS KNOWLEDGE. SUSPENSION STAYED FOR PROBATION WITH FOLLOWING TERMS AND CONDITIONS: HIS MEDICAL PRACTICE SHALL BE MONITORED BY A BOARD-APPROVED TEXAS PHYSICIAN WHO SHALL PROVIDE QUARTERLY REPORTS TO THE BOARD IN PLACE OF THIS PROVISION MAY LIMIT HIS PRACTICE TO A BOARD-APPROVED INSTITUTIONAL OR GROUP PRACTICE; SHALL OBTAIN 10 HOURS PER YEAR OF AN ETHICS COURSE; WITHIN 1 YEAR SHALL TAKE AND PASS THE SPEX AND THE JURISPRUDENCE EXAM WITH A SCORE OF 75 OR ABOVE, WITHIN 3 ATTEMPTS; SHALL ATTEND 50 HOURS PER YEAR OF CONTINUING MEDICAL EDUCATION WITH 1 COURSE IN RISK MANAGEMENT; SHALL PERFORM 100 HOURS OF COMMUNITY SERVICE FOR A BOARD-APPROVED NON-PROFIT; SHALL MAINTAIN ADEQUATE MEDICAL RECORDS WHICH SHALL BE AVAILABLE FOR REVIEW; SHALL ADOPT OR ESTABLISH A SYSTEM OF PATIENT RECORD KEEPING AND BILLING TO ENSURE THAT ALL PATIENT RECORDS ACCURATELY REFLECT THE PATIENT'S NAME, SERVICE RENDERED, DATE OF SERVICE, AND AMOUNT CHARGED; SHALL CONTINUE TO RECEIVE CARE AND TREATMENT FROM SPECIFIED PHYSICIAN WITH QUARTERLY REPORTS TO THE BOARD; SHALL APPEAR BEFORE THE BOARD UPON REQUEST; SHALL COOPERATE WITH THE BOARD IN VERIFYING COMPLIANCE INCLUDING PROVIDING COPIES OF MEDICAL RELEASES UPON REQUEST; SHALL ADEQUATELY SUPERVISE ALL EMPLOYEES UNDER HIS SUPERVISION; SHALL GIVE A COPY OF THIS ORDER TO ANY HEALTH CARE ENTITY WHERE HE HAS PRIVILEGES; TIME SPENT OUT OF TEXAS DOES NOT COUNT TOWARD PROBATION; SHALL INFORM THE BOARD OF CHANGE OF ADDRESS WITHIN 10 DAYS OR IF HE LEAVES THE STATE; SHALL NOT SEEK MODIFICATION FOR ONE YEAR.

LOSTETTER, ALVIN CHARLES MD, LICENSE NUMBER D6070 OF LAREDO, TX, WAS DISCIPLINED BY TEXAS ON OCTOBER 15, 1999
DISCIPLINARY ACTION: SURRENDER OF LICENSE

NOTES: DUE TO HIS SERIOUS AND DECLINING HEALTH CONDITION, HE HAS BEEN UNABLE TO FULLY COMPLY WITH THE TERMS AND CONDITIONS OF THE 10/24/98 BOARD ORDER. VOLUNTARY SURRENDER.

LOVELACE, CHARLES RAY JR DO, DATE OF BIRTH NOVEMBER 1, 1954, LICENSE NUMBER 00G9871 OF 423 RIGGS CIRCLE, MESQUITE, TX, WAS DISCIPLINED BY TEXAS ON APRIL 30, 1993
DISCIPLINARY ACTION: 120-MONTH PROBATION; MONITORING OF PHYSICIAN PERFORMANCE
OFFENSE: SUBSTANCE ABUSE

NOTES: HAS A 10 YEAR HISTORY OF POLYSUBSTANCE ABUSE INCLUDING ALCOHOL, MARIJUANA, HYDROCODONE, XANAX, DIAZEPAM, ATIVAN AND FIORICET. UNDERWENT EIGHT WEEKS OF INPATIENT ADDICTION TREATMENT IN 1988; AFTER COMPLETING OUTPATIENT MONITORING HE RELAPSED AND IN ORDER TO OBTAIN CONTROLLED SUBSTANCES WROTE PRESCRIPTIONS IN THE NAMES OF OTHER PEOPLE AND HE DIVERTED THESE PRESCRIPTIONS FOR HIS OWN USE; AGREED TO ENTER INTO TREATMENT IN 6/92 AND COMPLETED IT IN 12/92; PRESENTLY UNDER A CONTINUING CARE CONTRACT AND HAS ADHERED TO ITS REQUIREMENTS. SUSPENSION STAYED. CONDITIONS OF PROBATION: SHALL COMPLY WITH THE TERMS OF HIS CONTINUING CARE CONTRACT WITH QUARTERLY REPORTS TO THE BOARD; SHALL ABSTAIN FROM THE CONSUMPTION OF ALCOHOL/DRUGS IN ANY FORM UNLESS PRESCRIBED BY ANOTHER PHYSICIAN FOR A LEGITIMATE AND THERAPEUTIC PURPOSE; SHALL SUBMIT HIMSELF FOR EVALUATION AND TREATMENT TO A BOARD-APPROVED PSYCHIATRIST TO WHOM HE WILL PROVIDE A COPY OF THIS ORDER; SHALL SUBMIT HIMSELF FOR APPROPRIATE EXAMS INCLUDING DRUG OR ALCOHOL SCREENS; SHALL CONTINUE TO PARTICIPATE IN AA NOT LESS THAN 3 TIMES A WEEK WITH QUARTERLY REPORTS TO THE BOARD; SHALL NOT TREAT OR OTHERWISE SERVE AS PHYSICIAN, PRESCRIBE, DISPENSE OR ADMINISTER DRUGS THAT MAY BE SUBJECT TO ABUSE TO HIMSELF OR ANY MEMBER OF HIS FAMILY; SHALL NOT POSSESS, PRESCRIBE, DISPENSE OR ADMINISTER CONTROLLED SUBSTANCES EXCEPT TO HOSPITALIZED PATIENTS AND THEN ONLY WHEN MEDICALLY INDICATED AND IN THERAPEUTIC DOSES; SHALL KEEP A SEPARATE FILE OF SUCH PRESCRIPTIONS SUBJECT TO INSPECTION; SHALL BE MONITORED BY A BOARD-APPROVED PHYSICIAN WITH QUARTERLY REPORTS TO THE BOARD; SHALL ATTEND AT LEAST 50 HOURS PER YEAR OF CONTINUING MEDICAL EDUCATION; SHALL APPEAR BEFORE THE BOARD TWICE A YEAR; SHALL GIVE A COPY OF THIS ORDER TO ANY HEALTH CARE ENTITY WHERE HE HAS PRIVILEGES; SHALL COOPERATE WITH THE BOARD IN VERIFYING COMPLIANCE; SHALL INFORM THE BOARD OF A CHANGE OF ADDRESS WITHIN 1O DAYS OR IF HE LEAVES THE STATE; TIME SPENT OUT OF TEXAS DOES NOT COUNT TOWARD PROBATION. SHALL NOT SEEK MODIFICATION OF THIS ORDER FOR ONE YEAR. ON 5/11/95 ORDER MODIFIED SO HIS REQUIREMENTS TO

COMPLY WITH TERMS AND CONDITIONS OF HIS CONTINUING CARE CONTRACT AND HAVE THEM PROVIDE QUARTERLY REPORTS ARE DELETED; SHALL PERSONALLY APPEAR BEFORE THE BOARD ANNUALLY; ALL OTHER CONDITIONS REMAIN IN FULL EFFECT. ON 5/15/96 HIS PETITION FOR TERMINATION WAS DENIED, HOWEVER, ORDER MODIFIED AS FOLLOWS: THE REQUIREMENT THAT HE NOT POSSESS, PRESCRIBE, DISPENSE OR ADMINISTER CONTROLLED SUBSTANCES EXCEPT TO HOSPITALIZED PATIENTS IS DELETED; SEPARATE FROM PATIENT RECORDS, HE SHALL MAINTAIN A FILE CONSISTING OF A COPY OF EVERY PRESCRIPTION WRITTEN BY HIM FOR CONTROLLED SUBSTANCES OR DANGEROUS DRUGS WITH ADDICTIVE POTENTIAL OR POTENTIAL FOR ABUSE WHICH SHALL BE AVAILABLE FOR INSPECTION; HE SHALL NOT TELEPHONE TO A PHARMACY ANY PRESCRIPTION OR REFILL OF SUCH DRUGS; ALL OTHER PROVISIONS OF THIS ORDER REMAIN IN EFFECT. ON 8/22/98 ORDER TERMINATED.

LOVELACE, CHARLES RAY DO OF 3737 NORTH TOWN EAST BLVD., MESQUITENIO, TX, WAS DISCIPLINED BY DEA ON APRIL 23, 1996
DISCIPLINARY ACTION: RESTRICTION PLACED ON CONTROLLED SUBSTANCE LICENSE
OFFENSE: SUBSTANCE ABUSE

NOTES: HISTORY OF SUBSTANCE ABUSE.

LUHAR, HARASHADA K MD, LICENSE NUMBER 00G9872 OF AUSTIN, TX, WAS DISCIPLINED BY TEXAS ON NOVEMBER 3, 1994
DISCIPLINARY ACTION: REPRIMAND
OFFENSE: LOSS OR RESTRICTION OF HOSPITAL PRIVILEGES

NOTES: ON 12/28/93 THE QUALITY ASSURANCE COMMITTEE AT ONE HOSPITAL RECOMMENDED THE FOLLOWING IN REGARDS TO ONE CASE; OFFICIAL WARNING OF FAILURE TO MEET STANDARD OF CARE, RECOMMENDATION OF ADDITIONAL CONTINUING MEDICAL EDUCATION IN NEONATAL INTENSIVE CARE, MANDATORY CONSULTATION ON THE NEXT 12 CASES PRESENTING WITH SIGNIFICANT RESPIRATORY IMPAIRMENT; THE BOARD FOUND THAT SHE MISHANDLED THIS PATIENT'S RESPIRATORY ACIDOSIS BY HER FAILURE TO PROMPTLY INTUBATE THE PATIENT AND BY TREATING THE PATIENT WITH BICARBONATE IN LIEU OF INTUBATION AND WITHOUT ADEQUATE INDICATION.

LUKER, JOHN ALONZO MD, LICENSE NUMBER 00E2689 OF BASTROP, TX, WAS DISCIPLINED BY TEXAS ON JUNE 12, 1990
DISCIPLINARY ACTION: 120-MONTH PROBATION; RESTRICTION PLACED ON CONTROLLED SUBSTANCE LICENSE

NOTES: STIPULATED ORDER. CONDITIONS OF PROBATION INCLUDE: APPEAR BEFORE BOARD SEMI-ANNUALLY, SUBMIT FOR APPROPRIATE EXAMINATIONS TO DETERMINE FREEDOM FROM DRUGS AND ALCOHOL, NOT TREAT OR OTHERWISE SERVE AS PHYSICIAN, PRESCRIBE, DISPENSE OR ADMINISTER CONTROLLED SUBSTANCES OR OTHER DRUGS SUBJECT TO ABUSE, OR WRITE PRESCRIPTIONS FOR CONTROLLED SUBSTANCES OR DRUGS SUBJECT TO ABUSE, FOR HIMSELF OR ANY MEMBER OF HIS IMMEDIATE FAMILY, AND ADMINISTER TO HIMSELF OR HIS IMMEDIATE FAMILY ONLY SUCH DRUGS AS PRESCRIBED BY OTHER PHYSICIANS; NOT POSSESS, ADMINISTER, DISPENSE OR PRESCRIBE ANY CONTROLLED SUBSTANCE BUT MAY ORDER SUCH CONTROLLED SUBSTANCE TO BE ADMINISTERED TO HOSPITAL OR NURSING HOME PATIENTS FOR MEDICAL NEEDS; SUBMIT FOR PSYCHIATRIC EVALUATION AND FOLLOW RECOMMENDATIONS, IF ANY, REGARDING CONTINUING CARE AND TREATMENT; PARTICIPATE IN AA/NARCOTICS ANONYMOUS; CONTINUE CONTINUING MEDICAL EDUCATION. ON 8/19/94 ORDER MODIFIED AS FOLLOWS: HE IS GRANTED PERMISSION TO REAPPLY TO THE DRUG ENFORCEMENT ADMINISTRATION AND THE TEXAS DEPARTMENT OF PUBLIC SAFETY FOR SCHEDULES III, IV AND V CONTROLLED SUBSTANCES AUTHORITY; SHALL NOT ATTEMPT TO REGISTER FOR SCHEDULES II, IIN OR IIIN WITHOUT FIRST OBTAINING WRITTEN AUTHORITY FROM THE BOARD; SHALL NOT TREAT OR OTHERWISE SERVE AS PHYSICIAN, PRESCRIBE, DISPENSE OR ADMINISTER CONTROLLED SUBSTANCES OR ANY OTHER DRUGS THAT MAY BE SUBJECT TO ABUSE TO HIMSELF OR A MEMBER OF HIS FAMILY; MAY ADMINISTER TO HIS FAMILY ONLY SUCH DRUGS AS PRESCRIBED BY OTHER PHYSICIANS, AND IN COMPLIANCE WITH THEIR ORDERS AND DIRECTIONS; SEPARATE FROM PATIENT RECORDS, HE SHALL MAINTAIN A FILE CONSISTING OF A COPY OF EVERY PRESCRIPTION WRITTEN FOR CONTROLLED SUBSTANCES OR DANGEROUS DRUGS WHICH HAVE A POTENTIAL FOR ABUSE, BY DATE ISSUED WHICH SHALL BE AVAILABLE FOR INSPECTION BY THE BOARD; SHALL NOT TELEPHONE ANY PRESCRIPTION TO A PHARMACY FOR CONTROLLED SUBSTANCES OR DANGEROUS DRUGS; SHALL SURRENDER ALL CONTROLLED SUBSTANCES AND DANGEROUS DRUGS, INCLUDING SAMPLES, TO REPRESENTATIVES OF THE BOARD OR A REPRESENTATIVE OF THE TEXAS DEPARTMENT OF PUBLIC SAFETY NARCOTIC SERVICE. IN THE FUTURE, HE MAY NOT POSSESS ANY CONTROLLED SUBSTANCES OR DANGEROUS DRUGS EXCEPT AS OTHERWISE PROVIDED FOR IN THE BOARD ORDER AS MODIFIED. ON 10/5/96 THE BOARD DENIED HIS PETITION FOR TERMINATION. ON 8/22/98 ORDER TERMINATED.

LUNCEFORD, TENNIE MAE MD, LICENSE NUMBER C1428, WAS DISCIPLINED BY TEXAS ON JANUARY 18, 1997

NOTES: ALLEGATIONS OF VIOLATIONS OF THE MEDICAL PRACTICE ACT; NO DETERMINATIONS OF THESE ALLEGATIONS HAVE BEEN MADE. SHE RETIRED FROM PRACTICE DUE TO HEALTH REASONS. DUE TO PHYSICAL DISABILITY AND RETIREMENT, SHE SHALL NOT PRACTICE MEDICINE IN TEXAS WITHOUT BOARD PERMISSION IN WRITING UPON A PERSONAL APPEARANCE AND PRESENTATION OF EVIDENCE, INCLUDING BUT NOT LIMITED TO PASSING THE SPEX, THAT INDICATES THAT SHE IS PHYSICALLY, MENTALLY, AND OTHERWISE COMPETENT.

LUTHERER, BERTA DEL CARMEN MD, LICENSE NUMBER 00E1030 OF LUBBOCK, TX, WAS DISCIPLINED BY TEXAS ON APRIL 10, 1992
DISCIPLINARY ACTION: REPRIMAND

NOTES: PROFESSIONAL FAILURE TO PRACTICE MEDICINE IN AN ACCEPTABLE MANNER CONSISTENT WITH PUBLIC HEALTH AND WELFARE.

LUU, KHAM NGOC MD, DATE OF BIRTH AUGUST 2, 1957 OF 14315 ARBOR CREST STREET, HOUSTON, TX, WAS DISCIPLINED BY MEDICARE ON MAY 9, 1995
DISCIPLINARY ACTION: EXCLUSION FROM THE MEDICARE AND/OR MEDICAID PROGRAM
OFFENSE: NONCOMPLIANCE WITH A PROFESSIONAL RULE

NOTES: DEFAULTED ON PUBLIC HEALTH SERVICE EDUCATION LOAN. REINSTATED ON 7/30/96.

LYNN, ROBERT J MD, LICENSE NUMBER 0015188, WAS DISCIPLINED BY MINNESOTA ON NOVEMBER 17, 1990

DISCIPLINARY ACTION: LICENSE REVOCATION

LYNN, ROBERT J MD, DATE OF BIRTH JUNE 26, 1923, LICENSE NUMBER 0014121 OF 512 E BLUEBRIAR, GRANITE SHOALS, TX, WAS DISCIPLINED BY IOWA ON NOVEMBER 19, 1992
DISCIPLINARY ACTION: LICENSE REVOCATION
OFFENSE: PROFESSIONAL MISCONDUCT

NOTES: FRAUDULENT APPLICATION.

LYNN, WILLIAM SANFORD JR MD OF UNIV TEXAS MEDICAL BRANCH, GALVESTON, TX, WAS DISCIPLINED BY DEA ON AUGUST 27, 1990
DISCIPLINARY ACTION: SURRENDER OF CONTROLLED SUBSTANCE LICENSE
OFFENSE: OVERPRESCRIBING OR MISPRESCRIBING DRUGS

NOTES: WROTE EXCESSIVE PRESCRIPTIONS FOR TUSSIONEX SUSPENSION AND PERCODAN FROM 01/31/87 TO 07/13/90.

MABATID, HEIDI F MD, LICENSE NUMBER 0144665 OF 12984 LAKE WILDWOOD DRIVE, PENN VALLEY, CA, WAS DISCIPLINED BY NEW YORK ON DECEMBER 6, 1996
DISCIPLINARY ACTION: LICENSE REVOCATION
OFFENSE: CRIMINAL CONVICTION OR PLEA OF GUILTY, NOLO CONTENDERE, OR NO CONTEST TO A CRIME

NOTES: CONVICTED AFTER A GENERAL COURT MARTIAL HELD BY THE U.S. AIR FORCE OF NEGLIGENT DERELICTION OF DUTY; SIGNING A FALSE DOCUMENT ALLOWING HER DIVORCED HUSBAND TO CONTINUE TO USE HIS MILITARY DEPENDENT'S CARD TO RECEIVE MEDICAL TREATMENT; AND LARCENY.

MABATID, HEIDI F MD, DATE OF BIRTH DECEMBER 26, 1948, LICENSE NUMBER 038333L OF 12984 LAKE WILDWOOD DRIVE, PENN VALLEY, CA, WAS DISCIPLINED BY PENNSYLVANIA ON APRIL 6, 1998
DISCIPLINARY ACTION: LICENSE SUSPENSION
OFFENSE: DISCIPLINARY ACTION BY ANOTHER STATE OR AGENCY

NOTES: DISCIPLINARY ACTION TAKEN IN NEW YORK (FOR CONVICTION OF A GENERAL COURT MARTIAL- US AIR FORCE). LICENSE INDEFINITELY SUSPENDED UNTIL SUCH TIME AS HER NEW YORK LICENSE IS REINSTATED WITHOUT RESTRICTION.

MABATID, HEIDI FLORES MD, LICENSE NUMBER A38090 OF PENN VALLEY, CA, WAS DISCIPLINED BY CALIFORNIA ON NOVEMBER 6, 1997
DISCIPLINARY ACTION: LICENSE REVOCATION
OFFENSE: DISCIPLINARY ACTION BY ANOTHER STATE OR AGENCY

NOTES: DISCIPLINED BY NEW YORK FOR CONVICTION OF VIOLATIONS OF THE UNIFORM CODE OF MILITARY JUSTICE AND UNPROFESSIONAL CONDUCT. WHILE IN THE AIR FORCE SHE WILLFULLY AND WITH INTENT TO DECEIVE, FALSELY SIGNED A BASIC ALLOWANCE FOR QUARTERS AND COST OF LIVING ALLOWANCE RECERTIFICATION LISTING HER MOTHER AS A DEPENDENT WHEN IN FACT HER MOTHER WAS DECEASED.

MABATID, HEIDI FLORES MD, DATE OF BIRTH DECEMBER 26, 1948 OF 8115 CHESTNUT BARR, CONVERSE, TX, WAS DISCIPLINED BY MEDICARE ON AUGUST 20, 1998
DISCIPLINARY ACTION: EXCLUSION FROM THE MEDICARE AND/OR MEDICAID PROGRAM
OFFENSE: DISCIPLINARY ACTION BY ANOTHER STATE OR AGENCY

NOTES: LICENSE REVOKED, SUSPENDED, SURRENDERED OR OTHERWISE LOST FOR REASONS BEARING ON PROFESSIONAL PERFORMANCE, PROFESSIONAL COMPETENCE OR FINANCIAL INTEGRITY.

MABRAY, CHARLES R MD, LICENSE NUMBER 00D3325, WAS DISCIPLINED BY TEXAS ON AUGUST 17, 1996
DISCIPLINARY ACTION: REPRIMAND
OFFENSE: SUBSTANDARD CARE, INCOMPETENCE OR NEGLIGENCE

NOTES: FROM 1992 THROUGH 1995 PROVIDED THYROID MEDICATIONS TO VARIOUS FEMALE PATIENTS WITHOUT ADEQUATE BASELINE TESTING, AND WITHOUT ADEQUATE FOLLOW-UP TESTING AND ASSESSMENT; REPORTS IMPLEMENTING PRACTICE CHANGES TO ADDRESS THESE MATTERS.

MACELUCH, JOHN J DO, LICENSE NUMBER 00E5151 OF PANAMA CITY, FL, WAS DISCIPLINED BY TEXAS ON AUGUST 18, 1990

NOTES: STIPULATED ORDER. AGREED SETTLEMENT WHEREBY HE MUST OBTAIN APPROVAL OF THE BOARD BEFORE RETURNING TO PRACTICING IN TEXAS.

MACELUCH, JOHN J DO, DATE OF BIRTH AUGUST 26, 1941, LICENSE NUMBER 0001460 OF 600 N COVE BLVD, PANAMA CITY, FL, WAS DISCIPLINED BY IOWA ON JUNE 29, 1992

NOTES: BEFORE RETURNING TO IOWA TO PRACTICE MEDICINE HE MUST REQUEST A PERSONAL INTERVIEW WITH THE BOARD AND OBTAIN WRITTEN PERMISSION TO PRACTICE IN IOWA.

MACHEN, ROBERT N MD, LICENSE NUMBER 00C5781 OF DALLAS, TX, WAS DISCIPLINED BY TEXAS ON MARCH 31, 1990
DISCIPLINARY ACTION: RESTRICTION PLACED ON CONTROLLED SUBSTANCE LICENSE

NOTES: STIPULATED ORDER. MUST REFRAIN FROM DISPENSING, PRESCRIBING, OR ADMINISTERING CERTAIN MEDICATIONS TO PATIENTS SEEKING TREATMENT FOR WEIGHT CONTROL.

MADAN, VEENA MD, DATE OF BIRTH NOVEMBER 11, 1944, LICENSE NUMBER 0022595 OF DENVER, CO, WAS DISCIPLINED BY COLORADO ON FEBRUARY 21, 1993
DISCIPLINARY ACTION: 60-MONTH PROBATION; MONITORING OF PHYSICIAN PERFORMANCE
OFFENSE: SUBSTANDARD CARE, INCOMPETENCE OR NEGLIGENCE

NOTES: SUBSTANDARD CARE. PROBATION INCLUDES RESIDENCY TRAINING AND PRACTICE MONITORING.

MADAN, VEENA MD, DATE OF BIRTH NOVEMBER 11, 1944, LICENSE NUMBER 00F1768 OF PLANO, TX, WAS DISCIPLINED BY TEXAS ON AUGUST 19, 1994
DISCIPLINARY ACTION: RESTRICTION PLACED ON LICENSE; REQUIRED TO TAKE ADDITIONAL MEDICAL EDUCATION
OFFENSE: DISCIPLINARY ACTION BY ANOTHER STATE OR AGENCY

NOTES: ON 2/12/93 ENTERED INTO A STIPULATION AND ORDER WITH THE COLORADO BOARD RESTRICTED COLORADO LICENSE. CONDITIONS ON TEXAS LICENSE: SHALL NOT INDEPENDENTLY TREAT ANY PATIENT UNTIL SHE COMPLETES A BOARD-APPROVED THREE MONTH REFRESHER MINI-RESIDENCY IN ANESTHESIOLOGY AND PERSONALLY APPEARS BEFORE THE BOARD AND PROVIDES SUFFICIENT INFORMATION WHICH SHOWS THAT SHE IS ABLE TO SAFELY PRACTICE. ON 5/13/95 BOARD GRANTED HER PETITION REQUESTING TERMINATION OF ORDER SINCE SHE HAD SATISFIED ALL CONDITIONS.

MAES, MYRON L MD, LICENSE NUMBER J3348 OF BALTIMORE, MD, WAS DISCIPLINED BY TEXAS ON SEPTEMBER 20, 1997
DISCIPLINARY ACTION: FINE; REPRIMAND
OFFENSE: NONCOMPLIANCE WITH A PROFESSIONAL RULE

NOTES: FAILED TO SUBMIT 12 HOURS OF REQUIRED CONTINUING MEDICAL EDUCATION FOR HIS ANNUAL REGISTRATION FOR 1996; WAS GIVEN A 90 DAY EXTENSION BUT STILL FAILED TO OBTAIN OR PROVIDE PROOF OF CONTINUING MEDICAL EDUCATION; HIS LICENSE HAS BEEN IN "DELINQUENT" STATUS SINCE 8/30/96. HE WILL BE REQUIRED TO OBTAIN ALL PAST DUE CONTINUING MEDICAL EDUCATION HOURS FOR 6/1/95 THROUGH 5/31/96 BEFORE HE WILL BE ISSUED A CURRENT PHYSICIAN'S PERMIT. $100 FINE; SHALL COOPERATE WITH THE BOARD IN VERIFYING COMPLIANCE.

MAES, MYRON LEE MD, LICENSE NUMBER 0D46542 OF 2201 ROGENE DRIVE #T2, BALTIMORE, MD, WAS DISCIPLINED BY MARYLAND ON JULY 15, 1996
DISCIPLINARY ACTION: FINE
OFFENSE: PRACTICING WITHOUT A VALID LICENSE

NOTES: PRACTICED FOR APPROXIMATELY THREE MONTHS WITH A LAPSED LICENSE. $1,000 FINE.

MAGEE, DOUGLAS L MD OF 8484 WILL CLAYTON PARKWAY, HUMBLE, TX, WAS DISCIPLINED BY DEA ON OCTOBER 5, 1994
DISCIPLINARY ACTION: SURRENDER OF CONTROLLED SUBSTANCE LICENSE

NOTES: IMPAIRED PHYSICIAN. IN LIEU OF PUBLIC INTEREST REVOCATION.

MAGEE, DOUGLAS LEE MD, LICENSE NUMBER 00H4511 OF HUMBLE, TX, WAS DISCIPLINED BY TEXAS ON MARCH 4, 1995
DISCIPLINARY ACTION: LICENSE SUSPENSION
OFFENSE: SUBSTANCE ABUSE

NOTES: SUBSTANCE ABUSE BEGINNING IN 1991; IN 8/93, SOUGHT PSYCHIATRIC HELP AND WAS ADMITTED FOR INPATIENT TREATMENT FOR ONE MONTH; RELAPSED SIX WEEKS AFTER DISCHARGE; IN 6/94, RECEIVED FOUR WEEKS OF INPATIENT TREATMENT AND RELAPSED SIX DAYS AFTER DISCHARGE; IN 1994, OBTAINED HYDROCODONE AND SOMA BY MEANS OF FALSE AND FICTITIOUS PRESCRIPTIONS WRITTEN IN THE NAME OF A RELATIVE FOR HIS OWN USE; IN 1/95, CONSUMED VICODIN AND XANAX WITHOUT A LEGITIMATE MEDICAL PURPOSE; REPORTS ATTENDING AA MEETINGS AN AVERAGE OF THREE TIMES PER WEEK, RECEIVING CONTINUING CARE FROM A PSYCHIATRIST ON A WEEKLY BASIS AND MEETING WITH A MEDICAL SOCIETY MONITOR AN AVERAGE OF TWICE A MONTH IN REGARD TO HIS RECOVERY. SUSPENSION UNTIL HE REQUESTS TO HAVE SUSPENSION STAYED OR LIFTED AND APPEARS BEFORE THE BOARD WITH SUFFICIENT EVIDENCE WHICH INDICATES THAT HE IS PHYSICALLY, MENTALLY AND OTHERWISE COMPETENT TO SAFELY PRACTICE, INCLUDING AT A MINIMUM A 96-HOUR COMPLETE MEDICAL ASSESSMENT WITH PSYCHOLOGICAL AND NEUROPSYCHIATRIC EVALUATIONS WITH REPORTS TO THE BOARD. ON 8/9/97 ORDER MODIFIED AS FOLLOWS: FOLLOW-UP CARE AND COUNSELING AT LEAST ONCE EACH YEAR QUARTERLY; PARTICIPATION IN AA NO LESS THAN THREE TIME PER WEEK; ALLOWED TO APPLY FOR DEA AND DEPARTMENT OF PUBLIC SAFETY REGISTRATION CERTIFICATES FOR CONTROLLED SUBSTANCES IN SCHEDULES III, IV AND V, AND MAINTAIN A LOGBOOK, SEPARATE FROM PATIENT RECORDS, OF ALL PRESCRIPTIONS ISSUED FOR CONTROLLED SUBSTANCES OR DANGEROUS DRUGS WITH ADDICTIVE POTENTIAL OR POTENTIAL FOR ABUSE.

MAGEE, DOUGLAS LEE MD, LICENSE NUMBER 00H4511, WAS DISCIPLINED BY TEXAS ON JUNE 28, 1995
DISCIPLINARY ACTION: 60-MONTH PROBATION; REQUIRED TO TAKE ADDITIONAL MEDICAL EDUCATION

NOTES: SUSPENSION OF 3/04/95 LIFTED. PROBATION UNDER TERMS AND CONDITIONS: SHALL ABSTAIN FROM THE CONSUMPTION OF ALCOHOL/DRUGS IN ANY FORM UNLESS PRESCRIBED BY ANOTHER PHYSICIAN FOR A LEGITIMATE AND THERAPEUTIC PURPOSE; SHALL SUBMIT HIMSELF FOR APPROPRIATE EXAMS INCLUDING ALCOHOL AND DRUG SCREENS; SHALL SUBMIT HIMSELF FOR EVALUATION AND TREATMENT TO A BOARD-APPROVED PSYCHIATRIST WHO HE SHALL SEE AT LEAST ONCE A MONTH AND WHO SHALL SUBMIT REPORTS TO THE BOARD; SHALL PARTICIPATE IN AA'S PROGRAM NOT LESS THAN FIVE TIMES PER WEEK WITH QUARTERLY REPORTS TO THE BOARD; SHALL REQUEST A MEETING WITH THE HARRIS COUNTY MEDICAL SOCIETY PHYSICIANS COUNSELING COMMITTEE AND SHALL PARTICIPATE IN THEIR ACTIVITIES AND ATTEND WEEKLY MEETINGS WITH QUARTERLY REPORTS; SHALL COMPLY WITH THE TERMS OF HIS CONTINUED CARE CONTRACT WITH THE DESIGNATED PSYCHIATRIST WHO SHALL SUBMIT QUARTERLY REPORTS TO THE BOARD; SHALL COMPLY WITH THE TERMS AND CONDITIONS OF ANY AGREEMENT FOR HOSPITAL PRIVILEGES AND SHALL REPORT TO THE BOARD ANY DISCIPLINE IN REGARD TO ANY HOSPITAL PRIVILEGES; SHALL NOT POSSESS ALCOHOL, CONTROLLED SUBSTANCES, OR DANGEROUS DRUGS WITH ADDICTIVE POTENTIAL OR POTENTIAL FOR ABUSE; SHALL SURRENDER ALL SUCH DRUGS INCLUDING SAMPLES; SHALL NOT TREAT OR OTHERWISE SERVE AS PHYSICIAN, PRESCRIBE, DISPENSE OR ADMINISTER DRUGS THAT MAY BE SUBJECT TO ABUSE TO HIMSELF OR TO ANY MEMBER OF HIS FAMILY; SHALL NOT TELEPHONE HIMSELF OR PERMIT ANY INDIVIDUAL UNDER HIS SUPERVISION TO TELEPHONE TO A PHARMACY A PRESCRIPTION OR REFILL FOR CONTROLLED SUBSTANCES OR DANGEROUS DRUGS WITH ADDICTIVE POTENTIAL OR POTENTIAL FOR ABUSE; SHALL SURRENDER HIS DEA CONTROLLED SUBSTANCE REGISTRATION CERTIFICATE AND TEXAS DEPARTMENT OF PUBLIC SAFETY CONTROLLED SUBSTANCE REGISTRATION CERTIFICATE; SHALL SURRENDER TO THE BOARD ANY UNUSED TRIPLICATE PRESCRIPTION FORMS AND SHALL NOT ATTEMPT TO ORDER MORE; HIS MEDICAL PRACTICE, INCLUDING ANY OFFICE OR SURGICAL PRACTICE SHALL BE MONITORED BY A BOARD APPROVED TEXAS PHYSICIAN WHO SHALL SUBMIT REPORTS TO THE BOARD; SHALL MAINTAIN ADEQUATE MEDICAL RECORDS WHICH SHALL BE AVAILABLE FOR REVIEW; SHALL OBTAIN AT LEAST 50 HOURS OF CONTINUING MEDICAL EDUCATION AND SUBMIT PROOF OF ATTENDANCE TO THE BOARD; SHALL PERSONALLY APPEAR BEFORE THE BOARD AT LEAST TWO TIMES PER YEAR OR UPON REQUEST; SHALL COOPERATE WITH THE BOARD IN VERIFYING COMPLIANCE INCLUDING PROVIDING COPIES OF MEDICAL RELEASES AND PEER REVIEW RECORDS UPON REQUEST; SHALL GIVE A COPY OF THIS ORDER TO ANY HEALTH CARE ENTITY WHERE HE HAS PRIVILEGES; SHALL PROVIDE A COPY OF THIS ORDER TO ANYONE REQUESTING IT WITHIN 10 DAYS; TIME PERIOD OUT OF TEXAS DOES NOT COUNT TOWARD PROBATION; SHALL INFORM THE BOARD OF CHANGE OF ADDRESS WITHIN 10 DAYS OF IF HE LEAVES THE STATE; SHALL NOT SEEK MODIFICATION FOR ONE

YEAR. ON 8/9/97 PETITION TO MODIFY ORDER GRANTED REDUCING PSYCHIATRIC FOLLOW-UP CARE AND COUNSELING FROM MONTHLY TO QUARTERLY; REDUCING AA PARTICIPATION FROM FIVE TIMES A WEEK TO THREE; SHALL BE ALLOWED TO APPLY FOR DEA AND DEPARTMENT OF PUBLIC SAFETY REGISTRATION CERTIFICATES FOR CONTROLLED SUBSTANCES IN SCHEDULES III, IV, AND V, AND MAINTAIN A LOGBOOK OF ALL PRESCRIPTIONS ISSUED FOR CONTROLLED SUBSTANCES OR DANGEROUS DRUGS WITH ADDICTIVE POTENTIAL OR POTENTIAL FOR ABUSE. ON 2/7/98 ORDER MODIFIED DELETING THE REQUIREMENT OF PARTICIPATION IN THE HARRIS COUNTY MEDICAL SOCIETY PHYSICIANS COUNSELING COMMITTEE. ON 8/22/98 ORDER MODIFIED TO REQUIRE NO LESS THAN ONE APPEARANCE PER YEAR BEFORE THE BOARD AND DELETING SEVERAL REQUIREMENTS ALTHOUGH A TERMINATION REQUEST WAS DENIED. ON 10/15/99 ORDER TERMINATED.

MAHAFFEY, GENE F DO OF 2465 S DOWNING #103, DENVER, CO, WAS DISCIPLINED BY DEA ON MARCH 12, 1990
DISCIPLINARY ACTION: SURRENDER OF CONTROLLED SUBSTANCE LICENSE
OFFENSE: DISCIPLINARY ACTION BY ANOTHER STATE OR AGENCY

NOTES: REVOCATION OF STATE LICENSE DUE TO CONTINUING TO PRESCRIBE AMPHETAMINES AND DIURETICS WITHOUT MEDICAL INDICATION AND PRACTICING MEDICINE WHILE STATE LICENSE SUSPENDED.

MAHAFFEY, GENE F DO, DATE OF BIRTH OCTOBER 13, 1927 OF 3537 SOUTH HILLCREST DR, DENVER, CO, WAS DISCIPLINED BY MEDICARE ON JULY 26, 1990
DISCIPLINARY ACTION: EXCLUSION FROM THE MEDICARE AND/OR MEDICAID PROGRAM
OFFENSE: DISCIPLINARY ACTION BY ANOTHER STATE OR AGENCY

NOTES: LICENSE REVOCATION OR SUSPENSION.

MAHAFFEY, GENE F DO OF DENVER, CO, WAS DISCIPLINED BY MISSOURI ON JANUARY 25, 1991
DISCIPLINARY ACTION: LICENSE REVOCATION
OFFENSE: DISCIPLINARY ACTION BY ANOTHER STATE OR AGENCY

NOTES: REVOCATION OF COLORADO LICENSE BASED ON VIOLATION OF COLORADO BOARD STIPULATION/ORDER BY PRESCRIBING DRUGS RESTRICTED BY THE BOARD'S ORDER AND FAILING TO MEET WITH PATIENTS; FAILING TO KEEP CHARTS AND ADEQUATELY SUPERVISE STAFF IN THE TREATMENT OF ONE PATIENT; PRACTICING MEDICINE WHILE UNDER ORDER OF SUMMARY SUSPENSION.

MAHAFFEY, GENE FRANCIS DO, LICENSE NUMBER 00C3141 OF DENVER, CO, WAS DISCIPLINED BY TEXAS ON JULY 1, 1990
DISCIPLINARY ACTION: SURRENDER OF LICENSE

NOTES: LICENSE CANCELED WITH PROVISIONS; EARLIER BOARD ORDER (LICENSE REVOCATION, STAY OF REVOCATION, THREE YEAR PROBATION) TO BE REINSTATED SHOULD PHYSICIAN APPLY FOR LICENSE REINSTATEMENT. IF HE APPLIES FOR REINSTATEMENT FIVE YEARS FROM 1/27/90, HE MUST ALSO PASS A SPECIAL PURPOSE EXAMINATION.

MAJORS, IRVING R MD, DATE OF BIRTH SEPTEMBER 8, 1926 OF PO BOX 671, TROUP, TX, WAS DISCIPLINED BY MEDICARE ON MARCH 16, 1995
DISCIPLINARY ACTION: EXCLUSION FROM THE MEDICARE AND/OR MEDICAID PROGRAM
OFFENSE: DISCIPLINARY ACTION BY ANOTHER STATE OR AGENCY

NOTES: LICENSE REVOKED FOR REASONS BEARING ON PROFESSIONAL PERFORMANCE.

MAJORS, IRVING RICHARD MD, DATE OF BIRTH SEPTEMBER 8, 1926 OF TROUP, TX, WAS DISCIPLINED BY LOUISIANA ON MARCH 26, 1993
DISCIPLINARY ACTION: REVOCATION OF CONTROLLED SUBSTANCE LICENSE; 36-MONTH LICENSE SUSPENSION
OFFENSE: SUBSTANDARD CARE, INCOMPETENCE OR NEGLIGENCE

NOTES: PROFESSIONAL OR MEDICAL INCOMPETENCE; PRESCRIBING, DISPENSING, OR ADMINISTERING CONTROLLED SUBSTANCES IN OTHER THAN A LEGAL OR LEGITIMATE MANNER. MUST PASS SPEX EXAMINATION AND APPEAR BEFORE THE BOARD AS A CONDITION OF REINSTATEMENT. PROHIBITED FOR LIFE FROM PRESCRIBING CONTROLLED SUBSTANCES, AND ORDERED TO PAY FINE OF $5,000 AND COSTS OF ADMINISTRATIVE PROCEEDING.

MAJORS, IRVING RICHARD MD, DATE OF BIRTH SEPTEMBER 8, 1926, LICENSE NUMBER 00C2718 OF P.O. BOX 671, TROUP, TX, WAS DISCIPLINED BY TEXAS ON JULY 9, 1993
DISCIPLINARY ACTION: EMERGENCY SUSPENSION
OFFENSE: DISCIPLINARY ACTION BY ANOTHER STATE OR AGENCY

NOTES: AVAILABLE EVIDENCE AND INFORMATION INDICATES THAT HE ENGAGED IN ILLEGAL POSSESSION OF A CONTROLLED DANGEROUS DRUG, CONSPIRACY TO ILLEGALLY DISTRIBUTE A CONTROLLED DANGEROUS DRUG AND DISTRIBUTION OF A CONTROLLED DANGEROUS DRUG; ARKANSAS LICENSE WAS SUSPENDED ON 3/26/92 PENDING FINAL DISCIPLINARY ACTION AND LOUISIANA LICENSE WAS SUSPENDED FOR THREE YEARS ON 4/28/93 AS A RESULT OF THESE CHARGES; HOSPITAL PRIVILEGES REVOKED ON 1/6/92 DUE TO OFFENSIVE NATURE WITH STAFF AND PATIENTS; FAILING TO CONDUCT ADEQUATE EXAMS AND TESTS LEADING TO INAPPROPRIATE TREATMENT; LACK OF JUDGMENT IN PERFORMING CPR; REFUSING TO SEE PATIENTS IN EMERGENCY ROOM; LEAVING EMERGENCY ROOM PRIOR TO THE END OF HIS PERIOD OF COVERAGE.

MAJORS, IRVING RICHARD MD, DATE OF BIRTH SEPTEMBER 8, 1926, LICENSE NUMBER 00C2718 OF TROUP, TX, WAS DISCIPLINED BY TEXAS ON JANUARY 14, 1994
DISCIPLINARY ACTION: LICENSE REVOCATION
OFFENSE: DISCIPLINARY ACTION BY ANOTHER STATE OR AGENCY

NOTES: ILLEGALLY PRESCRIBED NARCOTICS TO AN UNDERCOVER AGENT IN LOUISIANA; LOUISIANA AND ARKANSAS LICENSES SUSPENDED BASED ON THESE CHARGES AND HOSPITAL PRIVILEGES WERE REVOKED IN TEXAS DUE TO THE DEATH OF A PATIENT UNDER HIS CARE. CONTINUED PRACTICE IS AN IMMINENT PERIL TO THE PUBLIC HEALTH, SAFETY, AND WELFARE REQUIRING IMMEDIATE EFFECT TO AN ORDER REVOKING HIS LICENSE.

MAJORS, IRVING RICHARD MD OF TROUP, TX, WAS DISCIPLINED BY LOUISIANA ON JULY 21, 1994
DISCIPLINARY ACTION: LICENSE REVOCATION
OFFENSE: DISCIPLINARY ACTION BY ANOTHER STATE OR AGENCY

NOTES: PROVIDING FALSE SWORN INFORMATION TO THE BOARD; DISCIPLINARY ACTION BY ARKANSAS; VIOLATION OF PREVIOUS BOARD ORDER.

MALABANAN, BEN C MD, LICENSE NUMBER 00E0258 OF DALLAS, TX, WAS DISCIPLINED BY TEXAS ON JANUARY 6, 1995

DISCIPLINARY ACTION: 60-MONTH PROBATION; FINE
OFFENSE: SUBSTANDARD CARE, INCOMPETENCE OR NEGLIGENCE

NOTES: FROM 1988 TO 1989 WORKED ON A SALARY BASIS FOR A CLINIC OWNED BY A NON-PHYSICIAN AND PROVIDED MEDICAL CARE TO PATIENTS ESTABLISHED UNDER THEIR GUIDELINES; A REVIEW OF PATIENT RECORDS FOUND INADEQUACIES INCLUDING, LACK OF DOCUMENTATION TO INDICATE A PHYSICAL WAS PERFORMED OR A HISTORY OBTAINED, OBTAINED NUMEROUS LAB STUDIES WITHOUT THE PATIENT BEING FIRST SEEN BY A PHYSICIAN, COMMITTING TO VAGUE, UNSUPPORTED OR BORDERLINE DIAGNOSIS, OMITTING THE DIAGNOSIS OF OBESITY WHEN CLEARLY IT SHOULD HAVE BEEN INCLUDED; PLACED AN INSULIN DEPENDENT DIABETIC ON A STRINGENT WEIGHT LOSS DIET WHILE STOPPING HER INSULIN WITHOUT CLOSE MONITORING, AND ALLOWED OTHERS TO LIST ERRONEOUS DIAGNOSES WITH INTENT TO DEFRAUD INSURANCE CARRIERS; NEITHER ADMITS NOR DENIES ALLEGATIONS. CONDITIONS OF PROBATION: SHALL PASS THE SPEX EXAM WITHIN ONE YEAR AND THE TEXAS MEDICAL JURISPRUDENCE EXAM; PRACTICE SHALL BE MONITORED BY A BOARD-APPROVED PHYSICIAN WITH QUARTERLY REPORTS; SHALL MAINTAIN ADEQUATE MEDICAL RECORDS ON ALL PATIENT OFFICE VISITS WHICH SHALL BE AVAILABLE FOR INSPECTION; SHALL NOT SIGN ANY PATIENT RECORD UNLESS HE HAS PERSONALLY EXAMINED THE PATIENT OR CLEARLY NOTES IN THE RECORD THAT HE DID NOT; SHALL PERSONALLY EXAMINE AND/OR TREAT PATIENTS IN ANY INSTANCE IN WHICH AN INITIAL DIAGNOSIS OR EXAM IS PERFORMED; SHALL OBTAIN AT LEAST 50 HOURS PER YEAR OF CONTINUING MEDICAL EDUCATION AND 10 HOURS PER YEAR OF AN ETHICS COURSE OR PROGRAM; SHALL PERFORM 100 HOURS PER YEAR OF COMMUNITY SERVICE; SHALL PAY A $2,500 ADMINISTRATIVE PENALTY WITHIN FOUR MONTHS; SHALL APPEAR BEFORE THE BOARD ONCE A YEAR OR UPON REQUEST; SHALL COOPERATE WITH THE BOARD IN VERIFYING COMPLIANCE; SHALL ADEQUATELY SUPERVISE THOSE UNDER HIS SUPERVISION; SHALL GIVE A COPY OF THIS ORDER TO ANY HEALTH CARE ENTITY WHERE HE HAS OR APPLIES FOR PRIVILEGES AND ANYONE ELSE WHO ASKS FOR IT; SHALL ENSURE ANY INQUIRIES REGARDING HIS TEXAS LICENSURE STATUS ARE ANSWERED BY REFERENCING THIS ORDER; SHALL INFORM BOARD OF CHANGE OF ADDRESS WITHIN 10 DAYS OR IF HE LEAVES THE STATE; TIME SPENT OUT OF TEXAS DOES NOT COUNT TOWARD PROBATION. SHALL NOT SEEK MODIFICATION FOR ONE YEAR.

MALABANAN, BEN CARPIO MD, LICENSE NUMBER E0258, WAS DISCIPLINED BY TEXAS ON MARCH 1, 1997
DISCIPLINARY ACTION: SURRENDER OF LICENSE

NOTES: VIOLATED TERMS OF 1/6/95 ORDER BY FAILING TO TAKE AND PASS THE SPEX BY 1/6/96. ON 3/25/96 HIS LICENSE WAS SUSPENDED FOR THIS NONCOMPLIANCE. BY VIRTUE OF A PLEA AGREEMENT ENTERED INTO WITH THE US DISTRICT COURT, HE AGREED TO SURRENDER HIS LICENSE AND NEVER TO PRACTICE MEDICINE IN THE U.S. AGAIN. THE BOARD HAS RECEIVED ALLEGATIONS INVOLVING ACTIONS WHICH IF PROVEN WOULD CONSTITUTE VIOLATIONS OF THE MEDICAL PRACTICE ACT. VOLUNTARY AND PERMANENT SURRENDER OF HIS LICENSE AND HIS RETIREMENT FROM MEDICINE IN TEXAS IN LIEU OF FURTHER INVESTIGATION OR HEARINGS.

MALABANAN, BEN CARPIO MD, DATE OF BIRTH MAY 20, 1935 OF PO BOX 9300 #27966-077, TEXARKANA, TX, WAS DISCIPLINED BY MEDICARE ON JULY 6, 1997
DISCIPLINARY ACTION: 72-MONTH EXCLUSION FROM THE MEDICARE AND/OR MEDICAID PROGRAM
OFFENSE: CRIMINAL CONVICTION OR PLEA OF GUILTY, NOLO CONTENDERE, OR NO CONTEST TO A CRIME

NOTES: CONVICTED OF A CRIME RELATED TO THE DELIVERY OF HEALTH CARE OR FINANCIAL MISCONDUCT INVOLVING A GOVERNMENT-OPERATED PROGRAM.

MALAMUD, KENNETH L MD, LICENSE NUMBER 00G1707 OF GEORGETOWN, TX, WAS DISCIPLINED BY TEXAS ON MAY 11, 1995
DISCIPLINARY ACTION: REPRIMAND; REQUIRED TO TAKE ADDITIONAL MEDICAL EDUCATION
OFFENSE: PROFESSIONAL MISCONDUCT

NOTES: IN 5/89, OBTAINED CONSENT FROM A PATIENT FOR AN OPHTHALMOLOGICAL PROCEDURE WHICH HE DID NOT PERFORM; INSTEAD PERFORMED A DIFFERENT PROCEDURE WITHOUT A PROPER CONSENT FORM; HIS DOCUMENTATION OF PROCEDURE WAS INADEQUATE; ADMITS TO ALTERING MEDICAL RECORD AND PLACING ADDENDUMS TO IT IN AN INCORRECT FORMAT; HAS INSTITUTED MEASURES TO CORRECT DEFICIENCIES. REQUIREMENTS AND REMEDIAL MEASURES FOR TWO YEARS: SHALL MAINTAIN ADEQUATE OPHTHALMOLOGICAL MEDICAL RECORDS WHICH SHALL BE AVAILABLE FOR REVIEW AND SHALL ADOPT A SYSTEM OF PATIENT RECORD KEEPING AND BILLING; SHALL NOT SIGN OR INDICATE IN ANY MANNER IN PATIENT RECORDS THAT HE HAS SEEN PATIENTS UNLESS HE ACTUALLY HAS SEEN AND EXAMINED THE PATIENT UNLESS IT IS CLEARLY NOTED THAT HE DID NOT PERSONALLY EXAMINE THE PATIENT; SHALL NOT PERFORM ANY MEDICAL PROCEDURE ON A PATIENT UNLESS HE HAS EXPLAINED THE PROCEDURE AND OBTAINED CONSENT FROM THE PATIENT; WITHIN ONE YEAR SHALL OBTAIN AT LEAST 50 HOURS OF CONTINUING MEDICAL EDUCATION, AT LEAST 10 OF WHICH SHALL BE IN ETHICS; SHALL APPEAR BEFORE THE BOARD AT LEAST ONCE A YEAR OR AT BOARD REQUEST; SHALL COOPERATE WITH BOARD IN VERIFYING COMPLIANCE; SHALL GIVE A COPY OF THIS ORDER TO ANY HEALTH CARE ENTITY WHERE HE HAS PRIVILEGES; SHALL PROVIDE A COPY OF THIS ORDER TO ANYONE REQUESTING IT WITHIN 10 DAYS; TIME PERIOD OUT OF TEXAS DOES NOT COUNT TOWARD THIS ORDER; SHALL INFORM BOARD OF CHANGE OF ADDRESS WITHIN 10 DAYS OR IF HE LEAVES THE STATE. SHALL NOT SEEK MODIFICATION FOR ONE YEAR.

MALAMUD, KENNETH L MD, LICENSE NUMBER 0132330 OF SAN GABRIEL EYE CENTER, GEORGETOWN, TX, WAS DISCIPLINED BY NEW YORK ON MAY 28, 1996
DISCIPLINARY ACTION: 12-MONTH PROBATION; REPRIMAND
OFFENSE: DISCIPLINARY ACTION BY ANOTHER STATE OR AGENCY

NOTES: ACTION IN TEXAS FOR FAILING TO MAINTAIN ADEQUATE PATIENT RECORDS. PROBATION UPON COMMENCEMENT OF PRACTICE IN NEW YORK.

MANION, ROBERT A MD, LICENSE NUMBER 00G6806 OF GRAND PRAIRIE, TX, WAS DISCIPLINED BY TEXAS ON NOVEMBER 19, 1993
DISCIPLINARY ACTION: 60-MONTH PROBATION; MONITORING OF PHYSICIAN PERFORMANCE
OFFENSE: SUBSTANCE ABUSE

NOTES: SUFFERS FROM ALCOHOLISM AND UNDERWENT INPATIENT TREATMENT IN 7/91 BUT LEFT AGAINST MEDICAL ADVICE; HAS CONSUMED ALCOHOL SINCE THEN ON MORE THAN ONE OCCASION AND AS RECENTLY AS 8/11/93. SUSPENSION STAYED.

CONDITIONS OF PROBATION: SHALL ABSTAIN FROM THE CONSUMPTION OF ALCOHOL/CHEMICAL SUBSTANCES IN ANY FORM UNLESS PRESCRIBED BY ANOTHER PHYSICIAN FOR A LEGITIMATE AND THERAPEUTIC PURPOSE; SHALL NOT TREAT OR OTHERWISE SERVE AS PHYSICIAN, PRESCRIBE, DISPENSE OR ADMINISTER DRUGS THAT MAY BE SUBJECT TO ABUSE TO HIMSELF OR ANY MEMBER OF HIS FAMILY; SEPARATE FROM PATIENT RECORDS SHALL MAINTAIN A FILE OF EVERY PRESCRIPTION WRITTEN FOR CONTROLLED SUBSTANCES OR DANGEROUS DRUGS WHICH SHALL BE AVAILABLE FOR INSPECTION; SHALL SUBMIT HIMSELF FOR EVALUATION AND TREATMENT TO A BOARD-APPROVED ADDICTIONOLOGIST WITH QUARTERLY REPORTS; SHALL PARTICIPATE IN ACTIVITIES OF A PHYSICIAN HEALTH AND REHABILITATION COMMITTEE AND ATTEND WEEKLY MEETINGS WITH QUARTERLY REPORTS; SHALL PARTICIPATE IN AA'S PROGRAM NOT LESS THAN THREE TIMES A WEEK WITH QUARTERLY REPORTS; SHALL FURNISH QUARTERLY REPORTS TO THE BOARD REGARDING HIS MEDICAL CONDITION AND COMPLIANCE WITH THIS ORDER; SHALL SUBMIT HIMSELF FOR APPROPRIATE EXAMS INCLUDING DRUG OR ALCOHOL SCREENS; SHALL APPEAR BEFORE THE BOARD ONCE A YEAR; SHALL GIVE A COPY OF THIS ORDER TO ANY HEALTH CARE ENTITY WHERE HE HAS PRIVILEGES; SHALL COOPERATE WITH THE BOARD IN VERIFYING COMPLIANCE; SHALL INFORM BOARD OF CHANGE OF ADDRESS WITHIN 10 DAYS OR IF HE LEAVES THE STATE; TIME SPENT OUT OF TEXAS DOES NOT COUNT TOWARD PROBATION. SHALL NOT SEEK MODIFICATION FOR ONE YEAR. ON 7/31/95 ORDER MODIFIED WITH ADDITION OF TERMS AND CONDITIONS AS FOLLOWS: SHALL MAINTAIN ADEQUATE MEDICAL RECORDS WHICH SHALL BE AVAILABLE FOR REVIEW; SHALL ADOPT OR ESTABLISH A SYSTEM OF PATIENT RECORD KEEPING AND BILLING TO ENSURE THAT ALL PATIENT RECORDS REFLECT THE PATIENT'S NAME, THE SERVICE RENDERED, THE DATE OF SERVICE AND THE AMOUNT CHARGED; SHALL OBTAIN AT LEAST 50 HOURS PER YEAR OF CONTINUING MEDICAL EDUCATION.

MANION, ROBERT A MD, LICENSE NUMBER G6806 OF JUNCTION, TX, WAS DISCIPLINED BY TEXAS ON NOVEMBER 22, 1997
DISCIPLINARY ACTION: 24-MONTH PROBATION; REQUIRED TO TAKE ADDITIONAL MEDICAL EDUCATION
OFFENSE: FAILURE TO COMPLY WITH PREVIOUS BOARD ORDER

NOTES: SUFFERS FROM ALCOHOLISM AND UNDERWENT INPATIENT TREATMENT IN 7/91; LICENSE PLACED ON PROBATION WITH CONDITIONS ON 11/19/93; ON 10/20/97 HE VIOLATED THAT ORDER BY TREATING HIMSELF WITH AN EXPECTORANT THAT WAS NOT PRESCRIBED BY ANOTHER PHYSICIAN FOR A LEGITIMATE AND THERAPEUTIC PURPOSE. SUSPENSION STAYED WITH FOLLOWING TERMS AND CONDITIONS OF PROBATION: SHALL ABSTAIN FROM THE CONSUMPTION OF ALCOHOL/DRUGS IN ANY FORM UNLESS PRESCRIBED BY ANOTHER PHYSICIAN FOR A LEGITIMATE AND THERAPEUTIC PURPOSE; SHALL SUBMIT HIMSELF FOR APPROPRIATE EXAMS INCLUDING DRUG OR ALCOHOL SCREENS; SHALL SUBMIT THE NAMES OF THREE ADDICTIONOLOGISTS FOR THE BOARD'S APPROVAL, AND UPON APPROVAL, SHALL SUBMIT HIMSELF FOR EVALUATION AND TREATMENT WITHIN 45 DAYS; SHALL PARTICIPATE IN THE ACTIVITIES OF A PHYSICIAN HEALTH AND REHABILITATION COMMITTEE AND ATTEND WEEKLY MEETINGS WITH QUARTERLY REPORTS; SHALL PARTICIPATE IN AA'S PROGRAM NOT LESS THAN THREE TIMES A WEEK; SHALL REPORT ON HIS ATTENDANCE; SEPARATE FROM PATIENT RECORDS, SHALL MAINTAIN A FILE OF EVERY PRESCRIPTION WRITTEN BY HIM FOR DANGEROUS DRUGS WITH ADDICTIVE POTENTIAL WHICH SHALL BE MADE AVAILABLE FOR REVIEW; SHALL UNDERGO EXAMINATIONS BY AN ALLERGIST AND A CARDIOLOGIST WITHIN 30 DAYS, BOTH OF WHOM WILL SUBMIT MONTHLY REPORTS; SHALL MAINTAIN ADEQUATE MEDICAL RECORDS WHICH SHALL BE AVAILABLE FOR REVIEW; SHALL OBTAIN 50 HOURS PER YEAR OF CONTINUING MEDICAL EDUCATION; SHALL APPEAR BEFORE THE BOARD AT LEAST TWICE A YEAR; SHALL COOPERATE WITH THE BOARD IN VERIFYING COMPLIANCE INCLUDING PROVIDING COPIES OF MEDICAL RELEASES UPON REQUEST; SHALL GIVE A COPY OF THIS ORDER TO ANY HEALTH CARE ENTITY WHERE HE HAS PRIVILEGES; SHALL PROVIDE A COPY OF THIS ORDER TO ANYONE REQUESTING IT WITHIN 10 DAYS; TIME SPENT OUT OF TEXAS DOES NOT COUNT TOWARD PROBATION; SHALL INFORM THE BOARD OF CHANGE OF ADDRESS WITHIN 10 DAYS OR IF HE LEAVES THE STATE; SHALL NOT SEEK MODIFICATION FOR ONE YEAR.

MANN, PAUL MICHAEL MD, LICENSE NUMBER 00D7443 OF HUMBLE, TX, WAS DISCIPLINED BY TEXAS ON DECEMBER 4, 1991

NOTES: BOARD ALLEGES THAT THE FOLLOWING DELEGATED OPHTHALMOLOGIC PROCEDURES ARE NOT IN THE BEST INTERESTS OF THE PATIENT: THE PERFORMANCE OF SCLERAL GROOVES; CREATION OF THE SCLERAL BED; CLOSING AND SUTURING OF THE EYE WOUND; AND PARACENTESIS PROCEDURES. NO FORMAL COMPLAINT HAS BEEN BROUGHT. HE NEITHER ADMITS NOR DENIES ALLEGATIONS, AND DENIES ANY VIOLATION OF THE MEDICAL PRACTICE ACT. AGREED THAT HE WILL NOT DELEGATE THESE PROCEDURES TO NONPHYSICIANS. ON 3/5/94 ORDER TERMINATED.

MARASIGAN, FREDDIE P MD, LICENSE NUMBER F6021 OF AMARILLO, TX, WAS DISCIPLINED BY TEXAS ON AUGUST 9, 1997
DISCIPLINARY ACTION: FINE
OFFENSE: SUBSTANDARD CARE, INCOMPETENCE OR NEGLIGENCE

NOTES: WHILE COVERING FOR ANOTHER PEDIATRICIAN, HE FAILED TO PROPERLY EXAMINE AND TREAT A SIX-YEAR-OLD CHILD WHO SUFFERS FROM ASTHMA BY TRYING TO ASSESS THE CHILD OVER THE PHONE. SHALL PAY A $1000 ADMINISTRATIVE PENALTY.

MARCOM, RALPH ANSON DO, LICENSE NUMBER 00D3644, WAS DISCIPLINED BY TEXAS ON AUGUST 17, 1996
DISCIPLINARY ACTION: 60-MONTH PROBATION; RESTRICTION PLACED ON CONTROLLED SUBSTANCE LICENSE
OFFENSE: NONCOMPLIANCE WITH A PROFESSIONAL RULE

NOTES: HIS RECORDS FOR TWO PATIENTS WHICH HE TREATED BETWEEN 8/88 AND 1/94 FOR CHRONIC AND SEVERE HEADACHES REVEAL NO HISTORY OR PHYSICAL EXAMINATION, AND CONTAIN NO RECORDED OBJECTIVE OR SUBJECTIVE ASSESSMENTS; PRESCRIBED LARGE AMOUNTS OF DARVOCET N WITHOUT A MEDICAL DIAGNOSIS FOR THE PRESCRIPTIONS RECORDED IN EITHER PATIENT'S MEDICAL RECORDS; THE RECORDS DO NOT DOCUMENT WHETHER EITHER PATIENT WAS EXAMINED BEFORE THE DRUGS WERE PRESCRIBED. CONDITIONS FOR PROBATION: WITHIN ONE YEAR SHALL TAKE AND PASS THE SPECIAL PURPOSE EXAMINATION AND THE MEDICAL JURISPRUDENCE EXAMINATION; SHALL MAINTAIN ADEQUATE MEDICAL RECORDS WHICH SHALL BE AVAILABLE UPON BOARD

REQUEST; SHALL NOT SIGN OR INDICATE IN ANY MANNER IN ANY PATIENT RECORDS, THAT HE HAS SEEN AND EXAMINED THE PATIENT UNLESS IT IS CLEARLY NOTED THAT HE DID NOT PERSONALLY EXAMINE THE PATIENT; HIS MEDICAL PRACTICE, INCLUDING ANY OFFICE AND SURGICAL PRACTICE, SHALL BE MONITORED BY A BOARD APPROVED TEXAS PHYSICIAN WHO SHALL SUBMIT QUARTERLY REPORTS TO THE BOARD; SHALL NOT TELEPHONE A PHARMACY A PRESCRIPTION OR REFILL FOR CONTROLLED SUBSTANCES OR DANGEROUS DRUGS WITH ADDICTIVE POTENTIAL OR POTENTIAL FOR ABUSE OR PERMIT ANY INDIVIDUAL UNDER HIS SUPERVISION TO DO SO; SHALL SURRENDER HIS CONTROLLED SUBSTANCE CERTIFICATES TO THE DEA AND THE DPS; SHALL NOT ATTEMPT TO REGISTER HIS CONTROLLED SUBSTANCE CERTIFICATES WITHOUT PRIOR BOARD APPROVAL; SHALL MAINTAIN A LOGBOOK OF ALL PRESCRIPTIONS FOR DANGEROUS DRUGS WITH ADDICTIVE POTENTIAL OR POTENTIAL FOR ABUSE AND MAKE IT AVAILABLE UPON BOARD REQUEST; SHALL OBTAIN AT LEAST 50 HOURS PER YEAR OF CONTINUING MEDICAL EDUCATION AT LEAST 25 HOURS IN RECORD KEEPING, RISK MANAGEMENT, PAIN MANAGEMENT, AND PHARMACOLOGY, AND SUBMIT PROOF TO THE BOARD; SHALL APPEAR BEFORE THE BOARD AT LEAST TWICE PER YEAR; SHALL COOPERATE WITH THE BOARD IN VERIFYING COMPLIANCE; SHALL GIVE A COPY OF THIS ORDER TO ANY HEALTH CARE ENTITY WHERE HE HAS PRIVILEGES; SHALL PROVIDE A COPY OF THIS ORDER TO ANYONE REQUESTING IT WITHIN 10 DAYS. TIME PERIOD OUT OF TEXAS DOES NOT COUNT TOWARD PROBATION; SHALL INFORM THE BOARD OF CHANGE OF ADDRESS WITHIN 10 DAYS OF IF HE LEAVES THE STATE; SHALL NOT SEEK MODIFICATION FOR ONE YEAR.

MARES, ALBERTO MD, LICENSE NUMBER 00F9774 OF SAN ANTONIO, TX, WAS DISCIPLINED BY TEXAS ON AUGUST 21, 1992
DISCIPLINARY ACTION: LICENSE REVOCATION
OFFENSE: OVERPRESCRIBING OR MISPRESCRIBING DRUGS

NOTES: NONTHERAPEUTIC PRESCRIBING; FAILURE TO PRACTICE MEDICINE IN AN ACCEPTABLE MANNER CONSISTENT WITH PUBLIC HEALTH AND WELFARE; UNPROFESSIONAL OR DISHONORABLE CONDUCT LIKELY TO DECEIVE, DEFRAUD OR INJURE THE PUBLIC. HE OBTAINED A TEMPORARY RESTRAINING ORDER FROM THE COURTS AND THE REVOCATION OF HIS LICENSE HAS BEEN LIFTED. ON 2/16/95 ORDER VACATED AND REMANDED BACK TO THE BOARD.

MARES, ALBERTO MD OF 111 LEXINGTON AVENUE, SAN ANTONIO, TX, WAS DISCIPLINED BY DEA ON AUGUST 15, 1995
DISCIPLINARY ACTION: SURRENDER OF CONTROLLED SUBSTANCE LICENSE
OFFENSE: PROFESSIONAL MISCONDUCT

NOTES: ILLEGAL DISPENSING.

MARES, ALBERTO MD, LICENSE NUMBER 00F9774 OF SAN ANTONIO, TX, WAS DISCIPLINED BY TEXAS ON JANUARY 27, 1996
DISCIPLINARY ACTION: LICENSE REVOCATION
OFFENSE: CRIMINAL CONVICTION OR PLEA OF GUILTY, NOLO CONTENDERE, OR NO CONTEST TO A CRIME

NOTES: ON 6/5/95 CONVICTED FOR FELONIES OF MAIL FRAUD AND OF DISPENSATION OF A CONTROLLED SUBSTANCE AND IMPRISONED FOR 33 MONTHS ON EACH OFFENSE TO BE SERVED CONCURRENTLY. SHALL BE ALLOWED TO SEEK REINSTATEMENT.

MARKSTROM, CARL ERIC MD, DATE OF BIRTH FEBRUARY 13, 1932, LICENSE NUMBER 00D1463 OF SEAGOVILLE, TX, WAS DISCIPLINED BY TEXAS ON AUGUST 18, 1990
DISCIPLINARY ACTION: REQUIRED TO ENTER AN IMPAIRED PHYSICIAN PROGRAM OR SUBSTANCE ABUSE TREATMENT; MONITORING OF PHYSICIAN PERFORMANCE
OFFENSE: SUBSTANCE ABUSE

NOTES: STIPULATED ORDER. MUST SUBMIT FOR PSYCHIATRIC EVALUATION AND FOLLOW RECOMMENDATIONS, IF ANY, REGARDING TREATMENT, PARTICIPATE IN DALLAS COUNTY MEDICAL SOCIETY'S COMMITTEE ON PHYSICIAN HEALTH AND REHABILITATION, ENTER INTO A DRUG REHABILITATION PROGRAM; SUBMIT FOR APPROPRIATE EXAMINATIONS TO DETERMINE FREEDOM FROM DRUGS AND ALCOHOL, AND REFRAIN FROM USE OF, AND NOT ADMINISTER OR PRESCRIBE TO SELF, DANGEROUS DRUGS OR CONTROLLED SUBSTANCES UNLESS SUCH ARE PRESCRIBED, ADMINISTERED OR DISPENSED BY ANOTHER PHYSICIAN TREATING HIM FOR LEGITIMATE MEDICAL NEED. RESTRICTIONS MODIFIED EFFECTIVE 6/17/92. ORDER TERMINATED ON 6/15/93; LICENSE FREE AND CLEAR OF ANY RESTRICTIONS.

MARKUS, GEORGE M MD, LICENSE NUMBER 00F6905, WAS DISCIPLINED BY TEXAS ON AUGUST 17, 1996
DISCIPLINARY ACTION: 60-MONTH RESTRICTION PLACED ON LICENSE; REQUIRED TO TAKE ADDITIONAL MEDICAL EDUCATION
OFFENSE: SEXUAL ABUSE OF OR SEXUAL MISCONDUCT WITH A PATIENT

NOTES: ALLEGATIONS THAT FROM ABOUT NOVEMBER 1991 TO NOVEMBER 1993 ENGAGED IN A SEXUAL RELATIONSHIP WITH AN ADULT FEMALE PATIENT; ADMITS TO HAVING ENGAGED IN SEXUAL INTERCOURSE WITH THIS FEMALE PRIOR TO HER BECOMING HIS PATIENT, DENIES SEXUAL MISCONDUCT WHILE SHE WAS HIS PATIENT; PRESCRIBED DIAZEPAM, TO HER WITHOUT DOCUMENTING IT IN HER MEDICAL RECORD WITH THE MEDICAL RATIONALE FOR SUCH PRESCRIBING; IN OCTOBER 1993 WENT TO HER PLACE OF EMPLOYMENT AND ENGAGED IN A PHYSICAL ALTERCATION; AS A RESULT HE WAS CHARGED WITH ASSAULT, ENTERED A PLEA OF NO CONTEST, AND RECEIVED DEFERRED ADJUDICATION, PROBATION, AND A FINE; SELF PRESCRIBED VARIOUS MEDICATIONS WITHOUT ADEQUATELY DOCUMENTING THE TYPE, FREQUENCY, AND QUANTITY OF THE DRUG PRESCRIBED; SELF-PRESCRIBED ON MULTIPLE OCCASIONS FOR DEPRESSION, PROZAC, WITHOUT ADEQUATE DOCUMENTATION OF THE FREQUENCY AND QUANTITY PRESCRIBED; WAS UNDER THE CARE OF A PSYCHOLOGIST FOR TREATMENT OF HIS DEPRESSION WHO WAS AWARE OF HIS SELF-PRESCRIBING OF PROZAC. DOES NOT ADMIT VIOLATION. RESTRICTED UNDER TERMS AND CONDITIONS FOR FIVE YEARS: SHALL SUBMIT HIMSELF FOR EVALUATION AND TREATMENT BY A BOARD-APPROVED PSYCHIATRIST AT LEAST ONCE A MONTH WHO SHALL SUBMIT REPORTS; ANYTIME HE PERFORMS A PHYSICAL EXAMINATION ON A FEMALE PATIENT, SHALL HAVE A CHAPERONE PRESENT WHO SHALL MAKE A NOTATION ON THE PATIENT'S CHARTS; SHALL NOT TREAT OR OTHERWISE SERVE AS PHYSICIAN, PRESCRIBE, DISPENSE, OR ADMINISTER DRUGS THAT MAY BE SUBJECT TO ABUSE TO HIMSELF OR ANY MEMBER OF HIS FAMILY; SHALL REFRAIN FROM THE PRESCRIPTION OR ADMINISTRATION OF ANY DRUG FOR ANY PATIENT UNLESS THE DRUG IS MEDICALLY INDICATED AND PRESCRIBED IN THERAPEUTIC DOSES; SHALL CONDUCT ADEQUATE FOLLOW-UP EXAMINATIONS ON ALL PATIENTS TO

DETERMINE WHETHER THE COURSE OF TREATMENT, INCLUDING THE PRESCRIBING OF DRUGS, IS APPROPRIATE; SHALL MAINTAIN ADEQUATE MEDICAL RECORDS WHICH SHALL BE AVAILABLE FOR REVIEW; WITHIN ONE YEAR SHALL OBTAIN SIX HOURS OF ETHICS THROUGH BOARD APPROVED COURSES OR PROGRAMS AND A BOARD APPROVED COURSE IN THE AREA OF RISK MANAGEMENT AND SHALL SUBMIT PROOF TO THE BOARD; SHALL COOPERATE WITH THE BOARD IN VERIFYING COMPLIANCE INCLUDING PROVIDING COPIES OF MEDICAL RELEASES AND PEER REVIEW RECORDS UPON REQUEST; SHALL PERSONALLY APPEAR BEFORE THE BOARD AT LEAST TWO TIMES PER YEAR OR UPON REQUEST; SHALL GIVE A COPY OF THIS ORDER TO ANY HEALTH CARE ENTITY WHERE HE HAS PRIVILEGES; SHALL PROVIDE A COPY OF THIS ORDER TO ANYONE REQUESTING IT WITHIN 10 DAYS; TIME PERIOD OUT OF TEXAS DOES NOT COUNT TOWARD RESTRICTION; SHALL INFORM THE BOARD OF CHANGE OF ADDRESS WITHIN 10 DAYS OF IF HE LEAVES THE STATE; SHALL NOT SEEK MODIFICATION FOR ONE YEAR. ON 4/4/98 PETITION FOR MODIFICATION OF ORDER DENIED. ON 10/15/99 ORDER TERMINATED.

MARON, BARRY R MD, DATE OF BIRTH NOVEMBER 30, 1938, LICENSE NUMBER 0020300 OF IA, WAS DISCIPLINED BY ARIZONA ON APRIL 15, 1993

NOTES: BOARD HAS INVESTIGATED INFORMATION THAT HE HAS BIPOLAR DISORDER AND SELF MEDICATES HIMSELF. CURRENTLY PRACTICING IN IOWA. SHALL NOT PRACTICE MEDICINE IN ARIZONA UNTIL HE HAS FIRST ADVISED THE BOARD OF HIS INTENTION TO DO SO AND RECEIVED AUTHORIZATION.

MARON, BARRY R MD, DATE OF BIRTH NOVEMBER 30, 1938, LICENSE NUMBER 0021140 OF BOX 1707, BORGER, TX, WAS DISCIPLINED BY NEW JERSEY ON NOVEMBER 2, 1994

NOTES: AGREES TO COMPLY WITH ALL REQUIREMENTS OF AN ORDER DATED 06/16/93 ISSUED BY THE BOARD OF MEDICAL EXAMINERS OF ARIZONA. SHALL PROVIDE NOTICE TO NEW JERSEY OF ANY CHANGE IN ANY OF THE TERMS OF THE ARIZONA AGREEMENT OR HIS MEDICAL CONDITION. PRIOR TO ENGAGING IN ACTIVE PRACTICE IN NEW JERSEY, SHALL APPEAR BEFORE THE BOARD OR A COMMITTEE OF THE BOARD TO RESPOND TO QUESTIONS CONCERNING HIS STATUS, HEALTH AND PLANS.

MARON, BARRY R MD, LICENSE NUMBER 0G16120 OF ALBUQUERQUE, NM, WAS DISCIPLINED BY CALIFORNIA ON MAY 19, 1995
DISCIPLINARY ACTION: 60-MONTH PROBATION
OFFENSE: DISCIPLINARY ACTION BY ANOTHER STATE OR AGENCY

NOTES: ARIZONA ORDER RESTRICTING RESUMPTION OF PRACTICE WITH PRECONDITIONS, SUCH AS PSYCHIATRIC EVALUATION FOR SAFE PRACTICE. REVOCATION STAYED.

MARON, BARRY R MD, DATE OF BIRTH NOVEMBER 30, 1938, LICENSE NUMBER 0028935 OF 408 NORTH MAIN STREET, WARSAW, NY, WAS DISCIPLINED BY IOWA ON AUGUST 8, 1996

NOTES: AGREED THAT HE WILL NOT RETURN TO PRACTICE IN IOWA UNLESS HE GIVES THE BOARD 30 DAYS NOTICE IN WRITING AND IF HE DOES RETURN SHALL ENTER INTO A CONSENT AGREEMENT PLACING ANY RESTRICTIONS ON HIS LICENSE THAT THE BOARD DEEMS NECESSARY.

MARRACK, DAVID MD, LICENSE NUMBER 00D1318 OF HOUSTON, TX, WAS DISCIPLINED BY TEXAS ON MARCH 6, 1992
DISCIPLINARY ACTION: 36-MONTH PROBATION
OFFENSE: PROFESSIONAL MISCONDUCT

NOTES: AIDING OR ABETTING, DIRECTLY OR INDIRECTLY, THE PRACTICE OF MEDICINE BY ANY PERSON, PARTNERSHIP, ASSOCIATION, OR CORPORATION NOT DULY LICENSED TO PRACTICE MEDICINE BY THE BOARD. LICENSE SUSPENDED, SUSPENSION STAYED; PROBATION UNDER TERMS AND CONDITIONS.

MARRACK, DAVID MD, LICENSE NUMBER 00D1318 OF HOUSTON, TX, WAS DISCIPLINED BY TEXAS ON APRIL 15, 1994
DISCIPLINARY ACTION: RESTRICTION PLACED ON LICENSE
OFFENSE: FAILURE TO COMPLY WITH PREVIOUS BOARD ORDER

NOTES: VIOLATED TERMS OF 3/6/92 ORDER IN THAT HE FAILED TO PROVIDE IN A TIMELY MANNER, UPON REQUEST, EVIDENCE RELATING TO HIS CURRENT EMPLOYMENT SITUATION WHICH WOULD DEMONSTRATE COMPLIANCE WITH THE PROVISION THAT HE WOULD NOT ACCEPT EMPLOYMENT OR ENTER INTO CONTRACTUAL RELATIONSHIPS WHERE HE WAS PAID TO TREAT PATIENTS BY ANYONE OTHER THAN LICENSED PHYSICIANS. THE FOLLOWING PROVISION WAS ADDED TO THAT ORDER: SHALL PROVIDE TO THE BOARD UPON REQUEST WRITTEN DOCUMENTATION TO ESTABLISH THE TERMS OF ANY EMPLOYMENT AGREEMENT HE ENTERS INTO. IF NO WRITTEN CONTRACT OF EMPLOYMENT EXISTS HE SHALL PROVIDE THE BOARD A WRITTEN NARRATIVE OF THE TERMS OF SUCH AGREEMENT. HE WILL NOTIFY THE BOARD WITHIN 10 DAYS OF ANY MODIFICATION OF THE TERMS OF THE AGREEMENT; ALL OTHER TERMS AND CONDITIONS OF THE 3/92 ORDER ARE IN EFFECT. SHALL NOT SEEK MODIFICATION FOR ONE YEAR.

MARTIN, ALLAN B MD, LICENSE NUMBER 0128864 OF 2991 EAST CHESTNUT AVE #8A, VINELAND, NJ, WAS DISCIPLINED BY NEW YORK ON JULY 6, 1992
DISCIPLINARY ACTION: SURRENDER OF LICENSE
OFFENSE: PROVIDING FALSE INFORMATION TO THE BOARD OR OTHER HEALTH AGENCY

NOTES: DID NOT CONTEST CHARGES THAT HE PRACTICED THE PROFESSION FRAUDULENTLY BY PROVIDING FALSE INFORMATION TO THE NEW JERSEY BOARD OF MEDICAL EXAMINERS.

MARTIN, ALLAN BRADLEY MD, DATE OF BIRTH JULY 17, 1947, LICENSE NUMBER 0034654 OF 2991 E CHESTNUT AVE #8A, VINELAND, NJ, WAS DISCIPLINED BY NEW JERSEY ON SEPTEMBER 16, 1992
DISCIPLINARY ACTION: LICENSE SUSPENSION; REQUIRED TO ENTER AN IMPAIRED PHYSICIAN PROGRAM OR SUBSTANCE ABUSE TREATMENT

NOTES: MAY PETITION FOR PARTIAL OR COMPLETE REINSTATEMENT OF LICENSE UPON DEMONSTRATION THAT HE HAS SUCCESSFULLY COMPLETED INPATIENT TREATMENT FOR ALCOHOLISM, AND THAT HE HAS FULLY COOPERATED WITH THE PHYSICIANS' HEALTH PROGRAM REGARDING HIS IMPAIRMENT PROBLEM.

MARTIN, ALLAN BRADLEY MD, DATE OF BIRTH JULY 17, 1947, LICENSE NUMBER 0034654 OF 2991 EAST CHESTNUT AVE, #8A, VINELAND, NJ, WAS DISCIPLINED BY NEW JERSEY ON JULY 14, 199[illegible]
DISCIPLINARY ACTION: RESTRICTION PLACED ON LICENSE; MONITORING OF PHYSICIAN PERFORMANCE

NOTES: LICENSE RESTORED WITH CONDITIONS: MAY BE EMPLOYED AS A SURGICAL ASSISTANT UNDER THE

SPECIFIC CIRCUMSTANCES DESCRIBED IN THE BOARD ORDER AND SHALL UNDERTAKE NO OTHER MEDICAL POSITION OR EMPLOYMENT WITHOUT WRITTEN APPROVAL FROM THE BOARD. SHALL CONTINUE TO COOPERATE WITH THE PHYSICIANS HEALTH PROGRAM AND SHALL AUTHORIZE AND CAUSE QUARTERLY REPORTS FROM THE CHIEF OF SURGERY AND MEDICAL DIRECTOR AT PERTH AMBOY GENERAL HOSPITAL AND OLD BRIDGE HOSPITAL RELATIVE TO EMPLOYMENT. ORDER MODIFIED ON 5/01/95: SHALL CONTINUE WITH PARTICIPATION IN THE AFTERCARE PROGRAM AS REQUIRED BY THE PHYSICIANS' HEALTH PROGRAM; MAY SEEK ALTERNATIVE EMPLOYMENT WITHIN AN INSTITUTIONAL SETTING IN A GEOGRAPHIC LOCATION CLOSER TO HIS PLACE OF RESIDENCE; SHALL NOTIFY THE BOARD OF HIS ACCEPTANCE OF ALTERNATE EMPLOYMENT; SHALL IMMEDIATELY NOTIFY THE BOARD OF ANY CHANGE IN SUBSEQUENT EMPLOYMENT; SHALL REFRAIN FROM ANY AND ALL ASPECTS OF THE PRIVATE PRACTICE OF MEDICINE PRIOR TO RECEIPT OF EXPRESS WRITTEN AUTHORITY FROM THE BOARD TO ENGAGE IN SUCH PRACTICE.

MARTIN, ALLAN BRADLEY MD, DATE OF BIRTH JULY 17, 1947, LICENSE NUMBER 00G2769 OF VINELAND, NJ, WAS DISCIPLINED BY TEXAS ON JUNE 22, 1994
DISCIPLINARY ACTION: SURRENDER OF LICENSE
OFFENSE: DISCIPLINARY ACTION BY ANOTHER STATE OR AGENCY

NOTES: ON 9/16/92 LICENSE WAS SUSPENDED WITH ADDITIONAL CONDITIONS BY THE NEW JERSEY BOARD BASED ON ALLEGATIONS THAT HE DELIBERATELY LIED IN WRITTEN MATERIALS SUBMITTED TO THE BOARD; A NEW JERSEY HOSPITAL SUSPENDED HIS PRIVILEGES BECAUSE OF CONCERN ABOUT ALCOHOL ABUSE. TEXAS LICENSE SURRENDERED IN LIEU OF FURTHER INVESTIGATION; SHALL NOT PETITION FOR REINSTATEMENT OF LICENSE.

MARTIN, ALLAN BRADLEY MD, DATE OF BIRTH JULY 17, 1947, LICENSE NUMBER 34654 OF 1416 SOUTH STATE STREET, VINELAND, NJ, WAS DISCIPLINED BY NEW JERSEY ON OCTOBER 22, 1999
DISCIPLINARY ACTION: PROBATION; RESTRICTION PLACED ON LICENSE
OFFENSE: SUBSTANCE ABUSE

NOTES: ON 3/17/99 LICENSE VOLUNTARILY SUSPENDED BASED UPON ALCOHOL ABUSE. LICENSE RESTORED WITH FOLLOWING RESTRICTIONS: SHALL BE EMPLOYED BY CORRECTIONAL HEALTH SERVICES; SHALL UNDERTAKE NO OTHER MEDICAL POSITION OR EMPLOYMENT WITHOUT PRIOR NOTICE AND APPROVAL OF THE BOARD; SHALL ATTEND THREE DOCUMENTED AA MEETINGS PER WEEK AND SUBMIT WEEKLY DOCUMENTATION OF HIS ATTENDANCE TO THE PHYSICIANS HEALTH PROGRAM (PHP); SHALL CONTINUE TO COOPERATE WITH THE PHP, INCLUDING TWICE WEEKLY RANDOM URINE TESTING, MONTHLY MEETINGS AND INGESTION OF ANTABUSE AS DIRECTED AND MONITORED BY THE PHP; SHALL SUPPLY HIS EMPLOYER WITH A COPY OF THE ORDER.

MARTIN, MARY ANNE MD, LICENSE NUMBER 00D5094 OF MESQUITE, TX, WAS DISCIPLINED BY TEXAS ON DECEMBER 17, 1991
DISCIPLINARY ACTION: LICENSE REVOCATION
OFFENSE: NONCOMPLIANCE WITH A PROFESSIONAL RULE

NOTES: VIOLATION OF SEVERAL SECTIONS OF THE MEDICAL PRACTICE ACT, INCLUDING INABILITY TO PRACTICE MEDICINE WITH REASONABLE SKILL AND SAFETY TO PATIENTS.

MARTIN, THOMAS STERLING MD, LICENSE NUMBER 00C5160 OF EL PASO, TX, WAS DISCIPLINED BY TEXAS ON APRIL 15, 1994
DISCIPLINARY ACTION: 12-MONTH PROBATION
OFFENSE: FAILURE TO COMPLY WITH PREVIOUS BOARD ORDER

NOTES: VIOLATED ORDER OF 6/13/89 IN THAT HE FAILED TO HAVE QUARTERLY REPORTS SUBMITTED TO THE BOARD FROM THE PHYSICIAN HEALTH AND REHABILITATION COMMITTEE AND HIS RECOVERING ABUSE SPONSOR. THE PROBATION AND OTHER CONDITIONS OF THAT ORDER WILL BE EXTENDED ONE YEAR; ALL OTHER TERMS AND CONDITIONS REMAIN IN EFFECT. SHALL NOT SEEK MODIFICATION FOR ONE YEAR.

MARTIN, WILLIAM CLYDE MD, LICENSE NUMBER 00D4213 OF WEATHERFORD, TX, WAS DISCIPLINED BY TEXAS ON MARCH 31, 1990
DISCIPLINARY ACTION: REPRIMAND; REQUIRED TO TAKE ADDITIONAL MEDICAL EDUCATION

NOTES: STIPULATED ORDER. ON 5/10/97 BOARD GRANTED HIS PETITION FOR TERMINATION OF THIS ORDER BASED ON COMPLIANCE WITH CONDITIONS.

MARTINEZ, ALBERTO NOE MD, LICENSE NUMBER 00G5337 OF JUNCTION, TX, WAS DISCIPLINED BY TEXAS ON JANUARY 27, 1996
DISCIPLINARY ACTION: 60-MONTH PROBATION; REQUIRED TO TAKE ADDITIONAL MEDICAL EDUCATION
OFFENSE: SUBSTANCE ABUSE

NOTES: INTEMPERATE USE OF ALCOHOL OR DRUGS: IN 1992 MEDICAL SOCIETY ATTEMPTED AN INTERVENTION WHEN HE DENIED HE HAD A SUBSTANCE ABUSE PROBLEM; ON 3/21/95 POLICE OFFICERS REPORTED HIM TO BE EXTREMELY INTOXICATED AT HOME; ON 3/29/95 AN INTERVENTION WAS CONDUCTED BY BEXAR COUNTY MEDICAL SOCIETY'S COMMITTEE ON PHYSICIAN HEALTH AND REHABILITATION; ADMITTED INTO ANCHOR HOSPITAL AND THE TALBOTT-MARSH RECOVERY CAMPUS AND WAS DISCHARGED ON 8/05/95 AFTER COMPLETION OF TREATMENT FOR ALCOHOL ABUSE; REPORTS A SOBRIETY DATE OF 3/25/95; CURRENTLY RECEIVING REGULAR COUNSELING FROM A PSYCHIATRIST AND A FAMILY THERAPIST; ATTENDS AA FIVE TIMES PER WEEK. HAS ENTERED INTO A RECOVERY CONTRACT. PROBATION UNDER TERMS AND CONDITIONS: SHALL ABSTAIN FROM THE CONSUMPTION OF ALCOHOL/DRUGS IN ANY FORM UNLESS PRESCRIBED BY ANOTHER PHYSICIAN FOR A LEGITIMATE AND THERAPEUTIC PURPOSE; SHALL SUBMIT HIMSELF FOR APPROPRIATE EXAMS, INCLUDING DRUG OR ALCOHOL SCREENS; SHALL SUBMIT HIMSELF FOR EVALUATION AND TREATMENT BY A BOARD-APPROVED PSYCHIATRIST WHOM HE SHALL SEE AT LEAST ONCE A MONTH AND WHO SHALL SUBMIT REPORTS TO THE BOARD; SHALL PARTICIPATE IN AA'S PROGRAM NOT LESS THAN THREE TIMES PER WEEK WITH QUARTERLY REPORTS TO THE BOARD; SHALL PARTICIPATE IN THE ACTIVITIES OF A PHYSICIAN HEALTH AND REHABILITATION COMMITTEE AND ATTEND WEEKLY MEETINGS WITH QUARTERLY REPORTS; SHALL COMPLY WITH THE TERMS AND CONDITIONS OF HIS CONTINUING CARE CONTRACTS AND SHALL REQUEST IN WRITING THAT THEY PROVIDE QUARTERLY REPORTS TO THE BOARD; SHALL COMPLY WITH THE TERMS AND CONDITIONS OF ANY CONTRACT OR AGREEMENT ENTERED FOR HOSPITAL PRIVILEGES AND SHALL REPORT IN WRITING TO THE BOARD ANY

DISCIPLINARY ACTION TAKEN; SHALL MAINTAIN ADEQUATE MEDICAL RECORDS WHICH SHALL BE AVAILABLE FOR REVIEW; SHALL OBTAIN AT LEAST 50 HOURS PER YEAR OF CONTINUING MEDICAL EDUCATION; SHALL APPEAR BEFORE THE BOARD AT LEAST ONCE PER YEAR; SHALL COOPERATE WITH THE BOARD IN VERIFYING COMPLIANCE INCLUDING PROVIDING COPIES OF MEDICAL RELEASES AND PEER REVIEW RECORDS UPON REQUEST; SHALL GIVE A COPY OF THIS ORDER TO ANY HEALTH CARE ENTITY WHERE HE HAS PRIVILEGES; SHALL PROVIDE A COPY OF THIS ORDER TO ANYONE REQUESTING IT WITHIN 10 DAYS; TIME PERIOD OUT OF TEXAS DOES NOT COUNT TOWARD PROBATION; SHALL INFORM THE BOARD OF CHANGE OF ADDRESS WITHIN 10 DAYS OR IF HE LEAVES THE STATE; SHALL NOT SEEK MODIFICATION FOR ONE YEAR. ON 5/10/97 PETITION FOR MODIFICATION OF ORDER DENIED.

MARTINEZ, DANIEL J MD, LICENSE NUMBER E8695 OF SAN ANTONIO, TX, WAS DISCIPLINED BY TEXAS ON NOVEMBER 22, 1997
DISCIPLINARY ACTION: REQUIRED TO ENTER AN IMPAIRED PHYSICIAN PROGRAM OR SUBSTANCE ABUSE TREATMENT; MONITORING OF PHYSICIAN PERFORMANCE
OFFENSE: LOSS OR RESTRICTION OF HOSPITAL PRIVILEGES

NOTES: IN 3/95 HE BEGAN USING COCAINE AND ON OCCASION ABUSED LORTAB, ESGIC PLUS, AND ETHANOL; ON 2/1/96 SOUTHWEST TEXAS METHODIST HOSPITAL SUMMARILY SUSPENDED PRIVILEGES; WHEN HOSPITAL WAS INFORMED THAT HE WAS SEEKING TREATMENT FOR IMPAIRMENT, HIS SUSPENSION WAS TERMINATED AND HE WAS GRANTED A MEDICAL LEAVE OF ABSENCE; ON OR ABOUT 8/18/96 HE ENTERED TREATMENT AND WAS DISCHARGED ON 1/13/97 WITH A DIAGNOSIS OF COCAINE AND ALCOHOL DEPENDENCE; HE AGAIN ENTERED TREATMENT AT ST. JUDE'S RECOVERY CENTER ON 1/13/97 AND COMPLETED THE PROGRAM IN 9/97. LICENSE LIMITED FOR FIVE YEARS AS FOLLOWS: SHALL ABSTAIN FROM THE CONSUMPTION OF ALCOHOL/DRUGS IN ANY FORM UNLESS PRESCRIBED BY ANOTHER PHYSICIAN FOR A LEGITIMATE AND THERAPEUTIC PURPOSE; SHALL SUBMIT HIMSELF FOR APPROPRIATE EXAMS INCLUDING DRUG OR ALCOHOL SCREENS; SHALL NOMINATE THREE CERTIFIED PSYCHIATRISTS FOR BOARD SELECTION OF A THERAPIST AND SHALL EXPEDITIOUSLY SUBMIT HIMSELF TO EVALUATION AND TREATMENT BY THE APPROVED PRACTITIONER; SHALL COOPERATE WITH THE BOARD IN VERIFYING COMPLIANCE INCLUDING PROVIDING COPIES OF MEDICAL RELEASES UPON REQUEST; SHALL PARTICIPATE IN THE ACTIVITIES OF A PHYSICIAN HEALTH AND REHABILITATION COMMITTEE AND ATTEND WEEKLY MEETINGS WITH QUARTERLY REPORTS; SHALL PARTICIPATE IN AA'S PROGRAM NOT LESS THAN THREE TIMES A WEEK; SHALL REPORT ON HIS ATTENDANCE; SHALL NOT TREAT OR OTHERWISE SERVE AS PHYSICIAN, PRESCRIBE, DISPENSE OR ADMINISTER DRUGS THAT MAY BE SUBJECT TO ABUSE TO HIMSELF OR TO ANY MEMBER OF HIS FAMILY; SHALL COMPLY WITH TERMS OF HIS CONTINUING CARE CONTRACT WITH QUARTERLY REPORTS; SEPARATE FROM PATIENT RECORDS, SHALL MAINTAIN A LOGBOOK OF EVERY PRESCRIPTION WRITTEN BY HIM FOR DANGEROUS DRUGS WITH ADDICTIVE POTENTIAL WHICH SHALL BE MADE AVAILABLE FOR REVIEW; SHALL GIVE A COPY OF THIS ORDER TO ANY HEALTH CARE ENTITY WHERE HE HAS PRIVILEGES; TIME SPENT OUT OF TEXAS DOES NOT COUNT TOWARD RESTRICTION; SHALL INFORM THE BOARD OF CHANGE OF ADDRESS WITHIN 10 DAYS OR IF HE LEAVES THE STATE; SHALL APPEAR BEFORE THE BOARD ONCE A YEAR; SHALL NOT SEEK MODIFICATION FOR ONE YEAR.

MARTINEZ, DANIEL J MD, LICENSE NUMBER E8695 OF SAN ANTONIO, TX, WAS DISCIPLINED BY TEXAS ON AUGUST 22, 1998
DISCIPLINARY ACTION: 60-MONTH PROBATION; REQUIRED TO ENTER AN IMPAIRED PHYSICIAN PROGRAM OR SUBSTANCE ABUSE TREATMENT
OFFENSE: FAILURE TO COMPLY WITH PREVIOUS BOARD ORDER

NOTES: VIOLATED 11/22/97 BOARD ORDER BY INGESTING COCAINE; ON OR ABOUT 5/8/98 HE ADMITTED INGESTING COCAINE DURING THE PREVIOUS 5 WEEKS AND WAS ADMITTED TO A HOSPITAL WITH A PROVISIONAL DIAGNOSIS OF CRACK ADDICTION/WITHDRAWAL, AND REMOTE USE OF ALCOHOL AND AMPHETAMINES; HE REMAINED IN TREATMENT UNTIL HIS DISCHARGE ON 7/6/98. SUSPENSION STAYED FOR PROBATION WITH THE FOLLOWING TERMS AND CONDITIONS: SHALL ABSTAIN FROM THE CONSUMPTION OF ALCOHOL/DRUGS IN ANY FORM UNLESS PRESCRIBED BY ANOTHER PHYSICIAN FOR A LEGITIMATE AND THERAPEUTIC PURPOSE; SHALL SUBMIT HIMSELF FOR APPROPRIATE EXAMS INCLUDING DRUG OR ALCOHOL SCREENS; SHALL NOMINATE THREE CERTIFIED PSYCHIATRISTS AND THREE PSYCHOTHERAPISTS FOR BOARD SELECTION OF A THERAPIST AND SHALL EXPEDITIOUSLY SUBMIT HIMSELF TO EVALUATION AND TREATMENT BY THE APPROVED PRACTITIONERS; SHALL COOPERATE WITH THE BOARD IN VERIFYING COMPLIANCE INCLUDING PROVIDING COPIES OF MEDICAL RELEASES UPON REQUEST; SHALL PARTICIPATE IN THE ACTIVITIES OF A PHYSICIAN HEALTH AND REHABILITATION COMMITTEE AND ATTEND WEEKLY MEETINGS WITH QUARTERLY REPORTS; SHALL CONTINUE TO PARTICIPATE IN AA'S PROGRAM NOT LESS THAN FIVE TIMES A WEEK; SHALL REPORT ON HIS ATTENDANCE; SHALL BE TESTED RANDOMLY WITH URINE DRUG SCREENS NO LESS THAN 5 TIMES PER MONTH; SHALL NOT TREAT OR OTHERWISE SERVE AS PHYSICIAN, PRESCRIBE, DISPENSE OR ADMINISTER DRUGS THAT MAY BE SUBJECT TO ABUSE TO HIMSELF OR TO ANY MEMBER OF HIS FAMILY; SHALL COMPLY WITH TERMS OF CONTINUING CARE CONTRACT; SEPARATE FROM PATIENT RECORDS, SHALL MAINTAIN A LOGBOOK OF EVERY PRESCRIPTION WRITTEN BY HIM FOR DANGEROUS DRUGS WITH ADDICTIVE POTENTIAL WHICH SHALL BE MADE AVAILABLE FOR REVIEW; SHALL GIVE A COPY OF THIS ORDER TO ANY HEALTH CARE ENTITY WHERE HE HAS PRIVILEGES; TIME SPENT OUT OF TEXAS DOES NOT COUNT TOWARD PROBATION; SHALL INFORM THE BOARD OF CHANGE OF ADDRESS WITHIN 10 DAYS OR IF HE LEAVES THE STATE; SHALL APPEAR BEFORE THE BOARD AT LEAST ONCE A YEAR; SHALL NOT SEEK MODIFICATION FOR ONE YEAR.

MARTINEZ, DANIEL J MD, LICENSE NUMBER E8695 OF SAN ANTONIO, TX, WAS DISCIPLINED BY TEXAS ON OCTOBER 14, 1998
DISCIPLINARY ACTION: LICENSE REVOCATION
OFFENSE: FAILURE TO COMPLY WITH PREVIOUS BOARD ORDER

NOTES: VIOLATED 8/22/98 BOARD ORDER.

MARTINEZ, DIONISIO F MD OF VERNON, TX, WAS DISCIPLINED BY MISSOURI ON JUNE 25, 1990
DISCIPLINARY ACTION: 1-MONTH LICENSE SUSPENSION
OFFENSE: SUBSTANDARD CARE, INCOMPETENCE OR NEGLIGENCE

NOTES: ALSO PRESCRIPTION VIOLATIONS AND NONCOMPLIANCE: FAILURE TO INFORM BOARD OF ADDRESS CHANGE.

MARTINEZ, MANUEL A JR MD, LICENSE NUMBER 00D4214 OF DEL RIO, TX, WAS DISCIPLINED BY TEXAS ON MARCH 31, 1990
DISCIPLINARY ACTION: REQUIRED TO TAKE ADDITIONAL MEDICAL EDUCATION

NOTES: STIPULATED ORDER.

MARTINEZ, MANUEL A JR MD OF 1120 SOUTH MAIN, DEL RIO, TX, WAS DISCIPLINED BY DEA ON JULY 29, 1994
DISCIPLINARY ACTION: SURRENDER OF CONTROLLED SUBSTANCE LICENSE

NOTES: IN LIEU OF PUBLIC INTEREST REVOCATION.

MARTINEZ, MANUEL A JR MD, LICENSE NUMBER 00D4214 OF DEL RIO, TX, WAS DISCIPLINED BY TEXAS ON AUGUST 19, 1994
DISCIPLINARY ACTION: 60-MONTH PROBATION; RESTRICTION PLACED ON LICENSE
OFFENSE: SUBSTANDARD CARE, INCOMPETENCE OR NEGLIGENCE

NOTES: SUBSTANDARD TREATMENT IN THE CARE OF SEVERAL PATIENTS BETWEEN 9/87 AND 2/90 INCLUDING: ORDERING GLYCERIN SUPPOSITORIES FOR AN INFANT ALTHOUGH THERE WAS NO INDICATION FOR THEM; DID NOT PLACE A PAP SMEAR IN SOLUTION SOON ENOUGH AFTER IT WAS TAKEN. CYTOLOGY RESULTS WERE NEGATIVE AND THE PAP SMEAR WAS NOT REPEATED, ANOTHER PAP SMEAR WAS DONE BY ANOTHER DOCTOR THREE MONTHS LATER WHICH REVEALED AN ENDOCERVICAL TUMOR MASS WHICH WAS MALIGNANT; THE PATIENT DIED FIVE MONTHS LATER; GIVING A 4 MONTH OLD PATIENT COMPAZINE AND TERRAMYCIN FOR VOMITING AND GASTROENTERITIS THE USE OF WHICH IS CONTRAINDICATED IN PATIENTS OF THIS AGE; GAVE A 2 MONTH OLD INFANT TERRAMYCIN WHICH IS NOT INDICATED FOR A CHILD THIS AGE -- NO DOCUMENTATION THAT AN ABDOMINAL EXAM WAS DONE ALTHOUGH HE SAID THAT ONE WAS PERFORMED; FAILED TO DOCUMENT ANY VITAL SIGNS IN THE COURSE OF TREATING PATIENT FOR HYPERTENSION FOR 12 MONTHS. SUSPENSION STAYED. CONDITIONS OF PROBATION: SHALL APPEAR BEFORE THE BOARD TWICE A YEAR; SHALL CONTINUE TO ATTEND AT LEAST 50 HOURS PER YEAR OF CONTINUING MEDICAL EDUCATION WITH AT LEAST ONE COURSE PER YEAR IN RISK MANAGEMENT AND ONE IN PHARMACOLOGY WITH AN EMPHASIS ON ANTIBIOTICS; SHALL BE SUPERVISED BY A BOARD-APPROVED PHYSICIAN WITH QUARTERLY REPORTS; SHALL MAINTAIN ADEQUATE MEDICAL RECORDS ON ALL PATIENT OFFICE VISITS WHICH SHALL BE AVAILABLE FOR INSPECTION; SHALL NOT SIGN ANY PATIENT RECORD UNLESS HE HAS PERSONALLY EXAMINED THE PATIENT OR CLEARLY NOTES IN THE RECORD THAT HE DID NOT; SHALL TAKE AND PASS THE 9/13/94 SPEX EXAM; SHALL NOT PRACTICE OBSTETRICS OR TREAT PATIENTS UNDER TWO YEARS OF AGE; SHALL GIVE A COPY OF THIS ORDER TO ANY HEALTH CARE ENTITY WHERE HE HAS PRIVILEGES; SHALL COOPERATE WITH THE BOARD IN VERIFYING COMPLIANCE; SHALL INFORM BOARD OF CHANGE OF ADDRESS WITHIN 10 DAYS OR IF HE LEAVES THE STATE; TIME SPENT OUT OF TEXAS DOES NOT COUNT TOWARD PROBATION. SHALL NOT SEEK MODIFICATION FOR ONE YEAR.

MARTINEZ, MANUEL A JR MD, LICENSE NUMBER 00D4214 OF DEL RIO, TX, WAS DISCIPLINED BY TEXAS ON AUGUST 18, 1995
DISCIPLINARY ACTION: SURRENDER OF LICENSE

NOTES: VOLUNTARY AND PERMANENT SURRENDER OF HIS LICENSE.

MARTINEZ-O'HARA, JOSEPH J MD OF 500 PAREDES LINE ROAD SUITE 2, BROWNSVILLE, TX, WAS DISCIPLINED BY DEA ON APRIL 22, 1996
DISCIPLINARY ACTION: SURRENDER OF CONTROLLED SUBSTANCE LICENSE
OFFENSE: CRIMINAL CONVICTION OR PLEA OF GUILTY, NOLO CONTENDERE, OR NO CONTEST TO A CRIME

NOTES: DRUG CONVICTION.

MARTINEZ-O'HARA, JOSEPH J MD, LICENSE NUMBER D24049 OF 500 PAREDES LINE ROAD, BROWNSVILLE, TX, WAS DISCIPLINED BY MARYLAND ON MAY 28, 1997
DISCIPLINARY ACTION: LICENSE REVOCATION
OFFENSE: CRIMINAL CONVICTION OR PLEA OF GUILTY, NOLO CONTENDERE, OR NO CONTEST TO A CRIME

NOTES: ON 3/18/96 PLED GUILTY TO BEING IN POSSESSION OF A CONTROLLED DANGEROUS SUBSTANCE, DIAZEPAM, BY FRAUD AND HE WAS PLACED ON COMMUNITY SUPERVISION FOR 10 YEARS.

MARTINEZ-O'HARA, JOSEPH JOHN MD, LICENSE NUMBER 00F7833 OF BROWNSVILLE, TX, WAS DISCIPLINED BY TEXAS ON MAY 15, 1996
DISCIPLINARY ACTION: 84-MONTH PROBATION; MONITORING OF PHYSICIAN PERFORMANCE
OFFENSE: LOSS OR RESTRICTION OF HOSPITAL PRIVILEGES

NOTES: ON 12/15/94 HIS MEDICAL PRACTICE PRIVILEGES AT A HOSPITAL WERE SUSPENDED BASED ON SELF-PRESCRIBING OF BENZODIAZEPINES USING PRESCRIPTIONS BEARING THE FORGED SIGNATURE OF ANOTHER PHYSICIAN; IN 4/95 HE WAS ARRESTED AND CHARGED WITH POSSESSION OR ATTEMPTS TO POSSESS A CONTROLLED SUBSTANCE THROUGH MISREPRESENTATION, FRAUD, FORGERY, DECEPTION OR SUBTERFUGE; ADMITS TO HAVING A PRIOR HISTORY OF DEPENDENCY ON BENZODIAZEPINES FROM 1978 TO 1983; IN 1983 HE UNDERWENT REHABILITATION IN ASSOCIATION WITH THE MARYLAND MEDICAL SOCIETY; CLAIMS COMPLETE SOBRIETY FROM 1983 TO 1994; ADMITS THAT IN THE FALL OF 1994 HE RELAPSED INTO INTEMPERATE USE OF BENZODIAZEPINES UPON MOVING AWAY FROM HIS FAMILY AND OTHER SUPPORT; REPORTS A SOBRIETY DATE OF 12/15/94 AND REPORTS REGULAR PARTICIPATION IN THE ACTIVITIES OF A PHYSICIANS HEALTH AND REHABILITATION COMMITTEE. SUSPENSION STAYED. PROBATION WITH TERMS AND CONDITIONS: SHALL ABSTAIN FROM THE CONSUMPTION OF ALCOHOL/DRUGS IN ANY FORM UNLESS PRESCRIBED BY ANOTHER PHYSICIAN FOR A LEGITIMATE AND THERAPEUTIC PURPOSE; SHALL SUBMIT HIMSELF FOR APPROPRIATE EXAMS INCLUDING DRUG OR ALCOHOL SCREENS; SHALL SUBMIT HIMSELF FOR EVALUATION AND TREATMENT BY A BOARD-APPROVED PSYCHIATRIST WHOM HE SHALL SEE AT LEAST ONCE A MONTH AND WHO SHALL SUBMIT REPORTS TO THE BOARD; SHALL CONTINUE TO PARTICIPATE IN AA'S PROGRAM NOT LESS THAN FIVE TIMES A WEEK WITH QUARTERLY REPORTS TO THE BOARD; SHALL PARTICIPATE IN THE ACTIVITIES OF A PHYSICIANS' HEALTH AND REHABILITATION COMMITTEE AND ATTEND WEEKLY MEETINGS WITH QUARTERLY REPORTS; SHALL NOT TREAT OR OTHERWISE SERVE AS PHYSICIAN, PRESCRIBE, DISPENSE OR ADMINISTER DRUGS THAT MAY BE SUBJECT TO ABUSE TO HIMSELF OR TO ANY MEMBER OF HIS FAMILY; SHALL APPEAR BEFORE BOARD AT LEAST TWO TIMES A YEAR; SHALL COOPERATE WITH BOARD IN VERIFYING COMPLIANCE INCLUDING PROVIDING COPIES OF MEDICAL

RELEASES UPON REQUEST; TIME SPENT OUT OF TEXAS DOES NOT COUNT TOWARD PROBATION; SHALL INFORM THE BOARD OF CHANGE OF ADDRESS WITHIN 10 DAYS OR IF HE LEAVES THE STATE. SHALL NOT SEEK MODIFICATION FOR ONE YEAR. ON 11/22/97 PETITION TO MODIFY ORDER GRANTED REDUCING AA PARTICIPATION FROM FIVE TO THREE TIMES PER WEEK.

MASHRU, PRAVINKUMAR K MD, LICENSE NUMBER G0470 OF MT. LAUREL, NJ, WAS DISCIPLINED BY TEXAS ON AUGUST 22, 1998
DISCIPLINARY ACTION: FINE; REPRIMAND
OFFENSE: NONCOMPLIANCE WITH A PROFESSIONAL RULE

NOTES: FAILED TO OBTAIN 12 HOURS OF CONTINUING MEDICAL EDUCATION DURING 8/31/96 - 8/31/97 AS REQUIRED FOR RENEWAL OF HIS LICENSE ON 11/30/97; WAS GRANTED A 90 DAY EXTENSION BUT STILL DID NOT OBTAIN THE REQUIRED HOURS; HIS LICENSE HAS BEEN IN A "DELINQUENT" STATUS SINCE 11/30/97; ON OR ABOUT 9/30/97 HE WAS ASSESSED A $100 PENALTY FEE; ON OR ABOUT 11/30/97 HE WAS ASSESSED A $50 FEE FOR A TEMPORARY LICENSE; BEFORE HE IS ISSUED A CURRENT PERMIT HE WILL BE REQUIRED TO PAY THE ANNUAL REGISTRATION, PENALTY, AND TEMPORARY LICENSE FEES AND OBTAIN ALL PAST DUE CONTINUING MEDICAL EDUCATION. $100 FINE; SHALL COOPERATE WITH THE BOARD IN VERIFYING COMPLIANCE.

MASON, EDWARD J JR MD, LICENSE NUMBER 00G6181 OF DALLAS, TX, WAS DISCIPLINED BY CALIFORNIA ON JUNE 10, 1992
DISCIPLINARY ACTION: LICENSE REVOCATION
OFFENSE: DISCIPLINARY ACTION BY ANOTHER STATE OR AGENCY

NOTES: DISCIPLINE BY TEXAS BOARD. DEFAULT DECISION.

MASON, JAMES EDWARD JR MD, LICENSE NUMBER 00C8755 OF DALLAS, TX, WAS DISCIPLINED BY TEXAS
OFFENSE: DIED

MASON, WALTER LEE MD, LICENSE NUMBER 00F1139 OF ALLEN, TX, WAS DISCIPLINED BY TEXAS ON AUGUST 20, 1992
DISCIPLINARY ACTION: 36-MONTH RESTRICTION PLACED ON LICENSE
OFFENSE: PROFESSIONAL MISCONDUCT

NOTES: OVERTREATING. ON 9/30/94 ORDER TERMINATED.

MASSAD, EUGENE MASSAD MD, LICENSE NUMBER C3144 OF DALLAS, TX, WAS DISCIPLINED BY TEXAS ON AUGUST 22, 1998
DISCIPLINARY ACTION: 60-MONTH PROBATION; RESTRICTION PLACED ON LICENSE
OFFENSE: OVERPRESCRIBING OR MISPRESCRIBING DRUGS

NOTES: A BOARD CONSULTANT FOUND HIS RECORD KEEPING TO BE ILLEGIBLE, POORLY ORGANIZED, AND GROSSLY INADEQUATE; HE CONTINUED TO PRESCRIBE VALIUM TO A PATIENT EVEN AFTER HE LEARNED THAT THE PATIENT HAD FORGED A PRESCRIPTION; HIS TREATMENT OF THIS PATIENT INVOLVED THE OVERPRESCRIBING OF VALIUM AND WAS BELOW THE STANDARD TREATMENT OF CHRONIC PAIN; HIS MEDICAL RECORDS FOR THE TREATMENT OF HIS FAMILY WITH APPETITE SUPPRESSANTS WERE BELOW STANDARD; HE TREATED ANOTHER PATIENT WITH VICODIN AND XANAX IN AN INAPPROPRIATE AND NONTHERAPEUTIC MANNER; HIS TREATMENT OF ANOTHER PATIENT'S OVERWEIGHT PROBLEMS IGNORED THE PATIENT'S HYPERTRIGLYCERIDEMIA AND ABNORMAL LIVER FUNCTION; HE MAINTAINS THAT THE PATIENT WAS AN ALCOHOLIC AND THAT HE ASSISTED HIM IN GAINING SUBSTANCE ABUSE TREATMENT; HE MAINTAINS THAT SINCE THE TIME OF HIS TREATMENTS OF THESE PATIENTS, HE HAS LIMITED HIS PRACTICE TO INDUSTRIAL/OCCUPATIONAL MEDICINE UNDER THE SUPERVISION OF ANOTHER PHYSICIAN, AND THAT HE NOW KEEPS WELL-ORGANIZED AND COMPLETE MEDICAL RECORDS AS A MATTER OF COURSE. SUSPENSION STAYED FOR PROBATION WITH THE FOLLOWING TERMS AND CONDITIONS: SHALL LIMIT HIS PRACTICE TO OCCUPATIONAL MEDICINE, FAMILY PRACTICE OR A PRACTICE IN A BOARD-APPROVED FACILITY; HIS PRACTICE OF BARIATRIC MEDICINE SHALL INCLUDE AN APPROPRIATE PHYSICAL AND PSYCHOLOGICAL EVALUATION, LAB TESTING, DISCUSSION OF TREATMENT RISK FACTORS WITH THE PATIENT, FOLLOW-UP CARE, MONITORED PRESCRIBING, AND MAINTENANCE OF PROPER MEDICAL RECORDS; SHALL ATTEND 50 HOURS PER YEAR OF CONTINUING MEDICAL EDUCATION WITH 1 COURSE IN RISK MANAGEMENT; SHALL MAINTAIN ADEQUATE MEDICAL RECORDS WHICH SHALL BE AVAILABLE FOR REVIEW; SEPARATE FROM PATIENT RECORDS, SHALL MAINTAIN A LOGBOOK OF EVERY PRESCRIPTION WRITTEN BY HIM FOR DANGEROUS DRUGS WITH ADDICTIVE POTENTIAL WHICH SHALL BE MADE AVAILABLE FOR REVIEW; SHALL NOT TREAT OR OTHERWISE SERVE AS PHYSICIAN, PRESCRIBE, DISPENSE OR ADMINISTER DRUGS THAT MAY BE SUBJECT TO ABUSE TO HIMSELF OR TO ANY MEMBER OF HIS FAMILY; SHALL APPEAR BEFORE THE BOARD ONCE A YEAR; SHALL COOPERATE WITH THE BOARD IN VERIFYING COMPLIANCE; SHALL GIVE A COPY OF THIS ORDER TO ANY HEALTH CARE ENTITY WHERE HE HAS PRIVILEGES; TIME SPENT OUT OF TEXAS DOES NOT COUNT TOWARD PROBATION; SHALL INFORM THE BOARD IF HE LEAVES THE STATE.

MASSEY, CHARLES R JR MD, LICENSE NUMBER 00G5341 OF FREDERICKSBURG, TX, WAS DISCIPLINED BY TEXAS ON AUGUST 24, 1991
DISCIPLINARY ACTION: 60-MONTH PROBATION; MONITORING OF PHYSICIAN PERFORMANCE
OFFENSE: SUBSTANCE ABUSE

NOTES: SUSPENSION STAYED; CONDITIONS OF PROBATION INCLUDE: SHALL CONTINUE TO PARTICIPATE IN AA AND CO-DEPENDENCY GROUP; SHALL SUBMIT FOR ALCOHOL OR DRUG SCREENS; SHALL CONTINUE TREATMENT FROM BOARD-DESIGNATED PHYSICIAN; SHALL APPEAR BEFORE THE BOARD ONE TIME A YEAR.

MATHIS, JAMES EDWARD MD, DATE OF BIRTH MARCH 10, 1930, LICENSE NUMBER 00C5162 OF 11300 HARWIN, HOUSTON, TX, WAS DISCIPLINED BY TEXAS ON APRIL 30, 1993
DISCIPLINARY ACTION: REPRIMAND
OFFENSE: NONCOMPLIANCE WITH A PROFESSIONAL RULE

NOTES: FAILED TO SUBMIT A COMPLETED MEDICAL PRACTICE ACT QUESTIONNAIRE AND LIABILITY CLAIM INFORMATION ON FOUR PATIENTS AFTER SEVERAL REQUESTS BY A BOARD INVESTIGATOR. SHALL GIVE A COPY OF THIS ORDER TO ANY HEALTH CARE ENTITY WHERE HE HAS PRIVILEGES.

MATSUSAKI, RONALD MD, LICENSE NUMBER G6344, WAS DISCIPLINED BY TEXAS ON MARCH 1, 1997
DISCIPLINARY ACTION: FINE; MONITORING OF PHYSICIAN PERFORMANCE
OFFENSE: PROFESSIONAL MISCONDUCT

NOTES: DURING 1994, ENTERED INTO A BUSINESS

ARRANGEMENT WITH NON-PHYSICIANS WHICH VIOLATED THE PROHIBITION AGAINST THE CORPORATE PRACTICE OF MEDICINE. HE DID NOT MAINTAIN CONTROL OVER THE CLINICS AND WAS INSTRUCTED BY A NON-PHYSICIAN TO PROVIDE PRE-SIGNED BLANK PRESCRIPTIONS TO NON-LICENSED INDIVIDUALS, WHO WERE TREATING PATIENTS. SHALL PAY AN ADMINISTRATIVE PENALTY OF $7500; SHALL COOPERATE WITH THE BOARD IN VERIFYING COMPLIANCE; SHALL INFORM THE BOARD OF CHANGE OF ADDRESS WITHIN 10 DAYS.

MATTHEIS, KENNETH ROBERT MD, DATE OF BIRTH MAY 1, 1939, LICENSE NUMBER 3696 OF 107 GREENBRIAR CIRCLE, KERRVILLE, TX, WAS DISCIPLINED BY NORTH DAKOTA ON JANUARY 8, 1999
DISCIPLINARY ACTION: RESTRICTION PLACED ON LICENSE
OFFENSE: SUBSTANDARD CARE, INCOMPETENCE OR NEGLIGENCE

NOTES: ENGAGED IN A CONTINUED PATTERN OF INAPPROPRIATE CARE INVOLVING INAPPROPRIATE TREATMENT/DIAGNOSIS. SUSPENSION STAYED; SHALL NOT DIRECTLY, OR IN A SUPERVISORY CAPACITY, PERFORM ANY MEDICAL SERVICES, NOR HAVE ANY PATIENT CONTACT RELATING TO THE EXAMINATION, DIAGNOSIS, OR TREATMENT OF ANY PERSON AFFLICTED WITH A DISEASE OR INJURY.

MAURER, ANNE R MD, LICENSE NUMBER 00H3493 OF LEXINGTON, KY, WAS DISCIPLINED BY TEXAS ON APRIL 20, 1991
DISCIPLINARY ACTION: 60-MONTH PROBATION; MONITORING OF PHYSICIAN PERFORMANCE

NOTES: UPON RETURN TO PRACTICE IN TEXAS, SHALL UNDERGO COMPLETE PSYCHIATRIC EXAM AND FOLLOW RECOMMENDATIONS; SUBMIT TO ALCOHOL OR DRUG SCREENS.

MAUSKAR, ANANT N MD OF HOUSTON, TX, WAS DISCIPLINED BY DEA ON APRIL 20, 1998
DISCIPLINARY ACTION: RESTRICTION PLACED ON CONTROLLED SUBSTANCE LICENSE; MONITORING OF PHYSICIAN PERFORMANCE
OFFENSE: DISCIPLINARY ACTION BY ANOTHER STATE OR AGENCY

NOTES: ON 11/1/93 DEA REGISTRATION WAS REVOKED BASED ON THREE OCCASIONS IN 1990 AND 1991 WHEN HE PRESCRIBED TO AN UNDERCOVER OFFICER FOR NO LEGITIMATE PURPOSE; THE DEA DECISION WAS UPHELD BY THE COURT OF APPEALS ON 8/25/94. ON 10/21/94 SUBMITTED AN APPLICATION FOR REREGISTRATION IN SCHEDULES II THROUGH V; TESTIFIED SINCE THE PREVIOUS PROCEEDING HE HAS TAKEN COURSES TO MAINTAIN HIS CONTINUING MEDICAL EDUCATION INCLUDING COURSES IN PAIN MANAGEMENT WHICH ADDRESSED THE PROPER HANDLING OF CONTROLLED SUBSTANCES; TEXAS HAS REISSUED ALL CONTROLLED SUBSTANCES PRESCRIBING PRIVILEGES EXCEPT SCHEDULE II NARCOTICS. DEA REGISTRATION SHALL NOT INCLUDE SCHEDULE II NARCOTICS AND HE SHALL SUBMIT QUARTERLY LOGS OF ALL HIS HANDLING OF CONTROLLED SUBSTANCES.

MAUSKAR, ANANT NILKANTH MD OF 8300 HOMESTEAD ROAD #5, HOUSTON, TX, WAS DISCIPLINED BY DEA ON NOVEMBER 16, 1993
DISCIPLINARY ACTION: REVOCATION OF CONTROLLED SUBSTANCE LICENSE
OFFENSE: OVERPRESCRIBING OR MISPRESCRIBING DRUGS

NOTES: ARRESTED 01/23/92 IN HOUSTON, TEXAS FOR ILLEGALLY PRESCRIBING CODEINE. ALIAS ANANT MAUSKER, ANAN MAUSKAUR.

MAZIQUE, EMORY E MD, LICENSE NUMBER 00D3647 OF HOUSTON, TX, WAS DISCIPLINED BY TEXAS ON AUGUST 24, 1991
DISCIPLINARY ACTION: SURRENDER OF CONTROLLED SUBSTANCE LICENSE; 36-MONTH PROBATION
OFFENSE: OVERPRESCRIBING OR MISPRESCRIBING DRUGS

NOTES: NONTHERAPEUTIC PRESCRIBING. SUSPENSION STAYED; CONDITIONS OF PROBATION: SHALL COMPLETE A TWO WEEK PRECEPTORSHIP ON THE PREVENTION AND TREATMENT OF DRUG ABUSE; SHALL ISSUE NO PRESCRIPTIONS FOR, NOR DISTRIBUTE OR DISPENSE, SCHEDULE II THROUGH V CONTROLLED SUBSTANCES WITHOUT ANOTHER PRACTITIONER'S APPROVAL; SHALL NOT POSSESS ANY SUCH SUBSTANCES; SHALL MAINTAIN COPIES OF ALL PRESCRIPTIONS ISSUED BY THE CONCURRING MEDICAL PRACTITIONER ON HIS BEHALF FOR PATIENTS FOR ALL DRUGS; SHALL SURRENDER DEA AND DPS CONTROLLED SUBSTANCES CERTIFICATES AND SHALL NOT ATTEMPT TO REREGISTER WITHOUT PRIOR BOARD APPROVAL; SHALL APPEAR BEFORE THE BOARD TWICE A YEAR.

MCAFEE, ALPHONSO C III MD, LICENSE NUMBER 00G5963 OF SPRING, TX, WAS DISCIPLINED BY TEXAS ON AUGUST 20, 1992
DISCIPLINARY ACTION: REPRIMAND
OFFENSE: PROFESSIONAL MISCONDUCT

NOTES: OVERTREATING OF PATIENTS. ON 8/22/98 ORDER TERMINATED.

MCALLEN, CULLEN A MD, DATE OF BIRTH NOVEMBER 15, 1960, LICENSE NUMBER 0030764 OF DECATUR, GA, WAS DISCIPLINED BY COLORADO ON OCTOBER 12, 1994
DISCIPLINARY ACTION: 60-MONTH PROBATION; MONITORING OF PHYSICIAN PERFORMANCE
OFFENSE: SUBSTANCE ABUSE

NOTES: HABITUAL INTEMPERANCE OR EXCESSIVE USE OF ANY HABIT-FORMING DRUG OR CONTROLLED SUBSTANCE. FIVE YEAR PROBATION INCLUDING PRACTICE AND TREATMENT MONITORING IN ABEYANCE PENDING HIS RELOCATION TO COLORADO TO PRACTICE MEDICINE.

MCALLEN, CULLEN A MD, LICENSE NUMBER 00H3827 OF ATLANTA, GA, WAS DISCIPLINED BY TEXAS ON MAY 11, 1995
DISCIPLINARY ACTION: 60-MONTH PROBATION; RESTRICTION PLACED ON LICENSE
OFFENSE: DISCIPLINARY ACTION BY ANOTHER STATE OR AGENCY

NOTES: ON 10/12/94, COLORADO LICENSE PLACED ON PROBATION WITH RESTRICTIONS DUE TO THE ABUSE OF HALOTHANE AND ALCOHOL; REPORTS A SOBRIETY DATE OF 11/21/93; REPORTS ATTENDING AN AVERAGE OF THREE AA MEETINGS PER WEEK; RECEIVED INPATIENT SUBSTANCE ABUSE TREATMENT AT A COLORADO HOSPITAL FROM 11/2O/93 TO 12/6/93; RECEIVED OUTPATIENT TREATMENT FROM THE HOSPITAL BETWEEN 12/7/93 AND 3/9/94. SUSPENSION STAYED. PROBATION WITH TERMS: SHALL NOT PRACTICE MEDICINE IN TEXAS INVOLVING DIRECT PATIENT CARE UNTIL HE HAS TAKEN AND PASSED THE SPECIAL PURPOSE EXAMINATION; SHALL NOT PRACTICE ANESTHESIA UNTIL HE PERSONALLY APPEARS BEFORE THE BOARD AND ASKS PERMISSION; SHALL ABSTAIN FROM THE CONSUMPTION OF ALCOHOL/DRUGS IN ANY FORM UNLESS PRESCRIBED BY ANOTHER PHYSICIAN FOR A LEGITIMATE AND THERAPEUTIC PURPOSE; SHALL SUBMIT HIMSELF FOR APPROPRIATE EXAMS INCLUDING DRUG OR ALCOHOL SCREENS; SHALL SUBMIT HIMSELF FOR EVALUATION AND TREATMENT BY A BOARD-APPROVED PSYCHIATRIST AT LEAST

MONTHLY WHO SHALL SUBMIT REPORTS; SHALL PARTICIPATE IN AA'S PROGRAM NOT LESS THAN THREE TIMES A WEEK WITH QUARTERLY REPORTS TO THE BOARD; SHALL PARTICIPATE IN ACTIVITIES OF AN IMPAIRED PHYSICIAN'S GROUP AND ATTEND WEEKLY MEETINGS WITH QUARTERLY REPORTS; SHALL NOT POSSESS ALCOHOL OR CONTROLLED SUBSTANCES EXCEPT AS PROVIDED FOR BY TERMS OF THIS ORDER; SHALL SURRENDER CONTROLLED SUBSTANCES AND, ANY DRUG SAMPLES IN HIS POSSESSION; SHALL NOT TREAT OR OTHERWISE SERVE AS A PHYSICIAN, PRESCRIBE, DISPENSE OR ADMINISTER DRUGS WITH POTENTIAL FOR ABUSE TO HIMSELF OR ANY MEMBER OF HIS FAMILY; SHALL NOT TELEPHONE TO A PHARMACY A PRESCRIPTION OR REFILL FOR CONTROLLED SUBSTANCES OR ALLOW ANY INDIVIDUAL UNDER HIS SUPERVISION TO DO SO; SHALL KEEP A SEPARATE LOG OF ALL PRESCRIPTIONS WHICH SHALL BE SUBJECT TO REVIEW; SHALL MAINTAIN ADEQUATE MEDICAL RECORDS WHICH SHALL BE AVAILABLE FOR REVIEW; SHALL OBTAIN AT LEAST 50 HOURS PER YEAR OF CONTINUING MEDICAL EDUCATION; SHALL COMPLY WITH TERMS OF THE COLORADO ORDER; SHALL APPEAR BEFORE BOARD AT LEAST ONCE A YEAR OR AT BOARD REQUEST; SHALL COOPERATE WITH BOARD IN VERIFYING COMPLIANCE INCLUDING PROVIDING COPIES OF MEDICAL RELEASES UPON REQUEST; SHALL PROVIDE A COPY OF THIS ORDER TO ANYONE REQUESTING IT WITHIN 10 DAYS; SHALL GIVE A COPY OF THIS ORDER TO ANY HEALTH CARE ENTITY WHERE HE HAS PRIVILEGES; TIME PERIOD OUT OF TEXAS DOES NOT COUNT TOWARD PROBATION; SHALL INFORM BOARD OF ANY CHANGE OF ADDRESS WITHIN 10 DAYS OR IF HE LEAVES THE STATE. SHALL NOT SEEK MODIFICATION FOR ONE YEAR. ON 2/7/98 PETITION TO MODIFY ORDER GRANTED; SHALL BE ALLOWED TO PRACTICE ANESTHESIA PROVIDED THAT THERE IS A BOARD-APPROVED MONITOR ON-SITE; HIS PSYCHIATRIST SHALL DETERMINE THE TREATMENT SCHEDULE; CONTINUING MEDICAL EDUCATION HOURS IN EXCESS OF FIFTY HOURS PER YEAR SHALL BE CARRIED FORWARD FOR TWELVE MONTHS. 1/29/99 ORDER TERMINATED.

MCCALL, VICTOR EUGENE MD, LICENSE NUMBER 00D3509 OF DUNCANVILLE, TX, WAS DISCIPLINED BY TEXAS ON FEBRUARY 22, 1991
DISCIPLINARY ACTION: 120-MONTH PROBATION; REQUIRED TO TAKE ADDITIONAL MEDICAL EDUCATION

NOTES: MUST COMPLETE COURSE IN GENERAL PHARMACOLOGY; COMPLETE COURSE IN ADVANCED CARDIAC LIFE SUPPORT; RESEARCH AND WRITE A PAPER SUITABLE FOR PUBLICATION REGARDING RADIOLOGICAL TECHNICIANS AND THE PROCEDURES OR TREATMENTS THAT CAN BE DELEGATED FROM A PHYSICIAN TO A TECHNICIAN; MAINTAIN ADEQUATE MEDICAL RECORDS FOR A RADIOLOGIST ON ALL PATIENT OFFICE VISITS; ADEQUATELY SUPERVISE ALL "EMPLOYEES OR DELEGATES"; APPEAR FOR SEMIANNUAL REPORTS TO BOARD. ON 11/3/94 PROBATION TERMINATED.

MCCALL, VICTOR EUGENE MD, LICENSE NUMBER 0015667 OF 6236 INDIAN CREEK DRIVE, FORT WORTH, TX, WAS DISCIPLINED BY OKLAHOMA ON SEPTEMBER 9, 1994
DISCIPLINARY ACTION: 60-MONTH PROBATION; MONITORING OF PHYSICIAN PERFORMANCE
OFFENSE: DISCIPLINARY ACTION BY ANOTHER STATE OR AGENCY

NOTES: ON 2/22/91 THE TEXAS BOARD ISSUED AN ORDER PLACING LICENSE ON PROBATION FOR 10 YEARS WITH CONDITIONS FOR DELEGATING TO A RADIOLOGIC TECHNICIAN THE RESPONSIBILITY FOR CALCULATING A DOSAGE FOR CHLORAL HYDRATE WHICH WAS INCORRECTLY CALCULATED AND LED TO THE DEATH OF THE PATIENT. EXPECTS TEXAS TO VACATE ITS ORDER; AGREES TO SUBMIT TO PROBATION IN OKLAHOMA. CONDITIONS OF PROBATION: SHALL PROVIDE THE BOARD WITH ANY DOCUMENTATION REQUESTED RELATED TO HIS PRACTICE AND SHALL PAY COSTS.

MCCALLUM, MICHAEL H MD, LICENSE NUMBER 00G6128 OF AUSTIN, TX, WAS DISCIPLINED BY TEXAS ON AUGUST 18, 1990
DISCIPLINARY ACTION: 60-MONTH PROBATION; MONITORING OF PHYSICIAN PERFORMANCE
OFFENSE: SUBSTANCE ABUSE

NOTES: STIPULATED ORDER. MUST APPEAR BEFORE BOARD OR BOARD COMMITTEE ANNUALLY, PARTICIPATE IN AA, SUBMIT FOR APPROPRIATE EXAMINATIONS TO DETERMINE FREEDOM FROM DRUGS AND ALCOHOL, AND COMPLY WITH TERMS OF AFTER-CARE AGREEMENT WITH SUBSTANCE ABUSE CENTER.

MCCALLUM, MICHAEL H MD, LICENSE NUMBER 00G6128 OF NEW BRAUNFELS, TX, WAS DISCIPLINED BY TEXAS ON DECEMBER 4, 1991
DISCIPLINARY ACTION: 120-MONTH PROBATION; RESTRICTION PLACED ON LICENSE
OFFENSE: FAILURE TO COMPLY WITH PREVIOUS BOARD ORDER

NOTES: ON 3/23/91 HE WAS RELIEVED FROM DUTY FOR THE DAY AT BRACKENRIDGE HOSPITAL FOR BEING ON DUTY WHILE UNDER THE INFLUENCE OF ALCOHOL, AND HIS CONTRACT WITH EMCARE WAS TERMINATED IN MARCH OR EARLY APRIL, 1991; THE HOSPITAL SUSPENDED HIS PRIVILEGES; ALCOHOL USE VIOLATED TERMS OF 8/17/90 BOARD ORDER; RELAPSE WAS IN 1/91; ENTERED TREATMENT ON 3/26/91, WAS TRANSFERRED TO A DIFFERENT PROGRAM ON 4/15/91, AND WAS DISCHARGED ON 8/3/91; ALSO EXECUTED A TWO YEAR CONTINUING CARE CONTRACT WITH TALBOTT/MARSH RECOVERY CENTER AND ANOTHER WITH THE TRAVIS COUNTY MEDICAL SOCIETY. SUSPENSION STAYED; CONDITIONS OF PROBATION: SHALL CONTINUE TO PARTICIPATE IN IMPAIRED PHYSICIANS PROGRAM, WITH WRITTEN QUARTERLY REPORTS TO BOARD; SHALL CONTINUE WITH AA OR OTHER BOARD APPROVED PROGRAM, AND ATTEND AT LEAST FIVE TIMES A WEEK, WITH QUARTERLY REPORTS TO BOARD; TREATING PHYSICIAN SHALL SUBMIT QUARTERLY REPORTS TO THE BOARD; SHALL PARTICIPATE IN BIOLOGICAL ALCOHOL/DRUG SCREENS AS DIRECTED BY TREATING PHYSICIAN; FOR FIRST SIX MONTHS SHALL SUBMIT TO BODILY FLUID SCREENS AT LEAST ONCE WEEKLY, THEREAFTER SCREENS SHALL BE RANDOM; PRACTICE LIMITED TO MCKENNA HOSPITAL, WITH A SUPERVISING PHYSICIAN AND QUARTERLY REPORTS TO THE BOARD; SHALL COMPLY WITH TERMS OF CONTINUING AND AFTERCARE CONTRACTS; SHALL APPEAR BEFORE THE BOARD TWICE A YEAR; SHALL GIVE A COPY OF THIS ORDER TO ANY INSTITUTION WHERE HE HAS PRIVILEGES; SHALL COOPERATE WITH BOARD IN VERIFYING COMPLIANCE; SHALL ADVISE THE BOARD OF ANY CHANGE OF ADDRESS WITHIN 10 DAYS; TIME SPENT OUT OF TEXAS DOES NOT COUNT TOWARDS PROBATION; SHALL NOT SEEK MODIFICATION OF THE ORDER FOR ONE YEAR. ON 1/14/94 ORDER MODIFIED AS FOLLOWS: HE SHALL REQUEST A MEETING, MEET PERIODICALLY AND

PARTICIPATE IN ACTIVITIES RECOMMENDED BY A SPECIFIED MEDICAL SOCIETY COMMITTEE AND HAVE QUARTERLY WRITTEN REPORTS SUBMITTED TO THE BOARD; SHALL PARTICIPATE IN BIOLOGICAL ALCOHOL/DRUG SCREENS WHICH SHALL BE MADE AVAILABLE TO THE BOARD UPON REQUEST; HIS MEDICAL PRACTICE SHALL BE LIMITED TO TEACHING EMERGENCY MEDICINE AT LBJ AND HERMAN HOSPITALS IN HOUSTON, TEXAS; HE SHALL NOT MAINTAIN AN OFFICE PRACTICE; IF HE DOES RECEIVE APPROVAL TO PRACTICE AT ANOTHER HOSPITAL, HIS MEDICAL PRACTICE, RECORD KEEPING AND PATIENT CHARTS SHALL BE MONITORED BY A PHYSICIAN ACCEPTABLE TO THE BOARD.

MCCALLUM, MICHAEL H MD, LICENSE NUMBER G6128 OF SPRING, TX, WAS DISCIPLINED BY TEXAS ON AUGUST 9, 1997
DISCIPLINARY ACTION: 120-MONTH PROBATION; RESTRICTION PLACED ON LICENSE
OFFENSE: FAILURE TO COMPLY WITH PREVIOUS BOARD ORDER

NOTES: HIS 3/97 ALCOHOL RELAPSE VIOLATES THE 12/4/91 BOARD ORDER; HE MAINTAINS HE DID NOT PRACTICE WHILE UNDER THE INFLUENCE; HAS SUCCESSFULLY COMPLETED A REHABILITATION PROGRAM. SUSPENSION STAYED FOR PROBATION WITH FOLLOWING TERMS AND CONDITIONS: SHALL ABSTAIN FROM THE CONSUMPTION OF ALCOHOL/DRUGS IN ANY FORM UNLESS PRESCRIBED BY ANOTHER PHYSICIAN FOR A LEGITIMATE AND THERAPEUTIC PURPOSE; SHALL SUBMIT HIMSELF FOR APPROPRIATE EXAMS INCLUDING DRUG OR ALCOHOL SCREENS; SHALL NOMINATE THREE CERTIFIED PSYCHIATRISTS FOR BOARD SELECTION OF A THERAPIST AND SHALL EXPEDITIOUSLY SUBMIT HIMSELF TO EVALUATION AND TREATMENT BY THE APPROVED PRACTITIONER; SHALL CONTINUE TO RECEIVE TREATMENT FROM SPECIFIED PHYSICIAN; SHALL BE LIMITED TO TEACHING EMERGENCY MEDICINE AT SPECIFIED HOSPITALS; SHALL NOT MAINTAIN AN OFFICE PRACTICE; SHALL PARTICIPATE IN THE ACTIVITIES OF A PHYSICIAN HEALTH AND REHABILITATION COMMITTEE WITH QUARTERLY REPORTS; SHALL CONTINUE TO PARTICIPATE IN AA OR SIMILAR PROGRAM APPROVED BY THE BOARD NO LESS THAN 5 TIMES A WEEK; SHALL NOT TREAT OR OTHERWISE SERVE AS PHYSICIAN, PRESCRIBE, DISPENSE OR ADMINISTER DRUGS THAT MAY BE SUBJECT TO ABUSE TO HIMSELF OR TO ANY MEMBER OF HIS FAMILY; SHALL APPEAR BEFORE THE BOARD AT LEAST TWICE A YEAR; SHALL COOPERATE WITH THE BOARD IN VERIFYING COMPLIANCE INCLUDING PROVIDING COPIES OF MEDICAL RELEASES; SHALL GIVE A COPY OF THIS ORDER TO ANY HEALTH CARE ENTITY WHERE HE HAS PRIVILEGES; SHALL PROVIDE A COPY OF THIS ORDER TO ANYONE REQUESTING IT WITHIN 10 DAYS; TIME SPENT OUT OF TEXAS DOES NOT COUNT TOWARD PROBATION; SHALL INFORM THE BOARD OF CHANGE OF ADDRESS WITHIN 10 DAYS OR IF HE LEAVES THE STATE; SHALL NOT SEEK MODIFICATION FOR ONE YEAR.

MCCASKILL, BERNIE L MD, LICENSE NUMBER 00E9799 OF DALLAS, TX, WAS DISCIPLINED BY TEXAS ON AUGUST 20, 1992
DISCIPLINARY ACTION: REPRIMAND

NOTES: PROFESSIONAL FAILURE TO PRACTICE MEDICINE IN AN ACCEPTABLE MANNER CONSISTENT WITH PUBLIC HEALTH AND WELFARE.

MCCLELLAN, DAVID MARK MD, DATE OF BIRTH OCTOBER 30, 1953, LICENSE NUMBER 00G0476 OF 5911 FM 2100, CROSBY, TX, WAS DISCIPLINED BY TEXAS ON JANUARY 29, 1993
DISCIPLINARY ACTION: 120-MONTH PROBATION; RESTRICTION PLACED ON LICENSE
OFFENSE: SEXUAL ABUSE OF OR SEXUAL MISCONDUCT WITH A PATIENT

NOTES: FROM 9/4/91 THROUGH 9/9/91 HE BEHAVED INAPPROPRIATELY TOWARDS ONE PATIENT IN THAT HE MADE SEXUAL ADVANCES BY CALLING HER HOME ON TWO OCCASIONS. SUSPENSION STAYED. CONDITIONS OF PROBATION: SHALL SUBMIT HIMSELF FOR EVALUATION AND TREATMENT TO A BOARD APPROVED PSYCHIATRIST WITHIN 30 DAYS WITH MONTHLY REPORTS TO THE BOARD; WILL FURNISH A COPY OF THIS ORDER TO THE PSYCHIATRIST; SHALL ATTEND AT LEAST 50 HOURS PER YEAR OF CONTINUING MEDICAL EDUCATION, 10 OF WHICH SHALL BE IN RISK MANAGEMENT AND ETHICS COMBINED; SHALL APPEAR BEFORE THE BOARD TWICE A YEAR; SHALL HAVE A CHAPERONE IN ATTENDANCE AT ALL TIMES THAT HE EXAMINES FEMALE PATIENTS; SHALL GIVE A COPY OF THIS ORDER TO ANY HEALTH CARE ENTITY WHERE HE HAS PRIVILEGES; SHALL COOPERATE WITH THE BOARD IN VERIFYING COMPLIANCE; SHALL INFORM BOARD OF ADDRESS CHANGE WITHIN 10 DAYS OR IF HE LEAVES THE STATE; TIME SPENT OUT OF TEXAS DOES NOT COUNT TOWARD PROBATION. SHALL NOT SEEK MODIFICATION FOR FIVE YEARS. ON 3/5/94 ORDER MODIFIED SUCH THAT HE SUBMITS TO FOLLOW-UP TREATMENT AND EVALUATION ONCE A YEAR AND SHALL FOLLOW PSYCHIATRIST'S RECOMMENDATIONS REGARDING FURTHER CARE AND TREATMENT. ON 6/28/95 REQUEST FOR TERMINATION OF THIS ORDER DENIED. ON 1/18/97 PROBATION, WHILE NOT SUPPORTING HIS CONDUCT, BOARD ORDERED PROBATION TERMINATED BASED ON COMPLIANCE WITH CONDITIONS.

MCCLINTOCK, LAURA LEIGH DO, LICENSE NUMBER J9755 OF FORT WORTH, TX, WAS DISCIPLINED BY TEXAS ON MAY 14, 1999
DISCIPLINARY ACTION: REPRIMAND; REQUIRED TO TAKE ADDITIONAL MEDICAL EDUCATION
OFFENSE: PROFESSIONAL MISCONDUCT

NOTES: IN 2/98 SHE MET WITH A PATIENT AND HIS FATHER, AND MADE INITIAL DIAGNOSES OF DEPRESSION AND SUBSTANCE ABUSE; DURING AN INTERVIEW SHE DETERMINED THAT HE NEEDED A PERIOD OF SEPARATION AND INPATIENT TREATMENT; SHE DETERMINED THAT IT WAS IMPERATIVE THAT THE PATIENT MAINTAIN SEPARATION FROM HIS MOTHER TO ENCOURAGE GROWTH DIRECTED MALE RELATIONSHIPS; AFTER THE PATIENT WAS DISCHARGED FROM THE HOSPITAL AND AFTER HE AND HIS FAMILY HAD BEEN UNABLE TO FIND A LIVING ARRANGEMENT FOR HIM ELSEWHERE, SHE PERMITTED HIM TO LIVE AT HER RESIDENCE; SHE CONTENDS THAT THE PHYSICIAN-PATIENT RELATIONSHIP CEASED UPON HIS DISCHARGE; HOWEVER, NO TERMINATION LETTER WAS SENT AND MEDICAL RECORDS INDICATE THAT ON DISCHARGE, ON 3/9/98, FOLLOW UP WITH HER WAS REINFORCED; EXHIBITED A BREACH OF THERAPEUTIC BOUNDARIES, BY PERMITTING HER PATIENT TO STAY AT HER HOME AND JEOPARDIZED HIS RECOVERY. LICENSE LIMITED AS FOLLOWS: WITHIN 1 YEAR SHALL RESEARCH AND WRITE A PAPER SUITABLE FOR PUBLICATION OF NO LESS THAN 20 PAGES REGARDING PHYSICIAN-PATIENT BOUNDARIES AND INAPPROPRIATE INTERPERSONAL RELATIONSHIPS BETWEEN PHYSICIANS AND PATIENTS; WITHIN 1 YEAR SHALL OBTAIN A COURSE IN PATIENT BOUNDARIES OR PATIENT TRANSFERENCE ISSUES OF AT LEAST 10 HOURS IN LENGTH; SHALL COOPERATE WITH THE

BOARD IN VERIFYING COMPLIANCE; TIME SPENT OUT OF TEXAS DOES NOT COUNT TOWARD RESTRICTION; SHALL INFORM THE BOARD OF CHANGE OF ADDRESS WITHIN 10 DAYS OR IF SHE LEAVES THE STATE; SHALL NOT SEEK MODIFICATION FOR ONE YEAR.

MCCOIG, EDWARD LLOYD MD, LICENSE NUMBER F4258 OF OUSTON, TX, WAS DISCIPLINED BY TEXAS ON AUGUST 9, 1997
DISCIPLINARY ACTION: FINE
OFFENSE: NONCOMPLIANCE WITH A PROFESSIONAL RULE

NOTES: FAILED TO RESPOND TO BOARD STAFF'S REQUESTS FOR MEDICAL RECORDS AND OTHER INFORMATION RELEVANT TO A BOARD INVESTIGATION AFTER SEVERAL REQUESTS FROM 5/96 THROUGH 10/96; RECORDS WERE TURNED OVER ON 2/21/97. $500 FINE; SHALL COOPERATE WITH THE BOARD IN VERIFYING COMPLIANCE.

MCCORKLE, ALLAN JAMES MD, LICENSE NUMBER 00J0110, WAS DISCIPLINED BY TEXAS ON AUGUST 17, 1996
DISCIPLINARY ACTION: 60-MONTH PROBATION; RESTRICTION PLACED ON CONTROLLED SUBSTANCE LICENSE
OFFENSE: SUBSTANCE ABUSE

NOTES: AS RECENTLY AS SEPTEMBER 1995 ENGAGED IN THE DIVERSION AND CONSUMPTION, WITHOUT A LEGITIMATE MEDICAL PURPOSE, OF PRESCRIPTION MEDICATIONS INCLUDING HYDROCODONE AND VARIOUS BENZODIAZEPINES; HAS A PRIOR HISTORY OF POLYSUBSTANCE ABUSE INCLUDING ALCOHOL AND AMPHETAMINE ABUSE; OBTAINED INPATIENT TREATMENT FOR SUBSTANCE ABUSE DURING SEPTEMBER AND OCTOBER OF 1995 FOR ABOUT 12 DAYS FOLLOWED BY 38 DAYS OF OUTPATIENT TREATMENT; REPORTS A SOBRIETY DATE OF 10/03/95; REPORTS REGULAR PARTICIPATION IN THE PHYSICIAN'S HEALTH AND REHABILITATION PROGRAM AND REGULAR ATTENDANCE AT AA MEETINGS; UNDER THE CARE OF A PSYCHIATRIST. SUSPENSION, STAYED. PROBATION UNDER TERMS AND CONDITIONS: SHALL ABSTAIN FROM THE CONSUMPTION OF DRUGS IN ANY FORM UNLESS PRESCRIBED BY ANOTHER PHYSICIAN FOR A LEGITIMATE AND THERAPEUTIC PURPOSE; SHALL SUBMIT HIMSELF TO APPROPRIATE EXAMS INCLUDING DRUG AND ALCOHOL SCREENS; SHALL CONTINUE TO RECEIVE CARE AND TREATMENT FROM HIS TREATING PSYCHIATRIST NO LESS THAN ONCE PER MONTH WHO SHALL PROVIDE QUARTERLY REPORTS TO THE BOARD; SHALL PARTICIPATE IN AA'S PROGRAM NOT LESS THAN THREE TIMES PER WEEK WITH QUARTERLY REPORTS TO THE BOARD; SHALL PARTICIPATE IN THE ACTIVITIES OF A PHYSICIAN HEALTH AND REHABILITATION COMMITTEE AND ATTEND WEEKLY MEETINGS WITH QUARTERLY REPORTS; SHALL COMPLY WITH THE TERMS OF ANY CONTRACT FOR HOSPITAL PRIVILEGES AND SHALL REPORT TO THE BOARD ANY RESTRICTIONS; SHALL NOT POSSESS, ALCOHOL, CONTROLLED SUBSTANCES OR DANGEROUS DRUGS WITH ADDICTIVE POTENTIAL OR POTENTIAL FOR ABUSE; SHALL SURRENDER TO THE BOARD ALL SUCH SUBSTANCES INCLUDING SAMPLES; SHALL NOT TREAT OR OTHERWISE SERVE AS PHYSICIAN, PRESCRIBE, DISPENSE OR ADMINISTER DRUGS THAT MAY BE SUBJECT TO ABUSE TO HIMSELF OR TO ANY MEMBER OF HIS FAMILY; SHALL NOT PERSONALLY TELEPHONE A PHARMACY A PRESCRIPTION OR REFILL FOR CONTROLLED SUBSTANCES OR DANGEROUS DRUGS WITH ADDICTIVE POTENTIAL OR POTENTIAL FOR ABUSE OR PERMIT ANY INDIVIDUAL UNDER HIS SUPERVISION TO DO SO; SEPARATE FROM PATIENT RECORDS, SHALL MAINTAIN A COPY OF EVERY PRESCRIPTION WRITTEN FOR CONTROLLED SUBSTANCES OR DANGEROUS DRUGS WITH ADDICTIVE POTENTIAL OR POTENTIAL FOR ABUSE AND MAKE IT AVAILABLE UPON BOARD REQUEST; HIS MEDICAL PRACTICE INCLUDING ANY OFFICE AND SURGICAL PRACTICE, SHALL BE MONITORED BY A BOARD APPROVED TEXAS PHYSICIAN WHO SHALL COUNSEL HIM ON ANY PERCEIVED DEFICIENCIES, AND MAKE QUARTERLY REPORTS TO THE BOARD; SHALL MAINTAIN ADEQUATE MEDICAL RECORDS WHICH SHALL BE AVAILABLE FOR REVIEW; SHALL ATTEND AT LEAST 50 HOURS PER YEAR OF CONTINUING MEDICAL EDUCATION AT LEAST 10 OF WHICH SHALL BE IN RISK MANAGEMENT AND SUBMIT PROOF TO THE BOARD; SHALL APPEAR BEFORE THE BOARD AT LEAST TWICE PER YEAR OR UPON BOARD REQUEST; SHALL COOPERATE WITH THE BOARD IN VERIFYING COMPLIANCE INCLUDING PROVIDING COPIES OF MEDICAL RELEASES AND PEER REVIEW RECORDS UPON REQUEST; SHALL GIVE A COPY OF THIS ORDER TO ANY HEALTH CARE ENTITY WHERE HE HAS PRIVILEGES; SHALL PROVIDE A COPY OF THIS ORDER TO ANYONE REQUESTING IT WITHIN 10 DAYS; TIME PERIOD OUT OF TEXAS DOES NOT COUNT TOWARD PROBATION; SHALL INFORM THE BOARD OF CHANGE OF ADDRESS WITHIN 10 DAYS OF IF HE LEAVES THE STATE; SHALL NOT SEEK MODIFICATION FOR ONE YEAR. ON 4/4/98 ORDER MODIFIED AS FOLLOWS: TREATMENT BY HIS PHYSICIAN IS CHANGED TO REQUIRE CARE BY A BOARD-APPROVED PSYCHIATRIST;

MCCORKLE, ALLAN JAMES MD, LICENSE NUMBER J0110 OF AMARILLO, TX, WAS DISCIPLINED BY TEXAS ON AUGUST 22, 1998
DISCIPLINARY ACTION: FINE
OFFENSE: FAILURE TO COMPLY WITH PREVIOUS BOARD ORDER

NOTES: VIOLATED 8/17/96 BOARD ORDER BY NOT BEING MONITORED BY A PHYSICIAN APPROVED BY THE BOARD; ON 3/6/98 WAS INSTRUCTED TO BE IN COMPLIANCE WITHIN 30 DAYS BUT BY 6/5/98 WAS STILL NOT IN COMPLIANCE. $2,000 FINE; THE 8/17/96 ORDER REMAINS IN FULL FORCE AND EFFECT.

MCCORKLE, BRANDT HALBERT DO, DATE OF BIRTH NOVEMBER 14, 1953, LICENSE NUMBER 00F4260 OF 104 DOGWOOD LOOP, MINEOLA, TX, WAS DISCIPLINED BY TEXAS ON AUGUST 6, 1993
DISCIPLINARY ACTION: EMERGENCY SUSPENSION
OFFENSE: SUBSTANCE ABUSE

NOTES: ON 2/15/93 HE ATTEMPTED SUICIDE; DURING SUBSEQUENT HOSPITAL STAY HE UNDERWENT A PSYCHIATRIC EVALUATION IN WHICH HE ADMITTED THAT HE WAS EXPERIENCING SEVERE MOOD SWINGS FOR SEVERAL YEARS; PRIOR MEDICAL HISTORY DENOTES HISTORY OF TOURETTE'S SYNDROME FOR WHICH HE WAS TREATED WITH HALDOL; WAS HOSPITALIZED BY HIS NEUROLOGIST AND TREATED WITH TALWIN FOR ANALGESIA; BECAME HABITUATED TO THIS DRUG AND CONTINUED TO ABUSE IT; SELF MEDICATED HIMSELF WITH TENORMIN AND DYNACIRC FOR HYPERTENSION AND PROSOM FOR INSOMNIA; ON 4/29/93 HIS DOCTOR'S IMPRESSION WAS RELAPSE IN MAJOR DRUG ABUSE AND REFERRED HIM FOR INPATIENT DETOXIFICATION; ALSO PRESCRIBED MEDICATIONS TO PATIENTS HE KNEW WERE ADDICTED; THEIR RECORDS WERE VERY POOR AND DID NOT DENOTE A HISTORY AND PHYSICAL OR OTHER WORKUP.

MCCORKLE, BRANDT HALBERT DO, DATE OF BIRTH NOVEMBER 14, 1953, LICENSE NUMBER 00F4260 OF 104 DOGWOOD LOOP,

MINEOLA, TX, WAS DISCIPLINED BY TEXAS ON AUGUST 20, 1993
DISCIPLINARY ACTION: LICENSE SUSPENSION
OFFENSE: SUBSTANCE ABUSE

NOTES: INDEFINITE SUSPENSION. PRIOR TO PRACTICING SHALL OBTAIN APPROVAL OF THE BOARD; SHALL SUBMIT TO A FULL PSYCHIATRIC, PSYCHOLOGICAL AND NEUROLOGICAL EXAM PRIOR TO SEEKING APPROVAL.

MCCORKLE, BRANDT HALBERT DO, DATE OF BIRTH NOVEMBER 14, 1953 OF 1060 N PACIFIC, MINEOLA, TX, WAS DISCIPLINED BY DEA ON SEPTEMBER 27, 1993
DISCIPLINARY ACTION: SURRENDER OF CONTROLLED SUBSTANCE LICENSE
OFFENSE: DISCIPLINARY ACTION BY ANOTHER STATE OR AGENCY

NOTES: MEDICAL LICENSE SUSPENDED ON 08/06/93 IN TEXAS AND SUSPENDED INDEFINITELY ON 08/20/93. VOLUNTARY SURRENDER OF REGISTRATION ON 09/09/93.

MCCORKLE, BRANDT HALBERT DO, LICENSE NUMBER 00F4260 OF MINEOLA, TX, WAS DISCIPLINED BY TEXAS ON MARCH 3, 1995
DISCIPLINARY ACTION: 120-MONTH PROBATION; RESTRICTION PLACED ON LICENSE
OFFENSE: SUBSTANCE ABUSE

NOTES: ACTION DUE TO INTEMPERATE USE OF ALCOHOL OR DRUGS AND PRESCRIBING OR DISPENSING TO A HABITUAL USER. HAS SATISFIED THE MINIMUM REQUIREMENTS OF 8/20/93 ORDER INCLUDING A FAVORABLE REPORT FROM HIS PSYCHIATRIST, CONTINUING MEDICAL EDUCATION AND POSSIBLE EMPLOYMENT. SUSPENSION STAYED. PROBATION WITH TERMS: SHALL NOT PRACTICE MEDICINE EXCEPT AS REQUIRED FOR DUTIES AS A PHYSICIAN FOR THE COUNTY DEPARTMENT OF HEALTH OR OTHER SIMILAR INSTITUTIONAL PROGRAM IN THE DISCRETION OF THE BOARD; HIS PRACTICE SHALL BE MONITORED BY A BOARD APPROVED PHYSICIAN WHO SHALL SUBMIT QUARTERLY REPORTS TO THE BOARD; SHALL OBTAIN AT LEAST 50 HOURS PER YEAR OF CONTINUING MEDICAL EDUCATION, AT LEAST EIGHT OF WHICH SHALL BE IN ADDICTIONOLOGY/PHARMACOLOGY; SHALL APPEAR BEFORE BOARD AT LEAST TWO TIMES EACH YEAR; SHALL ABSTAIN FROM THE CONSUMPTION OF ALCOHOL/DRUGS IN ANY FORM UNLESS PRESCRIBED BY ANOTHER PHYSICIAN FOR A LEGITIMATE AND THERAPEUTIC PURPOSE; SHALL SUBMIT HIMSELF FOR APPROPRIATE EXAMS INCLUDING DRUG OR ALCOHOL SCREENS; SHALL SUBMIT HIMSELF FOR EVALUATION AND TREATMENT BY A BOARD-APPROVED PSYCHIATRIST AT LEAST ONCE A MONTH WHO SHALL SEND REPORTS TO THE BOARD; SHALL PARTICIPATE IN AA'S PROGRAM NOT LESS THAN THREE TIMES A WEEK WITH QUARTERLY REPORTS TO THE BOARD; SHALL PARTICIPATE IN ACTIVITIES OF AN IMPAIRED PHYSICIAN'S GROUP WITH QUARTERLY REPORTS; SHALL NOT TREAT OR OTHERWISE SERVE AS PHYSICIAN, PRESCRIBE, DISPENSE OR ADMINISTER DRUGS THAT MAY BE SUBJECT TO ABUSE TO HIMSELF OR ANY MEMBER OF HIS FAMILY; SHALL COOPERATE WITH THE BOARD IN VERIFYING COMPLIANCE INCLUDING PROVIDING COPIES OF MEDICAL RELEASES UPON REQUEST; TIME PERIOD OUT OF TEXAS DOES NOT COUNT TOWARD PROBATION; SHALL INFORM THE BOARD OF CHANGE OF ADDRESS WITHIN 10 DAYS OR IF HE LEAVES THE STATE. SHALL NOT SEEK MODIFICATION FOR ONE YEAR. ON 5/10/97 PETITION TO MODIFY ORDER GRANTED TO REQUIRE THAT HE SEE HIS TREATING PSYCHIATRIST ON A QUARTERLY BASIS RATHER THAN MONTHLY. ON 10/24/98 PETITION TO TERMINATE ORDER DENIED; ORDER MODIFIED DELETING LIMITATIONS OF HIS PRACTICE ONLY TO THE DALLAS COUNTY DEPARTMENT OF HEALTH, AND THAT HIS PRACTICE BE MONITORED; DELETION OF 8 HOUR REQUIREMENT OF ADDICTIONOLOGY/PHARMACOLOGY CONTINUING EDUCATION REQUIREMENTS; SHALL RECEIVE CARE AT INTERVALS RECOMMENDED BY HIS TREATING PSYCHIATRIST; SHALL BE REQUIRED TO PARTICIPATE IN AA BUT WITH NO MINIMUM TIMES OF ATTENDANCE; DELETION OF REQUIREMENT TO PARTICIPATE IN THE TEXAS OSTEOPATHIC MEDICAL ASSOCIATION PHYSICIANS ASSISTANCE PROGRAM; AND DELETION OF LIMITATIONS ON PRESCRIBING AUTHORITY.

MCCORKLE, CARTER W DO OF MINEOLA, TX, WAS DISCIPLINED BY MISSOURI ON AUGUST 2, 1990
OFFENSE: DISCIPLINARY ACTION BY ANOTHER STATE OR AGENCY

NOTES: MUST APPEAR BEFORE BOARD BEFORE RETURNING TO PRACTICE IN MISSOURI.

MCCORKLE, RICKY ALLEN MD, LICENSE NUMBER 00G7286, WAS DISCIPLINED BY TEXAS ON AUGUST 17, 1996
DISCIPLINARY ACTION: 60-MONTH RESTRICTION PLACED ON LICENSE; REQUIRED TO TAKE ADDITIONAL MEDICAL EDUCATION
OFFENSE: OVERPRESCRIBING OR MISPRESCRIBING DRUGS

NOTES: BETWEEN 1989 AND 1995 PRESCRIBED LARGE AND EXCESSIVE QUANTITIES OF CONTROLLED SUBSTANCES AND DANGEROUS DRUGS TO SOME PATIENTS, INCLUDING, BUT NOT LIMITED TO FAMILY MEMBERS AND AN EMPLOYEE, WITHOUT DOCUMENTING PROPER MEDICAL ASSESSMENTS OR WITHOUT ADEQUATELY REASSESSING THE PATIENTS TO DETERMINE WHAT EFFECTS THE PRESCRIBED MEDICATIONS WERE HAVING, AND IN SOME INSTANCES, WITHOUT ADEQUATE MEDICAL INDICATIONS AND PROPER MEDICAL DOCUMENTATION TO SUPPORT THE PRESCRIBING OF THE DRUGS; SOME OF THESE PATIENTS WERE KNOW ABUSERS OF NARCOTIC DRUGS, CONTROLLED SUBSTANCES, OR DANGEROUS DRUGS; FAILED TO CREATE AN ADEQUATE MEDICAL RECORD REGARDING THE CARE HE RENDERED TO HIS SPOUSE; ON 6/01/95 AND 11/14/95 BOARD DRUG AUDITS REVEALED SOME DEFICIENCIES WITH RESPECT TO INADEQUATE DOCUMENTATION OF THE RECEIPT AND DISPENSING OF PHARMACEUTICAL SAMPLES AND THE STORAGE OF CONTROLLED SUBSTANCES SAMPLES IN AN UNSECURED MANNER; IMPROPERLY ORDERED RITALIN FOR USE IN HIS OFFICE BY WRITING A PRESCRIPTION IN HIS NAME INSTEAD OF USING THE APPROPRIATE DEA FORM FOR SUCH USE; ADMITTED TO HAVING USED MARIJUANA ON AN INFREQUENT BASIS IN THE PAST AND NOT TO THE POINT OF INTOXICATION AND WITHOUT MEDICAL PURPOSE; REPORTED THAT HE DISCONTINUED HIS USE OF MARIJUANA IN AUGUST 1995. RESTRICTED UNDER TERMS AND CONDITIONS FOR FIVE YEARS; SHALL ABSTAIN FROM THE USE OF MARIJUANA OR ANY OTHER ILLEGAL SUBSTANCES; SHALL SUBMIT HIMSELF TO APPROPRIATE EXAMS, INCLUDING SCREENING FOR MARIJUANA OR OTHER ILLEGAL SUBSTANCES; SHALL NOT TREAT OR OTHERWISE SERVE AS PHYSICIAN, PRESCRIBE, DISPENSE, OR ADMINISTER DRUGS WITH POTENTIAL FOR ABUSE, TO HIMSELF OR HIS FAMILY AND OFFICE STAFF; SHALL ABSTAIN FROM THE CARE AND TREATMENT OF PATIENTS WHOSE PRIMARY COMPLAINT IS INTRACTABLE PAIN; SHALL MAINTAIN A LOGBOOK OF ALL PRESCRIPTIONS WRITTEN BY HIMSELF FOR DRUGS WITH ADDICTIVE POTENTIAL AND MAKE IT

AVAILABLE UPON BOARD REQUEST; SHALL REFRAIN FROM THE PRESCRIPTION OR ADMINISTRATION OF ANY DRUG FOR ANY PATIENT UNLESS THE DRUG IS MEDICALLY INDICATED AND IS PRESCRIBED IN THERAPEUTIC DOSES; SHALL CONDUCT ADEQUATE FOLLOW-UP EXAMINATIONS ON ALL PATIENTS TO DETERMINE WHETHER THE COURSE OF TREATMENT, INCLUDING THE PRESCRIBING OF DRUGS, IS APPROPRIATE; SHALL MAINTAIN ADEQUATE MEDICAL RECORDS WHICH SHALL BE AVAILABLE FOR REVIEW; SHALL OBTAIN AT LEAST 60 HOURS PER YEAR OF CONTINUING MEDICAL EDUCATION INCLUDING AT LEAST 10 HOURS IN RISK MANAGEMENT AND 10 HOURS ON ETHICS AND SUBMIT PROOF TO THE BOARD; SHALL COOPERATE WITH THE BOARD IN VERIFYING COMPLIANCE INCLUDING PROVIDING COPIES OF MEDICAL RELEASES AND PEER REVIEW RECORDS UPON REQUEST; SHALL GIVE A COPY OF THIS ORDER TO ANY HEALTH CARE ENTITY WHERE HE HAS PRIVILEGES; SHALL PROVIDE A COPY OF THIS ORDER TO ANYONE REQUESTING IT WITHIN 10 DAYS; SHALL PERSONALLY APPEAR BEFORE THE BOARD AT LEAST ONCE PER YEAR OR UPON REQUEST; TIME PERIOD OUT OF TEXAS DOES NOT COUNT TOWARD RESTRICTION; SHALL INFORM THE BOARD OF CHANGE OF ADDRESS WITHIN 10 DAYS OF IF HE LEAVES THE STATE; SHALL NOT SEEK MODIFICATION FOR ONE YEAR.

MCCORKLE, RICKY ALLEN MD, LICENSE NUMBER G7286 OF SHERMAN, TX, WAS DISCIPLINED BY TEXAS ON MAY 16, 1998
DISCIPLINARY ACTION: 60-MONTH PROBATION; RESTRICTION PLACED ON LICENSE
OFFENSE: FAILURE TO COMPLY WITH PREVIOUS BOARD ORDER

NOTES: VIOLATED 8/17/96 BOARD ORDER IN THAT HE FAILED TO OBTAIN CONTINUING MEDICAL EDUCATION REQUIRED BY THE ORDER BETWEEN 8/96 AND 8/97. SUSPENSION STAYED FOR PROBATION WITH FOLLOWING TERMS AND CONDITIONS: SHALL NOMINATE THREE CERTIFIED PSYCHIATRISTS FOR BOARD SELECTION OF A THERAPIST AND SHALL EXPEDITIOUSLY SUBMIT HIMSELF TO EVALUATION AND TREATMENT BY THE APPROVED PRACTITIONER; SHALL ABSTAIN FROM THE CONSUMPTION OF MARIJUANA OR ANY OTHER ILLEGAL SUBSTANCES; SHALL SUBMIT HIMSELF FOR APPROPRIATE EXAMS INCLUDING DRUG OR ALCOHOL SCREENS; SHALL NOT TREAT OR OTHERWISE SERVE AS PHYSICIAN, PRESCRIBE, DISPENSE OR ADMINISTER DRUGS THAT MAY BE SUBJECT TO ABUSE TO HIMSELF OR TO ANY MEMBER OF HIS FAMILY; SHALL NOT CARE FOR PATIENTS WHOSE PRIMARY COMPLAINT IS INTRACTABLE PAIN; SEPARATE FROM PATIENT RECORDS, SHALL MAINTAIN A LOGBOOK OF EVERY PRESCRIPTION WRITTEN BY HIM FOR DANGEROUS DRUGS WITH ADDICTIVE POTENTIAL WHICH SHALL BE MADE AVAILABLE FOR REVIEW; SHALL MAINTAIN ADEQUATE MEDICAL RECORDS WHICH SHALL BE AVAILABLE FOR REVIEW; SHALL OBTAIN 60 HOURS OF CONTINUING MEDICAL EDUCATION, WITH 10 HOURS IN RISK MANAGEMENT AND 10 HOUR ON ETHICS PER YEAR; SHALL COOPERATE WITH THE BOARD IN VERIFYING COMPLIANCE INCLUDING PROVIDING COPIES OF MEDICAL RELEASES AND PEER REVIEW RECORDS UPON REQUEST; SHALL GIVE A COPY OF THIS ORDER TO ANY HEALTH CARE ENTITY WHERE HE HAS PRIVILEGES; SHALL PROVIDE A COPY OF THIS ORDER TO ANYONE REQUESTING IT WITHIN 10 DAYS; TIME SPENT OUT OF TEXAS DOES NOT COUNT TOWARD PROBATION; SHALL INFORM THE BOARD OF CHANGE OF ADDRESS WITHIN 10 DAYS OR IF HE LEAVES THE STATE; SHALL NOT SEEK MODIFICATION FOR ONE YEAR; SHALL APPEAR BEFORE THE BOARD AT LEAST ONCE A YEAR.

MCCORKLE, RICKY ALLEN MD, LICENSE NUMBER G7286 OF SHERMAN, TX, WAS DISCIPLINED BY TEXAS ON AUGUST 28, 1999
DISCIPLINARY ACTION: 12-MONTH PROBATION; FINE
OFFENSE: FAILURE TO COMPLY WITH PREVIOUS BOARD ORDER

NOTES: VIOLATED 5/16/98 ORDER BY FAILING TO SUBMIT HIMSELF FOR EVALUATION AND TREATMENT BY A BOARD-APPROVED PSYCHIATRIST. PROBATION EXTENDED; $2,500 FINE.

MCDANIEL, BRIAN D DO, LICENSE NUMBER J0999 OF VICTORIA, TX, WAS DISCIPLINED BY TEXAS ON NOVEMBER 22, 1997
DISCIPLINARY ACTION: 60-MONTH RESTRICTION PLACED ON CONTROLLED SUBSTANCE LICENSE; REQUIRED TO ENTER AN IMPAIRED PHYSICIAN PROGRAM OR SUBSTANCE ABUSE TREATMENT
OFFENSE: SUBSTANCE ABUSE

NOTES: IN 1995 HE BEGAN USING HYDROCODONE AS TREATMENT FOR A PULLED MUSCLE; HE WROTE PRESCRIPTIONS FOR HYDROCODONE UNDER FICTITIOUS NAMES FOR PERSONAL USE; ACCORDING TO HIS DRUG TREATMENT RECORDS, BY 11/96 HE WAS TAKING UP TO 30 TO 40 TABLETS IN 24 HOURS; HE COMPLETED TREATMENT AND AGREED TO A 5 YEAR MONITORING CONTRACT WITH THE BEXAR COUNTY IMPAIRED PHYSICIANS COMMITTEE ON 4/24/97; HIS DISCHARGE DIAGNOSIS WAS HYDROCODONE DEPENDENCE. LICENSE LIMITED AS FOLLOWS: SHALL ABSTAIN FROM THE CONSUMPTION OF ALCOHOL/DRUGS IN ANY FORM UNLESS PRESCRIBED BY ANOTHER PHYSICIAN FOR A LEGITIMATE AND THERAPEUTIC PURPOSE; SHALL SUBMIT HIMSELF FOR APPROPRIATE EXAMS INCLUDING DRUG OR ALCOHOL SCREENS; SHALL NOMINATE THREE CERTIFIED PSYCHIATRISTS FOR BOARD SELECTION OF A THERAPIST AND SHALL EXPEDITIOUSLY SUBMIT HIMSELF TO EVALUATION AND TREATMENT BY THE APPROVED PRACTITIONER; SHALL PARTICIPATE IN THE ACTIVITIES OF A PHYSICIAN HEALTH AND REHABILITATION COMMITTEE AND ATTEND WEEKLY MEETINGS WITH QUARTERLY REPORTS; SHALL PARTICIPATE IN AA'S PROGRAM NOT LESS THAN THREE TIMES A WEEK; SHALL REPORT ON HIS ATTENDANCE; SHALL COMPLY WITH TERMS OF HIS CONTINUING CARE CONTRACT WITH QUARTERLY REPORTS; SHALL NOT TREAT OR OTHERWISE SERVE AS PHYSICIAN, PRESCRIBE, DISPENSE OR ADMINISTER DRUGS THAT MAY BE SUBJECT TO ABUSE TO HIMSELF OR TO ANY MEMBER OF HIS FAMILY; IS AUTHORIZED TO REAPPLY TO THE DEA AND THE TEXAS DEPARTMENT OF PUBLIC SAFETY FOR SCHEDULE II THROUGH V DRUGS; SHALL NOT POSSESS, ADMINISTER, DISPENSE OR PRESCRIBE ANY DRUGS WITH ADDICTIVE POTENTIAL EXCEPT FOR INPATIENTS IN A HOSPITAL SETTING; SHALL APPEAR BEFORE THE BOARD AT LEASE TWICE A YEAR; SHALL COOPERATE WITH THE BOARD IN VERIFYING COMPLIANCE INCLUDING PROVIDING COPIES OF MEDICAL RELEASES AND PEER REVIEW RECORDS UPON REQUEST; SHALL GIVE A COPY OF THIS ORDER TO ANY HEALTH CARE ENTITY WHERE HE HAS PRIVILEGES; TIME SPENT OUT OF TEXAS DOES NOT COUNT TOWARD RESTRICTION; SHALL INFORM THE BOARD OF CHANGE OF ADDRESS WITHIN 10 DAYS OR IF HE LEAVES THE STATE; SHALL NOT SEEK MODIFICATION FOR ONE YEAR.

MCDANIEL, BRIAN DEAN DO OF 2709 HOSPITAL BLVD., GRAND PRAIRIE, TX, WAS DISCIPLINED BY DEA ON DECEMBER 16, 1996
DISCIPLINARY ACTION: SURRENDER OF CONTROLLED SUBSTANCE

LICENSE

MCDONALD, HERBERT B MD, LICENSE NUMBER E5843 OF COUPEVILLE, WA, WAS DISCIPLINED BY TEXAS ON AUGUST 9, 1997
DISCIPLINARY ACTION: FINE
OFFENSE: NONCOMPLIANCE WITH A PROFESSIONAL RULE

NOTES: FAILED TO OBTAIN THE FULL 24 HOURS OF CONTINUING MEDICAL EDUCATION FROM 6/1/96 THROUGH 5/31/97 AS A PREREQUISITE TO THE ANNUAL REGISTRATION OF HIS LICENSE. HE REPORTED THAT FAILURE WAS A RESULT OF INATTENTIVENESS TO CHANGES IN THE TEXAS LAW, AND HIS MISUNDERSTANDING THE NEED FOR CREDITS. SINCE HIS DISCOVERY OF HIS DEFICIENCY, HE HAS REPORTED COMPLETION OF TEN HOURS EARNED DURING 6/27-6/28/97 AND HAS REPORTED HIS SCHEDULED ATTENDANCE FOR 17 MORE HOURS ON 9/25-9/27/97. SHALL PAY AN ADMINISTRATIVE PENALTY OF $500 AND HE WILL BE REQUIRED TO COMPLETE ALL PAST DUE CREDITS BEFORE FUTURE ISSUANCE OF A CURRENT PHYSICIAN'S PERMIT. SHALL COOPERATE WITH THE BOARD IN VERIFYING COMPLIANCE.

MCELROY, DELMER GUINN MD, LICENSE NUMBER C5792 OF NEW CANEY, TX, WAS DISCIPLINED BY TEXAS ON DECEMBER 12, 1998
DISCIPLINARY ACTION: RESTRICTION PLACED ON CONTROLLED SUBSTANCE LICENSE
OFFENSE: OVERPRESCRIBING OR MISPRESCRIBING DRUGS

NOTES: PRESCRIBED WITHOUT ADEQUATE MEDICAL INDICATION AND IN MOST CASES IN A NONTHERAPEUTIC MANNER TO SIX PATIENTS, INCLUDING ONE HABITUAL USER; FAILED TO KEEP COMPLETE AND ACCURATE MEDICAL RECORDS REGARDING THE CARE PROVIDED TO THESE PATIENTS. LICENSE LIMITED AS FOLLOWS: SHALL NOT TREAT OR OTHERWISE SERVE AS PHYSICIAN, PRESCRIBE, DISPENSE OR ADMINISTER DRUGS THAT MAY BE SUBJECT TO ABUSE TO HIMSELF OR TO ANY MEMBER OF HIS FAMILY; SHALL NOT TELEPHONE TO A PHARMACY A PRESCRIPTION OR REFILL FOR CONTROLLED SUBSTANCES OR DANGEROUS DRUGS WITH ADDICTIVE POTENTIAL OR POTENTIAL FOR ABUSE OR PERMIT ANY INDIVIDUAL UNDER HIS SUPERVISION TO DO SO; SHALL IMMEDIATELY SURRENDER HIS DEA AND TEXAS DEPARTMENT OF PUBLIC SAFETY CONTROLLED SUBSTANCE CERTIFICATES AND ALL UNUSED TRIPLICATE PRESCRIPTION FORMS; SHALL APPEAR BEFORE THE BOARD UPON REQUEST; SHALL COOPERATE WITH THE BOARD IN VERIFYING COMPLIANCE; SHALL PROVIDE A COPY OF THIS ORDER TO ANYONE REQUESTING IT WITHIN 10 DAYS; SHALL INFORM THE BOARD OF CHANGE OF ADDRESS WITHIN 10 DAYS.

MCFARLAND, BRUCE ROBIN MD, LICENSE NUMBER H3353 OF CORPUS CHRISTI, TX, WAS DISCIPLINED BY TEXAS ON AUGUST 9, 1997
DISCIPLINARY ACTION: REPRIMAND; REQUIRED TO TAKE ADDITIONAL MEDICAL EDUCATION
OFFENSE: SUBSTANCE ABUSE

NOTES: ENGAGED IN THE INTEMPERATE USE OF ALCOHOL AND DRUGS. IN 7/93, HE WAS ARRESTED FOR DWI BY THE CORPUS CHRISTI POLICE DEPARTMENT. IN 1993, HE HAD BEEN THE SUBJECT OF AN INTERVENTION BY A COUNTY MEDICAL SOCIETY'S COMMITTEE FOR PHYSICIAN HEALTH AND REHABILITATION. IN RESPONSE TO THE INTERVENTION, IN 8/93, HE ADMITTED HIMSELF TO A HOSPITAL. DRUG SCREENS WERE POSITIVE FOR CANNABINOIDS AND OPIATES. HE WAS RELEASED AFTER FOUR DAYS WITH RECOMMENDATIONS TO WORK WITH THE COUNTY MEDICAL SOCIETY COMMITTEE AND RECEIVE FOLLOW-UP CARE. MEDICAL SOCIETY COMMITTEE DISCHARGED HIM ON 7/14/94 WITH THE OPINION THAT HE WAS NOT COMMITTED ENOUGH TO WORK WITH. HE IS NOT CURRENTLY RECEIVING ANY CARE OR TREATMENT AND CANNOT RECALL A SOBRIETY DATE. LICENSE RESTRICTED FOR FIVE YEARS UNDER THE FOLLOWING TERMS: SHALL ABSTAIN FROM THE CONSUMPTION OF ALCOHOL/DRUGS IN ANY FORM UNLESS PRESCRIBED BY ANOTHER PHYSICIAN FOR A LEGITIMATE AND THERAPEUTIC PURPOSE; SHALL SUBMIT HIMSELF FOR APPROPRIATE EXAMS INCLUDING DRUG OR ALCOHOL SCREENS; SHALL NOMINATE THREE CERTIFIED PSYCHIATRISTS FOR BOARD SELECTION OF A THERAPIST AND SHALL EXPEDITIOUSLY SUBMIT HIMSELF TO EVALUATION AND TREATMENT BY THE APPROVED PRACTITIONER; SHALL PARTICIPATE IN THE ACTIVITIES OF A PHYSICIAN HEALTH AND REHABILITATION COMMITTEE AND ATTEND WEEKLY MEETINGS WITH QUARTERLY REPORTS; SHALL PARTICIPATE IN AA'S PROGRAM NOT LESS THAN THREE TIMES A WEEK; SHALL REPORT ON HIS ATTENDANCE; SHALL NOT TREAT OR OTHERWISE SERVE AS PHYSICIAN, PRESCRIBE, DISPENSE OR ADMINISTER DRUGS THAT MAY BE SUBJECT TO ABUSE TO HIMSELF OR TO ANY MEMBER OF HIS FAMILY; SEPARATE FROM PATIENT RECORDS, SHALL MAINTAIN A FILE OF EVERY PRESCRIPTION WRITTEN BY HIM FOR DANGEROUS DRUGS WITH ADDICTIVE POTENTIAL WHICH SHALL BE MADE AVAILABLE FOR REVIEW; HIS MEDICAL PRACTICE SHALL BE MONITORED BY A BOARD APPROVED TEXAS PHYSICIAN WHO SHALL PROVIDE QUARTERLY REPORTS TO THE BOARD; SHALL OBTAIN AT LEAST 50 HOURS PER YEAR OF CONTINUING MEDICAL EDUCATION; WITHIN SIX MONTHS HE SHALL SUCCESSFULLY COMPLETE AN APPROVED COURSE IN PHARMACOLOGY; SHALL COOPERATE WITH THE BOARD IN VERIFYING COMPLIANCE INCLUDING PROVIDING COPIES OF MEDICAL RELEASES UPON REQUEST; SHALL APPEAR BEFORE THE BOARD UPON REQUEST; SHALL GIVE A COPY OF THIS ORDER TO ANY HEALTH CARE ENTITY WHERE HE HAS PRIVILEGES; TIME SPENT OUT OF TEXAS DOES NOT COUNT TOWARD RESTRICTION; SHALL INFORM THE BOARD OF CHANGE OF ADDRESS WITHIN 10 DAYS OR IF HE LEAVES THE STATE; SHALL NOT SEEK MODIFICATION FOR ONE YEAR.

MCFARLAND, BRUCE ROBIN MD, LICENSE NUMBER H3353 OF CORPUS CHRISTI, TX, WAS DISCIPLINED BY TEXAS ON AUGUST 28, 1999
DISCIPLINARY ACTION: 120-MONTH PROBATION; REQUIRED TO TAKE ADDITIONAL MEDICAL EDUCATION
OFFENSE: FAILURE TO COMPLY WITH PREVIOUS BOARD ORDER

NOTES: ON OR ABOUT 1/25/99 HIS URINE SPECIMEN TESTED POSITIVE FOR BENZODIAZEPINES; ON 1/27/99 HE PROVIDED NO EXPLANATION AND DENIED ANY USE OF ALCOHOL, CONTROLLED SUBSTANCES OR DANGEROUS DRUGS IN VIOLATION OF HIS 8/9/97 ORDER; ON 12/12/98 HE HAD A HAIR RESTORATION PROCEDURE IN WHICH HE WAS PROVIDED WITH VALIUM, DARVOCET, AND HYDROCODONE; HE DID NOT ADVISE THE DOCTOR WHO PERFORMED THE PROCEDURE OF HIS HISTORY OF SUBSTANCE ABUSE, AND DID NOT REQUEST THAT THE DOCTOR REPORT HIS TREATMENT TO THE BOARD; ON 1/28/99 THE DOCTOR CONFIRMED THE 12/12/98 PROCEDURE AND THE MEDICATIONS PROVIDED, AND REPORTED THAT HE WAS UNAWARE OF THE DOCTOR'S HISTORY OF SUBSTANCE ABUSE; ON 1/29/99 HE WAS ADMITTED

TO A CHEMICAL DEPENDENCE TREATMENT FACILITY. REVOCATION STAYED FOR PROBATION WITH FOLLOWING TERMS AND CONDITIONS: SHALL ABSTAIN FROM THE CONSUMPTION OF ALCOHOL/DRUGS IN ANY FORM UNLESS PRESCRIBED BY ANOTHER PHYSICIAN FOR A LEGITIMATE AND THERAPEUTIC PURPOSE; SHALL SUBMIT HIMSELF FOR APPROPRIATE EXAMS INCLUDING DRUG OR ALCOHOL SCREENS; SHALL NOMINATE THREE CERTIFIED PSYCHIATRISTS FOR BOARD SELECTION OF A THERAPIST AND SHALL EXPEDITIOUSLY SUBMIT HIMSELF TO EVALUATION AND TREATMENT BY THE APPROVED PRACTITIONER; SHALL PARTICIPATE IN THE ACTIVITIES OF A PHYSICIAN HEALTH AND REHABILITATION COMMITTEE AND ATTEND WEEKLY MEETINGS WITH QUARTERLY REPORTS; SHALL PARTICIPATE IN AA'S PROGRAM NOT LESS THAN THREE TIMES A WEEK; SHALL REPORT ON HIS ATTENDANCE; SHALL NOT TREAT OR OTHERWISE SERVE AS PHYSICIAN, PRESCRIBE, DISPENSE OR ADMINISTER DRUGS THAT MAY BE SUBJECT TO ABUSE TO HIMSELF OR TO ANY MEMBER OF HIS FAMILY; SEPARATE FROM PATIENT RECORDS, SHALL MAINTAIN A LOGBOOK OF EVERY PRESCRIPTION WRITTEN BY HIM FOR DANGEROUS DRUGS WITH ADDICTIVE POTENTIAL WHICH SHALL BE MADE AVAILABLE FOR REVIEW; BEGINNING NO LATER THAN 60 DAYS, HIS MEDICAL PRACTICE SHALL BE MONITORED BY A BOARD APPROVED TEXAS PHYSICIAN WHO SHALL PROVIDE QUARTERLY REPORTS TO THE BOARD; SHALL OBTAIN 50 HOURS PER YEAR OF CONTINUING MEDICAL EDUCATION WHICH SHALL INCLUDE COURSES IN RISK MANAGEMENT, ADDICTION, AND PHARMACOLOGY; SHALL COOPERATE WITH THE BOARD IN VERIFYING COMPLIANCE INCLUDING PROVIDING COPIES OF MEDICAL RELEASES UPON REQUEST; SHALL APPEAR BEFORE THE BOARD UPON REQUEST; WITHIN 60 DAYS, SHALL GIVE A COPY OF THIS ORDER TO ANY HEALTH CARE ENTITY WHERE HE HAS PRIVILEGES; TIME SPENT OUT OF TEXAS DOES NOT COUNT TOWARD PROBATION; SHALL INFORM THE BOARD OF CHANGE OF ADDRESS WITHIN 10 DAYS OR IF HE LEAVES THE STATE; SHALL NOT SEEK MODIFICATION FOR ONE YEAR.

MCFAUL, ROBERT B DO, LICENSE NUMBER F9800 OF SAN ANTONIO, TX, WAS DISCIPLINED BY TEXAS ON NOVEMBER 22, 1997
DISCIPLINARY ACTION: FINE

NOTES: ALLEGATIONS RAISED BY STAFF OF THE BOARD THAT WHEN THERE WAS SOME QUESTION WHERE IN THE LUNGS A CARCINOMA WAS LOCATED, HE SHOULD HAVE CANCELED A SURGERY AFTER A REVIEW OF A MEDICAL CHART; BONA FIDE DISPUTES AND CONTROVERSIES EXIST, BOTH AS TO THE FACTS AND EXTENT OF ANY ALLEGED VIOLATION, IF ANY; HE DENIES ANY WRONGDOING. $5,000 FINE; SHALL COOPERATE WITH THE BOARD IN VERIFYING COMPLIANCE.

MCFAUL, ROBERT BENTON DO, LICENSE NUMBER 3285 OF SAN ANTONIO, TX, WAS DISCIPLINED BY OHIO ON APRIL 26, 1999
DISCIPLINARY ACTION: REPRIMAND
OFFENSE: DISCIPLINARY ACTION BY ANOTHER STATE OR AGENCY

NOTES: FAILURE TO ADVISE OHIO MEDICAL BOARD ON LICENSE RENEWAL APPLICATION THAT DISCIPLINARY ACTION HAD BEEN INITIATED AGAINST HIM BY TEXAS BOARD RESULTING IN A MONETARY PENALTY.

MCGINNESS, JOHN E III MD, LICENSE NUMBER H3913 OF HOUSTON, TX, WAS DISCIPLINED BY TEXAS ON AUGUST 22, 1998
DISCIPLINARY ACTION: LICENSE SUSPENSION
OFFENSE: SUBSTANCE ABUSE

NOTES: IN 1988, AT THE TIME OF THE ISSUANCE OF HIS LICENSE, THE BOARD REQUESTED HIM TO SIGN AN AFFIDAVIT DUE TO CONCERNS REGARDING HIS USE OF ALCOHOL; HE ADMITS HE'S BEEN AN ALCOHOLIC SINCE 1988, HAS MADE SEVERAL ATTEMPTS TO ABSTAIN, AND ATTENDED AA UNTIL 1/94 AT WHICH TIME HE RELAPSED AND BEGAN TO DRINK ON A DAILY BASIS; IN 1997 HE RELAPSED AND BEGAN TO DRINK HEAVILY, UP TO 12 16-OUNCE CANS OF BEER DAILY; HE WAS UNABLE TO WORK DUE TO ALCOHOL CONSUMPTION AND DEPRESSION; IN 7/97 HE ENTERED TREATMENT; BETWEEN 11/97 & 2/98 HE TESTED POSITIVE FOR ALCOHOL ON 3 CONSECUTIVE DRUG SCREENS; ON 2/4/98 HE APPEARED BEFORE THE MEDICAL SOCIETY PHYSICIAN COUNSELING COMMITTEE IN AN INTOXICATED STATE; ON 3/25/98 WHILE STILL A PATIENT IN THE TRANSITIONAL LIVING PROGRAM, HE WAS CONFRONTED BY A COUNSELOR WHO DETECTED ALCOHOL ON HIS BREATH; ON 3/26/98 HE WAS DISCHARGED FROM THE TREATMENT CENTER DUE TO NONCOMPLIANCE; ON 5/29/98 HE SUBMITTED HIMSELF FOR TREATMENT AT THE MEN'S CENTER. SUSPENSION UNTIL HE REQUESTS TO HAVE HIS SUSPENSION STAYED OR APPEARS BEFORE THE BOARD WITH SUFFICIENT EVIDENCE THAT HE IS PHYSICALLY, MENTALLY AND OTHERWISE COMPETENT TO SAFELY PRACTICE MEDICINE INCLUDING AT A MINIMUM COMPLETE COPIES OF MEDICAL RECORDS AND REPORTS OF PSYCHOLOGICAL AND NEUROPSYCHIATRIC EVALUATIONS, INCLUDING A 96 HOUR INPATIENT EVALUATION CONDUCTED BY A BOARD-APPROVED CERTIFIED PSYCHIATRIST; SHALL COOPERATE WITH THE BOARD IN VERIFYING COMPLIANCE INCLUDING PROVIDING COPIES OF MEDICAL RELEASES UPON REQUEST; SHALL INFORM THE BOARD OF CHANGE OF ADDRESS WITHIN 10 DAYS; SHALL NOT SEEK MODIFICATION FOR ONE YEAR.

MCGONAGLE, MARTIN E MD, LICENSE NUMBER G6563 OF BROWNWOOD, TX, WAS DISCIPLINED BY TEXAS ON AUGUST 9, 1997
DISCIPLINARY ACTION: FINE; REPRIMAND
OFFENSE: NONCOMPLIANCE WITH A PROFESSIONAL RULE

NOTES: FAILED TO ADEQUATELY DOCUMENT THE MEDICAL CARE HE PROVIDED TO 11 PATIENTS; FAILED TO KEEP A PROPER DRUG INVENTORY; FAILED TO MAINTAIN COMPLETE AND ACCURATE RECORDS OF PURCHASES AND DISPOSALS OF DRUGS; AND FAILED TO MAINTAIN A PROPER CRASH CART IN HIS OFFICE. $10,000 FINE; SHALL GIVE A COPY OF THIS ORDER TO ANY HEALTH CARE ENTITY WHERE HE HAS PRIVILEGES.

MCGREGOR, SCOTT DUNCAN DO, DATE OF BIRTH SEPTEMBER 5, 1953 OF 2211 DANIEL WAY, CARROLLTON, TX, WAS DISCIPLINED BY MEDICARE ON SEPTEMBER 5, 1993
DISCIPLINARY ACTION: EXCLUSION FROM THE MEDICARE AND/OR MEDICAID PROGRAM
OFFENSE: NONCOMPLIANCE WITH A PROFESSIONAL RULE

NOTES: DEFAULTED ON HEALTH EDUCATION ASSISTANCE LOAN. REINSTATED ON 4/3/95.

MCGUIRE, TERENCE F MD, LICENSE NUMBER 00E5845 OF EDMONDS, WA, WAS DISCIPLINED BY TEXAS ON MARCH 4, 1995
DISCIPLINARY ACTION: REPRIMAND
OFFENSE: PROFESSIONAL MISCONDUCT

NOTES: BETWEEN 1989 AND 1991, FAILED TO MAINTAIN APPROPRIATE PHYSICIAN-PATIENT BOUNDARIES IN THE COURSE OF PSYCHIATRIC CARE OF AN ADULT

FEMALE PATIENT: ALLOWED A PERSONAL RELATIONSHIP TO DEVELOP AND CONTINUE WHICH HAD AN ADVERSE IMPACT ON PATIENT CARE AND INCLUDED INAPPROPRIATE PHYSICAL CONTACT; OVER THE COURSE OF SEVERAL YEARS, FAILED TO KEEP ADEQUATE RECORDS OF PSYCHIATRIC CARE AND COUNSELING OF VARIOUS PATIENTS; HE REPORTS HIS LACK OF DOCUMENTATION WAS INTENTIONAL IN AN EFFORT TO PROTECT THE CONFIDENTIALITY OF PATIENTS AND FAMILY MEMBERS INVOLVED IN CRITICAL WORK FOR THE GOVERNMENT.

MCINTYRE, ROBERT F MD, DATE OF BIRTH MARCH 28, 1951, LICENSE NUMBER 0033349 OF GARLAND, TX, WAS DISCIPLINED BY COLORADO ON JANUARY 20, 1994
DISCIPLINARY ACTION: 12-MONTH PROBATION; RESTRICTION PLACED ON LICENSE
OFFENSE: PHYSICAL OR MENTAL ILLNESS INHIBITING THE ABILITY TO PRACTICE WITH SKILL AND SAFETY
NOTES: PHYSICAL OR MENTAL DISABILITY ISSUES. APPLICATION FOR LICENSURE. PROBATION FOR AT LEAST ONE YEAR INCLUDING PRACTICE MONITORING; AND STIPULATION FOR PERMANENT PRACTICE RESTRICTION (LIMITED TO DISABILITY EVALUATIONS AND NONCLINICAL RISK MANAGEMENT ACTIVITIES). PROBATION IN ABEYANCE PENDING HIS RELOCATION TO COLORADO MEDICAL PRACTICE.

MCLAUGHLIN, BLAINE EDMUND MD, DATE OF BIRTH NOVEMBER 15, 1914, LICENSE NUMBER 00D7856 OF 6201 GREENWAY, FORT WORTH, TX, WAS DISCIPLINED BY TEXAS ON MARCH 26, 1993
DISCIPLINARY ACTION: SURRENDER OF LICENSE
OFFENSE: PHYSICAL OR MENTAL ILLNESS INHIBITING THE ABILITY TO PRACTICE WITH SKILL AND SAFETY
NOTES: RETIREMENT IS PERMANENT; SHALL NOT SEEK TO REACTIVATE LICENSE.

MCLAUGHLIN, BLAINE EDMUND MD, DATE OF BIRTH NOVEMBER 15, 1914 OF 800 8TH AVENUE SUITE 316, FORT WORTH, TX, WAS DISCIPLINED BY DEA ON JULY 19, 1993
DISCIPLINARY ACTION: SURRENDER OF CONTROLLED SUBSTANCE LICENSE
OFFENSE: DISCIPLINARY ACTION BY ANOTHER STATE OR AGENCY
NOTES: VOLUNTARY SURRENDER RESULTING FROM BOARD ACTION. ILL HEALTH OF PRACTITIONER.

MCLAUGHLIN, RICHARD A DR OF HOUSTON, TX, WAS DISCIPLINED BY ILLINOIS ON OCTOBER 1, 1991
DISCIPLINARY ACTION: LICENSE SUSPENSION
OFFENSE: DISCIPLINARY ACTION BY ANOTHER STATE OR AGENCY
NOTES: TEXAS LICENSE WAS DISCIPLINED FOR INADEQUATE CHARTING. INDEFINITE SUSPENSION.

MCLAUGHLIN, RICHARD A MD, DATE OF BIRTH SEPTEMBER 19, 1932, LICENSE NUMBER 00E3063 OF MARLOW HEIGHTS, MD, WAS DISCIPLINED BY TEXAS ON NOVEMBER 9, 1991
DISCIPLINARY ACTION: EMERGENCY SUSPENSION
OFFENSE: CRIMINAL CONVICTION OR PLEA OF GUILTY, NOLO CONTENDERE, OR NO CONTEST TO A CRIME
NOTES: CONVICTED IN A DISTRICT COURT OF HARRIS COUNTY, TEXAS, ON 9/10/91 OF RAPE OF A 34 YEAR OLD FEMALE PATIENT DURING A GYNECOLOGICAL EXAM IN HIS OFFICE; WAS SENTENCED TO FOUR YEARS IN THE TEXAS DEPARTMENT OF CORRECTIONS BEGINNING 9/20/91; AT THE TRIAL ANOTHER PATIENT ALSO TESTIFIED SHE HAD BEEN SEXUALLY ASSAULTED DURING A GYNECOLOGICAL EXAM. HE GAVE NOTICE OF APPEAL ON 9/20/91.

MCLAUGHLIN, RICHARD A MD, DATE OF BIRTH SEPTEMBER 19, 1932, LICENSE NUMBER 00E3063 OF MARLOW HEIGHTS, MD, WAS DISCIPLINED BY TEXAS ON AUGUST 21, 1992
DISCIPLINARY ACTION: LICENSE REVOCATION
OFFENSE: CRIMINAL CONVICTION OR PLEA OF GUILTY, NOLO CONTENDERE, OR NO CONTEST TO A CRIME
NOTES: CONVICTION OF FELONY INVOLVING MORAL TURPITUDE.

MCLAUGHLIN, RICHARD A JR MD, LICENSE NUMBER 0107914 OF 1301 FRANKLIN, HOUSTON, TX, WAS DISCIPLINED BY NEW YORK ON DECEMBER 17, 1993
DISCIPLINARY ACTION: LICENSE REVOCATION
OFFENSE: DISCIPLINARY ACTION BY ANOTHER STATE OR AGENCY
NOTES: CONVICTED OF SEXUALLY ASSAULTING A PATIENT; FOUND GUILTY OF MISCONDUCT BY THE TEXAS BOARD.

MCLAUGHLIN, RICHARD A MD, LICENSE NUMBER E3063, WAS DISCIPLINED BY TEXAS ON APRIL 2, 1998
DISCIPLINARY ACTION: DENIAL OF LICENSE REINSTATEMENT
OFFENSE: CRIMINAL CONVICTION OR PLEA OF GUILTY, NOLO CONTENDERE, OR NO CONTEST TO A CRIME
NOTES: ON 9/10/91 CONVICTED OF SEXUAL ASSAULT ON A FEMALE PATIENT, A SECOND DEGREE FELONY, DURING A GYNECOLOGICAL EXAM ON 10/25/85; DURING THE TRIAL, TWO OTHER FEMALE PATIENTS TESTIFIED THAT THEY HAD BEEN SEXUALLY ASSAULTED BY HIM DURING GYNECOLOGICAL EXAMS; HE WAS SENTENCED TO 4 YEARS IN PRISON AND SERVED 4 MONTHS IN JAIL WITH THE REMAINING TIME ON PROBATION; HE SATISFIED THE TERMS OF HIS PROBATION; HE HAS NOT PRACTICED MEDICINE IN ANY CAPACITY SINCE 1992; HE WAS UNWILLING TO TAKE THE SPEX TO DEMONSTRATE HIS COMPETENCY IN MEDICINE; SINCE TAKEN OFF PAROLE, HE HAS NOT SOUGHT ANY COUNSELING, GROUP THERAPY, OR TAKEN ANY PSYCHIATRIC OR PSYCHOLOGICAL EXAM; HAS NO RETRAINING ON PRESCRIPTION OR SURGICAL PROCEDURES.

MCLAUGHLIN, RICHARD AUSTEN MD, DATE OF BIRTH SEPTEMBER 19, 1932 OF 8701 HAMMERLY BLVD, APT 124, HOUSTON, TX, WAS DISCIPLINED BY MEDICARE ON OCTOBER 29, 1996
DISCIPLINARY ACTION: 60-MONTH EXCLUSION FROM THE MEDICARE AND/OR MEDICAID PROGRAM
OFFENSE: CRIMINAL CONVICTION OR PLEA OF GUILTY, NOLO CONTENDERE, OR NO CONTEST TO A CRIME
NOTES: CONVICTED OF A CRIME RELATED TO PATIENT ABUSE OR NEGLECT.

MCLEAN, JAMES R JR DO, LICENSE NUMBER 00D6496 OF DALLAS, TX, WAS DISCIPLINED BY TEXAS ON MAY 15, 1996
DISCIPLINARY ACTION: REQUIRED TO TAKE ADDITIONAL MEDICAL EDUCATION; MONITORING OF PHYSICIAN PERFORMANCE
OFFENSE: OVERPRESCRIBING OR MISPRESCRIBING DRUGS
NOTES: FROM APPROXIMATELY 5/93 THROUGH APPROXIMATELY 12/94, HE PRESCRIBED HYDROCODONE AND DIDREX TO AN ADULT MALE PATIENT WITHOUT ADEQUATE MEDICAL INDICATIONS AND DOCUMENTATION FOR THE AMOUNT OF MEDICATIONS PRESCRIBED; HE ACKNOWLEDGES THAT THE CARE AND RECORD KEEPING WERE DEFICIENT AND HAS STATED THAT IN RETROSPECT THE PATIENT-PHYSICIAN RELATIONSHIP SHOULD HAVE BEEN TERMINATED AND THE PATIENT

DISMISSED DUE TO NONCOMPLIANCE; MAINTAINS THAT THIS CASE AND RELATED RECORD KEEPING ARE NOT REPRESENTATIVE OF HIS USUAL PRACTICE. LICENSE RESTRICTED FOR TWO YEARS WITH TERMS AND CONDITIONS: SHALL MAINTAIN ADEQUATE MEDICAL RECORDS WHICH SHALL BE AVAILABLE FOR REVIEW; SHALL OBTAIN AT LEAST 50 HOURS PER YEAR OF CONTINUING MEDICAL EDUCATION INCLUDING AT LEAST 20 HOURS PER YEAR IN RISK MANAGEMENT/RECORD KEEPING; SHALL APPEAR BEFORE BOARD AT LEAST ONCE A YEAR; SHALL COOPERATE WITH BOARD IN VERIFYING COMPLIANCE; SHALL GIVE A COPY OF THIS ORDER TO ANY HEALTH CARE ENTITY WHERE HE HAS PRIVILEGES; SHALL PROVIDE A COPY OF THIS ORDER TO ANYONE REQUESTING IT WITHIN 10 DAYS; TIME SPENT OUT OF TEXAS DOES NOT COUNT TOWARD RESTRICTION; SHALL INFORM BOARD OF CHANGE OF ADDRESS WITHIN 10 DAYS OR IF HE LEAVES THE STATE. SHALL NOT SEEK MODIFICATION FOR ONE YEAR.

MCLEAN, JAMES R JR DO, LICENSE NUMBER D6496 OF DALLAS, TX, WAS DISCIPLINED BY TEXAS ON APRIL 4, 1998
DISCIPLINARY ACTION: 60-MONTH PROBATION; FINE
OFFENSE: PROFESSIONAL MISCONDUCT

NOTES: FAILED TO DOCUMENT THE MEDICAL RECORDS OF VARIOUS PATIENTS WHO WERE GIVEN TAKE-HOME INJECTIONS OF B-1, B-6 AND ADENOSINE PHOSPHATE FOR WEIGHT LOSS; FAILED TO DOCUMENT INSTRUCTIONS REGARDING THE INJECTIONS; FAILED TO ADEQUATELY DOCUMENT HISTORIES AND PHYSICALS; AND FAILED TO DOCUMENT VITAL SIGNS; HE STATES THAT ADENOSINE PHOSPHATE IS NO LONGER AVAILABLE FROM ANY MANUFACTURER AND WAS NOT AVAILABLE AT PHARMACIES; FAILED TO ADEQUATELY INFORM PATIENTS THE TREATMENT WAS EXPERIMENTAL; HE CONTENDS THAT HIS WEIGHT LOSS TREATMENT HAS NEVER PRODUCED ANY ADVERSE SIDE EFFECTS AND HAS BENEFITED CERTAIN PATIENTS WHO HAVE FOLLOWED HIS PROGRAM. SUSPENSION STAYED FOR PROBATION WITH FOLLOWING TERMS AND CONDITIONS: WITHIN 1 YEAR, SHALL TAKE AND PASS THE SPEX; SHALL OBTAIN 50 HOURS PER YEAR OF CONTINUING MEDICAL EDUCATION, AT LEAST 50 OF WHICH WILL BE IN FAMILY PRACTICE; $5,000 FINE; SHALL MAINTAIN ADEQUATE MEDICAL RECORDS WHICH SHALL BE AVAILABLE FOR REVIEW; SHALL INFORM PATIENTS OF ANY TREATMENT PROTOCOLS WHICH THE BOARD DETERMINES TO BE EXPERIMENTAL IN NATURE; SHALL APPEAR BEFORE THE BOARD ONCE A YEAR; SHALL COOPERATE WITH THE BOARD IN VERIFYING COMPLIANCE; SHALL GIVE A COPY OF THIS ORDER TO ANY HEALTH CARE ENTITY WHERE HE HAS PRIVILEGES; TIME SPENT OUT OF TEXAS DOES NOT COUNT TOWARD PROBATION; SHALL INFORM THE BOARD OF CHANGE OF ADDRESS WITHIN 10 DAYS OR IF HE LEAVES THE STATE; SHALL NOT SEEK MODIFICATION FOR ONE YEAR.

MCLEAN, JAMES R JR DO, LICENSE NUMBER D6496 OF DALLAS, TX, WAS DISCIPLINED BY TEXAS ON APRIL 8, 1999
DISCIPLINARY ACTION: LICENSE SUSPENSION
OFFENSE: FAILURE TO COMPLY WITH PREVIOUS BOARD ORDER

NOTES: FAILURE TO TAKE AND PASS THE SPEX AS REQUIRED BY 4/4/98 BOARD ORDER.

MCLEAN, PAUL EUGENE II MD, LICENSE NUMBER 00E2719 OF CORPUS CHRISTI, TX, WAS DISCIPLINED BY TEXAS ON AUGUST 19, 1994
DISCIPLINARY ACTION: SURRENDER OF CONTROLLED SUBSTANCE LICENSE; PROBATION
OFFENSE: SUBSTANCE ABUSE

NOTES: HE HAS SUFFERED FROM A LONG HISTORY OF CHEMICAL DEPENDENCY AND HAS SOUGHT TREATMENT SINCE 1980; LICENSE WAS SUSPENDED ON 6/11/86 AND HE SURRENDERED CONTROLLED SUBSTANCES CERTIFICATES; REQUESTED TERMINATION OF THE SUSPENSION ON 2/26/88 AND WAS DENIED; CONTINUED TO SUFFER RELAPSES FROM 1988 TO 1994; COMPLETED TREATMENT ON 2/5/93 AND HAS SINCE RETURNED FOR CONTINUING CARE VISITS, REGULARLY ATTENDS AA MEETINGS, AND FOLLOWS TWO AFTERCARE CONTRACTS; AS REQUIRED BY THE 6/11/86 ORDER HE HAS PROVIDED SUFFICIENT EVIDENCE THAT HE IS ABLE TO PRACTICE IN A MANNER CONSISTENT WITH PUBLIC WELFARE. SUSPENSION IMPOSED BY THE 1986 ORDER STAYED. CONDITIONS OF INDEFINITE PROBATION: PRACTICE RESTRICTED TO A SIX-MONTH MINI-FELLOWSHIP OR MINI-RESIDENCY WITH A BOARD-APPROVED SUPERVISOR WITH BIMONTHLY REPORTS TO THE BOARD; WITHIN ONE YEAR SHALL PASS THE SPEX EXAM; SHALL ABSTAIN FROM THE CONSUMPTION OF ALCOHOL/CHEMICAL SUBSTANCES IN ANY FORM UNLESS PRESCRIBED BY ANOTHER PHYSICIAN FOR A LEGITIMATE AND THERAPEUTIC PURPOSE; SHALL SURRENDER DEA AND TEXAS CONTROLLED SUBSTANCES CERTIFICATES AND ALL UNUSED TRIPLICATE PRESCRIPTION FORMS; SHALL NOT ATTEMPT TO REREGISTER WITHOUT PERMISSION; SEPARATE FROM PATIENT RECORDS SHALL MAINTAIN A FILE OF EVERY PRESCRIPTION WRITTEN FOR DANGEROUS DRUGS WHICH SHALL BE AVAILABLE FOR INSPECTION; SHALL NOT TREAT OR OTHERWISE SERVE AS PHYSICIAN, PRESCRIBE, DISPENSE OR ADMINISTER ANY DRUGS THAT MAY BE SUBJECT TO ABUSE TO HIMSELF OR ANY MEMBER OF HIS FAMILY; SHALL PARTICIPATE IN THE ACTIVITIES OF A PHYSICIAN HEALTH AND REHABILITATION COMMITTEE AND ATTEND WEEKLY MEETINGS WITH QUARTERLY REPORTS; SHALL FOLLOW ANY AFTERCARE CONTRACT HE HAS ENTERED INTO; SHALL CONTINUE TO PARTICIPATE IN AA'S PROGRAM NOT LESS THAN THREE TIMES A WEEK WITH QUARTERLY REPORTS TO THE BOARD; SHALL SUBMIT HIMSELF FOR APPROPRIATE EXAMS INCLUDING DRUG OR ALCOHOL SCREENS; WITHIN 30 DAYS SHALL UNDERGO A COMPLETE PHYSICAL EXAM FROM A BOARD-APPROVED PHYSICIAN AND SHALL PLACE HIMSELF UNDER THE CARE OF THIS PHYSICIAN FOR TREATMENT OF ANY CONDITION; SHALL SUBMIT HIMSELF FOR EVALUATION AND TREATMENT TO A BOARD-APPROVED PSYCHIATRIST WITH REPORTS TO THE BOARD; SHALL APPEAR BEFORE THE BOARD TWICE A YEAR; SHALL ATTEND AT LEAST 50 HOURS PER YEAR OF CONTINUING MEDICAL EDUCATION; SHALL GIVE A COPY OF THIS ORDER TO ANY HEALTH CARE ENTITY WHERE HE HAS PRIVILEGES; SHALL COOPERATE WITH THE BOARD IN VERIFYING COMPLIANCE; SHALL INFORM BOARD OF CHANGE OF ADDRESS WITHIN 10 DAYS OR IF HE LEAVES THE STATE; TIME SPENT OUT OF TEXAS SHALL NOT COUNT TOWARD PROBATION. SHALL NOT SEEK MODIFICATION FOR ONE YEAR. ON 10/13/95 ORDER MODIFIED AS FOLLOWS: HE IS AUTHORIZED TO REAPPLY TO THE DEA AND THE TEXAS DEPARTMENT OF PUBLIC SAFETY TO OBTAIN FULL PRESCRIBING AUTHORITY FOR CONTROLLED SUBSTANCES; SEPARATE FROM PATIENT RECORDS, SHALL MAINTAIN A FILE OF EVERY PRESCRIPTION WRITTEN FOR CONTROLLED SUBSTANCES WHICH SHALL BE AVAILABLE FOR REVIEW; SHALL SUBMIT HIMSELF FOR EVALUATION AND TREATMENT BY A BOARD

APPROVED PSYCHIATRIST AND FOLLOW THE PSYCHIATRIST'S RECOMMENDATIONS AND SEE HIM/HER AT LEAST MONTHLY; ALL OTHER CONDITIONS REMAIN IN EFFECT.

MCMAHAN, GRADY MARK DO OF 3400 W. WHEATLAND RD, DALLAS, TX, WAS DISCIPLINED BY DEA ON SEPTEMBER 26, 1994
DISCIPLINARY ACTION: SURRENDER OF CONTROLLED SUBSTANCE LICENSE

NOTES: IN LIEU OF PUBLIC INTEREST REVOCATION.

MCNEILL, ARCHIBALD J MD, LICENSE NUMBER 00B4282 OF DALLAS, TX, WAS DISCIPLINED BY TEXAS ON JUNE 17, 1992
DISCIPLINARY ACTION: SURRENDER OF LICENSE
OFFENSE: PHYSICAL OR MENTAL ILLNESS INHIBITING THE ABILITY TO PRACTICE WITH SKILL AND SAFETY

NOTES: INABILITY TO PRACTICE MEDICINE WITH REASONABLE SKILL AND SAFETY TO PATIENTS BY REASON OF ILLNESS. LICENSE PERMANENTLY AND VOLUNTARILY RETIRED.

MEALY, KATHERINE E MD, LICENSE NUMBER C041436 OF SAN JOSE, CA, WAS DISCIPLINED BY CALIFORNIA ON AUGUST 15, 1991
DISCIPLINARY ACTION: 2-MONTH LICENSE SUSPENSION; 58-MONTH PROBATION
OFFENSE: SUBSTANDARD CARE, INCOMPETENCE OR NEGLIGENCE

NOTES: GROSS NEGLIGENCE, INCOMPETENCE, REPEATED NEGLIGENT ACTS, EXCESSIVE USE OF DIAGNOSTIC SERVICES AT CENTER FOR WOMEN'S DISORDERS AND WEIGHT CONTROL. REVOCATION STAYED.

MEALY, KATHERINE E MD, LICENSE NUMBER 00G7688 OF SAN JOSE, CA, WAS DISCIPLINED BY TEXAS ON APRIL 10, 1992
DISCIPLINARY ACTION: SURRENDER OF LICENSE

NOTES: LICENSE VOLUNTARILY SURRENDERED IN LIEU OF FURTHER DISCIPLINARY ACTION.

MEDINA, MATIAS R MD, LICENSE NUMBER 00E9803 OF HOUSTON, TX, WAS DISCIPLINED BY TEXAS ON JANUARY 14, 1994
DISCIPLINARY ACTION: REPRIMAND; REQUIRED TO TAKE ADDITIONAL MEDICAL EDUCATION
OFFENSE: PROFESSIONAL MISCONDUCT

NOTES: FAILED TO ADEQUATELY SUPERVISE AN ACUPUNCTURIST UNDER HIS SUPERVISION; SEVERED THE RELATIONSHIP WHEN HE WAS INFORMED THERE WAS A PROBLEM. SHALL GIVE A COPY OF THIS ORDER TO ANY HEALTH CARE ENTITY WHERE HE HAS PRIVILEGES; SHALL TERMINATE ANY CURRENT SUPERVISION OF ACUPUNCTURISTS AND MUST PETITION FOR PERMISSION TO SUPERVISE ACUPUNCTURISTS IN THE FUTURE; SHALL TAKE AN ETHICS COURSE WITHIN THE NEXT YEAR; SHALL PASS THE TEXAS MEDICAL JURISPRUDENCE EXAM.

MEDINA, MATIAS R MD, LICENSE NUMBER 00E9803 OF HOUSTON, TX, WAS DISCIPLINED BY TEXAS ON JUNE 28, 1995
DISCIPLINARY ACTION: FINE; REPRIMAND
OFFENSE: PROFESSIONAL MISCONDUCT

NOTES: FAILING TO ADEQUATELY SUPERVISE THE ACTIVITIES OF THOSE ACTING UNDER HIS SUPERVISION IN THAT IN 1993 AND 1994 HE ALLOWED ANOTHER PHYSICIAN TO FILE MEDICARE/MEDICAID CLAIMS USING HIS PROVIDER NUMBER FOR PATIENTS SEEN PURPORTEDLY ONLY BY THE OTHER PHYSICIAN; PHYSICIAN USING HIS PROVIDER NUMBER DID NOT ALWAYS PERSONALLY SEE AND TREAT THE PATIENTS WHOSE PURPORTED CARE FORMED THE BASIS FOR CLAIMS FILED WITH MEDICARE/MEDICAID. SHALL PAY $5,000 FINE; SHALL PROVIDE A COPY OF THIS ORDER TO ANYONE REQUESTING IT WITHIN 10 DAYS.

MEHARRY, ROGER ALVIN MD, LICENSE NUMBER 00E5172 OF RUSK, TX, WAS DISCIPLINED BY TEXAS ON FEBRUARY 22, 1991
DISCIPLINARY ACTION: 60-MONTH PROBATION; REQUIRED TO TAKE ADDITIONAL MEDICAL EDUCATION

NOTES: MUST NOT PRESCRIBE OR ADMINISTER ANY DRUG FOR ANY PATIENT UNLESS SUCH DRUG IS THERAPEUTIC IN THE MANNER SUCH DRUG IS PRESCRIBED; LEARN AND UNDERSTAND THE POTENTIAL FOR ABUSE OF CONTROLLED SUBSTANCES AND OTHER PRESCRIPTION DRUGS; CONDUCT ADEQUATE FOLLOW-UP EXAMINATION ON ALL PATIENTS; NOT PERMIT ANY PERSON NOT LICENSED BY THIS BOARD TO TELEPHONE A PRESCRIPTION TO ANY PHARMACY ON HIS BEHALF WITHOUT FIRST PERFORMING A MEDICALLY APPROPRIATE EXAMINATION AND ARRIVING AT A DIAGNOSIS; MAINTAIN SEPARATE FILE OF EVERY PRESCRIPTION FOR CONTROLLED SUBSTANCES OR DANGEROUS DRUGS BY DATE ISSUED; COMPLETE PRECEPTORSHIP ON PREVENTION AND TREATMENT OF DRUG ABUSE; MAINTAIN ADEQUATE MEDICAL RECORDS ON ALL PATIENT OFFICE VISITS; ATTEND CONTINUING MEDICAL EDUCATION COURSES; NOT ATTEMPT TO REREGISTER FOR CONTROLLED SUBSTANCE REGISTRATION CERTIFICATES FROM DEA AND TDPS WITHOUT WRITTEN AUTHORITY FROM THE BOARD.

MEHARRY, ROGER ALVIN MD, LICENSE NUMBER 00E5172 OF RUSK, TX, WAS DISCIPLINED BY TEXAS ON JUNE 17, 1992
DISCIPLINARY ACTION: REPRIMAND
OFFENSE: NONCOMPLIANCE WITH A PROFESSIONAL RULE

NOTES: SEVERAL VIOLATIONS OF THE MEDICAL PRACTICE ACT.

MEHARRY, ROGER ALVIN MD, DATE OF BIRTH APRIL 8, 1936, LICENSE NUMBER 0031117 OF POST OFFICE BOX 516, RUSK, TX, WAS DISCIPLINED BY MICHIGAN ON JUNE 16, 1993
DISCIPLINARY ACTION: 32-MONTH PROBATION
OFFENSE: SUBSTANDARD CARE, INCOMPETENCE OR NEGLIGENCE

NOTES: NEGLIGENCE/INCOMPETENCE.

MEHARRY, ROGER ALVIN MD, LICENSE NUMBER 00E5172 OF RUSK, TX, WAS DISCIPLINED BY TEXAS ON AUGUST 19, 1994
DISCIPLINARY ACTION: 24-MONTH PROBATION; FINE
OFFENSE: SUBSTANDARD CARE, INCOMPETENCE OR NEGLIGENCE

NOTES: FAILED TO KEEP ADEQUATE RECORDS REFLECTIVE OF HIS CARE AND TREATMENT, REFERRAL AND FOLLOW-UP OF TWO PATIENTS; CONDITIONS OF THE 2/22/91 ORDER ARE EXTENDED AN ADDITIONAL TWO YEARS WITH THESE ADDITIONS: SHALL MAINTAIN ADEQUATE MEDICAL RECORDS ON ALL PATIENT OFFICE VISITS WHICH SHALL BE AVAILABLE FOR INSPECTION; SHALL PERSONALLY EXAMINE PATIENTS WHENEVER A FORM CERTIFIES A PERSONAL EXAM HAS BEEN PERFORMED, WHERE STATE LAW REQUIRES THIS OR WHERE AN INITIAL DIAGNOSIS OF PROBABLE DISEASE OR INJURY HAS BEEN MADE; SHALL PERSONALLY EXAMINE THE PATIENT DURING THE FIRST VISIT; SHALL NOT SIGN ANY PATIENT RECORD UNLESS HE HAS PERSONALLY EXAMINED THE PATIENT OR CLEARLY NOTES IN THE RECORD THAT HE HAS NOT; SHALL ATTEND AT LEAST 50 HOURS PER YEAR OF CONTINUING MEDICAL EDUCATION INCLUDING AN ADDITIONAL 10 HOURS IN

RISK MANAGEMENT AND 25 HOURS IN PHARMACOLOGY/ADDICTIONOLOGY DURING THE FIRST YEAR; SHALL APPEAR BEFORE THE BOARD ONCE A YEAR; SHALL PAY A $500 ADMINISTRATIVE PENALTY; SHALL GIVE A COPY OF THIS ORDER TO ANY HEALTH CARE ENTITY WHERE HE HAS PRIVILEGES; SHALL COOPERATE WITH THE BOARD IN VERIFYING COMPLIANCE; SHALL INFORM BOARD OF ADDRESS CHANGE WITHIN 10 DAYS OR IF HE LEAVES THE STATE; TIME SPENT OUT OF TEXAS DOES NOT COUNT TOWARD PROBATION. SHALL NOT SEEK MODIFICATION FOR ONE YEAR. ON 8/18/95 ORDER MODIFIED SO HE IS AUTHORIZED TO REAPPLY TO THE DEA AND THE TEXAS DEPARTMENT OF PUBLIC SAFETY TO OBTAIN FULL PRESCRIBING AUTHORITY FOR CONTROLLED SUBSTANCES; ALL OTHER CONDITIONS REMAIN IN EFFECT. ON 8/17/96 PROBATION TERMINATED.

MEHARRY, ROGER ALVIN MD, DATE OF BIRTH APRIL 8, 1936, LICENSE NUMBER 1031117 OF PO BOX 516, RUSK, TX, WAS DISCIPLINED BY MICHIGAN ON JULY 19, 1995
DISCIPLINARY ACTION: SURRENDER OF LICENSE
OFFENSE: FAILURE TO COMPLY WITH PREVIOUS BOARD ORDER

NOTES: PROBATION VIOLATION OF 5/93 MICHIGAN ORDER; FAILURE TO REPORT 8/19/94 TEXAS ACTION. PERMANENT SURRENDER OF LICENSE.

MEHDI, MUZAFFAR MD, LICENSE NUMBER E8071 OF DALLAS, TX, WAS DISCIPLINED BY TEXAS ON AUGUST 9, 1997
DISCIPLINARY ACTION: REPRIMAND
OFFENSE: PROVIDING FALSE INFORMATION TO THE BOARD OR OTHER HEALTH AGENCY

NOTES: BEFORE 1991 HE UTILIZED DIAGNOSTIC PROCEDURES AND ORDERED DIAGNOSTIC TESTS WITHOUT ANY OR ADEQUATE INDICATION; HE MADE DIAGNOSES OF TWO PATIENTS' CONDITIONS WITHOUT ADEQUATE INDICATION OR DOCUMENTATION IN THE PATIENTS' FILES; BILLED FOR SERVICES EITHER NOT PERFORMED OR NOT DOCUMENTED IN PATIENT FILES; HE IMPROPERLY BILLED FOR HIS SERVICES BY REPORTING SEPARATE BILLING CODES FOR SERVICES PROVIDED TO A PATIENT WHICH WERE PART OF A SINGLE PROCEDURE, BILLED A PATIENT FOR SERVICES IN EXCESS OF MEDICARE REIMBURSEMENT AFTER HAVING AGREED TO ACCEPT MEDICARE ASSIGNMENT; HE CONTENDS THAT HE HAS CORRECTED ALL OF THE DEFICIENCIES DESCRIBED ABOVE; IN 1991 HE WAS EXPELLED FROM THE DALLAS COUNTY MEDICAL SOCIETY FOR ALLEGED IMPROPER BILLING PRACTICES; SINCE 9/93 HE HAS COMPLETED 121.5 HOURS OF CONTINUING MEDICAL EDUCATION, AVERAGING 40.5 HOURS PER YEAR, INCLUDING 6 HOURS OF MEDICARE BILLING CONTINUING MEDICAL EDUCATION; HE MAINTAINS THAT HIS PRESENT EMPLOYER REQUIRES 50 HOURS PER YEAR OF CONTINUING MEDICAL EDUCATION, AND ALSO MONITORS HIS CHARTS, DAILY; HE ALSO MAINTAINS THAT HE DOES NOT HANDLE BILLING IN HIS PRESENT PROFESSIONAL CAPACITY; IN 9/92 HE ANSWERED "NO" TO THE QUESTION OF WHETHER THERE WAS ANY INVESTIGATION OR PENDING CHALLENGES TO HIS LICENSE ON HIS APPLICATION FOR REAPPOINTMENT AT CHILDREN'S MEDICAL CENTER, WHEN IN FACT HE WAS UNDER INVESTIGATION BY THE TEXAS BOARD FOR ALLEGED IMPROPER BILLING PRACTICES AND EXPULSION FROM THE DALLAS COUNTY MEDICAL SOCIETY; HE CONTENDS THAT THE QUESTION WAS MULTIFARIOUS, UNCLEAR, AND CONFUSING, PROVIDING FOR TWO DISTINCTLY DIFFERENT QUESTIONS REQUIRING A SINGLE "YES" OR "NO" ANSWER.

MEISNER, CARL ROGER MD, LICENSE NUMBER 00F0256 OF STAFFORD, TX, WAS DISCIPLINED BY TEXAS ON MAY 11, 1995
DISCIPLINARY ACTION: REPRIMAND
OFFENSE: PROFESSIONAL MISCONDUCT

NOTES: DURING 1993, HE IMPROPERLY DELEGATED MEDICAL TASKS AND DID NOT ADEQUATELY SUPERVISE AN INDIVIDUAL WHO, WHILE UNDER HIS SUPERVISION, WROTE PRESCRIPTIONS, MADE DIAGNOSES AND REFERRALS AND TREATED PATIENTS; INDIVIDUAL WAS NOT A LICENSED PHYSICIAN NOR AUTHORIZED TO PRACTICE AS A PHYSICIAN ASSISTANT; HE MAINTAINS THAT VIOLATIONS WERE DUE TO HIS MISUNDERSTANDING OF THE LAW AND INCORRECT LEGAL ADVICE. WITHIN ONE YEAR, SHALL TAKE AND PASS THE MEDICAL JURISPRUDENCE EXAMINATION.

MELCH, HERBERT R MD, LICENSE NUMBER C5450 OF FORT WORTH, TX, WAS DISCIPLINED BY TEXAS ON APRIL 10, 1999
DISCIPLINARY ACTION: RESTRICTION PLACED ON CONTROLLED SUBSTANCE LICENSE; REQUIRED TO TAKE ADDITIONAL MEDICAL EDUCATION
OFFENSE: OVERPRESCRIBING OR MISPRESCRIBING DRUGS

NOTES: A DRUG AUDIT CONDUCTED IDENTIFIED SEVERAL DEFICIENCIES: HE DID NOT HAVE AN INVENTORY OF THE CONTROLLED SUBSTANCES WHICH WERE MAINTAINED IN THE OFFICE, NOR DID HE HAVE A RECORD OF DISBURSEMENT OF ANY DRUGS; HE DID KEEP THE CONTROLLED SUBSTANCES IN A SECURED LOCKED CABINET, BUT KEPT THEM IN AN UNLOCKED SHELF BEHIND HIS DESK; HE WAS UNABLE TO PROVIDE THE MEDICAL RECORDS OF TWO PATIENTS WHO WERE IDENTIFIED BY THE INVESTIGATOR AS HAVING PRESENTED NUMEROUS PRESCRIPTIONS FOR CONTROLLED SUBSTANCES AT A PHARMACY; HE PRESCRIBED CONTROLLED SUBSTANCES TO BOTH PATIENTS OVER A PROLONGED PERIOD OF TIME; HE CLAIMS THAT THESE TWO PATIENTS STOLE THEIR MEDICAL RECORDS AND THAT HE REPORTED THE THEFTS TO THE POLICE; THE FORT WORTH POLICE WERE UNABLE TO CONFIRM A REPORT BY HIM ABOUT THE THEFTS; HE ALSO CLAIMED THAT AN OFFICE NURSE HAD PREVIOUSLY STOLEN PRESCRIPTION PADS AND THAT HE FIRED HER; AGAIN, NO POLICE REPORT EXISTED; A BOARD CONSULTANT REVIEWED THE MEDICAL RECORDS OF TWO OTHER PATIENTS WHO HAD BEEN PRESCRIBED CONTROLLED SUBSTANCES AND CONCLUDED THAT HIS MONITORING OF THE USE OF SCHEDULE II DRUGS FOR ONE OF THESE PATIENTS WAS SUBSTANDARD, AND THAT THE NUMBER AND FREQUENCY OF REFILLS AS WELL AS THE TOTAL AMOUNT FOR THE OTHER PATIENT'S PRESCRIPTIONS SEEMED TO BE EXCESSIVE. LICENSE LIMITED FOR FIVE YEARS AS FOLLOWS: SHALL NOT POSSESS, ADMINISTER, DISPENSE, OR PRESCRIBE SCHEDULE II CONTROLLED SUBSTANCES, EXCEPT AS IS MEDICALLY NECESSARY FOR TREATMENT OF INPATIENTS IN A HOSPITAL SETTING WHERE HE HAS PRIVILEGES OR PRACTICES MEDICINE; SHALL IMMEDIATELY SURRENDER ALL UNUSED TRIPLICATE PRESCRIPTION FORMS; SEPARATE FROM PATIENT RECORDS, SHALL MAINTAIN A LOGBOOK OF EVERY PRESCRIPTION WRITTEN BY HIM FOR DANGEROUS DRUGS WITH ADDICTIVE POTENTIAL WHICH SHALL BE MADE AVAILABLE FOR REVIEW; SHALL OBTAIN 50 HOURS PER YEAR OF CONTINUING MEDICAL EDUCATION; SHALL TAKE AND PASS THE SPEX WITH A SCORE OF 75 OR ABOVE WITHIN ONE YEAR; SHALL MAINTAIN ADEQUATE MEDICAL RECORDS WHICH SHALL BE

AVAILABLE FOR REVIEW; SHALL APPEAR BEFORE THE BOARD AT LEAST TWICE A YEAR FOR THE FIRST YEAR AND ONCE A YEAR THEREAFTER; SHALL COOPERATE WITH THE BOARD IN VERIFYING COMPLIANCE; SHALL ADEQUATELY SUPERVISE ALL OF HIS EMPLOYEES AND OTHERS UNDER HIS SUPERVISION; SHALL GIVE A COPY OF THIS ORDER TO ANY HEALTH CARE ENTITY WHERE HE HAS PRIVILEGES; TIME SPENT OUT OF TEXAS DOES NOT COUNT TOWARD RESTRICTION; SHALL INFORM THE BOARD OF CHANGE OF ADDRESS WITHIN 10 DAYS OR IF HE LEAVES THE STATE; SHALL NOT SEEK MODIFICATION FOR ONE YEAR.

MENDOZA, SAMUEL MD, LICENSE NUMBER 00C3777 OF ALVIN, TX, WAS DISCIPLINED BY TEXAS ON JUNE 28, 1995
DISCIPLINARY ACTION: SURRENDER OF LICENSE
OFFENSE: NONCOMPLIANCE WITH A PROFESSIONAL RULE

NOTES: ALLEGATIONS THAT HE VIOLATED THE MEDICAL PRACTICE ACT; DOES NOT ADMIT THIS. HAS NOT PRACTICED MEDICINE SINCE 1993. VOLUNTARY AND PERMANENT SURRENDER OF LICENSE IN LIEU OF FURTHER PROCEEDINGS.

MESSER, DALE L MD, LICENSE NUMBER D2740 OF ALVIN, TX, WAS DISCIPLINED BY TEXAS ON FEBRUARY 7, 1998
DISCIPLINARY ACTION: REPRIMAND; REQUIRED TO TAKE ADDITIONAL MEDICAL EDUCATION
OFFENSE: CRIMINAL CONVICTION OR PLEA OF GUILTY, NOLO CONTENDERE, OR NO CONTEST TO A CRIME

NOTES: ARRESTED AND CHARGED WITH FOUR COUNTS OF PRESCRIBING DIHYDROCODONE A SCHEDULE III NARCOTIC, FOR OTHER THAN VALID PURPOSES, AS A RESULT OF A U.S. DEA UNDERCOVER OPERATION DURING MAY, JUNE & AUGUST 1996; RECEIVED DEFERRED ADJUDICATION FOR THIS MATTER. LICENSE LIMITED FOR FIVE YEARS AS FOLLOWS: SHALL MAINTAIN ADEQUATE MEDICAL RECORDS WHICH SHALL BE AVAILABLE FOR REVIEW; SHALL NOT TREAT OR OTHERWISE SERVE AS PHYSICIAN, PRESCRIBE, DISPENSE OR ADMINISTER DRUGS THAT MAY BE SUBJECT TO ABUSE TO HIMSELF OR TO ANY MEMBER OF HIS FAMILY; SEPARATE FROM PATIENT RECORDS, SHALL MAINTAIN A LOGBOOK OF EVERY PRESCRIPTION WRITTEN BY HIM FOR DANGEROUS DRUGS WITH ADDICTIVE POTENTIAL WHICH SHALL BE MADE AVAILABLE FOR REVIEW; HIS MEDICAL PRACTICE SHALL BE MONITORED BY A BOARD APPROVED TEXAS PHYSICIAN WHO SHALL PROVIDE QUARTERLY REPORTS TO THE BOARD; SHALL OBTAIN 50 HOURS PER YEAR OF CONTINUING MEDICAL EDUCATION; SHALL COOPERATE WITH THE BOARD IN VERIFYING COMPLIANCE INCLUDING PROVIDING COPIES OF PEER REVIEW RECORDS UPON REQUEST; SHALL GIVE A COPY OF THIS ORDER TO ANY HEALTH CARE ENTITY WHERE HE HAS PRIVILEGES; SHALL PROVIDE A COPY OF THIS ORDER TO ANYONE REQUESTING IT WITHIN 10 DAYS; TIME SPENT OUT OF TEXAS DOES NOT COUNT TOWARD RESTRICTION; SHALL INFORM THE BOARD OF CHANGE OF ADDRESS WITHIN 10 DAYS OR IF HE LEAVES THE STATE; SHALL NOT SEEK MODIFICATION FOR ONE YEAR; SHALL APPEAR BEFORE THE BOARD UPON REQUEST. ON 4/10/99 THE REQUEST FOR TERMINATION OF THE ORDER WAS DENIED.

MESSINA, JOEL MICHAEL DO, LICENSE NUMBER 0002531 OF BRANDON, FL, WAS DISCIPLINED BY FLORIDA ON JUNE 1, 1990
DISCIPLINARY ACTION: RESTRICTION PLACED ON LICENSE

NOTES: CONDITIONS AND RESTRICTIONS PLACED ON LICENSE.

MESSINA, JOEL MICHAEL DO, DATE OF BIRTH SEPTEMBER 5, 1929, LICENSE NUMBER 00C5180 OF 500 VONDERBURG, BOX 1329, BRANDON, FL, WAS DISCIPLINED BY TEXAS ON JANUARY 29, 1993
DISCIPLINARY ACTION: RESTRICTION PLACED ON LICENSE
OFFENSE: DISCIPLINARY ACTION BY ANOTHER STATE OR AGENCY

NOTES: ON 7/27/90 FLORIDA BOARD RESTRICTED HIS LICENSE SUCH THAT HE COULD NOT PRACTICE OBSTETRICS OR TERMINATE PREGNANCIES FOR TWO YEARS, REPRIMANDED HIM AND FINED HIM $2,000; HE WAS ALSO PLACED UNDER SUPERVISION OF A MONITORING PHYSICIAN FOR TWO YEARS. TEXAS RESTRICTED HIS LICENSE INDEFINITELY SUCH THAT HE SHALL NOT TREAT ANY PATIENTS FOR OBSTETRICAL MATTERS OR TERMINATE PREGNANCIES; PRIOR TO PRACTICING IN TEXAS HE SHALL APPEAR BEFORE THE BOARD; SHALL GIVE A COPY OF THIS ORDER TO ANY HEALTH CARE ENTITY WHERE HE HAS PRIVILEGES; SHALL COOPERATE WITH THE BOARD IN VERIFYING COMPLIANCE; SHALL INFORM BOARD OF CHANGE OF ADDRESS WITHIN 10 DAYS OR IF HE LEAVES THE STATE; TIME SPENT OUT OF TEXAS DOES NOT COUNT TOWARD RESTRICTION.

MEZA, ALFONSO MD, LICENSE NUMBER 00E9308 OF PORT ARTHUR, TX, WAS DISCIPLINED BY TEXAS ON FEBRUARY 16, 1990
DISCIPLINARY ACTION: REQUIRED TO TAKE ADDITIONAL MEDICAL EDUCATION

NOTES: STIPULATED ORDER. SHALL PERFORM PATIENT EVALUATIONS THAT ARE CLINICALLY ADEQUATE TO SUPPORT DIAGNOSES AND MAKE TREATMENT DECISIONS AFTER DIAGNOSTIC INFORMATION OBTAINED. ORDER EFFECTIVE FOR ONE YEAR.

MICHAELIS, MICHAEL L MD OF 3555 KNICKERBOCKER ROAD, SAN ANGELO, TX, WAS DISCIPLINED BY DEA ON AUGUST 31, 1995
DISCIPLINARY ACTION: SURRENDER OF CONTROLLED SUBSTANCE LICENSE
OFFENSE: DISCIPLINARY ACTION BY ANOTHER STATE OR AGENCY

NOTES: STATE BOARD.

MICHAELIS, MICHAEL LYNN MD, LICENSE NUMBER 00H7190 OF SAN ANGELO, TX, WAS DISCIPLINED BY TEXAS ON JUNE 28, 1995
DISCIPLINARY ACTION: SURRENDER OF CONTROLLED SUBSTANCE LICENSE
OFFENSE: SUBSTANCE ABUSE

NOTES: INTEMPERATE USE OF CONTROLLED SUBSTANCES, SPECIFICALLY VICODIN. INDEFINITELY RESTRICTED FROM PRACTICING MEDICINE IN TEXAS; PRIOR TO PRACTICING IN TEXAS, SHALL APPEAR BEFORE BOARD WITH SUFFICIENT EVIDENCE THAT HE IS PHYSICALLY, MENTALLY AND OTHERWISE COMPETENT TO SAFELY PRACTICE MEDICINE INCLUDING AT A MINIMUM COPIES OF MEDICAL RECORDS AND REPORTS OF PSYCHOLOGICAL AND NEUROPSYCHIATRIC EVALUATIONS BY A BOARD-APPROVED PSYCHIATRIST; SHALL COOPERATE WITH THE BOARD IN VERIFYING COMPLIANCE INCLUDING PROVIDING COPIES OF ANY MEDICAL RELEASES UPON REQUEST; SHALL INFORM BOARD OF CHANGE OF ADDRESS WITHIN 10 DAYS; SHALL SURRENDER HIS DEA/DPS CONTROLLED SUBSTANCES CERTIFICATES; SHALL SURRENDER ALL UNUSED TRIPLICATE PRESCRIPTION FORMS AND SHALL NOT ATTEMPT TO ORDER MORE.

MICKISH, ALAN B MD, LICENSE NUMBER 00E1059 OF FORT WORTH, TX, WAS DISCIPLINED BY TEXAS ON OCTOBER 9, 1992
DISCIPLINARY ACTION: 36-MONTH PROBATION
OFFENSE: PROFESSIONAL MISCONDUCT

NOTES: COMMITTED SEVERAL VIOLATIONS OF THE MEDICAL PRACTICE ACT, INCLUDING AIDING AND ABETTING, DIRECTLY OR INDIRECTLY, THE PRACTICE OF MEDICINE BY ANY PERSON, PARTNERSHIP, ASSOCIATION, OR CORPORATION NOT DULY LICENSED TO PRACTICE MEDICINE BY THE BOARD. SUSPENSION STAYED. PROBATION ON TERMS AND CONDITIONS.

MICKISH, ALAN B MD, DATE OF BIRTH JANUARY 2, 1947, LICENSE NUMBER 0021568 OF IRVING, TX, WAS DISCIPLINED BY COLORADO ON AUGUST 20, 1993
DISCIPLINARY ACTION: REPRIMAND

MIKESKY, GREGORY R MD, DATE OF BIRTH MARCH 21, 1959 OF 511 SUMMIT STREET, SCHULENBURG, TX, WAS DISCIPLINED BY MEDICARE ON JUNE 12, 1993
DISCIPLINARY ACTION: EXCLUSION FROM THE MEDICARE AND/OR MEDICAID PROGRAM
OFFENSE: NONCOMPLIANCE WITH A PROFESSIONAL RULE

NOTES: DEFAULTED ON HEALTH EDUCATION ASSISTANCE LOAN.

MILAM, ROBERT W MD, LICENSE NUMBER GFE5383 OF CORPUS CHRISTI, TX, WAS DISCIPLINED BY CALIFORNIA ON MARCH 14, 1996
DISCIPLINARY ACTION: LICENSE REVOCATION
OFFENSE: DISCIPLINARY ACTION BY ANOTHER STATE OR AGENCY

NOTES: RESTRICTION OF HIS AUTHORITY TO PRACTICE MEDICINE BY THE UNITED STATES NAVY. DEFAULT ACTION.

MILES, PATRICK KELLY DO, LICENSE NUMBER 00D8037 OF ABELINE, TX, WAS DISCIPLINED BY TEXAS ON OCTOBER 27, 1993
DISCIPLINARY ACTION: EMERGENCY SUSPENSION
OFFENSE: PHYSICAL OR MENTAL ILLNESS INHIBITING THE ABILITY TO PRACTICE WITH SKILL AND SAFETY

NOTES: HISTORICALLY SUFFERS FROM CONFIRMED BIPOLAR DISORDER AND PROBABLE CYCLOTHYMIC DISORDER WHICH IS NOT ADEQUATELY CONTROLLED AS REPRESENTED BY BEHAVIORS AND ACTIVITIES INCLUDING THE FOLLOWING: ON 9/16/93 ATTEMPTED TO HAVE A PATIENT RELEASED WHO HAD BEEN INVOLUNTARILY COMMITTED TO A STATE HOSPITAL BECAUSE OF A CASE INVOLVING THE CHARGE OF MURDER AGAINST THE PATIENT; FROM INVOLUNTARY COMMITMENT BECAUSE OF A CASE INVOLVING MURDER; FALSE REPRESENTATIONS TO MEMBERS OF THE MEDICAL COMMUNITY AND OTHERS REGARDING HIS PROFESSIONAL EXPERIENCE AND ASSOCIATIONS; REPRESENTATIONS TO MEMBERS OF THE MEDICAL COMMUNITY WHICH DEMONSTRATE FAILURE TO MAINTAIN ADEQUATE BOUNDARIES IN PHYSICIAN-PATIENT RELATIONSHIPS; EXTREME AND INAPPROPRIATE REACTION TO NORMAL EVENTS AND CIRCUMSTANCES.

MILES, PATRICK KELLY DO, LICENSE NUMBER 00D8037 OF ABILENE, TX, WAS DISCIPLINED BY TEXAS ON MARCH 5, 1994
DISCIPLINARY ACTION: 60-MONTH PROBATION; RESTRICTION PLACED ON LICENSE
OFFENSE: PHYSICAL OR MENTAL ILLNESS INHIBITING THE ABILITY TO PRACTICE WITH SKILL AND SAFETY

NOTES: AFTER 10/27/93 EMERGENCY SUSPENSION, HE WAS EVALUATED BY A BOARD APPROVED PSYCHIATRIST ON 1/26/94 WHO MADE A DIAGNOSIS OF AN ATYPICAL CYCLOTHYMIA AND SIGNIFICANT ANXIETY BUT FELT THAT DR. MILES' CONDITION DID NOT PREVENT HIM FROM PRACTICING ALTHOUGH WITH RESTRICTIONS. FIVE YEAR SUSPENSION STAYED. CONDITIONS OF PROBATION: PRACTICE RESTRICTED TO THAT ASSOCIATED WITH A BOARD-APPROVED INSTITUTIONAL OR RESEARCH SETTING; SUPERVISOR WILL MAKE QUARTERLY REPORTS TO THE BOARD; SHALL CONTINUE TO RECEIVE TREATMENT FROM A PSYCHIATRIST WITH QUARTERLY REPORTS; SHALL APPEAR BEFORE THE BOARD ONCE A YEAR; SHALL GIVE A COPY OF THIS ORDER TO ANY HEALTH CARE ENTITY WHERE HE HAS PRIVILEGES; SHALL COOPERATE WITH THE BOARD IN VERIFYING COMPLIANCE; SHALL INFORM BOARD OF CHANGE OF ADDRESS WITHIN 10 DAYS OR IF HE LEAVES THE STATE; TIME SPENT OUT OF TEXAS DOES NOT COUNT TOWARD PROBATION. SHALL NOT SEEK MODIFICATION FOR ONE YEAR. ON 2/7/98 PETITION TO TERMINATE ORDER DENIED.

MILES, PATRICK KELLY DO, LICENSE NUMBER 0001579, WAS DISCIPLINED BY OKLAHOMA ON MARCH 17, 1994
DISCIPLINARY ACTION: 60-MONTH PROBATION; RESTRICTION PLACED ON LICENSE
OFFENSE: DISCIPLINARY ACTION BY ANOTHER STATE OR AGENCY

NOTES: ON 3/05/94 TEXAS LICENSE SANCTIONED WITH FIVE YEAR SUSPENSION STAYED AS PROBATION. IN OKLAHOMA FIVE YEAR SUSPENSION, STAYED AS PROBATION: SHALL NOT PETITION THE BOARD FOR MODIFICATION FOR AT LEAST ONE YEAR; SHALL SUBMIT TO PSYCHIATRIC EVALUATION AND TREATMENT, SHALL COMPLY WITH SAID PSYCHIATRIST'S RECOMMENDATIONS, IF ANY, REGARDING CONTINUING CARE AND TREATMENT, AND SHALL FURNISH THE BOARD WITH A COPY OF THESE RECOMMENDATIONS AND AUTHORIZE THE PSYCHIATRIST TO MAKE REPORTS TO THE BOARD; HIS PRACTICE SHALL BE RESTRICTED TO A BOARD APPROVED INSTITUTION OR RESEARCH SETTING UNDER THE SUPERVISION OF THE A MEDICAL DIRECTOR WHO SHALL MAKE QUARTERLY REPORTS; SHALL FURNISH THE BOARD WITH WRITTEN REPORTS REGARDING HIS MEDICAL CONDITION AND COMPLIANCE WITH THIS ORDER; SHALL NOTIFY THE BOARD IN WRITING OF ANY CHANGE OF ADDRESS, EMPLOYMENT, EMPLOYMENT TERMINATION OR HOSPITAL PRIVILEGE RESTRICTION AND ANY ADMINISTRATIVE PROCEEDING INITIATED AGAINST HIM BY ANY OTHER STATE OR FEDERAL REGULATORY BODY WITHIN 14 DAYS; SHALL APPEAR BEFORE THE BOARD UPON REQUEST; AGREES TO RANDOM, UNANNOUNCED VISITS FROM THE BOARD FOR OBSERVATION AND ACCESS TO ANY APPROPRIATE RECORDS, HOWEVER, THESE VISITS WILL NOT INTERRUPT HIS MEDICAL SERVICES; THE TIME PERIOD OF PROBATION SHALL NOT INCLUDE ANY PERIODS OF RESIDENCE OR PRACTICE OUTSIDE OF OKLAHOMA; SHALL INFORM THE BOARD IF HE LEAVES OKLAHOMA. ADMINISTRATIVE COSTS $435.

MILLER, VERLYN MICHAEL MD, DATE OF BIRTH APRIL 19, 1927, LICENSE NUMBER 0019579 OF P.O. BOX 381668, DUNCANVILLE, TX, WAS DISCIPLINED BY IOWA ON OCTOBER 7, 1993
DISCIPLINARY ACTION: LICENSE SUSPENSION
OFFENSE: PROFESSIONAL MISCONDUCT

NOTES: MAKING MISLEADING, DECEPTIVE, AND UNTRUE REPRESENTATION IN HIS PRACTICE OF MEDICINE. INDEFINITE SUSPENSION. REINSTATEMENT DENIED. IN 1/95 HE FILED AN APPLICATION FOR REINSTATEMENT; IN 4/95 THE BOARD ISSUED ITS PROPOSED DECISION; HE FILED AN APPEAL OF THE PROPOSED DECISION; IN LATE 2/96 HE DISMISSED THE APPEAL WHICH ALLOWED THE PROPOSED DECISION

TO BECOME A FINAL DECISION OF THE BOARD.

MIMS, ROBERT LEWIS MD, DATE OF BIRTH JUNE 11, 1955, LICENSE NUMBER 00F9827 OF 3221 OMEGA DRIVE, ARLINGTON, TX, WAS DISCIPLINED BY TEXAS ON MARCH 26, 1993
DISCIPLINARY ACTION: 60-MONTH PROBATION; REQUIRED TO TAKE ADDITIONAL MEDICAL EDUCATION
OFFENSE: SUBSTANDARD CARE, INCOMPETENCE OR NEGLIGENCE
NOTES: FROM 4/87 TO 10/90 EXCESSIVELY PRESCRIBED LOMOTIL (AVERAGE OF 200 DOSAGE UNITS PER DAY) TO A PATIENT WITHOUT ADEQUATE CONSULTATION WITH A GASTROENTEROLOGIST; ALSO FAILED TO HOSPITALIZE THE PATIENT. 5 YEAR SUSPENSION STAYED. CONDITIONS OF PROBATION: SHALL APPEAR BEFORE THE BOARD ONCE A YEAR; SHALL ATTEND AT LEAST 50 HOURS PER YEAR OF CONTINUING MEDICAL EDUCATION AND SHALL LEARN AND UNDERSTAND THE POTENTIAL FOR ABUSE OF CERTAIN PRESCRIPTION DRUGS; SHALL GIVE A COPY OF THIS ORDER TO ANY HEALTH CARE ENTITY WHERE HE HAS PRIVILEGES; SHALL COOPERATE WITH THE BOARD IN VERIFYING COMPLIANCE; SHALL INFORM BOARD OF CHANGE OF ADDRESS WITHIN 10 DAYS OR IF HE LEAVES THE STATE; TIME SPENT OUT OF TEXAS DOES NOT COUNT TOWARD PROBATION. SHALL NOT SEEK MODIFICATION FOR ONE YEAR. ON 5/11/95 BOARD GRANTED HIS PETITION FOR TERMINATION OF THIS ORDER BASED ON COMPLIANCE WITH THE TERMS OF THE ORDER.

MINOR, OFELIA M MD, LICENSE NUMBER 00D1738 OF HOUSTON, TX, WAS DISCIPLINED BY TEXAS ON MAY 17, 1994
DISCIPLINARY ACTION: SURRENDER OF LICENSE
NOTES: RETIREMENT IS PERMANENT AND SHE WILL NOT PETITION FOR REINSTATEMENT OF HER LICENSE.

MINOR, OFELIA M MD OF 2505 DORRINGTON STREET SUITE A, HOUSTON, TX, WAS DISCIPLINED BY DEA ON JULY 25, 1994
DISCIPLINARY ACTION: SURRENDER OF CONTROLLED SUBSTANCE LICENSE
OFFENSE: DISCIPLINARY ACTION BY ANOTHER STATE OR AGENCY
NOTES: STATE BOARD.

MINTON, CECIL LLOYD MD, LICENSE NUMBER C7713 OF DALLAS, TX, WAS DISCIPLINED BY TEXAS ON AUGUST 22, 1998
DISCIPLINARY ACTION: MONITORING OF PHYSICIAN PERFORMANCE
OFFENSE: NONCOMPLIANCE WITH A PROFESSIONAL RULE
NOTES: FAILED TO ADEQUATELY DOCUMENT IN A PATIENT'S CHART THE PRESCRIBING OF CONTROLLED SUBSTANCES AND THE MEDICAL INDICATION FOR SUCH DRUGS. LICENSE LIMITED FOR THREE YEARS AS FOLLOWS: SHALL NOT TREAT OR OTHERWISE SERVE AS PHYSICIAN, PRESCRIBE, DISPENSE OR ADMINISTER DRUGS THAT MAY BE SUBJECT TO ABUSE TO HIMSELF OR TO ANY MEMBER OF HIS FAMILY; WITHIN 30 DAYS SHALL TERMINATE THE PHYSICIAN-PATIENT RELATIONSHIP WITH THE PATIENT MENTIONED ABOVE, REFER HIM TO ANOTHER PHYSICIAN, AND PROVIDE SUCH SUBSEQUENT TREATING PHYSICIAN WITH A COPY OF THE BOARD ORDER; SHALL MAINTAIN ADEQUATE MEDICAL RECORDS WHICH SHALL BE AVAILABLE FOR REVIEW; SHALL COOPERATE WITH THE BOARD IN VERIFYING COMPLIANCE; TIME SPENT OUT OF TEXAS DOES NOT COUNT TOWARD RESTRICTION; SHALL INFORM THE BOARD OF CHANGE OF ADDRESS WITHIN 10 DAYS OR IF HE LEAVES THE STATE; SHALL NOT SEEK MODIFICATION FOR ONE YEAR.

MIRANDA, ROBERTO MD, LICENSE NUMBER E2740 OF SMITHVILLE, TX, WAS DISCIPLINED BY TEXAS ON MAY 14, 1999
DISCIPLINARY ACTION: 36-MONTH RESTRICTION PLACED ON LICENSE; REQUIRED TO TAKE ADDITIONAL MEDICAL EDUCATION
OFFENSE: LOSS OR RESTRICTION OF HOSPITAL PRIVILEGES
NOTES: ON 1/11/92 HE MADE A LAPAROTOMY INCISION 60 SECONDS AFTER THE ANESTHESIOLOGIST CLAIMED THAT HE PRONOUNCED THE PATIENT DEAD; HE DID NOT HAVE PERMISSION TO PERFORM AN AUTOPSY; ALSO SHOULD NOT HAVE PERFORMED THE LAPAROTOMY SINCE FAMILY HAD ASKED FOR NO RESUSCITATION; ON 2/24/92 HE WAS SUMMARILY SUSPENDED BY THE HOSPITAL FOR THE PERFORMANCE OF SURGERY AFTER PATIENT'S DEATH; SUSPENSION WAS LATER CHANGED TO A REPRIMAND; ON 4/1/93 HIS MEDICAL STAFF PRIVILEGES WERE TERMINATED AT ANOTHER HOSPITAL FOR FAILURE TO MEET AN ACCEPTABLE STANDARD OF MEDICAL PRACTICE AFTER A REVIEW OF HIS CHARTS FROM 8/92 THROUGH 3/93; ON 1/3/94, DURING SURGERY, HE CAUSED AN INJURY WHICH REQUIRED EXTENSIVE SURGICAL REPAIR; SUBSEQUENTLY, ON 2/21/94 HIS SURGICAL PRIVILEGES WERE RESTRICTED AT ANOTHER HOSPITAL AND REQUIRED THE PRESENCE OF ANOTHER SURGEON DURING ALL BILIARY CASES FOR 12 MONTHS, OR A LONGER TIME PERIOD THAT WOULD ALLOW FOR 12 CASES TO BE PROCTORED; ON 9/25/95 HE PERFORMED A BILATERAL INQUINAL HERNIA REPAIR; SUBSEQUENT TO SURGERY THE PATIENT DEVELOPED BILATERAL LOWER EXTREMITY EMBOLI; THE PATIENT'S LEGS WERE PALE IMMEDIATELY AFTER SURGERY, BUT UPON EXAMINATION BY HIM, THE LEGS WERE WARM ALL OF THE WAY TO THE FOOT; THE PATIENT WAS TRANSFERRED AND SUBSEQUENTLY REQUIRED AN AMPUTATION ABOVE THE RIGHT KNEE; THE CARE OF THE PATIENT DEMONSTRATED A LACK OF ATTENTION TO DETAILS; HE MAINTAINS THAT HE WAS NOT NOTIFIED OF THE PATIENT'S CONDITION AND AS SOON AS HE PERSONALLY OBSERVED THE PATIENT HE IMMEDIATELY TRANSFERRED THE PATIENT TO ANOTHER HOSPITAL; REVIEW OF OTHER CHARTS CONCERNING HIS SURGICAL PRACTICE INDICATES A PATTERN OF INADEQUATE DOCUMENTATION; HE INDICATES HE IS NO LONGER PRACTICING AS A SURGEON, BUT WORKS AS AN EMERGENCY ROOM PHYSICIAN. LICENSE LIMITED AS FOLLOWS: SHALL NOT PRACTICE SURGERY EXCEPT AS ALLOWED BY EMERGENCY ROOM PRIVILEGES OR OFFICE-BASED SURGICAL PROCEDURES; SHALL OBTAIN 50 HOURS PER YEAR OF CONTINUING MEDICAL EDUCATION WITH 25 HOURS IN THE AREA OF PRACTICE SPECIALTY; 25 HOURS MAY BE IN ANY COMBINATION OF GRAND ROUNDS, CASE CONFERENCES, OR ATTENDANCE AT HOSPITAL LECTURES AND SHALL NOT INCLUDE INFORMAL SELF-STUDY; WITHIN 1 YEAR SHALL TAKE AND SUCCESSFULLY COMPLETE AN ADVANCED CARDIAC LIFE SUPPORT COURSE AND AN ADVANCED TRAUMA LIFE SUPPORT COURSE AND OBTAIN CERTIFICATION; SHALL APPEAR BEFORE THE BOARD AT LEAST ONCE A YEAR; SHALL MAINTAIN ADEQUATE MEDICAL RECORDS WHICH SHALL BE AVAILABLE FOR REVIEW; SHALL COOPERATE WITH THE BOARD IN VERIFYING COMPLIANCE; TIME SPENT OUT OF TEXAS DOES NOT COUNT TOWARD RESTRICTION; SHALL INFORM THE BOARD OF CHANGE OF ADDRESS WITHIN 10 DAYS OR IF HE LEAVES THE STATE; SHALL NOT SEEK MODIFICATION FOR ONE YEAR.

MIRON, MORTON A MD, DATE OF BIRTH APRIL 30, 1938 OF 404 WEST BERLIN, TERRELL, TX, WAS DISCIPLINED BY MEDICARE ON AUGUST 17, 1994

DISCIPLINARY ACTION: EXCLUSION FROM THE MEDICARE AND/OR MEDICAID PROGRAM
OFFENSE: DISCIPLINARY ACTION BY ANOTHER STATE OR AGENCY

NOTES: LICENSE REVOKED FOR REASONS BEARING ON PROFESSIONAL PERFORMANCE.

MIRON, MORTON ARTHUR MD, DATE OF BIRTH APRIL 30, 1938, LICENSE NUMBER 00D2534 OF TERRELL, TX, WAS DISCIPLINED BY TEXAS ON AUGUST 28, 1992
DISCIPLINARY ACTION: EMERGENCY SUSPENSION
OFFENSE: PROFESSIONAL MISCONDUCT

NOTES: ALLEGATIONS OF UNPROFESSIONAL OR DISHONORABLE CONDUCT LIKELY TO DECEIVE, DEFRAUD, OR INJURE THE PUBLIC.

MIRON, MORTON ARTHUR MD, DATE OF BIRTH APRIL 30, 1938, LICENSE NUMBER 00D2534 OF 404 WEST BRIN, TERRELL, TX, WAS DISCIPLINED BY TEXAS ON JANUARY 14, 1994
DISCIPLINARY ACTION: LICENSE REVOCATION
OFFENSE: SEXUAL ABUSE OF OR SEXUAL MISCONDUCT WITH A PATIENT

NOTES: IN THE CASE OF TWO PATIENTS HE ENGAGED IN INAPPROPRIATE TOUCHING OF A SEXUAL NATURE; ACTIONS WERE INDIVIDUALLY AND COLLECTIVELY INAPPROPRIATE AND WITHOUT SUFFICIENT MEDICAL JUSTIFICATION; ONE PATIENT ARRANGED WITH TV CAMERAS TO VIDEOTAPE A 6/3/92 VISIT. ORDER WILL BECOME FINAL WHEN ALL APPEALS HAVE BEEN EXHAUSTED. HE HAS 20 DAYS TO FILE A MOTION FOR REHEARING.

MIRZATUNY, ARDASHES MD, LICENSE NUMBER 00F9830 OF TERRELL, TX, WAS DISCIPLINED BY TEXAS ON AUGUST 18, 1990
DISCIPLINARY ACTION: 72-MONTH PROBATION; RESTRICTION PLACED ON LICENSE

NOTES: STIPULATED ORDER. MUST APPEAR BEFORE BOARD TWICE ANNUALLY, CONTINUE PSYCHIATRIC TREATMENT UNTIL RELEASED BY PSYCHIATRIST, AND LIMIT HIS PRACTICE TO ADULTS.

MITCHELL, RODERICK LEE MD, LICENSE NUMBER 00F9834 OF MARSHALL, TX, WAS DISCIPLINED BY TEXAS ON JUNE 10, 1991
DISCIPLINARY ACTION: RESTRICTION PLACED ON LICENSE

NOTES: SHALL REFRAIN FROM ACCEPTING EMPLOYMENT OR ENTERING INTO CONTRACTUAL RELATIONSHIPS WHEREIN HE WOULD BE COMPENSATED TO DIAGNOSE AND/OR TREAT PATIENTS BY A LAYPERSON, CORPORATION, OR OTHER ENTITY NOT COMPRISED EXCLUSIVELY OF LICENSED PHYSICIANS, AND WHEREIN SAID PERSON OR ENTITY THEN WOULD RECEIVE AND RETAIN THE FEES PAID BY OR ON BEHALF OF PATIENTS FOR THE PHYSICIAN'S PROFESSIONAL SERVICES. ON 11/3/94 ORDER TERMINATED.

MOAYAD, HAMID DO, LICENSE NUMBER H4562 OF BEDFORD, TX, WAS DISCIPLINED BY TEXAS ON NOVEMBER 22, 1997
DISCIPLINARY ACTION: 36-MONTH RESTRICTION PLACED ON LICENSE; REQUIRED TO TAKE ADDITIONAL MEDICAL EDUCATION
OFFENSE: SUBSTANDARD CARE, INCOMPETENCE OR NEGLIGENCE

NOTES: FAILED TO ADEQUATELY TREAT AND MANAGE 7 PATIENTS SUFFERING FROM LYME DISEASE AND CHRONIC PAIN; FAILED TO INITIALLY MAKE THE DRUG LOGBOOK AVAILABLE DURING A DRUG AUDIT; FAILED TO MAINTAIN SCHEDULED DRUGS IN A LOCKED LOCATION; VARIOUS SCHEDULED DRUGS NOT ACCOUNTED FOR WERE NOTED IN THE LOGBOOK BUT NOT FOUND; HIS LOGBOOK WAS FOUND TO HAVE A NUMBER OF PAGES MISSING AND 40 MISSING BOTTLES OF TALWIN; ALL OF HIS CRASH CART DRUGS WERE EXPIRED. LICENSE LIMITED AS FOLLOWS: SHALL SEEK A SECOND OPINION ON ALL LYME DISEASE PATIENTS; SHALL NOT TREAT ANY INTRACTABLE PAIN PATIENTS; SHALL OBTAIN 50 HOURS PER YEAR OF CONTINUING MEDICAL EDUCATION WITH 10 HOURS IN LYME DISEASE OR RELATED SUBJECTS AND THE REMAINING HOURS IN NEUROLOGY; SEPARATE FROM PATIENT RECORDS, SHALL MAINTAIN A LOGBOOK OF EVERY PRESCRIPTION WRITTEN BY HIM FOR DANGEROUS DRUGS WITH ADDICTIVE POTENTIAL WHICH SHALL BE MADE AVAILABLE FOR REVIEW; SHALL APPEAR BEFORE THE BOARD AT LEAST ONCE A YEAR; SHALL COOPERATE WITH THE BOARD IN VERIFYING COMPLIANCE; SHALL GIVE A COPY OF THIS ORDER TO ANY HEALTH CARE ENTITY WHERE HE HAS PRIVILEGES; TIME SPENT OUT OF TEXAS DOES NOT COUNT TOWARD RESTRICTION; SHALL INFORM THE BOARD OF CHANGE OF ADDRESS WITHIN 10 DAYS OR IF HE LEAVES THE STATE; SHALL NOT SEEK MODIFICATION FOR ONE YEAR. ON 10/24/98 THE REQUEST FOR TERMINATION OF THE ORDER WAS DENIED; MODIFICATION OF THE ORDER WAS MADE SUCH THAT REQUESTS FOR MODIFICATION MAY BE MADE ONCE EVERY 6 MONTHS, RATHER THAN THE INITIAL 12 MONTH REQUIREMENT; ALL OTHER PROVISIONS OF THE ORDER REMAIN IN FULL EFFECT UNTIL SUPERSEDED BY A SUBSEQUENT BOARD ORDER.

MOISE, HAROLD E MD OF SAN ANTONIO, TX, WAS DISCIPLINED BY SOUTH CAROLINA ON DECEMBER 8, 1997
DISCIPLINARY ACTION: FINE; REPRIMAND
OFFENSE: OVERPRESCRIBING OR MISPRESCRIBING DRUGS

NOTES: INAPPROPRIATE PRESCRIBING FOR ONE PATIENT. $5000 FINE AND TERMS AND CONDITIONS PRIOR TO REACTIVATION.

MOISE, HAROLD EDWIN MD, DATE OF BIRTH OCTOBER 18, 1950, LICENSE NUMBER 0008476 OF 15915 WOLF CREEK, SAN ANTONIO, TX, WAS DISCIPLINED BY SOUTH CAROLINA ON JUNE 3, 1996
DISCIPLINARY ACTION: PROBATION; FINE
OFFENSE: FAILURE TO COMPLY WITH PREVIOUS BOARD ORDER

NOTES: FAILED TO SUBMIT A SPECIMEN AS REQUIRED BY INTERIM AGREEMENT. INDEFINITE SUSPENSION, STAYED AND PLACED ON PROBATION AFTER PAYMENT OF $1,000.00 FINE. TERMS AND CONDITIONS ON LICENSE.

MOLLIGAN, PATRICK FRANK MD OF LUBBOCK, TX, WAS DISCIPLINED BY LOUISIANA ON JANUARY 29, 1997
DISCIPLINARY ACTION: MONITORING OF PHYSICIAN PERFORMANCE
OFFENSE: DISCIPLINARY ACTION BY ANOTHER STATE OR AGENCY

NOTES: FRAUD, DECEIT OR PERJURY IN OBTAINING A LICENSE. PROHIBITED FROM PRACTICING MEDICINE IN LOUISIANA FOR TWO YEARS; REQUIRED TO COMPLY WITH TERMS IMPOSED ON HIS TEXAS MEDICAL LICENSE BY THE TEXAS BOARD WITH REPORTS TO THE BOARD; MUST APPEAR BEFORE THE BOARD AND PROVIDE WRITTEN NOTICE PRIOR TO FUTURE RELOCATION TO LOUISIANA.

MOLNAR, EUGENE M MD, LICENSE NUMBER 00D7193 OF NEWPORT BEACH, CA, WAS DISCIPLINED BY TEXAS ON AUGUST 24, 1991
DISCIPLINARY ACTION: 60-MONTH PROBATION
OFFENSE: DISCIPLINARY ACTION BY ANOTHER STATE OR AGENCY

NOTES: REVOCATION STAYED. BEFORE PRACTICING IN TEXAS

SHALL APPEAR BEFORE AND RECEIVE APPROVAL FROM THE TEXAS BOARD.

MOLNAR, EUGENE MICHAEL MD, LICENSE NUMBER 0015405, WAS DISCIPLINED BY ARIZONA ON APRIL 12, 1991
DISCIPLINARY ACTION: LICENSE REVOCATION
OFFENSE: DISCIPLINARY ACTION BY ANOTHER STATE OR AGENCY

NOTES: CALIFORNIA LICENSE WAS REVOKED ON 7/28/89 WITH REVOCATION STAYED TO 5 YEARS PROBATION, ALLEGING IMPROPER SURGICAL PROCEDURES AND INSURANCE FRAUD, AIDING THREE PERSONS IN THE UNAUTHORIZED PRACTICE OF NURSING, AND LYING ON A NEVADA REGISTRATION APPLICATION. ON 10/10/91 HIS REQUEST FOR A REHEARING WAS DENIED.

MOLNAR, EUGENE MICHAEL MD OF NEWPORT BEACH, CA, WAS DISCIPLINED BY ILLINOIS ON SEPTEMBER 1, 1991
DISCIPLINARY ACTION: LICENSE SUSPENSION
OFFENSE: DISCIPLINARY ACTION BY ANOTHER STATE OR AGENCY

NOTES: DISCIPLINED BY CALIFORNIA. INDEFINITE SUSPENSION.

MONROE, ELLIOT F MD OF 4000 THIRD ST, PANAMA CITY, FL, WAS DISCIPLINED BY DEA ON JULY 2, 1992
DISCIPLINARY ACTION: REVOCATION OF CONTROLLED SUBSTANCE LICENSE
OFFENSE: DISCIPLINARY ACTION BY ANOTHER STATE OR AGENCY

NOTES: ON 06/13/89 FLORIDA SUSPENDED HIS MEDICAL LICENSE AND ON 12/30/91 REVOKED IT, THEREBY TERMINATING HIS AUTHORITY TO PRESCRIBE, DISPENSE, ADMINISTER OR OTHERWISE HANDLE CONTROLLED SUBSTANCES. CURRENTLY LICENSED TO PRACTICE MEDICINE IN TEXAS.

MONROE, ELLIOT F MD OF 2236 DOGWOOD, PAMPA, TX, WAS DISCIPLINED BY DEA ON MARCH 30, 1993
DISCIPLINARY ACTION: DENIAL OF NEW LICENSE
OFFENSE: DISCIPLINARY ACTION BY ANOTHER STATE OR AGENCY

NOTES: ON 12/30/91 FLORIDA BOARD REVOKED HIS MEDICAL LICENSE DUE TO FINDINGS OF UNPROFESSIONAL CONDUCT, INCOMPETENCE AND NEGLIGENCE. ON 12/2/92 FOUND GUILTY OF KNOWINGLY AND INTENTIONALLY FURNISHING FALSE AND FRAUDULENT INFORMATION ON HIS DEA APPLICATIONS AND WAS SENTENCED TO A TERM OF THREE MONTHS INCARCERATION TO BE FOLLOWED BY A TERM OF SUPERVISED RELEASE FOR A PERIOD OF ONE YEAR.

MONROE, ELLIOT FAIL MD, LICENSE NUMBER 0019670 OF PANAMA CITY, FL, WAS DISCIPLINED BY FLORIDA ON SEPTEMBER 23, 1991
DISCIPLINARY ACTION: LICENSE REVOCATION
OFFENSE: SUBSTANDARD CARE, INCOMPETENCE OR NEGLIGENCE

NOTES: FAILURE TO PRACTICE WITH AN ACCEPTABLE LEVEL OF CARE AND SKILL; FAILING TO KEEP MEDICAL RECORDS JUSTIFYING THE COURSE OF TREATMENT OF A PATIENT.

MONROE, ELLIOT FAIL MD, LICENSE NUMBER 0019670 OF PANAMA CITY, FL, WAS DISCIPLINED BY FLORIDA ON DECEMBER 30, 1991
DISCIPLINARY ACTION: LICENSE REVOCATION
OFFENSE: SUBSTANDARD CARE, INCOMPETENCE OR NEGLIGENCE

NOTES: PRESCRIBING, DISPENSING, ADMINISTERING, MIXING, OR OTHERWISE PREPARING A LEGEND DRUG OTHER THAN IN THE COURSE OF PROFESSIONAL PRACTICE; FAILING TO PRACTICE MEDICINE WITH AN ACCEPTABLE LEVEL OF CARE AND SKILL; FAILING TO KEEP MEDICAL RECORDS JUSTIFYING THE COURSE OF TREATMENT OF A PATIENT; IMMORAL OR UNPROFESSIONAL CONDUCT, INCOMPETENCE, NEGLIGENCE, OR WILLFUL MISCONDUCT.

MONROE, ELLIOTT FAIL MD, DATE OF BIRTH JUNE 26, 1943, WAS DISCIPLINED BY MISSISSIPPI ON JULY 19, 1990
DISCIPLINARY ACTION: DENIAL OF NEW LICENSE

NOTES: LICENSE BY RECIPROCITY DENIED.

MONROE, ELLIOTT FAIL MD, DATE OF BIRTH JUNE 26, 1943 OF 2709 ARDEN AVENUE, PANAMA CITY, FL, WAS DISCIPLINED BY MEDICARE ON FEBRUARY 10, 1992
DISCIPLINARY ACTION: EXCLUSION FROM THE MEDICARE AND/OR MEDICAID PROGRAM
OFFENSE: DISCIPLINARY ACTION BY ANOTHER STATE OR AGENCY

NOTES: LICENSE REVOCATION OR SUSPENSION.

MONROE, ELLIOTT FAIL MD, DATE OF BIRTH JUNE 26, 1943, LICENSE NUMBER 00G2436 OF P.O. BOX 108, CLINTON, AL, WAS DISCIPLINED BY TEXAS ON MARCH 27, 1993
DISCIPLINARY ACTION: LICENSE REVOCATION
OFFENSE: DISCIPLINARY ACTION BY ANOTHER STATE OR AGENCY

NOTES: DISCIPLINARY ACTION BY ANOTHER STATE; UNPROFESSIONAL CONDUCT. APPLICATION FOR REINSTATEMENT MAY NOT BE MADE FOR ONE YEAR FROM THE DATE THIS ORDER BECOMES FINAL. ORDER WILL BECOME FINAL WHEN ALL APPEALS HAVE BEEN EXHAUSTED.

MONROE, ELLIOTT FAIL MD, WAS DISCIPLINED BY ALABAMA ON SEPTEMBER 29, 1993
DISCIPLINARY ACTION: DENIAL OF LICENSE REINSTATEMENT
OFFENSE: DISCIPLINARY ACTION BY ANOTHER STATE OR AGENCY

NOTES: FLORIDA LICENSE REVOKED IN 12/91 ON GROUNDS RELATED TO MEDICAL COMPETENCY; FAILED TO DEMONSTRATE COMPLIANCE WITH AN ADEQUATE AFTERCARE PROGRAM FOR ALCOHOLISM AND CHEMICAL DEPENDENCY. DENIAL OF APPLICATION FOR REINSTATEMENT OF ALABAMA LICENSE, WHICH WAS REVOKED ON 6/22/88.

MONTERO, KARIN E MD, LICENSE NUMBER H2158 OF AUSTIN, TX, WAS DISCIPLINED BY TEXAS ON APRIL 4, 1998
DISCIPLINARY ACTION: FINE
OFFENSE: NONCOMPLIANCE WITH A PROFESSIONAL RULE

NOTES: FAILED TO TIMELY RESPOND TO A BOARD REQUEST AND SUBPOENA FOR THE MEDICAL RECORDS OF THREE PATIENTS. $2,500 FINE; SHALL COOPERATE WITH THE BOARD IN VERIFYING COMPLIANCE.

MONTOYA, JUAN S MD, LICENSE NUMBER 00E2745 OF PASADENA, TX, WAS DISCIPLINED BY TEXAS ON MAY 15, 1996
DISCIPLINARY ACTION: 60-MONTH RESTRICTION PLACED ON LICENSE; REPRIMAND
OFFENSE: SEXUAL ABUSE OF OR SEXUAL MISCONDUCT WITH A PATIENT

NOTES: FROM 1986 THROUGH 1994, HE TREATED AN ADULT FEMALE IN THE COURSE OF HIS OBSTETRICAL AND GYNECOLOGICAL PRACTICE WITH WHOM HE MAINTAINED AN INAPPROPRIATE RELATIONSHIP OF A SEXUAL NATURE OUTSIDE THE PRACTICE SETTING; AT NO TIME FROM 1986 TO 1994 DID HE FORMALLY TERMINATE HIS RELATIONSHIP WITH THE PATIENT. LICENSE RESTRICTION WITH TERMS AND CONDITIONS: SHALL UNDERGO A COMPLETE EXAMINATION BY A BOARD-APPROVED PHYSICIAN

WHOM HE SHALL SEE FOR CONTINUING CARE AND TREATMENT FOR ANY CONDITION WHICH COULD ADVERSELY AFFECT HIS ABILITY TO SAFELY PRACTICE MEDICINE WITH MONTHLY REPORTS TO THE BOARD; SHALL HAVE A CHAPERONE PRESENT DURING THE EXAMINATION OF ANY FEMALE PATIENT AND SHALL NOTE THIS IN THE PATIENT'S CHART; SHALL OBTAIN AT LEAST 50 HOURS PER YEAR OF CONTINUING MEDICAL EDUCATION; WITHIN ONE YEAR SHALL OBTAIN 12 HOURS OF ETHICS THROUGH BOARD-APPROVED PROGRAMS OR COURSES; SHALL APPEAR BEFORE BOARD AT LEAST ONCE A YEAR OR UPON REQUEST; SHALL COOPERATE WITH BOARD IN VERIFYING COMPLIANCE INCLUDING PROVIDING MEDICAL RELEASES UPON REQUEST; SHALL GIVE A COPY OF THIS ORDER TO ANY HEALTH CARE ENTITY WHERE HE HAS PRIVILEGES; SHALL PROVIDE A COPY OF THIS ORDER TO ANYONE REQUESTING IT WITHIN 10 DAYS; TIME SPENT OUT OF TEXAS DOES NOT COUNT TOWARD RESTRICTION; SHALL INFORM BOARD OF CHANGE OF ADDRESS WITHIN 10 DAYS OR IF HE LEAVES THE STATE. SHALL NOT SEEK MODIFICATION FOR ONE YEAR. ON 5/10/97 PETITION TO TERMINATE ORDER DENIED. ON 5/16/98 ORDER TERMINATED.

MOORE, ANTHONY J MD, DATE OF BIRTH MARCH 21, 1944, LICENSE NUMBER 0019520 OF WILMINGTON, NC, WAS DISCIPLINED BY NORTH CAROLINA ON JUNE 1, 1992
DISCIPLINARY ACTION: SURRENDER OF LICENSE

MOORE, ANTHONY JOSEPH MD OF DURHAM, NC, WAS DISCIPLINED BY NORTH CAROLINA ON JANUARY 25, 1990
DISCIPLINARY ACTION: SURRENDER OF LICENSE

MOORE, ANTHONY JOSEPH MD OF DURHAM, NC, WAS DISCIPLINED BY NORTH CAROLINA ON OCTOBER 16, 1990
DISCIPLINARY ACTION: LICENSE REINSTATEMENT

NOTES: TEMPORARY LICENSE ISSUED WITH CONDITIONS.

MOORE, ANTHONY JOSEPH MD, LICENSE NUMBER 00C9232 OF BUTNER, NC, WAS DISCIPLINED BY TEXAS ON OCTOBER 5, 1991
DISCIPLINARY ACTION: 60-MONTH PROBATION
OFFENSE: DISCIPLINARY ACTION BY ANOTHER STATE OR AGENCY

NOTES: INTEMPERATE USE OF ALCOHOL OR DRUGS. LICENSE SUSPENDED, SUSPENSION STAYED; PROBATION UNDER TERMS AND CONDITIONS.

MOORE, JOSEPH W MD, LICENSE NUMBER F9848 OF AUSTIN, TX, WAS DISCIPLINED BY TEXAS ON DECEMBER 11, 1999
DISCIPLINARY ACTION: SURRENDER OF LICENSE
OFFENSE: OVERPRESCRIBING OR MISPRESCRIBING DRUGS

NOTES: FROM 8/17/97-3/98 PROVIDED COUPLE'S COUNSELING FOR A PAIR OF PATIENTS; FROM 3/98-9/98 CONTINUED TO TREAT THE PATIENTS INDIVIDUALLY; IN 8/98 HE SUB-LET A ROOM IN THE HOME OF ONE OF THE PATIENT'S AND MOVED IN FOR A MONTH THEREBY BREACHING BOUNDARIES OF PATIENT-PHYSICIAN RELATIONSHIP; HIS MEDICAL RECORDS ARE INADEQUATE IN THAT THEY FAIL TO PROPERLY RECORD THE PSYCHOSOCIAL HISTORY OF ONE OF THE PATIENTS; HE INAPPROPRIATELY PRESCRIBED ATIVAN FOR ONE OF THE PATIENT'S WITHOUT OBTAINING A COMPLETE HISTORY, WITHOUT ADEQUATELY MONITORING THE NUMBER OF PRESCRIPTIONS GIVEN TO THE PATIENT, AND PRIOR TO ATTEMPTING TREATMENT OF A DRUG WITHOUT ADDICTIVE POTENTIAL. VOLUNTARY AND PERMANENT SURRENDER OF LICENSE.

MOORE, M J MD, LICENSE NUMBER 00D4531 OF ORANGE, TX, WAS DISCIPLINED BY TEXAS ON NOVEMBER 3, 1994
DISCIPLINARY ACTION: SURRENDER OF CONTROLLED SUBSTANCE LICENSE; 120-MONTH PROBATION
OFFENSE: SUBSTANCE ABUSE

NOTES: HAS PRESCRIBED TO HIS RELATIVES, PEOPLE HE LIVES WITH AND HIMSELF; STATED TO AN INVESTIGATOR ON 6/16/93 THAT HE DID NOT DRINK AND THAT HE HAD TAKEN PAIN MEDICATIONS OCCASIONALLY AFTER OPEN HEART SURGERY; DID NOT HAVE MEDICAL RECORDS FOR THE PEOPLE HE PRESCRIBED FOR REFERENCED ABOVE AND SAID HE MAY HAVE DESTROYED THEM; AGREED TO SURRENDER HIS CONTROLLED SUBSTANCES REGISTRATION SCHEDULES II THROUGH V BY 9/3/93 BASED UPON ALLEGATIONS OF NON-THERAPEUTIC PRESCRIBING OF DARVOCET N-1OO TO AN UNDERCOVER AGENT; DR. MOORE HAS RECEIVED TREATMENT RELATED TO HIS ABUSE OF MEDICATIONS; SOBRIETY DATE IS 9/10/93; IS CURRENTLY UNDER THE CARE OF A PSYCHIATRIST AND ATTENDS AA. SUSPENSION STAYED. CONDITIONS OF PROBATION: SHALL SURRENDER HIS DEA AND TEXAS CONTROLLED SUBSTANCES CERTIFICATES, ALL UNUSED TRIPLICATE PRESCRIPTION FORMS AND ALL CONTROLLED SUBSTANCES IN HIS POSSESSION INCLUDING SAMPLES; SHALL NOT ATTEMPT TO REREGISTER WITHOUT PERMISSION; SHALL ABSTAIN FROM THE CONSUMPTION OF ALCOHOL/CHEMICAL SUBSTANCES IN ANY FORM UNLESS PRESCRIBED BY ANOTHER PHYSICIAN FOR A LEGITIMATE AND THERAPEUTIC PURPOSE; SHALL SUBMIT HIMSELF FOR APPROPRIATE EXAMS INCLUDING DRUG OR ALCOHOL SCREENS; SHALL SUBMIT HIMSELF FOR EVALUATION AND TREATMENT TO A BOARD-APPROVED PSYCHIATRIST WITH REPORTS TO THE BOARD; SHALL CONTINUE TO PARTICIPATE IN AA'S PROGRAM NOT LESS THAN THREE TIMES A WEEK WITH QUARTERLY REPORTS TO THE BOARD; SEPARATE FROM PATIENT RECORDS SHALL MAINTAIN A LOG OF EVERY PRESCRIPTION WRITTEN FOR DANGEROUS DRUGS WHICH SHALL BE AVAILABLE FOR INSPECTION; SHALL NOT TELEPHONE TO A PHARMACY ANY PRESCRIPTION FOR DANGEROUS DRUGS WITH A POTENTIAL FOR ABUSE; SHALL NOT TREAT OR OTHERWISE SERVE AS PHYSICIAN, PRESCRIBE, DISPENSE OR ADMINISTER DRUGS THAT MAY BE SUBJECT TO ABUSE TO HIMSELF OR ANY MEMBER OF HIS FAMILY; SHALL BE SUPERVISED BY A BOARD-APPROVED PHYSICIAN WITH QUARTERLY REPORTS; SHALL MAINTAIN A LIST OF ALL PRESCRIPTIONS FOR CONTROLLED SUBSTANCES OR DANGEROUS DRUGS PRESCRIBED BY HIS PHYSICIAN WHICH HE SHALL PROVIDE TO EACH PRESCRIBING PHYSICIAN AT EACH VISIT FOR THEM TO INITIAL; SHALL GIVE A COPY OF THIS ORDER TO ANY HEALTH CARE ENTITY WHERE HE HAS PRIVILEGES; SHALL COOPERATE WITH THE BOARD IN VERIFYING COMPLIANCE; SHALL INFORM BOARD OF CHANGE OF ADDRESS WITHIN 10 DAYS OR IF HE LEAVES THE STATE; TIME SPENT OUT OF TEXAS DOES NOT COUNT TOWARD PROBATION. SHALL NOT SEEK MODIFICATION FOR ONE YEAR.

MOORE, MILTON DONALD JR MD, LICENSE NUMBER G7692 OF HOUSTON, TX, WAS DISCIPLINED BY TEXAS ON MAY 14, 1999
DISCIPLINARY ACTION: FINE
OFFENSE: PROFESSIONAL MISCONDUCT

NOTES: ON 3/5/97 HE WAS NOT PRESENT IN HIS OFFICE AS HE WAS OUT-OF-TOWN; HIS STAFF ATTEMPTED TO

CANCEL PATIENTS SCHEDULED FOR THAT DAY, BUT 14 PATIENTS PRESENTED AT THE OFFICE BECAUSE APPARENTLY THEY DID NOT RECEIVE THE NOTIFICATION; A MEDICAL ASSISTANT WHO WAS WORKING FOR HIM SAW THE PATIENTS, BOTH NEW AND ESTABLISHED, AND ASSESSED THEIR CONDITIONS AND RECOMMENDED TREATMENT FOR THE PATIENTS WITHOUT THE SUPERVISION OF THE DOCTOR, INCLUDING THE DISPENSING OF PRESCRIPTION DRUGS AND WRITING PRESCRIPTIONS; HE ASSERTS THAT THE MEDICAL ASSISTANT PERFORMED THESE ACTS WITHOUT HIS PRIOR KNOWLEDGE OR CONSENT AND WAS SUBSEQUENTLY TERMINATED FROM HIS EMPLOY. SHALL PAY $1,000 FINE; SHALL INFORM THE BOARD OF CHANGE OF ADDRESS WITHIN 10 DAYS.

MOORE, MILTON JOE MD OF ORANGE, TX, WAS DISCIPLINED BY LOUISIANA ON FEBRUARY 15, 1990
OFFENSE: DISCIPLINARY ACTION BY ANOTHER STATE OR AGENCY

NOTES: DISCIPLINED BY TEXAS, ALSO INVESTIGATION OF SUSPECTED DISPENSING OF CONTROLLED SUBSTANCES IN OTHER THAN A LEGITIMATE MANNER; MUST COMPLY WITH TERMS AND CONDITIONS MANDATED BY TEXAS, MUST INFORM BOARD OF INTENT TO RELOCATE TO LOUISIANA.

MOORE, MILTON JOE MD OF 1309 WEST PARK, ORANGE, TX, WAS DISCIPLINED BY DEA ON SEPTEMBER 7, 1993
DISCIPLINARY ACTION: SURRENDER OF CONTROLLED SUBSTANCE LICENSE
OFFENSE: CRIMINAL CONVICTION OR PLEA OF GUILTY, NOLO CONTENDERE, OR NO CONTEST TO A CRIME

NOTES: SURRENDERED DEA REGISTRATION IN PLEA BARGAIN. SEARCH WARRANT EXECUTED ON 08/19/93 IN ORANGE, TX TO OBTAIN MEDICAL RECORDS. JUDGMENT FILED AGAINST HIM FOR UNLAWFUL DISPENSING OF CONTROLLED SUBSTANCE. ORDERED TO PAY FINE.

MOORE, MILTON JOE MD OF ORANGE, TX, WAS DISCIPLINED BY LOUISIANA ON MAY 26, 1995
OFFENSE: DISCIPLINARY ACTION BY ANOTHER STATE OR AGENCY

NOTES: DISCIPLINARY ACTION BY TEXAS; HABITUAL OR RECURRING ABUSE OF MOOD-ALTERING DRUGS; PRESCRIBING, DISPENSING OR ADMINISTERING CONTROLLED SUBSTANCES IN OTHER THAN A LEGAL OR LEGITIMATE MANNER. SUSPENSION STAYED. PROHIBITION OF PRACTICE IN LOUISIANA UNTIL AUTHORIZED BY THE BOARD; MUST COMPLETELY SATISFY THE TERMS OF THE TEXAS ORDER AND RECEIVE REINSTATEMENT OF UNRESTRICTED LICENSURE IN THAT STATE; REINSTATEMENT OF LOUISIANA LICENSE TO BE ON PROBATION FOR FIVE YEARS SUBJECT TO PRIOR NOTICE TO BOARD OF INTENT TO RELOCATE TO LOUISIANA.

MOOREHEAD, WILL EARL MD, DATE OF BIRTH OCTOBER 26, 1943, LICENSE NUMBER 0013230 OF 5600 S WILLOW SUITE 206, HOUSTON, TX, WAS DISCIPLINED BY GEORGIA ON JULY 17, 1991
DISCIPLINARY ACTION: LICENSE SUSPENSION; FINE
OFFENSE: DISCIPLINARY ACTION BY ANOTHER STATE OR AGENCY

NOTES: DUE TO REVOCATION OF LICENSE IN CALIFORNIA. $1500 FINE MUST BE PAID WITHIN 60 DAYS.

MORAN, PAUL AUSTIN DO, LICENSE NUMBER D6301 OF COLEMAN, TX, WAS DISCIPLINED BY TEXAS ON APRIL 10, 1999
DISCIPLINARY ACTION: 60-MONTH PROBATION; RESTRICTION PLACED ON CONTROLLED SUBSTANCE LICENSE
OFFENSE: PROFESSIONAL MISCONDUCT

NOTES: BETWEEN 2/5/97 AND 1/5/98 HIS RELATIVE PRESENTED AT LEAST 74 PRESCRIPTIONS DR. MORAN HAD WRITTEN FOR CONTROLLED SUBSTANCES TO 13 PHARMACIES IN 6 WEST TEXAS CITIES; DOCUMENTS SUBMITTED BY HIM AS REPRESENTING THE COMPLETE MEDICAL RECORD FOR THE RELATIVE FAIL TO PROVIDE OBJECTIVE DATA TO JUSTIFY THE NUMEROUS PRESCRIPTIONS FOR CONTROLLED SUBSTANCES AND, IN THE OPINION OF A BOARD CONSULTANT, ARE POSSIBLY FABRICATED AFTER THE FACT AND THEREFORE QUESTIONABLE AS VALID MEDICAL RECORDS; THE BOARD CONSULTANT CONCLUDED THAT THE NOTES WRITTEN BY HIM APPEAR TO BE A DESPERATE ATTEMPT TO COVER UP THE RELATIVE'S OBVIOUS NARCOTIC ADDICTION, AND THAT HIS STATEMENTS TO THE BOARD APPEAR TO BE THOSE OF AN INDIVIDUAL IN DENIAL WHO IS MAKING EXCUSES FOR HIS PATIENT'S BEHAVIOR. SUSPENSION STAYED FOR PROBATION AND PUBLIC REPRIMAND WITH FOLLOWING TERMS AND CONDITIONS: SHALL ATTEND 50 HOURS PER YEAR OF CONTINUING MEDICAL EDUCATION WITH 1 COURSE IN THE AREAS OF RISK MANAGEMENT AND ADDICTIONOLOGY; SHALL OBTAIN ONE ETHICS COURSE IN TRANSFERENCE OF PATIENTS, TREATMENT OF FAMILY MEMBERS OR A SIMILAR ETHICS PROGRAM PER YEAR; SHALL IMMEDIATELY REQUEST MODIFICATION OF HIS DEA AND TEXAS DEPARTMENT OF PUBLIC SAFETY CONTROLLED SUBSTANCES REGISTRATION CERTIFICATE TO ELIMINATE SCHEDULES II AND III; SHALL MAINTAIN ADEQUATE MEDICAL RECORDS WHICH SHALL BE AVAILABLE FOR REVIEW; SEPARATE FROM PATIENT RECORDS, SHALL MAINTAIN A LOGBOOK OF EVERY PRESCRIPTION WRITTEN BY HIM FOR DANGEROUS DRUGS WITH ADDICTIVE POTENTIAL WHICH SHALL BE MADE AVAILABLE FOR REVIEW; SHALL NOT TREAT OR OTHERWISE SERVE AS PHYSICIAN, PRESCRIBE, DISPENSE OR ADMINISTER DRUGS THAT MAY BE SUBJECT TO ABUSE TO HIMSELF OR TO ANY MEMBER OF HIS FAMILY; SHALL APPEAR BEFORE THE BOARD ONCE A YEAR; SHALL COOPERATE WITH THE BOARD IN VERIFYING COMPLIANCE; WITHIN 1 YEAR SHALL TAKE AND SUCCESSFULLY COMPLETE AN ADVANCED CARDIAC LIFE SUPPORT COURSE AND OBTAIN CERTIFICATION, AND AN ADVANCED TRAUMA LIFE SUPPORT COURSE AND OBTAIN CERTIFICATION; TIME SPENT OUT OF TEXAS DOES NOT COUNT TOWARD PROBATION; SHALL INFORM THE BOARD OF CHANGE OF ADDRESS WITHIN 10 DAYS OR IF HE LEAVES THE STATE; SHALL NOT SEEK MODIFICATION FOR ONE YEAR.

MORAN, WILMER JR MD, LICENSE NUMBER 00E1684 OF HOUSTON, TX, WAS DISCIPLINED BY TEXAS ON AUGUST 19, 1994
DISCIPLINARY ACTION: FINE; REPRIMAND
OFFENSE: PROFESSIONAL MISCONDUCT

NOTES: AIDED AND ABETTED THE UNLICENSED PRACTICE OF MEDICINE IN THAT HE ENGAGED IN THE CORPORATE PRACTICE OF MEDICINE BY VIRTUE OF HIS EMPLOYMENT BY GALLERIA DIAGNOSTIC SERVICE ON A SALARY BASIS IN THE FALL OF 1991; CEASED PRACTICE AS SOON AS HE LEARNED IT WAS ILLEGAL. SHALL NOT ACCEPT EMPLOYMENT OR ENTER INTO CONTRACTUAL RELATIONSHIPS WHERE HE WOULD BE COMPENSATED BY ANY ENTITY NOT COMPRISED EXCLUSIVELY OF TEXAS LICENSED PHYSICIANS WHERE THEY WOULD RECEIVE AND RETAIN THE FEES; SHALL PAY A $1,000 ADMINISTRATIVE PENALTY; SHALL GIVE A COPY OF THIS ORDER TO ANY HEALTH

CARE ENTITY WHERE HE HAS PRIVILEGES; SHALL COOPERATE WITH THE BOARD IN VERIFYING COMPLIANCE; SHALL INFORM BOARD OF CHANGE OF ADDRESS WITHIN 10 DAYS.

MORAN, WILMER JR MD, LICENSE NUMBER E1684 OF HOUSTON, TX, WAS DISCIPLINED BY TEXAS ON AUGUST 9, 1997
DISCIPLINARY ACTION: FINE; REPRIMAND
OFFENSE: NONCOMPLIANCE WITH A PROFESSIONAL RULE

NOTES: FAILED TO OBTAIN 24 HOURS OF CONTINUING MEDICAL EDUCATION AS REQUIRED FOR RENEWAL OF HIS LICENSE ON 12/1/95, EVEN AFTER OBTAINING AN EXTENSION; OWED MONEY FOR FINE AND LICENSURE FEES. $100 FINE.

MORGAN, MICKEY D MD, LICENSE NUMBER 00H3121 OF ALLEN, TX, WAS DISCIPLINED BY TEXAS ON JUNE 28, 1995
DISCIPLINARY ACTION: 60-MONTH PROBATION; RESTRICTION PLACED ON CONTROLLED SUBSTANCE LICENSE
OFFENSE: SUBSTANCE ABUSE

NOTES: IN 1/95 ARRESTED FOR DRIVING WHILE INTOXICATED AND LATER IN THE SAME DAY WAS CHARGED WITH PUBLIC INTOXICATION IN A SEPARATE INCIDENT; SELF-PRESCRIBED HYDROCODONE FOR SEVERAL MONTHS; EVALUATED BY A PHYSICIAN IN 1/95 WHO RECOMMENDED TREATMENT WITH ANTABUSE AND ZOLOFT FOR DEPRESSION; RECEIVED INPATIENT TREATMENT AND WAS DISCHARGED 1/27/95 AND IS CURRENTLY RECEIVING OUTPATIENT TREATMENT; REPORTS THAT HE IS ATTENDING WEEKLY GROUP PSYCHOTHERAPY SESSIONS, AA MEETINGS AND DAILY IMPAIRED PHYSICIAN MEETINGS; CURRENTLY UNDER A TREATMENT CONTRACT WITH TWO HOSPITALS WHERE HE HAS PRIVILEGES. SUSPENSION STAYED. PROBATION WITH TERMS: SHALL ABSTAIN FROM THE CONSUMPTION OF ALCOHOL/DRUGS IN ANY FORM UNLESS PRESCRIBED BY ANOTHER PHYSICIAN FOR A LEGITIMATE AND THERAPEUTIC PURPOSE; SHALL SUBMIT HIMSELF FOR APPROPRIATE EXAMS INCLUDING DRUG OR ALCOHOL SCREENS; SHALL SUBMIT HIMSELF FOR EVALUATION AND TREATMENT BY BOARD-APPROVED PSYCHIATRIST WHOM HE SHALL SEE AT LEAST ONCE A MONTH AND WHO SHALL SUBMIT REPORTS TO THE BOARD; SHALL PARTICIPATE IN AA'S PROGRAM NOT LESS THAN FIVE TIMES A WEEK WITH QUARTERLY REPORTS TO THE BOARD; SHALL COMPLY WITH THE TERMS OF HIS CONTINUING CARE CONTRACT WITH TWO HOSPITALS WITH QUARTERLY REPORTS; SHALL NOT POSSESS ALCOHOL, CONTROLLED SUBSTANCES OR DRUGS WITH ADDICTIVE POTENTIAL OR POTENTIAL FOR ABUSE; SHALL SURRENDER ANY SUCH DRUGS STILL IN HIS POSSESSION; SHALL NOT TREAT OR OTHERWISE SERVE AS PHYSICIAN, PRESCRIBE, DISPENSE, OR ADMINISTER DRUGS THAT MAY BE SUBJECT TO ABUSE TO HIMSELF OR ANY MEMBER OF HIS FAMILY; SHALL MAINTAIN A FILE WITH A COPY OF EVERY PRESCRIPTION WRITTEN FOR CONTROLLED SUBSTANCES AND DRUGS WITH ADDICTIVE POTENTIAL WHICH SHALL BE AVAILABLE FOR REVIEW; SHALL NOT TELEPHONE THE PHARMACY WITH PRESCRIPTIONS FOR THESE DRUGS; SHALL MAINTAIN ADEQUATE MEDICAL RECORDS WHICH SHALL BE AVAILABLE FOR REVIEW; SHALL OBTAIN AT LEAST 50 HOURS OF CONTINUING MEDICAL EDUCATION PER YEAR; SHALL APPEAR BEFORE BOARD AT LEAST ONCE A YEAR OR AT BOARD REQUEST; SHALL COOPERATE WITH THE BOARD IN VERIFYING COMPLIANCE INCLUDING PROVIDING COPIES OF MEDICAL RELEASES OR PEER REVIEW RECORDS UPON REQUEST; SHALL GIVE A COPY OF THIS ORDER TO ANY HEALTH CARE ENTITY WHERE HE HAS PRIVILEGES; SHALL PROVIDE A COPY OF THIS ORDER TO ANYONE REQUESTING IT WITHIN 10 DAYS; TIME PERIOD OUT OF TEXAS DOES NOT COUNT TOWARD PROBATION; SHALL INFORM BOARD OF CHANGE OF ADDRESS WITHIN 10 DAYS OR IF HE LEAVES THE STATE. SHALL NOT SEEK MODIFICATION FOR ONE YEAR. ON 8/22/98 PETITION TO TERMINATE ORDER DENIED; ORDER MODIFIED DELETING THE FOLLOWING REQUIREMENTS: PSYCHIATRIC TREATMENT; FORBIDDING UNILATERAL WITHDRAWAL FROM TREATMENT; SUBMISSION TO DRUG SCREENS ORDERED BY TREATING PHYSICIANS; NOTIFICATION OF THE BOARD UPON DISCONTINUATION OF TREATMENT; COMPLIANCE WITH CONTINUING CARE CONTRACTS WITH PRESBYTERIAN HOSPITAL AND HCA MEDICAL CENTER; CONTRACT FOR ABSTINENCE WITH ANY HOSPITAL GRANTING PRIVILEGES; FORBIDDING POSSESSION OF ALCOHOL, CONTROLLED SUBSTANCES, OR DANGEROUS DRUGS WITH POTENTIAL FOR ABUSE; FORBIDDING HIS TREATING HIS IMMEDIATE FAMILY; SEPARATE FILE OF COPIES OF PRESCRIPTIONS WRITTEN AND FORBIDDEN TELEPHONE PRESCRIPTIONS; FIFTY HOURS OF CONTINUING MEDICAL EDUCATION; AA PARTICIPATION MODIFIED TO NO LESS THAN THREE TIMES PER WEEK; ON 5/14/99 ORDER TERMINATED.

MORGAN, RICHARD DOUGLAS DO, LICENSE NUMBER 00H4565 OF BRADY, TX, WAS DISCIPLINED BY TEXAS ON APRIL 15, 1994
DISCIPLINARY ACTION: 60-MONTH PROBATION; REQUIRED TO TAKE ADDITIONAL MEDICAL EDUCATION
OFFENSE: DISCIPLINARY ACTION BY ANOTHER STATE OR AGENCY

NOTES: IN 8/93 DISCIPLINED BY THE U.S. AIR FORCE FOR THEFT OF STADOL, FALSE OFFICIAL STATEMENTS AND DERELICTION OF DUTIES FOR SELF-PRESCRIBING OF STADOL; SELF-ADMINISTERED STADOL BEFORE (FOR HEADACHES) AND AFTER HIS CAR ACCIDENT IN 6/92; USED STADOL FOR LOCAL ANESTHETIC PURPOSES WHICH WAS FOUND TO BE INAPPROPRIATE; PATIENT NAMES WERE USED TO DOCUMENT THAT STADOL WAS RECEIVED WHEN IN FACT THE PATIENTS DID NOT RECEIVE THE DRUGS; FALSIFIED MEDICAL RECORDS AND PHARMACY ACCOUNTING FORMS; PRESCRIBED STADOL TO HIS FATHER; HOSPITAL PRIVILEGES WERE SUSPENDED BASED ON THESE FINDINGS; AFTER SEPARATION FROM AIR FORCE HAS SUBMITTED TO THE CARE OF A FAMILY PHYSICIAN. SUSPENSION STAYED. CONDITIONS OF PROBATION: SHALL APPEAR BEFORE THE BOARD TWICE A YEAR; SHALL ATTEND AT LEAST 50 HOURS PER YEAR OF CONTINUING MEDICAL EDUCATION INCLUDING 20 HOURS IN PHARMACOLOGY/ADDICTIONOLOGY DURING THE FIRST YEAR; SHALL BE SUPERVISED BY A BOARD-APPROVED PHYSICIAN WITH QUARTERLY REPORTS; SHALL MAINTAIN ADEQUATE MEDICAL RECORDS ON ALL PATIENT OFFICE VISITS WHICH SHALL BE AVAILABLE FOR REVIEW; SHALL NOT PERSONALLY USE, POSSESS, ADMINISTER OR PRESCRIBE ANY PRESCRIPTION DRUG UNLESS PRESCRIBED, ADMINISTERED OR DISPENSED BY ANOTHER PHYSICIAN FOR A LEGITIMATE MEDICAL NEED; SHALL NOT TREAT OR OTHERWISE SERVE AS PHYSICIAN, PRESCRIBE, DISPENSE OR ADMINISTER DRUGS THAT MAY BE SUBJECT TO ABUSE TO HIMSELF OR ANY MEMBER OF HIS FAMILY; SEPARATE FROM PATIENT RECORDS, SHALL MAINTAIN A FILE OF EVERY PRESCRIPTION WRITTEN FOR CONTROLLED SUBSTANCES OR DANGEROUS DRUGS WHICH SHALL BE AVAILABLE FOR INSPECTION; SHALL ABSTAIN FROM THE CONSUMPTION OF ALCOHOL/CHEMICAL SUBSTANCES IN ANY FORM UNLESS PRESCRIBED BY ANOTHER PHYSICIAN FOR A LEGITIMATE MEDICAL

PURPOSE; SHALL SUBMIT HIMSELF FOR APPROPRIATE EXAMS INCLUDING DRUG AND ALCOHOL SCREENS; WITHIN 60 DAYS SHALL ENTER AN IN-PATIENT BOARD-APPROVED PAIN MANAGEMENT PROGRAM WITH REPORTS TO THE BOARD; SHALL UNDERGO A COMPLETE EXAMINATION BY A BOARD APPROVED PHYSICIAN UPON REQUEST; IN COMPLIANCE WITH CONDITIONS SET OUT BY SHANNON MEDICAL CENTER SHALL NOT POSSESS A KEY OR HAVE ACCESS TO ANY MEDICINE CABINET CONTAINING CONTROLLED SUBSTANCES OR DANGEROUS DRUGS AND SHALL SUBMIT TO ANY DRUG SCREENS ORDERED; SHALL GIVE A COPY OF THIS ORDER TO ANY HEALTH CARE ENTITY WHERE HE HAS PRIVILEGES; SHALL COOPERATE WITH THE BOARD IN VERIFYING COMPLIANCE; SHALL INFORM BOARD OF CHANGE OF ADDRESS WITHIN 10 DAYS OR IF HE LEAVES THE STATE; TIME SPENT OUT OF TEXAS DOES NOT COUNT TOWARD PROBATION. SHALL NOT SEEK MODIFICATION FOR ONE YEAR. ON 6/28/95 ORDER MODIFIED AS FOLLOWS: SHALL BE ALLOWED TO TELEPHONE PRESCRIPTIONS TO A PHARMACY FOR DRUGS SCHEDULES III, IV AND V AND FOR THESE DRUGS; SEPARATE FROM PATIENT RECORDS, SHALL MAINTAIN A FILE OF EVERY PRESCRIPTION WRITTEN FOR CONTROLLED SUBSTANCES WITH ADDICTIVE POTENTIAL OR POTENTIAL FOR ABUSE. ON 11/16/96 PROBATION TERMINATED.

MORGAN, TOMMY DAN MD, DATE OF BIRTH AUGUST 23, 1956, LICENSE NUMBER 0013066 OF 4846 SHERIDAN DRIVE, JACKSON, MS, WAS DISCIPLINED BY MISSISSIPPI ON NOVEMBER 18, 1993
DISCIPLINARY ACTION: PROBATION; MONITORING OF PHYSICIAN PERFORMANCE

NOTES: SUSPENSION OF FIVE YEARS STAYED; CONSENT AGREEMENT EXECUTED WITH TERMS AND CONDITIONS TO INCLUDE: RANDOM, UNANNOUNCED AND WITNESSED URINE SCREENS BY BOARD.

MORGAN, TOMMY DAN MD, DATE OF BIRTH AUGUST 23, 1956, LICENSE NUMBER 0013066 OF 206 RACHELLE DRIVE, OXFORD, MS, WAS DISCIPLINED BY MISSISSIPPI ON SEPTEMBER 21, 1995
DISCIPLINARY ACTION: 12-MONTH LICENSE SUSPENSION; PROBATION

NOTES: AFTER ONE YEAR SUSPENSION STAYED SUBJECT TO TERMS AND CONDITIONS.

MORGAN, TOMMY DAN MD OF 206 RACHELLE DRIVE, OXFORD, MS, WAS DISCIPLINED BY DEA ON NOVEMBER 14, 1995
DISCIPLINARY ACTION: SURRENDER OF CONTROLLED SUBSTANCE LICENSE
OFFENSE: DISCIPLINARY ACTION BY ANOTHER STATE OR AGENCY

NOTES: STATE BOARD.

MORGAN, TOMMY DAN MD, LICENSE NUMBER 0D42709 OF 206 RACHELLE DR, OXFORD, MS, WAS DISCIPLINED BY MARYLAND ON FEBRUARY 13, 1996
DISCIPLINARY ACTION: LICENSE SUSPENSION
OFFENSE: DISCIPLINARY ACTION BY ANOTHER STATE OR AGENCY

NOTES: RECIPROCAL JURISDICTION BASED ON A MISSISSIPPI ORDER PERTAINING TO A VIOLATION OF THE RULES AND REGULATIONS FOR PRESCRIBING, ADMINISTERING AND DISPENSING MEDICATION. INDEFINITE SUSPENSION UNTIL HIS MISSISSIPPI LICENSE IS REINSTATED.

MORGAN, TOMMY DAN MD, DATE OF BIRTH AUGUST 23, 1956, LICENSE NUMBER 13066 OF 1513 SOUTH LEE, ALVIN, TX, WAS DISCIPLINED BY MISSISSIPPI ON JANUARY 16, 1997
DISCIPLINARY ACTION: SURRENDER OF LICENSE

NOTES: HE VOLUNTARILY AND UNCONDITIONALLY SURRENDERED HIS LICENSE TO PRACTICE MEDICINE IN MISSISSIPPI TO AVOID A DISCIPLINARY HEARING.

MORRILL, THOMAS R DO, DATE OF BIRTH JANUARY 28, 1949 OF 550 E QUAIL RUN, ROCKWALL, TX, WAS DISCIPLINED BY MEDICARE ON JANUARY 5, 1997
DISCIPLINARY ACTION: EXCLUSION FROM THE MEDICARE AND/OR MEDICAID PROGRAM
OFFENSE: NONCOMPLIANCE WITH A PROFESSIONAL RULE

NOTES: DEFAULTED ON PUBLIC HEALTH SERVICE EDUCATION LOAN. REINSTATED ON 6/19/97.

MORRIS, BROCK A MD, LICENSE NUMBER 00E4548, WAS DISCIPLINED BY TEXAS ON AUGUST 17, 1996
DISCIPLINARY ACTION: 36-MONTH RESTRICTION PLACED ON LICENSE; 36-MONTH MONITORING OF PHYSICIAN PERFORMANCE
OFFENSE: SEXUAL ABUSE OF OR SEXUAL MISCONDUCT WITH A PATIENT

NOTES: ALLEGATIONS THAT PRIOR TO 1991 ENGAGED IN INAPPROPRIATE PHYSICAL CONTACT WITH FOUR ADULT FEMALE PATIENTS TO INCLUDE SEXUAL INTERCOURSE IN AT LEAST ONE INSTANCE; NONE OF THE PATIENTS INITIATED A COMPLAINT WITH THE BOARD; AND EACH PATIENT SUFFERS FROM OR HAS SUFFERED FROM A SIGNIFICANT PSYCHIATRIC CONDITION WHICH MAY DETRACT FROM THE CREDIBILITY OF ANTICIPATED TESTIMONY; BOARD REVIEW CONCLUDED THAT "INCONSISTENCIES MAKE IT IMPOSSIBLE TO ACCEPT THE CLAIMS AS FACTUAL;" HE DENIES THE ALLEGATIONS; ENTERED INTO AN AGREED ORDER. RESTRICTED UNDER TERMS AND CONDITIONS FOR THREE YEARS: SHALL NOT ENGAGE IN OR OTHERWISE CONDUCT EXCLUSIVELY PSYCHOTHERAPY ON ANY NEW FEMALE PATIENT, HOWEVER HE MAY ENGAGE IN MEDICATION MANAGEMENT AND RELATED THERAPY FOR ALL SUCH NEW PATIENTS; SHALL CONTINUE TO MAINTAIN A WINDOW IN HIS OFFICE DOOR PROVIDING CLEAR VIEW OF THE OFFICE; SHALL CONTINUE TO HAVE OFFICE STAFF PRESENT IN THE ADJOINING BUSINESS OFFICE DURING ALL TIMES IN WHICH HE IS IN SESSION OR COUNSELING WITH A FEMALE PATIENT; SHALL HAVE A CHAPERONE PRESENT IN THE ROOM WHILE PERFORMING A PHYSICAL EXAMINATION ON FEMALE PATIENTS WHO SHALL MAKE A NOTATION ON THE PATIENTS' CHARTS; HIS MEDICAL PRACTICE, INCLUDING ANY OFFICE AND HOSPITAL PRACTICE, SHALL BE MONITORED BY A BOARD APPROVED TEXAS PHYSICIAN WHO SHALL SUBMIT QUARTERLY REPORTS TO THE BOARD; SHALL SUBMIT HIMSELF FOR EVALUATION TO A BOARD APPROVED PSYCHIATRIST WHO SHALL SUBMIT REPORTS; SHALL MAINTAIN ADEQUATE RECORDS WHICH SHALL BE AVAILABLE FOR REVIEW; SHALL APPEAR BEFORE THE BOARD AT LEAST ONCE PER YEAR OR UPON BOARD REQUEST; SHALL COOPERATE WITH THE BOARD IN VERIFYING COMPLIANCE INCLUDING PROVIDING COPIES OF PEER REVIEW RECORDS UPON REQUEST; SHALL GIVE A COPY OF THIS ORDER TO ANY HEALTH CARE ENTITY WHERE HE HAS PRIVILEGES; SHALL OBTAIN AT LEAST EIGHT HOURS PER YEAR OF CONTINUING MEDICAL EDUCATION IN THE AREAS OF ADDRESSING CARE AND TREATMENT CONSIDERATIONS FOR BORDERLINE PERSONALITY DISORDERS, PHYSICIAN-PATIENT BOUNDARY ISSUES, AND TRANSFERENCE/COUNTER-TRANSFERENCE ISSUES AND SUBMIT PROOF TO THE BOARD; TIME PERIOD OUT OF TEXAS DOES NOT COUNT TOWARD

RESTRICTION; SHALL INFORM THE BOARD OF CHANGE OF ADDRESS WITHIN 10 DAYS OF IF HE LEAVES THE STATE; SHALL NOT SEEK MODIFICATION FOR ONE YEAR. ON 4/4/98 ORDER TERMINATED.

MORRIS, DARELD R DO, LICENSE NUMBER 0002938 OF 3501 B SOUTH GEORGIA, AMARILLO, TX, WAS DISCIPLINED BY FLORIDA ON FEBRUARY 5, 1999
DISCIPLINARY ACTION: FINE; RESTRICTION PLACED ON LICENSE

NOTES: $1,000 FINE; PERMANENT RESTRICTION ON PRACTICE; SHALL APPEAR BEFORE THE BOARD PRIOR TO RESUMPTION OF PRACTICE IN FLORIDA; SHALL NOTIFY THE BOARD WITHIN 1O DAYS OF CHANGE OF ADDRESS.

MORRIS, DARELD RAY DO, LICENSE NUMBER C8589 OF AMARILLO, TX, WAS DISCIPLINED BY TEXAS ON AUGUST 9, 1997
DISCIPLINARY ACTION: REPRIMAND
OFFENSE: PROFESSIONAL MISCONDUCT

NOTES: IN OR ABOUT 1994 HE ENTERED INTO A BUSINESS ARRANGEMENT WITH NON-PHYSICIANS; HE DID NOT MAINTAIN CONTROL OVER THE CLINIC, BUT RATHER THE NON-LICENSED INDIVIDUALS DID.

MORRIS, WILFORD JR DO OF SEALY, TX, WAS DISCIPLINED BY KANSAS ON JUNE 22, 1990

NOTES: STIPULATION AND ENFORCEMENT ORDER.

MORRISON, RICHARD FRANK MD, LICENSE NUMBER 00F4308 OF DALLAS, TX, WAS DISCIPLINED BY TEXAS ON MARCH 5, 1994
DISCIPLINARY ACTION: 60-MONTH PROBATION; MONITORING OF PHYSICIAN PERFORMANCE
OFFENSE: SUBSTANCE ABUSE

NOTES: IN 1983 AND 1991 WAS CONVICTED OF DRIVING WHILE INTOXICATED; IS CURRENTLY UNDER TREATMENT FOR DEPRESSION. FIVE YEAR SUSPENSION STAYED. CONDITIONS OF PROBATION: SHALL APPEAR BEFORE THE BOARD TWICE A YEAR; SHALL CONTINUE TO RECEIVE TREATMENT FOR DEPRESSION WITH QUARTERLY REPORTS TO THE BOARD; SHALL ABSTAIN FROM THE CONSUMPTION OF ALCOHOL OR OTHER DRUGS IN ANY FORM UNLESS PRESCRIBED BY ANOTHER PHYSICIAN FOR A LEGITIMATE MEDICAL PURPOSE; SHALL SUBMIT HIMSELF FOR APPROPRIATE EXAMS INCLUDING DRUG OR ALCOHOL SCREENS; SHALL NOT TREAT OR OTHERWISE SERVE AS PHYSICIAN, PRESCRIBE, DISPENSE OR ADMINISTER DRUGS THAT MAY BE SUBJECT TO ABUSE TO HIMSELF OR FOR ANY MEMBER OF HIS FAMILY; SHALL FURNISH WRITTEN REPORTS TO THE BOARD VERIFYING COMPLIANCE; SHALL GIVE A COPY OF THIS ORDER TO ANY HEALTH CARE ENTITY WHERE HE HAS PRIVILEGES; SHALL COOPERATE WITH THE BOARD IN VERIFYING COMPLIANCE; SHALL INFORM BOARD OF CHANGE OF ADDRESS WITHIN 10 DAYS OR IF THE LEAVES THE STATE; TIME SPENT OUT OF TEXAS DOES NOT COUNT TOWARD PROBATION. SHALL NOT SEEK MODIFICATION FOR ONE YEAR. ON 5/10/97 BOARD GRANTED HIS PETITION FOR TERMINATION OF THIS ORDER BASED ON COMPLIANCE WITH CONDITIONS.

MOTLAGH, FAKHRADDIN MD, LICENSE NUMBER 00E0264 OF SAN DIEGO, CA, WAS DISCIPLINED BY TEXAS ON AUGUST 18, 1995
DISCIPLINARY ACTION: LICENSE REVOCATION
OFFENSE: DISCIPLINARY ACTION BY ANOTHER STATE OR AGENCY

NOTES: CALIFORNIA BOARD REVOKED THEN STAYED THE REVOCATION AND PLACED HIM ON PROBATION FOR FIVE YEARS ALLEGING THAT HE HAD LEFT A CHEST RETRACTOR BLADE IN A SURGICAL PATIENT, KNEW HE HAD DONE SO, FAILED TO REMOVE THE BLADE AND FAILED TO INFORM THE PATIENT OR FAMILY OF THE PROBLEM.

MOWATT, IBRAHIM GARCIA JR MD, LICENSE NUMBER G2599, WAS DISCIPLINED BY TEXAS ON MARCH 1, 1997
DISCIPLINARY ACTION: 60-MONTH RESTRICTION PLACED ON LICENSE; REPRIMAND
OFFENSE: OVERPRESCRIBING OR MISPRESCRIBING DRUGS

NOTES: ON FOUR SEPARATE OCCASIONS IN 1994, HE PRESCRIBED CONTROLLED SUBSTANCES, NAMELY TYLENOL NO. 4 WITH CODEINE, AND DANGEROUS DRUGS, NAMELY SOMA, TO AN ADULT MALE PATIENT WITHOUT PERFORMING PROPER MEDICAL ASSESSMENTS, WITHOUT FORMULATING A PROPER RESPECTIVE MEDICAL TREATMENT PLAN AND RATIONALE, WITHOUT ADEQUATELY REASSESSING THE PATIENT TO DETERMINE WHAT EFFECT(S) THE MEDICATION WAS HAVING, AND WITHOUT ADEQUATE MEDICAL INDICATIONS AND DOCUMENTATION TO SUPPORT THIS PRESCRIPTION. HE STATES HE BELIEVED THERE WAS A MEDICAL NECESSITY FOR PRESCRIBING THESE DRUGS AND MAINTAINS THE SAME WAS INDICATED ON THE PATIENT'S CHART. FOLLOWING TERMS: SHALL MAINTAIN ADEQUATE MEDICAL RECORDS WHICH SHALL BE AVAILABLE FOR REVIEW; SEPARATE FROM PATIENT RECORDS, SHALL MAINTAIN A FILE OF EVERY PRESCRIPTION WRITTEN BY HIM FOR DANGEROUS DRUGS WITH ADDICTIVE POTENTIAL WHICH SHALL BE MADE AVAILABLE FOR REVIEW; SHALL OBTAIN AT LEAST 50 HOURS OF CONTINUING MEDICAL EDUCATION PER YEAR; WITHIN ONE YEAR SHALL SUCCESSFULLY COMPLETE AN APPROVED COURSE IN THE AREA OF RISK MANAGEMENT; SHALL COOPERATE WITH THE BOARD IN VERIFYING COMPLIANCE INCLUDING PROVIDING COPIES OF PEER REVIEW RECORDS UPON REQUEST; SHALL GIVE A COPY OF THIS ORDER TO ANY HEALTH CARE ENTITY WHERE HE HAS PRIVILEGES; SHALL PROVIDE A COPY OF THIS ORDER TO ANYONE REQUESTING IT WITHIN 10 DAYS; SHALL APPEAR BEFORE THE BOARD UPON REQUEST; TIME SPENT OUT OF TEXAS DOES NOT COUNT TOWARD RESTRICTION; SHALL INFORM THE BOARD OF CHANGE OF ADDRESS WITHIN 10 DAYS OR IF HE LEAVES THE STATE; SHALL NOT SEEK MODIFICATION FOR ONE YEAR. ON 4/4/98 AND 4/10/99 PETITIONS TO HAVE THE ORDER TERMINATED WERE DENIED.

MUELLER, LYNDA L MD, LICENSE NUMBER 0019565 OF 4611 WINDCASTLE DRIVE #1028, ARLINGTON, TX, WAS DISCIPLINED BY OKLAHOMA ON DECEMBER 12, 1996
DISCIPLINARY ACTION: 60-MONTH PROBATION; RESTRICTION PLACED ON CONTROLLED SUBSTANCE LICENSE
OFFENSE: SUBSTANCE ABUSE

NOTES: ESTABLISHED A PATTERN OF ABUSE OF ALCOHOL AND DRIVING UNDER THE INFLUENCE ARRESTS; ON 9/15/95 ENTERED INTO A WRITTEN AGREEMENT WITH THE BOARD; ON 1/04/96 ENTERED FULL-TIME IN-PATIENT TREATMENT AT COPAC; AND DISCHARGED FROM COPAC ON 4/12/96 UNDER A CONTINUING CARE ADVOCACY CONTRACT. TIMING OF PROBATION SHALL START WHEN SHE REPORTS TO THE BOARD REGARDING HER PRACTICE OF MEDICINE AND SURGERY IN OKLAHOMA; SHALL NOT PRESCRIBE, ADMINISTER, OR DISPENSE ANY MEDICATIONS FOR HER PERSONAL USE, TO SPECIFICALLY INCLUDE CONTROLLED DANGEROUS SUBSTANCES; SHALL TAKE NO MEDICATION UNLESS AUTHORIZED BY A PHYSICIAN FOR A LEGITIMATE MEDICAL NEED; SHALL

SUBMIT BIOLOGICAL FLUID SPECIMENS; SHALL PRESENT HERSELF TO A PHYSICAL AND/OR PSYCHIATRIC EXAMINATION BY A BOARD APPROVED DOCTOR WITH A REPORT SUBMITTED TO THE BOARD; SHALL COMPLY WITH ALL TERMS AND CONDITIONS OF HER CONTINUING CARE ADVOCACY CONTRACT; SHALL NOT PRESCRIBE, ADMINISTER, OR DISPENSE ANY SCHEDULE DRUGS OR CONTROLLED DANGEROUS SUBSTANCES UNTIL AUTHORIZED BY THE BOARD; SHALL FURNISH THE BOARD WITH ADDRESS/CHANGE OF ADDRESS; SHALL APPEAR BEFORE THE BOARD UPON REQUEST AND SUBMIT ANY REQUIRED REPORTS; SHALL PAY COSTS; AND SHALL FURNISH EACH STATE IN WHICH SHE HOLDS OR APPLIES FOR LICENSURE AND ALL HEALTH CARE ENTITIES WHERE SHE HAS PRIVILEGES A COPY OF THIS ORDER. ON 4/10/98 REQUEST TO WAIVE THE TERMS AND CONDITIONS OF PROBATION AND RESTORE TO HER A FULL AND UNRESTRICTED LICENSE IS DENIED. ON 5/6/99 REQUEST TO MODIFY TERMS OF HER PROBATION IS GRANTED ALLOWING HER TO PRESCRIBE CONTROLLED SUBSTANCES IN SCHEDULES II-V, USING DUPLICATE, SERIALLY NUMBERED PRESCRIPTION PADS TO BE MADE AVAILABLE TO THE BOARD UPON REQUEST; SHALL COMPLY WITH ALL TERMS AND CONDITIONS OF HER CONTRACT WITH THE PHYSICIANS RECOVERY NETWORK.

MULLEN, JOHN P MD, DATE OF BIRTH OCTOBER 11, 1940, LICENSE NUMBER 0027156 OF 1614 COLQUITT, SAN ANTONIO, TX, WAS DISCIPLINED BY NEW JERSEY ON APRIL 15, 1992

NOTES: SHALL APPEAR BEFORE A PRELIMINARY EVALUATION COMMITTEE OF THE BOARD OF MEDICAL EXAMINERS PRIOR TO COMMENCING THE PRACTICE OF MEDICINE IN NEW JERSEY. BOARD RESERVES THE RIGHT TO IMPOSE A REASSESSMENT OF HIS SKILLS AND REEDUCATION AT THAT TIME.

MUNCRIEF, KIM I DO, LICENSE NUMBER 2425, WAS DISCIPLINED BY OKLAHOMA ON SEPTEMBER 17, 1998
DISCIPLINARY ACTION: 60-MONTH PROBATION

MUNCRIEF, KIM IVAN DO, LICENSE NUMBER 00G7284 OF COLBERT, OK, WAS DISCIPLINED BY TEXAS ON JANUARY 27, 1990
DISCIPLINARY ACTION: PROBATION
OFFENSE: DISCIPLINARY ACTION BY ANOTHER STATE OR AGENCY

NOTES: STIPULATED ORDER. REVOCATION STAYED, INDEFINITE PROBATION. SHALL COMPLY WITH CONDITIONS OF OKLAHOMA BOARD ORDER, SUBMIT REPORTS TO TEXAS BOARD AS SUBMITTED TO OKLAHOMA BOARD, AND MUST SECURE BOARD APPROVAL BEFORE PRACTICING. PROBATION TERMINATED EFFECTIVE 1/9/92; LICENSE FREE OF ANY RESTRICTION OR LIMITATION.

MUNRO, IAN R MD, LICENSE NUMBER H1162 OF DALLAS, TX, WAS DISCIPLINED BY TEXAS ON AUGUST 28, 1999
DISCIPLINARY ACTION: FINE; REPRIMAND
OFFENSE: NONCOMPLIANCE WITH A PROFESSIONAL RULE

NOTES: FAILED TO PROVIDE PROOF OF CONTINUING MEDICAL EDUCATION WITH HIS MOST RECENT LICENSE RENEWAL APPLICATION; HE NO LONGER PRACTICES MEDICINE AND DOES NOT KEEP UP TO DATE WITH CONTINUING MEDICAL EDUCATION, BUT WOULD LIKE TO RETAIN THE RIGHT TO PRESCRIBE. $100 FINE; SHALL GIVE A COPY OF THIS ORDER TO ANY HEALTH CARE ENTITY WHERE HE HAS PRIVILEGES.

MURPHY, FRANK S DO OF 5201 ALPHA DRIVE, THE COLONY, TX, WAS DISCIPLINED BY DEA ON JUNE 14, 1994
DISCIPLINARY ACTION: SURRENDER OF CONTROLLED SUBSTANCE LICENSE
OFFENSE: DISCIPLINARY ACTION BY ANOTHER STATE OR AGENCY

NOTES: STATE BOARD.

MURPHY, FRANK STUART DO, DATE OF BIRTH JUNE 30, 1959, LICENSE NUMBER 00J3167 OF THE COLONY, TX, WAS DISCIPLINED BY TEXAS ON APRIL 15, 1994
DISCIPLINARY ACTION: LICENSE SUSPENSION
OFFENSE: LOSS OR RESTRICTION OF HOSPITAL PRIVILEGES

NOTES: IN 3/93 BEGAN TO CONDUCT PSYCHOTHERAPY WITH A FEMALE PATIENT SUFFERING FROM BIPOLAR DISORDER WHICH LASTED FOR SIX THERAPY SESSIONS OVER TWO WEEKS; REPORTED TO HIS SUPERVISOR THAT HE EXPERIENCED STRONG FEELINGS OF COUNTERTRANSFERENCE AND THERAPY WAS TERMINATED; HE THEN INITIATED A SEXUAL RELATIONSHIP WITH HIS FORMER PATIENT; HAD ADMITTED TO A HISTORY OF POLYSUBSTANCE ABUSE AS RECENTLY AS 6/93; ENGAGED IN THE ABUSE OF STREET DRUGS WITH HIS FORMER PATIENT; HOSPITAL PRIVILEGES WERE SUSPENDED ON 6/17/93; WAS DISCHARGED FROM TREATMENT ON 12/15/93; CLAIMS A SOBRIETY DATE OF 6/13/93. SUSPENSION UNTIL SUCH TIME AS HE APPEARS BEFORE THE BOARD AND PROVIDES SUFFICIENT EVIDENCE THAT HE IS PHYSICALLY, MENTALLY OR OTHERWISE COMPETENT TO SAFELY PRACTICE MEDICINE INCLUDING AT A MINIMUM, BUT SHALL NOT BE LIMITED TO, COMPLETE MEDICAL RECORDS AND REPORTS OF PSYCHOLOGICAL AND NEUROPSYCHIATRIC EVALUATIONS.

MURPHY, FRANK STUART DO, DATE OF BIRTH JUNE 13, 1959, LICENSE NUMBER 00J3167 OF DALLAS, TX, WAS DISCIPLINED BY TEXAS ON AUGUST 19, 1994
DISCIPLINARY ACTION: SURRENDER OF CONTROLLED SUBSTANCE LICENSE; 120-MONTH PROBATION
OFFENSE: SUBSTANCE ABUSE

NOTES: LICENSE SUSPENDED 4/15/94 DUE TO INTEMPERATE USE OF DRUGS OR ALCOHOL AND UNPROFESSIONAL OR DISHONORABLE CONDUCT. HAS SATISFIED THE MINIMUM REQUIREMENTS AS SET OUT IN THE 4/15/94 ORDER AND SUSPENSION IS NOW STAYED. CONDITIONS OF PROBATION: SHALL ABSTAIN FROM THE CONSUMPTION OF ALCOHOL/CHEMICAL SUBSTANCES IN ANY FORM UNLESS PRESCRIBED BY ANOTHER PHYSICIAN FOR A LEGITIMATE AND THERAPEUTIC PURPOSE; SHALL SUBMIT HIMSELF FOR APPROPRIATE EXAMS INCLUDING DRUG OR ALCOHOL SCREENS; SHALL NOT TREAT OR OTHERWISE SERVE AS PHYSICIAN, PRESCRIBE, DISPENSE OR ADMINISTER DRUGS THAT MAY BE SUBJECT TO ABUSE FOR HIMSELF OR ANY MEMBER OF HIS FAMILY; SHALL SURRENDER DEA AND TEXAS CONTROLLED SUBSTANCES CERTIFICATES, ALL UNUSED TRIPLICATE PRESCRIPTION FORMS AND ALL CONTROLLED SUBSTANCES IN HIS POSSESSION INCLUDING SAMPLES; SHALL NOT SEEK TO REREGISTER WITHOUT APPROVAL; SEPARATE FROM PATIENT RECORDS, SHALL MAINTAIN A FILE OF EVERY PRESCRIPTION WRITTEN FOR DANGEROUS DRUGS WHICH SHALL BE AVAILABLE FOR INSPECTION; SHALL PARTICIPATE IN THE ACTIVITIES OF A PHYSICIAN ASSISTANCE PROGAM AND ABIDE BY THEIR AFTERCARE PROGRAM CONTRACT WITH QUARTERLY REPORTS TO THE BOARD; SHALL PARTICIPATE IN AA'S PROGRAMS NOT LESS THAN THREE TIMES A WEEK WITH QUARTERLY REPORTS TO THE BOARD; SHALL

SUBMIT HIMSELF TO EVALUATION AND TREATMENT BY A BOARD-APPROVED PSYCHIATRIST WITH QUARTERLY REPORTS; SHALL ATTEND AT LEAST 50 HOURS PER YEAR OF CONTINUING MEDICAL EDUCATION; SHALL APPEAR BEFORE THE BOARD TWICE A YEAR; SHALL GIVE A COPY OF THIS ORDER TO ANY HEALTH CARE ENTITY WHERE HE HAS PRIVILEGES; SHALL COOPERATE WITH THE BOARD IN VERIFYING COMPLIANCE; SHALL INFORM BOARD OF CHANGE OF ADDRESS WITHIN 10 DAYS OR IF HE LEAVES THE STATE; TIME SPENT OUT OF TEXAS DOES NOT COUNT TOWARD PROBATION. SHALL NOT SEEK MODIFICATION FOR ONE YEAR. ON 1/27/96 HIS REQUEST FOR TERMINATION DENIED BUT ORDER MODIFIED AS FOLLOWS: HE IS AUTHORIZED TO REAPPLY TO THE DEA AND THE TEXAS DEPARTMENT OF PUBLIC SAFETY TO OBTAIN FULL PRESCRIBING AUTHORITY FOR CONTROLLED SUBSTANCES; NO LONGER REQUIRED TO SURRENDER ALL UNUSED TRIPLICATE PRESCRIPTION FORMS AND MAY ORDER MORE FORMS; SEPARATE FROM PATIENT RECORDS, HE SHALL MAINTAIN A COPY OF EVERY PRESCRIPTION WRITTEN FOR CONTROLLED SUBSTANCES OR DANGEROUS DRUGS WITH ADDICTIVE POTENTIAL OR POTENTIAL FOR ABUSE WHICH SHALL BE AVAILABLE FOR REVIEW; ALL OTHER CONDITIONS REMAIN IN EFFECT. ON 4/4/98 ORDER TERMINATED.

MURPHY, FRANK STUART DO, LICENSE NUMBER 0188414 OF 755 1/2 DUDLEY DRIVE, SHREVEPORT, LA, WAS DISCIPLINED BY NEW YORK ON NOVEMBER 7, 1995
DISCIPLINARY ACTION: 60-MONTH PROBATION
OFFENSE: DISCIPLINARY ACTION BY ANOTHER STATE OR AGENCY

NOTES: ACTION IN TEXAS FOR THE HABITUAL USE OF DRUGS AND ALCOHOL. FIVE YEAR SUSPENSION, STAYED WITH PROBATION UPON THE COMMENCEMENT OF PRACTICE IN NEW YORK.

MURPHY, JAMES M MD, LICENSE NUMBER 00G6219 OF DALLAS, TX, WAS DISCIPLINED BY TEXAS ON MARCH 2, 1996
DISCIPLINARY ACTION: FINE
OFFENSE: LOSS OR RESTRICTION OF HOSPITAL PRIVILEGES

NOTES: IN AN INPATIENT SURGERY ON 2/16/94, DID NOT ADEQUATELY COMMUNICATE PATIENT STATUS TO A RECOVERY ROOM NURSE PRIOR TO LEAVING THE ROOM TO ENGAGE IN A SECOND PROCEDURE; IN REVIEWED CASES DID NOT ADEQUATELY DOCUMENT WASTAGE OF ANESTHESIA DRUGS IN A MANNER CONSISTENT WITH HOSPITAL POLICY; IN 3/94 METHODIST HOSPITAL OF DALLAS, TEXAS, SUMMARILY SUSPENDED HIS PRIVILEGES ON GROUNDS WHICH INCLUDED INADEQUATE DOCUMENTATION OF WASTAGE OF ANESTHESIA DRUGS. SHALL PAY A $2,000 ADMINISTRATIVE PENALTY; SHALL COOPERATE WITH THE BOARD IN VERIFYING COMPLIANCE.

MURPHY, JAMES MARK MD, LICENSE NUMBER G6219 OF MESQUITE, TX, WAS DISCIPLINED BY TEXAS ON AUGUST 28, 1999
DISCIPLINARY ACTION: FINE
OFFENSE: NONCOMPLIANCE WITH A PROFESSIONAL RULE

NOTES: FAILED TO TIMELY PROVIDE COMPLETE MEDICAL RECORDS TO THE BOARD FOR THREE PATIENTS. $5,000 FINE; TIME SPENT OUT OF TEXAS DOES NOT COUNT TOWARD RESTRICTION; SHALL INFORM THE BOARD OF CHANGE OF ADDRESS WITHIN 10 DAYS OR IF HE LEAVES THE STATE; SHALL NOT SEEK MODIFICATION FOR ONE YEAR.

MURRAY, DUBOSE MD, LICENSE NUMBER R1652 OF CLARKSVILLE, TX, WAS DISCIPLINED BY ARKANSAS ON JUNE 10, 1999
DISCIPLINARY ACTION: SURRENDER OF LICENSE

MURRAY, ROBERT VINCENT JR MD, LICENSE NUMBER 00B8502 OF AUSTIN, TX, WAS DISCIPLINED BY TEXAS ON APRIL 15, 1994
DISCIPLINARY ACTION: 60-MONTH PROBATION; REQUIRED TO TAKE ADDITIONAL MEDICAL EDUCATION
OFFENSE: SUBSTANDARD CARE, INCOMPETENCE OR NEGLIGENCE

NOTES: FAILED TO FOLLOW UP ON LAB VALUES INDICATING A PATIENT WAS ANEMIC; ALTHOUGH HE STATES HE DOES MAKE HOME VISITS, HE FAILED TO VISIT OR INSIST AN 86 YEAR OLD PATIENT COME INTO THE OFFICE TO BE EVALUATED FOR ONSET SEIZURES, INSTEAD PRESCRIBING DILANTIN OVER THE PHONE; FAILED TO ADDRESS EXCEPT IN A PALLIATIVE MANNER A PATIENT'S COMPLAINT OF EXTREME SHORTNESS OF BREATH AND CHEST X-RAY SHOWING LUNG INFILTRATE EVEN THOUGH PATIENT HAD A HISTORY OF BREAST CANCER; FAILED TO RECOGNIZE SIGNS AND SYMPTOMS OF POSSIBLE PULMONARY EMBOLUS IN ANOTHER PATIENT; AFTER THIS PATIENT DIED HOSPITAL COMMITTEE SUGGESTED SEVERAL PROCEDURES SHOULD HAVE BEEN DONE. SUSPENSION STAYED. CONDITIONS OF PROBATION: SHALL WITHIN ONE YEAR COMPLETE A BOARD APPROVED INTERNAL MEDICINE COURSE; SHALL ATTEND AT LEAST 50 HOURS PER YEAR OF CONTINUING MEDICAL EDUCATION; SHALL APPLY FOR BOARD APPROVAL TO TAKE 6/94 SPEX EXAM; IF HE FAILS LICENSE WILL IMMEDIATELY BE SUSPENDED; IF HE PASSES MAY PETITION BOARD FOR EARLY TERMINATION OR MODIFICATION OF THIS ORDER; SHALL APPEAR BEFORE THE BOARD ONCE A YEAR; SHALL GIVE A COPY OF THIS ORDER TO ANY HEALTH CARE ENTITY WHERE HE HAS PRIVILEGES; SHALL COOPERATE WITH THE BOARD IN VERIFYING COMPLIANCE; SHALL INFORM BOARD OF CHANGE OF ADDRESS WITHIN 10 DAYS OR IF HE LEAVES THE STATE; TIME SPENT OUT OF TEXAS DOES NOT COUNT TOWARD PROBATION. SHALL NOT SEEK MODIFICATION FOR ONE YEAR. ON 11/03/94 ORDER WAS TERMINATED.

MURTHA, CARROLL E MD, LICENSE NUMBER 00C0429 OF ABILENE, TX, WAS DISCIPLINED BY TEXAS ON MARCH 31, 1990
DISCIPLINARY ACTION: 36-MONTH RESTRICTION PLACED ON CONTROLLED SUBSTANCE LICENSE; REQUIRED TO TAKE ADDITIONAL MEDICAL EDUCATION

NOTES: STIPULATED ORDER. MUST COMPLETE PRECEPTORSHIP ON PREVENTION AND TREATMENT OF DRUG ABUSE, PASS SPECIAL PURPOSE EXAMINATION, MUST NOT PRESCRIBE, DISPENSE, ADMINISTER OR POSSESS CERTAIN AMPHETAMINE-LIKE ACTION DRUGS OR ANORECTIC AGENTS.

NACOL, WILLIAM S JR MD, LICENSE NUMBER 00C5814 OF BATON ROUGE, LA, WAS DISCIPLINED BY TEXAS ON MAY 24, 1990
DISCIPLINARY ACTION: SURRENDER OF LICENSE

NOTES: STIPULATED ORDER.

NACOL, WILLIAM S JR MD OF BATON ROUGE, LA, WAS DISCIPLINED BY LOUISIANA ON NOVEMBER 15, 1990
DISCIPLINARY ACTION: LICENSE REVOCATION
OFFENSE: DISCIPLINARY ACTION BY ANOTHER STATE OR AGENCY

NOTES: CHARGED WITH CONVICTION OF A FELONY; PRESCRIBING, DISPENSING, OR ADMINISTERING CONTROLLED SUBSTANCES IN OTHER THAN A LEGAL OR LEGITIMATE MANNER; DISPENSATION OF

MEDICATIONS WITHOUT CURRENT REGISTRATION; PROFESSIONAL AND MEDICAL INCOMPETENCY; DISCIPLINED BY ANOTHER STATE.

NACOL, WILLIAM S JR MD, DATE OF BIRTH DECEMBER 2, 1925 OF 12509 COURSEY BLVD, BATON ROUGE, LA, WAS DISCIPLINED BY MEDICARE ON MARCH 16, 1992
DISCIPLINARY ACTION: 120-MONTH EXCLUSION FROM THE MEDICARE AND/OR MEDICAID PROGRAM
OFFENSE: CRIMINAL CONVICTION OR PLEA OF GUILTY, NOLO CONTENDERE, OR NO CONTEST TO A CRIME
NOTES: CONVICTION RELATING TO CONTROLLED SUBSTANCES.

NACOL, WILLIAM SAMUEL JR MD OF 3703 TWIN CITY HIGHWAY, PORT ARTHUR, TX, WAS DISCIPLINED BY DEA ON APRIL 30, 1990
DISCIPLINARY ACTION: SURRENDER OF CONTROLLED SUBSTANCE LICENSE
OFFENSE: CRIMINAL CONVICTION OR PLEA OF GUILTY, NOLO CONTENDERE, OR NO CONTEST TO A CRIME
NOTES: MEDICAL LICENSE REVOKED BY TEXAS BOARD OF MEDICAL EXAMINERS FOR INDISCRIMINATE PRESCRIBING OF HORMONES. CONSPIRED TO OBTAIN 100,000 DOSAGE UNITS PYRIBENZAMINE 10/82 TO 11/82 FOR DISTRIBUTING IN BEAUMONT AND HOUSTON TEXAS. INDICTED 04/03/87 FOR DISTRIBUTION, CONSPIRACY, UNLAWFUL USES OF COMMUNICATION AND UNLAWFUL REMOVAL OF A SYMBOL OF CONTROLLED SUBSTANCES. INVOLVED IN ILLEGAL DISTRIBUTION OF PYRIBENZAMINE AND TALWIN IN PORT ARTHUR AND BRIDGE CITY TEXAS AREAS. PLED GUILTY 03/90 IN JEFFERSON COUNTY TEXAS AND AGREED TO SURRENDER OF MEDICAL LICENSE AND REGISTRATION FOR TALWIN DISTRIBUTION. PLED GUILTY 03/08/90 IN TEXAS TO CONSPIRACY TO DISTRIBUTE AND POSSESSION WITH INTENT TO DISTRIBUTE TALWIN. SENTENCED 04/27/90 TO 1000 HOURS COMMUNITY SERVICE, FIVE YEARS PROBATION, $5000 FINE AND SURRENDERED CONTROLLED SUBSTANCE REGISTRATION VOLUNTARILY. INVOLVED IN DISPENSING ANORECTICS WITHOUT MEDICAL JUSTIFICATION. MEDICAL LICENSE REVOKED. VOLUNTARY SURRENDER OF REGISTRATION 02/05/91; CHARGES DISMISSED 08/22/91 IN TEXAS.

NAINI, GNANA S R MD, LICENSE NUMBER 00H6902 OF PLANO, TX, WAS DISCIPLINED BY TEXAS ON JANUARY 27, 1996
DISCIPLINARY ACTION: FINE
OFFENSE: PROFESSIONAL MISCONDUCT
NOTES: ENGAGED IN VERBALLY ABUSIVE BEHAVIOR WITH MULTIPLE PATIENTS REFERRED FOR DISABILITY EVALUATIONS BY THE TEXAS REHABILITATION COMMISSION; AND REQUIRED THEM TO UNDERGO EXAMINATIONS CONDUCTED IN A DEMEANING, INAPPROPRIATE, AND POTENTIALLY HARMFUL MANNER; SHE DENIES THE CHARGES. $2,500 FINE.

NAJERA, MIGUEL E MD, LICENSE NUMBER E4559 OF LAREDO, TX, WAS DISCIPLINED BY TEXAS ON APRIL 4, 1998
DISCIPLINARY ACTION: FINE
OFFENSE: SUBSTANDARD CARE, INCOMPETENCE OR NEGLIGENCE
NOTES: IN 5/90 WHILE TREATING A PATIENT FOR A HEART ATTACK, AN EMERGENCY ROOM PHYSICIAN LEFT A METAL GUIDE WIRE IN THE PATIENT WHICH WAS EVIDENT IN X-RAYS TAKEN AFTER THE PROCEDURE; FOR APPROXIMATELY 17 DAYS THE WIRE REMAINED IN THE PATIENT AND WAS REMOVED ON 5/23/90 BY DR. NAJERA; INSTEAD OF SENDING THE WIRE FOR CULTURE OR TO PATHOLOGY IT WAS THROWN AWAY; THE PATIENT DIED NEARLY 3 WEEKS AFTER THE OPERATION; THE FAMILY OF THE PATIENT DID NOT REQUEST AN AUTOPSY BECAUSE THEY WERE UNAWARE OF ANY COMPLICATIONS, AND LATER REFUSED TO CONSENT TO AN AUTOPSY; HE FAILED TO INFORM THE PATIENT AND/OR PATIENT'S FAMILY OF THE EXISTENCE OF THE GUIDE WIRE. $2,500 FINE; SHALL COOPERATE WITH THE BOARD IN VERIFYING COMPLIANCE.

NEESE, WILLIAM D MD, DATE OF BIRTH SEPTEMBER 12, 1935 OF 198 INDIES DRIVE, SOUTH, MARATHON, FL, WAS DISCIPLINED BY MEDICARE ON JULY 6, 1995
DISCIPLINARY ACTION: 120-MONTH EXCLUSION FROM THE MEDICARE AND/OR MEDICAID PROGRAM
OFFENSE: CRIMINAL CONVICTION OR PLEA OF GUILTY, NOLO CONTENDERE, OR NO CONTEST TO A CRIME
NOTES: CONVICTED OF A CRIME INVOLVING THE MEDICARE, MEDICAID, MATERNAL AND CHILD HEALTH SERVICES BLOCK GRANT OR BLOCK GRANTS TO STATES FOR SOCIAL SERVICES PROGRAMS.

NEESE, WILLIAM DEAN DO, LICENSE NUMBER 00E5869 OF ATLANTIC BEACH, FL, WAS DISCIPLINED BY TEXAS ON JANUARY 24, 1992
DISCIPLINARY ACTION: SURRENDER OF LICENSE
NOTES: LICENSE VOLUNTARILY SURRENDERED IN LIEU OF FURTHER DISCIPLINARY ACTION.

NEESE, WILLIAM DEAN DO, LICENSE NUMBER 0003968 OF JACKSONVILLE, FL, WAS DISCIPLINED BY FLORIDA ON APRIL 5, 1995
DISCIPLINARY ACTION: 12-MONTH LICENSE SUSPENSION; 36-MONTH PROBATION
OFFENSE: DISCIPLINARY ACTION BY ANOTHER STATE OR AGENCY
NOTES: CHARGED WITH HAVING DISCIPLINARY ACTION TAKEN AGAINST LICENSE BY ANOTHER JURISDICTION; BEING CONVICTED OF OR ENTERING A PLEA OF NOLO CONTENDERE TO A CRIME RELATED TO THE PRACTICE OF MEDICINE. $6,000 FINE; AND PROBATION WITH TERMS SET UPON REINSTATEMENT; REPRIMAND.

NELSON, STUART L MD, LICENSE NUMBER 00E7688 OF ALVARADO, TX, WAS DISCIPLINED BY TEXAS ON AUGUST 18, 1990
DISCIPLINARY ACTION: REPRIMAND; REQUIRED TO TAKE ADDITIONAL MEDICAL EDUCATION
NOTES: STIPULATED ORDER. MUST OBTAIN CONTINUING MEDICAL EDUCATION, PREPARE LIST OF PATIENTS BEING REIMBURSED UNDER WORKERS' COMPENSATION INSURANCE AND ALLOW INSPECTION BY BOARD REPRESENTATIVES OF SUCH PATIENTS' MEDICAL RECORDS. ORDER EFFECTIVE FOR THREE YEARS.

NELSON, STUART L MD, LICENSE NUMBER 00E7688 OF ALVARADO, TX, WAS DISCIPLINED BY TEXAS ON JULY 1, 1995
DISCIPLINARY ACTION: SURRENDER OF LICENSE
OFFENSE: NONCOMPLIANCE WITH A PROFESSIONAL RULE
NOTES: IN LIEU OF FURTHER INVESTIGATION INTO ALLEGATIONS THAT HE MAY HAVE VIOLATED THE MEDICAL PRACTICE ACT. SHALL NOT PETITION FOR REINSTATEMENT.

NELSON, STUART LEMUEL MD OF 208 EAST PURDOM, ALVARADO, TX, WAS DISCIPLINED BY DEA ON AUGUST 8, 1995
DISCIPLINARY ACTION: SURRENDER OF CONTROLLED SUBSTANCE

LICENSE
OFFENSE: DISCIPLINARY ACTION BY ANOTHER STATE OR AGENCY

NOTES: STATE BOARD.

NESSMAN, LAWRENCE DO, LICENSE NUMBER D1244 OF WAYNE, NJ, WAS DISCIPLINED BY TEXAS ON AUGUST 9, 1997
OFFENSE: DISCIPLINARY ACTION BY ANOTHER STATE OR AGENCY

NOTES: ON OR ABOUT 3/6/97 HIS MEDICAL LICENSE WAS REVOKED BY THE NEW JERSEY BOARD WHICH STATED THAT FROM AT LEAST 1990 TO 1995 HE ALLEGEDLY ENGAGED IN A WIDESPREAD PATTERN OF ECONOMIC FRAUD INVOLVING HUNDREDS OF PATIENTS AT HIS OFFICES IN NEW JERSEY. TEXAS LICENSE LIMITED AS FOLLOWS: SHALL NOT PRACTICE IN TEXAS UNTIL HE REQUESTS PERMISSION IN WRITING TO RESUME PRACTICE, PERSONALLY APPEARS BEFORE THE BOARD TO ORALLY PETITION FOR PERMISSION TO RESUME PRACTICE, AND PROVIDES SUFFICIENT EVIDENCE THAT HE IS PHYSICALLY, MENTALLY OR OTHERWISE COMPETENT TO PRACTICE SAFELY; SHALL COOPERATE WITH THE BOARD IN VERIFYING COMPLIANCE INCLUDING PROVIDING COPIES OF ANY MATERIALS THAT HE HAS SUBMITTED TO OR RECEIVED FROM THE NEW JERSEY BOARD; SHALL GIVE A COPY OF THIS ORDER TO ANY HEALTH CARE ENTITY WHERE HE HAS PRIVILEGES; SHALL INFORM THE BOARD OF CHANGE OF ADDRESS WITHIN 10 DAYS; SHALL NOT SEEK MODIFICATION FOR ONE YEAR. ON 4/4/98 THE REQUEST TO HAVE THE ORDER MODIFIED WAS DENIED.

NEUFELD, NEWTON D DO OF SPRINGFIELD, MO, WAS DISCIPLINED BY MISSOURI ON MARCH 11, 1991
DISCIPLINARY ACTION: 12-MONTH SURRENDER OF CONTROLLED SUBSTANCE LICENSE; 36-MONTH PROBATION
OFFENSE: OVERPRESCRIBING OR MISPRESCRIBING DRUGS

NOTES: WHILE LICENSED IN TEXAS, HE WROTE CONTROLLED DRUG PRESCRIPTIONS FOR A MISSOURI PATIENT; THE PRESCRIPTION DID NOT MEET ALL OF THE TECHNICAL REQUIREMENTS OF TEXAS LAW; HE DID NOT HAVE THE AUTHORITY TO PRESCRIBE CONTROLLED DRUGS IN MISSOURI; TEXAS ISSUED AN ORAL REPRIMAND.

NEUFELD, NEWTON D DO, LICENSE NUMBER 00C2895 OF SPRINGFIELD, MO, WAS DISCIPLINED BY TEXAS ON AUGUST 24, 1991
DISCIPLINARY ACTION: SURRENDER OF LICENSE

NOTES: SURRENDER IN LIEU OF FURTHER DISCIPLINARY ACTION.

NEUFELD, NEWTON D DO OF MOUNT VERNON, MO, WAS DISCIPLINED BY MISSOURI ON APRIL 28, 1993
DISCIPLINARY ACTION: 24-MONTH PROBATION
OFFENSE: DISCIPLINARY ACTION BY ANOTHER STATE OR AGENCY

NOTES: DISCIPLINE TAKEN BY TEXAS WHERE HE SURRENDERED HIS TEXAS MEDICAL LICENSE WITHOUT ADMITTING ANY VIOLATION OF TEXAS ADMINISTRATIVE PROCEDURES. PROBATION TIME ADDED TO PREVIOUS PROBATION.

NEWMAN, NICK J MD OF 1900 S COULTER, SUITE H, AMARILLO, TX, WAS DISCIPLINED BY DEA ON JANUARY 25, 1994
DISCIPLINARY ACTION: RESTRICTION PLACED ON CONTROLLED SUBSTANCE LICENSE
OFFENSE: SUBSTANCE ABUSE

NOTES: MEDICAL LICENSE SUSPENDED AROUND 7/89 FOR CHEMICAL DEPENDENCY IMPAIRMENT. USED XANAX SAMPLES TAKEN FROM PLACE OF EMPLOYMENT AROUND 6/93. REQUEST FOR SURRENDER OF REGISTRATION 10/20/93. REGISTRATION EXPIRED 10/31/93.

NEWMAN, NICK JAY MD, LICENSE NUMBER 00H8284, WAS DISCIPLINED BY TEXAS ON DECEMBER 4, 1991
DISCIPLINARY ACTION: MONITORING OF PHYSICIAN PERFORMANCE
OFFENSE: SUBSTANCE ABUSE

NOTES: ON 8/18/90 THE BOARD TERMINATED INDEFINITE SUSPENSION AND PLACED HIM ON PROBATION FOR THREE YEARS PROVIDING IN PART: SHALL SUBMIT FOR SCREENS OF BODILY FLUIDS; SHALL BE MONITORED BY BOARD APPROVED PHYSICIAN WITH QUARTERLY REPORTS TO THE BOARD. HE NOW DESIRES TO RELOCATE AND FINDS THE MONITORING REQUIREMENTS BURDENSOME, AS WELL AS A BARRIER TO ADMISSION TO A RESIDENCY PROGRAM; THERE IS NO EVIDENCE THAT PRIOR INTEMPERATE USE CAUSED ANY PROBLEMS WITH PATIENT CARE; HE IS IN COMPLIANCE WITH EARLIER BOARD ORDER AND MONITORING PHYSICIAN FINDS HE CONTINUES TO FUNCTION WITHOUT DIFFICULTY. PREVIOUS ORDER MODIFIED SUCH THAT HE IS PLACED ON PROBATION FOR REMAINDER OF THREE YEAR PERIOD; MUST REFRAIN FROM USE OF CONTROLLED SUBSTANCES AND GIVE HIS TREATING PHYSICIAN A COPY OF THE ORDER; SHALL SUBMIT TO RANDOM BODILY FLUID SCREENS; SHALL PARTICIPATE IN AA OR OTHER BOARD APPROVED PROGRAM, FREQUENCY DEPENDING ON AVAILABILITY OF PROGRAM WHERE HE RESIDES, WITH QUARTERLY REPORTS TO THE BOARD; SHALL GIVE A COPY OF THIS ORDER TO ALL INSTITUTIONS WHERE HE HAS PRIVILEGES; SHALL COOPERATE WITH THE BOARD IN VERIFYING COMPLIANCE; SHALL ADVISE THE BOARD OF ANY ADDRESS CHANGE WITHIN 10 DAYS; TIME SPENT OUT OF TEXAS DOES NOT COUNT TOWARDS PROBATION; SHALL NOT SEEK MODIFICATION OF THE ORDER FOR ONE YEAR.

NEWMAN, NICK JAY MD, LICENSE NUMBER 00H8284 OF TEMPLE, TX, WAS DISCIPLINED BY TEXAS ON OCTOBER 1, 1993
DISCIPLINARY ACTION: LICENSE SUSPENSION; REQUIRED TO ENTER AN IMPAIRED PHYSICIAN PROGRAM OR SUBSTANCE ABUSE TREATMENT
OFFENSE: FAILURE TO COMPLY WITH PREVIOUS BOARD ORDER

NOTES: VIOLATED 8/18/90 AND 12/4/91 BOARD ORDERS IN THAT HE CONSUMED TWO SAMPLES OF XANAX THAT HE TOOK FROM THE MEDICINE CABINET OF THE FACILITY WHERE HE WAS EMPLOYED IN 6/93; APPEARED TO BE IMPAIRED WHILE PERFORMING MEDICAL DUTIES; ENTERED A CHEMICAL ABUSE PROGRAM AND WAS DISCHARGED 7/26/93. IN LIEU OF AN EMERGENCY SUSPENSION HEARING HE AGREED TO THE VOLUNTARY SUSPENSION OF HIS LICENSE PENDING COMPLETION OF SATISFACTORY INPATIENT TREATMENT AND SUBSEQUENT PROOF THAT HE IS COMPETENT TO PRACTICE; SHALL GIVE A COPY OF THIS ORDER TO ANY HEALTH CARE ENTITY WHERE HE HAS PRIVILEGES; SHALL COOPERATE WITH THE BOARD IN VERIFYING COMPLIANCE; SHALL INFORM THE BOARD OF CHANGE OF ADDRESS WITHIN 10 DAYS.

NEWMAN, NICK JAY MD, LICENSE NUMBER 00H8284, WAS DISCIPLINED BY TEXAS ON JANUARY 5, 1995
DISCIPLINARY ACTION: 120-MONTH PROBATION; RESTRICTION PLACED ON CONTROLLED SUBSTANCE LICENSE
OFFENSE: SUBSTANCE ABUSE

NOTES: HAS SATISFIED THE MINIMUM REQUIREMENTS AS SET

OUT IN THE 10/93 ORDER. PREVIOUS SUSPENSION STAYED, PROBATION UNDER FOLLOWING TERMS AND CONDITIONS: SHALL ABSTAIN FROM THE CONSUMPTION OF ALCOHOL/DRUGS IN ANY FORM UNLESS PRESCRIBED BY ANOTHER PHYSICIAN FOR A LEGITIMATE AND THERAPEUTIC PURPOSE; SHALL CONTINUE TO RECEIVE CARE AND TREATMENT FROM A BOARD APPROVED PHYSICIAN WHO HE SHALL SEE AT LEAST ONCE A MONTH AND WHO SHALL PROVIDE QUARTERLY REPORTS; SHALL PARTICIPATE IN ACTIVITIES OF PHYSICIAN'S HEALTH AND REHABILITATION COMMITTEE AND ATTEND WEEKLY MEETINGS WITH QUARTERLY REPORTS; SHALL SUBMIT HIMSELF FOR APPROPRIATE EXAMS INCLUDING DRUG OR ALCOHOL SCREENS; SHALL PARTICIPATE IN AA'S PROGRAM NOT LESS THAN FIVE TIMES A WEEK WITH QUARTERLY REPORTS TO THE BOARD; SHALL COMPLY WITH THE TERMS AND CONDITIONS OF HIS CONTINUING CARE CONTRACT WITH QUARTERLY REPORTS; SHALL NOT POSSESS ALCOHOL, CONTROLLED SUBSTANCES OR DRUGS WITH POTENTIAL FOR ABUSE; SHALL SURRENDER ANY SUCH DRUGS INCLUDING SAMPLES; SHALL NOT TREAT OR OTHERWISE SERVE AS PHYSICIAN, PRESCRIBE, DISPENSE OR ADMINISTER DRUGS THAT MAY BE SUBJECT TO ABUSE TO HIMSELF OR TO ANY MEMBER OF HIS FAMILY; SHALL NOT PERMIT ANYONE UNDER HIS SUPERVISION TO TELEPHONE A PHARMACY A PRESCRIPTION OR REFILL FOR SUCH DRUGS; SHALL SURRENDER HIS DEA AND TEXAS CONTROLLED SUBSTANCES CERTIFICATES, AND TRIPLICATE PRESCRIPTION FORMS; HIS MEDICAL PRACTICE INCLUDING ANY OFFICE AND SURGICAL PRACTICE SHALL BE MONITORED BY A BOARD APPROVED TEXAS PHYSICIAN WHO SHALL SUBMIT QUARTERLY REPORTS; SHALL MAINTAIN ADEQUATE MEDICAL RECORDS WHICH SHALL BE AVAILABLE FOR REVIEW; SHALL COMPLY WITH CONDITIONS REQUIRED FOR HOSPITAL PRIVILEGES; SHALL APPEAR BEFORE THE BOARD TWICE A YEAR OR UPON REQUEST; SHALL GIVE A COPY OF THIS ORDER TO ANY HEALTH CARE ENTITY WHERE HE HAS PRIVILEGES; SHALL COOPERATE WITH THE BOARD IN VERIFYING COMPLIANCE INCLUDING PROVIDING COPIES OF MEDICAL RELEASES UPON REQUEST; SHALL OBTAIN AT LEAST 50 HOURS PER YEAR OF CONTINUING MEDICAL EDUCATION; SHALL PROVIDE A COPY OF THIS ORDER TO ANYONE REQUESTING IT WITHIN 10 DAYS; SHALL INFORM BOARD OF CHANGE OF ADDRESS WITHIN 10 DAYS OR IF HE LEAVES THE STATE; TIME SPENT OUF OF TEXAS DOES NOT COUNT TOWARD PROBATION. SHALL NOT SEEK MODIFICATION FOR ONE YEAR.

NEWMAN, NICK JAY MD, LICENSE NUMBER 00H8284 OF TEMPLE, TX, WAS DISCIPLINED BY TEXAS ON AUGUST 29, 1995
DISCIPLINARY ACTION: EMERGENCY SUSPENSION
OFFENSE: FAILURE TO COMPLY WITH PREVIOUS BOARD ORDER

NOTES: ON 8/19/95 DURING A COMPLIANCE INTERVIEW REQUIRED BY 2/2/95 PROBATION TERMS HE INDICATED THAT WITHIN THE PAST THREE WEEKS HE HAD TAKEN CHLORPHENIRAMINE AND PSEUDOEPHEDRINE, TWO OVER THE COUNTER MEDICATIONS, AND HYDROCODONE, A DANGEROUS DRUG, WHICH HE WAS ALLEGEDLY TAKING FOR AN EYE INJURY; WHEN REQUESTED TO SUBMIT A URINE SAMPLE FOR TESTING HE FRAUDULENTLY PROVIDED A SAMPLE OF HIS DAUGHTER'S URINE; SUBSEQUENT TO THE SCREEN HE ADMITTED TO INGESTING A HYDROCODONE TABLET EARLIER IN THE MORNING AND INGESTING VARIOUS QUANTITIES OF HYDROCODONE TABLETS OVER THE PAST FOUR MONTHS; AFTER FURTHER INTERVIEW HE SURRENDERED A BOTTLE WITH 22 TABLETS WHICH HE ASSERTED TO BE HYDROCODONE TABLETS. TEMPORARY SUSPENSION TO REMAIN IN EFFECT UNTIL IT IS SUPERSEDED BY A SUBSEQUENT BOARD ORDER.

NIMCHAN, RALPH MD, LICENSE NUMBER E3075 OF LAREDO, TX, WAS DISCIPLINED BY TEXAS ON APRIL 4, 1998
DISCIPLINARY ACTION: FINE
OFFENSE: SUBSTANDARD CARE, INCOMPETENCE OR NEGLIGENCE

NOTES: ON 5/6/90 A GUIDE WIRE WAS LEFT IN A PATIENT AFTER RESUSCITATIVE EFFORTS BY AN EMERGENCY ROOM TREATING PHYSICIAN; DR. NIMCHAN WAS CALLED IN TO CONSULT THE NEXT DAY; HE DID NOT DOCUMENT THE FACT THAT THE GUIDE WIRE WAS LEFT IN THE PATIENT, AND DID NOT INFORM THE PATIENT AND/OR THE PATIENT'S FAMILY OF THE WIRE'S EXISTENCE; HE BELIEVED THAT THE PATIENT'S FAMILY HAD BEEN MADE AWARE OF THE EXISTENCE OF THE GUIDE WIRE. $5,000 FINE.

NIX, DARRYL D DO, LICENSE NUMBER 00F9883 OF ARLINGTON, TX, WAS DISCIPLINED BY TEXAS ON JANUARY 6, 1995
DISCIPLINARY ACTION: REPRIMAND; 36-MONTH REQUIRED TO TAKE ADDITIONAL MEDICAL EDUCATION
OFFENSE: NONCOMPLIANCE WITH A PROFESSIONAL RULE

NOTES: FAILED TO KEEP ADEQUATE RECORDS OF HIS CARE AND TREATMENT OF ONE PATIENT; AGREED TO THIS ORDER IN LIEU OF FURTHER INVESTIGATION. CONDITIONS ON LICENSE FOR THREE YEARS: SHALL MAINTAIN ADEQUATE MEDICAL RECORDS ON ALL PATIENT OFFICE VISITS WHICH SHALL BE AVAILABLE FOR INSPECTION; SHALL OBTAIN AT LEAST 50 HOURS PER YEAR OF CONTINUING MEDICAL EDUCATION INCLUDING AT LEAST 25 HOURS IN RISK MANAGEMENT AND GENERAL OR ADDICTIVE PHARMACOLOGY; SHALL APPEAR BEFORE THE BOARD ONCE A YEAR; SHALL COOPERATE WITH THE BOARD IN VERIFYING COMPLIANCE; SHALL GIVE A COPY OF THIS ORDER TO ANY HEALTH CARE ENTITY WHERE HE HAS OR APPLIES FOR PRIVILEGES OR ANY ONE ELSE WHO REQUESTS IT; SHALL ENSURE ANY INQUIRIES REGARDING HIS TEXAS LICENSURE STATUS ARE ANSWERED BY REFERENCING THIS ORDER; SHALL INFORM BOARD OF CHANGE OF ADDRESS WITHIN 10 DAYS OR IF HE LEAVES THE STATE; TIME SPENT OUT OF TEXAS DOES NOT COUNT TOWARD RESTRICTION. SHALL NOT SEEK MODIFICATION FOR ONE YEAR.

NIX, DARRYL D DO, LICENSE NUMBER F9883 OF ARLINGTON, TX, WAS DISCIPLINED BY TEXAS ON DECEMBER 11, 1999
DISCIPLINARY ACTION: 60-MONTH PROBATION; REQUIRED TO TAKE ADDITIONAL MEDICAL EDUCATION
OFFENSE: SUBSTANDARD CARE, INCOMPETENCE OR NEGLIGENCE

NOTES: SUBSTANDARD CLINICAL RECORDS FAILED TO DOCUMENT ISSUES NECESSARY FOR ONE PATIENT THAT SUFFERED FROM MULTIPLE ILLNESSES SUCH AS INSOMNIA, A FINGER INJURY, ASTHMATIC BRONCHITIS, NIGHT SWEATS, LUMBAR STRAIN/PAIN, NECK PAIN, HEADACHES, ABDOMINAL PAIN, SINUS INFECTION, AND RESPIRATORY INFECTION; FAILED TO PURSUE A MULTIDISCIPLINARY CHRONIC PAIN MANAGEMENT APPROACH; REQUESTED BUT FAILED TO INSIST THAT PATIENT SEE A PAIN SPECIALIST; RECORDS SHOW NO INDICATION THAT HE REFERRED THIS CHRONIC PAIN PATIENT TO A PSYCHIATRIST AND/OR A PSYCHOLOGIST FOR TREATMENT; INAPPROPRIATELY PRESCRIBED "PHEN-FEN" TO THIS PATIENT WITHOUT PROPER INDICATION.

SUSPENSION STAYED FOR PROBATION WITH FOLLOWING TERMS AND CONDITIONS: SHALL TAKE AND PASS THE MEDICAL JURISPRUDENCE EXAM WITHIN ONE YEAR; PRIOR TO TREATING A PATIENT WITH CHRONIC PAIN, SHALL OBTAIN A WRITTEN CONSULTATION FROM A BOARD-APPROVED LICENSED TEXAS PHYSICIAN; MEDICAL RECORDS SHALL BE REVIEWED BY BOARD-APPROVED PHYSICIAN; SHALL MAINTAIN ADEQUATE MEDICAL RECORDS WHICH SHALL BE AVAILABLE FOR REVIEW; SHALL OBTAIN 50 HOURS PER YEAR OF CONTINUING MEDICAL EDUCATION WITH 10 HOURS IN CHRONIC PAIN AND 10 HOURS IN RISK MANAGEMENT; SHALL MAKE ANNUAL APPEARANCES BEFORE THE BOARD; TIME SPENT OUT OF TEXAS DOES NOT COUNT TOWARD PROBATION; SHALL INFORM THE BOARD OF CHANGE OF ADDRESS WITHIN 10 DAYS OR IF HE LEAVES THE STATE; SHALL COOPERATE WITH THE BOARD IN VERIFYING COMPLIANCE; SHALL GIVE A COPY OF THIS ORDER TO ANY HEALTH CARE ENTITY WHERE HE HAS PRIVILEGES; SHALL PROVIDE A COPY OF THIS ORDER TO ANYONE REQUESTING IT WITHIN 10 DAYS; SHALL NOT SEEK MODIFICATION FOR ONE YEAR.

NKONGHO, ANDREW L LACHE II MD, LICENSE NUMBER 00G4365 OF TEANECK, NJ, WAS DISCIPLINED BY TEXAS ON OCTOBER 1, 1993
DISCIPLINARY ACTION: 24-MONTH PROBATION; MONITORING OF PHYSICIAN PERFORMANCE
OFFENSE: DISCIPLINARY ACTION BY ANOTHER STATE OR AGENCY

NOTES: ON 11/9/92 NEW YORK PLACED LICENSE ON PROBATION BASED ON 4 CASES OF INAPPROPRIATE OR INCORRECT SURGERY IN 1984 AND 1985 DURING OR AFTER WHICH THE PATIENTS DIED; ALSO IN 1986 PRACTICED WHILE IMPAIRED BY ALCOHOL; TEXAS LICENSE SUSPENSION STAYED. PLACED ON PROBATION UNDER THE TERMS AND CONDITIONS OF NEW YORK ORDER; ADDITIONAL PROBATIONARY CONDITIONS; PRIOR TO PRACTICING IN TEXAS SHALL OBTAIN PERMISSION FROM THE BOARD; ANYTIME SPENT OUTSIDE NEW YORK OR TEXAS DOES NOT COUNT TOWARD PROBATION; WHEN NEW YORK REMOVES RESTRICTIONS HE MAY APPLY TO HAVE TEXAS RESTRICTIONS REMOVED. SHALL NOT SEEK MODIFICATION FOR ONE YEAR.

NOAMAN, ABDUL GALIL A MD, LICENSE NUMBER 00F0273, WAS DISCIPLINED BY TEXAS ON AUGUST 17, 1996
DISCIPLINARY ACTION: SURRENDER OF LICENSE
OFFENSE: NONCOMPLIANCE WITH A PROFESSIONAL RULE

NOTES: ALLEGATIONS OF VIOLATIONS OF THE MEDICAL PRACTICE ACT. DOES NOT ADMIT VIOLATION. VOLUNTARY AND PERMANENT SURRENDER.

NOAMAN, ABDUL GALIL AHMAD MD OF 321 N. HIGHLAND SUITE 100, SHERMAN, TX, WAS DISCIPLINED BY DEA ON DECEMBER 5, 1996
DISCIPLINARY ACTION: SURRENDER OF CONTROLLED SUBSTANCE LICENSE

NOTES: IN LIEU OF PUBLIC INTEREST REVOCATION.

NORDLUND, PAUL CLEMENS MD, LICENSE NUMBER 00D4247 OF UPLAND, CA, WAS DISCIPLINED BY TEXAS ON JUNE 17, 1992
DISCIPLINARY ACTION: PROBATION
OFFENSE: DISCIPLINARY ACTION BY ANOTHER STATE OR AGENCY

NOTES: REVOCATION STAYED, PLACED ON PROBATION UNDER TERMS AND CONDITIONS FOR THE REST OF HIS LIFE.

NORRID, HENRY DO, LICENSE NUMBER E3077 OF AMARILLO, TX, WAS DISCIPLINED BY TEXAS ON AUGUST 9, 1997
DISCIPLINARY ACTION: REPRIMAND
OFFENSE: OVERPRESCRIBING OR MISPRESCRIBING DRUGS

NOTES: FROM 1992 TO APPROXIMATELY 1995 HE ALLEGEDLY NONTHERAPEUTICALLY PRESCRIBED CONTROLLED SUBSTANCES AND DANGEROUS DRUGS TO FIVE ADULT PATIENTS; HE DENIES ALLEGATION, BUT DOES NOT DENY THE FACT THAT HIS MEDICAL RECORD DOCUMENTATION FOR THE FIVE PATIENTS FAILS TO ADEQUATELY DOCUMENT HIS MEDICAL RATIONALE FOR THE PRESCRIPTIONS; THE INADEQUATE DOCUMENTATION INCLUDES PATIENT COMPLAINTS, APPROPRIATE SUBJECTIVE AND OBJECTIVE FINDINGS TO SUPPORT THE DRUGS PRESCRIBED, PHYSICAL EXAMS, FAILURE TO MENTION ACTUAL DRUG PRESCRIBED OR ITS QUANTITY AND DOSAGE, TREATMENT PLAN AND FOLLOW UP. SINCE BEING NOTIFIED IN 8/94 OF THE INVESTIGATION, HE HAS ATTENDED CONTINUING MEDICAL EDUCATION SEMINARS AND COURSES IN AN EFFORT TO PROACTIVELY ADDRESS THE BOARD'S CONCERNS.

NORRID, HENRY DO, LICENSE NUMBER 120718 OF 1422 SOUTH TYLER STREET, AMARILLO, TX, WAS DISCIPLINED BY NEW YORK ON APRIL 27, 1998
DISCIPLINARY ACTION: REPRIMAND
OFFENSE: DISCIPLINARY ACTION BY ANOTHER STATE OR AGENCY

NOTES: DISCIPLINED BY THE TEXAS BOARD FOR FAILURE TO MAINTAIN ADEQUATE PATIENT RECORDS.

NORTHAM, BEN DO OF 5101 ROSS AVENUE, DALLAS, TX, WAS DISCIPLINED BY DEA ON MAY 2, 1999
DISCIPLINARY ACTION: SURRENDER OF CONTROLLED SUBSTANCE LICENSE
OFFENSE: DISCIPLINARY ACTION BY ANOTHER STATE OR AGENCY

NOTES: STATE BOARD.

NORTHAM, BEN L DO, LICENSE NUMBER D6510 OF DALLAS, TX, WAS DISCIPLINED BY TEXAS ON APRIL 4, 1998
DISCIPLINARY ACTION: 60-MONTH PROBATION; REQUIRED TO TAKE ADDITIONAL MEDICAL EDUCATION
OFFENSE: PROFESSIONAL MISCONDUCT

NOTES: FAILED TO DOCUMENT THE MEDICAL RECORDS OF VARIOUS PATIENTS WHO WERE GIVEN TAKE-HOME INJECTIONS OF B-1, B-6 AND ADENOSINE PHOSPHATE FOR WEIGHT LOSS; FAILED TO DOCUMENT INSTRUCTIONS REGARDING THE INJECTIONS; FAILED TO ADEQUATELY DOCUMENT HISTORIES AND PHYSICALS, AND FAILED TO DOCUMENT VITAL SIGNS; HE STATES THAT ADENOSINE PHOSPHATE IS NO LONGER AVAILABLE FROM ANY MANUFACTURER AND WAS NOT AVAILABLE AT PHARMACIES; HE FAILED TO ADEQUATELY INFORM THE PATIENTS THAT THE TREATMENT IS EXPERIMENTAL IN NATURE; HE CONTENDS THAT HIS WEIGHT LOSS TREATMENT HAS NEVER PRODUCED ANY ADVERSE SIDE EFFECTS AND HAS BENEFITED CERTAIN PATIENTS. SUSPENSION STAYED FOR PROBATION ON THESE TERMS; WITHIN 1 YEAR, SHALL TAKE AND PASS THE SPEX; SHALL OBTAIN 50 HOURS PER YEAR OF CONTINUING MEDICAL EDUCATION, 50 HOURS OF WHICH SHALL BE IN FAMILY PRACTICE; SHALL MAINTAIN ADEQUATE MEDICAL RECORDS WHICH SHALL BE AVAILABLE FOR REVIEW; SHALL INFORM PATIENTS OF ANY TREATMENT PROTOCOLS WHICH THE BOARD DETERMINES TO BE EXPERIMENTAL IN NATURE; SHALL APPEAR BEFORE THE BOARD AT LEAST ONCE A YEAR; SHALL COOPERATE WITH THE BOARD IN VERIFYING COMPLIANCE; SHALL GIVE A COPY OF THIS ORDER TO ANY HEALTH CARE ENTITY WHERE HE HAS

PRIVILEGES; TIME SPENT OUT OF TEXAS DOES NOT COUNT TOWARD PROBATION; SHALL INFORM THE BOARD OF CHANGE OF ADDRESS WITHIN 10 DAYS OR IF HE LEAVES THE STATE; SHALL NOT SEEK MODIFICATION FOR ONE YEAR.

NORTHAM, BEN L DO, LICENSE NUMBER D6510 OF DALLAS, TX, WAS DISCIPLINED BY TEXAS ON APRIL 8, 1999
DISCIPLINARY ACTION: LICENSE SUSPENSION
OFFENSE: FAILURE TO COMPLY WITH PREVIOUS BOARD ORDER

NOTES: FAILED TO TAKE AND PASS THE SPEX WITHIN 1 YEAR AS REQUIRED BY 4/4/98 BOARD ORDER.

NORTON, DEE HART JR MD, LICENSE NUMBER C7722 OF DALLAS, TX, WAS DISCIPLINED BY TEXAS ON APRIL 4, 1998
DISCIPLINARY ACTION: REPRIMAND
OFFENSE: LOSS OR RESTRICTION OF HOSPITAL PRIVILEGES

NOTES: ON 6/24/96 A PATIENT ADMITTED FOR TERM DELIVERY SIGNED A CONSENT FORM ALLOWING HIM TO PROVIDE EPIDURAL ANESTHESIA; HE ATTEMPTED SEVERAL EPIDURAL CATHETER PLACEMENTS WHICH INCLUDED A "WET TAP"; THE PATIENT DEVELOPED COMPLETE SPINAL BLOCK WITH RESPIRATORY DISTRESS; THE DECISION TO INTUBATE THE PATIENT WAS MADE BY THE CRNA WHILE HE WAS ABSENT TO OBTAIN ASSISTANCE FOR THE PATIENT; FETAL HEART TONES DROPPED TO 90 BEATS PER MINUTE; UPON HIS RETURN HE PERFORMED THE C-SECTION AND THE PATIENT AND CHILD DID WELL; FOLLOWING THIS INCIDENT, ON 7/8/96 DESPITE THE OB/GYN AT THE HOSPITAL ADVISORY COMMITTEE RECOMMENDATIONS TO TAKE NO ACTION, HIS EPIDURAL PRIVILEGES AT THE HOSPITAL WERE SUSPENDED; HE ASSERTS THAT HE LEFT THE PATIENT TO SEEK ASSISTANCE; THE BOARD FOUND THAT HE SHOULD HAVE REMAINED WITH THE PATIENT. SHALL COOPERATE WITH THE BOARD IN VERIFYING COMPLIANCE; SHALL GIVE A COPY OF THIS ORDER TO ANY HEALTH CARE ENTITY WHERE HE HAS PRIVILEGES.

NOVOSAD, CHARLES L JR MD, DATE OF BIRTH DECEMBER 19, 1930 OF PO BOX 3498, POJOAQUE, NM, WAS DISCIPLINED BY MEDICARE ON SEPTEMBER 15, 1996
DISCIPLINARY ACTION: EXCLUSION FROM THE MEDICARE AND/OR MEDICAID PROGRAM
OFFENSE: DISCIPLINARY ACTION BY ANOTHER STATE OR AGENCY

NOTES: LICENSE REVOKED FOR REASONS BEARING ON PROFESSIONAL PERFORMANCE.

NOVOSAD, CHARLES LOUIS JR MD OF 210 NORTH HIGHWAY 285, POJOAQUE, NM, WAS DISCIPLINED BY NEW MEXICO ON MAY 20, 1994
DISCIPLINARY ACTION: LICENSE REVOCATION
OFFENSE: OVERPRESCRIBING OR MISPRESCRIBING DRUGS

NOTES: UNPROFESSIONAL CONDUCT; INJUDICIOUS PRESCRIBING.

NOVOSAD, CHARLES LOUIS JR MD, LICENSE NUMBER 0008996, WAS DISCIPLINED BY OKLAHOMA ON SEPTEMBER 9, 1994
DISCIPLINARY ACTION: LICENSE REVOCATION
OFFENSE: DISCIPLINARY ACTION BY ANOTHER STATE OR AGENCY

NOTES: ON 5/20/94 NEW MEXICO BOARD REVOKED HIS LICENSE BASED ON OVER-PRESCRIPTION AND IMPROPER PRESCRIPTION OF CONTROLLED DANGEROUS SUBSTANCES.

NOVOSAD, CHARLES LOUIS JR MD, LICENSE NUMBER 00C4483 OF POJOAQUE, NM, WAS DISCIPLINED BY TEXAS ON JANUARY 6, 1995
OFFENSE: DISCIPLINARY ACTION BY ANOTHER STATE OR AGENCY

NOTES: ON 5/20/94 NEW MEXICO BOARD REVOKED HIS LICENSE ON THE GROUNDS OF INJUDICIOUS PRESCRIBING TO SEVERAL PATIENTS; PRESENTLY SEEKING JUDICIAL REVIEW OF THIS ORDER. SHALL NOT PRACTICE IN TEXAS UNTIL HE REQUESTS PERMISSION IN WRITING FROM THE TEXAS BOARD TO RESUME PRACTICE, PERSONALLY APPEARS BEFORE THE BOARD AND PROVIDES SUFFICIENT EVIDENCE THAT HE IS PHYSICALLY, MENTALLY AND OTHERWISE COMPETENT TO PRACTICE INCLUDING AT A MINIMUM CERTIFICATION OF REVERSAL OF THE NEW MEXICO REVOCATION; SHALL COOPERATE WITH THE BOARD IN VERIFYING COMPLIANCE; SHALL INFORM BOARD OF CHANGE OF ADDRESS WITHIN 10 DAYS.

NOVOSAD, CHARLES LOUIS JR MD OF POJOAQUE, NM, WAS DISCIPLINED BY DEA ON OCTOBER 11, 1995
DISCIPLINARY ACTION: REVOCATION OF CONTROLLED SUBSTANCE LICENSE
OFFENSE: DISCIPLINARY ACTION BY ANOTHER STATE OR AGENCY

NOTES: ON 5/20/94 NEW MEXICO BOARD ORDERED THE REVOCATION OF HIS LICENSE; ON 9/15/94 THE NEW MEXICO PHARMACY BOARD REVOKED HIS STATE REGISTRATION TO HANDLE CONTROLLED SUBSTANCES.

NUNNALLY, CLEON S MD, LICENSE NUMBER 00C6458, WAS DISCIPLINED BY TEXAS ON OCTOBER 5, 1991
DISCIPLINARY ACTION: REPRIMAND
OFFENSE: NONCOMPLIANCE WITH A PROFESSIONAL RULE

NOTES: PRESCRIBED DEMEROL TO HIS WIFE OUT OF OFFICE ACCOUNT, AND FAILED TO KEEP COMPLETE AND ACCURATE RECORDS TO SUPPORT THE USE OF DEMEROL IN HIS WIFE'S TREATMENT.

O'BRIEN, ROBERT BURNS MD, DATE OF BIRTH OCTOBER 2, 1927, LICENSE NUMBER 00C5818 OF 2600 N GESSNER SUITE 168, HOUSTON, TX, WAS DISCIPLINED BY TEXAS ON MARCH 26, 1993
DISCIPLINARY ACTION: LICENSE REVOCATION
OFFENSE: LOSS OR RESTRICTION OF HOSPITAL PRIVILEGES

NOTES: ALLOWED HIS BROTHER TO PRACTICE IN HIS PLACE AND AS A PHYSICIAN'S ASSISTANT AFTER THE BROTHER'S MEDICAL LICENSE HAD BEEN REVOKED. IN 1/91 MEMORIAL MEDICAL CENTER RESTRICTED HIS HOSPITAL PRIVILEGES IN THAT HE WAS REQUIRED TO INITIATE APPROPRIATE CONSULTATIONS WITHIN 24 HOURS OF ADMITTING PATIENTS; VOLUNTARILY PLACED HIS PRIVILEGES ON 90 DAY SUSPENSION AFTER HE FAILED TO OBTAIN THESE CONSULTATIONS; ALSO WITH RESPECT TO 1 PATIENT HE WAS GUILTY OF MISDIAGNOSIS, GROSS MISMANAGEMENT AND A DELAY IN TREATMENT; HE REFUSED TO COOPERATE WITH THE BOARD'S INVESTIGATION. ORDER WILL BECOME FINAL WHEN ALL APPEALS HAVE BEEN EXHAUSTED.

O'BRIEN, ROBERT BURNS MD, DATE OF BIRTH OCTOBER 2, 1927 OF 2600 N GESSNER SUITE 168, HOUSTON, TX, WAS DISCIPLINED BY MEDICARE ON AUGUST 30, 1994
DISCIPLINARY ACTION: EXCLUSION FROM THE MEDICARE AND/OR MEDICAID PROGRAM
OFFENSE: DISCIPLINARY ACTION BY ANOTHER STATE OR AGENCY

NOTES: LICENSE REVOKED FOR REASONS BEARING ON PROFESSIONAL COMPETENCE.

O'BRYAN, ROBERT KEENE MD, LICENSE NUMBER 00D9595 OF FORT SMITH, AR, WAS DISCIPLINED BY TEXAS ON MAY 11, 1995
DISCIPLINARY ACTION: REPRIMAND
OFFENSE: SUBSTANCE ABUSE

NOTES: ON 1/29/91 ADMINISTERED IV SEDATION TO A PATIENT AND DURING THE PROCEDURE THE PATIENT BECAME BRADYCARDIC, APNEIC AND HYPOTENSIVE; HE UNDERTOOK IMMEDIATE RESUSCITATIVE MECHANISMS, BUT THEY WERE INADEQUATE AND THE PATIENT EXPIRED; HE ADMITTED INCREASED USE OF ALCOHOL SUBSEQUENT TO PATIENT'S DEATH; REPORTS SOBRIETY DATE OF 7/22/91; IN 8/91, ADMITTED HIMSELF TO TALBOT-MARSH RECOVERY CENTER FOR TREATMENT OF SUBSTANCE ABUSE; REPORTS THAT HE ATTENDS AN AVERAGE OF SEVEN AA MEETINGS PER MONTH AND REGULAR PARTICIPATION IN THE ARKANSAS COMMITTEE FOR PHYSICIAN HEALTH AND REHABILITATION. SHALL NOT PRACTICE MEDICINE IN TEXAS UNTIL HE REQUESTS PERMISSION FROM THE BOARD AND PROVIDES SUFFICIENT EVIDENCE WHICH INDICATES THAT HE IS PHYSICALLY, MENTALLY AND OTHERWISE COMPETENT TO SAFELY PRACTICE MEDICINE INCLUDING AT A MINIMUM EVIDENCE OF CONTINUED SOBRIETY. DUE TO HIS SATISFYING THE MINIMUM REQUIREMENTS OF THIS ORDER, ON 11/14/96 BOARD GRANTED HIM PERMISSION TO RESUME MEDICAL PRACTICE IN TEXAS.

O'BRYAN, ROBERT KEENE MD, LICENSE NUMBER C35535 OF FORT SMITH, AR, WAS DISCIPLINED BY CALIFORNIA ON MAY 30, 1997
DISCIPLINARY ACTION: SURRENDER OF LICENSE

NOTES: WHILE CHARGES PENDING.

O'CONNOR, ANDREW M MD, LICENSE NUMBER E7690 OF DALLAS, TX, WAS DISCIPLINED BY TEXAS ON NOVEMBER 5, 1999
DISCIPLINARY ACTION: EMERGENCY SUSPENSION

NOTES: EVIDENCE THAT HIS CONTINUED PRACTICE WOULD CONSTITUTE A CONTINUING THREAT TO PUBLIC WELFARE.

O'DAY, MARY P MD, DATE OF BIRTH AUGUST 10, 1959 OF 701 ROSEDALE ST, APT G, HOUSTON, TX, WAS DISCIPLINED BY MEDICARE ON JULY 9, 1996
DISCIPLINARY ACTION: EXCLUSION FROM THE MEDICARE AND/OR MEDICAID PROGRAM
OFFENSE: NONCOMPLIANCE WITH A PROFESSIONAL RULE

NOTES: DEFAULTED ON PUBLIC HEALTH SERVICE EDUCATION LOAN. REINSTATED ON 10/7/96.

OCHOA, MIGUEL R MD, LICENSE NUMBER D4001, WAS DISCIPLINED BY TEXAS ON MAY 10, 1997
DISCIPLINARY ACTION: RESTRICTION PLACED ON LICENSE
OFFENSE: DISCIPLINARY ACTION BY ANOTHER STATE OR AGENCY

NOTES: ON 7/10/95 HE ENTERED INTO A CONSENT ORDER WITH THE ILLINOIS BOARD PLACING HIS LICENSE ON PROBATION BASED ON EXCESSIVE PRESCRIBING TO VARIOUS PATIENTS. HIS LICENSE IS HEREBY RESTRICTED UNTIL FURTHER ORDER OF THE BOARD; HE SHALL NOT PRACTICE MEDICINE IN TEXAS UNTIL SUCH TIME AS HE REQUESTS WRITTEN PERMISSION TO DO SO AND PERSONALLY APPEARS BEFORE THE BOARD AND PROVIDES SUFFICIENT EVIDENCE WHICH ADEQUATELY INDICATES THAT HE IS PHYSICALLY, MENTALLY, AND OTHERWISE COMPETENT TO ENGAGE IN THE PRACTICE OF MEDICINE. SUCH EVIDENCE SHALL INCLUDE AT A MINIMUM: NO PENDING ILLINOIS OR OTHER STATE LICENSURE ACTIONS/PROCEEDINGS; LIFTING OF ILLINOIS PROBATION; SHALL COOPERATE WITH THE BOARD IN VERIFYING COMPLIANCE; SHALL INFORM THE BOARD OF CHANGE OF ADDRESS WITHIN 10 DAYS; SHALL NOT SEEK MODIFICATION FOR ONE YEAR.

OEI, LIEM SOM MD OF SIOUX CITY, IA, WAS DISCIPLINED BY IOWA ON DECEMBER 18, 1997
DISCIPLINARY ACTION: FINE; RESTRICTION PLACED ON LICENSE
OFFENSE: SEXUAL ABUSE OF OR SEXUAL MISCONDUCT WITH A PATIENT

NOTES: CHARGED WITH HAVING ENGAGED IN IMPROPER SEXUAL CONTACT WITH THREE PATIENTS. $5000 CIVIL PENALTY; SEVERAL PRACTICE RESTRICTIONS WERE PLACED ON HIS LICENSE.

OEI, LIEM SOM MD, LICENSE NUMBER 3873, WAS DISCIPLINED BY SOUTH DAKOTA ON JUNE 2, 1998
DISCIPLINARY ACTION: RESTRICTION PLACED ON LICENSE; REQUIRED TO TAKE ADDITIONAL MEDICAL EDUCATION
OFFENSE: DISCIPLINARY ACTION BY ANOTHER STATE OR AGENCY

NOTES: ON 12/18/97 IOWA BOARD ENTERED INTO AN ORDER AND SETTLEMENT AGREEMENT WITH HIM. SOUTH DAKOTA LICENSE LIMITED AS FOLLOWS: SHALL ATTEND A PERSONALIZED CONTINUING MEDICAL EDUCATION PROGRAM ADDRESSING APPROPRIATE PHYSICIAN-PATIENT BOUNDARIES; SHALL HAVE A FEMALE CHAPERONE PRESENT AT ALL TIMES DURING EXAMINATIONS OF PATIENTS; SHALL NOT TREAT PATIENTS WHO MEET THE CRITERIA DESCRIBED IN SPECIFIED SECTIONS OF THE DIAGNOSTIC AND STATISTICAL MANUAL OF THE AMERICAN PSYCHIATRIC ASSOCIATION, EXCEPT IN EMERGENCY CASES; SHALL TAKE NINE HOURS OF CONTINUING MEDICAL EDUCATION WHICH ADDRESS THE CHARACTERISTICS OF MAJOR PSYCHIATRIC DISORDERS WITHIN ONE YEAR.

OEI, LIEM SOM MD, LICENSE NUMBER H1817 OF SIOUX CITY, IA, WAS DISCIPLINED BY TEXAS ON AUGUST 22, 1998
DISCIPLINARY ACTION: MONITORING OF PHYSICIAN PERFORMANCE
OFFENSE: DISCIPLINARY ACTION BY ANOTHER STATE OR AGENCY

NOTES: ON 12/18/97 THE IOWA BOARD PLACED RESTRICTIONS ON HIS LICENSE. TEXAS LICENSE LIMITED AS FOLLOWS: SHALL NOT PRACTICE IN TEXAS UNTIL HE APPEARS BEFORE THE BOARD WITH SUFFICIENT EVIDENCE AND INFORMATION THAT HE IS PHYSICALLY, MENTALLY AND OTHERWISE COMPETENT TO PRACTICE SAFELY INCLUDING AT A MINIMUM: SHALL PRESENT DOCUMENTATION OF HIS CURRENT LICENSURE STATUS IN OTHER STATES; SHALL PRESENT DOCUMENTATION FROM THE IOWA BOARD ATTESTING TO HIS COMPLIANCE WITH THE 1997 ORDER; SHALL APPEAR BEFORE THE BOARD UPON REQUEST; SHALL COOPERATE WITH THE BOARD IN VERIFYING COMPLIANCE INCLUDING PROVIDING COPIES OF PEER REVIEW RECORDS UPON REQUEST; SHALL PROVIDE COPIES OF ANY MATERIALS THAT HE HAS SUBMITTED TO OR RECEIVED FROM STATE MEDICAL BOARDS OF IOWA, NEBRASKA, NEW YORK, SOUTH DAKOTA, AND ARIZONA; SHALL PROVIDE A COPY OF THIS ORDER TO ANYONE REQUESTING IT WITHIN 10 DAYS; TIME SPENT OUT OF TEXAS DOES NOT COUNT TOWARD RESTRICTION; SHALL INFORM THE BOARD OF CHANGE OF ADDRESS WITHIN 10 DAYS OR IF HE LEAVES THE STATE; SHALL NOT SEEK MODIFICATION FOR ONE YEAR.

OEI, LIEM SOM MD, LICENSE NUMBER 128703 OF 1379 FOX RIDGE TRAIL, SIOUX CITY, IA, WAS DISCIPLINED BY NEW YORK ON

AUGUST 26, 1998
DISCIPLINARY ACTION: SURRENDER OF LICENSE
OFFENSE: DISCIPLINARY ACTION BY ANOTHER STATE OR AGENCY

NOTES: DISCIPLINED BY THE IOWA BOARD FOR PERFORMING INAPPROPRIATE PHYSICAL EXAMINATIONS AND ENGAGING IN SEXUAL CONTACT WITH TWO PATIENTS.

OFFUTT, DONALD NIXON MD, LICENSE NUMBER 00D5805 OF DALLAS, TX, WAS DISCIPLINED BY TEXAS ON APRIL 15, 1994
DISCIPLINARY ACTION: 60-MONTH PROBATION; REQUIRED TO TAKE ADDITIONAL MEDICAL EDUCATION
OFFENSE: SUBSTANCE ABUSE

NOTES: ADMITS HE IS AN ALCOHOLIC; VOLUNTARILY ADMITTED HIMSELF FOR INPATIENT TREATMENT ON 8/27/93; CURRENTLY MAINTAINING A HALF-TIME OUTPATIENT PSYCHIATRIC PRACTICE. SUSPENSION STAYED. CONDITIONS OF PROBATION: SHALL ABSTAIN FROM THE CONSUMPTION OF ALCOHOL/CHEMICAL SUBSTANCES IN ANY FORM UNLESS PRESCRIBED BY ANOTHER PHYSICIAN FOR A LEGITIMATE AND THERAPEUTIC PURPOSE; SHALL NOT TREAT OR OTHERWISE SERVE AS PHYSICIAN, PRESCRIBE, DISPENSE, OR ADMINISTER DRUGS THAT MAY BE SUBJECT TO ABUSE TO HIMSELF OR ANY MEMBER OF HIS FAMILY; SHALL PARTICIPATE IN AA'S PROGRAM NOT LESS THAN THREE TIMES A WEEK WITH QUARTERLY REPORTS TO THE BOARD AND SHALL INFORM THE BOARD OF HIS AA SPONSOR WITHIN 30 DAYS; SHALL SUBMIT HIMSELF FOR APPROPRIATE EXAMS INCLUDING DRUG OR ALCOHOL SCREENS; SHALL CONTINUE TO RECEIVE PSYCHIATRIC TREATMENT WITH QUARTERLY REPORTS; SHALL CONTINUE TO PARTICIPATE IN ACTIVITIES OF A PHYSICIAN HEALTH AND REHABILITATION COMMITTEE AND ATTEND WEEKLY MEETINGS WITH QUARTERLY REPORTS; SHALL ATTEND AT LEAST 50 HOURS PER YEAR OF CONTINUING MEDICAL EDUCATION INCLUDING COURSES IN ADDICTIONOLOGY AND SUBSTANCE ABUSE; SHALL PERFORM TWO HOURS PER MONTH OF COMMUNITY SERVICE FOR FIVE YEARS; PRIOR TO INCREASING HIS HOURS ABOVE HALFTIME OR ANY OTHER CHANGE IN THE NATURE OF HIS PRACTICE SHALL APPEAR BEFORE AND RECEIVE BOARD APPROVAL; SHALL APPEAR BEFORE THE BOARD FOUR TIMES A YEAR; SHALL GIVE A COPY OF THIS ORDER TO ANY HEALTH CARE ENTITY WHERE HE HAS PRIVILEGES; SHALL COOPERATE WITH THE BOARD IN VERIFYING COMPLIANCE; SHALL INFORM BOARD OF CHANGE OF ADDRESS WITHIN 10 DAYS OR IF HE LEAVES THE STATE; TIME SPENT OUT OF TEXAS DOES NOT COUNT TOWARD PROBATION. SHALL NOT SEEK MODIFICATION FOR ONE YEAR.

OFFUTT, DONALD NIXON MD, LICENSE NUMBER 00C3163 OF 403 B N. MORROW ST, HELENA, AR, WAS DISCIPLINED BY ARKANSAS ON MARCH 27, 1995
DISCIPLINARY ACTION: 60-MONTH PROBATION
OFFENSE: SUBSTANCE ABUSE

NOTES: HABITUAL INDULGENCE AND USE OF ALCOHOL WHICH RENDERS HIM INCAPABLE OF EXERCISING THE SKILL AND JUDGMENT NECESSARY TO TREAT HIS PATIENTS. FIVE YEAR SUSPENSION STAYED.

OFFUTT, DONALD NIXON MD, LICENSE NUMBER C3163 OF MENA, AR, WAS DISCIPLINED BY ARKANSAS ON MARCH 13, 1997
DISCIPLINARY ACTION: LICENSE REVOCATION

OGLE, ROBERT CURTIS DO, DATE OF BIRTH FEBRUARY 3, 1947 OF ROUTE 2 BOX 150, TENNESSEE COLONY, TX, WAS DISCIPLINED BY MEDICARE ON JULY 23, 1991
DISCIPLINARY ACTION: 240-MONTH EXCLUSION FROM THE MEDICARE AND/OR MEDICAID PROGRAM
OFFENSE: CRIMINAL CONVICTION OR PLEA OF GUILTY, NOLO CONTENDERE, OR NO CONTEST TO A CRIME

NOTES: CONVICTION RELATING TO FRAUD. REINSTATED ON 8/13/91.

OGLE, ROBERT CURTIS DO OF 406 HERITAGE, ROCKWALL, TX, WAS DISCIPLINED BY DEA ON NOVEMBER 16, 1993
DISCIPLINARY ACTION: RESTRICTION PLACED ON CONTROLLED SUBSTANCE LICENSE
OFFENSE: CRIMINAL CONVICTION OR PLEA OF GUILTY, NOLO CONTENDERE, OR NO CONTEST TO A CRIME

NOTES: DIVERTING 10,000+ DOSAGE UNITS OF CONTROLLED SUBSTANCES MONTHLY THROUGH PRESCRIPTIONS FOR NONMEDICAL PURPOSES. PLED GUILTY 08/17/83 TO DISPENSING QUAALUDE NOT FOR MEDICAL PURPOSE AND SURRENDERED BD. SENTENCED 09/28/83 TO PRISON, SPECIAL PAROLE AND FINE. PREVIOUS REGISTRATION VOLUNTARILY SURRENDERED AND RETIRED 07/31/84. WITHDRAWAL OF APPLICATION 02/24/89. APPROVAL OF APPLICATION; RESTRICTED TO SCHEDULES III, IIIN, IV AND V.

OLSON, DEAN R DO, DATE OF BIRTH APRIL 27, 1929, LICENSE NUMBER 1003999 OF 11970 SWEETWATER DR #5A, GRAND LEDGE, MI, WAS DISCIPLINED BY MICHIGAN ON JUNE 4, 1998
DISCIPLINARY ACTION: 12-MONTH PROBATION
OFFENSE: SUBSTANCE ABUSE

OLSON, DEAN RICHARD DO, LICENSE NUMBER C4487 OF GRAND LEDGE, MI, WAS DISCIPLINED BY TEXAS ON MAY 14, 1999
DISCIPLINARY ACTION: RESTRICTION PLACED ON LICENSE
OFFENSE: DISCIPLINARY ACTION BY ANOTHER STATE OR AGENCY

NOTES: HE IS UNDER A CONSENT ORDER FROM THE MICHIGAN BOARD FOR ALCOHOL IMPAIRMENT; ON 12/8/82 HE WAS FOUND GUILTY OF IMPAIRED DRIVING AND PLACED ON ONE YEAR PROBATION; ON 5/19/88 HE WAS CONVICTED OF OPERATING A MOTOR VEHICLE UNDER THE INFLUENCE OF ALCOHOL; HE CONTENDS THAT IN 1989 HE COMPLETED A 4 WEEK INPATIENT TREATMENT PROGRAM FOLLOWED BY 2 YEARS OF FORMAL AFTERCARE; IN ADDITION HE WAS TREATED IN A 14 DAY RESIDENCE PROGRAM IN 1996; ON 9/18/95 AN ADMINISTRATIVE COMPLAINT WAS FILED CHARGING HIM WITH VIOLATION OF THE MICHIGAN PUBLIC HEALTH CODE, CITING HIS PREVIOUS ARRESTS AS EVIDENCE THAT HE WAS IMPAIRED; ON 10/18/97 HE ENTERED INTO A RECOVERY MONITORING AGREEMENT FOR ONE YEAR. LICENSE LIMITED AS FOLLOWS: SHALL NOT PRACTICE UNTIL HE APPEARS BEFORE THE BOARD WITH EVIDENCE THAT HE IS PHYSICALLY, MENTALLY OR OTHERWISE COMPETENT TO PRACTICE SAFELY; SUCH EVIDENCE WILL INCLUDE: COMPLIANCE OR COMPLETION OF HIS MICHIGAN BOARD ORDER, AND DOCUMENTED SOBRIETY SUFFICIENT IN THE DISCRETION OF THE BOARD TO DEMONSTRATE ADEQUATE PROTECTION OF THE PUBLIC; SHALL COOPERATE WITH THE BOARD IN VERIFYING COMPLIANCE INCLUDING PROVIDING COPIES OF MEDICAL RELEASES UPON REQUEST; SHALL INFORM THE BOARD OF CHANGE OF ADDRESS WITHIN 10 DAYS; SHALL NOT SEEK MODIFICATION FOR ONE YEAR.

OOI, JAMES P MD, LICENSE NUMBER CO39127 OF SAN DIEGO, CA,

WAS DISCIPLINED BY CALIFORNIA ON OCTOBER 12, 1990
DISCIPLINARY ACTION: 60-MONTH PROBATION
OFFENSE: SUBSTANDARD CARE, INCOMPETENCE OR NEGLIGENCE

NOTES: GROSS NEGLIGENCE AND INCOMPETENCE IN MANAGING THERAPEUTIC ABORTIONS. REVOCATION STAYED.

OOI, JAMES PENG GUAN MD OF SAN DIEGO, CA, WAS DISCIPLINED BY LOUISIANA ON JUNE 20, 1991
DISCIPLINARY ACTION: PROBATION; RESTRICTION PLACED ON LICENSE
OFFENSE: DISCIPLINARY ACTION BY ANOTHER STATE OR AGENCY

NOTES: CHARGED WITH ACTION TAKEN BY THE LICENSING AUTHORITY OF CALIFORNIA. REVOCATION STAYED SUBJECT TO CONTINUING PROBATION ON SAME CONDITIONS AND FOR SAME DURATION AS IMPOSED BY CALIFORNIA, INCLUDING: SUCCESSFUL PASSING OF CLINICAL EXAMINATION IN FAMILY PRACTICE, PROHIBITION ON PERFORMING ANY ABORTION PROCEDURE PENDING SUCCESSFUL COMPLETION OF CLINICAL TRAINING PROGRAM, AND PRIOR NOTICE TO BOARD OF INTENT TO RELOCATE TO LOUISIANA.

OOI, JAMES PENG GWAN MD, LICENSE NUMBER 0033746 OF SAN DIEGO, CA, WAS DISCIPLINED BY WASHINGTON ON OCTOBER 6, 1995
DISCIPLINARY ACTION: DENIAL OF NEW LICENSE

NOTES: WOULD NOT CONSIDER ANOTHER APPLICATION UNTIL HE COMPLETED A TERM OF PROBATION IN CALIFORNIA, PASSED THE AMERICAN BOARD OF CERTIFICATION OF FAMILY PRACTICE AND PROVIDED UPDATED APPLICATION DOCUMENTATION. ON 5/15/96 THE BOARD TERMINATED ITS JURISDICTION AND HE WAS LICENSED IN WASHINGTON.

OOI, JAMES PENG MD, WAS DISCIPLINED BY TEXAS ON OCTOBER 5, 1996
DISCIPLINARY ACTION: RESTRICTION PLACED ON LICENSE; REQUIRED TO TAKE ADDITIONAL MEDICAL EDUCATION
OFFENSE: DISCIPLINARY ACTION BY ANOTHER STATE OR AGENCY

NOTES: ON 10/01/93 WAS DISCIPLINED IN CALIFORNIA BASED ON HIS CARE AND TREATMENT OF TWO PATIENTS UNDERGOING THERAPEUTIC ABORTIONS; HIS LICENSE WAS RESTORED TO CLEAR STATUS ON 11/02/95. LICENSES IN LOUISIANA AND WASHINGTON. PLACE IN A CONCURRENT PROBATIONARY STATUS BASED ON THE CALIFORNIA ACTION; BOTH RESTORED TO UNRESTRICTED STATUS IN 1996; IN 1990 HIS OBSTETRICAL PRIVILEGES AT SHARP MEMORIAL HOSPITAL WERE SUSPENDED AND A CO-ADMITTER WAS REQUIRED FOR ALL MAJOR AND INTENSIVE CARE UNIT CASES; AND IN 1996 THE REQUIREMENT FOR A CO-ADMITTER WAS DISCONTINUED, HOWEVER, THE SUSPENSION OF OBSTETRICAL PRIVILEGES REMAINED IN PLACE. RESTRICTED UNDER TERMS AND CONDITIONS FOR FIVE YEARS: SHALL NOT PERFORM ABORTIONS, INDEFINITELY AND IRRESPECTIVE OF THE FIVE YEAR TIME PERIOD; HIS MEDICAL PRACTICE, INCLUDING ANY OFFICE AND SURGICAL PRACTICE, SHALL BE MONITORED BY A BOARD APPROVED TEXAS PHYSICIAN WHO SHALL SUBMIT QUARTERLY REPORTS TO THE BOARD; WITHIN ONE YEAR SHALL TAKE AND PASS THE ADVANCED CARDIAC LIFE SUPPORT COURSE AND THE ADVANCED TRAUMA LIFE SUPPORT COURSE AND OBTAIN CERTIFICATION FOR BOTH; SHALL OBTAIN AT LEAST 50 HOURS PER YEAR OF CONTINUING MEDICAL EDUCATION ALL OF WHICH SHALL BE IN OBSTETRICS AND GYNECOLOGY, AND SUBMIT PROOF TO THE BOARD; SHALL APPEAR BEFORE THE BOARD AT LEAST TWICE PER YEAR OR UPON WRITTEN REQUEST; SHALL COOPERATE WITH THE BOARD IN VERIFYING COMPLIANCE INCLUDING PROVIDING COPIES OF PEER REVIEW RECORDS UPON REQUEST; SHALL COMPLY WITH ANY HOSPITAL RESTRICTIONS WHICH MAY BE IMPOSED AS A RESULT OF THIS ORDER; SHALL GIVE A COPY OF THIS ORDER TO ANY HEALTH CARE ENTITY WHERE HE HAS PRIVILEGES; SHALL PROVIDE A COPY OF THIS ORDER TO ANYONE REQUESTING IT WITHIN 10 DAYS; TIME PERIOD OUT OF TEXAS DOES NOT COUNT TOWARD RESTRICTION; SHALL INFORM THE BOARD OF CHANGE OF ADDRESS WITHIN 10 DAYS OR IF HE LEAVES THE STATE; SHALL NOT SEEK MODIFICATION FOR ONE YEAR.

ORLOWSKI, FRANCIS JOHN DO, LICENSE NUMBER 00C2088 OF BEDFORD, TX, WAS DISCIPLINED BY TEXAS ON JUNE 12, 1990
DISCIPLINARY ACTION: SURRENDER OF LICENSE

NOTES: STIPULATED ORDER. LICENSE IMMEDIATELY AND PERMANENTLY RETIRED IN LIEU OF INVESTIGATION AND SUBSEQUENT HEARING. MUST ALSO IMMEDIATELY SURRENDER CONTROLLED SUBSTANCE REGISTRATIONS AND TRIPLICATE PRESCRIPTION PADS.

ORO, FEBE LINDA MD, LICENSE NUMBER 00G4185 OF DENISON, TX, WAS DISCIPLINED BY TEXAS ON JUNE 28, 1995
DISCIPLINARY ACTION: FINE; REPRIMAND
OFFENSE: OVERCHARGING

NOTES: PROFESSIONAL FAILURE TO PRACTICE MEDICINE IN AN ACCEPTABLE MANNER CONSISTENT WITH PUBLIC HEALTH AND WELFARE; FAILED TO ADEQUATELY SUPERVISE THE ACTIVITIES OF THOSE UNDER HER SUPERVISION AND PERSISTENTLY OR FLAGRANTLY OVERCHARGED PATIENTS IN THAT DURING 1993 AND 1994 SHE, THROUGH HER OFFICE STAFF, BILLED VARIOUS PATIENTS FOR MORE TIME THAN SHE HAD ACTUALLY SPENT WITH THEM AND FOR MORE MEDICATION THAN PATIENTS ACTUALLY RECEIVED AND BILLED TREATMENTS AS OFFICE PROCEDURES WHEN THE PROCEDURES WERE ACTUALLY PERFORMED IN THE PATIENTS' HOMES; DURING 1993 AND 1994 FAILED TO KEEP ACCURATE MEDICAL RECORDS ON VARIOUS PATIENTS; REPORTS THAT CORRECTIVE MEASURES HAVE BEEN INSTITUTED WHICH SHALL ELIMINATE THE INACCURATE OVERBILLING AND INADEQUATE DOCUMENTATION. RESTRICTION FOR FIVE YEARS WITH TERMS: SHALL ENSURE HER HUSBAND IS NOT AN EMPLOYEE IN HER PRACTICE, IS NOT INVOLVED IN HER PRACTICE AND HAS NO AUTHORITY OVER PERSONNEL WITHIN HER OFFICE; SHALL MAINTAIN ADEQUATE RECORDS WHICH SHALL BE AVAILABLE FOR REVIEW; SHALL ADOPT OR ESTABLISH A SYSTEM OF PATIENT RECORD KEEPING AND BILLING; SHALL ATTEND AT LEAST 50 HOURS PER YEAR OF CONTINUING MEDICAL EDUCATION, DURING THE FIRST YEAR AT LEAST 20 HOURS SHALL BE IN RISK MANAGEMENT AND AT LEAST 10 HOURS SHALL BE IN ETHICS; SHALL OBTAIN AN OUTSIDE CONSULTANT WITHIN 30 DAYS TO AUDIT HER BILLING RECORDS; SHALL PAY FINE OF $10,000; SHALL APPEAR BEFORE BOARD AT LEAST TWO TIMES A YEAR; SHALL COOPERATE WITH THE BOARD IN VERIFYING COMPLIANCE; SHALL GIVE A COPY OF THIS ORDER TO ANY HEALTH CARE ENTITY WHERE SHE HAS PRIVILEGES; SHALL PROVIDE A COPY OF THIS ORDER TO ANYONE REQUESTING IT WITHIN 10 DAYS; TIME PERIOD OUT OF TEXAS DOES NOT COUNT TOWARD RESTRICTION; SHALL INFORM BOARD OF CHANGE OF ADDRESS WITHIN 10 DAYS OR IF SHE LEAVES STATE.

ORO, FEBE LINDA P MD, LICENSE NUMBER 0137616 OF PO BOX 64, DENNISON, TX, WAS DISCIPLINED BY NEW YORK ON JUNE 28, 1996
DISCIPLINARY ACTION: SURRENDER OF LICENSE
OFFENSE: DISCIPLINARY ACTION BY ANOTHER STATE OR AGENCY

NOTES: ACTION IN TEXAS FOR FAILING TO SUPERVISE ADEQUATELY THE ACTIVITIES OF THOSE UNDER HER SUPERVISION AND FOR OVERCHARGING OR EXCESSIVELY TREATING PATIENTS.

ORTEGA-MORA, JUAN ANTONIO MD, DATE OF BIRTH MARCH 6, 1943, LICENSE NUMBER 00E3593 OF PO BOX 111428, HOUSTON, TX, WAS DISCIPLINED BY TEXAS ON AUGUST 20, 1993
DISCIPLINARY ACTION: 36-MONTH PROBATION; REPRIMAND
OFFENSE: LOSS OR RESTRICTION OF HOSPITAL PRIVILEGES

NOTES: ON 5/29/92 HOSPITAL PRIVILEGES WERE RESTRICTED BASED UPON PEER REVIEW OF 18 MEDICAL CHARTS WHICH FOCUSED ON ON-CALL EMERGENCY ROOM PEDIATRIC PATIENTS. RECORDKEEPING FOR THESE PATIENTS REFLECTED INADEQUATE DOCUMENTATION OF DAILY EVALUATION, MEDICAL CARE OR TREATMENT PLANS; HE WAS ALSO SEVERAL MONTHS LATE IN COMPLETING DISCHARGE SUMMARIES; AS A RESULT OF THIS REVIEW HE AGREED TO TERMINATE FUTURE ON-CALL DUTIES FOR THE EMERGENCY ROOM AND TO A SIX MONTH PROCTORSHIP WHEREBY HIS ADMITTANCE OF PATIENTS WERE REVIEWED BY A PROCTOR; NO INJURY OR ILLNESSES RESULTED FROM LAPSES OF DOCUMENTATION. THREE YEAR SUSPENSION STAYED. CONDITIONS OF PROBATION: SHALL APPEAR BEFORE THE BOARD ONCE A YEAR; SHALL ATTEND AT LEAST 50 HOURS PER YEAR OF CONTINUING MEDICAL EDUCATION INCLUDING AT LEAST ONE COURSE IN RISK MANAGEMENT DURING THE FIRST YEAR; HOSPITAL PRACTICE SHALL BE MONITORED BY A BOARD-APPROVED SUPERVISOR WITH REPORTS TO THE BOARD EVERY FOUR MONTHS; SHALL ATTEND FIVE HOURS OF AN ETHICS COURSE FOR ONE YEAR; SHALL NOT SIGN ANY PATIENT RECORD UNLESS HE HAS PERSONALLY EXAMINED THE PATIENT OR CLEARLY NOTES IN THE RECORD THAT HE DID NOT. SHALL GIVE A COPY OF THIS ORDER TO ANY HEALTH CARE ENTITY WHERE HE HAS PRIVILEGES; SHALL COOPERATE WITH THE BOARD IN VERIFYING COMPLIANCE; SHALL INFORM BOARD OF CHANGE OF ADDRESS WITHIN 10 DAYS OR IF HE LEAVES THE STATE; TIME SPENT OUT OF TEXAS DOES NOT COUNT TOWARD PROBATION. SHALL NOT SEEK MODIFICATION FOR ONE YEAR.

OTERO, HUMBERTO MD, LICENSE NUMBER 00E3079 OF KENNER, LA, WAS DISCIPLINED BY TEXAS ON JULY 1, 1990
DISCIPLINARY ACTION: LICENSE REVOCATION
OFFENSE: DISCIPLINARY ACTION BY ANOTHER STATE OR AGENCY

NOTES: LOUISIANA LICENSE REVOKED.

OTTERSON, WARREN N MD, LICENSE NUMBER 00E8094, WAS DISCIPLINED BY TEXAS ON AUGUST 17, 1996
DISCIPLINARY ACTION: SURRENDER OF LICENSE
OFFENSE: NONCOMPLIANCE WITH A PROFESSIONAL RULE

NOTES: VIOLATED THE MEDICAL PRACTICE ACT. DOES NOT ADMIT VIOLATION. VOLUNTARY AND PERMANENT SURRENDER OF LICENSE IN LIEU OF FURTHER PROCEEDINGS.

OTTERSON, WARREN NELS MD, DATE OF BIRTH NOVEMBER 6, 1929 OF SHREVEPORT, LA, WAS DISCIPLINED BY LOUISIANA ON NOVEMBER 6, 1995
DISCIPLINARY ACTION: REVOCATION OF CONTROLLED SUBSTANCE LICENSE; 1-MONTH LICENSE SUSPENSION
OFFENSE: OVERPRESCRIBING OR MISPRESCRIBING DRUGS

NOTES: PRESCRIBED CONTROLLED SUBSTANCES WITHOUT LEGITIMATE MEDICAL JUSTIFICATION AND IN OTHER THAN A LEGAL OR LEGITIMATE MANNER; AND MAKING AND SUBMITTING FALSE, DECEPTIVE, OR UNFOUNDED CLAIMS. THREE YEAR PROBATION SUBJECT TO LIFETIME PROHIBITION ON PRESCRIPTION, DISPENSATION, OR ADMINISTRATION OF CONTROLLED SUBSTANCES AND OTHER SPECIFIED MEDICATIONS; AND COMPLETION OF SPECIFIED CONTINUING MEDICAL EDUCATION. $3,000 FINE.

OTTERSON, WARREN NELS MD OF PO BOX 33932 LSU MEDICAL CENTER, SHREVEPORT, LA, WAS DISCIPLINED BY DEA ON JANUARY 18, 1996
DISCIPLINARY ACTION: SURRENDER OF CONTROLLED SUBSTANCE LICENSE

NOTES: IN LIEU OF PUBLIC INTEREST REVOCATION.

OTTERSON, WARREN NELS MD, DATE OF BIRTH NOVEMBER 6, 1929, LICENSE NUMBER 0012134 OF 7370 BARKRIDGE DRIVE, SHREVEPORT, LA, WAS DISCIPLINED BY WISCONSIN ON JULY 24, 1996
DISCIPLINARY ACTION: SURRENDER OF LICENSE
OFFENSE: DISCIPLINARY ACTION BY ANOTHER STATE OR AGENCY

NOTES: ON 10/23/95 THE LOUISIANA BOARD IMPOSED DISCIPLINE UPON HIS LICENSE TO PRACTICE MEDICINE.

OVERTON, MARVIN C III MD, LICENSE NUMBER 00D3801 OF FORT WORTH, TX, WAS DISCIPLINED BY TEXAS ON MAY 15, 1996
DISCIPLINARY ACTION: SURRENDER OF LICENSE; RESTRICTION PLACED ON LICENSE
OFFENSE: SEXUAL ABUSE OF OR SEXUAL MISCONDUCT WITH A PATIENT

NOTES: ALLEGATIONS THAT HE INAPPROPRIATELY TOUCHED ONE ADULT FEMALE PATIENT DURING A MEDICAL EVALUATION AND WITHOUT A CHAPERONE BEING PRESENT. DOES NOT ADMIT VIOLATION. VOLUNTARY AND PERMANENT SURRENDER OF HIS LICENSE IN EFFECT AS OF 7/1/96; WHILE LICENSE IS STILL ACTIVE, HE SHALL HAVE A CHAPERONE PRESENT WHENEVER HE PERFORMS A PHYSICAL EXAMINATION OF A FEMALE PATIENT AND SHALL NOTE THIS IN THE PATIENT'S CHART; SHALL COOPERATE WITH BOARD IN VERIFYING COMPLIANCE.

OWENS, GUY MD, LICENSE NUMBER 00C4913 OF NEW BRITAIN, CT, WAS DISCIPLINED BY TEXAS ON JUNE 17, 1992
DISCIPLINARY ACTION: RESTRICTION PLACED ON LICENSE
OFFENSE: DISCIPLINARY ACTION BY ANOTHER STATE OR AGENCY

OWENS, RONALD HUBERT DO, LICENSE NUMBER 00C9475 OF DALLAS, TX, WAS DISCIPLINED BY TEXAS ON JANUARY 12, 1991
DISCIPLINARY ACTION: LICENSE SUSPENSION
OFFENSE: PHYSICAL OR MENTAL ILLNESS INHIBITING THE ABILITY TO PRACTICE WITH SKILL AND SAFETY

NOTES: MUST BEGIN AND CONTINUE PSYCHIATRIC EVALUATION AND TREATMENT; SUSPENSION TO CONTINUE UNTIL SUCH TIME AS HE CAN SHOW BOARD HE IS NO LONGER IMPAIRED BY MENTAL CONDITION AND CAN PRACTICE MEDICINE WITH REASONABLE SKILL AND SAFETY TO PATIENTS.

PANG, SHING YIP MD, DATE OF BIRTH OCTOBER 17, 1964 OF 2315 STENNETT DRIVE, ARLINGTON, TX, WAS DISCIPLINED BY

MEDICARE ON AUGUST 19, 1999
DISCIPLINARY ACTION: EXCLUSION FROM THE MEDICARE AND/OR MEDICAID PROGRAM
OFFENSE: CRIMINAL CONVICTION OR PLEA OF GUILTY, NOLO CONTENDERE, OR NO CONTEST TO A CRIME

NOTES: CONVICTED OF A CRIME INVOLVING THE MEDICARE, MEDICAID, MATERNAL AND CHILD HEALTH SERVICES BLOCK GRANT OR BLOCK GRANTS TO STATES FOR SOCIAL SERVICES PROGRAMS.

PARET, ROBERT W MD, LICENSE NUMBER 00D6915 OF OAK RIDGE, TN, WAS DISCIPLINED BY TEXAS ON MARCH 6, 1992
DISCIPLINARY ACTION: 48-MONTH PROBATION
OFFENSE: PROFESSIONAL MISCONDUCT

NOTES: UNPROFESSIONAL OR DISHONORABLE CONDUCT LIKELY TO DECEIVE, DEFRAUD OR INJURE THE PUBLIC. LICENSE SUSPENDED, SUSPENSION STAYED. ON 04/08/93, TERMINATION OF PROBATION GRANTED. LICENSE FREE AND CLEAR OF ANY RESTRICTIONS AND LIMITATIONS.

PARIANI, HARISH KUMAR MD, DATE OF BIRTH JULY 2, 1947 OF 20114 ATASCOSITA SHORES DRIVE, HUMBLE, TX, WAS DISCIPLINED BY MEDICARE ON AUGUST 20, 1998
DISCIPLINARY ACTION: 60-MONTH EXCLUSION FROM THE MEDICARE AND/OR MEDICAID PROGRAM
OFFENSE: CRIMINAL CONVICTION OR PLEA OF GUILTY, NOLO CONTENDERE, OR NO CONTEST TO A CRIME

NOTES: CONVICTED OF A CRIME INVOLVING THE MEDICARE, MEDICAID, MATERNAL AND CHILD HEALTH SERVICES BLOCK GRANT OR BLOCK GRANTS TO STATES FOR SOCIAL SERVICES PROGRAMS. REINSTATED ON 12/21/98.

PARIKH, KIRAN RAJEN MD, LICENSE NUMBER 00G5825 OF RICHMOND, TX, WAS DISCIPLINED BY TEXAS ON OCTOBER 5, 1991
DISCIPLINARY ACTION: 60-MONTH PROBATION; REQUIRED TO TAKE ADDITIONAL MEDICAL EDUCATION
OFFENSE: SUBSTANDARD CARE, INCOMPETENCE OR NEGLIGENCE

NOTES: FAILED TO REFER PATIENT TO AN OPHTHALMOLOGIST IN A TIMELY FASHION AND DEMONSTRATED EXTREMELY POOR DOCUMENTATION IN PATIENT'S CHART. FIVE YEAR SUSPENSION STAYED; CONDITIONS OF PROBATION: SHALL ATTEND REQUIRED CONTINUING MEDICAL EDUCATION WITH VERIFICATION TO BOARD; SHALL CONSULT WITH AN OPHTHALMOLOGIST WITHIN 7 DAYS OF ANY NONRESPONSIVE EYE PROBLEM; SHALL MAINTAIN ADEQUATE MEDICAL RECORDS ON ALL OFFICE VISITS AND MAKE THESE AVAILABLE TO BOARD; SHALL NOT MAKE ANY NOTES ON PATIENT RECORD UNLESS HAS PERSONALLY SEEN AND EXAMINED THE PATIENT UNLESS EXCEPTIONS ARE NOTED IN THE RECORD; SHALL PERSONALLY EXAMINE PATIENT DURING FIRST VISIT AND WHEN A DIAGNOSIS OF A NEW OR DIFFERENT DISEASE OR INJURY OCCURS; SHALL COOPERATE WITH BOARD IN VERIFYING COMPLIANCE; SHALL ADVISE BOARD OF ADDRESS CHANGE WITHIN 10 DAYS; TIME SPENT OUT OF TEXAS DOES NOT COUNT TOWARD PROBATION; SHALL APPEAR BEFORE THE BOARD TWICE A YEAR; SHALL NOT SEEK MODIFICATION OF THE ORDER FOR ONE YEAR. PROBATION TERMINATED ON 11/19/93.

PARKER, WAYLON M MD OF MARRERO, LA, WAS DISCIPLINED BY LOUISIANA ON APRIL 29, 1996
DISCIPLINARY ACTION: 16-MONTH LICENSE SUSPENSION
OFFENSE: DISCIPLINARY ACTION BY ANOTHER STATE OR AGENCY

NOTES: ACTION IN MISSISSIPPI. SURRENDER OF LICENSE IN TEXAS WHILE UNDER INVESTIGATION. MISREPRESENTATION AND DECEIT IN OBTAINING RENEWAL OF LICENSURE. APPLICATION FOR LICENSURE UPON COMPLETION OF PROBATION IMPOSED IN MISSISSIPPI; SHALL PAY ALL COSTS OF PROCEEDINGS.

PARKER, WAYLON M MD, WAS DISCIPLINED BY NEW MEXICO ON JANUARY 1, 1997
DISCIPLINARY ACTION: LICENSE REVOCATION
OFFENSE: DISCIPLINARY ACTION BY ANOTHER STATE OR AGENCY

NOTES: FAILURE TO INFORM BOARD OF SUSPENSION AND REVOCATION OF OTHER STATE LICENSES, AND HE MAY NEVER REAPPLY. AS OF 5/98, THE BOARD ACCEPTED PROPOSED ORDER TO WITHDRAW REVOCATION AND ALLOW HIM TO VOLUNTARILY SURRENDER NEW MEXICO LICENSE WITH CONDITION THAT HE MAY NEVER REAPPLY.

PARKER, WAYLON MORRIS MD, DATE OF BIRTH MAY 18, 1956, LICENSE NUMBER 00G7301 OF GULFPORT, MS, WAS DISCIPLINED BY TEXAS ON AUGUST 19, 1994
DISCIPLINARY ACTION: SURRENDER OF LICENSE
OFFENSE: OVERPRESCRIBING OR MISPRESCRIBING DRUGS

NOTES: ALLEGATIONS OF NON-THERAPEUTIC PRESCRIBING; HE DOES NOT ADMIT THIS BUT WISHES TO AVOID EXPENSE OF LITIGATION. SURRENDER IN LIEU OF FURTHER INVESTIGATION. SHALL NOT PETITION FOR REINSTATEMENT OF LICENSE.

PARKER, WAYLON MORRIS MD, DATE OF BIRTH MAY 18, 1956, LICENSE NUMBER 0012804 OF 4700 WICHERS DRIVE, SUITE 101, MARRERO, LA, WAS DISCIPLINED BY MISSISSIPPI ON SEPTEMBER 21, 1995
OFFENSE: DISCIPLINARY ACTION BY ANOTHER STATE OR AGENCY

NOTES: ON 8/15/94 TEXAS LICENSE SURRENDERED WHILE UNDER INVESTIGATION FOR NON-THERAPEUTIC PRESCRIBING TO A PATIENT HE HAD PREVIOUSLY IDENTIFIED AS HIS WIFE AND LATER SAID HE WAS TRYING TO PROTECT FROM SPOUSAL ABUSE. FIVE YEAR SUSPENSION STAYED SUBJECT TO CERTAIN CONDITIONS. ORDER MODIFIED ON 5/14/96 REQUIRING HIM TO RECEIVE PSYCHIATRIC TREATMENT/THERAPY FOR TWO YEARS WITH QUARTERLY REPORTS TO THE BOARD; SHALL COMPLETE THE COURSE "CLINICAL, LEGAL, AND ETHICAL ISSUES IN PRESCRIBING ABUSABLE DRUGS" OR AN EQUIVALENT BOARD APPROVED COURSE; PRACTICE LIMITED TO A GROUP SETTING WITH MONITORING; SHALL LIMIT PRACTICE TO PEDIATRICS AND SHALL NOT TREAT ADULTS OR FAMILY MEMBERS OR ANY SEXUALLY AND/OR PHYSICALLY ABUSED PATIENTS; CONTROLLED SUBSTANCES REGISTRATION CERTIFICATE LIMITED TO SCHEDULE V DRUGS WITH EXCEPTION OF BUPRENEX; ALSO CANNOT PRESCRIBE, ADMINISTER, DISPENSE OR POSSESS STADOL, NUBAIN, DALGEN, SOMA OR BUTALBITAL PRODUCTS.

PARKINSON, DAN W MD, DATE OF BIRTH MAY 27, 1954, LICENSE NUMBER 50655 OF 2802 CEDAR WOODS PLACE, HOUSTON, TX, WAS DISCIPLINED BY NEW JERSEY ON MAY 7, 1997
DISCIPLINARY ACTION: 12-MONTH LICENSE SUSPENSION; 48-MONTH PROBATION

NOTES: REMAINDER OF FIVE YEAR SUSPENSION STAYED. NO CREDIT SHALL BE TOWARD SUSPENSION FOR ANY PERIOD OF TIME HE ENGAGES IN PRACTICE OF MEDICINE OUTSIDE NEW JERSEY. ASSESSED PENALTY OF $100,000 AND COSTS. PRIOR TO RETURN

TO ACTIVE PRACTICE SHALL SUCCESSFULLY COMPLETE AN ETHICS COURSE AND APPEAR BEFORE THE BOARD.

PARKINSON, DAN W MD, LICENSE NUMBER 192297 OF 2802 CEDAR WOODS PLACE, HOUSTON, TX, WAS DISCIPLINED BY NEW YORK ON NOVEMBER 5, 1997
DISCIPLINARY ACTION: SURRENDER OF LICENSE
OFFENSE: DISCIPLINARY ACTION BY ANOTHER STATE OR AGENCY

NOTES: DISCIPLINED BY THE NEW JERSEY BOARD FOR SEEING PATIENTS FOR VISITS THAT LASTED NO MORE THAN FIVE MINUTES AND THEN BILLING THOSE VISITS AS "COMPLEX EVALUATIONS."

PARKINSON, DAN WEST MD, LICENSE NUMBER J5859 OF HOUSTON, TX, WAS DISCIPLINED BY TEXAS ON AUGUST 22, 1998
DISCIPLINARY ACTION: 60-MONTH PROBATION; REPRIMAND
OFFENSE: DISCIPLINARY ACTION BY ANOTHER STATE OR AGENCY

NOTES: ON 5/6/97 THE NEW JERSEY BOARD SUSPENDED HIS LICENSE; THE ORDER CRITICIZED HIS CIVILIAN PRACTICE WHICH RESULTED IN A LARGE NUMBER OF PATIENTS SEEN AND INACCURATE CODING; HE APPEALED THIS ACTION BASED UPON HIS DISAGREEMENT WITH THE ALLEGATIONS AND UPON THE FACT THAT NEW JERSEY HAD NOT AFFORDED HIM A HEARING; A BOARD CONSULTANT HAS DETERMINED THAT IT WAS UNREASONABLE FOR HIM TO HAVE EFFECTIVELY EVALUATED THE LARGE VOLUME OF PATIENTS HE SAW ON ONE SPECIFIED DAY; ON 10/19/97 HE SURRENDERED HIS NEW YORK LICENSE RATHER THAN CONTEST A DISCIPLINARY PROCEEDING BASED UPON THE NEW JERSEY ACTION. SUSPENSION STAYED FOR PROBATION WITH THE FOLLOWING TERMS AND CONDITIONS: SHALL OBTAIN 1 ETHICS COURSE PER YEAR FOR THE DURATION OF THE ORDER; SHALL PERFORM 100 HOURS OF COMMUNITY SERVICE PER YEAR FOR A BOARD-APPROVED NON-PROFIT; SHALL MAINTAIN ADEQUATE MEDICAL RECORDS WHICH SHALL BE AVAILABLE FOR REVIEW; SHALL ADOPT OR ESTABLISH A SYSTEM OF PATIENT RECORD KEEPING AND BILLING TO ENSURE THAT ALL PATIENT RECORDS ACCURATELY REFLECT THE PATIENT'S NAME, SERVICE RENDERED, DATE OF SERVICE AND AMOUNT CHARGED; HIS MEDICAL PRACTICE SHALL BE MONITORED BY A BOARD APPROVED TEXAS PHYSICIAN WHO SHALL PROVIDE QUARTERLY REPORTS TO THE BOARD; SHALL APPEAR BEFORE THE BOARD AT LEAST ONCE A YEAR; SHALL COOPERATE WITH THE BOARD IN VERIFYING COMPLIANCE INCLUDING PROVIDING COPIES OF ANY REPORTS SENT TO NEW JERSEY UPON REQUEST; SHALL ADEQUATELY SUPERVISE THE ACTIVITIES OF ALL HIS EMPLOYEES AND OTHERS UNDER HIS SUPERVISION; SHALL PERSONALLY PERFORM INITIAL EXAMINATIONS; SHALL GIVE A COPY OF THIS ORDER TO ANY HEALTH CARE ENTITY WHERE HE HAS PRIVILEGES; TIME SPENT OUT OF TEXAS DOES NOT COUNT TOWARD PROBATION; SHALL INFORM THE BOARD OF CHANGE OF ADDRESS WITHIN 10 DAYS OR IF HE LEAVES THE STATE; SHALL NOT SEEK MODIFICATION FOR ONE YEAR.

PARKINSON, DAN WEST MD, DATE OF BIRTH MAY 27, 1954, LICENSE NUMBER 044147E OF 2 PARTRIDGE LANE, CHERRY HILL, NJ, WAS DISCIPLINED BY PENNSYLVANIA ON AUGUST 22, 1999
DISCIPLINARY ACTION: LICENSE SUSPENSION
OFFENSE: DISCIPLINARY ACTION BY ANOTHER STATE OR AGENCY

NOTES: DISCIPLINED BY NEW JERSEY BOARD. PENNSYLVANIA LICENSE SUSPENDED UNTIL HE COMPLETES TERMS OF PROBATION IN NEW JERSEY AND LICENSE RESTORED WITHOUT RESTRICTION.

PARRY, DARRELL BOYD DO, LICENSE NUMBER H3278 OF PRESCOTT, AZ, WAS DISCIPLINED BY TEXAS ON OCTOBER 15, 1999
DISCIPLINARY ACTION: LICENSE SUSPENSION
OFFENSE: DISCIPLINARY ACTION BY ANOTHER STATE OR AGENCY

NOTES: ON 4/14/97 THE ARIZONA BOARD TEMPORARILY SUSPENDED HIS LICENSE DUE TO HIS MEDICAL CONDITION; HE SUFFERS FROM CHRONIC HEPATIC CELLULAR NECROSIS AND IS BEING TREATED BY A PHYSICIAN FOR LIVER NECROSIS CAUSED BY TYLENOL TOXICITY; HE HAS NOT PRACTICED SINCE 4/19/97; ON 4/22/97 HE VOLUNTARILY WITHDREW FROM THE PRACTICE OF MEDICINE DUE TO HIS EXTREME MEDICAL CONDITION. SUSPENSION UNTIL HE REQUESTS TO HAVE HIS SUSPENSION STAYED OR APPEARS BEFORE THE BOARD WITH SUFFICIENT EVIDENCE THAT HE IS PHYSICALLY, MENTALLY AND OTHERWISE COMPETENT TO SAFELY PRACTICE INCLUDING AT A MINIMUM COMPLETE COPIES OF MEDICAL RECORDS AND REPORTS OF MEDICAL EVALUATIONS; SHALL CONTINUE TO RECEIVE CARE AND TREATMENT FROM PRESENT PHYSICIAN WITH QUARTERLY REPORTS; SHALL COOPERATE WITH THE BOARD IN VERIFYING COMPLIANCE INCLUDING PROVIDING COPIES OF MEDICAL RELEASES AND ANY DOCUMENTS SENT TO OR RECEIVED FROM ARIZONA BOARD UPON REQUEST ; SHALL GIVE A COPY OF THIS ORDER TO ANY HEALTH CARE ENTITY WHERE HE HAS PRIVILEGES; SHALL PROVIDE A COPY OF THIS ORDER TO ANYONE REQUESTING IT WITHIN 10 DAYS; TIME SPENT OUT OF TEXAS DOES NOT COUNT TOWARD PROBATION/RESTRICTION; SHALL INFORM THE BOARD OF CHANGE OF ADDRESS WITHIN 10 DAYS OR IF HE LEAVES THE STATE; SHALL NOT SEEK MODIFICATION FOR ONE YEAR.

PARSONS, JAMES T MD, LICENSE NUMBER 00C6816 OF HOUSTON, TX, WAS DISCIPLINED BY TEXAS ON JANUARY 26, 1990
DISCIPLINARY ACTION: RESTRICTION PLACED ON LICENSE

NOTES: STIPULATED ORDER. MUST LIMIT PRACTICE OF MEDICINE TO OFFICE PRACTICE AND PERFORM NO ENDOSCOPIC PROCEDURES.

PARSONS, JAMES T MD, LICENSE NUMBER 0C24969 OF HOUSTON, TX, WAS DISCIPLINED BY CALIFORNIA ON APRIL 12, 1992
DISCIPLINARY ACTION: SURRENDER OF LICENSE

NOTES: VOLUNTARY SURRENDER WHILE CHARGES PENDING.

PARSONS, JAMES T MD, LICENSE NUMBER 00C6816 OF HOUSTON, TX, WAS DISCIPLINED BY TEXAS ON JUNE 22, 1994
DISCIPLINARY ACTION: 120-MONTH PROBATION; REQUIRED TO TAKE ADDITIONAL MEDICAL EDUCATION
OFFENSE: PROFESSIONAL MISCONDUCT

NOTES: ON 10/20/92 PERFORMED AN UNNECESSARY TENDON REPAIR ON ONE PATIENT; HIS OFFICE STAFF ERRONEOUSLY BILLED THE PATIENT FOR A SECOND PROCEDURE AS WELL; HE ALSO HAD NO MEDICAL RECORDS FOR TWO PATIENTS WHO PHARMACY RECORDS SHOW HAD PRESCRIPTIONS FROM HIM; HE HAD FAILED TO ADEQUATELY SUPERVISE ACTIVITIES OF HIS OFFICE NURSE, THEREBY ALLOWING HER TO CALL IN THE PRESCRIPTIONS USING HIS DEA NUMBER; FIRED THE NURSE UPON LEARNING OF THIS; 1/26/90 ORDER IS INDEPENDENT OF THIS ORDER; TEN YEAR SUSPENSION STAYED. CONDITIONS OF PROBATION: SHALL APPEAR BEFORE THE BOARD TWICE A YEAR; SHALL ATTEND AT LEAST 50 HOURS

PER YEAR OF CONTINUING MEDICAL EDUCATION FOR EACH YEAR OF PROBATION AND SIX HOURS PER YEAR OF AN ETHICS COURSE FOR TWO YEARS; SHALL ADEQUATELY SUPERVISE ALL OF HIS EMPLOYEES; SHALL PERFORM EIGHT HOURS PER MONTH OF COMMUNITY SERVICE FOR FOUR YEARS; WITHIN ONE YEAR SHALL PASS THE JURISPRUDENCE EXAM; SHALL GIVE A COPY OF THIS ORDER TO ANY HEALTH CARE ENTITY WHERE HE HAS PRIVILEGES; SHALL COOPERATE WITH THE BOARD IN VERIFYING COMPLIANCE; SHALL INFORM BOARD OF CHANGE OF ADDRESS WITHIN 10 DAYS OR IF HE LEAVES THE STATE; TIME SPENT OUT OF TEXAS DOES NOT COUNT TOWARD PROBATION. SHALL NOT SEEK MODIFICATION FOR ONE YEAR. ON 8/17/96 ORDER MODIFIED REDUCING HIS APPEARANCES BEFORE THE BOARD TO ONE TIME EACH YEAR; HIS REQUEST TO DROP COMMUNITY SERVICE REQUIREMENT DENIED; ALL OTHER CONDITIONS REMAIN IN EFFECT.

PASKOW, JAMES ANDREW MD, DATE OF BIRTH JANUARY 19, 1960, LICENSE NUMBER 00H8790 OF 38 DEERFERN PLACE, THE WOODLANDS, TX, WAS DISCIPLINED BY TEXAS ON APRIL 30, 1993
DISCIPLINARY ACTION: REPRIMAND
OFFENSE: PROFESSIONAL MISCONDUCT

NOTES: DURING THE SECOND YEAR IN A FAMILY PRACTICE PROGRAM ON 4/7/91 PERFORMED A C-SECTION ON A PATIENT DURING WHICH HORSEPLAY ENSUED; HE DISCHARGED A STAPLING GUN INTO HIS SUPERVISING PHYSICIAN'S ARM; CLAIMED THIS WAS AN ACCIDENT; AS A RESULT WAS NOT ALLOWED TO PERFORM C-SECTIONS FOR 3 MONTHS. HE UNDERSTANDS THE SERIOUSNESS OF THE INCIDENT AND ADMITS THAT THE INCIDENT DEMONSTRATED A LACK OF GOOD JUDGMENT. SHALL GIVE A COPY OF THIS ORDER TO ANY HEALTH CARE ENTITY WHERE HE HAS PRIVILEGES; SHALL COOPERATE WITH THE BOARD IN VERIFYING COMPLIANCE; SHALL INFORM BOARD OF CHANGE OF ADDRESS WITHIN 10 DAYS.

PATEL, ASHOK G MD, LICENSE NUMBER A39766 OF CEDAR HILL, TX, WAS DISCIPLINED BY CALIFORNIA ON SEPTEMBER 16, 1999
DISCIPLINARY ACTION: 60-MONTH PROBATION

NOTES: REVOCATION STAYED.

PATEL, ASHOKKUMAR G MD, LICENSE NUMBER F7367 OF CEDAR HILL, TX, WAS DISCIPLINED BY TEXAS ON AUGUST 22, 1998
DISCIPLINARY ACTION: 60-MONTH PROBATION; RESTRICTION PLACED ON LICENSE

NOTES: HE WAS A PARTICIPATING PHYSICIAN IN AN INSURANCE COMPANY'S PPO NETWORK; THE CARRIER REVIEWED RECORDS OF 6 PATIENTS SEEN BY HIM; THE BOARD RETAINED A CONSULTANT TO REVIEW THE RECORDS; THE CONSULTANT RAISED CERTAIN QUESTIONS RELATING TO THE CARE AND TREATMENT OF SUCH PATIENTS; THE DOCTOR HAS ASSERTED THAT BONA FIDE DISPUTES EXIST BOTH AS TO THE FACTS AND LAW AS TO WHETHER A VIOLATION HAS OCCURRED; DENIES ANY WRONGDOING. SUSPENSION STAYED FOR PROBATION WITH THE FOLLOWING TERMS AND CONDITIONS: SHALL NOT SEE MORE THAN 20 PATIENTS IN HIS OFFICE PRACTICE, EXCLUDING EMERGENCIES, ON ONE WORKING DAY; HIS MEDICAL PRACTICE SHALL BE MONITORED BY A BOARD APPROVED TEXAS PHYSICIAN WHO SHALL PROVIDE QUARTERLY REPORTS TO THE BOARD; SHALL MAINTAIN ADEQUATE MEDICAL RECORDS WHICH SHALL BE AVAILABLE FOR REVIEW; SHALL OBTAIN 100 HOURS PER YEAR OF CONTINUING MEDICAL EDUCATION WITH ONE HALF OF THE COURSES IN THE CARE AND TREATMENT OF PATIENTS WITH CARDIAC DISEASE OR DISORDERS OR HYPERTENSION; SHALL APPEAR BEFORE THE BOARD AT LEAST ONCE A YEAR; SHALL COOPERATE WITH THE BOARD IN VERIFYING COMPLIANCE; SHALL GIVE A COPY OF THIS ORDER TO ANY HEALTH CARE ENTITY WHERE HE HAS PRIVILEGES; SHALL PROVIDE A COPY OF THIS ORDER TO ANYONE REQUESTING IT WITHIN 10 DAYS; TIME SPENT OUT OF TEXAS DOES NOT COUNT TOWARD PROBATION; SHALL INFORM THE BOARD OF CHANGE OF ADDRESS WITHIN 10 DAYS OR IF HE LEAVES THE STATE; SHALL NOT SEEK MODIFICATION FOR ONE YEAR. ON 12/11/99 PETITION FOR THE TERMINATION OF THE ORDER DENIED BUT MODIFIED AS FOLLOWS: NUMBER OF PATIENTS HE IS ALLOWED TO SEE WAS INCREASED TO A MAXIMUM OF 40 PATIENTS IN HIS OFFICE PRACTICE, EXCLUDING EMERGENCIES, ON ONE WORKING DAY; SHALL ATTEND 200 HOURS OF CONTINUING EDUCATION IN THE NEXT TWO YEARS AND 50 HOURS PER YEAR AFTER THAT.

PATEL, PIYUSH V MD, LICENSE NUMBER G2452 OF MIDLAND, TX, WAS DISCIPLINED BY TEXAS ON AUGUST 28, 1999
DISCIPLINARY ACTION: FINE
OFFENSE: NONCOMPLIANCE WITH A PROFESSIONAL RULE

NOTES: AFTER EXAMINING SEVERAL PATIENT CASES THE BOARD FOUND BELOW STANDARD, INADEQUATE RECORD KEEPING FOR ONE PATIENT; SINCE THE TIME OF THE ABOVE PATIENT CARE, HE HAS SIGNIFICANTLY CHANGED HIS PRACTICE TO ALLOW FOR ADEQUATE RECORD KEEPING BY HIRING A BUSINESS MANAGER, FOUR REGISTERED NURSES, NEW INTERNIST PARTNERS, AND IS CONSOLIDATING HIS PRACTICE TO ONE LOCATION; HE HAS ENROLLED IN A CONTINUING MEDICAL EDUCATION COURSE TO IMPROVE HIS RECORD KEEPING AND HAS ARRANGED TO HAVE HIS INSURANCE CARRIER AUDIT HIS RECORD KEEPING PRACTICES. $2,500 FINE; TIME SPENT OUT OF TEXAS DOES NOT COUNT TOWARD RESTRICTION; SHALL INFORM THE BOARD OF CHANGE OF ADDRESS WITHIN 10 DAYS OR IF HE LEAVES THE STATE; SHALL NOT SEEK MODIFICATION FOR ONE YEAR.

PATEL, RAMESHBHAI F MD, DATE OF BIRTH DECEMBER 9, 1943 OF REG 10479039 FED CORR INST, FT WORTH, TX, WAS DISCIPLINED BY MEDICARE ON DECEMBER 3, 1991
DISCIPLINARY ACTION: 120-MONTH EXCLUSION FROM THE MEDICARE AND/OR MEDICAID PROGRAM
OFFENSE: CRIMINAL CONVICTION OR PLEA OF GUILTY, NOLO CONTENDERE, OR NO CONTEST TO A CRIME

NOTES: PROGRAM-RELATED CONVICTION.

PATEL, SURYAKANT J MD, DATE OF BIRTH APRIL 19, 1925, LICENSE NUMBER 0032396 OF 3703 MONTAGUE STREET, AMARILLO, TX, WAS DISCIPLINED BY NEW JERSEY ON MAY 7, 1996
OFFENSE: LOSS OR RESTRICTION OF HOSPITAL PRIVILEGES

NOTES: INFORMATION RECEIVED FROM VETERANS ADMINISTRATION MEDICAL CENTER THAT HE HAD BEEN SUBJECTED TO SUPERVISION OF HIS SURGERY OF THE CERVICAL SPINE FOR THREE MONTHS FOLLOWING REVIEW OF A MATTER IN WHICH A PATIENT WHO UNDERWENT SUCH SURGICAL CARE WAS RENDERED QUADRIPLEGIC. LICENSE TO PRACTICE SHALL REMAIN IN INACTIVE STATUS UNTIL HE APPEARS BEFORE THE REVIEW PANEL OF THE BOARD TO DISCUSS THESE CIRCUMSTANCES.

PATRICK, JOSEPH J MD, LICENSE NUMBER 0G41400 OF HOUSTON, TX, WAS DISCIPLINED BY CALIFORNIA ON SEPTEMBER 26, 1992
DISCIPLINARY ACTION: SURRENDER OF LICENSE

NOTES: VOLUNTARY SURRENDER WHILE CHARGES PENDING.

PATTEN, EDWARD L MD, DATE OF BIRTH JANUARY 16, 1949 OF 3332 SOUTHMORE BLVD & CIR, HOUSTON, TX, WAS DISCIPLINED BY MEDICARE ON MAY 24, 1991
DISCIPLINARY ACTION: 240-MONTH EXCLUSION FROM THE MEDICARE AND/OR MEDICAID PROGRAM
OFFENSE: CRIMINAL CONVICTION OR PLEA OF GUILTY, NOLO CONTENDERE, OR NO CONTEST TO A CRIME

NOTES: PROGRAM-RELATED CONVICTION.

PATTEN, EDWARD LEE MD, LICENSE NUMBER 00F0282 OF HOUSTON, TX, WAS DISCIPLINED BY TEXAS ON JANUARY 12, 1991
DISCIPLINARY ACTION: SURRENDER OF CONTROLLED SUBSTANCE LICENSE; PROBATION
OFFENSE: CRIMINAL CONVICTION OR PLEA OF GUILTY, NOLO CONTENDERE, OR NO CONTEST TO A CRIME

NOTES: PLACED ON PROBATION FOR THE PENDENCY OF HIS APPEAL FROM HIS U.S. DISTRICT COURT CONVICTION UNDER CONDITIONS INCLUDING: RESTRICTION OF MEDICAL LICENSE TO PRACTICE OF MEDICINE AT RIVERSIDE HOSPITAL, HOUSTON, TEXAS, BUT NOT TO PRACTICE SURGERY; SURRENDER CONTROLLED SUBSTANCES REGISTRATION CERTIFICATES AND NOT ATTEMPT TO REREGISTER OR OBTAIN REGISTRATIONS WITHOUT PRIOR WRITTEN AUTHORITY FROM BOARD; SUBMIT TO APPROPRIATE EXAMINATIONS TO DETERMINE FREEDOM FROM DRUGS AND ALCOHOL.

PATTEN, EDWARD LEE MD, LICENSE NUMBER 00F0282 OF HOUSTON, TX, WAS DISCIPLINED BY TEXAS ON OCTOBER 5, 1991
DISCIPLINARY ACTION: LICENSE SUSPENSION
OFFENSE: CRIMINAL CONVICTION OR PLEA OF GUILTY, NOLO CONTENDERE, OR NO CONTEST TO A CRIME

NOTES: ORDER OF PROBATION OF 1/12/91 EXPIRED WHEN HE WAS INCARCERATED ON ABOUT 3/11/91; IS SERVING A PRISON TERM OF 84 MONTHS. LICENSE SUSPENDED WHILE HE IS IN PRISON.

PATTEN, EDWARD LEE MD, LICENSE NUMBER 00F0282, WAS DISCIPLINED BY TEXAS ON NOVEMBER 16, 1996
DISCIPLINARY ACTION: 120-MONTH PROBATION; RESTRICTION PLACED ON LICENSE

NOTES: 10/5/91 SUSPENSION STAYED TO PROBATION WITH TERMS AND CONDITIONS: PRIOR TO PRACTICING IN TEXAS, SHALL TAKE AND PASS THE SPECIAL PURPOSE EXAMINATION WITH A SCORE OF 75 OR BETTER AND THE MEDICAL JURISPRUDENCE EXAM; HIS PRACTICE SHALL BE RESTRICTED TO AN INSTITUTIONAL OR SUPERVISED SETTING UNDER THE SUPERVISION OF A PHYSICIAN OR MEDICAL DIRECTOR ACCEPTABLE TO THE BOARD WHO SHALL PROVIDE QUARTERLY REPORTS; PRIOR TO PERFORMING ANY MAJOR SURGERY ON ANY PATIENT, SHALL BECOME BOARD CERTIFIED IN SURGERY; SHALL ABSTAIN FROM THE CONSUMPTION OF ALCOHOL/DRUGS IN ANY FORM UNLESS PRESCRIBED BY ANOTHER PHYSICIAN FOR A LEGITIMATE OR THERAPEUTIC PURPOSE; SHALL SUBMIT HIMSELF FOR APPROPRIATE EXAMS INCLUDING DRUG OR ALCOHOL SCREENS; SHALL SUBMIT HIMSELF FOR EVALUATION AND TREATMENT BY A BOARD-APPROVED PSYCHIATRIST WHOM HE SHALL SEE AT LEAST ONCE A MONTH AND WHO SHALL SUBMIT REPORTS TO THE BOARD; SHALL CONTINUE TO PARTICIPATE IN AA'S PROGRAM NOT LESS THAN THREE TIMES PER WEEK WITH QUARTERLY REPORTS TO THE BOARD; SHALL PARTICIPATE IN THE ACTIVITIES OF A PHYSICIAN'S HEALTH AND REHABILITATION COMMITTEE AND ATTEND WEEKLY MEETINGS WITH QUARTERLY REPORTS; SHALL NOT POSSESS ALCOHOL, CONTROLLED SUBSTANCES OR DANGEROUS DRUGS WITH ADDICTIVE POTENTIAL OR POTENTIAL FOR ABUSE AND SHALL SURRENDER ALL SUCH DRUGS INCLUDING SAMPLES; SHALL NOT TREAT OR OTHERWISE SERVE AS PHYSICIAN, PRESCRIBE, DISPENSE OR ADMINISTER DRUGS THAT MAY BE SUBJECT TO ABUSE TO HIMSELF OR TO ANY MEMBER OF HIS FAMILY; SHALL NOT TELEPHONE TO A PHARMACY A PRESCRIPTION OR REFILL FOR CONTROLLED SUBSTANCES OR DANGEROUS DRUGS WITH ADDICTIVE POTENTIAL OR POTENTIAL FOR ABUSE NOR ALLOW ANYONE UNDER HIS SUPERVISION TO DO SO; SHALL MAINTAIN A FILE WITH COPIES OF EVERY PRESCRIPTION WRITTEN BY HIM FOR THESE SUBSTANCES WHICH SHALL BE AVAILABLE FOR REVIEW; SHALL SURRENDER HIS DEA/DPS CONTROLLED SUBSTANCES REGISTRATION CERTIFICATES AND SHALL NOT ATTEMPT TO REREGISTER WITHOUT AUTHORITY FROM THE BOARD; SHALL SURRENDER ALL UNUSED TRIPLICATE FORMS AND SHALL NOT ATTEMPT TO ORDER MORE; HIS PRACTICE INCLUDING ANY OFFICE OR SURGICAL PRACTICE SHALL BE MONITORED BY A BOARD-APPROVED TEXAS PHYSICIAN WHO SHALL SUBMIT QUARTERLY REPORTS TO THE BOARD; SHALL MAINTAIN ADEQUATE MEDICAL RECORDS WHICH SHALL BE AVAILABLE FOR REVIEW; SHALL OBTAIN AT LEAST 50 HOURS PER YEAR OF CONTINUING MEDICAL EDUCATION; SHALL APPEAR BEFORE BOARD AT LEAST TWICE A YEAR; SHALL COOPERATE WITH THE BOARD IN VERIFYING COMPLIANCE INCLUDING PROVIDING ANY MEDICAL RELEASES UPON REQUEST; SHALL GIVE A COPY OF THIS ORDER TO ANY HEALTH CARE ENTITY WHERE HE HAS PRIVILEGES; SHALL PROVIDE A COPY OF THIS ORDER TO ANYONE REQUESTING IT WITHIN 10 DAYS; TIME SPENT OUT OF TEXAS DOES NOT COUNT TOWARD PROBATION; SHALL INFORM THE BOARD OF CHANGE OF ADDRESS WITHIN 10 DAYS OR IF HE LEAVES THE STATE. SHALL NOT SEEK MODIFICATION FOR ONE YEAR. ON 2/7/98 PETITION FOR MODIFICATION OF ORDER GRANTED ALLOWING SUCCESSFUL COMPLETION OF A MINI-RESIDENCY OR REMEDIAL COURSES IN SURGERY IN LIEU OF BOARD CERTIFICATION; ALLOWED TO APPLY FOR REGISTRATIONS FOR SUBSTANCES IN SCHEDULES III, IV AND V; PRESCRIPTIONS SHALL BE SERIALLY NUMBERED. ON 5/16/98 ORDER MODIFIED REDUCING PSYCHIATRIC VISITS FROM MONTHLY TO QUARTERLY, AND APPEARANCES BEFORE THE BOARD FROM TWO TO ONCE EACH YEAR. ON 5/14/99 ORDER MODIFIED DELETING REQUIREMENTS FOR PSYCHIATRIC CARE AND TREATMENT, AND PARTICIPATION WITH A LOCAL MEDICAL SOCIETY.

PATTON, GARRY MD, LICENSE NUMBER 0136992 OF PO BOX 712, MEXIA, TX, WAS DISCIPLINED BY NEW YORK ON APRIL 29, 1996
DISCIPLINARY ACTION: SURRENDER OF LICENSE
OFFENSE: DISCIPLINARY ACTION BY ANOTHER STATE OR AGENCY

NOTES: ACTION IN TEXAS FOR UNPROFESSIONAL AND FRAUDULENT CONDUCT AS WELL AS PRESCRIBING AND ADMINISTERING A DRUG IN A NON-THERAPEUTIC MANNER.

PATTON, GARRY J MD, LICENSE NUMBER 00G1746 OF MEXIA, TX, WAS DISCIPLINED BY TEXAS ON MARCH 4, 1995
DISCIPLINARY ACTION: 84-MONTH PROBATION; FINE

OFFENSE: PROVIDING FALSE INFORMATION TO THE BOARD OR OTHER HEALTH AGENCY

NOTES: SUBMITTED FALSE INFORMATION REGARDING HOSPITAL PRIVILEGES IN A BOARD QUESTIONNAIRE AND REGARDING AN INVESTIGATION BY THE LICENSING BOARD IN AN APPLICATION FOR HOSPITAL PRIVILEGES; FAILED TO TIMELY ATTEND TO AND APPROPRIATELY TREAT VARIOUS EMERGENCY ROOM PATIENTS FROM APPROXIMATELY 1990 THROUGH 1994 AND FAILED TO ADEQUATELY DOCUMENT THEIR PATIENT CARE; PRESCRIBED OR ADMINISTERED A DRUG OR TREATMENT THAT IS NONTHERAPEUTIC IN NATURE OR IN THE MANNER ADMINISTERED. NEITHER ADMITS OR DENIES ALLEGATIONS. SUSPENSION STAYED. PROBATION WITH TERMS: PRACTICE SHALL BE MONITORED BY A BOARD-APPROVED PHYSICIAN WHO SHALL SUBMIT QUARTERLY REPORTS; SHALL MAINTAIN ADEQUATE MEDICAL RECORDS WHICH SHALL BE AVAILABLE FOR INSPECTION UPON REQUEST OF THE BOARD; SHALL NOT SIGN OR INDICATE IN ANY MANNER IN PATIENT RECORDS THAT HE HAS SEEN PATIENTS UNLESS HE HAS ACTUALLY SEEN AND EXAMINED THE PATIENT UNLESS IT IS CLEARLY NOTED THAT HE DID NOT PERSONALLY EXAMINE THE PATIENT; SHALL EXAMINE ANY PATIENT WHO HAS A MORE SEVERE DIAGNOSIS OR A DIAGNOSIS DIFFERENT THAN THE ORIGINAL; SHALL ATTEND AT LEAST 50 HOURS PER YEAR OF CONTINUING MEDICAL EDUCATION AT LEAST 10 HOURS OF WHICH IS IN RISK MANAGEMENT; SHALL OBTAIN 10 HOURS OF AN ETHICS COURSE PER YEAR; WITHIN ONE YEAR, SHALL TAKE AND PASS THE SPECIAL PURPOSE EXAMINATION AND THE JURISPRUDENCE EXAMINATION; WITHIN SIX MONTHS, SHALL TAKE AND PASS AN ADVANCED CARDIAC LIFE SUPPORT COURSE (ACLS) AND ADVANCED TRAUMA LIFE SUPPORT COURSE (ATLS) AND OBTAIN CERTIFICATION FOR EACH, BEFORE HE FINISHES THESE TWO PROGRAMS; SHALL NOT PRACTICE EMERGENCY ROOM MEDICINE UNTIL OBTAINS CERTIFICATION; SHALL MAINTAIN ACLS AND ATLS CERTIFICATION THROUGHOUT PERIOD OF PROBATION; $2,500 FINE; SHALL APPEAR BEFORE BOARD AT LEAST TWO TIMES EACH YEAR OR UPON BOARD REQUEST; SHALL COOPERATE WITH BOARD IN VERIFYING COMPLIANCE INCLUDING PROVIDING COPIES OF ANY MEDICAL RELEASES UPON REQUEST; SHALL GIVE A COPY OF THIS ORDER TO ANY HEALTH CARE ENTITY WHERE HE HAS PRIVILEGES; TIME PERIOD OUT OF TEXAS DOES NOT COUNT TOWARD PROBATION; SHALL INFORM BOARD OF ANY CHANGE OF ADDRESS OR IF HE LEAVES THE STATE. SHALL NOT SEEK MODIFICATION FOR ONE YEAR.

PATTON, GARRY J MD, LICENSE NUMBER 00G1746, WAS DISCIPLINED BY TEXAS ON AUGUST 17, 1996
DISCIPLINARY ACTION: SURRENDER OF LICENSE
OFFENSE: FAILURE TO COMPLY WITH PREVIOUS BOARD ORDER

NOTES: ALLEGATIONS THAT HIS OFFICE STAFF, WITH AND WITHOUT HIS AUTHORIZATION, TELEPHONED NUMEROUS PRESCRIPTIONS TO LOCAL PHARMACIES. DOES NOT ADMIT VIOLATION. VOLUNTARY AND PERMANENT SURRENDER IN LIEU OF FURTHER PROCEEDINGS. SHALL RETIRE FROM THE PRACTICE OF MEDICINE; SHALL NOT DIAGNOSE, TREAT OR PRESCRIBE FOR ANY PATIENT, EITHER A FOR A FEE OR GRATUITOUSLY; AND SHALL NOT PETITION THE BOARD FOR REINSTATEMENT.

PAUL, RAJENDRA MD, DATE OF BIRTH FEBRUARY 11, 1945, LICENSE NUMBER 0028855 OF PO BOX 30826, SAVANNAH, GA, WAS DISCIPLINED BY GEORGIA ON SEPTEMBER 2, 1994
DISCIPLINARY ACTION: 60-MONTH PROBATION

NOTES: FAILURE TO PERFORM TO ACCEPTABLE AND PREVAILING MEDICAL PRACTICE.

PAUL, RAJENDRA MD, DATE OF BIRTH FEBRUARY 11, 1945, LICENSE NUMBER 00F3576 OF SAVANNAH, GA, WAS DISCIPLINED BY TEXAS ON JUNE 28, 1995
OFFENSE: DISCIPLINARY ACTION BY ANOTHER STATE OR AGENCY

NOTES: IN 9/94, GEORGIA BOARD PUT HIS LICENSE ON THREE YEARS' PROBATION WHICH INCLUDED A FINE FOR HIS FAILURE TO CONFORM TO THE MINIMAL STANDARDS OF ACCEPTABLE AND PREVAILING MEDICAL PRACTICE IN HIS TREATMENT OF SIX PLASTIC SURGERY PATIENTS. SHALL NOT PRACTICE MEDICINE IN TEXAS UNTIL HE APPEARS BEFORE THE BOARD WITH SUFFICIENT EVIDENCE WHICH ADEQUATELY INDICATES THAT HE IS PHYSICALLY, MENTALLY AND OTHERWISE COMPETENT TO SAFELY PRACTICE MEDICINE INCLUDING AT A MINIMUM COPIES OF COURT DOCUMENTS INDICATING THAT THE GEORGIA DISCIPLINARY ORDER HAS BEEN REVERSED OR OVERTURNED; OR COPIES OF GEORGIA BOARD RECORDS INDICATING THAT HE HAS FULFILLED THE TERMS OF HIS GEORGIA PROBATION AND THAT HIS LICENSE IS UNRESTRICTED; SHALL INFORM BOARD OF CHANGE OF ADDRESS WITHIN 10 DAYS. SHALL NOT SEEK MODIFICATION FOR ONE YEAR.

PAYNE, GERALD GENE MD, LICENSE NUMBER D1763 OF HEREFORD, TX, WAS DISCIPLINED BY TEXAS ON AUGUST 22, 1998
DISCIPLINARY ACTION: REPRIMAND; MONITORING OF PHYSICIAN PERFORMANCE
OFFENSE: PROFESSIONAL MISCONDUCT

NOTES: ON OR ABOUT 5/9/95, WHEN CALLED IN TO SEE A NEW PATIENT, HE WAS COVERED WITH WHITE SHOE POLISH AND WAS NOTED TO BE CONFUSED, DISORIENTED, AND UNABLE TO PERFORM A PROCEDURE ON THE PATIENT; THE INCIDENT RESULTED FROM A REACTION TO TAKING HYDROCODONE AND AMBIEN SIMULTANEOUSLY; HE OCCASIONALLY SELF-PRESCRIBES HYDROCODONE AND DURACT FOR BACK PAIN; FROM APPROXIMATELY 1993 - 1995 HE SELF-PRESCRIBED AMBIEN, A SLEEPING AGENT. LICENSE LIMITED FOR ONE YEAR AS FOLLOWS: SHALL NOT TREAT OR OTHERWISE SERVE AS PHYSICIAN, PRESCRIBE, DISPENSE OR ADMINISTER DRUGS THAT MAY BE SUBJECT TO ABUSE TO HIMSELF OR TO ANY MEMBER OF HIS FAMILY; SHALL ABSTAIN FROM THE CONSUMPTION OF ALCOHOL/DRUGS IN ANY FORM UNLESS PRESCRIBED BY ANOTHER PHYSICIAN FOR A LEGITIMATE AND THERAPEUTIC PURPOSE; SHALL SUBMIT HIMSELF FOR APPROPRIATE EXAMS INCLUDING DRUG OR ALCOHOL SCREENS; SHALL COOPERATE WITH THE BOARD IN VERIFYING COMPLIANCE INCLUDING PROVIDING COPIES OF MEDICAL RELEASES UPON REQUEST; SHALL APPEAR BEFORE THE BOARD AT LEAST TWICE A YEAR; SHALL GIVE A COPY OF THIS ORDER TO ANY HEALTH CARE ENTITY WHERE HE HAS PRIVILEGES; TIME SPENT OUT OF TEXAS DOES NOT COUNT TOWARD RESTRICTION; SHALL INFORM THE BOARD OF CHANGE OF ADDRESS WITHIN 10 DAYS OR IF HE LEAVES THE STATE; SHALL NOT SEEK MODIFICATION FOR ONE YEAR.

PAYNE, STEVEN M MD, LICENSE NUMBER J0184, WAS DISCIPLINED BY TEXAS ON FEBRUARY 17, 1997
DISCIPLINARY ACTION: RESTRICTION PLACED ON LICENSE
OFFENSE: SEXUAL ABUSE OF OR SEXUAL MISCONDUCT WITH A

PATIENT

NOTES: ON 1/24/97 HE WAS INDICTED ON FOUR COUNTS OF SEXUAL ASSAULT AGAINST PATIENTS OF HIS. ON 2/10/97 HE ENTERED AN ORDER AMENDING CONDITIONS OF BOND WHICH STIPULATES THAT HE MAY ONLY TREAT FEMALES IF OVER THE AGE OF 55, AND IF A BREAST OR VAGINAL EXAM IS NECESSARY, A CHAPERONE IS TO BE PRESENT DURING THE CONDUCTING OF SUCH EXAMS. HE DENIES ALL ALLEGATIONS MADE IN THE CRIMINAL COMPLAINTS AGAINST HIM. HE HAS VOLUNTARILY AGREED TO THE FOLLOWING ORDER: HIS PRACTICE OF MEDICINE SHALL BE RESTRICTED AS DESCRIBED ABOVE REGARDING FEMALE PATIENTS; HE SHALL COOPERATE WITH THE BOARD IN VERIFYING COMPLIANCE; SHALL ADVISE THE BOARD OF A CHANGE IN ADDRESS WITHIN 10 DAYS; THIS ORDER SHALL REMAIN IN EFFECT UNTIL FURTHER ACTION BY THE BOARD OR UNTIL THE BOND CONDITIONS IN THE CRIMINAL CASE ARE NO LONGER IN EFFECT.

PAYNE, STEVEN M MD, LICENSE NUMBER J0184 OF KATY, TX, WAS DISCIPLINED BY TEXAS ON MAY 16, 1998
DISCIPLINARY ACTION: 60-MONTH PROBATION; RESTRICTION PLACED ON LICENSE
OFFENSE: CRIMINAL CONVICTION OR PLEA OF GUILTY, NOLO CONTENDERE, OR NO CONTEST TO A CRIME

NOTES: PLED NO CONTEST TO ONE MISDEMEANOR CHARGE OF PUBLIC LEWDNESS WHICH INVOLVED A FEMALE PATIENT; ON 3/1/97 HE ENTERED INTO A BOARD ORDER PROHIBITING HIM FROM TREATING FEMALE PATIENTS UNDER THE AGE OF 55; HE SUBMITTED TO A 96 HOUR INPATIENT PSYCHIATRIC EVALUATION. SUSPENSION STAYED FOR PROBATION WITH FOLLOWING TERMS AND CONDITIONS: SHALL HAVE A CHAPERON PRESENT DURING PHYSICAL EXAMS ON A FEMALE PATIENT; SHALL NOT PERFORM PELVIC EXAMS ON ANY FEMALE PATIENT FOR THE FIRST 2 YEARS; SHALL NOT DATE OR SEEK TO DATE ANY OF HIS PATIENTS; SHALL CONTINUE TO RECEIVE CARE AND TREATMENT FROM HIS PSYCHIATRIST NO LESS THAN ONCE A MONTH FOR A PERIOD OF 6 MONTHS AND THEREAFTER AT LEAST EVERY THREE MONTHS; SHALL PARTICIPATE IN BI-WEEKLY GROUP THERAPY SESSIONS FOR A MINIMUM OF 3 MONTHS; SHALL MAINTAIN ADEQUATE MEDICAL RECORDS WHICH SHALL BE AVAILABLE FOR REVIEW; SHALL APPEAR BEFORE THE BOARD AT LEAST ONCE A YEAR; SHALL COOPERATE WITH THE BOARD IN VERIFYING COMPLIANCE INCLUDING PROVIDING COPIES OF MEDICAL RELEASES AND PEER REVIEW RECORDS UPON REQUEST; SHALL GIVE A COPY OF THIS ORDER TO ANY HEALTH CARE ENTITY WHERE HE HAS PRIVILEGES; SHALL PROVIDE A COPY OF THIS ORDER TO ANYONE REQUESTING IT WITHIN 10 DAYS; TIME SPENT OUT OF TEXAS DOES NOT COUNT TOWARD PROBATION; SHALL INFORM THE BOARD OF CHANGE OF ADDRESS WITHIN 10 DAYS OR IF HE LEAVES THE STATE; SHALL NOT SEEK MODIFICATION FOR ONE YEAR.

PEABODY, BRENDA K MD, LICENSE NUMBER H8316 OF OAKRIDGE, TN, WAS DISCIPLINED BY TEXAS ON AUGUST 22, 1998
DISCIPLINARY ACTION: FINE; REPRIMAND
OFFENSE: NONCOMPLIANCE WITH A PROFESSIONAL RULE

NOTES: FAILED TO SUBMIT REQUIRED CONTINUING MEDICAL EDUCATION ON HER ANNUAL REGISTRATION IN 2/97; A CONTINUING MEDICAL EDUCATION TEMPORARY LICENSE WAS ISSUED AND AFTER THAT EXPIRED SHE PROVIDED EVIDENCE OF HAVING TAKEN SOME CONTINUING MEDICAL EDUCATION, BUT WITH A BALANCE OF 3.5 HOURS; FOLLOW UP CALL WERE MADE 8/21/97, 9/2/97 AND 11/4/97 TO ALLOW HER TO DEMONSTRATE THE BALANCE OF THE REQUIRED CONTINUING MEDICAL EDUCATION; SHE WAS ADVISED THAT AN AFFIDAVIT WOULD SUFFICE TO REPRESENT (IF OBTAINED) THE BALANCE OF HOURS; SHE DID NOT SEND IN ANY ADDITIONAL INFORMATION UNTIL THE TIME OF THE INFORMAL SETTLEMENT CONFERENCE/SHOW COMPLIANCE PROCEEDING ON 4/22/98. $500 FINE.

PEARL, CONRAD R DO, DATE OF BIRTH DECEMBER 19, 1931, LICENSE NUMBER 0004524 OF 27676 CHERRY HILL ROAD, GARDEN CITY, MI, WAS DISCIPLINED BY MICHIGAN ON NOVEMBER 17, 1993
DISCIPLINARY ACTION: 6-MONTH SUSPENSION OF CONTROLLED SUBSTANCE LICENSE; FINE
OFFENSE: PROFESSIONAL MISCONDUCT

NOTES: DRUG RELATED. DRUG CONTROL LICENSE REVOKED; $2,500 FINE. ON 2/27/95 REINSTATEMENT OF CONTROLLED SUBSTANCE LICENSE DENIED.

PEARL, CONRAD R DO, DATE OF BIRTH DECEMBER 19, 1931, LICENSE NUMBER 0004524 OF 27676 CHERRY HILL ROAD, GARDEN CITY, MI, WAS DISCIPLINED BY MICHIGAN ON DECEMBER 2, 1993
DISCIPLINARY ACTION: 12-MONTH PROBATION; FINE
OFFENSE: SUBSTANDARD CARE, INCOMPETENCE OR NEGLIGENCE

NOTES: NEGLIGENCE/INCOMPETENCE. $2,500 FINE; LICENSE LIMITED.

PEARL, CONRAD R DO, LICENSE NUMBER 0002003 OF GARDEN CITY, MI, WAS DISCIPLINED BY FLORIDA ON JUNE 26, 1996
DISCIPLINARY ACTION: SURRENDER OF LICENSE
OFFENSE: DISCIPLINARY ACTION BY ANOTHER STATE OR AGENCY

NOTES: CHARGED WITH HAVING DISCIPLINARY ACTION TAKEN AGAINST LICENSE BY ANOTHER JURISDICTION. HE ACCEPTED RELINQUISHMENT OF LICENSE AGREEING NEVER AGAIN TO APPLY FOR LICENSURE IN FLORIDA.

PEARL, CONRAD R OF SOUTHFIELD, MI, WAS DISCIPLINED BY MISSOURI ON DECEMBER 3, 1996
DISCIPLINARY ACTION: SURRENDER OF LICENSE
OFFENSE: DISCIPLINARY ACTION BY ANOTHER STATE OR AGENCY

NOTES: BASED ON DISCIPLINE IN MICHIGAN AND VIOLATIONS OF THE DRUG RULES AND REGULATIONS. LICENSE WAS VOLUNTARILY SURRENDERED IN LIEU OF DISCIPLINARY ACTION.

PEARL, CONRAD ROBERT DO, LICENSE NUMBER 00D6842 OF GARDEN CITY, MI, WAS DISCIPLINED BY TEXAS ON JANUARY 6, 1995
DISCIPLINARY ACTION: SURRENDER OF LICENSE

NOTES: IN LIEU OF FURTHER INVESTIGATION OR A HEARING ON ALLEGATIONS THAT HE VIOLATED THE MEDICAL PRACTICE ACT. SHALL NOT PETITION FOR REINSTATEMENT.

PEARL, CONRAD ROBERT DO, LICENSE NUMBER 20A3851 OF GARDEN CITY, MI, WAS DISCIPLINED BY CALIFORNIA ON OCTOBER 6, 1995
DISCIPLINARY ACTION: LICENSE REVOCATION
OFFENSE: DISCIPLINARY ACTION BY ANOTHER STATE OR AGENCY

NOTES: ACTION TAKEN BY ANOTHER STATE.

PEARL, CONRAD ROBERT DO, LICENSE NUMBER 0000904 OF 27676 CHERRY HILL ROAD, GARDEN CITY, MI, WAS DISCIPLINED BY ARIZONA ON JULY 1, 1996
DISCIPLINARY ACTION: SURRENDER OF LICENSE

OFFENSE: DISCIPLINARY ACTION BY ANOTHER STATE OR AGENCY

NOTES: LICENSE REVOCATION IN CALIFORNIA ON 8/15/95 BASED ON ACTION IN MICHIGAN DUE TO NEGLIGENCE, INCOMPETENCE AND VIOLATION OF OR AIDING AND ABETTING A VIOLATION OF THE PUBLIC HEALTH CODE WHICH ON 12/07/93 PLACED HIS LICENSE ON ONE YEAR PROBATION AND HIS CONTROLLED DRUG LICENSE WAS REVOKED FOR A MINIMUM OF THREE YEARS DURING WHICH TIME HE IS UNABLE TO DISPENSE ANY CONTROLLED SUBSTANCES FROM HIS OFFICE; HIS CONTROLLED SUBSTANCE LICENSE WAS SUSPENDED FOR A MINIMUM OF SIX MONTHS AND ONE DAY DURING WHICH TIME HE IS UNABLE TO PRESCRIBE ANY CONTROLLED SUBSTANCES. SHALL DELIVER TO THE ARIZONA BOARD ALL DOCUMENTS THAT INDICATE THAT HE IS A LICENSEE OF THE BOARD.

PEARSON, LYNN L MD OF JASPER, TX, WAS DISCIPLINED BY DEA ON JULY 1, 1994
DISCIPLINARY ACTION: DENIAL OF NEW LICENSE
OFFENSE: CRIMINAL CONVICTION OR PLEA OF GUILTY, NOLO CONTENDERE, OR NO CONTEST TO A CRIME

NOTES: IN 5/86 CONVICTED OF TWO FELONY COUNTS OF THE UNLAWFUL DISPENSING OF PERCODAN, DILAUDID AND DOLOPHINE, ALL SCHEDULE II CONTROLLED SUBSTANCES. DEA REGISTRATION REVOKED 7/31/87; ON 2/8/88 TEXAS BOARD ORDERED THAT HIS MEDICAL LICENSE BE REVOKED, STAYED THAT REVOCATION, AND PLACED HIS LICENSE TO PRACTICE MEDICINE ON PROBATION FOR TWO YEARS. LIMITED HIM TO PRACTICE MEDICINE WITHOUT PAY AT A LOCAL COMMUNITY HEALTH CENTER AND PROHIBITED HIM FOR POSSESSING, DISPENSING OR PRESCRIBING ANY CONTROLLED SUBSTANCE; REISSUED CONTROLLED SUBSTANCE REGISTRATION 2/92 AND ABLE TO APPLY FOR SCHEDULE II THROUGH V.

PENCE, RONALD M MD, LICENSE NUMBER H2677 OF BEDFORD, TX, WAS DISCIPLINED BY TEXAS ON AUGUST 9, 1997
DISCIPLINARY ACTION: 48-MONTH PROBATION; FINE
OFFENSE: SEXUAL ABUSE OF OR SEXUAL MISCONDUCT WITH A PATIENT

NOTES: DURING 1993 AND 1994, HE DEVELOPED A ROMANTIC AND SEXUAL RELATIONSHIP WITH AN ADULT FEMALE REGISTERED NURSE. DURING THIS TIME, HE ALSO TREATED HER THROUGH INITIATION OF PRESCRIPTION MEDICATIONS INCLUDING PROZAC AND KLONOPIN, AND MODIFIED THE DOSAGE OF ESTROGEN MEDICATIONS. HE FAILED TO MAINTAIN MEDICAL RECORDS OF HIS CARE AND TREATMENT OF HER. ON ABOUT 4/26/94 SHE INGESTED AN OVERDOSE OF MEDICATIONS AND CALLED HIM FROM A LOCAL MOTEL. HE DROVE TO THE MOTEL AND TRANSPORTED HER TO A LOCAL HOSPITAL EMERGENCY ROOM. HE PROVIDED ALL INFORMATION OF WHICH HE WAS AWARE TO THE HOSPITAL STAFF REGARDING THE MEDICATIONS CONSUMED BY THE PATIENT. SUSPENSION IS FULLY PROBATED SUBJECT TO THE FOLLOWING TERMS AND CONDITIONS: SHALL COMPLY WITH THE APPROVED PSYCHIATRIST'S RECOMMENDATION TO RETURN FOR RE-EVALUATION IN THREE MONTHS AND TO CONTACT HIM SHOULD ANY SIGNIFICANT DETERIORATION OCCUR; HIS MEDICAL PRACTICE SHALL BE MONITORED BY A BOARD APPROVED TEXAS PHYSICIAN WHO SHALL PROVIDE QUARTERLY REPORTS TO THE BOARD; SHALL MAINTAIN ADEQUATE MEDICAL RECORDS WHICH SHALL BE AVAILABLE FOR REVIEW; SHALL ADOPT OR ESTABLISH A SYSTEM OF PATIENT RECORD KEEPING AND BILLING THAT ENSURES ACCURACY; SHALL OBTAIN AT LEAST 50 HOURS PER YEAR OF CONTINUING MEDICAL EDUCATION WITH AT LEAST FIVE HOURS IN ETHICS; WITHIN ONE YEAR, SHALL PASS THE JURISPRUDENCE EXAM; SHALL APPEAR BEFORE THE BOARD AT LEAST ONCE A YEAR; SHALL PAY AN ADMINISTRATIVE PENALTY OF $5000; SHALL COOPERATE WITH THE BOARD IN VERIFYING COMPLIANCE INCLUDING PROVIDING COPIES OF MEDICAL RELEASES AND PEER REVIEW RECORDS UPON REQUEST; SHALL GIVE A COPY OF THIS ORDER TO ANY HEALTH CARE ENTITY WHERE HE HAS PRIVILEGES; SHALL PROVIDE A COPY OF THIS ORDER TO ANYONE REQUESTING IT WITHIN 10 DAYS; TIME SPENT OUT OF TEXAS DOES NOT COUNT TOWARD PROBATION; SHALL INFORM THE BOARD OF CHANGE OF ADDRESS WITHIN 10 DAYS OR IF HE LEAVES THE STATE; SHALL NOT SEEK MODIFICATION FOR ONE YEAR. ON 10/15/99 THE ORDER WAS TERMINATED.

PENNINGTON, KAREN MD, LICENSE NUMBER 00E4592 OF KNOX CITY, TX, WAS DISCIPLINED BY TEXAS ON NOVEMBER 3, 1994
DISCIPLINARY ACTION: LICENSE SUSPENSION
OFFENSE: SUBSTANCE ABUSE

NOTES: ALLEGATIONS INVOLVING INTEMPERATE USE OF ALCOHOL OR DRUGS THAT COULD ENDANGER THE LIVES OF PATIENTS AND INABILITY TO PRACTICE WITH REASONABLE SKILL AND SAFETY; ON 9/21/94 AT HER REQUEST WAS TAKEN TO HOSPITAL WITH AN INITIAL DIAGNOSIS OF GASTROINTESTINAL BLEEDING, WEIGHT LOSS AND PNEUMONIA AND WAS CONSIDERED CRITICALLY ILL: ILLNESS IS A RESULT OF HER SELF-PRESCRIBING OF TYLENOL #4, DARVOCET AND PERCODAN WITHOUT A LEGITIMATE MEDICAL PURPOSE; STATES SHE BEGAN SELF-PRESCRIBING FOUR OR FIVE MONTHS AGO FOR ABDOMINAL PAIN; PREVIOUS SANCTIONS WERE 12/11/78 SUSPENSION FOR SELF-PRESCRIBING, 12/9/79 PROBATION, 8/28/82 REVOCATION DUE TO VIOLATION OF THE PROBATION; 5/24/90 LICENSE REINSTATED WITHOUT RESTRICTION. SUSPENSION UNTIL SHE PERSONALLY APPEARS BEFORE THE BOARD AND PROVIDES SUFFICIENT EVIDENCE THAT SHE IS PHYSICALLY, MENTALLY AND OTHERWISE COMPETENT TO SAFELY PRACTICE INCLUDING BUT NOT LIMITED TO MEDICAL RECORDS AND REPORTS OF PSYCHOLOGICAL AND NEUROPSYCHIATRIC EVALUATIONS.

PENNINGTON, KAREN MD OF 110 SOUTH SECOND BOX 99, KNOX CITY, TX, WAS DISCIPLINED BY DEA ON JANUARY 5, 1995
DISCIPLINARY ACTION: SURRENDER OF CONTROLLED SUBSTANCE LICENSE
OFFENSE: DISCIPLINARY ACTION BY ANOTHER STATE OR AGENCY

NOTES: STATE BOARD.

PEREZ, RAOUL MD, LICENSE NUMBER F5897 OF LIVINGSTON, TX, WAS DISCIPLINED BY TEXAS ON MAY 14, 1999
DISCIPLINARY ACTION: FINE
OFFENSE: PROFESSIONAL MISCONDUCT

NOTES: ON 11/12/91 A PATIENT TERMINATED THE PHYSICIAN/PATIENT RELATIONSHIP AS SHE WAS MOVING AWAY; SHE BEGAN CONTACTING THE DOCTOR SHORTLY THEREAFTER, SOLICITING A SOCIAL RELATIONSHIP; FIVE WEEKS AFTER THE 11/12/91 OFFICE VISIT HE FINALLY AGREED TO SEE HER SOCIALLY; HE FAILED TO DOCUMENT, IN WRITING, THE TERMINATION OF THE PHYSICIAN/PATIENT RELATIONSHIP; MEDICAL RECORDS INDICATE THAT ON 12/26/91 HE TREATED HER FOR ASTHMA AND PROVIDED SAMPLES OF THEODUR; HE MAINTAINS THAT HE DID NOT TREAT

HER ON 12/26/91 BUT THAT SHE CAME TO HIS OFFICE UNDER FALSE PRETENSES DEMANDING MONEY; MAINTAINS THAT CONTINUED RELATIONSHIP WAS COERCIVE BY HER. $7,500 FINE; SHALL COOPERATE WITH THE BOARD IN VERIFYING COMPLIANCE; SHALL INFORM THE BOARD OF CHANGE OF ADDRESS WITHIN 10 DAYS.

PETERSON, JON L MD, LICENSE NUMBER E8816 OF HOUSTON, TX, WAS DISCIPLINED BY TEXAS ON APRIL 10, 1999
DISCIPLINARY ACTION: FINE; REPRIMAND
OFFENSE: NONCOMPLIANCE WITH A PROFESSIONAL RULE

NOTES: INVOLVES AN UNREASONABLE FEE CHARGED BY HIM TO NEW YORK LIFE INSURANCE COMPANY FOR THE MEDICAL RECORDS OF A PATIENT; HE DENIES THAT HE IS GUILTY OF OVERCHARGING AND STATES THAT HIS PROFESSIONAL FEE FOR PULLING A PATIENT'S RECORD, FILLING OUT AN ATTENDING PHYSICIAN STATEMENT, AND ADDING COPIES OF PERTINENT LABORATORY OR TESTING DATA HAS ALWAYS BEEN $50; THE RECORD CONSISTED OF FOUR PAGES WITH NO SUMMARY. $100 FINE.

PETERSON, MARION G MD, LICENSE NUMBER 0A13817 OF MESA, AZ, WAS DISCIPLINED BY CALIFORNIA ON FEBRUARY 13, 1996
DISCIPLINARY ACTION: SURRENDER OF LICENSE

NOTES: WHILE CHARGES PENDING.

PETERSON, MARION G MD, LICENSE NUMBER C2089 OF MESA, AZ, WAS DISCIPLINED BY TEXAS ON MAY 16, 1998
DISCIPLINARY ACTION: SURRENDER OF LICENSE
OFFENSE: DISCIPLINARY ACTION BY ANOTHER STATE OR AGENCY

NOTES: VOLUNTARY SURRENDER ORDER WITH THE CALIFORNIA BOARD EFFECTIVE 2/13/96. VOLUNTARY AND PERMANENT SURRENDER.

PETTEY, THOMAS D MD, LICENSE NUMBER 00G9187 OF FORT WORTH, TX, WAS DISCIPLINED BY TEXAS ON AUGUST 18, 1990
DISCIPLINARY ACTION: 60-MONTH PROBATION; RESTRICTION PLACED ON LICENSE

NOTES: STIPULATED ORDER. MUST OBTAIN CONTINUING MEDICAL EDUCATION, ALLOW RANDOM REVIEW BY BOARD STAFF OF OFFICE PATIENT RECORDS TO ENSURE COMPLIANCE WITH ORDER AND TO ASCERTAIN THAT DOCUMENTATION HAS IMPROVED, AND REFRAIN FROM OBSTETRICS PRACTICE UNTIL PERMITTED TO DO SO BY BOARD (SUCH RESTRICTION INDEPENDENT OF AND SHALL SURVIVE PROBATIONARY PERIOD).

PETTEY, THOMAS DAVID MD, LICENSE NUMBER 0008789 OF FORT WORTH, TX, WAS DISCIPLINED BY MISSISSIPPI ON JANUARY 16, 1992
DISCIPLINARY ACTION: PROBATION
OFFENSE: DISCIPLINARY ACTION BY ANOTHER STATE OR AGENCY

NOTES: ACTION TAKEN IN TEXAS. FIVE-YEAR SUSPENSION, EFFECTIVE AUGUST 7, 1991, STAYED.

PETTY, PRESTON D MD, LICENSE NUMBER 0028630 OF ODESSA, TX, WAS DISCIPLINED BY FLORIDA ON OCTOBER 22, 1991
DISCIPLINARY ACTION: REQUIRED TO TAKE ADDITIONAL MEDICAL EDUCATION; RESTRICTION PLACED ON CONTROLLED SUBSTANCE LICENSE
OFFENSE: DISCIPLINARY ACTION BY ANOTHER STATE OR AGENCY

NOTES: IF EVER RETURNS TO PRACTICE MEDICINE IN FLORIDA, HIS LICENSE SHALL BE RESTRICTED IN THAT HE SHALL NOT PRESCRIBE, ADMINISTER, DISPENSE, MIX, OR ORDER SCHEDULED DRUGS UNTIL HE COMPLETES THE COURSE: "PROTECTING YOUR MEDICAL PRACTICE, CLINICAL, LEGAL, AND ETHICAL ISSUES IN PRESCRIBING ABUSABLE DRUGS", OR A BOARD APPROVED EQUIVALENT.

PHILLIPS, GREGGORY K MD, LICENSE NUMBER H6511 OF FORT WORTH, TX, WAS DISCIPLINED BY TEXAS ON OCTOBER 15, 1999
DISCIPLINARY ACTION: 60-MONTH PROBATION; RESTRICTION PLACED ON LICENSE
OFFENSE: SUBSTANCE ABUSE

NOTES: ON 10/28/97 & 11/4/97 HIS TRIPLICATE PRESCRIPTION RECORDS SHOW HIM PRESCRIBING FENTANYL TO AN INDIVIDUAL AT HIS HOME ADDRESS; ON 8/20/97 & 9/8/97 PHARMACY RECORDS INDICATE THAT HE PRESCRIBED LORTAB TO AN INDIVIDUAL AT HIS HOME ADDRESS; HIS MEDICAL RECORDS INDICATE THAT HE HAS ADMITTED TO PRESCRIBING UNIDENTIFIED DRUGS TO HIMSELF AND FAMILY MEMBERS, AS WELL AS TAKING UNIDENTIFIED DRUG SAMPLES FROM HIS OFFICE; FROM 10/13/98 - 3/5/99 HE VOLUNTARILY ADMITTED HIMSELF FOR CHEMICAL DEPENDENCY TREATMENT; HE REPORTS A SOBRIETY DATE OF 10/13/98; HIS AA MEETING ATTENDANCE HAS BEEN REPORTED BY HIM TO BE ON AN AVERAGE OF 5 TIMES PER WEEK. SUSPENSION STAYED FOR PROBATION WITH FOLLOWING TERMS AND CONDITIONS: SHALL NOT PRACTICE EMERGENCY MEDICINE UNLESS HE REQUESTS, IN WRITING, TO THE BOARD FOR APPROVAL TO RESUME PRACTICE; SHALL ABSTAIN FROM THE CONSUMPTION OF ALCOHOL/DRUGS IN ANY FORM UNLESS PRESCRIBED BY ANOTHER PHYSICIAN FOR A LEGITIMATE AND THERAPEUTIC PURPOSE; SHALL SUBMIT HIMSELF FOR APPROPRIATE EXAMS INCLUDING DRUG OR ALCOHOL SCREENS; SHALL NOMINATE THREE CERTIFIED PSYCHIATRISTS FOR BOARD SELECTION OF A THERAPIST AND SHALL EXPEDITIOUSLY SUBMIT HIMSELF TO EVALUATION AND TREATMENT BY THE APPROVED PRACTITIONER; SHALL PARTICIPATE IN THE ACTIVITIES OF A PHYSICIAN HEALTH AND REHABILITATION COMMITTEE AND ATTEND WEEKLY MEETINGS WITH QUARTERLY REPORTS; SHALL PARTICIPATE IN AA'S PROGRAM NOT LESS THAN THREE TIMES A WEEK; SHALL REPORT ON HIS ATTENDANCE; SHALL COMPLY WITH TERMS OF ANY CONTINUING CARE CONTRACT WITH QUARTERLY REPORTS; SHALL NOT TREAT OR OTHERWISE SERVE AS PHYSICIAN, PRESCRIBE, DISPENSE OR ADMINISTER DRUGS THAT MAY BE SUBJECT TO ABUSE TO HIMSELF OR TO ANY MEMBER OF HIS FAMILY; SHALL NOT PRESCRIBE, ADMINISTER OR DISPENSE DRUGS WITH POTENTIAL FOR ABUSE EXCEPT FOR INPATIENT TREATMENT; MAY PRESCRIBE SCHEDULE IV AND V CONTROLLED SUBSTANCES IN AN OUTPATIENT SETTING; SHALL SURRENDER ALL DRUGS WITH POTENTIAL FOR ABUSE IN HIS POSSESSION INCLUDING SAMPLES; SEPARATE FROM PATIENT RECORDS, SHALL MAINTAIN A LOGBOOK OF EVERY PRESCRIPTION WRITTEN BY HIM FOR DANGEROUS DRUGS WITH ADDICTIVE POTENTIAL WHICH SHALL BE MADE AVAILABLE FOR REVIEW; SHALL MAINTAIN ADEQUATE MEDICAL RECORDS WHICH SHALL BE AVAILABLE FOR REVIEW; SHALL OBTAIN 50 HOURS PER YEAR OF CONTINUING MEDICAL EDUCATION; SHALL APPEAR BEFORE THE BOARD AT LEAST TWICE A YEAR THE FIRST YEAR AND ONCE A YEAR THEREAFTER; SHALL COOPERATE WITH THE BOARD IN VERIFYING COMPLIANCE INCLUDING PROVIDING COPIES OF MEDICAL RELEASES UPON REQUEST; SHALL GIVE A COPY OF THIS ORDER TO ANY HEALTH CARE ENTITY WHERE HE HAS PRIVILEGES; TIME SPENT OUT OF TEXAS DOES NOT COUNT TOWARD PROBATION; SHALL INFORM THE

BOARD OF CHANGE OF ADDRESS WITHIN 10 DAYS OR IF HE LEAVES THE STATE; SHALL NOT SEEK MODIFICATION FOR ONE YEAR.

PHILLIPS, TREVOR DO, LICENSE NUMBER D3954 OF HOUSTON, TX, WAS DISCIPLINED BY TEXAS ON MAY 16, 1998
DISCIPLINARY ACTION: 36-MONTH RESTRICTION PLACED ON LICENSE; REQUIRED TO TAKE ADDITIONAL MEDICAL EDUCATION
OFFENSE: SUBSTANDARD CARE, INCOMPETENCE OR NEGLIGENCE

NOTES: INAPPROPRIATELY DIAGNOSED THYROID CONDITIONS AND INAPPROPRIATELY PRESCRIBED THYROID MEDICATION TO SEVERAL PATIENTS; FAILED TO ADEQUATELY DOCUMENT AND PERFORM PHYSICAL EXAMINATIONS DURING INITIAL VISITS AND FOLLOW-UP VISITS. SHALL OBTAIN 50 HOURS PER YEAR OF CONTINUING MEDICAL EDUCATION, WITH 25 HOURS IN NUTRITION AND 25 HOURS IN ENDOCRINOLOGY RELATED TOPICS; PRIOR TO TREATING ANY NEW ENDOCRINOPATHY, SHALL OBTAIN A WRITTEN CONSULTATION FROM A LICENSED TEXAS PHYSICIAN; SHALL MAINTAIN ADEQUATE MEDICAL RECORDS WHICH SHALL BE AVAILABLE FOR REVIEW; SHALL APPEAR BEFORE THE BOARD AT LEAST ONCE A YEAR; SHALL COOPERATE WITH THE BOARD IN VERIFYING COMPLIANCE; SHALL PROVIDE A COPY OF THIS ORDER TO ANYONE REQUESTING IT WITHIN 10 DAYS; TIME SPENT OUT OF TEXAS DOES NOT COUNT TOWARD RESTRICTION; SHALL INFORM THE BOARD OF CHANGE OF ADDRESS WITHIN 10 DAYS OR IF HE LEAVES THE STATE; SHALL NOT SEEK MODIFICATION FOR ONE YEAR.

PHUOC, HO TAN MD, LICENSE NUMBER 00F7052 OF HOUSTON, TX, WAS DISCIPLINED BY TEXAS ON AUGUST 24, 1991
DISCIPLINARY ACTION: RESTRICTION PLACED ON LICENSE

NOTES: MAY PERFORM CERTAIN PROCEDURES ON PATIENTS UNDER 12 ONLY IN HOSPITALS OR LICENSED SURGICAL CENTERS.

PIAZZA, KENNETH M MD OF 215 WATER STREET, JASPER, TX, WAS DISCIPLINED BY DEA ON SEPTEMBER 8, 1994
DISCIPLINARY ACTION: RESTRICTION PLACED ON CONTROLLED SUBSTANCE LICENSE
OFFENSE: PROFESSIONAL MISCONDUCT

NOTES: EXCESSIVE PURCHASES.

PIAZZA, KENNETH M MD OF 215 WATER STREET, JASPER, TX, WAS DISCIPLINED BY DEA ON JANUARY 29, 1998
DISCIPLINARY ACTION: SURRENDER OF CONTROLLED SUBSTANCE LICENSE

PIAZZA, KENNETH MICHAEL MD, LICENSE NUMBER E8112 OF JASPER, TX, WAS DISCIPLINED BY TEXAS ON MAY 14, 1999
DISCIPLINARY ACTION: SURRENDER OF LICENSE
OFFENSE: DISCIPLINARY ACTION BY ANOTHER STATE OR AGENCY

NOTES: ON 11/25/97 HE WAS ARRESTED FOR THE IMPROPER AND ILLEGAL DISPENSING AND PRESCRIBING OF CONTROLLED SUBSTANCES; HE PRESCRIBED COUGH SYRUP WITH CODEINE TO MANY OF HIS PATIENTS WHO WERE ON MEDICAID AND MEDICARE WHO DID NOT NEED THE MEDICATION AND WERE SELLING IT ON THE STREET; HE INDICATED TO THE BOARD THAT HE HAD TRIED PRESCRIBING DARVOCET, BUT THAT IT WAS NOT EFFECTIVE FOR PAIN IN HIS PATIENTS; IN 10/97 A DEA INVESTIGATOR INTERVIEWED SEVERAL FORMER EMPLOYEES OF HIS, AND EACH INDICATED THE MAJORITY OF HIS PATIENTS MENTIONED THAT THEY WERE NOT CONSUMING THE SYRUP, BUT SELLING ON THE STREET; ONE FORMER EMPLOYEE CLAIMED THAT SHE HAD QUESTIONED SEVERAL PATIENTS AND THEY TOLD HER THEY COULD TAKE THE SYRUP TO HOUSTON AND SELL IT FOR $250 ON THE STREET; ON 9/30/97, 10/20/97 AND 11/13/97 A DEA INVESTIGATOR AND OTHER AGENTS WENT TO HIS OFFICE IN AN UNDERCOVER CAPACITY AND OBTAINED PRESCRIPTIONS OF VALIUM AND PHENERGAN WITH CODEINE FOR A NON-MEDICAL PURPOSE; IN 1984 NEW YORK FINED HIM $5,000 AND HIS NEW YORK LICENSE WAS REVOKED FOR INCOMPETENCY, FRAUD, AND NEGLIGENT PRACTICES; IN 1988 HE WAS FINED $25,000 BY DEA AND SURRENDERED HIS DEA REGISTRATIONS FOR FAILING TO MAINTAIN ADEQUATE RECORDS FOR CONTROLLED SUBSTANCES; DEA LICENSE PARTIALLY REINSTATED IN 1994; ON 6/11/98 HE PLEADED GUILTY TO KNOWINGLY AND INTENTIONALLY HAVING DISPENSED A SCHEDULE IV CONTROLLED SUBSTANCE, DIAZEPAM, OUTSIDE THE SCOPE OF HIS PROFESSIONAL PRACTICE WITHOUT A LEGITIMATE MEDICAL REASON. VOLUNTARY AND PERMANENT SURRENDER.

PICKETT, JAN W MD, DATE OF BIRTH AUGUST 15, 1956 OF 4750 S COLONY BLVD, COLONY, TX, WAS DISCIPLINED BY MEDICARE ON MAY 9, 1995
DISCIPLINARY ACTION: EXCLUSION FROM THE MEDICARE AND/OR MEDICAID PROGRAM
OFFENSE: NONCOMPLIANCE WITH A PROFESSIONAL RULE

NOTES: DEFAULTED ON PUBLIC HEALTH SERVICE EDUCATION LOAN. REINSTATED ON 7/20/95.

PIERSON, ROBERT L MD, WAS DISCIPLINED BY NEBRASKA ON FEBRUARY 16, 1990
DISCIPLINARY ACTION: RESTRICTION PLACED ON LICENSE

PIERSON, ROBERT L MD OF 7709 CAMBRIDGE, HOUSTON, TX, WAS DISCIPLINED BY VERMONT ON JUNE 20, 1991
DISCIPLINARY ACTION: DENIAL OF NEW LICENSE
OFFENSE: DISCIPLINARY ACTION BY ANOTHER STATE OR AGENCY

NOTES: HAD CRIMINAL CONVICTIONS FOR FAILING TO KEEP DRUG RECORDS REQUIRED BY LAW AND FOR SHOPLIFTING; VOLUNTARILY SURRENDERED IOWA LICENSE AFTER INVESTIGATION REVEALED EVIDENCE OF SEXUAL INVOLVEMENT WITH PATIENTS AND PRESCRIBING DEPO-PROVERA, WHICH WAS NOT FDA APPROVED FOR PURPOSES OF BIRTH CONTROL; NEBRASKA LICENSE REVOKED IN 1986 AND REINSTATED IN 1990 WITH MULTIPLE CONDITIONS; NORTH DAKOTA THEN DENIED HIS LICENSE APPLICATION.

PIERSON, ROBERT L MD, WAS DISCIPLINED BY NEBRASKA ON JUNE 5, 1996
DISCIPLINARY ACTION: RESTRICTION PLACED ON LICENSE

NOTES: PETITION FOR REINSTATEMENT.

PIERSON, ROBERT LEROY MD, LICENSE NUMBER 0016506 OF GREENSBORO, AL, WAS DISCIPLINED BY ALABAMA ON JUNE 3, 1992
DISCIPLINARY ACTION: RESTRICTION PLACED ON LICENSE

NOTES: IN CONNECTION WITH LICENSURE APPLICATION. MUST ABIDE BY REQUIREMENTS OF PHYSICIANS RECOVERY NETWORK.

PIERSON, ROBERT LEROY MD, LICENSE NUMBER 16506, WAS DISCIPLINED BY ALABAMA ON AUGUST 6, 1997
DISCIPLINARY ACTION: PROBATION

NOTES: FAILED TO ABIDE BY VOLUNTARY RESTRICTIONS OF 6/3/92 AGREEMENT IN THAT HE FAILED TO ABIDE BY TERMS OF HIS ADVOCACY CONTRACT WITH PHYSICIANS RECOVERY NETWORK AND FAILED TO REMAIN UNDER THE CARE OF A PSYCHIATRIST. REVOCATION SUSPENDED. CONDITIONS OF PROBATION: SHALL NOT ACTIVELY PRACTICE IN ALABAMA UNLESS HE NOTIFIES THE BOARD AND GETS THEIR APPROVAL, OBTAINS A NEW EVALUATION BY THE PHYSICIANS RECOVERY NETWORK AND ENTERS INTO AN ADVOCACY CONTRACT WITH THEM.

PILISZEK, THEODORE S MD, LICENSE NUMBER 00G1149 OF HOUSTON, TX, WAS DISCIPLINED BY TEXAS ON AUGUST 18, 1995
DISCIPLINARY ACTION: FINE
OFFENSE: PROFESSIONAL MISCONDUCT

NOTES: FROM APPROXIMATELY 1990 THROUGH 7/94, HE ALLOWED THREE MEMBERS OF HIS OFFICE MEDICAL STAFF TO PERFORM RADIOLOGIC PROCEDURES ALTHOUGH THEY WERE NEITHER CERTIFIED BY THE DEPARTMENT OF HEALTH OR REGISTERED WITH THE BOARD TO PERFORM SUCH PROCEDURES. SHALL PAY $5,000 FINE; WITHIN ONE YEAR SHALL TAKE AND PASS THE MEDICAL JURISPRUDENCE EXAMINATION; SHALL GIVE A COPY OF THIS ORDER TO ANY HEALTH CARE ENTITY WHERE HE HAS PRIVILEGES; SHALL COOPERATE WITH THE BOARD IN VERIFYING COMPLIANCE.

PILLSBURY, CURTIS BRYANT MD, DATE OF BIRTH JANUARY 11, 1921, LICENSE NUMBER 00C2954 OF 2803 TAM OSHANTER, RICHARDSON, TX, WAS DISCIPLINED BY TEXAS ON APRIL 30, 1993
DISCIPLINARY ACTION: SURRENDER OF LICENSE
OFFENSE: FAILURE TO COMPLY WITH PREVIOUS BOARD ORDER

NOTES: HAS HAD PRACTICAL DIFFICULTIES IN FULLY COMPLYING WITH TERMS OF 5/89 ORDER. SURRENDER IS PERMANENT.

PINO, WILBERT B MD, DATE OF BIRTH OCTOBER 11, 1961 OF 3817 QUILL COURT, EL PASO, TX, WAS DISCIPLINED BY MEDICARE ON APRIL 16, 1994
DISCIPLINARY ACTION: EXCLUSION FROM THE MEDICARE AND/OR MEDICAID PROGRAM
OFFENSE: NONCOMPLIANCE WITH A PROFESSIONAL RULE

NOTES: DEFAULTED ON PUBLIC HEALTH SERVICE EDUCATION LOAN. REINSTATED ON 4/22/94.

PINSOF, LAWRENCE MD, LICENSE NUMBER 137628 OF 2016 MAIN STREET SUITE 2010, HOUSTON, TX, WAS DISCIPLINED BY NEW YORK ON JULY 3, 1998
DISCIPLINARY ACTION: LICENSE SUSPENSION; PROBATION
OFFENSE: DISCIPLINARY ACTION BY ANOTHER STATE OR AGENCY

NOTES: DISCIPLINED BY THE TEXAS BOARD FOR FAILING TO PRACTICE MEDICINE IN AN ACCEPTABLE MANNER; PROFESSIONAL INCOMPETENCE AND UNPROFESSIONAL CONDUCT. SUSPENSION UNTIL PROVEN FIT TO PRACTICE AND THE SUCCESSFUL COMPLETION OF ALL TERMS IMPOSED BY THE TEXAS BOARD; PROBATION FOR NO LESS THAN TWO YEARS.

PITTARD, CARLTON DUWAIN MD, DATE OF BIRTH DECEMBER 3, 1931, LICENSE NUMBER 00C6476 OF 1600 WEST COLLEGE SUITE 110, GRAPEVINE, TX, WAS DISCIPLINED BY TEXAS ON JUNE 15, 1993
DISCIPLINARY ACTION: 60-MONTH PROBATION; MONITORING OF PHYSICIAN PERFORMANCE
OFFENSE: NONCOMPLIANCE WITH A PROFESSIONAL RULE

NOTES: FAILED TO KEEP COMPLETE AND ACCURATE RECORDS OF THE PURCHASES AND DISPOSALS OF CONTROLLED SUBSTANCES, MAINTAIN AN INITIAL OR BIENNIAL INVENTORIES, MAINTAIN DISPENSATION CHARTS OF CONTROLLED SUBSTANCES, AND STORE SUCH DRUGS IN ACCORDANCE WITH FEDERAL AND STATE REQUIREMENTS; A 5/5/92 AUDIT NOTED MANY DEFICIENCIES IN THESE AREAS; IN 3/91 HE ORDERED SAMPLES OF TALWIN AND DISPENSED ENTIRE SUPPLY TO A PATIENT WHOSE SON USED THE DRUGS TO COMMIT SUICIDE; HAS SECURED THE ASSISTANCE OF A LAW FIRM IN BRINGING OFFICE INTO COMPLIANCE WITH STATE AND FEDERAL REGULATIONS. FIVE YEAR SUSPENSION STAYED. CONDITIONS OF PROBATION: SHALL MAINTAIN ADEQUATE MEDICAL RECORDS ON ALL PATIENT OFFICE VISITS AND MAKE THEM AVAILABLE FOR INSPECTION; SHALL COMPLY WITH ALL STATUTES, RULES AND REGULATIONS PERTAINING TO THE PRESCRIBING, ADMINISTERING, DISPENSING OR SUPPLYING OF DANGEROUS DRUGS OR CONTROLLED SUBSTANCES; SHALL ADEQUATELY SUPERVISE THE ACTIVITIES OF ALL EMPLOYEES; SHALL APPEAR BEFORE THE BOARD ONCE A YEAR; SHALL GIVE A COPY OF THIS ORDER TO ANY HEALTH CARE ENTITY WHERE HE HAS PRIVILEGES; SHALL COOPERATE WITH THE BOARD IN VERIFYING COMPLIANCE; SHALL INFORM BOARD OF CHANGE OF ADDRESS WITHIN 10 DAYS OR IF HE LEAVES THE STATE; TIME SPENT OUT OF TEXAS DOES NOT COUNT TOWARD PROBATION. SHALL NOT SEEK MODIFICATION FOR ONE YEAR. ON 8/19/94 REQUEST FOR TERMINATION WAS DENIED. ON 10/13/95 ORDER TERMINATED BASED ON COMPLIANCE WITH TERMS.

POAGE, MARY MARGARET MD, LICENSE NUMBER 00H8331 OF HOUSTON, TX, WAS DISCIPLINED BY TEXAS ON MARCH 4, 1995
DISCIPLINARY ACTION: 60-MONTH PROBATION; RESTRICTION PLACED ON LICENSE
OFFENSE: SUBSTANDARD CARE, INCOMPETENCE OR NEGLIGENCE

NOTES: IN 12/93, SHE FAILED TO FULLY ADDRESS THE SYMPTOMS OF AN INFANT WHO PRESENTED WITH A DIAGNOSIS OF SEPSIS AND MENINGITIS. EXHIBITED SIGNS OF EXCESSIVE STRESS AND ANXIETY DURING HER EFFORTS TO TREAT THE PATIENT DURING A CODE SITUATION; SHE CONTENDS THAT EMERGENCY ROOM FACILITIES WERE NOT PROPERLY PREPARED TO ADDRESS THE CHILD'S CONDITIONS; NEITHER ADMITS NOR DENIES THE ALLEGATIONS. SUSPENSION STAYED. PROBATION WITH TERMS: PRACTICE SHALL BE MONITORED BY BOARD-APPROVED MONITORING PHYSICIAN WHO SHALL SUBMIT QUARTERLY REPORTS; SHALL NOT PRACTICE MEDICINE IN A SOLO PRACTICE SETTING BUT IN AN INSTITUTIONAL OR GROUP PRACTICE APPROVED BY THE BOARD; SHALL NOT PRACTICE EMERGENCY ROOM MEDICINE UNLESS AUTHORIZED BY THE BOARD; SHALL OBTAIN AT LEAST 50 HOURS PER YEAR OF CONTINUING MEDICAL EDUCATION; SHALL SUBMIT TO EVALUATION AND TREATMENT BY A BOARD-APPROVED PSYCHIATRIST, WHOM SHE SHALL SEE MONTHLY FOR FOLLOW-UP CARE AND COUNSELING AND WHO SHALL SUBMIT REPORTS; SHALL APPEAR BEFORE BOARD AT LEAST ONCE A YEAR OR AT BOARD REQUEST; SHALL COOPERATE WITH THE BOARD IN VERIFYING COMPLIANCE INCLUDING PROVIDING COPIES OF MEDICAL RELEASES UPON REQUEST; SHALL GIVE A COPY OF THIS ORDER TO ANY HEALTH CARE ENTITY WHERE SHE HAS PRIVILEGES; SHALL PROVIDE A COPY OF THIS ORDER TO ANYONE REQUESTING IT WITHIN 10 DAYS; TIME PERIOD OUT OF TEXAS DOES NOT COUNT TOWARD PROBATION; SHALL INFORM THE BOARD OF CHANGE OF ADDRESS WITHIN 10 DAYS OF IF SHE LEAVES THE STATE; SHALL NOT SEEK MODIFICATION FOR ONE YEAR. ON 5/10/97 BOARD

GRANTED HER PETITION FOR TERMINATION OF THIS ORDER BASED ON COMPLIANCE WITH CONDITIONS.

POEHLMANN, KURT S MD, LICENSE NUMBER 00D1771 OF COMANCHE, TX, WAS DISCIPLINED BY TEXAS ON JUNE 22, 1994
DISCIPLINARY ACTION: RESTRICTION PLACED ON LICENSE; REQUIRED TO TAKE ADDITIONAL MEDICAL EDUCATION
OFFENSE: SUBSTANDARD CARE, INCOMPETENCE OR NEGLIGENCE

NOTES: RESIGNED FROM A HOSPITAL WHILE PRIVILEGE STATUS WAS UNDER INVESTIGATION; FAILED TO PRACTICE IN AN ACCEPTABLE MANNER ON EIGHT PATIENTS INVOLVING OBSTETRICS AND MYOCARDIAL INFARCTIONS; EXERCISED POOR JUDGEMENT IN ALLOWING PATIENTS TO MAKE THE DECISION FOR SURGERY. LICENSE IS RESTRICTED IN THAT HE SHALL NOT PRACTICE OBSTETRICS AND GYNECOLOGY EXCEPT THAT WHICH MAY ARISE IN EITHER AN EMERGENCY ROOM OR GENERAL FAMILY PRACTICE SETTING NOR SHALL HE PRACTICE INPATIENT SURGERY EXCEPT WHEN ASSISTING; SHALL ATTEND AT LEAST 50 HOURS PER YEAR OF CONTINUING MEDICAL EDUCATION INCLUDING AT LEAST 20 HOURS PER YEAR IN CARDIOLOGY COURSES; SHALL APPEAR BEFORE THE BOARD ONCE A YEAR; SHALL WITHIN THREE MONTHS UNDERGO A COMPLETE PHYSICAL EXAM INCLUDING BUT NOT LIMITED TO AN OPHTHALMOLOGICAL AND NEUROPSYCHOLOGICAL EVALUATION BY BOARD APPROVED PHYSICIANS; SHALL GIVE A COPY OF THIS ORDER TO ANY HEALTH CARE ENTITY WHERE HE HAS PRIVILEGES; SHALL COOPERATE WITH THE BOARD IN VERIFYING COMPLIANCE; SHALL INFORM BOARD OF CHANGE OF ADDRESS WITHIN 10 DAYS. SHALL NOT SEEK MODIFICATION FOR ONE YEAR. ON 4/4/98 ORDER TERMINATED.

POLINGER, IRIS SANDRA MD, LICENSE NUMBER 00E8117 OF STAFFORD, TX, WAS DISCIPLINED BY TEXAS ON JANUARY 24, 1992
DISCIPLINARY ACTION: PROBATION
OFFENSE: PROFESSIONAL MISCONDUCT

NOTES: SEVERAL VIOLATIONS OF THE MEDICAL PRACTICE ACT, INCLUDING PERSISTENTLY AND FLAGRANTLY OVERCHARGING OR OVERTREATING PATIENTS. THREE-YEAR SUSPENSION, STAYED; PROBATION UNDER TERMS AND CONDITIONS. ON 3/5/94 PROBATION TERMINATED.

POLLNOW, ROBERT E MD, DATE OF BIRTH JANUARY 30, 1946, LICENSE NUMBER 0027751 OF 4205 SQUIRE DRIVE, BETTENDORF, IA, WAS DISCIPLINED BY IOWA ON FEBRUARY 4, 1992
DISCIPLINARY ACTION: 60-MONTH PROBATION
OFFENSE: SUBSTANCE ABUSE

NOTES: ALLEGATIONS OF EXCESSIVE USE OF ALCOHOL.

POLLNOW, ROBERT EDWARD MD, DATE OF BIRTH JANUARY 30, 1946, LICENSE NUMBER 0018141, WAS DISCIPLINED BY OKLAHOMA ON JUNE 26, 1992
DISCIPLINARY ACTION: 60-MONTH PROBATION; RESTRICTION PLACED ON LICENSE
OFFENSE: SUBSTANCE ABUSE

NOTES: EVIDENCE INDICATED THAT HE PREVIOUSLY MISUSED ALCOHOL; HAS COMPLETED APPROPRIATE SUBSTANCE ABUSE TREATMENT; PRESENTLY IN RECOVERY. LICENSE GRANTED UNDER PROBATIONARY TERMS AND CONDITIONS: SHALL NOT PRESCRIBE, ADMINISTER OR DISPENSE ANY MEDICATIONS FOR HIS PERSONAL USE; SHALL TAKE NO MEDICATION UNLESS PRESCRIBED BY TREATING PHYSICIAN; SHALL ABSTAIN FROM ALCOHOL OR ANY SUBSTANCE WHICH WOULD ADVERSELY AFFECT HIS ABILITY TO PRACTICE; SHALL SUBMIT BIOLOGICAL FLUID SPECIMENS FOR ANALYSIS; SHALL MAINTAIN FORMAL RELATIONSHIP WITH PHYSICIAN RECOVERY COMMITTEE AND PARTICIPATE IN THEIR MEETINGS AND ACTIVITIES; SHALL NOT SUPERVISE A PHYSICIAN ASSISTANT; SHALL FURNISH BOARD WITH ADDRESS AND/OR CHANGE OF ADDRESS; SHALL APPEAR BEFORE BOARD UPON REQUEST; SHALL NOTIFY ANY HOSPITAL WHERE HE HOLDS STAFF PRIVILEGES OR CLINIC OR GROUP OF THE TERMS AND CONDITIONS. ON 8/9/96 HIS REQUEST FOR EARLY TERMINATION OF PROBATION DENIED.

POLLNOW, ROBERT EDWARD MD, DATE OF BIRTH JANUARY 30, 1946, LICENSE NUMBER 00E2321 OF 4205 SQUIRE DRIVE, BETTENDORF, IA, WAS DISCIPLINED BY TEXAS ON APRIL 30, 1993
DISCIPLINARY ACTION: 60-MONTH PROBATION; MONITORING OF PHYSICIAN PERFORMANCE
OFFENSE: DISCIPLINARY ACTION BY ANOTHER STATE OR AGENCY

NOTES: ON 1/23/92 PLACED ON PROBATION WITH CONDITIONS BY IOWA BOARD DUE TO ALCOHOL ABUSE; ON 7/2/92 HE WAS GRANTED LICENSURE BY OKLAHOMA ON PROBATION WITH CONDITIONS. FIVE YEAR SUSPENSION STAYED. CONDITIONS OF PROBATION: PRIOR TO PRACTICING IN TEXAS SHALL APPEAR BEFORE THE BOARD; SHALL PROVIDE THE TEXAS BOARD COPIES OF REPORTS SUBMITTED TO IOWA AND OKLAHOMA UPON REQUEST; SHALL PARTICIPATE IN ACTIVITIES OF A PHYSICIAN HEALTH AND REHABILITATION COMMITTEE AND ATTEND WEEKLY MEETINGS WITH QUARTERLY REPORTS; SHALL PARTICIPATE IN AA OR ANY SUBSTANTIALLY SIMILAR PROGRAM NOT LESS THAN TWICE A WEEK WITH QUARTERLY REPORTS TO THE BOARD; SHALL SUBMIT HIMSELF FOR APPROPRIATE EXAMS INCLUDING DRUG OR ALCOHOL SCREENS; SHALL SUBMIT HIMSELF FOR EVALUATION AND TREATMENT TO A BOARD-APPROVED PSYCHIATRIST; SHALL ABSTAIN FROM THE CONSUMPTION OF ALCOHOL/CHEMICAL SUBSTANCES IN ANY FORM; SHALL NOT TREAT OR OTHERWISE SERVE AS THE PHYSICIAN, PRESCRIBE, DISPENSE OR ADMINISTER DRUGS THAT MAY BE SUBJECT TO ABUSE FOR HIMSELF OR ANY MEMBER OF HIS FAMILY; SHALL FURNISH WRITTEN REPORTS TO THE BOARD REGARDING HIS MEDICAL CONDITION UPON REQUEST; SHALL GIVE A COPY OF THIS ORDER TO ANY HEALTH CARE ENTITY WHERE HE HAS PRIVILEGES; SHALL COOPERATE WITH THE BOARD IN VERIFYING COMPLIANCE; SHALL INFORM BOARD OF CHANGE OF ADDRESS WITHIN 10 DAYS OR IF HE LEAVES THE STATE; TIME SPENT OUT OF TEXAS DOES NOT COUNT TOWARD PROBATION. SHALL NOT SEEK MODIFICATION FOR ONE YEAR.

POLLNOW, ROBERT EDWARD MD, DATE OF BIRTH JANUARY 30, 1946, LICENSE NUMBER 0018141, WAS DISCIPLINED BY OKLAHOMA ON NOVEMBER 19, 1994
OFFENSE: FAILURE TO COMPLY WITH PREVIOUS BOARD ORDER

NOTES: CURRENTLY ON LEVEL II PROBATION WHICH REQUIRES HIM TO SUBMIT MONTHLY COMPLIANCE REPORTS ON A TIMELY BASIS; HAS FAILED TO SUBMIT REPORTS ON A TIMELY BASIS. LICENSE PLACED ON LEVEL I PROBATION AND SHALL BE REVIEWED IN SIX MONTHS.

POMONIS, NICK S DO, DATE OF BIRTH SEPTEMBER 17, 1956 OF 1610 BROWNING, ORANGE, TX, WAS DISCIPLINED BY MEDICARE ON FEBRUARY 8, 1995
DISCIPLINARY ACTION: EXCLUSION FROM THE MEDICARE AND/OR MEDICAID PROGRAM

OFFENSE: CRIMINAL CONVICTION OR PLEA OF GUILTY, NOLO CONTENDERE, OR NO CONTEST TO A CRIME

NOTES: PROGRAM-RELATED CONVICTION.

PORRES, RAFAEL MD, LICENSE NUMBER E4046 OF EL PASO, TX, WAS DISCIPLINED BY TEXAS ON MAY 16, 1998
DISCIPLINARY ACTION: 36-MONTH PROBATION; RESTRICTION PLACED ON LICENSE
OFFENSE: NONCOMPLIANCE WITH A PROFESSIONAL RULE

NOTES: THE BOARD REVIEWED 10 PATIENT RECORDS INVOLVING CALDWELL-LUC PROCEDURES AND FOUND: LIMITED HISTORIES OF PATIENTS' PROBLEMS WERE DOCUMENTED; PHYSICAL EXAM RECORDS OMITTED REFERENCES TO SALIENT SYMPTOMATOLOGY; OVERALL, DOCUMENTATION OF ONLY ONE PATIENT FULFILLED MINIMAL CRITERIA FOR SURGICAL TREATMENT FOR CHRONIC SINUSITIS; ALL PATIENTS EXCEPT ONE WERE REPORTED TO HAVE NASAL OBSTRUCTION AT THE INITIAL OFFICE VISIT, BUT NONE HAD DESCRIPTIONS OF THEIR TURBINATE CONGESTION, ALLERGIC SYMPTOMS, PAST OR PROPOSED ALLERGIC WORKUP; HE DID NOT PROPERLY CHART THE PRIOR HISTORIES, SYMPTOMS AND RADIOGRAPHIC FINDINGS; HE NO LONGER PERFORMS CALDWELL-LUC PROCEDURES AND REFERS THE ELIGIBLE PATIENTS FOR ENDOSCOPIC PROCEDURES. CONDITIONS OF PROBATION: SHALL OBTAIN 50 HOURS PER YEAR OF CONTINUING MEDICAL EDUCATION; SHALL MAINTAIN ADEQUATE MEDICAL RECORDS WHICH SHALL BE AVAILABLE FOR REVIEW; SHALL OBTAIN 10 HOURS OF AN ETHICS COURSE PER YEAR; PRIOR TO PERFORMING ANY SURGERY IN A HOSPITAL SETTING, SHALL OBTAIN A WRITTEN CONSULTATION FROM A LICENSED TEXAS PHYSICIAN; SHALL APPEAR BEFORE THE BOARD AT LEAST ONCE A YEAR; SHALL COOPERATE WITH THE BOARD IN VERIFYING COMPLIANCE; SHALL GIVE A COPY OF THIS ORDER TO ANY HEALTH CARE ENTITY WHERE HE HAS PRIVILEGES; TIME SPENT OUT OF TEXAS DOES NOT COUNT TOWARD PROBATION; SHALL INFORM THE BOARD OF CHANGE OF ADDRESS WITHIN 10 DAYS OR IF HE LEAVES THE STATE; SHALL NOT SEEK MODIFICATION FOR ONE YEAR.

PORTOCARRERO, MARIO JOSE MD, LICENSE NUMBER 00J9277, WAS DISCIPLINED BY TEXAS ON AUGUST 19, 1995
DISCIPLINARY ACTION: RESTRICTION PLACED ON LICENSE; MONITORING OF PHYSICIAN PERFORMANCE
OFFENSE: PHYSICAL OR MENTAL ILLNESS INHIBITING THE ABILITY TO PRACTICE WITH SKILL AND SAFETY

NOTES: HAD ATTENTION DEFICIT DISORDER AND WAS MEDICATED FOR IT DURING HIS FIRST YEAR OF RESIDENCY IN 1991 AND 1992 WHICH CAUSED PROBLEMS IN HIS FOCUSING ON MEDICAL PROBLEMS; WAS ON PROBATIONARY STATUS WITH THE PROGRAM IN 10-11/94; AFTER PROBATION REMAINED WITH THE PROGRAM IN GOOD STANDING. MUST PRACTICE UNDER THE FOLLOWING TERMS AND CONDITIONS FOR FIVE YEARS: SHALL SUBMIT HIMSELF FOR EVALUATION AND TREATMENT BY A BOARD-APPROVED PSYCHIATRIST AT LEAST MONTHLY WHO SHALL SUBMIT REPORTS; SHALL PROVIDE BOARD WITH WRITTEN REPORTS REGARDING ANY ASPECT OF HIS PHYSICAL OR MENTAL CONDITION WHEN REQUESTED; SHALL COMPLY WITH CONDITIONS REQUIRED FOR HOSPITAL PRIVILEGES; SHALL ONLY TREAT PATIENTS IN A GROUP/CLINIC SETTING AND SHALL ONLY ADMIT TO THE HOSPITAL ROUTINE PEDIATRIC PATIENTS OVER TWO YEARS OF AGE; SHALL NOT TREAT PATIENTS IN ANY INTENSIVE CARE-TYPE SETTING; PRACTICE SHALL BE MONITORED BY A LICENSED PHYSICIAN APPROVED BY THE BOARD WHO SHALL COUNSEL HIM ON ANY PERCEIVED DEFICIENCIES AND SUBMIT QUARTERLY REPORTS; SHALL PROVIDE A COPY OF THIS ORDER TO ANYONE REQUESTING IT WITHIN 10 DAYS; SHALL INFORM THE BOARD OF CHANGE OF ADDRESS WITHIN 10 DAYS OR IF HE LEAVES THE STATE; SHALL APPEAR BEFORE THE BOARD ONCE A YEAR; TIME SPENT OUT OF TEXAS DOES NOT COUNT TOWARD CONDITIONS; SHALL NOT SEEK MODIFICATION FOR ONE YEAR. ON 10/5/96 REQUEST FOR TERMINATION OF ORDER DENIED BUT ORDER MODIFIED AS FOLLOWS: ONLY REQUIRES FOLLOW-UP CARE AT LEAST ONCE EVERY THREE MONTHS CONCERNING PSYCHIATRIST CARE AND TREATMENT. ON 9/20/97 THE BOARD GRANTED HIS PETITION FOR TERMINATION OF THIS ORDER BASED ON COMPLIANCE WITH CONDITIONS.

PORTOCARRERO, MARIO JOSE MD, LICENSE NUMBER A54678 OF HOUSTON, TX, WAS DISCIPLINED BY CALIFORNIA ON JUNE 15, 1997
DISCIPLINARY ACTION: SURRENDER OF LICENSE

NOTES: WHILE CHARGES PENDING.

PRANGLE, ROBERT E DO, DATE OF BIRTH JANUARY 30, 1944, LICENSE NUMBER 00D9870 OF 13310 BEAMER #G, HOUSTON, TX, WAS DISCIPLINED BY TEXAS ON JANUARY 29, 1993
DISCIPLINARY ACTION: REPRIMAND
OFFENSE: OVERPRESCRIBING OR MISPRESCRIBING DRUGS

NOTES: NONTHERAPEUTICALLY PRESCRIBED EXCESSIVE AMOUNTS OF VICODIN AND FIORINAL TO A PATIENT WHEN HE KNEW SHE WAS HABITUATED TO THE MEDICATIONS AND FAILED TO KEEP ADEQUATE MEDICAL RECORDS FOR THIS PATIENT. SHALL GIVE A COPY OF THIS ORDER TO ANY HEALTH CARE ENTITY WHERE HE HAS PRIVILEGES; SHALL INFORM BOARD OF CHANGE OF ADDRESS WITHIN 10 DAYS.

PRATER, WILLIAM WARREN MD, LICENSE NUMBER 00F4390 OF PLANO, TX, WAS DISCIPLINED BY TEXAS ON AUGUST 19, 1994
DISCIPLINARY ACTION: EMERGENCY SUSPENSION
OFFENSE: SUBSTANCE ABUSE

NOTES: AVAILABLE EVIDENCE AND INFORMATION INDICATES: THAT HE IS CHEMICALLY DEPENDENT AND EXHIBITING BEHAVIOR WHICH CAUSES HIS CONTINUED PRACTICE TO CONSTITUTE A THREAT TO THE PUBLIC WELFARE; HAS ENGAGED IN THE USE OF VARIOUS MEDICATIONS INCLUDING NARCOTIC ANALGESICS, A STIMULANT, AN ANTIDEPRESSANT AND A BENZODIAZEPINE WITHOUT ANY LEGITIMATE MEDICAL OR THERAPEUTIC PURPOSE; HAS ENGAGED IN THE ILLEGAL USE OF VARIOUS STREET DRUGS INCLUDING COCAINE, MARIJUANA AND LSD; HAS ABANDONED HIS CARE OF ALL PATIENTS WITHOUT ADEQUATE NOTICE AND IN DOING SO MAY HAVE PUT THEM AT RISK; HAS WRITTEN FALSE OR FICTITIOUS PRESCRIPTIONS FOR DANGEROUS DRUGS IN THE NAMES OF OFFICE STAFF, PATIENTS, FRIENDS AND FAMILY WHICH HE DIVERTED FOR HIS OWN USE; FAILED TO KEEP ACCURATE RECORDS OF PURCHASES AND DISPOSALS OF LARGE QUANTITIES OF MEDICATIONS.

PRATER, WILLIAM WARREN MD OF 1212 COIT ROAD SUITE 109, PLANO, TX, WAS DISCIPLINED BY DEA ON SEPTEMBER 26, 1994
DISCIPLINARY ACTION: SURRENDER OF CONTROLLED SUBSTANCE LICENSE

NOTES: IN LIEU OF PUBLIC INTEREST REVOCATION.

PRATER, WILLIAM WARREN MD, LICENSE NUMBER 00F4390 OF PLANO, TX, WAS DISCIPLINED BY TEXAS ON OCTOBER 13, 1995
DISCIPLINARY ACTION: 2-MONTH LICENSE REVOCATION; LICENSE SUSPENSION
OFFENSE: SUBSTANCE ABUSE

NOTES: SINCE 8/94 EMERGENCY SUSPENSION, HE HAS UNDERGONE INPATIENT TREATMENT FROM 8/14/94 TO 3/2/95; FAVORABLE REPORT REGARDING HIS CURRENT RECOVERY STATUS HAS BEEN RECEIVED BY THE BOARD; REPORTED TO ATTEND AA AT LEAST FOUR TIMES A WEEK AND PHYSICIAN'S RECOVERY GROUP MEETINGS; HE REPORTS A SOBRIETY DATE OF 8/14/94; HAS ENTERED INTO A RECOVERY CONTRACT WITH PHYSICIAN'S REHABILITATION COMMITTEE AND IS BEING MONITORED AS PART OF CONTRACT; HAS SUBMITTED TO WEEKLY RANDOM DRUG SCREENS WHICH HAVE BEEN NEGATIVE. REINSTATEMENT OF LICENSE TO SUSPENSION FOLLOWING REVOCATION; SHALL NOT PRACTICE MEDICINE IN TEXAS UNTIL HE REQUESTS TO HAVE SUSPENSION STAYED OR LIFTED AND APPEARS BEFORE BOARD WITH EVIDENCE WHICH ADEQUATELY INDICATES THAT HE IS PHYSICALLY, MENTALLY OR OTHERWISE COMPETENT TO SAFELY PRACTICE MEDICINE INCLUDING AT A MINIMUM PROVIDING COPIES OF MEDICAL RECORDS AND REPORTS OF PSYCHOLOGICAL AND NEUROPSYCHIATRIC EVALUATIONS CONDUCTED BY A BOARD-APPROVED PSYCHIATRIST. ON 8/17/96 LICENSE PLACED ON PROBATION FOR 10 YEARS UNDER TERMS AND CONDITIONS. ON 1/29/99 PETITION FOR MODIFICATION OF ORDER GRANTED ALLOWING HIM TO REAPPLY FOR CONTROLLED SUBSTANCE REGISTRATION TO BE USED FOR INPATIENT TREATMENT ONLY; SHALL MAINTAIN A LOGBOOK OF ALL CONTROLLED SUBSTANCES PRESCRIBED WHICH SHALL BE MADE AVAILABLE FOR REVIEW BY THE BOARD.

PRATUMRAT, PAIROJ MD, LICENSE NUMBER G8748 OF GREENVILLE, TX, WAS DISCIPLINED BY TEXAS ON AUGUST 27, 1999
DISCIPLINARY ACTION: REPRIMAND

NOTES: PRACTICE INCONSISTENT WITH PUBLIC HEALTH AND WELFARE. ACTION WILL NOT BE FINAL UNTIL ALL APPEALS ARE EXHAUSTED.

PRICE, STEVEN L MD, LICENSE NUMBER E6571 OF HOUSTON, TX, WAS DISCIPLINED BY TEXAS ON SEPTEMBER 20, 1997
DISCIPLINARY ACTION: FINE; REPRIMAND
OFFENSE: PROFESSIONAL MISCONDUCT

NOTES: DURING 1994 HE PROVIDED TREATMENT IN THE NATURE OF PHYSICAL MODALITIES TO A PATIENT WITHOUT ADEQUATE MEDICAL NECESSITY; NO EVIDENCE OF HARM TO THE PATIENT HAS BEEN PROVIDED OR REPORTED TO THE BOARD. $1,000 FINE; SHALL COOPERATE WITH THE BOARD IN VERIFYING COMPLIANCE.

PRUETT, CHESTER E MD, LICENSE NUMBER G1752 OF SAN ANTONIO, TX, WAS DISCIPLINED BY TEXAS ON FEBRUARY 7, 1998
DISCIPLINARY ACTION: REQUIRED TO TAKE ADDITIONAL MEDICAL EDUCATION
OFFENSE: SEXUAL ABUSE OF OR SEXUAL MISCONDUCT WITH A PATIENT

NOTES: FROM APPROXIMATELY 5/12/96 TO 10/13/96, HE ENGAGED IN A ROMANTIC, SEXUAL RELATIONSHIP WITH A PATIENT. LICENSE LIMITED FOR THREE YEARS AS FOLLOWS: SHALL OBTAIN 50 HOURS PER YEAR OF CONTINUING MEDICAL EDUCATION; SHALL OBTAIN 15 HOURS OF AN ETHICS COURSE PER YEAR FOR 3 YEARS; WITHIN 1 YEAR SHALL TAKE AND PASS THE JURISPRUDENCE EXAM; SHALL APPEAR BEFORE THE BOARD ONCE A YEAR; SHALL COOPERATE WITH THE BOARD IN VERIFYING COMPLIANCE; SHALL GIVE A COPY OF THIS ORDER TO ANY HEALTH CARE ENTITY WHERE HE HAS PRIVILEGES; TIME SPENT OUT OF TEXAS DOES NOT COUNT TOWARD RESTRICTION; SHALL INFORM THE BOARD OF CHANGE OF ADDRESS WITHIN 10 DAYS; SHALL NOT SEEK MODIFICATION FOR ONE YEAR.

PUCEK, MARK DOUGLASS MD, DATE OF BIRTH JANUARY 5, 1956, LICENSE NUMBER 00G3707 OF 1414 S LOOP WEST #200, HOUSTON, TX, WAS DISCIPLINED BY TEXAS ON AUGUST 20, 1993
DISCIPLINARY ACTION: 60-MONTH PROBATION; RESTRICTION PLACED ON LICENSE
OFFENSE: PROFESSIONAL MISCONDUCT

NOTES: IN 1990 ENTERED INTO A VERBAL CONTRACT WITH GALLERIA DIAGNOSTIC SERVICES TO EVALUATE PERSONAL INJURY PATIENTS; HE BILLED THEM FOR SERVICES RENDERED; THEY THEN BILLED INSURANCE COMPANIES FOR PATIENT TREATMENT FOR SOME SERVICES USING HIS NAME; HE SAID HE DID NOT KNOW THEY HAD DONE THIS; TWO PATIENTS WERE GIVEN EXCESSIVE TREATMENT WITHOUT PHYSICIANS ORDERS AND BILLING WAS ALSO EXCESSIVE. FIVE YEAR SUSPENSION STAYED. CONDITIONS OF PROBATION: SHALL APPEAR BEFORE THE BOARD TWICE A YEAR; SHALL ATTEND SIX HOURS OF AN ETHICS COURSE PER YEAR FOR TWO YEARS; SHALL UTILIZE AN ACCURATE SYSTEM OF PATIENT RECORDKEEPING; SHALL NOT ACCEPT EMPLOYMENT OR ENTER INTO CONTRACTUAL RELATIONSHIPS WHEREIN HE WOULD BE COMPENSATED TO DIAGNOSE AND/OR TREAT PATIENTS BY A LAYPERSON, CORPORATION, OR OTHER ENTITY NOT COMPRISED EXCLUSIVELY OF TEXAS LICENSED PHYSICIANS AND WHEREIN THE PERSON OR ENTITY WOULD RECEIVE AND RETAIN THE FEES PAID BY OR ON BEHALF OF PATIENTS FOR THE PHYSICIAN'S PROFESSIONAL SERVICES; SHALL GIVE A COPY OF THIS ORDER TO ALL HEALTH CARE ENTITIES WHERE HE HAS PRIVILEGES; SHALL COOPERATE WITH THE BOARD IN VERIFYING COMPLIANCE; SHALL INFORM BOARD OF CHANGE OF ADDRESS WITHIN 10 DAYS OR IF HE LEAVES THE STATE; TIME SPENT OUT OF TEXAS DOES NOT COUNT TOWARD PROBATION. SHALL NOT SEEK MODIFICATION FOR ONE YEAR. ON 10/5/96 PROBATION TERMINATED.

PUGH, MARION MD, LICENSE NUMBER 0021586 OF DALLAS, TX, WAS DISCIPLINED BY COLORADO ON OCTOBER 10, 1990
DISCIPLINARY ACTION: SURRENDER OF LICENSE
OFFENSE: SUBSTANCE ABUSE

NOTES: HABITUAL INTEMPERANCE AND EXCESSIVE USE OF ALCOHOLIC BEVERAGES.

PUGH, MARION MD OF 1204A LAKEWAY DRIVE, LAKEWAY, TX, WAS DISCIPLINED BY DEA ON DECEMBER 16, 1999
DISCIPLINARY ACTION: SURRENDER OF CONTROLLED SUBSTANCE LICENSE

NOTES: IN LIEU OF PUBLIC INTEREST REVOCATION.

PUGH, MARION MD OF 9522 B WOODVALE, AUSTIN, TX, WAS DISCIPLINED BY DEA ON DECEMBER 16, 1999
DISCIPLINARY ACTION: SURRENDER OF CONTROLLED SUBSTANCE LICENSE

NOTES: IN LIEU OF PUBLIC INTEREST REVOCATION.

PUGH, MARION C JR MD, LICENSE NUMBER 00D5159 OF AUSTIN, TX, WAS DISCIPLINED BY TEXAS ON JANUARY 24, 1992
DISCIPLINARY ACTION: 60-MONTH PROBATION
OFFENSE: SUBSTANCE ABUSE

NOTES: INABILITY TO PRACTICE MEDICINE WITH REASONABLE SKILL AND SAFETY TO PATIENTS. LICENSE SUSPENDED, SUSPENSION STAYED; PROBATION UNDER TERMS AND CONDITIONS.

PULLIAM, ALBERT LEON MD, DATE OF BIRTH DECEMBER 29, 1939, LICENSE NUMBER 00E9340 OF HOUSTON, TX, WAS DISCIPLINED BY TEXAS ON MARCH 31, 1990
DISCIPLINARY ACTION: SURRENDER OF CONTROLLED SUBSTANCE LICENSE; 60-MONTH PROBATION

NOTES: STIPULATED ORDER. REVOCATION STAYED. MUST COMPLETE PRECEPTORSHIP ON PREVENTION AND TREATMENT OF DRUG ABUSE, APPEAR BEFORE BOARD SEMI-ANNUALLY, SURRENDER CONTROLLED SUBSTANCES REGISTRATIONS AND NOT REREGISTER WITHOUT BOARD AUTHORITY, AND COMPLY WITH TERMS OF CRIMINAL PROBATION. ON 4/30/93, MODIFICATION OF ORDER SO THAT HE MAY REAPPLY TO TEXAS DEPARTMENT OF PUBLIC SAFETY AND THE DRUG ENFORCEMENT ADMINISTRATION FOR REINSTATEMENT OF HIS CONTROLLED SUBSTANCE REGISTRATION IN ALL SCHEDULES AND FOR ISSUANCE OF TRIPLICATE PRESCRIPTION FORMS.

PULLIAM, ALBERT LEON MD, DATE OF BIRTH DECEMBER 29, 1939, LICENSE NUMBER 0036501 OF 6711 BELLFORT BOULEVARD #400, HOUSTON, TX, WAS DISCIPLINED BY MICHIGAN ON AUGUST 30, 1993
DISCIPLINARY ACTION: 6-MONTH LICENSE SUSPENSION
OFFENSE: PROFESSIONAL MISCONDUCT

NOTES: DIVERSION OR MISPRESCRIBING OF DRUGS.

PULLIAM, ALBERT LEON MD, DATE OF BIRTH DECEMBER 29, 1939 OF HOUSTON, TX, WAS DISCIPLINED BY DEA ON NOVEMBER 24, 1995
DISCIPLINARY ACTION: DENIAL OF NEW LICENSE
OFFENSE: OVERPRESCRIBING OR MISPRESCRIBING DRUGS

NOTES: ON 4/30/93 HE WAS GRANTED PERMISSION BY TEXAS BOARD TO REAPPLY FOR DEA PRIVILEGES. ON 11/11/93 HE RECEIVED HIS TEXAS CERTIFICATE TO DISPENSE CONTROLLED SUBSTANCES, AND THAT WAS RENEWED ON 3/31/94 FOR AN ADDITIONAL YEAR; IN 1988 HE HAD EXHIBITED AN INABILITY OR UNWILLINGNESS TO PROPERLY HANDLE CONTROLLED SUBSTANCES WHEN HE ISSUED PRESCRIPTIONS TO AN UNDERCOVER AGENT FOR OTHER THAN LEGITIMATE MEDICAL PURPOSES; FALSIFIED THE AGENT'S PATIENT RECORDS TO CONCEAL HIS ILLEGAL ACTIVITIES; RECEIVED A PURPORTEDLY "STOLEN" TELEVISION AND VCR FROM THE UNDERCOVER AGENT IN EXCHANGE FOR $150 AND PRESCRIPTIONS FOR CONTROLLED SUBSTANCES, BUT AT A HEARING IN 10/94 DENIED THIS FACT; HE OFFERED NO EVIDENCE OF REMEDIAL ACTIONS HE HAS TAKEN SINCE HIS 1989 CONVICTION TO REMEDY HIS PROBLEMS, FOR EXAMPLE REQUIRING ADDITIONAL EDUCATION, CONCERNING FALSIFYING PATIENT RECORDS AND FAILING TO CONDUCT MEDICAL EXAMINATIONS PRIOR TO DISPENSING MEDICATION.

PULLIAM, KATHY A MD, DATE OF BIRTH FEBRUARY 10, 1955, LICENSE NUMBER 0012699 OF 48 MEADOWOODS TERRACE, JACKSON, MS, WAS DISCIPLINED BY MISSISSIPPI ON SEPTEMBER 26, 1991
DISCIPLINARY ACTION: RESTRICTION PLACED ON LICENSE
OFFENSE: SUBSTANCE ABUSE

NOTES: RECENTLY SUFFERED A RELAPSE OF HER CHEMICAL DEPENDENCY. CONSENT AGREEMENT PROHIBITS THE PRACTICE OF MEDICINE IN MISSISSIPPI UNTIL SUCH TIME AS CERTAIN REQUIREMENTS ARE MET.

PULLIAM, KATHY A MD, DATE OF BIRTH FEBRUARY 10, 1955, LICENSE NUMBER 0012699 OF 48 MEADOWOODS TERRACE, JACKSON, MS, WAS DISCIPLINED BY MISSISSIPPI ON MARCH 19, 1992
DISCIPLINARY ACTION: RESTRICTION PLACED ON LICENSE; RESTRICTION PLACED ON CONTROLLED SUBSTANCE LICENSE

NOTES: PERMISSION TO RE-ENTER THE PRACTICE OF MEDICINE IN MISSISSIPPI SUBJECT TO TERMS AND CONDITIONS: PRACTICE LIMITED TO MISSISSIPPI STATE DEPARTMENT OF HEALTH; NO DRUG ENFORCEMENT ADMINISTRATION CERTIFICATE; PROHIBITED FROM ORDERING, MANUFACTURING, DISTRIBUTING, POSSESSING, DISPENSING, ADMINISTERING OR PRESCRIBING STADOL AND NUBAIN, OR THEIR GENERICS.

PULLIAM, KATHY A MD, LICENSE NUMBER 00F9982 OF JACKSON, MS, WAS DISCIPLINED BY TEXAS ON JUNE 17, 1992
DISCIPLINARY ACTION: 120-MONTH PROBATION
OFFENSE: SUBSTANCE ABUSE

NOTES: INABILITY TO PRACTICE MEDICINE WITH REASONABLE SKILL AND SAFETY TO PATIENTS BY REASON OF USE OF DRUGS. SUSPENSION STAYED.

PULLIAM, KATHY A MD, DATE OF BIRTH FEBRUARY 10, 1955, LICENSE NUMBER 0012699 OF 5613 BOGGS DRIVE, STONE MOUNTAIN, GA, WAS DISCIPLINED BY MISSISSIPPI ON JULY 16, 1992
DISCIPLINARY ACTION: LICENSE SUSPENSION
OFFENSE: FAILURE TO COMPLY WITH PREVIOUS BOARD ORDER

NOTES: SUFFERED RELAPSE OF HER CHEMICAL DEPENDENCY IN VIOLATION OF THE MARCH 19, 1992 BOARD ORDER. BOARD RATIFIED THE ORDER OF IMMEDIATE SUSPENSION OF HER MEDICAL LICENSE DATED JUNE 2, 1992, THE EFFECTIVE DATE OF THIS ORDER. ON 1/20/94 HER REQUEST FOR REINSTATEMENT WAS DENIED. AFTER ONE YEAR SHE MAY PETITION THE BOARD FOR RECONSIDERATION. ON 9/19/96 HER REQUEST FOR REINSTATEMENT WAS DENIED. ON 7/15/99 ORDER TERMINATED; UNRESTRICTED LICENSE; HOWEVER, IF SHE CHOOSES TO PRACTICE IN THE STATE, SHE SHALL ADVISE THE BOARD PRIOR TO INITIATION OF PRACTICE.

PULLIAM, KATHY A MD, LICENSE NUMBER 00F9982 OF JACKSON, MS, WAS DISCIPLINED BY TEXAS ON OCTOBER 9, 1992
DISCIPLINARY ACTION: 24-MONTH LICENSE SUSPENSION
OFFENSE: FAILURE TO COMPLY WITH PREVIOUS BOARD ORDER

NOTES: VIOLATED PREVIOUS ORDER OF 06/17/92.

PULLIAM, KATHY A MD, LICENSE NUMBER 00F9982, WAS DISCIPLINED BY TEXAS ON OCTOBER 13, 1995
DISCIPLINARY ACTION: 120-MONTH PROBATION; 120-MONTH RESTRICTION PLACED ON CONTROLLED SUBSTANCE LICENSE
OFFENSE: SUBSTANCE ABUSE

NOTES: IN 10/92 SHE ENTERED INTO A 20 MONTH AFTERCARE CONTRACT WITH METROPOLITAN ATLANTA RECOVERY RESIDENCIES AND ENTERED INTO AN EXTENDED AFTERCARE CONTRACT IN 6/94; IN 9/94 ENROLLED IN A PHYSICIAN'S WELL-BEING PROGRAM; HAS SATISFIED THE MINIMUM REQUIREMENTS OF 6/92 ORDER AS A PREREQUISITE FOR STAYING THE 10/92

SUSPENSION. SUSPENSION STAYED. PROBATION WITH TERMS: SHALL ABSTAIN FROM THE CONSUMPTION OF ALCOHOL/DRUGS IN ANY FORM UNLESS PRESCRIBED BY ANOTHER PHYSICIAN FOR A LEGITIMATE AND THERAPEUTIC PURPOSE; SHALL SUBMIT HERSELF FOR APPROPRIATE EXAMS INCLUDING DRUG OR ALCOHOL SCREENS; SHALL SUBMIT HERSELF FOR EVALUATION AND TREATMENT BY A BOARD-APPROVED PSYCHIATRIST WHOM SHE SHALL SEE FOR FOLLOW-UP CARE AND COUNSELING AT LEAST ONCE A MONTH AND WHO SHALL SUBMIT REPORTS TO THE BOARD; SHALL PARTICIPATE IN AA'S PROGRAM AT LEAST THREE TIMES A WEEK WITH QUARTERLY REPORTS TO THE BOARD; SHALL PARTICIPATE IN THE ACTIVITIES OF AN IMPAIRED PHYSICIAN'S GROUP AND ATTEND WEEKLY MEETINGS WITH QUARTERLY REPORTS; SHALL COMPLY WITH THE TERMS OF ANY CONTINUING CARE CONTRACT SHE ENTERS INTO AND SUBMIT QUARTERLY REPORTS TO THE BOARD; SHALL NOT POSSESS ALCOHOL, CONTROLLED SUBSTANCES OR DANGEROUS DRUGS WITH ADDICTIVE POTENTIAL OR POTENTIAL FOR ABUSE; SHALL SURRENDER ANY SUCH DRUGS IN HER POSSESSION; SHALL NOT TREAT OR OTHERWISE SERVE AS PHYSICIAN, PRESCRIBE, DISPENSE OR ADMINISTER DANGEROUS DRUGS THAT MAY BE SUBJECT TO ABUSE TO HERSELF OR ANY MEMBER OF HER FAMILY; SHALL NOT TELEPHONE TO A PHARMACY A PRESCRIPTION OR REFILL FOR THESE DRUGS AND SHALL NOT PERMIT ANYONE UNDER HER SUPERVISION TO DO SO; SHALL SURRENDER HER DEA AND DPS CONTROLLED SUBSTANCES REGISTRATION CERTIFICATE; SHALL SURRENDER ALL UNUSED TRIPLICATE PRESCRIPTION FORMS AND SHALL NOT ATTEMPT TO ORDER MORE; SHALL MAINTAIN A FILE WITH COPIES OF EVERY PRESCRIPTION WRITTEN BY HER FOR DANGEROUS DRUGS WITH ADDICTIVE POTENTIAL OR POTENTIAL FOR ABUSE THAT SHALL BE AVAILABLE FOR REVIEW; HER PRACTICE SHALL BE MONITORED BY A BOARD-APPROVED TEXAS PHYSICIAN WHO SHALL SUBMIT QUARTERLY REPORTS TO THE BOARD; SHALL MAINTAIN ADEQUATE MEDICAL RECORDS THAT SHALL BE AVAILABLE FOR REVIEW; SHALL OBTAIN AT LEAST 50 HOURS PER YEAR OF CONTINUING MEDICAL EDUCATION; SHALL APPEAR BEFORE BOARD AT LEAST TWICE A YEAR; SHALL COOPERATE WITH BOARD IN VERIFYING COMPLIANCE INCLUDING PROVIDING COPIES OF MEDICAL RELEASES UPON REQUEST; SHALL GIVE A COPY OF THIS ORDER TO ANY HEALTH CARE ENTITY WHERE SHE HAS PRIVILEGES; SHALL PROVIDE A COPY OF THIS ORDER TO ANYONE REQUESTING IT WITHIN 10 DAYS; TIME PERIOD OUT OF TEXAS DOES NOT COUNT TOWARD PROBATION; SHALL INFORM THE BOARD OF CHANGE OF ADDRESS WITHIN 10 DAYS OR IF SHE LEAVES THE STATE. SHALL NOT SEEK MODIFICATION FOR ONE YEAR. ON 5/10/97 PETITION FOR MODIFICATION OF ORDER GRANTED ALLOWING HER TO REAPPLY FOR SCHEDULES IV AND V, UPON PASSAGE OF AN EXAM FOR RECERTIFICATION IN PEDIATRICS; HER USE OF SCHEDULES IV AND V SHALL BE LIMITED TO PATIENTS IN INSTITUTIONAL OR HOSPITAL SETTINGS.

PULLIAM, KATHY ANN MD, LICENSE NUMBER 0010342 OF GA, WAS DISCIPLINED BY ALABAMA ON MARCH 2, 1993
DISCIPLINARY ACTION: LICENSE REVOCATION
OFFENSE: DISCIPLINARY ACTION BY ANOTHER STATE OR AGENCY

NOTES: UNABLE TO PRACTICE MEDICINE WITH REASONABLE SKILL AND SAFETY DUE TO EXCESSIVE USE OF DRUGS; MISSISSIPPI LICENSE HAD BEEN SUSPENDED DUE TO A VIOLATION OF A PREVIOUS CONSENT AGREEMENT.

PULLIAM, KATHY ANN MD OF STONE MOUNTAIN, GA, WAS DISCIPLINED BY LOUISIANA ON MARCH 22, 1993
DISCIPLINARY ACTION: LICENSE SUSPENSION
OFFENSE: DISCIPLINARY ACTION BY ANOTHER STATE OR AGENCY

NOTES: ACTION TAKEN BY BOTH MISSISSIPPI AND TEXAS; HABITUAL AND RECURRING ABUSE OF DRUGS, INCLUDING ALCOHOL; PROVIDING FALSE SWORN INFORMATION TO THE BOARD.

PULLIAM, KATHY ANN MD, LICENSE NUMBER 10342, WAS DISCIPLINED BY ALABAMA ON JUNE 4, 1997
DISCIPLINARY ACTION: DENIAL OF LICENSE REINSTATEMENT

QUENNEVILLE, KENNETH BRUCE MD, DATE OF BIRTH JANUARY 26, 1954, LICENSE NUMBER 00H1404 OF MIDLAND, TX, WAS DISCIPLINED BY TEXAS ON FEBRUARY 16, 1990
DISCIPLINARY ACTION: SURRENDER OF CONTROLLED SUBSTANCE LICENSE; EMERGENCY SUSPENSION
OFFENSE: SUBSTANCE ABUSE

NOTES: STIPULATED ORDER. LICENSE SUSPENDED UNTIL PSYCHIATRIST FINDS PHYSICIAN CAPABLE OF PRACTICING MEDICINE WITH REASONABLE SAFETY TO SELF AND PATIENTS. MUST PASS SPECIAL PURPOSE EXAMINATION. WHEN CONDITIONS SATISFIED, SUSPENSION TERMINATED AND LICENSE PROBATED WITH FOLLOWING TERMS: MUST SURRENDER CONTROLLED SUBSTANCES REGISTRATIONS AND NOT REREGISTER WITHOUT BOARD AUTHORITY, SURRENDER TRIPLICATE PRESCRIPTION FORMS AND NOT ORDER MORE UNTIL BOARD AUTHORIZES,
PARTICIPATE IN AA OR NARCOTICS ANONYMOUS, REPORT ANY INCIDENT IN WHICH HE PARTAKES OF ALCOHOL OR USES CONTROLLED SUBSTANCES NOT PRESCRIBED BY ANOTHER PHYSICIAN FOR LEGITIMATE, THERAPEUTIC CONDITION, AND SUBMIT FOR EXAMINATIONS TO DETERMINE FREEDOM FROM DRUGS AND ALCOHOL.

QUENNEVILLE, KENNETH BRUCE MD, DATE OF BIRTH JANUARY 26, 1954 OF 2300 WEST MICHIGAN AVENUE, MIDLAND, TX, WAS DISCIPLINED BY DEA ON SEPTEMBER 24, 1990
DISCIPLINARY ACTION: SURRENDER OF CONTROLLED SUBSTANCE LICENSE
OFFENSE: PRACTICING WITHOUT A VALID CONTROLLED SUBSTANCE LICENSE

NOTES: DISPENSING CONTROLLED DRUGS WITHOUT DEA REGISTRATION; SURRENDERED DEA REGISTRATION UPON ORDER FROM STATE OF TX; MEDICAL LICENSE SUSPENDED 02/16/90 FOR INTEMPERATE USE OF ALCOHOL AND DANGEROUS DRUGS. LICENSE REINSTATED 06/11/90 AND PLACED ON FIVE YEARS PROBATION.

QUENNEVILLE, KENNETH BRUCE MD, DATE OF BIRTH JANUARY 26, 1954, LICENSE NUMBER 00H1404 OF 411 S ORIENT STREET, STAMFORD, TX, WAS DISCIPLINED BY TEXAS ON JUNE 28, 1991
DISCIPLINARY ACTION: 60-MONTH PROBATION; REQUIRED TO TAKE ADDITIONAL MEDICAL EDUCATION

NOTES: TERMS OF PROBATION: SHALL CONTINUE TREATMENT FROM PHYSICIAN APPROVED BY BOARD; SHALL ATTEND AT LEAST 50 HOURS PER YEAR OF CONTINUING MEDICAL EDUCATION; SHALL APPEAR BEFORE THE BOARD ONCE A YEAR; SHALL PARTICIPATE FOUR TIMES A WEEK IN A 12-STEP PROGRAM OF AA OR NARCOTICS ANONYMOUS; SHALL IMMEDIATELY REPORT TO THE BOARD ANY USE OF

ALCOHOL OR CONTROLLED SUBSTANCE NOT PRESCRIBED BY ANOTHER PHYSICIAN FOR A LEGITIMATE AND THERAPEUTIC CONDITION; SHALL SUBMIT TO DRUG OR ALCOHOL SCREENS. PROBATION MODIFIED EFFECTIVE 4/11/92. PROBATION MODIFIED EFFECTIVE 8/20/92. ON 8/20/93 ORDER TERMINATED AND LICENSE FREE AND CLEAR OF ANY PREVIOUS RESTRICTIONS.

QUENNEVILLE, KENNETH BRUCE MD, LICENSE NUMBER H1404 OF EAGLE LAKE, TX, WAS DISCIPLINED BY TEXAS ON APRIL 4, 1998
DISCIPLINARY ACTION: 60-MONTH PROBATION; REQUIRED TO TAKE ADDITIONAL MEDICAL EDUCATION
OFFENSE: SUBSTANCE ABUSE

NOTES: ON 3/21/97 HE SELF-REPORTED HIS MOST RECENT RELAPSE INTO SUBSTANCE ABUSE INVOLVING HIS ABUSE OF XANAX BETWEEN 3/5/97-3/7/97; HE HAS A HISTORY OF SUBSTANCE ABUSE AND TREATMENT DATING BACK TO 1989 WHICH RESULTED IN SUSPENSION OF HIS TEXAS LICENSE ON 2/16/90 AND THE SUBSEQUENT REINSTATEMENT OF HIS LICENSE THROUGH A PROBATIONARY ORDER ENTERED BY THE BOARD ON 6/11/91; HIS HISTORY OF SUBSTANCE ABUSE INCLUDES THE INTEMPERATE USE OF ALCOHOL AND CONTROLLED SUBSTANCES, INCLUDING BENZODIAZEPINES AND COCAINE, AND HE HAS MULTIPLE ARRESTS FOR DRIVING WHILE INTOXICATED; AFTER TERMINATION OF THE PROBATIONARY ORDER IN 1993, HE RESUMED THE PERIODIC CONSUMPTION OF ALCOHOL WHICH LED TO FURTHER ABUSE OF CONTROLLED SUBSTANCES; SINCE RELAPSING AND SELF-REPORTING HIS DRUG CONSUMPTION TO THE BOARD, HE HAS REPORTEDLY OBTAINED A RECOVERY SPONSOR, ATTENDED AA MEETINGS 3-4 TIMES A WEEK, AND SUBMITTED TO RANDOM DRUG SCREENS WHICH HAVE SHOWN NO EVIDENCE OF FURTHER DRUG USE; NO EVIDENCE HAS BEEN RECEIVED OF PATIENT HARM RESULTING FROM HIS INTEMPERATE USE OF DRUGS. SUSPENSION STAYED FOR PROBATION WITH FOLLOWING TERMS AND CONDITIONS: SHALL ABSTAIN FROM THE CONSUMPTION OF ALCOHOL/DRUGS IN ANY FORM UNLESS PRESCRIBED BY ANOTHER PHYSICIAN FOR A LEGITIMATE AND THERAPEUTIC PURPOSE; SHALL SUBMIT HIMSELF FOR APPROPRIATE EXAMS INCLUDING DRUG OR ALCOHOL SCREENS; SHALL CONTINUE TO RECEIVE CARE AND TREATMENT FROM HIS PHYSICIAN ONCE A MONTH AND ARRANGE HIM TO PROVIDE QUARTERLY REPORTS TO THE BOARD; SHALL CONTINUE TO PARTICIPATE IN AA OR COMPARABLE PROGRAM 3 TIMES A WEEK; SHALL COMPLY WITH TERMS OF ANY CONTINUING CARE CONTRACT; SHALL NOT TREAT OR OTHERWISE SERVE AS PHYSICIAN, PRESCRIBE, DISPENSE OR ADMINISTER DRUGS THAT MAY BE SUBJECT TO ABUSE TO HIMSELF OR TO ANY MEMBER OF HIS FAMILY; SEPARATE FROM PATIENT RECORDS, SHALL MAINTAIN A LOGBOOK OF EVERY PRESCRIPTION WRITTEN BY HIM FOR DANGEROUS DRUGS WITH ADDICTIVE POTENTIAL WHICH SHALL BE MADE AVAILABLE FOR REVIEW; SHALL OBTAIN 50 HOURS PER YEAR OF CONTINUING MEDICAL EDUCATION; SHALL APPEAR BEFORE THE BOARD TWICE A YEAR; SHALL COOPERATE WITH THE BOARD IN VERIFYING COMPLIANCE INCLUDING PROVIDING COPIES OF MEDICAL RELEASES; TIME SPENT OUT OF TEXAS DOES NOT COUNT TOWARD PROBATION; SHALL INFORM THE BOARD OF CHANGE OF ADDRESS WITHIN 10 DAYS OR IF HE LEAVES THE STATE; SHALL NOT SEEK MODIFICATION FOR 36 MONTHS.

RAMAHI, MICHAEL RANDY DO OF 3404 YELLOWSTONE DRIVE, ARLINGTON, TX, WAS DISCIPLINED BY DEA ON MARCH 25, 1998
DISCIPLINARY ACTION: SURRENDER OF CONTROLLED SUBSTANCE LICENSE

RAMAHI, MICHAEL RANDY DO, LICENSE NUMBER J4462 OF ARLINGTON, TX, WAS DISCIPLINED BY TEXAS ON AUGUST 22, 1998
DISCIPLINARY ACTION: LICENSE SUSPENSION
OFFENSE: CRIMINAL CONVICTION OR PLEA OF GUILTY, NOLO CONTENDERE, OR NO CONTEST TO A CRIME

NOTES: PROVIDED FALSE INFORMATION ON HIS RE-APPLICATION FOR TEXAS LICENSURE FORM, DATED 8/17/97, RELATED TO THE OHIO ARREST AND CONVICTION OF ONE MISDEMEANOR COUNT OF OBTAINING PRESCRIPTIONS BY FRAUD; HE REPORTS THAT THE RESULTING CONVICTION WAS TO BE EXPUNGED UPON HIS SUCCESSFUL COMPLETION OF THE PROBATIONARY PERIOD; FROM 6/97 - 1/9/98 HE SELF-MEDICATED WITH VARIOUS DRUGS BY WRITING PRESCRIPTIONS IN THE NAME OF VARIOUS FAMILY MEMBERS AND HIMSELF; SEVERAL PHARMACISTS HAVE IDENTIFIED HIM AS THE PERSON PICKING UP THESE MEDICATIONS; HE HAS NOT PRACTICED MEDICINE IN TEXAS SINCE 11/97, AND VOLUNTARILY CEASED DUE TO INCAPACITATION FROM PAIN RELATED TO A CONGENITAL SPINAL CONJOINED NERVE ROOT ABNORMALITY AND HIS OWN CONCERNS ABOUT HIS PERCEIVED NEED TO SELF-PRESCRIBE FOR PAIN CONTROL FOR WHICH HE IS PRESENTLY GETTING TREATMENT; ON OR ABOUT 3/27/98 HE VOLUNTARILY SURRENDERED HIS DEA REGISTRATION; SUSPENSION UNTIL HE REQUESTS TO HAVE HIS SUSPENSION STAYED OR APPEARS BEFORE THE BOARD WITH SUFFICIENT EVIDENCE THAT HE IS PHYSICALLY, MENTALLY AND OTHERWISE COMPETENT TO SAFELY PRACTICE MEDICINE INCLUDING AT A MINIMUM COMPLETE COPIES OF MEDICAL RECORDS AND REPORTS OF PSYCHOLOGICAL AND NEUROPSYCHIATRIC EVALUATIONS, INCLUDING A 96 HOUR INPATIENT EVALUATION CONDUCTED BY A BOARD-APPROVED CERTIFIED PSYCHIATRIST; SHALL COOPERATE WITH THE BOARD IN VERIFYING COMPLIANCE INCLUDING PROVIDING COPIES OF MEDICAL RELEASES UPON REQUEST; SHALL INFORM THE BOARD OF CHANGE OF ADDRESS WITHIN 10 DAYS OR IF HE LEAVES THE STATE.

RAMAKRISHNAN, VASUKI MD, LICENSE NUMBER 00F5712 OF STAFFORD, TX, WAS DISCIPLINED BY TEXAS ON APRIL 15, 1994
DISCIPLINARY ACTION: 120-MONTH MONITORING OF PHYSICIAN PERFORMANCE
OFFENSE: PROFESSIONAL MISCONDUCT

NOTES: ON 10/5/93 PLACED ON PROBATION FOR ONE YEAR WITH DEFERRED ADJUDICATION FOR ENDANGERMENT OF HER SON IN DISTRICT COURT OF HARRIS COUNTY: REQUIRED TO CONTINUE COUNSELING AND PERFORM 100 HOURS OF COMMUNITY SERVICE; PREVIOUSLY HAD A HISTORY OF PSYCHOLOGICAL DIFFICULTIES COUPLED WITH INTERVENTION BY LAW ENFORCEMENT AND SOCIAL SERVICE AGENCIES; STRESS ARISES FROM SETTINGS OUTSIDE OF HER MEDICAL PRACTICE AND, AT THIS TIME, THE BOARD DOES NOT HAVE EVIDENCE THAT THERE HAS BEEN AN ADVERSE IMPACT ON HER PRACTICE; CURRENTLY RECEIVING CARE AND COUNSELING BY A PSYCHIATRIST. CONDITIONS OF MONITORING: SHALL CONTINUE TO RECEIVE CARE FROM HER CURRENT PSYCHIATRIST WITH QUARTERLY REPORTS; SHALL APPEAR BEFORE THE BOARD TWICE A YEAR; SHALL GIVE A COPY OF THIS ORDER TO ANY HEALTH CARE ENTITY WHERE SHE

HAS PRIVILEGES; SHALL COOPERATE WITH THE BOARD IN VERIFYING COMPLIANCE; SHALL INFORM BOARD OF CHANGE OF ADDRESS WITHIN 10 DAYS OR IF SHE LEAVES THE STATE; TIME SPENT OUT OF TEXAS DOES NOT COUNT TOWARD MONITORING. SHALL NOT SEEK MODIFICATION FOR ONE YEAR.

RAMAKRISHNAN, VASUKI MD, LICENSE NUMBER 00F5712, WAS DISCIPLINED BY TEXAS ON NOVEMBER 16, 1996
DISCIPLINARY ACTION: LICENSE SUSPENSION
OFFENSE: FAILURE TO COMPLY WITH PREVIOUS BOARD ORDER

NOTES: HAS NOT BEEN PRACTICING MEDICINE SINCE APPROXIMATELY 4/96; HAS FAILED TO CONTINUE TO RECEIVE CARE AND COUNSELING FROM HER BOARD-CERTIFIED PSYCHIATRIST AS REQUIRED BY 4/94 BOARD ORDER; HAS FAILED TO FULLY COOPERATE WITH HER BOARD COMPLIANCE OFFICER. SUSPENSION UNTIL SHE REQUESTS TO HAVE SUSPENSION STAYED OR LIFTED AND APPEARS BEFORE THE BOARD WITH EVIDENCE THAT INDICATES THAT SHE IS PHYSICALLY, MENTALLY AND OTHERWISE COMPETENT TO SAFELY PRACTICE MEDICINE INCLUDING AT A MINIMUM SUCCESSFUL PASSAGE OF THE SPECIAL PURPOSE EXAMINATION AND THE MEDICAL JURISPRUDENCE EXAMINATION AND COPIES OF MEDICAL RECORDS AND REPORTS OF PSYCHOLOGICAL AND NEUROPSYCHIATRIC EVALUATIONS CONDUCTED BY A BOARD-CERTIFIED PSYCHIATRIST. SHALL INFORM BOARD OF A CHANGE OF ADDRESS WITHIN 10 DAYS.

RAMESHWAR, ANTHONY B MD, LICENSE NUMBER 00G3059 OF THE WOODLANDS, TX, WAS DISCIPLINED BY TEXAS ON OCTOBER 5, 1991
DISCIPLINARY ACTION: 36-MONTH PROBATION; REQUIRED TO TAKE ADDITIONAL MEDICAL EDUCATION
OFFENSE: PROFESSIONAL MISCONDUCT

NOTES: IMPROPERLY BILLED FOR HOSPITAL VISITS AND PSYCHIATRIC SERVICES RENDERED TO ONE PATIENT. SUSPENSION STAYED; CONDITIONS OF PROBATION: SHALL ATTEND AT LEAST 10 HOURS CONTINUING MEDICAL EDUCATION PER YEAR IN RISK MANAGEMENT OR BILLING PROCEDURES AND SUBMIT PROOF TO THE BOARD; SHALL NOT SIGN OR INDICATE ANYTHING IN A PATIENT RECORD WITHOUT PERSONALLY SEEING AND EXAMINING THE PATIENT, UNLESS THE CHART CLEARLY REFLECTS THIS; SHALL NOT BACK DATE ANY ENTRY; SHALL UTILIZE A SYSTEM OF RECORDKEEPING THAT WILL INSURE ACCURACY; SHALL COOPERATE WITH THE BOARD IN VERIFYING COMPLIANCE; SHALL ADVISE THE BOARD OF ANY CHANGE OF ADDRESS WITHIN 10 DAYS; MAY NOT APPLY FOR REINSTATEMENT FOR AT LEAST A YEAR; TIME SPENT OUT OF TEXAS WILL NOT COUNT TOWARDS PROBATION. ON 1/14/94 PROBATION TERMINATED.

RAMEY, JOHN ALLEN MD, LICENSE NUMBER G12564 OF LA JOLLA, CA, WAS DISCIPLINED BY CALIFORNIA ON NOVEMBER 10, 1997
DISCIPLINARY ACTION: 24-MONTH PROBATION
OFFENSE: SUBSTANDARD CARE, INCOMPETENCE OR NEGLIGENCE

NOTES: GROSS NEGLIGENCE AND REPEATED NEGLIGENT ACTS IN HIS CARE AND TREATMENT, INCLUDING PERFORMING TWO SURGERIES WITHOUT MEDICAL INDICATION, OF A PATIENT SUFFERING FROM HEADACHES. REVOCATION STAYED. JUDICIAL REVIEW BEING PURSUED.

RAMEY, JOHN ALLEN MD, LICENSE NUMBER G12564 OF LA JOLLA, CA, WAS DISCIPLINED BY CALIFORNIA ON AUGUST 12, 1999
DISCIPLINARY ACTION: LICENSE REVOCATION

RAMEY, JOHN ALLEN MD, LICENSE NUMBER D3784 OF SAN DIEGO, CA, WAS DISCIPLINED BY TEXAS ON AUGUST 28, 1999
OFFENSE: DISCIPLINARY ACTION BY ANOTHER STATE OR AGENCY

NOTES: ON 11/10/97 THE CALIFORNIA BOARD PROBATED HIS LICENSE FOR 2 YEARS BASED ON HIS PERFORMANCE OF 2 SURGERIES WITHOUT THE NECESSARY MEDICAL INDICATION; ON 9/12/95 THE PATIENT WHO PRESENTED TO HIM HAD A HISTORY OF HEADACHES THAT WERE MANAGEABLE WITH ANTIHISTAMINES AND DECONGESTANTS; ON 10/4/95 HE PERFORMED AN ENDOSCOPY; ON 11/2/95 HE OPERATED, AND THEN PERFORMED A SIMILAR PROCEDURE ON 12/14/95; AFTER THE 2 SURGERIES THE PATIENT'S HEADACHES WORSENED; A BOARD CERTIFIED OTOLARYNGOLOGIST TESTIFIED THAT HIS CARE OF THE PATIENT FELL BELOW THE STANDARD OF CARE; THE PATIENT HAD CHRONIC ALLERGIC RHINITIS BY HISTORY, WHICH DID NOT CONSTITUTE AN INDICATION FOR SURGERY; ADDITIONALLY, THE 2 SURGERIES SHOULD HAVE BEEN PERFORMED AT ONE TIME. LICENSE LIMITED AS FOLLOWS: SHALL NOT PRACTICE IN TEXAS UNTIL HE APPEARS BEFORE THE BOARD WITH SUFFICIENT EVIDENCE THAT HE IS PHYSICALLY, MENTALLY OR OTHERWISE COMPETENT TO PRACTICE SAFELY; SHALL PROVIDE COPIES OF ANY REPORTS, DOCUMENTS, OR OTHER MATERIALS THAT HE HAS SUBMITTED TO OR RECEIVED FROM THE CALIFORNIA BOARD; SHALL COOPERATE WITH THE BOARD IN VERIFYING COMPLIANCE; SHALL GIVE A COPY OF THIS ORDER TO ANY HEALTH CARE ENTITY WHERE HE HAS PRIVILEGES; TIME SPENT OUT OF TEXAS DOES NOT COUNT TOWARD RESTRICTION; SHALL INFORM THE BOARD OF CHANGE OF ADDRESS WITHIN 10 DAYS OR IF HE LEAVES THE STATE; SHALL NOT SEEK MODIFICATION FOR ONE YEAR.

RAMIREZ, HUGO A MD, LICENSE NUMBER 031320L OF PASADENA, TX, WAS DISCIPLINED BY PENNSYLVANIA ON OCTOBER 11, 1990
DISCIPLINARY ACTION: LICENSE REVOCATION
OFFENSE: DISCIPLINARY ACTION BY ANOTHER STATE OR AGENCY

NOTES: LICENSE WAS REVOKED ON 7/24/87 BY THE TEXAS STATE BOARD OF MEDICAL EXAMINERS FOR UNPROFESSIONAL OR DISHONORABLE CONDUCT AND FOR NEGLIGENTLY FAILING TO PRACTICE MEDICINE IN AN ACCEPTABLE MANNER CONSISTENT WITH THE PUBLIC HEALTH AND WELFARE, WHICH RESULTED IN THE DEATH OF TWO PATIENTS. 10/31/90 ORDER GRANTED STAY OF HEARING EXAMINER'S ORDER OF REVOCATION PENDING REVIEW BY THE BOARD.

RAMIREZ, HUGO A MD, WAS DISCIPLINED BY TEXAS ON OCTOBER 5, 1991
DISCIPLINARY ACTION: DENIAL OF LICENSE REINSTATEMENT

NOTES: LICENSE REVOKED 8/21/87.

RAMIREZ, HUGO A MD OF ROLLING HILLS HOSP 60 E TOWNSHIP, ELKINS PARK, PA, WAS DISCIPLINED BY DEA ON MAY 11, 1992
DISCIPLINARY ACTION: DENIAL OF NEW LICENSE
OFFENSE: DISCIPLINARY ACTION BY ANOTHER STATE OR AGENCY

NOTES: MEDICAL LICENSE REVOKED BY PENNSYLVANIA EFFECTIVE 10/30/90 BASED ON PRIOR REVOCATION BY TEXAS ON 08/21/87. TEXAS ACTION DUE TO FINDING THAT HE FAILED TO INSURE A STERILE ENVIRONMENT DURING LIPOSUCTION PROCEDURES AND FAILED TO ORDER PROPER TESTS AND TO PROPERLY MONITOR PATIENTS AFTER THE PROCEDURES WERE COMPLETED. THEREFORE HE IS NOT AUTHORIZED TO

PRESCRIBE, DISPENSE, ADMINISTER OR OTHERWISE HANDLE CONTROLLED SUBSTANCES.

RAMIREZ, HUGO A MD, LICENSE NUMBER 0004225, WAS DISCIPLINED BY RHODE ISLAND ON FEBRUARY 17, 1993
DISCIPLINARY ACTION: DENIAL OF NEW LICENSE
OFFENSE: DISCIPLINARY ACTION BY ANOTHER STATE OR AGENCY

NOTES: REVOCATION OF LICENSE IN ANOTHER STATE; ACTIONS WOULD BE UNPROFESSIONAL CONDUCT IN RHODE ISLAND.

RAMIREZ, JAIME MD, LICENSE NUMBER 00G7422 OF PLANO, TX, WAS DISCIPLINED BY TEXAS ON JUNE 10, 1991
DISCIPLINARY ACTION: 60-MONTH PROBATION; RESTRICTION PLACED ON LICENSE
OFFENSE: LOSS OR RESTRICTION OF HOSPITAL PRIVILEGES

NOTES: SUBMITTED FALSE OR MISLEADING STATEMENT, DOCUMENT, OR CERTIFICATE TO BOARD IN AN APPLICATION FOR EXAMINATION OR LICENSURE; UNPROFESSIONAL OR DISHONORABLE CONDUCT LIKELY TO DECEIVE, DEFRAUD, OR INJURE THE PUBLIC; PROFESSIONAL FAILURE TO PRACTICE MEDICINE IN AN ACCEPTABLE MANNER CONSISTENT WITH PUBLIC HEALTH AND WELFARE; NONTHERAPEUTIC PRESCRIBING; LOSS OF HOSPITAL PRIVILEGES. SIX MONTH SUSPENSION STAYED; TERMS OF PROBATION: SHALL APPEAR BEFORE THE BOARD ONCE A YEAR; SHALL ATTEND AT LEAST 50 HOURS OF CONTINUING MEDICAL EDUCATION, AN ADVANCED TRAUMA LIFE SUPPORT COURSE, AND AN ADVANCED CARDIAC LIFE SUPPORT COURSE TO OBTAIN RECERTIFICATION IN THESE COURSES; SHALL NOT ACCEPT EMPLOYMENT OR ENTER INTO CONTRACTUAL RELATIONSHIPS WHEREIN HE WOULD BE COMPENSATED TO DIAGNOSE AND/OR TREAT PATIENTS BY A LAYPERSON, CORPORATION, OR OTHER ENTITY NOT COMPRISED EXCLUSIVELY OF LICENSED PHYSICIANS, AND WHEREIN SAID PERSON OR ENTITY THEN WOULD RECEIVE AND RETAIN THE FEES PAID BY OR ON BEHALF OF PATIENTS FOR THE PHYSICIAN'S PROFESSIONAL SERVICES.

RAMIREZ, JAIME MD OF 5540 DENTON DR CUTOFF, DALLAS, TX, WAS DISCIPLINED BY DEA ON JUNE 15, 1994
DISCIPLINARY ACTION: SURRENDER OF CONTROLLED SUBSTANCE LICENSE

NOTES: IN LIEU OF PUBLIC INTEREST REVOCATION.

RAMIREZ, JAIME MD, LICENSE NUMBER 00G7422 OF PLANO, TX, WAS DISCIPLINED BY TEXAS ON JUNE 22, 1994
DISCIPLINARY ACTION: FINE; REPRIMAND
OFFENSE: FAILURE TO COMPLY WITH PREVIOUS BOARD ORDER

NOTES: HAS ENGAGED IN THE CORPORATE PRACTICE OF MEDICINE IN VIOLATION OF A CONDITION OF 6/10/91 ORDER IN THAT HE ENTERED INTO AN AGREEMENT WITH THE OAK LAWN MEDICAL CENTER AGREEING TO PROVIDE PROFESSIONAL SERVICES FOR A SET RATE OF COMPENSATION; THIS WAS DONE FOR TAX PURPOSES. SHALL PAY A $5,000 ADMINISTRATIVE PENALTY WITHIN 90 DAYS; SHALL NOT ACCEPT EMPLOYMENT OR ENTER INTO CONTRACTUAL RELATIONSHIPS WHERE HE WOULD BE COMPENSATED TO DIAGNOSE AND/OR TREAT PATIENTS BY ANY ENTITY NOT COMPRISED EXCLUSIVELY OF TEXAS LICENSED PHYSICIANS; SHALL GIVE A COPY OF THIS ORDER TO ANY HEALTH CARE ENTITY WHERE HE HAS PRIVILEGES; SHALL COOPERATE WITH BOARD IN VERIFYING COMPLIANCE; SHALL INFORM BOARD OF CHANGE OF ADDRESS OR IF HE LEAVES THE STATE; TIME SPENT OUT OF TEXAS DOES NOT COUNT TOWARD RESTRICTION. SHALL NOT SEEK MODIFICATION FOR ONE YEAR.

RAMIREZ, JAIME MD, LICENSE NUMBER 00G7422 OF DALLAS, TX, WAS DISCIPLINED BY TEXAS ON NOVEMBER 1, 1995
DISCIPLINARY ACTION: 1-MONTH LICENSE SUSPENSION; 60-MONTH PROBATION
OFFENSE: PROVIDING FALSE INFORMATION TO THE BOARD OR OTHER HEALTH AGENCY

NOTES: IN 1994 HE SUBMITTED TO THE BOARD DOCUMENTATION FOR CONTINUING MEDICAL EDUCATION HOURS, ALL OF WHICH HE DID NOT ATTEND; FAILED TO KEEP ADEQUATE RECORDS REGARDING HIS PRESCRIBING AND ADMINISTERING OF CONTROLLED SUBSTANCES TO VARIOUS PATIENTS, SOME OF WHOM WERE ABUSERS OF CONTROLLED SUBSTANCES; IN 6/94 HE SURRENDERED HIS DEA CONTROLLED SUBSTANCES REGISTRATIONS AFTER AN AUDIT BY DEA. SUSPENSION TO BE STAYED AFTER 30 DAYS; PROBATION WITH TERMS: SHALL SURRENDER HIS DEA AND DPS CONTROLLED SUBSTANCES REGISTRATION CERTIFICATES AND ALL UNUSED TRIPLICATE PRESCRIPTION FORMS AND SHALL NOT ATTEMPT TO ORDER MORE; SHALL KEEP A LOG SUBJECT TO REVIEW OF ALL PRESCRIPTIONS WRITTEN FOR DANGEROUS DRUGS WITH ADDICTIVE POTENTIAL OR POTENTIAL FOR ABUSE; HIS PRACTICE SHALL BE MONITORED BY A BOARD-APPROVED PHYSICIAN WHO SHALL SUBMIT QUARTERLY REPORTS TO THE BOARD; SHALL MAINTAIN ADEQUATE MEDICAL RECORDS WHICH SHALL BE SUBJECT TO REVIEW; SHALL OBTAIN AT LEAST 50 HOURS OF CONTINUING MEDICAL EDUCATION; SHALL APPEAR BEFORE BOARD AT LEAST TWICE A YEAR; SHALL COOPERATE WITH BOARD IN VERIFYING COMPLIANCE; SHALL GIVE A COPY OF THIS ORDER TO ANY HEALTH CARE ENTITY WHERE HE HAS PRIVILEGES; SHALL PROVIDE A COPY OF THIS ORDER TO ANYONE REQUESTING IT WITHIN 10 DAYS; TIME SPENT OUT OF TEXAS DOES NOT COUNT TOWARD PROBATION; SHALL INFORM BOARD OF CHANGE OF ADDRESS WITHIN 10 DAYS OR IF HE LEAVES THE STATE. SHALL PAY $5,000 FINE. SHALL NOT SEEK MODIFICATION FOR ONE YEAR. THESE TERMS AND CONDITIONS ARE IN ADDITION TO TERMS AND CONDITIONS OF 6/10/91 ORDER; IN ANY INSTANCE WHERE BOTH ORDERS REQUIRE THE SAME ACTION MAY COMPLY BY PERFORMING THE REQUIRED ACTIONS PURSUANT TO EITHER ONE; UPON TERMINATION OF 6/10/91 ORDER WILL STILL BE REQUIRED TO COMPLY WITH ALL TERMS AND CONDITIONS OF THIS ORDER. ON 1/29/99 PETITION TO MODIFY ORDER GRANTED AUTHORIZING HIM TO REAPPLY FOR REGISTRATIONS IN SCHEDULES IV AND V; REDUCTION OF REPORTS FROM MONITORING PHYSICIAN FROM QUARTERLY TO TWICE PER YEAR.

RAMIREZ, JOHN P MD, LICENSE NUMBER 00H0743 OF HOUSTON, TX, WAS DISCIPLINED BY TEXAS ON JUNE 1, 1996
DISCIPLINARY ACTION: 1-MONTH LICENSE SUSPENSION; 60-MONTH PROBATION
OFFENSE: SEXUAL ABUSE OF OR SEXUAL MISCONDUCT WITH A PATIENT

NOTES: IN 1994 ON TWO SEPARATE DATES, HE ENGAGED IN SEXUAL ACTS, INCLUDING SEXUAL INTERCOURSE, WITH ONE ADULT FEMALE PATIENT AWAY FROM HIS OFFICE; SHORTLY AFTER ENGAGING IN SEXUAL INTERCOURSE WITH PATIENT ON THE SECOND OCCASION, HE ADMINISTERED THE DRUG PROVERA

TO HER WITHOUT ADEQUATE MEDICAL INDICATION AND WITHOUT DOCUMENTING THE ADMINISTRATION OF THE DRUG IN HER MEDICAL RECORD; WITH RESPECT TO THE SAME PATIENT, HE DISCLOSED HER MEDICAL CONDITION TO HER RELATIVE WITHOUT HER AUTHORIZATION; HE MAINTAINS THAT HE NEVER ENGAGED IN ANY SEXUAL IMPROPRIETY WITH ANY OTHER PATIENT. REMAINDER OF SUSPENSION STAYED. PROBATION WITH TERMS AND CONDITIONS: SHALL SUBMIT HIMSELF FOR EVALUATION AND TREATMENT BY A BOARD-APPROVED PSYCHIATRIST WHO SHALL SUBMIT REPORTS TO THE BOARD; SHALL HAVE A CHAPERONE PRESENT WHENEVER HE PERFORMS AN EXAMINATION OF A FEMALE PATIENT AND SHALL NOTE THIS IN THE PATIENTS CHART; SHALL MAINTAIN ADEQUATE MEDICAL RECORDS WHICH SHALL BE AVAILABLE FOR REVIEW; SHALL BECOME FAMILIAR WITH AND COMPLY WITH THE PROVISIONS FOR THE MAINTENANCE OF PATIENT CONFIDENTIALITY AND FOR RELEASING MEDICAL RECORDS; WITHIN SIX MONTHS, SHALL RESEARCH AND WRITE A PAPER OF RESEARCH QUALITY REGARDING PHYSICIAN-PATIENT BOUNDARIES AND INAPPROPRIATE INTERPERSONAL RELATIONSHIPS BETWEEN PHYSICIANS AND PATIENTS; WITHIN NINE MONTHS, SHALL TAKE AND PASS THE MEDICAL JURISPRUDENCE EXAMINATION; SHALL OBTAIN AT LEAST 50 HOURS PER YEAR OF CONTINUING MEDICAL EDUCATION; SHALL PERFORM 96 HOURS OF COMMUNITY SERVICE PER YEAR; SHALL NOT PRESCRIBE OR ADMINISTER ANY DRUG FOR ANY PATIENT UNLESS IT IS MEDICALLY INDICATED AND IS PRESCRIBED IN THERAPEUTIC DOSES; SHALL NOT TELEPHONE TO A PHARMACY A PRESCRIPTION OR REFILL FOR CONTROLLED SUBSTANCES OR DANGEROUS DRUGS WITH ADDICTIVE POTENTIAL OR POTENTIAL FOR ABUSE NOR ALLOW ANYONE UNDER HIS SUPERVISION TO DO SO; SHALL MAINTAIN A LOG OF ALL PRESCRIPTIONS WRITTEN FOR THESE SUBSTANCES WHICH SHALL BE AVAILABLE FOR REVIEW; SHALL NOT TREAT OR OTHERWISE SERVE AS PHYSICIAN, PRESCRIBE, DISPENSE OR ADMINISTER DRUGS THAT MAY BE SUBJECT TO ABUSE TO HIMSELF OR TO ANY MEMBER OF HIS FAMILY; SHALL COOPERATE WITH THE BOARD IN VERIFYING COMPLIANCE INCLUDING PROVIDING COPIES OF MEDICAL RELEASES AND PEER REVIEW RECORDS UPON REQUEST; SHALL GIVE A COPY OF THIS ORDER TO ANY HEALTH CARE ENTITY WHERE HE HAS PRIVILEGES; SHALL PROVIDE A COPY OF THIS ORDER TO ANYONE REQUESTING IT WITHIN 10 DAYS; SHALL APPEAR BEFORE BOARD AT LEAST TWO TIMES A YEAR OR AT BOARD REQUEST; TIME SPENT OUT OF TEXAS DOES NOT COUNT TOWARD PROBATION; SHALL INFORM BOARD OF CHANGE OF ADDRESS WITHIN 10 DAYS OR IF HE LEAVES THE STATE. SHALL NOT SEEK MODIFICATION FOR ONE YEAR. ON 8/9/97 PETITION TO TERMINATE ORDER DENIED. ON 8/22/98 PETITION TO TERMINATE ORDER DENIED. ON 5/14/99 PETITION TO TERMINATE ORDER DENIED; ORDER MODIFIED DELETING FORBIDDING TELEPHONE PRESCRIPTIONS, REQUIREMENT OF PRESCRIPTION LOGBOOK; REDUCTION OF APPEARANCES BEFORE THE BOARD FROM TWICE YEARLY TO ONCE A YEAR.

RAMON, ROGER G MD OF 3022 MCKINZIE RD SUITE A, CORPUS CHRISTI, TX, WAS DISCIPLINED BY DEA ON MAY 12, 1995
DISCIPLINARY ACTION: SURRENDER OF CONTROLLED SUBSTANCE LICENSE

NOTES: IN LIEU OF PUBLIC INTEREST REVOCATION.

RAMONET, JORGELINA G MD, LICENSE NUMBER 00G0802, WAS DISCIPLINED BY TEXAS ON AUGUST 17, 1996
DISCIPLINARY ACTION: FINE; REPRIMAND
OFFENSE: NONCOMPLIANCE WITH A PROFESSIONAL RULE

NOTES: FAILED TO OBTAIN 24 HOURS CONTINUING MEDICAL EDUCATION AS REQUIRED BY 3/1/95 FOR THE RENEWAL OF HER LICENSE; SHE WAS GRANTED AN EXTENSION UNTIL 3/29/96 WHICH SHE ALSO DID NOT MEET; STILL REQUIRED TO MEET CONTINUING MEDICAL EDUCATION REQUIREMENTS. SHALL COOPERATE WITH THE BOARD. $100 ADMINISTRATIVE PENALTY; SHALL COOPERATE WITH THE BOARD IN VERIFYING COMPLIANCE.

RAMPOLDI, JAMES MOSES MD, LICENSE NUMBER 00E3829 OF DENTON, TX, WAS DISCIPLINED BY TEXAS ON MARCH 5, 1994
DISCIPLINARY ACTION: 60-MONTH PROBATION; RESTRICTION PLACED ON LICENSE
OFFENSE: SUBSTANDARD CARE, INCOMPETENCE OR NEGLIGENCE

NOTES: FROM 1/90 THROUGH 8/91 HE FAILED TO ADEQUATELY DOCUMENT EVALUATIONS AND TREATMENT RENDERED TO A NURSING HOME PATIENT AND FAILED TO PERSONALLY EVALUATE HER ON A SUFFICIENTLY REGULAR BASIS TO ENABLE HIM TO RENDER ADEQUATE CARE TO HER. FIVE YEAR SUSPENSION STAYED. CONDITIONS OF PROBATION: SHALL MAINTAIN ADEQUATE MEDICAL RECORDS AND UTILIZE A SYSTEM TO INSURE THIS; SHALL NOT SIGN ANY PATIENT RECORD UNLESS HE HAS PERSONALLY EXAMINED THE PATIENT OR CLEARLY NOTES IN THE RECORD THAT HE DID NOT; SHALL PERSONALLY EXAMINE A PATIENT WHEN STATE LAW REQUIRES THAT A PHYSICIAN PERFORM THE EXAMINATION; SHALL ATTEND AT LEAST 50 HOURS PER YEAR OF CONTINUING MEDICAL EDUCATION IN FAMILY PRACTICE MEDICINE; SHALL RESPOND IN A TIMELY MANNER TO ALL BOARD REQUESTS FOR MEDICAL RECORDS OR OTHER INFORMATION; SHALL NOT SEE, TREAT OR SERVE AS A PHYSICIAN FOR NURSING HOME PATIENTS; SHALL APPEAR BEFORE THE BOARD ONCE A YEAR; SHALL GIVE A COPY OF THIS ORDER TO ANY HEALTH CARE ENTITY WHERE HE HAS PRIVILEGES; SHALL COOPERATE WITH THE BOARD IN VERIFYING COMPLIANCE; SHALL INFORM THE BOARD OF CHANGE OF ADDRESS WITHIN 10 DAYS OR IF HE LEAVES THE STATE; TIME SPENT OUT OF TEXAS DOES NOT COUNT TOWARD PROBATION. SHALL NOT SEEK MODIFICATION FOR ONE YEAR. ON 5/10/97 PETITION TO TERMINATE ORDER DENIED. ON 4/4/98 ORDER TERMINATED.

RANELLE, JOHN DO OF WOLFE CITY, TX, WAS DISCIPLINED BY MISSOURI ON AUGUST 22, 1990
OFFENSE: DISCIPLINARY ACTION BY ANOTHER STATE OR AGENCY

NOTES: ACTION TAKEN IN TEXAS BASED ON EXCESSIVE PRESCRIBING AND INADEQUATE PATIENT RECORDS. MUST APPEAR BEFORE BOARD BEFORE RETURNING TO PRACTICE IN MISSOURI. NO DATE LISTED BY DEA.

RANELLE, JOHN BARRY DO, LICENSE NUMBER 00E9349 OF WOLFE CITY, TX, WAS DISCIPLINED BY TEXAS ON FEBRUARY 16, 1990
DISCIPLINARY ACTION: 36-MONTH RESTRICTION PLACED ON CONTROLLED SUBSTANCE LICENSE; 36-MONTH MONITORING OF PHYSICIAN PERFORMANCE

NOTES: STIPULATED ORDER. SHALL APPEAR BEFORE BOARD EVERY SIX MONTHS, AUTHORIZE BOARD TO OBTAIN URINE OR BLOOD SAMPLES FOR DRUG AND ALCOHOL SCREENS, SURRENDER TRIPLICATE PRESCRIPTION FORMS AND NOT ORDER MORE UNTIL BOARD PERMITS, REQUEST MODIFICATION OF CONTROLLED SUBSTANCES REGISTRATIONS TO ELIMINATE

SCHEDULES II AND II-N AND NOT REREGISTER FOR SAME UNTIL BOARD APPROVAL, NOT PRESCRIBE, DISPENSE, ADMINISTER OR POSSESS SPECIFIC AMPHETAMINE-LIKE ACTION DRUGS OR ANORECTIC AGENTS, REFRAIN FROM CONSUMING PRESCRIPTION DRUGS UNLESS PRESCRIBED BY ANOTHER PHYSICIAN FOR VALID MEDICAL PURPOSES, MAINTAIN ADEQUATE MEDICAL RECORDS ON ALL PATIENT OFFICE VISITS TO INCLUDE CERTAIN INFORMATION, AND MAINTAIN SEPARATE FILE OF PRESCRIPTIONS FOR CONTROLLED SUBSTANCES.

RANELLE, JOHN BARRY DO, LICENSE NUMBER 00E9349 OF DALLAS, TX, WAS DISCIPLINED BY TEXAS ON MARCH 6, 1992
DISCIPLINARY ACTION: LICENSE SUSPENSION
OFFENSE: SUBSTANCE ABUSE

NOTES: UNPROFESSIONAL OR DISHONORABLE CONDUCT LIKELY TO DECEIVE, DEFRAUD OR INJURE THE PUBLIC, AND INTEMPERATE USE OF ALCOHOL OR DRUGS. LIFTING OF THE SUSPENSION WILL NOT BE CONSIDERED UNTIL CERTAIN MINIMUM REQUIREMENTS ARE MET. SUSPENSION TERMINATED ON 9/28/92.

RANELLE, JOHN BARRY DO, LICENSE NUMBER 00E9349 OF EULESS, TX, WAS DISCIPLINED BY TEXAS ON SEPTEMBER 28, 1992
DISCIPLINARY ACTION: 60-MONTH PROBATION

NOTES: SUSPENSION TERMINATED.

RANELLE, JOHN BARRY DO, LICENSE NUMBER 00E9349 OF EULESS, TX, WAS DISCIPLINED BY TEXAS ON JUNE 22, 1994
DISCIPLINARY ACTION: 60-MONTH PROBATION; RESTRICTION PLACED ON LICENSE
OFFENSE: FAILURE TO COMPLY WITH PREVIOUS BOARD ORDER

NOTES: ON 3/3/93 AND 7/30/93 PRESCRIBED DEMEROL A SCHEDULE II CONTROLLED SUBSTANCE AND FAILED TO ADEQUATELY DOCUMENT PRESCRIPTIONS IN PATIENT CHARTS IN VIOLATION OF 9/28/92 BOARD ORDER. SUSPENSION STAYED. CONDITIONS OF PROBATION; SHALL APPEAR BEFORE THE BOARD TWICE A YEAR; SHALL ABSTAIN FROM THE CONSUMPTION OF ALCOHOL/CHEMICAL SUBSTANCES IN ANY FORM UNLESS PRESCRIBED BY ANOTHER PHYSICIAN FOR A LEGITIMATE AND THERAPEUTIC PURPOSE; SHALL SUBMIT HIMSELF FOR APPROPRIATE EXAMS INCLUDING DRUG OR ALCOHOL SCREENS; SHALL SURRENDER DEA AND TEXAS CONTROLLED SUBSTANCES REGISTRATION CERTIFICATES, ALL UNUSED TRIPLICATE PRESCRIPTION FORMS AND ALL CONTROLLED SUBSTANCES IN HIS POSSESSION INCLUDING SAMPLES; SHALL NOT ATTEMPT TO REREGISTER WITHOUT PERMISSION; SHALL NOT PRESCRIBE, DISPENSE, ADMINISTER OR POSSESS ANY OF A LIST OF AMPHETAMINE-LIKE ACTION DRUGS UNDER ANY CIRCUMSTANCES; SHALL NOT TREAT OR OTHERWISE SERVE AS PHYSICIAN, PRESCRIBE, DISPENSE OR ADMINISTER DRUGS THAT MAY BE SUBJECT TO ABUSE FOR HIMSELF OR ANY MEMBER OF HIS FAMILY; SHALL MAINTAIN ADEQUATE MEDICAL RECORDS ON ALL PATIENT OFFICE VISITS WHICH SHALL BE AVAILABLE FOR INSPECTION; SEPARATE FROM PATIENT RECORDS SHALL MAINTAIN A FILE OF EVERY PRESCRIPTION WRITTEN FOR DANGEROUS DRUGS WHICH HAVE POTENTIAL FOR ABUSE WHICH SHALL BE AVAILABLE FOR INSPECTION; SHALL NOT TELEPHONE IN ANY PRESCRIPTIONS FOR DANGEROUS DRUGS; SHALL BE SUPERVISED BY A SPECIFIED PHYSICIAN WITH BIMONTHLY REPORTS; SHALL CONTINUE TO RECEIVE PSYCHIATRIC TREATMENT WITH QUARTERLY REPORTS; SHALL GIVE A COPY OF THIS ORDER TO ANY HEALTH CARE ENTITY WHERE HE HAS PRIVILEGES; SHALL COOPERATE WITH THE BOARD IN VERIFYING COMPLIANCE; SHALL INFORM BOARD OF CHANGE OF ADDRESS WITHIN 10 DAYS OR IF HE LEAVES THE STATE; TIME SPENT OUT OF TEXAS DOES NOT COUNT TOWARD PROBATION. THIS ORDER SUPERSEDES THAT OF 9/28/92. SHALL NOT SEEK MODIFICATION FOR ONE YEAR.

RANELLE, JOHN BARRY DO OF 1805 NORTH GARRETT, DALLAS, TX, WAS DISCIPLINED BY DEA ON OCTOBER 27, 1994
DISCIPLINARY ACTION: SURRENDER OF CONTROLLED SUBSTANCE LICENSE
OFFENSE: DISCIPLINARY ACTION BY ANOTHER STATE OR AGENCY

NOTES: STATE BOARD.

RANELLE, JOHN BARRY DO, LICENSE NUMBER 00E9349 OF FORT WORTH, TX, WAS DISCIPLINED BY TEXAS ON JUNE 28, 1995
DISCIPLINARY ACTION: LICENSE SUSPENSION
OFFENSE: FAILURE TO COMPLY WITH PREVIOUS BOARD ORDER

NOTES: SURRENDERED HIS DEA/DPS CONTROLLED SUBSTANCE REGISTRATION IN 8/94; BETWEEN 9/12/94 AND 9/14/94 PRESCRIBED FIORINAL, A SCHEDULE II CONTROLLED SUBSTANCE, TO THREE PATIENTS IN VIOLATION OF 6/22/94 BOARD ORDER; BETWEEN 6/28/94 AND 7/27/94, PRESCRIBED DARVOCET TO THREE PATIENTS ALSO A VIOLATION OF THE SAME ORDER; FAILED TO DOCUMENT PRESCRIPTION WRITTEN FOR DARVOCET IN THE MEDICAL RECORDS OF A PATIENT, IN VIOLATION OF BOARD ORDER. LICENSE SUSPENDED UNTIL HE REQUESTS TO HAVE SUSPENSION STAYED OR LIFTED AND APPEARS BEFORE BOARD WITH SUFFICIENT EVIDENCE THAT HE IS PHYSICALLY, MENTALLY AND OTHERWISE COMPETENT TO SAFELY PRACTICE MEDICINE INCLUDING AT A MINIMUM PROVIDING RECORDS AND MEDICAL REPORTS OF PSYCHOLOGICAL AND NEUROPSYCHIATRIC EVALUATIONS CONDUCTED BY BOARD-APPROVED PSYCHIATRIST. ON 1/18/97 PETITION TO LIFT SUSPENSION DENIED.

RANELLE, JOHN BARRY DO, DATE OF BIRTH JUNE 22, 1949 OF 305 DUNAWAY COURT, EULESS, TX, WAS DISCIPLINED BY MEDICARE ON OCTOBER 20, 1998
DISCIPLINARY ACTION: EXCLUSION FROM THE MEDICARE AND/OR MEDICAID PROGRAM
OFFENSE: DISCIPLINARY ACTION BY ANOTHER STATE OR AGENCY

NOTES: LICENSE REVOKED, SUSPENDED, SURRENDERED OR OTHERWISE LOST FOR REASONS BEARING ON PROFESSIONAL PERFORMANCE, PROFESSIONAL COMPETENCE OR FINANCIAL INTEGRITY.

RANELLE, JOHN BARRY DO, LICENSE NUMBER E9349, WAS DISCIPLINED BY TEXAS ON DECEMBER 11, 1999
DISCIPLINARY ACTION: 120-MONTH PROBATION; RESTRICTION PLACED ON LICENSE

NOTES: ON 6/4/99 HE UNDERWENT A PSYCHIATRIC EVALUATION, WHICH STATES THAT HE IS SAFE TO PRACTICE MEDICINE; ON 5/26/99 HE UNDERWENT A NEURO-PSYCHOLOGICAL EXAM WHICH STATES THAT HE CAN MAXIMALLY PRACTICE IF HE ENGAGES IN BEHAVIORAL THERAPY AND THERAPY FOR HIS DEPRESSION; ON 5/25/99 HE PASSED THE SPEX. SUSPENSION ENTERED 6/28/95 STAYED FOR PROBATION WITH FOLLOWING TERMS AND CONDITIONS: SHALL ABSTAIN FROM THE CONSUMPTION OF ALCOHOL/DRUGS IN ANY FORM UNLESS PRESCRIBED BY ANOTHER PHYSICIAN FOR A LEGITIMATE AND THERAPEUTIC PURPOSE; SHALL

SUBMIT HIMSELF FOR APPROPRIATE EXAMS INCLUDING DRUG OR ALCOHOL SCREENS; SHALL OBTAIN 50 HOURS PER YEAR OF CONTINUING MEDICAL EDUCATION; SHALL NOT HOLD PRIVILEGES AT ANY HOSPITAL; SHALL NOT POSSESS ALCOHOL, CONTROLLED SUBSTANCES, OR DANGEROUS DRUGS WITH ADDICTIVE POTENTIAL OR POTENTIAL FOR ABUSE; SHALL IMMEDIATELY SURRENDER HIS DEA AND TEXAS DEPARTMENT OF PUBLIC SAFETY CONTROLLED SUBSTANCES REGISTRATION CERTIFICATES AND ANY SAMPLES OF DRUGS STILL IN HIS POSSESSION; HIS MEDICAL PRACTICE SHALL BE MONITORED BY A BOARD APPROVED TEXAS PHYSICIAN WHO SHALL PROVIDE QUARTERLY REPORTS TO THE BOARD; SHALL MAINTAIN A LOGBOOK OF ALL PRESCRIPTIONS WRITTEN BY HIM FOR DANGEROUS DRUGS WITH ADDICTIVE POTENTIAL OR POTENTIAL FOR ABUSE WHICH SHALL BE AVAILABLE FOR REVIEW; SHALL LIMIT PRACTICE TO A GROUP OR AN INSTITUTIONAL SETTING; SHALL NOMINATE THREE CERTIFIED PSYCHIATRISTS FOR BOARD SELECTION OF A THERAPIST AND SHALL EXPEDITIOUSLY SUBMIT HIMSELF TO EVALUATION AND TREATMENT BY THE APPROVED PRACTITIONER; SHALL APPEAR BEFORE THE BOARD TWICE A YEAR; SHALL PARTICIPATE IN AA'S PROGRAM NOT LESS THAN THREE TIMES A WEEK; SHALL REPORT ON HIS ATTENDANCE; SHALL COOPERATE WITH THE BOARD IN VERIFYING COMPLIANCE; SHALL GIVE A COPY OF THIS ORDER TO ANY HEALTH CARE ENTITY WHERE HE HAS PRIVILEGES; SHALL PROVIDE A COPY OF THIS ORDER TO ANYONE REQUESTING IT WITHIN 10 DAYS; TIME SPENT OUT OF TEXAS DOES NOT COUNT TOWARD PROBATION; SHALL INFORM THE BOARD OF CHANGE OF ADDRESS WITHIN 10 DAYS OR IF HE LEAVES THE STATE; SHALL NOT SEEK MODIFICATION FOR ONE YEAR.

RANKIN, DOUGLAS HALL MD, LICENSE NUMBER 00F2867 OF AUSTIN, TX, WAS DISCIPLINED BY TEXAS ON DECEMBER 4, 1991
DISCIPLINARY ACTION: SURRENDER OF CONTROLLED SUBSTANCE LICENSE; 120-MONTH PROBATION
OFFENSE: SUBSTANCE ABUSE

NOTES: IS ADDICTED TO NUBAIN AND STADOL; HAS COMPLETED THE SOLUTIONS OUTPATIENT REHABILITATION AND IS CONTINUING IN WEEKLY AFTERCARE. SUSPENSION STAYED; CONDITIONS OF PROBATION: SHALL APPEAR BEFORE THE BOARD TWICE A YEAR TO VERIFY COMPLIANCE; SHALL NOT PETITION FOR MODIFICATION FOR AT LEAST ONE YEAR; SHALL SURRENDER HIS DEA AND TEXAS CONTROLLED SUBSTANCES REGISTRATIONS; SHALL SURRENDER ALL UNUSED TRIPLICATE PRESCRIPTION FORMS AND SHALL NOT ORDER MORE WITHOUT BOARD PERMISSION; SHALL SURRENDER ALL CONTROLLED SUBSTANCES, INCLUDING SAMPLES; SHALL REPORT TO THE BOARD WITHIN 24 HOURS IF HE PARTAKES OF ALCOHOL OR ANY OTHER CHEMICAL SUBSTANCES; SHALL ABSTAIN FROM CONSUMPTION OF ALCOHOL/CHEMICAL SUBSTANCES IN ANY FORM; SHALL PARTICIPATE IN THE IMPAIRED PHYSICIANS GROUP WEEKLY; SHALL PARTICIPATE IN AA, INCLUDING A 12-STEP PROGRAM, NOT LESS THAN 3 TIMES PER WEEK, WITH WRITTEN REPORTS TO THE BOARD EVERY 3 MONTHS; SHALL SUBMIT TO RANDOM SCREENS OF BODILY FLUIDS; SHALL CONTINUE TREATMENT WITH REPORTS TO THE BOARD FROM TREATING PHYSICIAN; SHALL COMPLY WITH RECOMMENDATIONS OF AFTERCARE PROGRAM; SHALL NOTIFY THE BOARD IMMEDIATELY IF HE DISCONTINUES MEDICAL CARE; SHALL SUPPLY WRITTEN REPORTS TO BOARD WHEN REQUESTED, AND COOPERATE WITH BOARD IN MONITORING COMPLIANCE; SHALL ADVISE THE BOARD OF ANY CHANGE OF ADDRESS WITHIN 10 DAYS; DURATION OF PROBATION NOT SERVED BY TIME SPENT OUT OF STATE; SHALL APPEAR BEFORE THE BOARD TWICE A YEAR. ON 1/14/94 ORDER MODIFIED AS FOLLOWS: HE IS GRANTED PERMISSION TO REAPPLY TO THE DRUG ENFORCEMENT ADMINISTRATION AND THE TEXAS DEPARTMENT OF PUBLIC SAFETY FOR SCHEDULES III, IV AND V ONLY; SEPARATE FROM PATIENT RECORDS, HE SHALL MAINTAIN A FILE CONSISTING OF A COPY OF EVERY PRESCRIPTION WRITTEN BY HIM FOR CONTROLLED SUBSTANCES OR DANGEROUS DRUGS BY DATE ISSUED WHICH SHALL BE AVAILABLE TO THE BOARD FOR INSPECTION; HE AND HIS STAFF SHALL NOT TELEPHONE ANY PRESCRIPTION TO A PHARMACY FOR CONTROLLED SUBSTANCES OR DANGEROUS DRUGS; SHALL NOT PRESCRIBE, DISPENSE, ADMINISTER, OR POSSESS STADOL, NUBAIN, SOMA OR THEIR GENERIC OR CHEMICAL EQUIVALENTS. ALL OTHER PROVISIONS OF THIS ORDER REMAIN IN EFFECT. ON 3/4/95 ORDER MODIFIED AS FOLLOWS: HE IS AUTHORIZED TO REAPPLY TO THE DEA AND THE TEXAS DEPARTMENT OF PUBLIC SAFETY TO OBTAIN AUTHORIZATION TO PRESCRIBE SCHEDULES II, IIN, III, IIIN, IV AND V; MAY NOT ADMINISTER, DISPENSE OR OTHERWISE PRESCRIBE BUT MAY ORDER SCHEDULES II, IIN AND IIIN CONTROLLED SUBSTANCES AS IS MEDICALLY NECESSARY FOR THE TREATMENT ON INPATIENTS IN A HOSPITAL SETTING WHERE HE HAS PRIVILEGES; SEPARATE FROM PATIENT RECORDS, HE SHALL MAINTAIN A FILE OF A COPY OF EVERY PRESCRIPTION WRITTEN FOR CONTROLLED SUBSTANCES WHICH SHALL BE AVAILABLE FOR REVIEW; MAY TELEPHONE TO A PHARMACY A PRESCRIPTION OR REFILL FOR SCHEDULES III, IV AND V CONTROLLED SUBSTANCES OR DRUGS WITH ADDICTIVE POTENTIAL OR POTENTIAL FOR ABUSE ONLY TO THE EXTENT NECESSARY TO MEET THE PATIENT'S IMMEDIATE NEEDS AND IN NO EVENT SHALL HE TELEPHONE A PRESCRIPTION OR REFILL FOR MORE THAN A THREE DAY SUPPLY; SHALL MAINTAIN A LOG FOR ALL PRESCRIPTIONS OR REFILLS TELEPHONED IN FOR CONTROLLED SUBSTANCES OR DRUGS WITH ADDICTIVE POTENTIAL OR POTENTIAL FOR ABUSE WHICH SHALL BE AVAILABLE FOR INSPECTION. ON 3/2/96 ORDER TERMINATED.

RAO, MOHAN KONAKONDRA MD, DATE OF BIRTH JANUARY 1, 1939 OF 3302 BILL OWENS PARKWAY, LONGVIEW, TX, WAS DISCIPLINED BY MEDICARE ON AUGUST 10, 1995
DISCIPLINARY ACTION: 60-MONTH EXCLUSION FROM THE MEDICARE AND/OR MEDICAID PROGRAM
OFFENSE: CRIMINAL CONVICTION OR PLEA OF GUILTY, NOLO CONTENDERE, OR NO CONTEST TO A CRIME

NOTES: CONVICTED OF A CRIME INVOLVING THE MEDICARE, MEDICAID, MATERNAL AND CHILD HEALTH SERVICES BLOCK GRANT OR BLOCK GRANTS TO STATES FOR SOCIAL SERVICES PROGRAMS.

RASKIN, MILTON MD, LICENSE NUMBER 0008865 OF 7908 PARKLAND STREET, EL PASO, TX, WAS DISCIPLINED BY GEORGIA ON FEBRUARY 8, 1990
DISCIPLINARY ACTION: NONRENEWAL OF LICENSE
OFFENSE: DISCIPLINARY ACTION BY ANOTHER STATE OR AGENCY

NOTES: DISCIPLINARY ACTION TAKEN BY MASSACHUSETTS.

RASKIN, MILTON MD, LICENSE NUMBER 00D4840 OF EL PASO, TX, WAS DISCIPLINED BY TEXAS ON JANUARY 6, 1995
DISCIPLINARY ACTION: SURRENDER OF LICENSE
OFFENSE: NONCOMPLIANCE WITH A PROFESSIONAL RULE

NOTES: ALLEGATIONS INCLUDE BILLING FOR SERVICES WITHOUT A DOCUMENTED INDICATION, BILLING FOR SERVICES WHICH THE RECORDS DO NOT INDICATE WERE PERFORMED, AND HAVING ENTERED INTO A CONTRACTUAL RELATIONSHIP WHICH WOULD CONSTITUTE A VIOLATION OF STATE STATUTES REGARDING ILLEGAL REMUNERATION AND/OR A VIOLATION OF THE CORPORATE PRACTICE OF MEDICINE PROHIBITION. SURRENDER IN LIEU OF FURTHER INVESTIGATION OR HEARING ON THE ALLEGATIONS. SHALL NOT PETITION FOR REINSTATEMENT.

RASKIN, MILTON MD OF 1891 LEE TREVINO STE #300, EL PASO, TX, WAS DISCIPLINED BY DEA ON MARCH 20, 1995
DISCIPLINARY ACTION: SURRENDER OF CONTROLLED SUBSTANCE LICENSE

NOTES: IN LIEU OF PUBLIC INTEREST REVOCATION.

RATLIFF, HUBERT WESLEY JR MD, LICENSE NUMBER 00D7662 OF PLANO, TX, WAS DISCIPLINED BY TEXAS ON MAY 11, 1995
DISCIPLINARY ACTION: 60-MONTH PROBATION; REQUIRED TO TAKE ADDITIONAL MEDICAL EDUCATION
OFFENSE: SUBSTANCE ABUSE

NOTES: ENGAGED IN THE INTEMPERATE USE OF ALCOHOL AND DRUGS; REPORTS SOBRIETY DATE OF 7/2/94; RECEIVED VOLUNTARY INPATIENT SUBSTANCE ABUSE TREATMENT IN TEXAS FROM 9/12/94 TO 10/11/94 AND VOLUNTARILY ADMITTED HIMSELF INTO A RESIDENTIAL SUBSTANCE ABUSE TREATMENT FACILITY IN MISSISSIPPI IN 11/94; REPORTS COMPLETING PROGRAM AND BEING DISCHARGED ON 3/10/95; ENTERED AN AFTERCARE RECOVERY CONTRACT; UNDER THE CARE OF A CERTIFIED ADDICTION MEDICINE SPECIALIST FOR CONTINUED SUBSTANCE ABUSE TREATMENT; REPORTS ATTENDING AN AVERAGE OF FOUR AA MEETINGS PER WEEK; DOES NOT ADMIT HE VIOLATED THE MEDICAL PRACTICE ACT, BUT AGREES TO COMPLY WITH THE CONDITIONS. SUSPENSION STAYED. PROBATION WITH TERMS: SHALL ABSTAIN FROM THE CONSUMPTION OF ALCOHOL/DRUGS IN ANY FORM UNLESS PRESCRIBED BY ANOTHER PHYSICIAN FOR A LEGITIMATE AND THERAPEUTIC PURPOSE; SHALL SUBMIT HIMSELF FOR APPROPRIATE EXAMS INCLUDING DRUG OR ALCOHOL SCREENS; SHALL CONTINUE TO RECEIVE CARE AND TREATMENT NO LESS THAN TWICE A WEEK FROM HIS ADDICTION PHYSICIAN WHO WILL SUBMIT QUARTERLY REPORTS; SHALL CONTINUE TO PARTICIPATE IN AA'S PROGRAM NOT LESS THAN FIVE TIMES A WEEK WITH QUARTERLY REPORTS TO THE BOARD; SHALL PARTICIPATE IN THE ACTIVITIES OF AN IMPAIRED PHYSICIAN'S GROUP AND ATTEND WEEKLY MEETINGS WITH QUARTERLY REPORTS; SHALL COMPLY WITH THE TERMS OF HIS CONTINUING CARE CONTRACT AND SHALL PROVIDE QUARTERLY REPORTS; SHALL COMPLY WITH TERMS OF ANY CONTRACT ENTERED INTO FOR HOSPITAL PRIVILEGES AND SHALL INFORM BOARD OF ANY DISCIPLINE; SHALL OBTAIN AT LEAST 50 HOURS PER YEAR OF CONTINUING MEDICAL EDUCATION; SHALL APPEAR BEFORE BOARD AT LEAST TWICE A YEAR OR AT BOARD REQUEST; SHALL COOPERATE WITH THE BOARD IN VERIFYING COMPLIANCE INCLUDING PROVIDING COPIES OF MEDICAL RELEASES OR PEER REVIEW RECORDS UPON REQUEST; SHALL GIVE A COPY OF THIS ORDER TO ANY HEALTH CARE ENTITY WHERE HE HAS PRIVILEGES; SHALL PROVIDE A COPY OF THE ORDER TO ANYONE REQUESTING IT WITHIN 10 DAYS; TIME PERIOD OUT OF TEXAS DOES NOT COUNT TOWARD PROBATION; SHALL INFORM BOARD OF CHANGE OF ADDRESS WITHIN 10 DAYS OR IF HE LEAVES THE STATE. SHALL NOT SEEK MODIFICATION FOR ONE YEAR. ON 5/15/96 ORDER MODIFIED SUCH THAT THE FREQUENCY OF MEETINGS WITH TREATING PHYSICIAN REDUCED TO NO LESS THAN TWICE A MONTH; AND WITH AA TO AT LEAST THREE TIMES A WEEK. ON 8/22/98 ORDER TERMINATED.

RAYMOND, DENNIS MICHAEL MD, LICENSE NUMBER G8362 OF DALLAS, TX, WAS DISCIPLINED BY TEXAS ON AUGUST 9, 1997
DISCIPLINARY ACTION: 60-MONTH RESTRICTION PLACED ON LICENSE; REQUIRED TO TAKE ADDITIONAL MEDICAL EDUCATION
OFFENSE: SEXUAL ABUSE OF OR SEXUAL MISCONDUCT WITH A PATIENT

NOTES: DURING 1993-1994 HE WAS TREATING AN ADULT FEMALE PSYCHIATRIC PATIENT WITH THERAPY; DURING 1994 HE PERFORMED PHYSICAL EXAMINATIONS ON HER AT HER REQUEST WHICH ARE NOT USUALLY PERFORMED BY A PSYCHIATRIST IN AN INPATIENT SETTING; DURING 1990-1994 HE ENGAGED IN SELF-DISCLOSURE OF PERSONAL INFORMATION TO A PATIENT AND PHYSICAL CONTACT WITH PATIENTS, SUCH AS HUGGING; DURING 1990-1994 HE FAILED TO ADEQUATELY DOCUMENT HIS CARE AND TREATMENT OF VARIOUS PATIENTS. LICENSE LIMITED AS FOLLOWS: SHALL HAVE A FEMALE CHAPERONE PRESENT WHEN EXAMINING FEMALE PATIENTS; SHALL MAINTAIN ADEQUATE MEDICAL RECORDS WHICH SHALL BE AVAILABLE FOR REVIEW; SHALL ATTEND AT LEAST 50 HOURS PER YEAR OF CONTINUING MEDICAL EDUCATION; SHALL COOPERATE WITH THE BOARD IN VERIFYING COMPLIANCE; SHALL GIVE A COPY OF THIS ORDER TO ANY HEALTH CARE ENTITY WHERE HE HAS PRIVILEGES; TIME SPENT OUT OF TEXAS DOES NOT COUNT TOWARD RESTRICTION; SHALL INFORM THE BOARD OF CHANGE OF ADDRESS WITHIN 10 DAYS OR IF HE LEAVES THE STATE; SHALL NOT SEEK MODIFICATION FOR ONE YEAR.

READING, WILLIAM H MD, LICENSE NUMBER 00G8363 OF VICTORIA, TX, WAS DISCIPLINED BY TEXAS ON AUGUST 20, 1992
DISCIPLINARY ACTION: 60-MONTH PROBATION
OFFENSE: SUBSTANDARD CARE, INCOMPETENCE OR NEGLIGENCE

NOTES: UNPROFESSIONAL OR DISHONORABLE CONDUCT THAT IS LIKELY TO DECEIVE, DEFRAUD OR INJURE THE PUBLIC; NONTHERAPEUTIC PRESCRIBING; OVERCHARGING OR OVERTREATING PATIENTS; FAILURE TO SUPERVISE ADEQUATELY THE ACTIVITIES OF THOSE ACTING UNDER THE SUPERVISION OF THE PHYSICIAN; PROFESSIONAL FAILURE TO PRACTICE MEDICINE IN AN ACCEPTABLE MANNER CONSISTENT WITH PUBLIC HEALTH AND WELFARE. LICENSE SUSPENDED, SUSPENSION STAYED. PROBATION UNDER TERMS AND CONDITIONS.

RECKENTHALER, KARL J MD, DATE OF BIRTH JANUARY 29, 1931, LICENSE NUMBER 0010766 OF GRANT MEMORIAL HOSPITAL, PETERSBURG, WV, WAS DISCIPLINED BY WEST VIRGINIA ON JANUARY 24, 1994
DISCIPLINARY ACTION: FINE; REPRIMAND
OFFENSE: PROFESSIONAL MISCONDUCT

NOTES: PERMITTED FABRICATION OF THE MINUTES OF THE MEETINGS OF THE RADIATION SAFETY COMMITTEE AT GRANT MEMORIAL HOSPITAL AND FAILED TO EXERCISE HIS RESPONSIBILITY AS RADIATION SAFETY OFFICER AND HOLD MEETINGS. ASSESSED A FINE OF $1,000 AND WITHIN FIVE DAYS MUST PROVIDE A COPY OF THIS ORDER TO ANY HEALTH CARE FACILITY WHERE HE HAS PRIVILEGES.

RECKENTHALER, KARL J MD, LICENSE NUMBER 00C7103 OF PETERSBURG, WV, WAS DISCIPLINED BY TEXAS ON JANUARY 6, 1995
DISCIPLINARY ACTION: SURRENDER OF LICENSE

NOTES: IN LIEU OF FURTHER INVESTIGATION OR A HEARING. SHALL NOT PETITION FOR REINSTATEMENT.

REDALEN, RICK R MD, LICENSE NUMBER 0002368, WAS DISCIPLINED BY HAWAII ON OCTOBER 20, 1993
DISCIPLINARY ACTION: 3-MONTH LICENSE SUSPENSION

REDALEN, RICK R DR, LICENSE NUMBER 0018790, WAS DISCIPLINED BY MINNESOTA ON MARCH 12, 1994

NOTES: STAYED SUSPENSION.

REDALEN, RICK RAY MD, DATE OF BIRTH MARCH 14, 1943, LICENSE NUMBER 0021025 OF ANKENY, IA, WAS DISCIPLINED BY IOWA ON OCTOBER 31, 1990
DISCIPLINARY ACTION: 24-MONTH PROBATION; FINE

NOTES: $1000 FINE. PROBATION TERMINATED ON 10/8/92; LICENSE RESTORED TO FULL PRIVILEGES.

REDALEN, RICK RAY MD, DATE OF BIRTH MARCH 14, 1943, LICENSE NUMBER 0021025 OF MONROE, LA, WAS DISCIPLINED BY IOWA ON MARCH 2, 1995
DISCIPLINARY ACTION: LICENSE REVOCATION
OFFENSE: NONCOMPLIANCE WITH A PROFESSIONAL RULE

NOTES: FAILED TO REPORT A MEDICAL MALPRACTICE JUDGMENT WHICH HAD BEEN RENDERED AGAINST HIM IN DUBUQUE COUNTY, IOWA, IN SEPTEMBER 1991.

REDALEN, RICK RAY MD OF BEDFORD, TX, WAS DISCIPLINED BY LOUISIANA ON OCTOBER 6, 1995
DISCIPLINARY ACTION: LICENSE REVOCATION
OFFENSE: DISCIPLINARY ACTION BY ANOTHER STATE OR AGENCY

NOTES: ACTION IN IOWA; RECURRING ABUSE OF ALCOHOL AND DRUGS WHICH AFFECT THE CENTRAL NERVOUS SYSTEM; DECEIT IN OBTAINING LICENSING; AND PROVIDING FALSE INFORMATION TO THE BOARD.

REDDIX-NORMAN, IRANCE E MD, DATE OF BIRTH OCTOBER 4, 1960 OF 1246 KINGS CREEK TRAIL, MISSOURI CITY, TX, WAS DISCIPLINED BY MEDICARE ON AUGUST 13, 1993
DISCIPLINARY ACTION: EXCLUSION FROM THE MEDICARE AND/OR MEDICAID PROGRAM
OFFENSE: NONCOMPLIANCE WITH A PROFESSIONAL RULE

NOTES: DEFAULTED ON HEALTH EDUCATION ASSISTANCE LOAN. REINSTATED ON 9/13/96.

REDDY, GADDUM J M MD OF ALEXANDRIA, LA, WAS DISCIPLINED BY LOUISIANA ON AUGUST 23, 1990
DISCIPLINARY ACTION: REQUIRED TO TAKE ADDITIONAL MEDICAL EDUCATION; 12-MONTH MONITORING OF PHYSICIAN PERFORMANCE
OFFENSE: SUBSTANDARD CARE, INCOMPETENCE OR NEGLIGENCE

NOTES: SUSPECTED CONTINUING OR RECURRING MEDICAL PRACTICE FAILING TO SATISFY PREVAILING AND USUALLY ACCEPTED STANDARDS OF PRACTICE. MUST PAY $1500 COSTS, COMPLETE CONTINUING MEDICAL EDUCATION, AND HAVE PRACTICE SUPERVISED FOR 12 MONTHS BY BOARD APPROVED PHYSICIAN.

REDDY, GADDUM J M MD, LICENSE NUMBER 0008168 OF TX, WAS DISCIPLINED BY ALABAMA ON JANUARY 23, 1991
DISCIPLINARY ACTION: PROBATION
OFFENSE: DISCIPLINARY ACTION BY ANOTHER STATE OR AGENCY

NOTES: LOUISIANA BOARD DISCIPLINED LICENSE BASED ON QUALITY OF CARE ISSUES. ON 10/12/92 PROBATION TERMINATED AFTER FINDING THAT LOUISIANA LICENSE HAD BEEN REINSTATED TO FULL, UNRESTRICTED STATUS AND ALL TERMS AND CONDITIONS HAD BEEN COMPLIED WITH.

REDDY, KALPANA Y MD, LICENSE NUMBER 00H3149 OF SHOREVIEW, MN, WAS DISCIPLINED BY TEXAS ON MARCH 7, 1992
DISCIPLINARY ACTION: LICENSE REVOCATION
OFFENSE: DISCIPLINARY ACTION BY ANOTHER STATE OR AGENCY

NOTES: SEVERAL VIOLATIONS OF THE MEDICAL PRACTICE ACT, INCLUDING DISCIPLINARY ACTION TAKEN BY A PEER REVIEW ENTITY.

REDELFS, JOHN W MD, LICENSE NUMBER C016552 OF SAN JOSE, CA, WAS DISCIPLINED BY CALIFORNIA ON JUNE 25, 1991
DISCIPLINARY ACTION: SURRENDER OF LICENSE

NOTES: VOLUNTARY SURRENDER WHILE CHARGES PENDING.

REDELFS, JOHN WRIGHT MD, LICENSE NUMBER 00C4867 OF SAN JOSE, CA, WAS DISCIPLINED BY TEXAS ON JANUARY 24, 1992
DISCIPLINARY ACTION: SURRENDER OF LICENSE

NOTES: LICENSE VOLUNTARILY SURRENDERED IN LIEU OF FURTHER DISCIPLINARY ACTION.

REECE, DOUGLAS L DO, DATE OF BIRTH JANUARY 26, 1942, LICENSE NUMBER 00E1398 OF LUBBOCK, TX, WAS DISCIPLINED BY TEXAS ON OCTOBER 26, 1990
DISCIPLINARY ACTION: 84-MONTH PROBATION; RESTRICTION PLACED ON LICENSE

NOTES: SUSPENSION STAYED; MUST LIVE AND PRACTICE IN LUBBOCK COUNTY UNLESS PRACTICE RELOCATION APPROVED BY BOARD; COMPLETE PRECEPTORSHIP RELATED TO DIAGNOSIS AND TREATMENT OF PATIENTS IN FAMILY PRACTICE, SPECIFICALLY INCLUDING PEDIATRICS; OBTAIN CONTINUING MEDICAL EDUCATION; SUBJECT TO MONITORING BY MEANS OF RETROSPECTIVE CHART REVIEW AND PERSONAL OBSERVATION; MUST NOT PRESCRIBE, ADMINISTER, OR DISPENSE DRUG WITH POTENTIAL OF ABUSE TO PERSON UNTIL SATISFIED OF LEGITIMATE MEDICAL AND THERAPEUTIC NEED, AFTER MEDICAL HISTORY AND EXAMINATION; CONDUCT ADEQUATE FOLLOW-UP EXAMINATION; MAINTAIN COPY OF PRESCRIPTIONS SEPARATE FROM PATIENTS' MEDICAL CHARTS AND MAKE COPIES AVAILABLE FOR INSPECTION BY PHYSICIANS MONITORING PRACTICE OR BY BOARD REPRESENTATIVES; NOT TREAT PATIENTS FOR WEIGHT CONTROL OR OBESITY WITH CONTROLLED SUBSTANCES OR OVER-THE-COUNTER DRUGS; NOT TREAT OBSTETRICAL PATIENTS; CONTINUE TO SEEK CARE FROM PSYCHOLOGIST OR PSYCHIATRIST AND FOLLOW ANY RECOMMENDATIONS; APPEAR BEFORE BOARD TWICE YEARLY.

REECE, DOUGLAS L DO, DATE OF BIRTH JANUARY 26, 1942 OF 2901 AVENUE Q, LUBBOCK, TX, WAS DISCIPLINED BY MEDICARE ON FEBRUARY 1, 1993
DISCIPLINARY ACTION: 60-MONTH EXCLUSION FROM THE MEDICARE AND/OR MEDICAID PROGRAM
OFFENSE: CRIMINAL CONVICTION OR PLEA OF GUILTY, NOLO CONTENDERE, OR NO CONTEST TO A CRIME

NOTES: CONVICTED AND SENTENCED TO 1O YEARS

PROBATION FOR MAKING A FALSE STATEMENT TO MEDICAID. REINSTATED ON 6/17/98.

REECE, DOUGLAS L DO, DATE OF BIRTH JANUARY 26, 1942, LICENSE NUMBER 00E1398 OF LUBBOCK, TX, WAS DISCIPLINED BY TEXAS ON OCTOBER 1, 1993
DISCIPLINARY ACTION: EMERGENCY SUSPENSION
OFFENSE: PHYSICAL OR MENTAL ILLNESS INHIBITING THE ABILITY TO PRACTICE WITH SKILL AND SAFETY

NOTES: AT A 9/17/93 MEETING BEFORE BOARD, PRESENTATION AND RESPONSE DEMONSTRATED A MARKED LACK OF CLARITY IN HIS MENTAL PROCESS; UNDERWENT A PSYCHIATRIC EVALUATION ON 9/23/93 WHICH REPORTED THAT HE DEMONSTRATED "COGNITIVE SLIPPAGE" AND THAT "JUDGMENT ABILITY AND INSIGHT SEEMED QUESTIONABLE."

REECE, DOUGLAS L DO OF 2901 AVENUE Q, LUBBOCK, TX, WAS DISCIPLINED BY DEA ON NOVEMBER 29, 1993
DISCIPLINARY ACTION: SURRENDER OF CONTROLLED SUBSTANCE LICENSE
OFFENSE: DISCIPLINARY ACTION BY ANOTHER STATE OR AGENCY

REECE, DOUGLAS L DO, DATE OF BIRTH JANUARY 26, 1942, LICENSE NUMBER 00E1398 OF LUBBOCK, TX, WAS DISCIPLINED BY TEXAS ON MARCH 5, 1994
DISCIPLINARY ACTION: 60-MONTH PROBATION; RESTRICTION PLACED ON LICENSE
OFFENSE: CRIMINAL CONVICTION OR PLEA OF GUILTY, NOLO CONTENDERE, OR NO CONTEST TO A CRIME

NOTES: ON 5/5/92 PLED GUILTY TO TAMPERING WITH GOVERNMENT RECORDS AND WAS SENTENCED TO 10 YEARS PROBATION UNDER AN ORDER FOR DEFERRED ADJUDICATION; ON 1/12/93 WAS EXCLUDED FROM MEDICARE PROGRAM FOR FIVE YEARS; APPEARED BEFORE BOARD IN SEPTEMBER AND EXHIBITED BEHAVIORS WHICH CAUSED CONCERN REGARDING HIS MENTAL CONDITION; ON 10/15/93 HE WAS EVALUATED BY A BOARD APPROVED PSYCHIATRIST WHO FELT HE COULD PRACTICE IN A STRUCTURED SUPERVISED SETTING. SUSPENSION STAYED. CONDITIONS OF PROBATION: PRACTICE RESTRICTED TO A BOARD APPROVED INSTITUTIONAL OR CLINICAL SETTING WITH SUPERVISOR MAKING QUARTERLY REPORTS; SHALL SUBMIT HIMSELF FOR EVALUATION AND TREATMENT TO A BOARD APPROVED PSYCHIATRIST WITH REPORTS; SHALL APPEAR BEFORE THE BOARD ONCE A YEAR; SHALL GIVE A COPY OF THIS ORDER TO ANY HEALTH CARE ENTITY WHERE HE HAS PRIVILEGES; SHALL COOPERATE WITH THE BOARD IN VERIFYING COMPLIANCE; SHALL INFORM BOARD OF CHANGE OF ADDRESS WITHIN 10 DAYS OR IF LEAVING THE STATE; TIME SPENT OUT OF TEXAS DOES NOT COUNT TOWARD PROBATION. SHALL NOT SEEK MODIFICATION FOR ONE YEAR. ON 5/10/97 PETITION TO TERMINATE ORDER DENIED; ORDER MODIFIED RESTRICTING HIS PRACTICE TO THAT OF A GROUP, INSTITUTIONAL, CLINICAL OR SUPERVISED SETTING; AND DELETING REQUIREMENT TO OBTAIN A BOARD-APPROVED TREATING PHYSICIAN. ON 4/4/98 ORDER TERMINATED.

REES, SEARLE B MD, LICENSE NUMBER 0026772 OF ROUTE 7, BOX 160, GILMER, TX, WAS DISCIPLINED BY MASSACHUSETTS ON NOVEMBER 9, 1994
DISCIPLINARY ACTION: NONRENEWAL OF LICENSE
OFFENSE: DISCIPLINARY ACTION BY ANOTHER STATE OR AGENCY

NOTES: DISCIPLINE BY TEXAS; CONTROLLED SUBSTANCE VIOLATION; FAILURE TO RESPOND TO BOARD. REVOCATION OF INCHOATE RIGHT TO RENEW LICENSE.

REES, SEARLE BEAUFORT MD, DATE OF BIRTH OCTOBER 7, 1927, LICENSE NUMBER 00G4434 OF 300 WEST UPSHUR STREET, GLADEWATER, TX, WAS DISCIPLINED BY TEXAS ON JANUARY 29, 1993
DISCIPLINARY ACTION: 60-MONTH PROBATION; RESTRICTION PLACED ON LICENSE
OFFENSE: OVERPRESCRIBING OR MISPRESCRIBING DRUGS

NOTES: PRESCRIBED FASTIN FOR SIX MONTHS AS THE SOLE WEIGHT CONTROL MEASURE FOR TWO PATIENTS; SUCH PRESCRIBING IS NONTHERAPEUTIC IN NATURE IN THE MANNER PRESCRIBED. 5 YEAR SUSPENSION STAYED. CONDITIONS OF PROBATION: SHALL APPEAR BEFORE THE BOARD TWICE A YEAR; SHALL ATTEND AT LEAST 50 HOURS PER YEAR OF CONTINUING MEDICAL EDUCATION INCLUDING AT LEAST 10 HOURS IN WEIGHT LOSS MANAGEMENT THE FIRST YEAR; SHALL NOT TREAT ANY PATIENT FOR WEIGHT CONTROL WITH ANY DRUGS; SHALL CONTINUE TO RECEIVE TREATMENT FROM HIS PRESENT DOCTOR; SHALL NOT TREAT OR OTHERWISE SERVE AS PHYSICIAN, PRESCRIBE, DISPENSE OR ADMINISTER DRUGS THAT MAY BE SUBJECT TO ABUSE TO HIMSELF OR ANY MEMBER OF HIS FAMILY; SHALL GIVE A COPY OF THIS ORDER TO ANY HEALTH CARE ENTITY WHERE HE HAS PRIVILEGES; SHALL COOPERATE WITH THE BOARD IN VERIFYING COMPLIANCE; SHALL NOTIFY BOARD OF CHANGE OF ADDRESS WITHIN 10 DAYS OR IF HE LEAVES THE STATE; TIME SPENT OUT OF TEXAS DOES NOT COUNT TOWARD PROBATION. SHALL NOT SEEK MODIFICATION FOR 1 YEAR.

REES, SEARLE BEAUFORT MD, DATE OF BIRTH OCTOBER 7, 1927, LICENSE NUMBER 00G4434 OF ROUTE 7 BOX 160, GILMER, TX, WAS DISCIPLINED BY TEXAS ON AUGUST 6, 1993
DISCIPLINARY ACTION: EMERGENCY SUSPENSION
OFFENSE: OVERPRESCRIBING OR MISPRESCRIBING DRUGS

NOTES: ON 1/29/93 ENTERED INTO AGREEMENT WITH BOARD RESULTING IN A STAYED SUSPENSION WITH FIVE YEAR PROBATION BASED ON NON-THERAPEUTIC PRESCRIBING OF FASTIN AS THE SOLE WEIGHT CONTROL MEASURE FOR TWO PATIENTS; BETWEEN 11/92 AND 3/93 AN UNDERCOVER NARCOTICS AGENT MADE SEVEN BUYS FROM HIM USING A FICTITIOUS PATIENT NAME; ON 2/26/93 DEA AGENTS RECEIVED PRESCRIPTIONS FOR TALWIN, VALIUM AND AXOTAL WITH NO PHYSICAL EXAMS AND NO MEDICAL NEED OR JUSTIFICATION; HE AND HIS WIFE WERE ARRESTED ON 3/16/93 FOR POSSESSION WITH INTENT TO DISTRIBUTE AND DISTRIBUTION OF SCHEDULE II, III AND IV CONTROLLED SUBSTANCES; SURRENDERED DEA AND TEXAS CONTROLLED SUBSTANCES REGISTRATIONS ON 3/29/93; HAS CONTINUED TO PRESCRIBE (OVER 80 PRESCRIPTIONS) SINCE THIS SURRENDER; ONE OF HIS PATIENTS OVERDOSED ON VALIUM AND ALCOHOL 5 DAYS AFTER HE PRESCRIBED/DISPENSED 100 TABLETS OF DEMEROL. HE SUFFERS FROM DEPRESSION, IS TAKING LITHIUM AND IS UNDER MEDICAL CARE.

REES, SEARLE BEAUFORT MD, DATE OF BIRTH OCTOBER 7, 1927, LICENSE NUMBER 00G4434 OF ROUTE 7 BOX 160, GILMER, TX, WAS DISCIPLINED BY TEXAS ON AUGUST 20, 1993
DISCIPLINARY ACTION: SURRENDER OF LICENSE
OFFENSE: PRACTICING WITHOUT A VALID CONTROLLED SUBSTANCE LICENSE

NOTES: CONTINUED TO PRESCRIBE CONTROLLED

SUBSTANCES TO NUMEROUS PATIENTS AFTER HE HAD SURRENDERED CONTROLLED SUBSTANCES REGISTRATION ON 3/29/93. SURRENDER IN LIEU OF FURTHER PROCEEDINGS.

REINER, MICHAEL DAVID MD, LICENSE NUMBER 0026184 OF HOUSTON, TX, WAS DISCIPLINED BY COLORADO ON OCTOBER 10, 1990
DISCIPLINARY ACTION: PROBATION
NOTES: REINSTATEMENT SOUGHT FROM SUSPENSION ORDER ENTERED ON 12/5/88. REINSTATEMENT SUBJECT TO PROBATIONARY TERMS AND CONDITIONS.

REISCHMANN, EDDY DO, LICENSE NUMBER 00D8603 OF PORTER, TX, WAS DISCIPLINED BY TEXAS ON MARCH 6, 1992
DISCIPLINARY ACTION: 60-MONTH PROBATION
OFFENSE: OVERPRESCRIBING OR MISPRESCRIBING DRUGS
NOTES: SEVERAL VIOLATIONS OF THE MEDICAL PRACTICE ACT, INCLUDING NONTHERAPEUTIC PRESCRIBING. LICENSE SUSPENDED, SUSPENSION STAYED; PROBATION UNDER TERMS AND CONDITIONS.

REISCHMANN, EDDY DO, LICENSE NUMBER 00D8603 OF PORTER, TX, WAS DISCIPLINED BY TEXAS ON NOVEMBER 14, 1992
DISCIPLINARY ACTION: LICENSE SUSPENSION
OFFENSE: FAILURE TO COMPLY WITH PREVIOUS BOARD ORDER
NOTES: FAILED TO PASS THE SPEX EXAMINATION AS REQUIRED BY THE PREVIOUS BOARD ORDER.

RENSHAW, RALPH R JR MD, LICENSE NUMBER C5846 OF SHERMAN, TX, WAS DISCIPLINED BY TEXAS ON AUGUST 28, 1999
DISCIPLINARY ACTION: 36-MONTH PROBATION; RESTRICTION PLACED ON LICENSE
OFFENSE: SUBSTANDARD CARE, INCOMPETENCE OR NEGLIGENCE
NOTES: SIX PATIENTS FILED LAWSUITS AGAINST HIM ALLEGING SUBSTANDARD CARE: ON 5/29/95 DURING SURGERY, A PATIENT SUFFERED SEVERE BURNS FROM THE INSIDE OUT OF HER LOWER RIGHT LEG WITH SUBSEQUENT INFECTION; THE CASE WAS NON-SUITED WITH NO PAYMENT MADE TO THE PATIENT; IN 7/92 PATIENT FILED A LAWSUIT ALLEGING THAT HE WAS NEGLIGENT IN IMPROPERLY PLACING THE NEEDLE FOR A NERVE BLOCK BY PLACING IT THROUGH THE PATIENT'S LUNG PLEURA AND FAILING TO DIAGNOSE PROPERLY AND TREAT THE PNEUMOTHORAX FOLLOWING THE NERVE BLOCK; THE CASE WAS SETTLED FOR $10,000; ON 7/9/93 AFTER PERFORMING A HIP REPLACEMENT, THE PATIENT NOTICED A DROP FOOT AND FILED A LAWSUIT ALLEGING THAT HE NEGLIGENTLY DAMAGED HER NERVES; ON 9/23/94 A PATIENT FILED A LAWSUIT ALLEGING THAT HE NEGLIGENTLY OPERATED AND FUSED THE WRONG LEVEL OF PATIENT'S NECK; THE CASE WAS SETTLED FOR $40,000; ON 3/4/94 HE WAS UNASSISTED BY A GENERAL/VASCULAR SURGEON DURING A PROCEDURE IN WHICH HE TORE A VEIN; HE REPORTEDLY ATTEMPTED TO STOP THE BLEEDING WITH THE USE OF LIGATURE CLIPS, WHICH CAUSED FURTHER INJURY AND BLEEDING; THE PATIENT LOST 4 UNITS OF BLOOD DURING THE ABORTED PROCEDURE AND WITHIN A FEW DAYS DEVELOPED DEEP VEIN THROMBOSIS; THE PATIENT FILED A LAWSUIT WHICH WAS SETTLED FOR $100,000; ON 2/11/89 A PATIENT SUED ALLEGING DR. RENSHAW WAS NEGLIGENT IN FAILING TO OBTAIN ADEQUATE CLOSED REDUCTION OF A FRACTURE; THE CASE WAS SETTLED FOR $35,000; THE DOCTOR DENIES THAT HIS CARE WAS BELOW STANDARD. PUBLIC REPRIMAND AND SUSPENSION STAYED FOR PROBATION WITH FOLLOWING TERMS AND CONDITIONS: SHALL NOT ACCEPT EMERGENCY ROOM CALL EFFECTIVE IMMEDIATELY; SHALL NOT PRACTICE SPINAL SURGERY EFFECTIVE 9/1/99; SHALL PHASE OUT ALL OTHER INPATIENT SURGERY BY 2/28/00; SHALL ONLY PERFORM OUTPATIENT SURGERY AFTER 2/28/00; SHALL ATTEND AT LEAST 50 HOURS OF CONTINUING MEDICAL EDUCATION WITH 1 COURSE IN THE AREA OF RISK MANAGEMENT; SHALL MAINTAIN ADEQUATE MEDICAL RECORDS WHICH SHALL BE AVAILABLE FOR REVIEW; SHALL COOPERATE WITH THE BOARD IN VERIFYING COMPLIANCE; SHALL APPEAR BEFORE THE BOARD AT LEAST ONCE A YEAR; TIME SPENT OUT OF TEXAS DOES NOT COUNT TOWARD PROBATION; SHALL INFORM THE BOARD OF CHANGE OF ADDRESS WITHIN 10 DAYS OR IF HE LEAVES THE STATE; SHALL NOT SEEK MODIFICATION FOR ONE YEAR.

RESTREPO, CHRISTIAN MD OF 5300 SAN JACINT #100, HOUSTON, TX, WAS DISCIPLINED BY DEA ON MARCH 29, 1996
DISCIPLINARY ACTION: SURRENDER OF CONTROLLED SUBSTANCE LICENSE
NOTES: IN LIEU OF PUBLIC INTEREST REVOCATION.

RETTIG, JEFFREY D DO, LICENSE NUMBER H4845 OF GROESBECK, TX, WAS DISCIPLINED BY TEXAS ON NOVEMBER 22, 1997
DISCIPLINARY ACTION: FINE
OFFENSE: PROFESSIONAL MISCONDUCT
NOTES: FROM 11/96 THROUGH AT LEAST 7/97 AIDED AND ABETTED THE UNLICENSED PRACTICE OF A PHYSICIAN ASSISTANT IN HIS OFFICE WHO SAW PATIENTS INDEPENDENTLY, MADE DIAGNOSES AND PROVIDED TREATMENT INCLUDING MEDICATIONS TO PATIENTS. LICENSE LIMITED AS FOLLOWS: $5,000 FINE TO BE PAID WITHIN 3 MONTHS; WITHIN 3 MONTHS SHALL TAKE AND PASS THE MEDICAL JURISPRUDENCE EXAM; SHALL COOPERATE WITH THE BOARD IN VERIFYING COMPLIANCE; TIME SPENT OUT OF TEXAS DOES NOT COUNT TOWARD RESTRICTION; SHALL INFORM THE BOARD OF CHANGE OF ADDRESS WITHIN 10 DAYS OR IF HE LEAVES THE STATE.

REYES, LUCIO A MD, DATE OF BIRTH APRIL 6, 1962 OF 4433 N STANTON STREET, #T16, EL PASO, TX, WAS DISCIPLINED BY MEDICARE ON MAY 4, 1995
DISCIPLINARY ACTION: 60-MONTH EXCLUSION FROM THE MEDICARE AND/OR MEDICAID PROGRAM
OFFENSE: CRIMINAL CONVICTION OR PLEA OF GUILTY, NOLO CONTENDERE, OR NO CONTEST TO A CRIME
NOTES: CONVICTED OF A CRIME RELATED TO PATIENT ABUSE OR NEGLECT.

REYES, LUCIO ARTURO MD, DATE OF BIRTH APRIL 6, 1912, LICENSE NUMBER 00J0787 OF CONROE, TX, WAS DISCIPLINED BY TEXAS ON OCTOBER 9, 1992
DISCIPLINARY ACTION: EMERGENCY SUSPENSION
OFFENSE: SUBSTANDARD CARE, INCOMPETENCE OR NEGLIGENCE
NOTES: UNPROFESSIONAL OR DISHONORABLE CONDUCT THAT IS LIKELY TO DECEIVE, DEFRAUD OR INJURE THE PUBLIC; AND PROFESSIONAL FAILURE TO PRACTICE MEDICINE IN AN ACCEPTABLE MANNER CONSISTENT WITH PUBLIC HEALTH AND WELFARE. LICENSE TEMPORARILY SUSPENDED PENDING A HEARING.

REYES, LUCIO ARTURO MD, DATE OF BIRTH APRIL 6, 1962, LICENSE NUMBER 00J0787 OF 1726 HAZELWOOD, CONROE, TX, WAS

DISCIPLINED BY TEXAS ON SEPTEMBER 30, 1994
DISCIPLINARY ACTION: LICENSE REVOCATION
OFFENSE: CRIMINAL CONVICTION OR PLEA OF GUILTY, NOLO CONTENDERE, OR NO CONTEST TO A CRIME

NOTES: ON 6/14/94 WAS CONVICTED IN THE DISTRICT COURT OF WALKER COUNTY, TEXAS OF SEXUAL ASSAULT COMMITTED ON 8/17/92 A SECOND DEGREE FELONY AND ATTEMPTED SEXUAL ASSAULT COMMITTED ON 9/19/92 A THIRD DEGREE FELONY; HE ENTERED GUILTY PLEAS TO BOTH OFFENSES.

REYNOLDS, JARRELL PAUL MD, LICENSE NUMBER 00H0755 OF COLEMAN, TX, WAS DISCIPLINED BY TEXAS ON MARCH 2, 1996
DISCIPLINARY ACTION: 60-MONTH PROBATION; RESTRICTION PLACED ON CONTROLLED SUBSTANCE LICENSE
OFFENSE: SUBSTANCE ABUSE

NOTES: IN THE FALL OF 1994 EVALUATED FOR ONE DAY FOR HYDROCODONE DEPENDENCE; FROM 1/11/95 UNTIL 1/18/95 RECEIVED INPATIENT TREATMENT AND FROM 1/18/95 UNTIL 2/04/95 HAD A PARTIAL ADMISSION; RELAPSED APPROXIMATELY JUNE/JULY 1995 AND BEGAN ABUSING DRUGS AGAIN; RECEIVED INPATIENT TREATMENT FROM 10/1/95 THROUGH 1/22/96; REPORTS ATTENDING AA FIVE TIMES A WEEK AND COUNSELING TWO TIMES PER WEEK; AND ENTERED INTO A CONTINUING CARE CONTRACT. SUSPENSION STAYED TO PROBATION UNDER TERMS AND CONDITIONS: SHALL NOT ACCEPT OR POSSESS SAMPLES OF CONTROLLED SUBSTANCES OR DANGEROUS DRUGS WITH ADDICTIVE POTENTIAL OR POTENTIAL FOR ABUSE AND SHALL IMMEDIATELY DESTROY HIS SAMPLES; WITHIN ONE YEAR SHALL SUCCESSFULLY COMPLETE AN ADVANCED CARDIAC LIFE SUPPORT COURSE (ACLS) AND AN ADVANCED TRAUMA LIFE SUPPORT COURSE (ATLS) AND OBTAIN CERTIFICATION FOR BOTH; SHALL ABSTAIN FROM THE CONSUMPTION OF ALCOHOL/DRUGS IN ANY FORM UNLESS PRESCRIBED BY ANOTHER PHYSICIAN FOR A LEGITIMATE AND THERAPEUTIC PURPOSE; SHALL SUBMIT HIMSELF FOR APPROPRIATE EXAMS INCLUDING DRUG OR ALCOHOL SCREENS; SHALL SUBMIT HIMSELF FOR EVALUATION AND TREATMENT TO A BOARD APPROVED PSYCHIATRIST WHO HE SHALL SEE AT LEAST ONCE A MONTH AND WHO SHALL SUBMIT REPORTS TO THE BOARD; SHALL PARTICIPATE IN AA'S PROGRAMS INITIALLY CONSISTING OF 90 MEETINGS IN 90 DAYS AND THEN NOT LESS THAN FIVE TIMES A WEEK FOR THE FIRST SIX MONTHS AND THEREAFTER THREE TIMES A WEEK WITH QUARTERLY REPORTS; SHALL MAINTAIN A DIARY OF HIS ACTIVITIES IN AA WHICH HE SHALL PROVIDE TO THE BOARD UPON REQUEST; SHALL PARTICIPATE IN THE ACTIVITIES OF A PHYSICIAN HEALTH AND REHABILITATION PROGRAM AND ATTEND WEEKLY MEETINGS WITH QUARTERLY REPORTS; SHALL NOT TREAT OR OTHERWISE SERVE AS PHYSICIAN, PRESCRIBE, DISPENSE, OR ADMINISTER CONTROLLED SUBSTANCES, DANGEROUS DRUGS THAT MAY BE SUBJECT TO ABUSE TO HIMSELF OR TO ANY MEMBER OF HIS FAMILY; SHALL COMPLY WITH THE TERMS AND CONDITIONS OF HIS CONTINUING CARE CONTRACTS WITH QUARTERLY REPORTS TO THE BOARD; HIS MEDICAL PRACTICE, INCLUDING ANY OFFICE AND SURGICAL PRACTICE, SHALL BE MONITORED BY A BOARD APPROVED TEXAS PHYSICIAN WHO SHALL SUBMIT QUARTERLY REPORTS TO THE BOARD; SHALL SURRENDER HIS DEA CONTROLLED SUBSTANCES REGISTRATION CERTIFICATE AND HIS TEXAS CONTROLLED SUBSTANCE REGISTRATION CERTIFICATE; SEPARATE FROM PATIENT RECORDS, SHALL MAINTAIN A FILE OF EVERY PRESCRIPTION WRITTEN BY HIM FOR DANGEROUS DRUGS WITH ADDICTIVE POTENTIAL OR POTENTIAL FOR ABUSE WHICH SHALL BE AVAILABLE FOR REVIEW; SHALL NOT TELEPHONE TO A PHARMACY ANY PRESCRIPTION OR REFILL OF SUCH DRUGS; SHALL OBTAIN AT LEAST 50 HOURS PER YEAR OF CONTINUING MEDICAL EDUCATION; SHALL COOPERATE WITH THE BOARD IN VERIFYING COMPLIANCE INCLUDING PROVIDING COPIES OF MEDICAL RELEASES UPON REQUEST; SHALL APPEAR BEFORE THE BOARD AT LEAST TWO TIMES EACH YEAR; SHALL GIVE A COPY OF THIS ORDER TO ANY HEALTH CARE ENTITY WHERE HE HAS PRIVILEGES; TIME PERIOD OUT OF TEXAS DOES NOT COUNT TOWARD PROBATION; SHALL INFORM THE BOARD OF CHANGE OF ADDRESS WITHIN 10 DAYS OR IF HE LEAVES THE STATE; SHALL NOT SEEK MODIFICATION FOR 24 MONTHS. ON 4/4/98 PETITION TO MODIFY ORDER GRANTED ALLOWING HIM TO APPLY FOR ALL CONTROLLED SUBSTANCE REGISTRATIONS BUT LIMIT HIS USE OF THESE TO THE ORDERING OF CONTROLLED SUBSTANCES FOR HOSPITALIZED INPATIENT USE ONLY. ON 4/10/99 PETITION TO TERMINATE ORDER DENIED; ORDER MODIFIED DELETING REQUIREMENTS RELATING TO HIS CONTROLLED SUBSTANCES REGISTRATION AND PRESCRIBING AUTHORITY, REQUIRED EDUCATION, CONTINUING PSYCHIATRIC CARE, PARTICIPATION IN AA AND THE COUNTY MEDICAL SOCIETY PHYSICIAN HEALTH AND REHABILITATION COMMITTEE, CONTINUING CARE CONTRACTS, AND MONITORING OF PRACTICE; MAY REQUEST MODIFICATION YEARLY; REDUCTION IN CONTINUING MEDICAL EDUCATION FROM FIFTY HOURS TO TWENTY-FIVE; AND REDUCTION IN APPEARANCES BEFORE THE BOARD FROM BIANNUAL TO ANNUAL.

REYNOLDS, JARRELL PAUL MD OF 310 SOUTH PECOS BOX 312, COLEMAN, TX, WAS DISCIPLINED BY DEA ON JUNE 13, 1996
DISCIPLINARY ACTION: SURRENDER OF CONTROLLED SUBSTANCE LICENSE

NOTES: IN LIEU OF ORDER TO SHOW CAUSE.

RHOADES, JOE WALKER DO, LICENSE NUMBER 00C3186 OF FORT WORTH, TX, WAS DISCIPLINED BY TEXAS ON JANUARY 6, 1995
DISCIPLINARY ACTION: REQUIRED TO TAKE ADDITIONAL MEDICAL EDUCATION; MONITORING OF PHYSICIAN PERFORMANCE
OFFENSE: OVERPRESCRIBING OR MISPRESCRIBING DRUGS

NOTES: OVER THE COURSE OF SEVERAL YEARS, HAS PRESCRIBED CONTROLLED SUBSTANCES TO TWO PATIENTS WITHOUT ADEQUATE DOCUMENTATION AND WITHOUT ADEQUATE FOLLOW-UP EVALUATIONS, REFERRAL OR DRUG COUNSELING; ACTION IN LIEU OF FURTHER INVESTIGATION. CONDITIONS OF THREE YEAR RESTRICTION: SEPARATE FROM PATIENT RECORDS SHALL MAINTAIN A FILE OF EVERY PRESCRIPTION WRITTEN FOR CONTROLLED SUBSTANCES OR DANGEROUS DRUGS WITH ADDICTIVE POTENTIAL WHICH SHALL BE AVAILABLE FOR INSPECTION; SHALL NOT TELEPHONE TO A PHARMACY ANY PRESCRIPTION OR REFILL FOR SUCH DRUGS; SHALL MAINTAIN ADEQUATE MEDICAL RECORDS ON ALL OFFICE VISITS WHICH SHALL BE AVAILABLE FOR INSPECTION; SHALL OBTAIN AT LEAST 50 HOURS PER YEAR OF CONTINUING MEDICAL EDUCATION; SHALL APPEAR BEFORE THE BOARD ONCE A YEAR OR UPON REQUEST; SHALL COOPERATE WITH THE BOARD IN VERIFYING COMPLIANCE; SHALL GIVE A COPY OF THIS ORDER TO ANY HEALTH CARE ENTITY WHERE HE HAS OR APPLIES FOR PRIVILEGES OR ANYONE ELSE WHO ASKS FOR IT; SHALL ENSURE INQUIRIES REGARDING

HIS TEXAS LICENSURE STATUS ARE ANSWERED BY REFERENCING THIS ORDER; SHALL INFORM BOARD OF CHANGE OF ADDRESS WITHIN 10 DAYS OR IF HE LEAVES THE STATE; TIME SPENT OUT OF TEXAS DOES NOT COUNT TOWARD RESTRICTION. SHALL NOT SEEK MODIFICATION FOR ONE YEAR.

RHODES, THOMAS P MD, LICENSE NUMBER G0007 OF CORPUS CHRISTI, TX, WAS DISCIPLINED BY TEXAS ON DECEMBER 4, 1998
DISCIPLINARY ACTION: EMERGENCY SUSPENSION

NOTES: ON 8/9/97 HE ENTERED INTO A NONDISCIPLINARY ORDER WITH THE BOARD BASED UPON SELF-REPORTING OF ABUSE OF MULTIPLE SUBSTANCES INCLUDING HYDROCODONE, AMPHETAMINES AND MORPHINE; IN 10/98 HE REPORTED THAT HE HAD RELAPSED BY INGESTING HYDROCODONE AND FASTING ON AT LEAST TWO OCCASIONS IN 7/98; AND BY INGESTING LORTAB AND FASTIN ON 7/23/98 & 7/24/98. ALSO ADMITTED TO NOT ATTENDING AA MEETINGS; MEDICAL SOCIETY REPORTED THAT HE HAS APPARENTLY ABANDONED HIS RECOVERY PROGRAM; BOARD ALSO HAS RECEIVED NEGATIVE REPORTS FROM HIS THERAPIST.

RHODES, THOMAS P MD OF 3560 S ALAMEDA, CORPUS CHRISTI, TX, WAS DISCIPLINED BY DEA ON MARCH 30, 1999
DISCIPLINARY ACTION: SURRENDER OF CONTROLLED SUBSTANCE LICENSE

NOTES: IN LIEU OF PUBLIC INTEREST REVOCATION.

RHODES, THOMAS P MD, LICENSE NUMBER G0007, WAS DISCIPLINED BY TEXAS ON APRIL 10, 1999
DISCIPLINARY ACTION: 120-MONTH PROBATION; RESTRICTION PLACED ON CONTROLLED SUBSTANCE LICENSE
OFFENSE: SUBSTANCE ABUSE

NOTES: ON OR ABOUT 11/19/98 HE RELAPSED BY INGESTING HYDROCODONE AND FASTIN AND LORCET, VIOLATING THE 8/9/97 CONFIDENTIAL NON-DISCIPLINARY REHABILITATION ORDER WITH THE BOARD BASED UPON HIS SELF-REPORTED HISTORY OF OPIOID DEPENDENCE; ON 11/19/98 HE ENTERED INPATIENT TREATMENT AND COMPLETED THE PROGRAM ON 12/14/98; ON 3/30/99 HE APPEARED BEFORE AN INFORMAL SETTLEMENT CONFERENCE PANEL AND REQUESTED THE LIFTING OF HIS EMERGENCY SUSPENSION. SUSPENSION STAYED FOR PROBATION WITH FOLLOWING TERMS AND RESTRICTIONS: SHALL IMMEDIATELY SURRENDER HIS DEA AND TEXAS DEPARTMENT OF PUBLIC SAFETY CONTROLLED SUBSTANCES REGISTRATION CERTIFICATES; SHALL ABSTAIN FROM THE CONSUMPTION OF ALCOHOL/DRUGS IN ANY FORM UNLESS PRESCRIBED BY ANOTHER PHYSICIAN FOR A LEGITIMATE AND THERAPEUTIC PURPOSE; SHALL SUBMIT HIMSELF FOR APPROPRIATE EXAMS INCLUDING DRUG OR ALCOHOL SCREENS; SHALL NOMINATE THREE CERTIFIED PSYCHIATRISTS FOR BOARD SELECTION OF A THERAPIST AND SHALL EXPEDITIOUSLY SUBMIT HIMSELF TO EVALUATION AND TREATMENT BY THE APPROVED PRACTITIONER; SHALL PARTICIPATE IN THE ACTIVITIES OF A PHYSICIAN HEALTH AND REHABILITATION COMMITTEE AND ATTEND WEEKLY MEETINGS WITH QUARTERLY REPORTS; SHALL PARTICIPATE IN AA'S PROGRAM NOT LESS THAN THREE TIMES A WEEK; SHALL REPORT ON HIS ATTENDANCE; SHALL NOT TREAT OR OTHERWISE SERVE AS PHYSICIAN, PRESCRIBE, DISPENSE OR ADMINISTER DRUGS THAT MAY BE SUBJECT TO ABUSE TO HIMSELF OR TO ANY MEMBER OF HIS FAMILY; SEPARATE FROM PATIENT RECORDS, SHALL MAINTAIN A LOGBOOK OF EVERY PRESCRIPTION WRITTEN BY HIM FOR DANGEROUS DRUGS WITH ADDICTIVE POTENTIAL WHICH SHALL BE MADE AVAILABLE FOR REVIEW; SHALL APPEAR BEFORE THE BOARD AT LEAST ONCE A YEAR; SHALL COOPERATE WITH THE BOARD IN VERIFYING COMPLIANCE INCLUDING PROVIDING COPIES OF MEDICAL RELEASES UPON REQUEST; SHALL GIVE A COPY OF THIS ORDER TO ANY HEALTH CARE ENTITY WHERE HE HAS PRIVILEGES; TIME SPENT OUT OF TEXAS DOES NOT COUNT TOWARD PROBATION; SHALL INFORM THE BOARD OF CHANGE OF ADDRESS WITHIN 10 DAYS OR IF HE LEAVES THE STATE; SHALL NOT SEEK MODIFICATION FOR ONE YEAR; HOWEVER, THIS ORDER SHALL NOT BE TERMINATED UNTIL THE 10 YEAR PROBATIONARY PERIOD HAS BEEN COMPLETED BY HIM.

RHODES, THOMAS P MD, LICENSE NUMBER G0007 OF CORPUS CHRISTI, TX, WAS DISCIPLINED BY TEXAS ON SEPTEMBER 28, 1999
DISCIPLINARY ACTION: EMERGENCY SUSPENSION

NOTES: EVIDENCE THAT HIS CONTINUED PRACTICE CONSTITUTES A CONTINUING THREAT TO PUBLIC WELFARE.

RICE, KARL WOODS MD, LICENSE NUMBER 00D9626 OF LONGVIEW, TX, WAS DISCIPLINED BY TEXAS ON AUGUST 20, 1992
DISCIPLINARY ACTION: 60-MONTH PROBATION
OFFENSE: SUBSTANCE ABUSE

NOTES: INTEMPERATE USE OF ALCOHOL. LICENSE SUSPENDED, SUSPENSION STAYED. PROBATION UNDER TERMS AND CONDITIONS. ON 9/30/94 PETITION FOR TERMINATION OF ORDER DENIED.

RICH, DOMINIC RICHARD DO, LICENSE NUMBER 00C4188 OF CORPUS CHRISTI, TX, WAS DISCIPLINED BY TEXAS ON OCTOBER 1, 1993
DISCIPLINARY ACTION: SURRENDER OF LICENSE

NOTES: IN LIEU OF FURTHER INVESTIGATION INTO ALLEGATIONS. SHALL NOT PETITION FOR REINSTATEMENT OF LICENSE.

RICHTER, JAMES K MD, LICENSE NUMBER 00C4518 OF SAN ANTONIO, TX, WAS DISCIPLINED BY TEXAS ON AUGUST 19, 1994
DISCIPLINARY ACTION: REQUIRED TO TAKE ADDITIONAL MEDICAL EDUCATION; MONITORING OF PHYSICIAN PERFORMANCE
OFFENSE: OVERPRESCRIBING OR MISPRESCRIBING DRUGS

NOTES: FROM 1989 THROUGH 1993 HE PRESCRIBED CONTROLLED STIMULANT MEDICATIONS FOR THE TREATMENT OF OBESITY TO MULTIPLE PATIENTS WITHOUT SUFFICIENTLY ESTABLISHING AND DOCUMENTING AN APPROPRIATE DIAGNOSIS AND BASIS FOR SUCH A DIAGNOSIS; ALSO FAILED TO ADEQUATELY DOCUMENT THE PRESCRIBING AND DISPENSING OF MEDICATIONS. CONDITIONS OF FIVE YEAR RESTRICTION: SHALL APPEAR BEFORE THE BOARD ONCE A YEAR; SHALL MAINTAIN ADEQUATE MEDICAL RECORDS ON ALL PATIENT OFFICE VISITS WHICH SHALL BE AVAILABLE FOR INSPECTION; SEPARATE FROM PATIENT RECORDS, SHALL MAINTAIN A FILE OF EVERY PRESCRIPTION WRITTEN FOR CONTROLLED SUBSTANCES OR DANGEROUS DRUGS WHICH SHALL BE AVAILABLE FOR INSPECTION; SHALL ATTEND AT LEAST 50 HOURS PER YEAR OF CONTINUING MEDICAL EDUCATION; PRIOR TO PRACTICING IN THE SPECIALTY OF FAMILY PRACTICE SHALL COMPLETE A BOARD-APPROVED MINI-RESIDENCY; WITHIN ONE YEAR SHALL PASS THE MEDICAL JURISPRUDENCE EXAM; SHALL GIVE A COPY

OF THIS ORDER TO ANY HEALTH CARE ENTITY WHERE HE HAS PRIVILEGES; SHALL COOPERATE WITH THE BOARD IN VERIFYING COMPLIANCE; SHALL INFORM BOARD OF CHANGE OF ADDRESS WITHIN 10 DAYS OR IF HE LEAVES THE STATE; TIME SPENT OUT OF TEXAS DOES NOT COUNT TOWARD RESTRICTION. SHALL NOT SEEK MODIFICATION FOR ONE YEAR.

RIEDWEG, EDWARD A MD OF 301 EAST DIVISION, GREENVILLE, TX, WAS DISCIPLINED BY DEA ON JULY 30, 1993
DISCIPLINARY ACTION: SURRENDER OF CONTROLLED SUBSTANCE LICENSE
OFFENSE: DISCIPLINARY ACTION BY ANOTHER STATE OR AGENCY

RIEDWEG, EDWARD ALBERT MD, DATE OF BIRTH NOVEMBER 26, 1941, LICENSE NUMBER 00E3757 OF DALLAS, TX, WAS DISCIPLINED BY TEXAS ON JUNE 17, 1992
DISCIPLINARY ACTION: 60-MONTH PROBATION
OFFENSE: SUBSTANCE ABUSE
NOTES: SEVERAL VIOLATIONS OF THE MEDICAL PRACTICE ACT, INCLUDING INTEMPERATE USE OF ALCOHOL OR DRUGS. LICENSE SUSPENDED, SUSPENSION STAYED. PROBATION UNDER TERMS AND CONDITIONS.

RIEDWEG, EDWARD ALBERT MD, DATE OF BIRTH NOVEMBER 26, 1941, LICENSE NUMBER 00E3757 OF 4401 A I-35 NORTH SUITE 210, DENTON, TX, WAS DISCIPLINED BY TEXAS ON APRIL 30, 1993
DISCIPLINARY ACTION: EMERGENCY SUSPENSION
OFFENSE: FAILURE TO COMPLY WITH PREVIOUS BOARD ORDER
NOTES: IN A 6/17/92 ORDER CONDITIONS OF PROBATION INCLUDED THAT HE ABSTAIN FROM CONSUMING ANY ALCOHOL OR OTHER DRUGS AND IF HE DID USE THEM WOULD REPORT THIS TO THE BOARD WITHIN 24 HOURS; ON 2/20/93 HE ADMITTED HE WAS DRINKING AND WAS RELIEVED OF HIS DUTIES IN THE EMERGENCY ROOM; WAS ADMITTED TO INPATIENT HOSPITALIZATION ON 3/22/93.

RIEDWEG, EDWARD ALBERT MD, DATE OF BIRTH NOVEMBER 26, 1941, LICENSE NUMBER 00E3757 OF 4401 AI35 NORTH SUITE 210, DENTON, TX, WAS DISCIPLINED BY TEXAS ON JUNE 15, 1993
DISCIPLINARY ACTION: LICENSE SUSPENSION; REQUIRED TO ENTER AN IMPAIRED PHYSICIAN PROGRAM OR SUBSTANCE ABUSE TREATMENT
OFFENSE: FAILURE TO COMPLY WITH PREVIOUS BOARD ORDER
NOTES: BY USING ALCOHOL WAS NOT COMPLYING WITH 6/17/92 ORDER. SUSPENSION FOR A MINIMUM OF ONE YEAR; SHALL THEN MAKE APPLICATION FOR REINSTATEMENT; BOARD SHALL REQUIRE AN INDEPENDENT MENTAL AND PHYSICAL EXAM; SHALL PROVIDE PROOF OF A DOCUMENTED AFTERCARE PROGRAM SATISFACTORY TO THE BOARD; SHALL INFORM BOARD OF CHANGE OF ADDRESS WITHIN 10 DAYS OR IF HE LEAVES THE STATE; TIME SPENT OUT OF TEXAS DOES NOT COUNT TOWARD SUSPENSION.

RIEDWEG, EDWARD ALBERT MD, DATE OF BIRTH NOVEMBER 26, 1941, LICENSE NUMBER 00E3757 OF KERRVILLE, TX, WAS DISCIPLINED BY TEXAS ON JULY 14, 1994
OFFENSE: SUBSTANCE ABUSE
NOTES: SINCE LICENSE SUSPENSION, HAS WORKED ON A VOLUNTEER BASIS ASSISTING IN UTILIZATION REVIEW; SIGNED A CONTINUING CARE CONTRACT WITH PHYSICIANS HEALTH AND REHABILITATION COMMITTEE; A PHYSICIAN HAS AGREED TO SUPERVISE HIS MEDICAL PRACTICE AND HE WAS EVALUATED BY A PSYCHIATRIST AND AN INTERNAL MEDICINE PHYSICIAN, NEITHER OF WHOM FOUND ANY PROBLEM THAT WOULD PREVENT HIM FOR PRACTICING MEDICINE. LICENSE REINSTATED FROM 6/3/93 SUSPENSION. HOWEVER, HE SHALL NOT PRACTICE MEDICINE UNTIL SUCH TIME AS HE UNDERGOES A 96 HOUR EVALUATION FOR CHEMICAL DEPENDENCY WHICH INDICATES HE IS ABLE TO SAFELY PRACTICE AND HE APPEARS BEFORE THE BOARD. UPON RETURN TO PRACTICE HE SHALL BE SUBJECT TO PROBATIONARY TERMS AND CONDITIONS.

RIEDWEG, EDWARD ALBERT MD, DATE OF BIRTH NOVEMBER 26, 1941, LICENSE NUMBER 00E3757 OF KERRVILLE, TX, WAS DISCIPLINED BY TEXAS ON AUGUST 20, 1994
DISCIPLINARY ACTION: SURRENDER OF CONTROLLED SUBSTANCE LICENSE; 120-MONTH PROBATION
OFFENSE: SUBSTANCE ABUSE
NOTES: LICENSE REINSTATED FROM SUSPENSION OF 6/3/93; ON 7/26/94 HE SUBMITTED TO A 96 HOUR MULTIDISCIPLINARY EVALUATION. THE EVALUATION INDICATED THAT HE IS ABLE TO SAFELY RETURN TO THE PRACTICE OF MEDICINE UNDER CERTAIN TERMS AND CONDITIONS. SUSPENSION STAYED. CONDITIONS OF PROBATION: SHALL APPEAR BEFORE THE BOARD TWICE A YEAR; PRACTICE SHALL BE SUPERVISED BY PRESENT SUPERVISOR WITH QUARTERLY REPORTS; SHALL ABSTAIN FROM THE CONSUMPTION OF ALCOHOL/CHEMICAL SUBSTANCES IN ANY FORM UNLESS PRESCRIBED BY ANOTHER PHYSICIAN FOR A LEGITIMATE AND THERAPEUTIC PURPOSE; SHALL CONTINUE TO PARTICIPATE WITH A PHYSICIANS HEALTH AND REHABILITATION COMMITTEE AND ATTEND WEEKLY MEETINGS WITH QUARTERLY REPORTS; SHALL CONTINUE TO PARTICIPATE IN AA'S PROGRAM NOT LESS THAN THREE TIMES A WEEK WITH QUARTERLY REPORTS TO THE BOARD; SHALL CONTINUE TO RECEIVE TREATMENT FROM CURRENT PSYCHIATRIST WITH QUARTERLY REPORTS; SHALL SUBMIT TO WEEKLY PSYCHOTHERAPY WITH A BOARD-APPROVED PSYCHOTHERAPIST WITH AT LEAST QUARTERLY REPORTS; SHALL SUBMIT HIMSELF FOR APPROPRIATE DRUG OR ALCOHOL SCREENS; SHALL NOT TREAT OR OTHERWISE SERVE AS PHYSICIAN, PRESCRIBE, DISPENSE OR ADMINISTER DRUGS THAT MAY BE SUBJECT TO ABUSE TO HIMSELF OR ANY MEMBER OF HIS FAMILY; SHALL ATTEND AT LEAST 50 HOURS PER YEAR OF CONTINUING MEDICAL EDUCATION INCLUDING AT LEAST 20 HOURS PER YEAR OF ADDICTIONOLOGY/PHARMACOLOGY; SHALL SURRENDER HIS DEA AND TEXAS CONTROLLED SUBSTANCES CERTIFICATE AND SHALL NOT ATTEMPT TO REREGISTER WITHOUT PERMISSION; SHALL GIVE A COPY OF THIS ORDER TO ANY HEALTH CARE ENTITY WHERE HE HAS PRIVILEGES; SHALL COOPERATE WITH THE BOARD IN VERIFYING COMPLIANCE; SHALL INFORM BOARD OF CHANGE OF ADDRESS WITHIN 10 DAYS OR IF HE LEAVES THE STATE; TIME SPENT OUT OF TEXAS DOES NOT COUNT TOWARD PROBATION. SHALL NOT SEEK MODIFICATION FOR ONE YEAR.

RIEDWEG, EDWARD ALBERT MD, DATE OF BIRTH NOVEMBER 26, 1941, LICENSE NUMBER 00E3757, WAS DISCIPLINED BY TEXAS ON AUGUST 17, 1996
DISCIPLINARY ACTION: LICENSE SUSPENSION
OFFENSE: FAILURE TO COMPLY WITH PREVIOUS BOARD ORDER
NOTES: ON 7/12/95 AND 11/23/95 SUFFERED A RELAPSE INTO THE USE OF ALCOHOL AND DRUGS IN VIOLATION OF AN 8/20/95 ORDER; FAILED TWICE TO IMMEDIATELY REPORT THIS TO THE BOARD; RECEIVED INPATIENT TREATMENT FROM 7/12/95 THROUGH 7/22/95 AND 11/23/95 THROUGH 12/22/95; HAS NOT PRACTICED

MEDICINE SINCE 11/23/95. SUSPENSION UNTIL HE REQUESTS TO THE BOARD IN WRITING TO HAVE THE SUSPENSION LIFTED AND APPEARS BEFORE THE BOARD WITH SUFFICIENT EVIDENCE AND INFORMATION THAT HE IS PHYSICALLY, MENTALLY, AND OTHERWISE COMPETENT TO SAFELY PRACTICE MEDICINE INCLUDING AT A MINIMUM AT LEAST ONE YEAR OF DOCUMENTED SOBRIETY AND COPIES OF RECORDS AND REPORTS OF PSYCHOLOGICAL AND NEUROPSYCHOLOGICAL EVALUATIONS OF A BOARD APPROVED PSYCHIATRIST. ON 8/22/98 PETITION TO LIFT SUSPENSION DENIED.

RIGGLE, KENNETH BURTON DO, LICENSE NUMBER 00C2963 OF PASADENA, TX, WAS DISCIPLINED BY TEXAS ON MARCH 6, 1992
DISCIPLINARY ACTION: SURRENDER OF LICENSE

NOTES: LICENSE RETIRED IN LIEU OF FURTHER DISCIPLINARY ACTION.

RINGER, B R DO, LICENSE NUMBER 00G0011, WAS DISCIPLINED BY TEXAS ON OCTOBER 18, 1996
DISCIPLINARY ACTION: 60-MONTH PROBATION; RESTRICTION PLACED ON LICENSE
OFFENSE: SEXUAL ABUSE OF OR SEXUAL MISCONDUCT WITH A PATIENT

NOTES: IN OCTOBER 1993 HE AGREED TO EXCHANGE LIPOSUCTION FOR DECORATING SERVICES IN HIS HOUSE; ON 1/13/94 HE MADE NUMEROUS INAPPROPRIATE COMMENTS AND TOUCHED THIS PATIENT IN AN ABUSIVE MANNER; HAD MADE INAPPROPRIATE COMMENTS TO ANOTHER PATIENT HE SAW IN 1/91. SUSPENSION, STAYED. CONDITIONS OF PROBATION: SHALL UNDERGO A COMPLETE PSYCHIATRIC EVALUATION BY A BOARD APPROVED PHYSICIAN WHO SHALL WRITE PERIODIC REPORTS NO LESS THAN ONCE EACH MONTH AND OTHER REPORTS UPON BOARD REQUEST; SHALL HAVE A CHAPERONE PRESENT IN THE ROOM DURING THE EXAMINATION OF A FEMALE PATIENT AND MAKE NOTATION IN THE PATIENT CHARTS THAT THE CHAPERONE WAS PRESENT; SHALL OBTAIN SIX HOURS OF AN ETHIC COURSE OR PROGRAM PER YEAR FOR FIVE YEARS AND SUBMIT PROOF TO THE BOARD; EVERY YEAR SHALL PERFORM 120 HOURS OF COMMUNITY SERVICE FOR A BOARD APPROVED NON-PROFIT CHARITABLE ORGANIZATION AND SUBMIT PROOF TO THE BOARD QUARTERLY; SHALL APPEAR BEFORE THE BOARD AT LEAST TWICE PER YEAR; SHALL COOPERATE WITH THE BOARD IN VERIFYING COMPLIANCE; TIME PERIOD OUT OF TEXAS DOES NOT COUNT TOWARD PROBATION; SHALL NOT SEEK MODIFICATION FOR ONE YEAR; REPRIMAND.

RINGER, B R JR DO, LICENSE NUMBER G0011 OF HOUSTON, TX, WAS DISCIPLINED BY TEXAS ON FEBRUARY 7, 1998
DISCIPLINARY ACTION: 60-MONTH PROBATION; RESTRICTION PLACED ON LICENSE
OFFENSE: SEXUAL ABUSE OF OR SEXUAL MISCONDUCT WITH A PATIENT

NOTES: ONE OF HIS PATIENTS FILED A CIVIL LAWSUIT AGAINST HIM DUE TO HER PAIN, DEPRESSION, AND ANGER RESULTING FROM HIS SEXUAL MISCONDUCT DURING ONE VISIT IN 1/13/94 WHEN HE ENGAGED IN NUMEROUS INCIDENTS OF SEXUAL COMMENTS AND TOUCHING. SUSPENSION STAYED FOR PROBATION WITH FOLLOWING TERMS AND CONDITIONS: SHALL UNDERGO A COMPLETE PSYCHIATRIC EVALUATION AND SUCH TREATMENT AS IS RECOMMENDED WITH MONTHLY REPORTS TO THE BOARD; SHALL COOPERATE WITH THE BOARD IN VERIFYING COMPLIANCE; SHALL HAVE A CHAPERONE ANYTIME HE PERFORMS A PHYSICAL EXAM ON A FEMALE PATIENT; SHALL OBTAIN 6 HOURS OF AN ETHICS COURSE PER YEAR FOR 5 YEARS; SHALL PERFORM 120 HOURS OF COMMUNITY SERVICE PER YEAR FOR A BOARD-APPROVED NON-PROFIT ORGANIZATION; SHALL APPEAR BEFORE THE BOARD TWICE A YEAR; TIME SPENT OUT OF TEXAS DOES NOT COUNT TOWARD PROBATION; SHALL NOT SEEK MODIFICATION FOR ONE YEAR; REPRIMAND.

RIVERA, RAUL MD, LICENSE NUMBER 0C27288 OF EL PASO, TX, WAS DISCIPLINED BY CALIFORNIA ON APRIL 8, 1992
DISCIPLINARY ACTION: 60-MONTH PROBATION
OFFENSE: DISCIPLINARY ACTION BY ANOTHER STATE OR AGENCY

NOTES: DISCIPLINE BY TEXAS BOARD FOR EXCESSIVE USE OF ALCOHOL. REVOCATION, STAYED. PROBATION WITH TERMS AND CONDITIONS.

RIVERA, RAUL MD, LICENSE NUMBER 00C8420 OF EL PASO, TX, WAS DISCIPLINED BY TEXAS ON JUNE 28, 1995
DISCIPLINARY ACTION: 120-MONTH PROBATION; REQUIRED TO TAKE ADDITIONAL MEDICAL EDUCATION
OFFENSE: FAILURE TO COMPLY WITH PREVIOUS BOARD ORDER

NOTES: BETWEEN 3/17/94 AND 5/31/94 HE INGESTED ALCOHOL AND DALMANE, A CONTROLLED SUBSTANCE, WITHOUT A LEGITIMATE MEDICAL REASON AND IN VIOLATION OF 10/27/89 BOARD ORDER; REPORTED RELAPSE TO BOARD ON 6/22/94; RECEIVED INPATIENT SUBSTANCE ABUSE TREATMENT FROM 6/1/94 TO 6/28/94; UNDER THE CARE OF A PSYCHIATRIST FOR ALCOHOLISM; HAS ENTERED AN AFTERCARE RECOVERY CONTRACT; REPORTS ATTENDING AA AN AVERAGE OF THREE TIMES PER WEEK AND REGULARLY PARTICIPATING IN ACTIVITIES OF MEDICAL SOCIETY COMMITTEE ON PHYSICIAN HEALTH AND REHABILITATION. SUSPENSION STAYED. PROBATION WITH TERMS: SHALL ABSTAIN FROM THE CONSUMPTION OF ALCOHOL/DRUGS IN ANY FORM UNLESS PRESCRIBED BY ANOTHER PHYSICIAN FOR A LEGITIMATE AND THERAPEUTIC PURPOSE; SHALL SUBMIT HIMSELF FOR APPROPRIATE EXAMS INCLUDING DRUG OR ALCOHOL SCREENS; SHALL SUBMIT HIMSELF FOR EVALUATION AND TREATMENT BY BOARD-APPROVED PSYCHIATRIST WHOM HE SHALL SEE AT LEAST ONCE A MONTH AND WHO SHALL SUBMIT REPORTS TO BOARD; SHALL CONTINUE TO PARTICIPATE IN AA'S PROGRAM NOT LESS THAN THREE TIMES A WEEK WITH QUARTERLY REPORTS TO THE BOARD; SHALL PARTICIPATE IN THE ACTIVITIES OF AN IMPAIRED PHYSICIAN'S GROUP AND ATTEND WEEKLY MEETINGS WITH QUARTERLY REPORTS; SHALL COMPLY WITH TERMS OF CONTINUING CARE CONTRACTS WITH QUARTERLY REPORTS; SHALL COMPLY WITH CONTRACTS FOR HOSPITAL PRIVILEGES AND SHALL REPORT ANY DISCIPLINARY ACTIONS TO THE BOARD; SHALL NOT TREAT OR OTHERWISE SERVE AS PHYSICIAN, PRESCRIBE, DISPENSE OR ADMINISTER DRUGS THAT MAY BE SUBJECT TO ABUSE TO HIMSELF OR TO A MEMBER OF HIS FAMILY; SHALL MAINTAIN A FILE WITH COPIES OF EVERY PRESCRIPTION WRITTEN FOR CONTROLLED SUBSTANCES OR DRUGS WITH ADDICTIVE POTENTIAL AND MAINTAIN A LOG OF ALL PRESCRIPTIONS TELEPHONED IN BY HIM OR AT HIS DIRECTION FOR THESE DRUGS BOTH OF WHICH SHALL BE AVAILABLE FOR REVIEW; SHALL NOT SIGN OR INDICATE IN ANY MANNER IN PATIENT RECORDS THAT HE HAS SEEN PATIENTS UNLESS HE ACTUALLY HAS SEEN AND EXAMINED THE PATIENT UNLESS IT IS CLEARLY NOTED THAT HE DID NOT PERSONALLY

EXAMINE THE PATIENT; SHALL MAINTAIN ADEQUATE MEDICAL RECORDS WHICH SHALL BE AVAILABLE FOR REVIEW; SHALL OBTAIN AT LEAST 50 HOURS PER YEAR OF CONTINUING MEDICAL EDUCATION; SHALL APPEAR BEFORE BOARD AT LEAST ONCE A YEAR OR AT BOARD REQUEST; SHALL COOPERATE WITH THE BOARD IN VERIFYING COMPLIANCE INCLUDING PROVIDING COPIES OF MEDICAL RELEASES UPON REQUEST; SHALL GIVE A COPY OF THIS ORDER TO ANY HEALTH CARE ENTITY WHERE HE HAS PRIVILEGES; SHALL PROVIDE A COPY OF THIS ORDER TO ANYONE REQUESTING IT WITHIN 10 DAYS; TIME PERIOD OUT OF TEXAS DOES NOT COUNT TOWARD PROBATION; SHALL INFORM BOARD OF CHANGE OF ADDRESS WITHIN 10 DAYS OR IF HE LEAVES THE STATE. MAY NOT SEEK MODIFICATION FOR ONE YEAR.

RIVERA, RAUL MD, LICENSE NUMBER 00C8420, WAS DISCIPLINED BY TEXAS ON JUNE 7, 1996
DISCIPLINARY ACTION: EMERGENCY SUSPENSION
OFFENSE: FAILURE TO COMPLY WITH PREVIOUS BOARD ORDER

NOTES: VIOLATED THE 6/28/95 ORDER IN THAT HE HAS ENGAGED IN THE FOLLOWING ACTIONS: ON OR ABOUT 5/29/96, HE INGESTED ALCOHOL; WHEN CONTACTED BY BOARD AND ADVISED TO SUBMIT A SPECIMEN FOR SCREENING, HE PROVIDED A BLOOD AND URINE SPECIMEN AND REPORTEDLY PRESENTED AT THE LAB WITH A STRONG ODOR OF ALCOHOL ON HIS BREATH, SHAKING HANDS AND COMMENTING THAT HE HAD TO VOMIT; RESULT OF SCREENING INDICATED THAT HE TESTED POSITIVE FOR ALCOHOL; FAILED TO IMMEDIATELY NOTIFY BOARD OF INGESTION OF ALCOHOL; FAILED TO ATTEND MEETINGS OF THE COUNTY MEDICAL SOCIETY IN 11/95 AND 2/96.

RIVERA, RAUL MD, LICENSE NUMBER C8420, WAS DISCIPLINED BY TEXAS ON JANUARY 16, 1997
DISCIPLINARY ACTION: 120-MONTH PROBATION; RESTRICTION PLACED ON LICENSE
OFFENSE: FAILURE TO COMPLY WITH PREVIOUS BOARD ORDER

NOTES: ON 5/29/96 HE RENDERED A BLOOD TEST POSITIVE FOR INGESTION OF ALCOHOL IN VIOLATION OF THE 6/28/95 ORDER. HE FAILED TO INFORM HIS COMPLIANCE OFFICER IMMEDIATELY, AND FAILED TO ATTEND REQUIRED MEETINGS BETWEEN 11/95 AND 2/96. A 6/22/96 ORDER SUSPENDED HIS LICENSE UNTIL SUCH TIME AS HE PERSONALLY APPEARED BEFORE THE BOARD AND SUBMITTED EVIDENCE THAT HE IS PHYSICALLY, MENTALLY, AND OTHERWISE COMPETENT TO PRACTICE. HE COMPLIED WITH ALL TERMS OF THE ORDER INCLUDING ALCOHOL DEPENDENCY TREATMENT AND PSYCHIATRIC EVALUATIONS. HE HAS SUBMITTED EVIDENCE OF AA ATTENDANCE, COOPERATED WITH THE BOARD STAFF, AND ENTERED INTO A CONTRACT WITH THE EL PASO MEDICAL SOCIETY PHYSICIAN HEALTH AND REHABILITATION COMMITTEE. SUSPENSION STAYED FOR PROBATION WITH TERMS AND CONDITIONS: MUST SUBMIT DOCUMENTATION OF ATTENDANCE AT AA FOR 90 CONSECUTIVE DAYS; SHALL ABSTAIN FROM THE CONSUMPTION OF ALCOHOL/DRUGS IN ANY FORM UNLESS PRESCRIBED BY ANOTHER PHYSICIAN FOR A LEGITIMATE AND THERAPEUTIC PURPOSE; SHALL SUBMIT HIMSELF FOR APPROPRIATE EXAMS INCLUDING DRUG OR ALCOHOL SCREENS; SHALL CONTINUE TO RECEIVE CARE AND TREATMENT FROM A SPECIFIED PHYSICIAN AT LEAST MONTHLY WITH QUARTERLY REPORTS; SHALL PARTICIPATE IN THE ACTIVITIES OF A PHYSICIAN HEALTH AND REHABILITATION COMMITTEE AND ATTEND WEEKLY MEETINGS WITH QUARTERLY REPORTS; SHALL PARTICIPATE IN AA'S PROGRAM NOT LESS THAN THREE TIMES A WEEK; SHALL REPORT ON HIS ATTENDANCE; SHALL COMPLY WITH TERMS OF HIS CONTINUING CARE CONTRACT; SEPARATE FROM PATIENT RECORDS, SHALL MAINTAIN A LOG BOOK OF EVERY PRESCRIPTION DRUG OR DANGEROUS DRUG WITH ADDICTIVE POTENTIAL WHICH SHALL BE MADE AVAILABLE FOR REVIEW; HIS MEDICAL PRACTICE SHALL BE MONITORED BY A BOARD APPROVED TEXAS PHYSICIAN WHO SHALL PROVIDE QUARTERLY REPORTS TO THE BOARD; SHALL NOT TREAT OR OTHERWISE SERVE AS PHYSICIAN, PRESCRIBE, DISPENSE OR ADMINISTER DRUGS THAT MAY BE SUBJECT TO ABUSE TO HIMSELF OR TO ANY MEMBER OF HIS FAMILY; HIS PRACTICE SHALL BE LIMITED TO AN OFFICE PRACTICE; SHALL PERSONALLY APPEAR BEFORE THE BOARD AT LEAST TWICE ANNUALLY FOR ONE YEAR AND ANNUALLY THEREAFTER; SHALL GIVE A COPY OF THIS ORDER TO ANY HEALTH CARE ENTITY WHERE HE HAS PRIVILEGES; SHALL PROVIDE A COPY OF THIS ORDER TO ANYONE REQUESTING IT WITHIN 10 DAYS; SHALL COOPERATE WITH THE BOARD IN VERIFYING COMPLIANCE INCLUDING PROVIDING COPIES OF MEDICAL RELEASES UPON REQUEST; TIME SPENT OUT OF TEXAS DOES NOT COUNT TOWARD PROBATION; SHALL INFORM THE BOARD OF CHANGE OF ADDRESS WITHIN 10 DAYS OR IF HE LEAVES THE STATE; SHALL NOT SEEK MODIFICATION FOR ONE YEAR.

RIVERA, RAUL MD, LICENSE NUMBER C8420 OF EL PASO, TX, WAS DISCIPLINED BY TEXAS ON JULY 24, 1998
DISCIPLINARY ACTION: EMERGENCY SUSPENSION
OFFENSE: FAILURE TO COMPLY WITH PREVIOUS BOARD ORDER

NOTES: VIOLATED 10/27/89, 6/28/95, & 1/16/97 BOARD ORDERS BY: INTEMPERATE USE OF ALCOHOL AND/OR DRUGS; UNPROFESSIONAL OR DISHONORABLE CONDUCT THAT IS LIKELY TO DECEIVE, DEFRAUD, OR INJURE THE PUBLIC; ON OR ABOUT 6/11/98 FAILED TO PROVIDE A RANDOM SCREEN; ON OR ABOUT 6/18/98 FAILED TO ATTEND MEETINGS OF THE MEDICAL SOCIETY'S HEALTH AND REHABILITATION COMMITTEE; ON OR ABOUT 7/6/98 TESTED POSITIVE FOR ALCOHOL AND ADMITTED TO BOARD THAT HE HAD INGESTED ALCOHOL, SPECIFICALLY 4 BEERS, THE MORNING OF 7/6/98.

RIVERA, RAUL MD, LICENSE NUMBER C8420 OF EL PASO, TX, WAS DISCIPLINED BY TEXAS ON JANUARY 29, 1999
DISCIPLINARY ACTION: LICENSE SUSPENSION
OFFENSE: FAILURE TO COMPLY WITH PREVIOUS BOARD ORDER

NOTES: INTEMPERATE USE OF ALCOHOL OR DRUGS IN VIOLATION OF PREVIOUS ORDERS. SUSPENSION UNTIL HE REQUESTS IN WRITING TO HAVE HIS SUSPENSION STAYED AND APPEARS BEFORE THE BOARD WITH SUFFICIENT EVIDENCE THAT HE IS PHYSICALLY, MENTALLY OR OTHERWISE COMPETENT TO PRACTICE SAFELY INCLUDING AT A MINIMUM: SHALL PROVIDE COPIES OF PSYCHOLOGICAL AND NEUROPSYCHIATRIC EVALUATIONS; SHALL COOPERATE WITH THE BOARD IN VERIFYING COMPLIANCE INCLUDING PROVIDING COPIES OF MEDICAL RELEASES UPON REQUEST; SHALL INFORM THE BOARD OF CHANGE OF ADDRESS WITHIN 10 DAYS; SHALL NOT SEEK MODIFICATION FOR ONE YEAR.

RIVERA, RAUL MD, LICENSE NUMBER C27288 OF EL PASO, TX, WAS DISCIPLINED BY CALIFORNIA ON OCTOBER 25, 1999
DISCIPLINARY ACTION: LICENSE REVOCATION

RIZOV, VLADIMIR Z MD, LICENSE NUMBER 00G4694 OF AUSTIN, TX, WAS DISCIPLINED BY TEXAS ON AUGUST 18, 1990
DISCIPLINARY ACTION: 60-MONTH PROBATION; REPRIMAND

NOTES: STIPULATED ORDER. MUST OBTAIN CONTINUING MEDICAL EDUCATION.

RIZOV, VLADIMIR Z MD, LICENSE NUMBER G4694 OF AUSTIN, TX, WAS DISCIPLINED BY TEXAS ON AUGUST 22, 1998
DISCIPLINARY ACTION: 36-MONTH PROBATION; FINE
OFFENSE: PROFESSIONAL MISCONDUCT

NOTES: FAILED TO ADEQUATELY SUPERVISE THE ACTIVITIES OF THOSE ACTING UNDER HIS SUPERVISION IN THAT IN 1995 AT PATIENTS' REQUEST SET UP A MORE CONVENIENT OFFICE LOCATION AND MADE ARRANGEMENTS WITH A NURSE TO CARRY OUT HIS DIRECT ORDERS; ALL BUT A FEW OF THE PATIENTS WERE INITIALLY SEEN BY HIM; HE SPECIFICALLY DENIES ANY VIOLATIONS OF THE MEDICAL PRACTICE ACT. REPRIMAND STAYED WITH FOLLOWING TERMS AND CONDITIONS: WITHIN 6 MONTHS SHALL OBTAIN 50 HOURS OF COURSES IN RISK MANAGEMENT OR PHARMACOLOGY AND SHALL TAKE AND PASS THE JURISPRUDENCE EXAM; SHALL OBTAIN 50 HOURS OF CONTINUING MEDICAL EDUCATION PER YEAR; SHALL MAINTAIN ADEQUATE MEDICAL RECORDS WHICH SHALL BE AVAILABLE FOR REVIEW; SHALL ADOPT OR ESTABLISH A SYSTEM OF PATIENT RECORD KEEPING AND BILLING TO ENSURE THAT ALL PATIENT RECORDS ACCURATELY REFLECT THE PATIENT'S NAME, SERVICE RENDERED, DATE OF SERVICE, AND AMOUNT CHARGED; $500 FINE; SHALL LIMIT HIS PRACTICE TO ONE CITY, NOT TO INCLUDE PRIVILEGES AT ANY HOSPITAL; SHALL APPEAR BEFORE THE BOARD UPON REQUEST; SHALL COOPERATE WITH THE BOARD IN VERIFYING COMPLIANCE; TIME SPENT OUT OF TEXAS DOES NOT COUNT TOWARD PROBATION; SHALL INFORM THE BOARD OF CHANGE OF ADDRESS WITHIN 10 DAYS OR IF HE LEAVES THE STATE; SHALL NOT SEEK MODIFICATION FOR ONE YEAR.

RO, KENNETH GENE MD, LICENSE NUMBER H7344 OF SUGAR LAND, TX, WAS DISCIPLINED BY TEXAS ON APRIL 4, 1998
DISCIPLINARY ACTION: REPRIMAND; REQUIRED TO TAKE ADDITIONAL MEDICAL EDUCATION
OFFENSE: PROFESSIONAL MISCONDUCT

NOTES: FROM 10/91 - 1/95 ENGAGED IN THE CORPORATE PRACTICE OF MEDICINE BY ALLOWING NONPHYSICIANS TO BILL FOR AND FINANCIALLY BENEFIT FROM HIS MEDICAL SERVICES; HE WAS PAID A FLAT FEE FOR HIS SERVICES IN EXCHANGE FOR TRANSFERRING REIMBURSEMENT TO A NONPHYSICIAN-OWNED CORPORATION. LICENSE LIMITED FOR THREE YEARS AS FOLLOWS: SHALL OBTAIN 10 HOURS OF AN ETHICS COURSE PER YEAR FOR 3 YEARS; WITHIN 6 MONTHS, SHALL TAKE AND PASS THE MEDICAL JURISPRUDENCE EXAM; SHALL APPEAR BEFORE THE BOARD ONCE A YEAR; SHALL COOPERATE WITH THE BOARD IN VERIFYING COMPLIANCE; SHALL GIVE A COPY OF THIS ORDER TO ANY HEALTH CARE ENTITY WHERE HE HAS PRIVILEGES; TIME SPENT OUT OF TEXAS DOES NOT COUNT TOWARD RESTRICTION; SHALL INFORM THE BOARD OF CHANGE OF ADDRESS WITHIN 10 DAYS OR IF HE LEAVES THE STATE; SHALL NOT SEEK MODIFICATION FOR ONE YEAR.

ROBERSON, FRED M MD OF ZUMBROTA, MN, WAS DISCIPLINED BY LOUISIANA ON DECEMBER 2, 1993
DISCIPLINARY ACTION: 36-MONTH PROBATION; MONITORING OF PHYSICIAN PERFORMANCE
OFFENSE: DISCIPLINARY ACTION BY ANOTHER STATE OR AGENCY

NOTES: ACTION TAKEN BY MINNESOTA; PRESCRIBING CONTROLLED SUBSTANCES IN OTHER THAN A LEGAL OR LEGITIMATE MANNER. LICENSE PLACED ON PROBATION FOR TERM CONCURRENT WITH ORDER PREVIOUSLY ENTERED BY MINNESOTA BOARD, SUBJECT TO COMPLIANCE WITH MINNESOTA ORDER, PROHIBITION ON MEDICAL PRACTICE IN LOUISIANA FOR THREE YEARS, PRIOR NOTICE TO BOARD OF INTENT TO RELOCATE TO LOUISIANA AFTER EXPIRATION OF THREE YEARS AND PROVISION OF QUARTERLY MEDICAL REPORTS TO THE BOARD.

ROBERSON, FRED M MD OF ZUMBROTA, MN, WAS DISCIPLINED BY LOUISIANA ON DECEMBER 8, 1994
DISCIPLINARY ACTION: LICENSE SUSPENSION; FINE
OFFENSE: DISCIPLINARY ACTION BY ANOTHER STATE OR AGENCY

NOTES: MAKING OR SUBMITTING FALSE, DECEPTIVE OR UNFOUNDED CLAIMS FOR THE PURPOSE OF OBTAINING COMPENSATION; PROFESSIONAL OR MEDICAL INCOMPETENCY; DISCIPLINARY ACTION BY MINNESOTA; VIOLATION OF PREVIOUS BOARD ORDER. REINSTATEMENT PRECLUDED FOR FIVE YEARS, CONDITIONED ON FULL COMPLIANCE WITH CONSENT ORDERS PREVIOUSLY ENTERED BY LOUISIANA AND MINNESOTA BOARDS. PROBATION UPON REINSTATEMENT, SUBJECT TO ADDITIONAL TERMS AND CONDITIONS AS IMPOSED BY BOARD AND PAYMENT OF $2,000 FINE WITHIN 30 DAYS.

ROBERSON, FRED MCRAE MD, LICENSE NUMBER 0033929, WAS DISCIPLINED BY MINNESOTA ON SEPTEMBER 12, 1992
DISCIPLINARY ACTION: RESTRICTION PLACED ON LICENSE

NOTES: AMENDED ORDERS ON 7/16/94, AND 11/18/95. ON 5/17/97 AMENDED ORDER. ON 11/14/98 UNCONDITIONAL LICENSE.

ROBERSON, FRED MCRAE MD, LICENSE NUMBER 00D4552 OF ZUMBROTA, MN, WAS DISCIPLINED BY TEXAS ON NOVEMBER 19, 1993
DISCIPLINARY ACTION: 60-MONTH PROBATION; MONITORING OF PHYSICIAN PERFORMANCE
OFFENSE: DISCIPLINARY ACTION BY ANOTHER STATE OR AGENCY

NOTES: ON 9/12/92 MINNESOTA BOARD RESTRICTED HIS LICENSE BASED ON THE FACT THAT HE SELF-PRESCRIBED NUMEROUS MEDICATIONS TO HIMSELF FROM 11/1/90 THROUGH 11/12/91 AVERAGING 3.7 TABLETS PER DAY OF PRIMARILY PAIN MEDICATION FOR TREATMENT RELATING TO AN ANKLE AND BACK INJURY; HE KEPT NO RECORD OF THE AMOUNT PRESCRIBED AND HAS BEEN SELF-PRESCRIBING INTERMITTENTLY SINCE 1979 OR 1980; BETWEEN 10/22/90 AND 7/5/91 PRESCRIBED NUMEROUS MEDICATIONS TO HIS WIFE FOLLOWING SURGERY FOR BREAST CANCER; HE KEPT NO RECORD OF THE AMOUNT PRESCRIBED; ADMITTED THAT ONE OF THESE PRESCRIPTIONS WAS FOR HIMSELF; MINNESOTA RESTRICTED HIS LICENSE SUCH THAT HE SHALL NOT PRESCRIBE OR SELF-ADMINISTER CONTROLLED SUBSTANCES FOR HIS OWN USE OR FOR THE USE OF HIS FAMILY; SHALL MAKE ARRANGEMENTS WITH A MONITORING/TREATING PHYSICIAN TO PROVIDE THE BOARD WITH QUARTERLY REPORTS REGARDING HIS PAIN MANAGEMENT. IN TEXAS FIVE YEAR SUSPENSION STAYED. CONDITIONS OF PROBATION: SAME TERMS AS MINNESOTA ORDER; PRIOR TO PRACTICING IN TEXAS SHALL APPEAR BEFORE THE BOARD; SHALL

INFORM THE BOARD IF HE LEAVES TEXAS OR MINNESOTA; TIME SPENT OUT OF TEXAS OR MINNESOTA SHALL NOT COUNT TOWARD PROBATION. SHALL NOT SEEK MODIFICATION FOR ONE YEAR.

ROBERTS, GARY F DO, DATE OF BIRTH NOVEMBER 27, 1963 OF 1522 HOLDERBY ROAD, HUNTINGTON, WV, WAS DISCIPLINED BY MEDICARE ON JULY 3, 1996
DISCIPLINARY ACTION: EXCLUSION FROM THE MEDICARE AND/OR MEDICAID PROGRAM
OFFENSE: NONCOMPLIANCE WITH A PROFESSIONAL RULE
NOTES: DEFAULTED ON PUBLIC HEALTH SERVICE EDUCATION LOAN. REINSTATED ON 7/15/96.

ROBERTS, GARY F MD, LICENSE NUMBER J1371 OF MESQUITE, TX, WAS DISCIPLINED BY TEXAS ON AUGUST 28, 1999
DISCIPLINARY ACTION: 60-MONTH RESTRICTION PLACED ON LICENSE; MONITORING OF PHYSICIAN PERFORMANCE
OFFENSE: SEXUAL ABUSE OF OR SEXUAL MISCONDUCT WITH A PATIENT
NOTES: ALLEGATIONS OF INAPPROPRIATE SEXUAL CONTACT WITH A MALE PATIENT ON 11/26/97; HE SOUGHT PSYCHIATRIC COUNSELING DURING 3 SESSIONS AND REPORTED THAT HE DID NOT SEEK ADDITIONAL COUNSELING BECAUSE HE HAD GAINED SUFFICIENT INSIGHT INTO HIS BEHAVIOR TO PREVENT FUTURE OCCURRENCES OF SUCH INCIDENCES IN H!S PRACTICE; HE HAS SELF-PRESCRIBED PROZAC AND DESYREL. LICENSE LIMITED AS FOLLOWS: SHALL NOMINATE THREE CERTIFIED PSYCHIATRISTS FOR BOARD SELECTION OF A THERAPIST AND SHALL EXPEDITIOUSLY SUBMIT HIMSELF TO EVALUATION AND TREATMENT BY THE APPROVED PRACTITIONER; SHALL NOT TREAT OR OTHERWISE SERVE AS PHYSICIAN, PRESCRIBE, DISPENSE OR ADMINISTER DRUGS THAT MAY BE SUBJECT TO ABUSE TO HIMSELF OR TO ANY MEMBER OF HIS FAMILY; SHALL HAVE A CHAPERONE PRESENT DURING EXAMS OF ANY PATIENTS; SHALL APPEAR BEFORE THE BOARD UPON REQUEST; TIME SPENT OUT OF TEXAS DOES NOT COUNT TOWARD RESTRICTION; SHALL INFORM THE BOARD OF CHANGE OF ADDRESS WITHIN 10 DAYS OR IF HE LEAVES THE STATE; SHALL NOT SEEK MODIFICATION FOR ONE YEAR.

ROBERTSON, GERALD MELVIN MD, LICENSE NUMBER 0005670 OF CALHOUN, LA, WAS DISCIPLINED BY MISSISSIPPI ON NOVEMBER 21, 1991
NOTES: IN VIEW OF THE LAPSED STATUS OF LICENSE, PENDING DISCIPLINARY ACTION WAS PLACED IN ABEYANCE WITH THE BOARD HAVING THE RIGHT TO ACTIVATE THE DISCIPLINARY ACTION IN THE EVENT HE ELECTS TO RENEW.

ROBERTSON, GERALD MELVIN MD, LICENSE NUMBER 00D9875 OF WEST MONROE, LA, WAS DISCIPLINED BY TEXAS ON AUGUST 20, 1992
DISCIPLINARY ACTION: RESTRICTION PLACED ON LICENSE
OFFENSE: DISCIPLINARY ACTION BY ANOTHER STATE OR AGENCY

ROBIN, SIDNEY THOMAS MD, LICENSE NUMBER E2824 OF AUSTIN, TX, WAS DISCIPLINED BY TEXAS ON JANUARY 29, 1999
DISCIPLINARY ACTION: FINE; REPRIMAND
OFFENSE: NONCOMPLIANCE WITH A PROFESSIONAL RULE
NOTES: FAILED TO OBTAIN 22 HOURS OF CONTINUING MEDICAL EDUCATION DURING 3/97 - 2/98, AS REQUIRED FOR RENEWAL OF HIS LICENSE ON 2/28/98. $100 FINE.

ROBINETT, KELLY EUGENE DO, LICENSE NUMBER 00G7576 OF BURLESON, TX, WAS DISCIPLINED BY TEXAS ON NOVEMBER 13, 1992
DISCIPLINARY ACTION: 60-MONTH PROBATION
OFFENSE: SUBSTANCE ABUSE
NOTES: UNPROFESSIONAL OR DISHONORABLE CONDUCT THAT IS LIKELY TO DECEIVE, DEFRAUD OR INJURE THE PUBLIC. LICENSE SUSPENDED, SUSPENSION STAYED. ON 11/3/94 ORDER MODIFIED AS FOLLOWS: SHALL ABSTAIN FROM THE CONSUMPTION OF ALCOHOL, DANGEROUS DRUGS, OR CONTROLLED SUBSTANCES IN ANY FORM UNLESS PRESCRIBED BY ANOTHER PHYSICIAN FOR A LEGITIMATE AND THERAPEUTIC PURPOSE; DANGEROUS DRUGS OR CONTROLLED SUBSTANCES FROM ANOTHER PHYSICIAN MUST BE REPORTED IMMEDIATELY TO THE BOARD CONCERNING THE MEDICAL CONDITION BEING TREATED AND THE SUBSTANCE PRESCRIBED, DISPENSED OR ADMINISTERED; SHALL SUBMIT HIMSELF FOR APPROPRIATE EXAMINATIONS, INCLUDING SCREENING FOR ALCOHOL OR DRUGS; SHALL CONTINUE TO PARTICIPATE IN THE ACTIVITIES OF COMMITTEE ON PHYSICIAN HEALTH AND REHABILITATION INCLUDING WEEKLY MEETINGS WITH QUARTERLY REPORTS; SHALL CONTINUE TO PARTICIPATE IN THE ACTIVITIES AND PROGRAMS OF ALCOHOLICS ANONYMOUS OR ANOTHER BOARD APPROVED PROGRAM ON A REGULAR BASIS OF NOT LESS THAN TWICE A WEEK WITH QUARTERLY REPORTS TO THE BOARD; HE IS GRANTED PERMISSION TO REAPPLY TO THE DRUG ENFORCEMENT ADMINISTRATION AND THE TEXAS DEPARTMENT OF PUBLIC SAFETY FOR SCHEDULES II, IIN, III, IIIN IV OR V; SEPARATE FROM PATIENT RECORDS SHALL MAINTAIN A COPY OF EVERY PRESCRIPTION WRITTEN FOR DANGEROUS DRUGS WHICH HAVE POTENTIAL FOR ABUSE BY DATE ISSUED WHICH SHALL BE AVAILABLE TO THE BOARD FOR INSPECTION; SHALL NOT TELEPHONE ANY PRESCRIPTION TO A PHARMACY FOR CONTROLLED SUBSTANCES OR DANGEROUS DRUGS; MAY ORDER CONTROLLED SUBSTANCES TO BE ADMINISTERED TO HOSPITAL OR NURSING HOME PATIENTS FOR THEIR MEDICAL NEEDS; SHALL NOT TREAT OR OTHERWISE SERVE AS PHYSICIAN, PRESCRIBE, DISPENSE OR ADMINISTER CONTROLLED SUBSTANCES OR ANY OTHER DRUGS THAT MAY BE SUBJECT TO ABUSE FOR HIMSELF OR ANY MEMBER OF HIS FAMILY; MAY ADMINISTER TO HIS IMMEDIATE FAMILY ONLY SUCH DRUGS AS ARE PRESCRIBED BY OTHER PHYSICIANS IN COMPLIANCE WITH THEIR ORDERS; SHALL SURRENDER ALL UNUSED TRIPLICATE PRESCRIPTION FORMS IN HIS POSSESSION; SHALL NOT ATTEMPT TO ORDER ANY MORE TRIPLICATE PRESCRIPTION FORMS UNTIL HE HAS BOARD AUTHORITY; SHALL APPEAR BEFORE THE BOARD ONCE A YEAR DURING EACH YEAR OF PROBATION TO REPORT ON HIS COMPLIANCE; SHALL GIVE A COPY OF THIS ORDER TO HEALTH CARE ENTITIES WHERE HE HAS PRIVILEGES; SHALL INFORM BOARD OF CHANGE OF ADDRESS WITHIN 10 DAYS OR IF HE LEAVES THE STATE; SHALL COOPERATE WITH BOARD IN VERIFYING COMPLIANCE; TIME SPENT OUT OF TEXAS DOES NOT COUNT TOWARD PROBATION; SHALL NOT SEEK MODIFICATION FOR ONE YEAR. ON 11/16/96 PROBATION TERMINATED.

ROBINSON, DANIEL D II MD, LICENSE NUMBER 00G3736, WAS DISCIPLINED BY TEXAS ON NOVEMBER 16, 1996
DISCIPLINARY ACTION: REPRIMAND
OFFENSE: SUBSTANDARD CARE, INCOMPETENCE OR NEGLIGENCE

NOTES: IN 1995, DID NOT ADEQUATELY MANAGE THE DIAGNOSTIC TESTING AND TREATMENT AND CARE OF AN 11 YEAR OLD PATIENT WHO PRESENTED WITH SYMPTOMS OF DIABETES; HE FAILED TO ADEQUATELY FOLLOW-UP WITH THE PATIENT'S FAMILY WHEN A URINALYSIS SHOWED POSITIVE FOR GLUCOSE AND TRACE KETONES.

ROBINSON, HERBERT J MD OF SAN ANTONIO, TX, WAS DISCIPLINED BY DEA ON MARCH 14, 1994
DISCIPLINARY ACTION: REVOCATION OF CONTROLLED SUBSTANCE LICENSE
OFFENSE: PROVIDING FALSE INFORMATION TO THE BOARD OR OTHER HEALTH AGENCY

NOTES: IN 1987, THE TEXAS BOARD SUBPOENAED PATIENT RECORDS FROM HIM WHICH HE REFUSED TO PROVIDE. ON 09/24/88 THE BOARD SUSPENDED HIS MEDICAL LICENSE INDEFINITELY UNTIL HE PROVIDED THE RECORDS IN QUESTION. SUSPENSION TERMINATED ON 1/12/91 AFTER HE PROVIDED THE RECORDS. IN A 1991 DEA APPLICATION HE LIED ABOUT THIS STATE LICENSE SUSPENSION.

ROBINSON, LUKE E MD, LICENSE NUMBER 00E4642 OF VICTORIA, TX, WAS DISCIPLINED BY TEXAS ON OCTOBER 5, 1991
DISCIPLINARY ACTION: 60-MONTH PROBATION; REQUIRED TO ENTER AN IMPAIRED PHYSICIAN PROGRAM OR SUBSTANCE ABUSE TREATMENT
OFFENSE: SUBSTANCE ABUSE

NOTES: FROM 1/90 THROUGH 12/12/90 HE ABUSED BENZODIAZEPAM AND ALCOHOL FOR NON-MEDICAL PURPOSES; PARTICIPATED IN A TREATMENT PROGRAM FOR TREATMENT OF CHEMICAL DEPENDENCY FROM 12/13/90 TO 1/25/91; EXECUTED A TWO YEAR CONTINUING CARE CONTRACT ON 1/25/91; IMPAIRMENT CAUSED HIM TO EXPERIENCE MEMORY BLACKOUTS AND CANCEL SCHEDULED SURGERIES AND APPOINTMENTS. SUSPENSION STAYED; CONDITIONS OF PROBATION: SHALL REFRAIN FROM CONSUMING ANY MOOD-ALTERING DRUGS, INCLUDING ALCOHOL; SHALL SUBMIT HIMSELF FOR RANDOM SCREENING OF BODILY FLUIDS; SHALL PARTICIPATE IN IMPAIRED PHYSICIANS PROGRAM WITH WEEKLY MEETINGS AND QUARTERLY REPORTS TO THE BOARD; SHALL PARTICIPATE IN AA, INCLUDING A 12-STEP PROGRAM, NOT LESS THAN TWICE A WEEK, WITH QUARTERLY REPORTS TO THE BOARD; SHALL COMPLY WITH CONDITIONS OF CONTINUING CARE CONTRACT; SHALL CONTINUE TO RECEIVE TREATMENT, WITH QUARTERLY REPORTS TO THE BOARD; SHALL APPEAR BEFORE THE BOARD TWICE A YEAR; SHALL COOPERATE WITH THE BOARD IN VERIFYING COMPLIANCE; SHALL ADVISE BOARD OF ANY CHANGE OF ADDRESS WITHIN 10 DAYS; TIME SPENT OUT OF TEXAS DOES NOT COUNT TOWARDS PROBATION; SHALL NOT PETITION FOR MODIFICATION FOR ONE YEAR. ON 4/15/94 REQUEST FOR TERMINATION OF THIS ORDER DENIED. ORDER MODIFIED AS FOLLOWS: APPEARANCES BEFORE BOARD REDUCED TO ONCE A YEAR DURING EACH YEAR OF PROBATION TO REPORT ON HIS COMPLIANCE; HE MAY REQUEST MODIFICATION OR TERMINATION OF THIS ORDER ONCE EVERY SIX MONTHS. ALL OTHER CONDITIONS OF THIS ORDER REMAIN IN EFFECT. ON 11/3/94 PROBATION TERMINATED.

ROBINSON, RALPH R MD, WAS DISCIPLINED BY WASHINGTON ON FEBRUARY 16, 1990
DISCIPLINARY ACTION: PROBATION; RESTRICTION PLACED ON CONTROLLED SUBSTANCE LICENSE
OFFENSE: DISCIPLINARY ACTION BY ANOTHER STATE OR AGENCY

NOTES: ON 12/6/89 BOARD ISSUED A STATEMENT OF CHARGES REGARDING FREQUENTLY PRESCRIBING, DISPENSING OR ADMINISTERING CONTROLLED SUBSTANCES FOR UNDIAGNOSED PAIN, FOR PROLONGED PERIODS OF TIME AND IN INAPPROPRIATE COMBINATIONS; HIS LICENSE HAS BEEN RESTRICTED IN KENTUCKY, ALABAMA, OKLAHOMA AND NORTH CAROLINA. THE FOLLOWING PROVISIONS OF THE KENTUCKY ORDER ARE ADOPTED BY WASHINGTON: UNABLE TO PRESCRIBE, ADMINISTER, OR DISPENSE SCHEDULE II, IIN, III, OR IIIN CONTROLLED DANGEROUS SUBSTANCES DURING PROBATION; MUST OBTAIN 15 HOURS PER YEAR OF CONTINUING MEDICAL EDUCATION IN PHARMACOLOGY FOR THE FIRST 2 YEARS OF PROBATION. WHEN HIS PRESCRIBING PRIVILEGES ARE REINSTATED IN COMMONWEALTH OF KENTUCKY, MAY APPLY FOR REINSTATEMENT IN WASHINGTON.

ROBINSON, RALPH R MD OF MIDDLESBORO, KY, WAS DISCIPLINED BY TENNESSEE ON MAY 14, 1990
DISCIPLINARY ACTION: 60-MONTH PROBATION; RESTRICTION PLACED ON CONTROLLED SUBSTANCE LICENSE
OFFENSE: DISCIPLINARY ACTION BY ANOTHER STATE OR AGENCY

NOTES: MAY NOT PRESCRIBE SCHEDULE II OR III DRUGS DURING PROBATION, HOWEVER, PHYSICIAN MAY REAPPLY FOR FULL DEA PRIVILEGES AFTER TWO YEARS. MUST COMPLETE CONTINUING MEDICAL EDUCATION COURSE IN PHARMACOLOGY.

ROBINSON, RALPH R MD, WAS DISCIPLINED BY WASHINGTON, D.C. ON SEPTEMBER 5, 1990
DISCIPLINARY ACTION: PROBATION
OFFENSE: DISCIPLINARY ACTION BY ANOTHER STATE OR AGENCY

NOTES: DISCIPLINED BY KENTUCKY FOR CONDUCT THAT WOULD BE GROUNDS FOR DISCIPLINARY ACTION IN THE DISTRICT OF COLUMBIA; FILED WITH THE BOARD A DOCUMENT HE KNEW OR SHOULD HAVE KNOWN WAS FALSE OR MISLEADING.

ROBINSON, RALPH R MD, LICENSE NUMBER C019518 OF MIDDLESBORO, KY, WAS DISCIPLINED BY CALIFORNIA ON JANUARY 10, 1991
DISCIPLINARY ACTION: SURRENDER OF LICENSE

NOTES: VOLUNTARY SURRENDER WHILE CHARGES PENDING.

ROBINSON, RALPH R MD OF MIDDLESBORO, KY, WAS DISCIPLINED BY VIRGINIA ON APRIL 9, 1991
DISCIPLINARY ACTION: PROBATION
OFFENSE: DISCIPLINARY ACTION BY ANOTHER STATE OR AGENCY

NOTES: DISCIPLINARY ACTION IN OTHER STATES.

ROBINSON, RALPH R MD, DATE OF BIRTH JULY 7, 1913, LICENSE NUMBER 0011914 OF BELL COUNTY, KY, WAS DISCIPLINED BY KENTUCKY ON MARCH 4, 1993
DISCIPLINARY ACTION: SURRENDER OF LICENSE

NOTES: IN LIEU OF INQUIRY CONCERNING MEDICAL PRACTICE.

ROBINSON, RALPH R MD, DATE OF BIRTH JULY 7, 1913, LICENSE NUMBER 0016797 OF MIDDLESBORO, KY, WAS DISCIPLINED BY VIRGINIA ON FEBRUARY 17, 1994
OFFENSE: DISCIPLINARY ACTION BY ANOTHER STATE OR AGENCY

NOTES: ON 2/18/93 KENTUCKY BOARD ACCEPTED HIS RETIREMENT FROM THE ACTIVE PRACTICE OF MEDICINE IN THAT JURISDICTION AND AGREED TO

TERMINATE INQUIRY INTO HIS PRESCRIBING OF CONTROLLED SUBSTANCES UNTIL HE REACTIVATES HIS KENTUCKY LICENSE. SURRENDER OF PRIVILEGE TO RENEW VIRGINIA LICENSE IN LIEU OF FURTHER ADMINISTRATIVE PROCEEDINGS.

ROBINSON, RALPH R MD OF 1032 18TH STREET SOUTH, BIRMINGHAM, AL, WAS DISCIPLINED BY DEA ON APRIL 7, 1995
DISCIPLINARY ACTION: RESTRICTION PLACED ON CONTROLLED SUBSTANCE LICENSE
OFFENSE: PROFESSIONAL MISCONDUCT

NOTES: ALLEGED CONTROLLED SUBSTANCE VIOLATIONS.

ROBINSON, RALPH ROLLIN MD, LICENSE NUMBER 00E7253 OF MIDDLESBORO, KY, WAS DISCIPLINED BY TEXAS ON DECEMBER 1, 1990
DISCIPLINARY ACTION: LICENSE REVOCATION

NOTES: PHYSICIAN, UNDER BOARD DISCIPLINARY ORDER, REQUESTED CANCELLATION OF LICENSE. IF HE REAPPLIES, BOARD DISCIPLINARY ORDER WILL BE REACTIVATED.

RODRIGUEZ, MARIO A MD, LICENSE NUMBER 00G9302 OF ARLINGTON, TX, WAS DISCIPLINED BY TEXAS ON APRIL 26, 1991
DISCIPLINARY ACTION: LICENSE REVOCATION
OFFENSE: PHYSICAL OR MENTAL ILLNESS INHIBITING THE ABILITY TO PRACTICE WITH SKILL AND SAFETY

NOTES: FAILURE TO PRACTICE MEDICINE WITH REASONABLE SAFETY AND SKILL NECESSARY BY REASON OF A MENTAL CONDITION.

RODRIGUEZ, SERGIO LUIS MD, LICENSE NUMBER 00D9276 OF LIBERTY, TX, WAS DISCIPLINED BY TEXAS ON APRIL 20, 1991
DISCIPLINARY ACTION: SURRENDER OF LICENSE

NOTES: LICENSE VOLUNTARILY SURRENDERED IN LIEU OF FURTHER DISCIPLINARY PROCEEDINGS.

RODRIGUEZ, SERGIO LUIS MD, LICENSE NUMBER 0C38767 OF LIBERTY, TX, WAS DISCIPLINED BY CALIFORNIA ON NOVEMBER 28, 1994
DISCIPLINARY ACTION: LICENSE REVOCATION
OFFENSE: DISCIPLINARY ACTION BY ANOTHER STATE OR AGENCY

NOTES: DISCIPLINED BY TEXAS BOARD FOR MENTAL IMPAIRMENT AFFECTING SAFE PRACTICES. DEFAULT DECISION.

RODRIGUEZ, VINCENT J MD, DATE OF BIRTH AUGUST 23, 1959 OF PO BOX 1, HUNT, TX, WAS DISCIPLINED BY MEDICARE ON DECEMBER 20, 1991
DISCIPLINARY ACTION: EXCLUSION FROM THE MEDICARE AND/OR MEDICAID PROGRAM
OFFENSE: DISCIPLINARY ACTION BY ANOTHER STATE OR AGENCY

NOTES: LICENSE REVOCATION OR SUSPENSION.

RODRIGUEZ, VINCENT J MD OF 704 NORTH THIRD STREET, PLAINVIEW, NE, WAS DISCIPLINED BY DEA ON MAY 8, 1995
DISCIPLINARY ACTION: SURRENDER OF CONTROLLED SUBSTANCE LICENSE

NOTES: IN LIEU OF ORDER TO SHOW CAUSE.

RODRIGUEZ, VINCENT JOHN MD, LICENSE NUMBER 0053547 OF TALLAHASSEE, FL, WAS DISCIPLINED BY FLORIDA ON FEBRUARY 6, 1990
DISCIPLINARY ACTION: EMERGENCY SUSPENSION
OFFENSE: OVERPRESCRIBING OR MISPRESCRIBING DRUGS

NOTES: INABILITY TO PRACTICE WITH REASONABLE SKILL BY REASON OF THE USE OF DRUGS OR AS A RESULT OF A MENTAL OR PHYSICAL CONDITION; PRESCRIBING TO HIMSELF.

RODRIGUEZ, VINCENT JOHN MD, LICENSE NUMBER 0028371 OF HUNT, TX, WAS DISCIPLINED BY COLORADO ON APRIL 10, 1991
DISCIPLINARY ACTION: LICENSE REVOCATION
OFFENSE: CRIMINAL CONVICTION OR PLEA OF GUILTY, NOLO CONTENDERE, OR NO CONTEST TO A CRIME

NOTES: ACTION BASED ON HABITUAL OR EXCESSIVE USE OF CONTROLLED SUBSTANCES AND FELONY CONVICTION FOR CARRYING A CONCEALED WEAPON.

RODRIGUEZ, VINCENT JOHN MD, LICENSE NUMBER 0053547 OF HUNT, TX, WAS DISCIPLINED BY FLORIDA ON MAY 6, 1991
DISCIPLINARY ACTION: LICENSE SUSPENSION; 60-MONTH

NOTES: CHARGED WITH BEING UNABLE TO PRACTICE BY REASON OF THE USE OF DRUGS OR AS A RESULT OF ANY MENTAL OR PHYSICAL CONDITION. IN LIEU OF FURTHER PROSECUTION, STIPULATED TO SUSPENSION UNTIL HE CAN PROVE HE IS ABLE TO PRACTICE WITH REASONABLE SKILL AND SAFETY, WHICH SHALL INCLUDE SATISFACTORY PSYCHIATRIC AND PHYSICAL EVALUATIONS; ACTIVE PHYSICIANS RECOVERY NETWORK CONTRACT; BOARD APPROVED PLAN FOR REENTRY TO PRACTICE. UPON REINSTATEMENT, PROBATION WITH TERMS AND CONDITIONS TO BE SET, WHICH SHALL INCLUDE CONTINUATION OF ACTIVE PHYSICIAN'S RECOVERY NETWORK CONTRACT.

RODRIGUEZ, VINCENT JOHN MD OF 9950 W 80TH AVENUE #16, ARVADA, CO, WAS DISCIPLINED BY DEA ON AUGUST 1, 1991
DISCIPLINARY ACTION: REVOCATION OF CONTROLLED SUBSTANCE LICENSE
OFFENSE: DISCIPLINARY ACTION BY ANOTHER STATE OR AGENCY

NOTES: ON 4/10/91 COLORADO REVOKED HIS LICENSE. IN HIS STATEMENT HE CONTENDS COLORADO ACTION WAS BASED ON FLORIDA'S EMERGENCY SUSPENSION OF HIS LICENSE ON 2/6/90 AND THAT HE HAD ENTERED INTO AN AGREEMENT WITH FLORIDA PERMITTING HIM TO SEEK REINSTATEMENT ON 5/6/91. DEA FOUND THESE FACTS IRRELEVANT TO THE FACT THAT HE DID NOT HAVE PRESCRIBING AUTHORITY IN COLORADO.

RODRIGUEZ, VINCENT JOHN MD, LICENSE NUMBER 0053547 OF PLAINVIEW, NE, WAS DISCIPLINED BY FLORIDA ON DECEMBER 29, 1995
DISCIPLINARY ACTION: LICENSE REVOCATION
OFFENSE: DISCIPLINARY ACTION BY ANOTHER STATE OR AGENCY

NOTES: VIOLATING BOARD RULE IN THAT HE FAILED TO NOTIFY THE BOARD OF THE ADDRESS OF HIS NEW PRIMARY PLACE OF PRACTICE; VIOLATING PREVIOUS BOARD ORDER IN THAT HE FAILED TO COMPLY WITH THE PHYSICIAN'S RECOVERY NETWORK CONTRACT AS REQUIRED; NEBRASKA BOARD ACCEPTED THE VOLUNTARY SURRENDER OF HIS LICENSE AND CONTROLLED SUBSTANCE REGISTRATION AFTER FILING A PETITION FOR DISCIPLINARY ACTION.

RODRIGUEZSILVA, MARIO A MD, LICENSE NUMBER 0049850 OF ARLINGTON, TX, WAS DISCIPLINED BY FLORIDA ON MAY 6, 1991
DISCIPLINARY ACTION: 24-MONTH LICENSE SUSPENSION; REQUIRED TO TAKE ADDITIONAL MEDICAL EDUCATION
OFFENSE: SUBSTANDARD CARE, INCOMPETENCE OR NEGLIGENCE

NOTES: CHARGED WITH FAILING TO PRACTICE MEDICINE WITH AN ACCEPTABLE LEVEL OF CARE AND SKILL; FAILING

TO KEEP WRITTEN MEDICAL RECORDS JUSTIFYING THE COURSE OF TREATMENT OF A PATIENT; PRESCRIBING, DISPENSING, ADMINISTERING, MIXING, OR OTHERWISE PREPARING LEGEND DRUGS NOT IN THE BEST INTEREST OF THE PATIENT. IN LIEU OF FURTHER PROSECUTION, STIPULATED TO ESTABLISH SATISFACTORY COMPLETION OF AN ACGME ACCREDITED RESIDENCY PROGRAM OF AT LEAST ONE YEAR. UPON REINSTATEMENT, BOARD MAY PLACE LICENSE ON PROBATION FOR A PERIOD NOT TO EXCEED 18 MONTHS WITH TERMS AND CONDITIONS.

ROGERS, CHERYL J MD, LICENSE NUMBER 1032007 OF PO BOX 292265, LOUISVILLE, TX, WAS DISCIPLINED BY INDIANA ON APRIL 17, 1990
DISCIPLINARY ACTION: 26-MONTH PROBATION; MONITORING OF PHYSICIAN PERFORMANCE
OFFENSE: SUBSTANCE ABUSE

NOTES: ABUSED DEMEROL WHICH SHE SELF-PRESCRIBED. EMERGENCY SUSPENSION LIFTED. THE FOLLOWING TERMS AND CONDITIONS WERE ATTACHED TO PROBATION WHICH FOLLOWED SUSPENSION: MUST SUBMIT COPIES OF RESULTS OF ANY AND ALL BLOOD AND/OR URINE SCREENS, MUST SUBMIT REPORTS CONCERNING ATTENDANCE AT AA, NARCOTICS ANONYMOUS AND CADUCEUS MEETINGS AND QUARTERLY REPORTS ON AFTERCARE PROGRAM. INDEFINITE PROBATION ISSUED AND STAYED, TO BEGIN 07/01/92, WHICH INCLUDES THE FOLLOWING TERMS AND CONDITIONS: POSSESSION OF AN UNLIMITED LICENSE TO PRACTICE MEDICINE DURING PROBATIONARY PERIOD, PROHIBITED FROM POSSESSING AN INDIANA CONTROLLED SUBSTANCE REGISTRATION PERMIT, PARTICIPATION IN AA OR NARCOTICS ANONYMOUS MEETINGS A MINIMUM OF THREE TIMES A WEEK, COMPLETION OF FOUR HOURS OF COMMUNITY SERVICE A WEEK FOR 46 WEEKS A YEAR, SUBMISSION TO RANDOM BLOOD AND URINE SCREENS. ASSESSED COSTS OF $150.

ROHLFING, JEFFREY W MD OF FRESNO, CA, WAS DISCIPLINED BY UTAH ON DECEMBER 11, 1997

NOTES: DISCIPLINARY ACTION TAKEN AGAINST HIS MEDICAL LICENSE IN CALIFORNIA. HE AGREED NOT TO PRACTICE MEDICINE IN UTAH BEFORE OR AFTER THE EXPIRATION DATE OF HIS LICENSES TO PRACTICE MEDICINE AND TO PRESCRIBE AND ADMINISTER CONTROLLED SUBSTANCES (WHICH IS 1/31/98). HE AGREED NOT TO RENEW HIS LICENSES. HE FURTHER AGREED THAT NO APPLICATION TO REAPPLY FOR LICENSURE WOULD BE CONSIDERED FOR AT LEAST FIVE YEARS FROM THE DATE OF THE ORDER.

ROHLFING, JEFFREY WILLIAM MD, LICENSE NUMBER C37481 OF FRESNO, CA, WAS DISCIPLINED BY CALIFORNIA ON FEBRUARY 17, 1997
DISCIPLINARY ACTION: 60-MONTH PROBATION
OFFENSE: SUBSTANCE ABUSE

NOTES: IMPAIRMENT DUE TO MENTAL ILLNESS, USE OF ALCOHOLIC BEVERAGES TO AN EXTENT THAT HIS ABILITY TO PRACTICE MEDICINE SAFELY WAS IMPAIRED; FAILURE TO COMPLY WITH THE BOARD'S DIVERSION PROGRAM. REVOCATION STAYED.

ROHLFING, JEFFREY WILLIAM MD, LICENSE NUMBER D9640 OF FRESNO, CA, WAS DISCIPLINED BY TEXAS ON APRIL 4, 1998
OFFENSE: DISCIPLINARY ACTION BY ANOTHER STATE OR AGENCY

NOTES: IN 12/96 THE CALIFORNIA BOARD PLACED HIS LICENSE ON PROBATION FOR EXHIBITING BIZARRE, IRRATIONAL, AND DELUSIONAL BEHAVIOR AND COMMUNICATIONS. LICENSE LIMITED AS FOLLOWS: SHALL NOT PRACTICE MEDICINE IN TEXAS UNTIL HE REQUESTS TO RESUME PRACTICING, APPEARS BEFORE THE BOARD WITH EVIDENCE THAT HE IS PHYSICALLY, MENTALLY AND OTHERWISE COMPETENT TO SAFELY PRACTICE; SHALL COMPLY WITH THE CALIFORNIA BOARD ORDER; SHALL SHOW THAT HE IS NOT THE SUBJECT OF ANY OTHER CIVIL, CRIMINAL OR ADMINISTRATIVE ACTION.

ROMAN, ERNEST T MD, LICENSE NUMBER 00H6938 OF MCALLEN, TX, WAS DISCIPLINED BY TEXAS ON JANUARY 6, 1995
DISCIPLINARY ACTION: 36-MONTH PROBATION; MONITORING OF PHYSICIAN PERFORMANCE
OFFENSE: PROFESSIONAL MISCONDUCT

NOTES: DURING 10/93 FAILED TO EXAMINE AND EVALUATE A PATIENT DURING THE PATIENT'S CARE AND TREATMENT INSTEAD DELEGATING AND RELYING ENTIRELY ON THE EVALUATION OF A MEDICAL ASSISTANT WHICH RESULTED IN A MISDIAGNOSIS; IN LIEU OF FURTHER INVESTIGATION. SUSPENSION STAYED. CONDITIONS OF PROBATION: SHALL ADEQUATELY SUPERVISE ALL INDIVIDUALS UNDER HIS CONTROL OR SUPERVISION OR IN WHICH HE HAS AN OWNERSHIP INTEREST; SHALL PERSONALLY EXAMINE AND OR TREAT PATIENTS WHEN A FORM REPRESENTS THIS OR ANY TIME AN INITIAL DIAGNOSIS OR EXAM IS PERFORMED; WITHIN SIX MONTHS SHALL PROVIDE A NOTARIZED REPORT DETAILING THE BILLING PRACTICES OF CLINICS UNDER HIS CONTROL OR SUPERVISION OR IN WHICH HE HAS AN OWNERSHIP INTEREST; SHALL APPEAR BEFORE THE BOARD ONCE A YEAR OR UPON REQUEST; SHALL COOPERATE WITH BOARD IN VERIFYING COMPLIANCE; SHALL GIVE A COPY OF THIS ORDER TO ANY HEALTH CARE ENTITY WHERE HE HAS OR APPLIES FOR PRIVILEGES OR ANYONE ELSE WHO ASKS; SHALL ENSURE ANY INQUIRIES REGARDING HIS TEXAS LICENSURE STATUS ARE ANSWERED BY REFERENCING THIS ORDER; SHALL INFORM BOARD OF CHANGE OF ADDRESS WITHIN 10 DAYS OR IF HE LEAVES THE STATE; TIME SPENT OUT OF TEXAS DOES NOT COUNT TOWARD PROBATION. SHALL NOT SEEK MODIFICATION FOR ONE YEAR.

ROMAN, ERNEST T MD, LICENSE NUMBER 0054514 OF PHARR, TX, WAS DISCIPLINED BY FLORIDA ON NOVEMBER 7, 1996
DISCIPLINARY ACTION: LICENSE SUSPENSION; FINE
OFFENSE: DISCIPLINARY ACTION BY ANOTHER STATE OR AGENCY

NOTES: ACTION BY ANOTHER STATE; FAILED TO REPORT DISCIPLINARY ACTION IN ANOTHER JURISDICTION; VIOLATING A BOARD RULE OR ORDER OR FAILING TO COMPLY WITH A LAWFUL SUBPOENA OF THE BOARD. SUSPENSION UNTIL HE DEMONSTRATES THAT HIS LICENSE TO PRACTICE MEDICINE IN TEXAS IS UNENCUMBERED; PROBATION UPON REINSTATEMENT; AND REPRIMAND. $1,000 FINE.

ROMEU, DELIO G MD, LICENSE NUMBER 00D5888 OF SAN ANTONIO, TX, WAS DISCIPLINED BY TEXAS ON MAY 15, 1996
DISCIPLINARY ACTION: FINE; 60-MONTH RESTRICTION PLACED ON LICENSE
OFFENSE: SEXUAL ABUSE OF OR SEXUAL MISCONDUCT WITH A PATIENT

NOTES: ALLEGATIONS HAVE BEEN RECEIVED CLAIMING THAT HE CONDUCTED AN INAPPROPRIATE BREAST EXAMINATION OF AN ADULT FEMALE WHOSE SIX YEAR OLD DAUGHTER WAS IN THE ROOM; MAINTAINS THAT

ALL ASPECTS OF HIS EXAMINATION WERE APPROPRIATE AND MEDICALLY INDICATED. RESTRICTION OF LICENSE WITH TERMS AND CONDITIONS: SHALL HAVE A CHAPERONE PRESENT WHENEVER HE EXAMINES A FEMALE PATIENT AND SHALL NOTE THIS IN THE PATIENT'S CHART; SHALL MAINTAIN ADEQUATE MEDICAL RECORDS WHICH SHALL BE AVAILABLE FOR REVIEW; SHALL ATTEND AT LEAST 50 HOURS PER YEAR OF CONTINUING MEDICAL EDUCATION, AT LEAST 10 HOURS OF WHICH SHALL BE IN RISK MANAGEMENT; SHALL APPEAR BEFORE BOARD AT LEAST ONCE A YEAR OR AT BOARD REQUEST; SHALL COOPERATE WITH BOARD IN VERIFYING COMPLIANCE; SHALL GIVE A COPY OF THIS ORDER TO ANY HEALTH CARE ENTITY WHERE HE HAS PRIVILEGES; SHALL PROVIDE A COPY OF THIS ORDER TO ANYONE REQUESTING IT WITHIN 10 DAYS; TIME SPENT OUT OF TEXAS DOES NOT COUNT TOWARD RESTRICTION; SHALL INFORM BOARD OF CHANGE OF ADDRESS WITHIN 10 DAYS OR IF HE LEAVES THE STATE. SHALL NOT SEEK MODIFICATION FOR ONE YEAR. SHALL PAY $500 FINE. ON 5/16/98 ORDER TERMINATED.

RORER, RICHARD S MD, DATE OF BIRTH NOVEMBER 1, 1963 OF 2312 MISTY RIDGE CIRCLE, ARLINGTON, TX, WAS DISCIPLINED BY MEDICARE ON APRIL 20, 1999
DISCIPLINARY ACTION: EXCLUSION FROM THE MEDICARE AND/OR MEDICAID PROGRAM
OFFENSE: NONCOMPLIANCE WITH A PROFESSIONAL RULE

NOTES: DEFAULTED ON PUBLIC HEALTH SERVICE EDUCATION LOAN.

ROSALES, ANNA MARIE MD, DATE OF BIRTH JANUARY 11, 1961 OF 3882 COUNTY ROAD #541, HONDO, TX, WAS DISCIPLINED BY MEDICARE ON MAY 20, 1998
DISCIPLINARY ACTION: EXCLUSION FROM THE MEDICARE AND/OR MEDICAID PROGRAM
OFFENSE: NONCOMPLIANCE WITH A PROFESSIONAL RULE

NOTES: DEFAULTED ON PUBLIC HEALTH SERVICE EDUCATION LOAN. REINSTATED ON 6/17/98.

ROSE, FRANK MD, LICENSE NUMBER 080718 OF ROSE CNTR 1520 NORTH FRAZIER ST, CONROE, TX, WAS DISCIPLINED BY NEW YORK ON JULY 2, 1997
DISCIPLINARY ACTION: 36-MONTH PROBATION; REPRIMAND
OFFENSE: DISCIPLINARY ACTION BY ANOTHER STATE OR AGENCY

NOTES: DISCIPLINED BY THE TEXAS BOARD FOR AIDING AND ABETTING THE UNLICENSED PRACTICE OF MEDICINE. PROBATION COMMENCING UPON PRACTICING IN NEW YORK.

ROSE, MARK RICHARD MD, LICENSE NUMBER J8112, WAS DISCIPLINED BY TEXAS ON AUGUST 9, 1997
DISCIPLINARY ACTION: 120-MONTH PROBATION; RESTRICTION PLACED ON LICENSE
OFFENSE: FAILURE TO COMPLY WITH PREVIOUS BOARD ORDER

NOTES: ON 5/11/95 THE BOARD GRANTED HIM A TEXAS LICENSE, UPON PASSAGE OF THE JURISPRUDENCE EXAM, AND PLACED HIM ON PROBATION FOR FIVE YEARS WITH TERMS BASED ON HIS HISTORY OF ALCOHOL ABUSE AND TREATMENT FOR SUCH. HE REPORTED A SOBRIETY DATE OF 2/10/93. ON 2/28/97 HE INGESTED ALCOHOL IN VIOLATION OF THE 5/11/95 ORDER AND WAS ARRESTED FOR DUI IN BOSSIER CITY, LOUISIANA. ON 3/3/97 HE REPORTED HIS RELAPSE TO HIS COMPLIANCE OFFICER. ON 3/5/97 HE ENTERED TREATMENT AT A SPECIFIED FACILITY. HE HAS ENTERED INTO AN AFTER-CARE CONTRACT WITH A COUNTY MEDICAL SOCIETY COMMITTEE ON PHYSICIAN HEALTH AND REHABILITATION. SUSPENSION STAYED FOR PROBATION UNDER THE FOLLOWING TERMS AND CONDITIONS: SHALL SUBMIT IN WRITING A PROPOSED PRACTICE ARRANGEMENT AND SETTING, INVOLVING NO MORE THAN 40 HOURS PER WEEK AND ONLY IN A GROUP OR INSTITUTIONAL SETTING; SHALL ABSTAIN FROM THE CONSUMPTION OF ALCOHOL/DRUGS IN ANY FORM UNLESS PRESCRIBED BY ANOTHER PHYSICIAN FOR A LEGITIMATE AND THERAPEUTIC PURPOSE; SHALL SUBMIT HIMSELF FOR APPROPRIATE EXAMS INCLUDING DRUG OR ALCOHOL SCREENS; SHALL NOMINATE THREE CERTIFIED PSYCHIATRISTS FOR BOARD SELECTION OF A THERAPIST AND SHALL EXPEDITIOUSLY SUBMIT HIMSELF TO EVALUATION AND TREATMENT BY THE APPROVED PRACTITIONER; SHALL PARTICIPATE IN THE ACTIVITIES OF A PHYSICIAN HEALTH AND REHABILITATION COMMITTEE AND ATTEND WEEKLY MEETINGS WITH QUARTERLY REPORTS; SHALL PARTICIPATE IN AA'S PROGRAM NOT LESS THAN FIVE TIMES A WEEK; SHALL REPORT ON HIS ATTENDANCE; SHALL COMPLY WITH HIS CONTINUING CARE CONTRACT WITH QUARTERLY REPORTS TO THE BOARD; SHALL APPEAR BEFORE THE BOARD UPON REQUEST; SHALL COMPLY WITH THE TERMS OF ANY CONTRACT OR AGREEMENT FOR HOSPITAL PRIVILEGES AND SHALL REPORT IN WRITING ANY ACTION AGAINST HIS PRIVILEGES; SHALL NOT TREAT OR OTHERWISE SERVE AS PHYSICIAN, PRESCRIBE, DISPENSE OR ADMINISTER DRUGS THAT MAY BE SUBJECT TO ABUSE TO HIMSELF OR TO ANY MEMBER OF HIS FAMILY; SHALL OBTAIN AT LEAST 50 HOURS PER YEAR OF CONTINUING MEDICAL EDUCATION; SHALL COOPERATE WITH THE BOARD IN VERIFYING COMPLIANCE INCLUDING PROVIDING COPIES OF MEDICAL RELEASES AND PEER REVIEW RECORDS UPON REQUEST; SHALL GIVE A COPY OF THIS ORDER TO ANY HEALTH CARE ENTITY WHERE HE HAS PRIVILEGES; SHALL PROVIDE A COPY OF THIS ORDER TO ANYONE REQUESTING IT WITHIN 10 DAYS; TIME SPENT OUT OF TEXAS DOES NOT COUNT TOWARD PROBATION; SHALL INFORM THE BOARD OF CHANGE OF ADDRESS WITHIN 10 DAYS OR IF HE LEAVES THE STATE; SHALL NOT SEEK MODIFICATION FOR ONE YEAR.

ROSE, TERRANCE L MD, LICENSE NUMBER 00G0028 OF RED OAK, TX, WAS DISCIPLINED BY TEXAS ON JANUARY 26, 1990
DISCIPLINARY ACTION: SURRENDER OF CONTROLLED SUBSTANCE LICENSE; 3-MONTH LICENSE SUSPENSION

NOTES: STIPULATED ORDER. REVOCATION STAYED. FOLLOWING LICENSE SUSPENSION, LICENSE REINSTATED UPON 10-YEAR PROBATION. MUST SUBMIT TO PSYCHIATRIC EVALUATION AND TREATMENT, SURRENDER CONTROLLED SUBSTANCES REGISTRATION CERTIFICATES AND UNUSED TRIPLICATE PRESCRIPTION FORMS AND NOT OBTAIN REGISTRATIONS WITHOUT BOARD PERMISSION, COMPLETE PRECEPTORSHIP ON PREVENTION AND TREATMENT OF DRUG ABUSE, APPEAR BEFORE BOARD ANNUALLY, OBTAIN CONTINUING MEDICAL EDUCATION, MAINTAIN ADEQUATE MEDICAL RECORDS ON PATIENT OFFICE VISITS, REFRAIN FROM ISSUING PRESCRIPTIONS AND FROM ADMINISTERING OR DISPENSING DANGEROUS DRUGS TO PATIENTS UNLESS PHYSICIAN CONCLUDED SUCH DRUG THERAPEUTIC FOR MEDICAL CONDITION, SHALL NOT PRESCRIBE, ADMINISTER, OR DISPENSE DRUGS WITH ABUSE POTENTIAL UNTIL SATISFIED OF LEGITIMATE MEDICAL AND THERAPEUTIC NEED AND AFTER EXAMINATION, AND MAINTAIN SEPARATE FILE OF PRESCRIPTIONS FOR DANGEROUS DRUGS. ON

6/28/95 ORDER MODIFIED AS FOLLOWS: HE IS AUTHORIZED TO REAPPLY TO THE DEA AND THE TEXAS DEPARTMENT OF PUBLIC SAFETY TO OBTAIN FULL PRESCRIBING AUTHORITY FOR CONTROLLED SUBSTANCES; SEPARATE FROM PATIENT RECORDS, SHALL MAINTAIN A FILE OF EVERY PRESCRIPTION WRITTEN FOR CONTROLLED SUBSTANCES WITH ADDICTIVE POTENTIAL AND MAINTAIN A LOG OF ALL PRESCRIPTIONS OR REFILLS TELEPHONED IN BY HIM FOR CONTROLLED SUBSTANCES WHICH SHALL BE AVAILABLE FOR INSPECTION; SHALL MAINTAIN ADEQUATE MEDICAL RECORDS WHICH SHALL BE AVAILABLE FOR REVIEW; SHALL INFORM THE BOARD OF CHANGE OF ADDRESS WITHIN 10 DAYS; ALL OTHER CONDITIONS REMAIN IN EFFECT.

ROSENKRANTZ, MILTON PAUL MD OF CHALMETTE, LA, WAS DISCIPLINED BY LOUISIANA ON JULY 19, 1990
DISCIPLINARY ACTION: 6-MONTH LICENSE SUSPENSION; 54-MONTH PROBATION
OFFENSE: SUBSTANDARD CARE, INCOMPETENCE OR NEGLIGENCE

NOTES: PRESCRIBING, DISPENSING, OR ADMINISTERING CONTROLLED SUBSTANCES WITHOUT LEGITIMATE MEDICAL JUSTIFICATION, PROFESSIONAL INCOMPETENCY, CONTINUING OR RECURRING MEDICAL PRACTICE FAILING TO SATISFY PREVAILING STANDARDS OF PRACTICE. PROBATION OF 4 1/2 YEARS AFTER MEDICAL LICENSE SUSPENSION TO INCLUDE THE FOLLOWING CONDITIONS: PROHIBITION ON PRESCRIPTION OF CONTROLLED SUBSTANCES FOR ONE YEAR; LIFETIME PROHIBITION ON PRESCRIPTION OF SCHEDULE II CONTROLLED SUBSTANCES; MAINTENANCE OF PRESCRIPTION LOG FOR DURATION OF PROBATION; COMPLETION OF SPECIFIED CONTINUING MEDICAL EDUCATION; 100 HOURS COMMUNITY SERVICE PER YEAR FOR FIVE YEARS; $5000 FINE.

ROSENKRANTZ, MILTON PAUL MD OF 401 W GENIE STREET, CHALMETTE, LA, WAS DISCIPLINED BY DEA ON SEPTEMBER 14, 1990
DISCIPLINARY ACTION: SURRENDER OF CONTROLLED SUBSTANCE LICENSE; FINE

NOTES: PAID $5,000 FINE; WITHDRAWAL OF APPLICATION.

ROSENKRANTZ, MILTON PAUL MD, LICENSE NUMBER 00E4646 OF NEW ORLEANS, LA, WAS DISCIPLINED BY TEXAS ON DECEMBER 3, 1990
DISCIPLINARY ACTION: 14-MONTH LICENSE SUSPENSION; PROBATION
OFFENSE: DISCIPLINARY ACTION BY ANOTHER STATE OR AGENCY

NOTES: ON 7/19/90 LOUISIANA BOARD SUSPENDED HIS LICENSE AND IMPOSED TERMS OF PROBATION AND FINE FOR PRESCRIBING CONTROLLED SUBSTANCES, PRIMARILY NARCOTIC ANALGESICS IN ALLEGEDLY EXCESSIVE QUANTITIES TO 19 PATIENTS. SUSPENSION UNTIL 2/15/91; MUST COMPLY WITH TERMS OF LOUISIANA ORDER; MUST RECEIVE PERMISSION FROM TEXAS BOARD BEFORE RETURNING TO PRACTICE IN TEXAS AND BE SUBJECT TO ANY TERMS IMPOSED. REQUEST TO PRACTICE IN TEXAS GRANTED 3/23/92; SHALL COMPLY WITH TERMS OF THIS ORDER, APPEAR ANNUALLY BEFORE THE BOARD AND PERFORM 100 HOURS PER YEAR OF COMMUNITY SERVICE.

ROTH, MAXIMO MD, LICENSE NUMBER 00C7757 OF TEXAS CITY, TX, WAS DISCIPLINED BY TEXAS ON MAY 15, 1996
DISCIPLINARY ACTION: FINE
OFFENSE: PROFESSIONAL MISCONDUCT

NOTES: IN 1/94, HIS MEDICAL ASSISTANT TREATED A PATIENT ON TWO OCCASIONS FOR A JOB-RELATED INJURY WITHOUT PHYSICIAN'S PRESENCE OR SUPERVISION INCLUDING HAVING AN X-RAY PERFORMED, CLEANING AND DRESSING A WOUND, A TETANUS BOOSTER, FAXING A PRESCRIPTION AND REMOVING A FOREIGN BODY FROM THE WOUND; REPORTS THAT THE ASSISTANT WAS REPRIMANDED AND INFORMED THAT SUCH BEHAVIOR WOULD NOT BE TOLERATED; A RANDOM REVIEW OF PATIENT RECORDS BY BOARD DID NOT REVEAL ANY SIMILAR UNSUPERVISED CARE BY THE MEDICAL ASSISTANT. SHALL PAY $1,000 FINE; SHALL COOPERATE WITH THE BOARD IN VERIFYING COMPLIANCE.

ROTHWELL, RICHARD O'NEILL MD, LICENSE NUMBER D9644 OF ABILENE, TX, WAS DISCIPLINED BY TEXAS ON AUGUST 22, 1998
DISCIPLINARY ACTION: FINE; REPRIMAND
OFFENSE: PROFESSIONAL MISCONDUCT

NOTES: IN 1990 HE FAILED TO PROPERLY TERMINATE THE PHYSICIAN-PATIENT RELATIONSHIP PRIOR TO ENGAGING IN A PERSONAL RELATIONSHIP WITH A PATIENT. $5,000 FINE.

ROUTH, LISA C MD, WAS DISCIPLINED BY ALASKA ON MAY 5, 1995
DISCIPLINARY ACTION: 6-MONTH PROBATION; FINE

NOTES: INFORMATION PROVIDED IN RELATION TO APPLICATION FOR ALASKA MEDICAL LICENSE. CONDITIONS OF PROBATION: PRACTICE MONITOR; CONSULTING PHYSICIAN MUST MEET WITH AND REVIEW SPECIFIC NUMBER OF CHARTS TO DISCUSS HANDLING AND MANAGEMENT OF PATIENTS AND PROVIDE REPORTS TO THE BOARD; MUST INFORM BOARD IF FORMAL CHARGES ARE FILED BY TEXAS STATE BOARD; $2500 FINE; A COPY OF THIS STIPULATION MUST GO TO MONITOR; MUST NOTIFY BOARD OF CURRENT ADDRESSES, EMPLOYER AND ALASKA HOSPITALS WHERE SHE IS ON STAFF.

ROUTH, LISA CAROLE MD, LICENSE NUMBER H2742 OF ANCHORAGE, AK, WAS DISCIPLINED BY TEXAS ON AUGUST 22, 1998
DISCIPLINARY ACTION: FINE; REPRIMAND
OFFENSE: DISCIPLINARY ACTION BY ANOTHER STATE OR AGENCY

NOTES: ALLEGATION THAT HER PROVISIONAL CLINICAL PRIVILEGES HAD BEEN TERMINATED, WHICH, IF TRUE, IS A REPORTABLE ACTION; SHE IS LICENSED TO PRACTICE IN TEXAS AND ALASKA, AND CURRENTLY PRACTICES IN ALASKA; SHE MAINTAINS THAT THE TERMINATION OF PRIVILEGES WAS A "DISPUTE" AND NOT DISCIPLINE, AND THAT HER ERRONEOUS ANSWERS ON HER ALASKA LICENSURE APPLICATION WERE THE RESULT OF A MISUNDERSTANDING; SHE MAINTAINS SHE DID NOT INTENTIONALLY ANSWER INCORRECTLY OR MISLEAD THE BOARD ON HER APPLICATION; ON 9/9/94 THE ALASKA BOARD CONTACTED THE TEXAS BOARD ABOUT THIS INVESTIGATION AS SHE WAS APPLYING FOR LICENSURE IN ALASKA AT THAT TIME; SHE HAD NOT DISCLOSED THE PENDING TEXAS INVESTIGATION ON APPROPRIATE LICENSING FORMS SUBMITTED TO THE ALASKA BOARD; SHE SAID SHE HAD NOT BEEN DISCIPLINED BY A HOSPITAL STAFF, INTERNSHIP OR RESIDENCY TRAINING PROGRAM ON HER ALASKA APPLICATION; HOWEVER, SHE WAS DISCIPLINED AT RICHARDSON MEDICAL CENTER AND TIMERLAWN PSYCHIATRIC HOSPITAL (BOTH FOR LATE REPORTS); ON 5/5/95 THE ALASKA BOARD DISCIPLINED HER LICENSE; SHE HAS COMPLETED HER PROBATIONARY PERIOD AND ALL OTHER REQUIREMENTS IN THE ALASKA ORDER AND PRESENTLY HOLDS AN

UNRESTRICTED LICENSE. $1,000 FINE.

ROYBAL-HAEN, MARIA E MD, DATE OF BIRTH NOVEMBER 17, 1952 OF 1101 PECAN BOULEVARD #131, MCALLEN, TX, WAS DISCIPLINED BY MEDICARE ON JANUARY 5, 1997
DISCIPLINARY ACTION: EXCLUSION FROM THE MEDICARE AND/OR MEDICAID PROGRAM
OFFENSE: NONCOMPLIANCE WITH A PROFESSIONAL RULE

NOTES: DEFAULTED ON PUBLIC HEALTH SERVICE EDUCATION LOAN.

ROYDER, JAMES O DO OF LANCASTER, TX, WAS DISCIPLINED BY MISSOURI ON JULY 15, 1997
DISCIPLINARY ACTION: 36-MONTH RESTRICTION PLACED ON LICENSE
OFFENSE: DISCIPLINARY ACTION BY ANOTHER STATE OR AGENCY

NOTES: ACTION BASED ON DISCIPLINE BY THE TEXAS BOARD FOR FAILURE TO COMPLY WITH STATE AND FEDERAL DRUG LAWS. LICENSE RESTRICTED FROM TREATING ANY PATIENTS FOR INTRACTABLE PAIN UNLESS FOR A LEGITIMATE MEDICAL PURPOSE IF BASED ON SCIENTIFIC KNOWLEDGE OF THE TREATMENT OF PAIN NOT IN CONTRAVENTION OF APPLICABLE STATE OR FEDERAL LAWS.

RUBENSTEIN, BARNEY MD OF SAN ANTONIO, TX, WAS DISCIPLINED BY DEA ON AUGUST 21, 1995
DISCIPLINARY ACTION: REVOCATION OF CONTROLLED SUBSTANCE LICENSE
OFFENSE: DISCIPLINARY ACTION BY ANOTHER STATE OR AGENCY

NOTES: ON 10/10/93 HIS MEDICAL LICENSE IN TEXAS WAS SUSPENDED, STAYED WITH SEVEN YEAR PROBATION BASED ON HIS PRESCRIBING PRACTICES IN AUTHORIZING PRESCRIPTIONS FOR HYDROCODONE AND TUSSIONEX TO HIMSELF AND MEMBERS OF HIS FAMILY. AS A CONDITION HE IS NO LONGER AUTHORIZED TO POSSESS, ADMINISTER, DISPENSE OR PRESCRIBE CONTROLLED SUBSTANCES.

RUBINSTEIN, BARNEY MD, LICENSE NUMBER 00C7116 OF SAN ANTONIO, TX, WAS DISCIPLINED BY TEXAS ON OCTOBER 1, 1993
DISCIPLINARY ACTION: 84-MONTH PROBATION; RESTRICTION PLACED ON CONTROLLED SUBSTANCE LICENSE
OFFENSE: OVERPRESCRIBING OR MISPRESCRIBING DRUGS

NOTES: ENGAGED IN EXCESSIVE PRESCRIBING OF VICODIN TO A MEMBER OF HIS FAMILY OVER TWO YEARS BEGINNING IN 1991 WITHOUT SUFFICIENT CLINICAL INDICATIONS TO JUSTIFY THE AMOUNT AND DURATION. SUSPENSION STAYED. CONDITIONS OF PROBATION: SHALL NOT POSSESS, ADMINISTER, DISPENSE OR PRESCRIBE ANY CONTROLLED SUBSTANCES UNLESS PRESCRIBED TO HIM BY ANOTHER PHYSICIAN; SHALL NOT TREAT OR OTHERWISE SERVE AS PHYSICIAN, PRESCRIBE, DISPENSE OR ADMINISTER DRUGS THAT MAY BE SUBJECT TO ABUSE TO HIMSELF OR HIS IMMEDIATE FAMILY; SHALL SURRENDER ALL UNUSED TRIPLICATE PRESCRIPTION FORMS; DURING FIRST YEAR OF PROBATION SHALL COMPLETE A BOARD-APPROVED COURSE IN CHRONIC PAIN MANAGEMENT AND 50 HOURS PER YEAR OF CONTINUING MEDICAL EDUCATION; SHALL APPEAR BEFORE THE BOARD ONCE A YEAR; SHALL GIVE A COPY OF THIS ORDER TO ANY HEALTH CARE ENTITY WHERE HE HAS PRIVILEGES; SHALL COOPERATE WITH THE BOARD IN VERIFYING COMPLIANCE; SHALL INFORM BOARD OF CHANGE OF ADDRESS WITHIN 10 DAYS OR IF HE LEAVES THE STATE; TIME SPENT OUT OF TEXAS DOES NOT COUNT TOWARD PROBATION. SHALL NOT SEEK MODIFICATION FOR ONE YEAR. ON 11/22/97 PETITION TO TERMINATE ORDER DENIED. ON 10/24/98 ORDER TERMINATED.

RUDY, ROBERT PATRICK MD, LICENSE NUMBER F1956 OF FRIENDSWOOD, TX, WAS DISCIPLINED BY TEXAS ON AUGUST 22, 1998
DISCIPLINARY ACTION: 60-MONTH PROBATION; RESTRICTION PLACED ON CONTROLLED SUBSTANCE LICENSE
OFFENSE: OVERPRESCRIBING OR MISPRESCRIBING DRUGS

NOTES: FROM 6/94 - 8/96 A PSYCHIATRIST PRESCRIBED NUMEROUS CONTROLLED SUBSTANCES TO A PATIENT; DR. RUDY ALSO PRESCRIBED CONTROLLED SUBSTANCES TO THE PATIENT, INCLUDING DEMEROL; HE CONTENDS THAT HE SHOULD BE ALLOWED TO PRESCRIBE CONTROLLED SUBSTANCES TO THIS PATIENT BECAUSE SHE HAS SEVERE HEADACHES; THE BOARD'S CONSULTANT OPINED THAT IT WAS NOT GOOD PRACTICE FOR HIM TO PRESCRIBE WITHOUT CONSULTING THE TREATING PSYCHIATRIST; THE CONSULTANT ALSO EXPRESSED CONCERNS ABOUT THE POTENTIAL FOR DRUG OVERDOSE IN THIS SITUATION; IN ADDITION, HE FAILED TO MAINTAIN MEDICAL RECORDS OF THE CARE AND TREATMENT OF THE PATIENT. SUSPENSION STAYED FOR PROBATION WITH THE FOLLOWING TERMS AND CONDITIONS: SHALL NOT TREAT OR OTHERWISE SERVE AS PHYSICIAN, PRESCRIBE, DISPENSE OR ADMINISTER DRUGS THAT MAY BE SUBJECT TO ABUSE TO HIMSELF OR TO ANY MEMBER OF HIS FAMILY; SHALL TERMINATE THE CARE AND TREATMENT OF SAID PATIENT IN WRITING TO THE PATIENT WITHIN 60 DAYS; SHALL MAINTAIN ADEQUATE MEDICAL RECORDS WHICH SHALL BE AVAILABLE FOR REVIEW; SHALL OBTAIN 50 HOURS PER YEAR OF CONTINUING MEDICAL EDUCATION WITH AT LEAST 50 HOURS IN PAIN MANAGEMENT; SHALL ATTEND AN ETHICS COURSE OR PROGRAM WITHIN 1 YEAR; SHALL LIMIT THE PRESCRIBING OF CONTROLLED SUBSTANCES OR DANGEROUS DRUGS WITH ADDICTIVE POTENTIAL OR POTENTIAL FOR ABUSE TO PATIENTS IN A HOSPICE OR HOSPITAL SETTING; SHALL OBTAIN A CONSULTATION WITHIN 60 DAYS OF THE ORDER FROM A LICENSED TEXAS PHYSICIAN, BOARD-APPROVED, PRIOR TO PRESCRIBING CONTROLLED SUBSTANCES OR DANGEROUS DRUGS WITH ADDICTIVE POTENTIAL FOR NEW PATIENTS; SEPARATE FROM PATIENT RECORDS, SHALL MAINTAIN A LOGBOOK OF EVERY PRESCRIPTION WRITTEN BY HIM FOR DANGEROUS DRUGS WITH ADDICTIVE POTENTIAL WHICH SHALL BE MADE AVAILABLE FOR REVIEW; SHALL APPEAR BEFORE THE BOARD AT LEAST ONCE A YEAR; SHALL COOPERATE WITH THE BOARD IN VERIFYING COMPLIANCE; SHALL GIVE A COPY OF THIS ORDER TO ANY HEALTH CARE ENTITY WHERE HE HAS PRIVILEGES; TIME SPENT OUT OF TEXAS DOES NOT COUNT TOWARD PROBATION; SHALL INFORM THE BOARD OF CHANGE OF ADDRESS WITHIN 10 DAYS OR IF HE LEAVES THE STATE; SHALL NOT SEEK MODIFICATION FOR ONE YEAR. ON 10/15/99 THE ORDER WAS MODIFIED BY DELETING RESTRICTIONS ON HIS PRESCRIBING PRIVILEGES.

RUNKE, LAWRENCE C MD, LICENSE NUMBER J5463, WAS DISCIPLINED BY TEXAS ON MAY 10, 1997
DISCIPLINARY ACTION: LICENSE SUSPENSION
OFFENSE: LOSS OR RESTRICTION OF HOSPITAL PRIVILEGES

NOTES: ON 7/14/95 HE WAS NOTIFIED BY THE HOSPITAL WHERE HE WORKED THAT A REVIEW ANALYSIS OF HIS CHARTS WAS TAKING PLACE WHICH REVEALED SEVERAL DEFICIENCIES, AND STAFF RECOMMENDED

THAT HE SHOULD HAVE A MANDATORY CONSULT FROM ONE OF HIS SURGICAL PEERS ON EACH AND EVERY SURGERY HE PERFORMS. HE WAS ALSO REQUESTED TO OBTAIN CONSULTS FROM OTHER SPECIALTIES AND TO IMPROVE HIS DOCUMENTATION AND HIS TIME MANAGEMENT. PROBLEMS INCLUDED INADEQUATE MEDICAL RECORDS, RECURRENT ERRORS IN JUDGMENT, DIFFICULTY WITH COMPLEX CASES, INCOMPLETE PLAN, ERRORS OR OMISSIONS, DIFFICULTY IN PRIORITIZING TIME FOR CASES BETWEEN TWO HOSPITALS. HE ALSO HAD STAFF PRIVILEGES AT HOSPITAL REMOVED. HE HAS APPLIED FOR LICENSURE IN OKLAHOMA, WHICH IS ON HOLD PENDING THE OUTCOME OF HIS TEXAS LICENSURE STATUS. HE INFORMED THE OKLAHOMA BOARD THAT HIS PRIVILEGES AT AN ARIZONA HOSPITAL HAVE ALSO BEEN REMOVED DUE TO DISRUPTIVE BEHAVIOR, THOUGH HIS ARIZONA LICENSE HAS NOT BEEN DISCIPLINED. SUSPENSION UNTIL HE REQUESTS TO HAVE THE SUSPENSION STAYED OR LIFTED, AND APPEARS BEFORE THE BOARD TO PROVIDE SUFFICIENT EVIDENCE THAT HE IS PHYSICALLY, MENTALLY, AND OTHERWISE COMPETENT TO SAFELY PRACTICE. SUCH EVIDENCE SHALL INCLUDE AT A MINIMUM THAT HE IS NOT THE SUBJECT OF ANY STATE OR FEDERAL DISCIPLINARY OR LICENSE INVESTIGATION, PROCEEDING, OR COMPLAINT. UPON ADEQUATE SHOWING THE SUSPENSION SHALL BE STAYED FOR PROBATION; SHALL COOPERATE WITH THE BOARD IN VERIFYING COMPLIANCE INCLUDING PROVIDING COPIES OF MEDICAL RELEASES UPON REQUEST; SHALL GIVE A COPY OF THIS ORDER TO ANY HEALTH CARE ENTITY WHERE HE HAS PRIVILEGES; SHALL INFORM THE BOARD OF CHANGE OF ADDRESS WITHIN 10 DAYS; SHALL NOT SEEK MODIFICATION FOR ONE YEAR.

RUNKE, LAWRENCE CARL MD, DATE OF BIRTH MAY 23, 1943 OF 480 31ST STREET SE, PARIS, TX, WAS DISCIPLINED BY MEDICARE ON OCTOBER 20, 1998
DISCIPLINARY ACTION: EXCLUSION FROM THE MEDICARE AND/OR MEDICAID PROGRAM
OFFENSE: DISCIPLINARY ACTION BY ANOTHER STATE OR AGENCY

NOTES: LICENSE REVOKED, SUSPENDED, SURRENDERED OR OTHERWISE LOST FOR REASONS BEARING ON PROFESSIONAL PERFORMANCE, PROFESSIONAL COMPETENCE OR FINANCIAL INTEGRITY.

RUSH, AVRIL BRICKLEY MD, LICENSE NUMBER G8390, WAS DISCIPLINED BY TEXAS ON MAY 10, 1997
DISCIPLINARY ACTION: LICENSE SUSPENSION; MONITORING OF PHYSICIAN PERFORMANCE
OFFENSE: SUBSTANCE ABUSE

NOTES: HAS A HISTORY OF SUBSTANCE ABUSE INCLUDING ABUSE OF AMBIEN. IN 6/94, HE WAS DIAGNOSED WITH MULTIPLE SCLEROSIS. HE HAS BEEN HOSPITALIZED ON SEVERAL OCCASIONS FOR DEPRESSION AND/OR CHEMICAL DEPENDENCY. IN 7/96, AFTER APPROXIMATELY SEVEN YEARS OF SOBRIETY, HE BEGAN TAKING AMBIEN RESULTING IN MEMORY LOSS AND BLACK-OUTS. ON 9/8/96, HE WAS ADMITTED FOR LONG TERM TREATMENT FOR FOUR MONTHS. HE REPORTS A SOBRIETY DATE OF 9/20/96. SUSPENSION FOR A MINIMUM OF SIX MONTHS OR UNTIL SUCH TIME AS HE REQUESTS A STAY AND PERSONALLY APPEARS BEFORE THE BOARD TO PROVIDE SUFFICIENT EVIDENCE THAT HE IS PHYSICALLY, MENTALLY, AND OTHERWISE COMPETENT TO PRACTICE MEDICINE. DURING THE SUSPENSION. SHALL ABSTAIN FROM THE CONSUMPTION OF ALCOHOL/DRUGS IN ANY FORM UNLESS PRESCRIBED BY ANOTHER PHYSICIAN FOR A LEGITIMATE AND THERAPEUTIC PURPOSE; SHALL SUBMIT HIMSELF FOR APPROPRIATE EXAMS INCLUDING DRUG OR ALCOHOL SCREENS; SHALL NOMINATE THREE CERTIFIED PSYCHIATRISTS FOR BOARD SELECTION OF A THERAPIST AND SHALL EXPEDITIOUSLY SUBMIT HIMSELF TO EVALUATION AND TREATMENT BY THE APPROVED PRACTITIONER; SHALL PARTICIPATE IN THE ACTIVITIES OF A PHYSICIAN HEALTH AND REHABILITATION COMMITTEE AND ATTEND WEEKLY MEETINGS WITH QUARTERLY REPORTS; SHALL PARTICIPATE IN NARCOTICS ANONYMOUS PROGRAM NOT LESS THAN THREE TIMES A WEEK; SHALL REPORT ON HIS ATTENDANCE; SHALL PERFORM 10 HOURS OF COMMUNITY SERVICE A WEEK AT A NON-PROFIT CHARITABLE ORGANIZATION. UPON ADEQUATE SHOWING BEFORE THE BOARD THAT HE IS ABLE TO SAFELY PRACTICE MEDICINE, THE SUSPENSION OF HIS LICENSE SHALL BE STAYED FOR PROBATION FOR FIVE YEARS UNDER SUCH TERMS AND CONDITIONS WHICH THE BOARD DEEMS NECESSARY.

RUSH, AVRIL BRICKLEY MD, LICENSE NUMBER G8390, WAS DISCIPLINED BY TEXAS ON NOVEMBER 22, 1997
DISCIPLINARY ACTION: 60-MONTH PROBATION; RESTRICTION PLACED ON LICENSE
OFFENSE: SUBSTANCE ABUSE

NOTES: HISTORY OF SUBSTANCE ABUSE MOST RECENTLY INCLUDING ABUSE OF AMBIEN; IN 6/94 SHE WAS DIAGNOSED WITH MULTIPLE SCLEROSIS AND HAS BEEN HOSPITALIZED ON SEVERAL OCCASIONS FOR DEPRESSION AND/OR CHEMICAL DEPENDENCY; IN 7/96 SHE BEGAN TAKING AMBIEN WHICH RESULTED IN MEMORY LOSS AND BLACKOUTS; ON 9/18/96 SHE WAS ADMITTED FOR DETOXIFICATION AND LONG TERM TREATMENT FOR 4 MONTHS; SHE REPORTS A SOBRIETY DATE OF 9/20/96. SUSPENSION ON LICENSE LIFTED; CONDITIONS OF PROBATION: SHALL ABSTAIN FROM THE CONSUMPTION OF ALCOHOL/DRUGS IN ANY FORM UNLESS PRESCRIBED BY ANOTHER PHYSICIAN FOR A LEGITIMATE AND THERAPEUTIC PURPOSE; SHALL SUBMIT HERSELF FOR APPROPRIATE EXAMS INCLUDING DRUG OR ALCOHOL SCREENS; SHALL NOMINATE THREE CERTIFIED PSYCHIATRISTS FOR BOARD SELECTION OF A THERAPIST AND SHALL EXPEDITIOUSLY SUBMIT HIMSELF TO EVALUATION AND TREATMENT BY THE APPROVED PRACTITIONER; SHALL PARTICIPATE IN THE ACTIVITIES OF A PHYSICIAN HEALTH AND REHABILITATION COMMITTEE AND ATTEND WEEKLY MEETINGS WITH QUARTERLY REPORTS; SHALL PARTICIPATE IN NARCOTICS ANONYMOUS PROGRAM NOT LESS THAN THREE TIMES A WEEK; SHALL REPORT ON HER ATTENDANCE; SEPARATE FROM PATIENT RECORDS, SHALL MAINTAIN A LOGBOOK OF EVERY PRESCRIPTION WRITTEN BY HER FOR DANGEROUS DRUGS WITH ADDICTIVE POTENTIAL WHICH SHALL BE MADE AVAILABLE FOR REVIEW; SHALL LIMIT PRACTICE TO A GROUP OR INSTITUTIONAL SETTING AND SHALL ONLY WORK 30 HOURS PER WEEK; MEDICAL PRACTICE SHALL BE MONITORED BY A BOARD APPROVED TEXAS PHYSICIAN WHO SHALL PROVIDE QUARTERLY REPORTS TO THE BOARD; SHALL NOT TREAT OR OTHERWISE SERVE AS PHYSICIAN, PRESCRIBE, DISPENSE OR ADMINISTER DRUGS THAT MAY BE SUBJECT TO ABUSE TO HERSELF OR TO ANY MEMBER OF HER FAMILY; SHALL APPEAR BEFORE THE BOARD UPON REQUEST; SHALL COOPERATE WITH THE BOARD IN VERIFYING COMPLIANCE INCLUDING PROVIDING COPIES OF MEDICAL RELEASES AND PEER REVIEW RECORDS UPON REQUEST; TIME SPENT OUT

OF TEXAS DOES NOT COUNT TOWARD PROBATION; SHALL INFORM THE BOARD OF CHANGE OF ADDRESS WITHIN 10 DAYS OR IF SHE LEAVES THE STATE; SHALL NOT SEEK MODIFICATION FOR SIX MONTHS. ON 8/22/98 THE REQUEST TO MODIFY THE ORDER WAS DENIED. ON 1/29/99 THE ORDER WAS MODIFIED AS FOLLOWS: REQUIREMENT OF MONTHLY VISIT WITH PSYCHIATRIST REDUCED TO ONCE EVERY TWO MONTHS AND 30 HOUR LIMIT ON PRACTICE INCREASED TO 40 HOURS; ALL OTHER PROVISIONS OF THE ORDER REMAIN IN FULL EFFECT UNTIL SUPERSEDED BY A SUBSEQUENT BOARD ORDER.

RUSSOL, FREDERICK JOSEPH MD, LICENSE NUMBER 00E8876 OF ODESSA, TX, WAS DISCIPLINED BY TEXAS ON JANUARY 14, 1994
DISCIPLINARY ACTION: REPRIMAND
OFFENSE: PROFESSIONAL MISCONDUCT

NOTES: AIDING AND ABETTING THE UNLICENSED PRACTICE OF MEDICINE IN THAT IN 1991 HE SERVED AS AN UNPAID MEDICAL DIRECTOR FOR A LAB OWNED AND OPERATED BY A NON-PHYSICIAN WHO PERFORMED ALLERGY TESTING AND TREATMENT OF ALLERGY WHICH INVOLVED INJECTIONS PURSUANT TO A PROTOCOL APPROVED BY DR. RUSSOL; PATIENTS WERE NOT REFERRALS FROM DR. RUSSOL AND SOME WERE NEVER EXAMINED BY HIM; LAB WAS NOT ASSOCIATED WITH HIS PRACTICE; DR. RUSSOL IS NO LONGER ASSOCIATED WITH THE LAB.

RYAN, ANDREW JACK MD, LICENSE NUMBER 00C5863, WAS DISCIPLINED BY TEXAS ON AUGUST 17, 1996
DISCIPLINARY ACTION: 84-MONTH PROBATION; RESTRICTION PLACED ON LICENSE
OFFENSE: SUBSTANCE ABUSE

NOTES: ON 5/2/94 VOLUNTARILY ENTERED SUBSTANCE ABUSE TREATMENT AND DISCHARGED WITH A DIAGNOSIS OF MAJOR DEPRESSION, ALCOHOL WITHDRAWAL SYNDROME, ALCOHOL DEPENDENCE DYSTHYMIC DISORDER; HAD PRIOR TREATMENT; ADMITTED HE DID NOT DRINK FOR 13 YEARS AFTER HIS SUBSTANCE ABUSE TREATMENT IN 1975 BUT HAD BEGUN DRINKING AGAIN IN 1988; REPORTS SOBRIETY DATE OF 5/03/94. BOARD ALSO INVESTIGATED ALLEGATION THAT HE ENGAGED IN INAPPROPRIATE PHYSICAL CONTACT WITH A 50 YEAR OLD MILDLY RETARDED MALE PATIENT; HE VIGOROUSLY DENIES ANY INAPPROPRIATE PHYSICAL CONTACT. SUSPENSION, STAYED. CONDITIONS OF PROBATION: SHALL ABSTAIN FROM THE CONSUMPTION OF ALCOHOL/DRUGS IN ANY FORM UNLESS PRESCRIBED BY ANOTHER PHYSICIAN FOR A LEGITIMATE AND THERAPEUTIC PURPOSE; HIS MEDICAL PRACTICE, INCLUDING ANY OFFICE AND SURGICAL PRACTICE, SHALL BE MONITORED BY A BOARD APPROVED TEXAS PHYSICIAN WHO SHALL SUBMIT QUARTERLY REPORTS TO THE BOARD; SHALL SUBMIT HIMSELF TO APPROPRIATE EXAMS, INCLUDING DRUG OR ALCOHOL SCREENS; SHALL SUBMIT HIMSELF FOR EVALUATION AND TREATMENT BY AND APPROVED PSYCHIATRIST, INCLUDING BUT NOT LIMITED TO PSYCHOLOGICAL/NEUROLOGICAL TESTING WHO HE SHALL SEE AT LEAST ONCE EACH MONTH AND WHO SHALL PROVIDE REPORTS; SHALL PARTICIPATE IN AA'S PROGRAM NOT LESS THAN THREE TIMES PER WEEK WITH QUARTERLY REPORTS TO THE BOARD; SHALL REQUEST A MEETING WITH THE HARRIS COUNTY MEDICAL SOCIETY PHYSICIANS COUNSELING COMMITTEE AND SHALL MEET PERIODICALLY WITH THE COMMITTEE AND PARTICIPATE IN THE ACTIVITIES RECOMMENDED BY THE COMMITTEE, INCLUDING PARTICIPATION IN WEEKLY MEETINGS, IF ANY AND SUBMIT PROOF TO THE BOARD; SHALL NOT POSSESS ALCOHOL, CONTROLLED SUBSTANCES, OR DANGEROUS DRUGS WITH ADDICTIVE POTENTIAL OR POTENTIAL FOR ABUSE; SHALL SURRENDER TO THE TEXAS DEPARTMENT OF PUBLIC SAFETY NARCOTIC SERVICE AND/OR THE BOARD ALL CONTROLLED SUBSTANCES AND DANGEROUS DRUGS WITH POTENTIAL FOR ABUSE, INCLUDING SAMPLES UNTIL SUCH POSSESSION IS AUTHORIZED BY THE BOARD; SHALL NOT TREAT OR OTHERWISE SERVE AS PHYSICIAN, PRESCRIBE, DISPENSE OR ADMINISTER DRUGS THAT MAY BE SUBJECT TO ABUSE TO HIMSELF OR TO ANY MEMBER OF HIS FAMILY; SEPARATE FROM PATIENT RECORDS, SHALL MAINTAIN A COPY OF EVERY PRESCRIPTION FOR CONTROLLED SUBSTANCES OR DANGEROUS DRUGS WITH ADDICTIVE POTENTIAL OR POTENTIAL FOR ABUSE AND MAKE IT AVAILABLE UPON BOARD REQUEST; SHALL MAINTAIN A LOGBOOK FOR ALL PRESCRIPTIONS OR REFILLS TELEPHONED IN BY HIM OR AT HIS DIRECTION FOR CONTROLLED SUBSTANCES OR DANGEROUS DRUGS WITH ADDICTIVE POTENTIAL OR POTENTIAL FOR ABUSE AND MAKE IT AVAILABLE UPON BOARD REQUEST; SHALL NOT DIAGNOSE, TREAT, OR OFFER TO TREAT ANY PATIENTS WHO HAVE BEEN ADJUDGED MENTALLY INCOMPETENT, BEEN APPOINTED A GUARDIAN OR ATTORNEY AD LITEM, IS A WARD OF THE STATE, IS UNDER 18 YEARS OF AGE, OR OTHERWISE REQUIRES CONSENT FOR TREATMENT BY A THIRD PARTY; SHALL OBTAIN AT LEAST 50 HOURS PER YEAR OF CONTINUING MEDICAL EDUCATION INCLUDING AT LEAST ONE COURSE PER YEAR IN PHYSICIAN/PATIENT TRANSFERENCE OR BOUNDARIES AND SUBMIT PROOF TO THE BOARD; WITHIN ONE YEAR, SHALL TAKE AND PASS THE MEDICAL JURISPRUDENCE EXAMINATION; SHALL APPEAR BEFORE THE BOARD AT LEAST TWICE PER YEAR AND UPON BOARD REQUEST; SHALL COOPERATE WITH THE BOARD IN VERIFYING COMPLIANCE INCLUDING PROVIDING COPIES OF MEDICAL RELEASES; SHALL GIVE A COPY OF THIS ORDER TO ANY HEALTH CARE ENTITY WHERE HE HAS PRIVILEGES; TIME PERIOD OUT OF TEXAS DOES NOT COUNT TOWARD PROBATION; SHALL INFORM THE BOARD OF CHANGE OF ADDRESS WITHIN 10 DAYS OF IF HE LEAVES THE STATE; SHALL NOT SEEK MODIFICATION FOR ONE YEAR.

SABATES, FELIX NABOR JR MD, LICENSE NUMBER 00J2773 OF HOUSTON, TX, WAS DISCIPLINED BY TEXAS ON JUNE 22, 1994
DISCIPLINARY ACTION: 60-MONTH PROBATION; REQUIRED TO TAKE ADDITIONAL MEDICAL EDUCATION
OFFENSE: SUBSTANCE ABUSE

NOTES: ON 10/15/93 VOLUNTARILY ADMITTED HIMSELF FOR EVALUATION DUE TO ALCOHOL AND COCAINE ABUSE AND A HISTORY OF A SUICIDE ATTEMPT IN 1992; HE WAS DISCHARGED FROM INPATIENT TREATMENT ON 12/93; IS UNDER PSYCHIATRIC TREATMENT AND HIS PSYCHIATRIST BELIEVES THAT HIS INVOLVEMENT WITH DRUGS WAS RELATED TO HIS PREVIOUSLY UNDIAGNOSED BIPOLAR DISORDER. SUSPENSION STAYED. CONDITIONS OF PROBATION: SHALL CONTINUE TREATMENT WITH HIS CURRENT PSYCHIATRIST WITH QUARTERLY REPORTS; SHALL ABSTAIN FROM THE CONSUMPTION OF ALCOHOL/CHEMICAL SUBSTANCES IN ANY FORM UNLESS PRESCRIBED BY A PHYSICIAN FOR A LEGITIMATE AND THERAPEUTIC PURPOSE; SHALL SUBMIT HIMSELF FOR APPROPRIATE EXAMS INCLUDING DRUG OR ALCOHOL SCREENS; SHALL PARTICIPATE IN AA'S PROGRAM NOT LESS THAN TWO TIMES A WEEK WITH QUARTERLY REPORTS; SHALL

NOT TREAT OR OTHERWISE SERVE AS PHYSICIAN, PRESCRIBE, DISPENSE OR ADMINISTER DRUGS THAT MAY BE SUBJECT TO ABUSE TO HIMSELF OR ANY MEMBER OF HIS FAMILY; SHALL ATTEND AT LEAST 50 HOURS PER YEAR OF CONTINUING MEDICAL EDUCATION; SEPARATE FROM PATIENT RECORDS, SHALL MAINTAIN A FILE OF EVERY PRESCRIPTION WRITTEN FOR CONTROLLED SUBSTANCES AND DANGEROUS DRUGS WHICH SHALL BE AVAILABLE FOR INSPECTION; SHALL PARTICIPATE IN CADUCEUS MEETINGS WEEKLY WITH QUARTERLY REPORTS; SHALL APPEAR BEFORE THE BOARD ONCE A YEAR; SHALL GIVE A COPY OF THIS ORDER TO ANY HEALTH CARE ENTITY WHERE HE HAS PRIVILEGES; SHALL COOPERATE WITH THE BOARD IN VERIFYING COMPLIANCE; SHALL INFORM BOARD OF CHANGE OF ADDRESS WITHIN 10 DAYS OR IF HE LEAVES THE STATE; TIME SPENT OUT OF TEXAS DOES NOT COUNT TOWARD PROBATION. SHALL NOT SEEK MODIFICATION FOR ONE YEAR. ON 8/9/97 BOARD GRANTED HIS PETITION TO TERMINATE THIS ORDER BASED ON COMPLIANCE WITH CONDITIONS.

SAIFEE, NAFEES FATIMA MD, LICENSE NUMBER E3762 OF FORT WORTH, TX, WAS DISCIPLINED BY TEXAS ON AUGUST 22, 1998
DISCIPLINARY ACTION: FINE
OFFENSE: NONCOMPLIANCE WITH A PROFESSIONAL RULE

NOTES: FAILED TO ADEQUATELY DOCUMENT HER ORDER FOR HOME PROGRAMS, HOME EXERCISE OR TENS HOME USE IN REGARD TO 3 PATIENTS WHO WERE PRESENTED TO HER OFFICE WITH INJURIES; SHE REPORTS SHE HAS REMEDIATED HER RECORD KEEPING DEFICIENCIES BY HIRING AN INDEPENDENT CONSULT TO REVIEW HER DOCUMENTATION. $5,000 FINE.

SALEH, WALEED MD, LICENSE NUMBER 00F2897 OF 2223 WEST STATE STREET, OLEAN, NY, WAS DISCIPLINED BY TEXAS ON AUGUST 17, 1996
DISCIPLINARY ACTION: LICENSE SUSPENSION
OFFENSE: DISCIPLINARY ACTION BY ANOTHER STATE OR AGENCY

NOTES: ON 12/31/93 TWO YEAR SUSPENSION STAYED TO PROBATION IN NEW YORK FOR ENGAGING IN UNPROFESSIONAL CONDUCT BY ORDERING TESTS, TREATMENT, OR USE OF TREATMENT FACILITIES NOT WARRANTED BY THE MEDICAL CONDITION OF FIVE PATIENTS; ON 5/01/95 ANOTHER NEW YORK ORDER FOUND HIM IN NONCOMPLIANCE WITH THIS ORDER FOR FAILING TO HAVE HIS PRACTICE MONITORED BY ANOTHER PHYSICIAN. TEXAS LICENSE ON SUSPENSION UNTIL HE APPEARS BEFORE THE BOARD AND ADEQUATELY INDICATES HIS COMPETENCE TO SAFELY PRACTICE MEDICINE INCLUDING AT A MINIMUM THAT HE HAS NO RESTRICTED LICENSE IN ANY OTHER JURISDICTION.

SAMBERSON, RANDALL RAY MD, DATE OF BIRTH MAY 22, 1951, LICENSE NUMBER 00E6598 OF AMARILLO, TX, WAS DISCIPLINED BY TEXAS ON SEPTEMBER 28, 1990
DISCIPLINARY ACTION: 36-MONTH RESTRICTION PLACED ON LICENSE; REQUIRED TO TAKE ADDITIONAL MEDICAL EDUCATION

NOTES: MAY PERFORM NO GYNECOLOGICAL SURGERY WITHOUT BOARD CERTIFIED OR BOARD ELIGIBLE OBSTETRICIAN-GYNECOLOGIST AS SURGICAL ASSISTANT. EFFECTIVE 4/30/93 LICENSE FREE OF ANY RESTRICTION OR LIMITATION.

SAMUELS, MICHAEL G DO, LICENSE NUMBER G3944, WAS DISCIPLINED BY TEXAS ON MAY 10, 1997
DISCIPLINARY ACTION: 60-MONTH PROBATION; FINE
OFFENSE: PROFESSIONAL MISCONDUCT

NOTES: ADMINISTERED SCIENTIFICALLY UNPROVEN AND NON-FDA APPROVED TREATMENTS WHICH HE TERMS "BLOOD IRRADIATION" TO ADULT PATIENTS WITHOUT INFORMING THE PATIENTS OF THE RISKS ASSOCIATED AND WITHOUT ADEQUATELY DOCUMENTING TREATMENT PROVIDED; MISLED THE PATIENTS RECEIVING BLOOD IRRADIATION THERAPY BY INFORMING THEM THAT IT COULD REDUCE THE VIRAL LOAD IN THE BLOOD OF AIDS/HIV PATIENTS AND THAT IT WOULD REDUCE THE AIDS VIRUS; BILLED THE PROCEDURES AS ALLERGY PHOTO PATCH TESTING, THEREBY MISLEADING INSURERS; PROVIDED HUMAN GROWTH HORMONE TO ADULT PATIENTS WITHOUT MEDICAL JUSTIFICATION AND IS CURRENTLY UNDER INVESTIGATION BY THE FDA FOR HIS USE OF THIS HORMONE; PROVIDED A "SPECIAL ANNOUNCEMENT" TO ALL HIS PATIENTS WHICH MADE THE SCIENTIFICALLY UNSUPPORTED CLAIM THAT ASLAN THERAPY COULD CURE CERTAIN ILLNESSES SUCH AS ALZHEIMER'S DISEASE, LUPUS, SCHIZOPHRENIA, AND DIABETES. HE DID NOT INFORM PATIENTS THAT THIS THERAPY IS EXPERIMENTAL AND UNAPPROVED BY THE FDA. SUSPENSION STAYED FOR PROBATION UNDER THE FOLLOWING TERMS: SHALL PROVIDE ADEQUATE INFORMED CONSENT FOR BLOOD IRRADIATION THERAPY AND ASLAN THERAPY THAT SHALL SPECIFY THAT THE TREATMENT IS UNPROVEN AND NOT FDA APPROVED; SHALL MAINTAIN ADEQUATE MEDICAL RECORDS WHICH SHALL BE AVAILABLE FOR REVIEW; SHALL ATTEND AT LEAST 50 HOURS OF CONTINUING MEDICAL EDUCATION PER YEAR, OF WHICH 10 HOURS SHALL BE IN ETHICS; SHALL PAY AN ADMINISTRATIVE PENALTY OF $10,000; SHALL COOPERATE WITH THE BOARD IN VERIFYING COMPLIANCE; SHALL APPEAR BEFORE THE BOARD AT LEAST ANNUALLY; SHALL GIVE A COPY OF THIS ORDER TO ANY HEALTH CARE ENTITY WHERE HE HAS PRIVILEGES; TIME SPENT OUT OF TEXAS DOES NOT COUNT TOWARD PROBATION; SHALL INFORM THE BOARD OF CHANGE OF ADDRESS WITHIN 10 DAYS OR IF HE LEAVES THE STATE; SHALL NOT SEEK MODIFICATION FOR ONE YEAR.

SAMUELS, MICHAEL G DO, LICENSE NUMBER G3944, WAS DISCIPLINED BY TEXAS ON AUGUST 9, 1997
DISCIPLINARY ACTION: SURRENDER OF LICENSE
OFFENSE: OVERPRESCRIBING OR MISPRESCRIBING DRUGS

NOTES: IN LIEU OF FURTHER INVESTIGATION REGARDING HIS NON-THERAPEUTIC PRESCRIBING, VOLUNTARY, PERMANENT SURRENDER OF LICENSE.

SANCHEZ, DANILO ABUD MD, DATE OF BIRTH JANUARY 18, 1952 OF 1891 NORTH LEE TREVINO, EL PASO, TX, WAS DISCIPLINED BY MEDICARE ON JULY 20, 1992
DISCIPLINARY ACTION: 48-MONTH EXCLUSION FROM THE MEDICARE AND/OR MEDICAID PROGRAM
OFFENSE: CRIMINAL CONVICTION OR PLEA OF GUILTY, NOLO CONTENDERE, OR NO CONTEST TO A CRIME

NOTES: CONVICTION RELATING TO FRAUD.

SANCHEZ, DANILO ABUD MD, LICENSE NUMBER A40289 OF LONG BEACH, CA, WAS DISCIPLINED BY CALIFORNIA ON FEBRUARY 17, 1997
DISCIPLINARY ACTION: LICENSE REVOCATION

SANCHEZ, DANILO ABUD MD, LICENSE NUMBER A40289 OF PARAMOUNT, CA, WAS DISCIPLINED BY CALIFORNIA ON JULY 29, 1997

DISCIPLINARY ACTION: LICENSE REVOCATION
OFFENSE: DISCIPLINARY ACTION BY ANOTHER STATE OR AGENCY

NOTES: FELONY CRIMINAL CONVICTION FOR MAKING FALSE, FICTITIOUS OR FRAUDULENT CLAIMS AND BILLING FOR SERVICES NOT RENDERED; DISCIPLINED BY TEXAS AND NEW MEXICO FOR ACTS RELATED TO CONVICTION.

SANCHEZ, DANILO ABUD MD, LICENSE NUMBER A40289 OF PARAMOUNT, CA, WAS DISCIPLINED BY CALIFORNIA ON JULY 29, 1997
DISCIPLINARY ACTION: LICENSE REVOCATION

SANCHEZ, DANILO ABUD MD, DATE OF BIRTH JANUARY 18, 1952, LICENSE NUMBER 038794L OF PO BOX 17524, LONG BEACH, CA, WAS DISCIPLINED BY PENNSYLVANIA ON NOVEMBER 22, 1999
DISCIPLINARY ACTION: LICENSE REVOCATION
OFFENSE: DISCIPLINARY ACTION BY ANOTHER STATE OR AGENCY

NOTES: MEDICAID/MEDICARE FELONY CONVICTION AND HAVING A DISCIPLINARY ACTION TAKEN BY TEXAS AND NEW MEXICO BOARDS. ALSO KNOWN AS DANILY ABUD.

SANCHEZ, MANUEL MD, LICENSE NUMBER 00F2899, WAS DISCIPLINED BY TEXAS ON NOVEMBER 16, 1996
DISCIPLINARY ACTION: FINE
OFFENSE: PROFESSIONAL MISCONDUCT

NOTES: FAILED TO ADEQUATELY SUPERVISE THE ACTIVITIES OF THOSE ACTING UNDER HIS SUPERVISION IN THAT DURING 1992 AND 1993 HE, THROUGH HIS OFFICE STAFF, BILLED FOR EVALUATIONS AND MEDICAL SERVICES WHICH WERE NOT REFLECTED IN THE PATIENT MEDICAL RECORDS. SHALL PAY $5,000 FINE; SHALL COOPERATE WITH THE BOARD IN VERIFYING COMPLIANCE; SHALL TAKE AND PASS THE MEDICAL JURISPRUDENCE EXAMINATION WITHIN 90 DAYS.

SANCHEZ-LEAL, HENRY R MD, LICENSE NUMBER 000T503 OF COLUMBIA, SC, WAS DISCIPLINED BY SOUTH CAROLINA ON MARCH 6, 1990
DISCIPLINARY ACTION: SURRENDER OF LICENSE

NOTES: NOT ELIGIBLE FOR REINSTATEMENT

SANCHEZ-LEAL, HENRY R MD, LICENSE NUMBER 00G0052 OF KERRVILLE, TX, WAS DISCIPLINED BY TEXAS ON SEPTEMBER 28, 1990
DISCIPLINARY ACTION: MONITORING OF PHYSICIAN PERFORMANCE

NOTES: MUST SUBMIT FOR APPROPRIATE EXAMINATIONS TO DETERMINE FREEDOM FROM DRUGS AND ALCOHOL; PARTICIPATE IN ALCOHOLICS/NARCOTICS ANONYMOUS; SUBMIT FOR PSYCHIATRIC EVALUATION AND FOLLOW ANY RECOMMENDATIONS REGARDING CARE.

SANDERS, LOY N DO, LICENSE NUMBER 00C5865 OF HOUSTON, TX, WAS DISCIPLINED BY TEXAS ON APRIL 1, 1996
DISCIPLINARY ACTION: SURRENDER OF LICENSE
OFFENSE: DISCIPLINARY ACTION BY ANOTHER STATE OR AGENCY

NOTES: ON 2/18/93 DEA CONDUCTED A COMPLETE AUDIT OF ALL SCHEDULED DRUGS AT HIS OFFICE AND CITED NINE SEPARATE VIOLATIONS OF FEDERAL REQUIREMENTS REGARDING RECORD KEEPING FOR INVENTORIES OF CONTROLLED SUBSTANCES. AGREED TO PAY $20,000 FOR THE VIOLATION. VOLUNTARY, PERMANENT SURRENDER IN LIEU OF FURTHER HEARINGS.

SANDERS, MARK ODELL MD, LICENSE NUMBER F4475 OF SUGARLAND, TX, WAS DISCIPLINED BY TEXAS ON DECEMBER 11, 1999
DISCIPLINARY ACTION: FINE
OFFENSE: NONCOMPLIANCE WITH A PROFESSIONAL RULE

NOTES: BOARD INVESTIGATED HIS CARE AND TREATMENT OF SIX CHRONIC PAIN PATIENTS AND FOUND THAT HE FAILED TO MAINTAIN ADEQUATE AND APPROPRIATE MEDICAL RECORDS WITHIN THE BOARD GUIDELINES; HE HAS UNDERTAKEN REVISIONS IN HIS DOCUMENTATION PROCESS AND HAS PRESENTED EXAMPLES OF THESE REVISIONS TO THE BOARD. $2,500 FINE; SHALL TAKE AND PASS THE MEDICAL JURISPRUDENCE EXAM WITHIN 90 DAYS AND WITHIN THREE ATTEMPTS.

SANDERS, MARK S MD, LICENSE NUMBER 00H0002 OF TEXAS CITY, TX, WAS DISCIPLINED BY TEXAS ON JANUARY 6, 1995
DISCIPLINARY ACTION: REPRIMAND
OFFENSE: SUBSTANDARD CARE, INCOMPETENCE OR NEGLIGENCE

NOTES: ON 2/11/93 HE PERFORMED A CARPAL TUNNEL RELEASE ON A PATIENT WHERE HE DEVIATED FROM THE STANDARD OF CARE BY PERFORMING THIS SURGERY WITHOUT ADEQUATE INTRAVENOUS ACCESS IN CASE ANY COMPLICATIONS AROSE; FAILED TO ADEQUATELY INFORM PATIENT AS TO THE NATURE OF THE PROCEDURE AND THEREFORE FAILED TO TRULY OBTAIN INFORMED CONSENT; NEITHER ADMITS NOR DENIES THE ALLEGATIONS. SHALL GIVE A COPY OF THIS ORDER TO ANY HEALTH CARE ENTITY WHERE HE HAS OR APPLIES FOR PRIVILEGES OR ANYONE ELSE WHO ASKS FOR IT. SHALL ENSURE ANY INQUIRIES REGARDING HIS TEXAS LICENSURE STATUS ARE ANSWERED BY REFERENCING THIS ORDER.

SANDS, LARRY REX MD, LICENSE NUMBER 00G0884 OF BROWNWOOD, TX, WAS DISCIPLINED BY TEXAS ON APRIL 21, 1990
DISCIPLINARY ACTION: 24-MONTH RESTRICTION PLACED ON LICENSE

NOTES: STIPULATED ORDER. WILL OBTAIN SPECIFIC INFORMATION FROM PATIENTS SEEKING WEIGHT LOSS TREATMENT, FOR THOSE WITH NO CONTRAINDICATION FOR SUCH TREATMENT, HE SHALL FOLLOW SPECIFICATIONS INCLUDING: PATIENTS RECEIVING CONTROLLED SUBSTANCE PRESCRIPTIONS SHALL RECEIVE WRITTEN INFORMATION DETAILING RISK OF HABITUATION; CONDUCT FOLLOWUP EXAMINATIONS. MAY USE TRAINED PERSONNEL FOR THIS PROVIDED HE DOES NOT DELEGATE DIAGNOSIS AND TREATMENT RESPONSIBILITIES TO UNLICENSED ASSISTANTS.

SANDS, LARRY REX MD, LICENSE NUMBER 00G0884 OF BROWNWOOD, TX, WAS DISCIPLINED BY TEXAS ON OCTOBER 1, 1993
DISCIPLINARY ACTION: 120-MONTH PROBATION; RESTRICTION PLACED ON LICENSE
OFFENSE: CRIMINAL CONVICTION OR PLEA OF GUILTY, NOLO CONTENDERE, OR NO CONTEST TO A CRIME

NOTES: ON 7/2/92 HE PLED GUILTY TO ONE COUNT OF MAIL FRAUD AND WAS PLACED ON PROBATION FOR FIVE YEARS, FINED AND ORDERED TO SUBMIT TO A HOME CONFINEMENT PROGRAM FOR NOT LONGER THAN 120 DAYS. TEN YEAR SUSPENSION STAYED. CONDITIONS OF PROBATION: SHALL APPEAR BEFORE THE BOARD TWICE A YEAR; SHALL ATTEND AT LEAST 50 HOURS PER YEAR OF CONTINUING MEDICAL EDUCATION AND SIX HOURS OF AN ETHICS COURSE OR PROGRAM PER

YEAR FOR 10 YEARS; SHALL BE SUPERVISED BY A BOARD APPROVED PHYSICIAN WITH THREE-TIMES-A-YEAR REPORTS TO THE BOARD; SHALL NOT PARTICIPATE IN THE BILLING PROCEDURE FOR ANY INDIVIDUAL OR THIRD-PARTY PAYER; SHALL SUBMIT HIMSELF FOR EVALUATION TO A BOARD APPROVED PSYCHIATRIST WITH REPORTS TO THE BOARD; SHALL PRACTICE ONLY IN A GROUP PRACTICE IN A MEDICALLY UNDER-SERVED AREA; SHALL NOT CHANGE THIS WITHOUT WRITTEN APPROVAL; SHALL INFORM THE BOARD IF HE LEAVES THE STATE; TIME SPENT OUT OF TEXAS DOES NOT COUNT TOWARD PROBATION; SHALL PERFORM 100 HOURS PER YEAR OF COMMUNITY SERVICE. ON 10/15/99 ORDER TERMINATED.

SANTIBANEZ, ALFREDO LUIS MD, LICENSE NUMBER E8234 OF HOUSTON, TX, WAS DISCIPLINED BY TEXAS ON DECEMBER 12, 1998
DISCIPLINARY ACTION: 60-MONTH PROBATION; FINE
OFFENSE: CRIMINAL CONVICTION OR PLEA OF GUILTY, NOLO CONTENDERE, OR NO CONTEST TO A CRIME

NOTES: IN 1992 PLED NOLO CONTENDERE TO A CRIMINAL CHARGE OF PUBLIC LEWDNESS INVOLVING AN ALLEGATION THAT HE EXPOSED HIS PENIS TO A PATIENT AND FORCED HER TO TOUCH IT; ALSO IN 1992 HE MADE LEWD AND INAPPROPRIATE SEXUAL REMARKS AS WELL AS INAPPROPRIATELY TOUCHED ANOTHER PATIENT; FROM 1986 - 1991 HE ENGAGED IN INAPPROPRIATE SEXUAL CONDUCT WITH ANOTHER PATIENT WHO WAS ALSO AN EMPLOYEE AT HIS OFFICE; IN 1997 HE ENGAGED IN LEWD AND INAPPROPRIATE SEXUAL REMARKS; DURING THE TIME OF THIS TREATMENT, HIS TEXAS LICENSE WAS INVALID; HE MAINTAINS THAT HE WAS NEVER ALONE WITH ANY OF THE PATIENTS REFERENCED ABOVE. SUSPENSION STAYED FOR PROBATION WITH FOLLOWING TERMS AND CONDITIONS: $10,000 FINE; PUBLIC REPRIMAND; SHALL OBTAIN 30 HOURS OF AN ETHICS COURSE BEFORE THE END OF THE FIRST YEAR THAT THE ORDER IS IN EFFECT; WITHIN 60 DAYS SHALL SUBMIT TO THE BOARD A DETAILED CORRECTIVE ACTION PLAN WHICH SPECIFICALLY ELABORATES STEPS WHICH HE CAN TAKE IN ORDER TO ELIMINATE OPPORTUNITIES FOR SEXUAL MISCONDUCT; SHALL HAVE A CHAPERONE PRESENT DURING PHYSICAL EXAMS OF FEMALE PATIENTS; DURING FIRST 2 YEARS OF ORDER, SHALL OBTAIN 75 HOURS PER YEAR OF CONTINUING MEDICAL EDUCATION WITH 50 HOURS IN FAMILY PRACTICE; SHALL COOPERATE WITH THE BOARD IN VERIFYING COMPLIANCE INCLUDING PROVIDING COPIES OF MEDICAL RELEASES UPON REQUEST; SHALL NOMINATE THREE CERTIFIED PSYCHIATRISTS FOR BOARD SELECTION OF A THERAPIST AND SHALL EXPEDITIOUSLY SUBMIT HIMSELF TO EVALUATION AND TREATMENT BY THE APPROVED PRACTITIONER; SHALL NOT TREAT OR OTHERWISE SERVE AS PHYSICIAN, PRESCRIBE, DISPENSE OR ADMINISTER DRUGS THAT MAY BE SUBJECT TO ABUSE TO HIMSELF OR TO ANY MEMBER OF HIS FAMILY; SHALL GIVE A COPY OF THIS ORDER TO ANY HEALTH CARE ENTITY WHERE HE HAS PRIVILEGES; TIME SPENT OUT OF TEXAS DOES NOT COUNT TOWARD PROBATION; SHALL INFORM THE BOARD OF CHANGE OF ADDRESS WITHIN 10 DAYS OR IF HE LEAVES THE STATE; SHALL NOT SEEK MODIFICATION FOR ONE YEAR. ON 4/10/99, HE WAS GRANTED A 90 DAY EXTENSION TO PAY FINE.

SANTOSCOY, ERNESTO MD, LICENSE NUMBER D3750 OF ANTHONY, TX, WAS DISCIPLINED BY TEXAS ON MAY 16, 1998
DISCIPLINARY ACTION: SURRENDER OF LICENSE

NOTES: ALLEGATIONS OF VIOLATIONS OF THE MEDICAL PRACTICE ACT. IN LIEU OF FURTHER PROCEEDINGS DUE TO HIS POOR HEALTH, VOLUNTARY AND PERMANENT SURRENDER.

SAPPINGTON, JOHN S MD, LICENSE NUMBER 0009034, WAS DISCIPLINED BY RHODE ISLAND
DISCIPLINARY ACTION: EMERGENCY SUSPENSION

NOTES: TEMPORARY SUSPENSION.

SAPPINGTON, JOHN S MD, LICENSE NUMBER 0188909 OF 490 ANGELL STREET APT 201A, PROVIDENCE, RI, WAS DISCIPLINED BY NEW YORK ON JANUARY 3, 1996
DISCIPLINARY ACTION: SURRENDER OF LICENSE
OFFENSE: SUBSTANCE ABUSE

NOTES: HE ADMITTED TO BEING A HABITUAL USER OF DRUGS AND TO HAVING A PSYCHIATRIC CONDITION WHICH IMPAIRS HIS ABILITY TO PRACTICE MEDICINE.

SAPPINGTON, JOHN S MD, LICENSE NUMBER 0009034, WAS DISCIPLINED BY RHODE ISLAND ON FEBRUARY 13, 1996
DISCIPLINARY ACTION: EMERGENCY SUSPENSION
OFFENSE: PROFESSIONAL MISCONDUCT

NOTES: IMMEDIATE DANGER TO THE PUBLIC; WILLFULLY MAKING AND FILING FALSE REPORTS OR RECORDS IN MEDICAL PRACTICE.

SAPPINGTON, JOHN S MD, LICENSE NUMBER 0009034, WAS DISCIPLINED BY RHODE ISLAND ON MARCH 13, 1996
DISCIPLINARY ACTION: SURRENDER OF LICENSE
OFFENSE: DISCIPLINARY ACTION BY ANOTHER STATE OR AGENCY

NOTES: DEPENDENCE UPON CONTROLLED SUBSTANCES. ACTS IN ANOTHER JURISDICTION WHICH ARE GROUNDS FOR DISCIPLINE IN RHODE ISLAND. ALSO SURRENDERED HIS TRAINING LICENSE.

SAPPINGTON, JOHN S MD, DATE OF BIRTH JANUARY 30, 1962 OF C/O 128 DORRANCE STREET, PROVIDENCE, RI, WAS DISCIPLINED BY MEDICARE ON AUGUST 13, 1996
DISCIPLINARY ACTION: EXCLUSION FROM THE MEDICARE AND/OR MEDICAID PROGRAM
OFFENSE: DISCIPLINARY ACTION BY ANOTHER STATE OR AGENCY

NOTES: LICENSE SURRENDERED FOR REASONS BEARING ON PROFESSIONAL COMPETENCE.

SAPPINGTON, JOHN S MD OF BARRINGTON, RI, WAS DISCIPLINED BY SOUTH CAROLINA ON MARCH 19, 1997
DISCIPLINARY ACTION: DENIAL OF NEW LICENSE

NOTES: COMMITTED ACTS WHICH WOULD BE GROUNDS FOR DISCIPLINE IN SOUTH CAROLINA.

SAPPINGTON, JOHN SHANNON DR, DATE OF BIRTH JANUARY 30, 1962, LICENSE NUMBER 00628 OF BAYTOWN, TX, WAS DISCIPLINED BY NORTH CAROLINA ON JANUARY 5, 1999
DISCIPLINARY ACTION: SURRENDER OF LICENSE

NOTES: VOLUNTARY SURRENDER.

SARGENT, MICHAEL G MD OF KATY, TX, WAS DISCIPLINED BY DEA ON JUNE 5, 1995
DISCIPLINARY ACTION: REVOCATION OF CONTROLLED SUBSTANCE LICENSE
OFFENSE: OVERPRESCRIBING OR MISPRESCRIBING DRUGS

NOTES: IN 7/91 DEA INVESTIGATORS IN HOUSTON, TEXAS RECEIVED AN ANONYMOUS COMPLAINT THAT HE WAS PRESCRIBING CONTROLLED SUBSTANCES TO

INDIVIDUALS WITHOUT A LEGITIMATE MEDICAL PURPOSE. SURVEYS ESTABLISHED THAT HE WAS PRESCRIBING TYLENOL #3 WITH CODEINE IN CONJUNCTION WITH VALIUM ON FIVE SEPARATE OCCASIONS TO TWO UNDERCOVER AGENTS WITHOUT A LEGITIMATE MEDICAL PURPOSE AND NOT IN THE USUAL COURSE OF PROFESSIONAL MEDICAL PRACTICE; HE DID NOT CONDUCT A COMPREHENSIVE PHYSICAL EXAMINATION OF EITHER AGENT; RECORDKEEPING PRACTICES, MEDICAL EXAMINATIONS AND PATIENT HISTORY PROCEDURES WERE EXTREMELY DEFICIENT.

SARGENT, MICHAEL G MD, LICENSE NUMBER 00F7910 OF KATY, TX, WAS DISCIPLINED BY TEXAS ON JUNE 28, 1995
DISCIPLINARY ACTION: 60-MONTH PROBATION; RESTRICTION PLACED ON CONTROLLED SUBSTANCE LICENSE
OFFENSE: OVERPRESCRIBING OR MISPRESCRIBING DRUGS

NOTES: FROM APPROXIMATELY 2/92 TO 1/94, PRESCRIBED LARGE AMOUNTS OF POTENTIALLY ADDICTIVE DRUGS, INCLUDING CONTROLLED SUBSTANCES, TO A PATIENT WITHOUT ADEQUATE INDICATION OR APPROPRIATE DOCUMENTATION TO SUPPORT THE PRESCRIBING; DID NOT KEEP ADEQUATE MEDICAL RECORDS CONCERNING HIS TREATMENT OF PATIENT. SUSPENSION STAYED. PROBATION WITH TERMS: SHALL SURRENDER HIS DEA/DPS CONTROLLED SUBSTANCES REGISTRATION CERTIFICATE; SHALL SURRENDER ALL UNUSED TRIPLICATE PRESCRIPTION FORMS AND SHALL NOT ATTEMPT TO ORDER MORE; SHALL MAINTAIN A FILE WITH COPIES OF EVERY PRESCRIPTION WRITTEN FOR DRUGS WITH ADDICTIVE POTENTIAL WHICH SHALL BE AVAILABLE FOR REVIEW; SHALL NOT TELEPHONE TO A PHARMACY ANY PRESCRIPTION FOR THESE DRUGS; SHALL MAINTAIN ADEQUATE MEDICAL RECORDS WHICH SHALL BE AVAILABLE FOR REVIEW; SHALL OBTAIN AT LEAST 50 HOURS PER YEAR OF CONTINUING MEDICAL EDUCATION WHICH SHALL INCLUDE AT LEAST ONE COURSE IN RISK MANAGEMENT AND ONE COURSE IN PAIN MANAGEMENT/ADDICTIONOLOGY; SHALL APPEAR BEFORE BOARD AT LEAST ONCE A YEAR OR AT BOARD REQUEST; SHALL COOPERATE WITH THE BOARD IN VERIFYING COMPLIANCE; SHALL GIVE A COPY OF THIS ORDER TO ANY HEALTH CARE ENTITY WHERE HE HAS PRIVILEGES; SHALL PROVIDE A COPY OF THIS ORDER TO ANYONE REQUESTING IT WITHIN 10 DAYS; TIME PERIOD OUT OF TEXAS SHALL NOT COUNT TOWARD PROBATION; SHALL INFORM BOARD OF CHANGE OF ADDRESS WITHIN 10 DAYS OR IF HE LEAVES THE STATE. SHALL NOT SEEK MODIFICATION FOR ONE YEAR. ON 8/22/98 ORDER TERMINATED.

SARIOL, OSCAR MD, LICENSE NUMBER 00E3765 OF FORT LAUDERDALE, FL, WAS DISCIPLINED BY TEXAS ON JANUARY 14, 1994
DISCIPLINARY ACTION: SURRENDER OF LICENSE

NOTES: WAIVES THE RIGHT TO A SHOW COMPLIANCE PROCEEDING. LICENSE IS PERMANENTLY CANCELED.

SAUCEDA, FRANCISCO B MD OF 226 BITTERS ROAD #100, SAN ANTONIO, TX, WAS DISCIPLINED BY DEA ON MARCH 27, 1998
DISCIPLINARY ACTION: SURRENDER OF CONTROLLED SUBSTANCE LICENSE

SAUCEDA, FRANCISCO BASIL MD, LICENSE NUMBER 00H8375 OF HOUSTON, TX, WAS DISCIPLINED BY TEXAS ON APRIL 10, 1992
DISCIPLINARY ACTION: 6-MONTH LICENSE SUSPENSION; 60-MONTH PROBATION
OFFENSE: SUBSTANCE ABUSE

NOTES: SUSPENSION SHALL REMAIN IN EFFECT UNTIL SUCH TIME AS HE IS EVALUATED BY AN APPROVED PSYCHIATRIST SPECIALIZING IN ADDICTIONOLOGY AND REPORTS ARE FURNISHED INDICATING THAT HE IS BOTH MENTALLY AND PHYSICALLY ABLE TO SAFELY PRACTICE MEDICINE. AFTER SUCH TIME, LICENSE IS SUSPENDED, SUSPENSION STAYED, AND PLACED ON PROBATION UNDER TERMS AND CONDITIONS. ON 10/14/93 ORDER MODIFIED AS FOLLOWS: HE MAY APPLY FOR DRUG ENFORCEMENT ADMINISTRATION AND TEXAS DEPARTMENT OF PUBLIC SAFETY CONTROLLED SUBSTANCES REGISTRATION CERTIFICATES; SEPARATE FROM PATIENT RECORDS, HE SHALL MAINTAIN A FILE CONSISTING OF A COPY OF EVERY PRESCRIPTION WRITTEN BY HIM FOR CONTROLLED SUBSTANCES AND DANGEROUS DRUGS BY DATE ISSUED WHICH SHALL BE AVAILABLE TO BOARD FOR INSPECTION; HE SHALL NOT TELEPHONE ANY PRESCRIPTION TO A PHARMACY FOR CONTROLLED SUBSTANCES OR DANGEROUS DRUGS. ALL OTHER PROVISIONS OF THIS ORDER REMAIN IN EFFECT.

SAUCEDA, FRANCISCO BASIL MD, LICENSE NUMBER H8375 OF SAN ANTONIO, TX, WAS DISCIPLINED BY TEXAS ON AUGUST 28, 1999
DISCIPLINARY ACTION: 60-MONTH PROBATION; RESTRICTION PLACED ON CONTROLLED SUBSTANCE LICENSE
OFFENSE: SUBSTANCE ABUSE

NOTES: ON 3/12/98 HE NOTIFIED THE BOARD OF HIS RELAPSE INTO OPIATE DEPENDENCY AND THE RESULTANT IMPAIRMENT OF HIS ABILITY TO PRACTICE MEDICINE; PREVIOUSLY ON 2/25/93 AND 10/19/95 HE HAD ENTERED INTO CONTRACTS WITH THE BEXAR COUNTY MEDICAL SOCIETY'S COMMITTEE ON PHYSICIAN HEALTH AND REHABILITATION; THE TERMS OF THESE CONTRACTS REQUIRED AA MEETINGS 4-5 TIMES PER WEEK AND RANDOM DRUG SCREENINGS; ON 3/5/98 HE WAS FOUND IN HIS HOME, DISORIENTED, UNABLE TO STAND AND EXHIBITING SLURRED SPEECH, HE WAS PRESENTED TO THE EMERGENCY DEPARTMENT OF A HOSPITAL AND SCREENED POSITIVE FOR OPIATES AND TRICYCLICS; HE WAS ADMITTED TO THE HOSPITAL FOR OBSERVATION BUT LEFT AGAINST MEDICAL ADVICE; ON 3/7/98 HE ADMITTED HIMSELF TO A HOSPITAL AND REPORTED HAVING USED HYDROCODONE FOR A MONTH AND A HALF FOR BACK PAIN AND THAT HE HAD ACCIDENTALLY OVERDOSED ON 3/5/98; HE WAS DETOXIFIED, TREATED FOR OPIATE DEPENDENCE AND DISCHARGED ON 3/7/98; HIS DIAGNOSIS ON DISCHARGE WAS HYDROCODONE ADDICTION/WITHDRAWAL, MORPHINE ADDICTION/WITHDRAWAL, KLONOPIN ADDICTION/WITHDRAWAL, AND DEPRESSION, SITUATIONAL. SUSPENSION STAYED FOR PROBATION WITH FOLLOWING TERMS AND CONDITIONS: SHALL ABSTAIN FROM THE CONSUMPTION OF ALCOHOL/DRUGS IN ANY FORM UNLESS PRESCRIBED BY ANOTHER PHYSICIAN FOR A LEGITIMATE AND THERAPEUTIC PURPOSE; SHALL SUBMIT HIMSELF FOR APPROPRIATE EXAMS INCLUDING DRUG OR ALCOHOL SCREENS; SHALL NOMINATE THREE CERTIFIED PSYCHIATRISTS FOR BOARD SELECTION OF A THERAPIST AND SHALL EXPEDITIOUSLY SUBMIT HIMSELF TO EVALUATION AND TREATMENT BY THE APPROVED PRACTITIONER; SHALL PARTICIPATE IN THE ACTIVITIES OF A PHYSICIAN HEALTH AND REHABILITATION COMMITTEE AND ATTEND WEEKLY MEETINGS WITH QUARTERLY REPORTS; SHALL PARTICIPATE IN AA'S PROGRAM NOT LESS THAN THREE TIMES A WEEK; SHALL REPORT ON HIS

ATTENDANCE; SHALL NOT TREAT OR OTHERWISE SERVE AS PHYSICIAN, PRESCRIBE, DISPENSE OR ADMINISTER DRUGS THAT MAY BE SUBJECT TO ABUSE TO HIMSELF OR TO ANY MEMBER OF HIS FAMILY; SHALL SURRENDER HIS DEA AND TEXAS DEPARTMENT OF PUBLIC SAFETY CONTROLLED SUBSTANCE CERTIFICATES AND ANY DRUGS WITH POTENTIAL FOR ABUSE IN HIS POSSESSION INCLUDING SAMPLES AND ANY UNUSED TRIPLICATE PRESCRIPTION FORMS; SEPARATE FROM PATIENT RECORDS, SHALL MAINTAIN A LOGBOOK OF EVERY PRESCRIPTION WRITTEN BY HIM FOR DANGEROUS DRUGS WITH ADDICTIVE POTENTIAL WHICH SHALL BE MADE AVAILABLE FOR REVIEW; SHALL OBTAIN 50 HOURS PER YEAR OF CONTINUING MEDICAL EDUCATION; SHALL APPEAR BEFORE THE BOARD UPON REQUEST; SHALL COOPERATE WITH THE BOARD IN VERIFYING COMPLIANCE INCLUDING PROVIDING COPIES OF MEDICAL RELEASES UPON REQUEST; SHALL GIVE A COPY OF THIS ORDER TO ANY HEALTH CARE ENTITY WHERE HE HAS PRIVILEGES; SHALL PROVIDE A COPY OF THIS ORDER TO ANYONE REQUESTING IT WITHIN 10 DAYS; TIME SPENT OUT OF TEXAS DOES NOT COUNT TOWARD PROBATION; SHALL INFORM THE BOARD OF CHANGE OF ADDRESS WITHIN 10 DAYS OR IF HE LEAVES THE STATE; SHALL NOT SEEK MODIFICATION FOR ONE YEAR.

SAVAGE, PATRICK JOSEPH MD, LICENSE NUMBER 00F7600 OF JONESBORO, AR, WAS DISCIPLINED BY TEXAS ON OCTOBER 26, 1990
DISCIPLINARY ACTION: REQUIRED TO ENTER AN IMPAIRED PHYSICIAN PROGRAM OR TREATMENT

NOTES: COMPLY WITH PROVISIONS OF AFTERCARE CONTRACT EXECUTED WITH PHYSICIANS' HEALTH COMMITTEE OF ARKANSAS MEDICAL SOCIETY; IF WISHING TO PRACTICE IN TEXAS, MUST DEMONSTRATE CAPACITY TO PRACTICE WITH REASONABLE SKILL AND SAFETY AND PROVIDE REPORT ON STATUS OF ARKANSAS LICENSE AND COMPLIANCE WITH AFTERCARE CONTRACT; IF GRANTED PERMISSION TO PRACTICE IN TEXAS, BOARD MAY IMPOSE CONDITIONAL TERMS AS DEEMED APPROPRIATE.

SAVAGE, PATRICK JOSEPH MD, DATE OF BIRTH JANUARY 21, 1949, LICENSE NUMBER 0008541 OF 1812 MACARTHUR PARK, JONESBORO, AR, WAS DISCIPLINED BY MISSISSIPPI ON NOVEMBER 15, 1990
DISCIPLINARY ACTION: PROBATION

NOTES: REVOCATION STAYED; CONSENT AGREEMENT.

SAYERS, STEPHEN C MD, LICENSE NUMBER G5574 OF CENTER, TX, WAS DISCIPLINED BY TEXAS ON APRIL 4, 1998
DISCIPLINARY ACTION: 60-MONTH PROBATION; RESTRICTION PLACED ON CONTROLLED SUBSTANCE LICENSE
OFFENSE: OVERPRESCRIBING OR MISPRESCRIBING DRUGS

NOTES: PROVIDED HYDROCODONE, A SCHEDULE III MEDICATION, TO A PATIENT FOR OTHER THAN THERAPEUTIC PURPOSES OVER A PERIOD OF 20 MONTHS; THE PATIENT, WHO WAS APPARENTLY A FRIEND OF HIS, WAS SEEN BY HIM FOR MIGRAINE HEADACHES AND BACK PAIN; OVER TIME, PRESCRIPTIONS WERE PROVIDED WITHOUT DOCUMENTATION OF MEDICAL NECESSITY; THE PATIENT ULTIMATELY BECAME ADDICTED TO LORCET TABLETS; THE DOCTOR WAS AWARE OF THE ADDICTION AND COUNSELED HIM, WHILE CONTINUING TO PRESCRIBE TO HIM. SUSPENSION STAYED FOR PROBATION WITH FOLLOWING TERMS AND CONDITIONS: SHALL ONLY POSSESS, ADMINISTER, DISPENSE OR PRESCRIBE DRUGS WITH POTENTIAL FOR ABUSE FOR TREATMENT OF INPATIENTS IN A HOSPITAL SETTING; SHALL IMMEDIATELY REQUEST MODIFICATION OF HIS DEA AND TEXAS DEPARTMENT OF PUBLIC SAFETY CONTROLLED SUBSTANCES CERTIFICATES TO ELIMINATE AUTHORITY TO PRESCRIBE OR DISPENSE SCHEDULE II DRUGS; SEPARATE FROM PATIENT RECORDS, SHALL MAINTAIN A LOGBOOK OF EVERY PRESCRIPTION WRITTEN BY HIM FOR DANGEROUS DRUGS WITH ADDICTIVE POTENTIAL WHICH SHALL BE MADE AVAILABLE FOR REVIEW; SHALL MAINTAIN ADEQUATE MEDICAL RECORDS WHICH SHALL BE AVAILABLE FOR REVIEW; SHALL NOMINATE THREE CERTIFIED PSYCHIATRISTS FOR BOARD SELECTION OF A THERAPIST AND SHALL EXPEDITIOUSLY SUBMIT HIMSELF TO EVALUATION AND TREATMENT BY THE APPROVED PRACTITIONER; SHALL OBTAIN 50 HOURS PER YEAR OF CONTINUING MEDICAL EDUCATION WITH 10 HOURS IN ADDICTIONOLOGY/PHARMACOLOGY; SHALL OBTAIN 10 HOURS OF AN ETHICS COURSE PER YEAR; SHALL APPEAR BEFORE THE BOARD ONCE A YEAR; SHALL COOPERATE WITH THE BOARD IN VERIFYING COMPLIANCE; TIME SPENT OUT OF TEXAS DOES NOT COUNT TOWARD PROBATION; SHALL INFORM THE BOARD OF CHANGE OF ADDRESS WITHIN 10 DAYS OR IF HE LEAVES THE STATE; SHALL NOT SEEK MODIFICATION FOR ONE YEAR. ON 4/10/99 MODIFICATIONS TO THE ORDER WERE MADE AS FOLLOWS: REQUIREMENT FOR PSYCHIATRIC VISIT REDUCED FROM ONCE A MONTH TO ONCE EVERY THREE MONTHS; ALL OTHER PROVISIONS OF THE ORDER REMAIN IN FULL EFFECT.

SCARLETT, MAXWELL CURTIS MD, LICENSE NUMBER 00E6910 OF FORT WORTH, TX, WAS DISCIPLINED BY TEXAS ON FEBRUARY 1, 1991
DISCIPLINARY ACTION: RESTRICTION PLACED ON LICENSE; REQUIRED TO TAKE ADDITIONAL MEDICAL EDUCATION
OFFENSE: LOSS OR RESTRICTION OF HOSPITAL PRIVILEGES

NOTES: DISCIPLINED BY HOSPITAL OR HOSPITAL MEDICAL STAFF INCLUDING REMOVAL, SUSPENSION, OR LIMITATION OF HOSPITAL PRIVILEGES OR OTHER DISCIPLINARY ACTIONS; FAILURE TO PRACTICE MEDICINE IN ACCEPTABLE MANNER CONSISTENT WITH PUBLIC HEALTH AND WELFARE. MUST PERFORM NO MAJOR SURGERY UNTIL AFTER COMPLETION OF APPROVED GENERAL SURGICAL RESIDENCY AND BOARD CERTIFICATION; COMPLETION OF 50 HOURS CONTINUING MEDICAL EDUCATION EACH YEAR WITH PROOF OF COMPLETION.

SCHACHAR, LESLIE MD, LICENSE NUMBER 00E6911 OF GAINESVILLE, TX, WAS DISCIPLINED BY TEXAS ON JUNE 28, 1995
DISCIPLINARY ACTION: 60-MONTH PROBATION; RESTRICTION PLACED ON LICENSE
OFFENSE: SUBSTANDARD CARE, INCOMPETENCE OR NEGLIGENCE

NOTES: FAILED TO PROVIDE SUFFICIENT EVIDENCE THAT HE ADEQUATELY DOCUMENTED THE CARE AND TREATMENT OF VARIOUS PATIENTS; FAILED TO PROVIDE SUFFICIENT EVIDENCE TO SHOW THAT HE OBTAINED ADEQUATE PREOPERATIVE EVALUATIONS OF VARIOUS PATIENTS PRIOR TO PERFORMING SURGERY; AND FAILED TO PROVIDE SUFFICIENT EVIDENCE THAT A PROCEDURE THAT HE PERFORMS IS THERAPEUTIC AND WITHIN THE STANDARD OF CARE FOR MACULAR DEGENERATION DISEASE. SUSPENSION STAYED. PROBATION WITH TERMS: SHALL CEASE PERFORMING VITRECTOMY WITH

SCLERAL TUCH SURGERY FOR MACULAR DEGENERATION EXCEPT AS APPROVED BY INSTITUTIONAL REVIEW BOARD AND AFTER OBTAINING APPROPRIATE INFORMED CONSENT FROM THE PATIENTS; SHALL OBTAIN APPROPRIATE INFORMED CONSENT ON ALL SURGERIES PERFORMED; SHALL OBTAIN AND MAINTAIN THE APPROPRIATE LICENSURE REQUIREMENTS FOR THE USE OF HIS MOBILE SURGICAL UNIT; SHALL PROVIDE APPROPRIATE PREOPERATIVE MEDICAL CLINICAL EVALUATION ON ALL SURGICAL PATIENTS AND LABORATORY TESTS AS REQUIRED; SHALL OBTAIN AND DOCUMENT ALL APPROPRIATE OCULAR EXAMINATION DATA PRIOR TO ANY OCULAR SURGICAL PROCEDURE; SHALL MAINTAIN ADEQUATE MEDICAL RECORDS WHICH SHALL BE AVAILABLE FOR REVIEW; SHALL APPEAR BEFORE BOARD AT LEAST TWICE A YEAR; SHALL GIVE A COPY OF THIS ORDER TO ANYONE REQUESTING IT WITHIN 10 DAYS; SHALL GIVE A COPY OF THIS ORDER TO ANY HEALTH CARE ENTITY WHERE HE HAS PRIVILEGES; TIME PERIOD OUT OF TEXAS DOES NOT COUNT TOWARD PROBATION; SHALL INFORM BOARD OF CHANGE OF ADDRESS WITHIN 10 DAYS OR IF HE LEAVES THE STATE. SHALL NOT SEEK MODIFICATION WITHIN ONE YEAR. ON 8/17/96 TERMINATION REQUEST DENIED; MODIFIED GIVEN HE WAS NOT PRESENTLY PRACTICING MEDICINE; ORDER MODIFIED REDUCING HIS APPEARANCES BEFORE THE BOARD TO ONCE A YEAR; ALL OTHER PROVISIONS OF THIS ORDER REMAIN IN EFFECT. ON 9/20/97 PETITION TO TERMINATE ORDER DENIED. ON 8/22/98 PETITION TO TERMINATE ORDER DENIED. ON 10/15/99 PETITION TO TERMINATE ORDER DENIED.

SCHACHAR, LESLIE MD, LICENSE NUMBER 0125650 OF 1925 NORTH GRAND, GAINESVILLE, TX, WAS DISCIPLINED BY NEW YORK ON SEPTEMBER 3, 1996
DISCIPLINARY ACTION: LICENSE REVOCATION
OFFENSE: DISCIPLINARY ACTION BY ANOTHER STATE OR AGENCY
NOTES: ACTION IN TEXAS FOR PERFORMING NONINDICATED EXPERIMENTAL EYE SURGERIES; FAILING TO MAINTAIN ADEQUATE PATIENT RECORDS; AND FAILING TO OBTAIN ADEQUATE PREOPERATIVE EVALUATIONS.

SCHARF, PAUL LLOYD MD, LICENSE NUMBER 00F1972, WAS DISCIPLINED BY TEXAS ON AUGUST 17, 1996
DISCIPLINARY ACTION: FINE; REPRIMAND
OFFENSE: NONCOMPLIANCE WITH A PROFESSIONAL RULE
NOTES: FAILED TO OBTAIN 24 HOURS OF CONTINUING MEDICAL EDUCATION AS REQUIRED BY 9/01/95 FOR THE RENEWAL OF HIS LICENSE; GIVEN AN EXTENSION TO 11/30/95 WHICH HE ALSO FAILED TO MEET. STILL REQUIRED TO MEET CONTINUING MEDICAL EDUCATION REQUIREMENTS; $100 ADMINISTRATIVE PENALTY; SHALL COOPERATE WITH THE BOARD IN VERIFYING COMPLIANCE.

SCHEFFEY, ERIC HESTON MD, LICENSE NUMBER 00E6607 OF HOUSTON, TX, WAS DISCIPLINED BY TEXAS ON MAY 25, 1995
DISCIPLINARY ACTION: 60-MONTH PROBATION; RESTRICTION PLACED ON LICENSE
OFFENSE: SUBSTANDARD CARE, INCOMPETENCE OR NEGLIGENCE
NOTES: HE PERSISTENTLY AND FLAGRANTLY OVERCHARGED OR OVERTREATED FOUR PATIENTS BETWEEN 1988 AND 1992 INCLUDING PERFORMING SURGERIES THAT WERE NOT INDICATED IN THREE OF THE CASES; UNSUPPORTED DIAGNOSIS IN TWO CASES; PERFORMING UNNECESSARY X-RAYS AND DIAGNOSTIC STUDIES IN ONE CASE AND OVERCHARGING IN ALL CASES. SUSPENSION STAYED. PROBATION WITH TERMS: SHALL NOT PERFORM ANY SURGERY WITHOUT FIRST OBTAINING A WRITTEN CONSULT FROM A BOARD-APPROVED PHYSICIAN AND AN ASSISTING SURGEON APPROVED BY THE BOARD; SHALL MAINTAIN ADEQUATE MEDICAL RECORDS WHICH SHALL BE AVAILABLE FOR REVIEW; SHALL ADOPT AND ESTABLISH A SYSTEM OF PATIENT RECORD KEEPING AND BILLING; HIS OFFICE AND SURGICAL PRACTICE SHALL BE MONITORED BY A BOARD-APPROVED PHYSICIAN WHO SHALL SUBMIT QUARTERLY REPORTS TO THE BOARD; SHALL OBTAIN AT LEAST 75 HOURS PER YEAR OF CONTINUING MEDICAL EDUCATION; IN ADDITION, SHALL SUCCESSFULLY COMPLETE 10 HOURS PER YEAR OF AN ETHICS COURSE; SHALL PERFORM 120 HOURS OF COMMUNITY SERVICE PER YEAR APPROVED BY THE BOARD; SHALL APPEAR BEFORE THE BOARD TWICE A YEAR; SHALL COOPERATE WITH THE BOARD IN VERIFYING COMPLIANCE; SHALL INFORM THE BOARD OF CHANGE OF ADDRESS WITHIN 10 DAYS OR IF HE LEAVES THE STATE; SHALL GIVE A COPY OF THIS ORDER TO ANY HEALTH CARE ENTITY WHERE HE HAS PRIVILEGES WITHIN 10 DAYS; TIME PERIOD OUT OF TEXAS DOES NOT COUNT TOWARD PROBATION. SHALL NOT SEEK MODIFICATION FOR ONE YEAR. ON 7/11/95 HE DISTRICT COURT STAYED THIS ORDER AND IT WILL NOT BE ENFORCED WHILE COURT DECISION PENDING. ON 8/3/95 DISTRICT COURT EXTENDED THIS STAY THROUGH 10/3/97 WHEN ORDER WAS ENFORCED. ON 2/7/98 PETITION TO MODIFY ORDER DENIED. ON 12/12/98 PETITION TO MODIFY ORDER DENIED. ON 12/11/99 PETITION TO MODIFY ORDER DENIED.

SCHEINER, JAMES J MD, LICENSE NUMBER D3974, WAS DISCIPLINED BY TEXAS ON MARCH 1, 1997
DISCIPLINARY ACTION: FINE; REPRIMAND
OFFENSE: DISCIPLINARY ACTION BY ANOTHER STATE OR AGENCY
NOTES: FALSIFIED RESPONSES ON HIS APPLICATION FOR STAFF PRIVILEGES AT A HOSPITAL IN CORSICANA. HE ANSWERED "NO" WHEN ASKED WHETHER ACTION HAD EVER BEEN TAKEN AGAINST HIS LICENSE IN ANOTHER JURISDICTION, AND WHETHER HIS PRIVILEGES AT ANY HOSPITAL HAD BEEN AFFECTED BY DISCIPLINARY ACTION. ACTION HAD BEEN TAKEN AGAINST HIS VIRGINIA LICENSE IN 1981 DUE TO A CONVICTION IN FEDERAL COURT FOR FALSIFYING DRUG RESEARCH RESULTS TO THE FDA. HIS PRIVILEGES AT A HOSPITAL IN VIRGINIA WERE REVOKED BASED ON THIS ACTION. ADMINISTRATIVE PENALTY OF $2500; HE SHALL GIVE A COPY OF THIS ORDER TO ANY HEALTH CARE ENTITY WHERE HE HAS PRIVILEGES; SHALL PROVIDE A COPY OF THIS ORDER TO ANYONE REQUESTING IT WITHIN 10 DAYS.

SCHMIDT, JOHN CHRISTOPHER DO, LICENSE NUMBER G5580, WAS DISCIPLINED BY TEXAS ON AUGUST 9, 1997
DISCIPLINARY ACTION: REPRIMAND; REQUIRED TO TAKE ADDITIONAL MEDICAL EDUCATION
OFFENSE: NONCOMPLIANCE WITH A PROFESSIONAL RULE
NOTES: FROM 1994 THROUGH 1996 ENGAGED IN PRESCRIBING OF NARCOTICS WITHOUT ADEQUATE DOCUMENTATION IN SEVEN PATIENT CHARTS; FAILED TO MAKE APPROPRIATE REFERRALS TO SPECIALISTS OR PHYSICAL THERAPY OR CHRONIC PAIN CLINICS, AS WOULD BE EXPECTED IF DEALING WITH PATIENTS WITH CHRONIC PAIN. SHALL OBTAIN AT LEAST 50 HOURS OF CONTINUING MEDICAL EDUCATION: 20 HOURS IN CHRONIC PAIN, 15 HOURS IN CONNECTIVE

TISSUE DISORDERS, AND 15 HOURS IN RISK MANAGEMENT; SEPARATE FROM PATIENT RECORDS, SHALL MAINTAIN A LOGBOOK OF EVERY PRESCRIPTION WRITTEN BY HIM FOR DANGEROUS DRUGS WITH ADDICTIVE POTENTIAL WHICH SHALL BE MADE AVAILABLE FOR REVIEW; SHALL MAINTAIN ADEQUATE MEDICAL RECORDS WHICH SHALL BE AVAILABLE FOR REVIEW; SHALL APPEAR BEFORE THE BOARD UPON REQUEST; SHALL COOPERATE WITH THE BOARD IN VERIFYING COMPLIANCE; SHALL GIVE A COPY OF THIS ORDER TO ANY HEALTH CARE ENTITY WHERE HE HAS PRIVILEGES; TIME SPENT OUT OF TEXAS DOES NOT COUNT TOWARD RESTRICTION; SHALL INFORM THE BOARD OF CHANGE OF ADDRESS WITHIN 10 DAYS OR IF HE LEAVES THE STATE; SHALL NOT SEEK MODIFICATION FOR ONE YEAR. ON 4/10/99 THE ORDER WAS TERMINATED.

SCHOENDIENST, STEVEN PAUL MD OF 22999 US HIGHWAY 59, KINGWOOD, TX, WAS DISCIPLINED BY DEA ON SEPTEMBER 4, 1997
DISCIPLINARY ACTION: SURRENDER OF CONTROLLED SUBSTANCE LICENSE

SCHOENDIENST, STEVEN PAUL MD, LICENSE NUMBER 17808 OF PO BOX 14544, OKLAHOMA CITY, OK, WAS DISCIPLINED BY OKLAHOMA ON FEBRUARY 11, 1998
DISCIPLINARY ACTION: 60-MONTH PROBATION; SURRENDER OF CONTROLLED SUBSTANCE LICENSE
OFFENSE: OVERPRESCRIBING OR MISPRESCRIBING DRUGS

NOTES: ON OR ABOUT 10/25/94 THROUGH 2/25/96 HE WRONGFULLY WROTE PRESCRIPTIONS FOR CONTROLLED DANGEROUS SUBSTANCES, WITHOUT MEDICAL NEED, TO PATIENTS WHO WERE NOT HIS PATIENTS, UPON WHOM HE PERFORMED NO PHYSICAL EXAMS AND FOR PURPOSES OTHER THAN THE RENDITION OF PROPER MEDICAL CARE. ADMITTED BOTH ORALLY AND IN WRITING THE VIOLATIONS OF STATE AND FEDERAL LAW AND OKLAHOMA BOARD RULES FOR THE IMPROPER WRITING OF PRESCRIPTIONS FOR CONTROLLED DANGEROUS SUBSTANCES TO PEOPLE OUTSIDE THE SCOPE OF THE DOCTOR/PATIENT RELATIONSHIP AND WITHOUT ESTABLISHED MEDICAL PROTOCOL OR NEED. CONDITIONS OF PROBATION AS FOLLOWS: SHALL NOT PRESCRIBE, ADMINISTER, OR DISPENSE ANY CONTROLLED AND DANGEROUS SUBSTANCES OR NARCOTICS IN SCHEDULES II THROUGH V; SHALL, ON 9/12/97, SURRENDER HIS REGISTRATION FOR STATE AND FEDERAL CONTROLLED DANGEROUS SUBSTANCES TO PROPER AUTHORITIES AND WILL NOT APPLY FOR REINSTATEMENT UNTIL THE TERM OF HIS PROBATION HAS EXPIRED UNLESS AUTHORIZED TO DO SO BY THE OKLAHOMA BOARD; SHALL PRACTICE IN A CONTROLLED ENVIRONMENT APPROVED BY THE BOARD LIMITED TO THE OKLAHOMA CITY VETERANS ADMINISTRATION HOSPITAL AND ASSOCIATED CLINICS; SHALL NOT ALLOW THE INDEPENDENT PRACTICE OF MEDICINE BY ANY PERSONNEL UNDER HIS SUPERVISION OR EMPLOY; SHALL REQUEST ALL HOSPITALS IN WHICH HE ANTICIPATES PRACTICING TO FURNISH A STATEMENT REGARDING MONITORING OF HIS PRACTICE; SHALL SUBMIT TO EVERY STATE IN WHICH HE HOLDS LICENSURE AND TO HOSPITALS, CLINICS OR OTHER INSTITUTIONS IN WHICH HE HOLDS OR ANTICIPATES HOLDING ANY FORM OF STAFF PRIVILEGE A COPY OF THIS ORDER; SHALL NOT SUPERVISE ALLIED HEALTH PROFESSIONALS; SHALL NOT PRESCRIBE, ADMINISTER OR DISPENSE ANY MEDICATIONS FOR HIS PERSONAL USE AND SHALL TAKE NONE UNLESS AUTHORIZED BY ANOTHER PHYSICIAN FOR A LEGITIMATE MEDICAL NEED; SHALL KEEP THE BOARD INFORMED OF HIS ADDRESS AND PAY COSTS.

SCHORSCH, MICHAEL E MD, LICENSE NUMBER 6680, WAS DISCIPLINED BY NEW HAMPSHIRE ON JUNE 15, 1995
DISCIPLINARY ACTION: PROBATION; MONITORING OF PHYSICIAN PERFORMANCE
OFFENSE: SUBSTANCE ABUSE

NOTES: LICENSE RESTRICTED TO REQUIRE MONITORING FOR SUBSTANCE ABUSE BASED ON VOLUNTARY ADMISSION TO TREATMENT PROGRAM. ON 9/18/97 RESTRICTIONS LIFTED.

SCHORSCH, MICHAEL E MD, LICENSE NUMBER 0006839 OF DALLAS, TX, WAS DISCIPLINED BY VERMONT ON AUGUST 7, 1996
DISCIPLINARY ACTION: MONITORING OF PHYSICIAN PERFORMANCE
OFFENSE: DISCIPLINARY ACTION BY ANOTHER STATE OR AGENCY

NOTES: DISCIPLINED BY NEW HAMPSHIRE BOARD FOR DRUG ABUSE. VERMONT LICENSE SUBJECT TO FOLLOWING CONDITIONS: SHALL NOT CONSUME, INJECT, OR OTHERWISE SELF-MEDICATE WITH ANY CONTROLLED SUBSTANCE OR LEGAL DRUG WHICH HAS NOT BEEN PRESCRIBED BY ANOTHER LICENSED PRACTITIONER FOR THERAPEUTIC OR MEDICALLY PROPER PURPOSES; SHALL UNDERGO COUNSELING WITH A BOARD-APPROVED THERAPIST ONCE PER MONTH FOR THREE YEARS; FOR THREE YEARS SHALL BE SUBJECT TO AT LEAST ONE WITNESSED RANDOM URINE OR BLOOD SCREEN EVERY THREE MONTHS ADMINISTERED BY A BOARD-APPROVED PHYSICIAN; SHALL ATTEND AA OR NARCOTICS ANONYMOUS MEETINGS ONCE A WEEK FOR THREE YEARS UNLESS THERAPIST REQUIRES MORE; SHALL NOTIFY BOARD OF ANY CHANGE IN PRACTICE. ON 12/3/97 CONDITIONS REMOVED FROM LICENSE.

SCHULTZ, FRED MICHAEL MD OF 2410 CROCKETT DRIVE, BROWNWOOD, TX, WAS DISCIPLINED BY DEA ON MARCH 10, 1995
DISCIPLINARY ACTION: RESTRICTION PLACED ON CONTROLLED SUBSTANCE LICENSE
OFFENSE: PROFESSIONAL MISCONDUCT

NOTES: ALLEGED CONTROLLED SUBSTANCE VIOLATIONS.

SCHULTZE, JORGE MD, LICENSE NUMBER 00D6164 OF SANTA CRUZ, BOLIVIA, WAS DISCIPLINED BY TEXAS ON DECEMBER 1, 1990
DISCIPLINARY ACTION: LICENSE REVOCATION
OFFENSE: CRIMINAL CONVICTION OR PLEA OF GUILTY, NOLO CONTENDERE, OR NO CONTEST TO A CRIME

NOTES: CONVICTION OF MISDEMEANOR INVOLVING MORAL TURPITUDE, USE OF ADVERTISING STATEMENT THAT WAS FALSE.

SCHULZ, ERIC H MD, DATE OF BIRTH JANUARY 12, 1960 OF 223 E RAINBOW RIDGE CIRCLE, SPRING, TX, WAS DISCIPLINED BY MEDICARE ON JANUARY 5, 1997
DISCIPLINARY ACTION: EXCLUSION FROM THE MEDICARE AND/OR MEDICAID PROGRAM
OFFENSE: NONCOMPLIANCE WITH A PROFESSIONAL RULE

NOTES: DEFAULTED ON PUBLIC HEALTH SERVICE EDUCATION LOAN.

SCHULZE, JOHN P MD, LICENSE NUMBER 00C5311 OF CORPUS CHRISTI, TX, WAS DISCIPLINED BY TEXAS ON JANUARY 6, 1995
DISCIPLINARY ACTION: 60-MONTH RESTRICTION PLACED ON CONTROLLED SUBSTANCE LICENSE; REQUIRED TO TAKE ADDITIONAL MEDICAL EDUCATION
OFFENSE: OVERPRESCRIBING OR MISPRESCRIBING DRUGS

NOTES: FROM 1987 THROUGH 7/1/92 PRESCRIBED DANGEROUS DRUGS AND CONTROLLED SUBSTANCES TO ONE PATIENT WITHOUT PERFORMING OR ADEQUATELY DOCUMENTING APPROPRIATE PHYSICAL EXAMS AND LAB STUDIES; FAILED TO APPROPRIATELY MONITOR THE PATIENT FOR HYPERTENSION AND WEIGHT LOSS AND CONDUCT APPROPRIATE FOLLOW-UP EXAMS; REPORTS HIS OFFICE STAFF IMPROPERLY ALLOWED THE PATIENT TO OBTAIN REFILLS OF MEDICATIONS WITHOUT REQUIRING HIM TO EXAMINE THE PATIENT; AGREED ORDER IN LIEU OF FURTHER INVESTIGATION OR A HEARING ON THE ALLEGATIONS. CONDITIONS OF FIVE YEAR RESTRICTION: SEPARATE FROM PATIENT RECORDS SHALL MAINTAIN A FILE OF EVERY PRESCRIPTION WRITTEN FOR CONTROLLED SUBSTANCES OR DANGEROUS DRUGS WHICH SHALL BE AVAILABLE FOR INSPECTION; SHALL NOT TELEPHONE A PRESCRIPTION TO A PHARMACY FOR SUCH DRUGS OR PERMIT ANY INDIVIDUAL TO DO SO ON HIS BEHALF; WITHIN 30 DAYS SHALL DEVELOP AND ENSURE COMPLIANCE WITH A WRITTEN OFFICE POLICY FOR PATIENT MONITORING AND FOLLOW-UP EXAMS WHICH SHALL BE DISTRIBUTED TO ALL OF HIS EMPLOYEES AND MADE AVAILABLE FOR REVIEW; SHALL MAINTAIN ADEQUATE MEDICAL RECORDS OF ALL OFFICE VISITS WHICH SHALL BE AVAILABLE FOR INSPECTION; SHALL NOT SIGN ANY PATIENT RECORD UNLESS HE HAS PERSONALLY EXAMINED THE PATIENT OR CLEARLY NOTES IN THE RECORD THAT HE DID NOT; SHALL PERSONALLY EXAMINE AND TREAT A PATIENT ANY TIME AN INITIAL DIAGNOSIS OR EXAM IS DONE; SHALL ADEQUATELY SUPERVISE THE ACTIVITIES OF ALL INDIVIDUALS UNDER HIS SUPERVISION; SHALL ATTEND AT LEAST 50 HOURS PER YEAR OF CONTINUING MEDICAL EDUCATION INCLUDING AT LEAST 15 HOURS IN RISK MANAGEMENT, MEDICAL RECORDKEEPING AND PHARMACOLOGY; SHALL APPEAR BEFORE THE BOARD ONCE A YEAR OR UPON REQUEST; SHALL COOPERATE WITH THE BOARD IN VERIFYING COMPLIANCE; SHALL EXECUTE ANY RELEASES NEEDED TO OBTAIN EMPLOYMENT RECORDS; SHALL GIVE A COPY OF THIS ORDER TO ANY HEALTH CARE ENTITY WHERE HE HAS OR HAS APPLIED FOR PRIVILEGES OR ANYONE ELSE WHO ASKS FOR IT; SHALL ENSURE INQUIRIES REGARDING HIS TEXAS LICENSURE STATUS ARE ANSWERED BY REFERENCING THIS ORDER; SHALL INFORM BOARD OF CHANGE OF ADDRESS WITHIN 10 DAYS OR IF HE LEAVES THE STATE; TIME SPENT OUT OF TEXAS DOES NOT COUNT TOWARD RESTRICTION. SHALL NOT SEEK MODIFICATION FOR ONE YEAR. ON 3/1/97 THE BOARD GRANTED HIS PETITION FOR TERMINATION OF THIS ORDER BASED ON COMPLIANCE WITH CONDITIONS.

SCHWARTZ, HAROLD R MD OF HOUSTON, TX, WAS DISCIPLINED BY DEA ON JANUARY 16, 1996
DISCIPLINARY ACTION: DENIAL OF NEW LICENSE
OFFENSE: OVERPRESCRIBING OR MISPRESCRIBING DRUGS

NOTES: ON MARCH 24, APRIL 7, AND APRIL 21, 1992, HE PRESCRIBED 24 TYLENOL NO. 4 AND 18 VALIUM 10 MG. TO AN UNDERCOVER OFFICER FOR NO LEGITIMATE MEDICAL REASON AND OUTSIDE THE USUAL COURSE OF PROFESSIONAL PRACTICE; FOLLOWING A FEDERAL SEARCH WARRANT ON 7/07/92, HE VOLUNTARILY SURRENDERED HIS DEA REGISTRATION BUT ADMITTED NO WRONGDOING; ON 2/01/93 HIS TEXAS PRIVILEGES TO PRESCRIBE CONTROLLED SUBSTANCES WAS REINSTATED; ON 4/14/94 HIS MEDICAL LICENSE WAS RESTRICTED FOR THREE YEARS FOR PRESCRIBING IN A NONTHERAPEUTIC MANNER; HE DID PROVIDE SOME EVIDENCE OF REHABILITATION, ACKNOWLEDGED HIS RECORDKEEPING FAILINGS.

SCHWARTZ, HAROLD ROBERT MD, LICENSE NUMBER 00B8522 OF HOUSTON, TX, WAS DISCIPLINED BY TEXAS ON JUNE 22, 1994
DISCIPLINARY ACTION: REQUIRED TO TAKE ADDITIONAL MEDICAL EDUCATION; MONITORING OF PHYSICIAN PERFORMANCE
OFFENSE: OVERPRESCRIBING OR MISPRESCRIBING DRUGS

NOTES: BETWEEN 3/24 AND 4/21/92 HE PRESCRIBED TO AN UNDERCOVER SHERIFF'S DEPARTMENT OFFICER TYLENOL #4 WITH CODEINE AND VALIUM ON THREE SEPARATE OCCASIONS WITHOUT ANY VALID MEDICAL JUSTIFICATION; MAINTAINED THAT HE PRESCRIBED THIS AS TREATMENT FOR DOCUMENTED HYPERTENSION ALTHOUGH ADMITS IT WAS POOR JUDGMENT PRESCRIBING IT WITH OTHER MEDICATIONS; VOLUNTARILY SURRENDERED DEA AND TEXAS CONTROLLED SUBSTANCES REGISTRATIONS; GRAND JURY CHOSE NOT TO PROCEED WITH CRIMINAL ACTION; TEXAS CONTROLLED SUBSTANCE REGISTRATION REINSTATED PRIOR TO THE DATE OF THIS ORDER. HIS DEA REGISTRATION HAS NOT BEEN REISSUED AS OF ORDER DATE. CONDITIONS OF THREE YEAR RESTRICTION ON LICENSE: SHALL ATTEND AT LEAST 50 HOURS PER YEAR OF CONTINUING MEDICAL EDUCATION SIX HOURS OF WHICH SHALL BE IN THE AREA OF RECORDKEEPING OR RISK MANAGEMENT; SHALL BE SUPERVISED BY A BOARD-APPROVED PHYSICIAN WITH QUARTERLY REPORTS; WITHIN ONE YEAR SHALL PASS THE SPEX EXAM; IN THE EVENT HE DOES NOT PASS THE SPEX EXAM WITHIN ONE YEAR HIS LICENSE SHALL BE IMMEDIATELY SUSPENDED; SHALL GIVE A COPY OF THIS ORDER TO ANY HEALTH CARE ENTITY WHERE HE HAS PRIVILEGES; SHALL COOPERATE WITH THE BOARD IN VERIFYING COMPLIANCE; SHALL INFORM BOARD OF CHANGE OF ADDRESS WITHIN 10 DAYS OR IF HE LEAVES THE STATE; TIME SPENT OUT OF TEXAS DOES NOT COUNT TOWARD RESTRICTION. SHALL NOT SEEK MODIFICATION FOR ONE YEAR.

SCHWARTZ, HAROLD ROBERT MD, LICENSE NUMBER 00B8522, WAS DISCIPLINED BY TEXAS ON AUGUST 30, 1995
DISCIPLINARY ACTION: LICENSE SUSPENSION
OFFENSE: FAILURE TO COMPLY WITH PREVIOUS BOARD ORDER

NOTES: FAILED TO TAKE AND PASS THE SPECIAL PURPOSE EXAMINATION (SPEX) BY 6/22/95 AS REQUIRED BY 6/22/94 ORDER IN THAT HE SAT FOR THE SPEX IN 3/95 AND OBTAINED A FAILING SCORE OF 60. SUSPENSION UNTIL HE TAKES AND PASSES THE SPEX AND APPEARS BEFORE THE BOARD WITH EVIDENCE THAT SHOWS HE HAS THE SKILLS AND KNOWLEDGE TO SAFELY PRACTICE MEDICINE AND IS OTHERWISE PHYSICALLY AND MENTALLY COMPETENT TO RESUME THE PRACTICE OF MEDICINE IN TEXAS.

SCONZERT, ALAN C MD, LICENSE NUMBER J3214 OF PASCO, WA, WAS DISCIPLINED BY TEXAS ON AUGUST 9, 1997
DISCIPLINARY ACTION: FINE; REPRIMAND
OFFENSE: DISCIPLINARY ACTION BY ANOTHER STATE OR AGENCY

NOTES: ON OR ABOUT 5/31/96 HE ENTERED INTO AN AGREED ORDER WITH THE STATE OF WASHINGTON BASED ON ALLEGATIONS THAT HE HAD DISPLAYED RUDE BEHAVIOR TOWARDS FOUR PATIENTS. $500 FINE; SHALL COMPLY WITH TERMS AND CONDITIONS IMPOSED BY THE WASHINGTON BOARD; SHALL COOPERATE WITH THE BOARD IN VERIFYING COMPLIANCE; SHALL NOT SEEK MODIFICATION OF

TEXAS ORDER FOR ONE YEAR.

SCONZERT, ALAN CARL MD, LICENSE NUMBER 0029514 OF PASCO, WA, WAS DISCIPLINED BY WASHINGTON ON MAY 31, 1996
DISCIPLINARY ACTION: REPRIMAND

NOTES: REQUIRED TO UNDERGO ANGER-MANAGEMENT THERAPY AND OTHER TERMS AND CONDITIONS. ON 12/4/97 REQUEST TO TERMINATE ORDER GRANTED; UNRESTRICTED LICENSE.

SCONZERT, ALAN CARL MD OF PASCO, WA, WAS DISCIPLINED BY LOUISIANA ON JULY 31, 1997
DISCIPLINARY ACTION: 36-MONTH PROBATION
OFFENSE: DISCIPLINARY ACTION BY ANOTHER STATE OR AGENCY

NOTES: DISCIPLINARY ACTION BY WASHINGTON. PROBATION SUBJECT TO TERMINATION UPON PETITION TO BOARD AND PROOF OF REINSTATEMENT OF UNRESTRICTED LICENSURE IN GOOD STANDING IN WASHINGTON.

SCOTT, HILLARD L MD OF NORMANDY, MO, WAS DISCIPLINED BY MISSOURI ON JULY 27, 1990
DISCIPLINARY ACTION: 1-MONTH LICENSE SUSPENSION; 36-MONTH PROBATION
OFFENSE: OVERPRESCRIBING OR MISPRESCRIBING DRUGS

NOTES: PROBATION RETROACTIVE TO 7/1/90.

SCOTT, HILLARD L MD, LICENSE NUMBER 00F7605 OF NORMANDY, MO, WAS DISCIPLINED BY TEXAS ON APRIL 20, 1991
DISCIPLINARY ACTION: 36-MONTH PROBATION
OFFENSE: DISCIPLINARY ACTION BY ANOTHER STATE OR AGENCY

NOTES: DISCIPLINED BY ANOTHER STATE FOR SIGNING BLANK PRESCRIPTION FORMS. PRIOR TO PRACTICING IN TEXAS SHALL APPEAR BEFORE AND RECEIVE APPROVAL OF BOARD.

SCRAGG, WILLIAM H MD, LICENSE NUMBER 00E5614, WAS DISCIPLINED BY TEXAS ON AUGUST 17, 1996
DISCIPLINARY ACTION: FINE
OFFENSE: NONCOMPLIANCE WITH A PROFESSIONAL RULE

NOTES: HIS MEDICAL RECORDS, CONCERNING THE CARE AND TREATMENT OF A PATIENT IN JULY 1994, DID NOT ADEQUATELY DOCUMENT HIS FINDINGS AND RECOMMENDATIONS TO THE PATIENT REGARDING HER NIPPLE RETRACTION, SPECIFICALLY THE NEED TO REFER THE PATIENT TO A SURGEON; HAS SUBMITTED A CORRECTIVE ACTION PLAN TO ADDRESS HIS RECORD-KEEPING AND REFERRAL OF PATIENTS IN BOTH THE OFFICE AND HOSPITAL SETTING. DOES NOT ADMIT VIOLATION. $1,000 FINE.

SEGGER, FRANZJOSEF MD, LICENSE NUMBER 00D7789 OF HOUSTON, TX, WAS DISCIPLINED BY TEXAS ON AUGUST 18, 1990
DISCIPLINARY ACTION: MONITORING OF PHYSICIAN PERFORMANCE; 60-MONTH
OFFENSE: SUBSTANCE ABUSE

NOTES: STIPULATED ORDER. MUST SUBMIT HIMSELF TO PSYCHIATRIST FOR EVALUATION AND TREATMENT AND FOLLOW RECOMMENDATIONS, IF ANY, SUBMIT FOR APPROPRIATE EXAMINATIONS TO DETERMINE FREEDOM FROM DRUGS AND ALCOHOL, AND PARTICIPATE IN HOUSTON DOCTOR'S GROUP, AN IMPAIRED PHYSICIANS PROGRAM. ON 1/6/95 ORDER TERMINATED.

SEGUROLA, JUAN IGNACIO MD, LICENSE NUMBER 0037730 OF CORAL GABLES, FL, WAS DISCIPLINED BY FLORIDA ON OCTOBER 12, 1994
DISCIPLINARY ACTION: FINE; REQUIRED TO TAKE ADDITIONAL MEDICAL EDUCATION
OFFENSE: SUBSTANDARD CARE, INCOMPETENCE OR NEGLIGENCE

NOTES: CHARGED WITH FAILURE TO PRACTICE MEDICINE WITH AN ACCEPTABLE LEVEL OF CARE AND SKILL; FAILING TO KEEP MEDICAL RECORDS JUSTIFYING THE COURSE OF TREATMENT OF A PATIENT. $6,000 FINE; SHALL COMPLETE 40 HOURS OF CONTINUING MEDICAL EDUCATION, 20 OF WHICH SHALL BE IN EMERGENCY MEDICINE WITHIN ONE YEAR.

SEGUROLA, JUAN IGNACIO MD, LICENSE NUMBER 00G2476 OF FORT LAUDERDALE, FL, WAS DISCIPLINED BY TEXAS ON MAY 11, 1995
DISCIPLINARY ACTION: SURRENDER OF LICENSE
OFFENSE: DISCIPLINARY ACTION BY ANOTHER STATE OR AGENCY

NOTES: LICENSE SANCTIONED IN FLORIDA IN 10/94 FOR GROSS OR REPEATED MALPRACTICE OR THE FAILURE TO PRACTICE MEDICINE WITH AN APPROPRIATE LEVEL OF CARE AND SKILL IN THAT HE FAILED TO DIAGNOSE A PATIENT'S ABDOMINAL AORTIC ANEURYSM BASED ON PATIENT'S SYMPTOMS, X-RAYS AND EXTERNAL EXAMINATION; PATIENT EXPIRED DUE TO RUPTURED ANEURYSM SEVERAL HOURS AFTER LEAVING THE EMERGENCY ROOM; FAILING TO KEEP WRITTEN MEDICAL RECORDS JUSTIFYING THE PATIENT'S COURSE OF TREATMENT; NEITHER ADMITTED NOR DENIED THESE CHARGES. VOLUNTARY SURRENDER; SHALL IMMEDIATELY RETIRE FROM THE PRACTICE OF MEDICINE IN TEXAS.

SEIFERT, JOHN D MD, LICENSE NUMBER 17495, WAS DISCIPLINED BY MINNESOTA ON NOVEMBER 13, 1999
DISCIPLINARY ACTION: RESTRICTION PLACED ON LICENSE

NOTES: CONDITIONED LICENSE.

SEIFERT, JOHN DUPONT MD, LICENSE NUMBER D4855 OF GARLAND, TX, WAS DISCIPLINED BY TEXAS ON OCTOBER 24, 1998
DISCIPLINARY ACTION: FINE
OFFENSE: NONCOMPLIANCE WITH A PROFESSIONAL RULE

NOTES: IN EARLY 1996 HE SUBMITTED ONE OR MORE HOSPITAL PRIVILEGE APPLICATIONS WHICH CONTAINED FALSE OR MISLEADING STATEMENTS PERTAINING TO A PAST ARREST AND/OR INVESTIGATION BY THE TEXAS BOARD; HE DENIES INTENTIONALLY OR KNOWINGLY SUBMITTING FALSE AND/OR MISLEADING STATEMENTS IN ANY HOSPITAL PRIVILEGE APPLICATION; AND THE INCORRECT ANSWER FIRST SUBMITTED REGARDING THE ISSUE OF A PAST ARREST WAS CORRECTED IMMEDIATELY AFTER DISCOVERY, WITH AN APPROPRIATE RESPONSE INDICATING A PAST ARREST HAD OCCURRED, PRIOR TO ANY REVIEW OF THE APPLICATION BY THE HOSPITAL CREDENTIALS COMMITTEE. $5000 FINE.

SERNAKER, HARRY L MD, LICENSE NUMBER D43515 OF 10701 POT SPRING ROAD, COCKEYSVILLE, MD, WAS DISCIPLINED BY MARYLAND ON SEPTEMBER 21, 1998
DISCIPLINARY ACTION: 6-MONTH LICENSE SUSPENSION; 36-MONTH PROBATION
OFFENSE: SUBSTANDARD CARE, INCOMPETENCE OR NEGLIGENCE

NOTES: FAILED TO MEET STANDARDS OF CARE IN HIS PRACTICE OF PAIN MANAGEMENT IN SEVEN OF THIRTEEN CASES REVIEWED. REMAINDER OF ONE-YEAR SUSPENSION STAYED. PROHIBITED FROM SURGICALLY IMPLANTING ANY PAIN MANAGEMENT DEVICES.

SERNAKER, HARRY L MD, LICENSE NUMBER J1385 OF MCALLEN, TX, WAS DISCIPLINED BY TEXAS ON AUGUST 28, 1999
DISCIPLINARY ACTION: 36-MONTH PROBATION; RESTRICTION PLACED ON LICENSE
OFFENSE: DISCIPLINARY ACTION BY ANOTHER STATE OR AGENCY

NOTES: IN 9/98 THE MARYLAND BOARD SUSPENDED HIS LICENSE FOR 6 MONTHS BASED ON 7 PATIENT CASES WHICH REVEALED NUMEROUS COMPLICATIONS INCLUDING MISHANDLED INFECTIONS, "RECYCLING" SPINAL CORD STIMULATORS AND MORPHINE PUMPS, AND OVERFILLING DRUG PUMPS. SUSPENSION STAYED FOR PROBATION WITH FOLLOWING TERMS AND CONDITIONS: WITHIN 6 MONTHS SHALL TAKE AND PASS WITH A SCORE OF 75 OR ABOVE, WITHIN 3 ATTEMPTS, THE MEDICAL JURISPRUDENCE EXAM; WITHIN 60 DAYS HIS MEDICAL PRACTICE SHALL BE MONITORED BY A BOARD APPROVED TEXAS PHYSICIAN WHO SHALL PROVIDE QUARTERLY REPORTS TO THE BOARD; SHALL LIMIT PRACTICE TO GROUP OR INSTITUTIONAL SETTING; SHALL APPEAR BEFORE THE BOARD UPON REQUEST; SHALL PROVIDE COPIES OF ALL MATERIALS SUBMITTED TO OR RECEIVED FROM THE MARYLAND BOARD; TIME SPENT OUT OF TEXAS DOES NOT COUNT TOWARD PROBATION; SHALL INFORM THE BOARD OF CHANGE OF ADDRESS WITHIN 10 DAYS OR IF HE LEAVES THE STATE; SHALL GIVE A COPY OF THIS ORDER TO ANY HEALTH CARE ENTITY WHERE HE HAS PRIVILEGES; SHALL PROVIDE A COPY OF THIS ORDER TO ANYONE REQUESTING IT WITHIN 10 DAYS; SHALL COOPERATE WITH THE BOARD IN VERIFYING COMPLIANCE; SHALL NOT SEEK MODIFICATION FOR ONE YEAR.

SERNAKER, HARRY LEWIS MD, LICENSE NUMBER G64996 OF MCALLEN, TX, WAS DISCIPLINED BY CALIFORNIA ON MAY 10, 1999
DISCIPLINARY ACTION: 36-MONTH PROBATION
OFFENSE: DISCIPLINARY ACTION BY ANOTHER STATE OR AGENCY

NOTES: DISCIPLINED BY MARYLAND BASED ON DEPARTURES FROM THE STANDARD OF CARE RELATED TO HIS IMPLANTATION OF PAIN MANAGEMENT DEVICES. REVOCATION STAYED.

SERNAKER, HARRY LEWIS MD, LICENSE NUMBER 141110 OF 12 IVY HILL COURT, COCKEYSVILLE, MD, WAS DISCIPLINED BY NEW YORK ON JUNE 8, 1999
DISCIPLINARY ACTION: LICENSE REVOCATION
OFFENSE: DISCIPLINARY ACTION BY ANOTHER STATE OR AGENCY

NOTES: DISCIPLINED BY THE MARYLAND BOARD FOR FAILING TO MEET APPROPRIATE STANDARDS FOR THE DELIVERY OF QUALITY MEDICAL AND SURGICAL CARE.

SERRANO, ANTONIO P MD, LICENSE NUMBER F1988 OF FORT WORTH, TX, WAS DISCIPLINED BY TEXAS ON SEPTEMBER 20, 1997
DISCIPLINARY ACTION: SURRENDER OF CONTROLLED SUBSTANCE LICENSE; 120-MONTH PROBATION
OFFENSE: SUBSTANCE ABUSE

NOTES: HE ADMITS SELF-MEDICATING AND SELF-PRESCRIBING FOR ANXIETY AND PAIN WITH XANAX, ATIVAN AND HYDROCODONE; DURING 1992 - 1994 HE WROTE PRESCRIPTIONS AND ORDERED MEDICATIONS FOR VARIOUS PATIENTS AND DIVERTED THE DRUGS FOR USE BY HIS WIFE, A KNOWN HABITUAL USER OF NARCOTIC DRUGS; HIS WIFE ADMITS TO CALLING IN PRESCRIPTIONS TO PHARMACIES FOR VARIOUS PATIENTS AND DIVERTING THE DRUGS FOR HER OWN USE; AND HE REMOVED CONTROLLED SUBSTANCES AND DANGEROUS DRUGS FROM THE MEDICATION STOCK AT THE CLINIC WHERE HE WORKED FOR HIS AND HIS WIFE'S USE; FAILED TO KEEP RECORDS OF HIS PURCHASES AND DISPOSALS OF MEDICATIONS; FAILED TO MAINTAIN SECURITY WITH REGARD TO HIS TRIPLICATE FORMS, WHICH IS A VIOLATION OF THE DRUG LAWS; IN 6/95 HE LEFT HIS PRACTICE LUBBOCK, TEXAS WITHOUT NOTIFYING PATIENTS OF THE CLOSURE OF HIS PRACTICE; HE CONTENDS THAT THE HOSPITAL BOUGHT THE CLINIC AND ASSUMED THE PRACTICE AND RESPONSIBILITY FOR NOTIFYING THE PATIENTS; ON 11/21/96 HE WAS DIAGNOSED WITH OPIATE AND BENZODIAZEPINE ABUSE, AND MIXED PERSONALITY DISORDER WITH NARCISSISTIC AND HISTRIONIC FEATURES. REVOCATION STAYED WITH FOLLOWING TERMS AND CONDITIONS: SHALL ABSTAIN FROM THE CONSUMPTION OF ALCOHOL/DRUGS IN ANY FORM UNLESS PRESCRIBED BY ANOTHER PHYSICIAN FOR A LEGITIMATE AND THERAPEUTIC PURPOSE; SHALL SUBMIT HIMSELF FOR APPROPRIATE EXAMS INCLUDING DRUG OR ALCOHOL SCREENS; SHALL NOMINATE THREE CERTIFIED PSYCHIATRISTS FOR BOARD SELECTION OF A THERAPIST AND SHALL EXPEDITIOUSLY SUBMIT HIMSELF TO EVALUATION AND TREATMENT BY THE APPROVED PRACTITIONER NO LESS THAN ONCE A MONTH; SHALL PARTICIPATE IN THE ACTIVITIES OF A PHYSICIAN HEALTH AND REHABILITATION COMMITTEE AND ATTEND WEEKLY MEETINGS WITH QUARTERLY REPORTS; SHALL PARTICIPATE IN AA'S PROGRAM NOT LESS THAN THREE TIMES A WEEK; SHALL REPORT ON HIS ATTENDANCE; SHALL NOT TREAT OR OTHERWISE SERVE AS PHYSICIAN, PRESCRIBE, DISPENSE OR ADMINISTER DRUGS THAT MAY BE SUBJECT TO ABUSE TO HIMSELF OR TO ANY MEMBER OF HIS FAMILY; SHALL SURRENDER HIS DEA CONTROLLED SUBSTANCES REGISTRATION CERTIFICATE AND HIS TEXAS CONTROLLED SUBSTANCES REGISTRATION, ANY DRUGS INCLUDING SAMPLES IN HIS POSSESSION AND ANY UNUSED TRIPLICATE PRESCRIPTION FORMS; SHALL MAINTAIN ADEQUATE MEDICAL RECORDS WHICH SHALL BE AVAILABLE FOR REVIEW; SHALL NOT SIGN OR INDICATE IN ANY MANNER IN PATIENT RECORDS THAT HE HAS SEEN PATIENTS UNLESS HE ACTUALLY HAS SEEN AND EXAMINED THE PATIENT UNLESS IT IS CLEARLY NOTED THAT HE DID NOT PERSONALLY EXAMINE THE PATIENT; SHALL PRACTICE MEDICINE ONLY IN A GROUP PRACTICE SETTING; HIS MEDICAL PRACTICE SHALL BE MONITORED BY A BOARD APPROVED TEXAS PHYSICIAN WHO SHALL PROVIDE QUARTERLY REPORTS TO THE BOARD; SHALL ATTEND 50 HOURS PER YEAR OF CONTINUING MEDICAL EDUCATION WITH AT LEAST FIVE HOURS IN RISK MANAGEMENT; WITHIN 1 YEAR, SHALL OBTAIN 10 HOURS OF ETHICS THROUGH COURSES OR PROGRAMS; AND, COMPLETE A TWO WEEK PRECEPTORSHIP ON THE PREVENTION AND TREATMENT OF DRUG ABUSE; AND, PASS THE MEDICAL JURISPRUDENCE EXAM; SHALL GIVE A COPY OF THIS ORDER TO ANY HEALTH CARE ENTITY WHERE HE HAS PRIVILEGES; SHALL APPEAR BEFORE THE BOARD AT LEAST ONCE A YEAR; SHALL COOPERATE WITH THE BOARD IN VERIFYING COMPLIANCE INCLUDING PROVIDING COPIES OF MEDICAL RELEASES UPON REQUEST; TIME SPENT OUT OF TEXAS DOES NOT COUNT TOWARD PROBATION; SHALL INFORM THE BOARD OF CHANGE OF ADDRESS WITHIN 10 DAYS OR IF HE LEAVES THE STATE; SHALL NOT SEEK MODIFICATION FOR ONE YEAR. ON 10/15/99 THE ORDER WAS MODIFIED AS FOLLOWS: HE IS HEREBY AUTHORIZED BY THE BOARD TO REAPPLY TO THE DEA AND TEXAS DEPARTMENT OF PUBLIC SAFETY TO OBTAIN CONTROLLED SUBSTANCE REGISTRATION FOR SCHEDULES IV AND V; SEPARATE FROM PATIENT RECORDS, SHALL MAINTAIN A LOGBOOK FILE OF EVERY PRESCRIPTION WRITTEN BY

HIM FOR DANGEROUS DRUGS WITH ADDICTIVE POTENTIAL WHICH SHALL BE MADE AVAILABLE FOR REVIEW; ALL OTHER PROVISIONS OF THE ORDER REMAIN IN FULL EFFECT.

SESSIONS, JOHN LAYTON DO, LICENSE NUMBER 00E3446 OF KIRBYVILLE, TX, WAS DISCIPLINED BY TEXAS ON AUGUST 18, 1995
DISCIPLINARY ACTION: FINE
OFFENSE: PROFESSIONAL MISCONDUCT

NOTES: BREACH OF PHYSICIAN-PATIENT CONFIDENTIALITY IN THAT DURING AN ADMINISTRATIVE HEARING BEFORE ANOTHER AGENCY HE INAPPROPRIATELY AND WITHOUT AUTHORIZATION REVEALED CONFIDENTIAL MEDICAL INFORMATION REGARDING A PATIENT WHO WAS NOT A SUBJECT OF THE HEARING. SHALL PAY $1,000 FINE; SHALL GIVE A COPY OF THIS ORDER TO ANY HEALTH CARE ENTITY WHERE HE HAS PRIVILEGES; SHALL GIVE A COPY OF THIS ORDER TO ANYONE REQUESTING IT WITHIN 10 DAYS.

SHAH, ARUNKUMAR J MD, LICENSE NUMBER 00F6323 OF HOUSTON, TX, WAS DISCIPLINED BY TEXAS ON FEBRUARY 22, 1991
DISCIPLINARY ACTION: 24-MONTH PROBATION; RESTRICTION PLACED ON CONTROLLED SUBSTANCE LICENSE

NOTES: MUST APPEAR BEFORE BOARD ANNUALLY; ATTEND CONTINUING MEDICAL EDUCATION COURSES; MAINTAIN ADEQUATE MEDICAL RECORDS ON ALL PATIENT OFFICE VISITS; NOT SIGN OR INDICATE IN ANY MANNER ON ANY PATIENT RECORD, ANY VISIT, EVALUATION, MEDICAL TREATMENT, MEDICAL OPINION, OR MEDICATION ORDER WITHOUT HAVING SEEN AND EXAMINED THE PATIENT, NOR MAKE ANY LATER ENTRY WITHOUT SO NOTING; REFRAIN FROM PRESCRIBING OR ADMINISTERING ANY DRUG FOR ANY PATIENT UNLESS IN HIS MEDICAL JUDGMENT SUCH DRUG IS THERAPEUTIC IN THE MANNER SUCH DRUG IS PRESCRIBED, NOR PRESCRIBE, ADMINISTER, OR DISPENSE ANY DRUG WITH A POTENTIAL FOR ABUSE TO ANY PERSON UNLESS SATISFIED THAT THERE IS A LEGITIMATE MEDICAL AND THERAPEUTIC NEED; MAINTAIN A FILE OF EVERY PRESCRIPTION WRITTEN FOR CONTROLLED SUBSTANCES OR DANGEROUS DRUGS BY DATE ISSUED; NOT ATTEMPT TO REREGISTER OR OTHERWISE OBTAIN CONTROLLED SUBSTANCE REGISTRATIONS WITHOUT PRIOR WRITTEN AUTHORITY FROM THE BOARD AFTER PERSONAL APPEARANCE BEFORE THE BOARD.

SHAH, ARUNKUMAR J MD OF HOUSTON, TX, WAS DISCIPLINED BY DEA ON FEBRUARY 5, 1993
DISCIPLINARY ACTION: DENIAL OF NEW LICENSE
OFFENSE: DISCIPLINARY ACTION BY ANOTHER STATE OR AGENCY

NOTES: ALLEGEDLY WROTE PRESCRIPTIONS TO UNDERCOVER OFFICERS WITHOUT A VALID MEDICAL INDICATION ON THREE OCCASIONS, SURRENDERED HIS TEXAS MEDICAL LICENSE AND CONTROLLED SUBSTANCE REGISTRATION AND HIS DEA CERTIFICATE OF REGISTRATION HAD BEEN PREVIOUSLY REVOKED.

SHAH, ARUNKUMAR JAYANTLAL MD OF 150 WEST PARKER ROAD SUITE 605, HOUSTON, TX, WAS DISCIPLINED BY DEA ON MAY 21, 1990
DISCIPLINARY ACTION: SURRENDER OF CONTROLLED SUBSTANCE LICENSE

NOTES: SURRENDERED MEDICAL LICENSE AND CEASED MEDICAL PRACTICE FOR ONE YEAR BEGINNING 07/31/89 AND PLACED IN PRE-TRIAL DIVERSION PROGRAM FOR ONE YEAR.

SHAH, DAULAT MD, LICENSE NUMBER 00G4399 OF HOUSTON, TX, WAS DISCIPLINED BY TEXAS ON AUGUST 19, 1994
DISCIPLINARY ACTION: LICENSE SUSPENSION; 60-MONTH PROBATION
OFFENSE: LOSS OR RESTRICTION OF HOSPITAL PRIVILEGES

NOTES: IN 2/94 HE ANSWERED NO TO A MEDICAL PRACTICE ACT QUESTIONNAIRE QUERY ASKING WHETHER HIS MEDICAL PRIVILEGES HAD EVER BEEN DISCIPLINED BY ANY HEALTH CARE FACILITY; IN 1985 HE WAS PLACED ON COURTESY PROBATION FOR ONE YEAR AT ONE HOSPITAL FOR FAILURE TO ATTEND MEETINGS AND FOR LACK OF ADMISSIONS; IN 6/88 HE WAS DENIED PRIVILEGES AT ONE HOSPITAL FOR FAILURE TO REVEAL THAT PRIVILEGES AT ANOTHER HOSPITAL HAD BEEN DENIED DUE TO FAILURE TO ATTEND SURGERY COMMITTEE MEETINGS; SUSPENDED FROM EMERGENCY ROOM CALL IN GENERAL SURGERY ON 5/19/93 AT ANOTHER HOSPITAL WHICH CONCLUDED THAT HE "SHOWED POOR JUDGMENT WITH REGARD TO TREATMENT" IN THE CASE OF ONE PATIENT AND AN INDEPENDENT REVIEW OF RECORDS INDICATED THAT HE DEVIATED FROM ACCEPTED STANDARDS OF CARE; HOSPITAL SUSPENSION WAS TO LAST UNTIL HE COMPLETED SPECIFIED CONTINUING MEDICAL EDUCATION WHICH HE HAS. SUSPENSION STAYED AFTER 14 DAYS. CONDITIONS OF PROBATION: SHALL ATTEND AT LEAST 50 HOURS PER YEAR OF CONTINUING MEDICAL EDUCATION AND DURING THE FIRST YEAR OF PROBATION SHALL SUCCESSFULLY COMPLETE ADVANCED CARDIAC LIFE SUPPORT AND ADVANCED TRAUMA LIFE SUPPORT TRAINING; WITHIN ONE YEAR SHALL PASS THE SPEX EXAM; SHALL APPEAR BEFORE THE BOARD ONCE A YEAR; SHALL GIVE A COPY OF THIS ORDER TO ANY HEALTH CARE ENTITY WHERE HE HAS PRIVILEGES; SHALL COOPERATE WITH THE BOARD IN VERIFYING COMPLIANCE; SHALL INFORM BOARD OF CHANGE OF ADDRESS WITHIN 10 DAYS OR IF HE LEAVES THE STATE; TIME SPENT OUT OF TEXAS DOES NOT COUNT TOWARD PROBATION. SHALL NOT SEEK MODIFICATION FOR ONE YEAR.

SHAH, DAULAT MD, LICENSE NUMBER 00G4399, WAS DISCIPLINED BY TEXAS ON AUGUST 19, 1995
DISCIPLINARY ACTION: LICENSE SUSPENSION
OFFENSE: FAILURE TO COMPLY WITH PREVIOUS BOARD ORDER

NOTES: FAILED TO TAKE AND PASS THE SPECIAL PURPOSE EXAMINATION (SPEX) BY 8/19/95 AS REQUIRED BY 8/94 ORDER IN THAT HE SAT FOR THE SPEX IN 12/94 AND OBTAINED A FAILING SCORE OF 69. SUSPENSION UNTIL HE TAKES AND PASSES THE SPEX AND APPEARS BEFORE BOARD WITH EVIDENCE WHICH INDICATES THAT HE HAS THE SKILLS AND KNOWLEDGE AND IS OTHERWISE PHYSICALLY AND MENTALLY COMPETENT TO RESUME THE SAFE PRACTICE OF MEDICINE IN TEXAS. ON 2/27/97 REQUEST TO HAVE SUSPENSION LIFTED DENIED. ON 5/16/98 ORDER TERMINATED.

SHAH, DAULAT MD, LICENSE NUMBER G4399, WAS DISCIPLINED BY TEXAS ON MAY 8, 1997
DISCIPLINARY ACTION: 48-MONTH PROBATION

NOTES: ON 8/19/94 THE BOARD SUSPENDED HIS MEDICAL LICENSE; 14 DAYS LATER THE SUSPENSION WAS STAYED AND HE WAS PLACED ON PROBATION FOR FIVE YEARS UNDER TERMS AND CONDITIONS, INCLUDING THE REQUIREMENT THAT HE PASS THE SPEX WITHIN ONE YEAR OR HIS LICENSE WOULD BE AUTOMATICALLY SUSPENDED. HE FAILED TO FULFILL THIS REQUIREMENT AND ON 8/19/95 HIS LICENSE WAS

SUSPENDED. HE HAS SINCE OBTAINED A PASSING SCORE ON THE SPEX, AND HAVING MET ALL OTHER REQUIREMENTS, HAS REQUESTED THE REINSTATEMENT OF HIS LICENSE. THE SUSPENSION IS THEREFORE STAYED FOR PROBATION SUBJECT TO THE TERMS OF THE 8/19/94 ORDER; SHALL NOT SEEK MODIFICATION FOR ONE YEAR.

SHARP, DOUGLAS ROBERT DO, DATE OF BIRTH MARCH 22, 1950, LICENSE NUMBER 00F1242 OF 6206 HWY 6 SOUTH, HOUSTON, TX, WAS DISCIPLINED BY TEXAS ON APRIL 30, 1993
DISCIPLINARY ACTION: SURRENDER OF CONTROLLED SUBSTANCE LICENSE; 120-MONTH PROBATION
OFFENSE: SUBSTANCE ABUSE
NOTES: ON 1/22/92 HE CONTACTED PHYSICIAN'S ASSISTANCE PROGRAM INFORMING THEM OF HIS SELF-MEDICATING FOR UPPER BACK AND NECK PAIN; MEDICATION ABUSE INCLUDED UP TO 40-50 LORTABS PER DAY AND DEMEROL INJECTIONS; WAS PLACED ON PROBATION FOR TWO YEARS FOR DRIVING WHILE INTOXICATED IN 1990; IN 9/92 RELAPSED AND ENTERED ANOTHER INPATIENT PROGRAM WHICH HE SUCCESSFULLY COMPLETED; IN 2/93 ENTERED A CONTINUING CARE CONTRACT WITH THE PHYSICIANS ASSISTANCE PROGRAM. REVOCATION STAYED. CONDITIONS OF PROBATION: SHALL APPEAR BEFORE THE BOARD TWICE A YEAR; SHALL SURRENDER DEA AND TEXAS CONTROLLED SUBSTANCES REGISTRATION CERTIFICATES AND SHALL NOT ATTEMPT TO REREGISTER WITHOUT BOARD PERMISSION; SHALL SURRENDER ALL CONTROLLED SUBSTANCES INCLUDING SAMPLES IN HIS POSSESSION; SHALL REFRAIN FROM THE PERSONAL USE OF AND NOT PERSONALLY POSSESS, ADMINISTER OR PRESCRIBE ANY CONTROLLED SUBSTANCE OR PRESCRIPTION DRUG UNLESS GIVEN BY ANOTHER PHYSICIAN FOR A LEGITIMATE AND THERAPEUTIC PURPOSE; SHALL NOT TREAT OR OTHERWISE SERVE AS PHYSICIAN, PRESCRIBE, DISPENSE OR ADMINISTER DRUGS THAT MAY BE SUBJECT TO ABUSE TO HIMSELF OR ANY MEMBER OF HIS FAMILY; SHALL ABSTAIN FROM THE CONSUMPTION OF ALCOHOL AND CHEMICAL SUBSTANCES IN ANY FORM; SHALL PARTICIPATE IN ACTIVITIES OF AN IMPAIRED PHYSICIAN COMMITTEE AND ATTEND WEEKLY MEETINGS WITH QUARTERLY REPORTS; SHALL PARTICIPATE IN AA MEETINGS NOT LESS THAN THREE TIMES A WEEK; SHALL SUBMIT HIMSELF FOR APPROPRIATE EXAMS INCLUDING DRUG OR ALCOHOL SCREENS; SHALL SUBMIT HIMSELF TO A BOARD-APPROVED PSYCHIATRIST FOR EVALUATION AND TREATMENT TO WHOM HE WILL PROVIDE COPIES OF THIS ORDER; THIS PSYCHIATRIST WILL SUBMIT REPORTS TO THE BOARD UPON REQUEST; SHALL FURNISH WRITTEN REPORTS TO THE BOARD REGARDING HIS MEDICAL CONDITION AND COMPLIANCE UPON REQUEST; SHALL COMPLY WITH THE TERMS OF HIS CONTRACT WITH THE TEXAS OSTEOPATHIC MEDICAL ASSOCIATION; SHALL LIMIT HIS PRACTICE TO THAT OF A BOARD-APPROVED GROUP SETTING; SHALL BE MONITORED OR SUPERVISED BY A BOARD-APPROVED SUPERVISOR WITH REPORTS TO THE BOARD EVERY FOUR MONTHS; SHALL GIVE A COPY OF THIS ORDER TO ANY HEALTH CARE ENTITY WHERE HE HAS PRIVILEGES; SHALL COOPERATE WITH THE BOARD IN VERIFYING COMPLIANCE; SHALL INFORM THE BOARD OF CHANGE OF ADDRESS WITHIN 10 DAYS OR IF HE LEAVES THE STATE; TIME SPENT OUT OF TEXAS DOES NOT COUNT TOWARD PROBATION. SHALL NOT SEEK MODIFICATION FOR ONE YEAR. ON 8/17/96 THE BOARD DENIED HIS PETITION FOR TERMINATION OF THIS ORDER. ON 2/7/98 PETITION TO TERMINATE ORDER DENIED; ORDER MODIFIED DELETING REQUIREMENTS FOR PARTICIPATION WITH THE IMPAIRED PHYSICIAN'S COMMITTEE, AND CONTINUING CARE BY A PSYCHIATRIST. ON 1/29/99 REQUEST TO TERMINATE ORDER DENIED.

SHARY, JOHN MD OF 2114 W SUNSET LANE, MISSION, TX, WAS DISCIPLINED BY DEA ON SEPTEMBER 14, 1999
DISCIPLINARY ACTION: SURRENDER OF CONTROLLED SUBSTANCE LICENSE
OFFENSE: DISCIPLINARY ACTION BY ANOTHER STATE OR AGENCY
NOTES: STATE BOARD.

SHARY, JOHN H III MD, LICENSE NUMBER 00E8903 OF EDINBERG, TX, WAS DISCIPLINED BY TEXAS ON MAY 15, 1996
DISCIPLINARY ACTION: LICENSE SUSPENSION; REQUIRED TO ENTER AN IMPAIRED PHYSICIAN PROGRAM OR SUBSTANCE ABUSE TREATMENT
OFFENSE: LOSS OR RESTRICTION OF HOSPITAL PRIVILEGES
NOTES: IN 4/96, HE INGESTED ALCOHOL AND COCAINE WHICH WAS CONFIRMED BY A POSITIVE URINE SCREEN IN VIOLATION OF THE 12/95 ORDER; ON OR ABOUT 5/1/96 HIS CLINICAL PRIVILEGES AT A HOSPITAL WERE SUSPENDED BASED ON HIS POSITIVE SCREEN; HE SELF-REPORTED HIS INGESTION OF COCAINE AND ALCOHOL TO THE BOARD ON 5/2/96. SUSPENSION UNTIL HE REQUESTS TO HAVE SUSPENSION STAYED OR LIFTED AND APPEARS BEFORE THE BOARD WITH SUFFICIENT EVIDENCE THAT INDICATES THAT HE IS PHYSICALLY, MENTALLY AND OTHERWISE COMPETENT TO SAFELY PRACTICE MEDICINE INCLUDING AT A MINIMUM SUCCESSFUL COMPLETION OF TREATMENT IN A BOARD-APPROVED INPATIENT DRUG REHABILITATION FACILITY WHOSE DIRECTOR OR PHYSICIAN IN CHARGE OF HIS CARE SHALL SUBMIT MONTHLY REPORTS DURING HIS TREATMENT.

SHARY, JOHN H III MD, LICENSE NUMBER 0159188 OF 2114 WEST SUNSET LANE, MISSION, TX, WAS DISCIPLINED BY NEW YORK ON OCTOBER 7, 1996
DISCIPLINARY ACTION: SURRENDER OF LICENSE
OFFENSE: DISCIPLINARY ACTION BY ANOTHER STATE OR AGENCY
NOTES: DISCIPLINED BY THE TEXAS BOARD FOR BEING A HABITUAL USER OF ALCOHOL OR DRUGS AND FOR VIOLATING THE TERMS OF PROBATION IMPOSED BY THE TEXAS BOARD.

SHARY, JOHN H III MD, LICENSE NUMBER 00E8903, WAS DISCIPLINED BY TEXAS ON NOVEMBER 14, 1996
DISCIPLINARY ACTION: 120-MONTH PROBATION; RESTRICTION PLACED ON CONTROLLED SUBSTANCE LICENSE
OFFENSE: SUBSTANCE ABUSE
NOTES: HAS RECEIVED INPATIENT TREATMENT IN MISSISSIPPI FROM 5/7/96 THROUGH 9/20/96 AND HAS REQUESTED THAT SUSPENSION BE LIFTED; HAS SATISFIED MINIMUM REQUIREMENTS FOR STAYING THE 5/15/96 SUSPENSION. PROBATION WITH TERMS AND CONDITIONS: SHALL ABSTAIN FROM THE CONSUMPTION OF ALCOHOL/DRUGS IN ANY FORM UNLESS PRESCRIBED BY ANOTHER PHYSICIAN FOR A LEGITIMATE AND THERAPEUTIC PURPOSE; SHALL SUBMIT HIMSELF FOR APPROPRIATE EXAMS INCLUDING DRUG OR ALCOHOL SCREENS; SHALL SUBMIT HIMSELF FOR EVALUATION AND TREATMENT BY A BOARD-CERTIFIED PSYCHIATRIST WHOM HE SHALL SEE AT LEAST ONCE A MONTH AND WHO SHALL SUBMIT REPORTS TO THE BOARD; SHALL CONTINUE TO PARTICIPATE IN AA'S PROGRAM NOT LESS THAN THREE TIMES A WEEK WITH QUARTERLY

REPORTS TO THE BOARD; SHALL PARTICIPATE IN THE ACTIVITIES OF A PHYSICIAN'S HEALTH AND REHABILITATION COMMITTEE AND ATTEND WEEKLY MEETINGS WITH QUARTERLY REPORTS; SHALL COMPLY WITH THE TERMS OF ANY CONTINUING CARE CONTRACT HE ENTERS INTO WITH QUARTERLY REPORTS; SHALL NOT TREAT OR OTHERWISE SERVE AS PHYSICIAN, PRESCRIBE, DISPENSE OR ADMINISTER DRUGS THAT MAY BE SUBJECT TO ABUSE TO HIMSELF OR TO ANY MEMBER OF HIS FAMILY; SHALL NOT TELEPHONE TO A PHARMACY A PRESCRIPTION OR REFILL FOR CONTROLLED SUBSTANCES OR DANGEROUS DRUGS WITH ADDICTIVE POTENTIAL OR POTENTIAL FOR ABUSE NOR SHALL HE ALLOW ANYONE UNDER HIS SUPERVISION TO DO SO; SHALL MAINTAIN A FILE CONSISTING OF EVERY PRESCRIPTION WRITTEN FOR THESE SUBSTANCES WHICH SHALL BE AVAILABLE FOR REVIEW; MAY REAPPLY TO THE DEA AND THE DPS TO OBTAIN AUTHORIZATION TO PRESCRIBE SCHEDULES III, III-N, IV AND V; HIS PRACTICE INCLUDING ANY OFFICE AND SURGICAL PRACTICE SHALL BE MONITORED BY A BOARD-APPROVED TEXAS PHYSICIAN WHO SHALL SUBMIT QUARTERLY REPORTS TO THE BOARD; SHALL MAINTAIN ADEQUATE MEDICAL RECORDS WHICH SHALL BE AVAILABLE FOR REVIEW; SHALL OBTAIN AT LEAST 50 HOURS PER YEAR OF CONTINUING MEDICAL EDUCATION; SHALL APPEAR BEFORE BOARD AT LEAST TWICE A YEAR; SHALL COOPERATE WITH THE BOARD IN VERIFYING COMPLIANCE INCLUDING PROVIDING ANY MEDICAL RELEASES UPON REQUEST; SHALL GIVE A COPY OF THIS ORDER TO ANY HEALTH CARE ENTITY WHERE HE HAS PRIVILEGES; SHALL PROVIDE A COPY OF THIS ORDER TO ANYONE REQUESTING IT WITHIN 10 DAYS; TIME SPENT OUT OF TEXAS DOES NOT COUNT TOWARD PROBATION; SHALL INFORM BOARD OF CHANGE OF ADDRESS WITHIN 10 DAYS OR IF HE LEAVES THE STATE. SHALL NOT SEEK MODIFICATION FOR ONE YEAR. ON 5/16/98 PETITION FOR MODIFICATION OF ORDER GRANTED DELETING MONTHLY PSYCHIATRIC TREATMENT; REDUCTION OF APPEARANCES BEFORE THE BOARD FROM BIANNUAL TO ANNUAL.

SHARY, JOHN H III MD, LICENSE NUMBER E8903 OF MISSION, TX, WAS DISCIPLINED BY TEXAS ON JULY 24, 1998
DISCIPLINARY ACTION: EMERGENCY SUSPENSION
OFFENSE: FAILURE TO COMPLY WITH PREVIOUS BOARD ORDER

NOTES: VIOLATED 11/96 BOARD ORDER IN THAT ON 7/14/98 TESTED POSITIVE FOR COCAINE METABOLITES; HE DENIED THAT HE HAD USED COCAINE OR ANY OTHER SUBSTANCE, BUT DECLINED TO SUBMIT ANOTHER URINE SAMPLE WHEN GIVEN THE OPPORTUNITY; ON 7/24/98 HE ADMITTED TO THE BOARD THAT HE HAD USED COCAINE ON 7/10/98 AND ON 7/23/98 AFTER HE SPOKE WITH THE BOARD; HE ALSO ADMITTED THAT HE TREATED PATIENTS ON 7/24/98 ALTHOUGH HE DID CANCEL SURGERIES; HE ALSO ADMITTED THAT HE HAD USED ALCOHOL ON 3 OCCASIONS.

SHARY, JOHN H III MD, LICENSE NUMBER E8903 OF MISSION, TX, WAS DISCIPLINED BY TEXAS ON AUGUST 22, 1998
DISCIPLINARY ACTION: LICENSE SUSPENSION
OFFENSE: SUBSTANCE ABUSE

NOTES: INTEMPERATE USE OF ALCOHOL OR DRUGS. SUSPENSION UNTIL HE REQUESTS TO HAVE HIS SUSPENSION STAYED OR APPEARS BEFORE THE BOARD WITH SUFFICIENT EVIDENCE THAT HE IS PHYSICALLY, MENTALLY AND OTHERWISE COMPETENT TO SAFELY PRACTICE MEDICINE INCLUDING AT A MINIMUM COMPLETE COPIES OF MEDICAL RECORDS AND REPORTS OF PSYCHOLOGICAL AND NEUROPSYCHIATRIC EVALUATIONS, INCLUDING A 96 HOUR INPATIENT EVALUATION CONDUCTED BY A BOARD-APPROVED CERTIFIED PSYCHIATRIST; SHALL COOPERATE WITH THE BOARD IN VERIFYING COMPLIANCE INCLUDING PROVIDING COPIES OF MEDICAL RELEASES UPON REQUEST; SHALL GIVE A COPY OF THIS ORDER TO ANY HEALTH CARE ENTITY WHERE HE HAS PRIVILEGES; SHALL INFORM THE BOARD OF CHANGE OF ADDRESS WITHIN 10 DAYS.

SHAUGHNESSY, DENNIS M MD, DATE OF BIRTH SEPTEMBER 9, 1941, LICENSE NUMBER 00F7913 OF 105 MANOR ROAD, SAN MARCOS, TX, WAS DISCIPLINED BY TEXAS ON APRIL 21, 1990
DISCIPLINARY ACTION: 120-MONTH RESTRICTION PLACED ON LICENSE; 120-MONTH MONITORING OF PHYSICIAN PERFORMANCE
OFFENSE: SUBSTANCE ABUSE

NOTES: STIPULATED ORDER. MUST IMMEDIATELY REPORT ANY INCIDENT IN WHICH HE CONSUMES ALCOHOL OR USES CONTROLLED SUBSTANCE NOT PRESCRIBED BY ANOTHER PHYSICIAN FOR VALID MEDICAL PURPOSE, CONTINUE TO PARTICIPATE IN AA, SUBMIT FOR APPROPRIATE EXAMINATIONS TO DETERMINE FREEDOM FROM DRUGS AND ALCOHOL, NOT RESUME PRACTICE OF GENERAL OR FAMILY MEDICINE, GENERAL SURGERY, OR WORK IN HOSPITAL EMERGENCY ROOMS UNLESS HE HAS PASSED SPECIAL PURPOSE EXAMINATION AND OBTAINED APPROVAL OF BOARD (BUT MAY PROVIDE SUBSTANCE ABUSE CARE AND TREATMENT AND/OR ADDICTIONOLOGY SERVICES FOR PATIENTS) AND APPEAR SEMI-ANNUALLY BEFORE BOARD. ON 3/26/93 MODIFICATION OF HIS ORDER REDUCING REQUIRED ATTENDANCE OF ALCOHOLICS ANONYMOUS MEETINGS FROM FOUR TO TWO WEEKLY. ALL OTHER TERMS OF THIS ORDER REMAIN IN EFFECT.

SHAUGHNESSY, DENNIS M MD, DATE OF BIRTH SEPTEMBER 9, 1941, LICENSE NUMBER 00F7913 OF 105 MANOR ROAD, SAN MARCOS, TX, WAS DISCIPLINED BY TEXAS ON AUGUST 20, 1993
OFFENSE: FAILURE TO COMPLY WITH PREVIOUS BOARD ORDER

NOTES: BY BOARD ORDER OF 4/21/90 HE IS RESTRICTED FROM CONSUMING ANY ALCOHOL AND THAT HE REPORT ANY USE IMMEDIATELY; ONCE IN 3/93 AND ONCE IN 6/93 CONSUMED ALCOHOL ON AN AIRPLANE ENROUTE TO A BUSINESS MEETING; DID NOT REPORT THESE INCIDENTS TO THE BOARD UNTIL SEVERAL DAYS AFTER THE SECOND INCIDENT. PREVIOUS ORDER MODIFIED SUCH THAT HE SHALL APPEAR BEFORE THE BOARD EVERY THREE MONTHS DURING EACH YEAR OF HIS REMAINING PROBATION.

SHAUGHNESSY, DENNIS M MD, DATE OF BIRTH SEPTEMBER 9, 1941, LICENSE NUMBER 00F7913 OF MIDLAND, TX, WAS DISCIPLINED BY TEXAS ON JUNE 22, 1994
DISCIPLINARY ACTION: LICENSE SUSPENSION
OFFENSE: CRIMINAL CONVICTION OR PLEA OF GUILTY, NOLO CONTENDERE, OR NO CONTEST TO A CRIME

NOTES: IN 4/21/90 ORDER WAS RESTRICTED FROM CONSUMING ALCOHOL; CONSUMED ALCOHOL ON 2/15/94 AND SUBSEQUENTLY PLEADED NOLO CONTENDERE TO DRIVING WHILE INTOXICATED; FINED AND PLACED ON PROBATION FOR ONE YEAR; HAD DISCONTINUED USE OF ANTABUSE PRIOR TO THIS INCIDENT; HAS RESUMED USE SINCE THEN. SUSPENSION UNTIL HE PERSONALLY APPEARS BEFORE BOARD AND PROVIDES SUFFICIENT EVIDENCE THAT HE IS PHYSICALLY, MENTALLY AND

OTHERWISE COMPETENT TO SAFELY PRACTICE MEDICINE.

SHAUGHNESSY, DENNIS M MD OF 105 MANOR DRIVE, SAN MARCOS, TX, WAS DISCIPLINED BY DEA ON AUGUST 12, 1994
DISCIPLINARY ACTION: SURRENDER OF CONTROLLED SUBSTANCE LICENSE
OFFENSE: DISCIPLINARY ACTION BY ANOTHER STATE OR AGENCY
NOTES: STATE BOARD.

SHAUGHNESSY, DENNIS M MD, DATE OF BIRTH SEPTEMBER 9, 1941, LICENSE NUMBER 00F7913 OF MIDLAND, TX, WAS DISCIPLINED BY TEXAS ON OCTOBER 10, 1994
DISCIPLINARY ACTION: SURRENDER OF CONTROLLED SUBSTANCE LICENSE; 120-MONTH PROBATION
OFFENSE: SUBSTANCE ABUSE
NOTES: SUSPENSION OF 6/22/94 STAYED. CONDITIONS OF PROBATION: SHALL ABSTAIN FROM THE CONSUMPTION OF ALCOHOL/CHEMICAL SUBSTANCES IN ANY FORM UNLESS PRESCRIBED BY ANOTHER PHYSICIAN FOR A LEGITIMATE AND THERAPEUTIC PURPOSE; SHALL SUBMIT HIMSELF FOR APPROPRIATE EXAMS INCLUDING DRUG OR ALCOHOL SCREENS; SHALL NOT TREAT OR OTHERWISE SERVE AS PHYSICIAN, PRESCRIBE, DISPENSE OR ADMINISTER DRUGS THAT MAY BE SUBJECT TO ABUSE TO HIMSELF OR ANY MEMBER OF HIS FAMILY; SHALL NOT USE, POSSESS, ADMINISTER OR PRESCRIBE ANY CONTROLLED SUBSTANCE OR DANGEROUS DRUGS UNLESS PRESCRIBED, ADMINISTERED OR DISPENSED BY ANOTHER PHYSICIAN WHO IS TREATING HIM FOR A LEGITIMATE MEDICAL NEED; SHALL SURRENDER DEA AND TEXAS CONTROLLED SUBSTANCES CERTIFICATES, ALL UNUSED TRIPLICATE PRESCRIPTION FORMS AND ALL CONTROLLED SUBSTANCES IN HIS POSSESSION INCLUDING SAMPLES; SHALL NOT REREGISTER WITHOUT PERMISSION; SEPARATE FROM PATIENT RECORDS SHALL MAINTAIN A FILE OF EVERY PRESCRIPTION WRITTEN FOR DANGEROUS DRUGS WHICH SHALL BE AVAILABLE FOR INSPECTION; SHALL NOT TELEPHONE ANY PRESCRIPTIONS TO A PHARMACY FOR DANGEROUS DRUGS THAT MAY BE HABIT-FORMING; SHALL BE SUPERVISED BY A BOARD-APPROVED PHYSICIAN WITH QUARTERLY REPORTS; SHALL CONTINUE TO PARTICIPATE IN AA'S PROGRAM NOT LESS THAN FOUR TIMES A WEEK WITH QUARTERLY REPORTS TO THE BOARD; SHALL SUBMIT HIMSELF FOR EVALUATION AND TREATMENT TO A BOARD-APPROVED PSYCHIATRIST WITH REPORTS TO THE BOARD; SHALL CONTINUE ANTABUSE TREATMENT UNTIL TREATMENT IS TERMINATED BY MONITORING PHYSICIAN OR TREATING PSYCHIATRIST; SHALL ATTEND AT LEAST 50 HOURS PER YEAR OF CONTINUING MEDICAL EDUCATION; SHALL ATTEND AT LEAST SIX HOURS OF CONTINUING EDUCATION ON THE SUBJECT OF ETHICS WITHIN 12 MONTHS; SHALL APPEAR BEFORE THE BOARD FOUR TIMES A YEAR; SHALL GIVE A COPY OF THIS ORDER TO ANY HEALTH CARE ENTITY WHERE HE HAS PRIVILEGES; SHALL COOPERATE WITH BOARD IN VERIFYING COMPLIANCE; SHALL INFORM BOARD OF CHANGE OF ADDRESS WITHIN 10 DAYS OR IF HE LEAVES THE STATE; TIME SPENT OUT OF TEXAS DOES NOT COUNT TOWARD PROBATION. SHALL NOT SEEK MODIFICATION FOR ONE YEAR. THIS ORDER TAKES THE PLACE OF THE 4/21/90 ORDER AS MODIFIED.

SHAUGHNESSY, DENNIS M MD, LICENSE NUMBER F7913 OF MIDLAND, TX, WAS DISCIPLINED BY TEXAS ON AUGUST 9, 1997
DISCIPLINARY ACTION: LICENSE SUSPENSION
OFFENSE: FAILURE TO COMPLY WITH PREVIOUS BOARD ORDER
NOTES: ON 6/12/97 HE INGESTED ALCOHOL IN VIOLATION OF HIS 9/30/94 ORDER OF PROBATION, CONFIRMED BY A URINE SAMPLE TAKEN THAT DAY. HE ADMITS CONSUMING ALCOHOL IN VIOLATION OF A BOARD ORDER. SUSPENSION UNTIL HE APPEARS BEFORE THE BOARD WITH SUFFICIENT EVIDENCE THAT HE IS PHYSICALLY, MENTALLY AND OTHERWISE COMPETENT TO SAFELY PRACTICE MEDICINE. SUCH EVIDENCE SHALL INCLUDE AT A MINIMUM: COMPLETE MEDICAL RECORDS AND REPORTS OF PSYCHOLOGICAL AND NEUROPSYCHIATRIC EVALUATIONS CONDUCTED BY AN APPROVED, BOARD CERTIFIED PSYCHIATRIST; SHALL INFORM THE BOARD OF CHANGE OF ADDRESS WITHIN 10 DAYS; SHALL COOPERATE WITH THE BOARD IN VERIFYING COMPLIANCE. ON 8/22/98 REQUEST TO HAVE THE SUSPENSION LIFTED DENIED.

SHAUGHNESSY, DENNIS M MD, LICENSE NUMBER F7913 OF MIDLAND, TX, WAS DISCIPLINED BY TEXAS ON JANUARY 29, 1999
DISCIPLINARY ACTION: 120-MONTH PROBATION; REQUIRED TO TAKE ADDITIONAL MEDICAL EDUCATION
OFFENSE: SUBSTANCE ABUSE
NOTES: HAS HAD A HISTORY OF ALCOHOLISM DATING FROM 1981; HE HAS UNDERGONE HOSPITAL TREATMENT FOR ALCOHOLISM ON SEVERAL OCCASIONS DURING THE INTERVENING YEARS. SUSPENSION IMPOSED ON 8/9/97 STAYED FOR PROBATION WITH THE FOLLOWING TERMS AND CONDITIONS: SHALL ABSTAIN FROM THE CONSUMPTION OF ALCOHOL/DRUGS IN ANY FORM UNLESS PRESCRIBED BY ANOTHER PHYSICIAN FOR A LEGITIMATE AND THERAPEUTIC PURPOSE; SHALL SUBMIT HIMSELF FOR APPROPRIATE EXAMS INCLUDING DRUG OR ALCOHOL SCREENS; SHALL NOMINATE THREE CERTIFIED PSYCHIATRISTS FOR BOARD SELECTION OF A THERAPIST AND SHALL EXPEDITIOUSLY SUBMIT HIMSELF TO EVALUATION AND TREATMENT BY THE APPROVED PRACTITIONER; SHALL ENGAGE IN GROUP/MARITAL COUNSELING WITH HIS SPOUSE ON AT LEAST A MONTHLY BASIS; SHALL CONTINUE TO RECEIVE CARE AND TREATMENT FROM HIS BOARD-APPROVED APPROVED PHYSICIAN NO LESS THAN ONCE EVERY THREE MONTHS WITH QUARTERLY REPORTS; SHALL PARTICIPATE IN THE ACTIVITIES OF A PHYSICIAN HEALTH AND REHABILITATION COMMITTEE AND ATTEND WEEKLY MEETINGS WITH QUARTERLY REPORTS; SHALL PARTICIPATE IN AA'S PROGRAM NOT LESS THAN FIVE TIMES A WEEK; SHALL REPORT ON HIS ATTENDANCE; SHALL NOT TREAT OR OTHERWISE SERVE AS PHYSICIAN, PRESCRIBE, DISPENSE OR ADMINISTER DRUGS THAT MAY BE SUBJECT TO ABUSE TO HIMSELF OR TO ANY MEMBER OF HIS FAMILY; SHALL OBTAIN 50 HOURS PER YEAR OF CONTINUING MEDICAL EDUCATION; SHALL APPEAR BEFORE THE BOARD UPON REQUEST; SHALL COOPERATE WITH THE BOARD IN VERIFYING COMPLIANCE INCLUDING PROVIDING COPIES OF MEDICAL RELEASES UPON REQUEST; SHALL GIVE A COPY OF THIS ORDER TO ANY HEALTH CARE ENTITY WHERE HE HAS PRIVILEGES; TIME SPENT OUT OF TEXAS DOES NOT COUNT TOWARD PROBATION; SHALL INFORM THE BOARD OF CHANGE OF ADDRESS WITHIN 10 DAYS OR IF HE LEAVES THE STATE; SHALL NOT SEEK MODIFICATION FOR ONE YEAR.

SHERP, GARY ALLAN MD, LICENSE NUMBER 00F3335 OF DALLAS, TX, WAS DISCIPLINED BY TEXAS ON AUGUST 24, 1991
DISCIPLINARY ACTION: 60-MONTH PROBATION; MONITORING OF PHYSICIAN PERFORMANCE

OFFENSE: LOSS OR RESTRICTION OF HOSPITAL PRIVILEGES

NOTES: SUBSTANCE ABUSE AND LOSS OF HOSPITAL PRIVILEGES. SUSPENSION STAYED; TERMS OF PROBATION: SHALL PARTICIPATE IN AN IMPAIRED PHYSICIANS PROGRAM WITH WRITTEN REPORTS TO BOARD; SHALL PARTICIPATE IN AA; SHALL SUBMIT TO DRUG OR ALCOHOL SCREENS; SHALL APPEAR BEFORE THE BOARD TWICE A YEAR.

SHERP, GARY ALLAN MD, LICENSE NUMBER 00F3335, WAS DISCIPLINED BY TEXAS ON NOVEMBER 9, 1991
DISCIPLINARY ACTION: EMERGENCY SUSPENSION
OFFENSE: SUBSTANCE ABUSE

NOTES: PERFORMED ANESTHESIOLOGY WHILE UNDER THE INFLUENCE OF SUFENTA IV FOR NON-MEDICAL PURPOSES, AND WAS SEEN DOZING DURING SURGERY ON ONE OR MORE OCCASIONS; ON AT LEAST ONE OCCASION, HE FAILED TO PROVIDE ADEQUATE ANESTHESIA TO A PATIENT, WHICH RESULTED IN THE PATIENT BEING AROUSABLE DURING SURGERY; ON ONE OR MORE OCCASIONS HE USED SUFENTA IV IMMEDIATELY BEFORE AND OR DURING SURGERY; THESE ACTS COULD HAVE ENDANGERED PATIENTS LIVES; DRUGS WERE OBTAINED THROUGH DIVERTING DRUGS INTENDED FOR HIS PATIENTS AND RECORDS SUBSEQUENTLY FALSIFIED BY HIM.

SHERP, GARY ALLAN MD, LICENSE NUMBER 00F3335 OF DALLAS, TX, WAS DISCIPLINED BY TEXAS ON JANUARY 24, 1992
DISCIPLINARY ACTION: LICENSE REVOCATION
OFFENSE: FAILURE TO COMPLY WITH PREVIOUS BOARD ORDER

NOTES: VIOLATION OF PREVIOUS BOARD ORDER FOR FAILURE TO PRACTICE MEDICINE IN AN ACCEPTABLE MANNER CONSISTENT WITH PUBLIC HEALTH AND WELFARE.

SHERP, GARY ALLAN MD, LICENSE NUMBER 00F3335, WAS DISCIPLINED BY TEXAS ON MAY 15, 1996
DISCIPLINARY ACTION: LICENSE REINSTATEMENT; RESTRICTION PLACED ON LICENSE

NOTES: PREVIOUS REVOCATION STAYED. UPON REINSTATEMENT, WITHIN SIX MONTHS: SHALL TAKE AND PASS THE SPECIAL PURPOSE EXAMINATION; SHALL COMPLETE A SIX MONTH MINI-RESIDENCY PROGRAM APPROVED BY THE BOARD; SHALL TAKE AND PASS THE TEXAS MEDICAL JURISPRUDENCE EXAMINATION WITHIN THREE ATTEMPTS. SHALL NOT PRACTICE ANESTHESIA AT ANY TIME SUBSEQUENT TO LICENSE REINSTATEMENT AND HIS LICENSE SHALL BE SUBJECT TO THE FOLLOWING TERMS FOR 10 YEARS: SHALL NOT PRACTICE MEDICINE IN TEXAS UNTIL HE APPEARS BEFORE BOARD TO PETITION FOR PERMISSION TO RESUME PRACTICE AND PROVIDES SUFFICIENT EVIDENCE WHICH INDICATES THAT HE IS PHYSICALLY, MENTALLY AND OTHERWISE COMPETENT TO SAFELY PRACTICE MEDICINE INCLUDING AT A MINIMUM THE COMPLETION OF A BOARD-APPROVED RESIDENCY PROGRAM IN AN AREA OF PRACTICE OTHER THAN ANESTHESIA; SHALL ABSTAIN FROM THE CONSUMPTION OF ALCOHOL/DRUGS IN ANY FORM UNLESS PRESCRIBED BY ANOTHER PHYSICIAN FOR A LEGITIMATE AND THERAPEUTIC PURPOSE; SHALL SUBMIT HIMSELF FOR APPROPRIATE EXAMS INCLUDING DRUG OR ALCOHOL SCREENS; SHALL PARTICIPATE IN AA'S PROGRAM AT LEAST THREE TIMES A WEEK WITH QUARTERLY REPORTS TO THE BOARD; SHALL PARTICIPATE IN THE ACTIVITIES OF A PHYSICIAN'S HEALTH AND REHABILITATION COMMITTEE AND ATTEND WEEKLY MEETINGS WITH QUARTERLY REPORTS; SHALL COMPLY WITH THE TERMS OF ANY CONTRACT ENTERED INTO FOR HOSPITAL PRIVILEGES; SHALL NOT POSSESS ALCOHOL, CONTROLLED SUBSTANCES OR DANGEROUS DRUGS WITH ADDICTIVE POTENTIAL OR POTENTIAL FOR ABUSE AND SHALL SURRENDER ALL SUCH DRUGS INCLUDING SAMPLES; SHALL NOT TREAT OR OTHERWISE SERVE AS PHYSICIAN, PRESCRIBE, DISPENSE OR ADMINISTER DRUGS THAT MAY BE SUBJECT TO ABUSE TO HIMSELF OR TO ANY MEMBER OF HIS FAMILY; SHALL SURRENDER HIS DEA/DPS CONTROLLED SUBSTANCES REGISTRATION CERTIFICATES AND SHALL NOT ATTEMPT TO REREGISTER WITHOUT PRIOR AUTHORITY FROM THE BOARD; SHALL MAINTAIN A FILE WITH COPIES OF EVERY PRESCRIPTION WRITTEN BY HIM FOR DANGEROUS DRUGS WITH ADDICTIVE POTENTIAL OR POTENTIAL FOR ABUSE WHICH SHALL BE AVAILABLE FOR REVIEW; HIS PRACTICE SHALL BE MONITORED BY A BOARD-APPROVED TEXAS PHYSICIAN WHO SHALL SUBMIT QUARTERLY REPORTS TO THE BOARD; SHALL MAINTAIN ADEQUATE MEDICAL RECORDS WHICH SHALL BE AVAILABLE FOR REVIEW; SHALL OBTAIN AT LEAST 50 HOURS PER YEAR OF CONTINUING MEDICAL EDUCATION, AT LEAST 25 OF WHICH SHALL BE IN ADDICTIONOLOGY; WITHIN ONE YEAR, SHALL TAKE AND COMPLETE AN ADVANCED CARDIAC LIFE SUPPORT COURSE AND AN ADVANCED TRAUMA LIFE SUPPORT COURSE AND OBTAIN CERTIFICATION IN BOTH; SHALL APPEAR BEFORE BOARD AT LEAST TWICE A YEAR; SHALL COOPERATE WITH THE BOARD IN VERIFYING COMPLIANCE INCLUDING PROVIDING COPIES OF MEDICAL RELEASES UPON REQUEST; SHALL GIVE A COPY OF THIS ORDER TO ANY HEALTH CARE ENTITY WHERE HE HAS PRIVILEGES; TIME SPENT OUT OF TEXAS DOES NOT COUNT TOWARD THIS ORDER; SHALL PROVIDE COPIES OF ANY REPORTS TO THE BOARD THAT HE HAS SUBMITTED TO OR RECEIVED FROM ANY OTHER STATE'S MEDICAL BOARD WHERE HE OBTAINS A LICENSE; SHALL INFORM BOARD OF CHANGE OF ADDRESS WITHIN 10 DAYS OR IF HE LEAVES THE STATE. SHALL NOT SEEK MODIFICATION FOR ONE YEAR.

SHIELDS, FREDERICK S MD, LICENSE NUMBER 00C7772 OF VICTORIA, TX, WAS DISCIPLINED BY TEXAS ON OCTOBER 5, 1991
DISCIPLINARY ACTION: SURRENDER OF LICENSE
OFFENSE: SUBSTANCE ABUSE

NOTES: HE PERFORMED A DILATION AND CURETAGE ON 7/8/88, DURING WHICH THE PATIENT STARTED HEMORRHAGING; SHE WAS TRANSFERRED TO A HOSPITAL FOR EMERGENCY CARE, WHERE SHE DIED. ALLEGED TO HAVE FAILED TO STOP DRINKING ALCOHOL, AS AGREED WITH THE EXECUTIVE COMMITTEE OF CITIZENS MEDICAL CENTER IN 3/90. EXECUTIVE COMMITTEE OF CITIZENS MEDICAL CENTER ACCEPTED HIS SURRENDER OF ADMITTING PRIVILEGES IN RESOLUTION OF A PEER REVIEW COMPLAINT ON 4/10/90.

SHIN, UN KYO MD OF 13910 JOSEY LANE, FARMERS BRANCH, TX, WAS DISCIPLINED BY DEA ON JULY 28, 1995
DISCIPLINARY ACTION: SURRENDER OF CONTROLLED SUBSTANCE LICENSE
OFFENSE: PROFESSIONAL MISCONDUCT

NOTES: PLED GUILTY TO ILLICIT DISTRIBUTION OF CONTROLLED SUBSTANCES.

SHIN, UN KYO MD, LICENSE NUMBER 00F1243 OF FARMERS BRANCH, TX, WAS DISCIPLINED BY TEXAS ON OCTOBER 13, 1995
DISCIPLINARY ACTION: LICENSE REVOCATION
OFFENSE: CRIMINAL CONVICTION OR PLEA OF GUILTY, NOLO

CONTENDERE, OR NO CONTEST TO A CRIME

NOTES: ON 6/9/95, PLED GUILTY TO THE FELONY OF UNLAWFULLY DISPENSING A CONTROLLED SUBSTANCE NOT IN THE USUAL COURSE OF PROFESSIONAL PRACTICE AND NOT FOR A LEGITIMATE MEDICAL PURPOSE.

SHINDER, THOMAS W MD, DATE OF BIRTH MARCH 28, 1959 OF 104 W ADKINS STREET, SEAGOVILLE, TX, WAS DISCIPLINED BY MEDICARE ON MARCH 18, 1999
DISCIPLINARY ACTION: EXCLUSION FROM THE MEDICARE AND/OR MEDICAID PROGRAM
OFFENSE: NONCOMPLIANCE WITH A PROFESSIONAL RULE

NOTES: DEFAULTED ON PUBLIC HEALTH SERVICE EDUCATION LOAN.

SHINDER, THOMAS WAYNE MD, LICENSE NUMBER 00N8397 OF LITTLE ROCK, AR, WAS DISCIPLINED BY ARKANSAS ON JULY 11, 1996
DISCIPLINARY ACTION: EMERGENCY SUSPENSION

NOTES: EXPIRATION DATE UPON COMPLIANCE OF TERMS.

SHIPKEY, FREDERICK H JR MD, LICENSE NUMBER 00D5474 OF JACKSON, MS, WAS DISCIPLINED BY TEXAS ON JANUARY 12, 1991
OFFENSE: DISCIPLINARY ACTION BY ANOTHER STATE OR AGENCY

NOTES: AGREED ORDER AS A RESULT OF HAVING BEEN DISCIPLINED BY MISSISSIPPI BOARD. MUST RECEIVE PERMISSION OF TEXAS BOARD BEFORE RETURNING TO PRACTICE MEDICINE IN TEXAS AND BE SUBJECT TO TERMS IMPOSED, IF ANY, INCLUDING A COMPLETE REPORT ON THE STATUS OF HIS MISSISSIPPI LICENSE.

SHORT, LUKE HENRY MD, LICENSE NUMBER 00C7145 OF 449 W NORTH STREET, MOUNTAIN HOME, AR, WAS DISCIPLINED BY ARKANSAS ON APRIL 8, 1994
DISCIPLINARY ACTION: EMERGENCY SUSPENSION

SHORT, LUKE HENRY MD, LICENSE NUMBER 00C7145 OF 449 W NORTH STREET, MOUNTAIN HOME, AR, WAS DISCIPLINED BY ARKANSAS ON JUNE 21, 1994
DISCIPLINARY ACTION: 24-MONTH PROBATION
OFFENSE: SUBSTANCE ABUSE

NOTES: EXCESSIVE USE OF NARCOTICS IN A HABITUAL, INTEMPERATE AND EXCESSIVE MANNER FOR NONMEDICAL REASONS; VIOLATION OF LAW REGULATING THE POSSESSION, DISTRIBUTION AND USE OF NARCOTICS AND CONTROLLED DRUGS. GRANTED TEMPORARY PERMIT TO PRACTICE 9/94. LICENSE RESTORED ON 6/8/95.

SHORT, LUKE HENRY MD, LICENSE NUMBER 00J3222 OF MOUNTAIN HOME, AR, WAS DISCIPLINED BY TEXAS ON JANUARY 6, 1995
DISCIPLINARY ACTION: SURRENDER OF LICENSE
OFFENSE: FAILURE TO COMPLY WITH PREVIOUS BOARD ORDER

NOTES: IN VIOLATION OF A 12/7/92 BOARD ORDER HE SUFFERED A RELAPSE THROUGH THE INGESTION OF FENTANYL IN 2/94; WAS ADMITTED FOR TREATMENT OF CHEMICAL DEPENDENCY; SELF-REPORTED THE RELAPSE TO THE BOARD; DISCHARGED FROM INPATIENT TREATMENT ON 6/25/94 AND ENTERED AFTERCARE. SHALL NOT PETITION FOR REINSTATEMENT.

SHORT, MARVIN JOHN II MD, LICENSE NUMBER 0006852 OF GREENVILLE, SC, WAS DISCIPLINED BY SOUTH CAROLINA ON AUGUST 11, 1992
DISCIPLINARY ACTION: SURRENDER OF CONTROLLED SUBSTANCE LICENSE; LICENSE SUSPENSION
OFFENSE: SUBSTANDARD CARE, INCOMPETENCE OR NEGLIGENCE

NOTES: INAPPROPRIATE PATIENT CARE. SUSPENSION STAYED AFTER PAYMENT OF $10,000 FINE AND SURRENDER OF CONTROLLED SUBSTANCES REGISTRATION; INDEFINITE PROBATION.

SHORT, MARVIN JOHN II MD, DATE OF BIRTH JULY 28, 1932, LICENSE NUMBER 00D1124 OF 604 GROVE ROAD, GREENVILLE, SC, WAS DISCIPLINED BY TEXAS ON JUNE 15, 1993
DISCIPLINARY ACTION: MONITORING OF PHYSICIAN PERFORMANCE
OFFENSE: DISCIPLINARY ACTION BY ANOTHER STATE OR AGENCY

NOTES: ON 8/11/92 SOUTH CAROLINA LICENSE PLACED ON INDEFINITE PROBATION AFTER A $10,000 FINE AND SURRENDER OF CONTROLLED SUBSTANCES REGISTRATIONS. PRIOR TO PRACTICING IN TEXAS SHALL APPEAR BEFORE THE BOARD TO OBTAIN APPROVAL; SHALL PROVIDE TEXAS WITH ANY REPORTS SUBMITTED TO SOUTH CAROLINA; SHALL GIVE A COPY OF THIS ORDER TO ANY HEALTH CARE ENTITY WHERE HE HAS PRIVILEGES; SHALL COOPERATE WITH THE BOARD IN VERIFYING COMPLIANCE; SHALL INFORM BOARD OF CHANGE OF ADDRESS WITHIN 10 DAYS. SHALL NOT SEEK MODIFICATION FOR ONE YEAR.

SILBERMAN, MICHAEL K MD, LICENSE NUMBER H5971 OF FORT WORTH, TX, WAS DISCIPLINED BY TEXAS ON NOVEMBER 22, 1997
DISCIPLINARY ACTION: LICENSE SUSPENSION; MONITORING OF PHYSICIAN PERFORMANCE
OFFENSE: CRIMINAL CONVICTION OR PLEA OF GUILTY, NOLO CONTENDERE, OR NO CONTEST TO A CRIME

NOTES: ON 5/17/96 HE PLEADED GUILTY TO A FELONY 2 CHARGE OF INDECENCY WITH A CHILD AND WAS FINED $174.00; ON 8/2/96 HE WAS FOUND GUILTY OF A 2ND DEGREE FELONY, INDECENCY WITH A CHILD, CONTACT AND A 3RD DEGREE FELONY, INDECENCY WITH A CHILD, EXPOSURE; HE WAS SENTENCED TO 8 AND 4 YEARS TO BE SERVED CONCURRENTLY; HE HAS FILED AN APPEAL AND IS CURRENTLY UNDER COMMUNITY SUPERVISION WHILE HIS APPEAL IS PENDING; THE CONDITIONS OF HIS APPEAL BOND INCLUDE: ELECTRONIC MONITORING AND REPORTING WEEKLY FOR URINALYSIS; NO CONTACT WITH MINORS OTHER THAN HIS OWN CHILDREN; ATTEND SEX OFFENDER TREATMENT; AND AVOID GOING TO CHILD ORIENTED UNSUPERVISED ESTABLISHMENTS; HE ALSO REPORTED THAT HIS PRIVILEGES HAD BEEN RESTRICTED WHILE HE WAS IN THE MILITARY DUE TO A CONVICTION OF CONDUCT UNBECOMING AN OFFICER AND WAS SENTENCED TO BE DISMISSED FROM THE U.S. AIR FORCE IN 5/94. SUSPENSION UNTIL HE REQUESTS TO HAVE HIS SUSPENSION STAYED OR APPEARS BEFORE THE BOARD WITH SUFFICIENT EVIDENCE THAT HE IS PHYSICALLY, MENTALLY AND OTHERWISE COMPETENT TO SAFELY PRACTICE MEDICINE INCLUDING AT A MINIMUM COMPLETE COPIES OF MEDICAL RECORDS AND REPORTS OF PSYCHOLOGICAL AND NEUROPSYCHIATRIC EVALUATIONS, INCLUDING A 96 HOUR INPATIENT EVALUATION CONDUCTED BY A BOARD-APPROVED CERTIFIED PSYCHIATRIST; SHALL DOCUMENT ADEQUATE MONITORING OF HIS PRACTICE AND THE STATUS OF HIS CRIMINAL APPEAL; SHALL COOPERATE WITH THE BOARD IN VERIFYING COMPLIANCE; SHALL GIVE A COPY OF THIS ORDER TO ANY HEALTH CARE ENTITY WHERE HE HAS PRIVILEGES; SHALL INFORM THE BOARD OF CHANGE OF ADDRESS WITHIN 10 DAYS; SHALL NOT SEEK MODIFICATION FOR ONE YEAR. HIS REQUEST ON THE

SAME DAY TO HAVE THE SUSPENSION LIFTED WAS DENIED.

SILBERMAN, MICHAEL K MD OF 1500 S MAIN, FORT WORTH, TX, WAS DISCIPLINED BY DEA ON FEBRUARY 23, 1998
DISCIPLINARY ACTION: SURRENDER OF CONTROLLED SUBSTANCE LICENSE

SILBERMAN, MICHAEL K MD, DATE OF BIRTH OCTOBER 11, 1958 OF 8700 CALMONT AVENUE #40, FORT WORTH, TX, WAS DISCIPLINED BY MEDICARE ON JUNE 18, 1998
DISCIPLINARY ACTION: EXCLUSION FROM THE MEDICARE AND/OR MEDICAID PROGRAM
OFFENSE: DISCIPLINARY ACTION BY ANOTHER STATE OR AGENCY

SILVA, MARCELINO S MD, LICENSE NUMBER E6173 OF LOCKHART, TX, WAS DISCIPLINED BY TEXAS ON AUGUST 9, 1997
DISCIPLINARY ACTION: 60-MONTH PROBATION; RESTRICTION PLACED ON LICENSE
OFFENSE: SUBSTANDARD CARE, INCOMPETENCE OR NEGLIGENCE
NOTES: BETWEEN 1991 AND 1993 HE ENGAGED IN INAPPROPRIATE BEHAVIOR WITH PATIENTS BY HIS COMMENTS OF A SEXUAL NATURE; HE CONTENDS THAT HIS COMMENTS WERE MISUNDERSTOOD BY HIS PATIENTS AND WERE NOT FOR PRURIENT PURPOSES; HE PRESCRIBED CONTROLLED SUBSTANCES ON 1-2 OCCASIONS TO A PATIENT HE SUSPECTED WAS ADDICTED, AND ON 3 OCCASIONS TO ANOTHER PATIENT AFTER HE SUSPECTED THE PATIENT WAS ADDICTED; FAILURE TO TIMELY DIAGNOSE A PATIENT'S ACUTE LYMPHOBLASTIC LEUKEMIA, CAUSING SUBOPTIMAL PAIN RELIEF DUE TO THE DELAY IN DIAGNOSIS; FAILURE TO TIMELY DIAGNOSE A PATIENT'S IMMUNE THROMBOCYTOPENIA AND LUPUS; THERE IS NO EVIDENCE OF ANY HARM CAUSED BY THE DELAY; FAILURE TO TIMELY DIAGNOSE A PATIENT'S ORTHOSTATIC HYPOTENSION; THERE IS NO EVIDENCE THAT ANY HARM WAS CAUSED BY THE DELAY. SUSPENSION STAYED FOR PROBATION WITH FOLLOWING TERMS AND CONDITIONS: SHALL NOMINATE THREE CERTIFIED PSYCHIATRISTS FOR BOARD SELECTION OF A THERAPIST AND SHALL EXPEDITIOUSLY SUBMIT HIMSELF TO EVALUATION AND TREATMENT BY THE APPROVED PRACTITIONER; SHALL HAVE A CHAPERONE PRESENT WHILE EXAMINING FEMALE OR MALE PATIENTS UNDER THE AGE OF 21; SHALL MAINTAIN ADEQUATE MEDICAL RECORDS WHICH SHALL BE AVAILABLE FOR REVIEW; SHALL OBTAIN AT LEAST 50 HOURS PER YEAR OF CONTINUING MEDICAL EDUCATION THAT SHALL INCLUDE ONE COURSE IN RISK MANAGEMENT AND ONE COURSE WHICH COVERS TRANSFERENCE, COUNTERTRANSFERENCE OR BOUNDARY ISSUES BETWEEN PATIENT AND PHYSICIAN; SHALL OBTAIN ONE ETHICS COURSE OR ATTEND ONE ETHICS PROGRAM PER YEAR; SHALL TAKE AND PASS THE SPEX WITHIN THREE MONTHS; SHALL APPEAR BEFORE THE BOARD TWICE A YEAR; SHALL COOPERATE WITH THE BOARD IN VERIFYING COMPLIANCE INCLUDING PROVIDING COPIES OF MEDICAL RELEASES UPON REQUEST; SHALL GIVE A COPY OF THIS ORDER TO ANY HEALTH CARE ENTITY WHERE HE HAS PRIVILEGES; SHALL PROVIDE A COPY OF THIS ORDER TO ANYONE REQUESTING IT WITHIN 10 DAYS; TIME SPENT OUT OF TEXAS DOES NOT COUNT TOWARD PROBATION; SHALL INFORM THE BOARD OF CHANGE OF ADDRESS WITHIN 10 DAYS OR IF HE LEAVES THE STATE; SHALL NOT SEEK MODIFICATION FOR ONE YEAR; REPRIMAND.

SILVA, MARCELINO S MD, LICENSE NUMBER E6173 OF LOCKHART, TX, WAS DISCIPLINED BY TEXAS ON NOVEMBER 22, 1997
DISCIPLINARY ACTION: LICENSE SUSPENSION
OFFENSE: FAILURE TO COMPLY WITH PREVIOUS BOARD ORDER
NOTES: VIOLATED 8/8/97 ORDER TO TAKE AND PASS THE SPEX

SILVA, MARCELINO S MD OF 1007 WEST SAN ANTONIO STREET, LOCKHART, TX, WAS DISCIPLINED BY DEA ON DECEMBER 30, 1997
DISCIPLINARY ACTION: SURRENDER OF CONTROLLED SUBSTANCE LICENSE
NOTES: IN LIEU OF PUBLIC INTEREST REVOCATION.

SILVA, MARCELINO S MD, DATE OF BIRTH JUNE 5, 1940 OF 1007 W SAN ANTONIO STREET, LOCKHART, TX, WAS DISCIPLINED BY MEDICARE ON JUNE 18, 1998
DISCIPLINARY ACTION: EXCLUSION FROM THE MEDICARE AND/OR MEDICAID PROGRAM
OFFENSE: DISCIPLINARY ACTION BY ANOTHER STATE OR AGENCY
NOTES: LICENSE REVOKED, SUSPENDED, SURRENDERED OR OTHERWISE LOST FOR REASONS BEARING ON PROFESSIONAL PERFORMANCE, PROFESSIONAL COMPETENCE OR FINANCIAL INTEGRITY.

SIMON, JEAN-CHARLES MD, LICENSE NUMBER 00G1776 OF SPRING, TX, WAS DISCIPLINED BY TEXAS ON NOVEMBER 3, 1994
DISCIPLINARY ACTION: 120-MONTH PROBATION; RESTRICTION PLACED ON LICENSE
OFFENSE: OVERPRESCRIBING OR MISPRESCRIBING DRUGS
NOTES: IN SIX CASES IN 1987 AND 1988 TESTS PERFORMED WITHOUT ADEQUATE INDICATION OR PRIOR TO ANY PHYSICAL EXAMINATION; IN FIVE CASES IN 1991 AND 1992 TREATMENTS AND CHARGES WERE EXCESSIVE IN RELATION TO THE INJURY AND THEIR MEDICAL RECORDS FAILED TO SUPPORT THE TREATMENT METHODS AND CHARGES OR TO DEMONSTRATE THAT ANY HOME SELF-CARE INSTRUCTION WAS GIVEN; IN SEVERAL CASES BETWEEN 1987 AND 1990 PATIENTS WERE PRESCRIBED MEDICATIONS WITHOUT EITHER ADEQUATE ASSESSMENT, FOLLOW-UP, OR DOCUMENTATION; SOME OF THESE PRESCRIPTIONS WERE REFILLED OR PRESCRIBED FOR LONG PERIODS OF TIME WITHOUT PROPER INDICATION; IN SOME CASES NO PROPER HISTORY OR PHYSICAL EXAM WAS PERFORMED AND IN ONE CASE THERE WAS INDICATION OF DRUG ABUSE; ENGAGED IN THE CORPORATE PRACTICE OF MEDICINE BY HIS SALARIED EMPLOYMENT AT A CLINIC OWNED AND OPERATED BY A NON-PHYSICIAN; SIGNED A MEMORANDUM OF AGREEMENT WITH THE DEA ON 3/21/94 REGARDING PREVIOUS SURRENDER OF CONTROLLED SUBSTANCES REGISTRATIONS. HE NEITHER ADMITS NOR DENIES THESE CHARGES. REVOCATION STAYED. CONDITIONS OF PROBATION: SHALL APPEAR BEFORE THE BOARD TWICE A YEAR; WITHIN ONE YEAR SHALL TAKE THE TEXAS MEDICAL JURISPRUDENCE EXAM; SHALL NOT ACCEPT EMPLOYMENT OR ENTER INTO CONTRACTUAL RELATIONSHIPS WHERE HE WOULD BE COMPENSATED TO DIAGNOSE OR TREAT PATIENTS BY ANY ENTITY NOT COMPOSED OF TEXAS LICENSED PHYSICIANS AND WHERE THE ENTITY WOULD RECEIVE AND RETAIN FEES PAID FOR THE PHYSICIAN'S PROFESSIONAL SERVICES; ORDER CONSTITUTES A PUBLIC REPRIMAND; SHALL PERSONALLY EXAMINE PATIENTS WHEN A FORM CERTIFIES THIS OR WHERE AN INITIAL DIAGNOSIS OF PROBABLE DISEASE OR INJURY HAS BEEN MADE; SHALL PERFORM 10 HOURS PER MONTH OF COMMUNITY SERVICE FOR TWO YEARS; SHALL FOLLOW TERMS OF AGREEMENT WITH DEA; SHALL

NOT ADMINISTER, DISPENSE, OR PRESCRIBE ANY SCHEDULE II OR IIN CONTROLLED SUBSTANCES ALTHOUGH MAY ORDER THESE CONTROLLED SUBSTANCES FOR HOSPITAL OR NURSING HOME PATIENTS; SHALL BE SUPERVISED BY A BOARD-APPROVED PHYSICIAN WITH QUARTERLY REPORTS; SHALL NOT TREAT ANY PATIENT FOR WEIGHT CONTROL OR OBESITY WITH ANY DRUGS; SEPARATE FROM PATIENT RECORDS, SHALL MAINTAIN A FILE OF EVERY PRESCRIPTION WRITTEN FOR CONTROLLED SUBSTANCES OR DANGEROUS DRUGS WHICH SHALL BE AVAILABLE FOR INSPECTION; SHALL NOT TELEPHONE ANY PRESCRIPTION FOR THESE DRUGS TO A PHARMACY; SHALL NOT PRESCRIBE, DISPENSE, ADMINISTER OR POSSESS ANY OF A SPECIFIED LIST OF AMPHETAMINE-LIKE DRUGS; SHALL NOT TREAT OR OTHERWISE SERVE AS PHYSICIAN, PRESCRIBE, DISPENSE OR ADMINISTER DRUGS THAT MAY BE SUBJECT TO ABUSE TO HIMSELF OR ANY MEMBER OF HIS FAMILY; SHALL NOT SIGN ANY PATIENT RECORD UNLESS HE HAS PERSONALLY EXAMINED THE PATIENT OR CLEARLY NOTES IN THE RECORD THAT HE DID NOT; SHALL MAINTAIN ADEQUATE MEDICAL RECORDS ON ALL PATIENT OFFICE VISITS WHICH SHALL BE AVAILABLE FOR INSPECTION; SHALL ATTEND SIX HOURS OF AN ETHICS COURSE OR PROGRAM PER YEAR FOR TWO YEARS AND SHALL ATTEND AT LEAST 75 HOURS OF CONTINUING MEDICAL EDUCATION INCLUDING 25 IN PHARMACOLOGY/ADDICTIONOLOGY; SHALL GIVE A COPY OF THIS ORDER TO ANY HEALTH CARE ENTITY WHERE HE HAS PRIVILEGES; SHALL COOPERATE WITH THE BOARD IN VERIFYING COMPLIANCE; SHALL INFORM BOARD OF CHANGE OF ADDRESS WITHIN 10 DAYS OR IF HE LEAVES THE STATE; TIME SPENT OUT OF TEXAS DOES NOT COUNT TOWARD PROBATION. SHALL NOT SEEK MODIFICATION FOR TWO YEARS. ON 10/5/96 THE BOARD DENIED HIS PETITION FOR MODIFICATION. ON 5/16/98 ORDER MODIFIED REDUCING APPEARANCES BEFORE THE BOARD FROM BIANNUAL TO ANNUAL.

SIMPSON, DON E MD, LICENSE NUMBER 00H8405, WAS DISCIPLINED BY TEXAS ON NOVEMBER 16, 1996
DISCIPLINARY ACTION: FINE; REPRIMAND
OFFENSE: NONCOMPLIANCE WITH A PROFESSIONAL RULE

NOTES: FAILED TO OBTAIN 24 HOURS OF CONTINUING MEDICAL EDUCATION AS REQUIRED FOR THE 2/29/96 RENEWAL OF HIS LICENSE; WAS ISSUED AN EXTENSION TO 5/29/96 WHICH HE ALSO FAILED TO MEET; IS STILL REQUIRED TO FULFILL CONTINUING MEDICAL EDUCATION REQUIREMENT. SHALL PAY $100 FINE; SHALL COOPERATE WITH THE BOARD IN VERIFYING COMPLIANCE.

SINCLARE, ROSS G MD, DATE OF BIRTH DECEMBER 31, 1930 OF 1703 MISSION SPRINGS, KATY, TX, WAS DISCIPLINED BY MEDICARE ON JULY 10, 1990
DISCIPLINARY ACTION: 60-MONTH EXCLUSION FROM THE MEDICARE AND/OR MEDICAID PROGRAM
OFFENSE: CRIMINAL CONVICTION OR PLEA OF GUILTY, NOLO CONTENDERE, OR NO CONTEST TO A CRIME

NOTES: PROGRAM-RELATED CONVICTION.

SINGH, JASBIR BHATIA MD, LICENSE NUMBER F7700 OF ABILENE, TX, WAS DISCIPLINED BY TEXAS ON APRIL 4, 1998
DISCIPLINARY ACTION: FINE
OFFENSE: SEXUAL ABUSE OF OR SEXUAL MISCONDUCT WITH A PATIENT

NOTES: IN 1995 HE PERFORMED BREAST EXAMS ON A PATIENT WHO ASSERTED THAT HIS EXAMS WERE INAPPROPRIATE; THE PATIENT ALSO ASSERTED THAT HE SLAPPED HER ON THE BUTTOCKS; HE FAILED TO DOCUMENT THE INDICATIONS FOR THE OCCURRENCE OR THE FINDINGS OF THE BREAST EXAMS OF THE PATIENT; HE CONTENDS THAT HE IS TRAINED IN FAMILY PRACTICE AND COMMONLY PERFORMS PHYSICAL EXAMS ON PATIENTS IN HIS OFFICE, AND THAT HE NO LONGER PERFORMS PHYSICAL EXAMS. $3,000 FINE TO BE PAID WITHIN 90 DAYS.

SJOBERG, WALTER EUGENE JR MD, LICENSE NUMBER 00C5884 OF AUSTIN, TX, WAS DISCIPLINED BY TEXAS ON APRIL 15, 1994
DISCIPLINARY ACTION: 60-MONTH RESTRICTION PLACED ON LICENSE; MONITORING OF PHYSICIAN PERFORMANCE
OFFENSE: LOSS OR RESTRICTION OF HOSPITAL PRIVILEGES

NOTES: HOSPITAL PRIVILEGES WERE RESTRICTED AS FOLLOWS IN 1993 FOR 12 MONTHS DUE TO USE OF ANTICOAGULANTS WITH A PATIENT WHO EXPIRED DUE TO AN INTRACRANIAL HEMORRHAGE: MANDATORY CONSULTATIONS ARE REQUIRED FOR ONE YEAR ON ALL ADMISSIONS INVOLVING ANTICOAGULANTS AND THE NEXT 20 CASES FOR ALL OTHER ADMISSIONS; THE CARE PROVIDED WAS DETERMINED BY THE HOSPITAL TO BE A SIGNIFICANT DEVIATION FROM THE STANDARD OF CARE. CONDITIONS OF RESTRICTIONS: OBTAIN MANDATORY CONSULTATION ON ALL HOSPITAL ADMISSIONS INVOLVING ANTICOAGULANTS AND ON THE NEXT 20 CASES FOR ALL HOSPITAL ADMISSIONS; SHALL COOPERATE WITH THE BOARD IN VERIFYING COMPLIANCE; SHALL INFORM BOARD OF CHANGE OF ADDRESS WITHIN 10 DAYS OR IF HE LEAVES THE STATE; TIME SPENT OUT OF TEXAS DOES NOT COUNT TOWARD RESTRICTION; SHALL APPEAR BEFORE THE BOARD ONCE A YEAR; SHALL GIVE A COPY OF THIS ORDER TO ANY HEALTH CARE ENTITY WHERE HE HAS PRIVILEGES; SHALL NOT SEEK MODIFICATION FOR ONE YEAR. ON 5/11/95 BOARD GRANTED HIS PETITION FOR TERMINATION OF THIS ORDER; RESTRICTIONS PLACED ON HOSPITAL PRIVILEGES HAVE BEEN TERMINATED.

SKARBOVIG, PETER JENS JR DO, LICENSE NUMBER 00F7174 OF KINGWOOD, TX, WAS DISCIPLINED BY TEXAS ON SEPTEMBER 28, 1990
DISCIPLINARY ACTION: SURRENDER OF LICENSE

NOTES: INABILITY TO PRACTICE MEDICINE WITH REASONABLE SKILL AND SAFETY TO PATIENTS BY REASON OF ILLNESS, DRUNKENNESS, EXCESSIVE USE OF DRUGS, NARCOTICS, CHEMICALS, OR ANY OTHER TYPE OF MATERIAL, OR AS RESULT OF ANY MENTAL OR PHYSICAL CONDITION. SURRENDER IN LIEU OF FUTURE DISCIPLINARY HEARING.

SLAHETKA, MARY FRANCES ANN MD, LICENSE NUMBER J1139 OF COVINGTON, LA, WAS DISCIPLINED BY TEXAS ON OCTOBER 14, 1999
DISCIPLINARY ACTION: LICENSE REVOCATION
OFFENSE: NONCOMPLIANCE WITH A PROFESSIONAL RULE

NOTES: FOR THE 1996 ANNUAL REGISTRATION PERIOD, SHE DID NOT PROVIDE SUFFICIENT EVIDENCE OF REQUIRED CONTINUING MEDICAL EDUCATION AND DID NOT COMPLETE THE REQUIRED HOURS. ACTION WILL NOT BE FINAL UNTIL ALL APPEALS ARE EXHAUSTED.

SLUSHER, KEVIN D MD, LICENSE NUMBER J7200 OF TYLER, TX, WAS DISCIPLINED BY TEXAS ON SEPTEMBER 28, 1999
DISCIPLINARY ACTION: EMERGENCY SUSPENSION

NOTES: EVIDENCE THAT HIS CONTINUED PRACTICE CONSTITUTES A CONTINUING THREAT TO PUBLIC WELFARE.

SLUSHER, KEVIN D MD, LICENSE NUMBER J7200 OF TYLER, TX, WAS DISCIPLINED BY TEXAS ON DECEMBER 11, 1999
DISCIPLINARY ACTION: LICENSE SUSPENSION
OFFENSE: SUBSTANCE ABUSE

NOTES: BOARD ENTERED A NONDISCIPLINARY, NON PUBLIC REHABILITATION ORDER ON 8/22/98 BASED ON HIS SELF-REPORTING POLYSUBSTANCE ABUSE AND THE SUSPENSION OF HIS HOSPITAL PRIVILEGES; VIOLATED THIS ORDER BY TESTING POSITIVE FOR NUBAIN ON 2/11/99; ON OR ABOUT 5/2/99 HE ADMITTED HIS VIOLATION AND STATED THAT FROM APPROXIMATELY 12/25/98-2/15/99 HE ABUSED CHEMICAL SUBSTANCES AND SELF PRESCRIBED NUBAIN AND BUPRENEX PRIOR TO THE SURRENDER OF HIS DEA REGISTRATION; VOLUNTARILY ADMITTED HIMSELF INTO A HALFWAY HOUSE AND WAS UNDER THE DIRECT CARE AND SUPERVISION OF A PHYSICIAN; IN 9/99 A BOARD INVESTIGATION OBTAINED SEVERAL HYDROCODONE PRESCRIPTIONS WRITTEN BY HIMSELF PRESCRIBING TO HIMSELF, AS WELL AS FICTITIOUS PERSONS; ON 9/17/99 HE ADMITTED TO THE RELAPSE, DETAILING AN ACCOUNT OF ALLEGEDLY FINDING A FENTANYL PATCH AND USING ITS CONTENTS TO GET HIGH, AND ALSO STEALING PRESCRIPTION PADS FROM HIS TREATING PHYSICIAN AND FORGING NUMEROUS PRESCRIPTIONS FOR LORTAB, OBTAINING DRUGS AND SELF-ADMINISTERING THE DRUGS. SUSPENSION UNTIL HE REQUESTS TO HAVE HIS SUSPENSION STAYED OR APPEARS BEFORE THE BOARD WITH SUFFICIENT EVIDENCE THAT HE IS PHYSICALLY, MENTALLY AND OTHERWISE COMPETENT TO SAFELY PRACTICE MEDICINE INCLUDING AT A MINIMUM COMPLETE COPIES OF MEDICAL RECORDS AND REPORTS OF PSYCHOLOGICAL AND NEUROPSYCHIATRIC EVALUATIONS.

SMALL, STUART D MD, LICENSE NUMBER E6921 OF PLANO, TX, WAS DISCIPLINED BY TEXAS ON APRIL 4, 1998
DISCIPLINARY ACTION: FINE; REPRIMAND
OFFENSE: NONCOMPLIANCE WITH A PROFESSIONAL RULE

NOTES: ADMINISTERED ANESTHESIA TO A SINGLE PATIENT DURING 1996 AT AN OUTPATIENT SURGERY FACILITY WITHOUT ADEQUATELY DOCUMENTING A PRE-ANESTHESIA EVALUATION PRIOR TO SURGERY. $1,000 FINE; SHALL COOPERATE WITH THE BOARD IN VERIFYING COMPLIANCE.

SMALL, STUART DAVID MD, LICENSE NUMBER G27024 OF PLANO, TX, WAS DISCIPLINED BY CALIFORNIA ON SEPTEMBER 10, 1998
DISCIPLINARY ACTION: REPRIMAND
OFFENSE: DISCIPLINARY ACTION BY ANOTHER STATE OR AGENCY

NOTES: DISCIPLINED BY TEXAS FOR FAILING TO ADEQUATELY DOCUMENT A PRE-SURGERY PRE-ANESTHESIA EVALUATION PRIOR TO ADMINISTERING ANESTHESIA.

SMILEY, EVELYN J K MD, LICENSE NUMBER 00C6518 OF LAMESA, TX, WAS DISCIPLINED BY TEXAS ON AUGUST 20, 1992
DISCIPLINARY ACTION: 60-MONTH PROBATION

NOTES: FAILURE TO PRACTICE MEDICINE IN AN ACCEPTABLE MANNER CONSISTENT WITH PUBLIC HEALTH AND WELFARE. LICENSE SUSPENDED, SUSPENSION STAYED. PROBATION UNDER TERMS AND CONDITIONS

SMILEY, EVELYN J K MD, LICENSE NUMBER 0C20354 OF LAMESA, TX, WAS DISCIPLINED BY CALIFORNIA ON JUNE 30, 1994
DISCIPLINARY ACTION: 60-MONTH PROBATION
OFFENSE: DISCIPLINARY ACTION BY ANOTHER STATE OR AGENCY

NOTES: DISCIPLINED BY THE TEXAS BOARD FOR FAILING TO PRACTICE MEDICINE IN AN ACCEPTABLE MANNER CONSISTENT WITH PUBLIC HEALTH AND WELFARE IN THE CARE AND TREATMENT OF THREE PATIENTS. ONE YEAR SUSPENSION STAYED.

SMITH, ART GLENN MD, DATE OF BIRTH NOVEMBER 28, 1958, LICENSE NUMBER 00H3344 OF SAN ANTONIO, TX, WAS DISCIPLINED BY TEXAS ON NOVEMBER 9, 1993
DISCIPLINARY ACTION: EMERGENCY SUSPENSION
OFFENSE: SEXUAL ABUSE OF OR SEXUAL MISCONDUCT WITH A PATIENT

NOTES: IN 8/93 ENGAGED IN ALLEGED INAPPROPRIATE AND UNPROFESSIONAL CONTACT WITH ONE PATIENT WHICH LED HER TO BELIEVE HE WAS ATTEMPTING TO INITIATE A SEXUAL RELATIONSHIP WITH HER; FROM 4/93 AND CONTINUING TO DATE OF ORDER HE HAS ENGAGED IN BEHAVIORS WHICH MAY BE INDICATIVE OF PSYCHIATRIC IMPAIRMENT SUCH AS STATEMENTS INDICATING PARANOID IDEATION, INAPPROPRIATE BEHAVIORS INCLUDING YELLING AND BEING ABUSIVE WITH STAFF AND PATIENTS OVER MINOR INCIDENTS AND CARRYING ON A CONVERSATION WITH A TELEPHONE WHICH WAS NOT CONNECTED TO ANY OTHER PARTY.

SMITH, ART GLENN MD, DATE OF BIRTH NOVEMBER 28, 1958, LICENSE NUMBER 00H3344 OF 1901 N LAMESA, BIG SPRING, TX, WAS DISCIPLINED BY TEXAS ON OCTOBER 13, 1995
DISCIPLINARY ACTION: 60-MONTH PROBATION; RESTRICTION PLACED ON LICENSE

NOTES: ON 3/03/95 UNDERWENT A BOARD RECOMMENDED EVALUATION BY A LICENSED PSYCHOLOGIST INDICATING HE WAS CAPABLE OF PRACTICING MEDICINE WITH REASONABLE SKILL AND SAFETY. SUSPENSION STAYED. PROBATION WITH TERMS: SHALL ABSTAIN FROM THE CONSUMPTION OF ALCOHOL/DRUGS IN ANY FORM UNLESS PRESCRIBED BY ANOTHER PHYSICIAN FOR A LEGITIMATE AND THERAPEUTIC PURPOSE; SHALL SUBMIT HIMSELF FOR APPROPRIATE EXAMS INCLUDING DRUG OR ALCOHOL SCREENS; SHALL CONTINUE TO RECEIVE CARE AND TREATMENT FROM PSYCHIATRIST/NEUROLOGIST AT LEAST ONCE A MONTH WITH QUARTERLY REPORTS TO THE BOARD; SHALL PRACTICE MEDICINE ONLY IN AN INSTITUTION OR GROUP PRACTICE SETTING APPROVED BY THE BOARD; HIS PRACTICE SHALL BE MONITORED BY A BOARD-APPROVED PHYSICIAN WHO SHALL SUBMIT QUARTERLY REPORTS TO THE BOARD; SHALL MAINTAIN ADEQUATE MEDICAL RECORDS WHICH SHALL BE AVAILABLE FOR REVIEW; SHALL OBTAIN AT LEAST 50 HOURS PER YEAR OF CONTINUING MEDICAL EDUCATION; SHALL APPEAR BEFORE THE BOARD AT LEAST TWICE A YEAR OR AT BOARD REQUEST; SHALL COOPERATE WITH THE BOARD IN VERIFYING COMPLIANCE INCLUDING PROVIDING MEDICAL REPORTS OR PEER REVIEW RECORDS UPON REQUEST; SHALL GIVE A COPY OF THIS ORDER TO ANY HEALTH CARE ENTITY WHERE HE HAS PRIVILEGES; SHALL PROVIDE A COPY OF THIS ORDER TO ANYONE REQUESTING IT WITHIN 10 DAYS; TIME SPENT OUT OF TEXAS DOES NOT COUNT TOWARD PROBATION; SHALL INFORM BOARD OF CHANGE OF ADDRESS WITHIN 10 DAYS OR IF HE LEAVES THE STATE. SHALL NOT SEEK MODIFICATION FOR ONE YEAR. ON 1/18/97 PETITION TO MODIFY ORDER GRANTED REDUCING CARE AND TREATMENT

FROM TREATING PHYSICIAN FROM ONCE PER MONTH TO ONCE EVERY SIX WEEKS. ON 11/22/97 PETITION TO TERMINATE ORDER DENIED; ORDER MODIFIED DELETING REQUIREMENTS FOR ABSTINENCE FROM ALCOHOL, DRUGS AND CONTROLLED SUBSTANCES, AND SUBMISSION TO AND PAYMENT FOR RANDOM DRUG SCREENS. ON 10/24/98 PETITION TO TERMINATE ORDER DENIED; ORDER MODIFIED TO REQUIRE QUARTERLY PSYCHIATRIC TREATMENT, AND DELETION OF MONITORING REQUIREMENT. ON 5/14/99 ORDER TERMINATED.

SMITH, DONALD W MD, LICENSE NUMBER 00D6870 OF SPRING, TX, WAS DISCIPLINED BY TEXAS ON OCTOBER 13, 1995
DISCIPLINARY ACTION: LICENSE SUSPENSION; MONITORING OF PHYSICIAN PERFORMANCE
OFFENSE: PHYSICAL OR MENTAL ILLNESS INHIBITING THE ABILITY TO PRACTICE WITH SKILL AND SAFETY
NOTES: INABILITY TO PRACTICE MEDICINE WITH REASONABLE SKILL AND SAFETY TO PATIENTS IN THAT IN 1994 HE BEGAN EXHIBITING MANIC BEHAVIOR AND IN 1/95 HIS PHYSICIAN ADVISED HIM THAT HE WAS ILL AND SHOULD NOT BE TREATING PATIENTS; INTEMPERATE USE OF ALCOHOL IN THAT DURING THIS PERIOD HE BEGAN DRINKING AGAIN; ON 5/18/95, TAKEN INTO PROTECTIVE CUSTODY UNDER A MENTAL HEALTH WARRANT AND TRANSPORTED TO A PSYCHIATRIC HOSPITAL FOR ADMISSION AND EVALUATION; ON 5/30/95 HE WAS DIAGNOSED AS MANIC DEPRESSIVE BY PHYSICIAN WHO PRESCRIBED LITHIUM; HE REPORTED THAT HE WAS TAKING WEEKLY LITHIUM LEVELS HIMSELF AND ALSO MONITORING HIS DIABETES FOR WHICH HE IS INSULIN DEPENDENT; ADMITS INGESTION OF ALCOHOL AS LATE AS 9/95; HE IS UNDER THE CARE OF A PSYCHIATRIST FOR MANIC DEPRESSION AND AN INTERNIST FOR DIABETES; REPORTS ATTENDING AA MEETINGS AN AVERAGE OF TWO TIMES A WEEK; PROFESSIONAL FAILURE TO PRACTICE MEDICINE IN AN ACCEPTABLE MANNER CONSISTENT WITH PUBLIC HEALTH AND WELFARE AND PRESCRIBING OR ADMINISTERING A DRUG OR TREATMENT THAT IS NONTHERAPEUTIC IN THE MANNER THE DRUG OR TREATMENT IS GIVEN IN THAT DUE TO HIS ILLNESS HE MADE ERRORS IN HIS TREATMENT REGIMEN AND HAD INAPPROPRIATELY AND/OR EXCESSIVELY ADMINISTERED MEDICATIONS TO ALL AGE GROUP PATIENTS FOR DIAGNOSES OF SINUSITIS, ALLERGIC RHINITIS AND UPPER RESPIRATORY INFECTIONS; INAPPROPRIATELY PRESCRIBED CONTROLLED SUBSTANCES TO FOUR PATIENTS. SUSPENSION UNTIL HE REQUESTS TO HAVE SUSPENSION STAYED OR LIFTED AND APPEARS BEFORE BOARD WITH EVIDENCE THAT INDICATES THAT HE IS PHYSICALLY, MENTALLY AND OTHERWISE COMPETENT TO SAFELY PRACTICE MEDICINE; EVIDENCE SHALL INCLUDE BUT NOT BE LIMITED TO COPIES OF MEDICAL RECORDS AND REPORTS OF PSYCHOLOGICAL AND NEUROPSYCHIATRIC EVALUATIONS, INCLUDING A 96-HOUR INPATIENT EVALUATION CONDUCTED BY A BOARD-APPROVED PSYCHIATRIST. ON 10/24/98 ORDER MODIFIED REDUCING APPEARANCES BEFORE THE BOARD FROM BIANNUAL TO ANNUAL.

SMITH, DONALD W MD, LICENSE NUMBER 00D6870, WAS DISCIPLINED BY TEXAS ON MAY 14, 1996
DISCIPLINARY ACTION: 120-MONTH PROBATION; RESTRICTION PLACED ON CONTROLLED SUBSTANCE LICENSE
NOTES: HAS SATISFIED THE MINIMUM REQUIREMENTS SET OUT IN 10/95 ORDER FOR REINSTATEMENT. SUSPENSION STAYED TO PROBATION WITH TERMS AND CONDITIONS: WITHIN 45 DAYS SHALL TAKE AND PASS THE SPECIAL PURPOSE EXAMINATION; SHALL ABSTAIN FROM THE CONSUMPTION OF ALCOHOL/DRUGS IN ANY FORM UNLESS PRESCRIBED BY ANOTHER PHYSICIAN FOR A LEGITIMATE AND THERAPEUTIC PURPOSE; SHALL SUBMIT HIMSELF FOR APPROPRIATE EXAMS INCLUDING DRUG OR ALCOHOL SCREENS; SHALL SUBMIT HIMSELF FOR EVALUATION AND TREATMENT BY A BOARD-APPROVED PSYCHIATRIST WHOM HE SHALL SEE AT LEAST ONCE A MONTH AND WHO SHALL SUBMIT REPORTS TO THE BOARD; SHALL PARTICIPATE IN AA'S PROGRAM NOT LESS THAN THREE TIMES A WEEK WITH QUARTERLY REPORTS TO THE BOARD; SHALL PARTICIPATE IN THE ACTIVITIES OF A PHYSICIAN'S COUNSELING COMMITTEE AND ATTEND WEEKLY MEETINGS WITH QUARTERLY REPORTS; SHALL NOT POSSESS ALCOHOL, CONTROLLED SUBSTANCES OR DANGEROUS DRUGS WITH ADDICTIVE POTENTIAL OR POTENTIAL FOR ABUSE AND SHALL SURRENDER ALL SUCH DRUGS INCLUDING SAMPLES; SHALL NOT TREAT OR OTHERWISE SERVE AS PHYSICIAN, PRESCRIBE, DISPENSE OR ADMINISTER DRUGS THAT MAY BE SUBJECT TO ABUSE TO HIMSELF OR TO ANY MEMBER OF HIS FAMILY; SHALL SEEK MODIFICATION OF HIS DEA/DPS CONTROLLED SUBSTANCES REGISTRATION CERTIFICATES TO ELIMINATE HIS AUTHORITY TO PRESCRIBE SCHEDULE II, IIN, III AND IIIN CONTROLLED SUBSTANCES AND SHALL NOT ATTEMPT TO REREGISTER WITHOUT BOARD AUTHORITY; SHALL MAINTAIN A FILE WITH COPIES OF EVERY PRESCRIPTION WRITTEN BY HIM FOR CONTROLLED SUBSTANCES OR DANGEROUS DRUGS WITH ADDICTIVE POTENTIAL OR POTENTIAL FOR ABUSE WHICH SHALL BE AVAILABLE FOR REVIEW; SHALL NOT PRESCRIBE OR ADMINISTER ANY DRUG FOR ANY PATIENT UNLESS IT IS MEDICALLY INDICATED AND PRESCRIBED IN THERAPEUTIC DOSES AND THERE IS A LEGITIMATE THERAPEUTIC NEED; HIS PRACTICE INCLUDING ANY OFFICE AND SURGICAL PRACTICE SHALL BE MONITORED BY A BOARD-APPROVED TEXAS PHYSICIAN WHO SHALL SUBMIT QUARTERLY REPORTS; SHALL MAINTAIN ADEQUATE MEDICAL RECORDS WHICH SHALL BE AVAILABLE FOR REVIEW; SHALL OBTAIN AT LEAST 50 HOURS PER YEAR OF CONTINUING MEDICAL EDUCATION; SHALL APPEAR BEFORE BOARD AT LEAST TWICE A YEAR; SHALL COOPERATE WITH THE BOARD IN VERIFYING COMPLIANCE INCLUDING PROVIDING ANY MEDICAL RELEASES UPON REQUEST; SHALL GIVE A COPY OF THIS ORDER TO ANY HEALTH CARE ENTITY WHERE HE HAS PRIVILEGES; TIME SPENT OUT OF TEXAS DOES NOT COUNT TOWARD PROBATION; SHALL INFORM BOARD OF CHANGE OF ADDRESS WITHIN 10 DAYS OR IF HE LEAVES THE STATE. SHALL NOT SEEK MODIFICATION FOR ONE YEAR.

SMITH, DONALD W MD, LICENSE NUMBER 0104078 OF 17907 KUYKENDAHL ROAD, SPRING, TX, WAS DISCIPLINED BY NEW YORK ON OCTOBER 15, 1996
DISCIPLINARY ACTION: LICENSE REVOCATION
OFFENSE: DISCIPLINARY ACTION BY ANOTHER STATE OR AGENCY
NOTES: DISCIPLINED BY THE TEXAS BOARD FOR HAVING A PSYCHIATRIC CONDITION WHICH IMPAIRS THE ABILITY TO PRACTICE MEDICINE; IMPROPERLY PRESCRIBING ANTIBIOTICS, CONTROLLED SUBSTANCES AND OTHER MEDICATIONS AND PRACTICING WHILE IMPAIRED BY ALCOHOL, DRUGS, PHYSICAL DISABILITY OR MENTAL DISABILITY.

SMITH, DONALD WILLARD MD OF 17907 KUYKENDAHL, SPRING, TX, WAS DISCIPLINED BY DEA ON DECEMBER 27, 1995

DISCIPLINARY ACTION: RESTRICTION PLACED ON CONTROLLED SUBSTANCE LICENSE
OFFENSE: DISCIPLINARY ACTION BY ANOTHER STATE OR AGENCY

NOTES: STATE BOARD.

SMITH, GEORGE ROBERT MD, LICENSE NUMBER 00H8411 OF DALLAS, TX, WAS DISCIPLINED BY TEXAS ON MARCH 4, 1995
DISCIPLINARY ACTION: 60-MONTH PROBATION; RESTRICTION PLACED ON CONTROLLED SUBSTANCE LICENSE
OFFENSE: SUBSTANCE ABUSE

NOTES: BEGINNING IN 1993, SELF-ADMINISTERED THE CONTROLLED SUBSTANCES HYDROCODONE AND CODEINE; IN 4/94, CLINICAL PRIVILEGES AT A HOSPITAL WERE SUMMARILY SUSPENDED DUE TO POSSIBLE SUBSTANCE ABUSE AS EVIDENCED BY BEHAVIORAL CHANGES AND FAILURE TO PROMPTLY RESPOND TO TELEPHONE CALLS AND HIS BEEPER; REPORTS SOBRIETY DATE OF 3/27/94; REPORTS THAT HE ATTENDS AA AN AVERAGE OF FIVE TIMES PER WEEK; UNDER THE CARE OF A PSYCHIATRIST FOR PSYCHIATRIC AND ADDICTION CARE; ENTERED INTO A RECOVERY CONTRACT WITH A COUNTY HOSPITAL; ENTERED INTO AN AFTERCARE RECOVERY CONTRACT WITH HIS PSYCHIATRIST; REPORTS REGULAR PARTICIPATION IN THE ACTIVITIES OF THE COMMITTEE ON PHYSICIAN HEALTH AND REHABILITATION. SUSPENSION STAYED. PROBATION WITH TERMS: SHALL ABSTAIN FROM THE CONSUMPTION OF ALCOHOL/DRUGS IN ANY FORM UNLESS PRESCRIBED BY ANOTHER PHYSICIAN FOR A LEGITIMATE AND THERAPEUTIC PURPOSE; SHALL SUBMIT HIMSELF FOR APPROPRIATE EXAMS INCLUDING DRUG OR ALCOHOL SCREENS; SHALL CONTINUE TO RECEIVE CARE AND TREATMENT FROM PSYCHIATRIST AT LEAST ONCE A MONTH WHO SHALL SUBMIT QUARTERLY REPORTS; SHALL CONTINUE TO PARTICIPATE IN AA'S PROGRAM NOT LESS THAN THREE TIMES A WEEK WITH QUARTERLY REPORTS TO THE BOARD; SHALL CONTINUE TO PARTICIPATE IN ACTIVITIES OF COMMITTEE ON PHYSICIAN HEALTH AND REHABILITATION AND ATTEND WEEKLY MEETINGS WITH QUARTERLY REPORTS; SHALL COMPLY WITH TERMS OF CONTINUING CARE CONTRACT WITH HIS PSYCHIATRIST; SHALL COMPLY WITH TERMS OF CONTRACT FOR HOSPITAL PRIVILEGES AND REPORT TO BOARD ANY DISCIPLINARY ACTION; SHALL NOT POSSESS ALCOHOL, CONTROLLED SUBSTANCES OR DRUGS WITH ADDICTIVE POTENTIAL; SHALL SURRENDER ANY CONTROLLED SUBSTANCE SAMPLES STILL IN HIS POSSESSION; SHALL NOT TREAT OR OTHERWISE SERVE AS A PHYSICIAN, PRESCRIBE, DISPENSE DRUGS THAT MAY BE SUBJECT TO ABUSE TO HIMSELF OR ANY MEMBER OF HIS FAMILY; SHALL NOT POSSESS, DISPENSE, ADMINISTER, PRESCRIBE OR OTHERWISE PROVIDE SCHEDULE II CONTROLLED SUBSTANCES TO ANY PATIENT, EXCEPT TO ORDER FOR HOSPITAL INPATIENTS ON A VENTILATOR AND FOR HOSPITAL INPATIENTS OR EMERGENCY ROOM PATIENTS WITH CONGESTIVE HEART FAILURE; SHALL MAINTAIN A LOG OF THESE PRESCRIPTIONS SUBJECT TO REVIEW; SHALL SURRENDER ALL UNUSED TRIPLICATE PRESCRIPTION FORMS AND SHALL NOT ATTEMPT TO ORDER MORE; SHALL MAINTAIN ADEQUATE MEDICAL RECORDS WHICH SHALL BE SUBJECT TO REVIEW; SHALL OBTAIN AT LEAST 50 HOURS PER YEAR OF CONTINUING MEDICAL EDUCATION; SHALL APPEAR BEFORE THE BOARD AT LEAST TWICE A YEAR OR AT BOARD REQUEST; SHALL COOPERATE WITH THE BOARD IN VERIFYING COMPLIANCE INCLUDING PROVIDING COPIES OF MEDICAL RELEASES AND PEER REVIEW RECORDS UPON REQUEST; SHALL GIVE A COPY OF ORDER TO ANY HEALTH CARE ENTITY WHERE HE HAS PRIVILEGES; SHALL PROVIDE A COPY TO ANYONE REQUESTING IT WITHIN 10 DAYS; TIME PERIOD OUT OF TEXAS DOES NOT COUNT TOWARD PROBATION; SHALL INFORM BOARD OF CHANGE OF ADDRESS WITHIN 10 DAYS OR IF HE LEAVES THE STATE. SHALL NOT SEEK MODIFICATION FOR ONE YEAR. ON 9/20/97 PETITION TO TERMINATE ORDER DENIED; ORDER MODIFIED DELETING REQUIREMENTS OF COMPLIANCE WITH CONTRACTS ENTERED INTO FOR HOSPITAL PRIVILEGES, RESTRICTION OF HIS SERVING AS A PHYSICIAN FOR HIMSELF OR HIS FAMILY, RESTRICTION FROM PRESCRIBING SCHEDULE II CONTROLLED SUBSTANCES, REQUIREMENT TO SURRENDER TRIPLICATE PRESCRIPTION FORMS, MAINTAINING A FILE COPY OF ALL PRESCRIPTIONS, AND MAINTENANCE OF MEDICAL RECORDS. ON 10/24/98 ORDER TERMINATED.

SMITH, JERRY W DO, LICENSE NUMBER 00C8065, WAS DISCIPLINED BY TEXAS ON NOVEMBER 16, 1996

NOTES: ALLEGATIONS OF VIOLATIONS OF THE MEDICAL PRACTICE ACT BUT NO DETERMINATION OF THESE VIOLATIONS HAS BEEN MADE; HE HAS BEEN RETIRED FROM THE ACTIVE PRACTICE OF MEDICINE, DUE TO HEALTH REASONS, SINCE 1/1/96. HAS NOT RENEWED HIS DEA OR DPA REGISTRATIONS. DOES NOT ADMIT VIOLATION. DUE TO HIS PHYSICAL DISABILITY AND RETIREMENT, SHALL NOT PRACTICE MEDICINE IN TEXAS UNTIL HE REQUESTS PERMISSION TO RESUME PRACTICE AND APPEARS BEFORE BOARD WITH SUFFICIENT EVIDENCE WHICH INDICATES THAT HE IS PHYSICALLY, MENTALLY AND OTHERWISE COMPETENT TO SAFELY PRACTICE MEDICINE, INCLUDING AT A MINIMUM PROOF OF A PASSING SCORE OF 75 OR HIGHER ON THE SPECIAL PURPOSE EXAMINATION.

SMITH, MONTE KEITH DO, LICENSE NUMBER 00H8413, WAS DISCIPLINED BY TEXAS ON AUGUST 17, 1996
DISCIPLINARY ACTION: 60-MONTH PROBATION; RESTRICTION PLACED ON LICENSE
OFFENSE: SUBSTANCE ABUSE

NOTES: IN 1993 BEGAN ABUSING PRESCRIPTION DRUGS, INCLUDING VICODIN, LORCET, AND HYDROCODONE, AS A RESULT OF THE STRESS AND BACK PAIN RELATED TO ESTABLISHING HIS PRACTICE AS AN INTERNIST; WROTE PRESCRIPTIONS TO HIS IMMEDIATE FAMILY TO DIVERT DRUGS TO HIMSELF; REPORTS A SOBRIETY DATE OF 8/22/95; ENTERED INPATIENT TREATMENT FOR HIS SUBSTANCE ABUSE IN AUGUST 1995 UNTIL SEPTEMBER 1995; ATTENDS AA ON AVERAGE FOUR TO FIVE TIMES PER WEEK; REPORTS REGULAR ATTENDANCE IN PHYSICIAN HEALTH AND REHABILITATION COMMITTEE AND HAS ENTERED INTO A CONTINUING CARE CONTRACT. SUSPENSION STAYED. PROBATION UNDER TERMS AND CONDITIONS: SHALL ABSTAIN FROM THE CONSUMPTION OF ALCOHOL/DRUGS IN ANY FORM UNLESS PRESCRIBED BY ANOTHER PHYSICIAN FOR A LEGITIMATE AND THERAPEUTIC PURPOSE; SHALL SUBMIT TO APPROPRIATE EXAMS, INCLUDING DRUG OR ALCOHOL SCREENS; SHALL CONTINUE TO RECEIVE CARE AND TREATMENT FROM HIS COUNSELORS NO LESS THAN ONCE A MONTH WHO SHALL PROVIDE QUARTERLY REPORTS TO THE BOARD; SHALL PARTICIPATE IN AA'S PROGRAM AT LEAST FOUR TIMES PER WEEK WITH QUARTERLY REPORTS TO THE BOARD; SHALL CONTINUE TO PARTICIPATE IN THE ACTIVITIES OF A PHYSICIAN

HEALTH AND REHABILITATION COMMITTEE, AND ATTEND WEEKLY MEETINGS WITH QUARTERLY REPORTS; SHALL COMPLY WITH THE TERMS OF HIS CONTINUING CARE CONTRACT AND AUTHORIZE THE CHAIRMAN TO REPORT QUARTERLY TO THE BOARD; SHALL NOT TREAT OR OTHERWISE SERVE AS PHYSICIAN, PRESCRIBE, DISPENSE OR ADMINISTER DRUGS THAT MAY BE SUBJECT TO ABUSE TO HIMSELF OR TO ANY MEMBER OF HIS FAMILY; SHALL CONTINUE TO PRACTICE MEDICINE AT HIS PRESENT PRACTICE LOCATION WITHIN THE PRISON SYSTEM AND OBTAIN BOARD APPROVAL BEFORE HE CHANGES; SHALL OBTAIN AT LEAST 50 HOURS PER YEAR OF CONTINUING MEDICAL EDUCATION AND PROVIDE PROOF TO THE BOARD; SHALL APPEAR BEFORE THE BOARD AT LEAST TWICE PER YEAR OR UPON BOARD REQUEST; SHALL COOPERATE WITH THE BOARD IN VERIFYING COMPLIANCE; SHALL GIVE A COPY OF THIS ORDER TO ANY HEALTH CARE ENTITY WHERE HE HAS PRIVILEGES; TIME PERIOD OUT OF TEXAS DOES NOT COUNT TOWARD PROBATION; SHALL INFORM THE BOARD OF CHANGE OF ADDRESS WITHIN 10 DAYS OF IF HE LEAVES THE STATE; SHALL NOT SEEK MODIFICATION FOR ONE YEAR. ON 8/22/98 ORDER MODIFIED MONTHLY PSYCHIATRIC TREATMENT TO ALLOW TREATMENT SCHEDULES TO BE ORDERED BY THE THERAPISTS, AND REDUCED APPEARANCES BEFORE THE BOARD FROM BIANNUAL TO ANNUAL. ON 10/15/99 ORDER TERMINATED.

SNYDER, JOHN T MD OF 1113 REDBUD, CHANNELVIEW, TX, WAS DISCIPLINED BY DEA ON JANUARY 29, 1990
DISCIPLINARY ACTION: SURRENDER OF CONTROLLED SUBSTANCE LICENSE
OFFENSE: PROFESSIONAL MISCONDUCT
NOTES: DISPENSED PHENTERMINE FOR ILLEGITIMATE MEDICAL PURPOSE.

SONIK, SIMON MD, DATE OF BIRTH JANUARY 22, 1931, LICENSE NUMBER 00F0318 OF 9660 HILLCROFT SUITE 550, HOUSTON, TX, WAS DISCIPLINED BY TEXAS ON JANUARY 29, 1993
DISCIPLINARY ACTION: REPRIMAND
OFFENSE: NONCOMPLIANCE WITH A PROFESSIONAL RULE
NOTES: FAILED TO KEEP ADEQUATE RECORDS OF THE MEDICAL CARE GIVEN TO A PATIENT. SHALL GIVE A COPY OF ORDER TO ANY HEALTH CARE ENTITY WHERE HE HAS PRIVILEGES; SHALL INFORM THE BOARD OF CHANGE OF ADDRESS WITHIN 10 DAYS.

SORIANO, SALVADOR L MD, LICENSE NUMBER 00D3405 OF DUNCANVILLE, TX, WAS DISCIPLINED BY TEXAS ON OCTOBER 5, 1991
DISCIPLINARY ACTION: 60-MONTH PROBATION; MONITORING OF PHYSICIAN PERFORMANCE
OFFENSE: SUBSTANCE ABUSE
NOTES: MADE HOSPITAL ROUNDS ON OR ABOUT 10/21/90 WHILE UNDER THE INFLUENCE OF A COMBINATION OF ALCOHOL AND AN ANTIDEPRESSANT, WHICH CAUSED HIS SPEECH TO BE SLURRED, EYES RED, AND UNABLE TO ACCURATELY COMMUNICATE INFORMATION ABOUT HIS PATIENT; HAD BEEN DEPRESSED SINCE 9/90; FAILED TO COMPLETE ADMISSION NOTES ON A PATIENT WITHIN 24 HOURS OF ADMISSION, LATER FALSIFIED RECORDS. DENIES THESE ALLEGATIONS BUT AGREED TO DISPOSE OF MATTER BY AGREED SETTLEMENT. SUSPENSION STAYED, PROBATION INCLUDES FOLLOWING CONDITIONS: SHALL SUBMIT HIMSELF FOR APPROPRIATE EXAMINATIONS, INCLUDING SCREENING FOR ALCOHOL OR DRUGS, THROUGH TESTS OF BODILY FLUIDS; SHALL SUBMIT IN WRITING TO BOARD THE NAMES OF THREE PSYCHIATRISTS FOR BOARD APPROVAL, AND SHALL EXPEDITIOUSLY SUBMIT HIMSELF FOR EVALUATION AND TREATMENT, FOLLOWING THE PSYCHIATRIST'S RECOMMENDATIONS, IF ANY, REGARDING CONTINUING CARE AND TREATMENT; SHALL APPEAR BEFORE THE BOARD TWICE A YEAR; MUST COOPERATE WITH THE BOARD IN VERIFYING COMPLIANCE; MUST ADVISE THE BOARD OF ANY CHANGE OF ADDRESS WITHIN 10 DAYS; TIME SPENT OUT OF TEXAS DOES NOT COUNT TOWARDS PROBATION.

SORRELS, WILLIAM F DO, LICENSE NUMBER 0001969, WAS DISCIPLINED BY SOUTH DAKOTA ON MARCH 2, 1994
DISCIPLINARY ACTION: 24-MONTH PROBATION; REQUIRED TO ENTER AN IMPAIRED PHYSICIAN PROGRAM OR SUBSTANCE ABUSE TREATMENT
OFFENSE: PROFESSIONAL MISCONDUCT
NOTES: UNPROFESSIONAL CONDUCT. TWO YEAR SUSPENSION, STAYED AS PROBATION UNDER TERMS AND CONDITIONS: SHALL PERMIT THE BOARD TO HAVE FREE ACCESS TO ALL RECORDS RELATING TO MEDICAL SERVICES PROVIDED BY HIM TO PATIENTS; SHALL COMPLY WITH BOARD REQUESTS; SHALL MAKE APPEARANCES BEFORE THE BOARD ANNUALLY AND/OR UPON REQUEST; SHALL NOT USE ALCOHOL OR ANY CONTROLLED SUBSTANCES UNLESS PRESCRIBED BY A LICENSED PHYSICIAN; SHALL PROVE TO THE BOARD THAT HE HAS NOT EXHIBITED HABITS OF ALCOHOL USE OR DRUG USE OR ALCOHOL OR DRUG ADDICTION; SHALL RECEIVE ALCOHOL AND CHEMICAL DEPENDENCY EVALUATION AND TREATMENT BY THE WORTHMORE TREATMENT CENTER OF ABERDEEN, SOUTH DAKOTA; SHALL PROVIDE THE BOARD WITH VERIFICATION OF TWO TIMES PER WEEK ATTENDANCE OF AA AND/OR NARCOTICS ANONYMOUS MEETINGS ON AT LEAST A MONTHLY BASIS; SHALL OBTAIN AFTERCARE COUNSELING ONE TIME PER WEEK FOR 12 WEEKS AND SHALL REQUIRE HIS AFTERCARE COUNSELOR TO PROVIDE THE BOARD WITH A REPORT REGARDING HIS SUCCESSFUL COMPLETION; SHALL SUBMIT TO RANDOM, WITNESSED BLOOD AND/OR URINALYSIS TESTS UPON BOARD REQUEST; PERIODS OF RESIDENCE OR PRACTICE OUTSIDE OF SOUTH DAKOTA SHALL NOT APPLY TO THE DURATION OF PROBATION; AND SHALL NOTIFY THE BOARD IN WRITING OF DATES OF DEPARTURE AND RETURN FROM SOUTH DAKOTA AND ANY CHANGES OF ADDRESS. ON 3/07/96 LICENSE REINSTATED TO UNRESTRICTED STATUS.

SORRELS, WILLIAM F DO, LICENSE NUMBER 00F7187 OF SD, WAS DISCIPLINED BY TEXAS ON SEPTEMBER 30, 1994
DISCIPLINARY ACTION: LICENSE SUSPENSION
OFFENSE: DISCIPLINARY ACTION BY ANOTHER STATE OR AGENCY
NOTES: ON 3/2/94 SIGNED AN AGREED DISPOSITION WITH THE SOUTH DAKOTA BOARD AGREEING TO A TWO YEAR STAYED SUSPENSION TO PROBATION; THERE HAD BEEN ALLEGATIONS OF UNLAWFUL USE OF COCAINE. SUSPENSION UNTIL HE PERSONALLY APPEARS BEFORE THE BOARD TO REQUEST PERMISSION TO PRACTICE AND PROVIDES SUFFICIENT EVIDENCE THAT HE IS PHYSICALLY, MENTALLY AND OTHERWISE COMPETENT TO SAFELY PRACTICE; SHALL GIVE A COPY OF THIS ORDER TO ANY HEALTH CARE ENTITY WHERE HE HAS PRIVILEGES; SHALL COOPERATE WITH THE BOARD IN VERIFYING COMPLIANCE; SHALL INFORM BOARD OF CHANGE OF ADDRESS WITHIN 10 DAYS; SHALL SURRENDER TEXAS CONTROLLED

SUBSTANCES CERTIFICATE AND ALL UNUSED TRIPLICATE PRESCRIPTION FORMS; SHALL NOT ATTEMPT TO REREGISTER WITHOUT PERMISSION; SHALL COMPLY WITH ALL TERMS OF THE SOUTH DAKOTA BOARD ORDER. ON 5/14/99 ORDER TERMINATED.

SORRELS, WILLIAM F DO OF 2200 NORTH KIMBALL SUITE 400, MITCHELL, SD, WAS DISCIPLINED BY DEA ON AUGUST 15, 1995
DISCIPLINARY ACTION: SURRENDER OF CONTROLLED SUBSTANCE LICENSE

NOTES: IN LIEU OF ORDER TO SHOW CAUSE.

SOTO-CORA, EDIBERTO MD, LICENSE NUMBER 00J0679 OF EL PASO, TX, WAS DISCIPLINED BY TEXAS ON MARCH 4, 1995
DISCIPLINARY ACTION: REPRIMAND
OFFENSE: LOSS OR RESTRICTION OF HOSPITAL PRIVILEGES

NOTES: PRIVILEGES TO PERFORM ILIAC ARTERY ANGIOPLASTY AND ILIAC STENT PLACEMENT WERE TEMPORARILY SUSPENDED BY ONE HOSPITAL FOR EIGHT DAYS PENDING PEER REVIEW EVALUATION; FOLLOWING PEER REVIEW, HIS PRIVILEGES WERE REINSTATED WITH A REPRIMAND: FOR SIX MONTHS HE WAS REQUIRED TO OBTAIN A CONSULTATION WITH A CARDIOLOGIST OR CARDIOVASCULAR SURGEON PRIOR TO PERFORMING PTCAS, PTAS, CORONARY ATHERECTOMIES, ILIAC STENTS AND CORONARY CATHETERIZATIONS AND HIS CHARTS WERE TO BE MONITORED FOR QUALITY OF CARE; APPEALED DECISION AND ON 11/19/92, HOSPITAL BOARD AMENDED THE RESTRICTIONS BY ELIMINATING THE REQUIREMENT TO OBTAIN CONSULTATION PRIOR TO DIAGNOSTIC CORONARY CATHETERIZATIONS. HE NEITHER ADMITS NOR DENIES FINDINGS. SHALL GIVE A COPY OF THIS ORDER TO ANY HEALTH CARE ENTITY WHERE HE HAS PRIVILEGES.

SOTO-CORA, EDIBERTO MD, LICENSE NUMBER 0058814 OF EL PASO, TX, WAS DISCIPLINED BY FLORIDA ON DECEMBER 24, 1996
DISCIPLINARY ACTION: FINE
OFFENSE: DISCIPLINARY ACTION BY ANOTHER STATE OR AGENCY

NOTES: CHARGED WITH HAVING A DISCIPLINARY ACTION TAKEN IN ANOTHER JURISDICTION AND FAILING TO REPORT THIS; VIOLATING A RULE OR A LAWFUL ORDER OF THE BOARD, OR FAILING TO COMPLY WITH A LAWFUL SUBPOENA OF THE BOARD. LETTER OF CONCERN; AND SHALL TAKE AND SUCCESSFULLY COMPLETE THE LAWS AND RULES EXAMINATION WITHIN 90 DAYS. $1,000 ADMINISTRATIVE FINE.

SOTOODEH, BAGHER MD, DATE OF BIRTH JULY 3, 1915, LICENSE NUMBER 00C5976 OF 105 E LAUREL STREET, SAN ANTONIO, TX, WAS DISCIPLINED BY TEXAS ON JANUARY 29, 1993
DISCIPLINARY ACTION: RESTRICTION PLACED ON LICENSE
OFFENSE: SUBSTANDARD CARE, INCOMPETENCE OR NEGLIGENCE

NOTES: HAD A HIGHER THAN AVERAGE COMPLICATION RATE AS WELL AS PROBLEMS IN SURGICAL TECHNIQUE IN PERFORMANCE OF CATARACT INTRAOCULAR LENS SURGERIES. SHALL NOT PERFORM ANY OF THE FOLLOWING MAJOR INVASIVE PROCEDURES OR ANY OTHER PROCEDURES NOT SPECIFIED IN THE ORDER AS MINOR PROCEDURES: CATARACT INTRAOCULAR LENS APPLICATION; GLAUCOMA FILTERING; LACERATION OF THE EYE; INTRAOCULAR FOREIGN BODY REMOVAL; MASTOIDECTOMY; STAPEDECTOMY; TYMPANOPLASTY; TONSILLECTOMY; LARYNGOSCOPY; RADIAL KERATOTOMY; ARGON PHOTO COAGULATION; AND YAG LASER IRIDOTOMY AND CAPSILOTOMY. SHALL GIVE A COPY OF THIS ORDER TO ANY HEALTH CARE ENTITY WHERE HE HAS PRIVILEGES; SHALL COOPERATE WITH THE BOARD TO VERIFY COMPLIANCE; SHALL INFORM BOARD OF CHANGE OF ADDRESS WITHIN 10 DAYS; TIME SPENT OUT OF TEXAS DOES NOT COUNT TOWARD RESTRICTION; SHALL NOT SEEK MODIFICATION TO THIS ORDER FOR 12 MONTHS. ON 8/17/96 HIS PETITION FOR TERMINATION OF THIS ORDER DENIED BUT ORDER MODIFIED ALLOWING HIM TO PERFORM PROCEDURES LISTED ABOVE IN THE CONTEXT OF A RESIDENCY PROGRAM; ALL OTHER CONDITIONS REMAIN IN EFFECT. ON 1/29/99 REQUEST TO TERMINATE ORDER DENIED.

SOUDA, ROBERT M MD, LICENSE NUMBER 00D1497 OF DALLAS, TX, WAS DISCIPLINED BY TEXAS ON NOVEMBER 30, 1994
DISCIPLINARY ACTION: SURRENDER OF LICENSE

NOTES: DENIES ALLEGATIONS CONCERNING POSSIBLE VIOLATIONS OF THE MEDICAL PRACTICE ACT BUT SURRENDERS LICENSE IN LIEU OF FURTHER INVESTIGATION. SHALL NOT PETITION FOR REINSTATEMENT OF LICENSE.

SOUDA, ROBERT M MD, LICENSE NUMBER 0011338 OF DALLAS, TX, WAS DISCIPLINED BY WASHINGTON ON MARCH 8, 1996
DISCIPLINARY ACTION: SURRENDER OF LICENSE
OFFENSE: DISCIPLINARY ACTION BY ANOTHER STATE OR AGENCY

NOTES: ACTION IN TEXAS. AGREED TO RETIRE.

SPAIN, MICHAEL MD OF 6603 FIRST PARK TEN, SAN ANTONIO, TX, WAS DISCIPLINED BY DEA ON FEBRUARY 3, 1998
DISCIPLINARY ACTION: SURRENDER OF CONTROLLED SUBSTANCE LICENSE

SPAIN, MICHAEL D MD, LICENSE NUMBER F7188 OF SAN ANTONIO, TX, WAS DISCIPLINED BY TEXAS ON MAY 16, 1998
DISCIPLINARY ACTION: SURRENDER OF LICENSE
OFFENSE: OVERPRESCRIBING OR MISPRESCRIBING DRUGS

NOTES: ON 8/18/97 VOLUNTARILY SURRENDERED HIS DEA REGISTRATIONS ON ALL SCHEDULED DRUGS, EXCEPT FOR SCHEDULE V; FAILED TO KEEP ADEQUATE MEDICAL RECORDS ON PATIENTS THAT HE IS PRESCRIBING NARCOTICS TO; FAILED TO MAINTAIN ADEQUATE DRUG RECORDS; HAS BEEN PRESCRIBING NARCOTICS TO PATIENTS WITHOUT INDICATION. VOLUNTARY SURRENDER.

SPALDING, MARSHA D MD, DATE OF BIRTH SEPTEMBER 20, 1957 OF 4848 NE STALLINGS DRIVE, NACOGDOCHES, TX, WAS DISCIPLINED BY MEDICARE ON DECEMBER 18, 1997
DISCIPLINARY ACTION: EXCLUSION FROM THE MEDICARE AND/OR MEDICAID PROGRAM
OFFENSE: NONCOMPLIANCE WITH A PROFESSIONAL RULE

NOTES: DEFAULTED ON PUBLIC HEALTH SERVICE EDUCATION LOAN. ALSO KNOWN AS MARSHA D. HUNT-RIVERA.

SPEAK, KENNETH EDWIN DO, LICENSE NUMBER 00C4555 OF KERENS, TX, WAS DISCIPLINED BY TEXAS ON JANUARY 11, 1991
DISCIPLINARY ACTION: 6-MONTH LICENSE SUSPENSION; REQUIRED TO TAKE ADDITIONAL MEDICAL EDUCATION
OFFENSE: SUBSTANDARD CARE, INCOMPETENCE OR NEGLIGENCE

NOTES: ADMINISTERED DRUG OR TREATMENT THAT WAS NONTHERAPEUTIC IN NATURE; FAILED PROFESSIONALLY TO PRACTICE MEDICINE IN ACCEPTABLE MANNER CONSISTENT WITH PUBLIC HEALTH AND WELFARE. SUSPENSION FOR AT LEAST

SIX MONTHS AND THEREAFTER UNTIL SUCCESSFUL COMPLETION OF MINI-RESIDENCY IN FAMILY PRACTICE AND SUCCESSFUL COMPLETION OF SPECIAL PURPOSE EXAMINATION. MOTION FOR REHEARING FILED.

SPENCER, JOHN P MD, LICENSE NUMBER E4948, WAS DISCIPLINED BY TEXAS ON MARCH 1, 1997
DISCIPLINARY ACTION: FINE; REPRIMAND
OFFENSE: PROFESSIONAL MISCONDUCT

NOTES: ON 12/12/94 AN ADULT FEMALE HOSPITAL INPATIENT OF 70 PLUS YEARS OF AGE, WAS SCHEDULED TO UNDERGO A STRESS TEST AT 9:30 AM CONDUCTED BY HIM; HE MAINTAINS THAT HE WAS NOT AWARE THAT HE WAS SCHEDULED TO PERFORM THE TEST UNTIL THAT MORNING, AND INFORMED A NURSE HE WOULD ARRIVE AS SOON AS POSSIBLE GIVEN THAT HE HAD SCHEDULED OFFICE VISITS FOR THAT MORNING. HE ARRIVED AT THE HOSPITAL AT APPROXIMATELY 1 PM AND ENGAGED IN HOSTILE VERBAL EXCHANGE AND PHYSICAL ALTERCATION WITH THE PATIENT'S HUSBAND, ALSO OF 70 PLUS YEARS; HE CAUSED THE HUSBAND TO FALL ONTO HIS SPOUSE, THE PATIENT, WHO WAS LYING ON A TABLE OR GURNEY. HE MAINTAINS THAT HE DID NOT STRIKE THE HUSBAND BUT PUSHED HIM AWAY WHEN HE BELIEVED HE WAS BEING THREATENED. PSYCHIATRIC EVALUATIONS AND DRUG TESTING RESULTED IN NEGATIVE FINDINGS. RESTRICTED AS FOLLOWS: WITHIN 14 DAYS, SHALL UNDERGO A PSYCHIATRIC EVALUATION WITH AN APPROVED PSYCHIATRIST WHO WILL REPORT TO THE BOARD ON HIS MENTAL FITNESS TO PRACTICE MEDICINE; ASSUMING HE IS ABLE TO PRACTICE, WITHIN ONE YEAR SHALL RESEARCH AND WRITE A PAPER SUITABLE FOR PUBLICATION OF NO LESS THAN 25 PAGES REGARDING ETHICAL ISSUES RELATING TO PHYSICIAN-PATIENT INTERACTION AND CONDUCT; SHALL OBTAIN 10 HOURS OF ETHICS COURSEWORK AND PERFORM 80 HOURS OF COMMUNITY SERVICE; SHALL PAY AN ADMINISTRATIVE PENALTY OF $1000; SHALL COOPERATE WITH THE BOARD IN VERIFYING COMPLIANCE INCLUDING PROVIDING COPIES OF MEDICAL RELEASES AND PEER REVIEW RECORDS UPON REQUEST; SHALL GIVE A COPY OF THIS ORDER TO ANY HEALTH CARE ENTITY WHERE HE HAS PRIVILEGES; SHALL PROVIDE A COPY OF THIS ORDER TO ANYONE REQUESTING IT WITHIN 10 DAYS; SHALL COOPERATE WITH THE BOARD IN VERIFYING COMPLIANCE; TIME SPENT OUT OF TEXAS DOES NOT COUNT TOWARD RESTRICTION; SHALL INFORM THE BOARD OF CHANGE OF ADDRESS WITHIN 10 DAYS OR IF HE LEAVES THE STATE; SHALL APPEAR PERSONALLY BEFORE THE BOARD AT LEAST TWICE YEARLY FOR THE FIRST YEAR AND ANNUALLY THEREAFTER IF UNDER CONTINUING CARE, OR AS REQUESTED; SHALL NOT SEEK MODIFICATION FOR ONE YEAR.

SPENCER, JOHN PAUL MD, LICENSE NUMBER N8004 OF HOUSTON, TX, WAS DISCIPLINED BY ARKANSAS ON JUNE 11, 1999
DISCIPLINARY ACTION: LICENSE REVOCATION

SPINKS, DAVID WAYNE DO, LICENSE NUMBER F4557, WAS DISCIPLINED BY TEXAS ON DECEMBER 11, 1999
DISCIPLINARY ACTION: REPRIMAND
OFFENSE: SUBSTANDARD CARE, INCOMPETENCE OR NEGLIGENCE

NOTES: IMPROPERLY DIAGNOSED A PATIENT WITH HYPOTHYROIDISM AND FAILED TO RECOGNIZE THE PROBABILITY THAT THE SYNTHETIC THYROID THERAPY HE WAS PRESCRIBING WAS CAUSING ADVERSE SIDE EFFECTS, INCLUDING TACHYCARDIA.

SPRINGER, GEORGE O MD, DATE OF BIRTH JULY 9, 1957 OF 3001 TYLER STREET, EL PASO, TX, WAS DISCIPLINED BY MEDICARE ON JANUARY 3, 1995
DISCIPLINARY ACTION: EXCLUSION FROM THE MEDICARE AND/OR MEDICAID PROGRAM
OFFENSE: NONCOMPLIANCE WITH A PROFESSIONAL RULE

NOTES: DEFAULTED ON PUBLIC HEALTH SERVICE EDUCATION LOAN. REINSTATED ON 1/3/95.

SPRINGER, TERRY W MD, LICENSE NUMBER G8434 OF ARLINGTON, TX, WAS DISCIPLINED BY TEXAS ON AUGUST 22, 1998
DISCIPLINARY ACTION: RESTRICTION PLACED ON CONTROLLED SUBSTANCE LICENSE; REQUIRED TO TAKE ADDITIONAL MEDICAL EDUCATION
OFFENSE: OVERPRESCRIBING OR MISPRESCRIBING DRUGS

NOTES: FROM APPROXIMATELY 10/93 - 1/95 HE PRESCRIBED CONTROLLED SUBSTANCES TO CERTAIN ADULT PATIENTS WITHOUT ADEQUATE MEDICAL INDICATION AND WITHOUT ADEQUATE MEDICAL DOCUMENTATION; FAILED TO REALIZE THE NUMBER OF TABLETS ACTUALLY PRESCRIBED TO THE PATIENTS DUE TO FAILING TO PROPERLY KEEP MEDICAL RECORDS AS TO THE AMOUNT AND FREQUENCY OF MEDICATION PRESCRIBED. LICENSE LIMITED FOR TWO YEARS AS FOLLOWS: SHALL NOT, EXCEPT IN AN EMERGENCY SITUATION, PRESCRIBE TO HIMSELF, ANY MEMBERS OF FAMILY, OR ANY MEMBER OF HIS STAFF; SEPARATE FROM PATIENT RECORDS, SHALL MAINTAIN A LOGBOOK OF EVERY PRESCRIPTION WRITTEN BY HIM FOR DANGEROUS DRUGS WITH ADDICTIVE POTENTIAL WHICH SHALL BE MADE AVAILABLE FOR REVIEW; SHALL NOT TELEPHONE TO A PHARMACY A PRESCRIPTION OR REFILL FOR CONTROLLED SUBSTANCES OR DANGEROUS DRUGS WITH ADDICTIVE POTENTIAL OR POTENTIAL FOR ABUSE, AND SHALL NOT PERMIT ANY INDIVIDUAL UNDER HIS SUPERVISION TO TELEPHONE SUCH A PRESCRIPTION OR REFILL TO A PHARMACY; SHALL MAINTAIN ADEQUATE MEDICAL RECORDS WHICH SHALL BE AVAILABLE FOR REVIEW; WITHIN 12 MONTHS SHALL SUCCESSFULLY COMPLETE A COURSE IN PHARMACOLOGY, A COURSE IN RISK MANAGEMENT, AND 5 HOURS OF ETHICS THROUGH COURSES OR PROGRAMS; SHALL COOPERATE WITH THE BOARD IN VERIFYING COMPLIANCE INCLUDING PROVIDING COPIES OF PEER REVIEW RECORDS UPON REQUEST; WITHIN 6 MONTHS SHALL SUCCESSFULLY COMPLETE AN ADVANCED TRAUMA LIFE SUPPORT COURSE AND OBTAIN CERTIFICATION; SHALL APPEAR BEFORE THE BOARD UPON REQUEST; TIME SPENT OUT OF TEXAS DOES NOT COUNT TOWARD RESTRICTION; SHALL INFORM THE BOARD OF CHANGE OF ADDRESS WITHIN 10 DAYS OR IF HE LEAVES THE STATE; SHALL NOT SEEK MODIFICATION FOR ONE YEAR.

SPROTT, MAXIE C II MD, LICENSE NUMBER G2230, WAS DISCIPLINED BY TEXAS ON MAY 10, 1997
DISCIPLINARY ACTION: REPRIMAND
OFFENSE: NONCOMPLIANCE WITH A PROFESSIONAL RULE

NOTES: FAILED TO RESPOND TO A BOARD REQUEST FOR MEDICAL RECORDS. SHALL GIVE A COPY OF THIS ORDER TO ANY HEALTH CARE ENTITY WHERE DR. SPROTT HAS PRIVILEGES.

SRIVATHANAKUL, SURAPHANDU MD, LICENSE NUMBER 00E7288 OF PALESTINE, TX, WAS DISCIPLINED BY TEXAS ON MARCH 4, 1995
DISCIPLINARY ACTION: FINE; REPRIMAND

OFFENSE: LOSS OR RESTRICTION OF HOSPITAL PRIVILEGES

NOTES: DURING 1993 AND 1994, FAILED TO MAKE ADEQUATE ARRANGEMENTS TO BE CONTACTED WHILE ON CALL WHICH RESULTED IN HIS UNAVAILABILITY WHEN NEEDED TO PROVIDE CARE TO TWO PATIENTS; IN 11/93, HE WAS NOTIFIED ABOUT A PATIENT'S WORSENING CONDITION AND GAVE TELEPHONIC ORDERS BUT FAILED TO PERSONALLY EXAMINE PATIENT AND WAS NOT ALWAYS READILY AVAILABLE WHEN HOSPITAL STAFF WAS ATTEMPTING TO COMMUNICATE PATIENT'S CONDITION; PATIENT WAS SUBSEQUENTLY DIAGNOSED BY ANOTHER PHYSICIAN AS HAVING MENINGITIS; MAINTAINS THAT THE PROBLEMS WERE RELATED TO A BEEPER MALFUNCTION; IN 12/93, PLACED ON SIX MONTHS PROBATION BY HOSPITAL; FOR THIS AND NOT TIMELY DOCUMENTING PATIENT RECORDS AND HIS CONTINUED UNRESPONSIVENESS TO STAFF ATTEMPTS TO CONTACT HIM. CONDITIONS IMPOSED ON PRIVILEGES INCLUDING CHART MONITORING; IN 3/94, RESIGNED HIS HOSPITAL PRIVILEGES IN LIEU OF A SUSPENSION WHEN THE HOSPITAL EXPRESSED CONCERNS THAT HE HAD NOT COMPLETED A HISTORY AND PHYSICAL IN A TIMELY MANNER. SHALL PAY $1,000 FINE.

STAFFORD, JOHN S MD, LICENSE NUMBER G5640 OF SANTA FE, TX, WAS DISCIPLINED BY TEXAS ON APRIL 4, 1998
DISCIPLINARY ACTION: FINE; REPRIMAND
OFFENSE: NONCOMPLIANCE WITH A PROFESSIONAL RULE

NOTES: FAILED TO OBTAIN THE REQUIRED 24 HOURS OF CONTINUING MEDICAL EDUCATION DURING THE REGULAR ANNUAL REPORTING PERIOD, 5/96 - 5/97, OR DURING THE 90 DAY EXTENSION UPON RENEWING HIS LICENSE; HE DID OBTAIN 70 HOURS OF CONTINUING MEDICAL EDUCATION BY 11/97. $100 FINE.

STANTON, JAMES MICHAEL MD, DATE OF BIRTH NOVEMBER 14, 1946, LICENSE NUMBER 00E3779 OF MISSOURI CITY, TX, WAS DISCIPLINED BY TEXAS ON OCTOBER 10, 1991
DISCIPLINARY ACTION: LICENSE REVOCATION
OFFENSE: FAILURE TO COMPLY WITH PREVIOUS BOARD ORDER

NOTES: ON 9/3/87 HE ENTERED INTO AN AGREEMENT WITH THE BOARD IN WHICH HE AGREED NOT TO PRESCRIBE, ADMINISTER, OR DISPENSE ANY CONTROLLED SUBSTANCES FOR HIMSELF OR HIS IMMEDIATE FAMILY EXCEPT IN EMERGENCIES; AGREEMENT WAS IN EFFECT UNTIL 9/30/90. HE ISSUED APPROXIMATELY 169 PRESCRIPTIONS OF CONTROLLED SUBSTANCES DURING THE PERIOD 1/4/89 THROUGH 9/2/90 IN THE NAME OF HIS MOTHER; HE SELF-ADMINISTERED THESE CONTROLLED SUBSTANCES. HE ISSUED APPROXIMATELY 201 PRESCRIPTIONS OF CONTROLLED SUBSTANCES IN THE NAME OF HIS MOTHER AND SELF-ADMINISTERED THEM DURING THE PERIOD 1/4/89 TO 11/29/90. PRESCRIPTIONS WRITTEN WERE FALSE AND FICTITIOUS.

STANTON, JAMES MICHAEL MD, DATE OF BIRTH NOVEMBER 14, 1946, LICENSE NUMBER 00E3779 OF 1201 BERING #99, HOUSTON, TX, WAS DISCIPLINED BY TEXAS ON NOVEMBER 30, 1992
DISCIPLINARY ACTION: SURRENDER OF CONTROLLED SUBSTANCE LICENSE; LICENSE REINSTATEMENT
OFFENSE: SUBSTANCE ABUSE

NOTES: SINCE 10/10/91 REVOCATION, HAS UNDERGONE OVER FIVE MONTHS OF IN-PATIENT TREATMENT FOR IMPAIRED PHYSICIANS; PROVIDED RESULTS OF URINE SCREENS CONDUCTED IN 1992 WHICH INDICATE THAT DRUGS OR THEIR METABOLITES WERE NOT DETECTED IN HIS URINE; PROVIDED FAVORABLE LETTERS REGARDING HIS PROFESSIONAL CHARACTER, ABILITIES AND REHABILITATION EFFORTS. PLACED ON TEN-YEAR PROBATION UNDER TERMS AND CONDITIONS: SHALL ATTEND AT LEAST 50 HOURS PER YEAR OF CONTINUING MEDICAL EDUCATION APPROVED FOR CREDITS; SHALL BE MONITORED OR SUPERVISED BY A BOARD-APPROVED PHYSICIAN WHO WILL MONITOR HIS MEDICAL PRACTICE, RECORD KEEPING AND PATIENT CHARTS AND WILL REPORT TO BOARD QUARTERLY; SHALL MAKE PATIENT MEDICAL RECORDS AVAILABLE FOR EVALUATION BY BOARD; SHALL ABSTAIN FROM CONSUMPTION OF ALCOHOL AND CHEMICAL SUBSTANCES IN ANY FORM, AND SHALL IMMEDIATELY REPORT TO BOARD ANY LAPSE; SHALL SURRENDER ALL CONTROLLED SUBSTANCES PRESENTLY IN HIS OFFICE OR POSSESSION AND MAY NOT POSSESS ANY IN THE FUTURE; SHALL NOT ATTEMPT TO REREGISTER FOR DEA CONTROLLED SUBSTANCES REGISTRATION CERTIFICATE WITHOUT PRIOR APPROVAL; SHALL CONTINUE TO PARTICIPATE IN ALCOHOLICS ANONYMOUS OR SIMILAR PROGRAM, AND IN A COUNTY IMPAIRED PHYSICIANS GROUP WITH QUARTERLY REPORTS; SHALL SUBMIT HIMSELF FOR APPROPRIATE EXAMINATIONS, INCLUDING URINE OR BLOOD SCREENINGS FOR ALCOHOL OR DRUGS; SHALL APPEAR BEFORE THE BOARD TWICE A YEAR; SHALL GIVE A COPY OF THE ORDER TO HOSPITALS WHERE HE HAS PRIVILEGES; SHALL COOPERATE WITH THE BOARD IN VERIFYING COMPLIANCE; SHALL ADVISE THE BOARD OF ANY ADDRESS CHANGE; TIME SPENT OUT OF THE STATE DOES NOT COUNT TOWARDS PROBATION; AFTER ONE YEAR MAY SEEK TERMINATION OR MODIFICATION OF THIS ORDER. BOARD DENIED HIS REQUEST FOR MODIFICATION OF THIS ORDER ON 6/22/94. ON 6/28/95 ORDER MODIFIED AS FOLLOWS: HE IS GIVEN AUTHORITY TO REAPPLY TO DEA AND TEXAS DEPARTMENT OF PUBLIC SAFETY FOR SCHEDULES IV AND V CONTROLLED SUBSTANCES PRESCRIBING; MUST MAINTAIN A LOG OF ALL PRESCRIPTIONS WRITTEN FOR CONTROLLED SUBSTANCES WHICH SHALL BE MADE AVAILABLE FOR INSPECTION. ON 8/17/96 ORDER MODIFIED AUTHORIZING HIM TO REAPPLY TO THE DEA AND THE TEXAS DEPARTMENT OF PUBLIC SAFETY TO OBTAIN FULL PRESCRIBING AUTHORITY FOR CONTROLLED SUBSTANCES; ALL OTHER CONDITIONS REMAIN IN EFFECT. ON 11/22/97 PETITION TO MODIFY ORDER GRANTED DELETING REQUIREMENT FOR PARTICIPATION IN THE ACTIVITIES OF A COUNTY IMPAIRED PHYSICIAN GROUP. ON 5/16/98 ORDER TERMINATED.

STANTON, JAMES MICHAEL MD, DATE OF BIRTH NOVEMBER 14, 1946 OF 1201 BERING DRIVE, HOUSTON, TX, WAS DISCIPLINED BY DEA ON DECEMBER 23, 1992
DISCIPLINARY ACTION: REVOCATION OF CONTROLLED SUBSTANCE LICENSE
OFFENSE: DISCIPLINARY ACTION BY ANOTHER STATE OR AGENCY

NOTES: THE TEXAS BOARD OF MEDICAL EXAMINERS FOUND THAT CONTROLLED SUBSTANCES PRESCRIBED AND ADMINISTERED BY HIM WERE NOT PRESCRIBED OR ADMINISTERED FOR A VALID MEDICAL REASON. FROM 01/04/89 TO 11/29/90 HE ISSUED 201 PRESCRIPTIONS OF CODEINE PRODUCTS IN HIS MOTHER'S NAME, WHICH WERE ACTUALLY FOR HIS PERSONAL USE. THE BOARD CONCLUDED THAT THE PUBLIC WAS PUT IN DANGER BY HIS SELF-ADMINISTRATION OF CONTROLLED SUBSTANCES AND THAT HE ENGAGED IN UNPROFESSIONAL OR DISHONORABLE CONDUCT THAT WAS LIKELY TO DECEIVE OR DEFRAUD OR

INJURE THE PUBLIC. MEDICAL LICENSE REVOKED IN TEXAS ON 10/10/91. THEREFORE, HE IS NOT AUTHORIZED TO HANDLE CONTROLLED SUBSTANCES.

STARNES, WILLIS L MD, DATE OF BIRTH AUGUST 1, 1940 OF 3204 N MACARTHUR BLVD #A, IRVING, TX, WAS DISCIPLINED BY MEDICARE ON FEBRUARY 8, 1995
DISCIPLINARY ACTION: EXCLUSION FROM THE MEDICARE AND/OR MEDICAID PROGRAM
OFFENSE: NONCOMPLIANCE WITH A PROFESSIONAL RULE

NOTES: DEFAULT ON HEALTH EDUCATION LOAN OR SCHOLARSHIP OBLIGATIONS. REINSTATED ON 3/1/96.

STARR, THOMAS PIERCE SR MD OF SAN ANTONIO, TX, WAS DISCIPLINED BY NORTH CAROLINA ON JULY 8, 1991
DISCIPLINARY ACTION: LICENSE REVOCATION

STAYER, DAVID SHELLENBERGE MD, LICENSE NUMBER 00D4900, WAS DISCIPLINED BY TEXAS ON AUGUST 17, 1996
DISCIPLINARY ACTION: SURRENDER OF LICENSE
OFFENSE: OVERPRESCRIBING OR MISPRESCRIBING DRUGS

NOTES: ALLEGED THAT HE PRESCRIBED CONTROLLED SUBSTANCES TO SEVERAL PATIENTS WITHOUT ANY OR ADEQUATE DOCUMENTED MEDICAL INDICATION AND DURING A PERIOD OF TIME WHEN HE DID NOT HAVE A CONTROLLED SUBSTANCES REGISTRATION CERTIFICATE FROM EITHER THE DEA OR THE TEXAS DPS. DOES NOT ADMIT VIOLATION. VOLUNTARY AND PERMANENT SURRENDER IN LIEU OF FURTHER PROCEEDINGS. SHALL RETIRE FROM THE PRACTICE OF MEDICINE.

STAYER, DAVID SHELLENBERGER MD, LICENSE NUMBER 00D4900 OF IRVING, TX, WAS DISCIPLINED BY TEXAS ON DECEMBER 4, 1991
DISCIPLINARY ACTION: REPRIMAND
OFFENSE: OVERPRESCRIBING OR MISPRESCRIBING DRUGS

NOTES: REFILLED PRESCRIPTION FOR WEIGHT CONTROL WITHOUT GIVING PATIENT A PHYSICAL EXAMINATION.

STEELE, JOHN GILBERT MD, LICENSE NUMBER 00C9149 OF IRVING, TX, WAS DISCIPLINED BY TEXAS ON JUNE 22, 1994
DISCIPLINARY ACTION: 60-MONTH PROBATION; MONITORING OF PHYSICIAN PERFORMANCE
OFFENSE: SUBSTANCE ABUSE

NOTES: HE ADMITS HE IS AN ALCOHOLIC; LAST SOBRIETY DATE STATED TO BE 1/3/92; HAS HAD NO DRUG/ALCOHOL SCREENS PERFORMED SINCE THEN; IS UNDER PSYCHIATRIC CARE AND ACTIVE IN AA; MAINTAINS AN OFFICE PRACTICE IN ORTHOPEDICS AND HAS NOT PERFORMED SURGERY FOR TWO YEARS. FIVE YEAR SUSPENSION STAYED. CONDITIONS OF PROBATION: SHALL CONTINUE PSYCHIATRIC TREATMENT WITH QUARTERLY REPORTS; SHALL PARTICIPATE IN AA'S PROGRAM NOT LESS THAN THREE TIMES A WEEK WITH QUARTERLY REPORTS TO THE BOARD; SHALL PARTICIPATE IN THE ACTIVITIES OF A PHYSICIAN HEALTH AND REHABILITATION COMMITTEE AND ATTEND WEEKLY MEETINGS WITH QUARTERLY REPORTS; SHALL SUBMIT HIMSELF FOR APPROPRIATE EXAMS INCLUDING DRUG OR ALCOHOL SCREENS; SHALL ABSTAIN FROM THE CONSUMPTION OF ALCOHOL/CHEMICAL SUBSTANCES IN ANY FORM UNLESS PRESCRIBED BY ANOTHER PHYSICIAN FOR A LEGITIMATE AND THERAPEUTIC PURPOSE; SHALL REFRAIN FROM THE PERSONAL USE OF AND SHALL NOT POSSESS OR ADMINISTER TO HIMSELF ANY PRESCRIPTION DRUG UNLESS PRESCRIBED, ADMINISTERED OR DISPENSED BY ANOTHER PHYSICIAN FOR A LEGITIMATE MEDICAL NEED; SHALL NOT TREAT OR OTHERWISE SERVE AS PHYSICIAN, PRESCRIBE, DISPENSE, OR ADMINISTER DRUGS THAT MAY BE SUBJECT TO ABUSE TO HIMSELF OR ANY MEMBER OF HIS FAMILY; SHALL SUBMIT HIMSELF FOR EVALUATION TO A BOARD-APPROVED NEUROPSYCHIATRIST; PRIOR TO PERFORMING SURGERY SHALL RECEIVE APPROVAL FROM BOARD AFTER SUBMITTING A PROPOSAL FOR A PERIOD OF ONLY ASSISTING AT SURGERY WITH BOARD-APPROVED SURGEON; SHALL APPEAR BEFORE THE BOARD TWICE A YEAR; SHALL GIVE A COPY OF THIS ORDER TO ALL HEALTH CARE ENTITIES WHERE HE HAS PRIVILEGES; SHALL COOPERATE WITH BOARD IN VERIFYING COMPLIANCE; SHALL INFORM BOARD OF CHANGE OF ADDRESS WITHIN 10 DAYS OR IF HE LEAVES THE STATE; TIME SPENT OUT OF TEXAS DOES NOT COUNT TOWARD PROBATION. SHALL NOT SEEK MODIFICATION FOR SIX MONTHS. ON 1/18/97 HIS PETITION FOR TERMINATION OF THIS ORDER WAS GRANTED BASED ON HIS COMPLIANCE WITH CONDITIONS.

STEGMAN, RONALD REGIS DO, DATE OF BIRTH OCTOBER 13, 1937, LICENSE NUMBER 00D2303 OF 12222 COIT ROAD, DALLAS, TX, WAS DISCIPLINED BY TEXAS ON JANUARY 29, 1993
DISCIPLINARY ACTION: LICENSE REVOCATION
OFFENSE: OVERPRESCRIBING OR MISPRESCRIBING DRUGS

NOTES: ON OR ABOUT 11/14/90 A BOARD INVESTIGATOR CONDUCTED A COMPLIANCE INSPECTION WITH DRUG RECORD AND INVENTORY LAWS OF DR. STEGMAN'S OFFICE; LARGE QUANTITIES OF CONTROLLED SUBSTANCES PREPACKAGED FOR DISPENSING WERE FOUND; HE DISPENSED PRESCRIPTION DRUGS/CONTROLLED SUBSTANCES FOR A SEPARATE FEE WITHOUT HAVING A PHARMACIST'S LICENSE; FAILED TO KEEP COMPLETE AND ACCURATE RECORDS OF ALL PURCHASES AND DISPOSALS OF CONTROLLED SUBSTANCES AS REQUIRED BY DEPARTMENT OF PUBLIC SAFETY DRUG RULES; PRESCRIBED 110 SHOTS OF DEMEROL TO A PATIENT WHICH WAS NONTHERAPEUTIC IN NATURE OR THE MANNER IN WHICH IT WAS ADMINISTERED; FAILED TO SUBMIT REQUIRED TRIPLICATE PRESCRIPTION FORMS FOR DEMEROL. SHALL SURRENDER TO THE BOARD HIS DEA AND TEXAS CONTROLLED SUBSTANCES CERTIFICATES. SHALL NOT SEEK REINSTATEMENT FOR ONE YEAR. ORDER APPEALED TO THE COURTS; WILL BECOME FINAL WHEN ALL APPEALS HAVE BEEN EXHAUSTED.

STEGMAN, RONALD REGIS DO, DATE OF BIRTH OCTOBER 13, 1937 OF 12222 C IT ROAD, DALLAS, TX, WAS DISCIPLINED BY MEDICARE ON FEBRUARY 28, 1994
DISCIPLINARY ACTION: EXCLUSION FROM THE MEDICARE AND/OR MEDICAID PROGRAM
OFFENSE: DISCIPLINARY ACTION BY ANOTHER STATE OR AGENCY

NOTES: LICENSE REVOKED FOR REASONS BEARING ON UNPROFESSIONAL AND DISHONORABLE CONDUCT AS A PHARMACIST PRACTICING WITHOUT A LICENSE.

STEGMAN, RONALD REGIS DO, DATE OF BIRTH OCTOBER 13, 1937, LICENSE NUMBER 002200L OF 12011 COIT ROAD SUITE 119, DALLAS, TX, WAS DISCIPLINED BY PENNSYLVANIA ON DECEMBER 12, 1996
DISCIPLINARY ACTION: LICENSE SUSPENSION
OFFENSE: DISCIPLINARY ACTION BY ANOTHER STATE OR AGENCY

NOTES: DISCIPLINARY ACTION TAKEN AGAINST HIM IN ANOTHER STATE. LICENSE SUSPENSION UNTIL HIS

TEXAS LICENSE IS REINSTATED.

STENGER, EARL MARTIN MD, LICENSE NUMBER 00D7315 OF SAN ANTONIO, TX, WAS DISCIPLINED BY TEXAS ON OCTOBER 13, 1995
DISCIPLINARY ACTION: LICENSE REVOCATION
OFFENSE: CRIMINAL CONVICTION OR PLEA OF GUILTY, NOLO CONTENDERE, OR NO CONTEST TO A CRIME

NOTES: DURING 11/94, PLED GUILTY TO ONE COUNT OF FRAUDULENT BILLING OF BIOFEEDBACK THERAPY AND ONE COUNT OF FEDERAL TAX FRAUD; ENTERED INTO A PLEA AGREEMENT THAT REQUIRES THAT HE BE IMPRISONED FROM 21 TO 27 MONTHS, PAY $200,000 IN RESTITUTION AND THAT HE NOT BILL FOR MEDICAL SERVICES ON HIS OWN BEHALF WHILE ON SUPERVISED RELEASE OR PROBATION; HE IS IN THE PROCESS OF SELLING HIS PRACTICE. SUSPENSION THROUGH 12/31/95. THEREAFTER, ON 1/1/96 HIS LICENSE SHALL BE REVOKED.

STENGER, EARL MARTIN JR MD OF 351 E HILDEBRAND, SAN ANTONIO, TX, WAS DISCIPLINED BY DEA ON NOVEMBER 5, 1997
DISCIPLINARY ACTION: SURRENDER OF CONTROLLED SUBSTANCE LICENSE

STENGER, EARL MARTIN MD, LICENSE NUMBER D7315, WAS DISCIPLINED BY TEXAS ON FEBRUARY 7, 1998
DISCIPLINARY ACTION: LICENSE REINSTATEMENT; 120-MONTH RESTRICTION PLACED ON LICENSE

NOTES: ON 1/1/96 HIS TEXAS LICENSE WAS REVOKED; SINCE 11/6/96 HE HAS BEEN EMPLOYED AS A "HEALTH COORDINATOR" BY EL CENTRO DEL BARRIO IN SAN ANTONIO, TEXAS; HE HAS BEEN EXTENDED AN OFFER TO WORK AS A PSYCHIATRIST AT EL CENTRO WHICH IS A NON-PROFIT HEALTH CLINIC WHICH SERVES A PREDOMINANTLY UNINSURED, MEDICALLY INDIGENT POPULATION; THE CLINIC DOES NOT CURRENTLY HAVE A PSYCHIATRIST ON STAFF. LICENSE LIMITED AS FOLLOWS: WITHIN 1 YEAR, SHALL TAKE AND PASS THE SPEX; MEDICAL PRACTICE SHALL BE LIMITED TO WORK AS A SALARIED EMPLOYEE OF A BOARD-APPROVED INSTITUTION; SHALL NOT APPLY FOR, POSSESS, OR RETAIN HOSPITAL PRIVILEGES, EITHER ACTIVE OR COURTESY; SHALL NOT PRESCRIBE, DISPENSE OR ADMINISTER DRUGS THAT MAY BE SUBJECT TO ABUSE AND SHALL SURRENDER ANY IN HIS POSSESSION INCLUDING SAMPLES; SHALL PERFORM 100 HOURS OF COMMUNITY SERVICE PER YEAR; SHALL OBTAIN 50 HOURS PER YEAR OF CONTINUING MEDICAL EDUCATION; WITHIN 1 YEAR SHALL OBTAIN 12 HOURS OF AN ETHICS COURSE; SHALL PROVIDE A COPY OF THIS ORDER TO HIS SUPERVISOR; HIS MEDICAL PRACTICE SHALL BE MONITORED BY A BOARD APPROVED TEXAS PHYSICIAN WHO SHALL PROVIDE QUARTERLY REPORTS TO THE BOARD; SHALL APPEAR BEFORE THE BOARD UPON REQUEST; SHALL COOPERATE WITH THE BOARD IN VERIFYING COMPLIANCE; SHALL PROVIDE A COPY OF THIS ORDER TO ANYONE REQUESTING IT WITHIN 10 DAYS; TIME SPENT OUT OF TEXAS DOES NOT COUNT TOWARD RESTRICTION; SHALL INFORM THE BOARD OF CHANGE OF ADDRESS WITHIN 10 DAYS OR IF HE LEAVES THE STATE; SHALL NOT SEEK MODIFICATION FOR ONE YEAR.

STENGER, EARL MARTIN MD, LICENSE NUMBER D7315 OF SAN ANTONIO, TX, WAS DISCIPLINED BY TEXAS ON FEBRUARY 9, 1999
DISCIPLINARY ACTION: LICENSE SUSPENSION
OFFENSE: FAILURE TO COMPLY WITH PREVIOUS BOARD ORDER

NOTES: FAILED TO TAKE AND PASS THE SPEX WITHIN 1 YEAR AS REQUIRED BY THE 2/7/98 BOARD ORDER. ON 4/10/99 A TYPOGRAPHICAL ERROR WAS MADE IN THE NAME ON THE 2/9/99 BOARD ORDER AND CORRECTED AS FOLLOWS: "ON THIS 2ND DAY FEBRUARY, 1999, IN THE MATTER OF THE LICENSE OF EARL MARTIN STENGER, MD., THE SECRETARY TREASURER, ACTING ON BEHALF OF THE BOARD, MAKES THE FOLLOWING FINDINGS OF FACT AND CONCLUSIONS OF LAW."; ALL OTHER PROVISIONS OF THE 2/9/99 ORDER REMAIN IN FULL EFFECT.

STENGER, EARL MARTIN MD, LICENSE NUMBER D7315 OF SAN ANTONIO, TX, WAS DISCIPLINED BY TEXAS ON APRIL 10, 1999
DISCIPLINARY ACTION: 120-MONTH PROBATION; RESTRICTION PLACED ON LICENSE
OFFENSE: FAILURE TO COMPLY WITH PREVIOUS BOARD ORDER

NOTES: FAILED TO PASS THE SPEX AS REQUIRED BY 2/7/98 BOARD ORDER AND LICENSE SUSPENDED ON 2/9/99; REQUESTING REINSTATEMENT AS HE IS THE ONLY PSYCHIATRIST AT A CLINIC WHICH SERVES PRIMARILY A MEDICALLY INDIGENT POPULATION. SUSPENSION STAYED FOR PROBATION WITH FOLLOWING TERMS AND CONDITIONS: WITHIN 2 YEARS SHALL TAKE AND PASS THE SPEX WITH A SCORE OF 75 OR ABOVE, WITHIN 3 ATTEMPTS OR OBTAIN BOARD CERTIFICATION IN PSYCHIATRY; SHALL NOT RETAIN OR APPLY FOR ANY HOSPITAL PRIVILEGES; MEDICAL PRACTICE SHALL BE LIMITED TO A BOARD-APPROVED INSTITUTIONAL SETTING; SEPARATE FROM PATIENT RECORDS, SHALL MAINTAIN A LOGBOOK OF EVERY PRESCRIPTION WRITTEN BY HIM FOR DANGEROUS DRUGS WITH ADDICTIVE POTENTIAL WHICH SHALL BE MADE AVAILABLE FOR REVIEW; SHALL OBTAIN 50 HOURS PER YEAR OF CONTINUING MEDICAL EDUCATION; HIS MEDICAL PRACTICE SHALL BE MONITORED BY A BOARD APPROVED TEXAS PHYSICIAN WHO SHALL PROVIDE QUARTERLY REPORTS TO THE BOARD; SHALL HAVE QUARTERLY REPORTS FROM HIS SUPERVISOR SUBMITTED TO THE BOARD; SHALL APPEAR BEFORE THE BOARD UPON REQUEST; SHALL COOPERATE WITH THE BOARD IN VERIFYING COMPLIANCE; SHALL PROVIDE A COPY OF THIS ORDER TO ANYONE REQUESTING IT WITHIN 10 DAYS; TIME SPENT OUT OF TEXAS DOES NOT COUNT TOWARD PROBATION; SHALL INFORM THE BOARD OF CHANGE OF ADDRESS WITHIN 10 DAYS OR IF HE LEAVES THE STATE; SHALL NOT SEEK MODIFICATION FOR ONE YEAR.

STERN, STEVEN E MD OF 17070 RED OAK DRIVE SUITE 201C, HOUSTON, TX, WAS DISCIPLINED BY DEA ON JANUARY 18, 1995
DISCIPLINARY ACTION: SURRENDER OF CONTROLLED SUBSTANCE LICENSE

NOTES: IN LIEU OF PUBLIC INTEREST REVOCATION.

STERN, STEVEN E MD OF 17070 RED OAK DRIVE SUITE 201C, HOUSTON, TX, WAS DISCIPLINED BY DEA ON MARCH 28, 1996
DISCIPLINARY ACTION: RESTRICTION PLACED ON CONTROLLED SUBSTANCE LICENSE

NOTES: MEMO OF UNDERSTANDING.

STERN, STEVEN E MD OF 17070 RED OAK DRIVE #201C, HOUSTON, TX, WAS DISCIPLINED BY DEA ON JANUARY 22, 1999
DISCIPLINARY ACTION: RESTRICTION PLACED ON CONTROLLED SUBSTANCE LICENSE

NOTES: MEMO OF UNDERSTANDING.

STERN, STEVEN EMERY MD, LICENSE NUMBER 00E4701 OF

HOUSTON, TX, WAS DISCIPLINED BY TEXAS ON NOVEMBER 19, 1993
DISCIPLINARY ACTION: REPRIMAND
OFFENSE: OVERPRESCRIBING OR MISPRESCRIBING DRUGS

NOTES: FROM 1/1/90 THROUGH 12/29/92 EXCESSIVELY PRESCRIBED FIORINAL WITH CODEINE #3 TO A FAMILY MEMBER IN AN EFFORT TO TREAT CHRONIC TENSION HEADACHES; WHEN HE BECAME AWARE THAT THIS PERSON HAD DEVELOPED A DEPENDENCE ON THE MEDICATION HE TERMINATED THE MEDICATION AND MADE ARRANGEMENTS FOR CARE BY ANOTHER PHYSICIAN; HAS HAD NO OTHER COMPLAINTS AGAINST HIM FILED WITH BOARD.

STERN, STEVEN EMERY MD, LICENSE NUMBER 00E4701 OF HOUSTON, TX, WAS DISCIPLINED BY TEXAS ON MARCH 2, 1996
DISCIPLINARY ACTION: FINE; REPRIMAND
OFFENSE: OVERPRESCRIBING OR MISPRESCRIBING DRUGS

NOTES: DEA ACTION. SUBSEQUENT TO A BOARD ORDER OF 11/93 HE RESUMED PRESCRIBING FIORINAL WITH CODEINE #3 TO THE SAME FAMILY MEMBER; FROM APPROXIMATELY JULY THROUGH DECEMBER 1994 WHILE THE RECIPIENT OF THE MEDICATION WAS UNDER THE CARE AND TREATMENT OF ANOTHER PHYSICIAN; THE RECORDS OF HIS CARE AND TREATMENT OF THE FAMILY MEMBER AND A MEMBER OF HIS OFFICE STAFF DID NOT ADEQUATELY DOCUMENT THE BASIS FOR THE CARE AND TREATMENT RENDERED; IN JANUARY 1995 AS THE RESULT OF A DEA INVESTIGATION, HE VOLUNTARILY SURRENDERED HIS DEA AND TEXAS CONTROLLED SUBSTANCE REGISTRATION; AND HIS TEXAS CONTROLLED SUBSTANCE REGISTRATION CERTIFICATE WAS SUBSEQUENTLY RETURNED. LICENSE RESTRICTED UNDER THE FOLLOWING TERMS AND CONDITIONS FOR TWO YEARS: SHALL NOT TREAT OR OTHERWISE SERVE AS PHYSICIAN, OR PRESCRIBE, DISPENSE OR ADMINISTER DRUGS THAT MAY BE SUBJECT TO ABUSE TO HIMSELF OR ANY MEMBER OF HIS FAMILY, EMPLOYEES, AND ANY MEMBERS OF HIS MEDICAL AND OFFICE STAFF; SHALL OBTAIN AT LEAST 50 HOURS PER YEAR OF CONTINUING MEDICAL EDUCATION OF WHICH AT LEAST 10 HOURS SHALL BE IN MEDICAL ETHICS; SHALL PERSONALLY APPEAR BEFORE THE BOARD AT LEAST ONE TIME PER YEAR AND UPON REQUEST; SHALL COOPERATE WITH THE BOARD IN VERIFYING COMPLIANCE INCLUDING PROVIDING COPIES OF PEER REVIEW RECORDS UPON REQUEST; SHALL GIVE A COPY OF THIS ORDER TO ANY HEALTH CARE ENTITY WHERE HE HAS PRIVILEGES; SHALL PROVIDE A COPY OF THIS ORDER TO ANYONE REQUESTING IT WITHIN 10 DAYS; TIME PERIOD OUT OF TEXAS DOES NOT COUNT TOWARD RESTRICTION; SHALL INFORM THE BOARD OF CHANGE OF ADDRESS WITHIN 10 DAYS OR IF HE LEAVES THE STATE; SHALL NOT SEEK MODIFICATION FOR ONE YEAR.$5,000 ADMINISTRATIVE PENALTY. THIS ORDER SUPERSEDES THE 11/19/93 ORDER.

STEWARD, ROBERT H MD, LICENSE NUMBER H3946 OF SANGER, TX, WAS DISCIPLINED BY TEXAS ON AUGUST 9, 1997
DISCIPLINARY ACTION: 84-MONTH PROBATION; REQUIRED TO TAKE ADDITIONAL MEDICAL EDUCATION
OFFENSE: LOSS OR RESTRICTION OF HOSPITAL PRIVILEGES

NOTES: HE ADMITS TO BEING AN ALCOHOLIC AND DRUG ADDICT WHOSE DRUGS OF CHOICE WERE "STREET DRUGS" INCLUDING METHAMPHETAMINES AND COCAINE; HE HAS BEEN IN TREATMENT SINCE 1996; IN 1996 WAS RELEASED FROM DUTIES AT DENTON MEDICAL CENTER DUE TO HIS BEHAVIOR AT WORK AND FAILURE TO MAINTAIN MALPRACTICE INSURANCE; HE CONTENDS IT WAS OVER WHETHER HE SHOULD HAVE TAKEN A LATE CASE; HIS EMPLOYMENT WAS TERMINATED FROM NORTH TEXAS ANESTHESIOLOGY EFFECTIVE 1/31/96 FOR NOT MEETING THEIR STANDARDS AND FAILING TO COMPLY WITH PREVIOUS CORRECTIONAL REQUESTS REGARDING UNPROFESSIONAL BEHAVIOR AT WORK; HE CONTENDS THAT HE WAS TERMINATED BECAUSE HE WAS NOT AMERICAN BOARD CERTIFIED IN ANESTHESIOLOGY AND HAD NOT TAKEN THE ORAL PART OF HIS BOARDS IN ORDER TO OBTAIN CERTIFICATION. PROBATION WITH FOLLOWING TERMS AND CONDITIONS: SHALL ABSTAIN FROM THE CONSUMPTION OF ALCOHOL/DRUGS IN ANY FORM UNLESS PRESCRIBED BY ANOTHER PHYSICIAN FOR A LEGITIMATE AND THERAPEUTIC PURPOSE; SHALL SUBMIT HIMSELF FOR APPROPRIATE EXAMS INCLUDING DRUG OR ALCOHOL SCREENS; SHALL NOMINATE THREE CERTIFIED PSYCHIATRISTS FOR BOARD SELECTION OF A THERAPIST AND SHALL EXPEDITIOUSLY SUBMIT HIMSELF TO EVALUATION AND TREATMENT BY THE APPROVED PRACTITIONER; SHALL PARTICIPATE IN THE ACTIVITIES OF A PHYSICIAN HEALTH AND REHABILITATION COMMITTEE AND ATTEND WEEKLY MEETINGS WITH QUARTERLY REPORTS; SHALL PARTICIPATE IN AA'S PROGRAM NOT LESS THAN THREE TIMES A WEEK; SHALL REPORT ON HIS ATTENDANCE; SHALL NOT TREAT OR OTHERWISE SERVE AS PHYSICIAN, PRESCRIBE, DISPENSE OR ADMINISTER DRUGS THAT MAY BE SUBJECT TO ABUSE TO HIMSELF OR TO ANY MEMBER OF HIS FAMILY; HIS MEDICAL PRACTICE SHALL BE MONITORED BY A BOARD APPROVED TEXAS PHYSICIAN WHO SHALL PROVIDE QUARTERLY REPORTS TO THE BOARD; SHALL OBTAIN AT LEAST 50 HOURS PER YEAR OF CONTINUING MEDICAL EDUCATION; SHALL APPEAR BEFORE THE BOARD UPON REQUEST; SHALL COOPERATE WITH THE BOARD IN VERIFYING COMPLIANCE INCLUDING PROVIDING COPIES OF MEDICAL RELEASES; SHALL GIVE A COPY OF THIS ORDER TO ANY HEALTH CARE ENTITY WHERE HE HAS PRIVILEGES; SHALL PROVIDE A COPY OF THIS ORDER TO ANYONE REQUESTING IT WITHIN 10 DAYS; TIME SPENT OUT OF TEXAS DOES NOT COUNT TOWARD PROBATION; SHALL INFORM THE BOARD OF CHANGE OF ADDRESS WITHIN 10 DAYS OR IF HE LEAVES THE STATE; SHALL NOT SEEK MODIFICATION FOR ONE YEAR.

STEWARD, ROBERT H MD, LICENSE NUMBER H3946, WAS DISCIPLINED BY TEXAS ON OCTOBER 21, 1999
DISCIPLINARY ACTION: EMERGENCY SUSPENSION

NOTES: EVIDENCE THAT HIS CONTINUED PRACTICE WOULD CONSTITUTE A CONTINUING THREAT TO PUBLIC WELFARE.

STILL, ROBERT LYLE JR MD, LICENSE NUMBER 00F7201 OF SAN ANTONIO, TX, WAS DISCIPLINED BY TEXAS ON JUNE 22, 1994
DISCIPLINARY ACTION: 60-MONTH PROBATION; REPRIMAND
OFFENSE: SUBSTANCE ABUSE

NOTES: ENTERED INPATIENT TREATMENT FOR ALCOHOLISM IN 9/90; CONTINUES TO ATTEND AA AND STATES A SOBRIETY DATE OF 9/27/90; VOLUNTARILY DISCLOSED THIS TO THE BOARD. SUSPENSION STAYED. CONDITIONS OF PROBATION: SHALL APPEAR BEFORE THE BOARD ONCE A YEAR; SHALL NOT TREAT OR OTHERWISE SERVE AS PHYSICIAN, PRESCRIBE, DISPENSE OR ADMINISTER DRUGS THAT MAY BE SUBJECT TO ABUSE TO HIMSELF OR ANY MEMBER OF HIS IMMEDIATE FAMILY; SHALL ABSTAIN FROM THE CONSUMPTION OF ALCOHOL/CHEMICAL SUBSTANCES

IN ANY FORM UNLESS PRESCRIBED BY ANOTHER PHYSICIAN FOR A LEGITIMATE AND THERAPEUTIC PURPOSE; SHALL SUBMIT HIMSELF FOR APPROPRIATE EXAMS INCLUDING DRUG OR ALCOHOL SCREENS; SHALL CONTINUE TO PARTICIPATE IN AA'S PROGRAM NOT LESS THAN THREE TIMES A WEEK WITH QUARTERLY REPORTS TO THE BOARD; SHALL CONTINUE TO PARTICIPATE IN ACTIVITIES OF A PHYSICIAN HEALTH AND REHABILITATION COMMITTEE AND PARTICIPATE IN WEEKLY MEETINGS WITH QUARTERLY REPORTS; SHALL ATTEND AT LEAST 50 HOURS PER YEAR OF CONTINUING MEDICAL EDUCATION; SHALL MAINTAIN ADEQUATE MEDICAL RECORDS ON ALL PATIENT OFFICE VISITS WHICH SHALL BE AVAILABLE FOR INSPECTION; SHALL NOT SIGN ANY PATIENT RECORD UNLESS HE HAS PERSONALLY EXAMINED THE PATIENT OR CLEARLY NOTES IN THE RECORD THAT HE DID NOT; SHALL GIVE A COPY OF THIS ORDER TO ANY HEALTH CARE ENTITY WHERE HE HAS PRIVILEGES; SHALL COOPERATE WITH THE BOARD IN VERIFYING COMPLIANCE; SHALL INFORM BOARD OF CHANGE OF ADDRESS WITHIN 10 DAYS OR IF HE LEAVES THE STATE; TIME SPENT OUT OF TEXAS DOES NOT COUNT TOWARD PROBATION. SHALL NOT SEEK MODIFICATION FOR ONE YEAR. ON 10/5/96 PROBATION TERMINATED.

STIVERS, ROBERT RUTHERFORD MD, DATE OF BIRTH AUGUST 31, 1934, LICENSE NUMBER 0012202 OF 2182 SPRING CREEK RD, ATLANTA, GA, WAS DISCIPLINED BY GEORGIA ON APRIL 5, 1991
DISCIPLINARY ACTION: EMERGENCY SUSPENSION
OFFENSE: SUBSTANCE ABUSE

NOTES: CHEMICAL DEPENDENCY (ALCOHOLISM) RELAPSE.

STIVERS, ROBERT RUTHERFORD MD, DATE OF BIRTH AUGUST 31, 1934, LICENSE NUMBER 0012202 OF 2182 SPRING CREEK RD, DECATUR, GA, WAS DISCIPLINED BY GEORGIA ON JUNE 1, 1992
DISCIPLINARY ACTION: 60-MONTH LICENSE SUSPENSION
OFFENSE: SUBSTANCE ABUSE

NOTES: PERSONAL USE OR ADDICTION (NARCOTIC VIOLATION), UNABLE TO PRACTICE MEDICINE WITH REASONABLE SKILL AND SAFETY TO THE PUBLIC BY REASON OF IMPAIRMENT. MAY PETITION FOR REINSTATEMENT AFTER TWO YEARS.

STIVERS, ROBERT RUTHERFORD MD, DATE OF BIRTH AUGUST 31, 1934, LICENSE NUMBER 00D4319 OF DECATUR, GA, WAS DISCIPLINED BY TEXAS ON APRIL 16, 1994
DISCIPLINARY ACTION: LICENSE REVOCATION
OFFENSE: DISCIPLINARY ACTION BY ANOTHER STATE OR AGENCY

NOTES: ON 4/5/91 GEORGIA BOARD ENTERED AN ORDER OF EMERGENCY SUSPENSION BECAUSE OF HIS RELAPSE INTO ALCOHOL DEPENDENCY; ON 6/1/92 GEORGIA SUSPENDED HIS LICENSE DUE TO HIS INABILITY TO PRACTICE MEDICINE WITH REASONABLE SKILL AND SAFETY BY REASON OF USE OF ALCOHOL; HE HAS NOT COMMUNICATED WITH TEXAS BOARD ABOUT THIS ACTION AND DID NOT APPEAR AT DISCIPLINARY HEARING CONCERNING THIS MATTER.

STOCKTON, ROBERT LOUIS MD, LICENSE NUMBER 00C8855 OF WACO, TX, WAS DISCIPLINED BY TEXAS ON JANUARY 26, 1990
DISCIPLINARY ACTION: 60-MONTH PROBATION; RESTRICTION PLACED ON LICENSE

NOTES: STIPULATED ORDER. MUST OBTAIN CONCURRING NEUROLOGICAL CONSULTATION PRIOR TO SURGERY ON ANY CASE WHICH HAS OR MAY HAVE NEUROSURGICAL IMPLICATIONS.

STOCKTON, ROBERT LOUIS MD, LICENSE NUMBER 0007457, WAS DISCIPLINED BY OKLAHOMA ON NOVEMBER 8, 1991
DISCIPLINARY ACTION: 60-MONTH PROBATION; MONITORING OF PHYSICIAN PERFORMANCE

NOTES: PROBATION RETROACTIVE TO 1/26/90 WITH FOLLOWING TERMS AND CONDITIONS: PRIOR TO PERFORMING SURGERY ON ANY CASE WHICH HAS OR MAY HAVE NEUROSURGICAL IMPLICATIONS, SHALL FIRST OBTAIN A WRITTEN CONCURRING NEUROLOGICAL CONSULTATION FROM AN ABMS BOARD-CERTIFIED NEUROSURGEON OR NEUROLOGIST; SHALL NOTIFY ANY HOSPITAL WHERE HE HOLDS STAFF PRIVILEGES OR CLINIC OR GROUP WHERE HE PRACTICES OF TERMS AND CONDITIONS; SHALL FURNISH BOARD WITH ADDRESS AND/OR CHANGE OF ADDRESS; SHALL APPEAR BEFORE BOARD UPON REQUEST. THIS PROBATION SHALL RUN CONCURRENTLY WITH THE EXISTING PROBATION TO THE TEXAS STATE BOARD OF MEDICAL EXAMINERS WITH REPORTS TO OKLAHOMA BOARD; SHALL APPEAR BEFORE OKLAHOMA BOARD BEFORE RESUMING PRACTICE IN THE STATE. ON 6/5/97 PROBATION TERMINATED AS HE RETIRED AND APPLIED FOR PHYSICIAN EMERITUS STATUS. IF REACTIVATE/REINSTATE LICENSE IN OKLAHOMA, TERMS OF PROBATION WOULD BE REINSTATED.

STOCKTON, ROBERT LOUIS MD, LICENSE NUMBER 00C8855 OF WACO, TX, WAS DISCIPLINED BY TEXAS ON JANUARY 14, 1994
DISCIPLINARY ACTION: SURRENDER OF LICENSE

NOTES: DOES NOT ADMIT ALLEGATIONS BUT SURRENDERS LICENSE IN LIEU OF FURTHER INVESTIGATION. SHALL NOT PETITION THE BOARD FOR REINSTATEMENT.

STOCKTON, ROBERT LOUIS MD OF 824 N 18TH STREET, WACO, TX, WAS DISCIPLINED BY DEA ON FEBRUARY 14, 1994
DISCIPLINARY ACTION: SURRENDER OF CONTROLLED SUBSTANCE LICENSE
OFFENSE: DISCIPLINARY ACTION BY ANOTHER STATE OR AGENCY

STOERMER, DIETRICH A MD, WAS DISCIPLINED BY NEVADA ON MARCH 5, 1993
DISCIPLINARY ACTION: RESTRICTION PLACED ON CONTROLLED SUBSTANCE LICENSE; REPRIMAND
OFFENSE: OVERPRESCRIBING OR MISPRESCRIBING DRUGS

NOTES: FAILED TO MAKE MEDICAL RECORDS AVAILABLE TO PATIENTS AND EXCESSIVE PRESCRIBING OF CONTROLLED SUBSTANCES. CONDITIONS: SUSPENDED FROM PRESCRIBING SCHEDULE II DRUGS UNTIL FURTHER ORDER OF THE BOARD; MUST COMPLETE CONTINUING MEDICAL EDUCATION ON CHRONIC PAIN MANAGEMENT INCLUDING INAPPROPRIATE WRITING OF PRESCRIPTIONS FOR CONTROLLED SUBSTANCES AND A COURSE ON APPROPRIATE MEDICAL RECORD KEEPING/DOCUMENTATION.

STOERMER, DIETRICH A MD, LICENSE NUMBER 0C39091 OF LAS VEGAS, NV, WAS DISCIPLINED BY CALIFORNIA ON SEPTEMBER 1, 1994
DISCIPLINARY ACTION: LICENSE REVOCATION
OFFENSE: DISCIPLINARY ACTION BY ANOTHER STATE OR AGENCY

NOTES: DISCIPLINED BY NEVADA BOARD FOR FAILURE TO MAKE MEDICAL RECORDS AVAILABLE TO PATIENTS FOR INSPECTION AND COPYING, AS REQUIRED BY LAW. DEFAULT DECISION.

STOERMER, DIETRICH ALBERT MD, LICENSE NUMBER 00E5952 OF

LAS VEGAS, NV, WAS DISCIPLINED BY TEXAS ON AUGUST 19, 1994
DISCIPLINARY ACTION: RESTRICTION PLACED ON CONTROLLED SUBSTANCE LICENSE; REQUIRED TO TAKE ADDITIONAL MEDICAL EDUCATION
OFFENSE: DISCIPLINARY ACTION BY ANOTHER STATE OR AGENCY

NOTES: LICENSE WAS DISCIPLINED BY ARIZONA BOARD ON 3/18/93. PRIOR TO PRACTICING IN TEXAS SHALL APPEAR BEFORE THE BOARD AND BE SUBJECT TO THE FOLLOWING RESTRICTIONS; SHALL NOT PRESCRIBE OR ADMINISTER SCHEDULE II CONTROLLED SUBSTANCES; SHALL ATTEND AT LEAST 50 HOURS PER YEAR OF CONTINUING MEDICAL EDUCATION INCLUDING AT LEAST 15 HOURS IN PAIN MANAGEMENT AND 6 HOURS IN RISK MANAGEMENT PER YEAR; SHALL GIVE A COPY OF THIS ORDER TO ANY HEALTH CARE ENTITY WHERE HE HAS PRIVILEGES; SHALL COOPERATE WITH THE BOARD IN VERIFYING COMPLIANCE; SHALL INFORM BOARD OF CHANGE OF ADDRESS WITHIN 10 DAYS. SHALL NOT SEEK MODIFICATION FOR ONE YEAR.

STOGRYN, RONALD S MD, LICENSE NUMBER F6123 OF SAN ANTONIO, TX, WAS DISCIPLINED BY TEXAS ON MAY 14, 1999
DISCIPLINARY ACTION: FINE; RESTRICTION PLACED ON CONTROLLED SUBSTANCE LICENSE
OFFENSE: LOSS OR RESTRICTION OF HOSPITAL PRIVILEGES

NOTES: HE WAS EXCLUDED AS A PROVIDER AT HUMANA HEALTH CARE DUE TO A DISCREPANCY IN HIS APPLICATION FOR REAPPOINTMENT; ON OR ABOUT 10/31/92 HUMANA TOOK MEDICAL PEER REVIEW ACTION AGAINST HIM; HUMANA HAD LEARNED THAT HE HAD LOST HIS PRIVILEGES AT A HOSPITAL IN ANOTHER CITY, BUT ON HIS APPLICATION HE DENIED ANY DISCIPLINARY ACTION BY THE HOSPITAL; HE AIDED AND ABETTED TWO SEPARATE INDIVIDUAL'S UNAUTHORIZED PRACTICE OF MEDICINE; HE WORKED AS A PHYSICIAN AT ADVANCED MEDICAL NUTRITION AND ENVIRONMENTAL HEALTH CENTER IN SAN ANTONIO FOR AN INDIVIDUAL WHO WAS NOT LICENSED AS A HEALTH CARE PROFESSIONAL BY A TEXAS AGENCY; HE REPORTS THAT HE WAS AWARE THAT THE AFOREMENTIONED INDIVIDUAL HAD ORDERED AND ADMINISTERED INTRAVENOUS CHELATION THERAPY TO PATIENTS THAT HE HAD NOT EXAMINED; HE WORKED AS A PHYSICIAN AT BROADWAY MEDICAL CLINIC WHICH WAS OWNED BY A NON-PHYSICIAN; HE APPROVED HIS DEA NUMBER FOR THE CLINIC TO PURCHASE APPETITE SUPPRESSANTS, DID NOT KNOW THE AMOUNT OF THE DRUGS OBTAINED UNDER HIS NAMES, NOR DID HE PAY FOR THEM, AND DID NOT APPROVE PURCHASES OR REVIEW INVOICES. PUBLIC REPRIMAND WITH FOLLOWING TERMS AND CONDITIONS FOR THREE YEARS: WITHIN 6 MONTHS SHALL TAKE AND PASS WITH A SCORE OF 75 OR ABOVE, WITHIN 3 ATTEMPTS, THE MEDICAL JURISPRUDENCE EXAM; $1,000 FINE; SHALL APPEAR AT LEAST ONCE A YEAR BEFORE THE BOARD; SHALL ADEQUATELY SUPERVISE THE ACTIVITIES OF ALL OF HIS EMPLOYEES AND OTHERS UNDER HIS SUPERVISION; SHALL EXAMINE AND/OR TREAT PATIENTS WHERE A FORM INDICATES HE HAS OR WHEN AN INITIAL DIAGNOSIS IS MADE; SHALL PERFORM 100 HOURS OF COMMUNITY SERVICE PER YEAR FOR A BOARD-APPROVED NON-PROFIT; SHALL ATTEND 50 HOURS PER YEAR OF CONTINUING MEDICAL EDUCATION WITH 1 COURSE IN THE AREA OF RISK MANAGEMENT AND AT LEAST 10 HOURS IN THE AREA OF ETHICS; SHALL SURRENDER HIS DEA AND TEXAS DEPARTMENT OF PUBLIC SAFETY CONTROLLED SUBSTANCES REGISTRATION CERTIFICATES; SHALL MAINTAIN ADEQUATE MEDICAL RECORDS WHICH SHALL BE AVAILABLE FOR REVIEW; SEPARATE FROM PATIENT RECORDS, SHALL MAINTAIN A LOGBOOK OF EVERY PRESCRIPTION WRITTEN BY HIM FOR DANGEROUS DRUGS WITH ADDICTIVE POTENTIAL WHICH SHALL BE MADE AVAILABLE FOR REVIEW; SHALL COOPERATE WITH THE BOARD IN VERIFYING COMPLIANCE; SHALL GIVE A COPY OF THIS ORDER TO ANY HEALTH CARE ENTITY WHERE HE HAS PRIVILEGES; TIME SPENT OUT OF TEXAS DOES NOT COUNT TOWARD RESTRICTION; SHALL INFORM THE BOARD OF CHANGE OF ADDRESS WITHIN 10 DAYS OR IF HE LEAVES THE STATE; SHALL NOT SEEK MODIFICATION FOR ONE YEAR.

STOWE, ROBERT HOMAN MD, LICENSE NUMBER 00H2814 OF EL PASO, TX, WAS DISCIPLINED BY TEXAS ON APRIL 15, 1994
DISCIPLINARY ACTION: 120-MONTH PROBATION; RESTRICTION PLACED ON LICENSE
OFFENSE: LOSS OR RESTRICTION OF HOSPITAL PRIVILEGES

NOTES: HAD A HISTORY OF ALCOHOL USE STARTING BACK IN HIGH SCHOOL; PERIODICALLY ABUSED ALCOHOL SINCE RESIDENCY; ADMITS THAT ON OCCASIONS HE PRACTICED MEDICINE WHEN HE WAS USING DRUGS OR UNDER THE INFLUENCE OF DRUGS; HOSPITAL PRIVILEGES WERE SUMMARILY SUSPENDED ON 3/3/93 PENDING THE OUTCOME OF DRUG TREATMENT AND REHABILITATION BASED ON A POSITIVE DRUG SCREEN; DISCHARGED FROM INPATIENT TREATMENT ON 7/13/93; IS CURRENTLY UNDER TREATMENT ON AN OUTPATIENT BASIS; SOBRIETY DATE 4/22/93; SINCE COMPLETION OF TREATMENT PROGRAM HAS BEEN ATTENDING AA ON A DAILY BASIS. TEN YEAR SUSPENSION STAYED. CONDITIONS OF PROBATION: SHALL ABSTAIN FROM THE CONSUMPTION OF ALCOHOL/CHEMICAL SUBSTANCES IN ANY FORM UNLESS PRESCRIBED BY ANOTHER PHYSICIAN FOR A LEGITIMATE AND THERAPEUTIC PURPOSE; SHALL NOT TREAT OR OTHERWISE SERVE AS PHYSICIAN, PRESCRIBE, DISPENSE OR ADMINISTER DRUGS THAT MAY BE SUBJECT TO ABUSE TO HIMSELF OR ANY MEMBER OF HIS FAMILY; SHALL PARTICIPATE IN ACTIVITIES OF A PHYSICIAN HEALTH AND REHABILITATION COMMITTEE AND ATTEND MEETINGS WITH QUARTERLY REPORTS; SHALL LIMIT HIS MEDICAL PRACTICE SOLELY TO THE PRACTICE OF ANESTHESIOLOGY IN HOSPITAL AND LICENSED AMBULATORY SURGERY SETTINGS; SHALL NOT POSSESS, ADMINISTER, DISPENSE OR PRESCRIBE ANY CONTROLLED SUBSTANCES EXCEPT TO ORDER THEM FOR HOSPITAL AND SURGICAL CENTER PATIENTS AND WHILE UNDER THE OBSERVATION OF A LICENSED PHYSICIAN OR REGISTERED NURSE; SHALL MAINTAIN A NOTEBOOK CONTAINING COPIES OF ALL PATIENT ANESTHESIA RECORDS AVAILABLE FOR INSPECTION; SHALL CONTINUE TO PARTICIPATE IN AA'S PROGRAM NOT LESS THAN THREE TIMES A WEEK WITH QUARTERLY REPORTS TO THE BOARD; SHALL SUBMIT HIMSELF FOR APPROPRIATE EXAMS INCLUDING DRUG OR ALCOHOL SCREENS; SHALL CONTINUE TO RECEIVE TREATMENT FROM A SPECIFIED PHYSICIAN WITH QUARTERLY REPORTS; SHALL HAVE RANDOM DRUG SCREENS BY HAIR ANALYSIS AT LEAST FOUR TIMES PER YEAR; SHALL APPEAR BEFORE THE BOARD TWICE A YEAR. ON 1/27/96 PROBATION MODIFIED LOOSENING THE RESTRICTIONS ON THE IMPAIRED PHYSICIANS PROGRAM HE SHALL PARTICIPATE WITH AND THE TREATMENT PHYSICIAN HE SHALL SEE; SHALL BE ABLE TO PRACTICE WITHIN A PSYCHIATRIC RESIDENCY EXCLUSIVELY AND SHALL BE ABLE TO ORDER CONTROLLED SUBSTANCES FOR PSYCHIATRIC PATIENTS AS PART OF THIS PROGRAM; DRUG SCREENS ARE REDUCED TO ONE PER YEAR;

SHALL APPEAR BEFORE THE BOARD ONCE A YEAR. ON 1/29/99 ORDER TERMINATED.

STRICKLAND, ALAN D MD, LICENSE NUMBER 00E2885 OF RICHARDSON, TX, WAS DISCIPLINED BY TEXAS ON DECEMBER 1, 1990
DISCIPLINARY ACTION: 24-MONTH PROBATION; RESTRICTION PLACED ON LICENSE
OFFENSE: PROFESSIONAL MISCONDUCT

NOTES: ADMINISTERED DRUG OR TREATMENT THAT WAS NONTHERAPEUTIC IN NATURE. FAILED PROFESSIONALLY TO PRACTICE MEDICINE IN ACCEPTABLE MANNER CONSISTENT WITH PUBLIC HEALTH AND WELFARE. RESTRICTIONS INCLUDE REFRAINING FROM RESEARCHING OR ADMINISTERING NONAPPROVED DRUGS WITHOUT INFORMED WRITTEN CONSENT AND REFRAINING FROM CONDUCTING EXPERIMENTS OR RESEARCH WITHOUT EXPRESS APPROVAL OF PROPER HOSPITAL AUTHORITY OR REVIEW COMMITTEE. MOTION FILED FOR REHEARING.

STRICKLAND, ANN ROBERTSHAW MD, DATE OF BIRTH JULY 29, 1951, LICENSE NUMBER 00F8330 OF 2476 BOLSOVER BOX 471, HOUSTON, TX, WAS DISCIPLINED BY TEXAS ON JUNE 15, 1993
DISCIPLINARY ACTION: LICENSE SUSPENSION
OFFENSE: PHYSICAL OR MENTAL ILLNESS INHIBITING THE ABILITY TO PRACTICE WITH SKILL AND SAFETY

NOTES: SUFFERS FROM A COMPLEX PARTIAL SEIZURE DISORDER, FIBROMYALGIA, AND OSTEOPOROSIS WITH ASSOCIATED FATIGUE AND PHYSICAL DIFFICULTIES AS WELL AS DEPRESSION AND CHRONIC POST TRAUMATIC STRESS DISORDER; AILMENTS ARE SO SEVERE SHE IS PRESENTLY UNABLE TO PRACTICE. LICENSE SUSPENDED UNTIL SHE PERSONALLY APPEARS BEFORE THE BOARD AND PROVIDES SUFFICIENT EVIDENCE TO SHOW THAT SHE IS PHYSICALLY, MENTALLY AND OTHERWISE COMPETENT TO PRACTICE INCLUDING PSYCHIATRIC REPORTS AND CURRENT PHYSICAL EXAMS; SHALL GIVE A COPY OF THIS ORDER TO ANY HEALTH CARE ENTITY WHERE SHE HAS PRIVILEGES; SHALL COOPERATE WITH THE BOARD IN VERIFYING COMPLIANCE; SHALL INFORM BOARD OF CHANGE OF ADDRESS.

STRINGER, DRENNON DURWOOD MD, LICENSE NUMBER 00F2953 OF DALLAS, TX, WAS DISCIPLINED BY TEXAS ON MARCH 5, 1994
DISCIPLINARY ACTION: REPRIMAND
OFFENSE: OVERPRESCRIBING OR MISPRESCRIBING DRUGS

NOTES: DISPENSED MEDICATIONS TO A PATIENT WHEN ACCESS TO A PHARMACY WAS POSSIBLE. SHALL GIVE A COPY OF THIS ORDER TO ANY HEALTH CARE ENTITY WHERE HE HAS PRIVILEGES.

STUBBLEFIELD, WAYNE MD, LICENSE NUMBER 00F2955 OF OKLAHOMA CITY, OK, WAS DISCIPLINED BY TEXAS ON AUGUST 18, 1990
OFFENSE: DISCIPLINARY ACTION BY ANOTHER STATE OR AGENCY

NOTES: STIPULATED ORDER. MUST COMPLY WITH TENNESSEE BOARD AGREED ORDER AND OKLAHOMA BOARD FINAL ORDER. IF DESIRING TO PRACTICE MEDICINE IN TEXAS, MUST DEMONSTRATE TO BOARD CAPACITY TO PRACTICE MEDICINE WITH REASONABLE SKILL AND SAFETY. IF AUTHORIZED TO PRACTICE IN TEXAS, MUST FOLLOW ANY ADDITIONAL TERMS OF PROBATION AS MAY BE IMPOSED.

SULLIVAN, BRIAN LOREN MD, LICENSE NUMBER 00E1946 OF AUSTIN, TX, WAS DISCIPLINED BY TEXAS ON APRIL 20, 1991
DISCIPLINARY ACTION: 24-MONTH PROBATION

NOTES: SHALL NOT TREAT OR OTHERWISE SERVE AS THE PHYSICIAN, PRESCRIBE, DISPENSE, OR ADMINISTER CONTROLLED SUBSTANCES OR ANY OTHER DRUGS THAT MAY BE SUBJECT TO ABUSE, OR WRITE PRESCRIPTIONS FOR CONTROLLED SUBSTANCES, FOR ANY MEMBER OF IMMEDIATE FAMILY; SHALL ADMINISTER TO IMMEDIATE FAMILY ONLY DRUGS THAT ARE PRESCRIBED BY OTHER PHYSICIANS; SHALL HAVE NO CONTROLLED SUBSTANCES, INCLUDING SAMPLES, IN HIS RESIDENCE UNLESS PRESCRIBED BY A PHYSICIAN OTHER THAN SELF AND ARE IN ORIGINAL CONTAINER AS DISPENSED; SHALL APPEAR BEFORE THE BOARD ANNUALLY.

SWARTZ, JOE M MD, DATE OF BIRTH OCTOBER 7, 1947, LICENSE NUMBER 0025956 OF BOULDER, CO, WAS DISCIPLINED BY COLORADO ON NOVEMBER 10, 1994
DISCIPLINARY ACTION: REPRIMAND

SWARTZ, JOE M MD, DATE OF BIRTH OCTOBER 7, 1947, LICENSE NUMBER 0025956, WAS DISCIPLINED BY COLORADO ON JUNE 8, 1995
DISCIPLINARY ACTION: REPRIMAND

SWARTZ, JOE M MD, LICENSE NUMBER 0C36167 OF BOULDER, CO, WAS DISCIPLINED BY CALIFORNIA ON FEBRUARY 13, 1996
DISCIPLINARY ACTION: REPRIMAND
OFFENSE: DISCIPLINARY ACTION BY ANOTHER STATE OR AGENCY

NOTES: ACTION IN COLORADO FOR UNJUSTIFIED USE OF NARCOTICS FOR MANAGEMENT OF PATIENT'S ABUSIVE MEMORY AND POST-TRAUMATIC STRESS DISORDER.

SWARTZ, JOE MATTHEW MD, LICENSE NUMBER 00E1145 OF BOULDER, CO, WAS DISCIPLINED BY TEXAS ON AUGUST 18, 1995
DISCIPLINARY ACTION: REPRIMAND
OFFENSE: DISCIPLINARY ACTION BY ANOTHER STATE OR AGENCY

NOTES: IN 10/91, COLORADO BOARD ISSUED HIM A LETTER OF ADMONITION BASED ON HIS PRESCRIBING CONTROLLED SUBSTANCES INCLUDING, BUT NOT LIMITED TO, HYDROCODONE, PERCOCET AND VICODIN TO A PATIENT WITHOUT ADEQUATE INDICATIONS OF A LEGITIMATE MEDICAL PURPOSE; MAINTAINS PRESCRIBING WAS MEDICALLY APPROPRIATE; IN APPROXIMATELY 1/95, HE ENTERED A PLEA OF GUILTY AND WAS CONVICTED FOR A FEDERAL CRIMINAL OFFENSE FOR MAKING A FALSE STATEMENT ON AN APPLICATION FOR MEDICARE PAYMENT. LICENSE RESTRICTED WITH TERMS: SHALL NOT PRACTICE MEDICINE IN TEXAS UNTIL HE APPEARS BEFORE BOARD WITH SUFFICIENT EVIDENCE WHICH INDICATES THAT HE IS PHYSICALLY, MENTALLY AND OTHERWISE COMPETENT TO SAFELY PRACTICE MEDICINE, HAS COMPLIED WITH ALL TERMS OF PROBATION AS SET FORTH IN COURT'S JUDGMENT AND HAS FULLY COMPLIED WITH AND SATISFIED ALL TERMS OF ANY ACTION TAKEN BY ANOTHER STATE; SHALL COOPERATE WITH BOARD IN VERIFYING COMPLIANCE; SHALL GIVE A COPY OF THIS ORDER TO ANY HEALTH CARE ENTITY WHERE HE HAS PRIVILEGES; TIME PERIOD OUT OF TEXAS DOES NOT COUNT TOWARD RESTRICTION; SHALL INFORM BOARD OF CHANGE OF ADDRESS WITHIN 10 DAYS OR IF HE LEAVES THE STATE. SHALL NOT SEEK MODIFICATION FOR ONE YEAR.

SWATE, TOMMY MD, LICENSE NUMBER R3011 OF SAN ANTONIO, TX, WAS DISCIPLINED BY ARKANSAS ON JANUARY 4, 1997
DISCIPLINARY ACTION: 120-MONTH PROBATION

NOTES: PROBATION IN CONJUNCTION WITH TEXAS.

SWATE, TOMMY ERNEST MD, LICENSE NUMBER 00E3781 OF HOUSTON, TX, WAS DISCIPLINED BY TEXAS ON JANUARY 24, 1992
DISCIPLINARY ACTION: 60-MONTH PROBATION
OFFENSE: SUBSTANDARD CARE, INCOMPETENCE OR NEGLIGENCE

NOTES: PROFESSIONAL FAILURE TO PRACTICE MEDICINE IN AN ACCEPTABLE MANNER CONSISTENT WITH PUBLIC HEALTH AND WELFARE, AND REPEATED OR RECURRING MERITORIOUS HEALTH-CARE LIABILITY CLAIMS. LICENSE SUSPENDED, SUSPENSION STAYED; PROBATION UNDER TERMS AND CONDITIONS.

SWATE, TOMMY ERNEST MD OF HOUSTON, TX, WAS DISCIPLINED BY LOUISIANA ON JANUARY 28, 1993
DISCIPLINARY ACTION: 48-MONTH PROBATION
OFFENSE: DISCIPLINARY ACTION BY ANOTHER STATE OR AGENCY

NOTES: ACTION TAKEN BY TEXAS. TERMS AND CONDITIONS OF PROBATION AS FOLLOWS: SUBJECT TO COMPLIANCE WITH TERMS AND CONDITIONS OF DISCIPLINARY ORDER OF TEXAS BOARD; PRIOR NOTIFICATION TO BOARD OF INTENT TO RELOCATE TO LOUISIANA.

SWATE, TOMMY ERNEST MD, LICENSE NUMBER 00E3781 OF ALPINE, TX, WAS DISCIPLINED BY TEXAS ON MARCH 2, 1996
DISCIPLINARY ACTION: 120-MONTH PROBATION; RESTRICTION PLACED ON LICENSE
OFFENSE: PROVIDING FALSE INFORMATION TO THE BOARD OR OTHER HEALTH AGENCY

NOTES: ON 1/20/94 A LOUISIANA ORDER PLACED HIM ON FOUR YEAR PROBATION SUBJECT TO COMPLIANCE WITH THE TEXAS ORDER OF 1992 WITH OTHER CONDITIONS; HAD FAILED TO REPORT 1992 TEXAS ORDER TO LOUISIANA; HAD TOLD LOUISIANA HAD NOT PRACTICED FOR THREE YEARS WHEN IN FACT HE HAD FUNCTIONED AS MEDICAL DIRECTOR OF TWO CLINICS IN TEXAS. DOES NOT ADMIT VIOLATION. SUSPENSION STAYED AS PROBATION WITH TERMS AND CONDITIONS ONE OF WHICH HE MAY SELECT: WITHIN ONE YEAR SHALL ENROLL IN AND SUCCESSFULLY COMPLETE A FULL TIME THREE YEAR RESIDENCY PROGRAM, IN WHICH CASE PROBATION SHALL BE REDUCED TO FIVE YEARS UPON SUCCESSFUL COMPLETION OF THE THREE YEAR PROGRAM; OR SHALL ENROLL IN AND SUCCESSFULLY COMPLETE A BOARD APPROVED SIX MONTH MINI-RESIDENCY IN WHICH CASE PROBATION SHALL BE REDUCED TO SEVEN YEARS; OR MAY PRACTICE MEDICINE IN A BOARD APPROVED INSTITUTIONAL SETTING OR MAY PRACTICE EMERGENCY ROOM MEDICINE IN CONJUNCTION WITH HIS REMEDIAL TRAINING, PROVIDED HOWEVER, THAT HE ATTEND AT LEAST 25 HOURS IN EMERGENCY MEDICINE AND NO REDUCTION IN PROBATIONARY TERM; THE FOLLOWING TERMS SHALL CONTINUE IN FULL FORCE REGARDLESS OF THE OPTION CHOSEN BY HIM UNLESS OTHERWISE SPECIFIED: SHALL NOT OPERATE A METHADONE CLINIC WITHIN TEXAS; SHALL MAINTAIN ADEQUATE MEDICAL RECORDS WHICH SHALL BE AVAILABLE FOR REVIEW; SHALL NOT SIGN ON ANY PATIENT RECORD THAT HE HAS SEEN THE PATIENT UNLESS HE HAS ACTUALLY SEEN THE PATIENT OR UNLESS THE PATIENT'S CHART CLEARLY REFLECTS THAT HE DID NOT; SHALL OBTAIN AT LEAST 50 HOURS PER YEAR OF CONTINUING MEDICAL EDUCATION; SHALL OBTAIN SIX HOURS OF AN ETHICS COURSE OR PROGRAM FOR EACH YEAR ON PROBATION; WITHIN ONE YEAR SHALL COMPLETE AN ADVANCED CARDIAC LIFE SUPPORT COURSE (ACLS) AND AN ADVANCED TRAUMA LIFE SUPPORT COURSE (ATLS) AND SHALL OBTAIN CERTIFICATION OF BOTH; WITHIN ONE YEAR SHALL TAKE AND PASS THE MEDICAL JURISPRUDENCE EXAMINATION; EACH YEAR SHALL PERFORM 120 HOURS OF COMMUNITY SERVICE FOR A BOARD APPROVED NON-PROFIT CHARITABLE ORGANIZATION AND SUBMIT PROOF OF COMPLETION TO THE BOARD; SHALL FOLLOW THE TERMS OF THE LOUISIANA ORDER AND SHALL PROVIDE THE BOARD WITH COPIES OF REPORTS SUBMITTED TO THE LOUISIANA BOARD; SHALL GIVE A COPY OF THIS ORDER TO ANY HEALTH CARE ENTITY WHERE HE HAS PRIVILEGES; SHALL COOPERATE WITH THE BOARD IN VERIFYING COMPLIANCE; TIME PERIOD OUT OF TEXAS DOES NOT COUNT TOWARD PROBATION EXCEPT IN FULFILLING RESIDENCY OPTIONS; SHALL INFORM THE BOARD OF CHANGE OF ADDRESS WITHIN 10 DAYS OF IF HE LEAVES THE STATE; SHALL NOT SEEK MODIFICATION FOR ONE YEAR.

SWERSKY, ERNEST DOUGLAS MD, LICENSE NUMBER 00F1263 OF DALLAS, TX, WAS DISCIPLINED BY TEXAS ON NOVEMBER 3, 1994
DISCIPLINARY ACTION: 60-MONTH PROBATION; RESTRICTION PLACED ON LICENSE
OFFENSE: PROFESSIONAL MISCONDUCT

NOTES: IN THE CASE OF FOUR PATIENTS FAILED TO DOCUMENT CARE AND TREATMENT IN THAT HE PROVIDED PSYCHOTHERAPY SESSIONS IN THE EVENING AFTER REGULAR OFFICE HOURS; DID NOT DOCUMENT IN THEIR RECORDS ANY INDICATIONS OF EMOTIONAL OR PSYCHOLOGICAL DIFFICULTIES OR ANY COUNSELING SESSIONS; DID NOT CHARGE THEM FOR THESE SESSIONS; FAILED TO MAINTAIN APPROPRIATE BOUNDARIES WITH ONE PATIENT BY DEVELOPING A PERSONAL AND SOCIAL RELATIONSHIP; ENGAGED IN PSYCHIATRIC COUNSELING OF PATIENTS WITHOUT APPROPRIATE TESTING, EVALUATION AND REFERRAL. SUSPENSION STAYED. CONDITIONS OF PROBATION: SHALL SUBMIT HIMSELF FOR EVALUATION AND TREATMENT BY A BOARD-APPROVED PSYCHIATRIST WITHIN 30 DAYS; SHALL REFRAIN FROM PERFORMING ANY PSYCHIATRIC COUNSELING; SHALL BE MONITORED BY A PHYSICIAN ACCEPTABLE TO THE BOARD; SHALL NOT PRESCRIBE ANY PSYCHOTROPIC DRUGS WITHOUT CONSULTATION WITH A BOARD-APPROVED PHYSICIAN; MONITORING PHYSICIAN SHALL SUBMIT REPORTS EVERY FOUR MONTHS; SHALL MAINTAIN ADEQUATE MEDICAL RECORDS ON ALL PATIENT OFFICE VISITS WHICH SHALL BE AVAILABLE FOR INSPECTION; SHALL NOT SIGN ANY PATIENT RECORD UNLESS HE HAS PERSONALLY EXAMINED THE PATIENT OR CLEARLY NOTES IN THE RECORD THAT HE DID NOT; SHALL ATTEND AT LEAST 50 HOURS PER YEAR OF CONTINUING MEDICAL EDUCATION; SHALL HAVE A CHAPERONE PRESENT ANY TIME HE PERFORMS A PHYSICAL EXAM ON A FEMALE PATIENT WITH THIS DOCUMENTED IN THE CHART; SHALL PERFORM 10 HOURS PER MONTH OF COMMUNITY SERVICE FOR A HOMELESS SHELTER OR OTHER SIMILAR PROGRAM; SHALL APPEAR BEFORE THE BOARD ONCE A YEAR; SHALL GIVE A COPY OF THIS ORDER TO ANY HEALTH CARE ENTITY WHERE HE HAS PRIVILEGES; SHALL COOPERATE WITH THE BOARD IN VERIFYING COMPLIANCE; SHALL INFORM BOARD OF CHANGE OF ADDRESS WITHIN 10 DAYS OR IF HE LEAVES THE STATE; TIME SPENT OUT OF TEXAS DOES NOT COUNT TOWARD PROBATION. SHALL NOT SEEK MODIFICATION FOR ONE YEAR. ON 3/1/97 PETITION TO MODIFY ORDER GRANTED DELETING REQUIREMENT

TO OBTAIN A TREATING PSYCHIATRIST AND SUBMIT TO FOLLOW-UP CARE AND COUNSELING AT LEAST TWICE MONTHLY. ON 11/22/97 PETITION FOR MODIFICATION OF ORDER GRANTED ALLOWING HIM TO PRESCRIBE PSYCHOTROPIC DRUGS AND CONDUCT PSYCHIATRIC COUNSELING. ON 10/24/98 ORDER TERMINATED.

SWICEGOOD, WILLIAM R II MD, LICENSE NUMBER 00F5132, WAS DISCIPLINED BY TEXAS ON AUGUST 17, 1996
DISCIPLINARY ACTION: 60-MONTH PROBATION; FINE
OFFENSE: PROFESSIONAL MISCONDUCT

NOTES: PRIOR TO 6/07/95 UTILIZED TELEPHONE DIRECTORY ADVERTISEMENTS AND BUSINESS CARDS WHICH DID NOT CONTAIN THE COMPLETE NAME OF THE SPECIALTY BOARD THROUGH WHICH HE WAS CERTIFIED AND COULD BE CONSTRUED TO IMPLY BOARD CERTIFICATION IN FAMILY PRACTICE WHEN HE HELD ONLY EMERGENCY MEDICINE CERTIFICATION IN VIOLATION OF ADVERTISING RULES; MAINTAINS THESE WERE ORDERED BY A NEW ASSISTANT AND ERRORS HAVE BEEN CORRECTED; AND FAILED TO KEEP COMPLETE AND ACCURATE RECORDS OF PURCHASES AND DISPOSALS OF DRUGS. SUSPENSION STAYED. CONDITIONS OF PROBATION: SHALL SUBMIT HIMSELF TO EVALUATION AND TREATMENT BY BOARD-APPROVED PSYCHIATRIST WHO HE SHALL SEE AT LEAST ONCE A MONTH FOR NOT LESS THAN ONE YEAR AND WHO SHALL PROVIDE REPORTS; SHALL CONTINUE HIS PRACTICE OF HAVING A CHAPERONE PRESENT IN THE ROOM DURING THE EXAMINATION OF A FEMALE PATIENT AND SHALL MAKE NOTATION IN THE PATIENT'S CHART; SHALL MAINTAIN ADEQUATE MEDICAL RECORDS WHICH SHALL BE AVAILABLE FOR REVIEW; SHALL OBTAIN AT LEAST 50 HOURS PER YEAR OF CONTINUING MEDICAL EDUCATION; SHALL OBTAIN 50 HOURS OF AN ETHICS COURSE OR PROGRAM FOR ONE YEAR AND SUBMIT PROOF TO THE BOARD; SHALL APPEAR BEFORE THE BOARD AT LEAST ONCE PER YEAR OR UPON BOARD REQUEST; SHALL COOPERATE WITH THE BOARD IN VERIFYING COMPLIANCE; SHALL GIVE A COPY OF THIS ORDER TO ANY HEALTH CARE ENTITY WITH SPECIFIED EXCLUSIONS WHERE HE HAS PRIVILEGES; SHALL PROVIDE A COPY OF THIS ORDER TO ANYONE REQUESTING IT WITHIN 10 DAYS; TIME PERIOD OUT OF TEXAS DOES NOT COUNT TOWARD PROBATION; SHALL INFORM THE BOARD OF CHANGE OF ADDRESS WITHIN 10 DAYS OF IF HE LEAVES THE STATE; SHALL NOT SEEK MODIFICATION FOR ONE YEAR. $5,000 ADMINISTRATIVE PENALTY; REPRIMAND.

SWIFT, LEON JOSEPH DO, LICENSE NUMBER H4739 OF ARLINGTON, TX, WAS DISCIPLINED BY TEXAS ON AUGUST 28, 1999
DISCIPLINARY ACTION: 60-MONTH RESTRICTION PLACED ON LICENSE; RESTRICTION PLACED ON CONTROLLED SUBSTANCE LICENSE
OFFENSE: FAILURE TO COMPLY WITH PREVIOUS BOARD ORDER

NOTES: VIOLATED 1/18/97 AGREED REHABILITATION ORDER BY FAILING TO ATTEND AA MEETINGS IN 7/98 AND 8/98 AND FAILING TO PROVIDE A TREATING PHYSICIAN A COPY OF HIS AGREED REHABILITATION ORDER; VOLUNTARILY DISCONTINUED HIS OFFICE PRACTICE FROM 7/1/98 THROUGH 10/11/98; ADVISED THE BOARD HE WAS TAKING HYDROCODONE FOR HIS NECK AND XANAX FOR DEPRESSION; HE REPORTS THAT HE HAS VOLUNTARILY NOT SEEN PATIENTS SINCE 12/98; HE REPORTS THAT HE CURRENTLY ATTENDS 6 AA MEETINGS PER WEEK AND THAT HIS INABILITY TO ATTEND 7-8/98 AA MEETINGS WAS DUE TO HIS ANXIETY DISORDER; HE REPORTS THAT HE HAS ABSTAINED FROM ANY DRUG OR ALCOHOL OTHER THAN AS PRESCRIBED BY HIS PHYSICIANS; HIS TREATING PHYSICIANS AND REPRESENTATIVES HAVE REPORTED TO THE BOARD THAT BASED ON THEIR CURRENT OBSERVATIONS, HE IS MENTALLY AND PHYSICALLY COMPETENT TO SAFELY PRACTICE UNDER CERTAIN CONDITIONS. LICENSE LIMITED AS FOLLOWS: SHALL NOT PRACTICE BEYOND 20 HOURS PER WEEK UNLESS HE APPEARS BEFORE THE BOARD DEMONSTRATING HIS COMPETENCE TO RESUME FULL TIME PRACTICE; SHALL ABSTAIN FROM THE CONSUMPTION OF ALCOHOL/DRUGS IN ANY FORM UNLESS PRESCRIBED BY ANOTHER PHYSICIAN FOR A LEGITIMATE AND THERAPEUTIC PURPOSE; SHALL SUBMIT HIMSELF FOR APPROPRIATE EXAMS INCLUDING DRUG OR ALCOHOL SCREENS; WITHIN 60 DAYS, SHALL NOMINATE THREE CERTIFIED PSYCHIATRISTS FOR BOARD SELECTION OF A THERAPIST AND SHALL EXPEDITIOUSLY SUBMIT HIMSELF TO EVALUATION AND TREATMENT BY THE APPROVED PRACTITIONER; WITHIN 60 DAYS, SHALL NOMINATE THREE CERTIFIED PHYSICIANS TO SERVE AS HIS PRIMARY CARE PHYSICIAN; SHALL PARTICIPATE IN THE ACTIVITIES OF A PHYSICIAN HEALTH AND REHABILITATION COMMITTEE AND ABIDE BY ANY AFTERCARE PROGRAM CONTRACT REQUIRED WITH QUARTERLY REPORTS; SHALL PARTICIPATE IN AA'S PROGRAM NO LESS THAN 90 TIMES IN 90 DAYS AND THEREAFTER ON A REGULAR BASIS ON NOT LESS THAN 5 TIMES EACH WEEK; SHALL REPORT ON HIS ATTENDANCE; SHALL SURRENDER ANY DRUGS WITH POTENTIAL FOR ABUSE IN HIS POSSESSION INCLUDING SAMPLES AND ALL UNUSED TRIPLICATE PRESCRIPTION FORMS; SHALL OBTAIN 50 HOURS PER YEAR OF CONTINUING MEDICAL EDUCATION; SHALL APPEAR BEFORE THE BOARD UPON REQUEST; SHALL COOPERATE WITH THE BOARD IN VERIFYING COMPLIANCE INCLUDING PROVIDING COPIES OF MEDICAL RELEASES UPON REQUEST; SHALL GIVE A COPY OF THIS ORDER TO ANY HEALTH CARE ENTITY WHERE HE HAS PRIVILEGES; SHALL PROVIDE A COPY OF THIS ORDER TO ANYONE REQUESTING IT WITHIN 10 DAYS; TIME SPENT OUT OF TEXAS DOES NOT COUNT TOWARD RESTRICTION; SHALL INFORM THE BOARD OF CHANGE OF ADDRESS WITHIN 10 DAYS OR IF HE LEAVES THE STATE.

SYRQUIN, ABRAHAM F MD, LICENSE NUMBER 0A26144 OF GRAND PRAIRIE, TX, WAS DISCIPLINED BY CALIFORNIA ON MARCH 8, 1996
DISCIPLINARY ACTION: REPRIMAND
OFFENSE: DISCIPLINARY ACTION BY ANOTHER STATE OR AGENCY

NOTES: ACTION IN TEXAS FOR FAILURE TO OBTAIN INFORMED CONSENT PRIOR TO REMOVING A SPONGE LEFT IN A PATIENT'S ABDOMEN FROM A PREVIOUS SURGERY AND CONCEALED THE SPONGE FOR SIX HOURS UNTIL CONFRONTED BY HOSPITAL OFFICIALS.

SYRQUIN, ABRAHAM FINKELBERG MD, LICENSE NUMBER 00D4325 OF GRAND PRAIRIE, TX, WAS DISCIPLINED BY TEXAS ON JUNE 26, 1992
DISCIPLINARY ACTION: REPRIMAND
OFFENSE: PROFESSIONAL MISCONDUCT

NOTES: UNPROFESSIONAL OR DISHONORABLE CONDUCT THAT IS LIKELY TO DECEIVE, DEFRAUD OR INJURE THE PUBLIC.

TABATABAI, JAFAR MD, LICENSE NUMBER 00D3792 OF STONE MOUNTAIN, GA, WAS DISCIPLINED BY TEXAS ON AUGUST 24, 1991
DISCIPLINARY ACTION: 60-MONTH PROBATION
OFFENSE: DISCIPLINARY ACTION BY ANOTHER STATE OR AGENCY

NOTES: SUSPENSION STAYED. SHALL COMPLY WITH TERMS OF GEORGIA BOARD ORDER; PRIOR TO PRACTICING IN TEXAS, SHALL APPEAR BEFORE AND RECEIVE APPROVAL OF TEXAS BOARD.

TABOADA, LUIS ENRIQUE MD, LICENSE NUMBER 00F2961 OF SAN ANTONIO, TX, WAS DISCIPLINED BY TEXAS ON NOVEMBER 3, 1994
DISCIPLINARY ACTION: FINE; REPRIMAND
OFFENSE: PROFESSIONAL MISCONDUCT

NOTES: FAILED TO MAINTAIN PROPER BOUNDARIES IN AN INTERPERSONAL RELATIONSHIP WITH AN ADULT FEMALE PATIENT WHOM HE INITIALLY MET IN A SOCIAL SETTING. $1,000 ADMINISTRATIVE PENALTY; SHALL WITHIN SIX MONTHS RESEARCH AND WRITE A PAPER ON APPROPRIATE AND INAPPROPRIATE INTERPERSONAL RELATIONSHIPS BETWEEN PHYSICIANS AND PATIENTS; SHALL GIVE A COPY OF THIS ORDER TO ANY HEALTH CARE ENTITY WERE HE HAS PRIVILEGES; SHALL COOPERATE WITH THE BOARD IN VERIFYING COMPLIANCE; SHALL INFORM BOARD OF CHANGE OF ADDRESS WITHIN 10 DAYS. SHALL NOT SEEK MODIFICATION FOR SIX MONTHS.

TACKER, WILLIS A MD, LICENSE NUMBER D7325, WAS DISCIPLINED BY TEXAS ON MAY 10, 1997
DISCIPLINARY ACTION: FINE; REPRIMAND
OFFENSE: NONCOMPLIANCE WITH A PROFESSIONAL RULE

NOTES: FAILED TO OBTAIN THE REQUIRED 24 HOURS OF CONTINUING MEDICAL EDUCATION FROM 6/1/95 TO 5/31/96 FOR THE RENEWAL OF HIS LICENSE ON 6/1/96. HE WAS ISSUED A TEMPORARY PERMIT WHICH GRANTED HIM 90 DAYS, OR UNTIL 8/30/96, TO OBTAIN THE 24 REQUIRED HOURS. HE FAILED TO OBTAIN THESE HOURS BY THE DEADLINE AND HIS LICENSE HAS BEEN IN "DELINQUENT" STATUS SINCE THEN. ON 8/30/96 HE WAS ASSESSED A PENALTY FEE OF $100 FOR LATE REGISTRATION AND HIS FAILURE TO COMPLETE EDUCATION CREDITS. ON 6/1/96 HE WAS ASSESSED A $50 FEE FOR THE TEMPORARY LICENSE. HE WILL BE REQUIRED TO OBTAIN ALL PAST DUE CONTINUING MEDICAL EDUCATION HOURS BEFORE HE WILL BE ISSUED A CURRENT PHYSICIAN'S PERMIT. SHALL ALSO PAY AN ADMINISTRATIVE PENALTY OF $100; SHALL COOPERATE WITH THE BOARD IN VERIFYING COMPLIANCE.

TAKASE, KOUJI MD, LICENSE NUMBER G1839 OF HOUSTON, TX, WAS DISCIPLINED BY TEXAS ON MAY 14, 1999
DISCIPLINARY ACTION: FINE
OFFENSE: NONCOMPLIANCE WITH A PROFESSIONAL RULE

NOTES: ALLEGATIONS OF INADEQUATE RECORD KEEPING FOR BARIATRIC PATIENTS. $1,500 FINE.

TALLANT, ARTHUR NILON MD OF 705 WEST HOPKINS, SAN MARCOS, TX, WAS DISCIPLINED BY DEA ON AUGUST 23, 1996
DISCIPLINARY ACTION: SURRENDER OF CONTROLLED SUBSTANCE LICENSE

NOTES: IN LIEU OF PUBLIC INTEREST REVOCATION.

TALMADGE, JOHN MILLS JR MD, LICENSE NUMBER E1948 OF DALLAS, TX, WAS DISCIPLINED BY TEXAS ON AUGUST 9, 1997
DISCIPLINARY ACTION: FINE; 60-MONTH RESTRICTION PLACED ON CONTROLLED SUBSTANCE LICENSE
OFFENSE: SUBSTANDARD CARE, INCOMPETENCE OR NEGLIGENCE

NOTES: FAILED TO ADEQUATELY DOCUMENT HIS CARE AND TREATMENT, INCLUDING DOCUMENTATION OF ASSESSMENT OF SUICIDE RISK PRIOR TO DISCHARGE, AND TO PROVIDE ONE-ON-ONE TREATMENT IN A TIMELY MANNER TO ONE PSYCHIATRIC PATIENT; FROM 6/12/95 TO 6/16/95 HE PRESCRIBED CONTROLLED SUBSTANCES TO ANOTHER PATIENT WHO WAS HOSPITALIZED AND DIAGNOSED AS SUFFERING FROM CHEMICAL DEPENDENCY AND SUBSTANCE ABUSE; HE FAILED TO NOTIFY THE BOARD IN WRITING OF HIS TREATMENT OF SAID PATIENT FOR SUBSTANCE ABUSE BEFORE PRESCRIBING CONTROLLED SUBSTANCES FOR HER. SHALL COMPLY WITH THE FOLLOWING TERMS AND CONDITIONS OVER THE NEXT 60 MONTHS: SEPARATE FROM PATIENT RECORDS, SHALL MAINTAIN A LOGBOOK OF EVERY PRESCRIPTION WRITTEN BY HIM FOR DANGEROUS DRUGS WITH ADDICTIVE POTENTIAL WHICH SHALL BE MADE AVAILABLE FOR REVIEW; SHALL REFRAIN FROM THE PRESCRIPTION OR ADMINISTRATION OF ANY DRUG FOR ANY PATIENT UNLESS THE DRUG IS MEDICALLY INDICATED AND IS PRESCRIBED IN THERAPEUTIC DOSES; SHALL OBTAIN AT LEAST 50 HOURS PER YEAR OF CONTINUING MEDICAL EDUCATION INCLUDING A COURSE IN PHARMACOLOGY ADDICTIONOLOGY WITHIN ONE YEAR; $2,500 FINE; SHALL COOPERATE WITH THE BOARD IN VERIFYING COMPLIANCE INCLUDING PROVIDING COPIES OF PEER REVIEW RECORDS UPON REQUEST; SHALL APPEAR BEFORE THE BOARD UPON REQUEST; SHALL GIVE A COPY OF THIS ORDER TO ANY HEALTH CARE ENTITY WHERE HE HAS PRIVILEGES; SHALL PROVIDE A COPY OF THIS ORDER TO ANYONE REQUESTING IT WITHIN 10 DAYS; TIME SPENT OUT OF TEXAS DOES NOT COUNT TOWARD PROBATION/RESTRICTION; SHALL INFORM THE BOARD OF CHANGE OF ADDRESS WITHIN 10 DAYS OR IF HE LEAVES THE STATE; SHALL NOT SEEK MODIFICATION FOR ONE YEAR. ON 10/15/99 ORDER TERMINATED.

TALMAGE, EDWARD ARTHUR MD, LICENSE NUMBER 00D2722 OF HOUSTON, TX, WAS DISCIPLINED BY TEXAS ON NOVEMBER 12, 199(
DISCIPLINARY ACTION: REPRIMAND
OFFENSE: LOSS OR RESTRICTION OF HOSPITAL PRIVILEGES

NOTES: DISCIPLINED BY HOSPITAL OR HOSPITAL MEDICAL STAFF INCLUDING REMOVAL, SUSPENSION, OR LIMITATION OF HOSPITAL PRIVILEGES OR OTHER DISCIPLINARY ACTIONS; PROFESSIONAL FAILURE TO PRACTICE MEDICINE IN ACCEPTABLE MANNER CONSISTENT WITH PUBLIC HEALTH AND WELFARE.

TALMAGE, EDWARD ARTHUR MD, LICENSE NUMBER D2722 OF HOUSTON, TX, WAS DISCIPLINED BY TEXAS ON AUGUST 9, 1997
DISCIPLINARY ACTION: REPRIMAND
OFFENSE: OVERPRESCRIBING OR MISPRESCRIBING DRUGS

NOTES: PRESCRIBING OR DISPENSING TO HABITUAL USER AND NONTHERAPEUTIC PRESCRIBING OR TREATMENT

TAMEZ, RICHARD JOSEPH DO, DATE OF BIRTH DECEMBER 12, 1928, LICENSE NUMBER 00C4571 OF 323 NW 24TH STREET, SAN ANTONIO, TX, WAS DISCIPLINED BY TEXAS ON AUGUST 20, 1993
DISCIPLINARY ACTION: 30-MONTH PROBATION; MONITORING OF PHYSICIAN PERFORMANCE
OFFENSE: SUBSTANCE ABUSE

NOTES: HAS SUFFERED FROM THE DISEASE OF ALCOHOLISM FOR APPROXIMATELY 10 YEARS AND HAS HAD SEVERAL RELAPSES THE LAST ONE TERMINATING IN 2/92 WHEN HE ENTERED INTO A TWO YEAR CONTRACT WITH THE PHYSICIAN HEALTH AND REHABILITATION COMMITTEE; RECEIVED INPATIENT TREATMENT IN 1987; CURRENTLY RECEIVING PSYCHIATRIC COUNSELING. SUSPENSION STAYED. CONDITIONS OF PROBATION: SHALL ABSTAIN FROM THE CONSUMPTION OF ALCOHOL/DRUGS IN ANY

FORM UNLESS PRESCRIBED BY ANOTHER PHYSICIAN FOR A LEGITIMATE MEDICAL PURPOSE; SHALL SUBMIT HIMSELF FOR APPROPRIATE EXAMS INCLUDING DRUG OR ALCOHOL SCREENS; SHALL PARTICIPATE IN ACTIVITIES OF A PHYSICIAN HEALTH AND REHABILITATION COMMITTEE AND ATTEND WEEKLY MEETINGS WITH QUARTERLY REPORTS; SHALL PARTICIPATE IN AA'S 12 STEP PROGRAM NOT LESS THAN TWICE A WEEK WITH QUARTERLY REPORTS TO THE BOARD; SHALL COMPLY WITH TERMS OF 2/92 CONTRACT; SHALL CONTINUE TO RECEIVE PSYCHIATRIC COUNSELING WITH QUARTERLY REPORTS TO THE BOARD; SHALL APPEAR BEFORE THE BOARD TWICE A YEAR; SHALL COOPERATE WITH THE BOARD IN VERIFYING COMPLIANCE; SHALL INFORM BOARD OF CHANGE OF ADDRESS WITHIN 10 DAYS OR IF HE LEAVES THE STATE; TIME SPENT OUT OF TEXAS DOES NOT COUNT TOWARD PROBATION. SHALL NOT SEEK MODIFICATION FOR ONE YEAR. ON 10/5/96 ORDER WAS TERMINATED.

TAN, EARL ENG-CHOW MD, DATE OF BIRTH APRIL 1, 1932 OF 6909 LYONS AVENUE, HOUSTON, TX, WAS DISCIPLINED BY MEDICARE ON JANUARY 2, 1994
DISCIPLINARY ACTION: 36-MONTH EXCLUSION FROM THE MEDICARE AND/OR MEDICAID PROGRAM
OFFENSE: OVERPRESCRIBING OR MISPRESCRIBING DRUGS

NOTES: PLED GUILTY TO DELIVERY OF A PRESCRIPTION WITHOUT A VALID PURPOSE.

TAN, EARL ENG-CHOW MD, LICENSE NUMBER 00F6196 OF HOUSTON, TX, WAS DISCIPLINED BY TEXAS ON MARCH 5, 1994
DISCIPLINARY ACTION: SURRENDER OF LICENSE
OFFENSE: NONCOMPLIANCE WITH A PROFESSIONAL RULE

NOTES: HE ADMITS HE VIOLATED THE MEDICAL PRACTICE ACT. VOLUNTARY SURRENDERS HIS LICENSE IN LIEU OF FURTHER INVESTIGATION OR A HEARING ON THE ALLEGATIONS. SHALL NOT PETITION FOR REINSTATEMENT.

TANNERYA, RICHARD GOAN MD, LICENSE NUMBER F5388 OF HOUSTON, TX, WAS DISCIPLINED BY TEXAS ON AUGUST 9, 1997
DISCIPLINARY ACTION: REPRIMAND
OFFENSE: PROFESSIONAL MISCONDUCT

NOTES: DELEGATED MEDICAL TASKS TO AN EMPLOYEE WHO WAS NOT ADEQUATELY TRAINED TO PERFORM THE TASK; FAILED TO ADEQUATELY SUPERVISE HIS ALLIED HEALTH OFFICE STAFF AS TO MEDICAL PROCEDURES AND FAILED TO ADEQUATELY SUPERVISE THE OFFICE STAFF AS TO THE MEDICAL BILLINGS. SHALL COOPERATE WITH THE BOARD IN VERIFYING COMPLIANCE; SHALL GIVE A COPY OF THIS ORDER TO ANY HEALTH CARE ENTITY WHERE HE HAS PRIVILEGES.

TANO, LEONEL MD, LICENSE NUMBER 00E7516 OF SAN ANTONIO, TX, WAS DISCIPLINED BY TEXAS ON AUGUST 18, 1990
DISCIPLINARY ACTION: RESTRICTION PLACED ON CONTROLLED SUBSTANCE LICENSE; REQUIRED TO TAKE ADDITIONAL MEDICAL EDUCATION

NOTES: STIPULATED ORDER. MUST REFRAIN FROM PRESCRIBING OR DISPENSING CONTROLLED SUBSTANCES TO KNOWN DRUG ABUSERS, INCLUDING METHADONE PATIENTS, AND COMPLETE RISK MANAGEMENT COURSE.

TANO, LEONEL MD OF SAN ANTONIO, TX, WAS DISCIPLINED BY DEA ON MAY 28, 1997
DISCIPLINARY ACTION: REVOCATION OF CONTROLLED SUBSTANCE LICENSE
OFFENSE: PROFESSIONAL MISCONDUCT

NOTES: IN 1987 IN A DEA INSPECTION OF A LOCAL NARCOTIC TREATMENT PROGRAM, IT WAS DISCOVERED THAT SOME OF THE CLIENTS TESTED POSITIVE FOR CONTROLLED SUBSTANCES OTHER THAN METHADONE WHICH THEY HAD RECEIVED FROM DR. TANO; IN 8/90 THE TEXAS BOARD ENTERED AN ORDER THAT FOUND HE PRESCRIBED CONTROLLED SUBSTANCES TO TWO CLIENTS IN THE PROGRAM WHO HE KNEW WERE HABITUAL USERS WITHOUT INFORMING THE BOARD; ORDER SAID HE COULD NOT PRESCRIBE CONTROLLED SUBSTANCES TO METHADONE PATIENTS; IN 1/92 AN INVESTIGATION OF HIS PRESCRIBING PRACTICES WAS INITIATED AND FOUR UNDERCOVER AGENTS MADE MULTIPLE VISITS TO HIS OFFICE; BETWEEN 2/92 AND 10/93 HE PRESCRIBED CONTROLLED SUBSTANCES WITH ONLY CURSORY EXAMINATIONS AND NO QUESTIONS ABOUT MEDICAL HISTORY OR CURRENT PROBLEMS; THESE SUBSTANCES INCLUDED XANAX AND HALCION TO STAY AWAKE, PHENTERMINE FOR WEIGHT LOSS, AND VICODIN FOR HEADACHES; ONE OF THE OFFICERS TRIED TO BUY XANAX ON THE STREET AND WAS TOLD SHE COULD GET IT FROM DR. TANO; DEA DETERMINED THAT HIS PRESCRIBING DEMONSTRATED A DISREGARD FOR HIS RESPONSIBILITIES AS A DEA REGISTRANT; THIS INVESTIGATION ALSO SHOWED THAT HE CONTINUED TO TREAT METHADONE PATIENTS IN SPITE OF THE TEXAS ORDER AND ISSUED A TOTAL OF 29 CONTROLLED SUBSTANCE PRESCRIPTIONS TO 21 DIFFERENT PATIENTS BETWEEN 2/91 AND 1/94 FROM ONE PROGRAM, 52 PRESCRIPTIONS TO SIX PATIENTS BETWEEN 9/90 AND 1/94 AND 50 PRESCRIPTIONS TO 18 PATIENTS BETWEEN 1/92 AND 2/94; EXCEPT FOR FIVE PATIENTS IT IS UNCLEAR WHETHER HE KNEW HE WAS PRESCRIBING TO INDIVIDUALS UNDERGOING METHADONE TREATMENT; HE HAD NO RECORDS INDICATING HE HAD NOTIFIED THE BOARD OF THESE PERSONS NAMES AS PER REGULATIONS; ON 11/30/94 ON A DEA APPLICATION FOR RENEWAL HE ANSWERED NO ON WHETHER HIS LICENSE HAD BEEN SANCTIONED BY ANOTHER STATE.

TAYLOR, ROOSEVELT JR MD, DATE OF BIRTH OCTOBER 11, 1938, LICENSE NUMBER 00D9896 OF AUSTIN, TX, WAS DISCIPLINED BY TEXAS ON JUNE 10, 1991
DISCIPLINARY ACTION: REPRIMAND; REQUIRED TO TAKE ADDITIONAL MEDICAL EDUCATION
OFFENSE: PROFESSIONAL MISCONDUCT

NOTES: ACTS WHICH CONSTITUTED UNPROFESSIONAL AND/OR DISHONORABLE CONDUCT LIKELY TO DECEIVE OR DEFRAUD THE PUBLIC, AND PROFESSIONAL FAILURE TO PRACTICE MEDICINE IN AN ACCEPTABLE MANNER CONSISTENT WITH PUBLIC HEALTH AND WELFARE. SHALL ATTEND FIVE HOURS OF AN ETHICS COURSE PER YEAR FOR FIVE YEARS.

TAYLOR, ROOSEVELT JR MD, DATE OF BIRTH OCTOBER 11, 1938, LICENSE NUMBER 0D11816, WAS DISCIPLINED BY MARYLAND ON JULY 22, 1992
DISCIPLINARY ACTION: REPRIMAND
OFFENSE: DISCIPLINARY ACTION BY ANOTHER STATE OR AGENCY

NOTES: ON JUNE 10, 1991, THE TEXAS STATE BOARD OF MEDICAL EXAMINERS REPRIMANDED HIM AND ORDERED HIM TO ATTEND 5 HOURS OF ETHICS COURSES EACH YEAR FOR FIVE YEARS AFTER FINDING HE HAD EXHIBITED "UNPROFESSIONAL OR DISHONORABLE CONDUCT." ON HIS MARYLAND

RENEWAL APPLICATION IN 1991 HE STATED THAT HE HAD NOT BEEN DISCIPLINED BY ANY OTHER BODY.

TAYLOR, ROOSEVELT JR MD, DATE OF BIRTH OCTOBER 11, 1938, LICENSE NUMBER 0023506 OF 1910 E MARTIN LUTHER KING JR BLV, AUSTIN, TX, WAS DISCIPLINED BY NEW JERSEY ON NOVEMBER 23, 1992
DISCIPLINARY ACTION: REPRIMAND
OFFENSE: PROFESSIONAL MISCONDUCT

NOTES: ENGAGED IN CONDUCT CONSTITUTING UNPROFESSIONAL OR DISHONORABLE CONDUCT IN TEXAS. PRIOR TO RESUMING PRACTICE IN NEW JERSEY, SHALL APPEAR BEFORE A COMMITTEE OF THE BOARD FOR A STATUS CONFERENCE.

TAYLOR, STANLEY KAY MD, LICENSE NUMBER 00D1079 OF ASPERMONT, TX, WAS DISCIPLINED BY TEXAS ON AUGUST 19, 1994
DISCIPLINARY ACTION: REPRIMAND; REQUIRED TO TAKE ADDITIONAL MEDICAL EDUCATION
OFFENSE: NONCOMPLIANCE WITH A PROFESSIONAL RULE

NOTES: FAILED TO ADEQUATELY DOCUMENT HIS CARE AND TREATMENT OF ONE PATIENT INCLUDING ADEQUATE DOCUMENTATION THAT THIS INITIAL DIAGNOSIS OF HEPATITIS A WAS A TENTATIVE WORKING DIAGNOSIS, THAT THE PATIENT PRESENTED MANAGEMENT DIFFICULTIES, THAT THE PATIENT WAS THOROUGHLY ADVISED OF HER CONDITION AND POSSIBLE COURSES OF ACTION AND THAT APPROPRIATE REFERRALS HAD BEEN MADE. SHALL MAINTAIN ADEQUATE MEDICAL RECORDS ON ALL PATIENT OFFICE VISITS WHICH SHALL BE AVAILABLE FOR INSPECTION; SHALL NOT "BACK DATE" ANY ENTRY OR RECORD OF PATIENT CARE; FOR FIVE YEARS SHALL ATTEND AT LEAST 50 HOURS PER YEAR OF CONTINUING MEDICAL EDUCATION; DURING THE FIRST YEAR 25 HOURS SHALL BE IN INTERNAL MEDICINE OR GASTROENTEROLOGY; SHALL GIVE A COPY OF THIS ORDER TO ANY HEALTH CARE ENTITY WHERE HE HAS PRIVILEGES; SHALL COOPERATE WITH THE BOARD IN VERIFYING COMPLIANCE; SHALL INFORM BOARD OF CHANGE OF ADDRESS WITHIN 10 DAYS OR IF HE LEAVES THE STATE; TIME SPENT OUT OF TEXAS DOES NOT COUNT TOWARDS RESTRICTION. SHALL NOT SEEK MODIFICATION FOR ONE YEAR. ON 10/13/95 ORDER TERMINATED BASED ON COMPLIANCE WITH CONDITIONS.

TEAGUE, ROBERT C MD, LICENSE NUMBER 0003925, WAS DISCIPLINED BY ARIZONA ON JULY 18, 1996
DISCIPLINARY ACTION: SURRENDER OF CONTROLLED SUBSTANCE LICENSE; 120-MONTH PROBATION
OFFENSE: OVERPRESCRIBING OR MISPRESCRIBING DRUGS

NOTES: PRESCRIBING, DISPENSING OR ADMINISTERING ANY CONTROLLED SUBSTANCE OR PRESCRIPTION-ONLY DRUG FOR OTHER THAN ACCEPTED THERAPEUTIC PURPOSES; BETWEEN 6/9/92 AND 11/4/92, HE PRESCRIBED A TOTAL OF 2,530 OF THE 15 MG SERAX, A SCHEDULE IV CONTROLLED SUBSTANCE, TO A 62-YEAR OLD PATIENT FOR AN AVERAGE DOSE OF MORE THAN 210 MG PER DAY, WHEN THE RECOMMENDED DOSE FOR ELDERLY PATIENTS IS NOT TO EXCEED 60 MG PER DAY; AS A CONSEQUENCE OF THE ABOVE FINDINGS, A PHARMACY SURVEY WAS UNDERTAKEN BY THE BOARD AND FROM PHARMACY PRINTOUTS BETWEEN 12/23/91 AND 1/6/93, IT WAS DETERMINED THAT ONE PATIENT RECEIVED 52 PRESCRIPTIONS OF PERCOCET FOR A TOTAL OF 1,956 DOSAGE UNITS AND ONE PRESCRIPTION OF ROXICET FOR 30 DOSAGE UNITS; A SECOND PATIENT RECEIVED 28 PRESCRIPTIONS OF ROXICET FOR A TOTAL OF 1,265 DOSAGE UNITS; PHYSICIAN WAS UNABLE TO ARTICULATE THE SPECIFIC USE FOR THE MEDICATIONS, BOTH OF WHICH ARE SCHEDULE II CONTROLLED SUBSTANCES. WITHIN 10 DAYS, SHALL SURRENDER HIS DRUG ENFORCEMENT ADMINISTRATION CERTIFICATE TO THE BOARD AND NOT PRESCRIBE ANY CONTROLLED SUBSTANCES THEREAFTER. ON 5/7/97 REQUEST TO TERMINATE ORDER DENIED. ON 11/19/98 REQUEST TO OBTAIN DEA CERTIFICATE DENIED. ON 7/29/99 REQUEST TO REINSTATE HIS DEA LICENSE UPON COMPLETION OF ADDITIONAL CONTINUING MEDICAL EDUCATION IN THE AREA OF PHARMACOLOGY GRANTED AS RESOLUTION OF SUPERIOR COURT CASE.

TEAGUE, ROBERT COLE MD, LICENSE NUMBER C5261 OF PHOENIX, AZ, WAS DISCIPLINED BY TEXAS ON APRIL 8, 1999
DISCIPLINARY ACTION: LICENSE REVOCATION; FINE
OFFENSE: DISCIPLINARY ACTION BY ANOTHER STATE OR AGENCY

NOTES: ON OR ABOUT 7/96 HE WAS PLACED ON 10 YEARS PROBATION BY THE ARIZONA BOARD FOR NON-THERAPEUTIC PRESCRIBING OF CONTROLLED SUBSTANCES IN 3 PATIENT CASES; IN 3/98 HE FAILED TO RESPOND TO THE TEXAS BOARD'S WRITTEN REQUEST FOR MEDICAL RECORDS AND HAD NOT DONE SO AS OF THE DATE OF THE ORDER. $50,000 FINE.

TEEL, THEODORE T MD, LICENSE NUMBER C3230, WAS DISCIPLINED BY TEXAS ON MAY 10, 1997
DISCIPLINARY ACTION: REQUIRED TO TAKE ADDITIONAL MEDICAL EDUCATION
OFFENSE: SUBSTANDARD CARE, INCOMPETENCE OR NEGLIGENCE

NOTES: FAILED TO ADEQUATELY DOCUMENT A PROPER EVALUATION ON A PATIENT WHO PRESENTED TO HIS OFFICE WITH SYMPTOMS OF "GAS ON THE STOMACH"; AND TO ADEQUATELY DOCUMENT A HISTORY AND PHYSICAL EXAMINATION ON THE PATIENT AS WELL. THE SAME PATIENT PRESENTED TO THE DOCTOR THREE ADDITIONAL TIMES AND HE FAILED TO PROPERLY DIAGNOSE COLON CANCER OR TO ORDER PROPER TESTS ON THE PATIENT WHEN HE FOUND BLOOD WHILE PERFORMING A RECTAL EXAM. LICENSE IS RESTRICTED FOR THREE YEARS AS FOLLOWS: SHALL UPDATE HIS PRACTICE BY SUBMITTING TO A CORRECTIVE ACTION PLAN ACCEPTABLE TO THE BOARD; SHALL MAINTAIN ADEQUATE MEDICAL RECORDS WHICH WILL BE AVAILABLE FOR REVIEW; SHALL OBTAIN AND CONSULT WITH AN APPROVED, PRIVATE CONSULTING FIRM FOR RISK MANAGEMENT IN HIS PRACTICE; SHALL ATTEND AT LEAST 100 HOURS OF CONTINUING MEDICAL EDUCATION THE FIRST YEAR AND AT LEAST 50 HOURS PER YEAR AFTER THAT WITH AT LEAST ONE COURSE IN FAMILY PRACTICE; SHALL APPEAR BEFORE THE BOARD ONCE A YEAR; SHALL COOPERATE WITH THE BOARD IN VERIFYING COMPLIANCE; SHALL GIVE A COPY OF THIS ORDER TO ANY HEALTH CARE ENTITY WHERE HE HAS PRIVILEGES; SHALL INFORM THE BOARD OF CHANGE OF ADDRESS WITHIN 10 DAYS; SHALL NOT SEEK MODIFICATION FOR ONE YEAR. ON 8/22/98 THE ORDER WAS TERMINATED.

TEKELL, GORDON SILAS MD, LICENSE NUMBER 0007235 OF YUMA, AZ, WAS DISCIPLINED BY ARIZONA ON JANUARY 21, 1993
DISCIPLINARY ACTION: RESTRICTION PLACED ON CONTROLLED SUBSTANCE LICENSE; REQUIRED TO TAKE ADDITIONAL MEDICAL EDUCATION
OFFENSE: OVERPRESCRIBING OR MISPRESCRIBING DRUGS

NOTES: ALLEGATIONS THAT HE HAD BEEN PRESCRIBING LARGE AMOUNTS OF SCHEDULED DRUGS. SHALL SUCCESSFULLY COMPLETE 40 HOURS OF CONTINUING MEDICAL EDUCATION ACCEPTABLE TO THE BOARD WITHIN SIX MONTHS OF THE EFFECTIVE DATE OF THIS ORDER IN THE SUBJECT OF THE USE OF NARCOTICS FOR PAIN CONTROL AND CHRONIC PAIN MANAGEMENT; CONSULT WITH AN INDEPENDENT ORGANIZATION ACCEPTABLE TO THE BOARD REGARDING THE PROPER CREATION, MANAGEMENT AND MAINTENANCE OF MEDICAL RECORDS; EFFECTIVE TWO WEEKS FROM 01/21/93, CEASE ANY AND ALL PRESCRIBING, DISPENSING, OR ADMINISTRATION OF ALL SCHEDULE II AND III CONTROLLED SUBSTANCES, EXCEPT FOR THOSE PATIENTS IN A RECOGNIZED HOSPICE PROGRAM. SUCCESSFULLY FULFILLED THE TERMS OF THIS STIPULATION AND ORDER, SO AS OF 07/15/93 THIS STIPULATION AND ORDER IS TERMINATED.

TEKELL, GORDON SILAS MD, LICENSE NUMBER 00C9159 OF YUMA, AZ, WAS DISCIPLINED BY TEXAS ON NOVEMBER 3, 1994
DISCIPLINARY ACTION: SURRENDER OF CONTROLLED SUBSTANCE LICENSE; LICENSE SUSPENSION
OFFENSE: DISCIPLINARY ACTION BY ANOTHER STATE OR AGENCY

NOTES: ARIZONA BOARD INITIATED DISCIPLINARY ACTION BASED ON ALLEGATIONS THAT HE HAD OVERPRESCRIBED VARIOUS PRESCRIPTION MEDICATIONS INCLUDING CONTROLLED SUBSTANCES; ENTERED INTO A WRITTEN STIPULATION WITH ARIZONA ON 3/18/93 WHICH REQUIRED HIM TO CEASE ANY PRESCRIBING OF SCHEDULE II AND III CONTROLLED SUBSTANCES EXCEPT IN A RECOGNIZED HOSPICE PROGRAM; THIS ORDER WAS TERMINATED ON 7/15/93. SUSPENSION UNTIL HE APPEARS BEFORE THE BOARD AND PROVIDES SUFFICIENT EVIDENCE THAT HE IS PHYSICALLY, MENTALLY AND OTHERWISE COMPETENT TO SAFELY PRACTICE; SHALL GIVE A COPY OF THIS ORDER TO ANY HEALTH CARE ENTITY WHERE HE HAS PRIVILEGES; SHALL COOPERATE WITH THE BOARD IN VERIFYING COMPLIANCE; SHALL INFORM BOARD OF CHANGE OF ADDRESS WITHIN 10 DAYS; SHALL SURRENDER TEXAS CONTROLLED SUBSTANCES CERTIFICATE AND ALL UNUSED TRIPLICATE PRESCRIPTION FORMS; SHALL NOT ATTEMPT TO REREGISTER WITHOUT PERMISSION.

TERRELL, WOODROW DR OF SEQUIN, TX, WAS DISCIPLINED BY ILLINOIS ON NOVEMBER 1, 1996
DISCIPLINARY ACTION: REPRIMAND
OFFENSE: PROFESSIONAL MISCONDUCT

NOTES: ALLEGEDLY PRE-SIGNED PRESCRIPTIONS WHICH WERE MISAPPROPRIATED BY AN EMPLOYEE.

TERRIAN, ROBERT JOSEPH DO, DATE OF BIRTH APRIL 12, 1949 OF 3500 CLIFFWOOD DRIVE, BEDFORD, TX, WAS DISCIPLINED BY MEDICARE ON NOVEMBER 19, 1998
DISCIPLINARY ACTION: EXCLUSION FROM THE MEDICARE AND/OR MEDICAID PROGRAM
OFFENSE: NONCOMPLIANCE WITH A PROFESSIONAL RULE

NOTES: DEFAULTED ON PUBLIC HEALTH SERVICE EDUCATION LOAN. REINSTATED ON 5/4/99.

TESSMER, JON F MD, DATE OF BIRTH NOVEMBER 21, 1946 OF 102 SOUTH PARK DRIVE, BROWNWOOD, TX, WAS DISCIPLINED BY MEDICARE ON MAY 9, 1995
DISCIPLINARY ACTION: EXCLUSION FROM THE MEDICARE AND/OR MEDICAID PROGRAM
OFFENSE: NONCOMPLIANCE WITH A PROFESSIONAL RULE

NOTES: DEFAULTED ON PUBLIC HEALTH SERVICE EDUCATION LOAN. REINSTATED ON 6/1/95.

TESSMER, JON F MD, LICENSE NUMBER 00G5685, WAS DISCIPLINED BY TEXAS ON AUGUST 17, 1996
DISCIPLINARY ACTION: 60-MONTH MONITORING OF PHYSICIAN PERFORMANCE
OFFENSE: LOSS OR RESTRICTION OF HOSPITAL PRIVILEGES

NOTES: PLACED ON MEDICAL LEAVE OF ABSENCE BY THE MEDICAL EXECUTIVE COMMITTEE (MEC) IN MAY AND JUNE 1993 FOR HIM TO RESOLVE CONTINUED DIFFICULTIES EXPERIENCED FROM THE ANTI-DEPRESSANTS AND OTHER STEROID WITHDRAWAL SIDE EFFECTS BROUGHT ABOUT BY TREATMENT FOR ASTHMA AND 1990 TREATMENT FOR A BACK INJURY; UPON HIS RETURN TO PRACTICE IN 6/93 MEC MONITORED HIS PRACTICE; IN APRIL 1994 HE AGAIN WAS PLACED ON MEDICAL LEAVE BY MEC AND RELIEVED OF ON-CALL REQUIREMENTS AND INDEPENDENT PRIVILEGES AT THE HOSPITAL UNTIL AFTER 6/01/94, RELATED TO THE DEVELOPMENT OF SOME MENTAL HEALTH AND PHYSICAL PROBLEMS AND APPARENT DIFFICULTIES WITH FUNCTIONING ON THE FLOOR BASED UPON CHART REVIEW AND MEDICAL STAFF/NURSING OBSERVATIONS; ON 7/21/94 ABLE TO RESUME STAFF FUNCTIONS WITH RESTRICTIONS; HAS WORKED VOLUNTARILY AND COOPERATIVELY WITH MEC IN HIS REHABILITATION PROGRAM; HAS BEEN WEANED OFF STEROIDS SINCE THE SUMMER OF 1994 AND CONTINUES TO PARTICIPATE IN ONGOING THERAPY FOR HIS DEPRESSION. RESTRICTED UNDER TERMS AND CONDITIONS FOR FIVE YEARS: SHALL NOT TREAT OR OTHERWISE SERVE AS PHYSICIAN, PRESCRIBE, DISPENSE, OR ADMINISTER DRUGS WITH POTENTIAL FOR ABUSE OR ALCOHOL TO HIMSELF OR ANY MEMBER OF HIS FAMILY; SHALL ABSTAIN FROM THE CONSUMPTION OF ALCOHOL/DRUGS IN ANY FORM UNLESS PRESCRIBED BY ANOTHER PHYSICIAN FOR A LEGITIMATE AND THERAPEUTIC PURPOSE; SHALL SUBMIT HIMSELF TO APPROPRIATE EXAMS, INCLUDING DRUG AND ALCOHOL SCREENS; SHALL SUBMIT HIMSELF FOR EVALUATION AND TREATMENT TO A BOARD APPROVED PSYCHIATRIST WHO HE SHALL SEE AT LEAST ONCE EACH MONTH AND WHO SHALL PROVIDE REPORTS; SHALL PARTICIPATE IN THE ACTIVITIES AND PROGRAMS OF A SUPPORT GROUP FOR FAMILY ISSUES/CHILDREN OF SUBSTANCE ABUSERS, OR ANY OTHER BOARD APPROVED SUBSTANTIALLY SIMILAR PROGRAM ON A REGULAR WEEKLY BASIS AND SUBMIT QUARTERLY REPORTS TO THE BOARD; HIS MEDICAL PRACTICE, INCLUDING ANY OFFICE AND SURGICAL PRACTICE, SHALL BE MONITORED BY THE MEC OR BY AN APPROVED LICENSED TEXAS PHYSICIAN WHO SHALL PROVIDE QUARTERLY REPORTS; SHALL PARTICIPATE IN A PHYSICIAN, HEALTH, AND REHABILITATION, GROUP AND ATTEND WEEKLY MEETINGS WITH QUARTERLY REPORTS TO THE BOARD; SHALL MAINTAIN A LOGBOOK OF ALL PRESCRIPTIONS FOR DRUGS WITH POTENTIAL FOR ABUSE WHICH SHALL BE AVAILABLE FOR BOARD INSPECTION; SHALL MAINTAIN ADEQUATE MEDICAL RECORDS WHICH SHALL BE AVAILABLE FOR REVIEW; SHALL APPEAR BEFORE THE BOARD AT LEAST ONCE A YEAR; SHALL COOPERATE WITH THE BOARD IN VERIFYING COMPLIANCE INCLUDING PROVIDING COPIES OF MEDICAL RELEASES AND PEER REVIEW RECORDS UPON REQUEST; SHALL GIVE A COPY OF THIS ORDER TO ANY HEALTH CARE ENTITY WHERE HE HAS PRIVILEGES; SHALL PROVIDE A COPY OF THIS ORDER TO ANYONE REQUESTING IT WITHIN 10 DAYS; TIME

PERIOD OUT OF TEXAS DOES NOT COUNT TOWARD RESTRICTION; SHALL INFORM THE BOARD OF CHANGE OF ADDRESS WITHIN 10 DAYS OF IF HE LEAVES THE STATE; SHALL NOT SEEK MODIFICATION FOR ONE YEAR. ON 5/14/99 REQUEST TO HAVE LICENSE REINSTATED DENIED.

TESSMER, JON F MD, LICENSE NUMBER G5685 OF HOUSTON, TX, WAS DISCIPLINED BY TEXAS ON FEBRUARY 7, 1998
DISCIPLINARY ACTION: 60-MONTH PROBATION
OFFENSE: FAILURE TO COMPLY WITH PREVIOUS BOARD ORDER

NOTES: VIOLATED 8/17/96 BOARD ORDER BY FAILING TO PARTICIPATE IN THE ACTIVITIES AND PROGRAMS OF A SUPPORT GROUP FOR FAMILY ISSUES/CHILDREN OF SUBSTANCE ABUSERS, OR OTHER COMPARABLE BOARD-APPROVED PROGRAM. SUSPENSION STAYED; ALL OTHER PROVISIONS OF THE 8/17/96 ORDER REMAIN IN FULL FORCE AND EFFECT; THE 5 YEAR TIME PERIOD IMPOSED FOR THIS ORDER SHALL SUPERSEDE THE TIME PERIOD IMPOSED BY THE 8/17/96 ORDER; SHALL NOT SEEK MODIFICATION FOR TWO YEARS.

TESSMER, JON F MD, LICENSE NUMBER G5685 OF HOUSTON, TX, WAS DISCIPLINED BY TEXAS ON OCTOBER 24, 1998
DISCIPLINARY ACTION: LICENSE SUSPENSION
OFFENSE: FAILURE TO COMPLY WITH PREVIOUS BOARD ORDER

NOTES: VIOLATED 8/17/96 AND 2/7/98 BOARD ORDERS BY: FAILING TO PAY OUTSTANDING COSTS OF DRUG SCREENS; FAILED TO PROVIDE ANY REPORTS RELATING TO THE NUMBER AND LOCATIONS OF MEETINGS ATTENDED OF A SUPPORT GROUP FOR FAMILY ISSUES/CHILDREN OF SUBSTANCE ABUSERS; FAILED TO REQUEST OR RECEIVE APPROVAL FROM THE BOARD TO ATTEND ANY PROGRAM SUBSTANTIALLY SIMILAR TO A SUPPORT GROUP FOR FAMILY ISSUES/CHILDREN OF SUBSTANCE ABUSERS; DID NOT ENSURE THAT QUARTERLY REPORTS WERE PROVIDED TO THE BOARD BY HIS MONITOR; ON 8/1/97 HE ADVISED THE BOARD THAT HIS MONITOR REFUSED TO CONTINUE AND THAT HE WAS WORKING AT THE MEDI-CLINIC AND COULD NOT AFFORD TO PAY A MONITOR; ON 5/6/98 HE WAS NOTIFIED THAT HE WAS TO APPEAR FOR A PERSONAL INTERVIEW ON 6/10/98; ON 6/10/98 HE ADVISED THE BOARD THAT HE HAD BEEN STUNG BY A WASP AND WOULD NOT BE ABLE TO ATTEND THE SCHEDULED APPEARANCE AS HE WAS ALLERGIC TO BEE STINGS; HE HAS PROVIDED NO DOCUMENTATION OF MEDICAL CARE RECEIVED FOR THE EMERGENT CONDITION HE REPORTED ON 6/10/98 NOR ANY DOCUMENTATION THAT HE WAS PHYSICALLY UNABLE TO ATTEND THE SCHEDULED APPEARANCE. SUSPENSION UNTIL HE REQUESTS TO HAVE HIS SUSPENSION STAYED OR APPEARS BEFORE THE BOARD WITH SUFFICIENT EVIDENCE THAT HE IS PHYSICALLY, MENTALLY AND OTHERWISE COMPETENT TO SAFELY PRACTICE MEDICINE INCLUDING AT A MINIMUM COMPLETE COPIES OF MEDICAL RECORDS AND REPORTS OF PSYCHOLOGICAL AND NEUROPSYCHIATRIC EVALUATIONS, INCLUDING A 96 HOUR INPATIENT EVALUATION CONDUCTED BY A BOARD-APPROVED CERTIFIED PSYCHIATRIST; SHALL PAY FOR ANY OUTSTANDING FEES FOR DRUG TESTS; SHALL PROVIDE DOCUMENTED EVIDENCE THAT HE HAS COMPLIED WITH ALL REQUIREMENTS OF THE 1996 ORDER; SHALL COOPERATE WITH THE BOARD IN VERIFYING COMPLIANCE INCLUDING PROVIDING COPIES OF MEDICAL RELEASES UPON REQUEST; SHALL INFORM THE BOARD OF CHANGE OF ADDRESS WITHIN 10 DAYS.

THEAGENE, SAMUEL M MD, LICENSE NUMBER J7690 OF SAN ANTONIO, TX, WAS DISCIPLINED BY TEXAS ON AUGUST 9, 1997
DISCIPLINARY ACTION: 24-MONTH RESTRICTION PLACED ON LICENSE; REQUIRED TO TAKE ADDITIONAL MEDICAL EDUCATION
OFFENSE: PROFESSIONAL MISCONDUCT

NOTES: IN 1995 HE ADMINISTERED TRIGGER POINT INJECTION TO AN ADULT FEMALE WHO WAS SEMI-DISROBED AT THE TIME. THE INJECTIONS WERE ADMINISTERED IN AN EXAMINATION ROOM WITH THE CURTAIN DRAWN CLOSED AND WITHOUT A CHAPERONE PRESENT. ALTHOUGH IT APPEARS THAT THE TREATMENT PROVIDED WAS CLINICALLY APPROPRIATE, HE DISPLAYED POOR JUDGMENT BY ADMINISTERING THE INJECTIONS TO A PARTIALLY CLAD FEMALE PATIENT WITHOUT A CHAPERONE. CONDITIONS ON LICENSE AS FOLLOWS: ANYTIME HE PERFORMS A PHYSICAL EXAM ON A FEMALE PATIENT, HE SHALL HAVE A CHAPERONE PRESENT IN THE ROOM TO OBSERVE HIM DIRECTLY; WITHIN TWO YEARS HE SHALL SUCCESSFULLY COMPLETE APPROVED COURSES IN THE AREAS OF RISK MANAGEMENT AND ETHICS; SHALL APPEAR BEFORE THE BOARD AT LEAST ANNUALLY; SHALL COOPERATE WITH THE BOARD IN VERIFYING COMPLIANCE INCLUDING PROVIDING COPIES OF PEER REVIEW RECORDS UPON REQUEST; TIME SPENT OUT OF TEXAS DOES NOT COUNT TOWARD RESTRICTION; SHALL INFORM THE BOARD OF CHANGE OF ADDRESS WITHIN 10 DAYS OR IF HE LEAVES THE STATE; SHALL NOT SEEK MODIFICATION FOR ONE YEAR. ON 10/24/98 THE REQUEST FOR TERMINATION OF THE ORDER WAS DENIED. ON 1/29/99 THE ORDER WAS TERMINATED.

THEAGENE, SAMUEL MICHAEL MD, DATE OF BIRTH FEBRUARY 13, 1958, LICENSE NUMBER 050961L OF 11146 VANCE JACKSON ROAD #4001, SAN ANTONIO, TX, WAS DISCIPLINED BY PENNSYLVANIA ON APRIL 1, 1998
DISCIPLINARY ACTION: PROBATION
OFFENSE: DISCIPLINARY ACTION BY ANOTHER STATE OR AGENCY

NOTES: DISCIPLINARY ACTION IN TEXAS. LICENSE PLACED ON PROBATION WITH CONDITIONS UNTIL SUCH TIME AS HIS TEXAS LICENSE IS REINSTATED WITHOUT RESTRICTION.

THOMAS, CLYDE E MD, DATE OF BIRTH NOVEMBER 1, 1913 OF 411 E 9TH ST PO BOX 2071, BIG SPRING, TX, WAS DISCIPLINED BY MEDICARE ON NOVEMBER 13, 1991
DISCIPLINARY ACTION: 120-MONTH EXCLUSION FROM THE MEDICARE AND/OR MEDICAID PROGRAM
OFFENSE: DISCIPLINARY ACTION BY ANOTHER STATE OR AGENCY

NOTES: PEER REVIEW ORGANIZATION RECOMMENDATION.

THOMAS, FITZGERALD M MD, LICENSE NUMBER 00H3635 OF ODESSA, TX, WAS DISCIPLINED BY TEXAS ON MAY 15, 1996
DISCIPLINARY ACTION: REQUIRED TO TAKE ADDITIONAL MEDICAL EDUCATION; MONITORING OF PHYSICIAN PERFORMANCE
OFFENSE: SUBSTANDARD CARE, INCOMPETENCE OR NEGLIGENCE

NOTES: IN 1/94 HE FAILED TO ADEQUATELY ASSESS AND TREAT THE CARDIAC CONDITION OF AN ADULT FEMALE WHOM HE ADMITTED TO THE HOSPITAL FOR COMPLAINTS OF CHEST PAIN, SHORTNESS OF BREATH AND LETHARGY; HE FAILED TO PERFORM CUSTOMARY TESTS WHICH ARE USED TO DETERMINE THE BASIS FOR SUCH COMPLAINTS; DISCHARGED PATIENT WITHOUT ADEQUATELY MANAGING HER MEDICAL CONDITION; SOON AFTER DISCHARGE, PATIENT DIED OF A HEART ATTACK; HE FAILED TO ADEQUATELY DOCUMENT HIS CARE OF PATIENT. LICENSE SUBJECT TO TERMS AND CONDITIONS FOR

THREE YEARS: SHALL OBTAIN AT LEAST 50 HOURS PER YEAR OF CONTINUING MEDICAL EDUCATION; IN ADDITION TO THE ABOVE REQUIREMENT, DURING THE FIRST YEAR OF ORDER HE SHALL OBTAIN AN ADDITIONAL 50 HOURS IN EITHER RISK MANAGEMENT OR TREATMENT OF CARDIAC PATIENTS OR A COMBINATION OF THESE TWO COURSES; SHALL GIVE A COPY OF THIS ORDER TO ANY HEALTH CARE ENTITY WHERE HE HAS PRIVILEGES; SHALL PROVIDE A COPY OF THIS ORDER TO ANYONE REQUESTING IT WITHIN 10 DAYS; SHALL COOPERATE WITH BOARD IN VERIFYING COMPLIANCE; SHALL APPEAR BEFORE BOARD AT LEAST ONCE A YEAR OR AT BOARD REQUEST; TIME SPENT OUT OF TEXAS DOES NOT COUNT TOWARD RESTRICTION; SHALL INFORM BOARD OF CHANGE OF ADDRESS WITHIN 10 DAYS OR IF HE LEAVES THE STATE. SHALL NOT SEEK MODIFICATION FOR ONE YEAR. ON 5/16/98 PETITION TO TERMINATE ORDER DENIED.

THOMAS, FRED BEHMAN DO, LICENSE NUMBER 00C7319 OF DALLAS, TX, WAS DISCIPLINED BY TEXAS ON JUNE 12, 1990
DISCIPLINARY ACTION: 36-MONTH RESTRICTION PLACED ON CONTROLLED SUBSTANCE LICENSE; REQUIRED TO TAKE ADDITIONAL MEDICAL EDUCATION
OFFENSE: PROFESSIONAL MISCONDUCT

NOTES: HAD FAILED TO KEEP RECORDS AND MAINTAIN INVENTORIES OF CONTROLLED SUBSTANCES DISPENSED AND DISPENSED AN ANORECTIC DRUG TO PATIENTS SEEKING TREATMENT FOR OBESITY IN QUANTITIES THAT EXCEEDED THOSE NECESSARY. HE HAS NEITHER DENIED OR ADMITTED THE CHARGES. STIPULATED ORDER. MUST COMPLETE PRECEPTORSHIP ON PREVENTION AND TREATMENT OF DRUG ABUSE, MAINTAIN ADEQUATE MEDICAL RECORDS ON PATIENT OFFICE VISITS. OTHER THAN SAMPLES, NOT DISPENSE MEDICATIONS TO PATIENTS IN QUANTITIES GREATER THAN NECESSARY FOR TREATMENT UNTIL ACCESS TO PHARMACY POSSIBLE. EXCEPT IN EMERGENCIES, MAY NOT ADMINISTER, PRESCRIBE, OR DISPENSE CONTROLLED SUBSTANCES TO SELF, MAINTAIN IN SEPARATE FILE COPY OF PRESCRIPTIONS WRITTEN FOR CONTROLLED SUBSTANCES, SUBMIT FOR PSYCHIATRIC EVALUATION AND FOLLOW RECOMMENDATIONS, IF ANY, REGARDING CONTINUING CARE AND TREATMENT AND APPEAR BEFORE BOARD SEMI-ANNUALLY. SHALL INFORM THE BOARD OF ADDRESS CHANGE. PROBATION MODIFIED, EFFECTIVE 3/6/92 REDUCING APPEARANCES BEFORE BOARD TO ANNUALLY.

THOMAS, JACK M MD, LICENSE NUMBER 00E4718 OF DENISON, TX, WAS DISCIPLINED BY TEXAS ON DECEMBER 4, 1991
DISCIPLINARY ACTION: LICENSE REVOCATION
OFFENSE: NONCOMPLIANCE WITH A PROFESSIONAL RULE

NOTES: ALLEGATIONS OF ILLEGAL DIVERSION TO UNKNOWN SOURCES OF QUANTITIES OF DILAUDID PRESCRIBED FOR PATIENTS; FAILURE TO KEEP COMPLETE AND ACCURATE RECORDS OF PURCHASES AND DISPOSALS OF CONTROLLED SUBSTANCES INCLUDING, BUT NOT LIMITED TO, DILAUDID; FAILURE TO COMPLY WITH A SUBPOENA RECEIVED IN HIS OFFICE ON 3/19/91; WRITING OF PRESCRIPTIONS DURING THE PERIOD OF 6/11/90 FOR PERCOCET, DEMEROL, AND DILAUDID TO A PERSON WHEN IN FACT SUCH PERSON WAS NOT A PATIENT DURING THE ABOVE PERIOD; CONTINUING MEDICAL DISABILITY AS REFLECTED BY HIS LAWYER'S ADMISSION DATED 9/12/91 COUPLED WITH HIS HOSPITALIZATION IN 3/91 FOR SEVERE DEPRESSION AND EPISODES REGARDING SUICIDAL THOUGHTS. HE WAS UNWILLING TO RESPOND TO ALLEGATIONS DUE TO HIS MENTAL IMPAIRMENT AND PENDING THE OUTCOME OF CRIMINAL CHARGES.

THOMAS, JACK M MD, LICENSE NUMBER E4718, WAS DISCIPLINED BY TEXAS ON MAY 14, 1999
DISCIPLINARY ACTION: LICENSE REINSTATEMENT

NOTES: HAS BEEN UNDER OUTPATIENT TREATMENT SINCE 12/4/91 REVOCATION. REQUEST FOR REINSTATEMENT GRANTED CONTIGENT UPON TAKING AND PASSING THE SPEX WITH A SCORE OF 75 OR ABOVE, WITHIN 3 ATTEMPTS WITHIN 1 YEAR; UPON REINSTATEMENT LICENSE ON PROBATION WITH SPECIFIED CONDITIONS.

THOMAS, JAMES H JR MD, LICENSE NUMBER 00G0199 OF HOUSTON, TX, WAS DISCIPLINED BY TEXAS ON MARCH 31, 1990
DISCIPLINARY ACTION: REPRIMAND

NOTES: STIPULATED ORDER.

THOMAS, JAMES H JR MD, LICENSE NUMBER G1099 OF HOUSTON, TX, WAS DISCIPLINED BY TEXAS ON APRIL 10, 1999
DISCIPLINARY ACTION: FINE; REPRIMAND
OFFENSE: LOSS OR RESTRICTION OF HOSPITAL PRIVILEGES

NOTES: ON OR ABOUT 11/23/93 HIS HOSPITAL PRIVILEGES WERE SUSPENDED FOR FAILURE TO PROVIDE ADEQUATE DOCUMENTATION OF TREATMENT. $1,000 FINE.

THOMAS, JOHN MAULDIN JR MD, DATE OF BIRTH JULY 16, 1950 OF ELLIS II UNIT, ROUTE 6, HUNTSVILLE, TX, WAS DISCIPLINED BY MEDICARE ON NOVEMBER 16, 1992
DISCIPLINARY ACTION: EXCLUSION FROM THE MEDICARE AND/OR MEDICAID PROGRAM
OFFENSE: CRIMINAL CONVICTION OR PLEA OF GUILTY, NOLO CONTENDERE, OR NO CONTEST TO A CRIME

NOTES: PROGRAM-RELATED CONVICTION.

THOMAS, STEPHEN C MD OF 22 WILLOWBREEZE, BUFFALO, NY, WAS DISCIPLINED BY DEA ON JANUARY 5, 1990
DISCIPLINARY ACTION: SURRENDER OF CONTROLLED SUBSTANCE LICENSE
OFFENSE: DISCIPLINARY ACTION BY ANOTHER STATE OR AGENCY

NOTES: SURRENDERED STATE MEDICAL LICENSE.

THOMAS, STEPHEN C MD, LICENSE NUMBER J5036 OF LUBBOCK, TX, WAS DISCIPLINED BY TEXAS ON NOVEMBER 10, 1998
DISCIPLINARY ACTION: EMERGENCY SUSPENSION
OFFENSE: SUBSTANCE ABUSE

NOTES: ON OR ABOUT 10/23/98 WAS ALLEGEDLY IN POSSESSION OF COCAINE; WROTE PRESCRIPTIONS FOR VALIUM AND DIAZEPAM FOR HIS FIANCEE AND HER BROTHER, AND THEN DIVERTED THESE MEDICATIONS FOR HIS OWN USE; HE DOES NOT MAINTAIN ANY MEDICAL RECORDS FOR EITHER HIS FIANCEE OR HER BROTHER; ON 10/28/98 HE ADMITTED TO THE BOARD THAT ON OCCASION HE RELAPSED TO THE USE OF COCAINE IN 8/98; HE STATED THAT HE HAS LIMITED HIS COCAINE USE TO THE WEEKENDS; HE IS CURRENTLY UNDER CONTRACT WITH A MEDICAL SOCIETY, AND THE CHAIRMAN REPORTED THAT ALL DRUG SCREENS HAVE BEEN NEGATIVE; HIS TEST SCREENS WOULD BE NEGATIVE DURING THE WEEK SINCE THE DRUG IS ONLY DETECTABLE FOR A SHORT PERIOD OF TIME.

THOMAS, STEPHEN C MD, LICENSE NUMBER 176191 OF 4905 76TH STREET, LUBBOCK, TX, WAS DISCIPLINED BY NEW YORK ON FEBRUARY 22, 1999
DISCIPLINARY ACTION: SURRENDER OF LICENSE
OFFENSE: DISCIPLINARY ACTION BY ANOTHER STATE OR AGENCY

NOTES: DISCIPLINED BY THE TEXAS BOARD FOR INAPPROPRIATELY PRESCRIBING CONTROLLED SUBSTANCES; ENGAGING IN THE INTEMPERATE USE OF DRUGS OR ALCOHOL; FAILING TO MAINTAIN PATIENT RECORDS.

THOMAS, STEPHEN C MD, LICENSE NUMBER J5036 OF LUBBOCK, TX, WAS DISCIPLINED BY TEXAS ON APRIL 10, 1999
DISCIPLINARY ACTION: LICENSE SUSPENSION
OFFENSE: SUBSTANCE ABUSE

NOTES: RELAPSED INTO COCAINE USE AS WELL AS DIVERTING VALIUM AND DIAZEPAM FOR HIS OWN USE. SUSPENSION UNTIL HE REQUESTS TO HAVE HIS SUSPENSION STAYED OR APPEARS BEFORE THE BOARD WITH SUFFICIENT EVIDENCE THAT HE IS PHYSICALLY, MENTALLY AND OTHERWISE COMPETENT TO SAFELY PRACTICE MEDICINE INCLUDING AT A MINIMUM COMPLETE COPIES OF MEDICAL RECORDS AND REPORTS OF PSYCHOLOGICAL AND NEUROPSYCHIATRIC EVALUATIONS, INCLUDING A 96 HOUR INPATIENT EVALUATION CONDUCTED BY A BOARD-APPROVED CERTIFIED PSYCHIATRIST; EVIDENCE THAT HE HAS MAINTAINED ONE YEAR OF SOBRIETY FROM HIS REPORTED SOBRIETY DATE OF 10/23/98; AND, RESOLVES ANY CURRENTLY PENDING CRIMINAL MATTER RELATED TO THE 10/23/98 ARREST, AND THE RESOLUTION OF THE CASE IS FINAL; SHALL COOPERATE WITH THE BOARD IN VERIFYING COMPLIANCE INCLUDING PROVIDING COPIES OF MEDICAL RELEASES; SHALL INFORM THE BOARD OF CHANGE OF ADDRESS WITHIN 10 DAYS; SHALL NOT SEEK MODIFICATION FOR ONE YEAR.

THOMAS, STEPHEN CROCKETT MD, LICENSE NUMBER 00J5036 OF LUBBOCK, TX, WAS DISCIPLINED BY TEXAS ON JUNE 22, 1994
DISCIPLINARY ACTION: 120-MONTH PROBATION; RESTRICTION PLACED ON CONTROLLED SUBSTANCE LICENSE
OFFENSE: DISCIPLINARY ACTION BY ANOTHER STATE OR AGENCY

NOTES: DURING HIS RESIDENCY IN NEW YORK STARTING IN 1987 HE ABUSED PRESCRIPTION MEDICATION WITH CODEINE, PERCOCET, PERCODAN AS WELL AS BENZODIAZEPINES; ON 12/19/89 AFTER BEING APPROACHED ABOUT THIS HE SURRENDERED HIS NEW YORK LICENSE; ENTERED INPATIENT AND OUTPATIENT TREATMENT PROGRAMS AT THIS TIME; WAS SUSPENDED FROM HIS RESIDENCY PROGRAM DURING TREATMENT AND IN 5/90 WAS REINSTATED ON PROBATION; NEW YORK LICENSE RESTORED ON 11/19/90 SUBJECT TO CONDITIONS; ON 6/2/92 DEA ISSUED HIM A CERTIFICATE WITH RESTRICTIONS; REMAINS IN PHYSICIANS HEALTH PROGRAM; GAVE INACCURATE ANSWERS ON APPLICATION FORMS REGARDING THESE ACTIONS BUT APPEARS TO HAVE CORRECTED THESE. CONDITIONS OF PROBATION: SHALL APPEAR BEFORE THE BOARD TWICE A YEAR; SHALL BE SUPERVISED BY A BOARD-APPROVED PHYSICIAN WITH REPORTS THREE TIMES A YEAR; SHALL COMPLETE A TWO WEEK PRECEPTORSHIP ON PREVENTION AND TREATMENT OF DRUG ABUSE; SHALL NOT APPLY FOR OR MAINTAIN DEA OR TEXAS CONTROLLED SUBSTANCES CERTIFICATES; SHALL NOT TREAT OR OTHERWISE SERVE AS PHYSICIAN, PRESCRIBE, DISPENSE OR ADMINISTER DRUGS THAT MAY BE SUBJECT TO ABUSE FOR HIMSELF OR ANY MEMBER OF HIS FAMILY; SHALL ABSTAIN FROM THE CONSUMPTION OF ALCOHOL/CHEMICAL SUBSTANCES IN ANY FORM UNLESS PRESCRIBED BY ANOTHER PHYSICIAN FOR A LEGITIMATE AND THERAPEUTIC PURPOSE; SHALL CONTINUE TO PARTICIPATE IN A PHYSICIAN HEALTH AND REHABILITATION GROUP AND ATTEND WEEKLY MEETING WITH QUARTERLY REPORTS; SHALL CONTINUE TO PARTICIPATE IN AA'S PROGRAM NOT LESS THAN THREE TIMES A WEEK WITH QUARTERLY REPORTS TO THE BOARD; SHALL SUBMIT HIMSELF FOR APPROPRIATE EXAMS INCLUDING DRUG OR ALCOHOL SCREENS; SHALL FURNISH WRITTEN REPORTS TO THE BOARD UPON REQUEST VERIFYING COMPLIANCE; SHALL INFORM BOARD OF CHANGE OF ADDRESS WITHIN 10 DAYS OR IF HE LEAVES THE STATE; TIME SPENT OUT OF TEXAS DOES NOT COUNT TOWARD PROBATION. SHALL NOT SEEK MODIFICATION FOR ONE YEAR. THIS ORDER TAKES THE PLACE OF 8/28/93 ORDER. ON 6/28/95 ORDER MODIFIED SO THAT HE SHALL NOT APPLY FOR OR MAINTAIN DEA CONTROLLED SUBSTANCES REGISTRATIONS OR CERTIFICATES IN TEXAS UNTIL BOARD GRANTS HIM APPROVAL TO REAPPLY; ALL OTHER CONDITIONS REMAIN IN EFFECT.

THOMPSON, ELIZABETH JANE MD OF 15321 SAN PEDRO #103, SAN ANTONIO, TX, WAS DISCIPLINED BY DEA ON NOVEMBER 25, 1996
DISCIPLINARY ACTION: SURRENDER OF CONTROLLED SUBSTANCE LICENSE

NOTES: IN LIEU OF PUBLIC INTEREST REVOCATION.

THOMPSON, FRANK WILLIAM DO, LICENSE NUMBER 00D3694 OF DALLAS, TX, WAS DISCIPLINED BY TEXAS ON APRIL 15, 1994
DISCIPLINARY ACTION: REPRIMAND
OFFENSE: OVERPRESCRIBING OR MISPRESCRIBING DRUGS

NOTES: NONTHERAPEUTIC PRESCRIBING IN THE MANNER IN WHICH A DRUG WAS USED IN THAT ON 2/14/89 HE FAILED TO OBTAIN RECORDS OF BASELINE STUDIES FOR ONE PATIENT PRIOR TO INITIATING TREATMENT OF HER PSORIASIS WITH METHOTREXATE, WHICH IS KNOWN TO HAVE SIDE EFFECTS AND COMPLICATIONS

THOMPSON, JAMES MD OF 9801 STONELAKE BLVD #1923, AUSTIN, TX, WAS DISCIPLINED BY DEA ON OCTOBER 15, 1999
DISCIPLINARY ACTION: RESTRICTION PLACED ON CONTROLLED SUBSTANCE LICENSE

NOTES: MEMO OF UNDERSTANDING.

THOMPSON, JAMES B MD OF 4214 FERNDALE, PORT ARTHUR, TX, WAS DISCIPLINED BY DEA ON JUNE 10, 1996
DISCIPLINARY ACTION: RESTRICTION PLACED ON CONTROLLED SUBSTANCE LICENSE

NOTES: MEMO OF UNDERSTANDING.

THOMPSON, LLOYD G MD, LICENSE NUMBER 00C9161 OF DALLAS, TX, WAS DISCIPLINED BY TEXAS ON JUNE 17, 1992
DISCIPLINARY ACTION: REPRIMAND
OFFENSE: NONCOMPLIANCE WITH A PROFESSIONAL RULE

NOTES: SEVERAL VIOLATIONS OF THE MEDICAL PRACTICE ACT, INCLUDING MISLEADING ADVERTISEMENT.

THOMPSON, LLOYD G MD, DATE OF BIRTH OCTOBER 15, 1934, LICENSE NUMBER 0016951, WAS DISCIPLINED BY COLORADO ON JULY 14, 1995
DISCIPLINARY ACTION: 24-MONTH LICENSE SUSPENSION

THOMPSON, LLOYD GILBERT MD, LICENSE NUMBER C9161 OF DALLAS, TX, WAS DISCIPLINED BY TEXAS ON AUGUST 28, 1999
DISCIPLINARY ACTION: 60-MONTH PROBATION; FINE
OFFENSE: CRIMINAL CONVICTION OR PLEA OF GUILTY, NOLO CONTENDERE, OR NO CONTEST TO A CRIME

NOTES: ON 8/7/96 HE PLED GUILTY TO ONE COUNT OF WIRE FRAUD IN THE U.S. DISTRICT COURT MIDDLE DISTRICT OF LOUISIANA; THE BOARD DETERMINED THAT HE FAILED TO MAINTAIN ADEQUATE MEDICAL RECORDS, USED NON-STANDARD ABBREVIATIONS AND FAILED TO RECORD VITAL SIGNS ON SOME OFFICE VISITS. SUSPENSION STAYED FOR PROBATION WITH FOLLOWING TERMS AND CONDITIONS: $5,000 FINE; SHALL OBTAIN 50 HOURS PER YEAR OF CONTINUING MEDICAL EDUCATION WITH 20 HOURS IN RISK MANAGEMENT AND/OR MEDICAL RECORD KEEPING; WITHIN 6 MONTHS SHALL SUCCESSFULLY COMPLETE A BOARD-APPROVED COURSE IN MEDICAL RECORD KEEPING; WITHIN 6 MONTHS SHALL IMPLEMENT A NEW MEDICAL RECORD FORMAT; SHALL APPEAR BEFORE THE BOARD AT LEAST TWICE A YEAR; TIME SPENT OUT OF TEXAS DOES NOT COUNT TOWARD PROBATION; SHALL INFORM THE BOARD OF CHANGE OF ADDRESS WITHIN 10 DAYS OR IF HE LEAVES THE STATE; SHALL NOT SEEK MODIFICATION FOR ONE YEAR.

THOMPSON, PEYTON L MD, LICENSE NUMBER 00D9687 OF HOUSTON, TX, WAS DISCIPLINED BY TEXAS ON JUNE 10, 1991
DISCIPLINARY ACTION: REPRIMAND
OFFENSE: PROFESSIONAL MISCONDUCT

NOTES: UNPROFESSIONAL OR DISHONORABLE CONDUCT LIKELY TO DECEIVE, DEFRAUD, OR INJURE THE PUBLIC.

THOMPSON, STEPHEN KELLY MD, DATE OF BIRTH JUNE 6, 1953, LICENSE NUMBER 00G2582 OF 1714 N HENDERSON, DALLAS, TX, WAS DISCIPLINED BY TEXAS ON MARCH 31, 1990
OFFENSE: DISCIPLINARY ACTION BY ANOTHER STATE OR AGENCY

NOTES: STIPULATED ORDER. MUST COMPLY WITH GEORGIA ORDER AND MUST DEMONSTRATE CAPACITY TO PRACTICE MEDICINE WITH REASONABLE SKILL AND SAFETY IF HE DESIRES TO PRACTICE IN TEXAS. IF GRANTED PERMISSION TO PRACTICE IN TEXAS WHILE GEORGIA ORDER EFFECTIVE, TEXAS BOARD MAY IMPOSE PROBATIONARY TERMS AS IT DEEMS APPROPRIATE. ON 8/20/93 ORDER TERMINATED AND LICENSE FREE AND CLEAR OF ANY RESTRICTIONS.

THOMPSON, WALTER FRED DO, LICENSE NUMBER 00E7301 OF KNOX CITY, TX, WAS DISCIPLINED BY TEXAS ON NOVEMBER 19, 1993
DISCIPLINARY ACTION: REPRIMAND
OFFENSE: SUBSTANDARD CARE, INCOMPETENCE OR NEGLIGENCE

NOTES: ON 9/24/91 HIS SON WAS INVOLVED IN AN AUTO ACCIDENT AT WHICH TIME DR. THOMPSON TRANSPORTED HIM TO THE FAMILY PHYSICIAN RATHER THAN TO A CLOSER HOSPITAL; DEMONSTRATES AN ERROR IN JUDGMENT; HE CONTENDS HE WAS EMOTIONALLY AFFECTED AT THE TIME. SHALL GIVE A COPY OF THIS ORDER TO ANY HEALTH CARE ENTITY WHERE HE HAS PRIVILEGES; SHALL COOPERATE WITH THE BOARD IN VERIFYING COMPLIANCE; SHALL INFORM BOARD OF CHANGE OF ADDRESS WITHIN 10 DAYS.

THOMSON, ALTON L JR MD, LICENSE NUMBER 0032275 OF STUART, FL, WAS DISCIPLINED BY FLORIDA ON OCTOBER 6, 1993
DISCIPLINARY ACTION: FINE; REQUIRED TO TAKE ADDITIONAL MEDICAL EDUCATION
OFFENSE: SUBSTANDARD CARE, INCOMPETENCE OR NEGLIGENCE

NOTES: CHARGED WITH FAILING TO PRACTICE MEDICINE WITH AN ACCEPTABLE LEVEL OF CARE AND SKILL. $4,500 FINE; SHALL COMPLETE 30 HOURS OF CONTINUING MEDICAL EDUCATION IN GYNECOLOGY AND DIAGNOSIS WITHIN TWO YEARS.

THOMSON, ALTON L JR MD, LICENSE NUMBER 00D8461 OF STUART, FL, WAS DISCIPLINED BY TEXAS ON SEPTEMBER 30, 1994
DISCIPLINARY ACTION: SURRENDER OF LICENSE
OFFENSE: NONCOMPLIANCE WITH A PROFESSIONAL RULE

NOTES: ALLEGATIONS THAT HE VIOLATED THE MEDICAL PRACTICE ACT; HE DID NOT ADMIT ALLEGATIONS. SURRENDER IN LIEU OF FURTHER INVESTIGATION. PERMANENT CANCELLATION.

THOMSON, MARY E MD, LICENSE NUMBER J2374 OF WAKE VILLAGE, TX, WAS DISCIPLINED BY TEXAS ON AUGUST 9, 1997
DISCIPLINARY ACTION: 120-MONTH PROBATION; RESTRICTION PLACED ON LICENSE
OFFENSE: CRIMINAL CONVICTION OR PLEA OF GUILTY, NOLO CONTENDERE, OR NO CONTEST TO A CRIME

NOTES: WAS EVALUATED IN JUNE 1996 AND DIAGNOSED WITH BIPOLAR II DISORDER, CURRENTLY IN DEPRESSED PHASE, AND OPIATE ABUSE CURRENTLY IN REMISSION. SHE IS BEING TREATED BY A LICENSED PHYSICIAN WITH PROZAC AND LITHIUM AND REPORTS SEEING THIS PRACTITIONER ON A MONTHLY BASIS. SHE IS ALSO INVOLVED IN INDIVIDUAL PSYCHOTHERAPY SINCE APRIL 1996, ON A WEEKLY OR TWICE WEEKLY SCHEDULE. PRIOR TO 6/28/95 SHE ENGAGED IN THE INTEMPERATE USE OF DEMEROL. SHE REPORTS ATTENDANCE AT A CADUCEUS AA GROUP AT LEAST TWICE WEEKLY. WHILE ENGAGED IN OPIATE ABUSE, SHE DIVERTED PATIENT PRESCRIPTIONS TO HERSELF; ON 6/7/97 SHE PLED GUILTY TO ONE COUNT OF OBTAINING CONTROLLED SUBSTANCES BY FRAUD IN US DISTRICT COURT AND WAS PLACED ON PROBATION FOR THREE YEARS. REVOCATION IS PROBATED AND SHE IS PLACED ON PROBATION UNDER THE FOLLOWING TERMS: SHE SHALL OBTAIN WRITTEN CONSENT FROM THE US DISTRICT COURT TO ALLOW HER TO BE EMPLOYED AS A PHYSICIAN DURING THE PROBATIONARY PERIOD PRIOR TO PRACTICING MEDICINE IN TEXAS; SHALL LIMIT HER PRACTICE TO AN APPROVED, INSTITUTIONAL SETTING; SHALL ABSTAIN FROM THE CONSUMPTION OF ALCOHOL, DANGEROUS DRUGS, OR CONTROLLED SUBSTANCES UNLESS PRESCRIBED BY ANOTHER PHYSICIAN FOR A LEGITIMATE AND THERAPEUTIC PURPOSE; SHALL SUBMIT HERSELF FOR APPROPRIATE EXAMS INCLUDING DRUG OR ALCOHOL SCREENS; SHALL NOMINATE THREE CERTIFIED PSYCHIATRISTS FOR BOARD SELECTION OF A THERAPIST AND SHALL EXPEDITIOUSLY SUBMIT HERSELF TO EVALUATION AND TREATMENT BY THE APPROVED PRACTITIONER, WHO WILL MONITOR THE DOCTOR'S LITHIUM LEVELS MONTHLY; SHALL COOPERATE WITH THE BOARD IN VERIFYING COMPLIANCE INCLUDING PROVIDING COPIES OF MEDICAL RELEASES UPON REQUEST; SHALL PARTICIPATE IN THE ACTIVITIES OF A PHYSICIAN HEALTH AND REHABILITATION COMMITTEE AND ATTEND WEEKLY MEETINGS WITH QUARTERLY REPORTS; SHALL PARTICIPATE IN AA'S PROGRAM NOT LESS THAN THREE TIMES A WEEK; SHALL REPORT ON HIS ATTENDANCE; EXCEPT AS OTHERWISE PROVIDED FOR BY THE TERMS OF THIS ORDER, SHE SHALL NOT POSSESS ALCOHOL, CONTROLLED SUBSTANCES, OR DANGEROUS DRUGS AND SHALL TURN OVER ANY IN

HER POSSESSION INCLUDING SAMPLES; SHALL NOT TREAT OR OTHERWISE SERVE AS PHYSICIAN, PRESCRIBE, DISPENSE OR ADMINISTER DRUGS THAT MAY BE SUBJECT TO ABUSE TO HERSELF OR TO ANY MEMBER OF HER FAMILY; SEPARATE FROM PATIENT RECORDS, SHALL MAINTAIN A FILE OF EVERY PRESCRIPTION WRITTEN BY HER FOR DANGEROUS DRUGS WITH ADDICTIVE POTENTIAL WHICH SHALL BE MADE AVAILABLE FOR REVIEW; HER MEDICAL PRACTICE SHALL BE MONITORED BY ONE OR MORE LICENSED TEXAS PHYSICIANS APPROVED BY THE BOARD WHO SHALL PROVIDE MONTHLY REPORTS TO THE BOARD; SHALL OBTAIN AT LEAST 50 HOURS PER YEAR OF CONTINUING MEDICAL EDUCATION; TIME SPENT OUT OF TEXAS DOES NOT COUNT TOWARD PROBATION; SHALL INFORM THE BOARD OF CHANGE OF ADDRESS WITHIN 10 DAYS OR IF SHE LEAVES THE STATE; SHALL NOT SEEK MODIFICATION FOR ONE YEAR.

THORNTON, THOMAS L MD, LICENSE NUMBER 00D4335 OF ALLEN, TX, WAS DISCIPLINED BY TEXAS ON APRIL 20, 1991

NOTES: LICENSE PLACED ON RETIRED STATUS IN LIEU OF DISCIPLINARY ACTION; IF DESIRES TO PRACTICE IN TEXAS, SHALL OBTAIN PRIOR APPROVAL FROM THE BOARD.

THURMAN, BENJAMIN H MD, LICENSE NUMBER F4604 OF SAN ANGELO, TX, WAS DISCIPLINED BY TEXAS ON AUGUST 22, 1998
DISCIPLINARY ACTION: FINE
OFFENSE: NONCOMPLIANCE WITH A PROFESSIONAL RULE

NOTES: ON OR ABOUT 10/9/97 THE BOARD REQUESTED 13 SPECIFIC PATIENT RECORDS TO BE SENT WITHIN 10 DAYS; ON OR ABOUT 10/20/97 HE ASKED FOR INDEXED INFORMATION BUT DID NOT COMMENT ON THE REQUESTED RECORDS; ON OR ABOUT 10/24/97 THE BOARD AGAIN REQUESTED THE RECORDS; ON OR ABOUT 10/31/97 THE BOARD RESPONDED TO HIS REQUEST FOR INFORMATION. $5,000 FINE; SHALL COOPERATE WITH THE BOARD IN VERIFYING COMPLIANCE.

TICAS, ROBERTO A MD, LICENSE NUMBER 00H8865 OF LAKE JACKSON, TX, WAS DISCIPLINED BY TEXAS ON JANUARY 6, 1995
DISCIPLINARY ACTION: 60-MONTH PROBATION; RESTRICTION PLACED ON CONTROLLED SUBSTANCE LICENSE
OFFENSE: SUBSTANCE ABUSE

NOTES: ON JULY 30 AND AUGUST 6 1994 EXHIBITED BEHAVIORAL CHANGES AND CONCERNS WERE RAISED THAT HIS CAPACITY TO FUNCTION AS A PHYSICIAN HAD BEEN REDUCED; REPORTED THAT HE SELF-MEDICATED FOR DEPRESSION AND ASTHMA AND CONSUMED BEER WHILE ON MEDICATIONS HE SELF-PRESCRIBED; AGREED TO A PHYSICAL AND MENTAL EXAM WHICH INDICATED HIS ABILITY WAS IMPAIRED BY ALCOHOL USE. SUSPENSION STAYED. CONDITIONS OF PROBATION: SHALL ABSTAIN FROM THE CONSUMPTION OF ALCOHOL/CHEMICAL SUBSTANCES IN ANY FORM UNLESS PRESCRIBED BY ANOTHER PHYSICIAN FOR A LEGITIMATE AND THERAPEUTIC PURPOSE; SHALL SUBMIT HIMSELF FOR APPROPRIATE EXAMS INCLUDING DRUG OR ALCOHOL SCREENS; SHALL SUBMIT HIMSELF TO A BOARD-APPROVED PSYCHIATRIST FOR EVALUATION AND TREATMENT WITH REPORTS TO THE BOARD; SHALL PARTICIPATE IN AA'S PROGRAM NOT LESS THAN THREE TIMES A WEEK WITH QUARTERLY REPORTS TO THE BOARD; SHALL PARTICIPATE IN ACTIVITIES OF A PHYSICIANS HEALTH AND REHABILITATION COMMITTEE INCLUDING WEEKLY MEETINGS WITH QUARTERLY REPORTS; SHALL COMPLY WITH CONDITIONS OF ANY AGREEMENT ENTERED INTO FOR HOSPITAL PRIVILEGES AND SHALL REPORT THESE TO THE BOARD; SHALL NOT POSSESS ALCOHOL OR DRUGS WITH POTENTIAL FOR ABUSE EXCEPT AS OTHERWISE PROVIDED IN THIS ORDER; SHALL SURRENDER ALL SUCH SUBSTANCES IN HIS POSSESSION INCLUDING SAMPLES; SHALL NOT TELEPHONE A PRESCRIPTION FOR CONTROLLED SUBSTANCES OR DANGEROUS DRUGS TO A PHARMACY; SEPARATE FROM PATIENT RECORDS SHALL MAINTAIN A FILE OF EVERY PRESCRIPTION WRITTEN FOR CONTROLLED SUBSTANCES OR DANGEROUS DRUGS WHICH SHALL BE AVAILABLE FOR INSPECTION; SHALL NOT POSSESS, ADMINISTER OR DISPENSE ANY DANGEROUS DRUGS OR CONTROLLED SUBSTANCES BUT MAY PRESCRIBE SUCH DRUGS FOR OUTPATIENTS AND MAY ORDER SUCH DRUGS FOR HOSPITAL INPATIENTS; MEDICAL PRACTICE SHALL BE MONITORED BY A BOARD-APPROVED PHYSICIAN WITH QUARTERLY REPORTS; SHALL MAINTAIN ADEQUATE MEDICAL RECORDS ON ALL OFFICE VISITS WHICH SHALL BE AVAILABLE FOR INSPECTION; SHALL OBTAIN AT LEAST 50 HOURS PER YEAR OF CONTINUING MEDICAL EDUCATION; SHALL PASS THE SPEX EXAM WITHIN ONE YEAR; SHALL APPEAR BEFORE THE BOARD TWICE A YEAR AND WHEN REQUESTED; SHALL COOPERATE WITH THE BOARD IN VERIFYING COMPLIANCE; SHALL EXECUTE RELEASES NECESSARY TO OBTAIN MEDICAL TREATMENT RECORDS AND PEER REVIEW RECORDS; SHALL GIVE A COPY OF THIS ORDER TO ANY HEALTH CARE ENTITY WHERE HE HAS OR APPLIES FOR PRIVILEGES OR ANYONE ELSE WHO REQUESTS IT; SHALL ENSURE INQUIRIES REGARDING HIS TEXAS LICENSURE STATUS ARE ANSWERED BY REFERENCING THIS ORDER; SHALL INFORM BOARD OF CHANGE OF ADDRESS WITHIN 10 DAYS OR IF HE LEAVES THE STATE; TIME SPENT OUT OF TEXAS DOES NOT COUNT TOWARD PROBATION. SHALL NOT SEEK MODIFICATION FOR ONE YEAR.

TICAS, ROBERTO A MD, LICENSE NUMBER 00H8865 OF LAKE JACKSON, TX, WAS DISCIPLINED BY TEXAS ON OCTOBER 14, 1995
DISCIPLINARY ACTION: EMERGENCY SUSPENSION
OFFENSE: FAILURE TO COMPLY WITH PREVIOUS BOARD ORDER

NOTES: AVAILABLE EVIDENCE AND INFORMATION INDICATE THE FOLLOWING: ON OR AROUND 5/30/95 HE INGESTED ALCOHOL IN VIOLATION OF 1/95 ORDER AND WAS ARRESTED AND SUBSEQUENTLY CHARGED WITH PUBLIC INTOXICATION; IN A 9/95 REPORT HIS TREATING PSYCHIATRIST REPORTED THAT HE SUFFERED A RELAPSE INTO THE USE OF ALCOHOL DURING MIDSUMMER OF 1995; FAILED TO REPORT HIS ALCOHOL INGESTION TO THE BOARD AS REQUIRED BY 1/95 ORDER; FROM 2/95 TO 4/95 HE PRESCRIBED 140 VICODIN, A SCHEDULE III CONTROLLED SUBSTANCE, AND 10 XANAX, A SCHEDULE IV CONTROLLED SUBSTANCE, TOGETHER WITH REFILLS FOR THE SAME AMOUNTS TO AN UNDERCOVER AGENT AND WITHOUT A VALID MEDICAL PURPOSE AND ALLEGEDLY ALTERED MEDICAL RECORDS TO ATTEMPT TO VALIDATE THESE PRESCRIPTIONS. IN 7/95 INDICTED ON FOUR COUNTS OF FRAUDULENT DELIVERY OF A CONTROLLED SUBSTANCE. SUSPENSION OF LICENSE UNTIL IT IS SUPERSEDED BY A SUBSEQUENT BOARD ORDER. ALLEGATIONS RELATED TO SUSPENSION WILL BE THE SUBJECT OF A DISCIPLINARY HEARING AS SOON AS CAN BE ACCOMPLISHED.

TICAS, ROBERTO A MD, LICENSE NUMBER 0181100 OF 201 OAK

DRIVE S SUITE 203B, LAKE JACKSON, TX, WAS DISCIPLINED BY NEW YORK ON DECEMBER 12, 1995
DISCIPLINARY ACTION: LICENSE SUSPENSION
OFFENSE: DISCIPLINARY ACTION BY ANOTHER STATE OR AGENCY

NOTES: ACTION IN TEXAS FOR HIS HABITUAL USE OF ALCOHOL AND/OR DRUGS. LICENSE SUSPENSION UNTIL SATISFACTORY COMPLETION OF CONDITIONS IMPOSED BY THE TEXAS BOARD.

TICAS, ROBERTO ARMANDO MD, LICENSE NUMBER 0181100 OF 600 TRAVIS SUITE 3000, HOUSTON, TX, WAS DISCIPLINED BY NEW YORK ON APRIL 29, 1996
DISCIPLINARY ACTION: SURRENDER OF LICENSE
OFFENSE: DISCIPLINARY ACTION BY ANOTHER STATE OR AGENCY

NOTES: ACTION IN TEXAS FOR VIOLATING THE TERMS OF HIS PREVIOUS AGREED ORDER BY INGESTING ALCOHOL AND PRESCRIBING EXCESSIVE AMOUNTS OF CONTROLLED SUBSTANCES FOR NON-THERAPEUTIC PURPOSES.

TINSLEY, MARK S MD, LICENSE NUMBER 0014907, WAS DISCIPLINED BY ARIZONA ON JUNE 8, 1990
OFFENSE: FAILURE TO COMPLY WITH PREVIOUS BOARD ORDER

NOTES: VIOLATED BOARD ORDER OF 10/7/88 BY USING ILLICIT DRUGS AND FAILING TO RESPOND TO A REQUEST FOR A URINE SPECIMEN. LICENSE PLACED ON INACTIVE STATUS IN ORDER FOR HIM TO ENTER A LONG-TERM DRUG DEPENDENCY PROGRAM.

TINSLEY, MARK S MD, LICENSE NUMBER 0014907, WAS DISCIPLINED BY ARIZONA ON JUNE 19, 1991
DISCIPLINARY ACTION: 60-MONTH PROBATION; RESTRICTION PLACED ON CONTROLLED SUBSTANCE LICENSE
OFFENSE: SUBSTANCE ABUSE

NOTES: ON 1/15/88 BOARD RECEIVED INFORMATION HE HAD BEEN TERMINATED FROM HIS SURGICAL RESIDENCY FOR FAILURE TO PERFORM IN ACCORDANCE WITH HIS CONTRACT AND FOR CONCERNS REGARDING HIS CLINICAL ABILITIES. ON 6/9/88 HE ENTERED AN INPATIENT CHEMICAL DEPENDENCY TREATMENT PROGRAM WHICH HE SUCCESSFULLY COMPLETED ON 09/29/88. ON 4/13/89 THE BOARD ISSUED A LETTER OF CONCERN REGARDING A MALPRACTICE COMPLAINT FOR FAILURE TO CORRECTLY DIAGNOSE TORSION OF THE PATIENT'S TESTICLE. IN EARLY 1990 HE WAS FIRED FROM HIS POSITION AS AN EMERGENCY ROOM PHYSICIAN. IN MAY 1990 HE ACKNOWLEDGED MISUSING DRUGS BETWEEN 4/7/90 AND 5/17/90. IN JUNE 1990 HE REQUESTED THE BOARD PLACE HIS LICENSE ON INACTIVE STATUS. ENTERED INPATIENT CHEMICAL DEPENDENCY TREATMENT ON 7/15/90 AND COMPLETED THE PROGRAM ON 8/17/90. ENTERED A SECOND INPATIENT CHEMICAL DEPENDENCY TREATMENT PROGRAM ON 8/29/90 AND WAS DISCHARGED ON 3/30/91. ON 6/19/91 HE ASKED THE BOARD TO RETURN HIS LICENSE TO ACTIVE STATUS. CONDITIONS OF PROBATION: SHALL SURRENDER HIS DEA REGISTRATION FOR SCHEDULE II SUBSTANCES AND SHALL NOT APPLY FOR REINSTATEMENT WITHOUT BOARD APPROVAL; SHALL PARTICIPATE IN THE ARIZONA MEDICAL ASSOCIATION'S MONITORED AFTERCARE TREATMENT PROGRAM; MUST HAVE THERAPIST SUBMIT QUARTERLY REPORTS TO THE BOARD AND OPEN HIS RECORDS TO THE BOARD; MUST ATTEND A MINIMUM OF 90 MEETINGS OF A 12 STEP RECOVERY PROGRAM WITHIN 90 DAYS AND THREE MEETINGS PER WEEK AFTER THAT; MUST OBTAIN ONE BOARD-APPROVED TREATING PHYSICIAN; MUST ABSTAIN FROM ALCOHOL AND OTHER DRUGS; MUST COMPLY WITH REQUESTS FOR RANDOM SCREENING OF BODILY FLUIDS; MUST MAINTAIN A LOG OF ALL MEDICATION; MUST SUBMIT TO MENTAL, PHYSICAL OR MEDICAL COMPETENCY EXAMS AS REQUESTED BY BOARD; MUST SUBMIT TO ANY THERAPY ORDERED BY BOARD; MUST APPEAR BEFORE BOARD FOR INTERVIEWS UPON REQUEST AND INFORM THE BOARD IF HE CHANGES ADDRESS OR WILL BE AWAY FOR MORE THAN FIVE DAYS. ON 1/25/92 BOARD GAVE WRITTEN PERMISSION FOR HIM TO REAPPLY FOR DEA CONTROLLED SUBSTANCES REGISTRATION FOR SCHEDULE II NARCOTICS DUE TO HIS ONGOING REHABILITATION EFFORTS. EFFECTIVE 10/16/93 HIS REQUEST TO CHANGE SUPPORT GROUPS WAS APPROVED. EFFECTIVE 4/16/94 PROBATION TERMINATED AND HE MUST ENTER INTO A STIPULATION WITH THE SAME TERMS AS HIS PROBATIONARY ORDER. ON 4/8/95 ORDER TERMINATED.

TINSLEY, MARK STANLY MD, LICENSE NUMBER 00G5693 OF PHOENIX, AZ, WAS DISCIPLINED BY TEXAS ON MARCH 6, 1992
DISCIPLINARY ACTION: 60-MONTH PROBATION
OFFENSE: DISCIPLINARY ACTION BY ANOTHER STATE OR AGENCY

NOTES: DISCIPLINARY ACTION TAKEN BY ANOTHER STATE BOARD FOR INTEMPERATE USE OF ALCOHOL OR DRUGS. LICENSE SUSPENDED, SUSPENSION STAYED; PROBATION UNDER TERMS AND CONDITIONS.

TITUS, PATRICK A MD, LICENSE NUMBER C8730 OF HOUSTON, TX, WAS DISCIPLINED BY TEXAS ON AUGUST 28, 1999
DISCIPLINARY ACTION: 60-MONTH RESTRICTION PLACED ON CONTROLLED SUBSTANCE LICENSE; REQUIRED TO TAKE ADDITIONAL MEDICAL EDUCATION
OFFENSE: OVERPRESCRIBING OR MISPRESCRIBING DRUGS

NOTES: IN 1992 & 1993 HE PRESCRIBED NUMEROUS PRESCRIPTIONS FOR SOMA, WITH OR WITHOUT FIORINAL TO VARIOUS PATIENTS ON A MONTHLY BASIS; HE DID NOT ADEQUATELY DOCUMENT HISTORY AND PHYSICAL EXAMS OR OTHER TREATMENT MODALITIES AS ALTERNATIVES FOR THESE PATIENTS, INCLUDING BIOFEEDBACK, RELAXATION, THERAPY, OR TRICYCLIC ANTIDEPRESSANTS; A BOARD CONSULTANT QUESTIONED WHETHER HE WAS OVER-PRESCRIBING SOMA AND FIORINAL, PARTICULARLY DUE TO THE LACK OF ADEQUATE DOCUMENTATION IN THE PATIENT'S MEDICAL RECORDS. LICENSE LIMITED AS FOLLOWS: SHALL SURRENDER DEA AND TEXAS DEPARTMENT OF PUBLIC SAFETY CONTROLLED SUBSTANCES REGISTRATION CERTIFICATES; SEPARATE FROM PATIENT RECORDS, SHALL MAINTAIN A LOGBOOK OF EVERY PRESCRIPTION WRITTEN BY HIM FOR DANGEROUS DRUGS WITH ADDICTIVE POTENTIAL WHICH SHALL BE MADE AVAILABLE FOR REVIEW; SHALL OBTAIN 50 HOURS PER YEAR OF CONTINUING MEDICAL EDUCATION; WITHIN 3 MONTHS SHALL SUCCESSFULLY COMPLETE A COURSE IN THE AREA OF PREVENTION AND TREATMENT OF DRUG ABUSE; SHALL APPEAR BEFORE THE BOARD AT LEAST TWICE A YEAR TO ADDRESS ISSUES RELATING TO COMPLIANCE; TIME SPENT OUT OF TEXAS DOES NOT COUNT TOWARD RESTRICTION; SHALL INFORM THE BOARD OF CHANGE OF ADDRESS WITHIN 10 DAYS OR IF HE LEAVES THE STATE; SHALL NOT SEEK MODIFICATION FOR ONE YEAR.

TIZARD, GARY T MD, LICENSE NUMBER 0012551 OF 394 WEST MAIN STREET, HENDERSONVILLE, TN, WAS DISCIPLINED BY TENNESSEE ON JULY 17, 1990
DISCIPLINARY ACTION: EMERGENCY SUSPENSION; RESTRICTION PLACED ON LICENSE

OFFENSE: PROFESSIONAL MISCONDUCT

NOTES: ALLEGED SEXUAL MISCONDUCT, PERSON UNSPECIFIED. ON 6/2/95 THIS ORDER SHALL REMAIN IN FULL FORCE AND EFFECT; HE DOES NOT WISH TO PURSUE THE MATTER AND THE CASE IS RETIRED FOR ADMINISTRATIVE PURPOSES ONLY.

TIZARD, GARY T MD, LICENSE NUMBER 00D7334 OF HENDERSONVILLE, TN, WAS DISCIPLINED BY TEXAS ON OCTOBER 26, 1990
DISCIPLINARY ACTION: LICENSE SUSPENSION
OFFENSE: DISCIPLINARY ACTION BY ANOTHER STATE OR AGENCY

NOTES: SUSPENDED PENDING OUTCOME OF FINAL HEARING BEFORE TENNESSEE BOARD; MUST AUTHORIZE TENNESSEE BOARD TO RELEASE INFORMATION TO TEXAS AS TO STATUS AND COMPLIANCE WITH PROBATION; RECEIVE APPROVAL OF TEXAS BOARD PRIOR TO PRACTICING MEDICINE IN TEXAS.

TIZARD, GARY T MD, WAS DISCIPLINED BY ARIZONA ON JANUARY 23, 1992
DISCIPLINARY ACTION: LICENSE REVOCATION
OFFENSE: DISCIPLINARY ACTION BY ANOTHER STATE OR AGENCY

NOTES: LICENSE WAS SUSPENDED IN TENNESSEE FOR UNPROFESSIONAL CONDUCT. TEXAS ENTERED INTO AN AGREED ORDER WITH DOCTOR TIZARD'S SURRENDERING HIS TEXAS LICENSE AS A RESULT OF ACTIONS TAKEN IN TENNESSEE. DR. TIZARD SIGNED A CANCELLATION OF HIS ARIZONA LICENSE WITH CAUSE WHICH REQUIRES BOARD ACTION.

TIZARD, GARY TIFFANY MD, DATE OF BIRTH JUNE 17, 1944 OF 111 WILLIAM SHY DR, HENDERSONVILLE, TN, WAS DISCIPLINED BY MEDICARE ON AUGUST 18, 1991
DISCIPLINARY ACTION: EXCLUSION FROM THE MEDICARE AND/OR MEDICAID PROGRAM
OFFENSE: DISCIPLINARY ACTION BY ANOTHER STATE OR AGENCY

NOTES: LICENSE REVOCATION OR SUSPENSION.

TJONG, PIANG S MD, LICENSE NUMBER 0117930 OF 9F, 136 HSIN YI ROAD, TOUFEN MIAOLI, TAIWAN, WAS DISCIPLINED BY NEW YORK ON NOVEMBER 27, 1996
DISCIPLINARY ACTION: SURRENDER OF LICENSE
OFFENSE: DISCIPLINARY ACTION BY ANOTHER STATE OR AGENCY

NOTES: ACTION IN CALIFORNIA FOR NEGLIGENCE ON MORE THAN ONE OCCASION INVOLVING EIGHT PATIENTS.

TJONG, PIANG S MD, LICENSE NUMBER F2481 OF FRESNO, CA, WAS DISCIPLINED BY TEXAS ON FEBRUARY 7, 1998
DISCIPLINARY ACTION: LICENSE SUSPENSION
OFFENSE: DISCIPLINARY ACTION BY ANOTHER STATE OR AGENCY

NOTES: IN 12/95 CALIFORNIA BOARD PUT LICENSE ON PROBATION FOR FAILURE TO TIMELY OR ADEQUATELY TREAT CONGESTIVE HEART FAILURE, GASTROINTESTINAL BLEEDING, SEPTIC SHOCK AND MYOCARDIAL INFARCTION; IN 11/96 HE SURRENDERED HIS NEW YORK LICENSE BASED ON THE ACTION TAKEN AGAINST HIM IN CALIFORNIA. INDEFINITE SUSPENSION; SHALL NOT PRACTICE IN TEXAS UNTIL HE REQUESTS IN WRITING TO RESUME PRACTICE, AND APPEARS BEFORE THE BOARD TO ORALLY PETITION FOR PERMISSION TO RESUME SUCH PRACTICE AND PROVIDES SUFFICIENT EVIDENCE OF HIS COMPETENCE INCLUDING BUT NOT LIMITED TO COMPLYING WITH CALIFORNIA BOARD ORDER.

TJONG, PIANG SIOE MD, LICENSE NUMBER 0A32475 OF FRESNO, CA, WAS DISCIPLINED BY CALIFORNIA ON DECEMBER 7, 1995
DISCIPLINARY ACTION: 60-MONTH PROBATION
OFFENSE: SUBSTANDARD CARE, INCOMPETENCE OR NEGLIGENCE

NOTES: REPEATED NEGLIGENT ACTS IN THE CARE AND TREATMENT OF PATIENTS AS A PRIMARY CARE PHYSICIAN. REVOCATION, STAYED.

TODD, EUGENE RAY MD, LICENSE NUMBER 00C7144 OF DALLAS, TX, WAS DISCIPLINED BY TEXAS ON JUNE 22, 1994
DISCIPLINARY ACTION: REQUIRED TO TAKE ADDITIONAL MEDICAL EDUCATION; MONITORING OF PHYSICIAN PERFORMANCE
OFFENSE: NONCOMPLIANCE WITH A PROFESSIONAL RULE

NOTES: TREATED A FAMILY MEMBER WITH PAIN MEDICATIONS; FAILED TO KEEP ANY MEDICAL RECORDS REGARDING THIS; AUDITED BY DEA WHICH FOUND THAT HIS RECORD KEEPING FOR STEROIDS WAS INADEQUATE. LICENSE RESTRICTED FOR THREE YEARS WITH THE FOLLOWING CONDITIONS: SHALL ATTEND AT LEAST 50 HOURS PER YEAR OF CONTINUING MEDICAL EDUCATION WITH AT LEAST 10 OF THESE IN RISK MANAGEMENT OR RECORDKEEPING COURSES; SHALL MAINTAIN ADEQUATE MEDICAL RECORDS ON ALL PATIENT OFFICE VISITS WHICH SHALL BE AVAILABLE FOR INSPECTION; SHALL NOT SIGN ANY PATIENT RECORD UNLESS HE HAS PERSONALLY EXAMINED THE PATIENT OR CLEARLY NOTES IN THE RECORD THAT HE DID NOT; SHALL NOT TREAT OR OTHERWISE SERVE AS PHYSICIAN, PRESCRIBE, DISPENSE OR ADMINISTER DRUGS THAT MAY BE SUBJECT TO ABUSE TO HIMSELF OR ANY MEMBER OF HIS FAMILY; SHALL APPEAR BEFORE THE BOARD ONCE A YEAR; SHALL GIVE A COPY OF THIS ORDER TO ANY HEALTH CARE ENTITY WHERE HE HAS PRIVILEGES; SHALL COOPERATE WITH THE BOARD IN VERIFYING COMPLIANCE; SHALL INFORM BOARD OF CHANGE OF ADDRESS WITHIN 10 DAYS OR IF HE LEAVES THE STATE; TIME SPENT OUT OF TEXAS DOES NOT COUNT TOWARD RESTRICTION. SHALL NOT SEEK MODIFICATION FOR ONE YEAR. PROBATION TERMINATED ON 5/15/96.

TODD, WILLIAM D MD, DATE OF BIRTH JANUARY 23, 1946, LICENSE NUMBER 0017077 OF KERRVILLE, TX, WAS DISCIPLINED BY KENTUCKY ON OCTOBER 20, 1994
DISCIPLINARY ACTION: SURRENDER OF LICENSE

TODD, WILLIAM DAVID MD, LICENSE NUMBER 00E2093 OF BIG SPRING, TX, WAS DISCIPLINED BY TEXAS ON MARCH 5, 1994
DISCIPLINARY ACTION: 60-MONTH PROBATION; REQUIRED TO TAKE ADDITIONAL MEDICAL EDUCATION
OFFENSE: DISCIPLINARY ACTION BY ANOTHER STATE OR AGENCY

NOTES: ON 9/1/93 KENTUCKY BOARD PLACED LICENSE ON A FIVE YEAR PROBATION WHICH REQUIRES PARTICIPATION WITH KENTUCKY IMPAIRED PHYSICIANS COMMITTEE AND AA, AND SHALL SUBMIT TO RANDOM BIOLOGICAL FLUID TESTING; HE IS AN ALCOHOLIC; CURRENTLY WORKING IN A HOSPITAL AS A PSYCHIATRIST AND IS SUPERVISED. FIVE YEAR SUSPENSION STAYED. CONDITIONS OF PROBATION: SHALL ABSTAIN FROM THE CONSUMPTION OF DRUGS/CHEMICAL SUBSTANCES IN ANY FORM UNLESS PRESCRIBED BY ANOTHER PHYSICIAN FOR A LEGITIMATE AND THERAPEUTIC PURPOSE; SHALL NOT TREAT OR OTHERWISE SERVE AS PHYSICIAN, PRESCRIBE, DISPENSE, OR ADMINISTER DRUGS SUBJECT TO ABUSE TO HIMSELF OR ANY MEMBER OF HIS FAMILY; SHALL PARTICIPATE IN AA'S PROGRAMS NOT LESS THAN THREE TIMES A WEEK WITH QUARTERLY REPORTS TO THE BOARD; SHALL SUBMIT

HIMSELF FOR APPROPRIATE EXAMS INCLUDING BLOOD OR ALCOHOL SCREENS; SHALL SUBMIT HIMSELF FOR EVALUATION AND TREATMENT BY A BOARD-APPROVED PSYCHIATRIST WITH QUARTERLY REPORTS; SHALL CONTINUE TO BE MONITORED BY HIS SUPERVISOR WITH QUARTERLY REPORTS; SHALL ATTEND AT LEAST 50 HOURS PER YEAR OF CONTINUING MEDICAL EDUCATION AT LEAST FIVE HOURS PER YEAR SHALL BE IN THE AREA OF SUBSTANCE ABUSE; SHALL PERFORM EIGHT HOURS PER MONTH OF COMMUNITY SERVICE FOR FIVE YEARS; SHALL APPEAR BEFORE THE BOARD FOUR TIMES A YEAR FOR THE FIRST YEAR AND TWICE A YEAR AFTER THAT; SHALL GIVE A COPY OF THIS ORDER TO ANY HEALTH CARE ENTITY WHERE HE HAS PRIVILEGES; SHALL COOPERATE WITH THE BOARD IN VERIFYING COMPLIANCE; SHALL INFORM BOARD OF CHANGE OF ADDRESS WITHIN 10 DAYS OR IF HE LEAVES THE STATE; TIME SPENT OUT OF TEXAS DOES NOT COUNT TOWARD PROBATION. SHALL NOT SEEK MODIFICATION FOR ONE YEAR.

TODD, WILLIAM DAVID MD, LICENSE NUMBER 00E2093 OF KERRVILLE, TX, WAS DISCIPLINED BY TEXAS ON MAY 11, 1995
DISCIPLINARY ACTION: LICENSE SUSPENSION
OFFENSE: FAILURE TO COMPLY WITH PREVIOUS BOARD ORDER

NOTES: IN 2/95, DRUG SCREEN REVEALED INGESTION OF A BENZODIAZEPINE (OXAZEPAM), A CONTROLLED SUBSTANCE WITHOUT LEGITIMATE MEDICAL REASON AND IN VIOLATION OF 3/94 BOARD ORDER. SUSPENSION UNTIL HE REQUESTS TO HAVE THE SUSPENSION STAYED OR LIFTED AND APPEARS BEFORE THE BOARD WITH SUFFICIENT EVIDENCE WHICH INDICATES THAT HE IS PHYSICALLY, MENTALLY AND OTHERWISE COMPETENT TO SAFELY PRACTICE MEDICINE INCLUDING AT A MINIMUM COPIES OF MEDICAL RECORDS AND REPORTS OF PSYCHOLOGICAL AND NEUROPSYCHIATRIC EVALUATIONS, INCLUDING A 96-HOUR INPATIENT EVALUATION CONDUCTED BY A BOARD-APPROVED PSYCHIATRIST.

TODD, WILLIAM DAVID MD OF 315 RUNNELS STREET, BIG SPRING, TX, WAS DISCIPLINED BY DEA ON AUGUST 14, 1995
DISCIPLINARY ACTION: SURRENDER OF CONTROLLED SUBSTANCE LICENSE
OFFENSE: DISCIPLINARY ACTION BY ANOTHER STATE OR AGENCY

NOTES: STATE BOARD.

TODD, WILLIAM DAVID MD, LICENSE NUMBER 00E2093 OF KERRVILLE, TX, WAS DISCIPLINED BY TEXAS ON AUGUST 18, 1995
DISCIPLINARY ACTION: 120-MONTH PROBATION; RESTRICTION PLACED ON CONTROLLED SUBSTANCE LICENSE
OFFENSE: SUBSTANCE ABUSE

NOTES: HAS SATISFIED THE MINIMUM REQUIREMENTS AS SET OUT IN 5/95 ORDER FOR REINSTATEMENT OF LICENSE. SUSPENSION STAYED. PROBATION UNDER TERMS AND CONDITIONS: SHALL ABSTAIN FROM THE CONSUMPTION OF ALCOHOL/DRUGS IN ANY FORM UNLESS PRESCRIBED BY ANOTHER PHYSICIAN FOR A LEGITIMATE AND THERAPEUTIC PURPOSE; SHALL SUBMIT HIMSELF FOR CARE AND TREATMENT TO A BOARD APPROVED PSYCHIATRIST WHO HE SHALL SEE AT LEAST MONTHLY AND WHO SHALL SUBMIT REPORTS TO THE BOARD; SHALL PARTICIPATE IN PHYSICIAN'S HEALTH AND REHABILITATION PROGRAM AND ATTEND WEEKLY MEETINGS WITH QUARTERLY REPORTS; SHALL SUBMIT HIMSELF FOR APPROPRIATE EXAMS INCLUDING DRUG OR ALCOHOL SCREENS; SHALL PARTICIPATE IN AA'S PROGRAM NOT LESS THAN FIVE TIMES A WEEK WITH QUARTERLY REPORTS TO THE BOARD; SHALL COMPLY WITH THE TERMS AND CONDITIONS OF ANY CONTINUING CARE CONTRACT WITH QUARTERLY REPORTS; SHALL NOT POSSESS ALCOHOL, CONTROLLED SUBSTANCES OR DRUGS WITH POTENTIAL FOR ABUSE AND SHALL SURRENDER ALL SUCH DRUGS INCLUDING SAMPLES; SHALL NOT TREAT OR OTHERWISE SERVE AS PHYSICIAN, PRESCRIBE, DISPENSE OR ADMINISTER DRUGS THAT MAY BE SUBJECT TO ABUSE TO HIMSELF OR TO ANY MEMBER OF HIS FAMILY; SHALL NOT PERMIT ANY INDIVIDUAL UNDER HIS SUPERVISION TO TELEPHONE A PHARMACY A PRESCRIPTION OR A REFILL FOR SUCH DRUGS; SHALL MAINTAIN A LOG OF ALL PRESCRIPTIONS FOR SUCH DRUGS WHICH SHALL BE AVAILABLE FOR REVIEW; HIS MEDICAL PRACTICE, INCLUDING ANY OFFICE AND SURGICAL PRACTICE SHALL BE MONITORED BY A BOARD APPROVED TEXAS PHYSICIAN WHO SHALL SUBMIT QUARTERLY REPORTS; SHALL MAINTAIN ADEQUATE MEDICAL RECORDS WHICH SHALL BE AVAILABLE FOR REVIEW; SHALL OBTAIN AT LEAST 50 HOURS OF CONTINUING MEDICAL EDUCATION PER YEAR; SHALL APPEAR BEFORE THE BOARD TWICE A YEAR; SHALL GIVE A COPY OF THIS ORDER TO ANY HEALTH CARE ENTITY WHERE HE HAS PRIVILEGES; SHALL COOPERATE WITH THE BOARD IN VERIFYING COMPLIANCE INCLUDING PROVIDING COPIES OF MEDICAL RELEASES UPON REQUEST; SHALL INFORM BOARD OF CHANGE OF ADDRESS WITHIN 10 DAYS OR IF HE LEAVES THE STATE; TIME SPENT OUT OF TEXAS DOES NOT COUNT TOWARD PROBATION. SHALL NOT SEEK MODIFICATION FOR ONE YEAR. ON 10/5/96 ORDER MODIFIED SO HE IS ONLY REQUIRED TO PARTICIPATE IN AA 3 TIMES PER WEEK. ON 8/22/98 ORDER MODIFIED DELETING MONITORING OF PRACTICE, AND REDUCING APPEARANCES BEFORE THE BOARD FROM BIANNUAL TO UPON BOARD'S REQUEST.

TOLON, EDWIN J T MD, LICENSE NUMBER D6878, WAS DISCIPLINED BY TEXAS ON JUNE 10, 1996
DISCIPLINARY ACTION: 60-MONTH PROBATION; REQUIRED TO TAKE ADDITIONAL MEDICAL EDUCATION
OFFENSE: NONCOMPLIANCE WITH A PROFESSIONAL RULE

NOTES: IN 1994 FAILED TO DOCUMENT HIS CARE AND TREATMENT OF VARIOUS PATIENTS; MEDICAL RECORDS ALSO FAIL TO SUPPORT THE TREATMENT OF THESE VARIOUS PATIENTS. SUSPENSION STAYED FOR PROBATION WITH FOLLOWING TERMS AND CONDITIONS: SHALL OBTAIN FIFTY HOURS OF CONTINUING MEDICAL EDUCATION PER YEAR WITH ONE COURSE IN RISK MANAGEMENT AND THE REMAINING HOURS IN FAMILY PRACTICE; SHALL MAINTAIN ADEQUATE MEDICAL RECORDS WHICH SHALL BE AVAILABLE FOR REVIEW; WITHIN THREE MONTHS SHALL TAKE AND PASS THE SPEX; HIS PRACTICE SHALL BE MONITORED BY A LICENSED TEXAS PHYSICIAN; SHALL COOPERATE WITH THE BOARD IN VERIFYING COMPLIANCE INCLUDING PROVIDING COPIES OF PEER REVIEW RECORDS UPON REQUEST; SHALL ADEQUATELY SUPERVISE ALL HIS EMPLOYEES AND ALL OTHER INDIVIDUALS UNDER HIS SUPERVISION; SHALL NOT SERVE AS A SUPERVISOR FOR A PHYSICIAN ASSISTANT OR AN ADVANCED PRACTICE NURSE; SHALL PERSONALLY EXAMINE AND/OR TREAT PATIENTS IN WHICH A FORM, RECORD, OR OTHER REPRESENTATION INDICATES THAT A PERSONAL EXAMINATION OR TREATMENT OF A PATIENT BY HIM HAS TAKEN PLACE; SHALL APPEAR BEFORE THE BOARD AT LEAST TWICE EACH YEAR; SHALL GIVE A COPY OF THIS ORDER TO ANY HEALTH CARE ENTITY WHERE HE HAS PRIVILEGES; SHALL

PROVIDE A COPY OF THIS ORDER TO ANYONE REQUESTING IT WITHIN 10 DAYS; TIME SPENT OUT OF TEXAS DOES NOT COUNT TOWARD PROBATION; SHALL INFORM THE BOARD OF CHANGE OF ADDRESS WITHIN 10 DAYS OR IF HE LEAVES THE STATE; SHALL NOT SEEK MODIFICATION FOR ONE YEAR.

TOLON, EDWIN J T MD, LICENSE NUMBER D6878, WAS DISCIPLINED BY TEXAS ON NOVEMBER 25, 1996
DISCIPLINARY ACTION: LICENSE SUSPENSION
OFFENSE: FAILURE TO COMPLY WITH PREVIOUS BOARD ORDER
NOTES: VIOLATED 6/22/96 ORDER BY FAILING TO TAKE AND PASS THE SPEX BY 9/22/96. UPON REINSTATEMENT SUSPENSION STAYED FOR PROBATION UNDER THE 6/22/96 ORDER'S TERMS AND CONDITIONS. ON 3/1/97 REQUEST TO HAVE SUSPENSION LIFTED DENIED.

TOMASEVIC, MIRA MD, LICENSE NUMBER 00G8764 OF ASPERMONT, TX, WAS DISCIPLINED BY TEXAS ON APRIL 10, 1992
DISCIPLINARY ACTION: 60-MONTH PROBATION
OFFENSE: DISCIPLINARY ACTION BY ANOTHER STATE OR AGENCY
NOTES: UNPROFESSIONAL OR DISHONORABLE CONDUCT LIKELY TO DECEIVE, DEFRAUD OR INJURE THE PUBLIC, AND DISCIPLINARY ACTION BY A PEER REVIEW ENTITY. LICENSE REVOKED, REVOCATION STAYED; PROBATION UNDER TERMS AND CONDITIONS. ON 10/1/93 ORDER MODIFIED SO THAT WITHIN SIX MONTHS SHE SHALL ENROLL IN, BEGIN PARTICIPATION IN, AND SUBSEQUENTLY COMPLETE A PHARMACOLOGY RETRAINING COURSE ACCEPTABLE TO THE BOARD.

TOVAR, JOSE A MD OF 3 ALPINE COURT, BELLAIRE, TX, WAS DISCIPLINED BY DEA ON DECEMBER 28, 1998
DISCIPLINARY ACTION: SURRENDER OF CONTROLLED SUBSTANCE LICENSE
NOTES: IN LIEU OF PUBLIC INTEREST REVOCATION.

TOVAR, T JOSE ANTONIO MD, LICENSE NUMBER D7339, WAS DISCIPLINED BY TEXAS ON MAY 10, 1997
DISCIPLINARY ACTION: 120-MONTH PROBATION; RESTRICTION PLACED ON LICENSE
OFFENSE: LOSS OR RESTRICTION OF HOSPITAL PRIVILEGES
NOTES: ON 7/17/95 ADMINISTERED ANESTHESIA TO A FIVE-YEAR-OLD PATIENT. HE FAILED TO ADEQUATELY MONITOR THE PATIENT'S RESPIRATORY STATUS AND VITAL SIGNS, PROPERLY AND ADEQUATELY PROVIDE VENTILATORY ASSISTANCE TO THE PATIENT, OR TO RECOGNIZE SEVERE HYPOVENTILATION. HE DID NOT ADEQUATELY FOLLOW GUIDELINES IN THE RESUSCITATION OF A PEDIATRIC PATIENT. ON 7/18/95 HOSPITAL SUMMARILY SUSPENDED HIS HOSPITAL PRIVILEGES. ON 7/25/95 A BRAIN FLOW SCAN PERFORMED ON THE PATIENT SHOWED NO BLOOD FLOW, CONSISTENT WITH BRAIN DEATH. THE PATIENT SUBSEQUENTLY DIED DUE TO GLOBAL, HYPOXIC ISCHEMIC ENCEPHALOPATHY. REVOCATION STAYED FOR PROBATION UNDER THE FOLLOWING TERMS: HE SHALL NO LONGER ENGAGE IN ANESTHESIOLOGY, NOR ADMINISTER ANY TYPE OF ANESTHESIA MEDICATION; SHALL PRACTICE MEDICINE ONLY IN A GROUP PRACTICE SETTING; SHALL ATTEND AT LEAST 50 HOURS OF CONTINUING MEDICAL EDUCATION PER YEAR WITH AT LEAST FIVE HOURS IN RISK MANAGEMENT; SHALL APPEAR BEFORE THE BOARD AT LEAST TWICE A YEAR; HIS MEDICAL PRACTICE SHALL BE MONITORED BY A BOARD APPROVED TEXAS PHYSICIAN WHO SHALL PROVIDE QUARTERLY REPORTS TO THE BOARD; SHALL MAINTAIN ADEQUATE MEDICAL RECORDS WHICH SHALL BE AVAILABLE FOR REVIEW; SHALL PASS THE SPEX AND THE JURISPRUDENCE EXAM WITHIN ONE YEAR; SHALL SUCCESSFULLY COMPLETE AN ADVANCED CARDIAC LIFE SUPPORT COURSE AND OBTAIN CERTIFICATION WITHIN SIX MONTHS; SHALL COOPERATE WITH THE BOARD IN VERIFYING COMPLIANCE; SHALL GIVE A COPY OF THIS ORDER TO ANY HEALTH CARE ENTITY WHERE HE HAS PRIVILEGES; TIME SPENT OUT OF TEXAS DOES NOT COUNT TOWARD PROBATION; SHALL INFORM THE BOARD OF CHANGE OF ADDRESS WITHIN 10 DAYS OR IF HE LEAVES THE STATE; SHALL NOT SEEK MODIFICATION FOR ONE YEAR; REPRIMAND. ON 5/16/98 THE ORDER WAS MODIFIED REDUCING THE REQUIREMENT TO APPEAR BEFORE THE BOARD FROM TWICE A YEAR TO ONCE A YEAR; ALL OTHER PROVISIONS OF THE ORDER REMAIN IN FULL FORCE.

TOVAR, T JOSE ANTONIO MD, LICENSE NUMBER D7339 OF BELLAIRE, TX, WAS DISCIPLINED BY TEXAS ON MAY 29, 1998
DISCIPLINARY ACTION: LICENSE SUSPENSION
OFFENSE: FAILURE TO COMPLY WITH PREVIOUS BOARD ORDER
NOTES: VIOLATED 5/10/97 ORDER BY FAILING TO PASS THE SPEX BY 5/11/98 AS REQUIRED; HE PASSED THE JURISPRUDENCE EXAM.

TOVAR, T JOSE ANTONIO MD, LICENSE NUMBER D7339 OF BELLAIRE, TX, WAS DISCIPLINED BY TEXAS ON AUGUST 22, 1998
DISCIPLINARY ACTION: REPRIMAND
OFFENSE: PROFESSIONAL MISCONDUCT
NOTES: IN 1995 HE ALLOWED THE HEALTH TOUCH CLINIC OF HOUSTON TO ENGAGE IN THE UNLICENSED PRACTICE OF MEDICINE BY USE OF HIM AS AN OSTENSIBLE INDEPENDENT CONTRACTOR; THE CLINIC BILLED FOR SERVICES USING HIS NAME AND FOR WHICH HE NEVER SAW PATIENTS. SHALL GIVE A COPY OF THIS ORDER TO ANY HEALTH CARE ENTITY WHERE HE HAS PRIVILEGES.

TOWNSEND-PARCHMAN, WALLACE MD, LICENSE NUMBER F7683 OF CARROLLTON, TX, WAS DISCIPLINED BY TEXAS ON NOVEMBER 22, 1997
DISCIPLINARY ACTION: 60-MONTH RESTRICTION PLACED ON LICENSE; MONITORING OF PHYSICIAN PERFORMANCE
OFFENSE: SEXUAL ABUSE OF OR SEXUAL MISCONDUCT WITH A PATIENT
NOTES: ON OR ABOUT 10/95 HE EXHIBITED INAPPROPRIATE BEHAVIOR TOWARDS A PATIENT, INCLUDING SEXUAL INNUENDO, GIVING GIFTS OR FAVORS TO THE PATIENT, AND DISCUSSING HIS OWN PERSONAL AND PSYCHIATRIC PROBLEMS; IN 6/89 HE WAS DIAGNOSED WITH BIPOLAR DISORDER AND IS CURRENTLY UNDER THE CARE OF A TEXAS PSYCHIATRIST; HE IS CURRENTLY ON LITHIUM CARBONATE AND OCCASIONAL ANTIDEPRESSANTS, AND IS SEEING A CLINICAL PSYCHOLOGIST FOR COUNSELING; HE NOW REALIZES THE INAPPROPRIATENESS OF HIS TREATMENT WITH THE PATIENT. LICENSE LIMITED TO FIVE YEARS AS FOLLOWS: SHALL NOT TREAT OR OTHERWISE SERVE AS PHYSICIAN, PRESCRIBE, DISPENSE OR ADMINISTER DRUGS THAT MAY BE SUBJECT TO ABUSE TO HIMSELF OR TO ANY MEMBER OF HIS FAMILY; SHALL NOMINATE THREE CERTIFIED PSYCHIATRISTS FOR BOARD SELECTION OF A THERAPIST AND SHALL EXPEDITIOUSLY SUBMIT HIMSELF TO EVALUATION AND TREATMENT BY THE APPROVED PRACTITIONER; SHALL CONTINUE TO SEE SPECIFIED PSYCHOLOGIST WITH QUARTERLY REPORTS; SHALL NOT PERFORM PSYCHOTHERAPY

ON PATIENTS; SHALL APPEAR BEFORE THE BOARD ONCE A YEAR; SHALL COOPERATE WITH THE BOARD IN VERIFYING COMPLIANCE INCLUDING PROVIDING COPIES OF MEDICAL RELEASES UPON REQUEST; SHALL GIVE A COPY OF THIS ORDER TO ANY HEALTH CARE ENTITY WHERE HE HAS PRIVILEGES; TIME SPENT OUT OF TEXAS DOES NOT COUNT TOWARD RESTRICTION; SHALL INFORM THE BOARD OF CHANGE OF ADDRESS WITHIN 10 DAYS OR IF HE LEAVES THE STATE; SHALL NOT SEEK MODIFICATION FOR ONE YEAR.

TOWNSEND-PARCHMAN, WALLACE MD, LICENSE NUMBER F7683 OF CARROLLTON, TX, WAS DISCIPLINED BY TEXAS ON APRIL 10, 1999
DISCIPLINARY ACTION: 60-MONTH PROBATION; RESTRICTION PLACED ON LICENSE
OFFENSE: FAILURE TO COMPLY WITH PREVIOUS BOARD ORDER

NOTES: VIOLATED 11/22/97 BOARD ORDER BY THE PROVIDING OF PSYCHOTHERAPY, OR THE BILLING FOR PSYCHOTHERAPY NOT PERFORMED IN THAT HE HAS BILLED BLUE CROSS/BLUE SHIELD FOR PSYCHOTHERAPY SINCE THE PREVIOUS BOARD ORDER; HE REPORTS THAT HE HAS PROVIDED NO PSYCHOTHERAPY IN VIOLATION OF THE ORDER, AND THAT THE BILLING WAS ERRONEOUS, AND DONE AS A RESULT OF HIS STAFF'S MISUNDERSTANDING OF PROPER BILLING CODES. SUSPENSION STAYED FOR PROBATION WITH TERMS AND CONDITIONS: SHALL NOT TREAT OR OTHERWISE SERVE AS PHYSICIAN, PRESCRIBE, DISPENSE OR ADMINISTER DRUGS THAT MAY BE SUBJECT TO ABUSE TO HIMSELF OR TO ANY MEMBER OF HIS FAMILY; SHALL NOMINATE THREE CERTIFIED PSYCHIATRISTS FOR BOARD SELECTION OF A THERAPIST AND SHALL EXPEDITIOUSLY SUBMIT HIMSELF TO EVALUATION AND TREATMENT BY THE APPROVED PRACTITIONER; SHALL CONTINUE TO RECEIVE CARE AND TREATMENT FROM HIS PSYCHOLOGIST, AND SHALL ARRANGE THAT THE PSYCHOLOGIST PROVIDE QUARTERLY REPORTS TO THE BOARD; SHALL NOT PERFORM PSYCHOTHERAPY ON PATIENTS; HIS MEDICAL PRACTICE SHALL BE MONITORED BY A BOARD APPROVED TEXAS PHYSICIAN WHO SHALL PROVIDE QUARTERLY REPORTS TO THE BOARD; WITHIN 1 YEAR SHALL COMPLETE A BOARD- APPROVED RISK MANAGEMENT COURSE; SHALL APPEAR BEFORE THE BOARD AT LEAST ONCE A YEAR; SHALL COOPERATE WITH THE BOARD IN VERIFYING COMPLIANCE INCLUDING PROVIDING COPIES OF MEDICAL RELEASES UPON REQUEST; SHALL GIVE A COPY OF THIS ORDER TO ANY HEALTH CARE ENTITY WHERE HE HAS PRIVILEGES; TIME SPENT OUT OF TEXAS DOES NOT COUNT TOWARD PROBATION; SHALL INFORM THE BOARD OF CHANGE OF ADDRESS WITHIN 10 DAYS OR IF HE LEAVES THE STATE; SHALL NOT SEEK MODIFICATION FOR ONE YEAR.

TRAN, PAUL MD OF 2918 MILAM STREET, HOUSTON, TX, WAS DISCIPLINED BY DEA ON JUNE 30, 1999
DISCIPLINARY ACTION: SURRENDER OF CONTROLLED SUBSTANCE LICENSE

TRAN, PAUL CHI TIEN MD, LICENSE NUMBER 00G2081, WAS DISCIPLINED BY TEXAS ON AUGUST 17, 1996
DISCIPLINARY ACTION: REPRIMAND
OFFENSE: SUBSTANDARD CARE, INCOMPETENCE OR NEGLIGENCE

NOTES: IN 1992, 1993, AND 1994 EXCESSIVELY PRESCRIBED AND ADMINISTERED PASSIVE PHYSICAL THERAPY MODALITIES IN THE TREATMENT OF SOFT TISSUE INJURIES SUSTAINED BY THREE ADULT PATIENTS FROM VEHICULAR ACCIDENTS. SHALL GIVE A COPY OF THIS ORDER TO ANY HEALTH CARE ENTITY WHERE HE HAS PRIVILEGES.

TRAN, PAUL CHI TIEN MD, LICENSE NUMBER A35347 OF HOUSTON, TX, WAS DISCIPLINED BY CALIFORNIA ON MARCH 4, 1997
DISCIPLINARY ACTION: REPRIMAND
OFFENSE: DISCIPLINARY ACTION BY ANOTHER STATE OR AGENCY

NOTES: DISCIPLINED BY TEXAS FOR PRESCRIBING AND ADMINISTERING EXCESSIVE PASSIVE PHYSICAL THERAPY IN THE TREATMENT OF SOFT TISSUE INJURIES SUSTAINED BY THREE PATIENTS.

TRAN, PAUL CHI TIEN MD, LICENSE NUMBER G2081 OF HOUSTON, TX, WAS DISCIPLINED BY TEXAS ON DECEMBER 11, 1999
DISCIPLINARY ACTION: LICENSE SUSPENSION; FINE
OFFENSE: CRIMINAL CONVICTION OR PLEA OF GUILTY, NOLO CONTENDERE, OR NO CONTEST TO A CRIME

NOTES: PRESCRIBED CONTROLLED SUBSTANCES TO A PATIENT FOR NON-THERAPEUTIC PURPOSES, WITHOUT PERFORMING A PHYSICAL EXAM OF THE PATIENT AND WITHOUT OBTAINING A PATIENT HISTORY; ON 12/6/98 PLED NOLO CONTENDERE TO THE CHARGE OF FRAUDULENT DELIVERY OF A PRESCRIPTION FOR A NON-MEDICAL PURPOSE. $5,000 FINE; SUSPENSION FOR AT LEAST 30 DAYS UNTIL HE REQUESTS TO HAVE HIS SUSPENSION STAYED OR APPEARS BEFORE THE BOARD WITH SUFFICIENT EVIDENCE THAT HE IS PHYSICALLY, MENTALLY AND OTHERWISE COMPETENT TO SAFELY PRACTICE MEDICINE INCLUDING AT A MINIMUM: SHALL TAKE AND PASS THE JURISPRUDENCE EXAM AND THE SPEX WITHIN THREE ATTEMPTS IN 90 DAYS; SHALL TAKE 30 HOURS OF CONTINUING MEDICAL EDUCATION IN THE AREAS OF MEDICAL ETHICS, PAIN MANAGEMENT AND/OR SUBSTANCE ABUSE AND DRUG SEEKING BEHAVIOR. SUSPENSION WILL BE FOLLOWED BY PROBATION UNDER SPECIFIED CONDITIONS.

TREVINO, RODOLFO MD, LICENSE NUMBER 00G6112, WAS DISCIPLINED BY TEXAS ON AUGUST 17, 1996
DISCIPLINARY ACTION: RESTRICTION PLACED ON LICENSE; MONITORING OF PHYSICIAN PERFORMANCE
OFFENSE: SEXUAL ABUSE OF OR SEXUAL MISCONDUCT WITH A PATIENT

NOTES: CRIMINAL COMPLAINTS HAVE BEEN FILED ALLEGING THAT HE HAS ENGAGED IN ACTS CONSTITUTING SEXUAL IMPROPRIETY AGAINST ADULT FEMALES WHO WERE HIS PATIENTS; DENIES ALL OF THE ALLEGATIONS MADE. AGREES TO THIS INTERIM AGREEMENT PENDING A FINAL BOARD RULING. CONDITIONS PLACED ON LICENSE: SHALL HAVE A CHAPERONE PRESENT IN THE ROOM DURING THE EXAMINATION OF ANY FEMALE PATIENT AND SHALL MAKE NOTATION ON THE PATIENT'S CHARTS INDICATING THE CHAPERONE WAS PRESENT; UPON BOARD REQUEST, SHALL PROVIDE REPORTS REGARDING HIS COMPLIANCE WITH THIS ORDER; EVERY 90 DAYS SHALL PROVIDE WRITTEN REPORTS TO THE BOARD INDICATING THE STATUS OF ANY CRIMINAL PROCEEDINGS; SHALL COOPERATE WITH THE BOARD IN VERIFYING COMPLIANCE; SHALL INFORM THE BOARD IN WRITING OF ANY CHANGE IN OFFICE OR MAILING ADDRESS WITHIN 10 DAYS; AND NONCOMPLIANCE SHALL CONSTITUTE FURTHER BOARD DISCIPLINARY ACTION.

TREVINO, VICTOR DANIEL MD, LICENSE NUMBER G7898 OF LAREDO, TX, WAS DISCIPLINED BY TEXAS ON APRIL 4, 1998

DISCIPLINARY ACTION: FINE

NOTES: PROFESSIONAL FAILURE TO PRACTICE IN AN ACCEPTABLE MANNER. $2,500 FINE; SHALL COOPERATE WITH THE BOARD IN VERIFYING COMPLIANCE.

TRIMBLE, ROBERT H MD, LICENSE NUMBER 00D1087 OF HOUSTON, TX, WAS DISCIPLINED BY TEXAS ON JUNE 17, 1992
DISCIPLINARY ACTION: REPRIMAND

NOTES: ADVISED NOT TO ENGAGE IN THE CORPORATE PRACTICE OF MEDICINE.

TROWBRIDGE, JOHN PARKS MD, LICENSE NUMBER F0052 OF HUMBLE, TX, WAS DISCIPLINED BY TEXAS ON AUGUST 22, 1998
DISCIPLINARY ACTION: REPRIMAND
OFFENSE: NONCOMPLIANCE WITH A PROFESSIONAL RULE

NOTES: HE USED TESTIMONIALS FROM HIS PATIENTS FOR ADVERTISING.

TRUMAN, MICHAEL ERNEST DO, LICENSE NUMBER 00D8836, WAS DISCIPLINED BY TEXAS ON AUGUST 17, 1996
DISCIPLINARY ACTION: 60-MONTH RESTRICTION PLACED ON LICENSE; 60-MONTH RESTRICTION PLACED ON CONTROLLED SUBSTANCE LICENSE
OFFENSE: PROFESSIONAL MISCONDUCT

NOTES: DURING 1995 ALLOWED HIS OBJECTIVITY AS A PHYSICIAN TO BE COMPROMISED BY HIS PERSONAL RELATIONSHIP WITH A FEMALE PATIENT WITH WHOM HE HAD BEEN FRIENDS FOR APPROXIMATELY 20 YEARS AND DEVELOPED MULTIPLE CONFLICTS OF INTEREST IN HIS CARE OF BOTH THIS FEMALE AND A MALE PATIENT DUE TO OVERLAPS OF THE PHYSICIAN-PATIENT RELATIONSHIPS AND THE SOCIAL RELATIONSHIPS BETWEEN THE PATIENTS AND HIMSELF; FAILED TO MAINTAIN APPROPRIATE PHYSICIAN-PATIENT BOUNDARIES; IN 12/95 INJECTED THE MALE PATIENT WITH THORAZINE IN AN ATTEMPT TO SEDATE HIM; THIS INCIDENT WAS WITHOUT ADEQUATE MEDICAL BASIS. RESTRICTED UNDER TERMS AND CONDITIONS FOR FIVE YEARS: WITHIN 30 DAYS SHALL ARRANGE FOR THE REFERRAL AND TRANSFER OF CARE FOR ANY PATIENT RECEIVING PSYCHIATRIC TREATMENT OR MENTAL HEALTH SERVICES FROM HIMSELF FOR MAJOR OR SEVERE PSYCHIATRIC ILLNESS OR MENTAL HEALTH CONDITION AND SHALL NOT PROVIDE FURTHER CARE TO SUCH PATIENTS AS DESIGNATED IN THE ORDER; SHALL REFER TO A PSYCHIATRIST ANY PATIENT WHO IS UNRESPONSIVE TO CONSERVATIVE THERAPY PROVIDED BY HIMSELF FOR MILD DEPRESSION, ANXIETY, PANIC ATTACKS OR PANIC DISORDERS, OR MOOD DISORDERS; SHALL NOT TREAT OR OTHERWISE SERVE AS PHYSICIAN, PRESCRIBE, ORDER, DISPENSE, OR ADMINISTER DRUGS, OR ALCOHOL TO HIS FAMILY OR ANY MEMBER OF HIS HOUSEHOLD; SHALL NOT PRESCRIBE, ADMINISTER, ORDER, OR DISPENSE ANTIPSYCHOTIC DRUGS FOR THE TREATMENT OF ANY MAJOR PSYCHIATRIC ILLNESS OR MENTAL HEALTH CONDITION; SHALL MAINTAIN A LOGBOOK OF ALL PRESCRIPTIONS WRITTEN OR TELEPHONED IN BY HIMSELF FOR CONTROLLED SUBSTANCES OR DANGEROUS DRUGS WITH ADDICTIVE POTENTIAL OR POTENTIAL FOR ABUSE WHICH SHALL BE AVAILABLE UPON BOARD REQUEST WHICH SHALL BE AVAILABLE FOR INSPECTION; SHALL MAINTAIN ADEQUATE MEDICAL RECORDS WHICH SHALL BE AVAILABLE FOR REVIEW; SHALL SUBMIT HIMSELF FOR EVALUATION AND TREATMENT TO A BOARD-APPROVED PSYCHIATRIST WHO SHALL MAKE REPORTS; SHALL COOPERATE WITH THE BOARD IN VERIFYING COMPLIANCE INCLUDING PROVIDING COPIES OF MEDICAL RELEASES AND PEER REVIEW RECORDS UPON REQUEST; SHALL PERSONALLY APPEAR BEFORE THE BOARD AT LEAST ONCE PER YEAR OR UPON BOARD REQUEST; SHALL GIVE A COPY OF THIS ORDER TO ANY HEALTH CARE ENTITY WHERE HE HAS PRIVILEGES; SHALL PROVIDE A COPY OF THIS ORDER TO ANYONE REQUESTING IT WITHIN 10 DAYS; TIME PERIOD OUT OF TEXAS DOES NOT COUNT TOWARD RESTRICTION; SHALL INFORM THE BOARD OF CHANGE OF ADDRESS WITHIN 10 DAYS OF IF HE LEAVES THE STATE; SHALL NOT SEEK MODIFICATION FOR ONE YEAR. ON 9/20/97 THE BOARD GRANTED HIS PETITION FOR TERMINATION OF THIS ORDER BASED ON A FAVORABLE PSYCHIATRIC EVALUATION AND HIS COMPLIANCE WITH CONDITIONS.

TSENG, ANGELA MD, LICENSE NUMBER 00G1566 OF MCKINNEY, TX, WAS DISCIPLINED BY TEXAS ON MARCH 2, 1996
DISCIPLINARY ACTION: FINE
OFFENSE: NONCOMPLIANCE WITH A PROFESSIONAL RULE

NOTES: ON 5/5/95 UNINTENTIONALLY FAILED TO PROVIDE COMPLETE AND ACCURATE INFORMATION IN HER MEDICAL PRACTICE QUESTIONNAIRE TO THE BOARD. SHALL PAY A $2,000 ADMINISTRATIVE PENALTY.

TSENG, MAO HSUNG MD, LICENSE NUMBER 0160199 OF 242 WENHUARD, CHIA YI CITY, TAIWAN, WAS DISCIPLINED BY NEW YORK ON JUNE 19, 1996
DISCIPLINARY ACTION: LICENSE REVOCATION
OFFENSE: SUBSTANDARD CARE, INCOMPETENCE OR NEGLIGENCE

NOTES: GUILTY OF GROSS NEGLIGENCE, GROSS INCOMPETENCE AND NEGLIGENCE, AND INCOMPETENCE ON MORE THAN ONE OCCASION INVOLVING HIS TREATMENT OF SEVERAL SURGICAL PATIENTS.

TSENG, MAO HSUNG MD, LICENSE NUMBER F0335 OF GOWANDA, NY, WAS DISCIPLINED BY TEXAS ON FEBRUARY 7, 1998
DISCIPLINARY ACTION: LICENSE REVOCATION
OFFENSE: DISCIPLINARY ACTION BY ANOTHER STATE OR AGENCY

NOTES: THE NEW YORK BOARD REVOKED HIS LICENSE DUE TO NEGLIGENCE, INCOMPETENCE AND GROSS NEGLIGENCE AND INCOMPETENCE INVOLVING FOUR PATIENTS HE SAW BETWEEN 4/89 AND 7/92 INCLUDING SURGERY THAT WAS NOT INDICATED AND PRESCRIBING IN EXCESSIVE AMOUNTS. ACTION WILL NOT BE FINAL UNTIL ALL APPEALS HAVE BEEN EXHAUSTED.

TUCKER, DONALD TOMMY MD, LICENSE NUMBER G4063 OF AUSTIN, TX, WAS DISCIPLINED BY TEXAS ON NOVEMBER 22, 1997
DISCIPLINARY ACTION: FINE
OFFENSE: OVERPRESCRIBING OR MISPRESCRIBING DRUGS

NOTES: FAILED TO ADEQUATELY MONITOR HIS PRESCRIBING OF CONTROLLED SUBSTANCES TO 9 CHRONIC PAIN PATIENTS; WAS EMPLOYED BY A CLINIC OWNED BY A CORPORATION IN VIOLATION OF THE MEDICAL PRACTICE ACT. $1,000 FINE; SHALL COOPERATE WITH THE BOARD IN VERIFYING COMPLIANCE.

TUCKER, THOMAS ANDREW MD, LICENSE NUMBER D1837, WAS DISCIPLINED BY TEXAS ON JANUARY 18, 1997
DISCIPLINARY ACTION: 60-MONTH PROBATION; RESTRICTION PLACED ON CONTROLLED SUBSTANCE LICENSE
OFFENSE: SUBSTANDARD CARE, INCOMPETENCE OR NEGLIGENCE

NOTES: FROM 1993 THROUGH 1995 HE DID NOT ADEQUATELY

MANAGE PHARMACOTHERAPY OF AT LEAST THREE ADULT PATIENTS. HE DID NOT ADEQUATELY DOCUMENT THE CARE AND TREATMENT HE PROVIDED. HE PROVIDED ADDICTIVE PRESCRIPTION MEDICATIONS, INCLUDING CONTROLLED SUBSTANCES, WHICH COULD HAVE JEOPARDIZED THE HEALTH OF PATIENTS HE KNEW OR SHOULD HAVE KNOWN WERE ABUSERS OF SUCH DRUGS. ON 3/12/96 A HOSPITAL FILED AN ACTION REPORT WITH THE NATIONAL PRACTITIONERS DATA BANK STATING THAT HE HAD RESIGNED AND SURRENDERED HIS CLINICAL PRIVILEGES WHILE UNDER INVESTIGATION FOR POSSIBLE PROFESSIONAL INCOMPETENCE REGARDING PHARMACOTHERAPY. UPON INQUIRY, HE RESPONDED THAT HE RESIGNED DUE TO PROFESSIONAL CONFLICT WITH THE COMMITTEE MEMBERS. SUSPENSION STAYED IN FAVOR OF PROBATION UNDER THE FOLLOWING TERMS AND CONDITIONS: WITHIN ONE YEAR SHALL PASS THE SPEX AND THE MEDICAL JURISPRUDENCE EXAMINATION GIVEN BY THE TEXAS BOARD; SHALL OBTAIN AT LEAST 50 HOURS PER YEAR OF CONTINUING MEDICAL EDUCATION WITH AN ADDITIONAL 50 HOURS DURING THE FIRST YEAR IN PAIN MANAGEMENT AND PSYCHOPHARMACOLOGY; IF HE HAS NOT ALREADY DONE SO, SHALL IMMEDIATELY REQUEST MODIFICATION OF HIS DRUG ENFORCEMENT ADMINISTRATION CONTROLLED SUBSTANCES REGISTRATION CERTIFICATE AND HIS TEXAS DEPARTMENT OF PUBLIC SAFETY CONTROLLED SUBSTANCES REGISTRATION CERTIFICATE TO ELIMINATE HIS AUTHORITY TO PRESCRIBE OR DISPENSE SCHEDULE II; SHALL NOT ATTEMPT TO RE-REGISTER WITHOUT FIRST OBTAINING WRITTEN DISCRETIONARY AUTHORITY FROM THE BOARD; IF IN POSSESSION OF ANY UNUSED TRIPLICATE PRESCRIPTION FORMS, SHALL SURRENDER TO THE TEXAS DPS AND SHALL NOT ATTEMPT TO ORDER MORE; SEPARATE FROM PATIENT RECORDS, SHALL MAINTAIN A COPY OF EVERY PRESCRIPTION WRITTEN FOR CONTROLLED SUBSTANCES TO BE MADE AVAILABLE FOR INSPECTION; SHALL NOT TELEPHONE TO A PHARMACY PRESCRIPTION OR REFILL OF SUCH DRUGS; ALL RECORDS SHALL BE MADE AVAILABLE FOR INSPECTION; HIS MEDICAL PRACTICE SHALL BE MONITORED BY A TEXAS PHYSICIAN WHO SHALL PROVIDE QUARTERLY REPORTS; SHALL APPEAR BEFORE THE BOARD UPON REQUEST; SHALL MAINTAIN ADEQUATE MEDICAL RECORDS WHICH SHALL BE MADE AVAILABLE TO THE BOARD FOR REVIEW; SHALL COOPERATE WITH THE BOARD IN VERIFYING COMPLIANCE INCLUDING PROVIDING COPIES OF MEDICAL RELEASES AND PEER REVIEW RECORDS UPON REQUEST; SHALL GIVE A COPY OF THIS ORDER TO ANY HEALTH CARE ENTITY WHERE HE HAS PRIVILEGES; SHALL PROVIDE A COPY OF THIS ORDER TO ANYONE REQUESTING IT WITHIN 10 DAYS; TIME SPENT OUT OF TEXAS DOES NOT COUNT TOWARD PROBATION; SHALL INFORM THE BOARD OF CHANGE OF ADDRESS WITHIN 10 DAYS OR IF HE LEAVES THE STATE. ON 4/4/98 THE TERMINATION REQUEST WAS DENIED; BUT THE ORDER WAS MODIFIED BY DELETING THE REQUIREMENT THAT HIS PRACTICE BE MONITORED.

TYLER, JOHN M JR MD, DATE OF BIRTH MAY 2, 1959, LICENSE NUMBER 30232, WAS DISCIPLINED BY COLORADO ON MARCH 20, 1997
DISCIPLINARY ACTION: 60-MONTH PROBATION; MONITORING OF PHYSICIAN PERFORMANCE
OFFENSE: PHYSICAL OR MENTAL ILLNESS INHIBITING THE ABILITY TO PRACTICE WITH SKILL AND SAFETY

NOTES: MENTAL DISABILITY. TERMS OF PROBATION INCLUDE: MUST AGREE TO REMAIN ABSTINENT FROM ADDICTIVE SUBSTANCES, TREATMENT MONITORING AND PRACTICE MONITORING.

TYLER, JOHN M JR MD, LICENSE NUMBER H2853 OF COLORADO SPRINGS, CO, WAS DISCIPLINED BY TEXAS ON MAY 16, 1998
DISCIPLINARY ACTION: MONITORING OF PHYSICIAN PERFORMANCE
OFFENSE: DISCIPLINARY ACTION BY ANOTHER STATE OR AGENCY

NOTES: ON OR ABOUT 3/20/97 HE ENTERED INTO AN AGREED ORDER WITH THE COLORADO BOARD, WHICH STIPULATED THAT FROM APPROXIMATELY 5/96- 8/96 HE CONSUMED 1-2 ALCOHOLIC DRINKS OVER LUNCH ONCE OR TWICE WEEKLY; HE WAS DIAGNOSED WITH ALCOHOL ABUSE IN EARLY REMISSION; THE COLORADO BOARD PLACED HIM ON PROBATIONARY STATUS FOR 5 YEARS. SHALL NOT PRACTICE IN TEXAS UNTIL HE APPEARS BEFORE THE BOARD WITH SUFFICIENT EVIDENCE THAT HE IS PHYSICALLY, MENTALLY AND OTHERWISE COMPETENT TO SAFELY PRACTICE INCLUDING AT A MINIMUM: SHALL ABSTAIN FROM THE CONSUMPTION OF ALCOHOL/DRUGS IN ANY FORM UNLESS PRESCRIBED BY ANOTHER PHYSICIAN FOR A LEGITIMATE AND THERAPEUTIC PURPOSE; SHALL PROVIDE EVIDENCE THAT HE HAS COMPLETED THE TERMS OF HIS COLORADO BOARD ORDER; SHALL COOPERATE WITH THE BOARD IN VERIFYING COMPLIANCE INCLUDING PROVIDING COPIES OF REPORTS SENT TO COLORADO; SHALL INFORM THE BOARD OF CHANGE OF ADDRESS WITHIN 10 DAYS OR IF HE LEAVES THE STATE; SHALL NOT SEEK MODIFICATION FOR ONE YEAR.

TYLER, MICHAEL EARL MD, LICENSE NUMBER E7525 OF SAN ANTONIO, TX, WAS DISCIPLINED BY TEXAS ON AUGUST 28, 1999
DISCIPLINARY ACTION: FINE
OFFENSE: PROFESSIONAL MISCONDUCT

NOTES: ALLEGATION THAT HE FAILED TO PROPERLY TERMINATE THE PHYSICIAN-PATIENT RELATIONSHIP PRIOR TO ENGAGING IN A PERSONAL RELATIONSHIP WITH A PATIENT; HE MAINTAINS THAT, ALTHOUGH NOT IN WRITING, HE DID TERMINATE THE PHYSICIAN-PATIENT RELATIONSHIP; HE IS NOW MARRIED TO THE PATIENT; ALLEGATIONS THAT HE ENGAGED IN ONE OR MORE TELEPHONE CONVERSATIONS WITH A PATIENT WHICH INCLUDED PERSONAL THREATS BY HIM AND PATIENT; BY THESE CONVERSATIONS, IT IS ALLEGED THAT HE UNNECESSARILY BLURRED PROFESSIONAL BOUNDARIES WITHOUT TERMINATING THE PHYSICIAN-PATIENT RELATIONSHIP; ALLEGATION THAT HE FAILED TO KEEP ADEQUATE MEDICAL RECORDS FOR PRESCRIPTIONS; HE DENIES ANY VIOLATION. $5,000 FINE.

TYSON, SAMUEL TILDEN II MD, LICENSE NUMBER H2185, WAS DISCIPLINED BY TEXAS ON AUGUST 9, 1997
DISCIPLINARY ACTION: REPRIMAND
OFFENSE: SUBSTANDARD CARE, INCOMPETENCE OR NEGLIGENCE

NOTES: IN TWO CASES HIS CARE AND TREATMENT OF PATIENTS WAS INADEQUATE; IN 1994 HE ADMINISTERED ANESTHESIA OF 8 MG. OF MORPHINE OVER 1 HOUR TO A 32 LB., TWO AND A HALF YEAR OLD BOY FOR TREATMENT OF LACERATION OF THE BOY'S TONGUE; THE MORPHINE WAS ADMINISTERED IN CONJUNCTION WITH VERSED AND BENADRYL; THE PATIENT LATER EXPIRED; AN AUTOPSY REPORT FOUND THE CAUSE OF DEATH AS A RESULT OF SEQUELAE OF LACERATION OF THE TONGUE AND SUBSEQUENT MEDICAL THERAPY; THE AUTOPSY FOUND NO VERSED AND SUB-THERAPEUTIC LEVELS

OF MORPHINE IN THE BLOODSTREAM AT THE TIME OF DEATH; THE PHARMACOKINETICS OF THE BENADRYL AS ADMINISTERED BY HIM DO NOT FIT THE LEVELS NOTED AT AUTOPSY; IN 1995 HE FAILED TO DIAGNOSE AND TREAT A PATIENT'S PNEUMONIA; THE PATIENT EXPIRED FIVE DAYS LATER DUE TO COMPLICATIONS FROM STREP PNEUMONIA. SHALL GIVE A COPY OF THIS ORDER TO ANY HEALTH CARE ENTITY WHERE HE HAS PRIVILEGES.

ULDRICH, DENNIS MD OF 124 DALLAS, SAN ANTONIO, TX, WAS DISCIPLINED BY DEA ON DECEMBER 27, 1999
DISCIPLINARY ACTION: SURRENDER OF CONTROLLED SUBSTANCE LICENSE
NOTES: IN LIEU OF PUBLIC INTEREST REVOCATION.

ULDRICH, DENNIS A MD, LICENSE NUMBER 0051767 OF BARNEGAT LIGHT, NJ, WAS DISCIPLINED BY OHIO ON JULY 18, 1995
DISCIPLINARY ACTION: LICENSE SUSPENSION; 120-MONTH PROBATION
OFFENSE: FAILURE TO COMPLY WITH PREVIOUS BOARD ORDER
NOTES: VIOLATION OF CONDITIONS OF LIMITATION IMPOSED BY 8/13/93 CONSENT AGREEMENT DUE TO FAILURE TO TIMELY NOTIFY THE OHIO BOARD OF HIS RELAPSE; IMPAIRMENT OF ABILITY TO PRACTICE ACCORDING TO ACCEPTABLE AND PREVAILING STANDARDS OF CARE BECAUSE OF HABITUAL OR EXCESSIVE USE OR ABUSE OF DRUGS, ALCOHOL OR OTHER SUBSTANCES. PERMANENT REVOCATION STAYED; INDEFINITE SUSPENSION FOR A MINIMUM OF 90 DAYS; CONDITIONS FOR REINSTATEMENT.

ULDRICH, DENNIS A MD, DATE OF BIRTH JULY 27, 1955 OF 124 DALLAS STREET, SAN ANTONIO, TX, WAS DISCIPLINED BY NEW JERSEY ON AUGUST 19, 1998
DISCIPLINARY ACTION: DENIAL OF NEW LICENSE
OFFENSE: DISCIPLINARY ACTION BY ANOTHER STATE OR AGENCY
NOTES: BOARD IS NOT SATISFIED THAT HE HAS BEEN HONEST ABOUT HIS HISTORY AND NOTES THAT HE HAS OFFERED MORE THAN ONE EXPLANATION FOR HIS ORIGINAL ADDICTION AND TREATMENT. BOARD ALSO FOUND HE HAD NOT BEEN TRUTHFUL WHEN HE STATED HIS LICENSES IN OHIO AND TEXAS HAD BEEN RESTORED. BOARD DOES NOT GRANT A LICENSE TO AN APPLICANT WHO'S LICENSE IN ANOTHER STATE IS SUSPENDED OR REVOKED. LICENSE IN TEXAS HAS TWICE BEEN SUSPENDED, AND IN OHIO IT HAS BEEN BOTH SUSPENDED AND REVOKED. HIS LICENSE IN OHIO IS PRESENTLY UNDER STAYED SUSPENSION OR REVOCATION AND ANY PRACTICE IN OHIO WOULD BE VERY RESTRICTED. HE MAY PRACTICE IN TEXAS ONLY UNDER THE TERMS OF A TEN-YEAR PROBATION AND SUBJECT TO MANY STRICT RESTRICTIONS.

ULDRICH, DENNIS A MD, LICENSE NUMBER H7841 OF SAN ANTONIO, TX, WAS DISCIPLINED BY TEXAS ON OCTOBER 15, 1999
DISCIPLINARY ACTION: LICENSE SUSPENSION
OFFENSE: FAILURE TO COMPLY WITH PREVIOUS BOARD ORDER
NOTES: ON 5/21/99 VIOLATED 5/15/96 ORDER BY SELF-REPORTING THAT HE HAD RELAPSED BY SELF-MEDICATING HIS PANIC ATTACKS WITH ALCOHOL AND XANAX; HE ADMITTED HIMSELF FOR TREATMENT; ON OR ABOUT 8/8/99 WHILE ON TRANSITIONAL PASS FROM TREATMENT HE RELAPSED BY DRINKING HEAVILY FOR FIVE OR SIX DAYS. SUSPENSION UNTIL HE REQUESTS TO HAVE HIS SUSPENSION STAYED OR APPEARS BEFORE THE BOARD WITH SUFFICIENT EVIDENCE THAT HE IS PHYSICALLY, MENTALLY AND OTHERWISE COMPETENT TO SAFELY PRACTICE MEDICINE INCLUDING AT A MINIMUM COMPLETE COPIES OF MEDICAL RECORDS AND REPORTS OF PSYCHOLOGICAL AND NEUROPSYCHIATRIC EVALUATIONS CONDUCTED WITHIN 60 DAYS PRIOR TO REQUEST TO STAY OR LIFT SUSPENSION; DOCUMENTED EVIDENCE THAT, FOR NO LESS THAN 12 CONSECUTIVE MONTHS IMMEDIATELY PRECEDING HIS REQUEST, THAT HE HAS MAINTAINED SOBRIETY AND ABSTINENCE FROM ALCOHOL, DANGEROUS DRUGS, OR CONTROLLED SUBSTANCES UNLESS PRESCRIBED BY ANOTHER PHYSICIAN FOR THERAPEUTIC PURPOSES; SHALL COOPERATE WITH THE BOARD IN VERIFYING COMPLIANCE; SHALL PROVIDE A COPY OF THIS ORDER TO ANYONE REQUESTING IT WITHIN 10 DAYS; SHALL INFORM THE BOARD OF CHANGE OF ADDRESS WITHIN 10 DAYS.

ULDRICH, DENNIS ALAN MD, DATE OF BIRTH JULY 27, 1955, LICENSE NUMBER 00H7841 OF 647 CYPRESS GREEN, SAN ANTONIO, TX, WAS DISCIPLINED BY TEXAS ON JANUARY 29, 1993
DISCIPLINARY ACTION: SURRENDER OF CONTROLLED SUBSTANCE LICENSE; 60-MONTH PROBATION
OFFENSE: SUBSTANCE ABUSE
NOTES: DURING 1/92 AND PRECEDING MONTHS, HE HAD INGESTED THE DRUGS PHENERGAN, ATIVAN, BENADRYL AND FENTANYL ON MULTIPLE OCCASIONS WITHOUT A VALID MEDICAL REASON; ON 1/20/92 WAS FOUND UNCONSCIOUS AND CYANOTIC DUE TO DRUG ABUSE; RECEIVED INPATIENT TREATMENT FOR DRUG DEPENDENCE IN 1/92 AND 3/92 AT AN AIR FORCE HOSPITAL AND FROM 3/92 THROUGH 6/92 AT AN ARMY HOSPITAL; HE FULLY COOPERATED WITH BOARD IN ITS INVESTIGATION; ON 7/14/92 ENTERED A MONITORED TREATMENT PROGRAM CONTRACT IN WHICH HE ACKNOWLEDGED HIS CHEMICAL DEPENDENCE. SUSPENSION STAYED. CONDITIONS OF PROBATION: SHALL ATTEND 50 HOURS PER YEAR OF CONTINUING MEDICAL EDUCATION APPROVED FOR CATEGORY I CREDITS; SHALL BE EVALUATED AND TREATED BY A BOARD-APPROVED PSYCHIATRIST TO WHOM HE WILL PROVIDE A COPY OF THIS ORDER WITH REPORTS TO THE BOARD; SHALL ABSTAIN FROM THE CONSUMPTION OF ALCOHOL OR OTHER DRUGS IN ANY FORM; SHALL SURRENDER ALL CONTROLLED SUBSTANCES INCLUDING SAMPLES; SHALL SURRENDER DEA AND TEXAS CONTROLLED SUBSTANCES REGISTRATION; SHALL NOT ATTEMPT TO REREGISTER FOR THESE WITHOUT BOARD AUTHORIZATION; SHALL PARTICIPATE IN ACTIVITIES OF A COUNTY IMPAIRED PHYSICIANS GROUP AND ATTEND WEEKLY MEETINGS WITH QUARTERLY REPORTS; SHALL SUBMIT HIMSELF FOR APPROPRIATE EXAMS INCLUDING DRUG OR ALCOHOL SCREENS; SHALL APPEAR BEFORE THE BOARD AT LEAST ONCE A YEAR; SHALL GIVE A COPY OF THIS ORDER TO ANY HEALTH CARE ENTITY WHERE HE HAS PRIVILEGES; SHALL COOPERATE WITH THE BOARD IN VERIFYING COMPLIANCE; SHALL INFORM BOARD OF CHANGE OF ADDRESS WITHIN 10 DAYS OR IF HE LEAVES THE STATE; TIME SPENT OUT OF TEXAS DOES NOT COUNT TOWARD PROBATION; SHALL COMPLY WITH ALL PROVISIONS OF TREATMENT CONTRACT ENTERED 7/14/92. SHALL NOT SEEK MODIFICATION FOR 1 YEAR OR UNTIL HE IS DISCHARGED FROM THE AIR FORCE WHICHEVER IS EARLIER. ON 1/14/94 THIS ORDER MODIFIED AS FOLLOWS: CONTINUING MEDICAL EDUCATION REQUIREMENT DROPPED FOR THE TIME HE IS IN A RESIDENCY TRAINING PROGRAM; HE MAY REAPPLY FOR CONTROLLED SUBSTANCES AUTHORITY IN SCHEDULES II THROUGH V BUT SHALL POSSESS, PRESCRIBE OR ADMINISTER THEM ONLY FOR PURPOSES OF RESIDENCY TRAINING; SEPARATE FROM OTHER RECORDS SHALL KEEP A LOG OF ALL

CONTROLLED SUBSTANCES ADMINISTERED, DISPENSED OR PRESCRIBED; SHALL GIVE A COPY OF THE ORIGINAL ORDER AND THIS MODIFICATION TO THE HEAD OF HIS RESIDENCY PROGRAM.

ULDRICH, DENNIS ALAN MD, LICENSE NUMBER 0051767 OF EL PASO, TX, WAS DISCIPLINED BY OHIO ON AUGUST 19, 1993
DISCIPLINARY ACTION: PROBATION; RESTRICTION PLACED ON LICENSE
OFFENSE: DISCIPLINARY ACTION BY ANOTHER STATE OR AGENCY

NOTES: PRIOR ACTION BY TEXAS BOARD WHICH WAS BASED ON HIS HISTORY OF SUBSTANCE ABUSE. AGREEMENT TO REMAIN IN EFFECT FOR A MINIMUM OF TWO YEARS PRIOR TO ANY REQUEST FOR TERMINATION.

ULDRICH, DENNIS ALAN MD, DATE OF BIRTH JULY 27, 1955, LICENSE NUMBER 00H7841 OF EL PASO, TX, WAS DISCIPLINED BY TEXAS ON AUGUST 19, 1994
DISCIPLINARY ACTION: EMERGENCY SUSPENSION
OFFENSE: FAILURE TO COMPLY WITH PREVIOUS BOARD ORDER

NOTES: AVAILABLE EVIDENCE AND INFORMATION INDICATE THAT: IN VIOLATION OF 1/29/93 ORDER HE INGESTED PROPOFOL ON 2/14/94 WHICH HE REPORTED TO THE BOARD; THE INGESTION WAS NOT PURSUANT TO A PRESCRIPTION FROM HIS PRIMARY CARE PHYSICIAN; ENTERED A RECOVERY PROGRAM AND WAS DISCHARGED ON 7/9/94 AND TRANSFERRED TO A TRANSITIONAL LIVING FACILITY; LEFT THE FACILITY ON 8/5/94 WITHOUT THE CONSENT OF THE STAFF.

ULDRICH, DENNIS ALAN MD, DATE OF BIRTH JULY 27, 1955, LICENSE NUMBER 00H7841 OF EL PASO, TX, WAS DISCIPLINED BY TEXAS ON MARCH 4, 1995
DISCIPLINARY ACTION: LICENSE SUSPENSION
OFFENSE: FAILURE TO COMPLY WITH PREVIOUS BOARD ORDER

NOTES: IN NONCOMPLIANCE WITH 1/29/93 ORDER IN THAT HE INGESTED PROPOFOL ON 2/14/94 NOT PURSUANT TO A PRESCRIPTION FROM HIS DOCTOR; SELF-REPORTED THIS; ENTERED INPATIENT TREATMENT IN 2/94 AND DISCHARGED IN 7/94; IN 8/94 LEFT A TREATMENT PROGRAM WITHOUT CONSENT. SUSPENSION UNTIL HE REQUESTS IN WRITING TO HAVE SUSPENSION STAYED OR LIFTED AND APPEARS BEFORE BOARD WITH SUFFICIENT EVIDENCE WHICH ADEQUATELY INDICATES THAT HE IS COMPETENT TO PRACTICE MEDICINE; EVIDENCE SHALL INCLUDE AT A MINIMUM 12 CONTINUOUS MONTHS OF ABSTINENCE FROM ALCOHOL, DANGEROUS DRUGS OR CONTROLLED SUBSTANCES UNLESS PRESCRIBED BY A PHYSICIAN FOR A LEGITIMATE AND THERAPEUTIC PURPOSE AND COPIES OF MEDICAL RECORDS AND REPORTS OF PSYCHOLOGICAL AND NEUROPSYCHIATRIC EVALUATIONS CONDUCTED BY A BOARD-APPROVED PSYCHIATRIST.

ULDRICH, DENNIS ALAN MD, DATE OF BIRTH JULY 27, 1955, LICENSE NUMBER 00H7841 OF EL PASO, TX, WAS DISCIPLINED BY TEXAS ON MAY 13, 1995
DISCIPLINARY ACTION: PROBATION

NOTES: HAS SATISFIED THE MINIMUM REQUIREMENTS AS SET OUT IN THE 3/95 ORDER FOR STAY OF SUSPENSION. SUSPENSION STAYED; PROBATION UNDER TERMS AND CONDITIONS: SHALL NOT PRACTICE MEDICINE IN TEXAS UNTIL HE REQUESTS TO RESUME PRACTICE, PERSONALLY APPEARING BEFORE THE BOARD GIVING EVIDENCE THAT HE IS PHYSICALLY, MENTALLY AND OTHERWISE COMPETENT TO SAFELY PRACTICE MEDICINE INCLUDING AT A MINIMUM CONTINUOUS ABSTINENCE FROM THE CONSUMPTION OF ALCOHOL, AND DANGEROUS DRUGS OR CONTROLLED SUBSTANCES IN ANY FORM. SHALL NOT SEEK MODIFICATION FOR ONE YEAR.

ULDRICH, DENNIS ALAN MD, DATE OF BIRTH JULY 27, 1955, LICENSE NUMBER 00H7841, WAS DISCIPLINED BY TEXAS ON MAY 15, 1996
DISCIPLINARY ACTION: 120-MONTH PROBATION; RESTRICTION PLACED ON LICENSE
OFFENSE: SUBSTANCE ABUSE

NOTES: HAS A SIGNIFICANT HISTORY OF SUBSTANCE ABUSE. HAS SATISFIED THE MINIMUM REQUIREMENTS OF 5/13/95 ORDER TO PRACTICE IN TEXAS. GRANTED PERMISSION TO RESUME PRACTICE IN TEXAS UNDER PROBATION WITH TERMS AND CONDITIONS: SHALL NOT PRACTICE ANESTHESIOLOGY; SHALL ABSTAIN FROM THE CONSUMPTION OF ALCOHOL/ DRUGS IN ANY FORM UNLESS PRESCRIBED BY ANOTHER PHYSICIAN FOR A LEGITIMATE AND THERAPEUTIC PURPOSE; SHALL SUBMIT HIMSELF FOR APPROPRIATE EXAMS INCLUDING DRUG OR ALCOHOL SCREENS; SHALL SUBMIT HIMSELF FOR EVALUATION AND TREATMENT BY BOARD-APPROVED PSYCHIATRIST WHOM HE SHALL SEE AT LEAST ONCE A MONTH AND WHO SHALL SUBMIT REPORTS TO THE BOARD; SHALL PARTICIPATE IN THE ACTIVITIES OF A HEALTH AND REHABILITATION COMMITTEE AND ATTEND WEEKLY MEETINGS WITH QUARTERLY REPORTS; SHALL PARTICIPATE IN AA'S PROGRAM NOT LESS THAN THREE TIMES A WEEK WITH QUARTERLY REPORTS TO THE BOARD; SHALL NOT TREAT OR OTHERWISE SERVE AS PHYSICIAN, PRESCRIBE, DISPENSE OR ADMINISTER DRUGS THAT MAY BE SUBJECT TO ABUSE TO HIMSELF OR TO ANY MEMBER OF HIS FAMILY; SHALL NOT POSSESS ALCOHOL, CONTROLLED SUBSTANCES OR DANGEROUS DRUGS WITH ADDICTIVE POTENTIAL OR POTENTIAL FOR ABUSE; SHALL SURRENDER ALL SUCH DRUGS INCLUDING SAMPLES; SHALL MAINTAIN A FILE WITH COPIES OF EVERY PRESCRIPTION WRITTEN FOR THESE DRUGS WHICH SHALL BE AVAILABLE FOR REVIEW; MAY REAPPLY TO THE DEA AND DPS TO OBTAIN FULL PRESCRIBING AUTHORITY FOR CONTROLLED SUBSTANCES; HIS PRACTICE, INCLUDING ANY OFFICE AND SURGICAL PRACTICE, SHALL BE MONITORED BY A BOARD-APPROVED TEXAS PHYSICIAN WHO SHALL SUBMIT QUARTERLY REPORTS TO THE BOARD; SHALL OBTAIN AT LEAST 50 HOURS PER YEAR OF CONTINUING MEDICAL EDUCATION; SHALL APPEAR BEFORE THE BOARD AT LEAST TWICE A YEAR OR AT BOARD REQUEST; SHALL GIVE A COPY OF THIS ORDER TO ANY HEALTH CARE ENTITY WHERE HE HAS PRIVILEGES; SHALL PROVIDE A COPY OF THIS ORDER TO ANYONE REQUESTING IT WITHIN 10 DAYS; SHALL COOPERATE WITH THE BOARD IN VERIFYING COMPLIANCE; TIME SPENT OUT OF TEXAS DOES NOT COUNT TOWARD PROBATION; SHALL INFORM BOARD OF CHANGE OF ADDRESS WITHIN 10 DAYS OR IF HE LEAVES THE STATE. SHALL NOT SEEK MODIFICATION FOR ONE YEAR. ON 5/16/98 PETITION FOR MODIFICATION OF ORDER GRANTED REDUCING REPORTING BY THE PHYSICIAN HEALTH AND REHABILITATION COMMITTEE AND HIS PRACTICE MONITOR FROM QUARTERLY TO BI-ANNUAL REPORTS, AND REDUCING APPEARANCES BEFORE THE BOARD FROM BIANNUAL TO ANNUAL. ON 5/14/99 PETITION TO MODIFY ORDER GRANTED REPLACING REQUIREMENT TO KEEP A COPY OF ALL PRESCRIPTIONS WITH A PRESCRIPTION LOGBOOK.

USSERY, FRED M III MD, LICENSE NUMBER E2908 OF HOUSTON, TX,

WAS DISCIPLINED BY TEXAS ON AUGUST 9, 1997
DISCIPLINARY ACTION: LICENSE SUSPENSION
OFFENSE: PHYSICAL OR MENTAL ILLNESS INHIBITING THE ABILITY TO PRACTICE WITH SKILL AND SAFETY

NOTES: ALLEGATIONS THAT HE MAY BE SUFFERING FROM PHYSICAL AND MENTAL IMPAIRMENTS WHICH WOULD RENDER HIM UNABLE TO SAFELY PRACTICE MEDICINE; IN 5/95 HE ATTEMPTED SUICIDE AND WAS SUBSEQUENTLY HOSPITALIZED; ON THE DAY OF RELEASE FROM HOSPITALIZATION, HE AGAIN ATTEMPTED SUICIDE VIA A CHEMICAL OVERDOSE AND WAS REHOSPITALIZED; NEUROPSYCHOLOGICAL/COGNITIVE EVALUATIONS CONDUCTED DURING THE HOSPITALIZATIONS CONCLUDED THAT HE IS SUFFERING FROM SIGNIFICANT COGNITIVE IMPAIRMENTS OF AN ORGANIC ETIOLOGY, FROM A MENTAL DISORDER NOT OTHERWISE SPECIFIED DUE TO A GENERAL MEDICAL CONDITION, AND FROM A RECURRENT MAJOR DEPRESSIVE DISORDER WITH PSYCHOTIC FEATURES IN REMISSION; THE EVALUATIONS ALSO FOUND HIM TO HAVE BOTH IMPAIRED MOTOR AND MENTAL SKILLS; AT THIS TIME, THE CONDITIONS HE IS SUFFERING MAY APPEAR TO BE PERMANENT IN NATURE. INDEFINITE SUSPENSION UNTIL HE REQUESTS TO HAVE HIS SUSPENSION STAYED OR APPEARS BEFORE THE BOARD WITH SUFFICIENT EVIDENCE THAT HE IS PHYSICALLY, MENTALLY AND OTHERWISE COMPETENT TO SAFELY PRACTICE INCLUDING AT A MINIMUM COMPLETE COPIES OF MEDICAL RECORDS AND REPORTS OF PSYCHOLOGICAL AND NEUROPSYCHIATRIC EVALUATIONS CONDUCTED BY A BOARD-APPROVED CERTIFIED PSYCHIATRIST.

USSERY, FRED M III MD, LICENSE NUMBER 5988 OF 305 SOUTH FIRST STREET, WEST MONROE, LA, WAS DISCIPLINED BY HAWAII ON MARCH 12, 1999
DISCIPLINARY ACTION: 60-MONTH LICENSE SUSPENSION
OFFENSE: DISCIPLINARY ACTION BY ANOTHER STATE OR AGENCY

NOTES: TEXAS SUSPENDED HIS LICENSE INDEFINITELY BASED UPON HIS MEDICAL CONDITION.

UY, SING DY MD, LICENSE NUMBER F8351 OF ODESSA, TX, WAS DISCIPLINED BY TEXAS ON MAY 16, 1998
DISCIPLINARY ACTION: REPRIMAND
OFFENSE: OVERPRESCRIBING OR MISPRESCRIBING DRUGS

NOTES: FROM 1989-1993 HE PRESCRIBED HALCION TO A PATIENT WITHOUT ADEQUATE INDICATION, FOLLOW-UP OR MONITORING; FAILED TO ADEQUATELY DOCUMENT THE INDICATIONS FOR HIS PRESCRIBING. SHALL GIVE A COPY OF THIS ORDER TO ANY HEALTH CARE ENTITY WHERE HE HAS PRIVILEGES.

VALDEZ, ANTHONY FRANCIS MD, LICENSE NUMBER H2862 OF EL PASO, TX, WAS DISCIPLINED BY TEXAS ON AUGUST 22, 1998
DISCIPLINARY ACTION: FINE
OFFENSE: NONCOMPLIANCE WITH A PROFESSIONAL RULE

NOTES: ALLEGATIONS THAT HE DID NOT ADEQUATELY DESCRIBE THE PROCEDURE UTILIZED RELATING TO A PATIENT NOR THE QUANTITY, THE ROUTE OF ADMINISTRATION, THE DURATIONS OF TREATMENT OR THE PATIENT'S RESPONSE; AND THAT HIS MEDICAL RECORDS DID NOT CONTAIN ADEQUATE PROGRESS NOTES OR GOALS OF TREATMENT FOR A PATIENT HE SAW FROM 8/95 THROUGH 2/96 FOR WHOM HE PRESCRIBED CODEINE OR HYDROCODONE; DENIES THAT HE VIOLATED MEDICAL PRACTICE ACT. $500 FINE; SHALL COOPERATE WITH THE BOARD IN VERIFYING COMPLIANCE.

VALDEZ, JOSEPH G MD, LICENSE NUMBER 00H2864 OF PASADENA, TX, WAS DISCIPLINED BY TEXAS ON MAY 11, 1995
DISCIPLINARY ACTION: FINE
OFFENSE: NONCOMPLIANCE WITH A PROFESSIONAL RULE

NOTES: PAID FOR A NEWSPAPER ADVERTISEMENT WHICH RAN TWICE BETWEEN 12/93 AND 1/94 THAT CLAIMED THAT NO DRUGS WOULD BE NECESSARY FOR NON-SURGICAL RELIEF THROUGH RECONSTRUCTIVE THERAPY AND THAT PATIENT MAY RETURN TO WORK RIGHT AFTER THE TREATMENT WHEN IN FACT NON-NARCOTIC DRUGS ARE REQUIRED FOR THE THERAPY AND NOT EVERY PATIENT IS ABLE TO RETURN TO WORK RIGHT AFTER THE TREATMENT; ALSO THE AD CONTAINED TESTIMONIALS WHICH ARE PROHIBITED; UPON BEING INFORMED OF THE LAW PROHIBITING SUCH ADVERTISING, HE IMMEDIATELY DISCONTINUED THE ADVERTISEMENT CONTAINING THE TESTIMONIALS. SHALL PAY $2,500 FINE; SHALL COOPERATE WITH THE BOARD IN VERIFYING COMPLIANCE.

VALVERDE, WILLIAM MARK MD, LICENSE NUMBER 00E1957 OF HOUSTON, TX, WAS DISCIPLINED BY TEXAS ON AUGUST 19, 1994
DISCIPLINARY ACTION: LICENSE SUSPENSION
OFFENSE: PHYSICAL OR MENTAL ILLNESS INHIBITING THE ABILITY TO PRACTICE WITH SKILL AND SAFETY

NOTES: ALLEGATIONS WHICH IF TRUE COULD INDICATE HE SUFFERS FROM AN INABILITY TO PRACTICE WITH REASONABLE SKILL AND SAFETY BECAUSE OF A MENTAL OR EMOTIONAL CONDITION; WHILE NOT ADMITTING THE ALLEGATIONS HE WISHES TO AVOID THE EXPENSE OF LITIGATION AND INSTEAD VOLUNTARILY UNDERGO A PSYCHIATRIC EVALUATION. SUSPENSION UNTIL SUCH TIME AS HE APPEARS BEFORE THE BOARD AND PROVIDES SUFFICIENT EVIDENCE THAT HE IS PHYSICALLY, MENTALLY AND OTHERWISE COMPETENT TO SAFELY PRACTICE; SHALL COOPERATE WITH THE BOARD IN VERIFYING COMPLIANCE; SHALL INFORM BOARD OF CHANGE OF ADDRESS WITHIN 10 DAYS. ON 2/7/98 PETITION TO TERMINATE ORDER DENIED.

VAN BOLDEN, VERNON II MD, LICENSE NUMBER 00G0854 OF NEW ORLEANS, LA, WAS DISCIPLINED BY TEXAS ON OCTOBER 9, 1992
DISCIPLINARY ACTION: LICENSE REVOCATION

NOTES: PROFESSIONAL FAILURE TO PRACTICE MEDICINE IN AN ACCEPTABLE MANNER CONSISTENT WITH PUBLIC HEALTH AND WELFARE.

VAN BOLDEN, VERNON II MD OF LUBBOCK, TX, WAS DISCIPLINED BY LOUISIANA ON JUNE 21, 1993
DISCIPLINARY ACTION: LICENSE REVOCATION
OFFENSE: DISCIPLINARY ACTION BY ANOTHER STATE OR AGENCY

NOTES: FRAUD, DECEIT OR PERJURY IN OBTAINING A LICENSE.

VANBUSKIRK, RONALD MD, LICENSE NUMBER 00F6338 OF MOUNT PLEASANT, TX, WAS DISCIPLINED BY TEXAS ON JUNE 17, 1992
DISCIPLINARY ACTION: 60-MONTH RESTRICTION PLACED ON LICENSE; REPRIMAND
OFFENSE: OVERPRESCRIBING OR MISPRESCRIBING DRUGS

NOTES: NONTHERAPEUTIC PRESCRIBING. LICENSE RESTRICTED UNDER TERMS AND CONDITIONS. ON 8/19/94 REQUEST FOR TERMINATION OF THIS ORDER WAS DENIED. ON 1/27/96 THE ORDER WAS TERMINATED.

VAUSE, DAVID DWIGHT MD, DATE OF BIRTH JANUARY 5, 1934, LICENSE NUMBER 00E3490 OF PO BOX 189, BLANCO, TX, WAS DISCIPLINED BY TEXAS ON APRIL 30, 1993
DISCIPLINARY ACTION: 60-MONTH PROBATION; REQUIRED TO TAKE ADDITIONAL MEDICAL EDUCATION
OFFENSE: SUBSTANDARD CARE, INCOMPETENCE OR NEGLIGENCE

NOTES: FAILED TO RELEASE MEDICAL RECORDS OF TWO PATIENTS OR TO RESPOND TO THE BOARD ABOUT SAME; FAILED TO ESTABLISH A PROTOCOL FOR TIMES WHEN HE IS ON CALL AS HE HAS NO ANSWERING SERVICE TO TAKE EMERGENCY CALLS; FAILED TO ADDRESS THE HIGH RISK PREGNANCY OF A 39 YEAR OLD PATIENT AND FAILED TO PROVIDE PROPER PRENATAL CARE WHICH COULD HAVE PREVENTED THE BIRTH OF HER STILLBORN CHILD; FAILED TO DIAGNOSE DIABETES IN TWO PATIENTS AND LEUKEMIA IN ONE; PRESCRIBED FASTIN FOR WEIGHT LOSS TO 3 PATIENTS WITHOUT TAKING A HISTORY AND PHYSICAL; KEPT AND USED DANGEROUS DRUGS AT HIS OFFICE WHICH WERE OUTDATED AND SHOULD HAVE BEEN DESTROYED; DISPENSED DRUGS OUT OF HIS OFFICE AFTER HE SUBSTITUTED AND RELABELED BOTTLES; HE NEITHER ADMITS NOR DENIES THE CHARGES. FIVE YEAR SUSPENSION STAYED. CONDITIONS OF PROBATION: SHALL TAKE THE SPEX EXAM ON 6/16/93; IF HE FAILS, HIS LICENSE WILL BE SUSPENDED UNTIL EXAM IS PASSED; SHALL WITHIN SIX MONTHS ENROLL IN AND SUBSEQUENTLY COMPLETE A PHARMACOLOGY RETRAINING COURSE; SHALL TAKE A BOARD-APPROVED PERSONALIZED CONTINUING MEDICAL EDUCATION ACUTE MINI-RESIDENCY AND COMPLETE WITHIN SIX MONTHS; SHALL ATTEND AT LEAST 75 HOURS PER YEAR OF CONTINUING MEDICAL EDUCATION; SHALL BE MONITORED OR SUPERVISED BY A BOARD-APPROVED PHYSICIAN WHO WILL MAKE BIMONTHLY REPORTS TO THE BOARD; SHALL MAINTAIN ADEQUATE MEDICAL RECORDS ON ALL PATIENT OFFICE VISITS; SHALL NOT SIGN ANY PATIENT RECORD UNLESS HE PERSONALLY SAW AND EXAMINED THE PATIENT AND THIS IS SO INDICATED IN THE RECORD; SHALL PERSONALLY EXAMINE PATIENTS DURING THEIR FIRST VISIT; SHALL PERFORM EIGHT HOURS PER MONTH OF COMMUNITY SERVICE; SHALL APPEAR BEFORE THE BOARD ONCE A YEAR; SHALL GIVE A COPY OF THIS ORDER TO ANY HEALTH CARE ENTITY WHERE HE HAS PRIVILEGES; SHALL COOPERATE WITH THE BOARD IN VERIFYING COMPLIANCE; SHALL INFORM BOARD OF CHANGE OF ADDRESS WITHIN 10 DAYS OR IF HE LEAVES THE STATE; TIME SPENT OUT OF TEXAS DOES NOT COUNT TOWARD PROBATION. SHALL NOT SEEK MODIFICATION FOR FIVE YEARS UNLESS FURTHER APPLICATION IS MADE TO THE BOARD.

VAUSE, DAVID DWIGHT MD, DATE OF BIRTH JANUARY 5, 1934, LICENSE NUMBER 00E3490 OF BLANCO, TX, WAS DISCIPLINED BY TEXAS ON AUGUST 18, 1995
DISCIPLINARY ACTION: LICENSE SUSPENSION; REQUIRED TO TAKE ADDITIONAL MEDICAL EDUCATION
OFFENSE: FAILURE TO COMPLY WITH PREVIOUS BOARD ORDER

NOTES: FAILED TO COMPLY WITH CONDITIONS OF 4/93 PROBATION: FAILED TO ENROLL IN AND SUBSEQUENTLY COMPLETE A PHARMACOLOGY RETRAINING COURSE WITHIN SIX MONTHS; FAILED TO TAKE PERSONALIZED CONTINUING MEDICAL EDUCATION ACUTE MINI-RESIDENCIES WITHIN ONE AND SIX MONTHS; FAILED TO ATTEND AT LEAST 75 HOURS PER YEAR OF CONTINUING MEDICAL EDUCATION; FAILED TO OBTAIN A BOARD-APPROVED MONITORING PHYSICIAN AND FAILED TO ENSURE THAT MONITORING PHYSICIAN CONDUCT A RETROSPECTIVE EVALUATION OF ALL OF HIS PATIENTS THE FIRST YEAR AND A 10 PERCENT REVIEW THEREAFTER; FAILED TO ENSURE THAT MONITORING PHYSICIAN SUBMIT REPORTS TO THE BOARD EVERY TWO MONTHS. SUSPENSION UNTIL HE REQUESTS TO HAVE SUSPENSION STAYED OR LIFTED AND APPEARS BEFORE BOARD WITH EVIDENCE WHICH ADEQUATELY INDICATES THAT HE IS PHYSICALLY, MENTALLY AND OTHERWISE COMPETENT TO SAFELY PRACTICE MEDICINE INCLUDING AT A MINIMUM: COMPLETION OF A PHARMACOLOGY RETRAINING COURSE; COMPLETION OF A PERSONALIZED CONTINUING MEDICAL EDUCATION ACUTE MINI-RESIDENCY; PROOF OF ATTENDING 150 HOURS OF CONTINUING MEDICAL EDUCATION SINCE 4/93; PROOF THAT HE HAS OBTAINED A BOARD-APPROVED MONITORING PHYSICIAN.

VEGA, JULIO MD, LICENSE NUMBER 00F5082 OF BUENA PARK, CA, WAS DISCIPLINED BY TEXAS ON MARCH 31, 1990
DISCIPLINARY ACTION: 120-MONTH PROBATION
OFFENSE: DISCIPLINARY ACTION BY ANOTHER STATE OR AGENCY

NOTES: STIPULATED ORDER. REVOCATION STAYED. BOUND BY CERTAIN CONDITIONS OF CALIFORNIA BOARD. MUST OBTAIN APPROVAL BEFORE PRACTICING MEDICINE IN TEXAS.

VEGGEBERG, KERMIT ROGER MD, LICENSE NUMBER 00D1172 OF HOUSTON, TX, WAS DISCIPLINED BY TEXAS ON AUGUST 19, 1994
DISCIPLINARY ACTION: 36-MONTH PROBATION; REQUIRED TO TAKE ADDITIONAL MEDICAL EDUCATION
OFFENSE: SUBSTANDARD CARE, INCOMPETENCE OR NEGLIGENCE

NOTES: HAD TREATED ONE PATIENT FOR A TOTAL HIP REPLACEMENT IN 1977 AND SUBSEQUENTLY PERFORMED SEVERAL REVISIONS; MADE ASSUMPTIONS ABOUT THE SIZES OF THE PROSTHETIC BALL AND CUP WHICH LED TO A MISMATCH WHICH RESULTED IN THE PATIENT EXPERIENCING MANY HIP DISLOCATIONS, EVENTUALLY NECESSITATING FURTHER SURGERIES WITH THE ATTENDANT PAIN AND RECOVERY PERIODS; HE WAS NOT IN THE HABIT OF DOCUMENTING PATIENTS' LEVELS OF PAIN. SUSPENSION STAYED. CONDITIONS OF PROBATION: SHALL ATTEND AT LEAST 100 HOURS OF CONTINUING MEDICAL EDUCATION DURING THE FIRST YEAR OF PROBATION AND 50 HOURS PER YEAR AFTER THAT; 75 HOURS OF THE FIRST YEAR SHALL BE IN THE AREA OF ORTHOPEDICS AND 25 SHALL BE IN THE AREA OF RADIOLOGY; SHALL BE MONITORED BY A BOARD-APPROVED PHYSICIAN WITH REPORTS THREE TIMES A YEAR; SHALL APPEAR BEFORE THE BOARD TWICE A YEAR; SHALL GIVE A COPY OF THIS ORDER TO ANY HEALTH CARE ENTITY WHERE HE HAS PRIVILEGES; SHALL COOPERATE WITH THE BOARD IN VERIFYING COMPLIANCE; SHALL INFORM BOARD OF CHANGE OF ADDRESS WITHIN 10 DAYS OR IF HE LEAVES THE STATE; TIME SPENT OUT OF TEXAS DOES NOT COUNT TOWARD PROBATION. SHALL NOT SEEK MODIFICATION FOR ONE YEAR. ON 10/13/95 REQUEST FOR TERMINATION DENIED BUT ORDER MODIFIED SO HE CAN PETITION FOR TERMINATION OR MODIFICATION ONCE EVERY SIX MONTHS; ALL OTHER CONDITIONS REMAIN IN EFFECT. ON 5/15/96 PROBATION TERMINATED.

VERDUZCO, RAFAEL MD, LICENSE NUMBER 00E2913 OF SUGARLAND, TX, WAS DISCIPLINED BY TEXAS ON AUGUST 18, 1995
DISCIPLINARY ACTION: 120-MONTH RESTRICTION PLACED ON LICENSE; REPRIMAND
OFFENSE: SUBSTANDARD CARE, INCOMPETENCE OR NEGLIGENCE

NOTES: IN 1986, HE FAILED TO PERFORM A TIMELY DELIVERY, FAILED TO GIVE IMPORT TO A NOTED MECONIUM STAIN AND FAILED TO EXPEDITE DELIVERY DESPITE NOTED INDICATIONS THAT THE FETUS WAS EXPERIENCING FETAL DISTRESS; CHILD SURVIVED AND ALLEGEDLY SUFFERS FROM SEVERAL DISABILITIES; PHYSICIAN HAS VOLUNTARILY DISCONTINUED HANDLING OBSTETRIC CASES. LICENSE RESTRICTED FOR 10 YEARS WITH TERMS: SHALL NOT ACT AS THE PRIMARY CARE PHYSICIAN FOR ANY OBSTETRIC PATIENT AND SHALL NOT PERFORM OR ASSIST IN PERFORMING ANY DELIVERY UNTIL HE REQUESTS PERMISSION TO RESUME THE PRACTICE OF OBSTETRICS, APPEARS BEFORE THE BOARD TO PETITION FOR PERMISSION AND PROVIDES SUFFICIENT EVIDENCE WHICH INDICATES THAT HE IS COMPETENT TO SAFELY PRACTICE OBSTETRICS INCLUDING AT A MINIMUM SUCCESSFUL COMPLETION OF A SIX MONTH MINI-RESIDENCY IN OBSTETRICS APPROVED BY THE BOARD; WITHIN ONE YEAR SHALL TAKE AND PASS THE CERTIFICATION EXAM ADMINISTERED BY THE AMERICAN BOARD OF MEDICAL SPECIALTIES IN FAMILY PRACTICE MEDICINE; SHALL OBTAIN AT LEAST 50 HOURS PER YEAR OF CONTINUING MEDICAL EDUCATION; DURING FIRST YEAR OF RESTRICTION SHALL PERFORM 100 HOURS OF COMMUNITY SERVICE; SHALL APPEAR BEFORE BOARD AT LEAST ONCE A YEAR OR AT BOARD REQUEST; SHALL COOPERATE WITH BOARD IN VERIFYING COMPLIANCE INCLUDING PROVIDING ANY PEER REVIEW RECORDS UPON REQUEST; SHALL GIVE A COPY OF THIS ORDER TO ANY HEALTH CARE ENTITY WHERE HE HAS PRIVILEGES; SHALL PROVIDE A COPY OF THIS ORDER TO ANYONE REQUESTING IT WITHIN 10 DAYS; TIME PERIOD OUT OF TEXAS DOES NOT COUNT TOWARD PROBATION; SHALL INFORM BOARD OF CHANGE OF ADDRESS WITHIN 10 DAYS OR IF HE LEAVES THE STATE. SHALL NOT SEEK MODIFICATION FOR ONE YEAR. ON 10/5/96 HIS PETITION FOR TERMINATION WAS DENIED. ON 11/22/97 PETITION TO TERMINATE ORDER DENIED; ORDER MODIFIED DELETING PARAGRAPH WHICH ESTABLISHES TERMS AND CONDITIONS FOR TEN YEARS, AND REQUIREMENTS THAT HE BECOME RECERTIFIED, AND PERFORM 100 HOURS OF COMMUNITY SERVICE. ON 4/10/99 ORDER TERMINATED.

VICKERS, FRANK ALLEN MD, LICENSE NUMBER 00C9172 OF HUNTSVILLE, TX, WAS DISCIPLINED BY TEXAS ON NOVEMBER 9, 1993
DISCIPLINARY ACTION: EMERGENCY SUSPENSION
OFFENSE: SUBSTANCE ABUSE

NOTES: IN 6/93 AND AS RECENTLY AS 11/5/93 ENGAGED IN THE INTEMPERATE USE OF DRUGS BY CONSUMING VARIOUS CONTROLLED SUBSTANCES INCLUDING STADOL, NUBAIN, DARVON, ATIVAN AND XANAX WITHOUT A LEGITIMATE MEDICAL REASON; DURING 10/93 HIS PHYSICAL AND MENTAL CONDITION HAS UNDERGONE A RAPID DETERIORATION CREATING AN INCREASE IN THE POTENTIAL FOR DANGER TO PATIENTS.

VICKERS, FRANK ALLEN MD, LICENSE NUMBER 00C9172 OF HOUSTON, TX, WAS DISCIPLINED BY TEXAS ON JUNE 22, 1994
DISCIPLINARY ACTION: LICENSE SUSPENSION
OFFENSE: SUBSTANCE ABUSE

NOTES: HE WAS TREATED FOR SUBSTANCE ABUSE AS AN INPATIENT FROM 8/83 THROUGH 12/83; REGULARLY ATTENDED MEETINGS OF AA AND A PHYSICIANS HEALTH AND REHABILITATION COMMITTEE UNTIL 1989; SUBSEQUENTLY RELAPSED AND RECEIVED INPATIENT TREATMENT IN 6/93; ON 11/5/93 WAS ARRESTED AND CHARGED WITH PUBLIC INTOXICATION THROUGH BEING UNDER THE INFLUENCE OF DRUGS; HAD IN HIS POSSESSION XANAX, ATIVAN, NUBAIN INJECTABLE, DARVON, AND PLACIDYL SUPPOSITORIES; WAS ADMITTED FOR INPATIENT TREATMENT ON 11/6/93 AND SINCE 2/4/94 HAS BEEN IN AN AFTERCARE RECOVERY AND SUPERVISION PROGRAM; HAS ADMITTED TO TAKING CONTROLLED SUBSTANCES AND DANGEROUS DRUGS WHICH HAVE POTENTIAL FOR ABUSE FROM SAMPLES LEFT IN HIS OFFICE, FROM SUPPLIES PURCHASED FOR OFFICE USE AND FROM UNUSED PORTIONS OF PRESCRIPTIONS LEFT IN HIS OFFICE BY PATIENTS; CLAIMS 11/5/93 AS A SOBRIETY DATE. SUSPENSION UNTIL SUCH TIME AS HE APPEARS BEFORE THE BOARD AND PROVIDES SUFFICIENT EVIDENCE THAT HE IS PHYSICALLY, MENTALLY AND OTHERWISE COMPETENT TO SAFELY PRACTICE.

VICKERS, FRANK ALLEN MD, LICENSE NUMBER 00C9172 OF HOUSTON, TX, WAS DISCIPLINED BY TEXAS ON NOVEMBER 23, 1994
DISCIPLINARY ACTION: SURRENDER OF CONTROLLED SUBSTANCE LICENSE; 120-MONTH PROBATION
OFFENSE: SUBSTANCE ABUSE

NOTES: HAS SATISFIED THE MINIMUM REQUIREMENTS OF 6/22/94 SUSPENSION AND SUSPENSION IS NOW STAYED. CONDITIONS OF PROBATION: PRACTICE RESTRICTED TO AN INSTITUTIONAL OR SUPERVISED SETTING WITH A BOARD-APPROVED SUPERVISOR WITH QUARTERLY REPORTS; SHALL ABSTAIN FROM THE CONSUMPTION OF ALCOHOL/CHEMICAL SUBSTANCES IN ANY FORM UNLESS PRESCRIBED BY ANOTHER PHYSICIAN FOR A LEGITIMATE AND THERAPEUTIC PURPOSE; SHALL SUBMIT HIMSELF FOR APPROPRIATE EXAMS INCLUDING DRUG OR ALCOHOL SCREENS; SHALL NOT TREAT OR OTHERWISE SERVE AS PHYSICIAN, PRESCRIBE DISPENSE OR ADMINISTER DRUGS THAT MAY BE SUBJECT TO ABUSE TO HIMSELF OR ANY MEMBER OF HIS FAMILY; SHALL SURRENDER DEA AND TEXAS CONTROLLED SUBSTANCES CERTIFICATES, ALL UNUSED TRIPLICATE PRESCRIPTION FORMS AND ALL CONTROLLED SUBSTANCES IN HIS POSSESSION INCLUDING SAMPLES; SHALL NOT SEEK TO REREGISTER WITHOUT PERMISSION; SEPARATE FROM PATIENT RECORDS, SHALL MAINTAIN A FILE OF EVERY PRESCRIPTION WRITTEN FOR DANGEROUS DRUGS WHICH SHALL BE AVAILABLE FOR INSPECTION; SHALL PARTICIPATE IN ACTIVITIES OF A PHYSICIANS COUNSELING COMMITTEE WITH QUARTERLY REPORTS; SHALL PARTICIPATE IN AA'S PROGRAM NOT LESS THAN THREE TIMES A WEEK WITH QUARTERLY REPORTS TO THE BOARD; SHALL ABIDE BY ALL TERMS OF 2/4/94 CONTRACT WITH HOSPITAL; SHALL SUBMIT HIMSELF FOR EVALUATION AND TREATMENT TO A BOARD-APPROVED PSYCHIATRIST; SHALL ATTEND AT LEAST 50 HOURS PER YEAR OF CONTINUING MEDICAL EDUCATION; SHALL APPEAR BEFORE THE BOARD TWICE A YEAR; SHALL GIVE A COPY OF THIS ORDER TO ANY HEALTH CARE ENTITY WHERE HE HAS PRIVILEGES; SHALL COOPERATE WITH THE BOARD IN VERIFYING COMPLIANCE; SHALL INFORM BOARD OF CHANGE OF ADDRESS WITHIN 10 DAYS OR IF HE LEAVES THE STATE; TIME SPENT OUT OF TEXAS DOES NOT COUNT TOWARD PROBATION. SHALL NOT SEEK MODIFICATION FOR ONE YEAR. ON 11/16/96 ORDER MODIFIED AS FOLLOWS: SHALL TAKE AND PASS THE SPECIAL PURPOSE EXAMINATION PRIOR TO PRACTICING MEDICINE IN TEXAS IN ORDER TO PRACTICE IN A GROUP SETTING; STILL MAY NOT PRACTICE IN A SOLO PRACTICE; HE IS AUTHORIZED TO REAPPLY TO THE DEA AND THE TEXAS

DEPARTMENT OF PUBLIC SAFETY TO OBTAIN FULL PRESCRIBING AUTHORITY FOR CONTROLLED SUBSTANCES; MEDICAL PRACTICE SHALL BE MONITORED BY A BOARD APPROVED PHYSICIAN WHO SHALL COUNSEL HIM ON ANY PERCEIVED DEFICIENCIES AND PROVIDE QUARTERLY REPORTS; ALL OTHER CONDITIONS REMAIN IN EFFECT. ON 11/22/97 REQUEST FOR TERMINATION DENIED. ON 8/22/98 ORDER MODIFIED REQUIRING BOARD APPEARANCES UPON REQUEST. ON 1/29/99 REQUEST FOR TERMINATION DENIED. ON 12/11/99 PETITION TO TERMINATE ORDER DENIED; ORDER MODIFIED DELETING ALL CONDITIONS WHICH DO NOT APPLY TO HIS SOBRIETY, RECOVERY, OR THE BOARD'S ABILITY TO MONITOR HIM.

VIGDERMAN, DAVID L DO, LICENSE NUMBER 00F7654 OF BIG SPRING, TX, WAS DISCIPLINED BY TEXAS ON JANUARY 25, 1992
DISCIPLINARY ACTION: 3-MONTH EMERGENCY SUSPENSION
OFFENSE: DISCIPLINARY ACTION BY ANOTHER STATE OR AGENCY

NOTES: LICENSE TEMPORARILY SUSPENDED. A FORMAL HEARING IS PENDING.

VIGDERMAN, DAVID L DO, LICENSE NUMBER 00F7654 OF BIG SPRING, TX, WAS DISCIPLINED BY TEXAS ON NOVEMBER 30, 1992
DISCIPLINARY ACTION: LICENSE REVOCATION
OFFENSE: DISCIPLINARY ACTION BY ANOTHER STATE OR AGENCY

NOTES: DISCIPLINARY ACTION TAKEN BY ANOTHER STATE BOARD FOR UNPROFESSIONAL OR DISHONORABLE CONDUCT LIKELY TO DECEIVE, DEFRAUD OR INJURE THE PUBLIC.

VIGIL, JACOB MD, DATE OF BIRTH JULY 7, 1955 OF 4251 BOY SCOUT LANE, EL PASO, TX, WAS DISCIPLINED BY MEDICARE ON MARCH 18, 1999
DISCIPLINARY ACTION: EXCLUSION FROM THE MEDICARE AND/OR MEDICAID PROGRAM
OFFENSE: NONCOMPLIANCE WITH A PROFESSIONAL RULE

NOTES: DEFAULTED ON PUBLIC HEALTH SERVICE EDUCATION LOAN.

VILLARREAL, CESAR Q MD, LICENSE NUMBER 27005 OF EL PASO, TX, WAS DISCIPLINED BY TEXAS ON JANUARY 29, 1999
DISCIPLINARY ACTION: FINE; REPRIMAND
OFFENSE: SEXUAL ABUSE OF OR SEXUAL MISCONDUCT WITH A PATIENT

NOTES: IN 9/97 HE ENGAGED IN INAPPROPRIATE CONDUCT BY TAKING A PATIENT HE WAS TREATING FOR DEPRESSION TO THE PATIENT'S APARTMENT; HE ADMITS TAKING THE PATIENT TO HER APARTMENT; THE PATIENT ALLEGED SEXUAL CONTACT WHICH HE DENIES; PLACED ON PAID SUSPENSION WITH UNIVERSITY BASED ON THE INCIDENT; CRIMINAL CHARGES WERE FILED AGAINST HIM AND LATER DISMISSED AFTER HE REACHED A MONETARY SETTLEMENT WITH THE PATIENT. $5,000 FINE; SHALL COOPERATE WITH THE BOARD IN VERIFYING COMPLIANCE.

VILLEGAS, LEO III DO OF 2162 TEXAS AVENUE, BRIDGE CITY, TX, WAS DISCIPLINED BY DEA ON SEPTEMBER 30, 1993
DISCIPLINARY ACTION: RESTRICTION PLACED ON CONTROLLED SUBSTANCE LICENSE
OFFENSE: OVERPRESCRIBING OR MISPRESCRIBING DRUGS

NOTES: PRESCRIBING LARGE QUANTITIES OF CONTROLLED SUBSTANCES WITHOUT LEGITIMATE MEDICAL REASONS. RESTRICTED 08/20/93 ORDER FROM SCHEDULES II AND III CONTROLLED SUBSTANCES. REGISTRATION MODIFIED 09/30/93.

VILLEGAS, LEO III DO OF 2162 TEXAS AVENUE, BRIDGE CITY, TX, WAS DISCIPLINED BY DEA ON JULY 19, 1994
DISCIPLINARY ACTION: RESTRICTION PLACED ON CONTROLLED SUBSTANCE LICENSE
OFFENSE: DISCIPLINARY ACTION BY ANOTHER STATE OR AGENCY

NOTES: STATE BOARD.

VILLEGAS, LEOPOLD III DO, LICENSE NUMBER 00G7763, WAS DISCIPLINED BY TEXAS ON AUGUST 20, 1993
DISCIPLINARY ACTION: 60-MONTH PROBATION; RESTRICTION PLACED ON CONTROLLED SUBSTANCE LICENSE
OFFENSE: SUBSTANCE ABUSE

NOTES: DIVERTED TYLOX PRESCRIPTIONS FOR HIS OWN USE; SUFFERS FROM POLIOMYELITIS RESIDUAL EFFECTS. FIVE YEAR SUSPENSION STAYED. CONDITIONS OF PROBATION: SHALL APPEAR BEFORE A COMMITTEE OF THE BOARD TWICE A YEAR; SHALL BE MONITORED BY A BOARD-APPROVED PHYSICIAN WHO SHALL REPORT TO THE BOARD THREE TIMES A YEAR; SHALL WITHIN 6 MONTHS ENROLL IN A TWO WEEK PRECEPTORSHIP ON THE PREVENTION AND TREATMENT OF DRUG ABUSE; ON 4/11/94, SINCE THE SPECIFIED COURSE WAS NOT OFFERED AT THIS TIME THIS PROVISION WAS DROPPED; SHALL NOT TREAT OR OTHERWISE SERVE AS PHYSICIAN, PRESCRIBE, DISPENSE OR ADMINISTER DRUGS THAT MAY BE SUBJECT TO ABUSE FOR HIMSELF OR ANY MEMBER OF HIS FAMILY; DEA AND CONTROLLED SUBSTANCES REGISTRATION LIMITED TO SCHEDULES IV AND V; SHALL ABSTAIN FROM THE CONSUMPTION OF ALCOHOL/CHEMICAL SUBSTANCES IN ANY FORM UNLESS PRESCRIBED BY ANOTHER PHYSICIAN FOR A LEGITIMATE AND THERAPEUTIC PURPOSE; SHALL ENTER A DRUG REHABILITATION PROGRAM WITHIN 20 DAYS WITH REPORTS TO THE BOARD; SHALL UNDERGO EXAMS AND ANY NECESSARY TREATMENT BY A BOARD-APPROVED NEUROLOGIST AND PSYCHIATRIST; SHALL FOLLOW THIS NEUROLOGIST'S RECOMMENDATIONS CONCERNING RESTRICTIONS ON HIS MEDICAL PRACTICE; SHALL PARTICIPATE IN THE ACTIVITIES OF AA NOT LESS THAN THREE TIMES A WEEK; SHALL PARTICIPATE IN ACTIVITIES OF A PHYSICIAN HEALTH AND REHABILITATION COMMITTEE AND ATTEND WEEKLY MEETINGS WITH QUARTERLY REPORTS; SHALL SUBMIT HIMSELF FOR APPROPRIATE EXAMS INCLUDING DRUG OR ALCOHOL SCREENS; SHALL GIVE A COPY OF THIS ORDER TO ANY HEALTH CARE ENTITY WHERE HE HAS PRIVILEGES; SHALL COOPERATE WITH THE BOARD IN VERIFYING COMPLIANCE; SHALL INFORM BOARD OF CHANGE OF ADDRESS WITHIN 10 DAYS OR IF HE LEAVES THE STATE; TIME SPENT OUT OF TEXAS DOES NOT COUNT TOWARD PROBATION. SHALL NOT SEEK MODIFICATION FOR ONE YEAR.

VILLEGAS, LEOPOLD III DO, LICENSE NUMBER 00G7763 OF ORANGE, TX, WAS DISCIPLINED BY TEXAS ON AUGUST 18, 1995
DISCIPLINARY ACTION: 48-MONTH PROBATION; RESTRICTION PLACED ON CONTROLLED SUBSTANCE LICENSE
OFFENSE: FAILURE TO COMPLY WITH PREVIOUS BOARD ORDER

NOTES: ON OR ABOUT 3/17/95, A POSITIVE TOXICOLOGY SCREEN OF A URINE SAMPLE CONFIRMED INGESTION OF BARBITURATES; HE ADMITTED INGESTING SAMPLES OF PANCOF-XP, A CONTROLLED SUBSTANCE, AND ESGIC-PLUS, A DANGEROUS DRUG WITH ADDICTIVE POTENTIAL, FOR HIS COLD SYMPTOMS AND NOT PURSUANT TO A PRESCRIPTION FROM A TREATING PHYSICIAN; INGESTION OF

SAMPLES WAS IN VIOLATION OF HIS 8/93 ORDER. SUSPENSION STAYED. PROBATION WITH TERMS: SHALL ABSTAIN FROM THE CONSUMPTION OF ALCOHOL/DRUGS IN ANY FORM UNLESS PRESCRIBED BY ANOTHER PHYSICIAN FOR A LEGITIMATE AND THERAPEUTIC PURPOSE; SHALL SUBMIT HIMSELF FOR APPROPRIATE EXAMS INCLUDING DRUG OR ALCOHOL SCREENS; SHALL CONTINUE TO RECEIVE CARE AND TREATMENT FROM HIS PHYSICIAN WHOM HE SHALL SEE NO LESS THAN ONCE A MONTH FOR CARE AND COUNSELING AND WHO SHALL SUBMIT QUARTERLY REPORTS TO THE BOARD; SHALL CONTINUE TO PARTICIPATE IN AA'S PROGRAM NOT LESS THAN THREE TIMES A WEEK WITH QUARTERLY REPORTS TO THE BOARD; SHALL CONTINUE TO PARTICIPATE IN THE ACTIVITIES OF AN IMPAIRED PHYSICIANS GROUP AND ATTEND WEEKLY MEETINGS WITH QUARTERLY REPORTS TO THE BOARD; SHALL NOT POSSESS ALCOHOL, CONTROLLED SUBSTANCES OR DANGEROUS DRUGS WITH ADDICTIVE POTENTIAL OR POTENTIAL FOR ABUSE; SHALL SURRENDER ANY SAMPLES IN HIS POSSESSION; SHALL NOT TREAT OR OTHERWISE SERVE AS PHYSICIAN, PRESCRIBE, DISPENSE OR ADMINISTER DRUGS THAT MIGHT BE SUBJECT TO ABUSE TO HIMSELF OR TO ANY MEMBER OF HIS FAMILY; SHALL IMMEDIATELY REQUEST MODIFICATION OF HIS DEA AND DPS CONTROLLED SUBSTANCES REGISTRATION CERTIFICATES TO ELIMINATE HIS AUTHORITY TO PRESCRIBE OR DISPENSE SCHEDULES II, II-N, III AND III-N; SHALL MAINTAIN A FILE WITH A COPY OF EVERY PRESCRIPTION WRITTEN BY HIM FOR CONTROLLED SUBSTANCES OR DANGEROUS DRUGS WITH ADDICTIVE POTENTIAL OR POTENTIAL FOR ABUSE AND A LOGBOOK FOR ALL PRESCRIPTIONS OR REFILLS TELEPHONED IN BY HIM FOR THESE DRUGS BOTH OF WHICH SHALL BE AVAILABLE FOR REVIEW; HIS MEDICAL PRACTICE SHALL CONTINUE TO BE MONITORED BY PHYSICIAN WHO WILL SUBMIT QUARTERLY REPORTS TO THE BOARD; SHALL MAINTAIN ADEQUATE MEDICAL RECORDS WHICH SHALL BE AVAILABLE FOR REVIEW; SHALL APPEAR BEFORE BOARD AT LEAST TWICE A YEAR; SHALL COOPERATE WITH THE BOARD IN VERIFYING COMPLIANCE; SHALL GIVE A COPY OF THIS ORDER TO ANY HEALTH CARE ENTITY WHERE HE HAS PRIVILEGES; TIME SPENT OUT OF TEXAS DOES NOT COUNT TOWARD PROBATION; SHALL INFORM BOARD OF CHANGE OF ADDRESS WITHIN 10 DAYS OR IF HE LEAVES THE STATE. SHALL NOT SEEK MODIFICATION FOR ONE YEAR. ON 5/10/97 PETITION TO TERMINATE ORDER DENIED; ORDER MODIFIED ALLOWING HIM TO REAPPLY FOR ALL CONTROLLED SUBSTANCE SCHEDULES. ON 4/4/98 ORDER TERMINATED.

VINSON, JACK R DO, LICENSE NUMBER 00C6109 OF DALLAS, TX, WAS DISCIPLINED BY TEXAS ON MAY 24, 1990
DISCIPLINARY ACTION: MONITORING OF PHYSICIAN PERFORMANCE

NOTES: STIPULATED ORDER. MUST MAINTAIN ADEQUATE MEDICAL RECORDS OF PATIENT OFFICE VISITS TO INCLUDE CERTAIN INFORMATION, ADEQUATELY ASCERTAIN LEGAL-MEDICAL STATUS OF PATIENTS, I.E. WHETHER OR NOT PATIENT HAS GUARDIAN OR SIGNED POWER OF ATTORNEY PRIOR TO INITIATING CERTAIN THERAPY, ASCERTAIN LEGAL CAPACITY AND AUTHORITY OF THOSE PERSONS WHO SIGN INFORMED CONSENT ON BEHALF OF PATIENT, AND OBTAIN CONSULTATION FROM BOARD-APPROVED INTERNIST FOR CERTAIN PATIENTS.

WADDINGHAM, RAND E MD, LICENSE NUMBER H5214 OF CRANE, TX, WAS DISCIPLINED BY TEXAS ON AUGUST 9, 1997
DISCIPLINARY ACTION: FINE; REQUIRED TO TAKE ADDITIONAL MEDICAL EDUCATION
OFFENSE: PROFESSIONAL MISCONDUCT

NOTES: HE TREATED A FAMILY MEMBER WHO HAD PREVIOUSLY ABUSED CONTROLLED SUBSTANCES, INSTEAD OF CONTACTING ANOTHER PHYSICIAN; HE FAILED TO KEEP ADEQUATE RECORDS CONCERNING HIS PRESCRIBING TO THIS PATIENT; HE PRESCRIBED AND ADMINISTERED CONTROLLED SUBSTANCES TO ANOTHER PATIENT WITH A POSSIBLE CHEMICAL DEPENDENCY; HE FAILED TO ADEQUATELY SUPERVISE A NURSE PRACTITIONER WHO IMPROPERLY ADMINISTERED PRESCRIPTION DRUGS TO ONE OF THESE TWO PATIENTS. SHALL ADHERE TO THE FOLLOWING CONDITIONS FOR TWO YEARS: SHALL OBTAIN AT LEAST 50 HOURS PER YEAR OF CONTINUING MEDICAL EDUCATION INCLUDING ONE COURSE IN RISK MANAGEMENT AND ONE COURSE IN PAIN MANAGEMENT; SHALL TAKE AND PASS THE MEDICAL JURISPRUDENCE EXAM WITHIN ONE YEAR; $2,500 FINE TO BE PAID; SHALL GIVE A COPY OF THIS ORDER TO ANY HEALTH CARE ENTITY WHERE HE HAS PRIVILEGES; SHALL PROVIDE A COPY OF THIS ORDER TO ANYONE REQUESTING IT WITHIN 10 DAYS; TIME SPENT OUT OF TEXAS DOES NOT COUNT TOWARD RESTRICTION; SHALL INFORM THE BOARD OF CHANGE OF ADDRESS WITHIN 10 DAYS OR IF HE LEAVES THE STATE; SHALL NOT SEEK MODIFICATION FOR ONE YEAR. ON 8/22/98 THE ORDER WAS TERMINATED.

WADDINGHAM, RAND EDWARD MD OF ANDREWS, TX, WAS DISCIPLINED BY UTAH ON JULY 1, 1998
DISCIPLINARY ACTION: PROBATION; CONTROLLED SUBSTANCE LICENSE PLACED ON PROBATION
OFFENSE: DISCIPLINARY ACTION BY ANOTHER STATE OR AGENCY

NOTES: DISCIPLINARY ACTION TAKEN AGAINST HIS MEDICAL LICENSE IN TEXAS. LICENSE TO PRACTICE MEDICINE IN UTAH CONDITIONED CONSISTENT WITH THE TERMS AND CONDITIONS PLACED ON HIS TEXAS LICENSE. ON 10/23/98 PROBATION ON LICENSES TO PRACTICE MEDICINE AND TO PRESCRIBE AND ADMINISTER CONTROLLED SUBSTANCES WAS TERMINATED AND SAID LICENSES WERE REINSTATED WITH FULL PRIVILEGES.

WALDEN, ARCHIE DON MD, DATE OF BIRTH NOVEMBER 23, 1933, LICENSE NUMBER 0016414 OF 546 GENERAL DISPENSARY, UNIT 29920 BOX 17 APO AE, WAS DISCIPLINED BY MINNESOTA ON NOVEMBER 14, 1992
DISCIPLINARY ACTION: FINE; REPRIMAND
OFFENSE: SEXUAL ABUSE OF OR SEXUAL MISCONDUCT WITH A PATIENT

NOTES: IMPROPER MANAGEMENT OF MEDICAL RECORDS; PRESCRIBING A DRUG OR DEVICE FOR OTHER THAN MEDICALLY ACCEPTED THERAPEUTIC PURPOSES; ENGAGING IN CONDUCT WITH A PATIENT WHICH IS SEXUAL OR MAY REASONABLY BE INTERPRETED BY THE PATIENT AS SEXUAL. SHALL PAY A CIVIL PENALTY OF $5,000.

WALDEN, ARCHIE DON MD, DATE OF BIRTH NOVEMBER 23, 1933, LICENSE NUMBER 00C7814 OF PEACHTREE CITY, GA, WAS DISCIPLINED BY TEXAS ON MARCH 5, 1994
DISCIPLINARY ACTION: REPRIMAND
OFFENSE: DISCIPLINARY ACTION BY ANOTHER STATE OR AGENCY

NOTES: ON 10/21/92 THE MINNESOTA BOARD SANCTIONED HIM FOR NUMEROUS CASES OF PATIENT TREATMENT IN WHICH LACK OF DOCUMENTATION OF MEDICATIONS, VITAL SIGNS, WEIGHTS, AND LABORATORY VALUES PROVIDED INADEQUATE INFORMATION FOR FOLLOW-

UP CARE AND MEDICAL MANAGEMENT OF PATIENTS WHICH RESULTED IN FRAGMENTED MEDICAL CARE. SHALL NOT PRACTICE MEDICINE IN TEXAS BEFORE APPEARING BEFORE BOARD AND PROVIDING INFORMATION THAT SHOWS HE IS ABLE TO SAFELY PRACTICE MEDICINE; BOARD MAY IMPOSE ADDITIONAL RESTRICTIONS AT THAT TIME.

WALKER, JONATHAN EDWARD MD, LICENSE NUMBER D2622 OF DALLAS, TX, WAS DISCIPLINED BY TEXAS ON AUGUST 22, 1998
DISCIPLINARY ACTION: REPRIMAND
OFFENSE: PROFESSIONAL MISCONDUCT

NOTES: ON OR ABOUT 4/25/96 ONE PATIENT WHOM HE HAD BEEN TREATING SINCE 1985 HAD GONE TO HIM EXPECTING CONVENTIONAL TREATMENT, AND INSTEAD RECEIVED WHAT HE CALLED "EASTERN HEALING TECHNIQUES"; ON 10/31/96 ANOTHER PATIENT, HAVING BEEN UNDER THE CARE OF NEUROLOGISTS FOR SEVERAL YEARS FOR MIGRAINE HEADACHES AND FAMILY HISTORY OF BRAIN CANCER, SAW HIM FOR THE FIRST TIME AND TOOK ALL HER MEDICAL RECORDS WITH HER; THE SAME PROCEDURE WAS PERFORMED ON HER AS THE FIRST PATIENT IN THAT THE DOCTOR CHOSE MEDICATIONS USING WHAT HE TERMED THE "CHINESE METHOD" OF DRUG SELECTION: BRINGING SEVERAL BASKETS OF MEDICATION IN AND PLACING THEM ON THE ABDOMENS OF THE PATIENTS AND DETERMINING WHICH MEDICATION TO USE BASED UPON A RESISTANCE TEST OF THEIR ARM; NOT INTERESTED IN USING THIS METHOD, SHE WAS PRESCRIBED FIORINAL EVEN THOUGH HER MEDICAL HISTORY STATED SHE WAS ALLERGIC TO IT; NEITHER HE NOR HIS ASSISTANT CONSULTED THE MEDICAL RECORDS THAT SHE'D BROUGHT WITH HER. AS A RESULT OF BOARD FINDINGS, HE HAS INCORPORATED THE FOLLOWING PROTOCOL INTO HIS PRACTICE: PRIOR TO OFFERING ADVICE ABOUT COMPLEMENTARY HEALTH CARE THERAPIES, HE WILL UNDERTAKE AN ASSESSMENT OF THE PATIENT; THE ASSESSMENT WILL FOLLOW CONVENTIONAL METHODS OF DIAGNOSIS AND WILL BE DOCUMENTED IN THE PATIENT'S CHART.

WALKER, LOUIS E JR MD, LICENSE NUMBER E1168, WAS DISCIPLINED BY TEXAS ON MAY 10, 1997
DISCIPLINARY ACTION: RESTRICTION PLACED ON CONTROLLED SUBSTANCE LICENSE; REQUIRED TO TAKE ADDITIONAL MEDICAL EDUCATION
OFFENSE: OVERPRESCRIBING OR MISPRESCRIBING DRUGS

NOTES: FROM APPROXIMATELY 8/94 TO 10/96, ON A CONTINUOUS AND FREQUENT BASIS, HE PRESCRIBED EXCESSIVE AMOUNTS OF CONTROLLED SUBSTANCES, NAMELY NARCOTIC PAIN KILLERS, SUCH AS DEMEROL, TO A FAMILY MEMBER WHILE AWARE THAT THE FAMILY MEMBER WAS RECEIVING MEDICAL CARE, INCLUDING THE PRESCRIBING OF SIMILAR SUBSTANCES FROM OTHER LICENSED TEXAS PHYSICIANS WHO WERE UNAWARE OF HIS DUPLICATIVE PRESCRIBING. HE LOST MEDICAL OBJECTIVITY WITH RESPECT TO HIS MEDICAL CARE OF THE FAMILY MEMBER. LICENSE RESTRICTED FOR FIVE YEARS UNDER THE FOLLOWING TERMS: INDEFINITELY RESTRICTED FROM PRESCRIBING ANY DRUG OR TREATMENT FOR ANY OF HIS FAMILY MEMBERS, INCLUDING ANY SELF-PRESCRIBING, OR PRESCRIBING TO HIS STAFF; SHALL IMMEDIATELY REQUEST MODIFICATION OF HIS DRUG ENFORCEMENT AGENCY AND TEXAS DEPARTMENT OF SAFETY CONTROLLED SUBSTANCES REGISTRATION CERTIFICATE TO ELIMINATE HIS AUTHORITY TO PRESCRIBE OR DISPENSE SCHEDULE II DRUGS; SEPARATE FROM PATIENT RECORDS, SHALL MAINTAIN A FILE OF EVERY PRESCRIPTION WRITTEN BY HIM FOR DANGEROUS DRUGS WITH ADDICTIVE POTENTIAL WHICH SHALL BE MADE AVAILABLE FOR REVIEW; SHALL NOMINATE THREE CERTIFIED PSYCHIATRISTS FOR BOARD SELECTION OF A THERAPIST AND SHALL EXPEDITIOUSLY SUBMIT HIMSELF TO EVALUATION AND TREATMENT BY THE APPROVED PRACTITIONER; SHALL COOPERATE WITH THE BOARD IN VERIFYING COMPLIANCE INCLUDING PROVIDING COPIES OF MEDICAL RELEASES UPON REQUEST; SHALL OBTAIN AT LEAST 50 HOURS PER YEAR OF CONTINUING MEDICAL EDUCATION INCLUDING AT LEAST 12 HOURS IN CHRONIC PAIN MANAGEMENT; SHALL GIVE A COPY OF THIS ORDER TO ANY HEALTH CARE ENTITY WHERE HE HAS PRIVILEGES; SHALL PROVIDE A COPY OF THIS ORDER TO ANYONE REQUESTING IT WITHIN 10 DAYS; TIME SPENT OUT OF TEXAS DOES NOT COUNT TOWARD RESTRICTION; SHALL INFORM THE BOARD OF CHANGE OF ADDRESS WITHIN 10 DAYS OR IF HE LEAVES THE STATE; SHALL NOT SEEK MODIFICATION FOR ONE YEAR. ON 10/24/98 THE REQUEST TO TERMINATE THE ORDER WAS DENIED BUT THE ORDER WAS MODIFIED AS FOLLOWS: DELETION OF REQUIREMENTS TO HAVE HIS CONTROLLED SUBSTANCE REGISTRATIONS MODIFIED, TO MAINTAIN A LOGBOOK OF PRESCRIPTIONS WRITTEN; AND, FOR REQUIREMENT FOR 12 CONTINUING MEDICAL EDUCATION HOURS IN THE AREA OF CHRONIC PAIN; ALL OTHER PROVISIONS OF THE ORDER REMAIN IN FULL EFFECT. ON 12/11/99 THE ORDER WAS TERMINATED.

WALLACE, C B JR MD, LICENSE NUMBER 0003656 OF KERRVILLE, TX, WAS DISCIPLINED BY TEXAS ON JANUARY 25, 1995
DISCIPLINARY ACTION: EMERGENCY SUSPENSION
OFFENSE: SUBSTANCE ABUSE

NOTES: INTEMPERATE USE OF ALCOHOL OR DRUGS.

WALSSON, ROMEO ROJAS MD, LICENSE NUMBER J8380, WAS DISCIPLINED BY TEXAS ON MAY 10, 1997
DISCIPLINARY ACTION: 60-MONTH PROBATION; FINE
OFFENSE: DISCIPLINARY ACTION BY ANOTHER STATE OR AGENCY

NOTES: ON 5/30/96 HE WAS DISCIPLINED BY THE COLLEGE OF PHYSICIANS AND SURGEONS OF SASKATCHEWAN IN CANADA, BASED UPON FINDINGS REGARDING AN INAPPROPRIATE SEXUAL RELATIONSHIP WITH A PATIENT BEGINNING IN JULY 1993 AND CONTINUING UNTIL THE SUMMER OF 1994. HAS BEEN DIAGNOSED WITH DEPRESSION AND IS BEING TREATED BY PSYCHIATRISTS IN SAN ANTONIO, TEXAS. SUSPENSION STAYED FOR PROBATION UNDER THE FOLLOWING TERMS: SHALL NOMINATE THREE CERTIFIED PSYCHIATRISTS FOR BOARD SELECTION OF A THERAPIST AND SHALL EXPEDITIOUSLY SUBMIT HIMSELF TO EVALUATION AND TREATMENT BY THE APPROVED PRACTITIONER; SHALL COOPERATE WITH THE BOARD IN VERIFYING COMPLIANCE INCLUDING PROVIDING COPIES OF MEDICAL RELEASES UPON REQUEST; SHALL ABSTAIN FROM THE CONSUMPTION OF ALCOHOL/DRUGS IN ANY FORM UNLESS PRESCRIBED BY ANOTHER PHYSICIAN FOR A LEGITIMATE AND THERAPEUTIC PURPOSE; SHALL SUBMIT HIMSELF FOR APPROPRIATE EXAMS INCLUDING DRUG OR ALCOHOL SCREENS; SHALL NOT TREAT OR OTHERWISE SERVE AS PHYSICIAN, PRESCRIBE, DISPENSE OR ADMINISTER DRUGS THAT MAY BE SUBJECT TO ABUSE TO HIMSELF OR TO ANY MEMBER OF HIS FAMILY; ANY TIME HE PERFORMS A PHYSICAL EXAMINATION ON A FEMALE PATIENT, HE

SHALL HAVE A CHAPERONE PRESENT IN THE ROOM WHO IS ABLE TO DIRECTLY OBSERVE HIM; SHALL OBTAIN AT LEAST 50 CONTINUING MEDICAL EDUCATION HOURS PER YEAR WITH AT LEAST TEN IN BOUNDARIES/TRANSFERENCE. SHALL OBTAIN EIGHT HOURS PER YEAR OF ETHICS COURSES FOR TWO YEARS; SHALL PAY AN ADMINISTRATIVE PENALTY OF $1000; SHALL APPEAR BEFORE THE BOARD AT LEAST TWICE YEARLY; SHALL GIVE A COPY OF THIS ORDER TO ANY HEALTH CARE ENTITY WHERE HE HAS PRIVILEGES; TIME SPENT OUT OF TEXAS DOES NOT COUNT TOWARD PROBATION; SHALL INFORM THE BOARD OF CHANGE OF ADDRESS WITHIN 10 DAYS OR IF HE LEAVES THE STATE; SHALL NOT SEEK MODIFICATION FOR ONE YEAR. ON 2/7/98 THE ORDER WAS AMENDED TO DESIGNATE THE PHYSICIAN FROM WHOM HE WAS TO RECEIVE CARE AND TREATMENT. ON 5/16/98 TERMINATION REQUEST WAS DENIED BUT MODIFICATIONS OF THE ORDER WERE MADE AS FOLLOWS: REQUIREMENTS THAT HE ABSTAIN FROM ALCOHOL, DANGEROUS DRUGS AND CONTROLLED SUBSTANCES AND SUBMIT TO RANDOM ALCOHOL AND DRUG SCREENS WERE DELETED; ALL OTHER PROVISIONS OF THE ORDER REMAIN IN FULL EFFECT. ON 5/14/99 TERMINATION REQUEST WAS DENIED.

WARE, STEPHEN HARRISON III MD, LICENSE NUMBER F3375 OF CORPUS CHRISTI, TX, WAS DISCIPLINED BY TEXAS ON FEBRUARY 7, 1998
DISCIPLINARY ACTION: 60-MONTH RESTRICTION PLACED ON LICENSE; REQUIRED TO TAKE ADDITIONAL MEDICAL EDUCATION
OFFENSE: SEXUAL ABUSE OF OR SEXUAL MISCONDUCT WITH A PATIENT

NOTES: FROM 1992-1995 ADMITTED TO BOUNDARY VIOLATIONS, INCLUDING SEXUAL RELATIONS WITH AT LEAST 16 PATIENTS; HE VOLUNTARILY REPORTED HIS MISCONDUCT TO THE BOARD ON 11/27/95 AFTER HE HAD VOLUNTARILY ENTERED MENTAL HEALTH TREATMENT FOR SEXUAL ADDICTION; ON 2/8/96 HE WAS DISCHARGED WITH A "GUARDED PROGNOSIS" AND SPECIFIED RECOMMENDATIONS; ON 2/14/96 HE ENTERED INTO A REHABILITATION CONTRACT AND MAINTAINS THAT HE HAS BEEN CONTINUALLY CHAPERONED IN HIS PRACTICE AND THAT HE HAS COMPLIED WITH THE TREATMENT TEAM RECOMMENDATIONS; ON 9/16/97 HE VOLUNTARILY SOUGHT POST-TREATMENT EVALUATION AND WAS DIAGNOSED WITH DEPRESSION IN REMISSION, ADJUSTMENT DISORDER WITH EMOTIONAL FEATURES, ESPECIALLY EXACERBATED SINCE RECENT ONSET OF BOARD ACTION, AND IMPULSE CONTROL DISORDER WITH ADDICTIVE FEATURES AS APPLIED TO SEXUAL CONDUCT AND BOUNDARIES IN MEDICAL PRACTICE. LICENSE LIMITED AS FOLLOWS: SHALL OBTAIN 12 HOURS OF AN ETHICS COURSE PER YEAR FOR EACH YEAR ORDER IS IN EFFECT; SHALL NOMINATE THREE CERTIFIED PSYCHIATRISTS FOR BOARD SELECTION OF A THERAPIST AND SHALL EXPEDITIOUSLY SUBMIT HIMSELF TO EVALUATION AND TREATMENT BY THE APPROVED PRACTITIONER; SHALL ABSTAIN FROM THE CONSUMPTION OF ALCOHOL/DRUGS IN ANY FORM UNLESS PRESCRIBED BY ANOTHER PHYSICIAN FOR A LEGITIMATE AND THERAPEUTIC PURPOSE; SHALL SUBMIT HIMSELF FOR APPROPRIATE EXAMS INCLUDING DRUG OR ALCOHOL SCREENS; SHALL PARTICIPATE IN AA'S PROGRAM NOT LESS THAN THREE TIMES A WEEK; SHALL REPORT ON HIS ATTENDANCE; SHALL PERFORM 200 HOURS OF COMMUNITY SERVICE PER YEAR FOR A BOARD-APPROVED NON-PROFIT ORGANIZATION; SHALL COMPLY WITH TERMS AND CONDITIONS OF HIS CONTINUING CARE CONTRACT WITH THE NUECES COUNTY IMPAIRED PHYSICIAN'S COMMITTEE WITH QUARTERLY REPORTS TO THE BOARD; SHALL HAVE A CHAPERONE PRESENT DURING THE EXAMINATION OF ANY FEMALE PATIENT; SHALL APPEAR BEFORE THE BOARD TWICE A YEAR; SHALL COOPERATE WITH THE BOARD IN VERIFYING COMPLIANCE INCLUDING PROVIDING COPIES OF MEDICAL RELEASES UPON REQUEST; SHALL GIVE A COPY OF THIS ORDER TO ANY HEALTH CARE ENTITY WHERE HE HAS PRIVILEGES; TIME SPENT OUT OF TEXAS DOES NOT COUNT TOWARD RESTRICTION; SHALL INFORM THE BOARD OF CHANGE OF ADDRESS WITHIN 10 DAYS OR IF HE LEAVES THE STATE; SHALL NOT SEEK MODIFICATION FOR ONE YEAR. ON 4/10/99 THE ORDER WAS MODIFIED AS FOLLOWS: REQUIREMENT THAT HE OBTAIN CONTINUING PSYCHIATRIC CARE MONTHLY SHALL BE MODIFIED TO REQUIRE CARE NO LESS OFTEN THAN QUARTERLY; REQUIREMENT TO PERFORM 200 HOURS OF COMMUNITY SERVICE LESSENED TO 100 HOURS PER YEAR; ALL OTHER PROVISIONS OF THE ORDER REMAIN IN FULL EFFECT.

WARE, STEVEN ALAN MD, LICENSE NUMBER F4652 OF HOUSTON, TX, WAS DISCIPLINED BY TEXAS ON AUGUST 9, 1997
DISCIPLINARY ACTION: FINE; REPRIMAND
OFFENSE: LOSS OR RESTRICTION OF HOSPITAL PRIVILEGES

NOTES: HIS PRIVILEGES WERE SUMMARILY SUSPENDED AND THEN SUSPENDED BY A HOSPITAL DUE TO HIS LACK OF AVAILABILITY, FAILURE TO ATTEND AND EVALUATE A PATIENT PRIOR TO RECOMMENDING DISCHARGE, AND NOT RESPONDING TO NOTIFICATION OF THE ACTION; HE MAINTAINS THAT HE DID NOT RECEIVE NOTICE OF A RIGHT TO A HEARING ON THE SUSPENSION OF HIS PRIVILEGES DUE TO A CHANGE OF PRACTICE ADDRESS, AND THEREFORE MAINTAINS THAT HE WAS UNABLE TO CONTEST THE HOSPITAL ACTION. $2,500 FINE.

WARREN, BRUCE HUNTINGTON MD, DATE OF BIRTH APRIL 14, 1927, LICENSE NUMBER 00D9316 OF 2391 NE LOOP 410, SAN ANTONIO, TX, WAS DISCIPLINED BY TEXAS ON OCTOBER 1, 1993
DISCIPLINARY ACTION: 60-MONTH PROBATION; REQUIRED TO TAKE ADDITIONAL MEDICAL EDUCATION
OFFENSE: SEXUAL ABUSE OF OR SEXUAL MISCONDUCT WITH A PATIENT

NOTES: VIOLATED THE BOUNDARIES OF THE DOCTOR-PATIENT RELATIONSHIP WITH ONE PATIENT WITH WHOM HE ENGAGED IN A PERSONAL RELATIONSHIP FROM 3/85 THROUGH 10/86 WHILE HE PROVIDED PSYCHIATRIC TREATMENT TO HER; GAVE HER MONEY ON SEVERAL OCCASIONS AND A GIFT ON AT LEAST ONE OCCASION; TOOK HER OUT TO LUNCH AND DINNER; THE PATIENT ALLEGES THEY HAD SEX ON AT LEAST TWO OCCASIONS WHICH HE DENIES. SUSPENSION STAYED. CONDITIONS OF PROBATION: SHALL ENROLL IN AND COMPLETE ONE BOARD-APPROVED ETHICS COURSE REGARDING SEXUAL ABUSE; SHALL SUBMIT HIMSELF FOR EVALUATION TO A BOARD APPROVED PSYCHIATRIST AND WILL FOLLOW TREATMENT RECOMMENDATIONS WITH REPORTS TO THE BOARD; SHALL APPEAR BEFORE THE BOARD ONCE A YEAR; SHALL COOPERATE WITH THE BOARD IN VERIFYING COMPLIANCE; SHALL INFORM BOARD OF CHANGE OF ADDRESS WITHIN 10 DAYS OR IF HE LEAVES THE STATE; TIME SPENT OUT OF TEXAS DOES NOT COUNT TOWARD PROBATION. SHALL NOT SEEK MODIFICATION FOR ONE YEAR.

WARREN, BRUCE HUNTINGTON MD OF 2914 WAR FEATHER DRIVE, SAN ANTONIO, TX, WAS DISCIPLINED BY DEA ON MARCH 1, 1994
DISCIPLINARY ACTION: SURRENDER OF CONTROLLED SUBSTANCE LICENSE

NOTES: IN LIEU OF PUBLIC INTEREST REVOCATION.

WARREN, BRUCE HUNTINGTON MD, DATE OF BIRTH APRIL 14, 1927, LICENSE NUMBER 00D9316 OF 2914 WAR FEATHER DRIVE, SAN ANTONIO, TX, WAS DISCIPLINED BY TEXAS ON NOVEMBER 7, 1995
DISCIPLINARY ACTION: SURRENDER OF LICENSE
OFFENSE: SEXUAL ABUSE OF OR SEXUAL MISCONDUCT WITH A PATIENT

NOTES: INAPPROPRIATE PERSONAL RELATIONSHIP BETWEEN HIM AND A PATIENT; DURING 1/94 OBSERVED ON GROUNDS OF A STATE HOSPITAL HOLDING HANDS AND KISSING HIS PATIENT. HE NEITHER ADMITS OR DENIES THESE ALLEGATIONS. VOLUNTARY AND PERMANENT SURRENDER TO AVOID THE EXPENSE OF LITIGATION; SHALL NOT PETITION THE BOARD FOR REINSTATEMENT OF HIS TEXAS MEDICAL LICENSE.

WASSERMAN, ALAN S MD, LICENSE NUMBER 00H5371 OF DENTON, TX, WAS DISCIPLINED BY TEXAS ON MAY 11, 1995
DISCIPLINARY ACTION: REPRIMAND; COMMUNITY SERVICE
OFFENSE: SUBSTANDARD CARE, INCOMPETENCE OR NEGLIGENCE

NOTES: IN 1993 HE TRANSPORTED AN UNSTABLE OBSTETRICS PATIENT TO ANOTHER LOCAL FACILITY IN HIS PERSONAL AUTOMOBILE; ALTHOUGH THERE WAS NOT AN ADVERSE OUTCOME HE EXERCISED POOR JUDGMENT; REPRIMANDED BY THE HOSPITAL IN PART FOR THIS; IN 3/93 PERFORMED A CIRCUMCISION WITH AN INSTRUMENT THAT WAS CHEMICALLY STERILIZED BUT NOT AUTOCLAVED. WITHIN ONE YEAR, SHALL PERFORM 100 HOURS OF COMMUNITY SERVICE FOR A NON-PROFIT CHARITABLE ORGANIZATION APPROVED BY THE BOARD; SHALL COOPERATE WITH THE BOARD IN VERIFYING COMPLIANCE; SHALL GIVE A COPY OF THIS ORDER TO ANY HEALTH CARE ENTITY WHERE HE HAS PRIVILEGES; SHALL PROVIDE A COPY OF THE ORDER TO ANYONE REQUESTING IT WITHIN 10 DAYS; SHALL INFORM BOARD OF CHANGE OF ADDRESS WITHIN 10 DAYS. ORDER SHALL REMAIN IN EFFECT FOR ONE YEAR.

WASSERMAN, ALAN S MD, LICENSE NUMBER 00H5371, WAS DISCIPLINED BY TEXAS ON AUGUST 17, 1996
DISCIPLINARY ACTION: 60-MONTH PROBATION; RESTRICTION PLACED ON LICENSE
OFFENSE: SUBSTANDARD CARE, INCOMPETENCE OR NEGLIGENCE

NOTES: ON 5/12/95 ATTEMPTED TO OVERSEE TWO PROCEDURES AT TWO DIFFERENT HOSPITALS, ONE A NON-EMERGENCY VAGINAL HYSTERECTOMY AND ONE AN INDUCED DELIVERY; HE INSTRUCTED THE DELIVERY OVER THE PHONE, THEN LEFT THE SURGERY TO ASSIST HER, RETURNING 30 MINUTES LATER TO COMPLETE SURGERY; NEITHER PATIENT SUFFERED ANY ADVERSE OUTCOME; HE HAS COMPLETED REQUIRED COMMUNITY SERVICE OF PREVIOUS ORDER. SUSPENSION, STAYED. PROBATIONS ON TERMS AND CONDITIONS: SHALL MAINTAIN MEDICAL STAFF PRIVILEGES AT NO MORE THAN ONE HOSPITAL AND SHALL NOT MAINTAIN ANY TYPE OF MEDICAL STAFF PRIVILEGES AT ANY OTHER HOSPITAL; SHALL REPORT TO THE BOARD WHERE HE WILL MAINTAIN HIS SOLE MEDICAL STAFF PRIVILEGES; PRIOR TO PERFORMING ANY SURGICAL PROCEDURE NOT INVOLVING OBSTETRICS, SHALL OBTAIN A WRITTEN CONSULTATION FROM A BOARD APPROVED LICENSED TEXAS PHYSICIAN WHICH SHALL BE INCLUDED IN THE PATIENT'S MEDICAL CHARTS AND MADE AVAILABLE UPON BOARD REQUEST; SHALL COMPLY WITH ANY RESTRICTIONS PLACED ON HIS MEDICAL STAFF PRIVILEGES AT ANY HOSPITAL; SHALL OBTAIN AT LEAST 50 HOURS PER YEAR OF CONTINUING MEDICAL EDUCATION; SHALL OBTAIN AN ADDITIONAL 25 HOURS EACH IN THE AREAS OF RISK MANAGEMENT AND HIGH RISK OBSTETRICS AND SUBMIT PROOF TO THE BOARD; SHALL COOPERATE WITH THE BOARD IN VERIFYING COMPLIANCE INCLUDING PROVIDING PEER REVIEW RECORDS; UPON REQUEST SHALL APPEAR BEFORE THE BOARD AT LEAST TWO TIMES PER YEAR OR UPON BOARD REQUEST; SHALL GIVE A COPY OF THIS ORDER TO ANY HEALTH CARE ENTITY WHERE HE HAS PRIVILEGES; SHALL PROVIDE A COPY OF THIS ORDER TO ANYONE REQUESTING IT WITHIN 10 DAYS; TIME PERIOD OUT OF TEXAS DOES NOT COUNT TOWARD PROBATION; SHALL INFORM THE BOARD OF CHANGE OF ADDRESS WITHIN 10 DAYS OF IF HE LEAVES THE STATE; SHALL NOT SEEK MODIFICATION FOR ONE YEAR. ON 9/20/97 PETITION TO MODIFY ORDER DENIED.

WASSERMAN, ALAN S MD OF DENTON, TX, WAS DISCIPLINED BY MISSOURI ON JANUARY 3, 1997
DISCIPLINARY ACTION: REPRIMAND
OFFENSE: DISCIPLINARY ACTION BY ANOTHER STATE OR AGENCY

NOTES: DISCIPLINED BY TEXAS BOARD FOR POOR JUDGMENT IN TRANSFERRING AN UNSTABLE OBSTETRIC PATIENT AND REVOCATION OF HOSPITAL PRIVILEGES AT SPECIFIED HOSPITAL. MUST NOTIFY THE BOARD 90 DAYS PRIOR TO RETURNING TO PRACTICE IN MISSOURI.

WATSON, JAMES R DO, DATE OF BIRTH JULY 6, 1944, LICENSE NUMBER 0001405 OF 1032 SOUTH W W WHITE, SAN ANTONIO, TX, WAS DISCIPLINED BY IOWA ON DECEMBER 23, 1991
DISCIPLINARY ACTION: PROBATION; FINE
OFFENSE: SEXUAL ABUSE OF OR SEXUAL MISCONDUCT WITH A PATIENT

NOTES: ACTION BASED ON ALLEGATIONS OF IMPROPER SEXUAL CONTACT WITH PATIENTS. CONDITION OF INDEFINITE PROBATION: SHALL NOT RETURN TO THE PRACTICE OF OSTEOPATHIC MEDICINE AND SURGERY THROUGH THE EXPIRATION OF HIS CURRENT LICENSE; SHALL NOT APPLY FOR RENEWAL OR REINSTATEMENT OF HIS LICENSE FOR FIVE YEARS; $5,000 CIVIL PENALTY ASSESSED.

WAYNE, BRYAN M MD OF 902 FROSTWOOD #246, HOUSTON, TX, WAS DISCIPLINED BY DEA ON MAY 12, 1995
DISCIPLINARY ACTION: SURRENDER OF CONTROLLED SUBSTANCE LICENSE

NOTES: IN LIEU OF PUBLIC INTEREST REVOCATION.

WAYNE, BRYAN MATTHEW MD, LICENSE NUMBER 00G8492 OF HOUSTON, TX, WAS DISCIPLINED BY TEXAS ON MAY 26, 1994
DISCIPLINARY ACTION: EMERGENCY SUSPENSION
OFFENSE: PROFESSIONAL MISCONDUCT

NOTES: AVAILABLE EVIDENCE AND INFORMATION INDICATE THE FOLLOWING: ON 3/11/94 DISCHARGED A WEAPON INTO HIS NEIGHBOR'S RESIDENCE AND DISCHARGED A SHOTGUN SEVERAL TIMES INTO THE AIR; THEN BARRICADED HIMSELF IN HIS RESIDENCE WHERE HE GAVE HIMSELF UP TO A SWAT TEAM THREE HOURS LATER; CHARGED WITH AGGRAVATED ASSAULT WITH A DEADLY WEAPON; HAS NOT PRACTICED MEDICINE SINCE 3/93 WHEN HE WAS DISCHARGED FROM HIS JOB; BOARD STAFF REQUESTED HIM TO SUBMIT TO A COMPLETE PSYCHIATRIC EXAM BY MAIL; HAS NOT RECEIVED A REPLY AND LETTER RETURNED TO BOARD MARKED UNCLAIMED.

WAYNE, BRYAN MATTHEW MD, LICENSE NUMBER 00G8492 OF HOUSTON, TX, WAS DISCIPLINED BY TEXAS ON AUGUST 19, 1994
DISCIPLINARY ACTION: LICENSE SUSPENSION
OFFENSE: PROFESSIONAL MISCONDUCT

NOTES: ON 3/11/94 HE WAS INVOLVED IN A DISTURBANCE WHICH RESULTED IN POLICE INTERVENTION; POLICE REPORT HE DISCHARGED A HAND HELD WEAPON INTO A NEIGHBORING BUSINESS AND DISCHARGED A SHOTGUN INTO THE AIR FOR UNKNOWN REASONS; THEY ALSO REPORT HE BARRICADED HIMSELF INSIDE HIS RESIDENCE FOR THREE HOURS UNTIL HE GAVE HIMSELF UP; WAS CHARGED WITH AGGRAVATED ASSAULT WITH A DEADLY WEAPON; HE STATES HE HAD PREVIOUS PROBLEMS WITH THE NEIGHBORING BUSINESS REGARDING DISRUPTIVE BEHAVIOR AND THAT HE TOLD THEM TWICE TO BE QUIET; THEN HE FIRED A BB PELLET GUN IN THEIR DIRECTION, WENT TO SLEEP AND AWOKE TO FIND A MESSAGE FROM THE POLICE ON HIS ANSWERING MACHINE; HE THEN TALKED TO THE POLICE AND AT THEIR REQUEST WENT OUTSIDE HIS RESIDENCE WHERE HE WAS ARRESTED; DENIES HE USED THE SHOTGUN OR THAT HE WAS BARRICADED; TRIAL DATE HAS BEEN POSTPONED. SUSPENSION UNTIL SUCH TIME AS HE PERSONALLY APPEARS BEFORE THE BOARD AND PROVIDES SUFFICIENT EVIDENCE THAT HE IS PHYSICALLY, MENTALLY AND OTHERWISE COMPETENT TO SAFELY PRACTICE MEDICINE.

WAYNE, BRYAN MATTHEW MD, LICENSE NUMBER 00G8492 OF HOUSTON, TX, WAS DISCIPLINED BY TEXAS ON OCTOBER 10, 1994
DISCIPLINARY ACTION: 60-MONTH PROBATION; MONITORING OF PHYSICIAN PERFORMANCE

NOTES: HE HAS SATISFIED THE MINIMUM REQUIREMENTS OF 8/19/94 ORDER SUSPENDING HIS LICENSE. THAT SUSPENSION NOW STAYED. CONDITIONS OF PROBATION: SHALL CONTINUE PSYCHIATRIC TREATMENT WITH QUARTERLY REPORTS; SHALL ABSTAIN FROM THE CONSUMPTION OF ALCOHOL/CHEMICAL SUBSTANCES IN ANY FORM UNLESS PRESCRIBED BY ANOTHER PHYSICIAN FOR A LEGITIMATE AND THERAPEUTIC PURPOSE; SHALL SUBMIT HIMSELF FOR APPROPRIATE EXAMS INCLUDING DRUG OR ALCOHOL SCREENS; SHALL APPEAR BEFORE THE BOARD ONCE A YEAR; SHALL GIVE A COPY OF THIS ORDER TO ANY HEALTH CARE ENTITY WHERE HE HAS PRIVILEGES; SHALL COOPERATE WITH THE BOARD IN VERIFYING COMPLIANCE; SHALL INFORM BOARD OF CHANGE OF ADDRESS WITHIN 10 DAYS OR IF HE LEAVES THE STATE; TIME SPENT OUT OF TEXAS DOES NOT COUNT TOWARD PROBATION. SHALL NOT SEEK MODIFICATION FOR ONE YEAR.

WAYNE, BRYAN MATTHEW MD, LICENSE NUMBER 00G8492 OF HOUSTON, TX, WAS DISCIPLINED BY TEXAS ON DECEMBER 20, 1994
DISCIPLINARY ACTION: EMERGENCY SUSPENSION

NOTES: EVIDENCE AND INFORMATION INDICATING THAT HE POSES A CONTINUING THREAT TO THE HEALTH AND WELFARE OF PATIENTS.

WEBB, PAUL C MD, LICENSE NUMBER E1442 OF KAUFMAN, TX, WAS DISCIPLINED BY TEXAS ON DECEMBER 11, 1999
DISCIPLINARY ACTION: FINE
OFFENSE: NONCOMPLIANCE WITH A PROFESSIONAL RULE

NOTES: DURING 6/97-5/98 REPORTED 31 HOURS OF CONTINUING MEDICAL EDUCATION; COULD ONLY SUBSTANTIATE ONE HOUR OF CONTINUING MEDICAL EDUCATION DURING THAT TIME PERIOD; SINCE 5/98 HAS SUBSTANTIATED 95.5 HOURS. $500 FINE.

WEBSTER, CHARLES L JR MD, LICENSE NUMBER 00D2313, WAS DISCIPLINED BY TEXAS ON OCTOBER 5, 1996
DISCIPLINARY ACTION: SURRENDER OF LICENSE
OFFENSE: SEXUAL ABUSE OF OR SEXUAL MISCONDUCT WITH A PATIENT

NOTES: ON 8/15/94 INDICTED ON FIVE COUNTS OF ALLEGED AGGRAVATED SEXUAL ASSAULT OF A CHILD AND FIVE COUNTS OF ALLEGED SEXUAL CONTACT OF A CHILD; CHARGES RELATED TO THREE CHILDREN UNDER 14; NEITHER ADMITS NOR DENIES CHARGES. VOLUNTARY AND PERMANENT SURRENDER; AND SHALL NOT PETITION THE BOARD FOR REINSTATEMENT.

WEHMER, RALPH E JR MD, DATE OF BIRTH JULY 29, 1948 OF 1007 WATER ST APT 102, BASTROP, TX, WAS DISCIPLINED BY MEDICARE ON AUGUST 10, 1990
DISCIPLINARY ACTION: 60-MONTH EXCLUSION FROM THE MEDICARE AND/OR MEDICAID PROGRAM
OFFENSE: CRIMINAL CONVICTION OR PLEA OF GUILTY, NOLO CONTENDERE, OR NO CONTEST TO A CRIME

NOTES: PROGRAM-RELATED CONVICTION.

WEHMER, RALPH EDWARD JR MD, LICENSE NUMBER 00G3899 OF BASTROP, TX, WAS DISCIPLINED BY TEXAS ON JUNE 10, 1991
DISCIPLINARY ACTION: 36-MONTH PROBATION
OFFENSE: PROFESSIONAL MISCONDUCT

NOTES: UNPROFESSIONAL OR DISHONORABLE CONDUCT LIKELY TO DECEIVE, DEFRAUD, OR INJURE THE PUBLIC. TERMS OF PROBATION: MUST APPEAR ONCE A YEAR BEFORE THE BOARD; MUST MAINTAIN ADEQUATE RECORDS ON ALL PATIENT OFFICE VISITS; MUST REFRAIN FROM NONTHERAPEUTIC PRESCRIBING; MUST CONDUCT ADEQUATE FOLLOW-UP EXAMS ON ALL PATIENTS TO DETERMINE WHETHER THE COURSE OF TREATMENT IS APPROPRIATE. ON 1/14/94 ORDER AMENDED TO INCLUDE ADDITION OF THE FOLLOWING: BEFORE THE DATE OF EXPIRATION OF THIS ORDER, HE MUST OBTAIN AT LEAST 50 HOURS OF CONTINUING MEDICAL EDUCATION IN THE AREAS OF EMERGENCY ROOM MEDICINE, DOCUMENTATION, CENTRAL INTRAVENOUS ACCESS, ADVANCED CARDIAC LIFE SUPPORT, AND ADVANCED TRAUMA LIFE SUPPORT AND SHALL SUBMIT PROOF OF SUCCESSFUL COMPLETION OF EACH COURSE.

WEISS, STEPHEN JOEL MD, LICENSE NUMBER 00E5985 OF HOUSTON, TX, WAS DISCIPLINED BY TEXAS ON JUNE 22, 1994
DISCIPLINARY ACTION: 60-MONTH PROBATION; REQUIRED TO TAKE ADDITIONAL MEDICAL EDUCATION
OFFENSE: PROFESSIONAL MISCONDUCT

NOTES: ON NUMEROUS PATIENTS BETWEEN 11/88 AND 9/92 HE: FAILED TO ACCURATELY INTERPRET AND RECORD DIAGNOSTIC FINDINGS; FAILED TO FORMULATE OR DOCUMENT APPROPRIATE TREATMENT PLANS OR CLINICAL RATIONALE FOR SUBSEQUENT TESTING; RECOMMENDED SURGICAL INTERVENTION EVEN THOUGH PATIENTS WERE POOR CANDIDATES; ORDERED UNNECESSARY REFERRALS; ORDERED PHYSICAL THERAPY FOR PERIODS OF MORE THAN A YEAR; CONSIDERED CHEMONUCLEOLYSIS AND PERFORMED MULTIPLE IMAGING STUDIES IN SPITE OF THE ABSENCE OF SUFFICIENT OBJECTIVE PHYSICAL FINDINGS, REPRODUCIBLE RADICULOPATHY AND PREVIOUS NEGATIVE TEST RESULTS; ASSESSED CONFLICTING IMPAIRMENT RATINGS; THESE ACTIONS CONSTITUTED FLAGRANT OVERCHARGING AND OVERTREATING

PATIENTS. SUSPENSION STAYED. CONDITIONS OF PROBATION: SHALL OBTAIN A WRITTEN SECOND OPINION ON EACH PATIENT FOR WHOM HE PRESCRIBES PHYSICAL THERAPY BEYOND SIX WEEKS FOR A 12-MONTH PERIOD; ALL DISCOGRAMS HE ORDERS SHALL BE PERFORMED AND READ BY A RADIOLOGIST; SHALL ATTEND AT LEAST 50 HOURS PER YEAR OF CONTINUING MEDICAL EDUCATION ONE-HALF OF WHICH SHALL BE IN THE AREA OF PAIN MANAGEMENT; SHALL MAINTAIN ADEQUATE MEDICAL RECORDS ON ALL PATIENT OFFICE VISITS WHICH SHALL BE AVAILABLE FOR INSPECTION; SHALL NOT SIGN ANY PATIENT RECORD UNLESS HE HAS PERSONALLY EXAMINED THE PATIENT OR CLEARLY NOTES IN THE RECORD THAT HE DID NOT; SHALL GIVE A COPY OF THIS ORDER TO ANY HEALTH CARE ENTITY WHERE HE HAS PRIVILEGES; SHALL COOPERATE WITH THE BOARD IN VERIFYING COMPLIANCE; SHALL INFORM BOARD OF CHANGE OF ADDRESS WITHIN 10 DAYS OR IF HE LEAVES THE STATE; TIME SPENT OUT OF TEXAS DOES NOT COUNT TOWARD PROBATION. SHALL NOT SEEK MODIFICATION FOR ONE YEAR.

WEISS, STEPHEN JOEL MD OF HOUSTON, TX, WAS DISCIPLINED BY LOUISIANA ON MARCH 2, 1995
DISCIPLINARY ACTION: 60-MONTH PROBATION; FINE
OFFENSE: DISCIPLINARY ACTION BY ANOTHER STATE OR AGENCY

NOTES: DISCIPLINARY ACTION BY ANOTHER STATE. PROHIBITION ON PRACTICE IN LOUISIANA DURING PROBATION, PRACTICE THEREAFTER CONDITIONED ON PRIOR NOTICE TO AND APPEARANCE BEFORE BOARD TO VERIFY COMPLIANCE WITH PROBATIONARY TERMS OF TEXAS ORDER AND SUCH ADDITIONAL TERMS AND CONDITIONS AS BOARD MAY DEEM APPROPRIATE; $1,000 FINE.

WEISS, STEPHEN JOEL MD, LICENSE NUMBER 0037217 OF HOUSTON, TX, WAS DISCIPLINED BY OHIO ON FEBRUARY 20, 1996
DISCIPLINARY ACTION: PROBATION; RESTRICTION PLACED ON LICENSE
OFFENSE: DISCIPLINARY ACTION BY ANOTHER STATE OR AGENCY

NOTES: PRIOR ACTION AGAINST HIS TEXAS MEDICAL LICENSE DUE TO HIS FAILURE TO ACCURATELY INTERPRET AND RECORD DIAGNOSTIC FINDINGS; FAILURE TO FORMULATE TREATMENT PLANS OR TESTING; RECOMMENDATIONS OF SURGICAL INTERVENTION ON POOR SURGICAL CANDIDATES AND ORDERING OF UNNECESSARY TREATMENT, CONSULTATIONS AND STUDIES. SIXTY DAY SUSPENSION STAYED TO PROBATIONARY TERMS AND CONDITIONS FOR AT LEAST FIVE YEARS. REQUIRED PROBATIONARY APPEARANCES REDUCED TO EVERY SIX MONTHS ON 12/04/96. ON 3/12/98 REQUEST TO REDUCE REQUIRED CHART REVIEW TO 10% GRANTED.

WEISS, STEPHEN JOEL MD, LICENSE NUMBER 0112493 OF 7333 NORTH FREEWAY SUITE 100, HOUSTON, TX, WAS DISCIPLINED BY NEW YORK ON JULY 30, 1996
DISCIPLINARY ACTION: LICENSE SUSPENSION; 12-MONTH PROBATION
OFFENSE: DISCIPLINARY ACTION BY ANOTHER STATE OR AGENCY

NOTES: ACTION IN TEXAS FOR ORDERING EXCESSIVE TESTS AND/OR TREATMENT NOT WARRANTED BY THE CONDITION OF THE PATIENT; NEGLIGENCE AND INCOMPETENCE ON MORE THAN ONE OCCASION. LICENSE SUSPENSION UNTIL THE SUCCESSFUL COMPLETION OF TEXAS PROBATION TERMS. PROBATION COMMENCING WHEN HE PRACTICES IN NEW YORK.

WEITZEL, ROBERT MD, LICENSE NUMBER H2895 OF SALT LAKE CITY, UT, WAS DISCIPLINED BY TEXAS ON OCTOBER 24, 1998
DISCIPLINARY ACTION: FINE; REPRIMAND
OFFENSE: DISCIPLINARY ACTION BY ANOTHER STATE OR AGENCY

NOTES: IN 1992 AFTER COMPLETING A PSYCHIATRY RESIDENCY IN CALIFORNIA AND TERMINATING HIS PHYSICIAN-PATIENT RELATIONSHIPS WITH ALL PATIENTS, HE RECEIVED A TELEPHONE CALL FROM A FORMER PATIENT WHOM HE HAD TREATED FOR DEPRESSION WHO WISHED TO BECOME INVOLVED IN A PERSONAL RELATIONSHIP WITH HIM; HE ENGAGED IN AN INTIMATE PERSONAL RELATIONSHIP WITHOUT ALLOWING SUFFICIENT TIME TO ELAPSE FROM THE DATE OF THE TERMINATION OF THE PHYSICIAN-PATIENT RELATIONSHIP TO THE ESTABLISHMENT OF THE PERSONAL RELATIONSHIP WHICH LASTED TWO YEARS; THE FORMER PATIENT FILED A LAWSUIT IN CALIFORNIA AGAINST HIM ALLEGING BOUNDARY VIOLATIONS IN THE CONTEXT OF THE PRIOR PHYSICIAN-PATIENT RELATIONSHIP WHICH HE HAS STEADFASTLY DENIED; LAWSUIT RESOLVED FOR WHAT HE CONSIDERED NUISANCE VALUE; HE SUBSEQUENTLY FAILED TO DISCLOSE THE MALPRACTICE SETTLEMENT AS WELL AS CALIFORNIA LICENSURE SURRENDER TO THE TEXAS BOARD, AND SUBMITTED AN INCORRECT RESPONSE TO A RELEVANT QUESTION ON HIS LICENSURE RENEWAL FORM FOR 1997; HAS ADMITTED THAT SUCH CONDUCT WAS IMPROPER; SINCE THE EVENTS WHICH LED TO HIS VOLUNTARY SURRENDER OF HIS CALIFORNIA LICENSE, HE HAS CEASED ENGAGING IN PSYCHOTHERAPY AND PRACTICES PSYCHIATRY WITH A PRIMARY FOCUS ON MEDICATION THERAPY. $3,500 FINE.

WERNER, MARK ALLEN MD, LICENSE NUMBER 00E6682 OF WEBSTER, TX, WAS DISCIPLINED BY TEXAS ON JUNE 10, 1991
DISCIPLINARY ACTION: SURRENDER OF CONTROLLED SUBSTANCE LICENSE
OFFENSE: DISCIPLINARY ACTION BY ANOTHER STATE OR AGENCY

NOTES: DISCIPLINARY ACTION TAKEN BY ANOTHER STATE DUE TO INTEMPERATE USE OF ALCOHOL OR DRUGS, AND UNPROFESSIONAL OR DISHONORABLE CONDUCT LIKELY TO DECEIVE, DEFRAUD, OR INJURE THE PUBLIC. MUST COMPLY WITH TERMS OF NEW MEXICO'S BOARD ORDER. ADDITIONAL TERMS AND CONDITIONS AS FOLLOWS: MUST REFRAIN FROM THE USE OF AND SHALL NOT POSSESS, ADMINISTER, OR PRESCRIBE ANY CONTROLLED SUBSTANCES OR ANY OTHER PRESCRIPTION MEDICATION UNLESS PRESCRIBED BY ANOTHER PHYSICIAN FOR A LEGITIMATE MEDICAL NEED; PRIOR TO PRACTICING IN TEXAS, SHALL RECEIVE BOARD APPROVAL; MUST SURRENDER ALL UNUSED TRIPLICATE PRESCRIPTION FORMS; SHALL NOT ATTEMPT TO ORDER MORE TRIPLICATE PRESCRIPTION FORMS UNTIL WRITTEN PERMISSION IS GRANTED; MUST SURRENDER DPS CONTROLLED SUBSTANCE REGISTRATION CERTIFICATE AND CANCEL DPS REGISTRATION; MUST NOT ATTEMPT TO REREGISTER CONTROLLED SUBSTANCES LICENSES WITHOUT PRIOR WRITTEN AUTHORITY FROM THE BOARD.

WEST, PATRICIA BEATY MD, LICENSE NUMBER 00C8019 OF VERNON, TX, WAS DISCIPLINED BY TEXAS ON AUGUST 24, 1991
DISCIPLINARY ACTION: 6-MONTH LICENSE SUSPENSION
OFFENSE: SUBSTANCE ABUSE

NOTES: INTEMPERATE USE OF ALCOHOL OR DRUGS AND INABILITY TO PRACTICE MEDICINE WITH REASONABLE SKILL AND SAFETY TO PATIENTS BY REASON OF ILLNESS AND DRUNKENNESS.

WESTBROOK, MARK DENTON MD, LICENSE NUMBER 00G3902 OF HOUSTON, TX, WAS DISCIPLINED BY TEXAS ON NOVEMBER 19, 1993
DISCIPLINARY ACTION: 60-MONTH MONITORING OF PHYSICIAN PERFORMANCE
OFFENSE: SUBSTANCE ABUSE

NOTES: HAS SUFFERED FROM ALCOHOLISM AND ABUSE OF HISTUSSIN IN RESPONSE TO HIS WIFE'S DIVING ACCIDENT FOLLOWED SHORTLY BY HIS MOTHER'S DEATH; HAS BEGUN ATTENDANCE AT AA AND HAS SOUGHT INDIVIDUAL AND GROUP PSYCHIATRIC TREATMENT ON HIS OWN INITIATIVE. LICENSE RESTRICTED UNDER THE FOLLOWING CONDITIONS: SHALL ABSTAIN FROM THE CONSUMPTION OF ALCOHOL/CHEMICAL SUBSTANCES IN ANY FORM UNLESS PRESCRIBED BY ANOTHER PHYSICIAN FOR A LEGITIMATE AND THERAPEUTIC PURPOSE; SHALL NOT TREAT OR OTHERWISE SERVE AS PHYSICIAN, PRESCRIBE, DISPENSE OR ADMINISTER DRUGS THAT MAY BE SUBJECT TO ABUSE TO HIMSELF OR ANY MEMBER OF HIS FAMILY; SHALL CONTINUE TO PARTICIPATE IN AA'S PROGRAM NOT LESS THAN THREE TIMES A WEEK WITH QUARTERLY REPORTS TO THE BOARD; SHALL CONTINUE TO PARTICIPATE IN INDIVIDUAL THERAPY AND THE SUNRISE PROGRAM WITH REPORTS TO THE BOARD; SHALL SUBMIT HIMSELF FOR APPROPRIATE EXAMS INCLUDING DRUG OR ALCOHOL SCREENS; SHALL COOPERATE WITH THE BOARD IN VERIFYING COMPLIANCE; SEPARATE FROM PATIENT RECORDS HE SHALL MAINTAIN A FILE OF EVERY PRESCRIPTION WRITTEN FOR DANGEROUS DRUGS WHICH SHALL BE AVAILABLE FOR INSPECTION; SHALL APPEAR BEFORE THE BOARD TWICE A YEAR; SHALL GIVE A COPY OF THIS ORDER TO ANY HEALTH CARE ENTITY WHERE HE HAS PRIVILEGES; SHALL INFORM BOARD OF CHANGE OF ADDRESS WITHIN 10 DAYS OR IF HE LEAVES THE STATE; TIME SPENT OUT OF TEXAS DOES NOT COUNT TOWARD RESTRICTION. SHALL NOT SEEK MODIFICATION FOR ONE YEAR.

WESTBROOK, MARK DENTON MD, LICENSE NUMBER 00G3902 OF HOUSTON, TX, WAS DISCIPLINED BY TEXAS ON AUGUST 19, 1994
DISCIPLINARY ACTION: 120-MONTH PROBATION; RESTRICTION PLACED ON CONTROLLED SUBSTANCE LICENSE
OFFENSE: FAILURE TO COMPLY WITH PREVIOUS BOARD ORDER

NOTES: ENTERED AN AGREED ORDER ON 11/19/93; BETWEEN 12/14/93 AND 1/19/94 HE SUFFERED A RELAPSE AND INGESTED ALCOHOL; SELF-REPORTED HIS RELAPSE ON 1/20/94; SINCE THEN HAS RECEIVED TREATMENT, IS IN INDIVIDUAL AND GROUP THERAPY AND IS UNDER THE CARE OF A PSYCHIATRIST. SUSPENSION STAYED. CONDITIONS OF PROBATION: SHALL ABSTAIN FROM THE CONSUMPTION OF ALCOHOL/CHEMICAL SUBSTANCES IN ANY FORM UNLESS PRESCRIBED BY ANOTHER PHYSICIAN FOR A LEGITIMATE AND THERAPEUTIC PURPOSE; SHALL NOT POSSESS SAMPLES OF DANGEROUS DRUGS WHICH HAVE POTENTIAL FOR ABUSE; SHALL SURRENDER ALL UNUSED TRIPLICATE PRESCRIPTION FORMS; SHALL NOT POSSESS, ADMINISTER DISPENSE OR PRESCRIBE ANY CONTROLLED SUBSTANCES BUT MAY ORDER THEM TO BE ADMINISTERED TO HOSPITAL OR NURSING HOME PATIENTS; SHALL NOT TREAT OR OTHERWISE SERVE AS PHYSICIAN, PRESCRIBE, DISPENSE OR ADMINISTER DRUGS THAT MAY BE SUBJECT TO ABUSE TO HIMSELF OR ANY MEMBER OF HIS FAMILY; SHALL CONTINUE TO PARTICIPATE IN AA'S PROGRAM NOT LESS THAN THREE TIMES A WEEK WITH QUARTERLY REPORTS TO THE BOARD; SHALL SUBMIT HIMSELF FOR APPROPRIATE EXAMS INCLUDING DRUG OR ALCOHOL SCREENS; SEPARATE FROM PATIENT RECORDS SHALL MAINTAIN A FILE CONSISTING OF EVERY PRESCRIPTION WRITTEN FOR DANGEROUS DRUGS WITH A POTENTIAL FOR ABUSE WHICH SHALL BE AVAILABLE FOR INSPECTION; SHALL NOT TELEPHONE ANY PRESCRIPTION TO A PHARMACY FOR DANGEROUS DRUGS; SHALL APPEAR BEFORE THE BOARD TWICE A YEAR; SHALL CONTINUE TO RECEIVE PSYCHIATRIC TREATMENT WITH QUARTERLY REPORTS; SHALL GIVE A COPY OF THIS ORDER TO ANY HEALTH CARE ENTITY WHERE HE HAS PRIVILEGES; SHALL COOPERATE WITH THE BOARD IN VERIFYING COMPLIANCE; SHALL INFORM BOARD OF CHANGE OF ADDRESS WITHIN 10 DAYS OR IF HE LEAVES THE STATE; TIME SPENT OUT OF TEXAS DOES NOT COUNT TOWARD PROBATION. SHALL NOT SEEK MODIFICATION FOR ONE YEAR. ORDER TAKES THE PLACE OF THE ORDER OF 11/19/93. ON 5/15/96 ORDER MODIFIED AS FOLLOWS: REQUIREMENTS THAT HE SURRENDER ALL UNUSED TRIPLICATE PRESCRIPTION FORMS, THAT HE NOT ATTEMPT TO ORDER ANY ADDITIONAL FORMS AND THAT HE NOT POSSESS, ADMINISTER, DISPENSE OR PRESCRIBE ANY CONTROLLED SUBSTANCES, EXCEPT FOR HOSPITALIZED OR NURSING HOME PATIENTS ARE DELETED. ON 4/4/98 ORDER MODIFIED DELETING REQUIREMENT FOR PSYCHIATRIC CARE. ON 1/29/99 ORDER TERMINATED. ON1/29/99 ORDER TERMINATED.

WHEELER, JAMES M MD, LICENSE NUMBER 00G3903, WAS DISCIPLINED BY TEXAS ON AUGUST 17, 1996
DISCIPLINARY ACTION: 36-MONTH RESTRICTION PLACED ON LICENSE; REQUIRED TO TAKE ADDITIONAL MEDICAL EDUCATION
OFFENSE: SEXUAL ABUSE OF OR SEXUAL MISCONDUCT WITH A PATIENT

NOTES: WITHOUT PROPER TERMINATION OF THE PHYSICIAN-PATIENT RELATIONSHIP ENGAGED IN A SOCIAL RELATIONSHIP WITH A PATIENT, WHICH INCLUDED SEXUALLY INTIMATE CONTACT OUTSIDE THE OFFICE; IN 7/93 CEASED PERFORMING ANY TYPE OF PHYSICAL EXAM ALTHOUGH HE CONTINUED TO SEE PATIENT IN HIS OFFICE UNTIL EARLY 1994; HE MAINTAINS THAT ON SEVERAL OCCASIONS HE ATTEMPTED TO TRANSFER THE PATIENT'S CARE TO ANOTHER PHYSICIAN, BUT WAS UNABLE TO DO SO COMPLETELY UNTIL EARLY 1994; HAS UNDERGONE THERAPY SINCE THIS EVENT. RESTRICTED UNDER CONDITIONS FOR THREE YEARS; SHALL MAINTAIN HIS CURRENT PRACTICE OF HAVING A CHAPERONE PRESENT IN THE ROOM DURING THE EXAMINATION OF A FEMALE PATIENT AND SHALL MAKE NOTATION ON THE PATIENT'S CHART INDICATING THE CHAPERONE WAS PRESENT; SHALL MAINTAIN ADEQUATE MEDICAL RECORDS WHICH SHALL BE AVAILABLE TO THE BOARD; SHALL OBTAIN AT LEAST 50 HOURS OF CONTINUING MEDICAL EDUCATION AND SHALL SUBMIT PROOF TO THE BOARD; WITHIN ONE YEAR SHALL OBTAIN 10 HOURS OF ETHICS THROUGH BOARD APPROVED COURSES OR PROGRAMS AND SUBMIT PROOF TO THE BOARD; WITHIN ONE YEAR SHALL TAKE AND PASS THE MEDICAL JURISPRUDENCE EXAMINATION AND PROVIDE PROOF TO THE BOARD; SHALL APPEAR BEFORE THE BOARD AT LEAST ONCE PER YEAR OR UPON BOARD REQUEST; SHALL COOPERATE WITH THE BOARD IN VERIFYING COMPLIANCE INCLUDING PROVIDING COPIES OF MEDICAL RELEASES UPON REQUEST; SHALL GIVE A COPY OF THIS ORDER TO ANY HEALTH CARE ENTITY WHERE HE HAS PRIVILEGES; SHALL PROVIDE A COPY OF THIS ORDER TO ANYONE REQUESTING IT WITHIN 10 DAYS; TIME PERIOD OUT OF TEXAS DOES NOT COUNT TOWARD RESTRICTION; SHALL INFORM THE BOARD OF CHANGE OF ADDRESS WITHIN 10 DAYS OF

IF HE LEAVES THE STATE; SHALL NOT SEEK MODIFICATION FOR ONE YEAR. ON 2/7/98 ORDER TERMINATED.

WHITAKER, JOHN F MD, LICENSE NUMBER C26847 OF DALLAS, TX, WAS DISCIPLINED BY CALIFORNIA ON JULY 7, 1999
DISCIPLINARY ACTION: REPRIMAND
OFFENSE: DISCIPLINARY ACTION BY ANOTHER STATE OR AGENCY

NOTES: VOLUNTARILY SURRENDERED HIS TEXAS MEDICAL LICENSE WHILE AN INVESTIGATION WAS PENDING.

WHITAKER, JOHN FREDRIC MD, LICENSE NUMBER D0347 OF DALLAS, TX, WAS DISCIPLINED BY TEXAS ON AUGUST 9, 1997
DISCIPLINARY ACTION: SURRENDER OF LICENSE

NOTES: VOLUNTARY AND PERMANENT SURRENDER IN LIEU OF FURTHER PROCEEDINGS.

WHITE, DEZRA MD, LICENSE NUMBER D5247, WAS DISCIPLINED BY TEXAS ON JANUARY 18, 1997
DISCIPLINARY ACTION: FINE; REPRIMAND
OFFENSE: SUBSTANDARD CARE, INCOMPETENCE OR NEGLIGENCE

NOTES: IN 12/90, HE BEGAN TREATMENT OF A PATIENT PREGNANT WITH TWINS. HE FOLLOWED THIS PATIENT AND PROVIDED CARE UNTIL 5/91, WHEN THE PATIENT SUFFERED ECLAMPSIA RESULTING IN THE FETAL DEMISE OF THE TWINS. PRIOR TO THIS EVENT, THE PATIENT HAD NOT INFORMED HIM OF ANY PREECLAMPTIC SYMPTOMS. THE PATIENT ALSO SUFFERED PERMANENT NEUROLOGICAL DEFICITS AND RESIDUAL BRAIN DAMAGE. HE ALTERED HER MEDICAL RECORDS TO CHANGE PATIENT BLOOD PRESSURE READINGS. A RELATED MALPRACTICE SUIT RESULTED IN DAMAGES IN FAVOR OF THE PATIENT OF $900,000. HE IS ASSESSED AN ADMINISTRATIVE PENALTY OF $10,000; SHALL OBTAIN 10 HOURS OF ETHICS THROUGH APPROVED COURSES WITHIN 6 MONTHS; SHALL GIVE A COPY OF THIS ORDER TO ANY HEALTH CARE ENTITY WHERE HE HAS PRIVILEGES; SHALL PROVIDE A COPY OF THIS ORDER TO ANYONE REQUESTING IT WITHIN 10 DAYS; SHALL COOPERATE WITH THE BOARD IN VERIFYING COMPLIANCE.

WHITE, JAMES HARRISON MD, LICENSE NUMBER C030449 OF NEWPORT BEACH, CA, WAS DISCIPLINED BY CALIFORNIA ON MAY 6, 1991
DISCIPLINARY ACTION: LICENSE REVOCATION
OFFENSE: CRIMINAL CONVICTION OR PLEA OF GUILTY, NOLO CONTENDERE, OR NO CONTEST TO A CRIME

NOTES: ACTION BASED ON CRIMINAL CONVICTION FOR ORAL COPULATION ON AN UNCONSCIOUS VICTIM AND FOR FAILURE TO APPEAR WHILE ON BAIL. DEFAULT DECISION.

WHITE, JAMES HARRISON MD, DATE OF BIRTH FEBRUARY 19, 1943 OF CA DEPT OF CORR POBOX 608 UNIT 2, TAHACHAPI, CA, WAS DISCIPLINED BY MEDICARE ON NOVEMBER 4, 1991
DISCIPLINARY ACTION: 240-MONTH EXCLUSION FROM THE MEDICARE AND/OR MEDICAID PROGRAM
OFFENSE: CRIMINAL CONVICTION OR PLEA OF GUILTY, NOLO CONTENDERE, OR NO CONTEST TO A CRIME

NOTES: CONVICTION FOR PATIENT ABUSE OR NEGLECT.

WHITE, JAMES HARRISON \ MD, LICENSE NUMBER 00D4357 OF CORONA DEL MAR, CA, WAS DISCIPLINED BY TEXAS ON NOVEMBER 13, 1992
DISCIPLINARY ACTION: LICENSE REVOCATION
OFFENSE: CRIMINAL CONVICTION OR PLEA OF GUILTY, NOLO CONTENDERE, OR NO CONTEST TO A CRIME

NOTES: CONVICTION OF FELONY INVOLVING MORAL TURPITUDE.

WHITELOCK, PAUL MD, LICENSE NUMBER D7364 OF DURANGO, CO, WAS DISCIPLINED BY TEXAS ON AUGUST 9, 1997
DISCIPLINARY ACTION: FINE; REPRIMAND
OFFENSE: NONCOMPLIANCE WITH A PROFESSIONAL RULE

NOTES: VIOLATION OF BOARD RULES RELATING TO MANDATORY COMPLETION AND REPORTING OF CONTINUING MEDICAL EDUCATION. $100 FINE.

WHITMAN, PAUL F JR MD OF 1000 N COCKRELL HILL ROAD, DESOTO, TX, WAS DISCIPLINED BY DEA ON AUGUST 10, 1993
DISCIPLINARY ACTION: SURRENDER OF CONTROLLED SUBSTANCE LICENSE
OFFENSE: SUBSTANCE ABUSE

NOTES: ADMITTED SELF ABUSE OF FENTANYL FROM HOSPITAL PHARMACY STOCKS.

WHITMAN, PAUL F JR MD, LICENSE NUMBER 00G8506 OF DESOTO, TX, WAS DISCIPLINED BY TEXAS ON JANUARY 14, 1994
DISCIPLINARY ACTION: 60-MONTH PROBATION; RESTRICTION PLACED ON LICENSE
OFFENSE: SUBSTANCE ABUSE

NOTES: PRIOR TO 7/7/93 ON NUMEROUS OCCASIONS DIVERTED FENTANYL FROM THE OPERATING ROOM WHERE HE SERVED AS AN ANESTHESIOLOGIST WHICH HE ADMINISTERED TO HIMSELF; AFTER INTERVENTION BY A HOSPITAL PHARMACIST HE VOLUNTARILY SURRENDERED HIS CONTROLLED SUBSTANCES CERTIFICATES; COMPLETED TREATMENT ON 11/6/93. SUSPENSION STAYED. CONDITIONS OF PROBATION: SHALL ABSTAIN FROM THE CONSUMPTION OF ALCOHOL/CHEMICAL SUBSTANCES IN ANY FORM UNLESS PRESCRIBED BY ANOTHER PHYSICIAN FOR A LEGITIMATE AND THERAPEUTIC PURPOSE; SHALL SUBMIT HIMSELF FOR APPROPRIATE EXAMS INCLUDING DRUG OR ALCOHOL SCREENS; SHALL LIMIT PRACTICE SOLELY TO THE PRACTICE OF ANESTHESIOLOGY IN A HOSPITAL SETTING; SHALL NOT POSSESS, ADMINISTER, DISPENSE OR PRESCRIBE ANY DANGEROUS DRUGS EXCEPT AS MEDICALLY NECESSARY FOR TREATMENT OF INPATIENTS; SHALL BE UNDER THE OBSERVATION OF A PHYSICIAN OR NURSE WHILE ADMINISTERING OR SUPERVISING THE ADMINISTRATION OF ANESTHESIA; SHALL CONTINUE TO RECEIVE TREATMENT FROM PSYCHIATRIST WITH QUARTERLY REPORTS; SHALL PARTICIPATE IN ACTIVITIES OF A PHYSICIAN HEALTH AND REHABILITATION COMMITTEE AND ATTEND WEEKLY MEETINGS WITH QUARTERLY REPORTS; SHALL ATTEND AT LEAST 50 HOURS PER YEAR OF CONTINUING MEDICAL EDUCATION; SHALL GIVE A COPY OF THIS ORDER TO ANY HEALTH CARE ENTITY WHERE HE HAS PRIVILEGES; SHALL COOPERATE WITH THE BOARD IN VERIFYING COMPLIANCE; SHALL INFORM BOARD OF CHANGE OF ADDRESS WITHIN 10 DAYS OR IF HE LEAVES THE STATE; TIME SPENT OUT OF TEXAS DOES NOT COUNT TOWARD PROBATION; SHALL APPEAR BEFORE THE BOARD ONCE A YEAR. SHALL NOT SEEK MODIFICATION FOR ONE YEAR. ON 11/3/94 ORDER MODIFIED AS FOLLOWS; LIMITATION OF PRACTICE OF ANESTHESIOLOGY TO A HOSPITAL SETTING AND TO PRESCRIBING CONTROLLED SUBSTANCES ONLY IN THAT SETTING MODIFIED TO ALLOW HIM TO PRACTICE PAIN MANAGEMENT IN A GROUP SETTING AND TO PRESCRIBE IN THIS SETTING; REQUIREMENT THAT HE BE OBSERVED

WHILE ADMINISTERING OR SUPERVISING THE ADMINISTRATION OF ANESTHESIA IS DROPPED; CONDITION ADDED THAT HE MAINTAIN A FILE OF PRESCRIPTIONS WRITTEN FOR CONTROLLED SUBSTANCES OR DANGEROUS DRUGS WHICH SHALL BE AVAILABLE FOR INSPECTION.

WHITNEY, RICHARD N MD, LICENSE NUMBER 00G1802 OF PLANO, TX, WAS DISCIPLINED BY TEXAS ON DECEMBER 3, 1990
DISCIPLINARY ACTION: 60-MONTH PROBATION; MONITORING OF PHYSICIAN PERFORMANCE

NOTES: MUST ATTEND AA MEETINGS ON A REGULAR BASIS; SUBMIT FOR APPROPRIATE EXAMINATIONS TO DETERMINE FREEDOM FROM DRUGS AND ALCOHOL; CONTINUE MONITORING BY SMITH COUNTY COMMITTEE FOR IMPAIRED PHYSICIANS; ABIDE BY CONTRACT WITH TALBOT RECOVERY SYSTEM; APPEAR BEFORE BOARD ONCE A YEAR.

WHITNEY, RICHARD N MD, LICENSE NUMBER 00C8175 OF 1708 E JOYCE ST, FAYETTEVILLE, AR, WAS DISCIPLINED BY ARKANSAS ON SEPTEMBER 23, 1995
DISCIPLINARY ACTION: 12-MONTH PROBATION; FINE
OFFENSE: OVERCHARGING

NOTES: FLAGRANT AND PERSISTENT OVER-CHARGING AND OVER-TREATING OF PATIENTS. $1,000 FINE PLUS BOARD EXPENSES OF $187.18, WITH ADDITIONAL RESTRICTIONS.

WHITTAKER, JOHN NORMAN MD, LICENSE NUMBER 00F1305 OF DE SOTO, TX, WAS DISCIPLINED BY TEXAS ON JANUARY 24, 1992
DISCIPLINARY ACTION: 24-MONTH RESTRICTION PLACED ON LICENSE; REPRIMAND
OFFENSE: PROFESSIONAL MISCONDUCT

NOTES: OVERTREATING OF PATIENTS.

WICOFF, JAMES S MD, DATE OF BIRTH APRIL 26, 1947 OF 2020 BABCOCK ROAD SUITE 29, SAN ANTONIO, TX, WAS DISCIPLINED BY MEDICARE ON DECEMBER 30, 1996
DISCIPLINARY ACTION: 36-MONTH EXCLUSION FROM THE MEDICARE AND/OR MEDICAID PROGRAM
OFFENSE: DISCIPLINARY ACTION BY ANOTHER STATE OR AGENCY

NOTES: SUSPENDED OR EXCLUDED BY A FEDERAL OR STATE HEALTH CARE PROGRAM FOR REASONS BEARING ON PROFESSIONAL PERFORMANCE.

WIGG, CINDY LOU MD, LICENSE NUMBER 00G7430, WAS DISCIPLINED BY TEXAS ON NOVEMBER 16, 1996
DISCIPLINARY ACTION: FINE
OFFENSE: SUBSTANDARD CARE, INCOMPETENCE OR NEGLIGENCE

NOTES: FROM 10/93 TO 12/93, SHE PRESCRIBED FOUR PRESCRIPTIONS FOR RITALIN, A SCHEDULE II CONTROLLED SUBSTANCE, TO A PATIENT SHE NEVER PHYSICALLY EXAMINED OR EVALUATED; SHE RELIED UPON THE HISTORY AS GIVEN BY THE PATIENT'S WIFE TO MAKE HER DIAGNOSIS OF ATTENTION DEFICIT HYPERACTIVITY DISORDER; SHE CONTENDS THAT SHE PRESCRIBED RITALIN IN ORDER TO FACILITATE THE PATIENT'S TREATMENT. SHALL PAY $2,000 FINE; SHALL GIVE A COPY OF THIS ORDER TO ANY HEALTH CARE ENTITY WHERE SHE HAS PRIVILEGES.

WILCOX, JAMES A DO OF EL PASO, TX, WAS DISCIPLINED BY IOWA ON JULY 1, 1996
DISCIPLINARY ACTION: SURRENDER OF LICENSE; FINE
OFFENSE: PROFESSIONAL MISCONDUCT

NOTES: ACCUSED OF HAVING A SEXUAL RELATIONSHIP WITH A FORMER PATIENT IN VIOLATION OF IOWA LAW AND PROFESSIONAL ETHICAL STANDARDS. PUBLIC LETTER OF WARNING AND REPRIMAND. $10,000 CIVIL PENALTY BEFORE SEEKING REINSTATEMENT OF HIS LICENSE.

WILCOX, JAMES A DO, LICENSE NUMBER H7253, WAS DISCIPLINED BY TEXAS ON MAY 10, 1997
DISCIPLINARY ACTION: REPRIMAND; REQUIRED TO TAKE ADDITIONAL MEDICAL EDUCATION
OFFENSE: DISCIPLINARY ACTION BY ANOTHER STATE OR AGENCY

NOTES: ON 4/4/96 A LETTER OF REPRIMAND FROM THE IOWA BOARD WAS ISSUED STATING THAT HE ENTERED INTO AN INTIMATE RELATIONSHIP WITH A FORMER PSYCHIATRIC PATIENT ONE MONTH AFTER TERMINATING PROFESSIONAL TREATMENT. THERE HAVE NEVER BEEN ANY ALLEGATIONS OR CLAIMS MADE AGAINST HIM OF IMPROPRIETIES DURING HIS PROFESSIONAL RELATIONSHIP WITH THE PATIENT. HE SURRENDERED HIS IOWA LICENSE EFFECTIVE 7/1/96; PRIOR TO FILING A PETITION SEEKING REINSTATEMENT OF HIS IOWA LICENSE, HE WILL HAVE TO PAY A CIVIL PENALTY OF $10,000. ON 3/27/96 AN ORDER WAS ENTERED BY THE IOWA DISTRICT COURT FINDING HIM IN VIOLATION OF IOWA CODE; AN APPEAL OF THIS ORDER IS PENDING. WITHIN SIX MONTHS SHALL PASS THE MEDICAL JURISPRUDENCE EXAM AND SHALL SUCCESSFULLY COMPLETE AN APPROVED COURSE IN ETHICS; SHALL COOPERATE WITH THE BOARD IN VERIFYING COMPLIANCE; SHALL APPEAR BEFORE THE BOARD UPON REQUEST; SHALL GIVE A COPY OF THIS ORDER TO ANY HEALTH CARE ENTITY WHERE HE HAS PRIVILEGES; TIME SPENT OUT OF TEXAS DOES NOT COUNT TOWARD RESTRICTION; SHALL INFORM THE BOARD OF CHANGE OF ADDRESS WITHIN 10 DAYS OR IF HE LEAVES THE STATE; SHALL NOT SEEK MODIFICATION FOR ONE YEAR.

WILCOX, JAMES ALLEN DO OF 505 EAST COLLEGE STREET, IOWA CITY, IA, WAS DISCIPLINED BY DEA ON DECEMBER 2, 1996
DISCIPLINARY ACTION: SURRENDER OF CONTROLLED SUBSTANCE LICENSE

NOTES: IN LIEU OF PUBLIC INTEREST REVOCATION.

WILCOX, LOUISE NELLIE MD, LICENSE NUMBER 00G1252 OF HOUSTON, TX, WAS DISCIPLINED BY TEXAS ON JUNE 17, 1992
DISCIPLINARY ACTION: REPRIMAND
OFFENSE: PROFESSIONAL MISCONDUCT

NOTES: INVOLVED IN THE CORPORATE PRACTICE OF MEDICINE.

WILKERSON, ROBERT GRAY JR MD OF 1305 GLOURIE, HOUSTON, TX, WAS DISCIPLINED BY DEA ON JUNE 5, 1996
DISCIPLINARY ACTION: RESTRICTION PLACED ON CONTROLLED SUBSTANCE LICENSE

NOTES: IN LIEU OF PUBLIC INTEREST REVOCATION.

WILKERSON, WILLIAM GEORGE MD, DATE OF BIRTH JANUARY 26, 1932, LICENSE NUMBER 00E0215 OF 1121 ELLIS AVENUE, LUFKIN, TX, WAS DISCIPLINED BY TEXAS ON MARCH 26, 1993
DISCIPLINARY ACTION: SURRENDER OF LICENSE

NOTES: LICENSE PERMANENTLY SURRENDERED IN LIEU OF FURTHER DISCIPLINARY ACTION; DOCTOR RETIRED FROM PRACTICE.

WILLIAMS, ALFRED VAUGHN MD, DATE OF BIRTH NOVEMBER 14, 1940, LICENSE NUMBER 00D4361 OF 4402 VANCE JACKSON, SUITE

100, SAN ANTONIO, TX, WAS DISCIPLINED BY TEXAS ON MAY 24, 1990
DISCIPLINARY ACTION: PROBATION; 60-MONTH MONITORING OF PHYSICIAN PERFORMANCE

NOTES: STIPULATED ORDER. MUST SUBMIT HIMSELF FOR PSYCHIATRIC EVALUATION AND FOLLOW ANY RECOMMENDATIONS REGARDING CARE, SUBMIT HIMSELF FOR APPROPRIATE EXAMINATIONS TO DETERMINE FREEDOM FROM DRUGS AND ALCOHOL, AND MAINTAIN SEPARATE FILE OF PRESCRIPTIONS WRITTEN FOR CONTROLLED SUBSTANCES. ON 8/20/93 BOARD MODIFIED ORDER GRANTING HIM PERMISSION TO REAPPLY TO THE DRUG ENFORCEMENT ADMINISTRATION AND TEXAS DEPARTMENT OF PUBLIC SAFETY FOR SCHEDULES II AND IIN CONTROLLED SUBSTANCES. SHOULD HE BE GRANTED THESE APPLICATIONS SCHEDULE II AND IIN ARE LIMITED TO HOSPITAL PATIENTS ONLY. ALL OTHER TERMS OF THIS ORDER REMAIN IN EFFECT.

WILLIAMS, ALFRED VAUGHN MD OF 4402 VANCE JACKSON, SAN ANTONIO, TX, WAS DISCIPLINED BY DEA ON AUGUST 24, 1990
DISCIPLINARY ACTION: RESTRICTION PLACED ON CONTROLLED SUBSTANCE LICENSE
OFFENSE: SUBSTANCE ABUSE

NOTES: PERSONAL USE OF DILAUDID.

WILLIAMS, ALFRED VAUGHN MD, LICENSE NUMBER D4361 OF SAN ANTONIO, TX, WAS DISCIPLINED BY TEXAS ON APRIL 4, 1998
DISCIPLINARY ACTION: SURRENDER OF LICENSE
OFFENSE: CRIMINAL CONVICTION OR PLEA OF GUILTY, NOLO CONTENDERE, OR NO CONTEST TO A CRIME

NOTES: ON 1/10/97 HE PLEADED GUILTY IN FEDERAL COURT TO BRIBERY OF AN IRS AGENT; IN 1990 THE BOARD PLACED HIM ON 5 YEARS PROBATION FOR ABUSING DILAUDID. VOLUNTARY AND PERMANENT SURRENDER.

WILLIAMS, ALFRED VAUGHN MD, DATE OF BIRTH NOVEMBER 14, 1940 OF 4402 VANCE JACKSON RD SUITE 100, SAN ANTONIO, TX, WAS DISCIPLINED BY MEDICARE ON DECEMBER 20, 1998
DISCIPLINARY ACTION: EXCLUSION FROM THE MEDICARE AND/OR MEDICAID PROGRAM
OFFENSE: DISCIPLINARY ACTION BY ANOTHER STATE OR AGENCY

NOTES: LICENSE REVOKED, SUSPENDED, SURRENDERED OR OTHERWISE LOST FOR REASONS BEARING ON PROFESSIONAL PERFORMANCE, PROFESSIONAL COMPETENCE OR FINANCIAL INTEGRITY.

WILLIAMS, AUBREY DUDLEY DO, LICENSE NUMBER 00D0756 OF PARKVILLE, MO, WAS DISCIPLINED BY TEXAS ON JUNE 10, 1991
DISCIPLINARY ACTION: SURRENDER OF LICENSE
OFFENSE: DISCIPLINARY ACTION BY ANOTHER STATE OR AGENCY

NOTES: DISCIPLINARY ACTION TAKEN BY ANOTHER STATE DUE TO UNPROFESSIONAL CONDUCT.

WILLIAMS, BARNEY KENNETH JR MD, LICENSE NUMBER 00C3911, WAS DISCIPLINED BY TEXAS ON AUGUST 20, 1993
DISCIPLINARY ACTION: 60-MONTH PROBATION; REQUIRED TO TAKE ADDITIONAL MEDICAL EDUCATION
OFFENSE: LOSS OR RESTRICTION OF HOSPITAL PRIVILEGES

NOTES: IN 1991 ENTERED INTO AN AGREEMENT WITH SID PETERSON MEMORIAL HOSPITAL FOR MEDICAL STAFF PRIVILEGES WHICH REQUIRED HIM TO BE MONITORED AND SCREENED FOR ALCOHOL CONSUMPTION; IN 11/92 RELAPSED WHILE ALONE ON A FISHING TRIP; HOSPITAL SUSPENDED PRIVILEGES ON 11/25/92 AND HE WAS REINSTATED ON 12/30/92 WITH A TWO YEAR SCREENING AND MONITORING CONTRACT. FIVE YEAR SUSPENSION STAYED. CONDITIONS OF PROBATION: SHALL ATTEND AT LEAST 50 HOURS PER YEAR OF CONTINUING MEDICAL EDUCATION; SHALL ABSTAIN FROM THE CONSUMPTION OF ALCOHOL/CHEMICAL SUBSTANCES IN ANY FORM; SHALL PARTICIPATE IN ACTIVITIES OF A PHYSICIAN HEALTH AND REHABILITATION COMMITTEE AND ATTEND WEEKLY MEETINGS WITH QUARTERLY REPORTS; SHALL PARTICIPATE IN AA NOT LESS THAN THREE TIMES A WEEK WITH QUARTERLY REPORTS; SHALL SUBMIT HIMSELF FOR APPROPRIATE EXAMS INCLUDING DRUG OR ALCOHOL SCREENS; SHALL APPEAR BEFORE THE BOARD ONCE A YEAR; SHALL NOT TREAT OR OTHERWISE SERVE AS PHYSICIAN, PRESCRIBE, DISPENSE OR ADMINISTER DRUGS THAT MAY BE SUBJECT TO ABUSE FOR HIMSELF OR ANY MEMBER OF HIS FAMILY; SHALL ABIDE BY THE TERMS OF HIS TWO YEAR CONTRACT WITH SID PETERSON MEMORIAL HOSPITAL; SHALL COOPERATE WITH THE BOARD IN VERIFYING COMPLIANCE; SHALL INFORM BOARD OF CHANGE OF ADDRESS WITHIN 1O DAYS OR IF HE LEAVES THE STATE; TIME SPENT OUT OF TEXAS DOES NOT COUNT TOWARD PROBATION. MAY NOT SEEK MODIFICATION FOR ONE YEAR. ON 9/30/94 BOARD DENIED A REQUEST TO TERMINATE PROBATION.

WILLIAMS, CONRAD R MD, WAS DISCIPLINED BY NEBRASKA ON AUGUST 13, 1999
DISCIPLINARY ACTION: 6-MONTH LICENSE SUSPENSION; RESTRICTION PLACED ON LICENSE
OFFENSE: PROFESSIONAL MISCONDUCT

NOTES: DISHONORABLE, UNPROFESSIONAL CONDUCT.

WILLIAMS, CONRAD REX MD, LICENSE NUMBER 00C7512 OF COLORADO SPRINGS, CO, WAS DISCIPLINED BY TEXAS ON MARCH 31, 1990
DISCIPLINARY ACTION: SURRENDER OF LICENSE

NOTES: STIPULATED ORDER.

WILLIAMS, CONRAD ROBERT MD, DATE OF BIRTH JANUARY 28, 1949, LICENSE NUMBER 0038690 OF 1115 RIVINGTON STREET, ROSELLE, NJ, WAS DISCIPLINED BY NEW JERSEY ON MARCH 8, 1990
DISCIPLINARY ACTION: SURRENDER OF LICENSE
OFFENSE: OVERPRESCRIBING OR MISPRESCRIBING DRUGS

NOTES: ACTION BASED ON QUESTIONABLE CONTROLLED DANGEROUS SUBSTANCE PRESCRIBING. SHALL NOT REAPPLY.

WILLIAMS, CONRAD ROBERT MD OF 44 ROOSEVELT AVE PO BOX 398, CARTERET, NJ, WAS DISCIPLINED BY DEA ON MAY 14, 1990
DISCIPLINARY ACTION: SURRENDER OF CONTROLLED SUBSTANCE LICENSE
OFFENSE: DISCIPLINARY ACTION BY ANOTHER STATE OR AGENCY

NOTES: LICENSE TO PRACTICE MEDICINE AND SURGERY IN NEW JERSEY PERMANENTLY SURRENDERED.

WILLIAMS, DEBRA N MD, LICENSE NUMBER 00F2116 OF BEAUMONT, TX, WAS DISCIPLINED BY TEXAS ON JANUARY 26, 1990
DISCIPLINARY ACTION: 60-MONTH PROBATION; RESTRICTION PLACED ON CONTROLLED SUBSTANCE LICENSE

NOTES: STIPULATED ORDER. REVOCATION STAYED. MUST REFRAIN FROM ACCEPTING CERTAIN EMPLOYMENT OR ENTERING INTO CONTRACTUAL RELATIONSHIPS, REFRAIN FROM ISSUING PRESCRIPTIONS, ADMINISTERING OR DISPENSING DRUGS TO PATIENTS

UNLESS THERAPEUTIC, MUST NOT PRESCRIBE, ADMINISTER, OR DISPENSE DRUGS WITH ABUSE POTENTIAL UNTIL SATISFIED OF LEGITIMATE MEDICAL AND THERAPEUTIC NEED AND AFTER EXAMINATION, MUST MAINTAIN COMPLETE AND ACCURATE RECORDS OF PURCHASES AND DISPOSALS OF CONTROLLED SUBSTANCES AND MAINTAIN SEPARATE FILE OF COPIES OF PRESCRIPTIONS FOR CONTROLLED SUBSTANCES OR DANGEROUS DRUGS, MUST NOT CALL IN CONTROLLED SUBSTANCES OR DANGEROUS DRUG PRESCRIPTIONS TO PHARMACIES AND MUST COMPLETE PRECEPTORSHIP ON PREVENTION AND TREATMENT OF DRUG ABUSE.

WILLIAMS, HARVEY E DO, DATE OF BIRTH APRIL 5, 1945, LICENSE NUMBER 0001258, WAS DISCIPLINED BY ARIZONA ON JANUARY 6, 1992
OFFENSE: PROFESSIONAL MISCONDUCT
NOTES: ADVERTISED IN A FALSE, DECEPTIVE, OR MISLEADING MANNER IN THAT A 100% GUARANTEE IN HIS ADVERTISEMENT OF 4/24/91 REGARDING BREAST AUGMENTATION WAS NOT EVER MEANT TO BE 100% MONEY BACK. CENSURED.

WILLIAMS, HARVEY E DO, DATE OF BIRTH APRIL 5, 1945, LICENSE NUMBER 0001258, WAS DISCIPLINED BY ARIZONA ON JULY 25, 1992
DISCIPLINARY ACTION: RESTRICTION PLACED ON LICENSE; REPRIMAND
OFFENSE: SUBSTANDARD CARE, INCOMPETENCE OR NEGLIGENCE
NOTES: SIX COMPLAINTS CONCERNING HIS INABILITY TO APPROPRIATELY PERFORM COSMETIC SURGERY PROCEDURES ON THE BREASTS OF FEMALE PATIENTS. PERMANENTLY RESTRICTED FROM PERFORMING ANY BREAST SURGERY MEANING ALL BREAST IMPLANTS, LIFTS, RECONSTRUCTION, OR OTHER SURGERIES RELATED TO THE BREAST AND PERFORMED EITHER ENTIRELY OR PARTIALLY FOR COSMETIC PURPOSES.

WILLIAMS, HARVEY E DO, DATE OF BIRTH APRIL 5, 1945, LICENSE NUMBER 00E5643 OF PO BOX 5673, SCOTTSDALE, AZ, WAS DISCIPLINED BY TEXAS ON JANUARY 29, 1993
DISCIPLINARY ACTION: RESTRICTION PLACED ON LICENSE
OFFENSE: DISCIPLINARY ACTION BY ANOTHER STATE OR AGENCY
NOTES: ON 7/25/92 ARIZONA BOARD RESTRICTED HIM FROM PERFORMING ANY BREAST SURGERY DEFINED AS ALL BREAST IMPLANTS, LIFTS, RECONSTRUCTION, OR OTHER SURGERIES RELATED TO THE BREAST AND PERFORMED EITHER ENTIRELY OR PARTIALLY FOR COSMETIC PURPOSES BASED ON HIS INABILITY TO APPROPRIATELY PERFORM SUCH SURGERY BASED ON SIX COMPLAINTS. HE IS PERMANENTLY RESTRICTED FROM PERFORMING SUCH SURGERY IN TEXAS; PRIOR TO PRACTICING IN TEXAS SHALL APPEAR BEFORE THE BOARD. SHALL NOT SEEK MODIFICATION FOR ONE YEAR.

WILLIAMS, HARVEY E D0, DATE OF BIRTH APRIL 5, 1945, LICENSE NUMBER 0001258, WAS DISCIPLINED BY ARIZONA ON MAY 12, 1993
DISCIPLINARY ACTION: PROBATION; REPRIMAND
OFFENSE: SUBSTANDARD CARE, INCOMPETENCE OR NEGLIGENCE
NOTES: ON 3/29/89 PERFORMED A BREAST IMPLANT PROCEDURE; FAILED TO MAINTAIN ADEQUATE RECORDS ON THE PATIENT; ON 8/5/89 A BACTERIAL CULTURE WAS OBTAINED WHICH WAS NOTED IN RECORDS; ALTHOUGH HE SHOULD HAVE BEEN AWARE OF IT, IMPLANT WAS NOT REMOVED UNTIL 4/24/90. MINIMUM TWO YEAR PROBATION UNDER TERMS AND CONDITIONS: SHALL COMPLETE A MINIMUM OF 10 HOURS OF BOARD APPROVED CONTINUING MEDICAL EDUCATION IN THE AREA OF RECORD KEEPING WITHIN ONE YEAR; SHALL MAKE HIS RECORDS OPEN FOR INSPECTION BY THE BOARD; SHALL MEET WITH THE BOARD UPON REQUEST TO REVIEW COMPLIANCE WITH THIS ORDER. ON 3/10/95 PROBATION SATISFIED IN FULL.

WILLIAMS, HARVEY E DO, DATE OF BIRTH APRIL 5, 1945, LICENSE NUMBER 00E5643 OF SCOTTSDALE, AZ, WAS DISCIPLINED BY TEXAS ON SEPTEMBER 30, 1994
DISCIPLINARY ACTION: SURRENDER OF LICENSE
OFFENSE: NONCOMPLIANCE WITH A PROFESSIONAL RULE
NOTES: ALLEGATIONS CONCERNING POSSIBLE VIOLATIONS OF THE MEDICAL PRACTICE ACT; DID NOT ADMIT ALLEGATIONS. SURRENDER IN LIEU OF FURTHER INVESTIGATION. SHALL NOT PETITION FOR REINSTATEMENT OF LICENSE.

WILLIAMS, HARVEY E DO, LICENSE NUMBER 20A3800 OF TUCSON, AZ, WAS DISCIPLINED BY CALIFORNIA ON MAY 13, 1996
DISCIPLINARY ACTION: LICENSE REVOCATION
OFFENSE: DISCIPLINARY ACTION BY ANOTHER STATE OR AGENCY
NOTES: ACTION IN ARIZONA FOR UNPROFESSIONAL CONDUCT.

WILLIAMS, PHILLIP EARLE JR MD, LICENSE NUMBER 00D2172 OF DALLAS, TX, WAS DISCIPLINED BY TEXAS ON APRIL 26, 1994
DISCIPLINARY ACTION: RESTRICTION PLACED ON LICENSE; REPRIMAND
OFFENSE: LOSS OR RESTRICTION OF HOSPITAL PRIVILEGES
NOTES: WAS THE SUBJECT OF DISCIPLINARY PROCEEDINGS AT A HOSPITAL WHICH RESULTED IN AN AGREEMENT THAT HIS PRACTICE BE RESTRICTED TO CERTAIN PROCEDURES THAT HE HAD ALREADY VOLUNTARILY RESTRICTED HIMSELF TO; WAS PLACED ON PROBATION BY THE HOSPITAL FOR ONE YEAR; HE HAS FULLY COMPLIED WITH THESE RESTRICTIONS; VEHEMENTLY DISAGREES THAT THE ACTION OF THE HOSPITAL WAS CORRECT BUT VOLUNTARILY ENTERS INTO THIS AGREEMENT. SURGICAL PRACTICE LIMITED TO THOSE PROCEDURES HE WAS CREDENTIALED FOR BY THE HOSPITAL AS OF 3/1/94; SHALL BE SUPERVISED BY CHIEF OF NEUROSURGERY AT HIS HOSPITAL WITH QUARTERLY REPORTS; SHALL ATTEND AT LEAST 50 HOURS PER YEAR OF CONTINUING MEDICAL EDUCATION; SHALL GIVE A COPY OF THIS ORDER TO ANY HEALTH CARE ENTITY WHERE HE HAS PRIVILEGES; SHALL COOPERATE WITH THE BOARD IN VERIFYING COMPLIANCE; SHALL INFORM BOARD OF CHANGE OF ADDRESS WITHIN 10 DAYS OR IF HE LEAVES THE STATE; TIME SPENT OUT OF TEXAS DOES NOT COUNT TOWARD RESTRICTION. SHALL NOT SEEK MODIFICATION FOR ONE YEAR.

WILLIAMSON, LINDA D MD, LICENSE NUMBER 00J3678 OF LAWTON, OK, WAS DISCIPLINED BY TEXAS ON JUNE 28, 1995
DISCIPLINARY ACTION: REPRIMAND
OFFENSE: DISCIPLINARY ACTION BY ANOTHER STATE OR AGENCY
NOTES: DISCIPLINED BY THE AIR FORCE WITH A FINE OF $750 FOR NOT TELLING THE TRUTH TO A SENIOR OFFICER ABOUT TAKING AND PASSING A PORTION OF THE NATIONAL MEDICAL BOARD EXAMINATION; SUBSEQUENT AIR FORCE REPORTS INDICATE THAT SHE RENDERED A HIGH QUALITY OF MEDICAL CARE AS A MILITARY PHYSICIAN; SHE WAS HONORABLY DISCHARGED FROM MILITARY SERVICE ON 6/30/94. SHALL GIVE A COPY OF THIS ORDER TO ANY HEALTH CARE ENTITY WHERE SHE HAS PRIVILEGES; SHALL INFORM BOARD OF CHANGE OF ADDRESS WITHIN 10

DAYS.

WILLIAMSON, MARK A MD, LICENSE NUMBER 00H4855 OF WEBSTER, TX, WAS DISCIPLINED BY TEXAS ON JANUARY 6, 1995
DISCIPLINARY ACTION: 60-MONTH PROBATION; REQUIRED TO TAKE ADDITIONAL MEDICAL EDUCATION
OFFENSE: SUBSTANCE ABUSE

NOTES: ADMITS TO POLYSUBSTANCE ABUSE FOR MANY YEARS INCLUDING BUT NOT LIMITED TO COCAINE AND ALCOHOL; REPORTS A SOBRIETY DATE OF 10/23/93; HAS BEEN ATTENDING AA AND ENTERED INTO AN AFTERCARE RECOVERY CONTRACT; RECEIVES OUTPATIENT AND PSYCHIATRIC TREATMENT. SUSPENSION STAYED. CONDITIONS OF PROBATION: SHALL ABSTAIN FROM THE CONSUMPTION OF ALCOHOL/CHEMICAL SUBSTANCES IN ANY FORM UNLESS PRESCRIBED BY ANOTHER PHYSICIAN FOR A LEGITIMATE AND THERAPEUTIC PURPOSE; SHALL SUBMIT HIMSELF FOR APPROPRIATE EXAMS INCLUDING DRUG OR ALCOHOL SCREENS; SHALL CONTINUE SUBSTANCE ABUSE TREATMENT WITH QUARTERLY REPORTS; SHALL PARTICIPATE IN AA'S PROGRAM NOT LESS THAN FIVE TIMES A WEEK WITH QUARTERLY REPORTS TO THE BOARD; SHALL PARTICIPATE WITH PHYSICIAN'S COUNSELING COMMITTEE AND ATTEND WEEKLY MEETINGS WITH QUARTERLY REPORTS; SHALL COMPLY WITH CONDITIONS OF CONTINUING CARE CONTRACT WITH THE HARRIS COUNTY MEDICAL SOCIETY WITH QUARTERLY REPORTS; SHALL COMPLY WITH CONDITIONS OF ANY AGREEMENT ENTERED INTO FOR HOSPITAL PRIVILEGES; SHALL NOT TREAT OR OTHERWISE SERVE AS PHYSICIAN, PRESCRIBE, DISPENSE OR ADMINISTER DRUGS THAT MAY BE SUBJECT TO ABUSE TO HIMSELF OR ANY MEMBER OF HIS FAMILY; SEPARATE FROM PATIENT RECORDS SHALL MAINTAIN A COPY OF EVERY PRESCRIPTION WRITTEN FOR CONTROLLED SUBSTANCES OR DANGEROUS DRUGS WHICH SHALL BE AVAILABLE FOR INSPECTION; SHALL MAINTAIN A LOGBOOK FOR ALL PRESCRIPTIONS OR REFILLS OF SUCH DRUGS TELEPHONED IN; SHALL OBTAIN AT LEAST 50 HOURS PER YEAR OF CONTINUING MEDICAL EDUCATION; SHALL APPEAR BEFORE THE BOARD ONCE A YEAR OR UPON REQUEST; SHALL COOPERATE WITH THE BOARD IN VERIFYING COMPLIANCE; SHALL EXECUTE RELEASES FOR RECORDS OF TREATMENT OR OF HIS PARTICIPATION WITH THE MEDICAL SOCIETY; SHALL GIVE A COPY OF THIS ORDER TO ANY HEALTH CARE ENTITY WHERE HE HAS OR HAS APPLIED FOR PRIVILEGES; SHALL ENSURE INQUIRIES REGARDING HIS TEXAS LICENSURE STATUS ARE ANSWERED BY REFERENCING THIS ORDER; SHALL INFORM BOARD OF CHANGE OF ADDRESS WITHIN 10 DAYS OR IF HE LEAVES THE STATE; TIME SPENT OUT OF TEXAS DOES NOT COUNT TOWARD PROBATION. SHALL NOT SEEK MODIFICATION FOR ONE YEAR. ON 1/18/97 BOARD GRANTED HIS PETITION FOR TERMINATION OF THIS ORDER BASED ON COMPLIANCE WITH CONDITIONS.

WILLIAMSON, THOMAS LEE MD, LICENSE NUMBER 21101, WAS DISCIPLINED BY ARIZONA ON JULY 26, 1997
DISCIPLINARY ACTION: LICENSE SUSPENSION
OFFENSE: FAILURE TO COMPLY WITH PREVIOUS BOARD ORDER

NOTES: HE VIOLATED THE TERMS OF THE REHABILITATION AND STIPULATION ORDER OF 1/31/97 BY RELAPSING WITH THE USE OF CHEMICAL SUBSTANCES. MAY NOT PRACTICE MEDICINE IN ARIZONA WHILE HIS LICENSE IS IN INACTIVE STATUS; MUST PAY ALL FEES PRIOR TO HIS LICENSE BEING PLACED ON INACTIVE STATUS; SHALL NOT REQUEST REACTIVATION OF HIS LICENSE UNTIL HE MEETS WITH THE BOARD AND COMPLIES WITH ALL REQUESTS OF THE BOARD WHICH MAY INCLUDE INPATIENT TREATMENT, PSYCHIATRIC AND PSYCHOMETRIC EVALUATION, PHYSICAL EXAMINATION AND TESTING, AND WRITTEN AND/OR ORAL COMPETENCY EXAMINATIONS. LICENSE PLACED ON INACTIVE STATUS.

WILLIAMSON, THOMAS LEE MD, LICENSE NUMBER H7105 OF PHOENIX, AZ, WAS DISCIPLINED BY TEXAS ON MAY 14, 1999
OFFENSE: DISCIPLINARY ACTION BY ANOTHER STATE OR AGENCY

NOTES: ON 1/31/97 HE WAS PLACED ON A NON-DISCIPLINARY REHABILITATION STIPULATION AND ORDER BY THE ARIZONA BOARD BASED UPON HIS HISTORY OF SUBSTANCE ABUSE; IN 6/97 HE RELAPSED; ON 7/26/97 HIS ARIZONA MEDICAL LICENSE WAS PLACED ON INACTIVE STATUS AFTER HE RELAPSED; ARIZONA MEDICAL LICENSE IS CURRENTLY ACTIVE; HE ADMITS THAT HE VIOLATED THE TERMS OF HIS REHABILITATION ORDER; HE STATES THAT AFTER A YEAR OF SOBRIETY HE FEELS HE CAN SAFELY RETURN TO THE PRACTICE OF MEDICINE AND PLANS TO PRACTICE IN PHOENIX; HE STATES THAT HE WILL CONTINUE TO BE MONITORED BY THE ARIZONA BOARD FOR 3-5 YEARS, INCLUDING RANDOM URINE DRUG SCREENS, REGULAR AA MEETINGS, AND THERAPY GROUPS. TEXAS LICENSE LIMITED AS FOLLOWS: SHALL NOT PRACTICE UNTIL HE APPEARS BEFORE THE BOARD TO ORALLY PETITION FOR PERMISSION TO RESUME PRACTICE AND PROVIDES EVIDENCE THAT HE IS PHYSICALLY, MENTALLY AND OTHERWISE COMPETENT TO PRACTICE SAFELY INCLUDING AT A MINIMUM: SHALL COMPLY WITH OR COMPLETE THE ARIZONA BOARD ORDER; SHALL HAVE DOCUMENTED SOBRIETY; SHALL COOPERATE WITH THE BOARD IN VERIFYING COMPLIANCE INCLUDING PROVIDING COPIES OF MEDICAL RELEASES UPON REQUEST; SHALL INFORM THE BOARD OF CHANGE OF ADDRESS WITHIN 10 DAYS; SHALL NOT SEEK MODIFICATION FOR ONE YEAR.

WILSON, GERALD T MD, LICENSE NUMBER 00E7321, WAS DISCIPLINED BY TEXAS ON NOVEMBER 16, 1996
DISCIPLINARY ACTION: RESTRICTION PLACED ON LICENSE; REQUIRED TO TAKE ADDITIONAL MEDICAL EDUCATION
OFFENSE: LOSS OR RESTRICTION OF HOSPITAL PRIVILEGES

NOTES: IN 1/95 HIS MEDICAL STAFF PRIVILEGES WERE SUMMARILY SUSPENDED BY A HOSPITAL WHERE HE HAD PRIVILEGES; IN 3/95, THIS HOSPITAL DENIED HIS REAPPOINTMENT TO ITS MEDICAL STAFF AND UPHELD THE SUMMARY SUSPENSION BASED ON A MEDICAL QUALITY OF CARE REVIEW OF HIS PATIENT CASES; IN 19 OF 26 CASES, HE WAS FOUND BY HOSPITAL'S MEDICAL CONSULTANT TO HAVE PRACTICED BELOW THE STANDARD OF CARE OF A PRUDENT TEXAS PHYSICIAN; HE REFUTES THE FINDINGS OF CONSULTANT AND REPORTS THAT HE CHOSE NOT TO CHALLENGE THE SUSPENSION BECAUSE OF FINANCIAL CONSIDERATIONS AND BECAUSE HE HAD PRIVILEGES AT OTHER HOSPITALS; HE REPORTS THAT HE DESIRES TO SLOW DOWN HIS PRACTICE AND HAS TAKEN SUCH STEPS BUT BELIEVES HE CAN STILL CONTRIBUTE TO THE CARE OF TEXAS PATIENTS; HE HAS MEDICAL STAFF PRIVILEGES AT THREE HOSPITALS AND HAS PROVIDED BOARD WITH LETTERS FROM HOSPITALS AND OTHER LICENSED PHYSICIANS IN SUPPORT OF HIS SKILLS. DOES NOT ADMIT VIOLATION. INDEFINITE RESTRICTION OF LICENSE WITH TERMS: SHALL NOT ACCEPT ANY NEW OBSTETRICAL CASES; SHALL NOT ACT AS THE PRIMARY SURGEON FOR ANY SURGICAL PROCEDURE

INVOLVING ONCOLOGY; SHALL TRANSFER ALL OF HIS CURRENT HIGH RISK OBSTETRICAL PATIENTS TO ANOTHER PHYSICIAN; SHALL POST A NOTICE IN ALL PATIENT AREAS INFORMING PATIENTS OF HIS RESTRICTED STATUS; SHALL SUBMIT HIMSELF FOR PHYSICAL EVALUATION AND TREATMENT BY A BOARD-APPROVED PHYSICIAN WHOM HE SHALL SEE AT LEAST ONCE EVERY THREE MONTHS AND WHO SHALL SUBMIT REPORTS TO THE BOARD; SHALL NOT ACT AS PHYSICIAN FOR HIMSELF OR HIS IMMEDIATE FAMILY; SHALL OBTAIN AT LEAST 50 HOURS PER YEAR OF CONTINUING MEDICAL EDUCATION; SHALL COOPERATE WITH THE BOARD IN VERIFYING COMPLIANCE INCLUDING PROVIDING COPIES OF MEDICAL RELEASES AND PEER REVIEW RECORDS UPON REQUEST; SHALL PROVIDE ANY RELEASES AS REQUESTED BY THE BOARD; SHALL APPEAR BEFORE BOARD AT LEAST TWICE A YEAR OR AT BOARD REQUEST; SHALL GIVE A COPY OF THIS ORDER TO ANY HEALTH CARE ENTITY WHERE HE HAS PRIVILEGES; SHALL PROVIDE A COPY OF THIS ORDER TO ANYONE REQUESTING IT WITHIN 10 DAYS; TIME SPENT OUT OF TEXAS DOES NOT COUNT TOWARD RESTRICTION; SHALL INFORM BOARD OF CHANGE OF ADDRESS WITHIN 10 DAYS OR IF HE LEAVES THE STATE. SHALL NOT SEEK MODIFICATION FOR ONE YEAR. ON 2/7/98 PETITION TO MODIFY ORDER GRANTED DELETING REQUIREMENT TO POST A NOTICE IN ALL PATIENT AREAS NOTING THAT HIS PRACTICE IS RESTRICTED BY THE TEXAS BOARD. ON 10/24/98 ORDER MODIFIED REDUCING APPEARANCES BEFORE THE BOARD FROM BIANNUAL TO ANNUAL. ON 12/11/99 PETITION TO TERMINATE ORDER DENIED.

WILSON, LARRY D MD, DATE OF BIRTH JANUARY 26, 1953, LICENSE NUMBER 00H1333 OF 6633 HWY 290E, SUITE 302, AUSTIN, TX, WAS DISCIPLINED BY TEXAS ON JANUARY 29, 1993
DISCIPLINARY ACTION: 36-MONTH PROBATION; RESTRICTION PLACED ON LICENSE
OFFENSE: PROFESSIONAL MISCONDUCT

NOTES: BETWEEN 3/89 AND 8/90 HE WAS THE MEDICAL DIRECTOR AT AN OUTPATIENT METHADONE THERAPY CLINIC FOR NARCOTIC DEPENDENT PERSONS; RECEIVED NO COMPENSATION FOR THESE SERVICES; FAILED TO MEET PROGRAM REQUIREMENTS RELATING TO REPORTING OF ADVERSE REACTIONS, WRITTEN JUSTIFICATION OF INCREASED DOSES OF MEDICATION, DOCUMENTATION OF PHYSICAL EXAMS, OBTAINING PROPER DOCUMENTATION FOR TRANSFER PATIENTS, DOCUMENTATION OF ADDICTION, AND REGULAR ATTENDANCE ON THE PREMISES OF THE PROGRAM; THESE FAILURES PERMITTED NON-QUALIFIED EMPLOYEES TO EXERCISE INDEPENDENT MEDICAL JUDGMENT WHICH CONSTITUTED IMPROPER DELEGATION OF RESPONSIBILITY AND PERMITTED THE PRACTICE OF MEDICINE BY A BUSINESS ENTITY NOT LICENSED TO DO SO; THIS MAY HAVE CONTRIBUTED TO ONE PATIENT'S DEATH. 3 YEAR SUSPENSION STAYED. CONDITIONS OF PROBATION: SHALL ATTEND AT LEAST 50 HOURS PER YEAR OF CONTINUING MEDICAL EDUCATION; SHALL NOT ACCEPT EMPLOYMENT OR ENTER INTO CONTRACTUAL RELATIONSHIPS WHERE HE WOULD BE COMPENSATED TO DIAGNOSE AND/OR TREAT PATIENTS BY A LAYPERSON, CORPORATION OR OTHER ENTITY NOT COMPRISED EXCLUSIVELY OF TEXAS LICENSED PHYSICIANS AND WHEREIN THE PERSON OR ENTITY WOULD RECEIVE AND RETAIN THE FEES PAID BY OR ON BEHALF OF PATIENTS FOR THE PHYSICIAN'S PROFESSIONAL SERVICES; SHALL PERFORM 12 HOURS PER MONTH OF COMMUNITY SERVICE FOR A NONPROFIT CHARITABLE ORGANIZATION FOR THE FIRST YEAR OF PROBATION; SHALL APPEAR BEFORE THE BOARD TWICE A YEAR; SHALL GIVE A COPY OF THIS ORDER TO ANY HEALTH CARE ENTITY WHERE HE HAS PRIVILEGES; SHALL COOPERATE WITH THE BOARD IN VERIFYING COMPLIANCE; SHALL INFORM BOARD OF CHANGE OF ADDRESS WITHIN 10 DAYS OR IF HE LEAVES THE STATE; TIME SPENT OUT OF TEXAS DOES NOT COUNT TOWARD PROBATION; SHALL NOT SEEK MODIFICATION FOR ONE YEAR. ON 6/22/94, BASED ON HISTORY OF COMPLIANCE AND EXEMPLARY COMMUNITY SERVICE THE ORDER WAS TERMINATED.

WILSON, MARK DANIEL MD, LICENSE NUMBER 00F4697 OF DENTON, TX, WAS DISCIPLINED BY TEXAS ON MARCH 31, 1990
DISCIPLINARY ACTION: RESTRICTION PLACED ON CONTROLLED SUBSTANCE LICENSE

NOTES: STIPULATED ORDER. MUST REFRAIN FROM PRESCRIPTION OR ADMINISTRATION OF ANY DRUG UNLESS IT IS THERAPEUTIC, MUST NOT PRESCRIBE, ADMINISTER OR DISPENSE DRUG WITH POTENTIAL OF ABUSE WITHOUT APPROPRIATE MEDICAL HISTORY AND CLINICALLY ADEQUATE EXAMINATION, MUST UNDERSTAND POTENTIAL FOR ABUSE OF CONTROLLED SUBSTANCES OR DANGEROUS DRUGS, SHALL NOT PRESCRIBE, DISPENSE, OR ADMINISTER DRUG OR MEDICATION HAVING ANORECTIC EFFECT WITHOUT PERMISSION FROM BOARD, MUST CONDUCT ADEQUATE FOLLOW-UP EXAMINATIONS ON PATIENTS TO DETERMINE WHETHER TREATMENT COURSE APPROPRIATE AND MUST MAINTAIN COPIES OF ANORECTIC AGENT PRESCRIPTIONS. RESTRICTIONS TERMINATED EFFECTIVE 6/16/92; LICENSE FREE OF ANY RESTRICTION OR LIMITATION.

WILSON, ROBERT S DO, DATE OF BIRTH AUGUST 20, 1949, LICENSE NUMBER 0027467, WAS DISCIPLINED BY COLORADO ON NOVEMBER 16, 1995
DISCIPLINARY ACTION: 60-MONTH PROBATION; MONITORING OF PHYSICIAN PERFORMANCE

NOTES: PRACTICE AND TREATMENT MONITORING.

WILSON, ROBERT STOREY DO, LICENSE NUMBER 00E4770 OF GRANBURY, TX, WAS DISCIPLINED BY TEXAS ON MAY 11, 1995
DISCIPLINARY ACTION: RESTRICTION PLACED ON CONTROLLED SUBSTANCE LICENSE; REQUIRED TO TAKE ADDITIONAL MEDICAL EDUCATION
OFFENSE: SUBSTANCE ABUSE

NOTES: IN 8/93 HE BEGAN SELF-ADMINISTERING DILAUDID WITHOUT A LEGITIMATE MEDICAL PURPOSE AND AS A RESULT OF EMOTIONAL HARDSHIP AND DEPRESSION HE EXPERIENCED DUE TO HIS WIFE'S MEDICAL CONDITION; WROTE FALSE AND FICTITIOUS PRESCRIPTIONS IN ORDER TO OBTAIN DILAUDID; IN 7/94, HE ENTERED AN INTERIM CONTRACT WITH THE TEXAS OSTEOPATHIC MEDICAL ASSOCIATION TO REFRAIN FROM THE PRACTICE OF MEDICINE UNTIL HE SUCCESSFULLY COMPLETED TREATMENT FOR SUBSTANCE ADDICTION; ENTERED A 24-MONTH AFTERCARE RECOVERY CONTRACT; VOLUNTARILY ENTERED A TREATMENT FACILITY IN 7/94 AND SUBSEQUENTLY VOLUNTARILY TRANSFERRED TO INPATIENT TREATMENT WHICH LASTED 97 DAYS; REPORTS SOBRIETY DATE OF 7/17/94; HAS BEEN IN COMPLIANCE WITH HIS AFTERCARE CONTRACT; REPORTS ATTENDING APPROXIMATELY FIVE AA OR NARCOTICS ANONYMOUS MEETINGS PER WEEK. LICENSE RESTRICTED FOR FIVE YEARS UNDER TERMS: SHALL ABSTAIN FROM THE CONSUMPTION OF ALCOHOL/DRUGS IN ANY FORM UNLESS PRESCRIBED BY ANOTHER PHYSICIAN FOR A LEGITIMATE AND

THERAPEUTIC PURPOSE; SHALL SUBMIT HIMSELF FOR APPROPRIATE EXAMS INCLUDING DRUG OR ALCOHOL SCREENS; SHALL SUBMIT HIMSELF FOR EVALUATION AND TREATMENT BY A BOARD-APPROVED PSYCHIATRIST AT LEAST ONCE A MONTH WHO WILL SUBMIT REPORTS TO THE BOARD; SHALL CONTINUE TO PARTICIPATE IN AA OR NARCOTICS ANONYMOUS PROGRAM NOT LESS THAN THREE TIMES A WEEK WITH QUARTERLY REPORTS TO THE BOARD; SHALL CONTINUE TO PARTICIPATE IN THE ACTIVITIES OF AN IMPAIRED PHYSICIAN'S GROUP AND ABIDE BY TERMS OF ANY AFTERCARE PROGRAM REQUIRED WITH QUARTERLY REPORTS; SHALL COMPLY WITH TERMS OF ANY CONTRACT ENTERED INTO FOR HOSPITAL PRIVILEGES AND SHALL INFORM BOARD OF ANY DISCIPLINE; EXCEPT AS OTHERWISE PROVIDED FOR BY THIS ORDER, SHALL NOT POSSESS ALCOHOL, CONTROLLED SUBSTANCES OR DRUGS WITH ADDICTIVE POTENTIAL; SHALL SURRENDER SAMPLES OF ANY SUCH DRUGS IN HIS POSSESSION; SHALL NOT OTHERWISE SERVE AS PHYSICIAN, PRESCRIBE, DISPENSE OR ADMINISTER DRUGS THAT MAY BE SUBJECT TO ABUSE TO HIMSELF OR TO ANY MEMBER OF HIS FAMILY; SHALL NOT TELEPHONE TO A PHARMACY A PRESCRIPTION FOR CONTROLLED SUBSTANCES NOR PERMIT ANYONE HE SUPERVISES TO TELEPHONE; MAY NOT POSSESS, ADMINISTER, DISPENSE, ORDER OR PRESCRIBE CONTROLLED SUBSTANCES EXCEPT ORDER FOR HOSPITAL INPATIENTS OR NURSING HOME PATIENTS; MAY PRESCRIBE RITALIN TO PEDIATRIC PATIENTS DIAGNOSED WITH ATTENTION DEFICIT ORDER; SHALL KEEP A SEPARATE LOG OF ALL PRESCRIPTIONS FOR CONTROLLED SUBSTANCES WHICH SHALL BE AVAILABLE FOR REVIEW; SHALL MAINTAIN ADEQUATE MEDICAL RECORDS WHICH SHALL BE AVAILABLE FOR REVIEW; SHALL OBTAIN AT LEAST 50 HOURS PER YEAR OF CONTINUING MEDICAL EDUCATION; SHALL APPEAR BEFORE BOARD AT LEAST ONCE A YEAR; SHALL COOPERATE WITH THE BOARD IN VERIFYING COMPLIANCE INCLUDING PROVIDING COPIES OF MEDICAL RELEASES OR PEER REVIEW RECORDS UPON REQUEST; SHALL GIVE A COPY OF THIS ORDER TO ANY HEALTH CARE ENTITY WHERE HE HAS PRIVILEGES; SHALL PROVIDE A COPY OF THE ORDER TO ANYONE REQUESTING IT WITHIN 10 DAYS; TIME PERIOD OUT OF TEXAS DOES NOT COUNT TOWARD PROBATION; SHALL INFORM BOARD OF CHANGE OF ADDRESS WITHIN 10 DAYS OR IF HE LEAVES THE STATE. SHALL NOT SEEK MODIFICATION FOR ONE YEAR. ON 5/10/97 PETITION TO TERMINATE ORDER DENIED. ON 8/10/97 PETITION TO TERMINATE ORDER DENIED. ON 8/22/98 ORDER TERMINATED.

WILSON, W BRAD MD, LICENSE NUMBER H3293, WAS DISCIPLINED BY TEXAS ON JANUARY 18, 1997
DISCIPLINARY ACTION: REPRIMAND
OFFENSE: OVERPRESCRIBING OR MISPRESCRIBING DRUGS

NOTES: FAILED TO KEEP ADEQUATE MEDICAL RECORDS CONCERNING HIS CARE, TREATMENT, AND PRESCRIBING FOR ONE PATIENT; HIS PRESCRIBING FOR THIS PATIENT WAS NON-THERAPEUTIC IN THAT HE FAILED TO SEEK OTHER PAIN MANAGEMENT OPTIONS FOR THIS PATIENT, WHO WAS AN ABUSER OF CONTROLLED SUBSTANCES, A FACT THAT HE KNEW OR SHOULD HAVE KNOWN. HE CONTINUED TO PRESCRIBE CONTROLLED SUBSTANCES TO THE PATIENT AFTER THE PATIENT'S OVERDOSE ON SUCH MEDICATION AND CONSEQUENT HOSPITALIZATION.

WIMBERLY, DAVID M MD, LICENSE NUMBER H5279, WAS DISCIPLINED BY TEXAS ON JANUARY 18, 1997
DISCIPLINARY ACTION: MONITORING OF PHYSICIAN PERFORMANCE
OFFENSE: SUBSTANCE ABUSE

NOTES: ON 4/26/96 HE WAS DISCOVERED IN AN UNCONSCIOUS STATE IN A HOSPITAL ROOM DUE TO SELF-ADMINISTRATION OF ANESTHESIA DRUGS WITHOUT A LEGITIMATE MEDICAL PURPOSE. PRIOR TO 4/26/96, HE HAD ENGAGED IN THE HABITUAL INTEMPERATE USE OF ALCOHOL TO THE POINT OF DEPENDENCY, AND IN EARLY 1996 BEGAN INJECTING HIMSELF WITH ANESTHESIA DRUGS WITHOUT A LEGITIMATE MEDICAL NEED. SHORTLY AFTER THE 4/26/96 INCIDENT HE VOLUNTARILY ENTERED A THREE-WEEK INPATIENT PROGRAM FOR SUBSTANCE ABUSE AND SATISFACTORILY COMPLETED IT. HE HAS BEEN ACTIVELY REHABILITATING SINCE THEN AND ALL MONITORING SHOWS EVIDENCE OF HIS CONTINUING SOBRIETY. HE ALSO MAINTAINS THAT HE NEVER DRANK ALCOHOL DURING THE DAY OR WHILE TAKING CARE OF PATIENTS; CONDITIONS ON LICENSE FOR FIVE YEARS: SHALL ABSTAIN FROM THE CONSUMPTION OF ALCOHOL/DRUGS IN ANY FORM UNLESS PRESCRIBED BY ANOTHER PHYSICIAN FOR A LEGITIMATE AND THERAPEUTIC PURPOSE; SHALL NOMINATE THREE CERTIFIED PSYCHIATRISTS FOR BOARD SELECTION OF A THERAPIST AND SHALL EXPEDITIOUSLY SUBMIT HIMSELF TO EVALUATION AND TREATMENT BY THE APPROVED PRACTITIONER; SHALL SUBMIT HIMSELF FOR APPROPRIATE EXAMS INCLUDING DRUG OR ALCOHOL SCREENS; SHALL PARTICIPATE IN THE ACTIVITIES OF A PHYSICIAN HEALTH AND REHABILITATION COMMITTEE AND ATTEND WEEKLY MEETINGS WITH QUARTERLY REPORTS; SHALL PARTICIPATE IN AA'S PROGRAM NOT LESS THAN THREE TIMES A WEEK; SHALL REPORT ON HIS ATTENDANCE; SHALL NOT TREAT OR OTHERWISE SERVE AS PHYSICIAN, PRESCRIBE, DISPENSE OR ADMINISTER DRUGS THAT MAY BE SUBJECT TO ABUSE TO HIMSELF OR TO ANY MEMBER OF HIS FAMILY; SHALL COOPERATE WITH THE BOARD IN VERIFYING COMPLIANCE INCLUDING PROVIDING COPIES OF MEDICAL RELEASES AND PEER REVIEW RECORDS UPON REQUEST; SHALL APPEAR BEFORE THE BOARD UPON REQUEST; SHALL GIVE A COPY OF THIS ORDER TO ANY HEALTH CARE ENTITY WHERE HE HAS PRIVILEGES; SHALL PROVIDE A COPY OF THIS ORDER TO ANYONE REQUESTING IT WITHIN 10 DAYS; TIME SPENT OUT OF TEXAS DOES NOT COUNT TOWARD RESTRICTION; SHALL INFORM THE BOARD OF CHANGE OF ADDRESS WITHIN 10 DAYS OR IF HE LEAVES THE STATE; SHALL NOT SEEK MODIFICATION FOR ONE YEAR. ON 1/29/99 TERMINATION REQUEST WAS DENIED; MODIFICATIONS OF THE ORDER WERE MADE AS FOLLOWS: DELETION OF REQUIREMENTS FOR ONGOING PSYCHIATRIC CARE AND COUNSELING, DRUG SCREENS ORDERED BY ANY TREATING PHYSICIAN, MANDATORY PARTICIPATION IN AA, AND COUNTY MEDICAL SOCIETY ACTIVITIES; AND THAT HE NOT SERVE AS A TREATING PHYSICIAN FOR HIS IMMEDIATE FAMILY; AND, LASTLY, THE REQUIREMENT OF 2 APPEARANCES PER YEAR BEFORE THE BOARD LESSENED TO 1 TIME EACH YEAR HE IS UNDER THE TERMS AND CONDITIONS OF THE ORDER; ALL OTHER PROVISIONS OF THE ORDER REMAIN IN FULL FORCE.

WIMBERLY, DAVID M MD, DATE OF BIRTH FEBRUARY 23, 1959, LICENSE NUMBER 032497 OF 405 DAVID STREET, FRIENDSWOOD, TX, WAS DISCIPLINED BY GEORGIA ON MARCH 6, 1998
DISCIPLINARY ACTION: PROBATION
OFFENSE: DISCIPLINARY ACTION BY ANOTHER STATE OR AGENCY

NOTES: TO RUN CONCURRENT WITH TEXAS ORDER OF WHICH PROBATIONARY TERMS BEGAN ON 1/18/97.

WIMPEE, MARC W MD, LICENSE NUMBER 00G5787 OF SAN ANGELO, TX, WAS DISCIPLINED BY TEXAS ON AUGUST 18, 1995
DISCIPLINARY ACTION: 60-MONTH PROBATION
OFFENSE: SUBSTANCE ABUSE

NOTES: INTEMPERATE USE OF ALCOHOL OR DRUGS. SUSPENSION STAYED. PROBATION UNDER TERMS AND CONDITIONS.

WIMPEE, MARC W MD, LICENSE NUMBER G5787, WAS DISCIPLINED BY TEXAS ON MAY 10, 1997
DISCIPLINARY ACTION: LICENSE SUSPENSION; REQUIRED TO ENTER AN IMPAIRED PHYSICIAN PROGRAM OR SUBSTANCE ABUSE TREATMENT
OFFENSE: FAILURE TO COMPLY WITH PREVIOUS BOARD ORDER

NOTES: VIOLATED THE TERMS OF THE 9/15/95 ORDER AS FOLLOWS: HE WAS REQUIRED TO ABSTAIN FROM THE USE OF CONTROLLED SUBSTANCES UNLESS PRESCRIBED BY ANOTHER PHYSICIAN FOR THERAPEUTIC PURPOSES; ON 9/23/96 HE TESTED POSITIVE FOR MORPHINE, A SCHEDULE II CONTROLLED SUBSTANCE. HE FAILED TO TIMELY PROVIDE A COPY OF THE ORDER TO SPECIFIED PHYSICIAN AND FAILED TO CAUSE TWO PHYSICIANS TO REPORT TO THE BOARD ON PRESCRIBING AS REQUIRED; HE DELAYED IN SEEKING A TREATING PSYCHIATRIST; DID NOT PROVIDE EVIDENCE OF HIS ATTENDANCE AT AA; HAS NOT OBTAINED A MONITORING PHYSICIAN; PRESCRIBED A CONTROLLED SUBSTANCE IN 10/95 DESPITE RESTRICTIONS; HAS NOT PROVEN HIS OBTAINING OF THE REQUIRED CONTINUING MEDICAL EDUCATION, AND HAS AT LEAST ONCE IN 11/95 REFUSED TO RELEASE RECORDS AS REQUIRED. SUSPENSION UNTIL HE REQUESTS TO HAVE HIS SUSPENSION STAYED OR APPEARS BEFORE THE BOARD WITH SUFFICIENT EVIDENCE THAT HE IS PHYSICALLY, MENTALLY AND OTHERWISE COMPETENT TO SAFELY PRACTICE MEDICINE INCLUDING AT A MINIMUM COMPLETE COPIES OF MEDICAL RECORDS AND REPORTS OF PSYCHOLOGICAL AND NEUROPSYCHIATRIC EVALUATIONS, INCLUDING A 96 HOUR INPATIENT EVALUATION CONDUCTED BY A BOARD-APPROVED CERTIFIED PSYCHIATRIST; PARTICIPATING IN AN AFTERCARE MONITORING CONTRACT AND AA; HAVING COMPLETED ALL THE BOARD'S CONTINUING MEDICAL EDUCATION REQUIREMENTS. UPON SUCH PROOF THE SUSPENSION SHALL BE STAYED FOR PROBATION OF UNDETERMINED LENGTH.

WIMPEE, MARC W MD OF 3023 GREEN MEADOW, SAN ANGELO, TX, WAS DISCIPLINED BY DEA ON JULY 14, 1997
DISCIPLINARY ACTION: SURRENDER OF CONTROLLED SUBSTANCE LICENSE

NOTES: IN LIEU OF PUBLIC INTEREST REVOCATION.

WINSLOW, DAVID EVERETT DO, DATE OF BIRTH APRIL 10, 1959, LICENSE NUMBER 00H4804 OF 2745 VALWOOD PARKWAY, DALLAS, TX, WAS DISCIPLINED BY TEXAS ON JANUARY 29, 1993
DISCIPLINARY ACTION: 120-MONTH PROBATION; RESTRICTION PLACED ON CONTROLLED SUBSTANCE LICENSE
OFFENSE: SUBSTANDARD CARE, INCOMPETENCE OR NEGLIGENCE

NOTES: FAILED TO KEEP ADEQUATE RECORDS OF WEIGHT CONTROL PATIENTS; FAILED TO DOCUMENT PHYSICAL EXAMS; FAILED TO ADEQUATELY ADDRESS PATIENT SYMPTOMS/COMPLAINTS. 10 YEAR SUSPENSION STAYED. SHALL APPEAR BEFORE THE BOARD ONCE A YEAR; SHALL ATTEND AT LEAST 50 HOURS PER YEAR OF CONTINUING MEDICAL EDUCATION; SHALL MAINTAIN ADEQUATE MEDICAL RECORDS ON ALL PATIENT OFFICE VISITS; SHALL NOT SIGN ANY PATIENT RECORD UNLESS HE HAS PERSONALLY SEEN AND EXAMINED THE PATIENT UNLESS THIS IS SO NOTED IN THE RECORD; SHALL TAKE THE SPEX EXAM WITHIN 1 YEAR; SHALL NOT TREAT ANY PATIENT FOR WEIGHT CONTROL WITH DRUGS; SHALL GIVE A COPY OF THIS ORDER TO ANY HEALTH CARE ENTITY WHERE HE HAS PRIVILEGES; SHALL COOPERATE WITH THE BOARD IN VERIFYING COMPLIANCE; SHALL INFORM BOARD OF ADDRESS CHANGE WITHIN 10 DAYS OR IF HE LEAVES THE STATE; TIME SPENT OUT OF TEXAS DOES NOT COUNT TOWARD PROBATION. ON 4/10/99 ORDER TERMINATED.

WINSLOW, JAMES R DO, LICENSE NUMBER 00C5930 OF DALLAS, TX, WAS DISCIPLINED BY TEXAS ON AUGUST 18, 1995
DISCIPLINARY ACTION: REPRIMAND; REQUIRED TO TAKE ADDITIONAL MEDICAL EDUCATION
OFFENSE: NONCOMPLIANCE WITH A PROFESSIONAL RULE

NOTES: HIS RECORD-KEEPING IN REGARD TO PRESCRIBING AND DISPENSING OF MEDICATIONS TO PATIENTS WAS INADEQUATE BY BOARD STANDARDS. RESTRICTION OF LICENSE WITH TERMS: ORDER SHALL REMAIN IN EFFECT UNTIL HE OFFICIALLY RETIRES FROM THE PRACTICE OF MEDICINE; SHALL ATTEND AT LEAST 50 HOURS PER YEAR OF CONTINUING MEDICAL EDUCATION, AT LEAST 10 HOURS OF WHICH SHALL BE IN PREVENTIVE MEDICINE; SHALL PERFORM 120 HOURS PER YEAR OF COMMUNITY SERVICE; SHALL APPEAR BEFORE BOARD AT LEAST ONCE A YEAR; SHALL COOPERATE WITH BOARD IN VERIFYING COMPLIANCE; SHALL GIVE A COPY OF THIS ORDER TO ANY HEALTH CARE ENTITY WHERE HE HAS PRIVILEGES; SHALL INFORM THE BOARD OF CHANGE OF ADDRESS WITHIN 10 DAYS. SHALL NOT SEEK MODIFICATION FOR ONE YEAR.

WINSTEAD, GLENN C MD, DATE OF BIRTH DECEMBER 17, 1944, LICENSE NUMBER 0006542 OF 2200 BOX ELDER, MILES CITY, MT, WAS DISCIPLINED BY MONTANA ON AUGUST 24, 1990
DISCIPLINARY ACTION: PROBATION
OFFENSE: CRIMINAL CONVICTION OR PLEA OF GUILTY, NOLO CONTENDERE, OR NO CONTEST TO A CRIME

NOTES: FEDERAL FELONY CONVICTION INVOLVING MORAL TURPITUDE - COUNTERFEITING. PROBATION UNTIL FURTHER ORDER OF THE BOARD WITH FOLLOWING TERMS AND CONDITIONS: SHALL UNDERGO REGULAR PSYCHOTHERAPY WITH QUARTERLY REPORTS TO THE BOARD; SHALL INSTITUTE AND MAINTAIN A RELATIONSHIP WITH A THIRD PARTY TO MANAGE ALL HIS FINANCIAL AFFAIRS, INCLUDING BOTH INCOMING AND OUTGOING MONIES; SHALL ENTER INTO AN AGREEMENT WITH THE PROFESSIONAL ASSISTANCE PROGRAM. ON 5/18/92 ORDER AMENDED ALLOWING HIS FIRST REPORT TO THE BOARD BE DUE ON 4/1/93, AND SHALL INSTRUCT HIS FINANCIAL MANAGER TO PROVIDE THE BOARD WITH ANNUAL REPORTS.

WINSTEAD, GLENN C MD, LICENSE NUMBER 00D9324 OF STEVENSVILLE, MT, WAS DISCIPLINED BY TEXAS ON FEBRUARY 22, 1991

NOTES: MUST APPEAR BEFORE TEXAS BOARD AND RECEIVE APPROVAL BEFORE PRACTICING IN TEXAS. ON 10/24/98 ORDER TERMINATED.

WINSTEAD, GLENN C MD, LICENSE NUMBER 0021097 OF GREAT FALLS, MT, WAS DISCIPLINED BY VIRGINIA ON APRIL 19, 1993
DISCIPLINARY ACTION: LICENSE REVOCATION
OFFENSE: CRIMINAL CONVICTION OR PLEA OF GUILTY, NOLO

CONTENDERE, OR NO CONTEST TO A CRIME

NOTES: BASED ON FELONY CONVICTION.

WINTEROWD, KEITH GENE DO, DATE OF BIRTH DECEMBER 28, 1934 OF PO BOX 1010, #26864-077, BASTROP, TX, WAS DISCIPLINED BY MEDICARE ON MARCH 16, 1997
DISCIPLINARY ACTION: EXCLUSION FROM THE MEDICARE AND/OR MEDICAID PROGRAM
OFFENSE: CRIMINAL CONVICTION OR PLEA OF GUILTY, NOLO CONTENDERE, OR NO CONTEST TO A CRIME

NOTES: CONVICTED OF A CRIME RELATED TO THE DELIVERY OF HEALTH CARE OR FINANCIAL MISCONDUCT INVOLVING A GOVERNMENT-OPERATED PROGRAM.

WINTEROWD, KEITH GENE DO, LICENSE NUMBER D1174 OF DESOTO, TX, WAS DISCIPLINED BY TEXAS ON AUGUST 9, 1997
DISCIPLINARY ACTION: SURRENDER OF LICENSE
OFFENSE: CRIMINAL CONVICTION OR PLEA OF GUILTY, NOLO CONTENDERE, OR NO CONTEST TO A CRIME

NOTES: ON OR ABOUT 12/95 THE U.S. DISTRICT COURT FOR THE NORTHERN DISTRICT OF TEXAS CONVICTED HIM OF 24 COUNTS OF MAIL FRAUD AND 5 COUNTS OF MAKING FALSE STATEMENTS TO A GOVERNMENT AGENCY. VOLUNTARY SURRENDER.

WITHERSPOON, ROBERT GLYNN JR MD, LICENSE NUMBER 00E4772 OF MOUNT PLEASANT, TX, WAS DISCIPLINED BY TEXAS ON JUNE 17, 1992
DISCIPLINARY ACTION: 60-MONTH PROBATION
OFFENSE: OVERPRESCRIBING OR MISPRESCRIBING DRUGS

NOTES: NONTHERAPEUTIC PRESCRIBING AND PROFESSIONAL FAILURE TO PRACTICE MEDICINE IN AN ACCEPTABLE MANNER CONSISTENT WITH PUBLIC HEALTH AND WELFARE. SUSPENSION STAYED.

WOLF, GARY DUKE DO, LICENSE NUMBER 00E9029 OF MANSFIELD, TX, WAS DISCIPLINED BY TEXAS ON JANUARY 6, 1995
DISCIPLINARY ACTION: REQUIRED TO TAKE ADDITIONAL MEDICAL EDUCATION; MONITORING OF PHYSICIAN PERFORMANCE
OFFENSE: OVERPRESCRIBING OR MISPRESCRIBING DRUGS

NOTES: FROM 1985 TO 1993 PRESCRIBED CONTROLLED SUBSTANCES TO VARIOUS PATIENTS WITHOUT ADEQUATE INDICATIONS AND SUFFICIENT MONITORING OR FOLLOW-UP; CARE AND TREATMENT APPEARS TO BE WELL DOCUMENTED AND HE REPORTS THAT PATIENTS HAVE BEEN WEANED OFF THE DRUGS PRESCRIBED; AGREEMENT IN LIEU OF FURTHER INVESTIGATION OR A HEARING. CONDITIONS OF THREE YEAR RESTRICTION: SHALL OBTAIN AT LEAST 50 HOURS PER YEAR OF CONTINUING MEDICAL EDUCATION INCLUDING 25 HOURS IN PHARMACOLOGY, SUBSTANCE ABUSE OR PAIN MANAGEMENT IN THE FIRST YEAR; SEPARATE FROM PATIENT RECORDS, SHALL MAINTAIN A FILE OF EVERY PRESCRIPTION WRITTEN FOR CONTROLLED SUBSTANCES OR DANGEROUS DRUGS WHICH SHALL BE AVAILABLE FOR INSPECTION; SHALL MAINTAIN A LOGBOOK FOR ALL PRESCRIPTIONS OR REFILLS OF SUCH DRUGS TELEPHONED IN, WHICH SHALL BE AVAILABLE FOR INSPECTION; SHALL APPEAR BEFORE THE BOARD ONCE A YEAR OR UPON REQUEST; SHALL COOPERATE WITH THE BOARD IN VERIFYING COMPLIANCE; SHALL EXECUTE RELEASES NECESSARY TO OBTAIN PEER REVIEW RECORDS; SHALL GIVE A COPY OF THIS ORDER TO ANY HEALTH CARE ENTITY WHERE HE HAS OR HAS APPLIED FOR PRIVILEGES OR ANYONE ELSE WHO REQUESTS IT; SHALL ENSURE INQUIRIES REGARDING HIS TEXAS LICENSURE STATUS ARE ANSWERED BY REFERENCING THIS ORDER; SHALL INFORM BOARD OF CHANGE OF ADDRESS WITHIN 10 DAYS OR IF HE LEAVES THE STATE; TIME SPENT OUT OF TEXAS DOES NOT COUNT TOWARD RESTRICTION. SHALL NOT SEEK MODIFICATION FOR ONE YEAR. ON 1/27/96 ORDER TERMINATED.

WOLF, GARY DUKE DO, LICENSE NUMBER 0002560, WAS DISCIPLINED BY OKLAHOMA ON JULY 14, 1995
DISCIPLINARY ACTION: 36-MONTH PROBATION; REQUIRED TO TAKE ADDITIONAL MEDICAL EDUCATION
OFFENSE: DISCIPLINARY ACTION BY ANOTHER STATE OR AGENCY

NOTES: THREE YEAR RESTRICTION PLACED ON LICENSE IN TEXAS UNDER TERMS AND CONDITIONS ON 1/06/95. OKLAHOMA LIMITED LICENSE: SHALL OBTAIN AT LEAST 50 HOURS PER YEAR OF CONTINUING MEDICAL EDUCATION DURING THE FIRST YEAR OF LIMITATION, AT LEAST 25 HOURS OF WHICH SHOULD BE IN PHARMACOLOGY, SUBSTANCE ABUSE OR PAIN MANAGEMENT; SHALL EACH YEAR SUBMIT PROOF TO THE BOARD OF THE PRIOR YEAR'S ATTENDANCE; SHALL REFRAIN FROM THE PRESCRIPTION OR ADMINISTRATION OF ANY DRUG UNLESS THE DRUG IS ISSUED TO HIS PATIENTS AND ONLY FOR THE EXPRESSED PURPOSE OF SERVING THE BEST INTERESTS AND PROMOTING THE WELFARE OF HIS PATIENTS; SHALL GIVE A COPY OF THIS ORDER TO ANY HEALTH CARE ENTITY WHERE HE HAS PRIVILEGES; SHALL NOTIFY THE BOARD IN WRITING OF ANY CHANGE IN ADDRESS, EMPLOYMENT, EMPLOYMENT TERMINATION OR HOSPITAL OR HEALTH CARE ENTITIES PRIVILEGE RESTRICTION OR ANY ADMINISTRATIVE PROCEEDING INITIATED AGAINST HIM BY ANY OTHER STATE OR FEDERAL REGULATORY BODY WITHIN 14 DAYS; SHALL APPEAR BEFORE THE BOARD BEFORE PRACTICING OSTEOPATHIC MEDICINE IN OKLAHOMA; $275.00 ADMINISTRATIVE COSTS. ON 12/10/98 PROBATION TERMINATED.

WOLF, GARY DUKE DO OF MANSFIELD, TX, WAS DISCIPLINED BY LOUISIANA ON AUGUST 24, 1995
DISCIPLINARY ACTION: 36-MONTH PROBATION
OFFENSE: DISCIPLINARY ACTION BY ANOTHER STATE OR AGENCY

NOTES: DISCIPLINARY ACTION BY TEXAS; PRESCRIBING, DISPENSING OR ADMINISTERING CONTROLLED SUBSTANCES IN OTHER THAN A LEGAL OR LEGITIMATE MANNER. CONDITIONS OF PROBATION: MUST COMPLY WITH TERMS OF PRIOR PROBATIONARY ORDER IMPOSED BY TEXAS; MUST COMPLETE TEXAS PROBATION AND APPEAR BEFORE BOARD PRIOR TO PRACTICING IN LOUISIANA.

WOLF, PHILIP L MD, DATE OF BIRTH JULY 13, 1955 OF 11202 FORREST RAIN, SAN ANTONIO, TX, WAS DISCIPLINED BY MEDICARE ON JANUARY 5, 1997
DISCIPLINARY ACTION: EXCLUSION FROM THE MEDICARE AND/OR MEDICAID PROGRAM
OFFENSE: NONCOMPLIANCE WITH A PROFESSIONAL RULE

NOTES: DEFAULTED ON PUBLIC HEALTH SERVICE EDUCATION LOAN.

WOLF, RENE JR MD, DATE OF BIRTH MARCH 8, 1949, LICENSE NUMBER 00F3672 OF DALLAS, TX, WAS DISCIPLINED BY TEXAS ON FEBRUARY 22, 1991

NOTES: MUST COMPLY WITH HAWAII BOARD ORDER; OBTAIN PERMISSION FROM TEXAS BOARD BEFORE PRACTICING MEDICINE IN TEXAS, AND FOLLOW SUCH TERMS AS MAY BE IMPOSED. ORDER TERMINATED ON

6/15/93; LICENSE FREE AND CLEAR OF RESTRICTIONS.

WOLF, RENE JR MD, DATE OF BIRTH MARCH 8, 1949, LICENSE NUMBER 00F3672 OF 4500 PEAR RIDGE #738, DALLAS, TX, WAS DISCIPLINED BY TEXAS ON DECEMBER 16, 1991
DISCIPLINARY ACTION: 24-MONTH PROBATION

NOTES: GRANTED PERMISSION TO PRACTICE IN TEXAS. PROBATION UNDER TERMS AND CONDITIONS. ON 1/29/93 MODIFICATION GRANTED SO THAT HE MAY REAPPLY FOR LIFTING OF PROBATIONARY CONDITIONS NO SOONER THAN 6/1/93 AND ALL OTHER TERMS IMPOSED BY THIS ORDER REMAIN IN EFFECT.

WOLFE, ALVIN E DO, LICENSE NUMBER 00D7715 OF WICHITA, KS, WAS DISCIPLINED BY TEXAS ON APRIL 21, 1990

NOTES: STIPULATED ORDER. MUST REQUEST PERSONAL INTERVIEW BEFORE BOARD TO DISCUSS PRESENT STATUS, LOCATION AND TYPE OF PRACTICE DESIRED TO ENTER INTO, AND RECEIVE APPROVAL PRIOR TO PRACTICING IN TEXAS.

WOLFE, ALVIN E DO, DATE OF BIRTH AUGUST 15, 1932, LICENSE NUMBER 0015428 OF WICHITA, KS, WAS DISCIPLINED BY COLORADO ON OCTOBER 18, 1991
DISCIPLINARY ACTION: SURRENDER OF LICENSE
OFFENSE: DISCIPLINARY ACTION BY ANOTHER STATE OR AGENCY

NOTES: ADMINISTERING, DISPENSING OR PRESCRIBING A HABIT FORMING DRUG NOT IN THE COURSE OF LEGITIMATE MEDICAL PRACTICE. PERMANENT SURRENDER OF COLORADO MEDICAL LICENSE. ACTION TAKEN BY KANSAS BOARD.

WOMACK, GROVER KENNETH MD, DATE OF BIRTH JULY 6, 1925, LICENSE NUMBER 00C5304 OF FORT WORTH, TX, WAS DISCIPLINED BY TEXAS ON JUNE 10, 1991
DISCIPLINARY ACTION: 60-MONTH PROBATION; MONITORING OF PHYSICIAN PERFORMANCE
OFFENSE: FAILURE TO COMPLY WITH PREVIOUS BOARD ORDER

NOTES: VIOLATED TERMS OF PREVIOUS BOARD ORDER; UNPROFESSIONAL OR DISHONORABLE CONDUCT LIKELY TO DECEIVE, DEFRAUD, OR INJURE THE PUBLIC. TERMS OF PROBATION: SHALL APPEAR ONCE A YEAR BEFORE THE BOARD; SHALL BE MONITORED BY BOARD APPROVED PHYSICIAN; SHALL ABSTAIN FROM CONSUMPTION OF ALCOHOL/CHEMICAL SUBSTANCES; SHALL IMMEDIATELY REPORT ANY USAGE OF ALCOHOL OR CHEMICAL SUBSTANCES NOT PRESCRIBED BY ANOTHER PHYSICIAN FOR A LEGITIMATE AND THERAPEUTIC CONDITION TO THE BOARD; SHALL PARTICIPATE IN AA; SHALL SUBMIT TO ALCOHOL OR DRUG SCREENS; SHALL CONTINUE TREATMENT WITH BOARD APPROVED PHYSICIAN; SHALL FURNISH WRITTEN REPORTS TO THE BOARD. ORDER TERMINATED ON 6/15/93; LICENSE FREE AND CLEAR OF ANY RESTRICTIONS.

WOMACK, JAMES C MD OF 1300 CEDAR, BANDERA, TX, WAS DISCIPLINED BY DEA ON FEBRUARY 5, 1993
DISCIPLINARY ACTION: DENIAL OF LICENSE REINSTATEMENT
OFFENSE: PRACTICING WITHOUT A VALID CONTROLLED SUBSTANCE LICENSE

NOTES: ON 12/16/91 HAD SURRENDERED DEA CERTIFICATE OF REGISTRATION BASED UPON PERSONAL ABUSE OF CONTROLLED SUBSTANCES; THEREFORE HE HAD NO AUTHORITY TO PRESCRIBE OR OTHERWISE HANDLE CONTROLLED SUBSTANCES, YET CONTINUED TO PRESCRIBE SUCH SUBSTANCES USING HIS FATHER'S DEA NUMBER. WHILE HE DID DEMONSTRATE REHABILITATION FROM SUBSTANCE ABUSE, HE FAILED TO DEMONSTRATE THAT HIS BEHAVIOR WAS IN ANY WAY JUSTIFIED OR THAT SUCH BEHAVIOR WAS NOT LIKELY TO RECUR. HOWEVER, GIVEN HIS REHABILITATION FROM SUBSTANCE ABUSE AND CONTRIBUTION IN MEDICALLY UNDERSERVED AREA, AN APPLICATION FOR DEA REGISTRATION MADE AFTER ONE YEAR WILL BE FAVORABLY CONSIDERED, PROVIDED NO ADDITIONAL EVIDENCE OF WRONGDOING.

WOMACK, JAMES CHANSLOR MD, LICENSE NUMBER G8516 OF BANDERA, TX, WAS DISCIPLINED BY TEXAS ON JANUARY 29, 1999
DISCIPLINARY ACTION: LICENSE SUSPENSION
OFFENSE: SUBSTANDARD CARE, INCOMPETENCE OR NEGLIGENCE

NOTES: ON 1/6/99 WAS ADMITTED TO THE EMERGENCY ROOM AND WAS TREATED FOR A CHEMICAL SUBSTANCE TOXICITY INCLUDING BUT NOT LIMITED TO ALCOHOL AND SOMA; ON OR APPROXIMATELY 1/18/99 HE SUBMITTED HIMSELF FOR ADMISSION FOR TREATMENT OF CHEMICAL DEPENDENCY AND DEPRESSION; HE HAS REPORTED TO THE BOARD THAT HE INTENDS TO FULLY COMPLETE EXTENSIVE TREATMENT FOR CHEMICAL DEPENDENCY AND DEPRESSION; ALSO ALLEGATIONS THAT HE FAILED TO SUPERVISE A PHYSICIAN ASSISTANT; FAILED TO MONITOR RESPONSES TO NARCOTIC ANALGESIA PRESCRIBED TO A PATIENT IN 9/98. SUSPENSION UNTIL HE REQUESTS TO HAVE THE SUSPENSION STAYED AND APPEARS BEFORE THE BOARD PROVIDING EVIDENCE THAT HE IS PHYSICALLY, MENTALLY AND OTHERWISE COMPETENT TO PRACTICE SAFELY INCLUDING BUT NOT LIMITED TO: SHALL HAVE COPIES OF PSYCHOLOGICAL ND NEUROPSYCHIATRIC EVALUATIONS CONDUCTED WITHIN 60 DAYS OF REQUEST TO HAVE SUSPENSION STAYED; SHALL COOPERATE WITH THE BOARD IN VERIFYING COMPLIANCE INCLUDING PROVIDING COPIES OF MEDICAL RELEASES UPON REQUEST; SHALL INFORM THE BOARD OF CHANGE OF ADDRESS WITHIN 10 DAYS; SHALL NOT SEEK MODIFICATION FOR ONE YEAR.

WOMACK, JAMES CHANSLOR MD OF 400 SHELBYVILLE STREET, CENTER, TX, WAS DISCIPLINED BY DEA ON MARCH 16, 1999
DISCIPLINARY ACTION: SURRENDER OF CONTROLLED SUBSTANCE LICENSE

NOTES: IN LIEU OF PUBLIC INTEREST REVOCATION.

WONNACOTT, JAMES BRIAN MD, LICENSE NUMBER 00F1313 OF PORTLAND, TX, WAS DISCIPLINED BY TEXAS ON JANUARY 6, 1995
DISCIPLINARY ACTION: REPRIMAND; REQUIRED TO TAKE ADDITIONAL MEDICAL EDUCATION
OFFENSE: PROFESSIONAL MISCONDUCT

NOTES: DESPITE RECEIVING WRITTEN REQUESTS, HE FAILED TO TIMELY PROVIDE MEDICAL RECORDS OF VARIOUS PATIENTS DURING OCTOBER THROUGH DECEMBER 1993 AND IN VARIOUS MONTHS IN 1994; DID NOT PROVIDE A WRITTEN EXPLANATION TO PATIENTS OR INCLUDE THIS IN THE WRITTEN RECORDS; MAINTAINS HE WAS UNABLE TO PROVIDE RECORDS DUE TO CHANGING OFFICE LOCATION AND IMPOUNDMENT OF RECORDS BY THE IRS IN 2/94; ALSO DURING THIS TIME PRESCRIBED VARIOUS MEDICATIONS OVER THE PHONE WITHOUT A PHYSICAL EXAM OR ACCESS TO THE MEDICAL RECORDS OF THE PATIENTS. CONDITIONS OF FIVE YEAR RESTRICTION: SHALL MAINTAIN ADEQUATE MEDICAL RECORDS ON ALL PATIENT OFFICE VISITS WHICH SHALL BE AVAILABLE FOR INSPECTION; SHALL BECOME FAMILIAR WITH AND

COMPLY WITH PROVISIONS OF THE MEDICAL PRACTICE ACT REGARDING TIMELY RELEASE OF MEDICAL RECORDS; SHALL ATTEND AT LEAST 50 HOURS PER YEAR OF CONTINUING MEDICAL EDUCATION INCLUDING AT LEAST 10 HOURS IN THE AREA OF RISK MANAGEMENT; WITHIN ONE YEAR SHALL TAKE AND PASS THE TEXAS MEDICAL JURISPRUDENCE EXAM; SHALL APPEAR BEFORE THE BOARD ONCE A YEAR OR UPON REQUEST; SHALL COOPERATE WITH THE BOARD IN VERIFYING COMPLIANCE; SHALL GIVE A COPY OF THIS ORDER TO ANY HEALTH CARE ENTITY WHERE HE HAS OR HAS APPLIED FOR PRIVILEGES OR ANYONE ELSE WHO REQUESTS IT; SHALL ENSURE INQUIRIES REGARDING HIS TEXAS LICENSURE STATUS ARE ANSWERED BY REFERENCING THIS ORDER; SHALL INFORM BOARD OF CHANGE OF ADDRESS WITHIN 10 DAYS OR IF HE LEAVES THE STATE; TIME SPENT OUT OF TEXAS DOES NOT COUNT TOWARD RESTRICTION. SHALL NOT SEEK MODIFICATION FOR ONE YEAR.

WONNACOTT, JAMES BRIAN MD, LICENSE NUMBER 00F1313 OF PORTLAND, TX, WAS DISCIPLINED BY TEXAS ON JANUARY 11, 1996
DISCIPLINARY ACTION: LICENSE SUSPENSION
OFFENSE: FAILURE TO COMPLY WITH PREVIOUS BOARD ORDER

NOTES: NONCOMPLIANCE TO AN ORDER DATED 1/06/95 BY FAILING TO SIT FOR THE MEDICAL JURISPRUDENCE EXAMINATION BEFORE 1/06/96. SUSPENSION UNTIL HE TAKES AND PASSES THE JURISPRUDENCE EXAMINATION AND THEREAFTER APPEARS BEFORE THE BOARD AND PROVIDES SUFFICIENT EVIDENCE TO SHOW THAT HE POSSESSES THE SKILLS AND KNOWLEDGE TO SAFELY PRACTICE MEDICINE.

WOOD, MARY JEAN MD OF 223 NORTHILL, SAN ANTONIO, TX, WAS DISCIPLINED BY DEA ON JUNE 26, 1998
DISCIPLINARY ACTION: SURRENDER OF CONTROLLED SUBSTANCE LICENSE

NOTES: IN LIEU OF PUBLIC INTEREST REVOCATION.

WOODBURN, RICHARD MD, LICENSE NUMBER 0A26567 OF SAN ANTONIO, TX, WAS DISCIPLINED BY CALIFORNIA ON JANUARY 9, 1995
DISCIPLINARY ACTION: SURRENDER OF LICENSE

NOTES: VOLUNTARY SURRENDER OF LICENSE WHILE CHARGES PENDING.

WOODBURN, RICHARD MD, DATE OF BIRTH MARCH 4, 1939, LICENSE NUMBER 1035788 OF 115 WESTCOURT LANE, SAN ANTONIO, TX, WAS DISCIPLINED BY MICHIGAN ON OCTOBER 20, 1995
DISCIPLINARY ACTION: 6-MONTH LICENSE SUSPENSION
OFFENSE: DISCIPLINARY ACTION BY ANOTHER STATE OR AGENCY

NOTES: FAILURE TO REPORT/COMPLY.

WOODBURN, RICHARD MD, DATE OF BIRTH MARCH 4, 1939 OF 115 WESTCOURT LANE, SAN ANTONIO, TX, WAS DISCIPLINED BY MEDICARE ON MARCH 3, 1996
DISCIPLINARY ACTION: EXCLUSION FROM THE MEDICARE AND/OR MEDICAID PROGRAM
OFFENSE: DISCIPLINARY ACTION BY ANOTHER STATE OR AGENCY

NOTES: SUSPENDED OR EXCLUDED BY A FEDERAL OR STATE HEALTH CARE PROGRAM FOR REASONS BEARING ON PROFESSIONAL COMPETENCE.

WOODS, THOMAS ALAN MD, LICENSE NUMBER 00D0354 OF DALLAS, TX, WAS DISCIPLINED BY TEXAS ON NOVEMBER 13, 1992
DISCIPLINARY ACTION: REPRIMAND
OFFENSE: PROFESSIONAL MISCONDUCT

NOTES: UNPROFESSIONAL OR DISHONORABLE CONDUCT THAT IS LIKELY TO DECEIVE, DEFRAUD OR INJURE THE PUBLIC.

WOODS, THOMAS ALAN MD, LICENSE NUMBER 00D0354 OF SPRINGFIELD, MO, WAS DISCIPLINED BY TEXAS ON MAY 15, 1996
DISCIPLINARY ACTION: SURRENDER OF LICENSE
OFFENSE: PROFESSIONAL MISCONDUCT

NOTES: ALLEGATIONS THAT HE HAS ENGAGED IN UNPROFESSIONAL AND DISHONORABLE CONDUCT LIKELY TO DECEIVE OR INJURE THE PUBLIC. VOLUNTARY AND PERMANENT SURRENDER OF LICENSE.

WOODWARD, ROBERT ALAN MD, DATE OF BIRTH FEBRUARY 28, 1957 OF MINDEN, LA, WAS DISCIPLINED BY LOUISIANA ON OCTOBER 22, 1992
DISCIPLINARY ACTION: LICENSE SUSPENSION; REQUIRED TO ENTER AN IMPAIRED PHYSICIAN PROGRAM OR SUBSTANCE ABUSE TREATMENT
OFFENSE: SUBSTANCE ABUSE

NOTES: HABITUAL OR RECURRING ABUSE OF DRUGS; PRESCRIBING, DISPENSING OR ADMINISTERING CONTROLLED SUBSTANCES WITHOUT LEGITIMATE MEDICAL JUSTIFICATION OR IN OTHER THAN A LEGAL OR LEGITIMATE MANNER. SUSPENDED PENDING SPECIFIED INPATIENT SUBSTANCE ABUSE TREATMENT. SUPERSEDING ORDER ENTERED 12/3/92 REINSTATING LICENSE ON PROBATION FOR FIVE YEARS SUBJECT TO CONTINUING AFTERCARE; PARTICIPATION IN IMPAIRED PHYSICIANS PROGRAM; ABSTINENCE FROM THE USE OF MOOD-ALTERING SUBSTANCES; LIFETIME PROHIBITION ON PRESCRIPTION, DISPENSATION OR ADMINISTRATION OF CONTROLLED SUBSTANCES; AND OBTAINING SPECIFIED CONTINUING MEDICAL EDUCATION.

WOODWARD, ROBERT ALAN MD, DATE OF BIRTH FEBRUARY 28, 1957, LICENSE NUMBER 00G8518 OF 211 CARROLLTON, SHREVEPORT, LA, WAS DISCIPLINED BY TEXAS ON JANUARY 29, 1993
DISCIPLINARY ACTION: 60-MONTH PROBATION; RESTRICTION PLACED ON CONTROLLED SUBSTANCE LICENSE
OFFENSE: DISCIPLINARY ACTION BY ANOTHER STATE OR AGENCY

NOTES: ACTION BASED ON THE 10/22/92 LOUISIANA ACTION FOR INTEMPERATE USE OF ALCOHOL OR DRUGS; UNPROFESSIONAL OR DISHONORABLE CONDUCT LIKELY TO DEFRAUD OR INJURE THE PUBLIC AND WRITING FALSE OR FICTITIOUS PRESCRIPTIONS FOR DANGEROUS DRUGS. 5 YEAR SUSPENSION STAYED. CONDITIONS OF PROBATION: WILL ABIDE BY THE CONDITIONS OF THE LOUISIANA PROBATION INCLUDING SHALL CONTINUE UNDER TREATMENT WITH QUARTERLY REPORTS; SHALL APPEAR BEFORE THE BOARD UPON REQUEST; LIFETIME PROHIBITION ON PRESCRIBING, DISPENSING OR ADMINISTERING ANY CONTROLLED SUBSTANCE EXCEPT FOR IN A HOSPITAL TO PROVIDE EMERGENCY SERVICES; LIFETIME ABSTINENCE FROM THE USE OF ANY MOOD-ALTERING SUBSTANCE EXCEPT AS PROVIDED BY ANOTHER PHYSICIAN FOR A LEGITIMATE MEDICAL PURPOSE; SHALL OBTAIN AT LEAST 50 HOURS WORTH OF CONTINUING MEDICAL EDUCATION PER YEAR. PRIOR TO PRACTICING IN TEXAS SHALL APPEAR BEFORE THE BOARD; SHALL INFORM THE BOARD IF HE LEAVES EITHER TEXAS OR LOUISIANA; TIME SPENT OUTSIDE THESE TWO STATES DOES NOT COUNT TOWARD PROBATION. SHALL NOT SEEK

MODIFICATION FOR 1 YEAR. ON 1/29/99 ORDER TERMINATED.

WOOLDRIDGE, DOUGLAS W MD, LICENSE NUMBER 0036792 OF 332 WASHINGTON ST, WELLESLEY, MA, WAS DISCIPLINED BY MASSACHUSETTS ON JUNE 12, 1996
DISCIPLINARY ACTION: REPRIMAND
OFFENSE: PROFESSIONAL MISCONDUCT

NOTES: LACK OF INFORMED CONSENT.

WOOLDRIDGE, DOUGLAS W MD, LICENSE NUMBER 36792 OF 332 WASHINGTON STREET, WELLESLEY, MA, WAS DISCIPLINED BY MASSACHUSETTS ON NOVEMBER 7, 1997
DISCIPLINARY ACTION: RESTRICTION PLACED ON LICENSE

NOTES: VOLUNTARY PRACTICE RESTRICTIONS.

WOOLDRIDGE, DOUGLAS W MD, LICENSE NUMBER 36792 OF 332 WASHINGTON STREET, WELLESLEY, MA, WAS DISCIPLINED BY MASSACHUSETTS ON MARCH 3, 1999
DISCIPLINARY ACTION: PROBATION
OFFENSE: SUBSTANDARD CARE, INCOMPETENCE OR NEGLIGENCE

NOTES: ENGAGED IN MISLEADING ADVERTISING; FAILED TO MAINTAIN MEDICAL RECORDS FOR THE REQUISITE TIME; PRESCRIBED SCHEDULE II CONTROLLED SUBSTANCES TO HIMSELF AND AN IMMEDIATE FAMILY MEMBER; ENGAGED IN CONDUCT WHICH PLACED INTO QUESTION HIS COMPETENCE TO PRACTICE MEDICINE BY ADMINISTERING CONSCIOUS SEDATION WITHOUT THE ASSISTANCE OF ADEQUATELY TRAINED PERSONNEL AND WITHOUT ADEQUATE DOCUMENTATION IN HIS SURGICAL RECORD; AND, USED LIQUID SILICONE SUBCUTANEOUSLY ON PATIENTS. SUSPENSION STAYED.

WOOLDRIDGE, DOUGLAS W ` MD, LICENSE NUMBER F0835 OF WELLESLEY, MA, WAS DISCIPLINED BY TEXAS ON AUGUST 28, 1999
DISCIPLINARY ACTION: SURRENDER OF LICENSE
OFFENSE: DISCIPLINARY ACTION BY ANOTHER STATE OR AGENCY

NOTES: ON 3/3/99 HE WAS DISCIPLINED BY THE MASSACHUSETTS BOARD FOR: MISLEADING ADVERTISING; INJECTING LIQUID SILICONE AT A TIME WHEN SUCH COURSE OF ACTION WAS UNAPPROVED BY THE FDA; ADMINISTERING INTRAVENOUS CONSCIOUS SEDATION WITHOUT EITHER PROPER ASSISTANCE OR PROPER DOCUMENTATION; IMPROPERLY PRESCRIBING DEMEROL TO HIS WIFE; FAILING TO MAINTAIN A PATIENT'S MEDICAL RECORDS FOR THE REQUISITE PERIOD OF TIME; AND PRACTICING MEDICINE WHILE HIS ABILITY TO PRACTICE WAS IMPAIRED BY DRUGS OR PHYSICAL DISABILITY. VOLUNTARY AND PERMANENT SURRENDER.

WOOLDRIDGE, DOUGLAS WAYNE MD, LICENSE NUMBER G47485 OF WELLESLEY, MA, WAS DISCIPLINED BY CALIFORNIA ON MAY 12, 1998
DISCIPLINARY ACTION: REPRIMAND
OFFENSE: PROFESSIONAL MISCONDUCT

NOTES: DISCIPLINED BY MASSACHUSETTS FOR TESTING A PATIENT FOR THE PRESENCE OF THE HTLV-III ANTIBODY OR ANTIGEN WITHOUT FIRST OBTAINING THE PATIENT'S WRITTEN INFORMED CONSENT.

WRIGHT, ARTHUR GLENN JR MD, DATE OF BIRTH JANUARY 16, 1929, LICENSE NUMBER 00C3922 OF 4225 DRIFTWOOD, CORPUS CHRISTI, TX, WAS DISCIPLINED BY TEXAS ON JANUARY 29, 1993
DISCIPLINARY ACTION: REPRIMAND
OFFENSE: NONCOMPLIANCE WITH A PROFESSIONAL RULE

NOTES: FROM 4/86 TO 4/92 FOR ONE PATIENT HE FAILED TO KEEP ADEQUATE RECORDS CONCERNING MEDICAL CONDITION OR PRESCRIBED MEDICATIONS; ALSO FAILED TO DOCUMENT WHETHER EFFORTS WERE MADE TO CONSULT OTHER PHYSICIANS CONCERNING THIS PATIENT'S INCONTINENCE, GASTRIC ULCERS, DUMPING SYNDROME OR SEVERE ARTHRITIS. SHALL GIVE A COPY OF THIS ORDER TO ANY HEALTH CARE ENTITY WHERE HE HAS PRIVILEGES; SHALL COOPERATE WITH THE BOARD IN VERIFYING COMPLIANCE; SHALL INFORM BOARD OF CHANGE OF ADDRESS WITHIN 10 DAYS.

WRIGHT, ARTHUR GLENN MD OF 4225 DRIFTWOOD, CORPUS CHRISTI, TX, WAS DISCIPLINED BY DEA ON MAY 8, 1996
DISCIPLINARY ACTION: RESTRICTION PLACED ON CONTROLLED SUBSTANCE LICENSE
OFFENSE: PROFESSIONAL MISCONDUCT

NOTES: ALLEGED CONTROLLED SUBSTANCE ACT VIOLATIONS.

WRIGHT, JOHN L JR MD, LICENSE NUMBER 00B8970 OF BIG LAKE, TX, WAS DISCIPLINED BY TEXAS ON JANUARY 24, 1992
DISCIPLINARY ACTION: SURRENDER OF LICENSE

NOTES: INABILITY TO PRACTICE MEDICINE WITH REASONABLE SKILL AND SAFETY TO PATIENTS. LICENSE PERMANENTLY RETIRED IN LIEU OF FURTHER DISCIPLINARY ACTION.

WYCKOFF, STUART M MD, WAS DISCIPLINED BY NEVADA ON JANUARY 19, 1991
DISCIPLINARY ACTION: RESTRICTION PLACED ON LICENSE; REPRIMAND
OFFENSE: SUBSTANDARD CARE, INCOMPETENCE OR NEGLIGENCE

NOTES: TREATED PATIENTS IN A MATTER NOT RECOGNIZED SCIENTIFICALLY AS BEING BENEFICIAL, FAILED TO EXERCISE SKILL OR DILIGENCE, SPECIFICALLY IN THE AREA OF ADOLESCENT PSYCHIATRY, REPEATED MALPRACTICE. CANNOT PROVIDE PSYCHIATRIC TREATMENT TO ANY PERSON UNDER 18; LICENSE STATUS INACTIVE FOR 3 YEARS SUBJECT TO CONDITIONS FOR REINSTATEMENT TO ACTIVE STATUS.

WYCKOFF, STUART M MD, LICENSE NUMBER 00E2955 OF FORT FAIRFIELD, ME, WAS DISCIPLINED BY TEXAS ON OCTOBER 5, 1991
DISCIPLINARY ACTION: 60-MONTH PROBATION; RESTRICTION PLACED ON LICENSE
OFFENSE: DISCIPLINARY ACTION BY ANOTHER STATE OR AGENCY

NOTES: MAINE BOARD FOUND THAT DURING HIS TREATMENT OF ADOLESCENT PATIENTS WHILE PRACTICING AS A PSYCHIATRIST IN THE STATE OF NEVADA, HE VIOLATED STANDARDS OF PROFESSIONAL BEHAVIOR IN THE PRACTICE OF PSYCHIATRY, INCLUDING THE INAPPROPRIATE USE OF PROFANITY, CONFRONTATIONAL STYLE, AND EXTREME AND INAPPROPRIATE DISCIPLINARY MEASURES; LICENSE RESTRICTED IN BOTH MAINE AND NEVADA. FIVE YEAR SUSPENSION STAYED, PROBATION ISSUED UNDER FOLLOWING CONDITIONS: SHALL TREAT NO INVOLUNTARY PATIENTS IN ANY PRACTICE SETTING; SHALL TREAT ONLY THOSE PATIENTS WHO SEEK HIS SERVICES INTENTIONALLY WITHOUT COERCION OF ANY KIND; SHALL NOT PROVIDE PROFESSIONAL TREATMENT TO ANY PERSON UNDER THE AGE OF 18 IN ANY PRACTICE SETTING EXCEPT UNDER CERTAIN CONDITIONS, INCLUDING GROUP OR FAMILY THERAPY; SUPERVISORY ROLE LIMITED TO ADMINISTRATIVE PERSONNEL; SHALL PROVIDE TEXAS

WITH COPIES OF REPORTS SENT TO MAINE; MUST APPEAR BEFORE BOARD BEFORE PRACTICING; TIME SPENT OUTSIDE OF TEXAS OR MAINE DOES NOT COUNT TOWARD PROBATION; SHALL COOPERATE WITH BOARD IN VERIFYING COMPLIANCE; SHALL APPEAR BEFORE BOARD ONCE A YEAR; MAY FILE FOR TERMINATION OF ORDER AFTER 8/1/92.

WYCKOFF, STUART MORELY MD, DATE OF BIRTH OCTOBER 13, 1949, LICENSE NUMBER 0013113 OF PO BOX 612, FORT FAIRFIELD, ME, WAS DISCIPLINED BY MAINE ON MAY 31, 1991
DISCIPLINARY ACTION: RESTRICTION PLACED ON LICENSE
OFFENSE: PROFESSIONAL MISCONDUCT

NOTES: ISSUED MODIFIED, CONDITIONAL LICENSE BASED ON UNPROFESSIONAL CONDUCT ALLEGED TO HAVE OCCURRED IN NEVADA.

YASHAR, JAMES J MD, LICENSE NUMBER 0003910 OF ONE RANDALL SQUARE, PROVIDENCE, RI, WAS DISCIPLINED BY RHODE ISLAND ON AUGUST 11, 1993
DISCIPLINARY ACTION: REPRIMAND; MONITORING OF PHYSICIAN PERFORMANCE
OFFENSE: LOSS OR RESTRICTION OF HOSPITAL PRIVILEGES

NOTES: VIOLATED A HOSPITAL OPEN HEART SURGERY GUIDELINE WHICH STATES THAT "ONE OF THE DESIGNATED CARDIAC SURGEONS WILL BE PHYSICALLY PRESENT IN THE HOSPITAL AFTER AN OPEN HEART SURGICAL CASE UNTIL THE PATIENT IS STABLE AND WILL REMAIN AVAILABLE FOR ANY EMERGENCY. THIS IN-HOUSE COVERAGE WILL BE CONTINUED WHEN THE PATIENT IS UNSTABLE, OR IF THE CARDIAC PHYSICIAN ASSISTANT IS UNAVAILABLE OR NEEDS ASSISTANCE IN CARING FOR A HEART PATIENT;" HOSPITAL SUSPENDED HIS PRIVILEGES FOR 20 DAYS AND SUBSEQUENTLY REACHED AN AGREEMENT WITH HIM TO REDEFINE HIS WORKLOAD. BOARD SHALL MONITOR COMPLIANCE WITH HOSPITAL AGREEMENT THROUGH QUARTERLY REPORTS WHICH MUST BE SENT TO THE BOARD BY THE HOSPITAL AND THE PHYSICIAN'S HEALTH COMMITTEE. MAY PETITION BOARD FOR RELIEF FROM RESTRICTIONS UPON SHOWING THAT AN ACCEPTABLE SURGICAL ASSISTANT HAS BEEN RECRUITED. ADMINISTRATIVE FEE OF $1,500 SHALL BE PAYABLE WITHIN 60 DAYS. ON 8/10/94 HE WAS GRANTED RELIEF FROM RESTRICTIONS.

YASHAR, JAMES J MD, LICENSE NUMBER 0035150 OF 1 RANDALL SQUARE, PROVIDENCE, RI, WAS DISCIPLINED BY MASSACHUSETTS ON NOVEMBER 30, 1994
DISCIPLINARY ACTION: REPRIMAND
OFFENSE: DISCIPLINARY ACTION BY ANOTHER STATE OR AGENCY

NOTES: DISCIPLINE BY RHODE ISLAND; MISCONDUCT, GENERAL.

YASHAR, JAMES JAMSHID MD, LICENSE NUMBER 00D4367 OF PROVIDENCE, RI, WAS DISCIPLINED BY TEXAS ON JANUARY 6, 1995
DISCIPLINARY ACTION: SURRENDER OF LICENSE
OFFENSE: DISCIPLINARY ACTION BY ANOTHER STATE OR AGENCY

NOTES: ON 4/30/93 ENTERED A CONSENT ORDER WITH RHODE ISLAND CONSTITUTING A PUBLIC REPRIMAND FOR FAILING TO MAINTAIN STANDARDS ESTABLISHED BY PEER REVIEW REQUIRING THAT AFTER AN OPEN HEART SURGICAL CASE, THE SURGEON WILL BE PHYSICALLY PRESENT IN THE HOSPITAL UNTIL THE PATIENT IS STABLE; HAS NO INTENTION OF PRACTICING IN TEXAS IN THE IMMEDIATE FUTURE; IN LIEU OF FURTHER INVESTIGATION OR HEARING. MAY PETITION FOR REINSTATEMENT.

YENTIS, RICHARD MD OF 1501 MERRIMAC CIRCLE #210, FORT WORTH, TX, WAS DISCIPLINED BY DEA ON JANUARY 6, 1998
DISCIPLINARY ACTION: SURRENDER OF CONTROLLED SUBSTANCE LICENSE

YENTIS, RICHARD D MD, LICENSE NUMBER 11392 OF FORT WORTH, TX, WAS DISCIPLINED BY FLORIDA ON SEPTEMBER 11, 1998
DISCIPLINARY ACTION: SURRENDER OF LICENSE
OFFENSE: CRIMINAL CONVICTION OR PLEA OF GUILTY, NOLO CONTENDERE, OR NO CONTEST TO A CRIME

NOTES: CHARGED WITH BEING FOUND GUILTY OF A CRIME DIRECTLY RELATING TO THE PRACTICE OF MEDICINE. VOLUNTARY SURRENDER WITH AGREEMENT NEVER TO REAPPLY FOR A FLORIDA LICENSE.

YENTIS, RICHARD D MD, LICENSE NUMBER C27959 OF FORT WORTH, TX, WAS DISCIPLINED BY CALIFORNIA ON MARCH 1, 1999
DISCIPLINARY ACTION: SURRENDER OF LICENSE

NOTES: WHILE CHARGES PENDING.

YENTIS, RICHARD DAVID MD, LICENSE NUMBER D5333 OF FORT WORTH, TX, WAS DISCIPLINED BY TEXAS ON AUGUST 9, 1997
DISCIPLINARY ACTION: LICENSE REVOCATION
OFFENSE: CRIMINAL CONVICTION OR PLEA OF GUILTY, NOLO CONTENDERE, OR NO CONTEST TO A CRIME

NOTES: ON OR ABOUT 1/13/97 HE WAS FOUND GUILTY OF 13 COUNTS OF FRAUD IN A SCHEME TO FILE FALSE INSURANCE CLAIMS; HE PLED "NOT GUILTY" AND IS APPEALING THE DECISION; THE COUNTS OF CONVICTION INVOLVE THE BILLING OF GOVERNMENT AND NONGOVERNMENT INSURANCE COMPANIES FOR LATE, CANCELED AND MISSED APPOINTMENTS.

YENTIS, RICHARD DAVID MD, DATE OF BIRTH JUNE 24, 1938 OF PO BOX 1500 #27500-077 FCI, EL RENO, TX, WAS DISCIPLINED BY MEDICARE ON OCTOBER 5, 1997
DISCIPLINARY ACTION: 96-MONTH EXCLUSION FROM THE MEDICARE AND/OR MEDICAID PROGRAM
OFFENSE: CRIMINAL CONVICTION OR PLEA OF GUILTY, NOLO CONTENDERE, OR NO CONTEST TO A CRIME

NOTES: CONVICTED OF A CRIME RELATED TO THE DELIVERY OF HEALTH CARE OR FINANCIAL MISCONDUCT INVOLVING A GOVERNMENT-OPERATED PROGRAM.

YENTIS, RICHARD DAVID MD, DATE OF BIRTH JUNE 24, 1938, LICENSE NUMBER 008581E OF 1501 MERRIMAC, FORT WORTH, TX, WAS DISCIPLINED BY PENNSYLVANIA ON NOVEMBER 18, 1997
DISCIPLINARY ACTION: SURRENDER OF LICENSE
OFFENSE: CRIMINAL CONVICTION OR PLEA OF GUILTY, NOLO CONTENDERE, OR NO CONTEST TO A CRIME

NOTES: FELONY CONVICTION FOR MAIL FRAUD AND/OR AIDING AND ABETTING IN MAIL FRAUD FOR FILING CLAIMS FOR SERVICES NOT RENDERED. VOLUNTARY SURRENDER.

YERGER, DAVID H MD, LICENSE NUMBER 0014447 OF PO BOX 5249, BILOXI, MS, WAS DISCIPLINED BY GEORGIA ON JULY 1, 1992
DISCIPLINARY ACTION: NONRENEWAL OF LICENSE
OFFENSE: DISCIPLINARY ACTION BY ANOTHER STATE OR AGENCY

NOTES: DISCIPLINARY ACTION IN AIR FORCE. ADMINISTRATIVE REVOCATION FOR FAILURE TO RENEW.

YERGER, DAVID H MD, DATE OF BIRTH DECEMBER 12, 1939, LICENSE NUMBER 0011884 OF HCR3, BOX 22 QUAIL RUN I, DEL RIO,

TX, WAS DISCIPLINED BY MISSISSIPPI ON JANUARY 21, 1993
OFFENSE: LOSS OR RESTRICTION OF HOSPITAL PRIVILEGES

NOTES: DISCIPLINARY ACTION TAKEN AGAINST STAFF PRIVILEGES AT KEESLER MEDICAL CENTER IN BILOXI, MS; ACTION IN CALIFORNIA. PROVISIONS INCLUDE: IF HE CHOOSES TO RETURN TO MISSISSIPPI TO PRACTICE MEDICINE, SHALL NOTIFY THE BOARD IN WRITING PRIOR TO DOING SO; SHALL APPEAR BEFORE THE BOARD. BOARD MAY PLACE ANY AND ALL RESTRICTIONS WHICH IT DEEMS NECESSARY TO DETERMINE HIS COMPETENCY TO PRACTICE MEDICINE AND TO PROTECT THE PUBLIC, INCLUDING BUT NOT LIMITED TO, LIMITATIONS ON LICENSEE'S SURGICAL PRACTICE/PRIVILEGES AND/OR RESTRICTIONS TO PRACTICE PRIMARY CARE.

YOUNG, ALAN W DO, DATE OF BIRTH AUGUST 8, 1954 OF SAN ANTONIO, TX, WAS DISCIPLINED BY IOWA ON AUGUST 1, 1990
DISCIPLINARY ACTION: DENIAL OF NEW LICENSE

NOTES: APPLICATION FOR LICENSURE DENIED DUE TO INELIGIBILITY.

ZAVALA, ALFONSO G MD, DATE OF BIRTH SEPTEMBER 8, 1952 OF 7665 PHOENIX #1127, HOUSTON, TX, WAS DISCIPLINED BY MEDICARE ON MAY 12, 1992
DISCIPLINARY ACTION: EXCLUSION FROM THE MEDICARE AND/OR MEDICAID PROGRAM
OFFENSE: NONCOMPLIANCE WITH A PROFESSIONAL RULE

NOTES: DEFAULT ON HEALTH EDUCATION LOAN OR SCHOLARSHIP OBLIGATIONS.

ZEPEDA, RUSSELL WAYNE MD, LICENSE NUMBER H0977 OF MAMMOTH SPRINGS, AR, WAS DISCIPLINED BY TEXAS ON MAY 14, 1999
DISCIPLINARY ACTION: 60-MONTH PROBATION; REQUIRED TO TAKE ADDITIONAL MEDICAL EDUCATION
OFFENSE: OVERPRESCRIBING OR MISPRESCRIBING DRUGS

NOTES: IN 6/97 THE BOARD RECEIVED INFORMATION THAT HE HAD WRITTEN AND CALLED IN PRESCRIPTIONS FOR DIET MEDICATIONS FOR FOUR INDIVIDUALS AT LEAST ONE OF WHOM HE HAD NOT SEEN; IN ONE CASE A PHARMACY REFUSED TO FILL A PRESCRIPTION FOR FASTIN; HE COULD NOT PRODUCE ANY MEDICAL RECORDS OR ADEQUATE MEDICAL DOCUMENTATION REGARDING ANY OF THESE PERSONS; HE CLAIMS THAT THE CLINIC WHERE THE RECORDS WERE KEPT HAS BEEN DISSOLVED, HOWEVER HE LEFT THE CLINIC IN 12/96 AND THE PRESCRIBING PERIOD IN QUESTION IS 1997; HE STATES THAT IT IS HIS PRACTICE TO NOT FILL IN THE DATE AND/OR PATIENT'S ADDRESS FOR A PRESCRIPTION AS HE EXPECTS THE ER NURSE TO PROPERLY FILL OUT THE PRESCRIPTION; HE ADMITS TO EXHIBITING POOR JUDGMENT, AND HAS PROVIDED INFORMATION REGARDING THE CRIMINAL BACKGROUND AND ACTIVITIES OF TWO OF THE INDIVIDUALS. SUSPENSION STAYED FOR PROBATION WITH THE FOLLOWING TERMS AND CONDITIONS: SHALL NOT TREAT OR OTHERWISE SERVE AS PHYSICIAN, PRESCRIBE, DISPENSE OR ADMINISTER DRUGS THAT MAY BE SUBJECT TO ABUSE TO HIMSELF OR TO ANY MEMBER OF HIS FAMILY; SEPARATE FROM PATIENT RECORDS, SHALL MAINTAIN A LOGBOOK OF EVERY PRESCRIPTION WRITTEN BY HIM FOR DANGEROUS DRUGS WITH ADDICTIVE POTENTIAL WHICH SHALL BE MADE AVAILABLE FOR REVIEW; SHALL OBTAIN 1 ETHICS COURSE PER YEAR FOR FIVE YEARS; WITHIN 1 YEAR SHALL TAKE AND PASS WITH A SCORE OF 75 OR ABOVE, WITHIN 3 ATTEMPTS, THE MEDICAL JURISPRUDENCE EXAM; SHALL EXAMINE AND/OR TREAT PATIENTS WHERE A FORM STATES THAT HE HAS OR WHEN AN INITIAL DIAGNOSIS IS MADE; SHALL OBTAIN 50 HOURS PER YEAR OF CONTINUING MEDICAL EDUCATION INCLUDING AT LEAST ONE COURSE IN RISK MANAGEMENT AND ONE IN ADDICTIONOLOGY; SHALL MAINTAIN ADEQUATE MEDICAL RECORDS WHICH SHALL BE AVAILABLE FOR REVIEW; SHALL COOPERATE WITH THE BOARD IN VERIFYING COMPLIANCE; SHALL APPEAR BEFORE THE BOARD AT LEAST ONCE A YEAR; TIME SPENT OUT OF TEXAS DOES NOT COUNT TOWARD PROBATION; SHALL INFORM THE BOARD OF CHANGE OF ADDRESS WITHIN 10 DAYS OR IF HE LEAVES THE STATE; SHALL NOT SEEK MODIFICATION FOR ONE YEAR.

ZINGERY, LEWIS W MD, LICENSE NUMBER 00F4724, WAS DISCIPLINED BY TEXAS ON AUGUST 17, 1996
DISCIPLINARY ACTION: 60-MONTH PROBATION; RESTRICTION PLACED ON CONTROLLED SUBSTANCE LICENSE
OFFENSE: OVERPRESCRIBING OR MISPRESCRIBING DRUGS

NOTES: HISTORY OF SUBSTANCE ABUSE INVOLVING ALCOHOL AND CODEINE COMPOUNDS WHICH RESULTED IN INPATIENT TREATMENT IN JANUARY 1991 AND FEBRUARY 1993; REPORTS A SOBRIETY DATE OF 1/13/93 AND FROM ABOUT FEBRUARY 1993 THROUGH OCTOBER 1994 PRESCRIBED VARIOUS MEDICATIONS TO MULTIPLE PATIENTS WITHOUT ADEQUATE INDICATIONS OR WITHOUT ADEQUATE DOCUMENTED INDICATIONS; MEDICATIONS PRESCRIBED INCLUDED CODEINE; SOME OF THE PATIENTS WERE MEMBERS OF HIS FAMILY. SUSPENSION STAYED. CONDITIONS OF PROBATION: SHALL ABSTAIN FROM THE CONSUMPTION OF ALCOHOL/DRUGS IN ANY FORM UNLESS PRESCRIBED BY ANOTHER PHYSICIAN FOR A LEGITIMATE AND THERAPEUTIC PURPOSE; SHALL SUBMIT HIMSELF TO APPROPRIATE EXAMS, INCLUDING DRUG OR ALCOHOL SCREENS; SHALL SUBMIT HIMSELF FOR EVALUATION AND TREATMENT TO A BOARD APPROVED PSYCHIATRIST WHO HE SHALL SEE AT LEAST ONCE A MONTH AND WHO SHALL MAKE REPORTS TO THE BOARD; SHALL PARTICIPATE IN AA'S PROGRAM NOT LESS THAN TWO TIMES PER WEEK WITH QUARTERLY REPORTS TO THE BOARD; SHALL NOT TREAT OR OTHERWISE SERVE AS PHYSICIAN, PRESCRIBE, DISPENSE OR ADMINISTER DRUGS THAT MAY BE SUBJECT TO ABUSE TO HIMSELF OR TO ANY MEMBER OF HIS FAMILY; EXCEPT FOR SCHEDULE IV AND V CONTROLLED SUBSTANCES, SHALL NOT PRESCRIBE, ADMINISTER, ORDER, OR DISPENSE CONTROLLED SUBSTANCES TO ANY PATIENT UNLESS THE MEDICATION IS PROVIDED IN A HOSPITAL SETTING OR FACILITY THAT HAS AN ORGANIZED MEDICAL STAFF AND IS LICENSED TO PROVIDE HOSPITAL OR OUT-PATIENT SURGERY AND ONLY FOR PREOPERATIVE AND POSTOPERATIVE PAIN RELIEF FOR GYNECOLOGY/OBSTETRICS PATIENTS OR FOR THE PURPOSES OF EMERGENCY CARE AND ONLY TO THE EXTENT NECESSARY TO ADDRESS THE IMMEDIATE NEEDS OF SUCH PATIENTS; SHALL MAINTAIN A LOG OF ALL CONTROLLED SUBSTANCES OR DANGEROUS DRUGS WITH ADDICTIVE POTENTIAL OR POTENTIAL FOR ABUSE HE PRESCRIBED WHICH SHALL BE MADE AVAILABLE UPON BOARD REQUEST; SHALL NOT TELEPHONE OR AUTHORIZE TELEPHONE PRESCRIPTIONS FOR THESE DRUGS; SHALL REFRAIN FROM THE PRESCRIPTION OR ADMINISTRATION OF ANY DRUG FOR ANY PATIENT UNLESS THE DRUG IS MEDICALLY INDICATED AND IS PRESCRIBED IN THERAPEUTIC DOSES; SHALL CONDUCT ADEQUATE FOLLOW-UP EXAMINATIONS ON ALL PATIENTS TO DETERMINE WHETHER THE COURSE OF TREATMENT, INCLUDING THE PRESCRIPTION OF DRUGS, IS APPROPRIATE; SHALL MAINTAIN ADEQUATE MEDICAL

RECORDS WHICH SHALL BE AVAILABLE FOR REVIEW; SHALL NOT SIGN OR INDICATE IN ANY MANNER IN PATIENT RECORDS THAT HE HAS SEEN PATIENTS UNLESS HE ACTUALLY HAS SEEN AND EXAMINED THE PATIENTS UNLESS IT IS CLEARLY NOTED THAT HE DID NOT PERSONALLY EXAMINE THE PATIENT; SHALL OBTAIN AT LEAST 50 HOURS PER YEAR OF CONTINUING MEDICAL EDUCATION AND SHALL SUBMIT PROOF TO THE BOARD; WITHIN SIX MONTHS SHALL ENROLL IN AND SUCCESSFULLY COMPLETE A BOARD APPROVED COURSE IN THE AREA OF APPROPRIATE PRESCRIBING OF CONTROLLED SUBSTANCES OR OTHER DRUGS WITH ADDICTIVE POTENTIAL AND SUBMIT PROOF TO THE BOARD; SHALL APPEAR BEFORE THE BOARD AT LEAST ONCE A YEAR OR UPON BOARD REQUEST; SHALL COOPERATE WITH THE BOARD IN VERIFYING COMPLIANCE INCLUDING PROVIDING COPIES OF MEDICAL RELEASES AND PEER REVIEW RECORDS UPON REQUEST; SHALL GIVE A COPY OF THIS ORDER TO ANY HEALTH CARE ENTITY WHERE HE HAS PRIVILEGES; TIME PERIOD OUT OF TEXAS DOES NOT COUNT TOWARD PROBATION; SHALL INFORM THE BOARD OF CHANGE OF ADDRESS WITHIN 10 DAYS OF IF HE LEAVES THE STATE; SHALL NOT SEEK MODIFICATION FOR ONE YEAR. ON 8/22/98 PETITION TO TERMINATE ORDER DENIED; ORDER MODIFIED DELETING LIMITATION OF HIS PRESCRIBING PRIVILEGES TO CONTROLLED SUBSTANCES IN SCHEDULES IV AND V. ON 10/15/99 PETITION TO TERMINATE ORDER DENIED; ORDER MODIFIED DELETING REQUIREMENTS OF CONTINUED PSYCHIATRIC TREATMENT AND A LOGBOOK OF CONTROLLED SUBSTANCE AND DANGEROUS DRUG PRESCRIPTIONS.

ZUAZU, GREGORIO B MD, LICENSE NUMBER 0039137 OF KINGWOOD, TX, WAS DISCIPLINED BY FLORIDA ON MAY 7, 1991
DISCIPLINARY ACTION: FINE; REPRIMAND
OFFENSE: PROVIDING FALSE INFORMATION TO THE BOARD OR OTHER HEALTH AGENCY

NOTES: FOUND GUILTY OF RENEWAL OF LICENSE BY FRAUDULENT MISREPRESENTATION IN THAT HE FALSELY CERTIFIED THAT HE COMPLETED THE CONTINUING MEDICAL EDUCATION REQUIREMENTS FOR LICENSE RENEWAL; VIOLATING A BOARD RULE IN THAT HE FAILED TO COMPLETE CONTINUING MEDICAL EDUCATION COURSES IN RESPONSE TO BOARD'S RANDOM AUDIT. MUST PAY $100O FINE AND SUBMIT DOCUMENTATION TO DEMONSTRATE COMPLETION OF ALL CONTINUING MEDICAL EDUCATION REQUIREMENTS FOR 1988-89 BIENNIUM WITHIN 6 MONTHS; DOCUMENT COMPLETION OF CONTINUING MEDICAL EDUCATION REQUIREMENTS WITH CERTIFICATES FOR 1990-91 BIENNIUM.

Public Citizen

Buyers Up • Congress Watch • Critical Mass • Global Trade Watch • Health Research Group • Litigation Group
Joan Claybrook, President

30+ Years of Consumer Activism

Dear Friend,

The year 2001 marks 30 years since a hardy group of enterprising young people came to the nation's capital to start an experiment in citizenship. The first "Nader's Raiders" showed special grit, integrity, and idealism that still serve us. You hold in your hands a book that is an example of the important work we do every day. Public Citizen is the only organization with the courage to write *Questionable Doctors*, because we are a completely independent organization representing citizens and consumers. I am writing to ask all buyers of *Questionable Doctors* to please help us continue this work by joining *Public Citizen* today.

When you join Public Citizen with a gift of $35 or more you'll get our monthly *Health Letter,* which will update you with new information important to your health and safety. You'll also receive our bi-monthly member publication *Public Citizen News*, which will keep you abreast of issues affecting citizens across the country.

We've helped purge cancer-producing additives from dozens of food products. We've pushed OSHA so that workplaces have fewer safety and health hazards. Many ineffective, unsafe drugs and medical devices have been forced from the market as a result of our tireless efforts. We have helped force government decision-making out of the smoke-filled back rooms. Still there is so much left to do.

We need to remove the flood of soft money polluting our political system, stop federal give-aways to corporate fat cats, rewrite unfair trade legislation that hurts American workers and weakens our environmental laws, pass new and improved laws to protect our health and safety, and compel federal agencies to enforce the laws we already have. *But we can't do it without you.*

To retain its independence, Public Citizen does not accept government or corporate funds. Our support comes from individual members who believe there should be full-time advocates of democratic principles working on their behalf and from foundation grants and publication sales. To remain effective, Public Citizen needs you. Please join us. As Ralph Nader reminds us, "together we *can* make a difference."

Sincerely,

Joan Claybrook

Joan Claybrook
President

Ralph Nader, Founder

1600 20th Street NW • Washington, DC 20009-1001 • (202) 588-1000
www.citizen.org

Public Citizen

Corporations, trade associations and other special interest groups send lobbyists to Washington, D.C., to advance their very particular agendas. Most speak for business or industry.

Public Citizen speaks for you—
before Congress
in the courts,
in the hallways and offices of
federal regulatory agencies

Ralph Nader founded Public Citizen to empower ordinary citizens with a voice in the halls of power and to protect the rights of consumers.

Public Citizen exposes threats to health and safety and presses for freedom of information and public disclosure. We've won important victories for citizens and consumers on issues concerning health care, injury prevention, campaign finance reform, cutting corporate subsidies, and fair trade.

Join together with thousands of other like-minded citizens, and you can help transform many issues at the national level.

"There can be no daily democracy without daily citizenship."

—Ralph Nader, founder of Public Citizen

1971

■ Public Citizen founded by Ralph Nader as an organization dedicated to protecting health, safety and democracy.

1972

■ Public Citizen files lawsuit resulting in new compensation system for airline passengers on overbooked flights.

■ Public Citizen plays key role in creation of Consumer Product Safety Commission.

1973

■ In response to Public Citizen's suit, President Nixon's firing of Watergate prosecutor Archibald Cox is ruled illegal.

1974

■ Public Citizen persuades Congress to override President Ford's veto and pass major improvements to Freedom of Information Act.

1975

■ Public Citizen wins Supreme Court ruling forbidding lawyers and other professionals from price fixing.

■ Public Citizen successfully lobbies Congress for energy conservation legislation, including fuel economy requirements for cars.

1976

■ FDA bans Red Dye No. 2 after Public Citizen's four-year campaign against the carcinogenic food dye.

■ Public Citizen petition leads to FDA ban on use of cancer-causing chloroform in cough medicines and toothpaste.

1977

■ Public Citizen mobilizes citizens who persuade President Carter to halt construction of Clinch River breeder reactor.

■ Public Citizen challenges airline industry's failure to provide adequate seating for nonsmokers.

1978

■ Congress passes Public Citizen's National Consumer Cooperative Bill authorizing $300 million in seed money for consumer cooperatives.

■ Public Citizen is instrumental in stopping the spraying of DDT in airline passenger cabins to control Japanese beetles on California-bound flights.

1979

■ Public Citizen petition leads to an Environmental Protection Agency ban on use of DBCP, a pesticide proven to cause sterility in men.

■ Public Citizen helps defeat legislation raising sugar price supports, thereby saving consumers $300 million a year.

1980

■ Public Citizen publishes best-selling *Pills That Don't Work*, a consumer guide to ineffective drugs.

■ Public Citizen plays critical role in passage of Superfund law, which requires cleanup of toxic waste sites.

■ Public Citizen lawsuit forces government to keep records of closed-door proceedings of Chrysler bailout.

1981

■ Public Citizen helps thwart President Reagan's attempts to dismantle Clean Air Act and to diminish authority of Consumer Product Safety Commission.

1982

■ The arthritis drug Oraflex is withdrawn from the market after Public Citizen exposes deaths and injuries caused by the drug.

■ After an extensive campaign, cancer-causing urea formaldehyde is banned in home insulation.

1983

■ Public Citizen wins historic separation of powers case; Supreme Court strikes down legislative veto.

■ *Over the Counter Pills That Don't Work* is published and becomes a national best-seller.

■ Public Citizen participates in landmark Supreme Court decision overturning President Reagan's revocation of auto safety standards for automatic restraints such as air bags.

1984

■ Following AT&T's divestiture, Public Citizen mounts nationwide "Campaign for Affordable Phones" to oppose rate hikes for residential customers.

■ Public Citizen wins court order forcing EPA to recall 700,000 GM cars with faulty emission controls.

1985

■ FDA requires a Reye's Syndrome warning for children on aspirin labels following three-year campaign by Public Citizen.

■ Public Citizen reveals the locations of more than 250 work sites nationwide where workers have been exposed to hazardous chemicals.

1986

■ Congress requires health warning labels on chewing tobacco and snuff, capping Public Citizen's two-year campaign.

■ Public Citizen wins court order forbidding President from stopping expenditure of appropriated funds without express authorization from Congress.

1987

■ Public Citizen helps persuade Congress to pass legislation restricting the time banks can hold checks.

1988

■ After seven years of litigation by Public Citizen, the Occupational Safety and Health Administration (OSHA) imposes standards for exposure to cancer-causing ethylene oxide.

■ Public Citizen sells 400,000 copies of *Worst Pills/Best Pills*, a consumer guide to dangerous and ineffective drugs and their preferable alternatives.

1989

■ Public Citizen and Ralph Nader stop the $45,500 congressional pay raise, forcing Congress to take a smaller raise and ban honoraria.

■ Public Citizen helps persuade California voters to shut down Rancho Seco nuclear plant.

■ Public Citizen obtains court order forcing the FDA to require labels warning women that high-absorbency tampons are more likely to cause Toxic Shock Syndrome.

1990

■ Public Citizen court victory forces the Nuclear Regulatory Commission to issue mandatory training requirements for nuclear plant workers.

■ Public Citizen publishes *Who Robbed America?*, a citizen's guide to the savings and loan scandal that cost taxpayers billions of dollars.

1991

■ Public Citizen plays key role in passage of new auto and truck safety law requiring air bags and head injury protections, and limiting the expansion of big rigs.

■ Public Citizen publishes *They Love To Fly ...And It Shows,* exposing House members who took nearly 4,000 privately-funded trips in 1989-90.

1992

■ Public Citizen's four-year campaign leads the FDA to severely restrict use of silicone gel breast implants.

■ OSHA imposes standard to protect workers from cadmium, linked to lung cancer and kidney damage, after Public Citizen wins court order.

1993

■ Public Citizen wins landmark court victory that prevents destruction of electronic records of the White House under Presidents Reagan, Bush and Clinton.

■ Public Citizen plays a leading role in opposing the North American Free Trade Agreement (NAFTA), launching a new citizens' trade movement.

1994

■ Public Citizen helps to enlist nearly 100 cosponsors for single-payer health care reform bill modeled after the Canadian system.

■ Public Citizen helps win legislation protecting consumers from home equity scams.

1995

■ Congressional gift ban and lobbying registration reform enacted after major Public Citizen campaign.

■ Public Citizen successfully defends tobacco industry whistle-blower who released key documents to Congress and the FDA, against civil damages and criminal contempt charges.

1996

■ Public Citizen wins Supreme Court decision upholding the right of people injured by defective medical devices to sue for compensation.

■ Public Citizen forges historic settlement to secure release of Nixon's White House tapes after 15 years of litigation.

■ Public Citizen successfully opposes legislation mandating temporary transport of nuclear waste to Nevada for storage.

1997

■ Public Citizen leads multi-year campaign that results in defeat of damaging Fast Track trade authority.

1998

■ Public Citizen protests and helps force redesign of unethical AIDS research in Africa, which would have denied known effective treatment to HIV-positive pregnant women.

■ Public Citizen helps lead a global citizens' campaign that results in the scuttling of the Multilateral Agreement on Investments, a proposed global investment treaty.

■ Public Citizen wins passage of legislation mandating safer air bags to protect women and children.

■ Public Citizen releases latest compilation of *16,638 Questionable Doctors*, the only publicly available, national compendium of disciplined doctors.

1999

■ Public Citizen publishes third edition of its best-selling *Worst Pills, Best Pills*, a consumer's guide to avoiding drug-induced death or illness.

■ Public Citizen wins release of historic grand jury records relating to the 1948 indictment of alleged Soviet agent Alger Hiss.

■ Public Citizen publishes *Whose Trade Organization? Corporate Globalization and the Erosion of Democracy*, a book exposing the WTO's five-year record of weakening health, safety, environmental and labor standards.

■ Public Citizen works successfully to pass major truck safety legislation, which creates the new Federal Motor Carrier Safety Administration.

■ Public Citizen leads global coalition to organize massive demonstrations in Seattle against the unaccountable, undemocratic World Trade Organization.

2000

■ Public Citizen petition leads to ban on diabetes drug Rezulin after 63 deaths from liver toxicity.

■ Public Citizen releases latest compilation of *Questionable Doctors*, a national compendium of disciplined doctors.

ORDER FORM

Public Citizen

1600 20th Street, NW, Washington, DC 20009-1001
www.citizen.org

Cut here to order or pass along to a friend.

Publications from Public Citizen

Qty.	Item Description	Price	Subtotal
	F6672 *Worst Pills/Best Pills* 1999 ed.	$16	
	FQON *Questionable Doctors* 4-volume National Edition	$407.50	
	2000 Edition Questionable Doctors Regional Editions		
	FQ001 Arkansas, Louisiana, Mississippi	$23.50	
	FQ002 Alaska, Idaho, Montana, Oregon, Washington, Wyoming	$23.50	
	FQ003 Arizona, Colorado, Nevada, New Mexico, Utah	$23.50	
	FQ004 California, Hawaii	$23.50	
	FQ005 Connecticut, Maine, Massachusetts, New Hampshire, Rhode Island, Vermont	$23.50	
	FQ006 Delaware, New Jersey	$23.50	
	FQ007 District of Columbia, Maryland, Virginia	$23.50	
	FQ008 Florida	$23.50	
	FQ009 Alabama, Georgia	$23.50	
	FQ010 Illinois, Indiana	$23.50	
	FQ011 Iowa, Missouri	$23.50	
	FQ012 New York	$23.50	
	FQ013 Kentucky, North Carolina, South Carolina, Tennessee	$23.50	
	FQ014 Kansas, Nebraska, North Dakota, South Dakota	$23.50	
	FQ015 Oklahoma, Texas	$23.50	
	FQ016 Minnesota, Wisconsin	$23.50	
	FQ017 Michigan, Ohio	$23.50	
	FQ018 Pennsylvania, West Virginia	$23.50	
Subtotal (1)			

Public Citizen Membership/Newsletter Subscription

	Price	Subtotal
Basic Membership (includes *PC News*)	$20	
Combination Membership with *Health Letter*	$35	
Special Introductory subscription to *Worst Pills, Best Pills News* for 12 months	$10	
I want to help even more with an additional contribution		
Subtotal (2)		
Add (1) and (2)	TOTAL	

Ordered By:

Name ______________________

Address (National Edition can only be shipped to a street address)

____

____

City ______________ State ______ Zip ________

E-mail ______________________

Phone number (___) ______________________

Please use an additional sheet of paper for gift orders.

❑ Payment enclosed (check or money order payable to "Public Citizen")

❑ Charge to credit card ❑ VISA ❑ MC ❑ AMEX ❑ Discover

Credit Card # ______________________

Exp. Date ______________________

Signature ______________________

U.S. orders only. Please allow 6-8 weeks for delivery.

BOQDBK

Public Citizen

Health Research Group Publications

Questionable Doctors

www.questionabledoctors.org

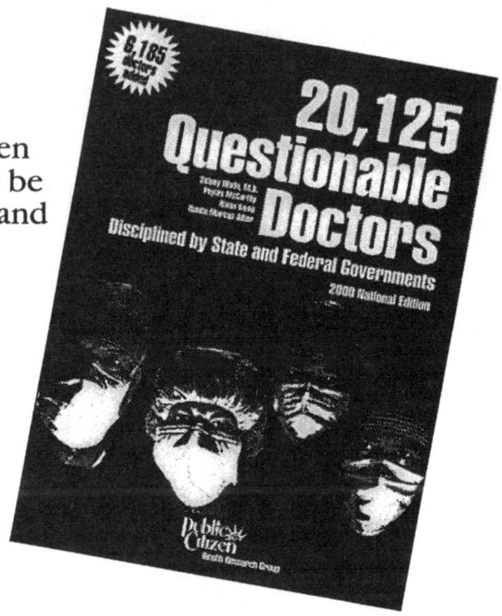

This is the only state-by-state listing of doctors who have been disciplined by state and federal agencies—doctors who may be continuing to treat unsuspecting patients. Order for friends and family.

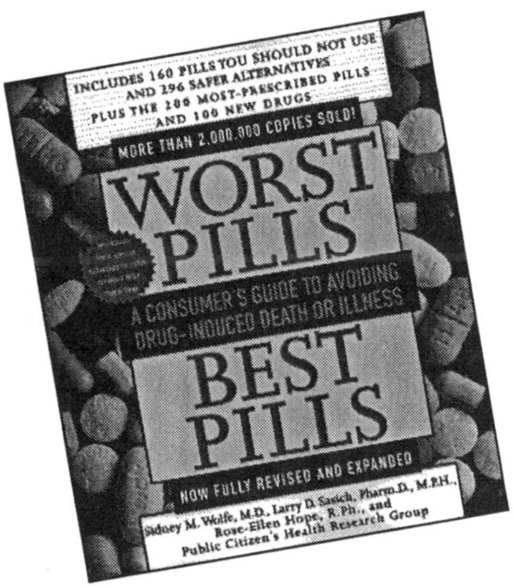

Worst Pills, Best Pills, 1999 edition

www.worstpills.org

What you can do to protect yourself and your loved ones from dangerous pharmaceuticals.

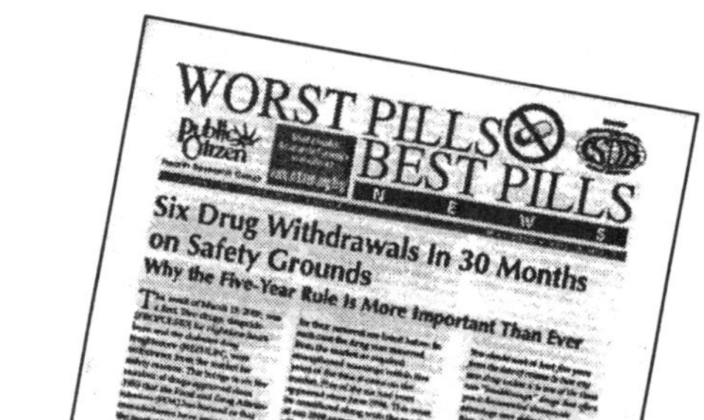

Worst Pills, Best Pills News

Pharmaceutical companies have gotten legislation passed to weaken FDA oversight of drug approvals. You can no longer be sure that just because a drug is on the market that it will be safe to use. *Worst Pills, Best Pills* is an excellent reference for you to find out which drugs are really safe, how to prevent adverse drug reactions, and which drugs should not be taken together. Every year, more and more drugs come onto the market. To stay up to date with the latest drugs, subscribe to *Worst Pills, Best Pills News.*

Get answers to your questions about the medical advice and care you receive—and how to ask your doctor important questions about the drugs prescribed for you. We are offering *Worst Pills, Best Pills News* at half price for new subscribers.

Order these publications by calling 1-877-747-1616 or use the form on the next page.